BLACKWELL'S FIVE-MINUTE VETERINARY CONSULT: EQUINE

THIRD EDITION

Blackwell's Five-Minute Veterinary Consult

EQUINE

THIRD EDITION

Edited by

Jean-Pierre Lavoie, DVM, Diplomate ACVIM

Professor
Associate Dean – Research
Faculté de Médecine Vétérinaire
Université de Montréal
St-Hyacinthe, Quebec, Canada

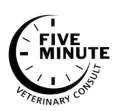

WILEY Blackwell

PREFACE

The concept for the Five-Minute Veterinary Consult was developed to provide concise and practical information for the diagnosis and treatment of equine diseases. The first *Five-Minute Veterinary Consult: Equine*, co-edited by Christopher M. Brown and Joseph Bertone, was published in 2002. It was an immediate success and the series was later expanded in both the veterinary and human fields.

The new third edition of the *Five-Minute Veterinary Consult: Equine* builds on the first and subsequent second edition of the book that was co-edited by Kenneth William Hinchcliff and myself. As in previous editions of the book, it provides brief, state-of-the-art summaries of more than 500 common medical conditions of horses. The goal is to offer equine clinicians and veterinary students a concise, yet comprehensive, up-to-date and easy-to-use overview of the causes, pathophysiology, clinical presentation, diagnosis, differential diagnosis, treatment, and prognosis of these conditions.

This book was made possible by the work of the 206 authors and the 24 section editors who summarized pertinent evidence-based, if available, information, or in situations with a paucity of published data, they shared their expert opinions.

Jean-Pierre Lavoie

CONSULTING EDITORS

JEAN-PIERRE LAVOIE, DVM
Diplomate ACVIM
Professor
Associate Dean – Research
Faculté de Médecine Vétérinaire
Université de Montréal
St-Hyacinthe, QC
Canada
Sports Medicine, Volume Editor

HEIDI BANSE, DVM, PhD
Diplomate ACVIM
Assistant Professor
Department of Veterinary Clinical Sciences
School of Veterinary Medicine
Lousiana State University
Baton Rouge, LA
USA
Endocrine

ASHLEY G. BOYLE, DVM
Diplomate ACVIM
Associate Professor
Department of Clinical Studies
New Bolton Center
School of Veterinary Medicine
University of Pennsylvania
Kennett Square, PA
USA
Infectious Diseases

CARLA L. CARLETON, DVM, MS
Diplomate ACT, Diplomate ACAW
Professor Emeritus
Department of Large Animal Clinical
Sciences
Veterinary Medical Center
College of Veterinary Medicine
Michigan State University
East Lansing, MI
USA
Theriogenology

ELIZABETH J. DAVIDSON, DVM
Diplomate ACVS, Diplomate ACVSMR
Associate Professor
Department of Clinical Studies—New Bolton
Center
School of Veterinary Medicine
University of Pennsylvania
Kennett Square, PA
USA
Musculoskeletal

STEVE ENSLEY, DVM, PhD
Clinical Professor
Department of Anatomy and Physiology
College of Veterinary Medicine
Kansas State University
Manhattan, KS
USA
Toxicology

CAROLINE N. HAHN, DVM, MSc, PhD
Diplomate ECVN, Diplomate ECEIM
Senior Lecturer
Royal (Dick) School of Veterinary Studies
The University of Edinburgh
Edinburgh
UK
Neurology

DAVID HODGSON, BVSc, PhD
Diplomate ACVIM
Professor Emeritus
Department of Large Animal Clinical
Sciences
Virginia-Maryland College of Veterinary
Medicine
Virginia Tech
Blacksburg, VA
USA
Hematopoietic

JENNIFER L. HODGSON, BVSc (Hons),
PhD
Diplomate ACVM
Professor
Department of Population Health Sciences
Virginia-Maryland College of Veterinary
Medicine
Virginia Tech
Blacksburg, VA
USA
Hematopoietic

DANIEL JEAN, DMV, PhD
Diplomate ACVIM
Professor
Department of Clinical Sciences
Faculté de Médecine Vétérinaire
Université de Montréal
St-Hyacinthe, QC
Canada
Respiratory

MATHILDE LECLÈRE, DVM, PhD
Diplomate ACVIM
Associate Professor
Department of Clinical Sciences
Faculté de Médecine Vétérinaire
Université de Montréal
St-Hyacinthe, QC
Canada
Respiratory

MICHEL LEVY, DVM
Diplomate ACVIM
Professor
Department of Production Animal Health
Faculty of Veterinary Medicine
University of Calgary
Calgary, AB
Canada
Endocrine

GWENDOLEN LORCH, DVM, MS, PhD
Diplomate ACVD
Associate Professor
Department of Veterinary Clinical Sciences
College of Veterinary Medicine
The Ohio State University
Columbus, OH
USA
Dermatology

CELIA M. MARR, BVMS, MVM, PhD, DEIM,
FRCVS
Diplomate ECEIM
Associate
Rossdales LLP
Newmarket
UK
Cardiology

HAROLD C. MCKENZIE, III, DVM, MS, MSc
(VetEd), FHEA, Diplomate ACVIM
Professor
Department of Veterinary Clinical Sciences
Virginia-Maryland College of Veterinary
Medicine
Virginia Tech
Blacksburg, VA
USA
Hematopoietic

vi

MARGARET C. MUDGE, VMD
Diplomate ACVS, ACVECC
Professor
Department of Veterinary Clinical Sciences
The Ohio State University
Columbus, OH
USA
Neonatology

OLIMPO OLIVER-ESPINOSA, DVM,
MSc, DVSc
Associate Professor
Clinica de Grandes Animales
Departamento de Salud Animal
Facultad de Medicina Veterinaria y
de Zootecnia
Universidad Nacional de Colombia
Bogota, DC
Colombia
Gastroenterology

VALÉRIE PICANDET, DVM
Diplomate ACVIM, Diplomate ECEIM
Centre Hospitalier Vétérinaire Equin de Livet
St Michel de Livet
France
Urinary

CARYN E. PLUMMER, DVM
Diplomate ACVO
Associate Professor
Departments of Large and Small Animal
Clinical Sciences
College of Veterinary Medicine
University of Florida
Gainesville, FL
USA
Ophthalmology

VIRGINIA B. REEF, DVM
Diplomate ACVIM (LAIM), DACVSMR
Associate Member ECVDI
Mark Whittier and Lila Griswold Allam
Professor of Medicine
Department of Clinical Studies—New Bolton
Center
University of Pennsylvania
Kennett Square, PA
USA
Cardiology

WILSON K. RUMBEIHA, BVM, PhD
Diplomate ABT, ABVT, Fellow ATS
Professor
Department of Molecular Biosciences
University of California – Davis
School of Veterinary Medicine
Davis, CA
USA
Toxicology

HENRY STÄMPFLI, DVM, DrMedVet
Diplomate ACVIM
Professor
Large Animal Medicine, Clinical Studies
Ontario Veterinary College
University of Guelph
Guelph, ON
Canada
Gastroenterology

SANDRA D. TAYLOR, DVM, PhD
Diplomate ACVIM
Associate Professor
Department of Veterinary Clinical Sciences
College of Veterinary Medicine
Purdue University
West Lafayette, IN
USA
Laboratory Tests

VICTORIA L. VOITH, DVM, MSc, MA, PhD
Diplomate ACVB
Professor
Animal Behavior Content Expert
College of Veterinary Medicine
Western University of Health Sciences
Pomona, CA
USA
Behavior

CONTRIBUTORS

MICHELLE ABRAHAM LINTON, BVMS, BSc
Diplomate ACVIM
Department of Internal Medicine
The University of Pennsylvania
New Bolton Center
Kennett Square, PA
USA

VERENA K. AFFOLTER, DMV, DECVP, PhD
Professor
Chief of Service Anatomic Pathology
Veterinary Medicine—PMI
University of California Davis
Davis, CA
USA

CLAIRE B. ANDREASEN, DVM, PhD
Diplomate ACVP
Professor
Department of Veterinary Pathology
College of Veterinary Medicine
Iowa State University
Ames, IA
USA

LIZ ARBITTIER, VMD, CVA
Assistant Professor
Section Field Service—Equine
Clinical Studies
New Bolton Center
University of Pennsylvania
Kennett Square, PA
USA

DEBRA C. ARCHER, BVMS, PhD, CertES
Diplomate ECVS
Professor of Equine Surgery
Philip Leverhulme Equine Hospital
Institute of Veterinary Science
University of Liverpool Leahurst Campus
Neston
UK

LUIS G. ARROYO, Lic Med Vet, DVSc, PhD
Diplomate ACVIM
Associate Professor
Department of Clinical Studies
Ontario Veterinary College
University of Guelph
Guelph, ON
Canada

JOHN D. BAIRD, BVSc, PhD
Professor Emeritus
Department of Clinical Studies
Ontario Veterinary College
University of Guelph
Guelph, ON
Canada

HEIDI BANSE, DVM, PhD
Diplomate ACVIM
Assistant Professor
Department of Veterinary Clinical Sciences
School of Veterinary Medicine
Lousiana State University
Baton Rouge, LA
USA

GIL BEN-SHLOMO, DVM, PhD
Diplomate ACVO, Diplomate ECVO
Associate Professor
Department of Clinical Sciences
College of Veterinary Medicine
Cornell University
Ithaca, NY
USA

EMILY H. BERRYHILL, DVM
Diplomate ACVIM
Staff Veterinarian
Department of Medicine and Epidemiology
School of Veterinary Medicine
University of California
Davis, CA
USA

FRANÇOIS-RENÉ BERTIN, DVM, MS, PhD
Diplomate ACVIM
Senior Lecturer
School of Veterinary Science
University of Queensland
Gatton, QLD
Australia

ANDREA S. BISCHOFBERGER, Dr Med Vet
Diplomate ACVS & ECVS
Senior Clinical Lecturer
Equine Department
Vetsuisse-Faculty
University of Zurich
Zurich
Switzerland

KATIE M. BOES, DVM, MS
Diplomate ACVP
Clinical Assistant Professor
Department of Biomedical Sciences &
Pathobiology
Virginia Polytechnic Institute and
State University
Blacksburg, VA
USA

LUDOVIC P. BOURÉ, DVM, MSc, DES
Diplomate ACVS, Diplomate ECVS
Preclinical Research Director—Global
Medical Director
Hernia—MITG Medtronic
North Haven, CT
USA

ASHLEY G. BOYLE, DVM
Diplomate ACVIM
Associate Professor
Department of Clinical Studies
New Bolton Center
School of Veterinary Medicine
University of Pennsylvania
Kennett Square, PA
USA

RANA BOZORGMANESH, BSc(Hons),
BVetMed(Hons)
Diplomate ACVIM, MRCVS
Internal Medicine Specialist
McGee Medicine Center
Hagyard Equine Medical Institute
Lexington, KY
USA

JOHAN BRÖJER, DVM, MSc, PhD
Diplomate ACVIM & ECEIM
Associate Professor
Department of Clinical Sciences
Swedish University of Agricultural Sciences
Uppsala
Sweden

BRANDY A. BURGESS, DVM, MSc, PhD
Diplomate ACVIM, Diplomate ACVPM
Assistant Professor
Department of Population Health
College of Veterinary Medicine
University of Georgia
Athens, GA
USA

TERESA A. BURNS, DVM, PhD
Diplomate ACVIM
Associate Professor
Department of Veterinary Clinical Sciences
College of Veterinary Medicine
The Ohio State University
Columbus, OH
USA

MARIA E. CADARIO, DVM, MV, MS
Diplomate ACT
Private Practice Equine
Reproduction Specialty Practice
Gainsville, FL
USA

CARLA L. CARLETON, DVM, MS
Diplomate ACT, Diplomate ACAW
Professor Emeritus
Department of Large Animal Clinical
Sciences
Veterinary Medical Center
College of Veterinary Medicine
Michigan State University
East Lansing, MI
USA

RUBIELA CASTAÑEDA-SALAZAR, DVM,
MSc
Assistant Professor
Departamento de Microbiología
Facultad de Ciencias
Pontificia Universidad Javeriana
Bogotá, DC
Colombia

STAN W. CASTEEL, DVM, PhD
Diplomate ABVT
Professor Emeritus
Department of Veterinary Pathobiology
College of Veterinary Medicine
University of Missouri
Columbia, MO
USA

YOUNG-HO CHOI, DVM, PhD
Diplomate ACT
Research Associate Professor
Department of Veterinary Physiology &
Pharmacology
College of Veterinary Medicine & Biomedical
Sciences
Texas A&M University
College Station, TX
USA

JOHN A. CHRISTIAN, DVM, PhD
Associate Professor
Department of Comparative Pathobiology
College of Veterinary Medicine
Purdue University
West Lafayette, IN
USA

SARA L. CONNOLLY, DVM, MS
Diplomate ACVP
Clinical Assistant Professor
Veterinary Diagnostic Laboratory
Department of Pathobiology
College of Veterinary Medicine
University of Illinois
Urbana, IL
USA

LAIS R.R. COSTA, MV, MS, PhD
Diplomate ACVIM & ABVP
Associate Veterinarian
The William R. Pritchard Veterinary Medical
Teaching Hospital
School of Veterinary Medicine
Davis, CA
USA

NATHALIE COTÉ, DMV, DVSc
Diplomate ACVS
Assistant Professor
Department of Clinical Studies
Ontario Veterinary College
University of Guelph
Guelph, ON
Canada

NICOLA C. CRIBB, MA, VetMB, DVSc
Diplomate ACVS
Adjunct Professor
Department of Clinical Studies
Ontario Veterinary College
University of Guelph
Guelph, ON
Canada

SHARON L. CROWELL-DAVIS, DVM, PhD
Diplomate ACVB
Professor
Department of Veterinary Biosciences and
Diagnostic Imaging
College of Veterinary Medicine
University of Georgia
Athens, GA
USA

ANTONIO M. CRUZ, LV, MVM, MSc, PhD
Diplomate ACVS, ECVS & ACVSMR
Equine Unit Director
Chief of Service
Veterinary Teaching Hospital
Department of Animal Medicine and Surgery
Faculty of Veterinary Medicine
Universidad Cardenal Herrera-CEU
CEU Universities
Valencia
Spain

ROBIN M. DABAREINER, DVM, PhD
Diplomate ACVS
Equine Lameness Specialist
Caldwell, TX
USA

BENJAMIN J. DARIEN, DVM, MS
Diplomate ACVIM
Associate Professor
Department of Medical Science
University of Wisconsin-Madison
Madison, WI
USA

FLORENT DAVID, DVM, MS
Diplomate ACVS, ECVS & ACVSMR, ECVDI
Associate
Head of Equine Surgery
Equine Veterinary Medical Center—
Al Shaqab
A Member of Qatar Foundation
Al Rayyan
Doha
Qatar

MARTIN DAVID, DMV, MS
Diplomate ACVP
Clinical Pathologist
IDEXX Laboratories
Westminster, CO
USA

ELIZABETH J. DAVIDSON, DVM
Diplomate ACVS, Diplomate ACVSMR
Associate Professor
Department of Clinical Studies—New Bolton
Center
School of Veterinary Medicine
University of Pennsylvania
Kennett Square, PA
USA

ELIZABETH DAVIS, DVM, PhD
Diplomate ACVIM
Professor and Interim Head
Department of Clinical Sciences
Kansas State University
College of Veterinary Medicine
Manhattan, NY
USA

NIKHITA P. DE BERNARDIS, DVM
Program Coordinator
International Programs and Special Projects
College of Veterinary Medicine
Cornell University
Ithaca, NY
USA

DEMIA J. DE TONNERRE, BVSc
Resident
Department of Large Animal Clinical
Sciences
College of Veterinary Medicine
University of Florida
Gainesville, FL
USA

THOMAS J. DIVERS, DVM
Diplomate ACVIM, ACVECC
Steffen Professor of Veterinary Medicine
Cornell University
Ithaca, NY
USA

ELAINE M.S. DORNELES, DVM, PhD
Adjunct Professor
Departmento de Medicina Veterinária
Universidade Federal de Lavras
Lavras, Minas Gerais
Brazil

PATRICIA M. DOWLING, DVM, MSc
Diplomate ACVIM & ACVCP
Professor
Co-Director, Canadian gFARAD
Western College of Veterinary Medicine
Saskatoon, SK
Canada

NORM G. DUCHARME, DVM, MSc
Diplomate ACVS
James Law Professor of Surgery
Cornell University Hospital for Animals
College of Veterinary Medicine
Cornell University
Ithaca, NY
USA

LAURA K. DUNBAR, DVM, MS
Diplomate ACVIM
Clinical Instructor
Department of Veterinary Clinical Sciences
College of Veterinary Medicine
The Ohio State University
Columbus, OH
USA

ROBERTA M. DWYER, DVM, MS
Diplomate ACVPM
Professor
Department of Animal and Food Sciences
College of Agriculture, Food and Environment
University of Kentucky
Lexington, KY
USA

STEVE ENSLEY, DVM, PhD
Clinical Professor
Department of Anatomy and Physiology
College of Veterinary Medicine
Kansas State University
Manhattan, KS
USA

KIRA L. EPSTEIN, DVM
Diplomate ACVS, ACVECC
Clinical Professor
Department of Large Animal Medicine
College of Veterinary Medicine
University of Georgia
Athens, GA
USA

KRISTA ESTELL, DVM
Diplomate ACVIM
Assistant Clinical Professor
Marion duPont Scott Equine Medical Center
Virginia Maryland College of
Veterinary Medicine
Leesburg, VA
USA

TIM J. EVANS, DVM
Diplomate ACT, Diplomate ABVT
Associate Professor
Department of Veterinary Pathobiology
College of Veterinary Medicine
University of Missouri
Columbia, MO
USA

M. JULIA B. FELIPPE, MedVet, MS, PhD
Diplomate ACVIM
Associate Professor
Department of Clinical Sciences
College of Veterinary Medicine
Cornell University
Ithaca, NY
USA

NICOLE J. FERNANDEZ, BSc, DVM, MVetSc
Diplomate ACVP
Associate Professor
Department of Veterinary Pathology
Western College of Veterinary Medicine
University of Saskatchewan
Saskatoon, SK
Canada

FRANCESCO FERRUCCI, DVM, PhD
Associate Professor
Department of Health, Animal Science and
Food Safety
School of Veterinary Medicine
Università Degli Studi di Milano
Milan
Italy

ANNA M. FIRSHMAN, BVSc, PhD
Diplomate ACVIM & ACVSMR
Associate Clinical Professor
Department of Veterinary Population
Medicine
College of Veterinary Medicine
University of Minnesota
Saint Paul, MN
USA

NICHOLAS FRANK, DVM, PhD
Diplomate ACVIM
Professor
Department of Clinical Sciences
Cummings School of Veterinary Medicine
Tufts University
North Grafton, MA
USA

MARY CATHERINE FURNESS, DVM, MSc,
DACVIM
Rockwood, ON
Canada

GONZALO GAJARDO AEDO, MV, MSc
Adjunct Professor
Clinical Science Specialist Equine Mention
Institute of Clinical Sciences
Universidad Austral de Chile
Valdivia
Chile

JOSÉ M. GARCÍA-LÓPEZ, VMD
Diplomate ACVS & ACVSMR
Associate Professor
Director of Equine Sports Medicine
Department of Clinical Sciences
Tufts University
Cummings School of Veterinary Medicine
North Grafton, MA
USA

ALISON K. GARDNER, DVM, MS
Diplomate ACVS
Clinical Instructor
Equine Emergency and Critical Care
College of Veterinary Medicine
The Ohio State University
Columbus, OH
USA

TAM GARLAND, DVM, PhD
Diplomate ABVT
Owner, Toxicologist
Garland, Bailey & Associates
College Station, TX
USA

CYNTHIA L. GASKILL, DVM, PhD
Diplomate ABVT
Associate Professor
Department of Veterinary Science
Veterinary Diagnostic Laboratory
University of Kentucky
Lexington, KY
USA

LIBERTY M. GETMAN, DVM, DACVS
Tennessee Equine Hospital
Thompson Station, TN
USA

JAMES R. GILKERSON, BVSc
BSc(Vet), PhD
Professor
Department of Veterinary Biosciences
Faculty of Veterinary and
Agricultural Sciences
The University of Melbourne
Melbourne, VIC
Australia

JENIFER R. GOLD, DVM
Diplomate ACVIM & ACVECC
Clinical Assistant Professor
Department of Clinical Sciences
College of Veterinary Medicine
Washington State University
Pullman, WA
USA

DIEGO GOMEZ-NIETO, DVM, MSc,
MVSc, PhD
Diplomate ACVIM
Clinical Assistant Professor
Department of Large Animal Clinical
Sciences
University of Florida
College of Veterinary Medicine
Gainesville, FL
USA

DYLAN GORVY, BSc, BVSc, PhD, CertES
(Soft Tissue), Diplomate ECVS
European Specialist in Equine Surgery
Head of Surgery
Mälaren Horse Clinic
Sigtuna
Sweden

SICILIA T. GRADY, DVM, MS, PhD
Resident
Department of Veterinary Physiology &
Pharmacology
College of Veterinary Medicine and
Biomedical Sciences
Texas A&M University
College Station, TX
USA

SHARI M. GREENBERG, DVM
Diplomate ACVO
New England Veterinary Center and
Cancer Care
Windsor, CT
USA

SHARON GWALTNEY-BRANT, DVM, PhD
Diplomate ABVT & ABT
Toxicology Consultant
Veterinary Information Network
Mahomet, IL
USA

CAROLINE N. HAHN, DVM, MSc, PhD
Diplomate ECVN, Diplomate ECEIM
Senior Lecturer
Royal (Dick) School of Veterinary Studies
The University of Edinburgh
Edinburgh
UK

JEFFERY O. HALL, DVM, PhD
Diplomate ABVT
Professor
Head, Diagnostic Veterinary Toxicology
Department of Animal, Dairy, and
Veterinary Sciences
College of Agriculture
Utah State University
Logan, UT
USA

KELSEY A. HART, DVM, PhD
Diplomate ACVIM
Assistant Professor
Department of Large Animal Medicine
University of Georgia
College of Veterinary Medicine
Athens, GA
USA

DIANA M. HASSEL, DVM, PhD
Diplomate ACVS & ACVECC
Associate Professor
Surgery and Critical Care
Department of Clinical Sciences
Colorado State University
Fort Collins, CO
USA

G. KENITRA HENDRIX, DVM, PhD
Diplomate ACVIM
Assistant Professor
Indiana Animal Disease Diagnostic
Laboratory
Department of Comparative Pathobiology
College of Veterinary Medicine
Purdue University
West Lafayette, IN
USA

JILL C. HIGGINS, DVM
Private Equine Practitioner/Consultant
Penryn, CA
USA

KATRIN HINRICHS, DVM, PhD
Diplomate ACT
Professor
Department of Veterinary Physiology and
Pharmacology
College of Veterinary Medicine &
Biomedical Sciences
Texas A&M University
College Station, TX
USA

DAVID HODGSON, BVSc, PhD
Diplomate ACVIM
Professor Emeritus
Department of Large Animal Clinical
Sciences
Virginia-Maryland College of Veterinary
Medicine
Virginia Tech
Blacksburg, VA
USA

JENNIFER L. HODGSON, BVSc (Hons),
PhD
Diplomate ACVM
Professor
Department of Population Health Sciences
Virginia-Maryland College of Veterinary
Medicine
Virginia Tech
Blacksburg, VA
USA

STEPHEN B. HOOSER, DVM, PhD
Diplomate ABVT
Professor
Department of Comparative Pathobiology
Head, Toxicology Section
Animal Disease Diagnostic Laboratory
College of Veterinary Medicine
Purdue University
West Lafayette, IN
USA

KATHERINE ALBRO HOUPT, VMD, PhD
Diplomate ACVB
Professor Emeritus
Department of Clinical Sciences
College of Veterinary Medicine
Cornell University
Ithaca, NY
USA

KRISTOPHER HUGHES, BVSc, FANZCVS
Diplomate ECEIM
Associate Professor
School of Animal and Veterinary Sciences
Charles Sturt University
New South Wales
Australia

SAMUEL D.A. HURCOMBE, BSc, BVMS, MS
Diplomate ACVIM, Diplomate ACVECC
Clinical Associate Professor
Cornell Ruffian Equine Specialists
Cornell University
College of Veterinary Medicine
Elmont, NY
USA

DANIEL JEAN, DMV, PhD
Diplomate ACVIM
Professor
Department of Clinical Sciences
Faculté de Médecine Vétérinaire
Université de Montréal
St-Hyacinthe, QC
Canada

EMILY E. JOHN, DVM, PhD
Diplomate ACVP
Associate Professor
Department of Pathobiology and Diagnostic
Investigation
College of Veterinary Medicine
Michigan State University
East Lansing, MI
USA

IMOGEN JOHNS, BVSc Diploma, ACVIM,
FHEA, MRCVS
B and W Equine Hospital
Breadstone
UK

AMY L. JOHNSON, DVM
Diplomate ACVIM
Assistant Professor
Department of Clinical Studies—New Bolton
Center
School of Veterinary Medicine
University of Pennsylvania
Kennett Square, PA
USA

PHILIP J. JOHNSON, BVSc(Hons), MS
Diplomate ACVIM, Diplomate ECEIM,
MRCVS
Professor
Department of Veterinary Medicine and
Surgery
College of Veterinary Medicine
University of Missouri
Columbia, MO
USA

EDUARD JOSE-CUNILLERAS, DVM, PhD
Diplomate ECEIM
Senior Lecturer
Department de Medicina i Cirurgia Animals
Facultat de Veterinaria
Universitat Autonoma de Barcelona
Bellaterra
Barcelona
Spain

GIGI KAY, BVM&S, MRCVS Cert (Eq Med)
Director
American Fondouk
Fes
Morocco

AUDREY A. KELLEMAN, DVM, DACT
Clinical Assistant Professor
Department of Large Animal Clinical
Sciences
University of Florida
College of Veterinary Medicine
Gainesville, FL
USA

DANIEL G. KENNEY, VMD
Diplomate ACVIM
Veterinarian
Ontario Veterinary College—Health Sciences
Centre
University of Guelph
Guelph, ON
Canada

DON KNOWLES, DVM, PhD
Diplomate ACVP
Research Leader and Professor
Animal Disease Research
Unit—ARS-USDA-PWA and
College of Veterinary Medicine
Washington State University
Pullman, WA
USA

JANICE KRITCHEVSKY, VMD, MS
Diplomate ACVIM
Professor, Large Animal Medicine
Department of Veterinary Clinical Sciences
School of Veterinary Medicine
Purdue University
West Lafayette, IN
USA

ANDREY P. LAGE, DVM, PhD
Associate Professor
Departamento de Medicina Veterinária
Preventiva
Escola de Veterinária
Universidade Federal de Minas Gerais
Belo Horizonte, Minas Gerais
Brazil

JEFFREY LAKRITZ, DVM, PhD
Diplomate ACVIM, Diplomate ACVCP
Professor
The Ohio State University College of
Veterinary Medicine
Columbus, OH
USA

SHEILA LAVERTY, MVB
Diplomate ACVS, Diplomate ECVS, FIOR
Professor
Département de Sciences Cliniques
Faculté de Médecine Vétérinaire
Université de Montréal
St-Hyacinthe, QC
Canada

JEAN-PIERRE LAVOIE, DVM
Diplomate ACVIM
Professor
Associate Dean – Research
Faculté de Médecine Vétérinaire
Université de Montréal
St-Hyacinthe, QC
Canada

MATHILDE LECLÈRE, DVM, PhD
Diplomate ACVIM
Associate Professor
Department of Clinical Sciences
Faculté de Médecine Vétérinaire
Université de Montréal
St-Hyacinthe, QC
Canada

LAURELINE LECOQ, DMV, MSc
Diplomate ACVIM
MedIAE_Equine Internal Medicine
Ambulatory Practice
Liège
Belgium

RENAUD LEGUILLETTE, DVM, MSc, PhD
Diplomate ACVIM, Diplomate ACVSMR
Calgary Chair in Equine Sports Medicine
Associate Professor
Department of Veterinary Clinical and
Diagnostic Sciences
Faculty of Veterinary Medicine (UCVM)
University of Calgary
Calgary, AL
Canada

SARAH S. LE JEUNE, DVM, DACVS,
DACVSMR, Cert Vet Acu/Chiro
Associate Professor
Integrative Sports Medicine and
Rehabilitation
Department of Surgical and Radiological
Sciences
School of Veterinary Medicine
University of California
Davis, CA
USA

MICHEL LEVY, DVM
Diplomate ACVIM
Professor
Department of Production Animal Health
Faculty of Veterinary Medicine
University of Calgary
Calgary, AB
Canada

RACHEL S. LIEPMAN, DVM, MS
Diplomate ACVIM
Equine Internal Medicine Specialist
Chaparral Veterinary Medical Center
Cave Creek, AZ
USA

JENNIFER K. LINTON, VMD
Diplomate ACT
Staff Veterinarian
Department of Clinical Studies
School of Veterinary Medicine
The University of Pennsylvania
Kennett Square, PA
USA

JANET LITTLEWOOD, MA, PhD,
GVSc(Hons), DVR, DVD, MRCVS
Veterinary Dermatology Referrals
Cambridge
UK

JEANNE LOFSTEDT, BVSc, MS
Diplomate ACVIM
Professor
Department of Health Management
Atlantic Veterinary College, UPEI
Charlottetown, PE
Canada

MAUREEN T. LONG, DVM, PhD
Diplomate ACVIM
Associate Professor
Department of Comparative, Diagnostic and
Population Medicine
College of Veterinary Medicine
University of Florida
Gainesville, FL
USA

GWENDOLEN LORCH, DVM, MS, PhD
Diplomate ACVD
Associate Professor
Department of Veterinary Clinical Sciences
College of Veterinary Medicine
The Ohio State University
Columbus, OH
USA

DANIELA LUETHY, DVM
Resident
New Bolton Center
School of Veterinary Medicine
University of Pennsylvania
Kennett Square, PA
USA

ROBERT J. MACKAY, BVSc(Dist), PhD
Diplomate ACVIM
Professor
Department of Large Animal Clinical
Sciences
College of Veterinary Medicine
University of Florida
Gainesville, FL
USA

JOHN E. MADIGAN, DVM, MS
Diplomate ACVIM, Diplomate ACAW
Distinguished Professor
Department of Medicine and Epidemiology
School of Veterinary Medicine
University of California
Davis, CA
USA

K. GARY MAGDESIAN, DVM
Diplomate ACVIM, Diplomate ACVECC,
Diplomate ACVCP
Henry Endowed Chair in Emergency
Medicine and Critical Care
Department of Medicine and Epidemiology
School of Veterinary Medicine
University of California
Davis, CA
USA

SOPHIE MAINGUY-SEERS, DMV
Resident
Department of Equine Internal Medicine
Faculté de Médecine Vétérinaire
Université de Montréal
St-Hyacinthe, QC
Canada

ERIN MALONE, DVM, PhD
Diplomate ACVS
Professor
Department of Veterinary Population
Medicine
University of Minnesota College of
Veterinary Medicine
St. Paul, MN
USA

CELIA M. MARR, BVMS, MVM, PhD, DEIM,
FRCVS
Diplomate ECEIM
Associate
Rossdales LLP
Newmarket
UK

ROSANNA MARSELLA, DVM, DACVD
Professor
College of Veterinary Medicine
University of Florida
Gainesville, FL
USA

BIANCA C. MARTINS, DVM, MS, PhD
Diplomate ACVO
Assistant Professor
Department of Veterinary Clinical Medicine
College of Veterinary Medicine
University of Illinois
Urbana, IL
USA

REBECCA S. MCCONNICO, DVM, PhD
Diplomate ACVIM
Professor
Department of Veterinary Clinical Sciences
School of Veterinary Medicine
Louisiana State University
Baton Rouge, LA
USA

SUE M. MCDONNELL, MA, PhD
Adjunct Professor and Clinical Associate
Section of Reproduction and Behavior
New Bolton Center
University of Pennsylvania School of
Veterinary Medicine
Kennett Square, PA
USA

BRUCE MCGORUM, BSc (Vet Pathol),
BVM&S, PhD, CEIM, DipECEIM, FRCVS
Head of Equine Section and RCVS and
European Specialist in Equine Medicine
Dick Vet Equine Hospital
Department of Veterinary Clinical Sciences
Royal (Dick) School of Veterinary Studies
and Roslin Institute
The University of Edinburgh
Edinburgh
UK

ERICA C. MCKENZIE, BSc, BVMS, PhD
Diplomate ACVIM, Diplomate ACVSMR
Professor
Department of Clinical Sciences
Carlson College of Veterinary Medicine
Oregon State University
Corvallis, OR
USA

HAROLD C. MCKENZIE, III, DVM, MS, MSc
(VetEd), FHEA, Diplomate ACVIM
Professor
Department of Veterinary Clinical Sciences
Virginia-Maryland College of Veterinary
Medicine
Virginia Tech
Blacksburg, VA
USA

RICHARD J. MCMULLEN, Jr. DMV
Diplomate ACVO, Diplomate ECVO, CAQ
Associate Professor
Department of Clinical Sciences
College of Veterinary Medicine
Auburn University
Auburn, AL
USA

CHARLOTTE MEANS, DVM, MLIS, DABVT,
DABT
Director of Toxicology
ASPCA Animal Poison Control Center
Urbana, IL
USA

NICOLA MENZIES-GOW, MA, VetMB, PhD
DipECEIM, CertEM(Int.med), FHEA, MRCVS
Senior Lecturer
Department of Clinical Science and Services
Royal Veterinary College
Hawkshead Lane
Hatfield
UK

DANIEL S. MILLS, BVSc, PhD, CBiol, FSB,
FHEA, CCAB, Dip ECAWBM(BM), FRCVS
Professor
European and RCVS Recognised Specialist
in Veterinary Behavioural Medicine
Joseph Banks Laboratories
School of Life Sciences
University of Lincoln
Lincoln
UK

MARTHA M. MISHEFF, DVM, MRCVS
Senior Veterinary Advisor
Sports Medicine, Lameness and Surgery
Sharjah Equine Hospital
Sharjah
United Arab Emirates

CAROLINE MONK, DVM
Diplomate ACVO
Staff Ophthalmologist
BluePearl Veterinary Partners
Atlanta, GA
USA

PETER R. MORRESEY, BVSc, MVM
Diplomate ACT, Diplomate ACVIM
Rood and Riddle Equine Hospital
Lexington, KY
USA

MARGARET C. MUDGE, VMD
Diplomate ACVS, ACVECC
Professor
Department of Veterinary Clinical Sciences
The Ohio State University
Columbus, OH
USA

RALF MUELLER, DVM
Diplomate ACVD, Fellow ANZCVSc,
Diplomate ECVD
Professor of Veterinary Dermatology
Centre for Clinical Veterinary Medicine
Faculty of Veterinary Medicine
LMU Munich
Munich
Germany

KATHLEEN R. MULLEN, DVM, MS
Diplomate ACVIM
Littleton Equine Medical Center
Littleton, CO
USA

AMELIA S. MUNSTERMAN, DVM, MS, PhD
Diplomate ACVS, Diplomate ACVECC
Certified Veterinary Acupuncturist
Clinical Assistant Professor
Department of Surgical Sciences
School of Veterinary Medicine
University of Wisconsin
Madison, WI
USA

SHANNON J. MURRAY, DVM, MS
Diplomate ACVS
Staff Surgeon
Littleton Equine Medical Center
Littleton, CO
USA

TIAS MUURLINK, BVSc(Hons), FANZCVSc
Director
Warwick Equine Veterinarians
Warwick, QLD
Australia

LIZ NELSON, BVSc
Resident
Department of Large Animal Clinical
Sciences
College of Veterinary Medicine
University of Florida
Gainesville, FL
USA

ROSE D. NOLEN-WALSTON, DVM
Diplomate ACVIM
Associate Professor
Department of Clinical Studies—New Bolton
School of Veterinary Medicine
University of Pennsylvania
Kennett Square, PA
USA

OLIMPO OLIVER-ESPINOSA, DVM,
MSc, DVSc
Associate Professor
Clinica de Grandes Animales
Departamento de Salud Animal
Facultad de Medicina Veterinaria y
de Zootecnia
Universidad Nacional de Colombia
Bogota, DC
Colombia

ERIC J. PARENTE, DVN, PhD
Diplomate ACVS
Professor of Surgery
Department of Clinical Studies—New
Bolton Center
University of Pennsylvania
Kennett Square, PA
USA

ERWIN G. PEARSON, DVM, MS
Diplomate ACVIM
Emeritus Professor
Large Animal Internal Medicine
College of Veterinary Medicine
Oregon State University
Corvallis, OR
USA

LISA K. PEARSON, DVM, MS, PhD
Diplomate ACT
Adjunct Faculty
College of Veterinary Medicine
Washington State University
Pullman, WA
USA

ANGELA M. PELZEL-MCCLUSKEY,
DVM, MS
Equine Epidemiologist
United States Department of Agriculture
Animal and Plant Health Inspection Service
Veterinary Services
Fort Collins, CO
USA

JEFFREY PHILLIPS, DVM, MSpVM, PhD
Diplomate ACVIM
Assistant Professor
College of Veterinary Medicine
Lincoln Memorial University
Harrogate, TN
USA

PERRINE PIAT, DVM
Diplomate ACVS, ECVS
Equine Surgeon and Practitioner
Clinique Equine de Provence
Saint Cannat
France

VALÉRIE PICANDET, DVM
Diplomate ACVIM, Diplomate ECEIM
Centre Hospitalier Vétérinaire Equin de Livet
St Michel de Livet
France

CARYN E. PLUMMER, DVM
Diplomate ACVO
Associate Professor
Departments of Large and Small Animal
Clinical Sciences
College of Veterinary Medicine
University of Florida
Gainesville, FL
USA

ROBERT H. POPPENGA, DVM, PhD
Diplomate ABVT
California Animal Health and Food Safety
Laboratory—Toxicology Section
School of Veterinary Medicine
University of California
West Health Sciences
Davis, CA
USA

BIRGIT PUSCHNER, DVM, PhD
Diplomate ABVT
Professor and Chair
Department of Molecular Biosciences
School of Veterinary Medicine
University of California
Davis, CA
USA

NICOLA PUSTERLA, DVM, PhD
Diplomate ACVIM
Professor
Department of Medicine and Epidemiology
School of Veterinary Medicine
University of California
Davis, CA
USA

SARAH M. RAABIS, DVM
Diplomate ACVIM
Clinical Instructor
Department of Medical Sciences
School of Veterinary Medicine
University of Wisconsin-Madison
Madison, WI
USA

KINDRA A. RADER, BS
Program Coordinator
Clinical Equine ICSI Program
Department of Veterinary Physiology and
Pharmacology
College of Veterinary Medicine and
Biomedical Sciences
Texas A&M University
College Station, TX
USA

SCOTT L. RADKE, DVM
Postdoctoral Research Associate
Department of Veterinary Diagnostic and
Production Animal Medicine
College of Veterinary Medicine
Iowa State University
Ames, IA
USA

ANN RASHMIR, DVM, MS, PGCVE
Diplomate ACVS
Associate Professor
College of Veterinary Medicine
Michigan State University
East Lansing, MI
USA

VIRGINIA B. REEF, DVM
Diplomate ACVIM (LAIM), DACVSMR
Associate Member ECVDI
Mark Whittier and Lila Griswold Allam
Professor of Medicine
Department of Clinical Studies—New Bolton
Center
University of Pennsylvania
Kennett Square, PA
USA

VERONICA L.H. ROBERTS, MA(Cantab),
VetMB, MA(Oxon), PGCert(HE)
Diplomate ECEIM, MRCVS
European and RCVS Specialist in Equine
Internal Medicine
Senior Clinical Fellow
School of Veterinary Clinical Sciences
University of Bristol
Langford
UK

ALEXANDER RODRIGUEZ-PALACIOS,
DVM, DVSc, PhD
Diplomate ACVS, Diplomate ECVS,
Diplomate ACVSMR, MRCVS
Senior Lecturer
Department of Equine Clinical Science
Institute of Veterinary Science
University of Liverpool
Neston
UK

MARIE-FRANCE ROY, DMV, PhD
Diplomate ACVIM
Assistant Professor
Department of Veterinary Clinical and
Diagnostic Sciences
Faculty of Veterinary Medicine
University of Calgary
Calgary, AL
Canada

LUIS RUBIO-MARTINEZ, DVM, DVSc, PhD
Diplomate ACVS, Diplomate ECVS,
Diplomate ACVSMR, MRCVS
Senior Lecturer
Department of Equine Clinical Science
Institute of Veterinary Science
University of Liverpool
Neston
UK

WILSON K. RUMBEIHA, BVM, PhD
Diplomate ABT, ABVT, Fellow ATS
Professor
Department of Molecular Biosciences
University of California – Davis
School of Veterinary Medicine
Davis, CA
USA

KAREN E. RUSSELL, DVM, PhD
Diplomate ACVP
Professor and Associate
Department Head for Clinical Services and
Residency Programs
Department of Veterinary Pathobiology
College of Veterinary Medicine and
Biomedical Sciences
Texas A&M University
College Station, TX
USA

ANGELIKA SCHOSTER, DVSc, PhD
Senior Clinical Lecturer
Equine Department
Vetsuisse Facility
University of Zurich
Zurich
Switzerland

HAROLD C. SCHOTT II, DVM, PhD
Diplomate ACVIM
Professor
Department of Large Animal Clinical
Sciences
College of Veterinary Medicine
Michigan State University
East Lansing, MI
USA

ERIC L. SCHROEDER, DVM, MS,
DACVECC, DACVIM
Assistant Professor
Department of Veterinary Clinical Sciences
The Ohio State University
College of Veterinary Medicine
Veterinary Medical Center
Columbus, OH
USA

JIM SCHUMACHER, DVM, MS, MRCVS,
Diplomate ACVS
Department of Large Animal Clinical
Sciences
College of Veterinary Medicine
University of Tennessee
Knoxville, TN
USA

KELLY P. SEARS, DVM, MS, PhD
Diplomate ACVIM
PhD Candidate, Immunology and Infectious
Disease
Department of Veterinary Microbiology
and Pathology
College of Veterinary Medicine
Washington State University
Pullman, WA
USA

DAVID SENTER, DVM
Diplomate ACVD
Adjunct Assistant Professor
The University of Missouri
College of Veterinary Medicine
Columbia, MO
USA

BARBARA L. SHERMAN, MS, PhD, DVM
Diplomate ACVB
Clinical Professor
Department of Clinical Sciences
College of Veterinary Medicine
North Carolina State University
Raleigh, NC
USA

JOANN SLACK, DVM, MS
Diplomate ACVIM
Associate Professor
Department of Clinical Studies
University of Pennsylvania—New
Bolton Center
Kennett Square, PA
USA

MARIANNE M. SLOET VAN
OLDRUITENBORGH-OOSTERBAAN,
DVM, PhD
Diplomate ECEIM, Specialist KNMvD Equine
Internal Medicine
Professor
Department of Equine Sciences
Faculty of Veterinary Medicine
Utrecht University
Utrecht
The Netherlands

KATIE J. SMITH, BVetMed Msc
Diplomate ACVS, MRCVS
University Equine Surgeon
Department of Veterinary Medicine
University of Cambridge
Cambridge
UK

ARYA SOBHAKUMARI, DVM, PhD
Diplomate ABT
Research Scientist
Global Quality and Applied Sciences
Nestle Purina PetCare
St. Louis, MO
USA

ALBERT SOLE-GUITART, DVM
Diplomate ACVS
Senior Lecturer
Equine Specialist Hospital
School of Veterinary Medicine
University of Queensland
Gatton, QLD
Australia

SHARON J. SPIER, DVM, PhD
Diplomate ACVIM
Professor
Department of Medicine and Epidemiology
School of Veterinary Medicine
University of California
Davis, CA
USA

BEATRICE T. SPONSELLER, DVM
Diplomate ABVP
Senior Clinician
Department of Veterinary Clinical Sciences
College of Veterinary Medicine
Iowa State University
Ames, IA
USA

BRETT SPONSELLER, DVM, PhD
Diplomate ACVIM
Associate Professor
Departments of Veterinary Microbiology &
Preventive Medicine and Veterinary Clinical
Sciences
College of Veterinary Medicine
Iowa State University
Ames, IA
USA

WENDY S. SPRAGUE, DVM, PhD
Veterinary Clinical Pathologist and Owner
Sprague Medical and Scientific
Communications, LLC
Fort Collins, CO
USA

HENRY STÄMPFLI, DVM, DrMedVet
Diplomate ACVIM
Professor
Large Animal Medicine, Clinical Studies
Ontario Veterinary College
University of Guelph
Guelph, ON
Canada

RAYMOND W. SWEENEY, VMD
Diplomate ACVIM
Professor
Department of Clinical Studies—New Bolton
Center
University of Pennsylvania
School of Veterinary Medicine
Kennett Square, PA
USA

CYPRIANNA SWIDERSKI, DVM, PhD
Diplomate ACVIM
Associate Professor
Department of Clinical Sciences
College of Veterinary Medicine
Mississippi State University
Mississippi State, MS
USA

SANDRA D. TAYLOR, DVM, PhD
Diplomate ACVIM
Associate Professor
Department of Veterinary Clinical Sciences
College of Veterinary Medicine
Purdue University
West Lafayette, IN
USA

FELIX THEISS, DrMedVet, DVM, PhD
Diplomate ECVS
Senior Clinical Lecturer
Equine Hospital
Division for Surgery
Justus-Liebig-University of Giessen
Giessen
Germany

JENNIFER S. THOMAS, DVM, PhD
Diplomate ACVP
Associate Professor
Department of Pathobiology and Diagnostics
College of Veterinary Medicine
Michigan State University
East Lansing, MI
USA

CRAIG A. THOMPSON, DVM
Diplomate ACVP
Clinical Assistant Professor
Department of Comparative Pathobiology
Purdue University
College of Veterinary Medicine
West Lafayette, IN
USA

LARRY J. THOMPSON, DVM, PhD
Diplomate ABVT
Senior Research Scientist
Nestlé Purina PetCare—PTC
St. Louis, MO
USA

AHMED TIBARY, DMV, MS, DSc, PhD
Diplomate ACT
Professor
Department of Veterinary Clinical Sciences
College of Veterinary Medicine
Washington State University
Pullman, WA
USA

PETER J. TIMONEY, MVB, MS, PhD, FRCVS
Frederick Van Lennep Chair in Equine
Veterinary Science
Maxwell H. Gluck Equine Research Center
Department of Veterinary Science
University of Kentucky
Lexington, KY
USA

RAMIRO TORIBIO, DVM, MS, PhD
Diplomate ACVIM
Professor
Department of Veterinary Clinical Sciences
College of Veterinary Medicine
The Ohio State University
Columbus, OH
USA

SUSAN J. TORNQUIST, DVM, MS, PhD
Diplomate ACVP
Professor
College of Veterinary Medicine
Oregon State University
Corvallis, OR
USA

ANDREW W. VAN EPS, BVSc, PhD,
MANZCVS
Diplomate ACVIM
Associate Professor
School of Veterinary Science
The University of Queensland
Gatton, QLD
Australia

EMMANUELLE VAN ERCK-WESTERGREN,
DVM, PhD
Diplomate ECEIM
Equine Sports Medicine Practice
Waterloo
Belgium

MODEST VENGUST, DVM, DVSc, PhD
Diplomate ACVIM, Diplomate ACVSMR and
Diplomate ECEIM
Associate Professor
University of Ljubljana
Veterinary Faculty
Ljubljana
Slovenia

ELISABETH-LIDWIEN J.M.M. VERDEGAAL, DVM
Diplomate ECEIM, Spec RNVA Eq Med
Senior Lecturer
Equine Health and Performance Centre
School of Animal and Veterinary Sciences
The University of Adelaide
Roseworthy Campus
Roseworthy, SA
Australia

ASHUTOSH VERMA, BVSc&AH, MVSc, PhD
Diplomate ACVM
Associate Professor
College of Veterinary Medicine
Lincoln Memorial University
Harrogate, TN
USA

LAURENT VIEL, DVM, MSc, PhD
Professor Emeritus
Ontario Veterinary College
University of Guelph
Guelph, ON
Canada

LINDA J. VOGELNEST, BVSc (Hons), MANZCVSc
Fellow ANZCVSc
Associate Lecturer
University of Sydney
Specialist Veterinary Dermatologist
Small Animal Specialist Hospital
North Ryde, NSW
Australia

VICTORIA L. VOITH, DVM, MSc, MA, PhD
Diplomate ACVB
Professor
Animal Behavior Content Expert
College of Veterinary Medicine
Western University of Health Sciences
Pomona, CA
USA

PETRA A. VOLMER, DVM, MS
Diplomate ABVP, Diplomate ABT
Senior Specialist, Drug Safety
Merck Animal Health
Madison, NJ
USA

JOHANNA L. WATSON, DVM, PhD
Diplomate ACVIM
Professor
Department of Medicine
University of California, Davis
Davis, CA
USA

JAMIE G. WEARN, BVSc, MS, DipVetClinStud
Diplomate ACVIM
Senior Lecturer
Discipline of Veterinary and Biomedical Sciences
College of Public Health, Medical and Veterinary Sciences
James Cook University
Townsville, QLD
Australia

J. SCOTT WEESE, DVM, DVSc
Diplomate ACVIM
Professor
Department of Pathobiology
Ontario Veterinary College
University of Guelph
Guelph, ON
Canada

STEPHEN D. WHITE, DVM
Diplomate ACVD
Professor
Department of Medicine and Epidemiology
School of Veterinary Medicine
University of California
Davis, CA
USA

ASHLEY WHITEHEAD, DVM, BSc, DVSc
Diplomate ACVIM
Instructor
Department of Veterinary Clinical and Diagnostic Sciences
Faculty of Veterinary Medicine
University of Calgary
Calgary, AL
USA

PAMELA A. WILKINS, DVM, MS, PhD
Diplomate ACVIM, Diplomate ACVECC
Professor
Department of Veterinary Clinical Medicine
University of Illinois College of Veterinary Medicine
Urbana, IL
USA

W. DAVID WILSON, BVMS, MS
Honorary Diplomate ACVIM
Professor Emeritus
Department of Medicine and Epidemiology
School of Veterinary Medicine
University of California-Davis
Davis, CA
USA

TINA WISMER, DVM, MS
Diplomate ABVT, Diplomate DABT
Medical Director
ASPCA Animal Poison Control Center
Urbana, IL
USA

SHARON G. WITONSKY, DVM, PhD, Diplomate ACVIM
Associate Professor
Department of Large Animal Clinical Sciences
Virginia Maryland College of Veterinary Medicine
Virginia Tech
Blacksburg, VA
USA

KAREN WOLFSDORF, DVM
Diplomate ACT
McGee Fertility Center
Hagyard Equine Medical Institute
Lexington, KT
USA

ABOUT THE COMPANION WEBSITE

This book is accompanied by a companion website:

www.fiveminutevet.com/equine

The website includes:

- Additional further reading lists not found in the book
- Client education handouts
- The figures from the book in PowerPoint
- Videos

CONTENTS

 *A client education handout for this topic is available at **www.fiveminutevet.com/equine** for you to download

*A client education handout for this topic is available at **www.fiveminutevet.com/equine** for you to download

*A client education handout for this topic is available at **www.fiveminutevet.com/equine** for you to download

*A client education handout for this topic is available at **www.fiveminutevet.com/equine** for you to download

*A client education handout for this topic is available at **www.fiveminutevet.com/equine** for you to download

*A client education handout for this topic is available at **www.fiveminutevet.com/equine** for you to download

*A client education handout for this topic is available at **www.fiveminutevet.com/equine** for you to download

*A client education handout for this topic is available at **www.fiveminutevet.com/equine** for you to download

*A client education handout for this topic is available at **www.fiveminutevet.com/equine** for you to download

*A client education handout for this topic is available at **www.fiveminutevet.com/equine** for you to download

*A client education handout for this topic is available at **www.fiveminutevet.com/equine** for you to download

CONTENTS *by Subject*

 *A client education handout for this topic is available at **www.fiveminutevet.com/equine** for you to download

DERMATOLOGY

ENDOCRINE

 *A client education handout for this topic is available at **www.fiveminutevet.com/equine** for you to download

GASTROENTEROLOGY

 *A client education handout for this topic is available at **www.fiveminutevet.com/equine**
for you to download

HEMATOPOIETIC

 *A client education handout for this topic is available at **www.fiveminutevet.com/equine** for you to download

INFECTIOUS DISEASES

 *A client education handout for this topic is available at **www.fiveminutevet.com/equine** for you to download

LABORATORY TESTS

 *A client education handout for this topic is available at **www.fiveminutevet.com/equine** for you to download

MUSCULOSKELETAL

NEONATOLOGY

 *A client education handout for this topic is available at **www.fiveminutevet.com/equine** for you to download

NEUROLOGY

OPHTHALMOLOGY

 *A client education handout for this topic is available at **www.fiveminutevet.com/equine** for you to download

RESPIRATORY

 *A client education handout for this topic is available at **www.fiveminutevet.com/equine** for you to download

SPORTS MEDICINE

THERIOGENOLOGY

 *A client education handout for this topic is available at **www.fiveminutevet.com/equine**
for you to download

TOXICOLOGY

 *A client education handout for this topic is available at **www.fiveminutevet.com/equine** for you to download

*A client education handout for this topic is available at **www.fiveminutevet.com/equine** for you to download

URINARY

 *A client education handout for this topic is available at **www.fiveminutevet.com/equine** for you to download

ABDOMINAL DISTENTION IN THE ADULT HORSE

BASICS

DEFINITION
Process by which the abdomen becomes enlarged, changing its normal contour and shape.

PATHOPHYSIOLOGY
The accumulation of fluid, gas, or ingesta in the peritoneal cavity, presence of abdominal masses, increased size of abdominal organs, or abdominal wall abnormalities such as edema may result in the distention and/or change in shape of the abdominal contour.

SYSTEMS AFFECTED
• GI—any condition, physical or functional, resulting in the vascular or nonvascular obstruction of the GI transit may lead to accumulation of gas and ingesta, resulting in abdominal distention
• Cardiovascular—secondary to GI obstruction, fluid sequestration and accumulation may lead to a hypovolemic shock. Vascular compromise of the GI tract leads to decreased GI protection, access of bacteria and/or toxins to the systemic circulation, and extravasation of a transudate/exudate into the peritoneal cavity. Intra-abdominal blood loss (hemoperitoneum) may occur from trauma or rupture of mesenteric or other (i.e. uterine, renal, ovarian) vessels due to increased traction or trauma (e.g. during foaling), from any other abdominal viscera (e.g. rupture of the spleen, liver, or ovarian follicle or cyst), or ascites secondary to heart failure. Electrolyte abnormalities from endotoxic shock or uroperitoneum may lead to secondary arrythmias and death. Alterations in oncotic or hydrostatic pressure may also lead to edema on the peritoneal cavity or intramurally in the intestinal wall
• Respiratory—abdominal distention may lead to increased pressure of the diaphragm, resulting in a shallow and fast respiratory pattern associated with atelectasis and hypoventilation due to failure of the alveoli to open. Occasionally rupture of the diaphragm resulting in internal entrapment and obstruction of the GI tract may be the initiating cause. In this case the presence of abdominal viscera in the thorax prevents the lungs from fully expanding, compounding the effects that pain and distention may have on the respiratory system
• Musculoskeletal/nervous/ophthalmic/skin— these systems may be injured through self-inflicted trauma secondary to abdominal pain. In cases of abdominal wall hernias, produced by trauma or lack of muscular tone with an eventual muscle rupture in older horses, the GI tract may become incarcerated, leading to its obstruction and potentially its vascular compromise, further promoting

abdominal distention. Lack of condition and fitness may over time lead to loss of abdominal muscular tone
• Reproductive—advanced pregnancy, either single or twin, will result in a marked change in the abdominal contour. Occasionally uterine torsion may be responsible for altered abdominal contour. Hydrops and ruptured of the prepubic tendon can be seen in pregnant mares and will manifest as change in the abdominal contour

SIGNALMENT
• All horses without exception may develop abdominal distention
• Pregnant mares may develop hydrops (any time during pregnancy), uterine torsion (mid-term), uroperitoneum (postpartum), or rupture of the mesocolon (postpartum), leading to hemoperitoneum and large colon torsion (peripartum)
• Rupture of the prepubic tendon occurs in older, sedentary mares in late pregnancy
• Miniature horses are predisposed to development of fecaliths, enteroliths, and small colon impactions
• Older horses are predisposed to pedunculating lipomas causing intestinal obstruction and are overrepresented in the incidence of tumors leading to hemoperitoneum, such as mesotheliomas, splenic hemangiosarcomas, and renal carcinomas
• Geographic distribution is important to consider the incidence of selected conditions such as ileal hypertrophy (southeast USA), enteroliths (south USA), and sand impactions (south USA)
• Uroperitoneum occurs mostly in male horses as a result of a ruptured bladder or urethra

SIGNS

Historical Findings
The clinical progression should help differentiate between vascular and nonvascular GI obstructions and other non-GI causes of distention.

Physical Examination Findings
A careful evaluation of clinical progression, historical facts, and of the horse including all systems may provide the information to determine the nature of the distention. Rectal examination, although practical, inexpensive, and quick, may not give a complete picture of the entire abdomen and may become less important if access to a good US machine and technique are possible.

CAUSES

Accumulation of Gas
• Functional obstruction—primary or secondary ileus. Primary ileus due to increased sympathetic drive. Secondary ileus due to pain (visceral or musculoskeletal), ischemic necrosis (e.g. verminous arteritis) post surgery, electrolyte abnormalities (e.g. endurance horses), dehydration,

inflammation of the bowel (enteritis) or abdominal cavity (peritonitis), and sedative or anesthetic drugs (e.g. α_2 agents, opioids)
• Physical obstruction: either vascular (large colon volvulus, mesenteric root volvulus, strangulating lipoma) or nonvascular (impaction, enteroliths, nephrosplenic entrapment)
• Cecal tympany from abnormal cecal motility patterns
• Excessive feed stuff fermentation—grain overload
• Free gas within the abdominal cavity secondary to trauma or anaerobic infections
• Colitis

Accumulation of Fluid
• Hemoperitoneum—ruptured viscera, vessel, ovarian cyst/follicle or tumor
• Uroperitoneum—ruptured bladder secondary to trauma, or obstructive urolithiasis
• Hydrops amnion or allantois
• Ascites—peritonitis, neoplasia, hypoproteinemia, right-sided heart failure
• Colitis or enteritis—secretory process leading to accumulation of fluid in lumen of large colon or small intestine
• Cecal impaction with fluid due to abnormal motility patterns
• Pyometra/mucometra

Solid Mass
• Abscess
• Neoplasia—lymphosarcoma, squamous cell carcinoma, mammary adenocarcinoma, mesothelioma, hemangiosarcoma, renal carcinoma, ovarian granulosa cell tumor

Body Wall Abnormality
• Hernia
• Prepubic tendon rupture

RISK FACTORS
• Cribbing predisposes horses to tympany of the colon and epiploic foramen entrapment
• Gastric ulcers predispose horses to gastric rupture
• Sudden exposure to large amounts of carbohydrate-rich feed or diets consisting of increased proportions of highly fermentable feedstuff (especially whole-grain corn) and decreased amounts of roughage can predispose to gastric, cecal, large colon tympany, and large colon displacement or volvulus
• Colonic impactions often occur in horses that are old or debilitated or that have poor dentition or in horses eating a diet with a large amount of fiber or following water deprivation
• Sudden change in physical activity or sudden stall rest imposed by another injury may lead to cecal or large colon impaction
• Sudden change of diet, even hay batch, has been associated with colic and abdominal gas distention
• Enterolithiasis occurs frequently in the states of California, Florida, and Indiana

• Sand impactions are seen frequently in the southern and coastal states
• Ileal hypertrophy has been associated with ingestion of Bermuda grass hay
• Periparturient mares are at increased risk of large colon volvulus, particularly if it has happened before
• Miniature horses are predisposed to small colon impactions
• Overconditioned and old horses are predisposed to strangulating lipomas

 DIAGNOSIS

DIFFERENTIAL DIAGNOSIS

Differentiating Similar Signs
Other conditions with the appearance of abdominal distention include:
• Marked subcutaneous edema along the ventral abdomen and thorax
• Pregnancy—diagnosis may be made via rectal palpation with or without ultrasonography
• "Hay belly"—may be diagnosed on history (malnourished, old, or nonfit horses or severely parasitized horses, diets high in poor quality roughage) and by fecal examination
• Pendulous abdomen secondary to pituitary adenoma and Cushing disease—usually accompanied by other distinctive signs, such as abnormal haircoat and failure to shed winter coat
• Extreme obesity—ribs not palpable, fat deposits evident along crest of neck, over tail-head, etc.
• Subcutaneous emphysema from penetrating chest wound, ruptured trachea, or subcutaneous anaerobic infection—characteristic crepitus noticed on palpation of the skin

Differentiating Causes
Signalment, history, physical examination, laboratory work, rectal palpation, and US examination findings often provide sufficient information to permit a tentative diagnosis. Some conditions are associated with characteristic findings:
• GI gas accumulation (bloat)—reduced GI sounds may be heard, and increased gaseous distention may be identified on percussion as a hyperresonant sound colloquially termed "ping"; depending on the inciting cause and the degree of distention present, various degrees of abdominal pain are present. Hypermotile sounds can also be auscultated in cases of spasmodic colic, which can be associated with an excessive amount of gas being produced
• Ascites from right-sided heart failure—tricuspid insufficiency results in findings including heart murmur, exercise intolerance, jugular distention and pulse, and

edema of the ventral abdomen, pectoral muscles, and distal limbs
• Ascites from intra-abdominal mesothelioma—because this tumor originates from the fluid-producing cells of the peritoneum, several liters of peritoneal fluid may be produced within a 24 h period; ascites may be more dramatic than is noted with other conditions
• Body wall defect from prepubic tendon rupture—one of the only causes of unilateral abdominal distention in the horse; also results in cranioventral positioning of the mammary gland, cranial tilting of the pelvis, and severe ventral abdominal swelling
• Presence of diarrhea may point towards colitis or enteritis. Evaluation of nasogastric reflux may be useful in this situation

CBC/BIOCHEMISTRY/URINALYSIS
Results are dependent on the cause. It is important to asses PCV, TP, and WBC, including a differential evaluation of WBC.

OTHER LABORATORY TESTS
• Abdominocentesis should be performed carefully in pregnant mares with intestinal distention, where the bowel may be torn easily by inadvertent penetration with a needle or teat cannula despite proper restraint.
 ◦ Abdominal lactate content when compared with systemic circulating lactate may offer valuable information toward the diagnosis of a vascular obstruction
 ◦ WBC count, TP level, and specific gravity of the peritoneal fluid should be measured, and the fluid should be assessed cytologically for evidence of degenerate neutrophils, neoplastic cells, bacteria, or plant material
 ◦ Other parameters such as Cr may also be measured in cases where uroperitoneum is suspected. In cases of uroperitoneum, Cr in the peritoneal fluid exceeds serum Cr levels by a ratio of > 2:1
 ◦ An increase in WBC count and TP levels and the appearance of degenerate neutrophils are indicative of increasing inflammation within the abdomen
 ◦ With hemoperitoneum, free-flowing blood may be evident from the needle or teat cannula during the centesis procedure. This should not be mistaken for puncture of the spleen during the procedure, in which case the PCV of the obtained sample is higher than the circulating blood

IMAGING
• Abdominal radiography may help to diagnose gas accumulation within bowel segments in small horses and ponies. Enteroliths or sand impactions may be evident in adult horses in the mid- to ventral abdomen on the lateral view
• US of the abdomen can be useful in skilled hands and can be used to identify the

location, amount, character, and echogenicity of peritoneal fluid and abdominal viscera, particularly thickness of the intestinal wall. It can also provide information on the condition of the heart, liver, spleen, kidney, and bladder, and can help identify the presence of intra-abdominal adhesions or masses

OTHER DIAGNOSTIC PROCEDURES
• Laparoscopy allows visualization of the abdominal cavity in the standing horse, and can be used to provide a definitive diagnosis of the cause of abdominal distention. It can be used in selected cases (i.e. peritonitis, ruptured bladder) to direct appropriate therapy and treatment. In the presence of GI distention the ability to identify the nature of the obstruction may be compromised
• Exploratory laparotomy through a flank incision in the standing horse is very limiting and should only be performed in selected cases as a therapeutic intervention if a confirmed diagnosis such as nephrosplenic entrapment or uterine torsion has been made
• Exploratory laparotomy through a ventral midline incision in the anesthetized horse should not be delayed unnecessarily as it may be a life-saving diagnostic and therapeutic tool if used appropriately

 TREATMENT

• Specific treatment is largely dependent on the cause of abdominal distention. Cardiovascular stabilization through rehydration and correction of electrolyte and acid–base abnormalities should be initiated prior to treatment of the primary disease process
• In horses with severe gaseous distention, trocarization of the cecum and/or large colon may be necessary to improve ventilation and comfort. Although the complications of this procedure are reportedly very low, it is associated with peritonitis and any horse that is trocarized should be treated preemptively with anti-inflammatory drugs and broad-spectrum antibiotic therapy to reduce and minimize the inherent risk of peritonitis
• Mares with hydrops or rupture of the prepubic tendon may require induction of parturition. Horses with abdominal distention should be confined to a stall and monitored continuously until a diagnosis has been made and appropriate treatment initiated
• Feed should be withheld from horses showing any signs of abdominal discomfort
• Prompt and adequate referral to a hospital facility may be required in cases requiring surgical intervention or prolonged nursing care

(CONTINUED) **ABDOMINAL DISTENTION IN THE ADULT HORSE**

MEDICATIONS

Drug therapy is dictated by the inciting cause.

FOLLOW-UP

Plans for monitoring are based on cause and treatment.

MISCELLANEOUS

ASSOCIATED CONDITIONS
N/A

AGE-RELATED FACTORS
N/A

PREGNANCY/FERTILITY/BREEDING
• Termination of pregnancy may be indicated in mares with hydrops or nonresolving uterine torsion
• Induction of parturition may be necessary in mares close to term that have experienced rupture of the prepubic tendon. These mares should be monitored carefully and parturition attended as they may require assistance with delivery due to their inability to perform effective abdominal press for fetal expulsion

SYNONYMS
Bloat

SEE ALSO
• Acute adult abdominal pain—acute colic
• Colic, chronic/recurrent
• Oral stereotypic behavior

ABBREVIATIONS
• Cr = creatinine
• GI = gastrointestinal
• PCV = packed cell volume
• TP = total protein
• US = ultrasonography, ultrasound
• WBC = white blood cell

Suggested Reading
Sanchez C. Disorders of the gastrointestinal system. In: Reed S, Bayly W, Sellon D, eds. Equine Internal Medicine, 4e. St. Louis, MO: Elsevier, 2017:709–715.

Author Antonio M. Cruz
Consulting Editors Henry Stämpfli and Olimpo Oliver-Espinosa

ABDOMINAL HERNIA IN ADULT HORSES

BASICS

OVERVIEW
Abdominal hernia is an exteriorization of internal organs through a defect or an anatomic opening in the abdominal wall. In adult horses, abdominal hernias include ventral, incisional, and acquired inguinal hernia.

SIGNALMENT
Ventral Hernia
Common in older, late-term pregnant mares. Draft breeds are predisposed.

Incisional Hernia
Complication of ventral midline celiotomy in 6–18% of horses.

Acquired Inguinal Hernia
• Refers to the passage of intestine (small intestine most commonly) and/or omentum through the vaginal ring into the inguinal canal and in the scrotum
• Particularly in the stallion
• Standardbred, draft breeds, Tennessee Walking, and Andalusian horses are predisposed

SIGNS
Ventral Hernia
Painful swelling is associated with a body wall defect.

Incisional Hernia
Incisional edema and swelling. Discharge from the incision and increase in drainage of peritoneal fluid are commonly observed prior to dehiscence.

Acquired Inguinal Hernia
Colic signs depending on degree of intestinal strangulation and scrotal swelling. The testis is usually cool due to vascular compromise.

CAUSES AND RISK FACTORS
Ventral Hernia
In pregnant mares, old broodmares, and twin gestation. Associated with trauma, hydrops (allantois and amnion).

Incisional Hernia
Incisional infection, edema and drainage, postoperative pain, re-laparotomy, and suture material and suture patterns. Older and heavy horses, type of incision, degree of surgical trauma, length of surgery, and difficulties during recovery. No stent bandage during recovery.

Acquired Inguinal Hernia
Often in stallions after copulation or strenuous exercise. Large vaginal rings may predispose to herniation.

DIAGNOSIS

DIFFERENTIAL DIAGNOSIS
Ventral Hernia
Prepubic tendon rupture (pelvis tilted cranioventrally, cranioventral displacement of the udder).

Incisional Hernia
Postoperative wound infection, severe peri-incisional edema, seroma, and sinus formation are easily differentiated from incisional hernias with the abdominal wall being intact on palpation and US examination.

Acquired Inguinal Hernia
Torsion of the spermatic cord, orchitis, testicular vasculature thrombosis, hydrocele, hematocele, and testicular neoplasia.

CBC/BIOCHEMISTRY/URINALYSIS
Unremarkable in absence of secondary intestinal strangulation.

IMAGING
Abdominal US
US is used to confirm herniation, to evaluate the extent of the abdominal wall defect, and to identify hernia contents.

OTHER DIAGNOSTIC PROCEDURES
External Palpation
To define the hernia ring and contents. To differentiate between reducible and nonreducible hernias. Palpation of inguinal regions and scrotum is mandatory in stallions with signs of colic.

Rectal Palpation
Rectal palpation of stallions with inguinal hernia reveals presence of distended intestine (small intestine most commonly) entering the vaginal ring.

TREATMENT

Ventral Hernia and Incisional Hernia
Small hernias are treated initially conservatively by supporting the ventral abdominal wall, decreasing the amount of local inflammation and edema, and preventing enlargement of the hernia. Rest, low-bulk diet, and monitoring for signs of intestinal obstruction. Anecdotal reports of incisional hernia healing using postsurgical commercially available abdominal bandage. Ventral or incisional hernia may resolve with conservative treatment, but surgical closure of the abdominal defect 8–12 weeks after its occurrence is usually required. In a recent report, herniorrhaphy was performed within 21 days for treating external traumatic abdominal hernias in horses and mules. Application of a mesh is based on the size of the wall defect and the surgeon's preference. Horses with acute severe incisional dehiscence (eventration) are emergency surgical candidates.

Acquired Inguinal Hernia
Treatment is usually surgical by performing a ventral midline celiotomy, resecting the nonviable small intestine, and castrating the horse. During the early phase, it may be possible to reduce the hernia using external inguinal/scrotal massages under general anesthesia in dorsal recumbency or using traction per rectum.

MEDICATIONS

DRUG(S) OF CHOICE
Ventral and Incisional Hernia
Anti-inflammatories to decrease inflammation and antibiotics to resolve infection to allow fibrous tissue to form at the hernial ring prior to herniorrhaphy.

FOLLOW-UP

• The prognosis for ventral hernia is guarded. Incisional and inguinal hernias warrant a favorable prognosis
• From 3 to 5 months of rest is required after surgical correction of both ventral and incisional hernias

ABBREVIATIONS
• US = ultrasonography, ultrasound

Suggested Reading
Azizi S, Hashemi-Asl SM, Torabi E. Early herniorrhaphy of large traumatic abdominal wounds in horses and mules. Equine Vet J 2016;48:434–437.
Dukti S, White N. Surgical complications of colic surgery. Vet Clin Equine 2009;24:515–534.
Schumacher J, Perkins J. Inguinal herniation and rupture in horses. Equine Vet Educ 2010;22:7–10.

Author Albert Sole-Guitart
Consulting Editors Henry Stämpfli and Olimpo Oliver-Espinosa

Client Education Handout available online

ABDOMINOCENTESIS—INCREASED PERITONEAL FLUID

BASICS

DEFINITION
• Procedure for sampling peritoneal fluid by collection through the abdominal wall
• Abdominocentesis is usually performed at the most dependent part of the abdominal wall. The site is clipped and prepared aseptically. Either a needle or a blunt-tipped cannula can be used to enter the abdominal cavity. Using a needle is usually faster and is associated with less bleeding from vessels in the skin; the cannula is less likely to result in inadvertent enterocentesis or laceration of the intestinal wall. When using a cannula, the site is first infused with local anesthesia and a small skin incision is made
• Transabdominal ultrasound may be used to locate fluid pockets
• Peritoneal fluid is collected into EDTA-containing tubes for assessment of the total nucleated cell count and cytology, and into a sterile clot tube for bacterial culture or biochemical tests
• Equine abdominal fluid normally appears clear and colorless to slightly yellow and does not clot
• Total protein commonly is assessed by refractometer and normally is < 2.5 g/dL
• The nucleated cells may be counted by hemocytometer or by using some hematology analyzers. The nucleated cell count in fluid from normal horses is < 5000 cells/µL, with a predominance of nondegenerative neutrophils (22–98%) and large mononuclear cells (1–68%), which include mesothelial cells and macrophages. Small lymphocytes may constitute 0–36% of the total cell count and eosinophils up to 7%; mast cells and basophils are rarely seen. Normally, few erythrocytes are present
• Biochemical measurements in addition to total protein may include lactate as an indicator of intestinal ischemia or hypoperfusion, glucose as an indicator of septic peritonitis and creatinine, and/or potassium to aid in diagnosis of uroabdomen

PATHOPHYSIOLOGY
• Normal peritoneal fluid is a dialysate of plasma; many of the low-molecular-weight substances in blood are present in the peritoneal fluid at similar concentrations
• High-molecular-weight molecules (e.g. proteins) normally are not present in abdominal fluid
• Cells in normal peritoneal fluid include mesothelial cells that line the abdominal cavity and cover visceral surfaces, and small numbers of cells from the blood and lymphatics
• Fluid circulates constantly through the abdominal cavity and is drained via lymphatic vessels. When fluid production exceeds drainage, effusion develops. This may occur with some systemic disorders (e.g. cardiovascular disease) or with local disorders of abdominal organs or mesothelium. Changes in peritoneal fluid protein, cell numbers, and cell types may reflect those disorders
• During inadequate intestinal perfusion and ischemia, anaerobic glycolysis can result in increased peritoneal fluid lactate concentration. A peritoneal fluid lactate concentration that is higher than the serum concentration provides evidence of intra-abdominal infection or ischemia
• When infection is present in the abdomen, the peritoneal fluid glucose concentration is usually < 30 mg/dL, as glucose is actively consumed by bacteria. It is also reported that a difference of > 50 mg/dL between the serum and peritoneal fluid is highly diagnostic for infection in the abdomen. The glucose measurement might be most useful when timely cytologic examination is not available
• A localized process in the abdomen, such as a walled-off abscess or a tumor, may not be reflected in a peritoneal fluid sample
• Repeated sampling of peritoneal fluid is necessary, in some cases, to follow the course of a disease or to monitor therapy, whether it is medical or surgical

SYSTEMS AFFECTED
• GI
• Hepatobiliary
• Hemic/lymphatic/immune
• Renal/urologic
• Cardiovascular
• Reproductive

GENETICS
N/A

INCIDENCE/PREVALENCE
N/A

GEOGRAPHIC DISTRIBUTION
N/A

SIGNALMENT
Any breed, age, or sex.

SIGNS
• Colic
• Chronic weight loss
• Abdominal distention
• Diarrhea
• Pyrexia

CAUSES
• Peritonitis caused by compromised gut wall
• Hemorrhage (hemoabdomen)
• Intra-abdominal neoplasia
• Intestinal parasitism and secondary thromboembolism
• Inflammation of abdominal organs
• Compromised venous return due to intestinal displacement, distention, etc.
• Breeding and foaling injuries
• Bile or urine leakage
• Postsurgical inflammation or other complications
• Abdominal abscess
• Decreased oncotic pressure
• Congestive heart failure

RISK FACTORS
• Abdominal surgery
• Pregnancy
• Hypoalbuminemia

DIAGNOSIS

DIFFERENTIAL DIAGNOSIS

Peritonitis
Peritonitis may be caused by a number of conditions, including a displaced or strangulated bowel, bowel necrosis, obstruction, bowel rupture, abscess, or thromboembolism.
• The fluid is an exudate with an increased nucleated cell count and a predominance of neutrophils
• The total protein usually is > 2.5 g/dL due to the presence of inflammatory proteins
• Bacteria are present in septic peritonitis and may be intracellular or extracellular. Degenerative changes in neutrophils are usually seen and the glucose concentration of the fluid is decreased
• With gut rupture, cells often are degenerate and mixed bacterial types, ciliated protozoa, and plant material may be seen
• Postsurgical peritonitis also produces an exudate with increased cell numbers and total protein within 24 h and lasting up to 2 weeks. Neutrophils generally are not degenerate and no bacteria are seen. Increased RBC numbers may be seen

Hemorrhage
• With a splenic tap, the PCV is higher in abdominal fluid than in blood, and small lymphocyte numbers may be increased
• With hemorrhage into the abdomen, the PCV of fluid is lower than that of blood. Platelets are absent, and erythrophagocytosis or macrophages containing hemoglobin-breakdown pigments may be seen
• With blood contamination at the time of sampling, fluid initially may look clear, with bloody streaks appearing during sampling. Phagocytosis of RBCs is not seen, and platelets may be present

Neoplasia
A diagnosis may be established on finding neoplastic cells in fluid but absence of neoplastic cells does not rule out neoplasia, because tumor cells may not exfoliate into fluid.

Parasitism
Migration of parasitic larvae may be associated with increased eosinophils, but this does not occur often and is not diagnostic for parasitism.

A

ABDOMINOCENTESIS—INCREASED PERITONEAL FLUID (CONTINUED)

Uroabdomen
• Typically, peritoneal fluid creatinine and potassium concentrations are increased compared with serum concentrations
• Hyperkalemia, marked hyponatremia, and hypochloremia are typical but are not present in all cases

Ascites
• A transudate with low cell numbers and low protein content may be present with hypoalbuminemia or lymphatic or vascular obstruction or stasis
• Serum biochemical profile and history contribute to this diagnosis

Congestive Heart Failure
Increased hydrostatic pressure within vessels may result in a modified transudate with a higher cell count and protein level than a transudate, but these values may be normal for equine abdominal fluid.

CBC/BIOCHEMISTRY/URINALYSIS
• Inflammatory causes of abdominal effusion may be associated with leukocytosis or hyperfibrinogenemia if disease is systemic
• Left shift or toxic changes in neutrophils indicate systemic inflammation
• Serum biochemistries help in assessing causes of transudate, e.g. panhypoproteinemia is consistent with GI protein loss; elevated liver enzymes suggest hepatic disease
• Serum electrolyte concentrations and comparison of serum and fluid creatinine concentrations aid in diagnosis of uroperitoneum

OTHER LABORATORY TESTS
Bacterial culture is helpful in some cases, such as abdominal abscess.

IMAGING
Ultrasonography
• May be useful in identifying a subjective increase in peritoneal fluid, hemoabdomen, GI distention or wall thickening, intussusception, masses, adhesions, abnormal liver/spleen/kidney, and enteroliths
• Ultrasonographic location of peritoneal fluid might help in performing abdominocentesis

Abdominal Radiography
In adult horses, may aid in establishing the diagnosis of diaphragmatic hernia, sand enteropathy, and enteroliths.

OTHER DIAGNOSTIC PROCEDURES
• Palpation per rectum might aid in the diagnosis of GI abnormalities or abdominal effusion

• Laparoscopy may be used to establish the diagnosis in cases of chronic colic or weight loss
• Gastroscopy can be useful in establishing the diagnosis of gastric ulcers, impaction, and neoplasia
• Exploratory laparotomy is necessary for definitive diagnosis in some cases

PATHOLOGIC FINDINGS
As described.

TREATMENT
Directed at the underlying cause.

MEDICATIONS
Based on the underlying cause.

FOLLOW-UP

PATIENT MONITORING
No specific monitoring procedures are indicated following an uncomplicated abdominocentesis.

PREVENTION/AVOIDANCE
N/A

POSSIBLE COMPLICATIONS
• Subcutaneous swelling at the site may be more commonly observed when a blunt cannula is used for the procedure
• Accidental enterocentesis is rarely associated with clinical disease but causes an increased nucleated cell count in abdominal fluid within 4 h. When the gut is tapped, there will be few, if any, cells, large numbers of bacteria, and plant material on cytologic examination. Also, the physical condition of the horse is relatively normal compared with one with a gut rupture
• Puncture of a compromised intestinal wall could cause leakage and rapid development of severe peritonitis. Sand impaction is associated with increased risk of intestinal puncture
• Accidental amniocentesis may occur in pregnant mares. This has not been reported to be associated with any specific sequelae

EXPECTED COURSE AND PROGNOSIS
Dependent on the underlying cause.

MISCELLANEOUS

AGE-RELATED FACTORS
Foals normally have peritoneal fluid protein concentrations similar to those of adults, but total nucleated cell counts (< 1500 cells/µL) that are lower than those of adults.

PREGNANCY/FERTILITY/BREEDING
There are no significant differences between fluid from mares that are pregnant or have recently foaled and fluid from nonperipartum mares.

SYNONYMS
• Abdominal paracentesis
• Belly tap
• Intraperitoneal tap

SEE ALSO
• Abdominal distention in the adult horse
• Acute adult abdominal pain—acute colic
• Peritonitis

ABBREVIATIONS
• GI = gastrointestinal
• PCV = packed cell volume
• RBC = red blood cell

Suggested Reading
Brownlow MA, Hutchins DR, Johnston KG. Reference values for equine peritoneal fluid. Equine Vet J 1981;13:127–130.
Duesterdieck-Zellmer KF, Richl JH, McKenzie EC, et al. Effects of abdominocentesis technique on peritoneal fluid and clinical variables in horses. Equine Vet Educ 2014;26:262–268.
Latson KM, Nieto JE, Beldomenico PM, Snyder JR. Evaluation of peritoneal fluid lactate as a marker of intestinal ischaemia in equine colic. Equine Vet J 2005;37:342–346.
Parry BW, Brownlow MA. Peritoneal fluid. In: Cowell RL, Tyler RD, eds. Cytology and Hematology of the Horse. Goleta, CA: American Veterinary Publications, 1992:121–151.
Van Hoogmoed L, Snyder JR, Christopher M, Vatistas N. Evaluation of peritoneal fluid pH, glucose concentration, and lactate dehydrogenase activity for detection of septic peritonitis in horses. J Am Vet Med Assoc 1999;214:1032–1036.

Author Susan J. Tornquist
Consulting Editor Sandra D. Taylor

BASICS

DEFINITION
• Estrus—period of sexual receptivity of the mare for the stallion
• Abnormal estrus interval—mare displays sexual behavior for longer or shorter periods than normal
• Abnormal interovulatory intervals result from altered estrus or diestrus lengths

PATHOPHYSIOLOGY
Mares are seasonally polyestrous with the ovulatory period in spring/summer:
• Average estrous cycle is 21 days
• Estrus length averages 5–7 days
• Diestrus length more consistently 14–15 days

Key Hormonal Events in the Equine Estrous Cycle
• FSH causes follicular growth
• Follicular estradiol (E_2) stimulates increased GnRH pulse frequency and LH secretion
• LH surge causes ovulation
• Progesterone (P_4) (CL origin) rises from basal levels (<1 ng/mL) at ovulation to > 4 ng/mL by 4–5 days post ovulation
• A second FSH surge in diestrus initiates another follicular wave
• Endometrial $PGF_{2\alpha}$ is released 14–15 days post ovulation, causing luteolysis and a decline in P4 levels

Sexual Behavior
• Absence of P_4 allows onset of estrus behavior even if E_2 is present in small quantities
• Conditions that eliminate P_4 and/or > E_2 concentrations are likely to induce estrus behavior (including bilateral ovariectomy)

SYSTEMS AFFECTED
• Reproductive
• Behavioral
• Endocrine

SIGNALMENT
• Mares of any age/breed
• Ponies have longer estrous cycles (average 24 days) than mares

SIGNS

Historical Findings
• Chief complaints—infertility, failure to show estrus, prolonged estrus, split estrus, or frequent estrus behavior
• Reproductive history—review breeding/teasing records, previous foaling data, urogenital infections/treatments, pharmaceutical interventions
• Seasonal influences—review time of year, individual variation (onset/duration/termination of cyclicity)

• Have clients log behaviors in a journal for persistent estrus cases to identify patterns

Physical Examination Findings
• Poor body condition/malnutrition or metabolic disease (pituitary pars intermedia dysfunction) may contribute to abnormal cyclicity
• Poor perineal conformation can result in pneumovagina, ascending infections, and/or urine pooling, anestrus/infertility
• Clitoral enlargement may relate to drug history (anabolic steroids) or intersex conditions
• TRP and US are essential for evaluation. Rule out pregnancy. Assess uterine size/tone, ovarian size/shape/location, and cervical relaxation. Serial TRP may be needed to completely define status
• Vaginal speculum examination to identify inflammation, urine pooling, cervical competency, conformational abnormalities

CAUSES

Shortened Estrus Duration
• Split heats often observed during transition periods (seasonality)
• Silent heat—mare with normal cyclic ovarian activity but minimal or no overt sexual receptivity
• Often behavior-based problem—nervousness, foal-at-side, maiden mare; possibly previous anabolic steroid use

Lengthened Estrus Duration
• May appear as persistent estrus behavior or split heats
• Persistent estrus behavior due to cystitis, vaginitis, urine pooling, ovarian neoplasia (GTCT), chromosomal abnormalities
• Split heats often observed during transition periods (seasonality)
• Up to 30% of bilaterally ovariectomized mares may show persistent estrus

Shortened Interestrus Interval
Premature luteolysis:
1. endometritis
2. endotoxemia (i.e. colic, colitis, laminitis)
3. iatrogenic due to intrauterine infusions, biopsy, administration of $PGF_{2\alpha}$

Lengthened Interestrus Interval
• Prolonged CL function—diestrus ovulation, persistent CL (due to idiopathic/spontaneous or uteropathic (pyometra) causes), pregnancy, early embryonic death after maternal recognition of pregnancy or endometrial cup formation, oxytocin treatment, placement of intrauterine marbles, use of deslorelin implants
• Suppression of estrus behavior by treatment with altrenogest or natural P_4
• Induction of anestrus via GnRH vaccination or bilateral ovariectomy

DIAGNOSIS

DIFFERENTIAL DIAGNOSIS

Differentiating Conditions with Similar Symptoms
• Behavior complaints must be investigated as to the inciting cause—physiologic, pathologic, or psychologic
• All mares should be submitted for physical and urogenital examination including TRP, US, and vaginal speculum examination
• Urinalysis, uterine culture, uterine cytology, and endometrial biopsy can provide specific diagnoses for persistent estrus behavior, endometritis
• Serial examination may be required to differentiate silent heat, split heat, transitional period, prolonged CL function
• GTCT may be suspected on US; confirm with serology
• Karyotype to diagnose chromosomal disorders

CBC/BIOCHEMISTRY/URINALYSIS
N/A

OTHER LABORATORY TESTS
• Serum progesterone
  ○ Basal < 1 ng/mL (no luteal tissue present)
• GTCT panel
  ○ Nonpregnant mare—AMH < 3.8 ng/mL, inhibin < 0.7 ng/mL, testosterone 20–45 pg/mL
  ○ GTCT if AMH > 8.0 ng/mL, inhibin > 0.7 ng/mL, testosterone > 100 pg/mL
• Karyotype

IMAGING
• Transrectal US of reproductive tract
• Hysteroscopy to diagnose uterine abnormalities

OTHER DIAGNOSTIC PROCEDURES
N/A

TREATMENT
• Serial monitoring of the mare's reproductive tract by TRP and US
• For persistent estrus:
  ○ Treat underlying endometritis, cystitis, vaginitis, urine pooling
  ○ Correct poor perineal conformation (Caslick's vulvoplasty, Gadd procedure, Pouret procedure)
• For prolonged diestrus:
  ○ Rule out pregnancy
  ○ Treat pyometra or other uterine disease, if present

- PGF$_{2\alpha}$ treatment
- Remove marble or deslorelin implant
- For anestrus:
  - Identify if mare is cyclic or truly anestrus
  - If cyclic, modify teasing/breeding management schemes. Breed based on TRP and US, if possible
  - Ovariectomy if GTCT diagnosed
  - If anestrus during the breeding season, identify and treat inciting cause, if possible
  - Consider artificial lighting schemes or pharmaceuticals to advance the vernal transition period in broodmares

MEDICATIONS

DRUG(S) OF CHOICE
- To induce luteolysis—PGF$_{2\alpha}$ (dinoprost tromethamine, Lutalyse (Pfizer) 10 mg IM) or analogs
- To induce ovulation in estrus—deslorelin 1.8 mg IM: ovulation within 48 h if follicle(s) > 30 mm; hCG 2500 IU IV: ovulation within 48 h if follicle(s) > 35 mm
- To hasten vernal transition:
  - Altrenogest (0.044 mg/kg PO daily ≥ 15 days) if follicles > 20 mm are present and mare is exhibiting behavioral estrus. PGF$_{2\alpha}$ is given on day 15
  - Combination P$_4$/E$_2$ treatments followed by PGF$_{2\alpha}$ are also used
  - Dopamine antagonists—domperidone 1.1 mg/kg PO daily or sulpiride 1.0 mg/kg or 200 mg/mare IM daily; often used in combination with artificial photoperiod
  - FSH—used experimentally
- To suppress estrus:
  - Oxytocin 60 IU IM daily 7–14 days post ovulation or for 29 days at any time during the cycle
  - Altrenogest 0.044 mg/kg PO daily
  - Natural P$_4$—available in several injectable formulations (short- or long-acting)

CONTRAINDICATIONS
PGF$_{2\alpha}$ and analogs—contraindicated with equine asthma/bronchoconstrictive disease.

PRECAUTIONS
- Horses
  - PGF$_{2\alpha}$ causes sweating/colic-like symptoms due to stimulation of smooth muscle. Symptomatic treatment if not resolved in 1–2 h
  - Antibodies to hCG can develop:
    - Limit use to < 2 or 3 times per breeding season

- Half-life of antibodies is 1 to several months
  - Deslorelin implants are associated with prolonged interovulatory periods in nonpregnant mares, if not removed soon after ovulation has been confirmed. Not available in the USA
  - Progesterone supplementation may be contraindicated in mares with a history of uterine infection
- Humans
  - PGF$_{2\alpha}$ should not be handled by pregnant women or persons with asthma/bronchial disease
  - Altrenogest should not be handled by pregnant women or persons with thrombophlebitis, thromboembolic disorders, cerebrovascular/coronary artery disease, breast cancer, estrogen-dependent neoplasia, undiagnosed vaginal bleeding, or tumors that developed with use of oral contraceptives or estrogen-containing products

POSSIBLE INTERACTIONS
N/A

ALTERNATIVE DRUGS
Cloprostenol sodium (Estrumate (Schering-Plough Animal Health) 250 µg/mL IM) is a PGF$_{2\alpha}$ analog. This product is used in similar fashion to dinoprost tromethamine and has been associated with fewer side effects. While it is not currently approved for use in horses, it is in broad use in the absence of an alternative.

FOLLOW-UP

PATIENT MONITORING
The mare should be examined serially until normal cyclicity or pregnancy is determined.

POSSIBLE COMPLICATIONS
Undesirable behavior, infertility, prolonged nonpregnant intervals.

MISCELLANEOUS

PREGNANCY/FERTILITY/BREEDING
PGF$_{2\alpha}$ administration to pregnant mares can cause luteolysis and abortion. Definitively rule out pregnancy before administering this drug or its analogs.

SYNONYMS
- Persistent estrus
- Prolonged CL function

SEE ALSO
- Aggression
- Anestrus
- Clitoral enlargement
- Disorders of sexual development
- Early embryonic death
- Endometritis
- Large ovary syndrome
- Ovulation failure
- Pneumovagina/pneumouterus
- Prolonged diestrus
- Pyometra
- Urine pooling/urovagina
- Vaginitis and vaginal discharge
- Vulvar conformation

ABBREVIATIONS
- AMH = anti-Müllerian hormone
- CL = corpus luteum
- E$_2$ = estradiol
- FSH = follicle-stimulating hormone
- GnRH = gonadotropin-releasing hormone
- GTCT = granulosa–theca cell tumor
- hCG = human chorionic gonadotropin
- LH = luteinizing hormone
- P$_4$ = progesterone
- PGF$_{2\alpha}$ = prostaglandin F$_{2\alpha}$
- TRP = transrectal palpation
- US = ultrasonography, ultrasound

Suggested Reading
Aurich C. Reproductive cycles of horses. Anim Reprod Sci 2011;124:220–228.
Ball BA, Almeida J, Conley AJ. Determination of serum anti-Müllerian hormone concentrations for the diagnosis of granulosa-call tumours in mares. Equine Vet J 2013;45:199–203.
Coffman EA, Pinto CR. A review on the use of prostaglandin F2a for controlling the estrous cycle in mares. J Equine Vet Sci 2016;40:34–40.
Schulman ML, Botha AE, Muenscher SB, et al. Reversibility of the effects of GnRH-vaccination used to suppress reproductive function in mares. Equine Vet J 2013;45:111–113.
Vanderwall DK, Parkinson KC, Rigas J. How to use oxytocin treatment to prolong corpus luteum function for suppressing estrus in mares. J Equine Vet Sci 2016;36:1–4.
Author Lisa K. Pearson
Consulting Editor Carla L. Carleton
Acknowledgment The author and editor acknowledge the prior contribution of Carole C. Miller.

ABNORMAL SCROTAL ENLARGEMENT

BASICS

DEFINITION
Clinically visible increased scrotal size due a process involving the scrotum or its content (testes, epididymides, blood supply). The enlargement may be bilateral or unilateral. Clinic and systemic signs are variable and depend on the cause.

PATHOPHYSIOLOGY
• The equine scrotum and associated contents are relatively well protected. The scrotum is almost symmetrical and covered with a think pliable skin with freely movable content
• Scrotal enlargement may appear acutely or progressively
• Acute scrotal enlargement is more common and often due to trauma (breeding accident, jumping), spermatic cord torsion, inguinal/scrotal herniation, or inflammatory processes (epididymitis, orchitis)
• Trauma can result in scrotal hemorrhage, edema, rupture of the tunica albuginea, hematocele
• Progressive enlargement of the scrotum is often due to vascular abnormalities or poor thermoregulation (poor lymphatic drainage, edema, hydrocele) or neoplasia
• Scrotal enlargement may be observed following abdominal surgery

SYSTEMS AFFECTED
Reproductive

GENETICS
N/A

INCIDENCE/PREVALENCE
Scrotal enlargement due to trauma is the most common presentation in breeding stallions.

SIGNALMENT
• Intact male horses
• Inguinal hernia is a common cause of scrotal enlargement in foals

SIGNS
Historical Findings
• Gross changes in the size of the scrotum (usually acute)
• Pain (generally colic-like symptoms)
• Reluctance to breed, jump, or walk
• Extreme environmental temperatures (hot or cold)

Physical Examination Findings
• Increased scrotal size (unilateral or bilateral)
• Abnormal testicular position
• Abnormal scrotal temperature (too warm or cold)
• Edema/engorgement of scrotum and/or contents
• Scrotal lesions (laceration, abscesses, neoplasia)
• Pain may be elicited on palpation (spermatic cord torsion, epididymitis, orchitis, rupture)

• Derangements in systemic parameters (elevated heart rate, respiratory rate, inappetence, CBC abnormalities)
• Any combination of abnormalities may be present and not all signs are present in every animal

CAUSES
• 3 most common:
  ○ Trauma; may include testicular hematoma/rupture
  ○ Inguinal/scrotal hernia
  ○ Torsion of the spermatic cord, also known as testicular torsion
• Inflammatory/infectious causes:
  ○ EIA
  ○ EVA/equine arteritis virus
  ○ Orchitis/epididymitis
• Neoplasia:
  ○ Primary scrotal—melanoma, sarcoid
  ○ Testicular neoplasia—seminoma, teratoma, interstitial cell tumor, Sertoli cell tumor
• Noninflammatory scrotal edema
• Hydrocele/hematocele
• Varicocele

RISK FACTORS
• Breeding activity
• Large internal inguinal rings
• Systemic illness
• Extremes of ambient temperature (hot or cold)

DIAGNOSIS

DIFFERENTIAL DIAGNOSIS
Differentiating Causes
• Duration of problem
  ○ Acute—traumatic injury, torsion of spermatic cord, herniation, infection
  ○ Chronic—neoplasia, temperature-induced hydrocele/edema, varicocele, infection
• History of recent breeding, semen collection, and/or trauma
• Palpation of the caudal ligament of the epididymis (attaches epididymal tail to caudal testis and aids in the determination of testicular orientation)
• Palpation of the inguinal rings
• US (see Imaging)

CBC/BIOCHEMISTRY/URINALYSIS
• Inflammatory or stress leukocyte response
• Increased fibrinogen
• Results of serum biochemistry profile and urinalysis are usually normal

OTHER LABORATORY TESTS
• EVA
  ○ Serum neutralization or complement fixation
  ○ Acute and convalescent serum samples
  ○ If stallion is seropositive, carrier state is determined with virus isolation
  ○ Virus isolation from serum and/or seminal plasma

  ○ Semen is the best sample for diagnosis (freeze portion of ejaculate and send to approved laboratory along with serum samples)
  ○ *Send samples to an approved laboratory*
• EIA
  ○ Agar gel immunodiffusion or ELISA, the Coggins test

IMAGING—SCROTAL US
Examination of scrotal contents may reveal:
• Bowel with inguinal/scrotal herniation
• Rupture of the testis/tunica albuginea
  ○ Accumulation of hypoechoic fluid in scrotum with loss of discrete hyperechoic tunica albuginea around testicular parenchyma
  ○ Hypoechoic appearance of contents will gradually contain echogenic densities with the formation of fibrin clots
• Engorgement of the pampiniform plexus and/or testicular congestion with torsion of the spermatic cord
  ○ Doppler can verify loss of blood flow to the testis
• Hypoechoic dilation of venous plexus of spermatic cord with varicocele
• Hypoechoic accumulation of fluid within the vaginal cavity with hydrocele
• Loss of homogeneity in testicular parenchyma with neoplasia
  ○ May see areas of increased or decreased echogenicity or be variable throughout

OTHER DIAGNOSTIC PROCEDURES
• Needle aspirate and cytology—to differentiate hydrocele from recent hemorrhage
• Neoplasia—diagnosed using fine needle aspirate and/or biopsy

PATHOLOGIC FINDINGS
Dependent on etiology.

TREATMENT
• Treatment is directed at the cause of scrotal enlargement
• Management of inflammation is a primary concern with abnormal scrotal enlargement
• Sexual rest is indicated for all causes of scrotal enlargement

APPROPRIATE HEALTH CARE
• Acute scrotal enlargement warrants hospitalization for treatment and care
• Chronic scrotal enlargement may or may not warrant hospitalization; etiology dependent

NURSING CARE
• Cold therapy (cold packs, ice water baths, water hose/hydrotherapy) for acute scrotal trauma is implemented only in the absence of testicular rupture
  ○ Testicular tunics *must* be intact
  ○ Cold therapy sessions should not exceed 20 min and can be repeated every 2 h

• Scrotal massage with emollient salve—useful to reduce scrotal edema and ischemic injury
• Fluid removal should be considered with a hydrocele
  ○ Use only an aseptically placed needle or an IV catheter
  ○ Excess fluid accumulation may cause thermal damage to the testes, acts as an insulator
• Administration of IV fluids is dependent on the systemic status of the horse

ACTIVITY
The need to restrict activity depends on the etiology of scrotal enlargement.

DIET
Diet modification is necessary only with secondary ileus or as a preoperative consideration.

CLIENT EDUCATION
• Fertility may be irreversibly impaired with acute scrotal trauma
• Semen evaluation should be performed 90 days after nonsurgical resolution of scrotal enlargement
• Compensatory semen production may occur in the remaining testis of a horse undergoing hemicastration
• Following removal of a neoplasia, examine carefully for evidence of metastatic tumor growth (serial examinations)

SURGICAL CONSIDERATIONS
• Hemicastration is the treatment of choice for:
  ○ Torsion of the spermatic cord, if the duration of vascular compromise has caused irreversible damage and/or gonadal necrosis
  ○ Unilateral inguinal/scrotal herniation
  ○ Testicular rupture
  ○ Unilateral neoplasia
  ○ Varicocele
  ○ Nonresponsive hydrocele/hematocele
• Primary repair of scrotal laceration is required to protect scrotal contents
  ○ Repair generally fails due to extensive scrotal edema associated with traumatic injury

MEDICATIONS
DRUG(S) OF CHOICE
• Anti-inflammatory therapy (phenylbutazone 2–4 mg/kg PO or IV BID or flunixin meglumine 1 mg/kg IV BID) is indicated in all cases
• Diuretics (furosemide 0.5–1 mg/kg IV) may be useful in managing scrotal edema
• Antibiotic therapy should be considered in cases of scrotal laceration or scrotal hemorrhage
• Tetanus toxoid should be administered for scrotal trauma or prior to surgery

CONTRAINDICATIONS
N/A

PRECAUTIONS
N/A

POSSIBLE INTERACTIONS
N/A

ALTERNATIVE DRUGS
N/A

FOLLOW-UP
PATIENT MONITORING
Semen collection and evaluation 90 days after complete resolution of cause and/or surgery.

PREVENTION/AVOIDANCE
Adequate management of breeding to avoid trauma.

POSSIBLE COMPLICATIONS
• Infertility
• Endotoxemia
• Laminitis
• Scrotal adhesions
• Death

EXPECTED COURSE AND PROGNOSIS
• Prognosis for survival and fertility are good in unilateral cases of trauma or spermatic cord torsion if managed quickly and correctly
• Recurrent severe hematocele; hydrocele may result in testicular degeneration and loss of fertility

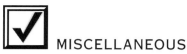

MISCELLANEOUS
ASSOCIATED CONDITIONS
N/A

AGE-RELATED FACTORS
N/A

ZOONOTIC POTENTIAL
N/A

PREGNANCY/FERTILITY/BREEDING
N/A

SYNONYMS
N/A

SEE ALSO
Abnormal testicular size

ABBREVIATIONS
• EIA = equine infectious anemia
• ELISA = enzyme-linked immunosorbent assay
• EVA = equine viral arteritis
• US = ultrasonography, ultrasound

Suggested Reading
Gonzalez M, Tibary A, Sellon DC, Daniels J. Unilateral orchitis and epididymitis caused by *Corynebacterium pseudotuberculosis* in a stallion. Equine Vet Educ 2008;20:30–36.
Morresey PR. The enlarged scrotum. Clin Tech Equine Pract 2007;6265–6270.
Threlfall WR, Carleton CL, Robertson J, et al. Recurrent torsion of the spermatic cord and scrotal testis in a stallion. J Am Vet Med Assoc 1990;196:1641–1643.
Tibary A, Chabchoub A, Sghiri A. Diagnostic procedures for an increase in volume of the scrotal bursa in stallion. Le Nouveau Praticien Veterinaire—Equine 2007;14:21–27.
Van der Velden MA. Surgical treatment of acquired inguinal hernia in the horse: a review of 51 cases. Equine Vet J 1988;20:173–177.

Author Ahmed Tibary
Consulting Editor Carla L. Carleton
Acknowledgment The author and editor acknowledge the prior contribution of Margo L. Macpherson.

BASICS

DEFINITION
Any significant deviation (increase or decrease) in the size of the testes. This may be unilateral or bilateral.

PATHOPHYSIOLOGY
- The testes and epididymides are positioned in a horizontal orientation and are freely movable within the scrotum
- Changes in testicular size are often first noticed as a variation in scrotal size
- Abnormal testicular size may be congenital or acquired
- Testicular hypoplasia is the most common congenital abnormality
  - It may be associated with incomplete or delayed testicular descent (cryptorchidism)
  - Hypoplastic testes are hard, dense, and have poor or arrested spermatogenic activity
- Acquired abnormal testicular size can be acute or progressive
- *Acute enlargement* of a testis occurs after trauma, torsion of the spermatic cord, or orchitis/epididymitis. Testicular neoplasia may be seen in some cases of acute enlargement
- Progressive enlargement of the testis is often due to *testicular neoplasia*
  - Seminoma, teratoma, Sertoli cell tumor, interstitial cell tumor
  - Of these, seminoma is the most frequently reported testicular tumor of the stallion
  - Most equine testicular tumors arise from germ cells, including seminomas and teratomas
  - The effect of neoplasia on testicular size (increase or decrease) may be insidious
- Reduction of testicular size, *testicular atrophy*, is often a consequence of testicular degeneration
- *Testicular degeneration* may arise from thermal injury, infection, trauma, vascular insult, hormonal disturbances, toxins, and age. Spermatogenesis is severely affected. Reduction or loss of fertility depends on the degree of compromise of spermatogenesis and whether the affection is bilateral or unilateral

SYSTEMS AFFECTED
- Reproductive
- Other systems (respiratory, gastrointestinal, lymphatic) may be affected subsequent to metastasis of primary testicular neoplasia

GENETICS
Cryptorchidism and testicular hypoplasia are suspected to have genetic components.

INCIDENCE/PREVALENCE
N/A

GEOGRAPHIC DISTRIBUTION
N/A

SIGNALMENT
- Intact male horses
- Any age

SIGNS
Historical Findings
- Recent history of breeding or semen collection
- Gross changes in the size of a testis
- Reduced fertility
- Pain (generally colic-like symptoms)
- Reluctance to breed, jump, or walk

Physical Examination Findings
- Increased or decreased scrotal size
- Increased or decreased testicular size
- Abnormal testicular texture (too soft or too firm)
- Abnormal testicular position
- Abnormal scrotal temperature (too warm or too cold)
- Edema/engorged scrotum and/or contents
- Derangements in systemic parameters (elevated heart rate, respiratory rate, inappetence, CBC abnormalities)

CAUSES
- Common causes of decreased testicular size
  - Cryptorchidism
  - Testicular degeneration, atrophy
- Common causes of increased testicular size
  - Trauma (testicular hematoma, rupture)
- Other causes of increased testicular size
  - Neoplasia (primarily seminoma)
  - Orchitis/epididymitis (bacterial infection, EIA, EVA, *Strongylus edentatus* infection, autoimmune)

RISK FACTORS
- Breeding activity
- Systemic illness
- Temperature extremes
- Anabolic steroid use

DIAGNOSIS

DIFFERENTIAL DIAGNOSIS
Differentiating Similar Signs
- Scrotal enlargement due to scrotal hydrocele/hematocele and scrotal or inguinal hernia may be confused with testicular enlargement
- US examination and measurement of the testes is the best means of differentiating the pathologies

Differentiating Causes
- Duration of problem
  - *Acute*—traumatic injury, infection
  - *Chronic*—cryptorchidism, neoplasia, infection, testicular degeneration/hypoplasia
- History of recent breeding and/or trauma
- Palpation of the caudal ligament of the epididymis (attaches epididymal tail to caudal testis and aids in the determination of testicular orientation)

- Testicular hypoplasia is usually congenital, while testicular degeneration is acquired
- US (see Imaging)

CBC/BIOCHEMISTRY/URINALYSIS
- Inflammatory or stress leukocyte response
- Eosinophilia may be an indicator of a parasitic infection
- Increased fibrinogen in peripheral blood
- Serum biochemistry profile and urinalysis are usually normal

OTHER LABORATORY TESTS
- EVA
  - Serum neutralization or complement fixation
  - Requires acute and convalescent serum samples
  - If stallion is seropositive, carrier state is determined with virus isolation
  - Semen is best sample for diagnosis (freeze portion of ejaculate and send to approved laboratory with serum samples)
  - *Send samples to an approved laboratory*
- EIA
  - Agar gel immunodiffusion or ELISA, the Coggins test
- Testicular degeneration
  - Endocrine profile (luteinizing hormone, FSH, testosterone, estrogens) from pooled samples obtained hourly for a minimum of 4 samples (due to pulsatile release of hormones)
  - Abnormal elevation of FSH and low total estrogen concentration are indicative of testicular degeneration

IMAGING—SCROTAL/TESTICULAR US
Testicular parenchyma should appear uniformly echogenic. Aberrations that may be identified by US include:
- Rupture of the testis/tunica albuginea
  - Hypoechoic fluid accumulates in the scrotum with loss of discrete hyperechoic tunica albuginea around testicular parenchyma
  - Hypoechoic appearance of contents will gradually be replaced with echogenic densities as fibrin clots form
- Engorgement of the pampiniform plexus and/or testicular congestion with torsion of the spermatic cord
  - Doppler can verify loss of blood flow to the testis
- Loss of homogeneity in testicular parenchyma with neoplasia
  - Neoplasia results in heterogeneity (usually a circumscribed area) in testicular parenchyma
  - May see areas of increased or decreased echogenicity or be variable throughout

OTHER DIAGNOSTIC PROCEDURES
- Needle aspirate and cytology—diagnose and/or differentiate recent hemorrhage or neoplasia
- Testicular biopsy (histopathology)—diagnose and/or differentiate neoplasia and testicular degeneration/hypoplasia

- Semen evaluation is useful in the diagnosis of testicular degeneration or hypoplasia:
  - Oligospermia
  - Azoospermia
  - Presence of round spermatids (spheroids)

PATHOLOGIC FINDINGS
- Testicular hypoplasia—round, small diameter seminiferous tubules, spermatogenic arrest
- Testicular degeneration—large, collapsed seminiferous tubules, vacuolization, poor or incomplete spermatogenesis
- Testicular neoplasia—depends on neoplasm

TREATMENT
Treatment is directed at the cause of testicular abnormality.

APPROPRIATE HEALTH CARE
Inpatient versus Outpatient
- Most causes of testicular enlargement require hospitalization for treatment/resolution
- Horses with testicular degeneration that are not systemically ill may be managed on the farm
- Horses with hypoplastic testes can be managed on an outpatient basis

NURSING CARE
- Cold therapy (cold packs, ice water baths, water hose/hydrotherapy) is indicated for acute orchitis/epididymitis
- Cold therapy sessions should not exceed 20 min and can be repeated every 2 h
- Sexual rest is indicated in most cases until resolution of the problem
- Administration of IV fluids is dependent on the systemic status of the horse

ACTIVITY
Restriction depends on the cause of the testicular aberration.

DIET
Modification is necessary only with cases of secondary ileus or as a preoperative consideration.

CLIENT EDUCATION
- Fertility may permanently be lowered
- Testicular degeneration results in various degrees of reduction in ejaculate quality
- Testicular hypoplasia is a permanent condition
- Horses with neoplasia should be examined carefully for evidence of metastatic tumor growth
- Compensatory sperm production may occur in the remaining testis of a horse undergoing hemicastration
- Serial semen evaluations are beneficial to monitor the fertility status of horses following testicular insult and treatment
  - Semen should be evaluated 75–90 days after complete resolution of testicular insult

SURGICAL CONSIDERATIONS
Hemicastration is the treatment of choice for:
- Torsion of the spermatic cord, if the duration of vascular compromise has caused irreversible damage and/or gonadal necrosis
- Testicular rupture
- Unilateral neoplasia or any condition causing irreparable damage to testis/es

MEDICATIONS
DRUG(S) OF CHOICE
- Anti-inflammatory therapy (phenylbutazone 2–4 mg/kg PO or IV BID or flunixin meglumine 1 mg/kg IV BID) is indicated in most cases
- Antibiotic therapy should be considered in cases of orchitis/epididymitis and testicular trauma
- Tetanus toxoid should be administered after testicular trauma and/or prior to surgery
- Antiparasitic therapy for *Strongylus edentatus* infection (ivermectin 0.2 mg/kg PO every 30 days until resolution of lesions)

CONTRAINDICATIONS
N/A

PRECAUTIONS
N/A

POSSIBLE INTERACTIONS
N/A

ALTERNATIVE DRUGS
N/A

FOLLOW-UP
PATIENT MONITORING
Semen collection and evaluation 90 days after complete resolution of testicular problem and/or surgery.

POSSIBLE COMPLICATIONS
- Infertility/subfertility
- Endotoxemia
- Laminitis
- Scrotal adhesions
- Death

EXPECTED COURSE AND PROGNOSIS
Dependent on etiology.

MISCELLANEOUS
ASSOCIATED CONDITIONS
- Cryptorchidism is commonly associated with testicular hypoplasia
- Male equine hybrids (mules or hinnies) often have hypoplastic testes

AGE-RELATED FACTORS
- Prepubertal testes are small and can be misdiagnosed as pathologically hypoplastic

- Testicular growth increases rapidly from 12 to 24 months of age in horses
- Testes may take 4–5 years to reach full size and maturity

ZOONOTIC POTENTIAL
N/A

PREGNANCY/FERTILITY/BREEDING
N/A

SYNONYMS
N/A

SEE ALSO
- Abnormal scrotal enlargement
- Cryptorchidism

ABBREVIATIONS
- EIA = equine infectious anemia
- ELISA = enzyme-linked immunosorbent assay
- EVA = equine viral arteritis
- FSH = follicle-stimulating hormone
- US = ultrasonography, ultrasound

Suggested Reading
Blanchard TL, Johnson L, Roser AJ. Increased germ cell loss rates and poor semen quality in stallions with idiopathic testicular degeneration. J Equine Vet Sci 2000;20:263–265.
Brito LFC, Englis JB, Turner RM, et al. Bilateral testicular mixed germ cell-sex cord-stromal tumours in a stallion. Reprod Dom Anim 2009;44:846–851.
Govaere J, Ducatelle R, Hoogewijs M, et al. Case of bilateral seminoma in a trotter stallion. Reprod Dom Anim 2010;45:537–539.
Pearson LK, Rodriguez JS, Tibary A. How to obtain a stallion testicular biopsy using a spring-loaded split needle biopsy instrument. Proc AAEP 2011;57:219–225.
Turner RM, Zeng W. The emerging pathophysiology of age-related testicular degeneration with a focus on the stallion and an update on potential therapies. Reprod Dom Anim 2012;47(Suppl. 4):178–186.

Author Ahmed Tibary
Consulting Editor Carla L. Carleton
Acknowledgment The author and editor acknowledge the prior contribution of Margo L. Macpherson.

BASICS

DEFINITION
Fetal loss after 40 days of gestation (term *stillbirth* may apply >300 days) involving maternal, placental, and/or fetal invasion by microorganisms.

PATHOPHYSIOLOGY
• Approximately 5–15% of abortions are infectious. • Abortion *storms* can occur, especially with EHV or MRLS when caterpillar populations are greatly increased. • Can involve viruses, bacteria, rickettsia, protozoa, fungi, or, with MRLS, ingestion of ETC. Some of the specific microorganisms associated with spontaneous, infectious equine abortions are listed below

Viruses
• EHV-1 (1P and 1B strains); EHV-4; rarely EHV-2. EHV abortions generally occur late in gestation; >7 months. • EVA (>3 months of gestation). • Equine infectious anemia (direct causal relationship not yet established). • Vesivirus: recent correlation between its antibodies and equine abortions

Bacteria
• Placentitis and possible, subsequent fetal infection by *Streptococcus* spp., *Actinobacillus* spp., *Escherichia coli*, *Pseudomonas* spp., *Klebsiella* spp., *Staphylococcus* spp., nocardioform actinomycetes, such as *Amycolatopsis* spp., *Cellulosimicrobium* spp., *Crossiella* spp., and *Rhodococcus* spp., *Taylorella equigenitalis* (rare, reportable), and *Leptospira* serovars. • Endotoxemia causes release of prostaglandin F2 alpha (especially <80 days of gestation (day 60 in many mares); may be factor later in gestation, if repeated exposure. • MRLS is closely associated with ETC, or, potentially, other species of caterpillars, the setae of which cause microscopic bowel puncture and subsequent bacteremic spread to the fetus and/or placenta; species of *Actinobacillus* and nonhemolytic *Streptococcus* are cultured approximately 65% of the time

Rickettsiae
Ehrlichia risticii (Potomac horse fever).

Fungi
Placentitis caused by *Aspergillus* spp., *Candida* spp., or *Histoplasma capsulatum.*

Protozoa
Sarcocystis neurona or, possibly, *Neospora* spp. in aborted fetuses from EPM-affected mares.

MRLS
1. A major concern in years when caterpillar populations are greatly increased; the geographic distribution, financial impact, and unusual pathogenesis of this syndrome make it a topic worthy of separate discussion.
2. Early (≈40–150 days of gestation) and late (>269 days of gestation) abortion syndromes.
3. Associated with greatly increased populations of ETCs.
4. Oral exposure to ETC setae in conjunction with MRLS; currently theorized to be associated with microscopic bowel puncture and bacteremic spread to fetus and/or placenta

Depending on the specific infectious cause, the pathophysiologic mechanisms of spontaneous infectious abortions can involve the following sequence of events: • Fetal death by microorganisms. • Fetal expulsion after placental infection, insufficiency, or separation. • Premature parturition induced by microbial toxins, fetal *stress*, or a combination of mechanisms. • Final result—fetal death followed by absorption, maceration, or autolysis; fetal death during the stress of delivery (*stillbirth*) or birth of a live fetus incapable of extrauterine survival.
• Some have suggested a caterpillar toxin-associated cause for the 2001–2002 outbreak of MRLS in central Kentucky and surrounding areas. • It is currently thought ingestion of ETC by pregnant mares is associated with penetration of intestinal mucosa by bacteria-contaminated, barbed caterpillar setae and their fragments. These migrate in blood vessels as septic setal emboli, deposited in vascular, immunologically susceptible targets, such as the early and late-term fetus and placenta

SYSTEMS AFFECTED
• Reproductive. • Other organ systems can be affected if there is maternal systemic disease

SIGNS

Historical Findings
One or more of the following: • Vaginal discharge, which can potentially be mucopurulent, hemorrhagic, or serosanguineous. • Premature udder development with dripping milk. • Anorexia or colic; GI disease. • Failure to deliver on expected due date. • *Recent* (1–16 weeks before presentation) systemic infectious disease or, similarly, recent introduction of infected *carrier* horses to the premises.
• Other, recently aborting mares. • Inadequate EHV-1 prophylaxis. • History of placentitis. • Previous history of dystocia, especially with perineal and/or cervical trauma. • Previous endometrial biopsy with moderate/severe endometritis or fibrosis. • None or excessive abdominal distention consistent with gestation length. • Behavioral estrus in a pregnant mare, which might be normal, depending on gestation length, time of year, gestation length at time of loss. • Climatic and environmental conditions favoring increased populations of ETC (*Malacosoma americanum*) or, possibly, other caterpillar species with setae and development of MRLS in early and late pregnant mares. • Possibly geographic location if suspect MRLS and nocardioform placentitis

Physical Examination Findings
• Early pregnancy loss is frequently unobserved and is described as *asymptomatic*.
• Unless complications occur, abortion may occur rapidly, with the sole sign being a relatively normal, previously pregnant mare later found open. • Signs range from none to multisystemic and life-threatening disease, especially if dystocia occurs during delivery or if maternal organs are infected. • Depending on microorganisms involved, multiple animals can be affected. • Most *symptomatic* spontaneous infectious abortions occur during the second half of gestation; characterized by one or more of the following findings on physical examination: ◦ Fetal parts/placental structures protruding through vulvar lips; abdominal straining or discomfort. ◦ Premature placental separation (*red bag*). ◦ Vulvar discharge (variable appearance), premature udder development, dripping milk. ◦ A previously documented pregnancy is not detected at the next examination. ◦ Evidence of fetal death by TRP, transrectal or transabdominal US. ◦ Anorexia, fever, signs of concurrent systemic disease, especially with endotoxemia, dystocia, RFM. ◦ Evidence of placental separation or echogenic allantoic fluid, especially in association with MRLS, as observed using transrectal or transabdominal US

RISK FACTORS
• Pregnant mares intermixed with young horses or horses in training are susceptible to EHV-1, EVA, or *E. risticii*. • Immunologically naive mares brought to premises with enzootic EHV-1, EVA, *E. risticii*, or *Leptospira* infections. • Pregnant mares traveling to horse shows or competitions. • Poor perineal conformation or dystocia with perineal lacerations or cervical trauma predisposes mares to ascending bacterial or fungal placentitis and, possibly, subsequent fetal infection. • Concurrent maternal GI disease or EPM. • Large numbers of ETCs in pastures with pregnant mares. • Geographic location with respect to MRLS and nocardioform placentitis

 DIAGNOSIS

DIFFERENTIAL DIAGNOSIS

Other Causes of Abortion
• Abortion, spontaneous, noninfectious.
• Twinning. • Fetal abnormalities/teratogenesis. • Umbilical cord abnormalities with excessive twisting and thrombosis.
• Placental pathology. • Maternal malnutrition or other noninfectious systemic disease. • Old mare, history of early embryonic death or abortion. • Old mare, poor endometrial biopsy. • Maternal exposure to: ◦ Endophyte-infected tall fescue pasture, exposure to ergotized grasses, small cereal

grains during last month of gestation; little or no mammary development (agalactia, if term is reached). ∘ Phytoestrogens. ∘ Other xenobiotics. • Iatrogenic or inappropriately timed induction of labor

Other Causes of Labor or Abdominal Discomfort
• Normal parturition. • Dystocia unassociated with abortion. • Prepartum uterine artery rupture. • Colic associated with uterine torsion. • Discomfort associated with hydrops of fetal membranes or prepubic tendon rupture. • Colic unassociated with reproductive disease

Other Causes of Vulvar Discharge
• Normal parturition. • Dystocia unassociated with abortion. • Normal estrus. • Endometritis. • Metritis or partial RFM. • Mucometra or pyometra

IMAGING
Transrectal and transabdominal US can evaluate fetal viability, placentitis, and alterations in appearance of amniotic and/or allantoic fluids, as well as other gestational abnormalities.

OTHER DIAGNOSTIC PROCEDURES
• Except for placentitis, abortions secondary to endotoxemia, and fetal expulsion associated with dystocia, most abortions are *asymptomatic*. The expelled fetus and fetal membranes vary in condition from intact to autolytic in appearance. • Definitive diagnosis of equine abortion in ≈50–60% of all cases. • Excluding twins and EHV-1, the diagnostic rate may only be 30%, especially if limited samples are submitted and are accompanied by moderate to severe fetal and placental autolysis with environmental contamination. • Laboratory testing to determine the cause of a spontaneous, potentially infectious abortion includes the following procedures: ∘ CBC, serum biochemistry for inflammatory or stress leukocyte response, or evidence of other organ system involvement. ∘ Suspected endotoxemia—maternal P_4 assay is indicated if the pregnancy is at risk prior to determining an infectious cause of an impending abortion. ELISA or RIA analyses for P_4 may be useful at <80 days of gestation (normal levels vary from >1 to >4 ng/mL, depending on reference laboratory). At >100 days, RIA detects both P_4 (very low > day 150) and cross-reacting 5α-pregnanes of uterofetoplacental origin. Acceptable levels of 5α-pregnanes vary with stage of gestation and the laboratory used. ∘ To aid in establishing a diagnosis of abortions caused by placentitis, a maternal uterine swab/uterine lavage sample or, as advocated by some, a uterine biopsy can provide samples for culture and cytology (swab or lavage) or histopathology (biopsy). ∘ Analyses for other maternal hormones can be performed. ∘ Maternal serologic testing can be useful in diagnosing infectious abortions (diagnostic for abortions by *Leptospira*

serovars; confirms EVA abortion). Serum samples should be collected in all cases of abortion in which cause is unknown (a paired sample collected 21 days later might be indicated). • The following samples should be collected from the fetus and the fetal membranes for histopathologic and cytologic evaluations, as well as microbiologic, serologic, and molecular testing procedures: ∘ Fresh/chilled fetal thoracic or abdominal fluid and serum from the fetal heart or cord blood. ∘ Fetal stomach contents. ∘ 10% neutral-buffered formalin-fixed and chilled/frozen fetal membranes (chorioallantois or allantochorion; amnion or allantoamnion), as well as fixed and chilled/frozen samples of fetal heart, lung, thymus, liver, kidney, lymph nodes, spleen, adrenal, skeletal muscle, and brain. ∘ Stained cytologic smears collected from fetal membranes

PATHOLOGIC FINDINGS
Viruses
• EHV ∘ Gross pleural effusion, ascites, fetal icterus, pulmonary congestion, and edema; 1 mm, yellowish-white spots on enlarged liver; relatively fresh fetus. ∘ Histopathologic findings for EHV-1 and -4 include areas of necrosis, prominent, eosinophilic, intranuclear inclusion bodies in lymphoid tissue, liver, adrenal cortex, lung, as well as a hyperplastic, necrotizing bronchiolitis. ∘ Fluorescent antibody staining of fetal tissues. ∘ Virus isolation from aborted fetus. ∘ PCR can be used for EHV-1/EHV-4, as well as, possibly, other viruses and microorganisms listed below, depending on the diagnostic laboratory. • EVA ∘ Few gross lesions. ∘ Autolyzed fetus. ∘ Placental/fetal vascular lesions. • Vesivirus ∘ Nonspecific lesions

Bacteria and Fungi
• Fetal infection and placentitis ∘ Gross pleural effusion, ascites with enlarged liver; rare plaques of mycotic dermatitis; placental edema and thickening with fibronecrotic exudate on the chorionic surface, especially at the *cervical star* in fungal infections. ∘ Histopathologic evidence of inflammatory disease; autolysis may make interpretation difficult. • Leptospirosis ∘ Gross fetal icterus and autolysis. ∘ Nonspecific histologic changes; mild, diffuse placentitis

Endotoxemia
Fetus minimally autolyzed.

Rickettsiae
• *Ehrlichia risticii* ∘ Gross placentitis. ∘ Typical histopathologic findings include colitis, periportal hepatitis, lymphoid hyperplasia, and necrosis

Protozoa
There are reports of *Sarcocystis neurona*-associated abortions in EPM-positive mares.

MRLS
Histopathologic findings similar to bacterial infections.

 ### TREATMENT
APPROPRIATE HEALTH CARE
• Except late-gestational placentitis (>270 days) and endotoxemia, no therapy indicated to preserve fetal viability with spontaneous, infectious abortion. • For mares that abort, there is only *prophylactic* therapy for metritis or endometritis. • Therapy is generally limited to intrauterine lavage with or without antibacterial therapy but might include a systemic component consisting of antibiotics, NSAIDs, and/or IV fluids, especially if septicemia, endotoxemia, and/or laminitis are suspected. • Preexisting GI disease and complications, such as laminitis, may warrant hospitalization and intensive care

NURSING CARE
Most affected horses require limited nursing care, except in instances of endotoxemia and Gram-negative septicemia, dystocia, RFM, metritis, laminitis.

ACTIVITY
There should be paddock exercise to permit observation, but this recommendation is subject to change if the mare exhibits clinical signs of laminitis.

DIET
Feed and water intake, as well defecation and urination, should be monitored, but no particular dietary changes should take place in the absence of GI disease or laminitis.

CLIENT EDUCATION
Inform owners of: • Availability of vaccines to prevent some types of viral abortion. • Increased risk for abortion in mares with a previous history of dystocia (especially those mares with perineal or cervical trauma) or placentitis. • Possible complications of abortion

SURGICAL CONSIDERATIONS
Indicated in instances of dystocia or GI disease requiring surgical intervention or repair of previous perineal lacerations, cervical trauma, or other structural abnormalities.

 ### MEDICATIONS
DRUG(S) OF CHOICE
• Altrenogest administered 0.044–0.088 mg/kg PO daily can be started later during gestation, continued longer, or used only for short periods of time, depending on serum P_4 levels during the first 80 days of gestation, clinical circumstances, risk factors, clinician preference. Note that serum levels reflect only endogenous P_4, not

exogenous, oral product. • If near term, altrenogest frequently is discontinued 7–14 days before the foaling date unless indicated otherwise by fetal maturity/viability, or actual gestational age is in question

PRECAUTIONS, POSSIBLE INTERACTIONS

• Altrenogest is only used to prevent abortion in cases of endotoxemia or placentitis (>270 days of gestation) if the fetus is viable. • Altrenogest is absorbed through skin; wear gloves and wash hands

ALTERNATIVE DRUGS

• Injectable P_4 (150–500 mg oil base) IM. • Newer, repository forms of P_4 are occasionally introduced; however, some evidence of efficacy should be provided prior to use

FOLLOW-UP

PATIENT MONITORING

• 7–10 days post abortion, TRP and US to monitor uterine involution. • Observation for signs of systemic disease, laminitis. • Assess genital tract health using vaginal speculum, hysteroscopy, uterine culture and cytology, and/or endometrial biopsy. • Base treatment on results of these testing procedures. Uterine culture <14 days postpartum or post abortion can be affected by contamination at the time of parturition (abortion)

PREVENTION/AVOIDANCE

Vaccines

• A killed-virus EHV-1 vaccine at 5, 7, and 9 months of gestation (some recommend vaccination at 3 months of gestation, as well); approved for abortion prevention in pregnant mares; 2 month interval due to short-lived vaccinal immunity. • Other EHV vaccines, including combinations of EHV-1 and -4, have been used off-label for abortion prevention, with some anecdotal reports of their efficacy for this purpose. • EVA vaccine not specifically labeled for abortion prevention; a modified live vaccine only to be administered to open mares 3 weeks before anticipated exposure to infected semen or in enzootic conditions. First-time vaccinated mares should be isolated for 3 weeks after exposure to infected semen. Note that some

countries forbid importation of horses with titers to EVA

Additional Prophylactic Steps

• Segregate pregnant mares from horses susceptible/exposed to infections. • Isolate immunologically naive individuals until immunity to enzootic infections is established and/or enhanced. Depending on infectious agent, protection may only be accomplished postpartum. • Limit transport of pregnant mares to exhibitions or competitions. • Careful observation of pregnant mares and monitor mammary development. • Use appropriate biosecurity protocols and isolate aborting mares, with proper disposal of contaminated fetal tissues. • Proper diagnostics to identify an infectious cause of abortion. • Correct structural abnormalities, such as poor perineal conformation, perineal lacerations, or cervical trauma, in order to prevent ascending placentitis. • Manage preexisting endometritis before next breeding. • Prevent pregnant mare exposure to ETCs until 7–8 weeks after ETC death. • Insecticides to control ETCs; consider toxicity of insecticide

POSSIBLE COMPLICATIONS

• Abortion in late pregnancy can be associated with dystocia and other potentially life-threatening conditions. • Future fertility and reproductive value can be impaired by dystocia, RFM, endometritis, laminitis, septicemia, trauma to genital tract

EXPECTED COURSE AND PROGNOSIS

• Most patients recover with appropriate treatment. • Complications can involve significant impact on mare's survivability and future fertility. • Prognosis is guarded for pregnancy maintenance with endotoxemia and placentitis. • Mares with placentitis, especially those with predisposing structural abnormalities, are more susceptible to future recurrence of this type of abortion

MISCELLANEOUS

SYNONYMS

• Abortion. • Spontaneous abortion. • Infectious abortion. • Bacterial abortion. • Viral abortion. • Fungal abortion. • Mycotic abortion. • Protozoal abortion. • Rickettsial abortion

SEE ALSO

• Abortion, spontaneous, noninfectious
• Contagious equine metritis (CEM)
• Dystocia
• Endometrial biopsy
• Endometritis
• Fetal stress/distress/viability
• High-risk pregnancy
• Placental insufficiency
• Placentitis
• Premature placental separation
• Retained fetal membranes

ABBREVIATIONS

• EHV = equine herpesvirus
• ELISA = enzyme-linked immunosorbent assay
• EPM = equine protozoal encephalomyelitis
• ETC = eastern tent caterpillar
• EVA = equine viral arteritis
• GI = gastrointestinal
• MRLS = mare reproductive loss syndrome
• NSAID = nonsteroidal anti-inflammatory drug
• P_4 = progesterone
• PCR = polymerase chain reaction
• RFM = retained fetal membranes/placenta
• RIA = radioimmunoassay
• TRP = transrectal palpation
• US = ultrasonography, ultrasound

Suggested Reading

Christensen BW, Roberts JF, Pozor MA, et al. Nocardioform placentitis with isolation of *Amycolatopsis* spp in Florida-bred mare. J Am Vet Med Assoc 2006;228:1234–1239.

McKinnon AO, Pycock JF. Maintenance of pregnancy. In: McKinnon AO, Squires EL, Vaala WE, Varner DD, eds. Equine Reproduction, 2e. Ames, IA: Wiley Blackwell, 2011:2410–2417.

Powell DG. Mare reproductive loss syndrome. In: McKinnon AO, Squires EL, Vaala WE, Varner DD, eds. Equine Reproduction, 2e. Ames, IA: Wiley Blackwell, 2011:2410–2417.

Timoney PJ. Equine herpes virus. In: McKinnon AO, Squires EL, Vaala WE, Varner DD, eds. Equine Reproduction, 2e. Ames, IA: Wiley Blackwell, 2011:2376–2390.

Troedsson MHT, Macpherson ML. Placentitis. In: McKinnon AO, Squires EL, Vaala WE, Varner DD, eds. Equine Reproduction, 2e. Ames, IA: Wiley Blackwell, 2011:2359–2367.

Webb BA, Barney WE, Dahlman DL, et al. Eastern tent caterpillars (*Malacosoma americanum*) cause mare reproductive loss syndrome. J Insect Physiol 2004;50:185–193.

Author Tim J. Evans
Consulting Editor Carla L. Carleton

ABORTION, SPONTANEOUS, NONINFECTIOUS

 BASICS

DEFINITION

Fetal loss >40 days (term *stillbirth* may apply >300 days) due to noninfectious conditions.

PATHOPHYSIOLOGY

Approximately 85–95% of abortions are noninfectious in nature. Some of the specific causes of spontaneous, noninfectious equine abortions are as follows.
- *Twin pregnancies* that persist >40 days, ≈70% end in abortion/stillbirth
- *Luteal insufficiency/early CL regression*
  ○ Anecdotal—decreased levels of luteal progesterone at <80 days of gestation
- *Placental abnormalities*
  ○ Umbilical cord torsion, as evidenced by vascular compromise, e.g. cord thrombus, can be associated with abortion
  ○ Torsion of the amnion
  ○ Long umbilical cord/cervical pole ischemia disorder
  ○ Confirmed body pregnancy
  ○ Placental separation
  ○ Villous atrophy, hypoplasia, or placental insufficiency (can also be associated with prolonged gestation)
  ○ Hydrops
  ○ Various placental abnormalities reported with foals resulting from SCNT
- *Fetal abnormalities*
  ○ Developmental abnormalities, such as hydrocephalus or anencephaly
  ○ Fetal trauma
  ○ Chromosomal abnormalities
- *Maternal abnormalities*
  ○ Concurrent maternal disease, such as PPID and EMS/IR
  ○ Trauma
  ○ Malnutrition/starvation; selenium deficiency
  ○ Anecdotal—severe maternal anxiety/stress and/or pain, such as severe laminitis
  ○ Moderate to severe endometritis and/or endometrial periglandular fibrosis
  ○ Lymphatic cysts—anecdotal
  ○ Chromosomal abnormalities
- *Xenobiotics*
  ○ Ergopeptine alkaloids associated with fescue toxicosis or ergotism can be associated with placental thickening and abortion, although prolonged gestation is more common
  ○ Phytoestrogens—anecdotal abortions early in spring
  ○ Xenobiotics causing maternal disease, such as cardiac glycosides, taxine alkaloids, carbamates, organophosphates
  ○ Originally proposed with mare reproductive loss syndrome, but *penetrating septic septal emboli* now suspected
  ○ Equine protozoal encephalomyelitis therapies during pregnancy

- Repeated large doses of corticosteroids during late gestation*Iatrogenic causes*
  ○ Prostaglandin F2 alpha to terminate a pregnancy
  ○ Procedures mistakenly done on a pregnant mare, such as artificial insemination, intrauterine infusions, samples taken for cytology, culture, or biopsy
  ○ Possible mechanisms can involve the sequence of events below:
    ▪ Fetal death/premature parturition—some intrinsic structural or functional defect or exposure to xenobiotics
    ▪ Fetal expulsion <80 days of gestation after CL loss, a result of endometritis or other factors
    ▪ Fetal death/expulsion by placental insufficiency or separation
    ▪ Fetal *stress*, dead twin fetus, maternal *stress*, or combination
    ▪ Fetal reabsorption, maceration, mummification, autolysis, death during delivery (stillbirth) or delivery of live fetus incapable of extrauterine survival

SYSTEMS AFFECTED
- Reproductive
- Other organ systems can be affected if there is maternal systemic disease

SIGNS

Historical Findings
One or more of the following:
- Signs consistent with labor at an unexpected stage of gestation
- Dystocia, birth of nonviable foal
- Previous history of abortion, dystocia, or birth of a nonviable foal
- Vaginal discharge, which is generally mucoid, hemorrhagic, or serosanguineous
- Premature udder development; dripping milk
- Anorexia or colic
- *Recent* systemic disease
- Moderate/severe endometritis and/or endometrial periglandular fibrosis
- None/excessive abdominal distention consistent with stage of gestation
- Behavioral estrus in pregnant mare, which might be normal for stage of gestation and is dependent on time of year and stage of pregnancy when pregnancy is lost

Physical Examination Findings
- Depends on the cause, time of fetal death, stage of gestation, duration of the condition, and whether pregnancy ended in dystocia or with RFM
- Abortion usually occurs rapidly and is unobserved
- Signs range from none to multisystemic and life-threatening disease
- Most *symptomatic* spontaneous noninfectious abortions occur during the second half of gestation, characterized by one or more of the following physical examination findings:

- Fetal/placental structures protruding through vulval lips; abdominal straining or discomfort
  ○ Premature placental separation (*red bag*)
  ○ Vulval discharge (variable appearance), premature udder development, dripping milk
  ○ Previously diagnosed pregnancy absent at next examination; fetal death determined by TRP or transrectal/transabdominal US
  ○ Twin fetuses
  ○ Placental separation or hydrops of fetal membranes
  ○ Signs of concurrent, systemic disease, dystocia, or RFM
- Note that signs are extremely variable. Mares pregnant at early check can remain *asymptomatic* but abort. Abortion can be unobserved early in gestation, may be rapid without signs

RISK FACTORS
- Often nonspecific
- See Pathophysiology

 DIAGNOSIS

DIFFERENTIAL DIAGNOSIS

Other Causes of Abortion
- Infectious, spontaneous abortion
- Placentitis

Other Causes of Signs of Labor or Abdominal Discomfort
- Normal parturition
- Dystocia unassociated with abortion
- Prepartum uterine artery rupture
- Colic associated with uterine torsion
- Discomfort associated with hydrops of fetal membranes or prepubic tendon rupture
- Colic unassociated with reproductive disease

Other Causes of Vulval Discharge
- Normal parturition
- Dystocia not associated with abortion
- Normal estrus
- Endometritis, metritis, or RFM, mucometra or pyometra

DIAGNOSTIC PROCEDURES
- *Asymptomatic* unless—placentitis, secondary to endotoxemia, fetal expulsion associated with twins or dystocia
- Definitive causative diagnosis of equine abortion occurs in ≈50–60% of all cases
- Excluding twins and equine herpesvirus 1, the diagnostic rate may be only 30%
- Note that unless the cause of the abortion is obvious, such as twins or iatrogenic, must rule out infectious causes, especially if multiple mares are affected or at risk:
  ○ CBC, serum biochemistry
  ○ Maternal P_4 may be useful at <80 days of gestation
  ○ Maternal estrogen concentrations
  ○ Decreased maternal relaxin concentration associated with abnormal placental function

○ Decreased maternal prolactin secretion during late gestation—associated with fescue toxicosis and ergotism
○ Anecdotal reports of lower triiodothyronine/thyroxine levels with history of conception failure, early embryonic death, or abortion. The significance of low T_4 levels is unknown and somewhat controversial
○ Test for PPID and EMS/IR
○ Cytogenetic studies—useful if maternal or fetal chromosomal abnormalities are suspected
○ Endometrial biopsy to assess endometrial inflammation and/or fibrosis
○ Vaginal speculum examination and hysteroscopy if structural cervical or uterine abnormalities are suspected
○ Xenobiotics—narrow testing to one or several potential xenobiotics in maternal and fetal samples. Might be very expensive, and unproductive. Feed or environmental analyses, for ergopeptine alkaloids, phytoestrogens, heavy metals, or fescue endophyte
○ Imaging with transrectal and transabdominal US can be used to evaluate fetal viability, placentitis, and alterations in appearance of amniotic and/or allantoic fluids, as well as other gestational abnormalities, such as hydrops
○ Collect samples for histopathology, cytology, microbiology, serology, and molecular testing procedures:
  ■ If available, fresh/chilled fetal thoracic or abdominal fluid and serum from the fetal heart or cord blood
  ■ Fetal stomach content
  ■ 10% formalin-fixed and chilled/frozen samples of fetal membranes fetal viscera

PATHOLOGIC FINDINGS
• Macroscopic and histological evidence of physical causes (see Pathophysiology)
• Twins—avillous chorionic membrane at point of contact between the fetal membranes
• Umbilical cord torsion should be confirmed by evidence of vascular compromise
• Villous atrophy or hypoplasia might suggest endometrial periglandular fibrosis and/or lymphatic cysts
• Placental edema, gross and histopathological, is consistent with equine fescue toxicosis
• Various placental abnormalities reported with foals resulting from SCNT cloning procedures

TREATMENT
APPROPRIATE HEALTH CARE
• Except in cases of late-gestational placentitis (>270 days) and endotoxemia, no therapy indicated to preserve fetal viability with spontaneous, infectious abortion

• For mares that abort, there is only *prophylactic* therapy for metritis or endometritis. Therapy is generally limited to intrauterine lavage, with or without antibacterial therapy
• Preexisting GI disease and complications, such as laminitis, might warrant hospitalization and intensive care

NURSING CARE
Most affected horses require limited nursing care, except in instances of complications, e.g. septicemia, dystocia, RFM, metritis, and laminitis.

ACTIVITY
There should be paddock exercise to permit observation; recommendation subject to change if the mare exhibits clinical signs of laminitis.

DIET
Monitor feed and water intake, defecation, and urination; no particular dietary changes in the absence of GI disease or laminitis.

CLIENT EDUCATION
• The increased survivability of twin foals has led some breeders and, even, veterinarians to be less concerned about twin pregnancies. However, the risk of abortion, dystocia, and neonatal complications associated with twins still warrants prevention and/or management and discussion of the inherent risks related to pregnancy ending in abortion or complicated delivery
• Periglandular fibrosis is irreversible
• Older mares or mares with preexisting systemic disease might be at increased risk of spontaneous abortion
• Embryo transfer—especially mares with a history of abortion or those with severe endometrial periglandular fibrosis or severe structural abnormalities
• Risks associated with ingestion of endophyte-infected fescue and/or ergotized grasses and grains
• Inform owners of the possible complications of abortion

SURGICAL CONSIDERATIONS
• Dystocia or GI disease requiring surgical intervention
• Reduction of twin pregnancies can involve surgical approaches for selected fetal decapitation or other means for elimination of one twin
• Hysteroscopic removal of lymphatic cysts to prevent future abortions

MEDICATIONS
DRUG(S) OF CHOICE
• Altrenogest administered 0.044–0.088 mg/kg PO daily can be started later during gestation, continued longer, or used only for short periods of time,

depending on serum P_4 levels during first 80 days of gestation, clinical circumstances, risk factors, clinician preference. Note that serum levels reflect only endogenous P_4, not exogenous, oral product
• If near term, altrenogest frequently is discontinued 7–14 days before foaling date, unless indicated otherwise by fetal maturity/viability, or actual gestational age is in question

PRECAUTIONS, POSSIBLE INTERACTIONS
• Altrenogest is only used to prevent abortion in cases of endotoxemia or placentitis (>270 days of gestation) if fetus is viable
• Altrenogest is absorbed through skin; wear gloves and wash hands

ALTERNATIVE DRUGS
• Injectable P_4 (150–500 mg oil base) IM
• Newer, repository forms of P_4 are occasionally introduced; however, some evidence of efficacy should be provided prior to use
• Medications for preexisting maternal disease

FOLLOW-UP
PATIENT MONITORING
• At 7–10 days post abortion monitor uterine involution
• Observe for any signs of systemic disease and laminitis
• Assess genital tract health— ± vaginal speculum, hysteroscopy, uterine culture and cytology, endometrial biopsy
• Base treatment on clinical results of these procedures
• Uterine culture <14 days postpartum or post abortion is affected by contamination at the time of parturition (abortion)

PREVENTION/AVOIDANCE
• Early recognition of at-risk mares
• Record double ovulations
• Early twin diagnosis (<25 days, as early as day 14 or 15)
• Selective embryonic/fetal reduction involving transrectal, transvaginal, or transabdominal US or, potentially, surgery and induced death of one fetus
• Manage preexisting endometritis before next breeding to minimize inflammation
• Careful observation of pregnant mares, monitor mammary gland development
• Remove mares from fescue pasture during last third of gestation (minimum 30 days)
• Domperidone (1.1 mg/kg PO daily) at earliest signs of equine fescue toxicosis or 10–14 days prior to due date; continue until parturition and development of normal mammary gland
• Injection with fluphenazine (25 mg IM in pony mares) on day 320 of gestation has been suggested for prophylaxis of fescue toxicosis

• Careful use of medications in pregnant mares
• Avoid exposure to known toxicants

POSSIBLE COMPLICATIONS
• Dystocia, other potentially life-threatening conditions
• Future fertility and reproductive value can be impaired by dystocia, RFM, endometritis, laminitis, septicemia, trauma to genital tract
• Potential complications associated with twin reduction increase the later in gestation they are attempted

EXPECTED COURSE AND PROGNOSIS
• Most patients recover with appropriate treatment
• Complications can involve significant impact on mare's survivability and future fertility
• Guarded prognosis for pregnancy maintenance with severe endometritis and endometrial periglandular fibrosis

 MISCELLANEOUS

SYNONYMS
• Abortion
• Spontaneous abortion

• Noninfectious abortion
• Twin abortion

SEE ALSO
• Abortion, spontaneous, infectious
• Dystocia
• Endometrial biopsy
• Endometritis
• Fetal stress/distress/viability
• High-risk pregnancy
• Placental insufficiency
• Placentitis
• Premature placental separation

ABBREVIATIONS
• CL = corpus luteum
• EMS = equine metabolic syndrome
• GI = gastrointestinal
• IR = insulin dysregulation
• P_4 = progesterone
• PPID = pituitary pars intermedia dysfunction
• RFM = retained fetal membranes/placenta
• SCNT = somatic cell nuclear transfer
• TRP = transrectal palpation
• US = ultrasonography, ultrasound

Suggested Reading
Burns TA. Effects of common equine endocrine diseases on reproduction. VCNA Eq Pract 2016;32(3):435–449.

Gupta RC, Evans TJ, Nicholson SS. Ergot and fescue toxicosis. In: Gupta RC, ed. Veterinary Toxicology: Basic and Clinical Principles, 3e. New York: Academic Press, 2018:995.
McKinnon AO. Origin and outcome of twin pregnancies. In: McKinnon AO, Squires EL, Vaala WE, Varner DD, eds. Equine Reproduction, 2e. Ames, IA: Wiley Blackwell, 2011:2350–2358.
Pozor MA, Sheppard B, Hinrichs K, et al. Placental abnormalities in equine pregnancies generated by SCNT from one donor horse. Theriogenology 2016;86(6):1573–1572.
Sebastian MM, Bernard WV, Riddle WT, et al. Review paper: mare reproductive loss syndrome. Vet Pathol 2008;45:710–722.
Troedsson MHT, Macpherson ML. Placentitis. In: McKinnon AO, Squires EL, Vaala WE, Varner DD, eds. Equine Reproduction, 2e. Ames, IA: Wiley Blackwell, 2011:2359–2367.

Author Tim J. Evans
Consulting Editor Carla L. Carleton

BASICS

OVERVIEW
• Results from the ingestion of wilted or dried *Acer rubrum* (red maple) leaves
• Most frequently reported in the eastern half of North America
• The specific toxin has not been identified. Pyrogallol and gallic acid, metabolites formed from intestinal bacterial metabolism of tannic acid found in wilted or dry leaves, have been suggested
• Clinical findings are consistent with oxidative injury to red blood cells, resulting in the formation of methemoglobin, Heinz bodies, and hemolytic anemia
• Affected organ systems include:
  ◦ Cardiovascular—tachycardia secondary to anemia
  ◦ Hemic—methemoglobinemia, hemolytic anemia, and Heinz bodies
  ◦ Renal—pigmenturia, hematuria, and proteinuria; renal failure secondary to hemoglobin deposition in the kidney
  ◦ Reproductive—abortion secondary to fetal hypoxia
  ◦ Respiratory—polypnea secondary to anemia

SIGNALMENT
No breed, gender, or age predilections.

SIGNS
• Acute death can result from rapid formation of methemoglobin. Alternatively, hemolytic crisis can develop over several days as the hemolysis and methemoglobinemia progressively worsen
• Lethargy, weakness, anorexia, and perhaps colic or fever. Yellow or brown mucous membranes, red or brown urine, tachycardia, polypnea, and dehydration

CAUSES AND RISK FACTORS
In summer and fall months after an event that results in leaf wilting such as tree pruning, fallen branches after a storm, or autumn leaves falling.

DIAGNOSIS

DIFFERENTIAL DIAGNOSIS
• All causes of hemolytic anemia
• Hemolytic anemia accompanied by Heinz bodies and/or methemoglobinemia indicates oxidant toxicosis. The most common causes in horses are onions, red maple, and phenothiazine anthelmintics, which can only be differentiated by a history of ingestion

CBC/BIOCHEMISTRY/URINALYSIS
• Interpretation may be difficult due to hemolysis
• Decreased packed cell volume, hemoglobin, and erythrocyte count confirm anemia, whereas increased mean corpuscular hemoglobin concentration and mean corpuscular hemoglobin support intravascular hemolysis with hemoglobinemia
• Heinz bodies are not present in all cases. They may be seen on routinely stained blood smears but are more apparent in new methylene blue-stained smears
• Serum bilirubin, especially unconjugated bilirubin, is increased because of hemolytic anemia and inappetence
• Urinalysis results include proteinuria and hemoglobinuria, with few or no intact erythrocytes
• Increased albumin and total protein result from dehydration
• Blood urea nitrogen and creatinine increase if a pigment nephropathy develops and causes acute renal failure
• Elevated liver enzymes and creatine phosphokinase may occur, probably secondary to cell damage caused by anemia-induced hypoxia
• Eccentrocytes and ghost cells have been reported

OTHER LABORATORY TESTS
The percentage of methemoglobin in the blood often is elevated.

PATHOLOGIC FINDINGS
• Gross findings include generalized icterus, enlarged spleen, and discolored kidneys. Petechiae and ecchymoses may be present
• Histopathologic findings include erythrophagocytosis by macrophages, renal pigment casts and sloughed epithelial cells, splenic and hepatic hemosiderin, and centrilobular hepatic lipidosis. Pulmonary thrombosis possible

TREATMENT
• Inpatient or outpatient according to severity
• IV fluids to maintain renal perfusion
• Blood transfusion with severe anemia
• Continuous nasal oxygen administration may be helpful

MEDICATIONS

DRUG(S) OF CHOICE
Ascorbic acid has been used for its antioxidant effects (30–50 mg/kg every 12 h added to IV fluids).

CONTRAINDICATIONS/POSSIBLE INTERACTIONS
• Do not treat methemoglobinemia with methylene blue because of its poor efficacy and it may increase Heinz body formation
• NSAIDs to control pain but can compromise renal function

FOLLOW-UP

PATIENT MONITORING
Monitor methemoglobinemia and anemia to adjust therapy.

PREVENTION/AVOIDANCE
Remove fallen branches immediately after storms or pruning.

EXPECTED COURSE AND PROGNOSIS
• Prognosis depends on the quantity of leaves ingested
• Death is attributed to severe methemoglobinemia, anemia, or to renal failure

MISCELLANEOUS

ASSOCIATED CONDITIONS
Laminitis can occur during or after the course of the disease.

PREGNANCY/FERTILITY/BREEDING
Anemia and methemoglobinemia can result in fetal hypoxia, followed by abortion.

ABBREVIATIONS
NSAID = nonsteroidal anti-inflammatory drug

Suggested Reading
Agrawal K, Ebel JG, Altier C, Bischoff K. Identification of prototoxins and a microbial basis for red maple (*Acer Rubrum*) toxicosis in equines. J Vet Diagn Invest 2013;25(1);112–119.
Alward A, Corriher CA, Barton MH, et al. Red maple (*Acer rubrum*) leaf toxicosis in horses: a retrospective study of 32 cases. J Vet Intern Med 2006;20;1197–1201.
Burrows GE, Tyrl RJ. Sapindaceae juss. In: Burrows GE, ed. Toxic Plants of North America, 2e. Ames, IA: Wiley, 2013:1110–1124.
Author Scott L. Radke
Consulting Editors Wilson K. Rumbeiha and Steve Ensley
Acknowledgment The author and editors acknowledge the prior contribution of Konnie H. Plumlee.

A

ACIDOSIS, METABOLIC

BASICS

DEFINITION
• A disruption of acid–base homeostasis producing increased H^+ concentration, which is reflected by acidemia (decreased blood pH) and low plasma HCO_3^- concentration
• Normal plasma HCO_3^- concentration is $\cong 24$ mEq/L
• Normal blood pH ranges from 7.35 to 7.45

PATHOPHYSIOLOGY
• H^+ is regulated by intracellular and extracellular buffering, respiratory buffering (i.e. variation of CO_2 levels via changes in ventilation), and regulation of HCO_3^- via renal excretion of H^+
• Renal H^+ excretion is accomplished by direct secretion of limited amounts of H^+, increased generation of ammonium ions, and titration to phosphates and urates (titratable acidity)
• Resorption of HCO_3^- occurs when H^+ is secreted, 90% in the proximal tubule and the remainder in the distal nephron
• Buffering of H^+ occurs rapidly and is accomplished by proteins, phosphates, and HCO_3^-
• The most important buffer is HCO_3^-
• Respiratory compensation responds within minutes
• Definitive regulation of H^+ and HCO_3^- concentrations is accomplished by the kidney
• Renal processing of acidosis begins within hours but may take days to normalize pH
• Inability to excrete H^+, loss of HCO_3^-, increased production of H^+, and accumulation of acids are the major mechanisms producing metabolic acidosis
• Hyperproteinemia (i.e. weak acids) and overhydration (i.e. dilutional acidosis) also produce metabolic acidosis via alteration of the balance between strong cations and anions

SYSTEMS AFFECTED
Respiratory
• Chemoreceptors sense low pH in blood or CSF and stimulate hyperventilation to increase elimination of CO_2 and increase pH
• Decreased respiratory muscle strength can lead to hypoventilation and worsening acidosis

Cardiovascular
• Hyperkalemia secondary to acidemia may cause arrhythmias and decreased cardiac contractility
• Vasodilation of arterioles; constriction of veins
• Vascular effects may be offset by catecholamine effects

Neuroendocrine
• CNS depression
• CSF acidosis in acute situations

Renal
The kidney responds to low arterial pH by increasing H^+ excretion and generating

increased concentrations of HCO_3^- to bring the systemic pH back to normal.

Metabolic
• Decreased affinity for O_2—hemoglobin binding, enhancing release of O_2 to tissues
• Increased protein catabolism
• Increased ionized Ca^{2+} concentration

GENETICS
Fanconi syndrome may be heritable in Quarter Horses.

SIGNALMENT
Any breed, age, or sex.

SIGNS
• Dependent on the underlying cause
• Weakness, depression, and tachypnea are clinical signs of metabolic acidosis

CAUSES
• Loss of HCO_3^- from the GI tract (e.g. colitis)
• RTA results in HCO_3^- loss both directly and indirectly, depending on the type of tubular dysfunction
• Aminoaciduria, lactic aciduria, and glucosuria is suggestive of Fanconi syndrome
• Renal failure results in an inability to excrete H^+ and accumulation of uremic acids
• Lactic acidosis can result from anaerobic metabolism, which occurs secondary to decreased tissue perfusion. Hypovolemia from severe dehydration (e.g. diarrhea, sweating, decreased intake), fluid sequestration (e.g. ascites, pleural effusion, internal diarrhea), or hemorrhage leads to decreased tissue perfusion. SIRS produces acidosis via several mechanisms, including hypotension (decreased tissue perfusion), decreased cardiac contractility, tissue ischemia, fluid shifts, hypoxemia, and hepatic damage
• Chronic causes of hypoxemia produce lactic acidosis
• Grain overload produces metabolic acidosis via production of lactic acid, fluid sequestration in the GI tract, and secretion into the GI tract
• High-intensity anaerobic exercise and rhabdomyolysis results in production of lactate, which can result in transient metabolic acidosis
• Malignant hyperthermia is uncommon but has occurred in anesthetized horses and results in severe lactic acidosis
• Acute or endstage hepatic failure may result in metabolic acidosis due to failure of the liver to metabolize lactic acid
• Asphyxia at parturition may decrease perfusion, which can result in lactic acidosis
• Ingestion of exogenous acids (e.g. salicylates, ethylene or propylene glycol) is uncommon
• Proteins are weak acids; conditions producing significant hyperproteinemia (e.g. chronic infection, immune-mediated disease, plasma cell myeloma, lymphoma) produce metabolic acidosis

• Total parenteral nutrition can lead to metabolic acidosis when cationic (e.g. lysine, arginine) or sulfur-containing amino acids are metabolized as H^+ is formed

RISK FACTORS
• Patients with chronic renal failure or chronic hypoxemia (e.g. severe equine asthma) may be at greater risk for acidosis with progression of their primary problem
• Horses on acetazolamide for hyperkalemic periodic paralysis may develop acidosis more readily, as acetazolamide is a carbonic anhydrase inhibitor that causes increased HCO_3^- excretion
• Highly anionic diets can induce metabolic acidosis in equids

DIAGNOSIS

DIFFERENTIAL DIAGNOSIS
• Some causes of metabolic acidosis can be identified on physical examination (e.g. diarrhea, hypovolemia, colic with ischemic lesions)
• Decreased HCO_3^- concentrations are also seen in conditions with chronic respiratory alkalosis; PCO_2 is low if compensation is occurring, but pH will be normal or mildly increased

LABORATORY FINDINGS
Drugs That May Alter Laboratory Results
• Excessive anticoagulant may falsely decrease results via dilution
• Excessive Na^+ heparin (acidic) may falsely decrease HCO_3^- concentrations

Disorders That May Alter Laboratory Results
With poor peripheral perfusion, results of blood gas analysis on samples taken from peripheral vessels may not reflect the overall systemic condition. Appropriate reference ranges must be used (venous vs. arterial).

CBC/BIOCHEMISTRY/URINALYSIS
• Measurement of serum electrolytes and protein concentrations is important to determine the cause and to guide treatment
• Calculation of the AG may be useful, especially in mixed acid–base disorders
• Proportionate changes in Na^+ and Cl^- concentrations occur with alterations of fluid balance
• Normal Na^+ concentrations with hypochloremia or hyperchloremia indicate acid–base imbalance
• Albumin/protein concentrations are not considered when calculating the AG; however, because proteins are weak acids, hyperproteinemia (e.g. dehydration, chronic inflammation, neoplasia) can contribute to metabolic acidosis
• Urinalysis and fractional excretion of electrolytes, in combination with serum creatinine and blood urea nitrogen

concentrations, are useful in cases of renal dysfunction

Horses with Hyperchloremia and Normal AG
- Loss of HCO_3^-—diarrhea, type 2 RTA, and primary respiratory alkalosis; however, severely affected colitis patients often are acidotic and low in Na^+, K^+, Cl^-, and HCO_3^- because of water intake after isotonic fluid loss
- Salt poisoning
- Cl^- retention—renal failure, type 1 or 4 RTA, and acetazolamide therapy

Horses with Increased AG
Accumulation of unmeasured anions, such as:
- Lactate—hypovolemia, hypotension from SIRS, hypoxemia, third space fluid loss, anaerobic exercise, rhabdomyolysis, liver failure, malignant hyperthermia
- Phosphates, sulfates, and organic acids—renal failure, toxic ingestion

OTHER LABORATORY TESTS

Total CO_2
- Closely approximates HCO_3^- concentration because most CO_2 is carried in the blood as HCO_3^-
- Respiratory alkalosis also decreases TCO_2; differentiation can only be made with blood gas analysis
- Analyze rapidly with minimal room-air exposure as CO_2 will decrease

Blood Gas Analysis
- Needed to determine primary change in blood pH
- Decreased blood pH indicates acidemia. A concurrent decrease in HCO_3^- indicates primary metabolic acidemia. An accompanying decrease in PCO_2 indicates respiratory compensation
- Decreased HCO_3^- with increased blood pH indicates compensation for a respiratory alkalosis
- Determine if hypoxemia is contributing to lactic acidemia
- Blood gas parameters must be assessed against appropriate reference ranges for the sample taken
- Blood lactate—elevation indicates contribution to metabolic acidemia

IMAGING
Ultrasonography can be useful in evaluating colitis, ascites, and pleural effusion, as well as cardiac, renal, and hepatic architecture.

PATHOLOGIC FINDINGS
Dependent on the underlying cause.

TREATMENT
Directed at the primary cause.

MEDICATIONS

DRUG(S) OF CHOICE
- Isotonic fluid therapy is usually sufficient to correct lactic acidosis from hypovolemia in mild cases
- With severe hypovolemia, therapy may include hypertonic saline, colloids, or blood transfusion followed by crystalloid fluid administration
- Alkalinizing therapy is reserved for patients with a pH < 7.2 that persists following rehydration
- $NaHCO_3^-$ is most frequently utilized
- $NaHCO_3^-$ deficit (mEq) is calculated as follows—base deficit × body weight (kg) × 0.3 (extracellular fluid space (0.5 in foals))
- A negative BE, or 24 minus HCO_3^-, can be used for the base deficit
- In acute cases, half the deficit can be given over 30 min, in fluids, or as a 5% solution to adults
- Isotonic HCO_3^- (1.3%) is a good choice in neonates or severely affected adults
- Correction to a pH > 7.2 and BE ≥ − 5 is usually adequate

PRECAUTIONS
- Use HCO_3^- therapy cautiously in patients with respiratory compromise, because the CO_2 that is generated may not be eliminated, causing a further decrease in pH
- Na^+ load may affect blood volume in neonates and patients with compromised renal, neurologic, or cardiac function
- Rebound alkalosis or cerebral acidosis is reported from overdose or rapid administration of HCO_3^- since both CO_2 and H_2CO_3 cross the blood–brain barrier

POSSIBLE INTERACTIONS
HCO_3^- cannot be mixed with Ca^{2+}.

ALTERNATIVE DRUGS
Oral rehydration solutions (4–8 L PO every 2 h in adults without ileus).

FOLLOW-UP

PATIENT MONITORING
Serial blood gas analysis to evaluate efficacy of therapy.

POSSIBLE COMPLICATIONS
- Hyperkalemia
- Cardiac arrhythmias, hypotension
- Severe, untreated metabolic acidosis with a pH < 7.0 may result in death

MISCELLANEOUS

ASSOCIATED CONDITIONS
- Hyperchloremia
- Hyperkalemia
- Respiratory alkalosis

AGE-RELATED FACTORS
- Asphyxia during parturition in neonates
- Conditions associated with premature neonates

PREGNANCY/FERTILITY/BREEDING
Metabolic acidosis may decrease uterine blood flow and result in placental insufficiency.

SEE ALSO
- Chloride, hyperchloremia
- *Clostridium difficile* infection
- Diarrhea, neonate
- Hypoxemia
- Idiopathic colitis
- Potassium, hyperkalemia
- Potomac horse fever (PHF)
- Septicemia, neonate

ABBREVIATIONS
- AG = anion gap
- BE = base excess
- CNS = central nervous system
- CSF = cerebrospinal fluid
- GI = gastrointestinal
- PCO_2 = partial pressure of carbon dioxide
- RTA = renal tubular acidosis
- SIRS = systemic inflammatory response syndrome
- TCO_2 = total carbon dioxide

Suggested Reading
Fielding L. Crystalloid and colloid therapy. Vet Clin North Am Equine Pract 2014;30(2):415–425.
Hall JE. Guyton and Hall: Textbook of Medical Physiology, 13e. Philadelphia, PA: Elsevier Inc., 2016:497–556.
Ohmes CM, Davis EG, Beard LA, et al. Transient Fanconi syndrome in Quarter Horses. Can Vet J 2014;55:147–151.

Author Sara L. Connolly
Consulting Editor Sandra D. Taylor
Acknowledgment The author and editor acknowledge the prior contribution of Jennifer G. Adams.

A

ACIDOSIS, RESPIRATORY

BASICS

DEFINITION
• Increase in blood PCO_2
• Homeostatic mechanisms maintain normal blood concentrations within a narrow range
• Arterial concentrations in the range 35–42 mmHg
• Venous concentrations in the range 43–49 mmHg

PATHOPHYSIOLOGY
• CO_2 is formed in all tissues during metabolic energy production and diffuses passively out of cells and into the blood in gaseous form
• Most of this CO_2 (65–70%) combines with water almost instantaneously to form carbonic acid, which then dissociates into HCO_3^- and H +
• Most CO_2 is transported in the blood as HCO_3^-. Some is bound to proteins, especially deoxygenated hemoglobin, and a small amount is dissolved directly into plasma
• In the lungs, the reverse occurs, and CO_2 passively diffuses out of capillaries into the alveoli
• These 3 forms of CO_2 exist in equilibrium in the blood, but PCO_2 as measured by blood gases depends on the dissolved portion
• The chemical components of the carbonic acid equilibrium are:

$$CO_2 + H_2O = H_2CO_3 = H^+ + HCO_3^-$$

• Alveolar CO_2 then is removed mechanically by ventilation as air moves in and out of the lungs
• Hypercapnia is present only when tissue production exceeds the capacity of normal lungs to eliminate CO_2 or when components of the respiratory system are abnormal
• Respiratory acidosis results from disease or alteration of the respiratory center in the brain, peripheral chemoreceptors that control respiration, mechanical components of respiration (chest wall, respiratory muscles), or the respiratory tract (airways, alveoli, pulmonary vasculature, lung parenchyma). This can result in hypoventilation, diffusion impairment, or V/Q mismatching
• Because CO_2 diffuses across alveolar membranes in direct proportion to ventilation, hypoventilation leads to increased blood CO_2 concentration
• Diffusion impairment (e.g. pneumonia) rarely results in hypercapnia given that CO_2 diffuses very readily across alveolar membranes
• Increased blood CO_2 concentration develops as a compensatory response of the lungs to metabolic alkalosis

SYSTEMS AFFECTED
Respiratory

GENETICS
N/A

INCIDENCE/PREVALENCE
N/A

GEOGRAPHIC DISTRIBUTION
N/A

SIGNALMENT
• Any breed, age or sex
• Neonatal foals with perinatal asphyxia
• Anesthetized patients develop some degree of hypercapnia when breathing spontaneously
• Because of their size, equids are predisposed to hypoventilation under anesthesia

SIGNS

Historical Findings
• Neonatal foals born from a dam with dystocia
• Respiratory noise may be heard, especially with exercise, in cases of upper airway obstruction

Physical Examination Findings
• None if minute ventilation is increased via increased tidal volume; if not, tachypnea may be present
• Decreased respiratory rate or an apneustic breathing pattern may be present in neonatal foals with perinatal asphyxia
• Decrease or absence of airway sounds may be found at auscultation in cases with damage or disease of the chest wall or thorax
• Abnormal sounds may be present with pulmonary disease

CAUSES
• Upper airway obstruction leading to hypoventilation. Specific causes—nasal edema, cyst, mass, or infection of the paranasal sinuses, laryngeal or pharyngeal paralysis or inflammation, soft palate displacement, pharyngeal or epiglottal cysts, and tracheal masses or collapse
• Hypoxia to the respiratory center of the brainstem in foals with perinatal asphyxia can cause hypoventilation
• Injury or disease of the thorax, diaphragm, or pleura may restrict movement of the chest wall or respiratory muscles. Tension pneumothorax may rapidly lead to death
• Large volumes of pleural or peritoneal fluid, as well as severe GI distention, may restrict diaphragmatic movement, leading to hypoventilation
• Paresis or paralysis of the respiratory muscles can be seen with neurologic diseases such as botulism, tetanus, encephalitis, or head trauma
• Respiratory muscle damage caused by box elder seeds (i.e. seasonal pasture myopathy)
• Severe pneumonia, pulmonary edema, or acute respiratory distress syndrome can cause diffusion impairment
• Premature foals with significant atelectasis (diffusion impairment) and weak thoracic muscles (hypoventilation)

• Hypoventilation caused by muscle relaxation and decreased sensitivity of the respiratory center to CO_2 occurs in all anesthetized horses. Heavy sedation also may produce temporary hypercapnia via muscle relaxation and respiratory center insensitivity
• Pregnant animals are more prone to hypoventilation under general anesthesia because of abdominal distention from the pregnant uterus
• Defective cellular metabolism of muscle is seen with malignant hyperthermia. This syndrome is very rare but has been seen in horses with inhalant anesthesia or succinyl choline administration. Abnormal metabolic processes in muscle cells are triggered, resulting in tremendous production of heat and CO_2, such that elimination mechanisms are overwhelmed and respiratory acidosis results
• Anaerobic exercise produces temporary respiratory acidosis because ventilation is limited when chest wall movement is linked to stride at high speeds

RISK FACTORS
• General anesthesia, heavy sedation
• Pregnancy
• Prolonged recumbency
• History of malignant hyperthermia in related individuals
• Prematurity, dystocia, asphyxia or sepsis, persistent fetal circulation, or pulmonary hypertension in neonates

DIAGNOSIS

DIFFERENTIAL DIAGNOSIS
• Physiologic states or disease processes that present with tachypnea (e.g. fever, hyperthermia, excitement, anxiety, painful conditions, hypoxemia, metabolic acidosis, and CNS derangements)
• Under anesthesia, tachypnea also may result from a light plane of anesthesia, hypoxemia, metabolic acidosis, or faulty anesthetic rebreathing systems
• Compensatory hypercapnia secondary to metabolic alkalosis caused by upper GI obstruction, early large colon impaction or simple obstruction, or supplementation with HCO_3^- or other alkalinizing agent. pH in these cases is often still higher than normal because compensatory hypoventilation is limited once hypoxemia develops

LABORATORY FINDINGS

Drugs That May Alter Laboratory Results
N/A

Disorders That May Alter Laboratory Results
• With poor peripheral perfusion, results of blood gas analysis on samples taken from peripheral vessels may not reflect the overall

systemic condition. Appropriate reference ranges must be used (venous vs. arterial)
• Prolonged exposure to room air may alter PCO_2 concentrations, because the sample equilibrates with the air
• Cellular metabolism of red blood cells continues after sampling; if not measured quickly, PCO_2 concentrations may be falsely elevated

CBC/BIOCHEMISTRY/URINALYSIS
N/A

OTHER LABORATORY TESTS
• Arterial blood gas analysis is necessary to evaluate adequacy of ventilation and gas exchange and to document hypercapnia
• Handheld analyzers are available and easy to use, and some require only small amounts of whole blood. Otherwise, pre-heparinized syringes are preferred or use syringes heparinized before sampling
• Perform sampling anaerobically. Immediately evacuate any air bubbles, and cap the needle with a rubber stopper
• Perform analysis within 15–20 min. If not possible, samples can be stored on ice, and results may be valid for 3–4 h when glass syringes or dedicated arterial blood gas syringes are used

IMAGING
N/A

OTHER DIAGNOSTIC PROCEDURES
• Capnography or capnometry to measure CO_2 indirectly from expired gases
• Samples of end-tidal gases reflect arterial PCO_2 concentrations, because this gas is essentially alveolar gas
• Continuous monitoring of anesthetized or ventilated patients
• V/Q mismatch is always present in anesthetized or recumbent patients, and end-tidal CO_2 concentrations may underestimate arterial concentrations by $\cong$ 10–15 mmHg

TREATMENT
• Emergency therapy occasionally may be necessary for upper airway obstructions (e.g. passage of a nasotracheal tube or tracheotomy). Stridor is usually present in affected horses
• Definitive therapy for hypercapnia involves resolution of the primary disease process affecting ventilation, diffusion, or gas exchange
• Avoid excessive anesthetic depth. If depth is adequate, controlled ventilation is necessary when hypoventilation persists and $PaCO_2$ is > 60 mmHg
• In neonates, postural therapy and coupage may improve gas exchange
• With botulism or severe lung disease, treat hypercapnia with controlled ventilation

MEDICATIONS
DRUG(S) OF CHOICE
Caffeine
Respiratory stimulant (10 mg/kg PO loading dose followed by 2.5 mg/kg PO every 12 h) for foals with perinatal asphyxia that do not have ileus.

Doxapram
• Respiratory stimulant (0.2–0.5 mg/kg IV or an infusion of 0.01–0.05 mg/kg/min) in foals with perinatal asphyxia or muscular weakness
• Anesthetized patients who are breathing poorly may respond temporarily to its effects, but controlled ventilation, decreasing depth, and anesthetic reversal are more specific and appropriate therapies
• Not indicated for healthy patients being weaned from controlled ventilation

CONTRAINDICATIONS
• Controlled ventilation may cause barotrauma in foals with meconium aspiration
• Partial obstruction of the small airways may lead to air trapping in alveoli, which may rupture

PRECAUTIONS
• Monitor ventilated patients continuously for airway obstruction caused by accumulation of secretions, kinking of tubing, hoses, etc.
• Oxygen toxicity can develop with inspired PO_2 > 50% or if PaO_2 > 100 mmHg is maintained for prolonged periods (10–12 h).

POSSIBLE INTERACTIONS
N/A

ALTERNATIVE DRUGS
N/A

FOLLOW-UP
PATIENT MONITORING
Use serial arterial blood gas analyses or capnometry to assess adequacy of ventilation and monitor progress, especially during weaning from ventilation.

PREVENTION/AVOIDANCE
N/A

POSSIBLE COMPLICATIONS
• Respiratory acidosis lowers systemic pH and may affect ionization of protein-bound drugs
• Acidosis decreases heart contractility and may cause or contribute to CNS depression

• Hypercapnia and resultant acidosis predispose patients to cardiac arrhythmias, especially under general anesthesia
• The $PaCO_2$ concentration greatly affects cerebral blood flow and cerebrospinal fluid pressure
• Severe or prolonged hypercapnia may contribute to brain damage or herniation in cases of head trauma

EXPECTED COURSE AND PROGNOSIS
Dependent on the underlying cause.

MISCELLANEOUS
ASSOCIATED CONDITIONS
Disorders that result in metabolic alkalosis.

AGE-RELATED FACTORS
Neonates with perinatal asphyxia or prematurity.

ZOONOTIC POTENTIAL
N/A

PREGNANCY/FERTILITY/BREEDING
See Risk Factors.

SYNONYMS
• Hypercapnia
• Hypercarbia

SEE ALSO
• Botulism
• Neonatal maladjustment syndrome

ABBREVIATIONS
• CNS = central nervous system
• GI = gastrointestinal
• $PaCO_2$ = partial pressure of carbon dioxide in arterial blood
• PaO_2 = partial pressure of oxygen in arterial blood
• PCO_2 = partial pressure of carbon dioxide
• PO_2 = partial pressure of oxygen
• V/Q = ventilation/perfusion

Suggested Reading
Hall JE. Guyton and Hall: Textbook of Medical Physiology, 13e. Philadelphia, PA: Elsevier Inc., 2016:497–556.
Moens Y. Mechanical ventilation and respiratory mechanics during equine anesthesia. Vet Clin North Am Equine Pract 2013;29(1):51–67.
Palmer JE. Ventilatory support of the critically ill foal. Vet Clin North Am Equine Pract 2005;21(2):457–486.

Author Sara L. Connolly
Consulting Editor Sandra D. Taylor
Acknowledgment The author and editor acknowledge the prior contribution of Jennifer G. Adams.

A

ACTINOBACILLOSIS

BASICS

OVERVIEW
- Acute rapidly progressive septicemia due to *Actinobacillus equuli* or *Actinobacillus suis*-like organisms in neonatal foals. Also known as "sleepy foal disease"
- *A. equuli*—Gram-negative coccobacillary to rod-shaped pleomorphic organism
- Normal inhabitant of the mucous membranes of the alimentary tract
- Fetal infection may follow transplacental infection
- Kidneys are a frequent site of neonatal infection
- Can have characteristic lesions including embolic nephritis, embolic pneumonia, lymphoid necrosis, multifocal hepatic necrosis, and septic arthritis. Subsp. *haemolyticus* appears to prefer the respiratory tract
- Adult infection frequently endogenous. Fecal contamination or spread from oral mucous membranes. Soft tissue abscesses, respiratory infections, and rarely conjunctival, urinary tract, joint, guttural pouch, skin, and genital tract infections

SIGNALMENT
- Foals < 2 days of age
- Adults—any age

SIGNS
Foals
- Acute onset, depression, diarrhea, recumbency, distended painful joints, sudden death
- Fever may not be present, hypothermia. May progress rapidly to septic shock
- Bone and joint infections may not be obvious for days to weeks and may be unaccompanied by signs of systemic disease

Adults
- Depends on affected organ system. Systemic actinobacillosis—rare and associated with underlying disease or another predisposing factor
- Primary peritonitis

CAUSES AND RISK FACTORS
Foals
- Commonly associated with failure of transfer of passive immunity
- Perinatal stress, prematurity, and/or unsanitary environmental conditions
- Portals of entry include respiratory tract, gastrointestinal tract, placenta, and umbilical remnant

Adults
- Pneumonia and pleuropneumonia secondary to viral infection or stressful events
- Trauma predisposes to abscess formation

DIAGNOSIS

DIFFERENTIAL DIAGNOSIS
Foals
- Other causes of bacterial, viral, and fungal neonatal sepsis
- Equine herpesvirus type 1, equine viral arteritis
- Perinatal hypoxic–ischemic anoxic or inflammatory insults

Adults
- Other causes of fever or peritonitis
- Other bacterial, viral, or fungal pneumonia or pleuropneumonia
- Other causes of respiratory distress, fever, coughing, and nasal discharge—sinusitis, guttural pouch empyema, heaves (recurrent airway obstruction), inflammatory airway disease, interstitial pneumonia, mycoplasma infections, neoplasia, dysphagia

CBC/BIOCHEMISTRY/URINALYSIS
Foals
- Leukocytosis or leukopenia
- Hyperfibrinogenemia at birth possible with in utero infections. Increases in fibrinogen and SAA common
- Increased creatinine and/or blood urea nitrogen with renal involvement
- Metabolic acidosis, hypoxemia, and hypercapnia may be observed in foals in septic shock
- Hypoglycemia may be present
- Frequent complete or partial failure of passive transfer (serum IgG <800 mg/dL)
- Urinalysis may be abnormal with renal involvement

Adults
- Leukocytosis and hyperfibrinogenemia possible
- Anemia of chronic disease in longstanding infection
- Other abnormalities depend on body system involved

IMAGING
Foals
- Radiographs—thorax, joints
- Ultrasonography—umbilicus, kidneys
- Computed tomography—pulmonary disease in neonatal foals

Adults
Radiographic and ultrasonographic evaluation of affected body system.

OTHER DIAGNOSTIC PROCEDURES
Foals
- Blood culture
- Synovial bacterial culture
- Kidneys—multifocal microabscesses at postmortem examination

Adults
- Culture/cytology of affected body system

- Normal inhabitant of equine gastrointestinal mucosa so results should be interpreted cautiously

TREATMENT
Foals
- Hospitalization
- Intranasal oxygen supplementation
- Early antimicrobial therapy

MEDICATIONS

DRUG(S) OF CHOICE
Foals
- Isotonic polyionic balanced fluids
- IV plasma based on IgG concentrations
- IV dextrose or parenteral nutrition
- Broad-spectrum antimicrobial therapy, gentamicin 12 mg/kg IV SID or amikacin 25–30 mg/kg IV SID and potassium penicillin 20 000 IU/kg IV QID or ceftiofur sodium 5–10 mg/kg IV BID–QID. Monitor plasma creatinine concentration. Therapeutic drug monitoring desirable
- Systemic inflammatory response syndrome or multiorgan dysfunction syndrome—intensive fluid management and inopressor therapy
- Severe respiratory disturbance—assisted ventilation
- Regional limb perfusion and/or direct instillation with antimicrobials for septic joints

Adults
Antimicrobial therapy based on culture/sensitivity.

MISCELLANEOUS
- Continue treatment until clinical signs have resolved and white blood count, differential, and fibrinogen/SAA concentration are within normal limits for 48 h
- Commonly isolated from foals lost to mare reproductive loss syndrome and adult horses affected by pericarditis during the same time period

ABBREVIATIONS
- IgG = immunoglobulin G
- SAA = serum amyloid A

Suggested Reading
Layman QD, Rezabek GB, Ramachandran A, et al. A retrospective study of equine actinobacillosis cases: 1999–2011. J Vet Diagn Invest 2014;26:365–375.

Author Pamela A. Wilkins
Consulting Editor Ashley G. Boyle

ACUTE ADULT ABDOMINAL PAIN—ACUTE COLIC

BASICS

DEFINITION
Signs are associated with discomfort originating within the abdominal cavity. May develop acutely or gradually. Considered chronic when persisting for more than 3–4 days.

PATHOPHYSIOLOGY
• Most acute abdominal pain originates from the GI tract but may also arise from other systems
• In the intestinal tract, pain may originate from increased intramural tension, tension on a mesentery, ischemia, inflammation, smooth muscle spasms, or a combination of any of these
• Causes can be divided into strangulating and nonstrangulating lesions. Nonstrangulating lesions include intraluminal lesions, extraluminal lesions, mural lesions, as well as spasmodic colic, intestinal displacement, ileus, and inflammatory bowel disease. Strangulating lesions, such as torsions and incarcerations, are usually associated with a compromise of local blood supply followed by intestinal necrosis. The necrosis may lead to cardiovascular shock

SYSTEMS AFFECTED
• Cardiovascular—dehydration and endotoxemia may lead to shock and result in organ failure
• GI—the large colon and the distal part of the small intestine are commonly involved
• Other systems can be involved (e.g. urinary system, reproductive tract, hepatobiliary, peritoneum and pleura)

SIGNALMENT
Nonspecific. There may be an age, breed, or sex predisposition for a specific problem.

SIGNS
General Comments
May be subtle and easily missed initially. As the disease progresses, changes in clinical parameters, rectal examination findings, transabdominal ultrasound findings, and laboratory data allow a more accurate localization.

Historical Findings
• Abdominal pain can appear acutely or following an episode of anorexia, depression, and/or decreased fecal output. Recent history of change in the exercise, diet, or availability of drinking water may also be present
• Mild abdominal pain—decrease in appetite and/or fecal output, mild depression, yawning, extended neck and rolling of the upper lip, teeth grinding, muscle fasciculation
• Moderate abdominal pain—frequent lying down, pawing, flank watching, groaning, posture for urinating with small quantities of urine passed, kicking the abdomen, attempts to roll
• Severe abdominal pain—walking in a tight circle, constantly getting up and down, rolling, traumatizing self and handlers, sweating, labored breathing

Physical Examination Findings
Depending on the stage of the disease signs may vary in severity:
• General findings—abdominal distention, sweating, increased respiratory rate, changes in body temperature, abnormal quality and quantity of feces
• Cardiovascular findings—tacky mucous membranes, increased capillary refill time, increased heart rate, dehydration, cold extremities. In endotoxemic shock, the cause of pain is likely due to a strangulating lesion or to a severe inflammatory process (colitis, peritonitis)
• GI findings—increase, decrease, or absence in gut motility, gas-filled resonant viscus on percussion, presence of net gastric reflux on passage of the nasogastric tube. Possible gastric reflux in stomach and small intestinal lesions. Abnormalities on rectal examination—gaseous distention of viscus by gas, liquid, or food; displacement of viscus; thickening of the intestinal wall; presence of tight bands, uterine or renal abnormalities

CAUSES
GI
• Nonstrangulated obstructive lesions:
  ○ Gastric—ulcers, distention, impaction, rupture, tumor. Small intestine—enterocolitis, ascarid impaction, ileal impaction, ileal hypertrophy, stricture, adhesions. Large colon—ulceration, colitis, impaction, gas distention, mild displacement, left dorsal and right displacement, enterolith, sand impactions. Cecum—impaction, gas distention. Small colon—impaction, enterolith
• Strangulating obstructive lesions:
  ○ Small intestine—incarceration into a space/rent in the mesentery/inguinal ring/gastrosplenic ligament/epiploic foramen, strangulation by lipoma, volvulus. Large colon—volvulus, incarceration, thromboembolic infarction. Cecum—intussusception, thromboembolic infarction, torsion. Small colon—strangulating lipoma, submucosal hematoma, thromboembolic infarction

Others
• Reproductive—uterine torsion, laceration, abortion, parturition, testicular torsion, hematoma in the broad ligament, trauma
• Renal/urologic—renal/ureteral/bladder/urethral calculi, cystitis, renal inflammatory processes
• Hepatobiliary—hepatitis, hepatobiliary calculi

RISK FACTORS
• No access to water
• Sudden change in diet
• Poor enteric parasite control
• Pregnancy
• Previous abdominal surgery
• Congenital abnormalities
• Certain medication

DIAGNOSIS

DIFFERENTIAL DIAGNOSIS
Other causes of pain that might mimic pain originating from the abdominal cavity include myositis, pleuropneumonia, hemorrhagic shock, rabies, and musculoskeletal injuries.

CBC/BIOCHEMISTRY/URINALYSIS
• Increase in packed cell volume and total protein with dehydration
• Possible hypoproteinemia secondary to GI protein loss
• Leukopenia in acute inflammation and endotoxemia or leukocytosis in chronic inflammation
• Metabolic acidosis and production of lactic acid in cardiovascular shock. Metabolic alkalosis and loss of chloride when large amount of gastric reflux is present. Increased lactate concentration in presence of endotoxemia, tissue hypoxia, liver disease
• Hypokalemia and hypocalcemia, especially if anorexia is present and in lactating mare
• Hypochloremia and hyponatremia (colitis)
• Alkaline phosphatase may be increased
• Azotemia in severe dehydration or acute renal failure

OTHER LABORATORY TESTS
Abdominal Paracentesis
• Normal fluid has a pale, clear yellow color
• Increase of the protein level and WBCs is indicative of primary peritonitis or secondary to morphologic change of the viscera
• Foul-smelling reddish-brown fluid with an increase in the RBCs, WBCs, and protein is indicative of necrotic bowel. Presence of plant materials suggests intestinal rupture
• Lactate concentration > 1 mmol/L may indicate intestinal ischemia

Urinalysis
A change in specific gravity, increase in leukocyte content, RBCs, and pH may be noticed in cases with renal disease.

IMAGING
Radiographs
May be useful in sand impactions or enteroliths in adults. In foals for localization of gas, fluid distention, impaction, or congenital abnormality (atresia coli).

Ultrasonography
• Evaluation of—amount and characteristics of abdominal fluid; motility, wall thickness, and diameter of small intestine and its location; motility and wall thickness of the large intestine; nephrosplenic space for presence of intestine; intussusceptions, abscesses, or mass
• Also useful in evaluating the stomach, kidneys, liver, spleen, uterus, etc.

Endoscopy
Gastroscopy—evaluation of the stomach for ulcers, impaction or tumor.
Cystoscopy—evaluation of the urethra, bladder, and opening of the ureters for inflammation or calculi.

OTHER DIAGNOSTIC PROCEDURES
Exploratory laparotomy/laparoscopy.

TREATMENT
• Horses should be taken off feed until diagnosis/resolution of the underlying problem
• The history, physical examination, and laboratory results will help differentiate between medical or surgical condition
• Reasons for exploratory laparotomy—moderate to severe abdominal pain, unresponsiveness to medical treatment, progressive increase in heart rate or heart rates above 60–70/min, cardiovascular compromise or deterioration, presence of moderate to severe gas distention or displacement of the large colon, gas distention of small intestine, gastric reflux, abnormal paracentesis findings
• Supportive treatment for medical and surgical cases includes pain management, IV fluids, gastric decompression if necessary, electrolyte replenishment, and control of the abdominal pain

MEDICATIONS
DRUG(S) OF CHOICE
• Analgesics—control the abdominal pain
  ○ NSAIDs initially—flunixin meglumine (0.5–1.1 mg/kg IV, IM every 8 h), α_2-blockers such as xylazine (0.25–0.5 mg/kg IV or IM), detomidine (5–10 μg/kg IV or IM), or romifidine (0.02–0.05 mg/kg IV or IM)
  ○ Narcotic analgesic butorphanol (0.02–0.075 mg/kg IV) in conjunction with the α_2-blockers

• Spasmolytics (indicated in spasmodic colic)—N-butylscopammonium bromide (0.3 mg/kg)
• Laxatives—mainly used for impactions:
  ○ Mineral oil—10 mL/kg via nasogastric tube
  ○ Osmotic laxative—disodium (0.5 g/kg) or magnesium sulfate (0.5–1 g/kg) in 4 L of warm water via nasogastric tube ideally followed by oral or IV fluid therapy. Dioctyl sodium sulfosuccinate (10–30 mg/kg of a 10% solution). Water, via an indwelling nasogastric tube, if there is no gastric reflux
• Parenteral fluid treatments—in cases of dehydration or moderate to severe impaction problems, IV fluid (100–150 mL/kg/day). If cardiovascular shock is present, hypertonic saline (2 L of 7% NaCl in an adult horse) prior to balanced electrolyte solutions may be given. Correction of electrolyte imbalances, especially hypokalemia and hypocalcemia, which are important for intestinal motility. Moderate to severe sodium bicarbonate deficit may be corrected as well as low plasma protein level (< 40 g/L)
• Treatment of endotoxemia—flunixin meglumine 0.25 mg/kg every 6 h
• Intestinal motility stimulants (see chapter Ileus)
• Antimicrobial therapy if peritonitis is suspected or surgery is performed

CONTRAINDICATIONS
Acepromazine is contraindicated due to its peripheral vasodilatory effect.

PRECAUTIONS
Repeat use of α_2-blockers and butorphanol causes prolonged ileus. Repeat dose of NSAIDs, especially in presence of dehydration, can result in gastric or large colon ulceration as well as renal damage.

FOLLOW-UP
PATIENT MONITORING
Monitor closely for deterioration of clinical signs and cardiovascular status until resolution of the abdominal pain. Following resolution of these signs, reintroduction to feed should be done gradually.

POSSIBLE COMPLICATIONS
• Endotoxemia
• Laminitis
• Circulatory shock
• Adhesions
• GI rupture
• Peritonitis

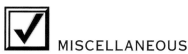

MISCELLANEOUS
ASSOCIATED CONDITIONS
N/A

AGE-RELATED FACTORS
Older horses are more predisposed to strangulated lipoma and epiploic foramen entrapment; younger horses are more predisposed to ulcer problems, intussusception, and ascarid impactions.

ZOONOTIC POTENTIAL
N/A

PREGNANCY/FERTILITY/BREEDING
Mares in late gestation or in the postpartum period are predisposed to large colon torsion. Parturition can present clinical signs similar to a GI accident.

SYNONYMS
Colic

ABBREVIATIONS
• GI = gastrointestinal
• NSAID = nonsteroidal anti-inflammatory drug
• RBC = red blood cell
• WBC = white blood cell

Suggested Reading
Hackett ES. Specific causes of colic. In: Southwood LL, ed. Practical Guide to Equine Colic. Ames, IA: Wiley Blackwell, 2013:204–230.
Mair T, Divers T, Ducharme N. Section 1: Diagnostic procedures in equine gastroenterology. In: Mair T, Divers T, Ducharme N (eds). Manual of Equine Gastroenterology. Philadelphia, PA: WB Saunders, 2002:3–46.
Mair T, Divers T, Ducharme N. Section 4: Colic. In: Mair T, Divers T, Ducharme N (eds). Manual of Equine Gastroenterology. Philadelphia, PA: WB Saunders, 2002:101–141.
Walton RM. Clinical laboratory data. In: Southwood LL, ed. Practical Guide to Equine Colic. Ames, IA: Wiley Blackwell, 2013:78–85.

Author Nathalie Coté
Consulting Editors Henry Stämpfli and Olimpo Oliver-Espinosa

BASICS

OVERVIEW
Epiglottiditis is a nonspecific inflammatory disease of the epiglottis.

SIGNALMENT
- Primarily racehorses (2–10 years) in active race training
- Occasionally seen in older horses (15–30 years) with inflammatory disease or neoplasia
- No known breed or sex predilection
- May be associated with epiglottic abscess or epiglottic chondritis

SIGNS
- Chief complaints—abnormal respiratory tract noise and exercise intolerance
- Coughing (eating) is fairly common
- Some horses act mildly pained when swallowing

CAUSES AND RISK FACTORS
- Cause—suspect viral or subepiglottic trauma or surgical trauma
- Repeated, strenuous exercise may induce inflammatory changes on the subepiglottic mucosal surface
- Inhaled particulate activities, bacterial or viral infections
- May be secondary to surgical trauma

 DIAGNOSIS

DIFFERENTIAL DIAGNOSIS
- The diagnosis is established based on endoscopy of the upper respiratory tract
- Occasionally, the endoscopic appearance of a swollen epiglottis is misinterpreted as epiglottic entrapment by the aryepiglottic folds
- May be associated with epiglottic abscess or chondritis

CBC/BIOCHEMISTRY/URINALYSIS
N/A

OTHER LABORATORY TESTS
N/A

IMAGING
Imaging is not usually performed.

OTHER DIAGNOSTIC PROCEDURES
- During endoscopy, the epiglottis may appear swollen and discolored (reddish-purplish), primarily along the lateral margins and ventral (lingual) mucosal surfaces. Epiglottis may appear more rounded and bulbous. The ventral mucosal surfaces

often are ulcerated, and in more chronic cases granulation tissue surrounded by fibrous connective tissue is seen
- If ulceration is seen at the rostral tip or dorsal surface of the epiglottic cartilage one should suspect associated epiglottic chondritis and abscessation
- Horses with epiglottiditis often intermittently or persistently displace the soft palate dorsally
- The caudal free margin of the soft palate may have a variable amount of inflammation, ulceration, or thickening

 TREATMENT

- Outpatient (stall-side) basis
- Discontinue exercise for a minimum of 7–21 days, depending on the extent of the problem
- If swallowing is difficult or stimulates coughing, hay may need to be eliminated completely or partially from the diet

 MEDICATIONS

DRUG(S) OF CHOICE
- Horses are initially treated with phenylbutazone (4.4 mg/kg IV) or flunixin meglumine (1.1 mg/kg IV) and dexamethasone (0.044 mg/kg IV). Spray 20 mL of a pharyngeal spray (140 mL of DMSO, 140 mL of glycerin, 266 mL of distilled water, and 14 mL of dexamethasone 4 mg/mL and often an antibiotic such as nitrofurazone) into the pharynx twice daily for 7–14 days through a 10 F catheter introduced via the nasal passages
- Antimicrobial therapy may be indicated if infection is suspected—procaine penicillin G (IM), trimethoprim–sulfamethoxazole (PO), ceftiofur (IM, IV) at usual recommended dosages for 5–7 days

CONTRAINDICATIONS/POSSIBLE INTERACTIONS
No contraindications.

 FOLLOW-UP

PATIENT MONITORING
Substantial improvement of the epiglottis and adjacent tissue and in pharyngeal function usually is seen at follow-up endoscopy after

about 1 week of therapy. Continue rest and therapy until healing is judged complete (repeated endoscopy performed at 1 week intervals).

PREVENTION/AVOIDANCE
Horses with more chronic-appearing inflammation or with associated epiglottic abscess and/or chondritis may require more protracted therapy (2–4 weeks), and complete resolution of thickening and cartilage deformity may not occur. Occasionally, epiglottic entrapment may develop.

POSSIBLE COMPLICATIONS
Healing may result in fibrosis or cicatrix on the lingual epiglottic surface sufficient to interfere with normal soft palate function. Endoscopy may reveal intermittent or persistent dorsal displacement of the soft palate, which may need surgical treatment.

EXPECTED COURSE AND PROGNOSIS
Epiglottiditis is a serious, potentially career-limiting or -ending problem in racehorses. Prognosis depends primarily on severity of the condition during the initial examination and the degree of involvement and resulting deformity of the epiglottic cartilage. Resolution of acute inflammation results in complete return to normal exercise tolerance.

 MISCELLANEOUS

SEE ALSO
- Dorsal displacement of the soft palate (DDSP)
- Inspiratory dyspnea

ABBREVIATIONS
DMSO = dimethylsulfoxide

Suggested Reading
Hawkins JF, Tulleners EP. Epiglottitis in horses: 20 cases (1988–1993). J Am Vet Med Assoc 1994;205:1577–1580.
Infernuso T, Watts AE, Ducharme NG. Septic epiglottic chondritis with abscessation in 2 young thoroughbred racehorses. Can Vet J 2006;47:1007–1010.
Ortved KF, Cheetham J, Mitchell LM, Ducharme NG. Successful treatment of persistent dorsal displacement of the soft palate and evaluation of laryngohyoid position in 15 racehorses. Equine Vet J 2010;42:23–29.

Author Norm G. Ducharme
Consulting Editors Daniel Jean and Mathilde Leclère

ACUTE HEPATITIS IN ADULT HORSES (THEILER DISEASE)

BASICS

OVERVIEW
The clinical disease (acute hepatitis, Theiler disease, serum hepatitis) is characterized by fulminant hepatic failure and encephalopathy in adult horses. There appear to be 3 separate epidemiologic diseases with identical clinical, clinicopathologic, and pathologic findings:
- Acute, often fulminant hepatitis in horses that have received equine-origin blood products approximately 4–10 weeks earlier and less severe to subclinical disease in other horses receiving the same product
- Acute, sometimes fulminant hepatitis occurring in a horse that was in contact with a blood product-inoculated Theiler disease horse, but that did not itself receive the equine-origin blood product
- Acute, fulminant hepatitis in horses (often broodmares on pasture in the fall) with no known equine-origin blood product administration. This last syndrome can occur as farm outbreaks

SIGNALMENT
Adult horses, particularly those with a history of receiving equine-origin serum (especially tetanus antitoxin) or plasma approximately 4–10 weeks earlier. May also be horses without recent history of equine blood product administration (nonbiologic origin acute hepatitis).

SIGNS
- Usually sudden in onset and rapidly progressive, with death occurring 2–6 days later in some cases
- Horses are often icteric and pass dark urine owing to the presence of bilirubin
- Many have signs of hepatic encephalopathy including acute blindness and aimless wandering around the stall or paddock
- Frequent yawning has been reported. Other neurologic signs may range from mild to severe depression or coma to maniacal behavior or seizures
- Hemolysis and hemoglobinuria may be present, are poor prognostic indicators, and are thought to be the result of damage to the red blood cells passing through the damaged sinusoids, oxidative damage resulting from liver failure, or release of large amounts of copper or iron from the diseased liver
- Some horses may have signs of photosensitivity and abdominal pain

CAUSES AND RISK FACTORS
- Most commonly associated with administration of an equine-origin blood product 4–10 weeks before the onset of signs. Some epidemiologic evidence suggests that some cases may result from an infectious agent
- Currently, there are at least 4 viruses that can establish chronic/persistent infection in

horses and are being studied for their possible association with liver disease. NPHV (also called equine hepacivirus [EHCV]), TDAV, and EPgV are from the family Flaviviridae, genus *Hepacivirus*, which also includes the human hepatitis C virus. The fourth virus, EqPV-H, is in the family Parvoviridae, genus unclassified

DIAGNOSIS

DIFFERENTIAL DIAGNOSIS
- Acute onset of icterus in adult horses has multiple causes—prehepatic, hepatic, or posthepatic; serum biochemistries and CBC assist in differentiating these causes:
  - Prehepatic—red maple or wild onion toxicity, equine infectious anemia, immune-mediated hemolytic anemia poisoning
  - Hepatic—anorexia, Theiler disease, *Clostridium novyi,* bacterial cholangiohepatitis, hepatotoxicity
  - Posthepatic—cholelithiasis and other causes of biliary obstruction
- Signs of HE can be very similar to those of several acute neurologic diseases—rabies, Eastern equine encephalomyelitis, Western equine encephalitis, and acute protozoal myeloencephalitis. Icterus and serum biochemical changes help in differentiating these problems
- Hematuria, hemoglobinuria, myoglobinuria, and bilirubinuria may cause pigmenturia; urinalysis and serum biochemistries aid in differentiation. Urine from horses with hepatic failure will have green-colored bubbles (bilirubinuria) when shaken and this can serve as a useful point-of-care test to differentiate liver failure and HE from other causes of encephalopathy including encephalitides

CBC/BIOCHEMISTRY/URINALYSIS
- CBC—usually normal, a small number of horses may have thrombocytopenia likely associated with disseminated intravascular coagulation
- Biochemistry—typical of acute, severe liver disease predominantly affecting hepatocellular function
- Marked increase in aspartate aminotransferase (often nearly 2000 IU/L; >4000 IU/L seems to be associated with a poor prognosis)
- Marked elevations in SDH and GLDH
- Moderate increases in biliary-derived enzymes (GGT usually increased to 100–300 IU/L). GGT continues to increase during initial recovery due to bile duct hyperplasia and this should not be interpreted as a poor prognostic indicator. GGT may remain elevated, although progressively decreasing values, for ≥2 weeks after clinical recovery

- Both conjugated and unconjugated bilirubin are increased with conjugating often constituting less than 20% of total bilirubin
- Increased anion gap
- Mild hyperglycemia, rarely hypoglycemia
- Urinalysis—bilirubinuria and hemoglobinuria. The latter is a poor prognostic indicator

OTHER LABORATORY TESTS
- Prolongation of prothrombin time and partial thromboplastin time
- Hyperlactatemia
- Hyperammonemia
- Elevated bile acids
- Equine hepatitis virus PCR panel is available for research and informational purposes. Panel includes PCR testing for TDAV, NPHV, EPgV, and EqPV-H. (Note that there is no evidence for EqPeg causing liver disease in horses and testing may not be warranted.) Submit serum, fresh or formalin-fixed paraffin-embedded liver, or equine biologic products to the Cornell University Animal Health Diagnostic Center

IMAGING
Ultrasonography may suggest the liver is smaller and more hypoechoic than normal. May appear otherwise unremarkable.

OTHER DIAGNOSTIC PROCEDURES
Liver biopsy is not indicated in horses with "classic" signs of Theiler disease as histologic data will likely not change therapy.

PATHOLOGIC FINDINGS
- The liver is almost always smaller than normal. In 13 cases of Theiler disease, liver weight in comparison with body weight was 1%. In healthy control horses, liver weight was 1.6% of body weight, suggesting a 40% decrease in hepatic size following disease
- Histologically, affected livers show severe centrilobular or massive liver necrosis/apoptosis with portal areas less severely affected but with a mononuclear cell infiltration and slight to moderate bile duct proliferation, with or without fibrosis. Vasculitis has occasionally been reported. Alzheimer type II astrocytes are present in the brain in virtually all of the cases

TREATMENT
- Goals of therapy are to treat or prevent HE, provide supportive care including IV fluids, nutritional support, and antioxidant, anti-inflammatory, and antibiotic therapies
- Restrict activity, and avoid sunlight
- In cases with HE, house the horse in a quiet place, preferably padded to prevent injury
- Fluid therapy—correct deficits using hypertonic saline (7.5%, 4 mL/kg) or balanced isotonic crystalloid fluid preferably with an acetate rather than a lactate buffer at

20–30 mL/kg for the first hours with 50 g dextrose and 20 mEq KCl added to each liter. Continue at maintenance rate in patients that are not eating and drinking. Multiple B vitamins can be added to the fluids
• Nutritional support—if the horse is still eating, a high-carbohydrate, low-protein diet is recommended. Highly palatable grass hay (fed at approximately 1.5% of body weight per day) along with small amounts of high glycemic feeds at <1.0 g/kg/day should be offered in 4–6 meals per day. The protein should be high in BCAAs. Sorghum or soaked beet pulp have high concentrations of BCAAs. Commercial BCAA pastes can be administered in patients that are not eating

MEDICATIONS
DRUG(S) OF CHOICE
• Control of HE includes decreasing GI-derived neurotoxins (predominantly ammonia), decreasing cerebral edema, correcting glucose, electrolyte, and acid–base abnormalities, and maintaining perfusion and oxygenation to the brain and other vital organs. Ideally, all sedation should be avoided, but to prevent injury detomidine (5–10 μg/kg IV) can be used. If more long-term sedation is required, gabapentin (5–12 mg/kg PO every 12 h) or pregabalin (2–4 mg/kg PO every 12 h) could be considered. Conversely, in horses with profound coma, sarmazenil (0.04 mg/kg IV) or flumazenil (0.01–0.02 mg/kg IV) may be useful GABA receptor antagonists
• Metronidazole (15 mg/kg PO every 12 h), Neomycin (10–20 mg/kg PO every 8 h) and/or lactulose (0.3–0.5 mL/kg PO or per rectum every 8 h) may help reduce ammonia production and absorption from the GI tract
• Anti-inflammatory treatment—pentoxifylline (7.5 mg/kg PO or IV

(compounded) every 8–12 h) to reduce systemic inflammation
• Antimicrobial therapy—bactericidal antibiotic (e.g. ceftiofur) to prevent bacterial translocation from GI tract to blood
• Antioxidant therapy—acetylcysteine by slow IV administration (up to 100 mg/kg) diluted in 5% dextrose. S-adenosyl methionine (10–15 mg/kg PO) to provide antioxidant effect

CONTRAINDICATIONS/POSSIBLE INTERACTIONS
• Neomycin should not be given for more than 24–36 h; it may induce severe diarrhea
• Avoid overly sedating horses with HE as excessive lowering of the head in the standing horse may induce cerebral edema
• Ideally, all oral medications should be given by dose syringe rather than nasogastric tube as nasal bleeding resulting from passage of a stomach tube can result in ingestion of considerable amounts of blood protein, which would likely increase blood ammonia production
• Because the liver metabolizes many drugs, their duration of action may be increased in acute hepatic disease

FOLLOW-UP
PATIENT MONITORING
Monitor liver enzymes and bilirubin every 2–3 days. Maintain adequate serum potassium levels to reduce hyperammonemia.

EXPECTED COURSE AND PROGNOSIS
• Horses with severe HE have a poor prognosis. Horses that continue to eat for 3 days and have supportive treatments may fully recover

• Decline in serum SDH and GLDH after 2–3 days of treatment along with concurrent improvement in clinical signs suggests a favorable prognosis
• There are no proven long-term consequences in horses that recover

MISCELLANEOUS
ABBREVIATIONS
• BCAA = branched-chain amino acid
• EPgV = equine pegivirus
• EqPV-H = equine parvovirus
• GI = gastrointestinal
• GGT = γ-glutamyltransferase
• GLDH = glutamate dehydrogenase
• HE = hepatic encephalopathy
• NPHV = nonprimate hepacivirus
• PCR = polymerase chain reaction
• SDH = sorbitol dehydrogenase (IDH)
• TDAV = Theiler disease-associated virus

Suggested Reading
Chandriani S, Skewes-Cox P, Zhong W, et al. Identification of a previously undescribed divergent virus from the Flaviviridae family in an outbreak of equine serum hepatitis. Proc Natl Acad Sci USA 2013;110(15):E1407–1415.
Divers TJ. The equine liver in health and disease. Proc Am Assoc Equine Pract 2015;61:81–103.

Authors Kathleen R. Mullen and Thomas J. Divers
Consulting Editors Michel Lévy and Heidi Banse
Acknowledgment The authors and editors acknowledge the prior contribution of Christopher M. Brown.

 Client Education Handout available online

A

ACUTE KIDNEY INJURY (AKI) AND ACUTE RENAL FAILURE (ARF)

 BASICS

DEFINITION
Both AKI and ARF are a consequence of an abrupt, sustained decrease in GFR, resulting in azotemia and disturbances in fluid, electrolyte, and acid–base homeostasis. The term AKI has been introduced to increase awareness of subclinical renal damage that may accompany many disease processes.

PATHOPHYSIOLOGY
• Most commonly due to combined hemodynamic and nephrotoxic insults
• Perpetuated by decreased GFR in damaged glomeruli and tubular obstruction with desquamated tubular epithelial cells and debris

SYSTEMS AFFECTED
• Renal/urologic—injury/failure
• Endocrine/metabolic—disturbances in electrolyte and acid–base homeostasis
• GI—inappetence, possible diarrhea, and increased risk of ulcers
• Nervous/neuromuscular—occasional ataxia or encephalopathy in severe cases
• Hemic/lymphatic/immune—altered hemostasis, increased susceptibility to infection
• Musculoskeletal—acute laminitis in severe cases

GENETICS
N/A

INCIDENCE/PREVALENCE
• Low for ARF
• AKI may be a common secondary problem with many disease processes

GEOGRAPHIC DISTRIBUTION
N/A

SIGNALMENT
Breed Predilections
None

Mean Age and Range
Foals <30 days of age (especially when receiving nephrotoxic medications, or affected with hypoxic–ischemic multiorgan damage or septicemia) may be at greater risk, but all ages can be affected.

Predominant Sex
None

SIGNS
Historical Findings
Horse are often presented for concurrent medical problems.

Physical Examination Findings
• Lethargy, anorexia, dehydration, edema, ulcers, or uremic odor in the oral cavity
• Severity of lethargy and anorexia often are greater than would be expected for the primary disease process
• Oliguria/anuria

• Rectal examination may reveal an enlarged, painful left kidney
• Markedly azotemic patients may have neurologic deficits—ataxia, hypermetria, and mental obtundation

CAUSES
• Hemorrhagic, hypovolemic, or endotoxic shock
• Pigmenturia
• Vasculitis
• Disseminated intravascular coagulation
• Use of nephrotoxic medications—aminoglycosides; NSAIDs
• Other nephrotoxins include heavy metals (e.g. mercury [in counterirritants or blisters], lead, cadmium), vitamins D and K3, and high doses of oxytetracycline, especially when administered to neonates
• In occasional cases, infectious agents—*Actinobacillus equuli* in neonates; *Leptospira* spp. in all age groups

RISK FACTORS
• Renal hypoperfusion
• Exposure to nephrotoxins or nephrotoxic drugs, particularly in patients with dehydration
• Colic, diarrhea, pleuritis, peritonitis, prolonged exercise, rhabdomyolysis, hemolysis, or septicemia/endotoxemia

 DIAGNOSIS

DIFFERENTIAL DIAGNOSIS
• Uroperitoneum
• Obstruction of lower urinary tract
• Chronic kidney disease
• Heart failure
• Gastric ulcers

CBC/BIOCHEMISTRY/URINALYSIS
• Normal to high PCV, variable leukogram, CBC changes reflect underlying primary disease process
• AKI may be reflected by minor increases in Cr (0.3 mg/dL or a 50% increase) that often do not exceed the upper limit of the reference range
• ARF is characterized by progressive increases in BUN (50–150 mg/dL; 18–54 mmol/L) and Cr (2.0–20 mg/dL; 177–1768 μmol/L)
• Variable hyponatremia, hypochloremia, hyperkalemia, hypocalcemia, and hyperphosphatemia
• Mild to moderate metabolic acidosis, severity varying with the underlying disease process; development of renal tubular acidosis may complicate recovery
• Mild to moderate hyperglycemia and hyperlactatemia
• Urine specific gravity—may remain high (>1.035) with AKI, low (<1.020) with ARF; best assessed during initial patient evaluation (before rehydration)

• ARF may be accompanied by mild to moderate proteinuria, glucosuria, pigmenturia, and increased RBCs and casts on sediment examination
• Urine pH—normal to acidic, especially with concurrent depletion of body potassium stores
• Myoglobinuria or hemoglobinuria/hematuria

OTHER LABORATORY TESTS
• Increased fractional clearances (i.e. excretions) of sodium and phosphorus; decreased clearance of potassium
• Enzymuria—urinary GGT:Cr ratio >25
• Rising titers to *Leptospira* spp. may be found in horses with ARF attributable to leptospirosis

IMAGING
Transabdominal/Transrectal Ultrasonography
• Kidneys may be enlarged (diameter >8 cm; length >15 cm), with increased echogenicity of renal cortices
• Rarely subcapsular/perirenal edema or hemorrhage
• Variable dilation of renal pelves
• Nephrolithiasis/ureterolithiasis would indicate underlying chronic kidney disease and possible "acute-on-chronic" exacerbation of renal failure

OTHER DIAGNOSTIC PROCEDURES
• Percutaneous renal biopsy with routine histopathologic, immunohistochemical, and electron microscopic evaluation of the sample may provide information regarding cause, severity, and prognosis. Proceed with caution, however, because life-threatening hemorrhage can be a complication
• CVP >8–10 mmHg indicates fluid overload

PATHOLOGIC FINDINGS
• Gross—enlargement of kidneys due to nephrosis and subcapsular and interstitial edema, causing tissue to bulge onto cut surfaces
• Histopathologic—glomeruli may be congested and have a cellular infiltrate; tubules have denuded or flattened epithelium and varying amounts of accumulated eosinophilic debris

 TREATMENT

APPROPRIATE HEALTH CARE
Properly recognize and treat all underlying primary disease processes, usually on an inpatient basis for continuous fluid therapy.

NURSING CARE
Fluid Therapy
• After initial measurement of body weight, judiciously correct estimated dehydration with normal (0.9%) saline or another potassium-poor electrolyte solution over 12–24 h

• Avoid overzealous fluid replacement (more than twice maintenance rate) unless a higher fluid administration rate is needed for primary disease process
• Fluids may be supplemented with calcium gluconate or sodium bicarbonate if hyperkalemia or acidosis requires specific correction
• Additional fluid replacement is no longer necessary once appetite and drinking return to normal (i.e. there is no benefit to continuing fluid therapy until Cr returns to a normal value)

Oral Electrolyte Supplementation
• Sodium chloride (30 g) can be administered in concentrate feed or as an oral slurry/paste every 6–12 h to encourage increased drinking and urine output
• Potassium chloride can be supplemented in nonhyperkalemic patients with total body potassium depletion—common with anorexia of ≥ 2 days

ACTIVITY
Stall rest, with limited hand-walking or small paddock for grazing grass if appetite is poor.

DIET
Encourage intake by offering a variety of concentrate feeds, bran mash, and hay types.

CLIENT EDUCATION
None

SURGICAL CONSIDERATIONS
N/A

MEDICATIONS
DRUG(S) OF CHOICE
• Judicious fluid therapy is the mainstay of treatment—see Nursing Care
• Furosemide—for oliguria/anuria (i.e. lack of urination during first 6 h of fluid therapy or urine output <0.5 mL/kg/h); this diuretic may be administered twice (1–2 mg/kg IV or IM) at 1 h intervals; if effective, urination should be observed within 1 h after the second dose; if ineffective, consider a furosemide constant rate infusion; if ineffective, discontinue treatment
• *Routine use of mannitol and dopamine in patients with ARF is no longer recommended*

CONTRAINDICATIONS
Avoid all nephrotoxic medications—gentamicin, tetracyclines, and NSAIDs.

PRECAUTIONS
• As little as 40 mL/kg of IV fluids (20 L per 500 kg horse) may produce increases in CVP and significant pulmonary edema in oliguric/anuric patients
• Furosemide—at repeated dosages can result in electrolyte derangements
• Reassess dosage schedule of drugs eliminated by urinary excretion

POSSIBLE INTERACTIONS
N/A

ALTERNATIVE DRUGS
Consider peritoneal dialysis or hemodialysis (foals only) in refractory cases.

FOLLOW-UP
PATIENT MONITORING
• Assess clinical status (emphasizing hydration), urine output, and body weight at least twice daily during the initial 24 h of treatment and at least daily thereafter
• Monitor for subcutaneous and pulmonary edema—increased respiratory rate and effort as evidence of overhydration
• Assess azotemia and electrolyte and acid–basis status at least daily for the initial 3 days of treatment
• Consider placing a central venous line to maintain CVP <8 cmH$_2$O in more critical patients and neonates

PREVENTION/AVOIDANCE
• Anticipate compromised renal function in patients with other diseases or undergoing prolonged anesthesia and surgery; institute appropriate treatment to minimize dehydration and potential renal damage
• Ensure adequate hydration status in patients receiving nephrotoxic medications, especially when combined (i.e. aminoglycosides and NSAIDs or tetracyclines)
• Avoid concurrent use of multiple anti-inflammatory drugs—NSAIDs

POSSIBLE COMPLICATIONS
• Pulmonary and peripheral edema; conjunctival edema may be dramatic
• Severe hyperkalemia accompanied by cardiac arrhythmias and death
• Laminitis—often rapidly progressive and refractory to supportive care
• Signs of neurologic impairment—ataxia; mental obtundation
• GI ulceration or bleeding
• Coagulopathy
• Sepsis

EXPECTED COURSE AND PROGNOSIS
• Prognosis for recovery varies with the underlying primary disease process
• ARF may complicate recovery, prolong hospitalization and treatment, and increase cost
• Prognosis for recovery from AKI/ARF usually is favorable if azotemia decreases by 25–50% after the initial 24 h of treatment; extent of recovery of renal function in patients with ARF may require 3–6 weeks to fully assess
• Guarded prognosis for patients with Cr >10 mg/dL at initial evaluation and when azotemia remains unchanged after the initial 24 h of treatment

• Poor prognosis for patients that have persistent anuria (>24 h), that have increased magnitude of azotemia after the initial 24 h of treatment, that rapidly develop edema, or that remain oliguric >72 h

MISCELLANEOUS
ASSOCIATED CONDITIONS
N/A

AGE-RELATED FACTORS
Neonates, especially premature or dysmature foals, may have markedly elevated Cr concentrations (approaching 25 mg/dL) due to placental insufficiency; this azotemia typically resolves in 2–3 days and should not be confused with ARF or uroperitoneum.

ZOONOTIC POTENTIAL
Leptospirosis has infectious and zoonotic potential; avoid direct contact with infective urine.

PREGNANCY/FERTILITY/BREEDING
N/A

SYNONYMS
• Acute nephrosis
• Acute tubular necrosis
• Vasomotor nephropathy

SEE ALSO
• Anuria/oliguria
• Chronic kidney disease (CKD)
• Pigmenturia (hematuria, hemoglobinuria, and myoglobinuria)

ABBREVIATIONS
• AKI = acute kidney injury
• ARF = acute renal failure
• BUN = blood urea nitrogen
• Cr = creatinine
• CVP = central venous pressure
• GFR = glomerular filtration rate
• GGT = γ-glutamyltransferase
• GI = gastrointestinal
• NSAID = nonsteroidal anti-inflammatory drug
• PCV = packed cell volume
• RBC = red blood cell

Suggested Reading
McLeland S. Diseases of the equine urinary system. Vet Clin NA: Equine Pract 2015;31(2):377–387.
Tyner GA, Nolen-Walston RD, Hall T, et al. A multicenter retrospective study of 151 renal biopsies in horses. J Vet Intern Med 2011;25:532–539.

Author Harold C. Schott II
Consulting Editor Valérie Picandet

A

ACUTE-PHASE RESPONSE

BASICS

OVERVIEW
• The APR is a highly conserved, nonspecific, innate response to damage- or danger-associated signals. APR enhances the body's response to infection and/or inflammation and aids in the restoration of homeostasis
• The physiology of the APR:
  ○ Activation of inflammatory response initiated by innate recognition of DAMPs (DNA, etc.) and/or PAMPs (endotoxin, lipoteichoic acids, etc.) by pattern recognition receptors
    ▪ May also occur secondary to physiologic stress and neural inputs
  ○ Inflammatory activation results in increased production of proinflammatory mediators, particularly cytokines such as IL-6, IL-1, and tumor necrosis factor
  ○ IL-6 is primarily responsible for altering the hepatic production of APPs, resulting in:
    ▪ Increased production of positive APPs (FIB, SAA, CRP, Hp, ceruloplasmin, hepcidin, α_1-antitrypsin, etc.)
    ▪ Decreased production of negative APPs (albumin, transferrin)
  ○ Extrahepatic production of some APPs may occur (SAA, Hp)
• APPs have numerous roles in the response to infection or injury:
  ○ Minimize ongoing tissue damage, interfere with the growth and reproduction of pathogenic organisms, facilitate wound repair and tissue healing, enhance phagocytosis
• APPs are divided into 3 groups:
  ○ Major APPs have very low plasma concentrations in normal animals and increase more than 100-fold during APR (SAA)
  ○ Moderate APPs are present at measurable levels in normal animals but increase 5–10-fold during APR (Hp)
  ○ Minor APPs increase gradually to ~2 × resting concentrations (FIB)
• Substantial interest exists in the utility of APPs as indicators of occult infection, injury, or inflammation
  ○ Monitoring APPs over time may aid in assessing response to treatment
  ○ APPs may have utility as prognostic markers in a number of diseases or conditions

SIGNALMENT
• No specific signalment, as this is an innate response that occurs in any individual at any stage of the life cycle
• Monitoring the APR may have utility in monitoring disease status and response to treatment, or in a herd situation by enabling the early identification of individuals with an occult inflammatory stimulus

SIGNS
• Activation of APR may be accompanied by physical changes consistent with systemic inflammation (fever, decreased appetite, lethargy, depression, and cachexia)
• Other signs are typically referable to the primary disease process, rather than the APR itself

CAUSES AND RISK FACTORS
Based upon the primary disease process.

DIAGNOSIS

DIFFERENTIAL DIAGNOSIS
• Because the APR is nonspecific it may be difficult to differentiate between initiating pathologies
• The pattern of the response may be the same regardless of initiating stimulus

CBC/BIOCHEMISTRY/URINALYSIS
• CBC changes in association with the APR include leukocytosis and anemia of inflammation
• Biochemistry changes include decreases in serum albumin, calcium, and iron concentrations

OTHER LABORATORY TESTS
Abnormalities of coagulation may be present.

IMAGING
N/A

OTHER DIAGNOSTIC PROCEDURES
• Increased APPs should initiate an investigation aimed at identifying the underlying etiology
• The failure of one or more APPs to decline over time may indicate the need for patient reevaluation
• Increasing APPs during treatment may indicate worsening of the patient's condition, requiring reevaluation of the patient

TREATMENT

Treatment should be directed towards resolution of the primary disease process and controlling the inflammatory response.

MEDICATIONS

DRUG(S) OF CHOICE
No specific treatment.

CONTRAINDICATIONS/POSSIBLE INTERACTIONS
N/A

FOLLOW-UP

PATIENT MONITORING
• Serial monitoring of APPs such as FIB, SAA, and Hp has demonstrated utility in detecting occult disease conditions and monitoring the response to treatment
• APR has proven less useful in prognostication

PREVENTION/AVOIDANCE
N/A

POSSIBLE COMPLICATIONS
N/A

EXPECTED COURSE AND PROGNOSIS
• Increased positive APP levels are expected while the primary inflammatory stimulus is present
• The rate at which APP levels return to normal is variable, with major APPs such as SAA decreasing rapidly and minor APPs such as FIB returning more slowly to normal

MISCELLANEOUS

SEE ALSO
Anemia, chronic disease

ABBREVIATIONS
• APP = acute phase protein
• APR = acute phase response
• CRP = C-reactive protein
• DAMP = damage-associated molecular pattern
• FIB = fibrinogen
• Hp = haptoglobin
• IL = interleukin
• PAMP = pathogen-associated molecular pattern
• SAA = serum amyloid A

Suggested Reading
Crisman MV, Scarratt WK, Zimmerman KL. Blood proteins and inflammation in the horse. Vet Clin North Am Equine Pract 2008;24:285–297, vi.
Schrödl W, Buchler R, Wendler S, et al. Acute phase proteins as promising biomarkers: perspectives and limitations for human and veterinary medicine. Proteomics Clin Appl 2016;10(11):1077–1092.
Author Harold C. McKenzie
Consulting Editors David Hodgson, Harold C. McKenzie, and Jennifer L. Hodgson

BASICS

OVERVIEW
• Fatal respiratory disease in Arabian foals with SCID
• May be a severe pathogen in Fell Pony foals affected by "Fell Pony syndrome"
• Other breeds may be affected as foals, but seldom succumb
• Approximately 25% of affected foals also have diarrhea
• A role for adenovirus in adult respiratory disease has been suggested

SIGNALMENT
• Usually older than 8–10 weeks when clinical signs become present unless FTPI is present
• Primarily Arabians; other breeds affected sporadically (Fell Ponies)
• SCID-affected foals are frequently clinically normal at birth

SIGNS
• Identical to other causes of foal pneumonia—fever, tachypnea, dyspnea, depression, and abnormalities on thoracic auscultation
• Mild to moderate diarrhea may also be present (EAdV-2 strains)

CAUSES AND RISK FACTORS
• Foals with SCID have a defect in lymphoid stem cells that may result from altered purine metabolism. The absence of an adaptive immune response causes these foals to be susceptible to even minor pathogens, such as adenovirus
• Owing to maternally derived immunity reaching a nadir at 1–2 months of age, these foals become unable to mount an appropriate immune response and deteriorate
• Foals that are immunosuppressed for other reasons, such as Fell Pony syndrome
• Adenovirus (EAdV-1) may predispose foals to bacterial pneumonia and may play a significant role in the pathogenesis of bacterial pneumonia in non-SCID foals
• Antigenically distinct adenovirus, EAdV-2, has been identified in non-SCID foals with diarrhea, usually associated with concurrent rotavirus infection. The role of EAdV-2 in foal diarrhea is not clear

DIAGNOSIS

DIFFERENTIAL DIAGNOSIS
Other viral and bacterial causes of pneumonia in immunocompromised foals:

• Equine herpesvirus type 1
• Equine influenza virus
• Equine arteritis virus
• *Streptococcus equi* var. *zooepidemicus*
• *Actinobacillus equuli*
• *Pasteurella* spp.
• *Klebsiella pneumoniae*
• *Salmonella* spp.
• *Bordetella bronchiseptica*
• *Rhodococcus equi*
• Other causes of diarrhea in foals—bacterial, viral, and parasitic

CBC/BIOCHEMISTRY/URINALYSIS
Antemortem diagnosis of SCID is supported by finding appropriate clinical signs in an Arabian foal of the appropriate age with persistent severe lymphopenia (≤500 cells/µL) and the absence of IgM on SRID (see Other Laboratory Tests).

OTHER LABORATORY TESTS
• Antibody titers—SCID foals do not demonstrate a 4-fold rise; non-SCID-affected foals develop a rise in 10 days
• Virus isolation/PCR—may be isolated/identified from normal and infected foals
• Histopathology—intranuclear inclusions can be detected in tissues. Antemortem—may demonstrate intranuclear inclusions in conjunctival and nasal epithelial cells. Postmortem—gross and histologic evidence of lymphoid hypoplasia of the thymus, spleen, and lymph nodes
• SRID—precolostral testing of SCID foals demonstrates an absence of IgM, but, as IgM is absorbed by the foal from colostrum, foals with adequate transfer of maternal antibody cannot be tested until IgM levels have waned, usually at ≥3 weeks of age
• Fell Pony syndrome—measurement of IgM after 4 weeks of age (concentration will be decreased) and demonstration of B-cell lymphopenia

IMAGING
• Radiographs—pneumonia
• Ultrasonography—lymphoid tissues may be suggestive of, but not diagnostic for, SCID

TREATMENT
• No specific treatment
• Non-SCID foals—supportive, with broad-spectrum antibiotics
• SCID and Fell Pony foals—treatment is not productive. Experimental treatment in SCID foals with bone marrow stem cell transplants

MEDICATIONS

DRUG(S) OF CHOICE
• Non-SCID foals—treat concurrent bacterial infection based on culture and sensitivity
• Foals with adenovirus associated with rotavirus—supportive therapy

CONTRAINDICATIONS/POSSIBLE INTERACTIONS
N/A

FOLLOW-UP

CLIENT EDUCATION
• SCID prevention—genetic testing for identification of carriers and removal from breeding programs
• Approximately 1 of 4 foals from the mating of 2 heterozygotes results in a SCID foal
• Arabian foals from parents of unknown SCID status—test at birth for IgM levels (presuckle) and lymphocyte count
• Fell Pony syndrome—recommendations not yet established. Future availability of testing for mutation in the sodium/myoinositol cotransporter gene possible

MISCELLANEOUS

ABBREVIATIONS
• EAdV = equine adenovirus type
• FTPI = failure of transfer of passive immunity
• Ig = immunoglobulin
• PCR = polymerase chain reaction
• SCID = severe combined immunodeficiency syndrome
• SRID = serial radial immunodiffusion

Suggested Reading
Fox-Clipsham LY, Carter SD, Goodhead I, et al. Identification of a mutation associated with fatal foal immunodeficiency syndrome in the Fell and Dales pony. PLoS Genet 2011;7:e1002133.
Thomas GW, Bell SC, Carter SD. Immunoglobulin and peripheral B-lymphocyte concentrations in Fell Pony foal syndrome. Equine Vet J 2005;37:48–52.

Author Pamela A. Wilkins
Consulting Editor Ashley G. Boyle

A

ADRENAL INSUFFICIENCY

BASICS

OVERVIEW
- Synonymous with hypoadrenocorticism and "adrenal exhaustion"
- Characterized by glucocorticoid (i.e. cortisol) and/or mineralocorticoid (i.e. aldosterone) deficiency caused by adrenal cortex destruction (primary AI), ACTH deficiency (secondary AI), or suppression of the HPA axis by exogenous steroid or ACTH administration
- May be permanent, complete AI ("Addison disease," rare), or transient, "relative" AI secondary to concurrent critical illness (RAI/CIRCI)

Systems Affected
- Endocrine
- Cardiovascular
- Renal
- Musculoskeletal
- Gastrointestinal
- Behavioral
- Immune

SIGNALMENT
Any age, sex, and breed. RAI/CIRCI is most common in neonatal foals, especially premature foals.

SIGNS
- Acute RAI/CIRCI—signs of septic shock, including fever or hypothermia, hyperemic mucous membranes, weakness, hypotension, hemoconcentration, cardiovascular collapse, and death
- Chronic cases—depression, anorexia, weight loss, poor hair coat, exercise intolerance, polyuria/polydipsia, mild abdominal pain, salt craving, and diarrhea

CAUSES AND RISK FACTORS
- Chronic administration of glucocorticoids, exogenous ACTH, or anabolic steroids
- HPA axis immaturity attributable to prematurity in neonatal foals
- HPA axis suppression and/or adrenal hemorrhage and necrosis subsequent to systemic inflammatory response or sepsis/septic shock

DIAGNOSIS

DIFFERENTIAL DIAGNOSIS
Renal failure, colitis, primary cardiovascular disease.

CBC/BIOCHEMISTRY/URINALYSIS
- Acute RAI/CIRCI—hemoconcentration, leukopenia (neutropenia), and hypoglycemia. If mineralocorticoid secretion is also affected, hyponatremia, hypochloremia, hyperkalemia, and decreased sodium–potassium ratio (reference range >27) may be seen, but this is uncommon

- Chronic cases—mineralocorticoid secretion is generally maintained, so serum electrolytes are usually within normal limits

OTHER LABORATORY TESTS
- Measure baseline plasma ACTH and cortisol concentrations. AI should be considered in ill or stressed animals with ACTH and cortisol concentrations below reference intervals, though this is not a sensitive test for AI
- ACTH stimulation testing—administer synthetic ACTH (1 μg/kg IV or IM, 100 μg IV for a neonatal foal). Measure serum cortisol before and 90–120 min after ACTH. An increase <2–4-fold is consistent with AI
- With insufficient aldosterone secretion, fractional excretion of sodium (reference range <1%) is increased despite a normal or low serum sodium concentration

IMAGING
N/A

OTHER DIAGNOSTIC PROCEDURES
N/A

TREATMENT

- Complete rest and avoidance of stress, particularly surgery, infection, and trauma
- Fluid, dextrose, and electrolyte support
- Treat the underlying primary cause
- If mineralocorticoid insufficiency, provide sodium supplementation (e.g. salt) and avoid potassium supplementation

MEDICATIONS

DRUG(S) OF CHOICE
- Glucocorticoid and, if necessary, mineralocorticoid replacement at physiologic doses equivalent to daily corticosteroid production rates
- For acute RAI/CIRCI in foals, low-dose hydrocortisone (1.3 mg/kg/day IV divided every 4–6 h) is recommended. This dose may also be effective in adult horses with RAI/CIRCI and acute AI, though it has not been well studied to date
- Avoid long-term or high-dose steroid supplementation as this can prolong HPA axis suppression. In acute RAI/CIRCI, a tapering course of hydrocortisone over 3–7 days is recommended
- For longer term therapy in adult horses with chronic AI, the maintenance dose of prednisolone is approximately 25 mg/day. However, exposure to stress dramatically increases corticosteroid requirements. During periods of stress, increase the dose by 2–10-fold and divide into 2 or 3 daily doses
- Mineralocorticoid replacement with fludrocortisone may be considered

CONTRAINDICATIONS/POSSIBLE INTERACTIONS
N/A

FOLLOW-UP

PATIENT MONITORING
- Monitor electrolytes, renal function, acid–base balance, blood glucose, and blood pressure
- Once the animal is stable, HPA axis recovery can be documented by repeating ACTH stimulation test

PREVENTION/AVOIDANCE
Avoid excessive use of exogenous glucocorticoids, ACTH, and anabolic steroids.

POSSIBLE COMPLICATIONS
Excessive glucocorticoid administration, especially with long-acting forms (e.g. triamcinolone), increases susceptibility to infections and may induce insulin dysregulation, which could increase the risk of laminitis.

EXPECTED COURSE AND PROGNOSIS
N/A

MISCELLANEOUS

ASSOCIATED CONDITIONS
N/A

AGE-RELATED FACTORS
N/A

ZOONOTIC POTENTIAL
N/A

PREGNANCY/FERTILITY/BREEDING
N/A

ABBREVIATIONS
- AI = adrenal insufficiency
- ACTH = adrenocorticotropin hormone
- CIRCI = critical illness-related corticosteroid insufficiency
- HPA = hypothalamic–pituitary–adrenal
- RAI = relative adrenal insufficiency

Suggested Reading
Hart KA. Adrenal glands. In: Smith BP, ed. Large Animal Internal Medicine, 5e. St. Louis, MO: Elsevier Mosby, 2015:1228–1233.

Author Kelsey A. Hart
Consulting Editor Michel Lévy and Heidi Banse
Acknowledgment The author and editors acknowledge the prior contribution of Laurent Couëtil.

 Client Education Handout available online

BASICS

OVERVIEW
- Intoxication by aflatoxins
- Diffuse liver disease is its hallmark with acute and chronic forms dictated by dose and duration of exposure
- Ingestion of aflatoxin-contaminated cereal grains, especially corn. Cereal-based pelleted feed can also be a source
- Drought conditions favor aflatoxin production on grains. Aflatoxin production by contaminating fungi is more likely in warm (>25°C) and humid (97–99% relative humidity) conditions
- Outbreaks of aflatoxicosis in horses are rarely reported and have been linked to the ingestion of aflatoxin-contaminated feed in the range of 58.4–200 μg/kg

SIGNALMENT
Younger horses are more susceptible.

SIGNS
- Clinical signs of aflatoxicosis in horses are principally referable to hepatocellular necrosis and may include inappetence, lethargy, fever, jaundice, weakness, weight loss, reduced growth, tremors, ataxia, and even death
- Experimental ponies given single lethal doses of aflatoxin (2 mg/kg) developed fever, elevated heart and respiratory rates, tenesmus, bloody feces, and tetanic convulsions with death occurring 3–32 days after dosing. Ponies administered high oral doses of aflatoxin (400 μg/kg for 5 days) were lethargic, anorectic, and slightly icteric on the 5th day. Signs of hepatic encephalopathy occur when blood ammonia levels are sufficiently elevated
- Chronic low-level exposure may present as an ill-defined loss of condition or mild diarrhea

CAUSES AND RISK FACTORS
The most likely contaminated diets are corn-based, while less likely exposure comes from diets containing peanut and cottonseed meals.

DIAGNOSIS

- Signs and lesions of aflatoxicosis reflect liver disease. None are pathognomonic for either acute or chronic aflatoxin poisoning
- Diagnosis of aflatoxicosis is supported by laboratory demonstration of aflatoxin concentrations in feed
- Demonstration of aflatoxins in liver (postmortem) or stomach contents may also be supportive of the diagnosis
- Hepatic biopsy—evidence of centrilobular necrosis in acute cases; periportal fibrosis, biliary hyperplasia, and Kupffer cell hemosiderosis may be evident in chronic cases
- Overt liver failure is a rare manifestation of aflatoxicosis in horses
- Elevated serum liver enzymes

DIFFERENTIAL DIAGNOSIS
Any causes of liver diseases.

CBC/BIOCHEMISTRY/URINALYSIS
- White blood cell counts, especially lymphocytes, are decreased and blood glucose may be decreased. Total serum/plasma lipid and cholesterol concentrations may be elevated
- Elevations of prothrombin time, serum/plasma aspartate aminotransferase, alkaline phosphatase, γ-glutamyltransferase, and bile acids are consistent with the severe liver necrosis and biliary hyperplasia seen postmortem

OTHER LABORATORY TESTS
- Chemical analysis of feed samples is necessary to confirm the presence of aflatoxin. The inability to obtain samples contemporary with the time of exposure might preclude detection of aflatoxin levels consistent with chronic intoxication
- Feed concentrations of aflatoxin necessary to induce acute intoxication typically exceed the FDA cut-off for safe aflatoxin levels (>20 μg/kg) in feed intended for horses
- Chemical analysis of gastric contents and tissues (postmortem) for aflatoxins may help support the diagnosis

IMAGING
Ultrasonographic images of aflatoxin-affected hepatic parenchyma have not been reported. Logically, generalized parenchymal hyperechogenicity might be identified in chronic cases (consequence of fibrosis).

OTHER DIAGNOSTIC PROCEDURES
- Necropsy findings include fatty liver, hemorrhagic enteritis, and pale swollen kidneys
- Histologic changes in the liver include fatty degeneration, centrilobular necrosis, periportal fibrosis, and bile duct hyperplasia

TREATMENT
Specific antidotes are unavailable. Removal of aflatoxin-contaminated feed should be undertaken. Symptomatic and supportive treatment for hepatic disease should be undertaken (Carlson 2015).

MEDICATIONS

DRUG(S) AND FLUIDS
Dextrose 5% should be given slowly IV to hypoglycemic animals. Balanced electrolyte solutions are given for maintenance.

CONTRAINDICATIONS/POSSIBLE INTERACTIONS
Drugs subject to hepatic clearance should be given cautiously.

FOLLOW-UP

PATIENT MONITORING
Liver enzymes should be monitored to evaluate liver status.

PREVENTION/AVOIDANCE
Test grain/feeds before feeding.

EXPECTED COURSE AND PROGNOSIS
Survival of acute intoxication does not guarantee complete recovery. Ponies have died from liver failure up to 30 days following a single toxic dose of aflatoxin.

MISCELLANEOUS

ABBREVIATIONS
FDA = United States Food and Drug Administration

Suggested Reading
Caloni F, Cortinovis C. Toxicological effects of aflatoxins in horses. Vet J 2011;188(3):270–273.
Carlson KL. Hepatic diseases in the horse. In: Sprayberry KA, Robinson NE, eds. Robinson's Current Therapy in Equine Medicine, 7e. St. Louis, MO: WB Saunders, 2015:287–293.

Authors Stan W. Casteel and Philip J. Johnson
Consulting Editors Wilson K. Rumbeiha and Steve Ensley

A

AFRICAN HORSE SICKNESS

BASICS

OVERVIEW
- Infectious disease affecting the cardiovascular and respiratory systems, characterized by fever and edema
- Not reported in the USA. Most commonly found on the African continent, with recent outbreaks investigated in South Africa, Zimbabwe, and Mozambique. India, Turkey, Iraq, Syria, Lebanon, Jordan, and Spain have reported outbreaks in the past
- Geographic range of the disease is limited by that of its principal vector, *Culicoides* spp. The disease is most prevalent in low-lying, moist, warm areas

SIGNALMENT
- All breeds of horses as well as other equids, such as donkeys and mules. Donkeys and zebras are more resistant than horses and infections may be subclinical
- There is no apparent breed, age, or sex predilection
- Dogs fed uncooked infected horse meat have developed AHS

SIGNS
- Fever (but not accompanied by inappetence)
- Pulmonary edema with coughing, frothy nasal discharge, dyspnea
- Subcutaneous edema of head and neck, edema of supraorbital fossa
- Colic

CAUSES AND RISK FACTORS
- Caused by the AHS virus, a viscerotropic RNA virus of the genus *Orbivirus*
- Transmitted by arthropod vectors, primarily *Culicoides* spp., but also mosquitos and ticks,
- Not transmitted with direct contact between equids
- Spread of the disease to uninfected countries can occur through travel of infected horses or movement of infected insect vectors in aircraft or heavy wind
- Virus affects vascular endothelium, resulting in the clinical sign of edema that predominates
- Disease occurs seasonally, during warm wet periods

DIAGNOSIS

DIFFERENTIAL DIAGNOSIS
- Equine infectious anemia, equine viral arteritis, purpura haemorrhagica, equine anaplasmosis, and equine piroplasmosis may have similar clinical presentation to AHS and may require laboratory testing to differentiate it
- Index of suspicion for AHS should be raised when there is a history of travel to countries known to harbor the disease
- Congestive heart failure may result in pulmonary and subcutaneous edema, but heart murmurs and/or venous distention should be present, and fever may not be present

CBC/BIOCHEMISTRY/URINALYSIS
N/A

OTHER LABORATORY TESTS
- Definitive diagnosis depends on identification of virus by PCR or virus isolation from whole blood or tissues (spleen, lung, lymph node), or antibodies to AHS virus in serum
- In the USA, if AHS is suspected, the federal area veterinarian in charge should be notified immediately so that appropriate samples can be forwarded for testing

IMAGING
- Thoracic radiography may reveal evidence of pulmonary edema
- Thoracic ultrasonography may reveal pleural effusion or pericardial effusion

PATHOLOGIC FINDINGS
- Pulmonary edema, with frothy fluid in the bronchi and trachea
- Pleural effusion
- Pericardial effusion
- Yellow gelatinous edema fluid in the musculature of the neck and jugular groove
- Petechial hemorrhages on endocardium, epicardium, and oral mucous membranes and tongue

TREATMENT

There is no specific treatment for AHS. Supportive nursing care and symptomatic treatment may improve outcome in some cases, but usually the course of the disease is not altered by treatment.

MEDICATIONS

DRUG(S) OF CHOICE
N/A

CONTRAINDICATIONS/POSSIBLE INTERACTIONS
N/A

FOLLOW-UP

PREVENTION/AVOIDANCE
- Vaccination is effective. However, nine serotypes of the virus exist, and vaccination with one strain does not result in immunity to heterologous strains, so polyvalent strains of vaccine should be used
- Vaccination should be combined with other measures aimed at limiting exposure to insect vectors, such as fly-proof stabling, pasturing only during daylight, use of insect repellents, and keeping horses on high ground away from low-lying, swampy, insect-infested areas
- Countries free of the disease restrict importation of horses from countries known to harbor the disease, or impose quarantine of at least 60 days in insect-proof housing. Zebras and donkeys, because of inapparent infection, are particularly dangerous

EXPECTED COURSE AND PROGNOSIS
- Mortality in horses generally is high, up to 90%. In mules and donkeys, mortality may be lower (50%)
- The incubation period ranges from 7 to 14 days. Once clinical signs are observed, the clinical progression is rapid. Death usually occurs within 4–5 days after the onset of fever
- Survivors do not harbor the virus. Survivors have life-long immunity to the homologous strain

MISCELLANEOUS

ZOONOTIC POTENTIAL
The disease does not affect humans.

ABBREVIATIONS
- AHS = African horse sickness
- PCR = polymerase chain reaction

Suggested Reading
Committee on Foreign and Emerging Diseases of the US Animal Health Association. Foreign Animal Diseases, 7e ("The Gray Book," online). Boca Raton, FL: Boca Publications Group Inc., 2008:103. https://www.aphis.usda.gov/emergency_response/downloads/nahems/fad.pdf
OIE—World Organisation for Animal Health. Information on aquatic and terrestrial animal diseases. http://www.oie.int/en/animal-health-in-the-world/animal-diseases

Author Raymond W. Sweeney
Consulting Editor Ashley G. Boyle

BASICS

DEFINITION
- Agalactia—failure of the mammary gland to secrete colostrum or milk after foaling
- Hypogalactia—also referred to as dysgalactia is subnormal milk production

PATHOPHYSIOLOGY
- Estrogens (equilin, equilenin, and estradiol-17β from the fetoplacental unit) in late gestation induce mammary duct development
- Progestagen (5β-pregnane) stimulates lobuloalveolar growth
- Lactogenesis is triggered by a decrease of progestagen and increase of prolactin in the last few days of pregnancy
- After initiation of lactation, prolactin is not required for maintenance
- Colostrogenesis is initiated a few days prior to parturition. Lactation peaks 30–60 days postpartum
- Milk production is 2.5–4% of body weight and requires nutritional demands of the dam are met
- Agalactia/hypogalactia may be caused by alterations of hormonal events (low prolactin level), defects in the mammary tissue itself (mammary disease), poor nutritional status, or presence of systemic illness or disease

SYSTEMS AFFECTED
- Reproductive
- Endocrine/metabolic

GENETICS
Milk production is likely determined by genetics.

INCIDENCE/PREVALENCE
Agalactia or dysgalactia is commonly seen in equine practice when predisposing factors are present.

GEOGRAPHIC DISTRIBUTION
- Fescue toxicosis—tall fescue infected by the fungus *Neotyphodium coenophialum* in central and southeast USA
- Black oat infected by *Claviceps purpurea* in Brazil
- Rye grass infected by *Neotyphodium lolii* in Argentina

SIGNALMENT
Mares of any breed or age may be affected.

SIGNS

Historical Findings
- Grazing endophyte-infected tall fescue or ergot-infected feeds prepartum
- Prolonged gestation, history of placentitis, dystocia, thickened fetal membranes, retained fetal membranes, and *red bag* (premature placental separation)
- Previous history—agalactia/hypogalactia or mammary gland disease

- Clinical evidence of systemic disease; known exposure to infectious disease

Physical Examination Findings
- Weak, septicemic foal—FTPI and/or inadequate nutrition
- Flaccid udder and secretion of a clear or thick, yellow-tinged fluid from the teats
- Mastitis—swollen, painful udder, warm to the touch, secretion of grossly or microscopically abnormal milk
- Distinct, palpable masses with mammary abscessation or neoplasia

CAUSES

Endocrinologic Disorders
- Ergot alkaloids (fescue toxicosis) depress prolactin secretion (dopamine DA_2 receptor agonists and serotonin antagonists)
- Abortion/premature birth affects normal progesterone, estrogen, and prolactin fluctuations necessary for lactation onset

Mammary Gland Disease
- Inflammation and/or infection
- Abscessation or fibrosis
- Neoplasia
- Trauma

Systemic Disease
- Any debilitating systemic disease or stress-producing disorder
- Malnutrition/nutritional deficiency

Others
- Poor nutrition
- Obesity

DIAGNOSIS

DIFFERENTIAL DIAGNOSIS

Differentiating Similar Signs
- Differentiate agalactia/hypogalactia from behavioral nursing problems:
  - Mare anxiety, pain, udder edema
  - Direct examination of udder and secretions
  - Observe interaction between mare and foal as its attempts to nurse
- Failure of milk letdown can occur in mares:
  - Oxytocin stimulates milk letdown, *not* milk secretion

DIFFERENTIATING CAUSES
- Indicators of fescue syndrome:
  - History of fescue ingestion
  - Prolonged gestation
  - Dystocia
  - Retained fetal membranes, thickened fetal membranes
  - Weak, dysmature foal; mare with agalactia
- Full physical examination to differentiate mastitis, mammary fibrosis, neoplasia, abscessation, traumatic injury, systemic illness

OTHER LABORATORY TESTS
Serum prolactin levels are decreased in fescue-induced agalactia.

OTHER DIAGNOSTIC PROCEDURES
- If mastitis is suspected
  - Cytology or culture of udder secretion
- If neoplasia is suspected
  - Fine needle aspirate—cytology
  - Biopsy—histopathology

TREATMENT

APPROPRIATE HEALTH CARE
- Promote lactation using selective D_2 dopamine receptor antagonists
- Mastitis
  - Local or systemic antibiotics based on culture/sensitivity
  - Frequent stripping of mammary gland
  - Heat packs or hydrotherapy
  - Correct nutritional deficiencies

NURSING CARE
- Foals at risk of FTPI need oral administration of colostrum from another mare
- Foals with FTPI need supportive treatment and IV administration of hyperimmune plasma

ACTIVITY
N/A

DIET
Supplementation of mare feed to meet lactation demand.

CLIENT EDUCATION
- Management of mares at risk of agalactia (remove from infected pastures)
- Close monitoring of periparturient mares for mammary gland development or overt edema
- Test colostrum quality upon parturition
- Observe foal nursing behavior

SURGICAL CONSIDERATIONS
N/A

MEDICATIONS

DRUG(S) OF CHOICE FOR FESCUE TOXICITY
- Domperidone (1.1 mg/kg PO daily)
  - Selective DA_2 dopamine receptor antagonist; reverses effects of fescue ingestion
  - Treat for minimum of 15 days prepartum; discontinue when/if lactation is observed at foaling
  - If the mare is agalactic at foaling and has not been treated prior to parturition, initiate treatment at foaling and continue for 5 days or until lactation ensues
- Thyrotropin-releasing hormone—2.0 mg, SC, BID, 5 days, begin day 1 postpartum
  - Increases serum prolactin, due to its action as a prolactin-releasing factor

AGALACTIA/HYPOGALACTIA   (CONTINUED)

CONTRAINDICATIONS
- Perphenazine, dopamine receptor antagonist; published, but:
  - Severe side effects in horses preclude its use
  - Sweating, colic, hyperesthesia, ataxia, posterior paresis
- Metoclopramide is used to treat agalactia of unknown origin
  - Significant risk for developing severe central nervous system side effects in horses
  - Its use is contraindicated

PRECAUTIONS
- Remove pregnant mares from endophyte-infected fescue pastures/hay minimum 30 days, preferably 60–90 days, prepartum
- If removal is not possible, treat with domperidone during last 2–4 weeks of gestation

ALTERNATIVE DRUGS
- Acepromazine maleate (20 mg IM TID)
  - Some dopamine antagonistic properties; tried as agalactia treatment
    - At least one report of it having no effect on lactation
  - Sedation is the primary side effect
- Reserpine (0.5–2.0 mg IM every 48 h or 0.01 mg/kg PO every 24 h)
  - Depletes serotonin, dopamine, and norepinephrine in the brain and other tissues
  - Gastrointestinal motility is greatly increased and can cause profuse diarrhea
  - Sedation—a common side effect
  - Not FDA approved for agalactia
- Sulpiride (3.3 mg/kg PO daily)
  - Dopamine antagonist to treat agalactia; less effective than domperidone
  - Not FDA approved for agalactia

FOLLOW-UP

PATIENT MONITORING
- If effective, most treatments stimulate milk production in 2–5 days
- In absence of other systemic signs, agalactia is not life-threatening
- Foals need intensive medical and nutritional management with prolonged agalactia

MISCELLANEOUS

ASSOCIATED CONDITIONS
Mare
Prolonged gestation, abortion, dystocia, uterine rupture, thickened placental membranes, red bag, retained fetal membranes, infertility, prolonged luteal function, early embryonic death, weak and dysmature foals.

Neonate
- FTPI
- Malnutrition
- Starvation

SEE ALSO
- Dystocia
- Failure of transfer of passive immunity (FTPI)
- Fescue toxicosis
- Mastitis
- Prolonged pregnancy
- Retained fetal membranes

ABBREVIATIONS
- FDA = United States Food and Drug Administration
- FTPI = failure of transfer of passive immunity

Suggested Reading
Cross DL, Reinmeyer CR, Prado JC, et al. Efficacy of domperidone gel in an induced model of fescue toxicosis in periparturient mares. Theriogenology 2012;78: 1361–1370.
Evans TJ, Youngquist RS, Loch WE, Cross DL. A comparison of the relative efficacies of domperidone and reserpine in treating equine "fescue toxicosis." Proc AAEP 1999;45:207–209.
Morresey PR. Agalactia, dysgalactia and nutrition of the postpartum mare. Proc AAEP 2012;58:370–374.
Tibary A. Mammary gland, lactation. In: Carleton CL, ed. Blackwell's Five Minute Veterinary Consult. Clinical Companion Equine Theriogenology. Ames, IA: Wiley Blackwell, 2011:348–354.
Tibary A. Mammary gland, mastitis. In: Carleton CL, ed. Blackwell's Five Minute Veterinary Consult. Clinical Companion Equine Theriogenology. Ames, IA: Wiley Blackwell, 2011:336–347.

Author Ahmed Tibary
Consulting Editor Carla L. Carleton
Acknowledgment The author and editor acknowledge the prior contribution of Carole C. Miller.

BASICS

DEFINITION
• Behaviors that do, or attempt to do, injury to another with the apparent motivation of causing harm
• Agonistic behaviors include threats, offensive aggressive behaviors, defensive behaviors, and submissive behaviors
• Aggression occurs in specific contexts or circumstances and is influenced by numerous variables, including internal states, external stimuli, learned experiences, etc
• It can be classified in numerous overlapping categories, e.g. according to the target, function, motivation, whether offensive or defensive

PATHOPHYSIOLOGY
• Aggression usually is a normal, species-typical behavior but can be triggered by anxiety, fear, and underlying pathophysiologic conditions that result in pain or endocrine and CNS abnormalities. Underlying conditions may be acute or chronic as well as intermittent. Consequently, corresponding aggression may vary in intensity and frequency
• "Grouchiness" or "irritability" may be related to low or moderate levels of pain
• Endocrine and gonad abnormalities, e.g., hypertestosteronism and ovarian and ovarian tumors in mares, retained testicles in males
• CNS disorders, e.g., encephalopathies, rabies, irritating or ablative lesions
• Low serum serotonin levels have been associated with aggressive behavior, stress, and illness

SYSTEMS AFFECTED
• Many physiologic and behavioral systems can be affected
• Musculoskeletal, skin, ophthalmic injuries may be incurred due to aggressive behaviors
• Reproductive behaviors may be interrupted
  ○ Horses may exhibit aggression towards members of the same sex to disrupt courtship and copulation. Some breeding stallions managed "in-hand" are aggressive to the mare and handlers
  ○ Some mares are aggressive towards their foals. In free-ranging situations the foal may not survive; in a controlled environment, successful intervention is possible. Some mares aggressively defend their foals against other animals, including people
• Aggressive outbursts can severely affect the human-animal bond and consequently impair a horse's welfare
• Frequent or prolonged states of aggression can result in chronic stress and result in changes in the hypothalamic–pituitary–cortical continuum. Chronic stress can affect immune function, body maintenance
• Interference with learning and performance

GENETICS
Genetics has been shown to influence specific types of aggressive behaviors in many species, but the mechanisms are unknown.

INCIDENCE/PREVALENCE
Unknown

GEOGRAPHIC DISTRIBUTION
Unknown

SIGNALMENT
Breed Predilections
Aggressive protection of foals is reported more often in Arabian mares.

Mean Age and Range
• Any age
• Playful aggression is most common in young horses and colts
• Intraspecific, intermale aggression is more common and intense in mature males

Predominant Sex
• Intact males are more likely to show aggression to other horses and people
• Self-mutilation is most likely to be exhibited by isolated stallions and geldings

SIGNS
General Comments
Aggressive behaviors range from mild threats to intense injurious acts.
• Mild forms include laying back of ears, lowering and extending head, nodding or swinging of head and neck, shifting of hindquarters toward another sometimes with mild pushing
• Moderate aggression adds threats to bite, strike or kick, tail switching, sometimes slight hopping motions with rear quarters, head and body bumping, harsh vocal squeals. There is an apparent restraint in intensity and effort
• High levels of aggression include serious efforts to bite, strike, or kick, severe bites, and attempts to knock opponent off balance. Rearing and striking with forelegs (boxing)
• Play aggression includes components of above but of low intensity, usually not causing any or serious harm between unshod horses
• Defensive behaviors include moving away and/or shifting rear quarters toward aggressor
• Offensive behaviors usually involve a head-on approach and threat
• Submissive behaviors include deferring to more dominant animal and "snapping" (jaw-waving, teeth-clamping, or *unterlegenheitgebärde*). Sometimes a slight sucking sound occurs. The ears are usually in a somewhat horizontal position
• Mares with elevated testosterone levels may show "stallion-like" behaviors, e.g. mounting other mares, vocalizing like a stallion, herding other mares, and aggression to other horses

Historical Findings
• Ask questions to identify exactly what behaviors are occurring. Determine when, where, how often they occur, when did they start and how did they progress, the targets of the aggression; the situations that tend to make it worse and situations when it does *not* occur; and what has been done thus far to deal with the problem. These answers form the basis for diagnosis, treatment, and risk assessment
• Aggressiveness associated with endocrine abnormalities is generally of gradual onset

Physical Examination Findings
• Examine carefully for pain. Chronic vertebral problems are often overlooked as a source of pain and aggression or grouchiness in riding horses
• Reproductive tract abnormalities, including retained testicles. Mares may have ovarian abnormalities, enlarged clitoris, blind vaginal sac, "cresty neck"

CAUSES
• Pain
• Fear/defense
• Play aggression usually is inhibited and causes few serious injuries among unshod horses of similar ages and weight; however, play can cause serious injury to people
• Protective—occurs in defense of other animals or people with whom the aggressor has a relationship and that are perceived to be under threat
• Dominance—hierarchies exist in groups of horses and are usually initially established via aggression, threats, and reciprocal deference. Once hierarchies are established and there is sufficient opportunity for the subordinate horse to defer, high levels of aggression rarely occur
• Resource guarding—food, preferred pasture partners, water, shelter, etc. Usually directed toward other horses but can be directed toward people
• Redirected—occurs during conflict situations in which a horse attacks another animal or person when access to the original target is blocked
• Redirected aggression occurs when a horse is motivated to be aggressive but is either physically or psychologically prevented from aggressing the eliciting stimuli and, instead, redirects the aggression to another target
• Infanticide—stallions may kill foals that are not theirs or are not recognized as theirs
• Sex related—occurs as part of courtship, copulation, or intrasexual competition
• Endocrine abnormalities
• CNS abnormalities such as encephalitis. Rabies may be manifested as "dumb," "furious," "paralytic," or any combination as well as other pathologic signs. These horses may be violent and, in attempts to control them, handlers are exposed to saliva and biting

RISK FACTORS
• Inappropriate use of punishment and mismanagement

AGGRESSION (CONTINUED)

- Small enclosures and poorly designed enclosures that prevent escape or deferral to threats
- Inadequate designs of water and feeding sites that result in fighting over access to resources
- Indiscriminate hand feeding treats can lead to "nipping"
- Adjacent stabling of horses that exhibit aggression toward each other
- Insufficient exercise
- Foals reared in isolation from other horses may not develop adequate social skills and may develop inappropriately rough play aggression with people

DIAGNOSIS

DIFFERENTIAL DIAGNOSIS
- Rule out pathologic conditions, before establishing solely a nonmedical behavioral diagnosis
- Aberrant, intense, steadily increasing aggressiveness or "grouchiness" warrants comprehensive medical workup
- Nonmedical diagnoses are based on circumstances and behavioral signs exhibited and ruling out medical causes
- Be aware that residual aggressive behaviors can persist after successful treatment of medical problems and management changes. Behavior modification may also be necessary

CBC/BIOCHEMISTRY/URINALYSIS
Dependent on clinical signs.

OTHER LABORATORY TESTS
- Dependent on clinical signs
- Testosterone, estrogen, and inhibin assays may be indicated
- Karyotyping of mares exhibiting stallion-like behaviors

IMAGING
Radiographs, endoscopic examinations, transrectal ultrasonography of reproductive organs.

OTHER DIAGNOSTIC PROCEDURES
- Rectal palpation
- Vaginal examination
- Lameness examination
- Visual recordings of the behavior to study and to monitor occurrence and intensity of the behavior

PATHOLOGIC FINDINGS
Dependent on etiology of aggression.

TREATMENT

AIMS
- Identify underlying reason for aggression and contributing factors
- Correct medical causes

- Specific treatments vary with the kind of aggression
- Most treatments of nonmedical conditions involve changing handling techniques, physical or social environments, and/or using behavior modification techniques to change the motivational state of the animal
- Behavior modification must be done precisely if it is to be safe and effective. Even stallions that are "unruly" when bred "in-hand" can be successfully retained using positive and negative reinforcement with very little or no punishment. It should always be remembered that the use of aversive stimuli comes with the risk of causing anxiety, fear, and aggression. Referral to an experienced and competent veterinary behaviorist, applied animal behaviorist, or trainer is often necessary to help the client implement the plan
- Assess the risks of treating and keeping a horse exhibiting aggression

APPROPRIATE HEALTH CARE
N/A

NURSING CARE
N/A

ACTIVITY
- Prevent or control access to targets of aggression
- Increase appropriate and safe types of exercise

DIET
Reduction of energy and protein intake is reported to reduce activity level and aggressiveness. However, numerous interventions (generally increased exercise and changes in environment) are usually also implemented simultaneously and it is difficult to assess the effect of the diet.

CLIENT EDUCATION
- Advise owner of risks involved with keeping the animal when considering treatment. Aggressive animals can deliver serious injury or cause death, and keeping an aggressive animal may place the client at risk of criminal and civil legal actions
- Advise owner that, even if underlying medical reasons are alleviated, there may be residual behavior patterns that require behavior modification and/or training

SURGICAL CONSIDERATIONS
- Removal of abnormal gonads in mares (ovarian tumors, aberrant testicular tissue) has a good prognosis
- Castration of stallions and colts usually reduces, but does not always eliminate, aggressive behaviors directed towards other horses and people. Age and experience of horse prior to castration are reported to be unrelated to effectiveness of castration
- Castration has been reported to completely improve self-mutilation in only 3 of 10 self-mutilating stallions

MEDICATIONS

DRUG(S) OF CHOICE
- No drug is approved by the FDA for the treatment of aggressive behaviors in horses
- Pain medications may help to reduce or eliminate pain-elicited aggression
- Anxiolytics or antidepressants may help with fear-motivated aggression
- Naturally occurring and synthetic progestins can inhibit aggression in domestic and wild equids. In larger doses progestins can reduce arousal and can be sedating

CONTRAINDICATIONS
- Benzodiazepines may increase aggressive behaviors
- Use of commercial synthetic progestins can affect testosterone levels, sperm production, and testicular morphology. There are few reported studies on the consequences of long-term use of exogenous progestins in horses
- Synthetic progestins are not disallowed when used to regulate the estrus cycle of performance mares. The drugs however are usually banned for use in other performance horses

PRECAUTIONS
- Inform clients that use of psychoactive drugs and progestins for aggression problems constitutes off-label and experimental use
- Inform clients regarding possible benefits, dangers, and side effects
- Obtain written informed consent before prescribing off-label medication

POSSIBLE INTERACTIONS
N/A

ALTERNATIVE DRUGS
N/A

FOLLOW-UP

PATIENT MONITORING
- Contact clients on a regular basis to check compliance with recommendations and to provide additional support
- Behavioral problems generally require intensive follow-up

PREVENTION/AVOIDANCE
- Avoid inappropriate use of punishment
- Rear foals with other horses. Ideally foals should remain with mother for 6 months and allowed access to other foals and (appropriate) horses as much as possible and for as long as possible
- Sufficient exercise and opportunities for appropriate play
- Adequate space to defer to dominant horses
- Strategic placement of critical resources, e.g. food, water, shelter, to alleviate competition

(CONTINUED)

• Ground work that results in the horse consistently and quickly yielding to the requests of the handler. Most easily accomplished with naive and young horses
• If the aggression is not pathophysiologic, at the first indication there might be an aggressive behavior problem advise clients to seek help from qualified, accomplished professionals who address such behaviors

POSSIBLE COMPLICATIONS
See Client Education.

EXPECTED COURSE AND PROGNOSIS
• Ovariectomies usually resolve aggressive and stallion-like behaviors of mares related to ovarian pathologies
• Removal of normal or retained testicles in males generally results in reduction of aggressive and typically masculine behaviors. Approximately one-third retain some aggressive behaviors to other horses and interest in mares. From 5% to 17% retain some aggressiveness toward people
• Successful treatment of nonmedical causes of aggression is dependent on many variables

MISCELLANEOUS

ASSOCIATED CONDITIONS
N/A

AGE-RELATED FACTORS
N/A

ZOONOTIC POTENTIAL
N/A

PREGNANCY/FERTILITY/BREEDING
N/A

SYNONYMS
N/A

SEE ALSO
• Excessive maternal behavior/foal stealing
• Fear
• Learning, training, and behavior problems
• Maternal foal rejection
• Self-mutilation
• Stallion sexual behavior problems

ABBREVIATIONS
• CNS = central nervous system
• FDA = United States Food and Drug Administration

Suggested Reading
Ayala I, Martos NF, Silvan G, et al. Cortisol, adrenocorticotropic hormone, serotonin, adrenaline and noradrenaline serum concentrations in relation to disease and stress in the horse. Res Vet Sci 2012;93:103–107.
Crowell-Davis SL. Normal behavior and behavior problems. In: Kobluk CN, Ames TR, Geor RJ, eds. The Horse: Diseases and Clinical Management. Philadelphia, PA: WB Saunders, 1995:1–21.
Dodman NH, Normile JA, Shuster L, Rand W. Equine self-mutilation syndrome (57 cases). JAVMA 1994;204(8): 1219–1223.
Fureix C, Menguy H, Hausberger M. Partners with bad temper: reject or cure? A study of chronic pain and aggression in horses. PLoS One 2010;5(8):e12434.
Goolsby HA, Brady HA, Prien DS. The off-label use of altrenogest in stallions: a survey. J Equine Vet Sci 2004;24(2):72–75.
Hinde RA. The Bases of Aggression in Animals. J Psychosom Res 1969;3(3): 213–219.
Houpt KA. Domestic Animal Behavior for Veterinarians and Animal Scientists, 5e. Ames, IA: Wiley Blackwell, 2011.
Long MT. Contagious neurological diseases. In: Furr M, Reed S, eds. Equine Neurology, 2e. Ames, IA: Wiley Blackwell, 2015:262–272.
McDonnell SM, Turner RM, Diehl NK. Modifying Unruly Breeding Behavior in Stallions. Compendium 1995;17(3): 411–417.
McDonnell SM. Abnormal Sexual Behavior. In: McKinnon AO, Squires EL, Vaala WE, Varner DD, eds. Equine Reproduction, 2e. Wiley-Blackwell, 2011:1407–1412.
McGreevy P. Equine Behaviour: A Guide for Veterinarians and Equine Scientists, 2e. Philadelphia, PA: WB Saunders, 2012.
Meral Y, Cakiroglu D, Sancak AA. Relationships between serum serotonin and serum lipid levels, and aggression in horses. Dtsch Tierarzti Wochenscher 2007;114: 30–32.
Mills DS, McDonnell S. Domestic Horse: The Origins, Development, and Management of Its Behaviour. New York, NY: Cambridge University Press, 2005.
Waring GH. Horse Behavior, 2e. Norwich, NY: Noyes Publications/William Andrew Publishing, 2003.

Author Victoria L. Voith
Consulting Editor Victoria L. Voith
Acknowledgment The author/editor acknowledges the prior contribution of Daniel Q. Estep.

ALKALINE PHOSPHATASE (ALP)

BASICS

DEFINITION
• Serum ALP concentration is mainly used as a marker for cholestasis. Although nonhepatic tissues may contribute to serum ALP concentration, the potential for significant contribution other than from bone is limited
• Reference intervals vary depending on the assay substrate employed; thus, comparisons across laboratories may not be valid

PATHOPHYSIOLOGY
• 2 genes produce distinct ALP isoenzymes—intestinal ALP and tissue-unspecific ALP
• Intestinal ALP is expressed only in the intestine and the tissue-unspecific ALP elsewhere; however, the equine kidney expresses both
• Post-translational modification (especially glycosylation) produces tissue-specific isoforms of ALP (e.g. bone, liver) and affects circulating half-life
• High tissue concentrations occur in kidney, intestine, liver, and bone; lower concentrations occur in placenta and other tissues
• Although intestine and kidney have much higher tissue concentrations than liver and bone, renal ALP is not released into blood, and intestinal ALP has a very short half-life of ≅8 min. Thus, serum concentrations consist mostly of liver and, to a lesser extent, bone ALP
• Liver ALP activity is greatest on the biliary canalicular membrane of hepatocytes. Increased blood activity results from increased synthesis (i.e. induction) or membrane release. The mechanism of release into the blood is proposed to involve membrane solubilization by bile salts, release of membrane fragments, or biliary regurgitation. A serum phospholipase contributes to cleavage of the enzyme from the membrane
• Cholestasis leads to increased serum ALP concentrations. Hepatocellular injury alone has little effect. Bile duct ligation leads to nearly 3-fold elevations within 10 days
• Serum ALP concentration rises with biliary hyperplasia, as seen with GGT
• Because increased ALP often involves enzyme induction, serum ALP increases in acute obstructive icterus may lag behind other markers such as conjugated bilirubin and bile salts

SYSTEMS AFFECTED
• Hepatobiliary—increases are associated with cholestasis
• Musculoskeletal—increases are associated with increased osteoblastic activity
• GI—severe GI disease can be associated with mild increases, the source of which is often unclear

• Reproductive—placental increases during pregnancy. Semen ALP comes mainly from the epididymis and testes. High semen ALP and few/no sperm confirms decreased sperm production versus ejaculatory failure or blockage

SIGNALMENT
• Neonates and foals—activity at days 1–3 of age is up to 20-fold above that of adults. Values decrease to < 5- to 10-fold by 2 weeks, and then taper to adult concentrations by 6 months to 1 year
• Pregnancy—equivocal impact on serum ALP concentration; some diseases associated with cholestasis and increased ALP are more common in pregnant mares (e.g. hyperlipemia, Theiler's disease)
• Ponies and donkeys—particularly susceptible to hyperlipemia and hepatic lipidosis

SIGNS
General Comments
Signs result from the underlying disease process.

Historical Findings
• Owners may report icterus, dark urine, anorexia, weight loss, lethargy, and behavioral changes associated with hepatic disease in conditions associated with cholestasis
• Abdominal pain (colic) may occur with acute hepatopathies or biliary obstructions

Physical Examination Findings
• Icterus
• Increased heart and respiratory rates, fever, photosensitization, weight loss, or obesity vary with the nature and severity of the underlying disease process

CAUSES
Hepatobiliary System
• Metabolic—secondary to severe anemia, hyperlipemia, or fasting (< 50% increase within 2–3 days, nonpathologic)
• Immune-mediated, infectious—chronic active hepatitis, Theiler's disease (i.e. serum hepatitis), amyloidosis, endotoxemia, viral (e.g. EIA, equine viral arteritis, equine herpesvirus in perinatal foals), bacterial (e.g. Tyzzer's disease, salmonellosis), fungal, protozoal (piroplasmosis), and parasitic (e.g. liver flukes, larval migrans)
• Nutritional—hepatic lipidosis
• Degenerative—cirrhosis; cholelithiasis
• Toxic—pyrrolizidine alkaloid-containing plants (e.g. *Senecio, Crotalaria*), alsike clover, aflatoxin, rubratoxin; chemical toxins (e.g. arsenic, chlorinated hydrocarbons, phenol, paraquat) primarily cause hepatocellular injury; cholestasis secondary to hepatocellular swelling or progression to a chronic hepatopathy may increase serum ALP concentration; some anesthetics (e.g. halothane) are associated with mild, transient increases

• Anomaly—biliary atresia; portovascular shunt
• Neoplastic—rare

Musculoskeletal System
• Rapid bone growth—juveniles
• Severe bony lesions

GI System
GI disease—enteritis, colitis, intestinal displacement.

Reproductive System
Pregnancy increases placental ALP, with mild increases in total serum ALP concentration possible.

Hematopoietic System
• Severe anemia (e.g. acute EIA, red maple leaf toxicity, onion toxicity, postparturient hemorrhage) leads to hypoxic injury and hepatocellular swelling, with subsequent cholestasis
• Hepatic lymphoma, leukemias, etc.

RISK FACTORS
Those associated with any disease leading to cholestasis.

DIAGNOSIS

DIFFERENTIAL DIAGNOSIS
• Increases caused by bone ALP mostly seen in growing animals. In adults, increased bone ALP likely involves lameness or obvious bony lesions. Increases from bone ALP are relatively mild
• Highest elevations generally associated with longstanding conditions involving severe cholestasis
• Concurrent obesity and high enzyme concentrations suggest hyperlipemia/lipidosis, whereas anorexia and weight loss are typical of most other differentials

LABORATORY FINDINGS
Drugs That May Alter Laboratory Results
• Arsenate, beryllium, cyanide, fluoride, manganese, phosphate, sulfhydryl compounds, and zinc may cause falsely low values
• Complexing anticoagulants (e.g. citrate, EDTA, oxalate) inhibit ALP and should not be used for sample collection

Disorders That May Alter Laboratory Results
• Extreme icterus, severe lipemia, and marked hemolysis may affect values
• Activity tends to increase with storage

Valid if Run in a Human Laboratory?
• Valid, but concentrations vary with the methodology used
• Equine reference intervals should be generated in-house or based on literature values using the same methodology

CBC/BIOCHEMISTRY/URINALYSIS
- No routine laboratory tests provide a causative or specific diagnosis for ALP increases
- Most suggest a process (e.g. injury, cholestasis, insufficiency, inflammatory) rather than a cause

Erythrocytes
- Nonregenerative anemia may be seen with liver disease
- Microcytosis is associated with portosystemic shunts
- Acanthocytes, schistocytes (hepatic microvascular disease) are associated with decreased RBC survival
- Severe hemolytic anemia can cause hypoxic injury leading to hepatocellular swelling and secondary cholestasis

Leukocytes
- Neutrophilia or neutropenia and monocytosis may occur with inflammatory liver disease
- Evidence of antigenic stimulation (e.g. lymphocytosis, reactive lymphoid cells) may be seen

Glucose
Postprandial hyperglycemia or fasting hypoglycemia may occur with hepatic insufficiency/shunts.

Albumin
- Decreased production with hepatic insufficiency may decrease serum concentrations; usually a late event
- Albumin is a negative acute-phase reactant; mild decreases may occur with inflammation

Blood Urea Nitrogen
Decreased concentrations (especially relative to creatinine) occur with hepatic insufficiency/shunts due to decreased conversion of ammonia to urea.

GGT
Increases with either injury or cholestasis.

Bilirubin
- Conjugated—increases with cholestasis
- Unconjugated—increases with increased RBC destruction or decreased hepatic uptake as with fasting or decreased function

Triglycerides
Increased with hyperlipemia.

Urinalysis
- Bilirubinuria indicates cholestasis
- Ammonia urates may be observed with hepatic insufficiency/shunt

OTHER LABORATORY TESTS
Bile Acids
- Sensitive indicator of hepatic disease but not specific for the type of process
- Assesses enterohepatic circulation, adequate hepatocellular perfusion, and hepatobiliary function
- More sensitive than ALP for cholestasis

Ammonia
Serum concentrations correlate inversely with hepatic functional mass.

Clearance Tests (Sulfobromophthalein, Indocyanine Green)
- Prolonged clearance intervals with decreased functional mass or cholestasis
- Accelerated clearance (possibly masking insufficiency) with hypoalbuminemia

Coagulation Tests
Prothrombin time; activated partial thromboplastin time; may be prolonged with hepatic insufficiency/shunting.

IMAGING
Ultrasonography—useful for assessing liver size, shape, position, and parenchymal texture.

OTHER DIAGNOSTIC PROCEDURES
Aspiration cytology or biopsy for microbiologic testing, cytologic imprints, and histopathologic evaluation.

TREATMENT
- Decision regarding outpatient versus inpatient treatment depends on the severity of disease, intensity of supportive care required, need for isolation of infectious conditions, etc.
- Avoid negative energy balance, especially in ponies and donkeys, to avoid/treat hyperlipemia and hepatic lipidosis
- A high-carbohydrate, low-protein diet reduces ammonia production
- Specific therapy depends on the underlying cause

MEDICATIONS
DRUG(S) OF CHOICE
Liver disease:
- Fluid and nutritional support may be needed
- Anorexic and hypoglycemic cases may benefit from IV 5% dextrose (2 mL/kg/h); otherwise, fluid support depends on specific electrolyte and acid–base abnormalities
- Lactulose (333 mg/kg PO every 8 h) by nasogastric tube is suggested to combat GI ammonia production/absorption but may cause diarrhea

CONTRAINDICATIONS
Dependent on the underlying cause.

PRECAUTIONS
- Dependent on the underlying cause
- With suspected hepatic insufficiency, assess coagulation profiles before invasive procedures

POSSIBLE INTERACTIONS
Dependent on the underlying cause.

ALTERNATIVE DRUGS
Dependent on the underlying cause.

FOLLOW-UP
PATIENT MONITORING
Serial chemistries can help to establish a prognosis by characterizing disease progression and identifying evidence of improvement.

PREVENTION/AVOIDANCE
Dependent on the underlying cause.

POSSIBLE COMPLICATIONS
Dependent on the underlying cause.

EXPECTED COURSE AND PROGNOSIS
- Dependent on the underlying cause
- Hypoglycemia or ALP > 900 IU/L with liver disease carries a guarded prognosis

MISCELLANEOUS
ASSOCIATED CONDITIONS
Dependent on the underlying cause.

AGE-RELATED FACTORS
See Signalment.

ZOONOTIC POTENTIAL
Dependent on the underlying cause.

PREGNANCY/FERTILITY/BREEDING
See Signalment.

SYNONYMS
N/A

SEE ALSO
See Causes.

ABBREVIATIONS
- ALP = alkaline phosphatase
- EIA = equine infectious anemia
- GGT = γ-glutamyltransferase
- GI = gastrointestinal
- RBC = red blood cell

Suggested Reading
Helene A, Perron MF, Sandersen C, et al. Prognostic value of clinical signs and blood parameters in equids suffering from hepatic diseases. J Equine Vet Sci 2005;25:18–25.
Smith GW, Davis JL. Diseases of the hepatobiliary system. In: Smith B, ed. Large Animal Internal Medicine, 5e. St. Louis, MO: Elsevier Mosby, 2015:843–872.

Author John A. Christian
Consulting Editor Sandra D. Taylor

A

ALKALOSIS, METABOLIC

BASICS

OVERVIEW
- A disruption of acid–base homeostasis producing decreased H^+ concentration, which is reflected by alkalemia (increased blood pH) and high plasma HCO_3^-
- Normal plasma HCO_3^- concentration is $\cong$ 24 mEq/L
- Normal blood pH ranges from 7.35 to 7.45
- Hypoventilation should increase CO_2 concentrations to lower pH; however, respiratory compensation is limited once hypoxemia develops

Pathophysiology
- The kidney normally is capable of responding to a high pH by excreting HCO_3^- into the urine. Metabolic alkalosis persists only when renal excretion of HCO_3^- is impaired or reabsorption is enhanced
- Excessive loss of H^+, retention of HCO_3^-, and contraction of extracellular fluid volume without loss of HCO_3^- (i.e. contraction alkalosis) are the common mechanisms that initiate metabolic alkalosis

Systems Affected
- Respiratory
  - Chemoreceptors sense high pH in blood or cerebrospinal fluid and depress ventilation to decrease removal of CO_2
- Cardiovascular
  - Cardiac arrhythmias
  - Arteriolar vasoconstriction
  - Decreased coronary and cerebral blood flow caused by vasoconstriction
- Metabolic
  - Increased affinity of O_2–hemoglobin binding, which inhibits release of O_2 to the tissues
  - Decreased ionized Ca^{2+} concentration
- Renal
  - The kidney responds to high pH by excreting HCO_3^-

SIGNALMENT
- Any breed, age, or sex
- Horses used for endurance exercise

SIGNS

Historical Findings
Recent participation in endurance event.

Physical Examination Findings
Dependent on the underlying cause.

CAUSES AND RISK FACTORS
- Gastrointestinal loss of H^+ and Cl^- is seen with gastric reflux that occurs with anterior enteritis and ileus
- Salivary loss of Cl^- (e.g. ptyalism, dysphagia, esophageal trauma/obstruction)
- Cl^- loss is seen with excessive sweating (e.g. endurance event) and diuretic therapy (furosemide). Equine sweat contains large amounts of Cl^- and K^+; fluid loss can be extreme with moderate intensity exercise, especially in warm, humid conditions
- K^+ depletion is associated with anorexia, renal failure, and diuretic therapy (acetazolamide)
- Iatrogenic HCO_3^- therapy in racehorses
- Hypoalbuminemia since proteins are weak acids

DIAGNOSIS

DIFFERENTIAL DIAGNOSIS
N/A

CBC/BIOCHEMISTRY/URINALYSIS
- Measurements of serum electrolytes, protein concentrations, and chemistries are important to determine the cause and to guide treatment
- Normal or elevated Na^+ concentrations with hypochloremia are suggestive of metabolic alkalosis
- K^+ and Cl^- are decreased in horses that sweat excessively; K^+ may be low because of the primary cause or as a response to the extracellular shift of H^+
- Ionized Ca^{2+} is decreased
- Mg^{2+} may be decreased, especially with sweat loss
- Urinalysis may reveal decreased urine pH

OTHER LABORATORY TESTS
- Many laboratories measure TCO_2, which closely approximates HCO_3^-
- TCO_2 must be analyzed rapidly and with minimal room-air exposure within the sample tube
- Increased blood pH indicates alkalemia. A concurrent increase in blood HCO_3^- concentration indicates metabolic alkalemia. An accompanying increase in PCO_2 concentration indicates respiratory compensation
- Increased HCO_3^- concentration with decreased blood pH indicates compensation for a respiratory acidosis
- The exacerbation of severe asthma is often associated with increased blood pH, increased PCO_2 concentration, and increased HCO_3^- concentration, suggesting excess compensation for a respiratory acidosis
- Blood gas parameters must be assessed against appropriate reference ranges for the sample taken

IMAGING
N/A

OTHER DIAGNOSTIC PROCEDURES
N/A

TREATMENT
Directed at the primary cause.

MEDICATIONS

DRUG(S) OF CHOICE
- Replacement of fluid losses with isotonic fluids may be sufficient to restore acid–base status in mild cases
- Address specific electrolyte losses
- Large volumes may be needed in some endurance athletes with excessive fluid losses from sweating or hyperthermia
- With hypochloremia, give fluids containing Cl^-, or the alkalosis will not be corrected even if hydration is restored
- 0.9% saline or isotonic crystalloids with added Ca^{2+} and KCl are the fluids of choice
- With excessive K^+ loss, IV supplementation is necessary if the horse remains anorexic

CONTRAINDICATIONS/POSSIBLE INTERACTIONS
Any alkalinizing therapy (e.g. lactated Ringer's solution) can worsen the alkalosis.

FOLLOW-UP

PATIENT MONITORING
Serial blood gas analysis and measurement of electrolytes are important in evaluating efficacy of therapy.

POSSIBLE COMPLICATIONS
- Hypokalemia
- Hypocalcemia

EXPECTED COURSE AND PROGNOSIS
Dependent on the underlying cause.

MISCELLANEOUS

ASSOCIATED CONDITIONS
- Hypochloremia
- Hypokalemia
- Respiratory acidosis

SEE ALSO
- Chloride, hypochloremia
- Hyperthermia
- Potassium, hypokalemia

ABBREVIATIONS
- PCO_2 = partial pressure of carbon dioxide
- TCO_2 = total carbon dioxide

Suggested Reading
Hinchcliff KW, ed. Fluids and electrolytes in athletic horses. Vet Clin North Am Equine Pract 1998;14(1):1–225.
Author Sara L. Connolly
Consulting Editor Sandra D. Taylor
Acknowledgment The author and editor acknowledge the prior contribution of Jennifer G. Adams.

BASICS

OVERVIEW
• Decrease in blood PCO_2 concentration
• Arterial concentrations in range 35-42 mmHg
• Venous concentrations in range 43-49 mmHg

Pathophysiology
• CO_2 is formed in all tissues during metabolic energy production and diffuses passively out of cells and into the blood in gaseous form
• Most (65–70%) CO_2 combines with water almost instantaneously to form carbonic acid, which then dissociates into HCO_3^- and H^+. Therefore, most CO_2 is transported in the blood as HCO_3^-, with some bound to proteins and a small amount dissolved directly into plasma
• In the lungs, the reverse occurs, and CO_2 passively diffuses out of capillaries into the alveoli
• These 3 forms of CO_2 exist in equilibrium in the blood, but PCO_2 as measured by blood gases depends on the dissolved portion
• Alveolar CO_2 is then removed mechanically by ventilation as air moves in and out of the lungs
• Respiratory alkalosis occurs with hyperventilation or when tissue production of CO_2 drops but ventilation remains unchanged

Systems Affected
• Brain (hypocapnia decreases cerebral blood flow)
• Alterations in pH affect acid–base balance, protein binding, and electrolyte levels directly in the blood and via effects on the kidney
• The kidney responds to high pH by generating more H^+ and excreting more HCO_3^-. It also reabsorbs Cl^- to maintain electroneutrality. Alkalosis decreases serum K^+ and ionized Ca^{2+} concentrations
• Severe alkalemia can cause venoconstriction and predispose to arrhythmias

SIGNALMENT
Any breed, age, or sex.

SIGNS
Tachypnea

CAUSES AND RISK FACTORS
Acute—Hyperventilation
• Exercise, fever, hyperthermia, pain, anxiety, excitement, or fear
• Stimulation of medullary respiratory center (e.g. central nervous system disorder, septicemia, acidosis, endotoxemia)
• Tissue hypoxia from anemia, hypovolemia, or hypoxemia

Chronic
• Chronic respiratory disease or chronic, painful conditions (e.g. laminitis)

• Overventilation with mechanical ventilators produces low PCO_2 concentrations in anesthetized patients and sick neonates
• Prolonged general anesthesia may lower tissue CO_2 production and produce respiratory alkalosis
• Compensatory response to primary metabolic acidosis

DIAGNOSIS

DIFFERENTIAL DIAGNOSIS
• Any condition that causes tachypnea
• Chronic respiratory alkalosis results in compensatory metabolic acidosis, in which HCO_3^- is low and pH should be normal, because compensation is very effective in this circumstance
• Primary acute metabolic acidosis; often, pH remains low in severe cases, because respiratory compensation rarely is complete

LABORATORY FINDINGS
Disorders That May Alter Laboratory Results
• With poor peripheral perfusion, results of blood gas analysis on samples taken from peripheral arteries may not reflect the overall systemic condition
• Prolonged exposure to room air may alter PCO_2 concentrations because the sample equilibrates with the air

CBC/BIOCHEMISTRY/URINALYSIS
N/A

OTHER LABORATORY TESTS
• Blood gas analysis. Abnormalities that indicate a primary respiratory alkalemia are elevated pH and decreased PCO_2. A concurrent decrease in HCO_3^- indicates metabolic compensation
• Venous samples may be adequate to identify the condition, but arterial samples are necessary to evaluate adequacy of pulmonary function as a cause. Samples must be evaluated against appropriate reference values
• Handheld analyzers require only small amounts of whole blood. Otherwise, use heparinized syringes
• Perform sampling anaerobically. Immediately evacuate any air bubbles and cap the needle with a rubber stopper
• Perform analysis within 15–20 min. If not possible, samples collected in syringes designed for arterial blood collection can be stored on ice, and results will be valid for 3–4 h

IMAGING
N/A

OTHER DIAGNOSTIC PROCEDURES
• Capnography or capnometry to measure CO_2 indirectly from expired gases
• Samples of end-tidal gases reflect arterial PCO_2 concentrations

• Continuous monitoring of anesthetized or ventilated patients
• V/Q mismatch is always present in anesthetized or recumbent patients, and end-tidal CO_2 concentrations may underestimate arterial concentrations by $\cong$10–15 mmHg

TREATMENT
Treat underlying cause.

MEDICATIONS
DRUG(S) OF CHOICE
N/A

CONTRAINDICATIONS/POSSIBLE INTERACTIONS
N/A

FOLLOW-UP
PATIENT MONITORING
Repeat blood gas analysis following resolution of clinical signs and/or treatment.

POSSIBLE COMPLICATIONS
Severe alkalemia can result in neurologic signs, muscular excitability, and cardiac arrhythmias.

MISCELLANEOUS
ASSOCIATED CONDITIONS
Disorders that result in metabolic acidosis.

PREGNANCY/FERTILITY/BREEDING
Late-term pregnant mares might hyperventilate because of decreased lung volume caused by abdominal distention.

SYNONYMS
• Hypocapnia
• Hypocarbia

SEE ALSO
• Acidosis, metabolic
• Chloride, hyperchloremia
• Potassium, hypokalemia

ABBREVIATIONS
• PCO_2 = partial pressure of carbon dioxide
• V/Q = ventilation–perfusion ratio

Suggested Reading
Viu J, Armengou L, Ríos J, et al. Acid base imbalances in ill neonatal foals and their association with survival. Equine Vet J 2017;49(1):51–57.

Author Sara L. Connolly
Consulting Editor Sandra D. Taylor
Acknowledgment The author and editor acknowledge the prior contribution of Jennifer G. Adams.

A

ALOPECIA

BASICS

DEFINITION
- Alopecia is characterized by an absolute decrease in the number of hairs per given area of body surface or hairs that are shorter than normal even though their number is within normal limits. Simply stated, it is a loss or lack of the hair from skin areas where it is normally present
- Alopecia may be congenital or acquired
- Congenital alopecia is rare in horses and represents changes in hair follicle quantity or quality
- Common etiologies of acquired alopecia are adnexal destruction or atrophy secondary to infection, physical trauma, immune-mediated reactions, nutritional supplements and deficiencies, toxicities, physiologic stressors, hypersensitivities, neoplasia, and various miscellaneous causes. Acquired alopecia can be subdivided into infectious and noninfectious causes

PATHOPHYSIOLOGY
- Acquired alopecia represents a disruption in the growth of the hair follicle with or without damage to the hair bulb, follicular wall, and/or hair shaft. The animal is born with a normal hair coat, has or had normal hair follicles at one time, and is or was capable of producing structurally normal hairs
- Congenital alopecia is the result of abnormal morphogenesis or lack of adnexal structures (therefore hair) in regions of the body where they normally are expected. Animals with congenital hypotrichosis may be born with varying degrees of hypotrichosis or a complete haircoat; however, if born with a complete haircoat a rapid onset of progressive permanent alopecia within the first few months of life ensues

SYSTEMS AFFECTED
Skin/exocrine

GENETICS
Congenital alopecia does not necessarily imply a genetic basis, although in most cases the disease is based on genetic abnormalities and thus is hereditary. The exact mode of inheritance is unknown.

INCIDENCE/PREVALENCE
True incidence is unknown.

GEOGRAPHIC DISTRIBUTION
Presumably worldwide.

SIGNALMENT
- Congenital hypotrichosis has been documented in certain Arabian lines and a blue roan Percheron
- Appaloosas with foundation bloodlines have hair dystrophy/thinning of the long mane and tail hair
- Acquired alopecia can occur in all breeds

- Appaloosas and Quarter Horses are predisposed to alopecia areata
- Both sexes are affected equally

SIGNS
General Comments
- May be an acute onset or slowly progressive
- Multifocal patches of circular alopecia are most commonly associated with bacterial folliculitis, dermatophytosis, or dermatophilosis
- Large diffuse areas of alopecia may indicate an immune-mediated etiology or congenital abnormality
- Congenital hypotrichosis may be regional, multifocal, or generalized. It might become clinically apparent only weeks after birth and usually does not continually progress with age

CAUSES
- Noncicatricial alopecia (nonscarring causes)
  - Mild to moderate inflammation of the hair follicle (folliculitis and furunculosis)
  - Defects in the hair shaft
  - Hair follicle dystrophies
  - Altered hair follicle function
  - Trauma (self-induced from pruritus)
- Cicatricial alopecia (scarring causes)
  - Physical, chemical, or thermal injury
  - Severe furunculosis
  - Neoplasia
  - Severe inflammatory disease such as in cutaneous onchocerciasis

Congenital Causes
- Congenital hypothyroidism may be a cause of congenital hypotrichosis and alopecia
- Trichorrhexis nodosa is a hair shaft defect that may be hereditary or acquired
- Congenital hypotrichosis
- Epidermolysis bullosa
- Mane and tail dystrophy
- Follicular dysgenesis

Acquired Causes
Infectious
- Bacterial
  - The most common bacterial infection is dermatophilosis. Folliculitis and furunculosis due to *Staphylococcus* spp. (common) and *Corynebacterium pseudotuberculosis* (uncommon). Other bacterial causes are abscesses due to *Fusiformis* and *Streptococcus* spp.
- Fungal
  - Dermatophytosis due to *Microsporum gypseum*, *M. equinum* or *M. canis* or *Trichophyton equinum* var. *equinum* cause alopecia. Other fungal causes are mycetoma and subcutaneous mycosis such as phycomycosis and pythiosis
  - Brittle tail syndrome caused by the contagious, keratolytic fungus *Equicapillimyces hongkongensis* is a newly described condition causing weakening and breakage only of the tail hairs
  - Piedra is a rare fungal infection caused by *Trichosporon beigelii* that causes white nodules on the hair shafts that cause

breakage of the shafts. The mane, tail, and distal limbs are most commonly affected
- Parasitic
  - Follicular parasitic infections of the follicle that result in alopecia are rare and include *Demodex equi* and *Pelodera strongyloides*. Other more common parasitic infections that cause alopecia are *Culicoides*, onchocerciasis, lice, ticks, oxyuriasis and mites (*Sarcoptes* spp., *Chorioptes* spp., *Psoroptes* spp., and Trombiculidae)
- Viral
  - Viral papillomas—congenital, cutaneous, or pinnal
Noninfectious
- Immune mediated
  - Cell-mediated autoimmune disease directed toward the hair follicle and adnexa
    - Alopecia areata
    - Hair follicle dystrophy—possible variant of alopecia areata
    - Sebaceous adenitis—rare, case reports in 2006 and 2013
  - Drug eruptions
  - Pemphigus foliaceus
  - Systemic lupus erythematosus
  - Sarcoidosis
- Physical
  - Burns from chemicals, hot, cold, or ropes
  - Scalding from exudate, urine, or feces
  - Tail and mane rubbing as stable vice
- Neoplasia
  - Sarcoids
  - Squamous cell carcinoma
- Miscellaneous
  - Symmetrical atrophy of hair follicles secondary to endocrine disorders is extremely rare to nonexistent
  - Anagen and telogen effluvium
  - Anhidrosis
  - Iodism
  - Selenium, mimosine, or mercury toxicities
  - Copper deficiency

RISK FACTORS
N/A

DIAGNOSIS

DIFFERENTIAL DIAGNOSIS
- Accurate diagnosis of alopecia requires a careful history and physical examination
- Key points in the history include recognition of breed predispositions for congenital alopecia; the duration and progression of lesions; the presence or absence of pruritus or evidence of contagion
- On physical examination, the distribution of lesions should be noted (focal, multifocal, generalized, or symmetrical), and the hairs examined to determine if they are being shed from the hair follicle or broken off. Signs of secondary infections or ectoparasites should be noted. The degree of crusts, scale, and exudate help prioritize the differentials

- Patchy, localized to multifocal
  - Bacterial folliculitis and furunculosis
  - Dermatophytosis
  - Dermatophilosis
  - Linear alopecia
  - Alopecia areata—results from selective and reversible damage to anagen hair follicles. Initial lesions may be focal or multifocal, well-circumscribed alopecia that progresses to diffuse alopecia. The mane, tail, and face are often involved and hoof dystrophies can occur. The alopecic skin has minimal or no visible inflammation. Prognosis varies, some cases spontaneously resolve, some respond to immunosuppressive doses of steroids, while others have no hair regrowth
- Generalized, symmetrical, and large patchy multifocal
  - Normal shed—"physiologic telogen effluvium"
  - Telogen effluvium—a reaction pattern characterized by widespread alopecia in response to severe metabolic stress. Serious illness, high fever, pregnancy, and adverse reaction to supplements are all potential inducers of telogen effluvium. Rapid premature cessation of anagen growth leads to abrupt synchronization of the follicular cycle such that hair follicles proceed in unison through catagen and telogen. This leads to hair loss of variable severity when old telogen hairs are forced out by new, synchronous anagen hairs. Hair loss usually occurs within 3–4 weeks after the insult but may occur up to 2 months later. Alopecia resolves spontaneously if the initiating factor is no longer present, and new anagen hairs grow
  - Anagen effluvium—a reaction pattern characterized by shedding during anagen arrest. Severe stresses such as high-dose cytotoxic therapy or infectious or metabolic disease halt anagen hair growth and result in hair loss within days to weeks of the insult. The hairs are lost due to structural weakness or dysplastic changes damaging the hair shaft

CBC/BIOCHEMISTRY/URINALYSIS
Useful to rule out metabolic causes.

OTHER LABORATORY TESTS
N/A

IMAGING
N/A

OTHER DIAGNOSTIC PROCEDURES
- Cytology should be obtained from pustules, papules, erosions, or ulcers. Neutrophilic exudate with intra- and/or extracellular cocci representative of a secondary folliculitis are easily identified if cytology is sampled from ruptured pustules or impression smears made from the underside of crusts or a fresh erosion or ulcer. Impression smears from the surface of lesions often do *not* show bacteria, but rather numbers of shed keratinocytes

- Direct hair examination (trichography)—hairs will have either anagen or telogen roots. Telogen hairs have uniform shaft diameters and slightly rough-surfaced, tapered, spear-shaped angular non-pigmented roots. Anagen hairs have rounded, smooth pigmented bulbs that bend. Distal ends of hair shafts may appear fractured from self-induced trauma. No normal animal should have all of its hairs in telogen but rather should have an admixture of anagen and telogen. Anagen defluxion reveals fragmented hair shafts with the absence of roots. Animals with alopecia areata may have short hairs with fractured distal ends and shafts that taper towards the proximal end (exclamation point hairs)
- Perform skin scrapings to rule out ectoparasites
- Perform bacterial and dermatophyte test medium cultures to determine bacterial species and susceptibility and/or dermatophyte infections
- Perform skin biopsies if the tests listed above do not identify or suggest an underlying cause. A biopsy evaluates hair follicles, adnexal structures, inflammation, and anagen/telogen ratios. Biopsies may reveal evidence for bacterial, parasitic, or fungal causes of alopecia but should *not* be considered as the definitive test for determination of alopecia caused by infectious agents. If cytologic identification reveals evidence of folliculitis, treat the patient with appropriate antimicrobials, parasiticides, or antifungals for a minimum of 3 weeks. If no improvement in the degree of alopecia is noted, obtain a biopsy for histopathology, preferably while the patient is still receiving treatment. Often biopsies submitted from patients with moderate to severe bacterial folliculitis make it difficult to determine and may mask the primary cause of alopecia. Submit biopsies from affected and nonaffected sites
- Definitive diagnosis of alopecia areata requires histologic confirmation. Multiple biopsies need to be collected as pathognomonic lesions can be sparse. Biopsy from newly developed areas of alopecia, rather than older lesions

PATHOLOGIC FINDINGS
- Biopsies of telogen effluvium are misleading, as they will demonstrate most follicles in the active growing (anagen) phase. Often the hair cycle has returned to normal by the time the decision to biopsy has been made
- Anagen effluvium findings include apoptosis and fragmented cell nuclei of the keratinocytes of the hair matrix of anagen follicles, as well as eosinophilic dysplastic hair shafts within the pilar canal
- Alopecia areata has 2 major histologic features. The first is hair follicle miniaturization and the second feature is lymphocytic bulbitis. The lymphocytic

bulbitis involves anagen follicles and is best found in recently developed areas of alopecia. A lymphocytic mural folliculitis affecting the follicular isthmus is possible. The bulbitis may be very difficult to demonstrate especially in chronic lesions where the inflammation may be nonexistent. Chronic lesions only exhibit small telogen follicles lacking hair shafts that may be somewhat atrophic
- Histologic findings of alopecia secondary to infectious organisms are covered in the appropriate dermatology sections

 TREATMENT

The clinical approach to alopecia is to identify the cause and, if the etiology is something that may benefit from pharmaceutical treatment, then therapy may resolve the clinical signs.

APPROPRIATE HEALTH CARE
Relevance equated to etiology; most require outpatient medical management.

NURSING CARE
Relevance equated to etiology.

ACTIVITY
Patients with multifocal to generalized hypotrichosis may be more susceptible to hypothermia and solar dermatoses.

DIET
Telogen effluvium has been associated with the administration of a feed supplement.

CLIENT EDUCATION
Relevance equated to etiology.

SURGICAL CONSIDERATIONS
N/A

 MEDICATIONS

DRUG(S) OF CHOICE
- Varies with cause
- Dermatophytosis—lime sulfur or enilconazole, miconazole/chlorhexidine rinses; systemic griseofulvin
- Dermatophilosis—topical antimicrobial therapy
- Bacterial folliculitis—systemic and topical antimicrobial therapy
- Pemphigus foliaceus—immunosuppressive therapy
- There are no hair growth-promoting pharmaceuticals for horses

CONTRAINDICATIONS
N/A

PRECAUTIONS
N/A

POSSIBLE INTERACTIONS
None

ALTERNATIVE DRUGS
None

FOLLOW-UP

PATIENT MONITORING
Varies with cause.

PREVENTION/AVOIDANCE
• Varies with cause
• Patients with documented congenital alopecia and their parents should not be used for breeding

POSSIBLE COMPLICATIONS
N/A

EXPECTED COURSE AND PROGNOSIS
• Prognosis is based on whether the alopecia is classified as noncicatricial or cicatricial
• Cicatricial alopecia is characterized by permanent destruction of the hair follicles and regrowth of hair will not occur
• In noncicatricial alopecia, future hair growth will occur if the causative factors are eliminated or corrected
• Telogen and post-anagen effluvium resolve upon identification and elimination of cause

MISCELLANEOUS

ASSOCIATED CONDITIONS
N/A

AGE-RELATED FACTORS
N/A

ZOONOTIC POTENTIAL
Dermatophytosis and dermatophilosis are zoonotic.

PREGNANCY/FERTILITY/BREEDING
• Postpartum telogen effluvium is thought to be due to the physiologic stress of pregnancy and lactation
• Avoid the use of griseofulvin to treat dermatophytosis in pregnant mares
• Mares that receive iodine-deficient diets give birth to weak or dead foals with no haircoat

SYNONYMS
• Alopecia = hypotrichosis
• Anagen effluvium = anagen defluxion or defluvium
• Telogen effluvium = telogen defluxion or defluvium

SEE ALSO
• Dermatophilosis
• Pemphigus foliaceus
• Sarcoid

Suggested Reading
Pascoe RRR, Knottenbelt DC. Manual of Equine Dermatology. London, UK WB Saunders, 1999:68.
Rosychuk R. Noninflammatory, nonpruritic alopecia of horses. Vet Clin North Am Equine Pract 2013;29:629–641.
von Tscharner C, Kunkle GA, Yager JA. Stannard's illustrated equine dermatology notes. Alopecia in the horse—an overview. Vet Dermatol 2000;11:191–203.

Author David Senter
Consulting Editor Gwendolen Lorch
Acknowledgment The author acknowledges the prior contribution of Gwendolen Lorch.

BASICS

OVERVIEW
- Amitraz, a formamide acaricide, is widely used for the control of mites and ticks in veterinary medicine
- Not approved for use in horses but intentional or accidental exposures have occurred
- Clinical signs are referable to the CNS or GI system
- Acts on α_2-adrenergic receptors in the CNS and on both α_1- and α_2-adrenergic receptors in the periphery. It is also believed to inhibit monaminoxidase, block prostaglandin E_2 synthesis, and cause a local anesthetic effect
- High doses cause depression while low doses result in hyperreactivity to external stimuli. Aggressive behavior possible
- Reduces smooth muscle activity in the GI tract
- Depresses respiratory rate centrally, probably by inhibiting respiratory neurons located in the ventral portion of the brain. α_2-Adrenergic agonists can accentuate amitraz-induced respiratory depression
- Inhibits antidiuretic hormone and thus may promote diuresis
- Induces hyperglycemia and hypoinsulinemia by inhibiting insulin secretion mediated by α_2-adrenergic receptors located within the pancreatic islets
- More slowly metabolized in ponies than in sheep, which may explain higher toxicity in equines

SIGNALMENT
N/A

SIGNS
Depression, ataxia, muscular incoordination, and impaction colic, which may persist for days. Facial swelling, tachypnea, and tachycardia have also been reported.

CAUSES AND RISK FACTORS
- Deliberate or accidental exposure for parasite control
- May be deliberately administered IV to alter performance in athletic horses due to its sedative/tranquilizing effects
- When in stored solutions, may break down to the highly toxic N-3,5-dimethylphenyl-N-methyl formadine derivative to more easily induce toxicosis
- No demonstrable adverse effects in a chronic low-dose toxicity study in horses

DIAGNOSIS

DIFFERENTIAL DIAGNOSIS
- Signs of colic can be due to many other disorders
- Signs of depression and ataxia can be due to viral encephalomyelitis, hepatoencephalopathy, meningitis, or brain abscess or tumor

CBC/BIOCHEMISTRY/URINALYSIS
- With acute intoxication, total protein and packed cell volume may increase due to dehydration and a mild acidosis may be seen
- Hyperglycemia and hypoinsulinemia result from inhibition of insulin release

OTHER LABORATORY TESTS
Drug-testing laboratories have methods for the detection of amitraz and its major metabolite in performance horses.

IMAGING
N/A

OTHER DIAGNOSTIC PROCEDURES
N/A

PATHOLOGIC FINDINGS
Experimental amitraz-treated horses had fecalith obstruction in the proximal small colon aboral to marked colonic impaction.

TREATMENT

- If dermal exposure to amitraz occurs, horses should be immediately bathed with soap and water to reduce further absorption
- If ingested, activated charcoal (1–4 g/kg PO in water slurry (1 g in 5 mL of water)) can be administered via nasogastric tube to reduce absorption
- Mineral oil per nasogastric tube may be used to manage feed impaction
- Oxygen and mechanical ventilation may be necessary if respiratory depression is severe
- IV or fluid therapy or fluids via nasogastric tube may be beneficial

MEDICATIONS

DRUG(S) OF CHOICE
- The α_2-adrenergic antagonists yohimbine and atipamezole are used for treatment of amitraz intoxication in dogs and cats, but their use has not been documented in horses

- Yohimbine has a high affinity for the α_2-adrenergic receptors α_2A, α_2B, and α_2C and a low affinity for the α_2D receptor. Yohimbine reverses amitraz-induced sedation in horses. A suggested dose for horses is 0.15 mg/kg IV slowly
- Atipamezole is a potent and selective α_2-adrenergic antagonist, is considered a new generation of α_2-adrenergic antagonists owing to its high selectivity for α_2-adrenergic receptors, like α_2A, α_2B, and α_2C receptors, and has a 100 times higher affinity for the α_2D receptor than yohimbine. Atipamezole is more efficacious in reversing amitraz toxicity in cats than yohimbine. A suggested dose for horses is 0.1 mg/kg IV
- Analgesics such as NSAIDs may be used to control GI pain

CONTRAINDICATIONS/POSSIBLE INTERACTIONS
- Atropine is contraindicated due to the known sensitivity of horses to the anticholinergic effects on GI motility
- Adverse drug interactions are possible with xylazine, benzodiazepines, and macrocyclic lactones (e.g. ivermectin)

FOLLOW-UP

EXPECTED COURSE AND PROGNOSIS
The impaction colic effects of amitraz toxicosis may persist for days, but the prognosis is good with supportive treatment. Once the impaction resolves, some horses may experience diarrhea transiently.

MISCELLANEOUS

ABBREVIATIONS
- CNS = central nervous system
- GI = gastrointestinal
- NSAID = nonsteroidal anti-inflammatory drug

Suggested Reading
Auer D, Seawright AA, Pollitt CC, et al. Illness in horses following spraying with amitraz. Aust Vet J 1984;61:257–259.
Queiroz-Neto A, Zamur G, Goncalves SC, et al. Characterization of the antinociceptive and sedative effect of amitraz in horses. J Vet Pharmacol Ther 1998;21:400–405.

Author Patricia M. Dowling
Consulting Editors Wilson K. Rumbeiha and Steve Ensley

AMMONIA, HYPERAMMONEMIA

 BASICS

DEFINITION
• Free ammonia (NH_3) is a nonprotein nitrogen compound that can permeate cells and result in hyperammonemia. At physiologic pH, almost all blood ammonia is the ammonium ion (NH_4^+), which is less permeable for cells. In order to eliminate waste nitrogen as ammonia, mammals convert it to an excretable form—urea. To a lesser extent, ammonia is eliminated by conversion to glutamine
• Reference intervals for plasma ammonia concentrations are dependent on the type of assay and reported units. Hyperammonemia occurs when concentrations exceed the established laboratory reference intervals

PATHOPHYSIOLOGY
• The major source of blood ammonia is derived primarily from dietary nitrogen via the GI tract bacterial proteases, ureases, and amine oxidases
• Ammonia also may be derived from catabolism of glutamine and protein, and skeletal muscle exertion
• Ammonia is delivered to the liver via the portal vein or hepatic artery, where functional hepatocytes remove ammonia to form urea by means of the Krebs–Henseleit urea cycle
• Often, 70% of the liver mass has inadequate function before serum hyperammonemia is detected. If functional liver mass is inadequate, ammonia is not converted to urea, and plasma ammonia concentration increases. Urea concentrations also rise when glomerular filtration is inadequate. Acid–base status affects the absorption of ammonia
• As blood pH increases, free ammonia (NH_3) increases and can permeate cells via nonionic diffusion to produce toxicity. Ammonia is one of the compounds responsible for clinical signs of hepatic encephalopathy
• Hyperammonemia has a toxic effect on neuron cell membranes by inhibition of ATP and alteration of the tricarboxylic acid cycle; both lead to neuronal cell energy depletion
• Other neurotoxins in hepatic encephalopathy are the result of—alterations in monoamine neurotransmitters due to altered aromatic amino acids, increased activity of GABA, glutamate receptor alterations, and increased endogenous benzodiazepine-like substances. Additionally, GI-derived neurotoxins are implicated, such as mercaptans, short-chain fatty acids, and phenols

SYSTEMS AFFECTED
• Nervous—ammonia is neurotoxic and the brain is affected by high plasma concentrations
• The degree of hyperammonemia does not necessarily correlate with the severity of

hepatic encephalopathy signs since other compounds are involved. Ammonia interferes with the blood–brain barrier, cerebral blood flow, cellular excitability, neurotransmitter metabolism, and ratios of neurotransmitter precursor amino acids
• Degenerative changes of the neurons and supporting cells have been observed in chronically affected animals

GENETICS
N/A

INCIDENCE/PREVALENCE
N/A

GEOGRAPHIC DISTRIBUTION
N/A

SIGNALMENT
• Portacaval shunts have been reported in foals (rare)
• Ponies/donkeys (hepatic lipidosis)

SIGNS
General Comments
• Clinical signs of hyperammonemia are primarily those of hepatic encephalopathy, although this is not the only substance responsible for clinical signs
• Signs may be sporadic, progressive, and worsen after feeding

Historical Findings
Ptyalism, behavior changes, visual deficits (blindness), compulsive circling, pacing, anxiety, head pressing, stupor, coma, unusual positions/posture, sudden falling to the ground, violent thrashing

Physical Examination Findings
Stunted growth, loss of body condition, poor hair coat, mentation changes and aberrant behavior. Similar findings as discussed in liver disease (e.g. icterus) may be observed, especially in horses with acute hepatitis. In animals affected chronically, neuronal degeneration occurs and signs become persistent.

CAUSES
• Liver disease resulting in inadequate functional mass. Hepatic encephalopathy is a prominent clinical feature of hepatic failure in the horse, and is associated with hepatitis and hepatic cirrhosis. Abnormalities of the urea cycle, abnormal portal blood flow, or any disorder that results in markedly impaired liver function can cause hyperammonemia
• Decreased functional hepatic mass can result from toxins such as pyrrolizidine alkaloids, excess iron, blue-green algae, mycotoxins, urea poisoning, ammonium salt fertilizers, and other hepatotoxic drugs or chemicals; infectious diseases such as Tyzzer's disease due to *Clostridium piliforme* in foals, virus-associated Theiler's disease; and syndromes including hyperlipidemia in ponies and occasionally in horses, with associated hepatic dysfunction
• Portosystemic shunts; acquired or congenital

• Intestinal hyperammonemia in the absence of liver disease is thought to occur when intestinal disease induces increased ammonia production by microflora and a concurrent increase in GI permeability

RISK FACTORS
• Horses in areas with hepatotoxic plants or toxins
• Administration of equine-derived biologics (e.g. plasma, tetanus anti-toxin)
• Feedstuffs contaminated with high levels of urea, nitrogen, ammonium salts, or mycotoxins
• Anorexia in overconditioned horses

 DIAGNOSIS

DIFFERENTIAL DIAGNOSIS
• Primary neurologic diseases such as inflammatory, degenerative, infectious, or neoplastic CNS diseases. Rabies should be a differential diagnosis for abnormal behavior
• Behavior-based problems
• Possible intestinal bacterial overgrowth resulting in transient hyperammonemia (proposed)
• Differentiation consists of evaluating the history, signalment, and results of serum biochemistry, hematology, urinalysis, and hepatic biopsy

CBC/BIOCHEMISTRY/URINALYSIS
• CBC—microcytosis may occur in animals with portosystemic shunts, but may be difficult to determine in the horse; red blood cell histograms may be useful
• Ammonia is labile in blood samples, limiting the diagnostic use
• Biochemistry—liver enzymes may be normal in animals with portosystemic shunts, but bile acid concentrations and ammonia concentrations will be elevated. Usually, other biochemical abnormalities are present, indicating hepatic dysfunction if the liver disease is severe enough to produce hepatic encephalopathy. Finding elevated liver enzymes (sorbitol dehydrogenase, glutamate dehydrogenase, alkaline phosphatase, γ-glutamyltransferase, or aspartate aminotransferase) and hyperbilirubinemia, hypoglycemia (not common), hyper- or hypocholesterolemia, or low blood urea nitrogen suggestive of end-stage hepatic failure support a diagnosis of liver disease
• Urinalysis—ammonium biurate crystals and low urine specific gravity due to underlying liver disease in some animals

OTHER LABORATORY TESTS
• Measurement of serum bile acid concentrations has largely replaced ammonia assays due to convenience of sampling. Of note, generally bile acid samples in horses are obtained at one time point and postprandial bile acid measurements are not performed,

since horses have continuous bile acid secretion due to the lack of a gallbladder and a weak common bile duct sphincter
• Coagulation factor production may be decreased in liver failure, resulting in prolonged prothrombin time and partial thromboplastin time

IMAGING
Ultrasonographic evaluation of the liver and portal vessels is advised.

OTHER DIAGNOSTIC PROCEDURES
Hepatic biopsy can determine lesions leading to inadequate functional hepatic mass, such as fibrosis, dysplasia, or microvascular shunts. Prior coagulation assessment is advised.

PATHOLOGIC FINDINGS
• Decreased functional hepatic mass; decreased liver size; microhepatica
• Portosystemic shunt
• Degenerative changes of the neurons and supporting cells have been observed in chronically affected animals
• Lesions of cutaneous photosensitivity/dermatitis in some cases of hepatic failure

TREATMENT

APPROPRIATE HEALTH CARE
• Prevent signs associated with hepatic encephalopathy
• Fluid administration is needed to correct dehydration and maintain tissue perfusion. It is important to maintain normal plasma potassium concentrations because low plasma potassium may increase the intracellular movement of ammonia

NURSING CARE
See Appropriate Health Care.

ACTIVITY
Restrict activity.

DIET
Feed a very low protein diet, or fast the patient initially, and then institute a protein-restricted diet when the patient is stable.

CLIENT EDUCATION
Discussion of the prognosis.

SURGICAL CONSIDERATIONS
Correction of hepatic shunts.

MEDICATIONS

DRUG(S) OF CHOICE
• Lactulose is an acidifying agent used to decrease ammonia absorption from the

intestine and lower plasma ammonia concentration in equine hyperammonemia. Lactulose acts as a cathartic laxative and maintains ammonia in its nonabsorbable ammonium ion form
• Antibiotics with a broad spectrum against intestinal flora have been used orally, such as the nonabsorbable aminoglycoside neomycin; however, neomycin is contraindicated in GI obstruction and can be nephrotoxic. Metronidazole has been used in horses with acute colitis, but caution should be used with this drug because decreased hepatic clearance can result in neurologic signs

CONTRAINDICATIONS
Any drugs that affect the CNS must be used with caution because of the common association of hyperammonemia with hepatic encephalopathy and possibly impaired hepatic metabolism. Barbiturates and benzodiazepine-like drugs are of particular concern.

PRECAUTIONS
• Sodium bicarbonate in fluids should be administered slowly, because rapid correction of acidosis may favor intracellular ammonia movement
• Ammonia tolerance testing is contraindicated in animals with baseline hyperammonemia

POSSIBLE INTERACTIONS
Because of impaired hepatic metabolism, any drugs that inhibit metabolism by the liver or are metabolized by the liver should be used with caution or the dosage should be adjusted.

ALTERNATIVE DRUGS
N/A

FOLLOW-UP

PATIENT MONITORING
Repeated assessment of plasma ammonia can be helpful. Monitoring of serum potassium and glucose concentrations is advised in critical patients.

PREVENTION/AVOIDANCE
N/A

POSSIBLE COMPLICATIONS
Inaccuracy due to the labile nature of ammonia in blood samples. Delay in processing results in falsely elevated readings of ammonia concentration.

EXPECTED COURSE AND PROGNOSIS
Guarded prognosis for most causes of hyperammonemia.

✓ MISCELLANEOUS

ASSOCIATED CONDITIONS
N/A

AGE-RELATED FACTORS
Congenital hepatic shunts are found in young animals versus acquired shunts that may occur at various ages.

ZOONOTIC POTENTIAL
N/A

PREGNANCY/FERTILITY/BREEDING
N/A

SYNONYMS
N/A

SEE ALSO
• Bile acids
• Hepatic encephalopathy
• Icterus (prehepatic, hepatic, posthepatic)
• Toxic hepatopathy

ABBREVIATIONS
• CNS = central nervous system
• GABA = γ-aminobutyric acid
• GI = gastrointestinal

Internet Resources
Cornell University College of Veterinary Medicine, Ammonia. http://www.eclinpath.com/chemistry/liver/liver-function-tests/ammonia

Suggested Reading
Bain PJ. Liver. In: Latimer KS, ed. Duncan & Prasse's Veterinary Laboratory Medicine: Clinical Pathology, 5e. Hoboken, NJ: Wiley Blackwell, 2011:221–223.
Barton MH. Disorders of the liver. In: Reed SM, Bayly WM, Sellon DC, eds. Equine Internal Medicine, 3e. St. Louis, MO: WB Saunders, 2010:944–949.
Meyer DJ, Walton RM. The liver. In: Walton RM, ed. Equine Clinical Pathology. Ames, IA: Wiley Blackwell, 2014:71–86.

Author Claire B. Andreasen
Consulting Editor Sandra D. Taylor

AMYLASE, LIPASE, AND TRYPSIN

 BASICS

OVERVIEW
• Serum amylase or lipase concentrations above laboratory reference interval in horses are suggestive of pancreatic disease
• Pancreatic disease and panniculitis (inflammation of adipose tissue) are rare in horses
• Reference range for serum activity of amylase and lipase are <35 IU/L and <87 IU/L, respectively
• Amylase and lipase are rarely measured in routine equine serum biochemical profiles
• Trypsin is released from damaged pancreatic cells

Pathophysiology
• Amylase in blood comes from a number of sources, including intestinal mucosa, liver, and pancreas
• Amylase is cleared from the blood by the kidneys, so renal dysfunction could lead to higher concentrations remaining in the blood
• Damage to pancreatic cells can cause leakage of amylase into the blood or peritoneal fluid, but this is not common in the horse
• Lipase is derived from the pancreas, gastrointestinal mucosa, and other tissues. Clinical serum assays detect all forms of lipase
• Although uncommon in the horse, damage to pancreatic cells can cause release of lipase into the blood or peritoneal cavity
• Panniculitis can result in abnormally high serum activity of amylase and lipase. This disease is often associated with pancreatitis
• Increased activity of trypsin in blood is a result of leakage from damaged pancreatic cells, usually in horses with colic

Systems Affected
Pancreas, peritoneum, peripheral adipose tissue.

SIGNALMENT
N/A

SIGNS
Varies with underlying cause:
• Pancreatitis—colic, gastric reflux, tachycardia, and signs of hypovolemic shock
• Hyperlipemia—depression, anorexia, lipemic serum
• Panniculitis—possible colic

CAUSES AND RISK FACTORS
• Proximal duodenitis-jejunitis (proximal enteritis) enteritis
• Hyperlipemia
• Glucocorticoid administration
• Heparin-induced lipoprotein lipase activity
• Obstruction to common bile and pancreatic ducts
• Renal disease
• Pancreatitis

 DIAGNOSIS

DIFFERENTIAL DIAGNOSIS
• Colic with small intestinal distention should lead a clinician to suspect inflammation and obstruction of the small intestine rather than pancreatic inflammation, although colic and ileus can be caused by peritonitis secondary to pancreatitis
• In a pony, donkey, or miniature horse, hyperlipemia should be considered

LABORATORY FINDINGS
Drugs That May Alter Laboratory Results
N/A

Disorders That May Alter Laboratory Results
• Hemolysis inhibits lipase activity
• Lipemia falsely decreases serum lipase activity measured by kinetic assays

CBC/BIOCHEMISTRY/URINALYSIS
• Peritoneal fluid amylase and lipase activities are usually less than those in blood except in pancreatitis
• GGT is concentrated in the pancreas as well as the liver, so increased serum activity could indicate pancreatitis as well as hepatitis or cholestasis, or elevations of GGT could be secondary to the proximity of the bile duct to an inflamed pancreatic duct

OTHER LABORATORY TESTS
• Serum triglyceride >500 mg/dL indicates hyperlipemia, and can interfere with insulin's ability to inhibit hormone-sensitive lipase and thus, increase lipolysis
• Nonesterified fatty acid concentrations >0.5 mEq/L could indicate hyperlipemia due to fat mobilization and can interfere with insulin's ability to inhibit hormone-sensitive lipase, thus increasing lipolysis
• Abdominocentesis to compare peritoneal fluid amylase and lipase concentrations with serum concentrations. Peritoneal fluid concentrations of amylase and lipase greater than serum concentrations suggest pancreatitis, but this also can be a nonspecific finding of peritonitis/serositis

DIAGNOSTIC PROCEDURES
Exploratory celiotomy may be indicated in cases of colic with undiagnosed causes of continued pain or indications of small intestinal obstruction. Abdominal fluid analysis should precede this invasive procedure.

 TREATMENT
Dependent on the underlying cause.

 MEDICATIONS

DRUG(S) OF CHOICE
Dependent on the underlying cause. There is no specific treatment for pancreatitis or panniculitis in horses.

CONTRAINDICATIONS/POSSIBLE INTERACTIONS
N/A

 FOLLOW-UP

PATIENT MONITORING
• Repeat measurements of blood and peritoneal fluid amylase, lipase, and trypsin
• Observe frequently for signs of colic

POSSIBLE COMPLICATIONS
• Small intestinal obstruction, pancreatitis, and hyperlipemia can cause death
• Leakage of amylase and lipase into the peritoneal cavity can induce nonseptic peritonitis

 MISCELLANEOUS

SEE ALSO
• Acute adult abdominal pain—acute colic
• Hyperlipidemia/hyperlipemia

ABBREVIATIONS
GGT = γ-glutamyltransferase

Suggested Reading
Parry BW, Crisman MV. Serum and peritoneal fluid amylase and lipase reference values in horses. Equine Vet J 1991;23: 390–391.
Watson TD, Burns L, Love S, et al. Plasma lipids, lipoproteins and post-heparin lipases in ponies with hyperlipaemia. Equine Vet J 1992;24(5):341–346.
Yamout SZ, Nieto JE, Anderson J, et al. Pathological evidence of pancreatitis in 43 horses. Equine Vet J Suppl 2012;43:45–50.

Author Jenifer R. Gold
Consulting Editor Sandra D. Taylor
Acknowledgment The author and editor acknowledge the prior contribution of Kenneth W. Hinchcliff.

BASICS

DEFINITION
Caused by bacteria that live and grow in the absence of molecular oxygen. Facultative—growing with or without oxygen; obligate (discussed here)—growing without oxygen.

PATHOPHYSIOLOGY
Dermal and mucosal surfaces serve as protective barriers to infection. A breach in this protective barrier allows normal flora or commensal bacteria to gain access and potentially allows an infection to become established. Contamination of a wound or an injection site by environmental organisms may lead to infection. Anaerobic organisms establish invasion through virulence factors, and release of enzymes and toxins. Anaerobic infections develop primarily in body sites where there is low oxygen tension, a low redox potential, or both.

SYSTEMS AFFECTED
Upper Respiratory Tract
• Apical abscesses. • Sinusitis. • Pharyngeal abscesses

Lower Respiratory Tract
• Pneumonia. • Pulmonary abscesses. • Pleuropneumonia

GI
• Sialadenitis. • Peritonitis. • Abdominal abscesses. • Enteritis. • Colitis

Musculoskeletal
• Soft tissue abscesses. • Foot abscesses. • Thrush. • Canker. • Osteomyelitis. • Sequestra. • Septic arthritis. • Clostridial myonecrosis

Neuromuscular
Primarily affected by the toxins of these bacteria

Vascular
• Omphalophlebitis/omphalitis. • Thrombophlebitis

Hematopoietic
Sepsis

Reproductive
Metritis

Ophthalmic
• Ulcerative keratitis. • Stromal abscess

GEOGRAPHIC DISTRIBUTION
Worldwide distribution.

SIGNS
Variable depending on what system and organism is involved.

Upper Respiratory Tract
• Nasal discharge. • Facial swelling and crepitation. • Malodorous exudates

Lower Respiratory Tract
• Cough. • Nasal discharge. • Malodorous breath, pleural fluid. • Fever. • Inappetence. • Abnormal lung sounds. • Lethargy

GI
• Dysphagia. • Abdominal discomfort. • Fever. • Diarrhea. • Inappetence. • Reflux

Musculoskeletal
• Swollen and painful muscles or joints. • Lameness. • Fever. • Crepitation over swollen muscles

Vascular
• Swollen and painful umbilicus. • Fever. • Lethargy. • Inappetence. • Swollen, hard, painful veins

Hematopoietic
• Fever. • Depression. • Tachycardia, ± arrhythmias. • Tachypnea, ± dyspnea. • Mucous membrane alterations. • Laminitis. • Abdominal discomfort

Reproductive
• Vaginal discharge. • Fever. • Lethargy. • Endotoxemia

Ocular
• Blepharospasm. • Epiphora. • Corneal opacity

CAUSES
The most common bacterial species involved in anaerobic infections include: • *Bacteroides* spp. • *Clostridium* spp. • *Fusobacterium* spp. • *Peptostreptococcus* spp. • *Prevotella* spp. • *Eubacterium* spp.

RISK FACTORS
Concurrent diseases, wounds, corticosteroid therapy, antibiotic therapy, immunosuppression, leukopenia, tissue anoxia, prior or concurrent aerobic infections, presence of a foreign body.

DIAGNOSIS

DIFFERENTIAL DIAGNOSIS
Upper Respiratory Tract
• Aerobic infection (*Streptococcus* spp., *Staphylococcus* spp.). • Fungal infection (*Cryptococcus neoformans, Coccidioides immitis*). • Granuloma. • Neoplasia (anaerobes may proliferate in necrotic neoplastic tissues)

Lower Respiratory Tract
• Aerobic infection (*Streptococcus* spp., *Staphylococcus* spp., *Escherichia coli, Klebsiella, Pasteurella, Bordetella* spp.). • Fungal infection (*Coccidioides, Cryptococcus, Histoplasma, Aspergillus, Candida* spp.). • *Mycoplasma* infection. • Thoracic trauma. • Esophageal rupture. • Neoplasia

GI
• Peritonitis—aerobic infection (*Streptococcus* spp., *E. coli*), neoplasia. • Abdominal abscesses—aerobic infection (*Streptococcus* spp., *Rhodococcus equi, Corynebacterium pseudotuberculosis*), neoplasia, granuloma. • Enteritis/colitis—*Salmonella* spp., Potomac horse fever, idiopathic, parasitic, antibiotic associated, NSAID drug toxicity, fungal infection. • Sialadenitis—botulism, oral foreign body, dental disease

Musculoskeletal
• Aerobic infection (*Staphylococcus aureus, Corynebacterium pseudotuberculosis*). • Fungal infection. • Neoplasia

Vascular
Aerobic infection (*Streptococcus* spp., *E. coli, Proteus* spp.).

Hematopoietic
Aerobic infection (*Streptococcus* spp., *Staphylococcus* spp., *E. coli, Actinobacillus* spp., *Salmonella* spp., *Klebsiella* spp.).

Reproductive
• Aerobic infection (*Streptococcus zooepidemicus, E. coli, Klebsiella* spp., *Staphylococcus* spp., *Proteus* spp., *Pseudomonas* spp., *Corynebacterium* spp.). • Fungal infection (*Candida* spp.). • Neoplasia

Ocular
Other causes of ulcerative keratitis, e.g. aerobic bacteria, fungi, viruses, immune mediated.

CBC/BIOCHEMISTRY/URINALYSIS
• Inflammatory leukogram. • Hyperfibrinogenemia, increased serum amyloid A concentration. • Elevated total protein. • ± Anemia of chronic disease. • Blood chemistry is usually normal unless there is secondary systemic involvement or severe disease

OTHER LABORATORY TESTS
• Direct cytology—all aspirated fluids should be Gram stained. • Anaerobic culture—aspirates/tissue specimens must be placed in the appropriate anaerobic bacterial transport medium and stored at room temperature with minimal exposure to oxygen. • Fluorescent antibody testing. • Direct immunofluorescence testing

IMAGING
• Radiographs of the affected anatomic region revealing abscessation, fluid line, areas of consolidation, or lytic bone changes. • Sonograms of the affected anatomic region revealing gas echoes, fluid, abscessation, areas of consolidation, or masses

PATHOLOGIC FINDINGS
Lesions are characterized by necrotic, edematous, emphysematous, and hyperemic tissues. Neutrophils, monocytes, and macrophages may accumulate in the tissue architecture, with bacteria interspersed.

ANAEROBIC BACTERIAL INFECTIONS (CONTINUED)

TREATMENT

AIMS
Elimination of infection—effective antimicrobial therapy, exposure to oxygen, drainage of purulent exudates, and debridement of necrotic tissue.

APPROPRIATE HEALTH CARE
• Initial hospitalization for intensive therapy, antimicrobials, and debridement/drainage.
• Hyperbaric oxygen therapy has been anecdotally utilized in areas with extensive tissue necrosis

NURSING CARE
Care may include staged debridement, frequent hot compress therapy, and/or bandaging. Intensive care of indwelling tubes for constant drainage of body cavities may be required. Supportive care includes IV fluids and/or total/partial parenteral nutrition.

ACTIVITY
Most likely decreased or restricted and will depend on the body system affected.

CLIENT EDUCATION
Some cases may be life-threatening depending on the extent of the illness and complications may arise. In cases with severe muscle necrosis requiring debridement or fasciotomies, a cosmetic appearance may not be likely.

SURGICAL CONSIDERATIONS
Surgery may be necessary to perform fasciotomies, to debride necrotic tissue, or to graft skin on large areas that sloughed tissue during active infection. Surgery may also be required for the placement of an indwelling catheter to allow for lavage and flushing.

MEDICATIONS

DRUG(S) OF CHOICE

Penicillin
First line of defense against anaerobic infections. Excellent activity against most anaerobic infections, except beta-lactamase-producing *Bacteroides*. Preferred drug for clostridial infections. Dose 22 000–44 000 IU/kg QID IV (aqueous) or BID IM (procaine).

Ampicillin
Comparable to penicillin in its spectrum. Dose 25–100 mg/kg IV QID.

Metronidazole
Consistently effective against obligate anaerobes including *Bacteroides fragilis*; not effective against facultative anaerobes or aerobes. Rapid oral absorption (bioavailability 75–85%). Distributes well into synovial fluid, peritoneal fluid, cerebrospinal fluid, and urine; poor endometrial concentrations. Use

orally in cases of diarrhea caused by *Clostridium* spp. Per rectum to horses that are anorexic or are refluxing (bioavailability 30%). Dose 15–25 mg/kg PO, IV, or per rectum QID–TID.

Tetracyclines
Can be used for anaerobic infections but penicillin-resistant *Bacteroides* spp. are demonstrating tetracycline resistance. Dose of oxytetracycline 5–7.5 mg/kg IV BID. Doxycycline is effective against most anaerobes, but, as with oxytetracycline, resistance to *Bacteroides* spp. is common. Dose 10–20 mg/kg PO BID. Higher doses have been associated with fatal colitis.

Chloramphenicol
All obligate anaerobes are susceptible. It has good tissue penetration into central nervous system, peritoneal, pleural, and synovial fluids. Absorption decreases with repeated oral administration; the result is lower concentrations with subsequent doses. Dose 45–60 mg/kg PO TID–QID.

Cephalosporins
In general, variable efficacy against most anaerobes for both ceftiofur and cefquinome.

Rifampin (rifampicin)
Usually not necessary in most anaerobic infections but it may be useful in polymicrobial infections in walled-off abscesses. Most strains of *Bacteroides* and *Clostridium* are sensitive to rifampin. Dose 5 mg/kg PO BID.

Trimethoprim–sulfonamides (TMS)
Trimethoprim and sulfa combinations are effective against some obligate anaerobes. Activity is unpredictable. Dose 30 mg/kg BID PO.

CONTRAINDICATIONS
Static drugs such as chloramphenicol are not recommended for immunocompromised patients.

PRECAUTIONS
Chloramphenicol can cause the development of aplastic anemia rarely in humans. Oral administration of metronidazole may cause anorexia but resolves when the drug is discontinued, or with mouth washes after treatments.

POSSIBLE INTERACTIONS
Chloramphenicol may affect the metabolism of other drugs.

FOLLOW-UP

PATIENT MONITORING
Response to therapy can be noted by monitoring changes in clinical signs. Hematologic and sonographic evaluations also help to establish the patient's response to therapy.

PREVENTION/AVOIDANCE
IM injections have been reported to cause severe necrotizing myonecrosis; avoid giving these injections of irritating drugs if possible or monitor injection sites closely after administration. Provide proper and immediate treatment of wounds to help prevent anaerobic infections.

POSSIBLE COMPLICATIONS
Severe infections may result in severe tissue sloughing, laminitis, endotoxemia, or death.

EXPECTED COURSE AND PROGNOSIS
Depends on the body system affected and the severity of the disease.

MISCELLANEOUS

ASSOCIATED CONDITIONS
Depends on the body system affected and the severity of the disease.

PREGNANCY/FERTILITY/BREEDING
Infection of the reproductive tract may result in breeding and conception problems.

ZOONOTIC POTENTIAL
Bacteria can cause disease in both humans and horses, but no direct transmission is likely unless there is severe immunocompromise or contamination of an open wound.

SEE ALSO
• Botulism
• Clostridial myositis
• Tetanus

ABBREVIATIONS
• GI = gastrointestinal.
• NSAID = nonsteroidal anti-inflammatory drug

Suggested Reading
Kinoshita Y, Niwa H, Katayama Y, Hariu K. Dominant obligate anaerobes revealed in lower respiratory tract infection in horses by 16S rRNA gene sequencing. J Vet Med Sci 2014;76:587–591.
Moore RM. Diagnosis and treatment of obligate anaerobic bacterial infections in horses. Compend Contin Educ Pract Vet 1993;15(7):989–994.
Wilson DA. Management of severely infected wounds. NAVC 2006;249–251.

Author Imogen Johns
Consulting Editor Ashley G. Boyle
Acknowledgment The author and editor acknowledge the prior contribution of Shannon B. Graham.

BASICS

DEFINITION
• Anaphylactic shock is an immediate (type 1) hypersensitivity reaction that is systemic and life-threatening
• Anaphylactoid reactions, which are not a hypersensitivity, may induce similar clinical signs and outcomes

PATHOPHYSIOLOGY
• Exposure to antigens (allergens) can result in synthesis of antigen-specific IgE
• IgE binds to, and sensitizes, tissue mast cells or circulating basophils
• Reexposure to antigen results in release of substances from sensitized cells that mediate type 1 hypersensitivities and, in severe cases, anaphylaxis
• Sensitization occurs ~10 days after first exposure, but can persist for years
• Anaphylactoid reactions usually involve activation of the complement system and degranulation of mast cells or basophils. These reactions do not require previous exposure and host sensitization with IgE

SYSTEMS AFFECTED
• Shock organs of the horse are the respiratory and gastrointestinal tracts
• The skin and hemic systems may also be involved

GENETICS
High levels of IgE are associated with certain ELA-DRB haplotypes.

INCIDENCE/PREVALENCE
Prevalence unknown, but 16% of blood transfusions reported allergic reactions in one study, and 6–10% of adverse drug reactions are reported to be allergic.

SIGNALMENT
There is no breed, sex, or age predilection.

SIGNS
General Comments
Mild, moderate, or severe clinical signs may occur depending on the dose and route of antigen challenge, organ system involved, and individual inflammatory responses of the patient.

Historical Findings
Possible exposure to antigens and/or agents associated with anaphylaxis.

Physical Examination Findings
• Mild cases may present with urticaria and rhinitis; moderate cases with angioedema, diarrhea, sweating, and colic; severe reactions with dyspnea and respiratory distress, tachypnea, pulmonary emphysema, coughing, hypotension, and collapse
• Pale mucous membranes, poor peripheral pulses, and cold extremities may be associated with cardiovascular collapse

CAUSES
• A wide range of antigens or agents may induce anaphylaxis or anaphylactoid reactions
• Reactions can occur at any time, including, rarely, after the first exposure to highly charged or osmotically active agents (e.g. iodinated radiocontrast medium, dextran)
• Implicated agents include insect venom, vaccines, whole blood or blood products, antimicrobials, anthelmintics, thiamine, vitamins (B, K, E/selenium), iron, copper, halothane, thiamylal, and guaifenesin, or inadvertent injection of products, e.g. milk
• The sensitizing agent is often not identified

RISK FACTORS
• Prior exposure to potential allergens
• Previous anaphylactic reactions
• Repeated parenteral administration of the same biologic preparation at high doses

DIAGNOSIS

• Diagnosis largely based on history and classical clinical presentation
• A *rule of twos* states that reactions begin from 2 min to 2 h following injection, infusion, ingestion, contact, or inhalation
• Response to treatment may support the diagnosis

DIFFERENTIAL DIAGNOSIS
• Acute pneumonia may resemble anaphylaxis, but horses are usually more toxemic and lung changes are prominent in ventral lobes compared with widespread involvement with anaphylaxis
• An inappropriate dose or route of drug administration (such as intracarotid injection) may result in collapse associated with neurologic deficits (e.g. blindness, seizures)

CBC/BIOCHEMISTRY/URINALYSIS
Hemoconcentration, leukopenia, thrombocytopenia, hyperkalemia, increases in hepatic and myocardial enzyme activities, and coagulation deficits are reported, although diagnostic relevance is uncertain.

OTHER LABORATORY TESTS
N/A

IMAGING
N/A

OTHER DIAGNOSTIC PROCEDURES
Provocative intradermal/conjunctival challenge testing with the suspected antigen may help confirm diagnosis, but value is questionable due to high rate of false negatives and risk of inducing anaphylaxis.

PATHOLOGIC FINDINGS
• Severe, diffuse pulmonary emphysema, and peribronchiolar edema at necropsy
• Widespread petechiae, edema, and extravasation of blood in the wall of the large bowel, subcutaneous edema, congestion of

the kidney, spleen, and liver, and evidence of laminitis

TREATMENT

AIMS
Immediate steps include (1) stop exposure to trigger if possible; (2) rapid assessment of patient status; (3) secure airway and check vital parameters; and (4) perform tracheotomy if necessary (e.g. respiratory distress).

APPROPRIATE HEALTH CARE
In severe cases, early recognition of clinical signs and immediate steps are critical for patient survival.

NURSING CARE
Oxygen Therapy
• High-flow oxygen therapy is indicated during systemic anaphylaxis to help improve tissue oxygenation
• Recommended flow rates are 5–10 L/min for foals and 10–15 L/min for adults directly into the nasal passage

Fluid Therapy
• Horses that remain hypotensive following epinephrine treatment should receive fluid therapy
• Crystalloids and colloid fluids may help restore intravascular fluid volume, cardiac output, and aerobic metabolism. Careful monitoring is required to evaluate for worsening of tissue edema that accompanies anaphylaxis, especially the upper airways, lungs, and neural tissues
• Volumes of crystalloids recommended in foals is 50–80 mL/kg divided into separate bolus doses; for adults 10–20 mL/kg/h
• Hypertonic (7.2%) saline solution may also be used in adult horses exhibiting shock at 2–4 mL/kg simultaneously with crystalloid fluids
• As a general rule ~10 L of crystalloids should be provided over time for each liter of hypertonic saline

DIET
• Oral intake should be discontinued until recovery from an anaphylactic event
• Diet should be evaluated to determine if components are potential cause of anaphylactic reaction

SURGICAL CONSIDERATIONS
Nasotracheal intubation or tracheotomy if severe respiratory distress to secure the airways prior to epinephrine treatments.

MEDICATIONS

DRUG(S) OF CHOICE
• Epinephrine is the most effective treatment for systemic anaphylaxis and shock

• Epinephrine should be administered immediately upon recognition of signs, even if there is doubt, and simultaneously during patient assessment
• In adult horses, recommended dose is 0.01 mg/kg of a 1:1000 dilution slowly IV, or 0.02 mg/kg IM when dyspnea and hypotension are mild
• When IV access is not possible, a higher dose may be administered via the intratracheal route (20 ml/450 kg horse)
• In foals 0.01–0.02 mg/kg given slowly IV is recommended
• Additional medications may be considered for severe cases, or for localized reactions

Vasopressors
• Vasopressors should be considered for horses with persistent hypotension refractory to epinephrine and volume replacement
• Dobutamine (50 mg diluted in 500 mL of 5% dextrose solution; 100 μg/mL; using 5–10 μg/kg/min over 10–20 min), dopamine (titrated as a continuous infusion at 1–20 μg/kg/min), norepinephrine (0.1–1.5 μg/kg/min), and vasopressin (0.01–0.04 μg/kg/min as a constant infusion for refractory hypotension or 0.3–0.6 μg/kg as a single dose for cardiovascular collapse)
• Drugs should be titrated to maintain a mean arterial blood pressure > 60–70 mmHg
• Cardiac monitoring is recommended as arrhythmias may develop

Bronchodilators
• May be used in horses exhibiting bronchospasm resistant to epinephrine
• Inhalation therapy with β_2-agonists (e.g. albuterol) (every 3–4 h via an inhaler; 720 μg or 8 puffs at 90 μg/puff) or nebulization (2–5 mL of a 0.5% solution diluted in sterile saline)

Furosemide
Furosemide (1 mg/kg IV) is indicated in horses with pulmonary edema.

Antihistamines
• Antihistamines may be used to control clinical signs such as urticaria and pruritus
• If cardiovascular status of horse is stable doxylamine succinate (0.5 mg/kg slowly IV or IM), pyrilamine maleate (1.0 mg/kg slowly IV, IM, or SC), tripelennamine hydrochloride (1 mg/kg IM not IV), or hydroxyzine hydrochloride (1–1.5 mg/kg PO) may be administered every 6-12 h

Glucocorticoids
• Systemic glucocorticoids are not useful in the acute phase, but are indicated to halt progressive inflammation, prevent recurrence of anaphylaxis, and prevent late-phase or protracted reactions
• Dexamethasone (0.2–0.5 mg/kg IV) is used for treating rapidly progressing edema
• Prednisolone sodium succinate (0.25–10 mg/kg IV) is preferred for systemic reactions
• Prednisolone (0.4–1.6 mg/kg PO SID) may be used for managing persistent urticaria

CONTRAINDICATIONS
The use of equine plasma and dextrans is contraindicated in anaphylaxis treatment owing to concerns with induction of subsequent anaphylactic events.

PRECAUTIONS
• Epinephrine may increase the risk of arrhythmia
• Dobutamine potentiates hypoxemia-induced cardiac arrhythmias
• Glucocorticoid administration has been associated with laminitis
• If antihistamines are given, slow IV administration is recommended to avoid adverse effects

POSSIBLE INTERACTIONS
Antihistamines enhance the effects of epinephrine on vascular resistance and, therefore, should be used separately.

ALTERNATIVE DRUGS
N/A

FOLLOW UP

PATIENT MONITORING
Biphasic, multiphasic, or protracted anaphylactic episodes may occur after the primary event despite therapy.

PREVENTION/AVOIDANCE
• Avoidance of known allergens/antigens
• If avoidance is not possible, pretreatment with flunixin meglumine and antihistamines or corticosteroids and antihistamines may be warranted
• Allergen-specific IgE testing may aid in detecting sensitivity to agents and facilitate avoidance
• Desensitization procedures have not been well documented in horses
• In horses with suspected drug reactions avoid drugs with immunologic or biochemical similarity
• Oral therapy versus parenteral should be considered if drug is required

• Horses with known history of anaphylaxis should be monitored for 20–30 min after giving agents of unknown sensitivity
• Cross-matching prior to transfusions may decrease risk of anaphylaxis
• Adverse reactions to procaine penicillin G are less likely with avoidance of repeated injected sites, slow drug administration, and proper drug storage. Reaction is more likely due to the excitatory effects of unbound procaine than anaphylaxis

POSSIBLE COMPLICATIONS
Complications can include laminitis, purpura haemorrhagica, subcutaneous edema, hemolytic anemia, and hemorrhagic colitis.

EXPECTED COURSE AND PROGNOSIS
• Prognosis depends on type and severity of the event; speed of disease onset and recognition by owners/veterinarians; response to treatment; and development of complications
• Local reactions are rarely life-threatening and the prognosis will largely reflect response to treatment
• Severe systemic reactions carry a considerable risk of death
• The risk of death increases when recognition of a systemic response, or subsequent emergency treatment, is delayed

MISCELLANEOUS

ASSOCIATED CONDITIONS
None

AGE-RELATED FACTORS
N/A

ZOONOTIC POTENTIAL
None

PREGNANCY/FERTILITY/BREEDING
N/A

SYNONYMS
None

SEE ALSO
Blood and plasma transfusion reactions

ABBREVIATIONS
Ig = immunoglobulin

Suggested Reading
Radcliffe RM. Anaphylaxis. In: Felippe MJB, ed. Equine Clinical Immunology. Ames, IA: Wiley Blackwell, 2016:31–38.

Author Jennifer L. Hodgson
Consulting Editors David Hodgson, Harold C. McKenzie, and Jennifer L. Hodgson

BASICS

DEFINITION
Decreased erythrocyte count or hemoglobin content as a consequence of a decrease in PCV, RBC count, or Hb concentration.

PATHOPHYSIOLOGY
• Anemia results from 1 or more of the following:
  ◦ Blood loss (internal or external hemorrhage)
  ◦ Increased RBC destruction (intravascular or extravascular hemolysis)
  ◦ Decreased or ineffective RBC production
• Characterization of anemia (regenerative vs. nonregenerative) is best done by examining bone marrow aspirates. Serial monitoring of PCV and plasma TP concentration may be useful
  ◦ Evaluation of immature RBCs and RBC indices in peripheral blood is unrewarding in horses, even during intense erythropoiesis
• The circulating RBC mass varies due to the effects of breed, age, activity, and splenic contraction, which can increase the RBCs by ~50%
• Nonregenerative anemia occurs when the rate of erythropoiesis is insufficient to replace aged RBCs, and develops slowly due to the long lifespan of equine RBCs (≈ 150 days)
• Mechanisms associated with nonregenerative anemia include:
  ◦ Diseases interfering with erythropoiesis (↓ erythrocyte life span or ↓ erythropoietin responsiveness)
  ◦ Deficiency or alterations in substances necessary for RBC production
  ◦ Diseases that damage or displace bone marrow elements and affect RBC precursors and/or all marrow precursors

SYSTEMS AFFECTED
Decreased circulating RBC mass, decreased oxygen-carrying capacity, and reduced blood viscosity are the main consequences of anemia, but severity is dependent on the magnitude and rate of development of anemia.

GENETICS
Hereditary disorders of hemostasis may contribute to blood loss anemia.

INCIDENCE/PREVALENCE
Dependent upon etiology.

GEOGRAPHIC DISTRIBUTION
See Anemia, Heinz body.

SIGNALMENT
There is no breed, sex, or age predilection.

SIGNS
General Comments
Clinical signs relate to the compensatory mechanisms activated in response to anemia as well as the primary disease process (often more prominent).

Historical Findings
• Dependent upon primary disease process
• Most common presenting complaints are exercise intolerance, signs of depression, and inappetence

Physical Examination Findings
• Horses with chronic anemia may be subclinical, but exercise may induce exaggerated tachycardia, weakness, and reduced performance
• In acute or severe cases, tachycardia, tachypnea, and low-grade holosystolic heart murmur are present at rest
• Pale mucous membranes
• Other signs depend on the primary disease process and may include:
  ◦ Icterus, fever, and pigmenturia (hemolysis)
  ◦ Weight loss, polyuria, and polydipsia (chronic renal failure)
  ◦ Weight loss, fever, and lethargy (chronic infectious, inflammatory, neoplastic, or immune-mediated processes)

CAUSES
Hemorrhage
External hemorrhage, epistaxis, hemothorax, hematuria, hemoperitoneum, GI hemorrhage, or coagulopathy.

Hemolysis
• Immune-mediated disease (secondary immune-mediated anemia, autoimmune hemolytic anemia or NI)
• Infectious diseases (piroplasmosis, anaplasmosis, and EIA)
• Oxidant induced (red maple, phenothiazines, and wild onions)
• Iatrogenic (hypotonic or hypertonic IV solutions)
• Other toxicities (IV DMSO, heavy metal toxicosis, bacterial toxins, snake bite)
• Miscellaneous (endstage hepatic disease, hemolytic uremic syndrome, hemangiosarcoma, and disseminated intravascular coagulation)

Nonregenerative Anemia
• Anemia of chronic disease associated with infectious, inflammatory, neoplastic, or endocrine disorders
• Iron deficiency due to chronic hemorrhage or nutritional deficiency
• Bone marrow failure (myelophthisis, myeloproliferative disease, bone marrow toxins, radiation, immune mediated)
• Miscellaneous (chronic renal disease, chronic hepatic disease, or recent hemorrhage/hemolysis)

RISK FACTORS
• Dependent on risk factors for the primary disease process
• Age (e.g. neoplasia, middle uterine artery rupture) and sex (e.g. idiopathic urethral hemorrhage in geldings)
• Any infectious or inflammatory disease
• Foals consuming incompatible colostrum are at risk for NI
• Inadequate preventative anthelmintic use or long-term high-dose NSAID administration
• Geographic location for exposure to infectious agents or toxic plants

DIAGNOSIS

DIFFERENTIAL DIAGNOSIS
• Identification of the basic mechanisms involved, using historical, clinical, hematologic, and biochemical findings
• Severe hemorrhage or hemolysis should be suspected with sudden onset of clinical signs or a history of trauma
• Chronic nonregenerative anemia secondary to infectious, inflammatory, or neoplastic conditions may be associated with fever and weight loss
• Laboratory error may result in a falsely low PCV or RBC count and falsely high MCH and MCHC

CBC/BIOCHEMISTRY/URINALYSIS
• PCV, RBC count, and (except in IV hemolysis) Hb concentrations below the lower limit of reference intervals
• Reticulocytes, nucleated RBCs, Howell–Jolly bodies, polychromasia, anisocytosis, and RBC indices are less useful for classification of anemia in horses
• A moderate increase in MCV (hemolytic anemia) and red cell distribution width (hemorrhagic anemia) may occur 2–3 weeks after onset of regenerative anemia
• Increased MCH values may indicate free Hb (hemolysis) while decreased MCH, MCHC, and mean cell volume may indicate iron deficiency anemia
• Heinz bodies may be observed with hemolytic anemia due to oxidative injury
• Rouleaux formation may complicate recognition of autoagglutination in immune-mediated hemolytic anemia
• Neoplastic cells may be observed in blood smears with myeloproliferative disorders
• Severe neutropenia and thrombocytopenia may accompany myelophthisis
• Blood loss usually results in concomitant decreases in PCV and TP
• Hemolytic anemia usually results in decreased PCV, normal TP, and marked increases in serum total direct bilirubin concentration with normal liver enzymes
• Nonregenerative anemia due to inadequate erythropoiesis may be accompanied by normal or increased TP (due to increased globulin and fibrinogen concentrations) and an inflammatory leukogram

OTHER LABORATORY TESTS
• Positive direct Coombs test is evidence for immune-mediated hemolytic anemia

• Microscopic examination of blood diluted with saline (1:4) aids in differentiating autoagglutination from rouleaux formation in horses with immune-mediated hemolytic anemia

• Serum Fe concentration usually is increased, total iron-binding capacity usually decreased, and storage iron usually increased in horses with anemia of chronic disease

• Serum iron concentration, percentage saturation of transferrin, and storage iron usually are decreased, while total iron-binding capacity usually is increased in iron deficiency anemia

• Coggins or C-ELISA test for diagnosis of EIA

• Serology for *Babesia, Theileria*, or *Anaplasma phagocytophilum*

• Identification of organisms in blood smears

IMAGING

As indicated for underlying disease processes.

OTHER DIAGNOSTIC PROCEDURES

• Bone marrow aspiration and core biopsy may show increased erythropoiesis and a decreased M:E ratio in horses with regenerative anemia or may reveal decreased erythropoiesis and an increased M:E ratio with nonregenerative anemia. Infiltration with abnormal cell types may be observed in myelodysplasia or myeloproliferative disorders

• Abdominocentesis or thoracocentesis to detect internal hemorrhage

• Fecal occult blood to detect GI hemorrhage, but this test lacks sensitivity and specificity

• Endoscopy to assist in detecting respiratory or GI hemorrhage

PATHOLOGIC FINDINGS

Associated with primary disease.

TREATMENT

AIMS

Aims of therapy are identification and elimination of primary cause of anemia, nursing care, minimizing physiologic stress, ensuring adequate tissue perfusion, and administering blood transfusions if indicated.

APPROPRIATE HEALTH CARE

• Large-volume isotonic or small-volume hypertonic saline fluid therapy if there are signs of hemorrhagic shock

• Whole blood or packed RBC transfusion if PCV decreases to < 8–12%, although transfusion may be required despite higher PCV (~20%) in cases of acute blood loss

  ○ Cross-matching is strongly recommended, particularly if the patient has received previous transfusions or has been pregnant

  ○ If cross matching is not possible a known Aa/Qa-negative donor should be used, if available

  ○ If a typed donor is not available then a gelding of the same breed that has never received a transfusion may be a reasonable alternative

NURSING CARE

• Close monitoring of vital signs, serial determination of PCV and TP, and adjustment of infusion rate are essential in horses receiving fluid therapy

• Monitor for renal failure induced by hemoglobinuria or hypoxia

ACTIVITY

• Horses with lethargy, intolerance to mild exercise, or a PCV < 15% should be restricted to stall rest

• Transport of severely anemic animals may cause clinical deterioration

DIET

• Ensure access to oxidative plant toxins is eliminated

• Oral iron supplementation in horses with confirmed iron deficiency anemia (rare)

CLIENT EDUCATION

Dependent upon etiology.

SURGICAL CONSIDERATIONS

May be indicated with significant uncontrolled internal hemorrhage, although this carries a high anesthetic risk. Loss of accumulated blood may be associated with clinical deterioration—consider autotransfusion.

MEDICATIONS

DRUG(S) OF CHOICE

Specific therapy of the primary disease process.

PRECAUTIONS

• Severe reactions to transfusions may occur and necessitate careful monitoring and prompt therapy

• Hypertonic saline should be used with caution in horses with uncontrolled bleeding as it may cause increased blood loss

• Parenteral administration of iron formulations is not recommended as iron deficiency is extremely rare and serious adverse reactions may occur

FOLLOW-UP

PATIENT MONITORING

Monitor PCV to assess regenerative responses. PCV should increase by an average of 0.5–1%

per day within 3–5 days of an acute hemorrhagic or hemolytic episode.

PREVENTION/AVOIDANCE

Dependent upon etiology.

POSSIBLE COMPLICATIONS

Hypoxia-associated injury to numerous tissues and organ systems, or death in severe cases.

EXPECTED COURSE AND PROGNOSIS

Highly dependent upon the cause, severity, and rapidity of onset.

MISCELLANEOUS

ASSOCIATED CONDITIONS

Dependent upon etiology.

AGE-RELATED FACTORS

Dependent upon etiology.

PREGNANCY/FERTILITY/BREEDING

For discussion of NI, see Anemia, immune mediated

SEE ALSO

• Blood and plasma transfusion reactions

• Myeloproliferative diseases

ABBREVIATIONS

• C-ELISA = competitive enzyme-linked immunosorbent assay

• DMSO = dimethylsulfoxide

• EIA = equine infectious anemia

• GI = gastrointestinal

• Hb = hemoglobin

• MCH = mean cell hemoglobin

• MCHC = mean cell hemoglobin concentration

• M:E = myeloid-to-erythroid

• NI = neonatal isoerythrolysis

• NSAID = nonsteroidal anti-inflammatory drug

• PCV = packed cell volume

• RBC = red blood cell

• TP = total protein

Suggested Reading
Satué K, Muñoz A, Gardón JC. Interpretation of alterations in the horse erythrogram. J Hematol Res 2014;1:1–10.

Author Harold C. McKenzie

Consulting Editors David Hodgson, Harold C. McKenzie, and Jennifer L. Hodgson

Acknowledgment The author and editors acknowledge the prior contribution of Nicholas Malikedes.

BASICS

OVERVIEW
- ACD is thought to be a protective response that limits the availability of iron for bacterial growth
- ACD, or "anemia of inflammatory disease," is associated with substantial, sustained activation of the immune system
- ACD typically presents as a mild to moderate, nonregenerative, normochromic, normocytic anemia
- ACD is characterized by low serum iron concentration and low to normal TIBC with normal to increased serum ferritin concentrations
- Proinflammatory cytokines induce hepcidin production by the liver
  - Hepcidin regulates systemic iron homeostasis and decreases serum iron and total body iron stores
  - Hepcidin reduces the function of ferroportin, the primary iron transporter molecule in duodenal enterocytes and macrophages
  - This leads to impaired enteric iron absorption (enterocytes) and increased iron retention (macrophages)
  - Anemia ensues due to decreased availability of iron for Hb production (*relative* iron deficiency)
- Impaired EPO responsiveness and decreased RBC survival also result from the action of proinflammatory cytokines and contribute to the development of anemia

SIGNALMENT
- Animals with chronic inflammation
- Older animals may be at increased risk, but there is no defined age, breed, or sex predilection for ACD

SIGNS
- Often subclinical, but exercise may induce exaggerated tachycardia, weakness, and reduced performance
- Pale mucous membranes, weakness, lethargy
- Fever, weight loss, or signs referable to primary disease process may be present
- Tachycardia, tachypnea, low-grade holosystolic heart murmur

CAUSES AND RISK FACTORS
Acute and chronic inflammatory conditions, such as infection, neoplasia, autoimmune disorders, or chronic kidney diseases.

DIAGNOSIS

DIFFERENTIAL DIAGNOSIS
- Chronic anemia due to insensible blood loss (GI or urogenital)
- Iron deficiency anemia
- Anemia associated with chronic renal disease (EPO deficiency)
- Myelodysplastic or myeloproliferative disorders
- Aplastic anemia (toxins, drugs)
- Pure red cell aplasia (recombinant human EPO exposure)

CBC/BIOCHEMISTRY/URINALYSIS
- PCV, total RBC count, and Hb concentrations below the lower limit of reference intervals
- Mild to moderate normochromic, normocytic anemia that may progress to hypochromic and microcytic
- Inflammatory leukogram, increased total protein, and hyperglobulinemia may be present due to chronic antigenic stimulation

OTHER LABORATORY TESTS
Hyperfibrinogenemia and increased serum amyloid A may indicate chronic antigenic stimulation.

IMAGING
As indicated for diagnosis of primary disease.

OTHER DIAGNOSTIC PROCEDURES
- Decreased serum iron concentration (range 120–150 μg/dL)
- Normal to decreased TIBC (range 200–262 μg/dL)
- Decreased transferrin saturation (range 20–52%)
- Normal to increased serum ferritin concentration (range 152 ± 54.6 μg/dL)
- Bone marrow aspiration or core biopsy may reveal decreased erythropoiesis and increased iron storage

TREATMENT

- Directed towards resolution of the primary disease process
- Treatments that decrease the production or activity of proinflammatory cytokines may aid in decreasing hepcidin production—pentoxifylline appeared to be of benefit in some human studies
- Treatments that inhibit the activity of hepcidin show potential benefit in human patients but are not available for equine patients

MEDICATIONS

DRUG(S) OF CHOICE
- Iron supplementation has been suggested but oral administration is unlikely to be effective due to impaired GI absorption
- Parenteral iron supplementation may be of more benefit than oral supplementation but carries increased risk of iron toxicity and is not recommended
- Recombinant human EPO should not be used owing to the risk of pure red cell aplasia

CONTRAINDICATIONS/POSSIBLE INTERACTIONS
N/A

FOLLOW-UP

PATIENT MONITORING
- Monitoring as indicated for management of primary disease process
- Serial monitoring of CBC to assess PCV and red blood cell indices (mean cell hemoglobin, mean cell hemoglobin concentration, mean cell volume, RBC distribution width) for evidence of a regenerative response

PREVENTION/AVOIDANCE
Effective treatment of primary disease, where possible, is the best form of prevention.

POSSIBLE COMPLICATIONS
- Most cases are subclinical, but affected animals may be susceptible to stress or exercise-induced tachycardia and tachypnea
- More severe consequences are rare, as the anemia is typically mild to moderate in nature

EXPECTED COURSE AND PROGNOSIS
ACD is expected to resolve in conjunction with resolution of the primary disease process.

MISCELLANEOUS

SEE ALSO
Anemia

AGE-RELATED FACTORS
N/A

ABBREVIATIONS
- ACD = anemia of chronic disease
- EPO = erythropoietin
- GI = gastrointestinal
- Hb = hemoglobin
- PCV = packed cell volume
- RBC = red blood cell
- TIBC = total iron-binding capacity

Suggested Reading
Carlson GP. Anemia of inflammatory disease. In: Smith BP, ed. Large Animal Internal Medicine, 5e. St. Louis, MO: Elsevier Mosby, 2015:1068.

Author Harold C. McKenzie
Consulting Editors David Hodgson, Harold C. McKenzie, and Jennifer L. Hodgson

ANEMIA, HEINZ BODY

BASICS

DEFINITION
• Heinz bodies are small, round, blue-black, refractile aggregations of oxidized, precipitated hemoglobin, present near the margin of RBCs
• Heinz body anemia occurs as a result of exposure to certain oxidizing agents
• Heinz bodies damage the RBC membrane, resulting in lysis (intravascular hemolysis) and removal of the damaged RBCs from the circulation by the reticuloendothelial system (extravascular hemolysis)

PATHOPHYSIOLOGY
• Mild oxidative stress is associated with normal oxygen transport within RBCs
• There are protective enzyme systems in place to counteract the oxidative stress; however Heinz body hemolytic anemia can result if these systems are overwhelmed
• Denatured hemoglobin precipitates to form Heinz bodies, which attach to the RBC membrane and cause increased cell fragility with resultant intravascular or extravascular hemolysis
• Many oxidant toxins also oxidize ferrous iron (Fe^{2+}) in the hemoglobin molecule to the ferric form (Fe^{3+}), resulting in methemoglobin production. Methemoglobin decreases the oxygen-carrying capacity of the blood, resulting in tissue hypoxia

SYSTEMS AFFECTED
• Hemic/lymphatic/immune—regenerative anemia with bone marrow RBC hyperplasia and splenomegaly. Release of hemoglobin and other products of hemolysis may result in pyrexia
• Cardiovascular and respiratory—tachycardia and tachypnea, holosystolic heart murmur, mucous membrane pallor
• Renal/urologic—intravascular hemolysis may result in hemoglobinuria, hemoglobinuric nephropathy, and acute anuric renal failure
• Hepatobiliary—hyperbilirubinemia and icterus, hypoxic hepatocellular damage
• Gastrointestinal—hypoxic damage to intestines may result in motility disorders and colic
• Musculoskeletal—hypoxic damage to laminae may result in laminitis

GENETICS
N/A

INCIDENCE/PREVALENCE
Data currently unavailable.

GEOGRAPHIC DISTRIBUTION
Acer rubrum (red maple) is widespread throughout eastern and central North America.

SIGNALMENT
Can occur in horses of any breed, age, or sex.

SIGNS

Historical Findings
• Exercise intolerance or sudden onset of dullness, lethargy, inappetence, and/or colic are common presenting signs
• Acute, apparently unexplained death
• There may be history of access to wilted or dried leaves or bark of red maple (*A. rubrum*) or other oxidative toxins (e.g. phenothiazine, wild onions)

Physical Examination Findings
• Weakness, pale or icteric mucous membranes, tachypnea, tachycardia, and holosystolic heart murmur. Pyrexia may be associated with hemolysis
• With concurrent methemoglobinemia there may be muddy-brown, cyanotic mucous membranes, and brownish blood
• Pigmenturia/hemoglobinuria and oliguria (or polyuria) may occur due to hemoglobin-induced nephropathy
• Rectal examination may reveal an enlarged spleen
• Severely affected horses may develop ataxia, and death may occur

CAUSES
• Ingestion of wilted or dried red maple leaves or bark, wild or domestic onions, members of the Brassica family
• Phenothiazine, methylene blue, or acetylphenylhydrazine toxicities
• Reported in a case of lymphoma possibly due to failure of the reticuloendothelial system to remove Heinz bodies
• Reported with EIA

RISK FACTORS
• Exposure to toxins (e.g. wilted or dried red maple leaves (more likely in the fall), onions)
• Lymphoma
• EIA infection
• When RBCs from a Saddlebred colt with glucose-6-phosphate dehydrogenase deficiency were exposed to acetylphenylhydrazine, more and smaller Heinz bodies were produced
• Thin horses may be at greater risk of phenothiazine toxicosis
• Selenium deficiency results in decreased glutathione peroxidase (involved in RBC counteraction of oxidative stress) and, therefore, may contribute to Heinz body formation
• Equine RBCs have less developed protective mechanisms to reverse the oxidation of hemoglobin

DIAGNOSIS

DIFFERENTIAL DIAGNOSIS
• Causes of anemia include hemorrhage, hemolysis, and decreased RBC production
• Hemorrhage is usually easily differentiated based on history and physical examination

findings. Hemorrhage is usually also associated with hypoalbuminemia as well as anemia (after the initial 12 h), which is not a feature of hemolysis
• Anemia of chronic inflammation may be associated with inflammatory, infectious, or neoplastic disorders, e.g. lymphosarcoma (usually a more complex history and other clinical signs associated with affected organ system) or purpura haemorrhagica (usually a history of respiratory disease)
• Horses with immune-mediated hemolytic anemia will be positive on flow cytometry for erythrocyte-bound immunoglobulins and may have a positive Coombs test (poor sensitivity)
• EIA cases will have a positive Coggins or C-ELISA test
• Piroplasmosis cases may have intracellular organisms on Giemsa- or new methylene blue-stained blood smears and/or be seropositive or seroconvert on convalescent titer
• Cases of anaplasmosis may have intracytoplasmic inclusion bodies in neutrophils on Giemsa-stained blood smears and/or a positive PCR result
• Envenomation and heavy metal toxicosis (e.g. chronic consumption of lead, copper, or selenium) must be differentiated based on history of exposure
• Familial methemoglobinemia has been described in Standardbreds
• Nitrate/nitrite toxicity can be differentiated based on history of exposure

CBC/BIOCHEMISTRY/URINALYSIS
• Variable anemia; PCV is often <20%
• Direct blood smears may reveal eccentrocytes, RBC fragments, and anisocytosis
• An inflammatory leukogram may be present (neutrophilia is common)
• Increased mean corpuscular hemoglobin reflects hemoglobinemia associated with intravascular hemolysis
• Biochemical abnormalities usually include increased total and indirect bilirubin, azotemia (associated with hemoglobinuric nephropathy), and increased hepatic enzyme activity (associated with hypoxic injury to the liver)
• Urinalysis may reveal bilirubinuria, hemoglobinuria (no microscopic hematuria), methemoglobinuria, and proteinuria

OTHER LABORATORY TESTS
• Heinz bodies will be visualized on crystal violet or new methylene blue-stained smears. Initially, a very high percentage of RBCs have Heinz body inclusions but later, as these are removed from the circulation, the number of affected cells decreases
• Increased RBC osmotic fragility
• Bone marrow aspiration may reveal a regenerative response with an myeloid to erythroid ratio <0.5

- Co-oximetry can be performed to ascertain methemoglobin content (normal is ≤1.77%)

IMAGING
Splenic/hepatic ultrasonography may be used to detect splenic/hepatic enlargement—may appear hyperechoic or hypoechoic with some loss of architecture due to increased fluid component.

OTHER DIAGNOSTIC PROCEDURES
A thorough diagnostic workup is indicated to ascertain underlying etiology.

PATHOLOGIC FINDINGS
- Gross—pale or icteric tissues, enlarged liver and spleen, renal congestion, possible signs of congestive heart failure
- Histopathology—renal tubular nephrosis with hemoglobin casts, centrilobular hepatic degeneration and necrosis, and phagocytized RBCs and hemosiderin in the spleen and liver

TREATMENT
APPROPRIATE HEALTH CARE
- In-hospital medical management may be necessary depending on the severity of the anemia and associated clinical signs
- Activated charcoal and mineral oil should be administered via nasogastric intubation to reduce further absorption of toxin
- IV fluid therapy with isotonic crystalloids should be initiated to improve perfusion, prevent hemoglobin-induced nephropathy, and promote diuresis (however excessive hemodilution should be avoided)
- Cross-matched blood or packed RBC transfusion should be considered if PCV decreases to <8–12%, or if there is persistent tachycardia, tachypnea, weak pulse pressure, or a poor response to isotonic fluid therapy
- Oxygen therapy is ineffective if oxygen-carrying capacity is decreased owing to methemoglobinemia

NURSING CARE
Close monitoring of vital signs, IV fluid rates (to avoid excessive hemodilution), CBC/biochemistry, urine output, and renal function is recommended.

ACTIVITY
Exercise and stress should be avoided to prevent increased oxygen demand.

DIET
Palatable and nutritious feeds should be provided to encourage voluntary intake.

CLIENT EDUCATION
Clients should be warned of the hazards of exposure to wilted red maple leaves (including red maple hybrids) and other toxins.

SURGICAL CONSIDERATIONS
Anemia and methemoglobinemia put these cases at increased anesthetic risk and therefore surgery should be postponed if possible (or blood transfusion may be required before an emergency procedure).

MEDICATIONS
DRUG(S) OF CHOICE
Treatment is largely supportive, as there is no specific therapy.

CONTRAINDICATIONS
- Methylene blue therapy may exacerbate Heinz body formation and has been associated with decreased survival
- Corticosteroid use has also been associated with decreased survival

PRECAUTIONS
N/A

POSSIBLE INTERACTIONS
N/A

ALTERNATIVE DRUGS
Vitamin C (ascorbic acid) (30 mg/kg twice daily, diluted in IV fluids) has been used for methemoglobin-associated conditions (no proven efficacy).

FOLLOW-UP
PATIENT MONITORING
- The PCV should be monitored closely and should remain stable or slowly increase over time (reflective of bone marrow regeneration and therapeutic response)
- Renal function and urine output should also be monitored, as well as for signs of laminitis

PREVENTION/AVOIDANCE
- Limiting access to potential toxins including wilted red maple leaves and onions
- Minimizing use of phenothiazines or, if absolutely necessary, attempt to use the minimum effective dose

POSSIBLE COMPLICATIONS
- Laminitis
- Nephropathy/renal failure
- Abortion, weak foals
- Coma and death

EXPECTED COURSE AND PROGNOSIS
- Prognosis is variable depending on the severity of the anemia and whether or not there is concurrent methemoglobinemia
- Horses with red maple toxicity have a guarded to poor prognosis, with a 60% fatality rate

MISCELLANEOUS
ASSOCIATED CONDITIONS
- Methemoglobinemia
- Pigment nephropathy

AGE-RELATED FACTORS
N/A

ZOONOTIC POTENTIAL
N/A

PREGNANCY/FERTILITY/BREEDING
Pregnant mares may abort or deliver a weak foal.

SYNONYMS
- Oxidant-induced hemolysis
- Oxidative hemoglobinemia

SEE ALSO
- Anemia
- Anemia, immune mediated
- Infectious anemia (EIA)
- Methemoglobin

ABBREVIATIONS
- C-ELISA = competitive enzyme-linked immunosorbent assay
- EIA = equine infectious anemia
- PCR = polymerase chain reaction
- PCV = packed cell volume
- RBC = red blood cell

Suggested Reading
Alward A, Corriher CA, Barton MH, et al. Red maple (*Acer rubrum*) leaf toxicosis in horses: a retrospective study of 32 cases. J Vet Intern Med 2006;20:1197–1201.
Carlson GP, Aleman A. Heinz body hemolytic anemia. In: Smith BP, ed. Large Animal Internal Medicine, 5e. St. Louis, MO: Elsevier Mosby, 2015:1062–1064.

Author Rana Bozorgmanesh
Consulting Editors David Hodgson, Harold C. McKenzie, and Jennifer L. Hodgson
Acknowledgment The author and editors acknowledge the prior contribution of Nicholas Malikides.

ANEMIA, IMMUNE MEDIATED

BASICS

DEFINITION
IMHA is a destruction of RBCs associated with immunoglobulin and/or complement attachment to either RBC antigens or foreign antigens coating the surface of RBCs.

PATHOPHYSIOLOGY
• Can be primary or secondary (most common)
• Primary IMHA occurs when the immune system produces specific autoantibodies to normal erythrocyte antigens (includes NI, or transfusion reaction)
• Secondary IMHA most commonly occurs as a result of agents that:
 ◦ Alter the RBC membrane, exposing antigens to which the host produces antibody (e.g. infectious agents, neoplasia)
 ◦ Form immune complexes that adsorb to the RBC and fix complement (e.g. infectious agents)
 ◦ Directly bind to the RBC and act as haptens that bind antibody (e.g. drugs)
 ◦ Stimulate the immune system, resulting in production of antibodies with cross-reactivity to RBCs (e.g. infectious agents, neoplasia)
• Antibody- and/or complement-coated RBCs are removed from the circulation by extravascular hemolysis (if removed by the reticuloendothelial system) and/or intravascular hemolysis (if complement mediated)

SYSTEMS AFFECTED
• Hemic/lymphatic/immune
• Cardiovascular/respiratory
• Hepatobiliary
• Renal
• Gastrointestinal

GENETICS
Foals born to multiparous dams known to be RBC antigen Aa or Qa negative are at increased risk of developing NI.

INCIDENCE/PREVALENCE
• Unknown
• Weak anecdotal evidence suggests IMHA is a rare consequence of other disease states in adult horses
• NI is reported in foals in most countries

GEOGRAPHIC DISTRIBUTION
N/A

SIGNALMENT
Any breed, age, or sex.

SIGNS
General Comments
Signs often reflect the primary, underlying disease process such as infection or neoplasia.
Historical Findings
• History generally reflects an underlying disease process and may include chronic

weight loss (e.g. neoplastic diseases) or signs of depression and inappetence (e.g. infectious diseases)
• Exercise intolerance, weakness, and lethargy
• There may be a history of exposure to blood transfusion(s) or certain drugs (typically in the previous 5–12 days)

Physical Examination Findings
• Signs of anemia—proportional to the degree of anemia
• Exercise intolerance, weakness, pale or icteric mucous membranes, fever, tachypnea, tachycardia, holosystolic heart murmur, abdominal pain, and hemoglobinuria
• Foals with NI typically present with acute-onset weakness and icterus during the first few days of life
• Severe debilitation and death may occur

CAUSES
Primary Immune Mediated
• NI
• Autoimmune hemolytic anemia
• Incompatible blood transfusion

Secondary Immune Mediated
• Infectious—e.g. acute viral infections, EIA, *Clostridium perfringens*, *Rhodococcus equi*, or streptococcal organisms
• Neoplastic—e.g. lymphoma
• Drug associated—e.g. penicillins, trimethoprim–sulfamethoxazole, and potentially cephalosporins, rifampin (rifampicin), chloramphenicol and various NSAIDs

RISK FACTORS
• Foals born to multiparous dams that have previously had a blood transfusion(s), or the mare is RBC antigen Aa or Qa negative, are at increased risk of developing NI
• Exposure to incompatible blood transfusion and certain drugs

DIAGNOSIS

DIFFERENTIAL DIAGNOSIS
• Other diseases causing anemia
• Hemorrhage (acute or chronic)
• Heinz body anemia

CBC/BIOCHEMISTRY/URINALYSIS
• PCV is often <0.20 L/L (<20%)
• May have neutrophilic leukocytosis
• RBC autoagglutination:
 ◦ May be observed due to the presence of antibodies and/or complement on the surface of the RBCs
 ◦ Must be distinguished from rouleaux formation. "In saline" agglutination test can be used to differentiate—place one drop of blood on slide, add 0.9% saline as 1:4 with blood. Normal RBCs disperse evenly on the slide, while agglutination results in clumping of cells
 ◦ Spherocytes may be observed in blood smears, but are more difficult to identify in

horses owing to the lack of central pallor in normal equine RBCs
• Increased mean corpuscular hemoglobin suggests intravascular hemolysis, which may also result in discolored plasma
• Increased serum total bilirubin concentration (indirect greater than direct)
• Bilirubinuria and hemoglobinuria may be observed in the rarer cases when intravascular hemolysis occurs

OTHER LABORATORY TESTS
• Positive direct antiglobulin (Coombs) test (detects presence of antibody on the surface of RBCs). False-negative results are possible, particularly if there has been prior corticosteroid therapy. False-positive results also can occur, emphasizing the need to use multiple methods to confirm the diagnosis of IMHA
• RBC osmotic fragility may be increased in IMHA, although this test can be positive with RBCs damaged by oxidant insults
• Bone marrow aspiration reveals a diffuse, regenerative erythron (myeloid to erythroid ratio is <0.5)
• Infectious causes of IMHA may have positive serology and/or evidence of hematologic parasites on direct or special stained blood smears:
 ◦ Horses with EIA will be seropositive for virus on Coggins or C-ELISA tests
 ◦ Horses with equine piroplasmosis may have organisms observed in Giemsa- or new methylene blue-stained blood smears, be seropositive or seroconvert on their convalescent titer, or be positive via PCR
 ◦ Horses with equine granulocytic ehrlichiosis may have granular inclusion bodies observed in cytoplasm of neutrophils in Giemsa-stained blood smears, be seropositive or seroconvert with acute and convalescent samples, or be positive via PCR

IMAGING
No specific imaging findings would be expected for IMHA itself—abnormalities identified are related to the original disease process.

OTHER DIAGNOSTIC PROCEDURES
A thorough diagnostic workup should be performed to rule out neoplasia and infectious causes of secondary IMHA.

PATHOLOGIC FINDINGS
• Necropsy findings may include an enlarged liver and spleen and pale or icteric tissues
• Findings referable to the initial disease process

TREATMENT
AIMS
• Treatment of IMHA involves identification and resolution (if possible) of any underlying

infection or disease, reduction of the immune response, and provision of supportive care
• Administration of any drugs should be discontinued as IMHA could be caused by an adverse drug reaction. If antimicrobial therapy is required, a molecularly dissimilar antibiotic should be used

APPROPRIATE HEALTH CARE
• Most cases of IMHA are treated in hospitals, especially if severe
• Balanced polyionic IV fluid therapy may be indicated to expand vascular volume if volume depleted, and to induce diuresis if significant hemoglobinuria is present
• Emergency medical therapy with cross-matched blood transfusion is indicated if there is evidence of tissue hypoxia (PCV < 8–12%). In foals, washed RBCs from the dam or appropriate blood-typed blood is optimal

NURSING CARE
• Serial analysis of PCV in order to monitor response to therapy should be performed
• Close monitoring of vital signs and adjustment of fluid rate is essential in horses receiving fluid therapy
• In foals with NI, provide adequate warmth and hydration, avoid stress, and confine mare and foal to restrict activity

ACTIVITY
Minimize or eliminate activity, but allow the animal access to fresh air and sunshine if possible.

DIET
• Make efforts to keep the horse eating a balanced diet, with good quality hay and grain
• Fresh water should be available ad libitum

CLIENT EDUCATION
• Clients should be made aware that horses with primary (or autoimmune) IMHA often require long-term corticosteroid therapy
• If an infectious cause is not identified, neoplasia is highly suspected, and the prognosis will be related to the neoplasia, rather than the IMHA
• Corticosteroid administration may be associated with the development of laminitis
• Clients should be educated in preventative measures for NI

SURGICAL CONSIDERATIONS
None

MEDICATIONS

DRUG(S) OF CHOICE
• In adults, corticosteroids (dexamethasone 0.1 mg/kg IV or IM every 24 h) are indicated until PCV ceases to decline. The dose may

then be decreased by 0.01 mg/kg/day until the total dose is 20 mg/day (for a 500 kg horse), after which alternate-day oral prednisolone is recommended. Alternatively, oral prednisolone (1 mg/kg) may be used in place of dexamethasone at any time during therapy, although anecdotally dexamethasone is more efficacious
• From 4 to 7 days often are needed for corticosteroids to have a therapeutic effect (with stabilization of PCV) and up to 10 weeks of treatment may be necessary
• Horses without clinical signs of anemia may not need immunosuppressive therapy if the initiating cause can be effectively treated

CONTRAINDICATIONS
Corticosteroids may exacerbate underlying infectious diseases so should be used only in horses that are EIA (Coggins) negative.

PRECAUTIONS
• Cross-match before blood transfusion
• Corticosteroid therapy may predispose horses to laminitis and should be used with caution in pregnant mares

POSSIBLE INTERACTIONS
N/A

ALTERNATIVE DRUGS
The immunosuppressive agent azathioprine (3 mg/kg PO once daily) has been used in horses nonresponsive to corticosteroids, or when corticosteroids were contraindicated (e.g. the development of laminitis).

FOLLOW-UP

PATIENT MONITORING
PCV should be carefully monitored during dexamethasone treatment. The frequency of dexamethasone administration can be increased to twice daily in horses initially on once a day treatment if the PCV does not stabilize within 24–48 h.

PREVENTION/AVOIDANCE
• Avoid drugs known to have caused secondary IMHA
• Provide alternate colostrum source in foals born to mares at risk of NI

POSSIBLE COMPLICATIONS
• Pigment nephropathy secondary to intravascular hemolysis
• Laminitis

EXPECTED COURSE AND PROGNOSIS
• If the primary cause can be identified and successfully treated, the prognosis for IMHA is good
• Red cell numbers recover as the immune-mediated response resolves, but may take several weeks

• Horses requiring constant corticosteroid treatment may have an incurable underlying disease such as neoplasia (e.g. lymphoma) or have true autoimmune hemolytic anemia. The prognosis for survival in these horses is poor

MISCELLANEOUS

ASSOCIATED CONDITIONS
• Pigment nephropathy
• Laminitis

AGE-RELATED FACTORS
• All ages can be affected
• Foals with NI will develop signs within the first few days of life

PREGNANCY/FERTILITY/BREEDING
Use corticosteroids cautiously in pregnant mares.

SYNONYMS
• Autoimmune hemolytic anemia
• Immune-mediated hemolytic disease

SEE ALSO
• Anemia
• Neonatal isoerythrolysis

ABBREVIATIONS
• C-ELISA = competitive–enzyme-linked immunosorbent assay
• EIA = equine infectious anemia
• IMHA = immune-mediated hemolytic anemia
• NI = neonatal isoerythrolysis
• NSAID = nonsteroidal anti-inflammatory drug
• PCV = packed cell volume
• PCR = polymerase chain reaction
• RBC = red blood cell

Suggested Reading
Kendall A, Pringle J. Immune-mediated haemolytic anaemia: drug induced or not? Equine Vet Educ 2014;26:234–236.
Sellon DC. Disorders of the hematopoietic system. In: Reed SM, Bayly WM, Sellon DC, eds. Equine Internal Medicine, 3e. St. Louis, MO: WB Saunders, 2010:730–776.

Author Imogen Johns
Consulting Editors David Hodgson, Harold C. McKenzie, and Jennifer L. Hodgson
Acknowledgment The author and editors acknowledge the prior contribution of Nicholas Malikides.

 Client Education Handout available online

A

ANEMIA, IRON DEFICIENCY

BASICS

OVERVIEW
• Iron deficiency results from chronic external loss of blood (adult horses) or dietary deprivation (usually young foals). Unless adult horses lack access to soil, pasture, or feed, inadequate Fe intake is unlikely
• Iron deficiency impairs Hb synthesis, impairs RBC maturation, and leads to anemia
• Anemia and reduced blood Hb concentration may compromise tissue oxygen delivery

SIGNALMENT
• No breed or sex predilection
• Rapid growth of foals is associated with high Fe demands. Mare's milk has low Fe concentrations and therefore deficiency may occur in foals with limited access to pasture, Fe-rich soils, forage, or grain

SIGNS
• Clinical signs may be absent or mild due to physiologic compensation
• Lethargy and exercise intolerance may be the first signs noted
• When PCV drops below 12%, tissue hypoxia can cause tachycardia, tachypnea, and signs of depression. Pale mucous membranes will be present, and a systolic heart murmur may be noted

CAUSES AND RISK FACTORS
Risk factors for chronic hemorrhage include inadequate anthelmintic use, NSAID administration, and toxin exposure.

Chronic, Low-Grade Hemorrhage
• Severe internal or external parasitism
• Bleeding gastrointestinal, respiratory, and urogenital lesions (e.g. gastroduodenal ulcers, NSAID toxicosis, neoplasia, hemorrhagic cystitis, guttural pouch mycosis, and ethmoid hematoma)
• Coagulopathies leading to chronic blood loss (e.g. heritable coagulopathies, warfarin toxicosis, moldy sweet clover)

Diet
Inadequate dietary Fe intake (foals).

DIAGNOSIS

DIFFERENTIAL DIAGNOSIS
• Causes of low-grade, hemolytic anemia include immune-mediated, oxidant-induced, and parasite-induced hemolysis
• Causes of decreased RBC production include anemia of chronic disease and aplastic anemia

CBC/BIOCHEMISTRY/URINALYSIS
• Initial normochromic, normocytic anemia may progress to a microcytic, hypochromic, nonregenerative anemia. Microcytosis often precedes hypochromasia
• Thrombocytosis may be observed
• Decreased plasma protein and albumin concentrations are typical with chronic hemorrhage

OTHER LABORATORY TESTS
Initial Stage
• Decreased stainable Fe in marrow macrophages
• Decreased serum ferritin concentration (reference range 152 ± 54.6 μg/dL) with serum ferritin < 45 ng/mL highly indicative of Fe deficiency

Later Stages
• Decreased serum iron concentration (reference range 120–150 μg/dL)
• Normal or increased TIBC (reference range 200–262 μg/dL)
• Decreased transferrin saturation (reference range 20–52%) with values < 16% reflecting insufficient iron available for erythropoiesis
• Decreased mean cell volume with decreased hemoglobin concentration (mean cell hemoglobin concentration)
• Serum iron, serum ferritin, and TIBC may be affected by conditions other than Fe deficiency including acute and chronic inflammation, renal disease, and corticosteroid therapy

IMAGING
N/A

OTHER DIAGNOSTIC PROCEDURES
• Bone marrow cytology may show predominant late rubricytes and metarubricytes, depletion of macrophage iron, and sideroblasts
• Diagnostic workup of causes of chronic hemorrhage is indicated

TREATMENT
• Horses with lethargy, intolerance to mild exercise, or a PCV < 15% should be restricted to stall rest
• Blood transfusion is rarely necessary unless PCV drops below 8% or there are clinical and laboratory signs of tissue hypoxia

MEDICATIONS

DRUG(S) OF CHOICE
• Appropriate treatment of causes of chronic blood loss
• Oral ferrous sulfate (1 g/450 kg body weight) is the safest Fe supplement
• Iron cacodylate (1 g/adult horse) may be given slowly IV, but must be used with caution owing to the possibility of anaphylaxis

CONTRAINDICATIONS/POSSIBLE INTERACTIONS
• Do not use iron dextrans because of idiosyncratic reactions (anaphylaxis and sudden death)
• Iatrogenic iron overload has been reported in adult horses
• Do not give foals iron-containing products during the first 2 days of life as fatal hepatopathies may occur

FOLLOW-UP

PATIENT MONITORING
• Monitor serum iron, TIBC, and percentage saturation at ≈2 week intervals
• Discontinue iron supplementation when values for PCV, serum iron, TIBC, and % saturation return to reference ranges

PREVENTION/AVOIDANCE
Nursing foals should have access to pasture and, when appropriate, forage and grain.

POSSIBLE COMPLICATIONS
May result in death if affected animals are left untreated.

EXPECTED COURSE AND PROGNOSIS
Prolonged iron supplementation may be required.

MISCELLANEOUS

AGE-RELATED FACTORS
Foals are at increased risk owing to high iron demands and limited dietary intake.

SEE ALSO
Anemia, chronic disease

ABBREVIATIONS
• Hb = hemoglobin
• NSAID = nonsteroidal anti-inflammatory drug
• PCV = packed cell volume
• RBC = red blood cell
• TIBC = total iron-binding capacity

Suggested Reading
Satué K, Muñoz A, Gardón JC. Interpretation of alterations in the horse erythrogram. J Hematol Res 2014;1:1–10.

Author Harold C. McKenzie
Consulting Editors David Hodgson, Harold C. McKenzie, and Jennifer L. Hodgson

Acknowledgment The author and editors acknowledge the prior contribution of Nicholas Malikedes.

BASICS

DEFINITION
Failure of mare to show estrus. Can be physiologic or pathologic.

PATHOPHYSIOLOGY
Mares are seasonally polyestrus with the ovulatory period in spring/summer; primarily regulated by photoperiod:
- Increasing day length decreases melatonin secretion (pineal gland), allowing increased production and release of GnRH, stimulating gonadotropin release (FSH and LH)
  - FSH promotes folliculogenesis
  - D_2 dopamine likely regulates ovarian function locally
- When sufficient LH is produced by dominant follicle(s), ovulation occurs, initiating cyclicity
- Average estrous cycle is 21 days; defined as the interval between 2 ovulations with progesterone > 1 ng/mL. Repeatable in individual mares
- Key hormonal events of equine estrous cycle:
  - FSH causes follicular growth
  - Follicular E_2 stimulates increased GnRH pulse frequency and LH secretion
  - LH surge causes ovulation
  - P_4 (CL origin) rises from basal levels (<1 ng/mL) at ovulation to > 4 ng/mL by 4–5 days post ovulation
  - A second FSH surge in diestrus initiates another follicular wave
  - Endometrial $PGF_{2\alpha}$ is released 14–15 days post ovulation causing luteolysis and decline in P_4 levels

SYSTEMS AFFECTED
- Reproductive
- Endocrine
- Behavioral

SIGNS

Historical Findings
- Chief complaint—failure of mare to show estrus or accept stallion
- Inadequate teasing
- Seasonal influences
- Reproductive history—estrous cycle length, teasing response, prior breeding/foaling data, previous genital tract injuries/infections
- Pharmaceuticals interfering with normal estrous cycle

Physical Examination Findings
- Poor body condition/malnutrition or metabolic disease (PPID)
- Poor perineal conformation can result in pneumovagina, ascending infections and/or urine pooling, anestrus/infertility
- Clitoral enlargement may relate to drug history (anabolic steroids) or intersex conditions
- TRP and US are essential for evaluation. Rule out pregnancy. Assess uterine size/tone, ovarian size/shape/location, and cervical

relaxation. Serial TRP and US may be needed to completely define status
- Vaginal speculum examination to identify inflammation, urine pooling, cervical competency, conformational abnormalities

CAUSES

Normal Physiologic
- Winter anestrus—≈30% of mares cycle year-round; most enter a period of anestrus
- 2 transitional phases occur yearly—fall transition (ovulatory to anestrus) and vernal transition (anestrus to cyclicity). Behavior and ovarian activity varies during transition
- Behavioral anestrus (silent heat)—mare has normal cycle but fails to demonstrate estrus
- Pregnancy
- Persistent endometrial cups—early embryonic death after formation of endometrial cups results in persistent CL activity
  - eCG (by endometrial cups, 35–150 days of pregnancy) is luteotropic, maintaining primary CL and formation of secondary CLs
- Postpartum anestrus—most mares reestablish cyclicity ≤ 20 days postpartum. Some fail to continue cycling after their first postpartum ovulation, due to ovarian factors, seasonal factors (foaling late in winter without artificial light supplementation), or lactational anestrus/poor body condition
- Age—puberty occurs at 12–24 months and mares > 25 years may develop ovarian senescence

Congenital Abnormalities
- Gonadal dysgenesis—no functional ovarian tissue; can result in anestrus, erratic estrus, or prolonged estrus
  - Behavioral estrus may be due to adrenal-origin steroid production and absence of progesterone
  - Typically flaccid, infantile uterus, hypoplastic endometrium, small, nonfunctional ovaries
  - Most common chromosomal defect—XO monosomy; most common intersex condition—XY sex reversal

Endocrine Disorders
- PPID—destruction of FSH/LH-secreting cells and/or overproduction of glucocorticoids
- Increased adrenal-origin androgens can suppress normal hypothalamic–pituitary–ovarian axis

Ovarian Abnormalities
- Ovarian hematoma, hemorrhagic anovulatory follicle, or ovarian abscess
- Ovarian neoplasia (most common—GTCT)

Uterine Abnormalities
Pyometra—can prevent formation and release of $PGF_{2\alpha}$, prolonging diestrus.

Iatrogenic/Pharmacologic
- GnRH vaccination—prevents ovarian activity

- Bilateral ovariectomy—although up to 30% of mares show constant estrus
- Drugs causing behavioral anestrus:
  - Anabolic steroids
  - Progesterone/progestins—inhibition of estrus behavior
  - Oxytocin treatment to prolong CL lifespan
- Placement of intrauterine marbles to prolong CL lifespan

RISK FACTORS
Foaling in late winter; poor body condition at foaling.

DIAGNOSIS

DIFFERENTIAL DIAGNOSIS

Differentiating Causes
- Review history/breeding/foaling records—medical/reproductive history, teasing methods
- Physical examination, serial TRP and US to determine reproductive status, cyclicity, uterine/ovarian abnormalities
- Vaginal examination

OTHER LABORATORY TESTS
- Serum progesterone
  - Basal < 1 ng/mL
- GTCT panel
  - Nonpregnant mare—AMH < 3.8 ng/mL, inhibin < 0.7 ng/mL, testosterone 20–45 pg/mL
  - GTCT if AMH > 8.0 ng/mL, inhibin > 0.7 ng/mL, testosterone 100 pg/mL
- Serum eCG—diagnosis of persistent endometrial cups
- PPID testing
- Karyotype

IMAGING
Transrectal US of reproductive tract. Hysteroscopy to diagnose uterine abnormalities.

OTHER DIAGNOSTIC PROCEDURES
Uterine cytology/culture/biopsy for diagnosis, treatment, and to monitor progression of pyometra/endometritis.

TREATMENT
- Alter management/teasing techniques to elicit a response from a mare and/or base timing of artificial insemination on TRP and US
- Advancement of the vernal transition:
  - Artificial lighting—expose mare to 14.5–16 h light/day or to additional 1–2 h light at 10 h after dusk (flash lighting). Duration of transition remains unchanged. Minimum of 60–90 days is needed to achieve cyclicity

○ Pharmaceuticals—combinations of FSH, dopamine antagonists, and P_4/E_2
• Mare due to foal in late winter—add supplemental lighting 2 months prior to parturition to improve postpartum cyclicity and decrease potential for anestrus
• Ovarian tumors
    ○ Removal of GTCT removes inhibin suppression of contralateral ovary, allowing cyclicity, often with longer interovulatory period. The time to cycle is affected by season:
        ▪ If in winter, following the solstice, cyclicity resumes as day length increases
        ▪ If in spring or summer, cyclicity may not resume until fall and significant decreases in day length
    ○ Some mares fail to cycle again
• Pyometra/endometritis—specific intrauterine therapies based on diagnostic testing

MEDICATIONS

DRUG(S) OF CHOICE
• To induce luteolysis:
    ○ $PGF_{2\alpha}$ (Lutalyse 10 mg IM) or analogs
• To induce ovulation in estrus:
    ○ Deslorelin 1.8 mg IM—ovulation usually within 48 h if follicle(s) > 30 mm
    ○ hCG 2500 IU IV—ovulation within 48 h if follicle(s) > 35 mm
• To hasten vernal transition:
    ○ Altrenogest (0.044 mg/kg PO daily ≥ 15 days) if follicles > 20 mm are present and mare is exhibiting behavioral estrus. $PGF_{2\alpha}$ is given on day 15
    ○ Combination P_4/E_2 treatments followed by $PGF_{2\alpha}$ are also used
    ○ Dopamine antagonists—domperidone 1.1 mg/kg PO daily or sulpiride 1.0 mg/kg or 200 mg/mare IM daily; often used in combination with artificial photoperiod

CONTRAINDICATIONS
$PGF_{2\alpha}$ and analogs—contraindicated with equine asthma/bronchoconstrictive disease.

PRECAUTIONS
• Horses:
    ○ $PGF_{2\alpha}$ causes sweating/colic-like symptoms due to stimulation of smooth muscle
    ○ Symptomatic treatment is recommended if it fails to resolve in 1–2 h

○ Antibodies to hCG can develop. Limit use to < 2 or 3 times per breeding season
○ Deslorelin implants are associated with FSH suppression in diestrus with prolonged interovulatory period in nonpregnant mares
○ Progesterone supplementation can decrease uterine clearance; use may be contraindicated in mares with a history of uterine infection
• Humans:
    ○ $PGF_{2\alpha}$ should not be handled by pregnant women or persons with asthma/bronchial disease
    ○ Altrenogest should not be handled by pregnant women or persons with thrombophlebitis, thromboembolic disorders, cerebrovascular/coronary artery disease, breast cancer, estrogen-dependent neoplasia, undiagnosed vaginal bleeding, or tumors that developed with use of oral contraceptives or estrogen-containing products

ALTERNATIVE DRUGS
Cloprostenol sodium (Estrumate 250 µg/mL IM) is a $PGF_{2\alpha}$ analog. This product is used in similar fashion to natural $PGF_{2\alpha}$ and has been associated with fewer side effects. Not currently approved for use in horses.

FOLLOW-UP

PATIENT MONITORING
• Serial TRP and US—establish diagnosis for etiology of anestrus
• Mares with persistent endometrial cups will return to cyclicity upon regression of endometrial cups, as eCG decreases (up to 150 days post ovulation)

POSSIBLE COMPLICATIONS
Infertility may result from intractable persistent anestrus.

MISCELLANEOUS

AGE-RELATED FACTORS
Postpartum anestrus occurs more often in old mares.

PREGNANCY/FERTILITY/BREEDING
$PGF_{2\alpha}$ administration to pregnant mares can cause luteolysis and abortion. Definitively rule out pregnancy before administering this drug or its analogs.

SYNONYMS
• Gonadal dysgenesis
• Gonadal hypoplasia
• Lactational anestrus
• Postpartum anestrus

SEE ALSO
• Abnormal estrus intervals
• Aggression
• Disorders of sexual development
• Early embryonic death
• Endometritis
• Large ovary syndrome
• Ovulation failure
• Pituitary pars intermedia dysfunction
• Prolonged diestrus
• Pyometra

ABBREVIATIONS
• AMH = anti-Müllerian hormone
• CL = corpus luteum
• E_2 = estradiol
• eCG = equine chorionic gonadotropin
• FSH = follicle-stimulating hormone
• GnRH = gonadotropin releasing hormone
• GTCT = granulosa–theca cell tumor
• hCG = human chorionic gonadotropin
• LH = luteinizing hormone
• P_4 = progesterone
• $PGF_{2\alpha}$ = prostaglandin $F_{2\alpha}$
• PPID = pituitary pars intermedia dysfunction
• TRP = transrectal palpation
• US = ultrasonography, ultrasound

Suggested Reading
Aurich C. Reproductive cycles of horses. Anim Reprod Sci 2011;124:220–228.
Donadeu FX, Watson ED. Seasonal changes in ovarian activity: lessons learnt from the horse. Anim Reprod Sci 2007;100:225–242.
Vanderwall DK, Parkinson KC, Rigas J. How to use oxytocin treatment to prolong corpus luteum function for suppressing estrus in mares. J Equine Vet Sci 2016;36:1–4.
Williams GL, Thorson JF, Prezotto LD, et al. Reproductive seasonality in the mare: neuroendocrine basis and pharmacologic control. Domest Anim Endocrinol 2012;43:103–115.

Author Lisa K. Pearson
Consulting Editor Carla L. Carleton
Acknowledgment The author and editor acknowledge the prior contribution of Carole C. Miller.

BASICS

DEFINITION
ALD is an abnormal deviation from the normal axis of the limb in the frontal plane, usually accompanied by an additional degree of axial rotation. Valgus is the lateral deviation, while varus is the medial deviation of the limb to the location of the deformity. The deformity is named by the joint around which the deviation is centered.

PATHOPHYSIOLOGY
Perinatal Factors
• Flaccidity of periarticular soft tissue structures and perinatal soft tissue trauma can lead to unstable joints, resulting in abnormal loading of the articular surfaces inducing ALD
• Anything to jeopardize the intrauterine environment of the foal (i.e. placentitis, twin foal) and premature birth (<315 days) may result in incomplete ossification (carpus and tarsus) at birth

Developmental Factors
• Unbalanced nutrition (i.e. "crib feeding" leading to excessive grain intake, unbalanced trace minerals) can result in disproportionate growth at the level of the physis, causing ALD
• Frequently observed in rapidly growing foals
• Can occur days to months after birth
• Excessive exercise and trauma can result in microfractures and crushing of the growth plate leading to early closure in severe cases (i.e. Salter–Harris type V fracture)

SYSTEMS AFFECTED
Musculoskeletal—one or more joints may be involved in the front limbs and/or hindlimbs, including the fetlock, carpus, and tarsus.

GENETICS
N/A

INCIDENCE/PREVALENCE
• Most foals are born with some form of angular limb deformity; however, most cases resolve within 4 weeks without intervention
• Prevalence of thoroughbred foals with ALD requiring intervention may be as high as 4.7%

GEOGRAPHIC DISTRIBUTION
N/A

SIGNALMENT
Most commonly encountered in neonatal foals.

Breed Predilections
Observed in all breeds, most commonly Thoroughbreds, Quarter Horses, and miniature horses.

Age and Range
May either be present at birth or develop days to months following birth.

Predominant Sex
N/A

SIGNS
General Comments
• Spontaneous correction of mild ALD may occur
• Foals with ALD must be monitored closely, as there is a limited surgical window prior to various physis closures
• Some degree of carpal valgus (up to 4°) is normal in foals. This will correct as the foal grows and the chest broadens

Historical Findings
• Prematurity/dysmaturity
• Placentitis or twinning in the mare
• Witnessed or suspected trauma at the physis
• Crib-feeding practices on the farm

Physical Examination Findings
• A valgus deformity results in what is termed "splay foot," which should not be confused with outward rotation of the entire limb ("toed out")
• A varus deformity results in what is termed "pigeon toed"

CAUSES
Perinatal Factors
• Prematurity/dysmaturity
• Ligamentous laxity
• Perinatal soft tissue trauma
• Intrauterine malpositioning

Developmental Factors
• Nutritional imbalances
• External trauma to the physis
• Overload of a limb

RISK FACTORS
N/A

DIAGNOSIS

DIFFERENTIAL DIAGNOSIS
• Laxity of periarticular soft tissues
• Incomplete ossification/collapse of the cuboidal bones
• Diaphyseal curvature (MCIII/MTIII)

CBC/BIOCHEMISTRY/URINALYSIS
N/A

LABORATORY TESTS
N/A

IMAGING
Radiography allows for determination of the location and the degree of the deformity, as well as concurrent physitis or physeal crushing or cuboidal bone crushing. Radiographs should be centered over the joint of interest, including the mid-diaphysis of the bones proximal and distal to the deformity.

OTHER DIAGNOSTIC PROCEDURES
• Examination of the limb in both a standing and a flexed position
• Observation of the foal at a walk
• Manipulation/palpation of the limb can help determine whether the deformity is related to soft tissue laxity or bony abnormality

PATHOLOGIC FINDINGS
• Asymmetric early closure of either the medial or lateral physis due to injuries or inflammation
• Delayed ossification

TREATMENT

AIMS
A straighter limb will allow for more even load-bearing and should reduce the incidence of athletic injury.

APPROPRIATE HEALTH CARE
N/A

NURSING CARE
Splints and Casts
• The purpose is to maintain the limb in proper alignment and to facilitate adequate weight-bearing for foals with incomplete ossification of the cuboidal bones and laxity of periarticular soft tissue structures
• Problems with casts and splints in foals include osteopenia and tendon/ligament laxity. Ending the cast/splint at the level of the fetlock can help prevent these problems
• Commercial splints/braces are available and may be easier for the owner to change safely
• Splints are contraindicated if the ALD is due to radial/tibial deformity rather than incomplete ossification or laxity of periarticular structures
• Splints should be changed every 3–4 days
• Casts should be changed every 10–14 days

Corrective Shoeing
• Application of glue-on/composite materials with an extension on the medial aspect (valgus deformities) or the lateral aspect (varus deformities) may assist in correction of the deformity
• Hoof trimming may also be performed—the outside of the hoof should be lowered for valgus deformity; the inside for varus deformity. It is important to not overtrim or create an abnormal hoof shape that will further alter normal weight-bearing. Corrective shoeing/trimming should only be attempted if the physis is still open; cosmetic farrierwork on a mature animal with an angular limb deformity will result in joint pathology

ACTIVITY
Stall Rest
• Effective treatment for newborn foals, specifically for incomplete ossification and straight limbs
• Foals with ALD due to disproportionate growth at the level of the physis (>10°) and diaphyseal deformities should be stall rested for 4–6 weeks

• Foals with laxity of the periarticular supporting structures require supervised exercise in addition to stall rest
• It is important not to prolong stall rest beyond 4–6 weeks

DIET
Balanced nutrition is very important.

CLIENT EDUCATION
The examination of a foal for ALD should begin shortly after birth, followed by examination once a week for 4 weeks, and once monthly for 6 months.

SURGICAL CONSIDERATIONS
Growth Acceleration (Periosteal Transection and Elevation)
• Periosteal transection is performed on the concave aspect of the limb (e.g. lateral aspect of the distal radial physis for a carpal valgus deformity) in order to accelerate growth
• The timing of surgery depends on the site of abnormal growth
• The maximum effect is observed within 2 months
• Overcorrection of the deformity has not been observed
• A bandage should be maintained for 10–14 days following surgery
• Stall rest for 2–3 weeks after surgery

Growth Retardation (Transphyseal Bridging)
• Performed in foals <3 months with severe ALD or foals with significant ALD following the rapid growth phase (MCIII/MTIII and proximal phalanx = 2 months, tibia = 4 months, and radius = 6 months)
• The goal is to retard growth by bridging the convex side of the limb, allowing the shorter side of the affected limb to keep growing
• Current techniques include 1 transphyseal screw across the physis or 2 screws with a figure-of-eight cerclage wire connecting the two. The one-screw transphyseal technique may result in more acceptable cosmesis, but carries an increased risk of physitis. Surgical staple techniques and small bone plates have also been described. Periosteal transection and elevation are often performed in combination with growth retardation techniques
• A bandage should be maintained for 10–14 days
• The foal should be stall rested for 2–3 days following surgery
• Implants need to be removed as soon as the deformity has been corrected, as overcorrection can occur

Corrective Osteotomy
• Osteotomies have been performed for correction of significant ALD in foals with closed growth plates
• Current techniques—closing wedge or step osteotomy
• Maintain a bandage and splint or cast for several weeks following surgery

MEDICATIONS
DRUG(S) OF CHOICE
• For foals that require splinting or casting, conservative doses of NSAIDs may be beneficial
• For surgical cases, NSAIDs and antibiotics may be given as needed perioperatively

CONTRAINDICATIONS
N/A

PRECAUTIONS
NSAIDs can have an ulcerogenic effect on foals. Ulcer prophylaxis may include omeprazole or ranitidine during NSAID administration.

POSSIBLE INTERACTIONS
N/A

ALTERNATIVE DRUGS
N/A

FOLLOW-UP
PATIENT MONITORING
• Foals with splints and casts should be assisted to nurse if unable to do so on their own
• Careful monitoring insures implant removal the instant correction has occurred in transphyseal bridging
• Foals with incomplete ossification should be evaluated at 2 week intervals to assess ossification progress

PREVENTION/AVOIDANCE
Balanced nutrition is very important.

POSSIBLE COMPLICATIONS
• Nonsurgical management—pressure sores, osteopenia, and tendon/ligament laxity from cast/splint application
• Surgical management—hematoma/seroma formation at surgery site, incisional infection, wound dehiscence, overcorrection
• Failure of transfer of passive immunity may result if foals are unable to nurse due to ALD following birth

EXPECTED COURSE AND PROGNOSIS
• Studies have indicated an improvement in approximately 80% of foals that have undergone a periosteal transection
• No significant difference in sales price or racing performance was seen between foals that were treated with a transphyseal screw for ALD and maternal siblings without ALD
• Foals with lameness or more than 30% collapse of the third and central tarsal bones associated with incomplete ossification have a poorer prognosis

MISCELLANEOUS
ASSOCIATED CONDITIONS
N/A

AGE-RELATED FACTORS
Timing of intervention is important.

ZOONOTIC POTENTIAL
N/A

PREGNANCY/FERTILITY/BREEDING
N/A

SYNONYMS
N/A

SEE ALSO
Flexural limb deformity

ABBREVIATIONS
• ALD = angular limb deformity
• MCIII = third metacarpal bone
• MTIII = third metatarsal bone
• NSAID = nonsteroidal anti-inflammatory drug

Suggested Reading
Auer JA. Angular limb deformities. In: Auer JA, Stick JA eds. Equine Surgery. St. Louis, MO: WB Saunders, 2012:1201–1221.
Baker WT, Slone DE, Lynch TM, et al. Racing and sales performance after unilateral or bilateral single transphyseal screw insertion for varus angular limb deformities of the carpus in 53 thoroughbreds. Vet Surg 2011;40(1):124–128.
Carlson ER, Bramlage LR, Stewart AA, et al. Complications after two transphyseal bridging techniques for treatment of angular limb deformities of the distal radius in 568 thoroughbred yearlings. Equine Vet J 2012;44(4):416–419.

Authors Alison K. Gardner and Shannon J. Murray
Consulting Editor Margaret C. Mudge

BASICS

OVERVIEW
• Anhidrosis (also known as dry coat disease, nonsweaters, or "dry puffers") is the inability to sweat effectively. The current theory is that overstimulation of sweat gland β_2 receptors downregulates sweating at first temporarily and then permanently
• Systems affected—skin/exocrine

SIGNALMENT
No coat color, age, or sex predilections. Warmbloods and Thoroughbreds are more commonly affected. Rare in Arabians. Up to 20% of horses may be affected when exercising in a hot, humid climate.

SIGNS
• Tachypnea at rest in warm conditions
• Extended tachypnea and hyperthermia after exercise
• Reduction or absence of sweating during or after exercise
• Brief bouts of excessive sweating may precede anhidrosis
• Dry and flaky skin with alopecia, especially on the face and neck, in chronic cases
• Lethargy and altered (decreased or increased) water intake in severe cases

CAUSES AND RISK FACTORS
• Heat-stressed horses may have increased circulating epinephrine, an adrenergic agonist, that may overstimulate the sweat gland β_2 receptors, resulting in downregulation or degradation
• Horses maintained in hot, humid climates are susceptible. Poor acclimatization after introduction from a cool climate, intense exercise during hot, humid conditions, water/salt restriction, and feeding a high-carbohydrate diet are suspected risk factors
• Treatment of foals with macrolide antibiotics causes temporary anhidrosis

DIAGNOSIS

DIFFERENTIAL DIAGNOSIS
Respiratory diseases that cause an increase in respiratory rate, especially heaves. Infectious diseases that cause an increase in rectal temperature.

CBC/BIOCHEMISTRY/URINALYSIS
Hyponatremia and hypochloremia in chronic severe cases. Decreased renal fractional excretion of chloride.

DIAGNOSTIC PROCEDURES
Intradermal injections, 0.1 mL/site, in the neck below the mane, of a drug with β_2-agonist activity (e.g. terbutaline sulfate, albuterol (salbutamol), epinephrine) using serial dilutions (0.001–1000 µg/mL) and a control (sterile saline)—read the results at 30 min. Sweat can be collected into absorbent pads taped over injection sites for more accurate results. Normal horses sweat in response to all dilutions. Anhidrotic horses have a decreased response to some or all.

PATHOLOGIC FINDINGS
Thickened basal laminae, thin myoepithelial and fundic epithelial cells, thickened connective tissues, and marked reduction of vesicles in the secretory cells. Luminal microvilli often are absent and the lumen of the duct is clogged with cellular debris.

TREATMENT
• Environmental management is the only reliable treatment option at present
• Horses exhibiting signs of heat stress should be immediately taken to a shaded environment, and cooled with cold water and fans
• Restrict to a stall with a fan and/or mister during hot periods of the day
• Minimize the feeding of carbohydrates
• Provide free-choice cool, fresh water and salt supplementation
• Inform clients that these horses will be prone to poor performance and will only improve once effective sweating has returned
• Discontinue use of β_2-agonists such as clenbuterol
• Keep foals that are treated with macrolides out of direct sunlight during and for a week after treatment

MEDICATIONS

DRUG(S) OF CHOICE
• Supplemental electrolytes, especially sodium salts
• Anecdotally, iodinated casein (10–15 g/day for 4–8 days) and with 1000–3000 IU PO of vitamin E (α-tocopherol) daily for 1 month, or amino acid supplements containing tyrosine

FOLLOW-UP

PATIENT MONITORING
Normally, a horse can reduce its body temperature to within normal limits approximately 30 min after exercise. Monitor respiration and rectal temperature post exercise.

PREVENTION/AVOIDANCE
• Carefully acclimatize horses to exercise in hot/humid conditions
• Keep foals treated with macrolides out of direct sunlight during and for a week after treatment
• Exercise during the cooler periods of the day
• Stall the horse in a cool environment (e.g. fan, water mister, air-conditioning) during the hotter periods of the day
• Anhidrosis is usually a lifelong problem, consider relocating the horse to a more temperate climate
• Avoid administration of β_2-agonists

POSSIBLE COMPLICATIONS
Heat stroke may occur if horses are exercised during the hotter periods of the day.

EXPECTED COURSE AND PROGNOSIS
• Most horses respond to a change in environment and begin to sweat normally after a few weeks
• Horses that have previously suffered from the disease will usually become anhidrotic if exposed to hot, humid conditions again

MISCELLANEOUS

ASSOCIATED CONDITIONS
Skin lesions—dry, flaky skin and alopecia, especially around the eyes and shoulders.

Suggested Reading
Hubert JD, Norwood G, Beadle RM. Equine anhidrosis. Vet Clin North Am Equine Pract 2002;18:355–369.

Author Robert J. MacKay
Consulting Editors Michel Lévy and Heidi Banse
Acknowledgment The author and editors acknowledge the prior contribution of Jeremy D. Hubert and Ralph E. Beadle.

ANOREXIA AND DECREASED FOOD INTAKE

 BASICS

DEFINITION
Anorexia is the loss of appetite or lack of desire for food. Some conditions may not lead to complete loss of appetite, but merely reduced food intake.

PATHOPHYSIOLOGY
Appetite Suppression
Anorexia is commonly a sign of systemic disease, including but not limited to GI disease. Reduced food intake can also be caused by various conditions affecting the lips, mouth, tongue, pharynx, esophagus, or stomach, and may include painful conditions, mechanical obstructions, or nervous or neuromuscular dysfunctions.
Anorexia appears to be the result of a modification of central regulation of feeding behavior in the hypothalamus. Many factors and substances may be involved in regulating feed intake. Anorexia associated with alterations of smell and taste has not been shown in the horse. Decreased food intake has been associated with parasitic infections, but the mechanism is unknown. Pain and depression appear to cause anorexia. Serotonin agonists decrease food intake, apparently via central histaminergic activity. The neurotransmitter neuropeptide Y and various cytokines may cause cancer anorexia–cachexia syndrome. Primary disease conditions, such as infection, inflammation, injury, toxins, immunologic reactions, and necrosis, may cause anorexia via cytokine release. In addition, a proteoglycan has been identified on the cell membranes of animals and has been named *satiomem*. It reduces food intake and may be a satiety or anorexigenic substance.

SIGNALMENT
Signalment depends on underlying disease; any horse can be affected.

SIGNS
Signs include a general lack of interest or a lack of interest in certain types of food only.

Physical Examination Findings
• Clinical signs depend on the cause of anorexia. They are highly variable and depend on the underlying disease when due to systemic disease
• Common clinical signs in association with anorexia due to difficulty or inability of prehension, chewing, or swallowing of food include:
  ◦ Increased salivation (ptyalism), often due to oral or dental disease or inability to swallow (CN IX, X, and XII), or intoxications
  ◦ CN abnormalities—hypoesthesia of the face (CN V), neurogenic atrophy of the masticatory muscles (CN V, motor component), bilateral paralysis of facial muscles (CN VII)
  ◦ Expulsion of partially chewed food ("quidding")
  ◦ Nasal discharge containing feed material
  ◦ Cough due to foreign material entering trachea; aspiration pneumonia can ensue
  ◦ Oral lesions
  ◦ Masses on the head in association with the mandibles and sinuses
  ◦ If anorexia or decreased food intake occurs for prolonged periods of time weight loss, muscle wasting, and poor hair coat are evident. Edema can occur if hypoproteinemia due to decreased protein intake is severe
  ◦ Slight jaundice

CAUSES
Anorexia
Anorexia can be a sign of systemic disease, commonly due to GI or abdominal disorders, including colic.
Anorexia commonly occurs after one of the following primary disease processes in any organ system—inflammation, infection (bacterial, viral, fungal, or parasitic), injury, intoxications, immunologic reactions, neoplasia, necrosis, dehydration, electrolyte imbalances, acid–base disorders, severe respiratory distress, uremia, cardiac disease, metabolic disorders, side effects of medications and pain.
Common specific causes include:
• gastric ulcers and pyloric stenosis
• primary GI colic
• peritonitis, colitis
• liver disease
• renal failure, renal tubular acidosis
• hypertriglyceridemia
• pneumonia and pleuropneumonia
• lymphoma and other malignant tumors
• neurologic disease
• cerebral disease
• laminitis
• endotoxemia, sepsis
• administration of metronidazole or valacyclovir (valaciclovir)
• prematurity and dysmaturity leading to muscle weakness in foals
• hypocalcemia, hypomagnesemia, hyponatremia
• congenital myotonia
Common causes of anorexia associated with inability to access, prehend, and swallow food include—pain (lips, tongue, mouth, teeth, mandibles, maxilla, sinuses, muscles, pharynx, esophagus, or temporomandibular joint), mechanical obstructions, and nervous dysfunction (lips, tongue, pharynx, esophagus).
Common specific causes include:
• Inability to access feed, e.g. neck pain preventing the horse from eating from the ground
• Swelling of the lips, e.g. bee stings or snake bites
• Mucosal lesions due to dental "points," virus-associated oral lesions (vesicular stomatitis), oral ulcers due to contact dermatitis, mechanical injury or phenylbutazone administration, oral lacerations, oral abscesses
• Tongue lacerations, tongue abscesses
• Neoplasia of the mouth or tongue
• Dental disease
• Postsurgical complication after head and neck surgery
• Guttural pouch disease (empyema, mycosis, neoplasia)
• Strangles
• Sinus disease (sinusitis, cysts, neoplasia)
• Neurologic disease affecting CN function, e.g. equine herpesvirus, equine protozoal myeloencephalitis, yellow star thistle poisoning, rabies, verminous encephalitis
• Tetanus, botulism, tick paralysis
• Temporomandibular joint disease
• Rhabdomyolysis affecting masseter muscles
• Mechanical obstruction in mouth, pharynx, or esophagus, e.g. foreign body, choke
• Pharyngitis
• Hyoid bone injury
• Esophageal disease (stricture, diverticulum, megaesophagus, neoplasia, choke, intramural inclusion cysts)
• Persistent right aortic arch, persistent dorsal displacement, epiglottic entrapment
• Compression of the pharynx (cysts—epiglottic, dorsal pharyngeal, aryepiglottic, soft palate, guttural pouch, or laryngeal neoplasia, strangles)
• Hyperkalemic periodic paralysis
• Muscle weakness (foals)
• Ruptured rectus capitus ventralis muscle
Unwillingness to eat can also be due to social factors such as anxiety owing to management problems (e.g. constant interruption, fear, low rank in herd).

RISK FACTORS
There are no specific risk factors for anorexia.

 DIAGNOSIS

DIFFERENTIAL DIAGNOSIS
• Anorexia due to unpalatable or wrong feed materials
• Anorexia due to inability to access, prehend, and swallow food (see Causes for list of differential diagnoses)
• Anorexia due to systemic disease (see Causes for list of differential diagnoses)

CBC/BIOCHEMISTRY/URINALYSIS
• Free (unconjugated or indirect) bilirubin elevations. In cachectic animals bilirubin levels may be normal
• Hypokalemia
• Hypoproteinemia and decreased blood urea nitrogen (urea) if longstanding
• Decreased creatine kinase if associated with weight loss

• Laboratory findings are consistent with the primary disease process (e.g. inflammation, internal organ damage) or secondary disease (e.g. aspiration pneumonia). Hematology, biochemistry (including renal and liver enzymes, albumin, globulin, triglycerides, and muscle enzymes), urinalysis, and evaluation of acute-phase proteins (fibrinogen, serum amyloid A) should be performed

OTHER LABORATORY TESTS
Based on suspected primary disease processes.

IMAGING
If the anorexia is associated with difficulties of food prehension and swallowing:
• Radiography of the head for evaluation of teeth, bones of the head, temporomandibular joint pharyngeal area, sinuses, and guttural pouches
• Radiography of the neck and thorax plus barium swallow or fluoroscopy for evaluation of the pharynx and esophagus
• Radiographs of the thorax to assess secondary complications such as aspiration pneumonia
• Ultrasonography of the tongue and pharynx
• Endoscopy of the oral cavity
• Endoscopy of the upper airways including nasal passage, pharynx, larynx, guttural pouches, and sinuses if necessary
If an underlying systemic disease is suspected:
• Abdominal and thoracic ultrasonography for primary inflammatory or neoplastic problems

OTHER DIAGNOSTIC PROCEDURES
• Examination of the food supply for evidence of contamination or spoilage
• Offering food to the patient and evaluating response, prehension, and swallowing
• Oral examination (under sedation using speculum and endoscope if available)
• Passage of a nasogastric tube to rule out a mechanical obstruction (e.g. choke)
• Neurologic examination
• Rectal examination for internal organ disease

TREATMENT
Dependent on primary disease.

ACTIVITY/DIET
Offer highly palatable and varied feed in easy to access locations in cases of anorexia. Supply feed that is easy to chew and swallow in cases of dysphagia. Force-feeding by nasogastric

intubation or parenteral nutrition may be required. Activity should be limited to stall rest or hand-walking in most cases.

MEDICATIONS
DRUG(S) OF CHOICE
• Depends on primary disease process
• Oral administration of 40 g KCl once or twice daily in anorectic patients

CONTRAINDICATIONS
KCl administration may be contraindicated in patients with abnormal renal function or those suspected of having hyperkalemic periodic paralysis.

FOLLOW-UP
PATIENT MONITORING
The patient should be monitored for dehydration, electrolyte imbalance, acid–base abnormalities, and weight loss, and, in cases of dysphagia, aspiration pneumonia.

POSSIBLE COMPLICATIONS
• Dehydration
• Hypokalemia
• Hypocalcemia
• Metabolic alkalosis with salivary loss
• Weight loss
• Aspiration pneumonia with dysphagia

EXPECTED COURSE AND PROGNOSIS
Dependent on the underlying cause.

MISCELLANEOUS
ASSOCIATED CONDITIONS
• Other primary disease conditions, such as infection, inflammation, injury, toxins, immunologic reactions, and necrosis
• Cancer-related anorexia–cachexia syndrome
• Dehydration, electrolyte imbalances (hypokalemia, hypocalcemia), or acid–base disorders as a result of lack of intake of fluid and electrolytes may exacerbate the anorexia
• Salivary loss of electrolytes leads to metabolic alkalosis and hypochloremia, primarily
• Aspiration pneumonia occurs secondary to dysphagia

AGE-RELATED FACTORS
Depends on primary disease process. Foals are affected by different disease than adults.

ZOONOTIC POTENTIAL
Rabies can cause anorexia or dysphagia. Precautions should be taken while examining and treating the patient.

SYNONYMS
Decreased appetite.

SEE ALSO
• Acute kidney injury (AKI) and acute renal failure (ARF)
• Aspiration pneumonia
• Botulism
• Chronic kidney disease (CKD)
• Colic, chronic/recurrent
• Esophageal obstruction (choke)
• Gastric ulcers and erosions (equine gastric ulcer syndrome, EGUS)
• Guttural pouch empyema
• Guttural pouch mycosis
• Guttural pouch tympany
• Head trauma
• Hendra virus
• Ileus
• Lead (Pb) toxicosis
• Monensin toxicosis
• Nigropallidal encephalomalacia
• Organophosphate and carbamate toxicosis
• Peritonitis
• Rabies
• Sinusitis (paranasal)
• Snake envenomation
• *Streptococcus equi* infection
• Tetanus
• Vesicular stomatitis

ABBREVIATIONS
• CN = cranial nerve
• GI = gastrointestinal

Suggested Reading
Magdesian KG. Parenteral nutrition in the mature horse. Equine Vet Educ 2010;22:364–371.
Stratton-Phelps M. Assisted enteral feeding in adult horses. Compend Cont Educ Pract Vet 2004;26:46–49.

Author Angelika Schoster
Consulting Editors Henry Stämpfli and Olimpo Oliver-Espinosa

 Client Education Handout available online

ANTHRAX

BASICS

OVERVIEW
• A fatal infectious disease that affects animals and humans caused by *Bacillus anthracis,* a Gram-positive spore-forming bacillus
• Worldwide distribution
• Mainly herbivores
• Most common form obtained after ingestion of soil, forage, or water contaminated with *B. anthracis* through wounds in the oral, pharyngeal, and GI mucosa, but the organisms may also be inhaled or inoculated by biting insects
• The organism passes to its vegetative form and produces exotoxins (lethal toxin and edema toxin) that impair phagocytosis and vascular integrity resulting in hemorrhage, edema, renal failure, shock, and almost invariably death. When *B. anthracis* is exposed to the environment, long-lasting spores (decades) are formed that are a potential source of infection for other animals

SIGNALMENT
• No gender, age, or breed predilections
• Grazing habits may affect signalment in some species

SIGNS
• Acute form—fever or hypothermia, depression, generalized muscle twitching, severe tachycardia and tachypnea, severe edema of the glottis, hypotonia of the anal sphincter, and death in less than 4 days; severe colic, bloody discharge from body orifices, and painful subcutaneous swellings
• Chronic form—pharyngeal edema, inspiratory stridor, head and neck swelling. Death up to 2 weeks after initial signs are noted
• Peracute form—death with few clinical signs, less common in horses

CAUSES AND RISK FACTORS
• Most common in tropical and subtropical climates; sporadic in temperate regions, usually in the summer
• Areas with soils high in calcium and with alkaline pH (>6.1) and with climate cycles of heavy rain and drought
• Overgrazing increases the ingestion of soil. Coarse forage causes erosions in the oral mucosa

DIAGNOSIS

DIFFERENTIAL DIAGNOSIS
Lightning strike, poisoning or intoxication by plants, colic, enteritis, purpura haemorrhagica, malignant edema.

CBC/BIOCHEMISTRY/URINALYSIS
Routine laboratory findings have not been reported.

OTHER LABORATORY TESTS
Bacterial culture of blood or exudate. Results may be negative early in disease or if antibiotics have been administered. If the carcass has been opened, use lymph nodes or spleen. Cultures should only be performed in a facility capable of containment to prevent infection of laboratory personnel.

DIAGNOSTIC PROCEDURES
• Gram-positive, encapsulated, blunt-ended bacilli, occurring singly or in short chains on microscopic examination of blood smear or edema fluid. Smears become unreliable about 24 h after death
• Immunofluorescence of blood or tissue is a rapid confirmatory test for *B. anthracis* in culture
• PCR

PATHOLOGIC FINDINGS
• Because of human health risk and danger of environmental contamination, necropsy should not be performed if anthrax is suspected. Diagnosis can be made without necropsy
• Dark, nonclotting blood from orifices; absence of rigor mortis; splenomegaly; and lymphadenopathy are hallmarks of anthrax. Edema in the submucosa of the digestive tract, ventral abdomen, and chest is often observed

TREATMENT
• The high mortality, rapid course of disease, and late referral in some geographic areas usually limit the opportunity for treatment. The prognosis is poor even with treatment
• Isolate affected and in-contact animals

MEDICATIONS

DRUG(S) OF CHOICE
• Penicillin G (40 000 IU/kg IV every 4–6 h), oxytetracycline (5–11 mg/kg IV every 12 h), or enrofloxacin (7.5 mg/kg IV every 24 h). Continue treatment for at least 5 days
• Anthrax antiserum may be useful but is not available in the USA

FOLLOW-UP
• Regulatory officials should be notified when anthrax is suspected and the premises placed under quarantine

• Carcasses should not be opened. Dispose of by burning or deep (>2 m) burial with lime. The area can be disinfected with 5% aqueous lye or 10% formaldehyde. Hypochlorite (10% bleach) is sporicidal, but surfaces should be very clean before its use
• Susceptible animals should be vaccinated. Avirulent live spore vaccine. Provides immunity in 1 week. Some recommend a second vaccination in 2–4 weeks. Annual boosters are required. Severe adverse reactions have been reported. No antibiotics should be administered within 5 days before or after vaccination

MISCELLANEOUS

ZOONOTIC POTENTIAL
Severe zoonosis; gloves and mask should be worn if it is necessary to contact infected material or animals. Three presentations have been described—cutaneous (most common), pulmonary, and GI. All can progress to systemic dissemination followed by septic shock and death. Antibiotic therapy is successful if diagnosed early; commonly used antibiotics include ciprofloxacin and doxycycline.

SYNONYMS
• Charbon
• Splenic fever
• Woolsorter's disease

ABBREVIATIONS
• GI = gastrointestinal
• PCR = polymerase chain reaction

Suggested Reading
Walker RL. Anthrax. In: Smith BP, ed. Large Animal Internal Medicine, 4e. St. Louis, MO: Mosby, 2009:1180–1183.

Author Gonzalo Gajardo Aedo
Consulting Editor Ashley G. Boyle
The author and editor acknowledge the prior contribution of Laura K Reilly.

BASICS

OVERVIEW
• ACRs are a commonly used class of rodenticides
• ACRs interfere with normal blood clotting and cause coagulopathy by inhibiting vitamin K epoxide reductase in liver and preventing formation of active clotting factors
• First-generation anticoagulants such as warfarin, coumafuryl, coumachlor, and coumatetralyl are short-acting, requiring multiple feedings to result in toxicosis
• Long-acting or second-generation ACRs include chlorophacinone, diphacinone, pindone, brodifacoum, bromadiolone, difethialone, difenacoum, and others. These are more toxic
• Most ACRs used today are second generation, with activity in the body lasting ~1 month or longer
• Minimum toxic dosage has not been established in horses. Coagulopathy has been reported in horses associated with a brodifacoum dosage of 0.125 mg/kg, and a diphacinone dosage of 0.2 mg/kg

SIGNALMENT
Poisoning can occur after accidental ingestion of bait or as a result of malicious intent.

SIGNS
• Hemorrhage of variable severity. Can be internal, external, or both, and can be focal or widespread
• Signs generally manifest within 2–5 days after ingestion and include pale mucous membranes, weakness, anorexia, dyspnea, tachycardia, hematomas and swellings, hematuria, bleeding from the mouth, and epistaxis
• Signs are delayed and do not occur until days after exposure, after existing clotting factors are depleted

CAUSES AND RISK FACTORS
• Careless bait placement
• Baits often contain ingredients that are attractive to horses

 DIAGNOSIS

DIFFERENTIAL DIAGNOSIS
• Dicoumarol toxicosis
• Other causes of coagulopathy

CBC/BIOCHEMISTRY/URINALYSIS
• Anemia and hypoproteinemia suggestive of blood loss possible
• Urinalysis may show the presence of red blood cells

OTHER LABORATORY TESTS
• Prolonged PT, aPTT, and activated coagulation time. aPTT is reported to increase before PT in horses

• Chemical analysis of serum, whole blood or liver tissue (postmortem) for specific ACR compounds

IMAGING
Chest radiographs may show evidence of fluid in the chest cavity or hemorrhage within the lungs.

PATHOLOGIC FINDINGS
Hemorrhages may occur in any part of the body and may be focal or widespread.

 TREATMENT

• Whole-blood or plasma transfusions to replace clotting factors if patient is actively bleeding. Whole blood is preferred with severe anemia
• Keep patient confined to stall rest
• Decontamination with AC and possibly a cathartic via nasogastric tube is appropriate if instituted soon after exposure (within several hours) and the patient is asymptomatic

 MEDICATIONS

DRUG(S) OF CHOICE
• Vitamin K1 (phytonadione) 2.5 mg/kg every 24 h or divided into twice daily dosing, given PO or SC and continuing for 3–5 weeks for long-acting ACRs, or 1–2 weeks for short-acting compounds. If ACR compound is unknown, treat as for a long-acting ACR
• PO administration of vitamin K1 formulated for injection is preferable to SC injection, unless AC has been administered. Mixing vitamin K1 with a small amount of a digestible fat increases absorption. Most injectable formulations of vitamin K1 are well absorbed orally and can be administered orally until compounded vitamin K1 oral solution can be obtained
• A day or longer may be required for new clotting factor synthesis

CONTRAINDICATIONS/POSSIBLE INTERACTIONS
• Do not use vitamin K3 (menadione) in horses. Vitamin K3 is ineffective and nephrotoxic
• Do not administer vitamin K1 IV as it can cause anaphylactic reaction
• NSAIDs and other drugs affecting coagulation are contraindicated

 FOLLOW-UP

PATIENT MONITORING
• Continued monitoring of coagulation times and blood loss until patient is stable
• Check clotting times 2–3 days and 5 days after the last dose of vitamin K1 to determine if additional treatment is necessary

PREVENTION/AVOIDANCE
• Prevent access to rodenticide baits
• Not all rodenticides are anticoagulant compounds. Verify active ingredient if possible before treatment

POSSIBLE COMPLICATIONS
If duration of vitamin K1 therapy is too short, recurrence of coagulopathy can occur.

EXPECTED COURSE AND PROGNOSIS
• The prognosis is good if treatment is instituted before coagulopathy occurs
• The prognosis in patients with active bleeding depends on the severity and speed of hemorrhage, and the site of hemorrhage. Bleeding into the lungs, chest cavity, brain, or cranium can result in rapid death

 MISCELLANEOUS

ASSOCIATED CONDITIONS
N/A

AGE-RELATED FACTORS
N/A

ZOONOTIC POTENTIAL
N/A

PREGNANCY/FERTILITY/BREEDING
• Lactating mares may excrete ACR in their milk
• Monitor foals for coagulopathy, and treat with vitamin K1 if clotting times are elevated. Alternatively, consider weaning the foal from the affected mare and providing an alternative milk supply

SEE ALSO
• Coagulation Defects Acquired
• Coagulation Defects, Inherited
• Dicoumarol (moldy sweet clover) toxicosis
• Disseminated Intravascular Coagulation

ABBREVIATIONS
• AC = activated charcoal
• ACR = anticoagulant rodenticide
• aPTT = activated partial thromboplastin time
• NSAID = nonsteroidal anti-inflammatory drug
• PT = prothrombin time

Suggested Reading
Boermans HJ, Johnstone I, Black WD, Murphy M. Clinical signs, laboratory changes and toxicokinetics of brodifacoum in the horse. Can J Vet Res 1991;55:21–27.
McConnico RS, Copedge K, Bischoff KL. Brodifacoum toxicosis in two horses. J Am Vet Med Assoc 1997;211:882–886.

Author Cynthia L. Gaskill
Consulting Editors Wilson K. Rumbeiha and Steve Ensley
Acknowledgment The author and editors acknowledge the prior contribution of Anita M. Kore.

ANURIA/OLIGURIA

BASICS

DEFINITION
• *Anuria*—lack of urine production
• *Oliguria*—decreased urine production (<0.5 mL/kg/h, or <250 mL/h in a 500 kg horse)
• Anuria or oliguria may be physiologic or pathologic
• This chapter will focus on intrinsic renal failure causing anuria and oliguria

PATHOPHYSIOLOGY
N/A

SYSTEMS AFFECTED
Renal/urologic

GENETICS
N/A

INCIDENCE/PREVALENCE
Unknown

GEOGRAPHIC DISTRIBUTION
None

SIGNALMENT
No age, sex, or breed predilection documented.

SIGNS
• No or insufficient urine production
• Repeated posturing to urinate, with no urine production, in case of urinary tract obstruction
• Abdominal distention in case of uroperitoneum
• Edema when persistent anuria

CAUSES
• Physiologic oliguria—hyperosmolality; any disease process leading to renal hypoperfusion (e.g. dehydration, hypotension, low cardiac output)
• Pathologic anuria/oliguria—intrinsic ARF; trauma to the lower urinary tract

RISK FACTORS
• Risk factors predisposing to ARF
• For trauma to lower urogenital tract—birth trauma (e.g. dystocia) would increase the risk of urinary tract disruption and uroperitoneum in neonates and their dams; penile trauma is more common in breeding stallions

DIAGNOSIS

DIFFERENTIAL DIAGNOSIS
Pathologic Anuria/Oliguria
• Intrinsic AKI/ARF, terminal CKD, lower urinary tract disruption resulting in uroperitoneum, and urinary tract obstruction consequent to urolithiasis
• Bladder displacement
• Progressive abdominal distention should increase suspicion of uroperitoneum

• Repeated posturing to urinate, with little urine passed, supports urinary tract obstruction

CBC/BIOCHEMISTRY/URINALYSIS
• Normal to high packed cell volume in most cases; mild to moderate anemia possible with terminal CKD
• Moderate to severe increases in blood urea nitrogen (59–150 mg/dL; 18–54 mmol/L) and Cr (2.0–20 mg/dL; 177–1768 μmol/L)
• Variable hyponatremia, hypochloremia, hyperkalemia, hypocalcemia, and hyperphosphatemia—hyperkalemia and hyperphosphatemia more common with intrinsic AKI/ARF; hyperkalemia most apparent with urinary tract disruption and development of uroperitoneum
• Mild to moderate metabolic acidosis—dependent on the underlying disease process
• Mild to moderate hyperglycemia—attributed to stress
• USG—high (>1.035) with physiologic oliguria, low (<1.020) with oliguria due to intrinsic AKI/ARF; USG best assessed in urine collected during initial patient evaluation (before rehydration) or while the horse is not receiving fluids
• Oliguria with intrinsic AKI/ARF may be accompanied by mild to moderate proteinuria, glucosuria, pigmenturia, and increased numbers of red blood cells and casts on sediment examination
• Urine pH—normal to acidic, especially with concurrent depletion of body potassium stores

OTHER LABORATORY TESTS
• Fractional clearances (i.e. excretions) of electrolytes in cases of ARF/CKD
• Increased urinary γ-glutamyltransferase to Cr ratio >25 in cases of ARF
• Increased urine protein to Cr ratio in cases of CKD

IMAGING
Transabdominal and Transrectal Ultrasonography
• Kidneys may be enlarged, with loss of detail of corticomedullary junction, in intrinsic AKI/ARF
• Kidneys typically are reduced in size, with increased parenchymal echogenicity, in CKD
• Accumulation of hypoechoic fluid in the peritoneal cavity in cases of uroperitoneum
• Urinary calculi can be identified as hyperechoic structures associated with a shadow cone and distended proximal urinary tract

Urethroscopy/Cystoscopy
Endoscopy of the lower urinary tract is indicated when there is suspicion of lower urinary tract obstruction.

DIAGNOSTIC PROCEDURES
• Abdominocentesis is indicated in cases of peritoneal effusion. Peritoneal Cr concentration over twice blood concentration in cases of uroperitoneum

• Measurement of glomerular filtration rate and renal biopsies are indicated in case of CKD/chronic renal failure
• Central venous pressure/arterial pressure measurements

PATHOLOGIC FINDINGS
See specific topics.

TREATMENT

APPROPRIATE HEALTH CARE
• *Treat anuria/oliguria as a medical emergency because persistent renal hypoperfusion may lead to ischemic AKI/ARF*
• If untreated, metabolic disturbances, most notably hyperkalemia, may lead to cardiac arrhythmias and death
• Once the patient is stabilized (largely with supportive treatment in the form of IV fluid therapy), pursue further diagnostic evaluation to determine if surgical intervention (for correction of uroperitoneum or relief of obstruction) is needed
• Proper recognition and treatment of all primary disease processes, usually on an inpatient basis for continuous fluid therapy, is warranted
• Avoid nephrotoxic medications

NURSING CARE
• Fluid therapy is a large part of supportive treatment
• Peritoneal drainage and urinary catheterization to remove urine from the abdomen is part of the treatment of uroperitoneum

ACTIVITY
Stall rest.

CLIENT EDUCATION
N/A

SURGICAL CONSIDERATIONS
Surgical intervention is indicated for uroperitoneum and urolithiasis. See specific topics.

MEDICATIONS

DRUG(S) OF CHOICE
• Fluid therapy to correct renal hypoperfusion—after initial measurement of body weight, correct estimated dehydration with isotonic (0.9%) saline or another potassium-poor electrolyte solution over 12–24 h; monitor closely for subcutaneous and pulmonary edema (i.e. increased respiratory rate and effort); conjunctival edema may develop rapidly in horses with intrinsic oliguric to anuric AKI/ARF; use maintenance fluid therapy judiciously in animals that are not clinically dehydrated; if hemorrhage is contributing to hypovolemia

and renal hypoperfusion, initial treatment with hypertonic saline and/or a blood transfusion may have value
• Severe hyperkalemia (>7.0 mEq/L) or cardiac arrhythmias—treat with agents that decrease serum potassium concentration (e.g. sodium bicarbonate (1–2 mEq/kg IV over 5–15 min)), or counteract the effects of hyperkalemia on cardiac conduction (e.g. calcium gluconate (0.5 mL/kg of a 10% solution by slow IV injection))
• Furosemide—this diuretic may be administered 2 times (1–2 mg/kg IV or IM) at 1–2 h intervals; if effective, urination should be observed within 1 h after administration of the second dose; if ineffective, discontinue
• Based on recent evidence in critically ill human patients *the routine use of mannitol or dopamine in equine patients with oliguria is no longer recommended*

CONTRAINDICATIONS
Avoid all nephrotoxic medications unless specifically indicated for the underlying disease process, and then modify dosage accordingly.

PRECAUTIONS
• Monitor response to fluid therapy closely—as little as 40 mL/kg of IV fluids (20 L to a 500 kg horse) may produce pulmonary edema
• Reassess dosage schedule of drugs eliminated by urinary excretion; consider discontinuing all nephrotoxic medications (especially gentamicin, tetracycline, and NSAIDs)

POSSIBLE INTERACTIONS
Use of multiple anti-inflammatory drugs (e.g. corticosteroids and one or more NSAIDs) will have additive negative effects on renal blood flow; avoid combined administration in azotemic patients.

ALTERNATIVE DRUGS
None

FOLLOW-UP

PATIENT MONITORING
• Assess clinical status (emphasizing hydration), urine output, and body weight frequently for the first 3 days
• Assess magnitude of azotemia and electrolyte and acid–basis status at least daily for the first 3 days of treatment
• Consider placing a central venous line to maintain central venous pressure <8 cmH$_2$O in more critical patients and neonates

PREVENTION/AVOIDANCE
See specific topics.

POSSIBLE COMPLICATIONS
• Severe hyperkalemia accompanied by cardiac arrhythmias and death
• Pulmonary and peripheral edema; conjunctival edema may be dramatic

EXPECTED COURSE AND PROGNOSIS
Dependent on underlying cause. Poor prognosis if diuresis is not rapidly restored.

MISCELLANEOUS

ASSOCIATED CONDITIONS
• Colic; enterocolitis
• Pleuritis; peritonitis; septicemia
• Exhausted horse syndrome—multiorgan failure

AGE-RELATED FACTORS
Neonates afflicted with hypoxic–ischemic multiorgan damage or septicemia may be at increased risk of anuric/oliguric AKI/ARF.

ZOONOTIC POTENTIAL
Leptospirosis has infectious and zoonotic potential; avoid direct contact with infective urine.

PREGNANCY/FERTILITY/BREEDING
None

SYNONYMS
None

SEE ALSO
• Acute kidney injury (AKI) and acute renal failure (ARF)
• Chronic kidney disease (CKD)
• Urolithiasis
• Uroperitoneum, neonate

ABBREVIATIONS
• AKI = acute kidney injury
• ARF = acute renal failure
• CKD = chronic kidney disease
• Cr = creatinine
• NSAID = nonsteroidal anti-inflammatory drug
• USG = urinary specific gravity

Suggested Reading
Bayly WM. Acute renal failure. In: Reed SM, Bayly WM, Sellon DC, eds. Equine Internal Medicine, 4e. St. Louis, MO: Elsevier, 2017:923–930.
Schott HC. Chronic kidney disease. In: Reed SM, Bayly WM, Sellon DC, eds. Equine Internal Medicine, 4e. St. Louis, MO: WB Saunders, 2017:930–946.

Author Harold C. Schott II
Consulting Editor Valérie Picandet

AORTIC REGURGITATION

BASICS

DEFINITION
Occurs when blood leaks from the aortic valve into the left ventricular outflow tract during diastole.

PATHOPHYSIOLOGY
• The aortic leaflets do not form a complete seal between the aorta and left ventricle
• During diastole, blood regurgitates into the left ventricular outflow tract, causing a left ventricular volume overload. As this volume overload worsens, stretching of the mitral annulus occurs, and MR often develops. MR compounds the severe left ventricular volume overload, and these horses often rapidly develop CHF
• Severe regurgitation results in decreased coronary artery blood flow and decreased myocardial perfusion
• Ventricular arrhythmias may develop secondary to decreased myocardial perfusion and increased myocardial oxygen demand during exercise

SYSTEMS AFFECTED
Cardiovascular

GENETICS
N/A

INCIDENCE/PREVALENCE
N/A

GEOGRAPHIC DISTRIBUTION
N/A

SIGNALMENT
Usually horses >10 years.

SIGNS
General Comments
Often an incidental finding during routine auscultation.

Historical Findings
• Poor performance
• Possibly CHF

Physical Examination Findings
• Grade 1–6/6, decrescendo or musical holodiastolic murmur with PMI in the aortic valve area radiating to the left apex and right side
• Bounding arterial pulses with moderate to severe regurgitation
• Other, less common findings—AF, ventricular premature complexes, accentuated third heart sounds, and CHF

CAUSES
• Degenerative changes of the aortic leaflets
• Aortic valve prolapse
• Nonvegetative valvulitis
• Fenestration of aortic leaflets
• Flail aortic leaflet
• Infective endocarditis
• Ventricular septal defect
• Congenital malformation
• Disease of the aortic root

RISK FACTORS
Old age.

DIAGNOSIS

DIFFERENTIAL DIAGNOSIS
Pulmonic regurgitation—rare; murmurs not usually detectable and should have PMI in the pulmonic valve area; differentiate echocardiographically.

CBC/BIOCHEMISTRY/URINALYSIS
May have neutrophilic leukocytosis, elevated serum amyloid A, and hyperfibrinogenemia with bacterial endocarditis.

OTHER LABORATORY TESTS
• Elevated cardiac troponin I or cardiac troponin T with concurrent myocardial disease
• Positive blood culture may be obtained with bacterial endocarditis

IMAGING
ECG
• Ventricular premature complexes may be present with severe regurgitation
• AF often develops with marked left ventricular volume overload and subsequent left atrial enlargement

Echocardiography
• Most affected horses have thickened aortic valve leaflets
• An echogenic band parallel to or a nodular thickening of the left coronary leaflet free edge are the most common findings
• Prolapse of an aortic leaflet (usually the noncoronary leaflet) into the left ventricular outflow tract frequently is detected
• Fenestration of the aortic leaflet, flail aortic leaflet, vegetations associated with infective endocarditis, or aortic root abnormalities are infrequently detected
• Left ventricle—enlarged and dilated, with a rounded apex and thinner left ventricular free wall and interventricular septum with pattern of left ventricular volume overload
• Increased septal-to-E point separation may be present
• Normal or decreased fractional shortening with left ventricular enlargement is consistent with myocardial dysfunction
• Dilatation of the aortic root occurs with longstanding regurgitation
• High-frequency vibrations on the mitral valve septal leaflet or interventricular septum usually are detected, created by turbulence in the left ventricular outflow tract
• High-frequency vibrations on the aortic leaflets usually are visualized in horses with musical holodiastolic murmurs
• Premature mitral valve closure may indicate more severe aortic insufficiency
• Decreasing aortic root diameter throughout diastole is another indication of increasing severity

• Pulsed-wave or color-flow Doppler reveals a jet or jets of regurgitation in the left ventricular outflow tract. Size of the jet at its origin and its size and extent in the left ventricle represent another means of semiquantitating its severity, as is strength of the regurgitation signal
• A steep slope and short pressure half-time of the continuous-wave Doppler spectral tracing of the regurgitation jet indicate more severe regurgitation

Thoracic Radiography
• Left-sided cardiac enlargement presents with moderate to severe regurgitation
• Pulmonary edema may be present with CHF

OTHER DIAGNOSTIC PROCEDURES
Cardiac Catheterization
• Right-sided catheterization may reveal elevated pulmonary capillary wedge pressures and pulmonary arterial pressures with severe regurgitation and concurrent MR
• Right ventricular and atrial pressures may be elevated with CHF
• Oxygen saturation of blood obtained from the right atrium, right ventricle, and pulmonary artery should be normal

Noninvasive Blood Pressure Measurement
Pulse pressure >60 mmHg—progression likely.

Exercising ECG
Should be performed in all horses with moderate to severe aortic regurgitation.

Continuous 24 h Holter Monitoring
Use if ventricular premature complexes suspected.

PATHOLOGIC FINDINGS
• Focal or diffuse thickening or distortion of one or more aortic leaflets (bands, nodules, plaques, and fenestrations) may be present
• Flail aortic leaflets, infective endocarditis, or congenital malformations of the aortic valve infrequently are detected
• Aortic root dilatation usually is present with severe, longstanding regurgitation
• Jet lesions usually are detected on the ventricular side of the mitral valve septal leaflet and, less frequently, on the interventricular septum
• Left ventricular enlargement and thinning of the left ventricular free wall and interventricular septum with significant regurgitation
• Atrial myocardial thinning with atrial dilatation has been documented in horses with AF and enlargement
• Inflammatory cell infiltrate has been detected with myocarditis and aortic regurgitation; however, most affected horses do not have significant underlying myocardial disease

TREATMENT

AIMS
• Management by intermittent monitoring in horses with aortic regurgitation that is mild or moderate in severity
• Palliative care in horses with severe aortic regurgitation

APPROPRIATE HEALTH CARE
• Most affected horses require no treatment and can be monitored on an outpatient basis
• Horses with moderate to severe regurgitation may benefit from long-term vasodilator therapy, particularly with ACE inhibitors
• Treat horses with severe regurgitation and CHF with positive inotropic drugs, vasodilators, and diuretics and monitor response to therapy

NURSING CARE
N/A

ACTIVITY
• Affected horses are safe to continue in full athletic work until the regurgitation becomes severe or ventricular arrhythmias develop
• Monitor horses with moderate to severe regurgitation by ECG during high-intensity exercise to ensure they are safe for ridden activities. These horses can be used for lower level athletic activities until they begin to develop CHF
• Horses with significant ventricular arrhythmias or pulmonary artery dilatation are no longer safe to ride

CLIENT EDUCATION
• Regularly palpate for bounding arterial pulses which indicate significant left ventricular volume overload and moderate to severe regurgitation
• Regularly monitor cardiac rhythm; any irregularities other than second-degree atrioventricular block should prompt ECG
• Carefully monitor for exercise intolerance, respiratory distress, prolonged recovery after exercise, increased resting respiratory rate or heart rate, or cough; if detected, seek a cardiac reexamination

SURGICAL CONSIDERATIONS
N/A

MEDICATIONS

DRUG(S) OF CHOICE
• Severe regurgitation—consider benazepril (1 mg/kg PO every 12 h)

• ACE inhibitors prolong the time to valve replacement in humans with moderate to severe regurgitation
• Some horses with moderate to severe regurgitation have experienced a decrease in left ventricular chamber size with ACE inhibitors
• Treatment of affected horses in heart failure includes digoxin, diuretics, and vasodilators

CONTRAINDICATIONS
ACE inhibitors and other vasodilators must be withdrawn before competition to comply with the medication rules of the various governing bodies of equine sports.

PRECAUTIONS
ACE inhibitors can cause hypotension; thus, do not give a large dose without time to accommodate to this treatment.

ALTERNATIVE DRUGS
Other ACE inhibitors and other vasodilatory drugs should have some beneficial effect in horses with moderate to severe regurgitation, but they may be less effective than benazepril.

FOLLOW-UP

PATIENT MONITORING
• Frequently monitor arterial pulses and cardiac rhythm
• Reexamine horses with mild to moderate regurgitation by echocardiography every year
• Reexamine horses with severe regurgitation by echocardiography and with exercising ECG every 6 months to monitor progression of valvular insufficiency and determine if the horse continues to be safe to ride or drive

POSSIBLE COMPLICATIONS
Chronic regurgitation—ventricular arrhythmias; AF; MR; CHF.

EXPECTED COURSE AND PROGNOSIS
• Most affected horses have a normal performance life and life expectancy
• Progression of regurgitation associated with degenerative valve disease usually is slow. With the typical onset of regurgitation that occurs in old horses, other problems are more likely to end a horse's performance career or shorten life expectancy
• Affected horses with CHF usually have severe underlying valvular and/or myocardial disease and a guarded to grave prognosis for life. Most affected horses being treated for CHF respond to the supportive therapy and improve. This improvement usually is short lived, however, and most are euthanized within 2–6 months of initiating treatment

MISCELLANEOUS

ASSOCIATED CONDITIONS
N/A

AGE-RELATED FACTORS
Old horses are more likely to be affected.

PREGNANCY/FERTILITY/BREEDING
• Affected mares should not experience any problems with pregnancy unless the regurgitation is severe
• Treat pregnant affected mares with CHF for the underlying cardiac disease with positive inotropic drugs and diuretics; ACE inhibitors are contraindicated because of potential adverse effects on the fetus

SYNONYMS
Aortic insufficiency

SEE ALSO
• Endocarditis, infective
• Ventricular septal defect (VSD)

ABBREVIATIONS
• ACE = angiotensin-converting enzyme
• AF = atrial fibrillation
• CHF = congestive heart failure
• MR = mitral regurgitation
• PMI = point of maximal intensity

Suggested Reading
Afonso T, Giguere S, Rapoport G, et al. Pharmacodynamic evaluation of 4 angiotensin-converting enzyme inhibitors in healthy adult horses. J Vet Intern Med 2013;27:1185–1192.
Reef VB, Spencer P. Echocardiographic evaluation of equine aortic insufficiency. Am J Vet Res 1987;48:904–909.
Reef VB, Bonagura J, Buhl R, et al. Recommendations for management of equine athletes with cardiovascular abnormalities. J Vet Intern Med 2014;28:749–761.
Ven S, Decloedt A, Van Der Veckens N, et al. Assessing aortic regurgitation severity from 2D, M-mode and Doppler echocardiographic measurements in horses. Vet J 2016;210:34–38.

Author Virginia B. Reef
Consulting Editors Celia M. Marr and Virginia B. Reef

AORTIC RUPTURE

BASICS

DEFINITION
A defect in the wall of the aorta at the aortic root, usually in the right sinus of Valsalva or the aortic arch.

PATHOPHYSIOLOGY
• Aortic rupture can result in dissecting aneurysm, exsanguination into the thoracic cavity, cardiac tamponade from hemopericardium; a shunt between the aorta and heart if the defect is located in the aortic root; or a shunt between the aorta and pulmonary artery if the defect is located in the aortic arch
• With an aortic rupture confined to the right sinus of Valsalva, an aorticocardiac fistula is created. Blood from the aorta shunts into the right side of the heart, at either the atrial or ventricular level, depending on the site of the rupture
• Subendocardial dissection of blood into the interventricular septum is common, with subsequent rupture into the right or left ventricle (more commonly, the rupture is into the right ventricle)
• Often associated with a unifocal ventricular tachycardia that may be associated with dissection of blood into the interventricular septum
• Aortic arch rupture leads to periaortic hematoma, aortopulmonary fistulation, and pseudoaneurysm

SYSTEMS AFFECTED
Cardiovascular

INCIDENCE/PREVALENCE
Rare

SIGNALMENT
• Aortic root rupture more frequently occurs in old horses, particularly males and often during or after breeding or other exercise
• The Friesian breed is predisposed to aortic arch rupture and signs occur in young adults

SIGNS
General Comments
Often interpreted by owners as colic, because the horse appears distressed, may be looking at its flanks, and acts uncomfortable.

Historical Findings
• Acute onset of colic or distress, particularly with aortic root rupture
• Subacute or chronic low-grade colic, particularly with aortic arch rupture
• Less commonly, exercise intolerance; syncope, CHF

Physical Examination Findings
• Tachycardia
• Tachypnea

• Continuous machinery murmur—usually loudest on the right side
• Bounding arterial pulses
• Other, less common findings—jugular pulses and distention, ventricular tachycardia (unifocal), and CHF

CAUSES
• A congenital aneurysm in the wall of the aortic root, usually in the right sinus of Valsalva, predisposes to aortic root rupture
• Necrosis and degeneration of the aortic media have been associated, especially in old breeding stallions
• Aberrant parasite migration in the ascending aorta is unlikely
• Hereditary connective tissue disorders suspected to be an underlying cause in Friesians

RISK FACTORS
• Aortic aneurysm
• Aortitis
• Friesian breed

DIAGNOSIS

DIFFERENTIAL DIAGNOSIS
Ventricular Septal Defect with Aortic Regurgitation
• Murmurs are systolic (band shaped and pansystolic) and diastolic (holodiastolic and decrescendo), not continuous
• Arterial pulses usually are not bounding, unless the associated aortic regurgitation is severe
• No history of acute colic or distress
• Differentiate echocardiographically

Patent Ductus Arteriosus
• No history of acute colic or distress
• No unifocal ventricular tachycardia
• Differentiate echocardiographically

CBC/BIOCHEMISTRY/URINALYSIS
Increased serum creatinine and blood urea nitrogen may occur because of impaired renal perfusion, which is associated with sustained ventricular tachycardia and blood loss.

OTHER LABORATORY TESTS
Serum cardiac troponin I can be elevated with significant myocardial cell injury.

IMAGING
ECG
Uniform ventricular tachycardia with a heart rate of >100 bpm may be present with aortic root rupture.

Echocardiography
• 2-dimensional echocardiography is diagnostic for a defect in the aortic root at the sinus of Valsalva or for a sinus of Valsalva aneurysm

• The rupture may be a small, irregular defect in the aortic wall (usually associated with the right aortic leaflet) or be visualized flailing in the right atrium or ventricle
• Anechoic to echoic fluid may be detected dissecting subendocardially into the interventricular septum, most frequently along the right ventricular side; however, dissection of blood subendocardially along the left side also occurs
• Use color-flow Doppler, pulsed-wave Doppler, or contrast echocardiography to localize the shunt associated with the aortic cardiac fistula
• Transthoracic echocardiography may demonstrate pulmonary artery dilation, displacement of the pulmonary artery, and aortopulmonary fistulation (best visualized from the left cranial window) with aortic arch rupture
• Transesophageal echocardiography is potentially useful with aortic arch rupture

Thoracic Radiography
• An enlarged cardiac silhouette should be present in horses with a large aorticocardiac shunt
• Pulmonary overcirculation and edema may be detected

OTHER DIAGNOSTIC PROCEDURES
Cardiac Catheterization
• Elevated right ventricular pressure, pulmonary arterial pressure, pulmonary capillary wedge pressure, and oxygen saturation of the blood are detected in horses with aorticocardiac fistula into the right ventricle
• With a shunt into the right atrium, right atrial pressures and oxygen saturation also are elevated

Arterial Blood Pressure
Demonstrates the wide difference between peak systolic pressure and end-diastolic pressure associated with continuous shunting of blood from the aorta into the heart.

PATHOLOGIC FINDINGS
• Postmortem examination confirms the site and extent of the rupture and the presence of aorticocardiac or aortopulmonary fistula
• Path of the dissection can be traced
• Dissecting tracts into the interventricular septum usually are lined with immature and mature fibrous tissue, and disruption of the conduction system has been detected
• Degeneration and necrosis of the aortic media have been reported in some horses with aortic rupture but not in other affected horses
• An absence of media in the right sinus of Valsalva was reported in one horse with a sinus of Valsalva (i.e. aortic root) aneurysm
• Fibrosis and scarring of the rupture site have been reported in old breeding stallions that died of unrelated causes

TREATMENT

AIMS
Palliative care.

APPROPRIATE HEALTH CARE
• Closely monitor affected horses with ventricular tachycardia if the tachycardia is uniform, the heart rate is <100 bpm, no R-on-T complexes are detected, and no clinical signs of cardiovascular collapse are observed
• If ventricular tachycardia is multiform, R-on-T complexes are detected, heart rate is >100 bpm, or with clinical signs of cardiovascular collapse, institute antiarrhythmic treatment on an inpatient basis
• If CHF also is present, institute treatment for CHF as well. Consider humane euthanasia, however, because the horse is no longer safe to use for athletic work

NURSING CARE
• Perform continuous ECG monitoring during the attempted conversion from ventricular tachycardia to sinus rhythm
• Keep horses quiet and unmoving during antiarrhythmic treatment

ACTIVITY
• Stall confinement until conversion to sinus rhythm has been successfully achieved
• Restrict athletic activity as much as possible once ventricular tachycardia has been converted

CLIENT EDUCATION
• Affected horses are not safe to ride or use for any type of athletic work because of the risk of sudden death associated with further aortic rupture or development of fatal ventricular arrhythmia
• If the horse is a breeding stallion and such continued use is desired, warn the stallion and mare handlers (and all other personnel involved) about the risk of sudden death
• Develop an emergency plan in the event the stallion becomes unsteady or unsafe to handle

SURGICAL CONSIDERATIONS
N/A

MEDICATIONS

DRUG(S) OF CHOICE
Antiarrhythmics
• Indicated with multiform ventricular tachycardia, R-on-T complexes, heart rate >120 bpm, or clinical signs of cardiovascular collapse

• Drug selection depends on severity of ventricular tachycardia and associated clinical signs
• Lidocaine (0.25 mg/kg IV slowly, can repeat in 5–10 min) is rapid acting and has a very short duration of action. However, it also has central nervous system effects in horses and, thus, must be used carefully
• Procainamide (1 mg/kg/min IV to total dose of 20 mg/kg) and quinidine gluconate (0.5–2.2 mg/kg IV every 10 min to total dose 10 mg/kg) have been effective in converting sustained, uniform ventricular tachycardia but have a slower onset of action
• Magnesium sulfate (2.2–4.4 mg/kg IV slowly, can repeat in 5 min to total dose of 55 mg/kg) has been successful in converting sustained ventricular tachycardia and is not arrhythmogenic

CONTRAINDICATIONS
Other vasodilators or antihypertensive drugs have the potential to adversely affect the stallion's libido, breeding performance, or fertility.

PRECAUTIONS
Affected horses could experience sudden death at any time; thus, everyone working around these horses must be aware of the safety issues involved.

POSSIBLE INTERACTIONS
Any antiarrhythmic drug has the potential to cause development of a more adverse arrhythmia as well as to convert to sinus rhythm.

ALTERNATIVE DRUGS
Propranolol
• The IV form is less likely to be effective but should be considered in affected horses with refractory ventricular tachycardia
• Lowers systolic blood pressure

FOLLOW-UP

PATIENT MONITORING
• Routine monitoring of heart rate and of respiratory rate and rhythm after conversion to sinus rhythm
• Persistent tachypnea, tachycardia, or new arrhythmias indicate deterioration in clinical status
• Return of venous distention and jugular pulsations or development of ventral edema or coughing indicate the onset of CHF and worsening of ventricular volume overload

PREVENTION/AVOIDANCE
• With intact aneurysms of the sinus of Valsalva, control of systemic blood pressure may prolong the time until rupture occurs

• With degenerative changes in the aortic media, antihypertensive drugs theoretically should have some benefit. However, identification of horses at risk has not yet been accomplished

POSSIBLE COMPLICATIONS
• Deterioration of uniform ventricular tachycardia into fatal ventricular arrhythmia
• Severe, acute CHF from massive right atrial or ventricular, left atrial, and left ventricular volume overload
• Tricuspid valve rupture, leading to massive tricuspid regurgitation and CHF
• Rupture of a chorda tendinea of the tricuspid or mitral valve, leading to massive tricuspid or mitral regurgitation, respectively, and acute right- or left-sided CHF
• Sudden death

EXPECTED COURSE AND PROGNOSIS
• Prognosis for life of affected horses is grave and sudden death is possible
• Although the condition is invariably fatal, some horses can live relatively comfortably for several months after diagnosis

MISCELLANEOUS

ASSOCIATED CONDITIONS
Aortic root aneurysm.

AGE-RELATED FACTORS
Old horses are more likely to be affected with aortic root rupture, but horses as young as 4 years have been diagnosed. Aortic arch rupture typically presents in horses <4 years old.

PREGNANCY/FERTILITY/BREEDING
• Rupture of a sinus of Valsalva aneurysm has been seen in one late-gestation pregnant mare. The volume expansion of late pregnancy may predispose pregnant mares to aortic rupture at this time
• Aortic root rupture has been seen in one mare during early pregnancy. This mare experienced acute onset of ventricular tachycardia and subendocardial dissection of blood into the interventricular septum but survived to have the foal

SYNONYMS
• Aortic cardiac fistula
• Aorticocardiac fistula

SEE ALSO
Ventricular arrhythmias

ABBREVIATIONS
CHF = congestive heart failure

A

AORTIC RUPTURE   (CONTINUED)

Suggested Reading

Lester GD, Lombard CW, Ackerman N. Echocardiographic detection of a dissecting aortic root aneurysm in a Thoroughbred stallion. Vet Radiol Ultrasound 1992;33:202–205.

Marr CM, Reef VB, Brazil T, et al. Clinical and echocardiographic findings in horses with aortic root rupture. Vet Radiol Ultrasound 1998;39:22–31.

Ploeg M, Saey V, van Loon G, Delesalle C. Thoracic aortic rupture in horses. Equine Vet J 2017;49(3):269–274.

Reef VB, Klump S, Maxson AD, et al. Echocardiographic detection of an intact aneurysm in a horse. J Am Vet Med Assoc 1990;197:752–755.

Roby KA, Reef VB, Shaw DP, Sweeney CR. Rupture of an aortic sinus aneurysm in a 15-year-old broodmare. J Am Vet Med Assoc 1986;189:305–308.

Author Celia M. Marr
Consulting Editors Celia M. Marr and Virginia B. Reef

Acknowledgment The author acknowledges the prior contribution of Virginia B. Reef.

BASICS

OVERVIEW
Aortoiliac thrombosis occurs when a thrombus forms at the aortic quadrification and terminal portions of the aorta. Depending on its size, it may involve 1 or more of the internal and external iliac arteries. Larger thrombi may extend into the coccygeal arteries. Clinical signs relate to occlusion of these vessels and compromise to blood supply.

Systems affected
• Cardiovascular
• Musculoskeletal

SIGNALMENT
Horses of any age can be affected and there are no known breed or sex predilections.

SIGNS
• Affected horses generally present with hindlimb lameness, which is typically chronic and insidious but can be more acute and severe
• Lameness usually becomes increasingly severe with exercise
• After exercise the affected limb may be cool with reduced pulse pressure
• The thrombus may be palpable on transrectal examination
• Ejaculatory failure has been reported

CAUSES AND RISK FACTORS
Specific causes and risk factors have not been identified. Parasites are unlikely to be involved.

DIAGNOSIS

DIFFERENTIAL DIAGNOSIS
There are numerous causes of hindlimb lameness. Clinical signs of aortoiliac thrombosis can be similar to those of exertional rhabdomyolysis.

LABORATORY TESTS
• Laboratory tests are not generally helpful and no link between aortoiliac thrombosis and coagulopathy has been documented
• Modest increases in serum creatine kinase and aspartate aminotransferase activity may occur and measurement of these enzymes may help rule out primary myopathy

IMAGING
• Transrectal ultrasonographic imaging will usually demonstrate the thrombus and allow the extent of blood vessel involvement to be defined; the femoral artery should also be evaluated transcutaneously
• First-pass radionucleotide imaging will also demonstrate reduction of blood flow in affected iliac arteries and scintigraphic studies are indicated in some horses presenting with hindlimb lameness to rule out other causes

TREATMENT
• Horses should be withdrawn from work and rested (stall or pasture). Some horses improve following treatment with aspirin (18 mg/kg PO every 48 h) or clopidogrel at 2 mg/kg PO every 24 hours

• Surgical thrombectomy has been successful in restoring athletic activity in approximately 65% of cases

FOLLOW-UP

PATIENT MONITORING
Transrectal ultrasonography will allow the size and extent of the thrombus to be determined.

POSSIBLE COMPLICATIONS
Platelet count should be monitored every 2–4 weeks in horses receiving long-term aspirin therapy.

EXPECTED COURSE AND PROGNOSIS
The prognosis is fair—some horses resolve completely following either medical management or surgical intervention. In others the condition is progressive and requires the horse to be retired from all forms of exercise.

Suggested Reading
Rijkenhuizen AB, Sinclair D, Jahn W. Surgical thrombectomy in horses with aortoiliac thrombosis: 17 cases. Equine Vet J 2009;41:754–758.
Warmerdam EPL. Ultrasonography of the femoral artery in 6 normal horses and three horses with thrombosis. Vet Radiol Ultrasound 1998;39:137–141.

Author Celia M. Marr
Consulting Editors Celia M. Marr and Virginia B. Reef

ARSENIC TOXICOSIS

BASICS

OVERVIEW
• Results from excessive exposure to arsenic-containing pesticides, arsenic-contaminated soils, burn piles, and water or feed
• Ashes from chromated copper arsenate-treated lumber are high in arsenic
• Toxicity depends on the form of arsenic ingested
• Trivalent inorganic forms (e.g. arsenic trioxide; sodium, potassium, and calcium salts of arsenite) are 10-fold more toxic than inorganic pentavalent forms (e.g. sodium, potassium, and calcium salts of arsenate)
• Trivalent inorganic arsenicals inhibit cellular respiration and damage capillaries, mostly of the GI tract
• Pentavalent inorganic arsenicals uncouple oxidative phosphorylation, leading to deficits in cellular energy

SIGNALMENT
No breed, age, or sex predilections.

SIGNS
• Peracute or acute syndromes are likely
• Peracute—patient often found dead; death caused by cardiovascular collapse
• Acute—intense abdominal pain, hypersalivation, severe watery diarrhea, decreased abdominal sounds, muscle tremors, weak and rapid pulse with signs of circulatory shock, ataxia, depression, and recumbency; if the animal survives for several days, oliguria and proteinuria secondary to renal damage
• Chronic—not described in horses but should be considered in regions of high water arsenic

CAUSES AND RISK FACTORS
Accidental exposure to old arsenic-containing pesticides or arsenic-contaminated soils, ashes, water, or feed.

DIAGNOSIS

DIFFERENTIAL DIAGNOSIS
• Lead toxicosis—evidence of neurologic dysfunction is likely; blood lead concentrations are indicative
• Mercury toxicosis
• NSAID toxicosis—history of previous prolonged use
• Cantharidin toxicosis—evidence of cystitis, history of feeding beetle-contaminated hay
• Salmonellosis
• Colitis X
• Acute cyathostomiasis
• Clostridial colitis

CBC/BIOCHEMISTRY/URINALYSIS
• Reflect circulatory shock and possible liver and kidney damage

• Hemoconcentration—elevated packed cell volume and plasma total protein
• Leukopenia with degenerative changes in peripheral blood neutrophils
• Azotemia
• Electrolytes—hypokalemia; hyponatremia; hypochloremia
• Hyperglycemia
• Hyperbilirubinemia
• Elevated lactate dehydrogenase and creatine kinase

OTHER LABORATORY TESTS
• Antemortem—measurement of arsenic in urine, whole blood, or GI contents
• Postmortem—measurement of arsenic in liver, kidney, or hair (chronic cases)
• Arsenic is rapidly excreted after exposure ceases

IMAGING
N/A

OTHER DIAGNOSTIC PROCEDURES
N/A

PATHOLOGIC FINDINGS
Gross
• GI hemorrhage, mucosal congestion, edema, and ulcers/erosion either localized or throughout the GI tract, which may be filled with watery, dark-green, black, or hemorrhagic ingesta and necrotic material from mucosal sloughing
• Pulmonary edema and epicardial and serosal hemorrhage
• Pale swollen kidneys

Histopathologic
Necrotizing, hemorrhagic typhlocolitis, with necrotizing vasculitis, submucosal edema, renal tubular necrosis, and hepatic fatty degeneration.

TREATMENT
• Urgent treatment is necessary
• Remove animal from known or potential source of exposure
• GI decontamination
• Treat circulatory shock, dehydration, acidosis, and colic

MEDICATIONS

DRUG(S) OF CHOICE
• Hasten elimination of absorbed arsenic with chelators
  ◦ Dimercaprol (British anti-Lewisite) is the classic arsenic chelator (loading dose of 4–5 mg/kg given by deep IM injection, followed by 2–3 mg/kg every 4 h for 24 h and then 1 mg/kg every 4 h for 2 days); adverse reactions include tremors, convulsions, and coma

  ◦ DMSA is a less toxic chelator (equine dose not established, but 10 mg/kg PO every 8 h is suggested)
• Control abdominal pain
  ◦ Flunixin meglumine (1.1 mg/kg IV or IM every 24 h for 5 days) or butorphanol tartrate (0.1 mg/kg IV every 3–4 h up to 48 h)
  ◦ Xylazine hydrochloride (0.5–1 mg/kg IV or IM) may be used in conjunction with butorphanol (0.02–0.03 mg/kg IV)
• Demulcents—mineral oil or kaolin–pectin

CONTRAINDICATIONS/POSSIBLE INTERACTIONS
• Dimercaprol should not be used in patients with renal impairment
• Use NSAIDs cautiously because of possible adverse GI and renal effects

FOLLOW-UP
• Monitor renal and hepatic function
• Provide a bland diet, containing reduced amounts of high-quality protein
• Identify source of exposure and properly dispose of source
• Expected course and prognosis depend on the severity of clinical signs
• If the animal survives, recovery should be complete

MISCELLANEOUS

ASSOCIATED CONDITIONS
N/A

AGE-RELATED FACTORS
N/A

ZOONOTIC POTENTIAL
N/A

PREGNANCY/FERTILITY/BREEDING
N/A

ABBREVIATIONS
• DMSA = 2,3-dimercaptosuccinic acid, succimer
• GI = gastrointestinal
• NSAID = nonsteroidal anti-inflammatory drug

Suggested Reading
Casteel SW. Metal toxicosis in horses. Vet Clin North Am Equine Pract 2001;17:517–527.
Pace LW, Turnquist SE, Casteel SW, et al. Acute arsenic toxicosis in five horses. Vet Pathol 1997;34:160–164.

Authors Arya Sobhakumari and Robert H. Poppenga
Consulting Editors Wilson K. Rumbeiha and Steve Ensley

ARTIFICIAL INSEMINATION

BASICS

DEFINITION
- Intrauterine placement of extended fresh, cooled, frozen semen; aseptic technique
- Standard AI—min. $300–1000 \times 10^6$ PMS, fresh/cooled transported semen; $200–250 \times 10^6$ PMS, frozen semen; deposited into *uterine body*
- DHI for standard or lower doses—$1–25 \times 10^6$ PMS; low volume deposited into *tip of uterine horn* (ipsilateral to DF)
- HI for LDI—$1–3 \times 10^6$ PMS to *tip of uterine horn* (ipsilateral to DF)

PATHOPHYSIOLOGY
Advantages
- Prevent stallion overuse
- Efficient use of ejaculate—breed more mares per season (AI, 120+; live cover, 40–80)
- Wider stud use—older with problems: musculoskeletal, behavioral
- Ship semen across all borders—eliminate mare and foal transport, ↓stallion injuries; ↓trauma to mares (recent genital surgery, genital abnormalities, rejecting stallion's advance)
- Extender antibiotics prevent many infections/transmission of VD
- Assess semen before AI
- LDI—stallion with limited availability/showing, large book/short supply, subfertile/poor quality, or costly (sex-sorted)
  - Divide frozen AI dose to produce more than one foal
  - Stallion is dead or epididymal spermatozoa collected at the time of castration or stallion's death

SYSTEMS AFFECTED
Reproductive

SIGNALMENT
- Thoroughbreds—only live cover
- Other breed registries allow AI

SIGNS
Historical Findings
Records of prior cycles/pregnancies—predict days in heat, time of ovulation, selection of stallion, and semen to be used.

Teasing and Physical Examination Findings
- Ovulation timing is critical
  - Predict by history, teasing record, previous TRP/US
  - During estrus—tease daily; min. every other day
  - On second day of estrus, daily or every other day TRP/US
  - Perform US, as needed, to determine optimal time to breed
- TRP—DF (35 + mm), ↓uterine and cervical tone

- Follicle size/growth rate, edema of endometrial folds (peaks preovulation 72–96 h, decreased/absent 24–48 h in young, normal mares)
- DF often pear-shaped 12–24 h preovulation
  - Low uterine edema plus DF (≥40 mm)—indicates ovulation is close
- Ovulation depression, corpus haemorrhagicum, corpus luteum—evidence of ovulation

DIAGNOSIS

PROCEDURAL ISSUES
Timing and Frequency of Breeding
- Semen longevity varies by stallion, preservation method
- Equine ova—short viability (8–18 h post ovulation)

Teasing and Examinations
- AI as close to ovulation as possible
- OIA—GnRH analog, hCG, or combination when DF is >35 mm induces ovulation
- US 4–6 h post AI for DUC (especially if using frozen semen) and ovulation
- Evaluate normal, fertile mares 24–48 h after AI for ovulation
- Oxytocin IM/IV 4–6 h post AI. Can be given by trained personnel to ensure uterine clearance

Fresh (Raw or Extended) Semen
- Routine breeding—every other day if not using OIA, stallion has a small book, or mare is normal
  - Begin day 2 or 3 of estrus until mare teases out or when a DF follicle is detected by TRP/US
  - Can use OIA
- Inseminate within 48 h preovulation (acceptable pregnancy rates)

Cooled Transported Semen
- More mare examinations; fertility of some cooled semen decreases markedly >24 h
- OIA when DF is ≥35 mm to induce ovulation; order semen
- Semen arrives 24 h after ovulatory drug administration and 12–18 h before expected ovulation
- AI ≤ 12–24 h preovulation, min. dose of 500×10^6 PMS for acceptable conception rates
- Semen with poor post-cooling fertility should be sent *counter to counter* (i.e. airline transport)
  - Use only one AI dose if good quality semen; mare is predisposed to DUC/PMIE
  - No advantage to keeping second AI dose to rebreed next day in normal mares; uterus is best incubator for sperm

Frozen Thawed Semen
- Precise timing of AI; post-thaw longevity is reduced to ≤12–24 h

- Mare management—serial, daily teasing, TRP/US
- 2 different protocols for AI depending if multiple doses or a single dose of semen; fertile mare or predisposed to DUC
- Timed AI:
  - OIA when DF ≥ 35 mm
  - AI at 24 h; repeat at 40 h after OIA; ensure viable sperm available during ovulatory period
  - Treat mare if intrauterine fluid 4–6 h after AI
- Alternatively:
  - OIA when DF ≥ 35 mm
  - TRP/US—TID–QID, ensure AI very close to preovulation, or, most important, ≤6–8 h post ovulation
  - Treat mare if intrauterine fluid 4–6 h after AI
- Pregnancy rate for timed AI (2 doses) is equal to a one-time AI 6–8 h post ovulation, less intensive labor, fewer mare examinations; trade-off is increased endometrial irritation
- Combined methods for AI—timed but using one dose
  - OIA when DF ≥ 35 mm at 8–10 PM (preferably combination of OIA and when follicle <40 mm to have more control over induction)
  - TRP/US only once or twice the next day and again at 8 AM, 34–36 h post induction to assure the presence of a DF
  - TRP/US 6 h later, 40–42 h post induction; >90% of mares ovulate within this window
  - If mare has ovulated, proceed to AI; if not, keep performing TRP/US every 6 h until ovulation
  - This method assures AI within 2–6 h of ovulation, limiting the waste of an AI dose if ovulation does not occur
  - Treat mare if DUC 4–6 h after AI

Low-Dose Insemination
- Allows use of a reduced dose of semen (fresh, cooled, frozen)
  - Acceptable pregnancy with doses as low as 25×10^6 PMS in volumes of 20–1000 μL (1 mL)
  - Deposit semen at UTJ, ipsilateral to DF
- Can be either HI or DHI
  - Similar pregnancy rates when using >5×10^6 PMS
  - HI may provide advantage when AI dose is $1–3 \times 10^6$ PMS
  - DHI is inexpensive; requires less personnel and skills
- Mare management varies according to method of semen preservation and severity of her endometrial inflammatory reaction

General Comments
- If ovulation has not occurred within recommended times for fresh (48 h), cooled (24 h), or frozen (6–12 h) semen, rebreed
  - Consider it may be an anovulatory follicle if mare is unresponsive to the OIA

ARTIFICIAL INSEMINATION   (CONTINUED)

• Older ova or semen, poor timing, percent EED increases

LABORATORY TESTS
Progesterone level of >1 ng/mL confirms ovulation.

IMAGING
US

OTHER DIAGNOSTIC PROCEDURES

Semen Analysis
• Min. parameters—volume, motility, concentration
• Morphology—optional, of particular use if stallion has fertility problems
• Small sample of cooled/frozen semen should be saved and warmed (37°C); evaluate immediately post AI
   ○ For DHI with frozen semen—after thawing straws, remove the sealed end, place one drop of semen on a slide for evaluation pre-AI
   ○ Pipet and stylet—completely empty straws unless purposely saving 10% of the last straw
• Slide, coverslip, pipet—prewarm to avoid cold shock
• Min. number of sperm—$300–1000 \times 10^6$ PMS (fresh/chilled); $200–250 \times 10^6$ PMS (frozen)

Stallion's Disease Status
Should be negative for equine infectious anemia, equine viral arteritis, contagious equine metritis, VD.

Mare Selection
• Her fertility matters even more if using frozen semen or its quality is poor
• Reproductive history ± normal estrous cycles, uterine cultures/cytology, DUC
• Fertility is best—normal, pluriparous/maidens; less, older pluriparous; older maiden/barren mare

Prebreeding Uterine Culture and Cytology of Mare
• All, except young maiden mares—at least one negative uterine culture and cytology prebreeding
   ○ Avoid disease transmission to the stallion
   ○ Early identification of possible problems
• Pregnancy rates lower, EED higher if treated for an infection in same cycle as AI

TREATMENT

Prebreeding
• Presence of ≥2 cm uterine fluid prebreeding, LRS uterine lavage up to 1 h before AI
• Use 10 IU oxytocin IV post lavage only if performed >4 h prebreeding
• Should not affect fertility

AI Technique
• Sterile, disposable equipment. Mare restrained, rectum free of manure, perineal area thoroughly cleansed (mild detergent/antiseptic solution/soap); min. three rinses to remove any residue
• Sterile sleeve; non-spermicidal lubricant applied to dorsum of gloved hand
   ○ 50–56 cm AI pipet carried in the gloved hand for fresh and cooled semen, less frequent for frozen semen
   ○ Index finger first passes through cervical lumen, serves as a guide by which the pipet can readily be advanced to a position no more than 2.5 cm into the uterine body
   ○ Syringe, non-spermicidal plastic plunger, e.g. Air-Tite, containing the extended semen is attached to the pipet, semen is slowly deposited into uterus; remaining semen in the pipet is rapidly delivered by using a small bolus of air (1–3 mL) in the syringe

Fresh Extended Semen
• AI immediately after collection
• Semen mixed with appropriate extender; immediate AI; semen-to-extender ratio (1:1 or 1:2), if small ejaculate volume and high concentration or mare predisposed to PMIE

Cooled Transported Semen
• Before first shipment, perform longevity test to determine best semen extender
• Collect, dilute in extender, cool to 4–6°C for 24–48 h. With transport, can be modest decrease of fertilizing capacity (stallion dependent)
• Semen-to-extender ratio of 1:3 or 1:4 is acceptable; may be as high as 1:15 (dependent on original concentration); semen longevity optimized by extending to $25–50 \times 10^6$ spermatozoa/mL
• Ship minimum 1×10^9 PMS; approx. 50% loss in shipment; so 500×10^6 PMS remain for AI at 24 h

Frozen Thawed Semen
• Frozen semen packed in 0.5, 2.5, or 5 mL straws; stored in liquid nitrogen
• A 5 mL straw contains $600–1000 \times 10^6$ sperm cells
• Dependent on post-freeze sperm motility and AI method, 1–4 + straws may be needed
• A 0.5 mL straw contains $200–800 \times 10^6$ sperm cells
   ○ Thawing protocols vary; reported best paired with a particular freezing method. Seek specific information regarding thawing. In absence of a recommended protocol, 37°C for 30–60 s may be an acceptable alternative
• Post thaw, semen should be in the mare within 5 min
• Methods of frozen semen AI:
   ○ Into uterine body, regular AI pipet
   ○ DHI—flexible pipet and stylet (0.5 mL straws, LDI flexible pipet, and inner catheter (2.5–5 mL straws))
   ○ HI (LDI, especially when $<1–3 \times 10^6$ PMS)
• Advantages of DHI and HI over *uterine body*—reduction in sperm transport time;

increased number of sperm to colonize the oviduct ipsilateral to the DF (77% vs. 54%)
• Post-AI uterine treatment, strongly recommended (high concentration of spermatozoa in thawed straw + absence of seminal plasma may induce an acute PMIE)
• No scientific evidence that reducing spermatozoa number decreases the PMIE

Procedures
• Sedation of the mare is recommended for HI but is rarely needed for DHI. Procedure should be performed quickly (≤10 min) to avoid inducing uterine trauma
• DHI—flexible 65–75 cm AI pipet through the cervix, to tip of the uterine horn ipsilateral to DF:
   ○ Attach 3 mL syringe to the external pipet end (avoid introducing air during the procedure)
   ○ Hold sterile pipet in a 45° curve before the procedure, the bend helps direct its tip into the desired horn
   ○ Once through the cervix, remove the AI hand from the vagina, place it in the rectum to transrectally guide the pipet tip rostral and slightly ventral into the uterine horn, toward its tip
   ○ Manual transrectal elevation of the uterine horn tip may help pipet passage
   ○ Insert the 0.5 mL straw into the pipet; a flexible steel stylet pushes the straw through the pipet to the nipple at the tip; deposit the semen close to or onto the UTJ. If more than one straw is used, remove the stylet, its bulbous end grabs the straw, the next straw is then introduced
• A similar pipet, without stylet, with an inner tube, is used for AI of frozen semen from 2.5–5 mL straws. This pipet also used for AI of cooled shipped semen after centrifugation (poor quality, very dilute)
• HI—introduction of an endoscope into the mare's uterus:
   ○ Approach and visualize the UTJ/oviductal papilla ipsilateral to DF
   ○ Pass small catheter loaded with semen through the channel, deposit semen slowly on the UTJ
   ○ Rapidly remove endoscope
   ○ No significant irritation if performed in <5 min
   ○ Volumes >1 mL tend to run down the air-distended uterine horn
• HI compared with DHI—↑expensive, ↑skill, ↑labor, ↑personnel. The method of choice if AI of $1–3 \times 10^6$ PMS

Post Breeding
• US 4–6 h after AI for DUC
   ○ If fluid, uterine lavage (sterile saline/LRS), followed by oxytocin 4–6 h after AI
   ○ Repeat oxytocin at 3–4 h intervals, if fluid persists; again at 12–24 h until inflammation resolves

MEDICATIONS

DRUG(S) OF CHOICE
• OIA most effective if follicle is ≥35 mm; within 36–42 h with:
  ◦ hCG (1500–3000 IU IV/IM; range 36–72 h)
  ◦ GnRH analog—Sucromate (deslorelin acetate 1.8 mg IM)
  ◦ *Compounded* GnRH analogs (deslorelin 1.5 mg IM, histrelin 1 mg IM)
  ◦ *Compounded* GnRH analog + hCG combo (deslorelin 1.5–2 mg + hCG 1500–2500 IU IM)
• Ecbolic drugs—to treat PMIE and DUC
• Prostaglandins—misoprostol for cervical relaxation

CONTRAINDICATIONS
See chapter Endometritis.

PRECAUTIONS
See chapter Endometritis.

FOLLOW-UP

PATIENT MONITORING
• Begin teasing by 11 days post ovulation
  ◦ Suspect endometritis if a shortened cycle; owing to endogenous prostaglandin release
• US for pregnancy 14–15 days post ovulation; rule out potential twins vs. lymphatic cyst
• Follow-up TRP/US—24–30 days (confirm embryo and heartbeat)
• Serial TRP examinations—45, 60, 90, 120 days gestation

POSSIBLE COMPLICATIONS
• Artificial vagina preparation, handling, maintenance
• Semen evaluation at collection—ship adequate AI dose and/or send correct number of semen straws
• Shipping methods—Equitainer, reusable box cooling containers, vapor tank
  ◦ Cooled shipments—entire breeding program is at mercy of airlines/couriers
• Operator skills
  ◦ To manipulate and place semen through the cervix, into the uterine lumen, or to the tip of the horn (proper and timely)
  ◦ Handling storage, straw transfer from main tank, water bath, vapor shipper, thawing and evaluation of frozen semen
• Misidentification of stallions/mares

MISCELLANEOUS

PREGNANCY/FERTILITY/BREEDING
Cooled Semen
Per cycle pregnancy rates almost equal to on-farm fresh semen AI (60–75%) if quality is good after cooling for 24 h at 5–6°C.

Frozen Semen
• Pregnancy rates per cycle using frozen semen are 5–10% lower than cooled shipped semen for most stallions
• Spermatozoa are stressed; loss of ≅50% at freezing and thawing
• First-cycle pregnancy rates 30–45% (range 0–70%); wide range between stallions
  ◦ Requires greatest management. Good quality of semen has positive impact on pregnancy rate

• Candidate selection for frozen semen breeding
  ◦ Most fertile—young pluriparous mares, young maidens
  ◦ Least fertile—old pluriparous mares, old maidens, barren mares
• Older eggs or semen due to poor timing—decreased conception rate, increased EED

SYNONYMS
Artificial breeding

SEE ALSO
• Conception failure
• Early embryonic death
• Endometritis
• Spermatogenesis and factors affecting sperm production

ABBREVIATIONS
• AI = artificial insemination
• DF = dominant follicle
• DHI = deep horn insemination
• DUC = delayed uterine clearance
• EED = early embryonic death
• GnRH = gonadotropin-releasing hormone
• hCG = human chorionic gonadotropin
• HI = hysteroscopic insemination
• LDI = low-dose AI
• LRS = lactated Ringer's solution
• OIA = ovulation induction agent
• PMIE = post-mating-induced endometritis
• PMS = progressively motile sperm
• TRP = transrectal palpation
• US = ultrasound
• UTJ = uterotubal junction
• VD = venereal disease

Author Maria E. Cadario
Consulting Editor Carla L. Carleton

ARYTENOID CHONDROPATHY

 BASICS

DEFINITION
• A septic inflammatory process of one or both arytenoid cartilages, resulting in the formation of luminal swelling, granulomas, and deformation with enlargement
• This interferes with the ability of the affected arytenoid cartilage to fully abduct during forced inspiration and/or to resist collapsing airway pressure during inspiration. In addition "kissing lesions" on the medial surface of the opposing arytenoid cartilage may be seen

SIGNALMENT
Racehorses are more commonly affected, although it can be observed in older horses of any breed or function.

SIGNS
• Upper respiratory noise, exercise intolerance, or both
• The disease usually worsens gradually, with progressive involvement of one or both arytenoid cartilages
• Can lead to ventilation interference proportional to the loss of abductory function and the mechanical size of the granulomas or affected arytenoid cartilages. The more intense the high-intensity exercise occurs, the earlier the effect of an obstruction is detected (the horse does not "finish" or close well)
• In show horses, loss of points during competition because of upper respiratory noise may be the main concern; this upper airway noise may resemble that of horses with laryngeal hemiplegia

CAUSES
• Physical trauma to the mucosa of the arytenoid cartilage caused by air turbulence or aspiration of track surface particles during exercise or severe coughing or intubation (e.g. endotracheal, nasogastric) procedures
• Upper airway infection leading to coughing and contact ulcers on the medial surface of the arytenoid cartilage dorsal to the vocal processes. If the inflammatory condition persists and infection develops, arytenoid cartilage sepsis occurs
• In many cases, the inciting cause is never found

 DIAGNOSIS

DIFFERENTIAL DIAGNOSIS
• Laryngeal hemiplegia
• Congenital malformation of the laryngeal cartilages (i.e. fourth branchial arch defect)

CBC/BIOCHEMISTRY/URINALYSIS
In active infection with abscessation, serum amyloid A and fibrinogen may be elevated.

OTHER LABORATORY TESTS
• Arterial blood gases during exercise
• Hypoventilation can be evaluated using arterial blood gases—typically at maximal exercise $PaCO_2$ can be >50 mmHg; PaO_2 may be <65 mmHg in affected horses

IMAGING
• Lateral radiography of the larynx may reveal enlarged laryngeal cartilages, sometimes with associated osseous metaplasia
• Ultrasonographic examination of the larynx using the mid-ventral and caudoventral windows to evaluate for abscess and the caudolateral window to assess the presence of disease in the lateral aspect of the arytenoid cartilage. MRI and CT are rarely indicated but may also reveal the extent of arytenoid cartilage involvement

OTHER DIAGNOSTIC PROCEDURES
• The diagnosis is established on the basis of videoendoscopic examination at rest:
  ○ The body of the arytenoid is irregular and thickened
  ○ A mass of granulation tissue may protrude from the medial surface of the arytenoid cartilage into the airway. The size or location of the protruding mass has no correlation with the amount of abduction remaining
  ○ The corniculate process may be deformed
  ○ Contact (i.e. "kissing") lesions may be observed on the contralateral arytenoid cartilage
• Eventually, the condition may lead to decreased or total inability of the affected arytenoid cartilage to abduct during inspiration

 TREATMENT

• Medical treatment is indicated only in acute cases with mucosal ulceration and swellings
• Consider endoscopically guided excision of intralaryngeal granulations if the affected arytenoid cartilage retains sufficient abductory function for intended athletic activity
• When arytenoid abduction is severely reduced, partial arytenoidectomy (excision of the body and corniculate process of affected arytenoid cartilage) is the treatment of choice to restore exercise capacity and to reduce upper airway noise
• Permanent tracheotomy can be used in countries where athletic competition is allowed with this procedure and to salvage the animal for breeding purposes

 MEDICATIONS

DRUG(S) OF CHOICE
• Acute case—broad-spectrum antibiotics and NSAIDs
• Chronic case—none, other than routine perioperative antimicrobial and anti-inflammatory agents
• Use of nasopharyngeal spray, consisting of various anti-inflammatory and antimicrobial agents (140 mL DMSO, 140 mL glycerin, 266 mL distilled water, and 14 mL dexamethasone 4 mg/mL and often an antibiotic such as nitrofurazone—makes 560 mL, enough for 2 weeks) can be applied (20 mL BID) using a soft rubber feeding tube
• If the airway is significantly compromised, a temporary tracheotomy may be needed until the swelling resolves

 FOLLOW-UP

PATIENT MONITORING
• Videoendoscopy of the upper airway 2–6 weeks after surgery to monitor patient response
• Final response to treatment or continuation of monitoring of affected horses is made on the basis of evaluating exercise tolerance and upper respiratory noise
• Laser resection of the unsupported ipsilateral aryepiglottic fold might be needed to improve airway patency

POSSIBLE COMPLICATIONS
• Horses undergoing removal of the corniculate and body of the arytenoid cartilage have a slightly increased risk of tracheal aspiration of feed during deglutition. In addition, these procedures do not fully restore the airway diameter, so a mild degree of airway obstruction persists, which may interfere with performance or result in upper airway noise during exercise. Postsurgery dynamic endoscopy is indicated if results are not satisfactory to identify if a soft tissue resection of collapsing tissue is needed
• Bilateral arytenoidectomy increases the risk for tracheal aspiration of feed during deglutition and for glottic stenosis because of webbing at the resection site

EXPECTED COURSE AND PROGNOSIS
• Horses with acute swelling of the arytenoid cartilage may respond favorably to NSAIDs, topical anti-inflammatory agents, and antibiotics
• Untreated horses exhibit a progressive increase in exercise intolerance and upper respiratory noise

• Horses with focal elevated granulations on the medial surface of the arytenoid cartilage that maintain abductory function may respond to simple "lumpectomy"; recurrence of granuloma is seen in approximately 20–30% of horses
• Horses with generalized involvement of an arytenoid cartilage and without surgical treatment often develop contralateral contact or "kissing" lesions
• Horses with unilateral lesions treated surgically have a fair prognosis (60%) for elimination or significant reduction of exercise intolerance; however, the prognosis is guarded (20%) in horses with bilateral lesions

 MISCELLANEOUS

SEE ALSO
• Dynamic collapse of the upper airways
• Laryngeal hemiparesis/hemiplegia (recurrent laryngeal neuropathy)

ABBREVIATIONS
• CT = computed tomography
• DMSO = dimethylsulfoxide
• MRI = magnetic resonance imaging
• NSAID = nonsteroidal anti-inflammatory drug
• $PaCO_2$ = partial pressure of carbon dioxide in arterial blood
• PaO_2 = partial pressure of oxygen in arterial blood

Suggested Reading
Hay WP, Tulleners E. Excision of intralaryngeal granulation tissue in 25 horses using a neodymium: YAG laser (1986 to 1991). Vet Surg 1993;22:129–134.
Haynes PF, Snider TG, McLure JR, McClure JJ. Chronic chondritis of the equine arytenoid cartilage. J Am Vet Med Assoc 1980;177:1135–1142.
Lumsden JM, Derksen FJ, Stick JA, et al. Evaluation of partial arytenoidectomy as a treatment for equine laryngeal hemiplegia. Equine Vet J 1994;26:92–93.
Parente EJ, Tulleners EP, Southwood LL. Long-term study of partial arytenoidectomy with primary mucosal closure in 76 Thoroughbred racehorses (1992-2006). Equine Vet J 2008;40:214–218.
Radcliffe CH, Woodie JB, Hackett RP, et al. A comparison of laryngoplasty and modified partial arytenoidectomy as treatments for laryngeal hemiplegia in exercising horses. Vet Surg 2006;35:643–652.
Tulleners EP, Harrison IW, Raker CW. Management of arytenoid chondropathy and failed laryngoplasty in horses: 75 cases (1979–1985). J Am Vet Med Assoc 1988;192:670–675.
Witte TH, Mohammed HO, Radcliffe CH, et al. Racing performance after combined prosthetic laryngoplasty and ipsilateral ventriculocordectomy or partial arytenoidectomy: 135 Thoroughbred racehorses competing at less than 2400 m (1997-2007). Equine Vet J 2009;41:70–75.

Author Norm G. Ducharme
Consulting Editors Daniel Jean and Mathilde Leclère

ASCARID INFESTATION

BASICS

DEFINITION
Roundworm infestation caused by *Parascaris equorum*.

PATHOPHYSIOLOGY
• Direct life cycle—fecal–oral route. • Adult horses, especially brood mares, and older foals—main reservoir of infection (eggs). • Eggs accumulate in the environment (highly resistant), sticking to different surfaces, including the mare's mammary gland. • After ingestion—embryonated eggs hatch in the host's small intestine, larvae migrate through the intestinal wall to the liver and lungs, larvae travel up the bronchial tree, are swallowed, and develop into 10–50 cm long mature adult ascarids in the duodenum and proximal jejunum. Prepatent period, 10–12 weeks. • SIO—associated with a large burden of parasites

SYSTEMS AFFECTED
• Gastrointestinal—colic, enteritis, maldigestion, and malabsorption. • Hepatobiliary—migrating larvae resulting in temporary liver damage. • Respiratory—tracheobronchitis

INCIDENCE/PREVALENCE
• Prevalence—31–61%. • Infection prevalence—up to 100% in tested farms and in 80% of foals. • Colic due to SIO—0.5% (25/5134 cases of colic)

GEOGRAPHIC DISTRIBUTION
Worldwide

SIGNALMENT
• Any ages—primarily foals. • Adult horses—debilitated and immunocompromised

SIGNS
• Ascarid infestation—lethargy, weakness, decreased weight gain, dull hair coat, and "pot-bellied" appearance. • Mild to moderate colic—intestinal phase of the infection. • SIO—severe colic, can be complicated with volvulus or intussusception. • Peritonitis—perforation of the intestine. • Coughing and mucopurulent nasal discharge with or without systemic illness—larval migration through the lungs

CAUSES
N/A

RISK FACTORS
• All foals are at risk. • Breeding farms—large yearly population of young horses grazing on same pasture. • Ascarid impaction and SIO—usually 24 h after anthelmintic therapy (72% of the cases)

DIAGNOSIS

DIFFERENTIAL DIAGNOSIS
• Other causes of delayed growth. • SIO—small intestine strangulating lesion

CBC/BIOCHEMISTRY/URINALYSIS
• Eosinophilia—during larval migration, 10–40 days post infection. • Leukopenia and mild anemia. • Hypoproteinemia—severe infestation

OTHER LABORATORY TESTS
N/A

IMAGING
Transabdominal ultrasonography—adult ascarids within the intestinal lumen or in the peritoneal cavity (perforation).

OTHER DIAGNOSTIC PROCEDURES
• Fecal flotation. • Eosinophils in tracheal wash—verminous lung disease

PATHOLOGIC FINDINGS
Adult forms in the intestinal lumen or free in the abdominal cavity (intestinal perforation).

TREATMENT

APPROPRIATE HEALTH CARE
Treatment indicated when fecal egg counts >100 eggs per gram.

CLIENT EDUCATION
Severe parasite burdens suspected—benzimidazoles are recommended. Avoid anthelmintics that result in paralysis of the parasites (e.g. pyrantel pamoate, piperazine, organophosphates, ivermectin).

SURGICAL CONSIDERATIONS
For removal of dead parasites and correction of secondary complications (intussusceptions and intestinal volvulus).

MEDICATIONS

DRUG(S) OF CHOICE
• Anthelmintics—do not eliminate migrating larvae. Preventative therapy should be given until 1 year of age. • Broodmares—deworm at monthly intervals in the last trimester of pregnancy. Reduce environmental contamination. • Fenbendazole—10 mg/kg every 24 h PO for 5 consecutive days (varies in effectiveness against ascarids). • Moxidectin—0.4 mg/kg PO and ivermectin 0.2 mg/kg PO. Advocated to be 100% efficient in eliminating ascarid infection in horses. Resistance to these and other macrocyclic lactone anthelmintics has been identified in Europe and North America

CONTRAINDICATIONS
See Client Education.

FOLLOW-UP

PATIENT MONITORING
Fecal floatation—conducted in 10% or more of foals every 4–6 months. If >10% of foals are positive indicates failure of the anthelmintic therapy or of the prevention and control strategies.

PREVENTION/AVOIDANCE
• Contaminated facilities—disinfection with a 5% phenolic compound. • Grazing of broodmares, foals, and weanlings on heavily contaminated pastures should be avoided. • *P. equorum* eggs—remain viable in the environment for years. • Frequent removal of manure from stalls and pastures

POSSIBLE COMPLICATIONS
Toxicosis—overdose of anthelmintic.

EXPECTED COURSE AND PROGNOSIS
• Prognosis—favorable in uncomplicated cases (delay in growth is common). • SIO—short-term (discharge from hospital) and long-term (>1 year) survival 64% and 27%, respectively. • Formation of adhesions—associated with nonsurvival

MISCELLANEOUS

ASSOCIATED CONDITIONS
• SIO. • Peritonitis

AGE-RELATED FACTORS
Primarily in foals.

ZOONOTIC POTENTIAL
Human infection—extremely rare.

PREGNANCY/FERTILITY/BREEDING
N/A

SYNONYMS
N/A

ABBREVIATIONS
SIO = small intestine obstruction

Suggested Reading
Cribb NC, Cote NM, Bouré LP, Peregrine AS. Acute small intestinal obstruction associated with *Parascaris equorum* infection in young horses: 25 cases (1985-2004). N Z Vet J 2006;54:338–343.

Author Diego Gomez-Nieto
Consulting Editors Henry Stämpfli and Olimpo Oliver-Espinosa
Acknowledgment The author and editors acknowledge the prior contribution of Carlos Medina-Torres.

ASPARTATE AMINOTRANSFERASE (AST)

BASICS

DEFINITION
- Catalyzes the transamination of L-aspartate and 2-oxoglutarate to oxaloacetate and glutamate. Requires pyridoxal 5′-phosphate as a cofactor
- AST is present in cytoplasm and in larger amounts in the mitochondria
- AST is present in skeletal muscle, cardiac muscle cells, hepatocytes, and erythrocytes
- Reported normal AST activity in horses varies from 48 to 456 IU/L

PATHOPHYSIOLOGY
- Increases in AST activity are typically indicative of hepatocellular and/or striated muscle injury; however, increases occur with hemolysis because of the high AST content in erythrocytes
- The degree of elevation of AST concentrations is proportional to the number of hepatocytes affected
- The magnitude of AST elevation with skeletal muscle injury is not necessarily proportional to the extent of tissue injury
- Increases above the reference range can occur with IM injections, recumbency, trauma, and long trailer rides
- AST is a sensitive indicator of hepatocellular and striated muscle injury; however, because it is present in many tissues, AST lacks specificity. Other biochemical parameters need to be examined concurrently with AST to localize the source of the increase (i.e. SDH for liver and CK for muscle)
- After tissue injury, AST activity increases slower and remains increased longer than SDH or CK
- Increased SDH concentration, with normal or increased AST concentration, indicates acute or ongoing hepatocellular injury. If serial serum biochemistry analyses reveal continuously or progressively increased activities of both enzymes, ongoing hepatocellular injury is likely. During treatment of hepatic disease, enzymes can be used to monitor progress and cessation of the insult. If, after documentation of recent hepatocellular injury, serial serum biochemistry analyses reveal increased AST and progressively decreasing or normal SDH activity, cessation of the original insult is likely. Because AST has a longer half-life, AST may increase even after cessation of original insult, and the activity may remain increased for weeks
- A similar interpretative approach is used when determining if muscle injury is present. Muscle and hepatocellular injury can occur concurrently, and increases in AST, CK, and SDH concentrations may be seen together

SYSTEMS AFFECTED
- Musculoskeletal
- Hepatobiliary
- Cardiovascular (myocardium)
- Hemic (erythrocytes)

GENETICS
- PSSM type 1—Quarter Horses, Paints, and draft horses are predisposed
- PSSM type 2—Quarter Horses and Warmbloods are predisposed

INCIDENCE/PREVALENCE
N/A

GEOGRAPHIC DISTRIBUTION
N/A

SIGNALMENT
- See Genetics
- Any breed, age, or sex

SIGNS
Historical Findings
- Dependent on the underlying cause
- Strenuous exercise or overtraining

Physical Examination Findings
- Dependent on the underlying cause
- Muscle disorders—reluctance or inability to move, stiffness, and recumbency
- Liver disorders—icterus, neurologic deficits, discolored urine, anorexia, colic, weight loss, photosensitization, and fever
- Clinical signs due to hepatic failure generally do not appear until 75% of the hepatic functional mass is lost

CAUSES
- Degenerative conditions—chronic active hepatitis, rhabdomyolysis, and cholelithiasis
- Anomaly, congenital or hereditary diseases—polysaccharide storage myopathy (PSSM), glycogen branching enzyme deficiency; biliary atresia
- Metabolic diseases—shock, hypovolemia, hypoxia caused by severe gastrointestinal disease, severe anemia, or general anesthesia
- Neoplastic or nutritional diseases—neoplasia, hepatic lipidosis, and vitamin E/selenium deficiency
- Infectious and immune-mediated diseases—hepatitis of various causes (e.g. viral, bacterial, protozoal, fungal, parasitic), Theiler's disease, amyloidosis, sepsis, endotoxemia, and immune-mediated myositis
- Toxic or trauma—pyrrolizidine alkaloid-containing plants, cottonseed, castor bean, oak, alsike clover, fungal toxins (e.g. aflatoxins, cyclopiazonic acid, fumonisin, phalloidin [mushrooms]), and chemical compounds/elements, such as ethanol, chlorinated hydrocarbons, carbon tetrachloride, monensin, copper, iron, and petroleum

RISK FACTORS
Dependent on the underlying cause.

DIAGNOSIS

DIFFERENTIAL DIAGNOSIS
See Causes.

CBC/BIOCHEMISTRY/URINALYSIS
CBC
- Erythrocytes—liver disease may cause nonregenerative anemia of chronic inflammation. Hemolytic anemia may increase serum AST activity, and anemia from any cause can cause hypoxic liver or muscle damage
- Leukocytes—leukocytosis or leukopenia may be seen with inflammatory diseases; morphologic changes of the leukocytes (e.g. neutrophil toxicity) also may be seen
- Platelets—quantitative decreases and increases may be seen with a variety of systemic diseases that may affect the liver or striated muscle

Biochemistry
- Glucose—decreased in endstage liver disease
- Blood urea nitrogen—increased in severe rhabdomyolysis from secondary renal injury (i.e. pigment nephropathy); decreased in liver insufficiency and endstage liver disease from decreased conversion of ammonia to urea
- Albumin—rarely decreased in endstage liver disease from decreased production
- Globulin—increased in endstage liver disease and with chronic antigenic stimulation
- SDH—increased with acute and ongoing hepatocellular injury
- Alkaline phosphatase—increased with cholestatic disease
- γ-Glutamyltransferase—increased with cholestatic disease
- CK—increased with acute or ongoing muscle injury
- Conjugated bilirubin—increased with cholestatic disease
- Unconjugated bilirubin—increased with anorexia and prehepatic cholestasis (e.g. massive in vivo hemolysis)
- Triglycerides—increases may be associated with hepatic lipidosis
- In vitro hemolysis falsely increases AST. Prolonged in vitro exposure of serum to erythrocytes falsely increases AST activity even before visible signs of hemolysis are present. To avoid this confounding factor, prompt separation of serum from the cellular components of blood is strongly recommended
- If laboratory analysis will not occur within 1–2 days, freeze the serum sample

Urinalysis
Bilirubinuria—conjugated bilirubin, detected by the commonly used dipstick and diazo tablet methods, indicates cholestatic disease.

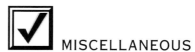

ASPARTATE AMINOTRANSFERASE (AST) (CONTINUED)

OTHER LABORATORY TESTS

SBAs
• Bile acids will increase in the circulation prior to total bilirubin in cases of liver disease. In the horse, SBAs are not affected by short-term fasting (<3 days). Postprandial increases are also not seen because of the lack of a gallbladder. SBAs are a good adjunct test when abnormal liver enzymes are detected. An increase in SBAs indicates liver dysfunction
• Congenital abnormalities of the portal circulation cause SBAs to bypass the liver, which results in increases in circulation. In contrast, total bilirubin will not be increased as a result of the shunt, but may be increased due to fasting

Plasma Ammonia Concentration
• Increases indicate hepatic insufficiency/decreased functional mass
• Plasma ammonia measurement requires special handling, which limits its general availability
• Consult reference laboratory for specific sample submission requirements

Coagulation Tests and Plasma Fibrinogen Concentration
• The liver manufactures many of the coagulation factors; therefore, significant decreases in liver function may lead to deficiencies in these factors and to coagulation abnormalities
• APTT and PT—decreased APTT and PT are seen when <30% of the activity of the factors is present

Cardiac Troponin I
Elevations indicate myocarditis.

Toxicology
Analysis of tissue biopsy, feed, ingesta, serum/plasma, or other body fluids may indicate presence of a toxin.

IMAGING

Transabdominal Ultrasonography
• Evaluate size, echogenicity, shape, and position of liver
• Useful for guidance when obtaining liver biopsy for cytology, histopathology, and microbiology

• Helpful in the evaluation of muscle and tendon injuries

OTHER DIAGNOSTIC PROCEDURES
Liver or muscle biopsy for cytology (impression smear) and histopathology.

PATHOLOGIC FINDINGS
Dependent on the underlying cause.

TREATMENT
Dependent on the underlying cause.

MEDICATIONS

DRUG(S) OF CHOICE
Dependent on the underlying cause.

CONTRAINDICATIONS
With suspected hepatic insufficiency, assess the relative safety/risk of performing invasive procedures (e.g. fine needle aspiration, tissue biopsy, laparoscopy, surgery) in light of coagulation panel results.

PRECAUTIONS
Dependent on the underlying cause.

POSSIBLE INTERACTIONS
Dependent on the underlying cause.

ALTERNATIVE DRUGS
Dependent on the underlying cause.

FOLLOW-UP

PATIENT MONITORING
Serial serum biochemistry analyses to monitor progression or improvement of the disease.

PREVENTION/AVOIDANCE
Dependent on the underlying cause.

POSSIBLE COMPLICATIONS
Dependent on the underlying cause.

EXPECTED COURSE AND PROGNOSIS
Dependent on the underlying cause.

✓ ## MISCELLANEOUS

ASSOCIATED CONDITIONS
Dependent on the underlying cause.

AGE-RELATED FACTORS
N/A

ZOONOTIC POTENTIAL
Dependent on the underlying cause.

PREGNANCY/FERTILITY/BREEDING
N/A

SYNONYMS
Previously known as glutamate oxaloacetate transaminase (SGOT).

SEE ALSO
Ammonia, hyperammonemia

ABBREVIATIONS
• APTT = activated partial thromboplastin time
• AST = aspartate aminotransferase
• CK = creatine kinase
• PT = prothrombin time
• SBA = serum bile acid
• SDH = sorbitol dehydrogenase

Suggested Reading
Divers TJ, Barton MH. Disorders of the liver. In: Reed SM, Bayly WM, Sellon DC, eds. Equine Internal Medicine, 4e. St. Louis, MO: Elsevier, 2018:843–887.
Meyer DJ, Walton RM. The liver. In: Walton RJ, ed. Equine Clinical Pathology. Ames, IA: Wiley Blackwell, 2014:71–86.
Smith GW, Davis JL. Diseases of the hepatobiliary system. In: Smith B, ed. Large Animal Internal Medicine, 5e. St. Louis, MO: Elsevier Mosby, 2015:843–871.
Valberg SJ. Diseases of muscle. In: Smith B, ed. Large Animal Internal Medicine, 5e. St. Louis, MO: Elsevier Mosby, 2015:1298–1307.

Author Jenifer R. Gold
Consulting Editor Sandra D. Taylor
Acknowledgment The author and editor acknowledge the prior contribution of Armando R. Irizarry-Rovira.

BASICS

OVERVIEW
• May develop after inhalation of foreign material and bacteria into the lower respiratory tract
• Causes include dysphagia, obstructive esophageal disorders, GI reflux, and accidental inhalation of foreign material (nasogastric intubation)

SIGNALMENT
Foals appear more prone to GI reflux and subsequent aspiration pneumonia.

SIGNS
Historical Findings
• Dysphagia, ptyalism, or discharge of food, water, or milk from the nostrils
• Recent history of drenching or nasogastric intubation

Physical Examination Findings
• Clinical signs—fever, depression, anorexia, cough, nasal discharge (may be serohemorrhagic), tachypnea, and dyspnea
• Foul-smelling breath or nasal discharge suggests strongly anaerobic infection
• Abnormal lung sounds (auscultation)

CAUSES AND RISK FACTORS
Dysphagia
• Neurologic diseases affecting cranial nerves IX and X—guttural pouch diseases, botulism, lead toxicity, and viral encephalitis
• Primary myopathies of pharyngeal and laryngeal muscles—white muscle disease and hyperkalemic periodic paralysis
• Pharyngeal obstruction—strangles, pharyngeal abscess, neoplasia, foreign body, dorsal displacement of soft palate
• Congenital—cleft palate and hypoplasia of the soft palate
• Iatrogenic causes—pharyngeal and laryngeal surgery

Esophageal Disorders
• Esophageal obstruction
• Esophageal diverticulum
• Esophageal fistula
• Megaesophagus

GI Reflux
Gastric outflow obstruction (foals).

Accidental Inhalation of a Foreign Body
Administration of fluids by drenching or nasogastric tube.

DIAGNOSIS

DIFFERENTIAL DIAGNOSIS
• Acute bronchopneumonia
• Pleuropneumonia
• Interstitial pneumonia
• Respiratory distress syndrome

CBC/BIOCHEMISTRY/URINALYSIS
• Hyperfibrinogenemia, hyperglobulinemia, and anemia are common with chronic pneumonia
• Elevated white blood cell count with neutrophilia may be observed

OTHER LABORATORY TESTS
• Increased blood and tissue concentrations of lead (lead toxicity)
• Decreased whole-blood selenium concentration and glutathione peroxidase activity with increased serum creatine kinase and aspartate aminotransferase (white muscle disease)
• Hyperkalemic periodic paralysis—genetic testing or finding hyperkalemia during clinical episodes

IMAGING
• Thoracic radiography commonly reveals ventral patchy opacity obscuring the cardiac silhouette
• Contrast radiography may help to identify esophageal diseases
• Thoracic ultrasonography may detect pleural effusion

OTHER DIAGNOSTIC PROCEDURES
• Tracheobronchial aspiration and/or thoracocentesis for cytology, Gram stain, and culture (both aerobic and anaerobic)
• Endoscopy of the respiratory and upper GI tracts may help to identify the primary cause

PATHOLOGIC FINDINGS
• Lung consolidation (ventral part)
• Acute cases—hemorrhagic and edematous areas
• Chronic cases—lungs with necrotic and purulent materials
• Pleural space—fibrinous exudate and adhesions

TREATMENT
• Restore airway patency, drain pleural effusion, etc.
• Nasal oxygen (6–10 L/min) if PaO_2 <60 mmHg
• Thoracocentesis or indwelling chest tubes can achieve drainage; a one-way valve prevents pneumothorax
• Treat primary disease
• Stall rest
• Dysphagic horses may be fed with a nasogastric tube
• Fluid therapy as needed

MEDICATIONS

DRUG(S) OF CHOICE
• Systemic administration of broad-spectrum antimicrobials. Preferred combinations include sodium or potassium penicillin (22 000–40 000 IU/kg IV every 6 h),

aminoglycoside (gentamicin (6.6–8.8 mg/kg IV every 24 h) or amikacin (15–20 mg/kg IV or IM every 24 h) for foals), and metronidazole (15–25 mg/kg IV or PO every 6–8 h)
• Other antimicrobial options include procaine penicillin G (22 000 IU/kg IM every 12 h), trimethoprim–sulfamethoxazole (30 mg/kg PO every 12 h), ceftiofur (1–5 mg/kg IV or IM every 12 h), or chloramphenicol (20–50 mg/kg PO every 6–8 h for adults and foals >1 week)
• NSAIDs—flunixin meglumine (1.1 mg/kg PO or IV every 12–24 h) or phenylbutazone (2.2–4.4 mg/kg PO or IV every 12 h)

CONTRAINDICATIONS/POSSIBLE INTERACTIONS
Use aminoglycosides and NSAIDs with caution in horses with renal dysfunction and/or dehydration.

FOLLOW-UP

PATIENT MONITORING
Follow progress of pulmonary lesions by radiography/ultrasonography.

PREVENTION/AVOIDANCE
Prevent or avoid exposure to primary causes.

POSSIBLE COMPLICATIONS
• Pleuritis, lung abscess
• Thrombophlebitis
• Laminitis
• Disseminated intravascular coagulation
• Septicemia

EXPECTED COURSE AND PROGNOSIS
• Prolonged treatment is often needed
• Prognosis is guarded

MISCELLANEOUS

SEE ALSO
• Hemorrhagic nasal discharge
• Pleuropneumonia
• Respiratory distress syndrome in foals

ABBREVIATIONS
• GI = gastrointestinal
• NSAID = nonsteroidal anti-inflammatory drug
• PaO_2 = partial pressure of oxygen in arterial blood

Suggested Reading
Ainsworth DM, Hackett R. Bacterial pneumonia. In: Reed SM, Bayly WM, Sellon DC, eds. Equine Internal Medicine, 3e. St. Louis, MO: WB Saunders, 2010:325–328.

Author Daniel Jean
Consulting Editors Daniel Jean and Mathilde Leclère

Acknowledgment The editors acknowledge the prior contribution of Laurent Couëtil.

A

ATHEROMA OF THE FALSE NOSTRIL

BASICS

OVERVIEW
• Epidermal inclusion cyst, epidermoid cyst, or infundibular follicular cyst of the false nostril (nasal diverticulum)
• The term "atheroma" is likely a misnomer as the term refers to a sebaceous cyst
• Often present at birth and becomes apparent with age as the cyst enlarges
• Usually a cosmetic issue only

SIGNALMENT
• Can be noticed at any age
• Usually becomes apparent between weaning and 3 years of age
• No known sex or breed predilections

SIGNS
• Soft to firm, spherical swelling covered by normal skin in the caudal dorsal to lateral aspect of the false nostril in the area of the nasomaxillary notch
• Typically unilateral, but can be bilateral
• Not painful on palpation
• Size increases with age and can reach up to 5 cm
• Usually not associated with respiratory compromise

CAUSES AND RISK FACTORS
• Congenitally aberrant epithelial tissue between the skin and mucous membrane of the false nostril
• Can slowly enlarge due to progressive exfoliation of keratinized material within the cyst

DIAGNOSIS
Characteristic location and physical features of the swelling.

DIFFERENTIAL DIAGNOSIS
• An abscess can be ruled out as there is no heat or pain associated with the cyst
• Cysts could become inflamed if keratinized material leaks into the surrounding tissue

CBC/BIOCHEMISTRY/URINALYSIS
N/A

OTHER LABORATORY TESTS
• Aspirated fluid is white to gray, milky to creamy in appearance, and odorless
• Cytologically the cyst fluid contains keratinized and nonkeratinized squamous epithelial cells
• Trichrome staining reveals squamous epithelial cells and keratinous debris
• Histologically the cyst lining comprises varying thickness of stratified squamous epithelium

IMAGING
Ultrasonographic findings consistent with cystic structure, usually unilocular, mostly homogeneous echogenicity.

OTHER DIAGNOSTIC PROCEDURES
• Palpation
• Ultrasonographic evaluation
• Centesis
• Histologic evaluation

TREATMENT
• None required/indicated. Usually not removed unless for cosmetic reasons or for airway noise or impairment from large swelling size
• If removed surgically, it is imperative to remove the entire cyst lining to prevent recurrence
• Total surgical removal can be done under general anesthesia or standing with sedation and local anesthesia of the infraorbital nerve
• The cyst can be approached surgically through the skin over the dorsum of the swelling. The cyst then is dissected in its entirety, and the wound is closed
• Another option is to open the cyst ventrally into the false nostril, drain the contents, and remove the lining using a burr instrument. In this technique, the wound is left open to heal by second intention
• Intralesional injection of neutral-buffered 10% formalin after aspirating the cyst content has been reported. Injection of formalin until leakage around the needle is seen (2–4.5 mL). There is transient swelling within 24 h of injecting the formalin. Desiccation of the cyst occurs after a few weeks

MEDICATIONS

DRUG(S) OF CHOICE
Draining and cauterizing or sclerosing the cyst has been done using tincture of iodine, silver nitrate, or both followed by packing; this requires daily treatment and carries a high risk of recurrence.

CONTRAINDICATIONS/POSSIBLE INTERACTIONS
Transient swelling if chemical ablation is used.

FOLLOW-UP
Usual precautions for tetanus prophylaxis and asepsis of the surgical site.

POSSIBLE COMPLICATIONS
• A cyst may become abscessed if infection is introduced during centesis
• Transient swelling after surgery
• Recurrence if lining not removed
• Infection at surgery site
• Scar formation
• White hair at surgery site

EXPECTED COURSE AND PROGNOSIS
Favorable prognosis for both leaving the cyst untouched and for surgical removal if needed.

MISCELLANEOUS

ASSOCIATED CONDITIONS
In addition to false nostril cysts, other congenital cutaneous cysts reported in horses are dentigerous cysts and, very rarely, dermoid cysts.

AGE-RELATED FACTORS
May increase in size with age.

ZOONOTIC POTENTIAL
None

PREGNANCY/FERTILITY/BREEDING
N/A

SEE ALSO
N/A

Suggested Reading
Frankeny RL. Intralesional administration of formalin for treatment of epidermal inclusion cysts in five horses. J Am Vet Med Assoc 2003;223:221–222.
Schumacher J, Dixon PM. Diseases of the nasal cavities. In: McGorum BC, Dixon PM, Robinson NE, Schumaker J. Equine Respiratory Medicine and Surgery. Philadelphia, PA: WB Saunders, 2006:372–373.
Scott DW, Miller Jr WH. Neoplasms, cysts, hamartomas, and keratoses. In: Scott DW, Miller Jr WH. Equine Dermatology, 2e. Maryland Heights, MO: Elsevier Saunders, 2011:468–516.
Tremaine WH, Clarke CJ, Dixon PM. Histopathological findings in equine sinonasal disorders. Equine Vet J 1999;31(4):296–303.

Author Mathilde Leclère
Consulting Editors Mathilde Leclère and Daniel Jean
Acknowledgment The editors acknowledge the prior contribution of Wendy Duckett.

BASICS

DEFINITION
AD is defined as a multifactorial disease in which a genetic predisposition leads to the development of a cutaneous IgE- and cell-mediated hypersensitivity, most commonly against environmental allergens, and, upon exposure to that allergen, to clinical signs in the patient.

PATHOPHYSIOLOGY
The pathophysiology of equine atopy is not well elucidated. In human and canine AD, deviations in T-cell development have been detected. Allergen-specific IgE has been identified in atopic horses and CD4+ CD25+ regulatory cells in horses with IH. Whether the exact pathomechanism is similar to dogs and humans, with an initial development of Th2 cells secreting IL-4, IL-5, and IL-13 leading to a switch to IgE production and cellular and humoral hyperreactivity against specific antigens, remains to be elucidated.

SYSTEMS AFFECTED
Skin/Respiratory
The skin is only one of the organs that can be affected. There is evidence that equine asthma (heaves, recurrent airway obstruction) may also be due to a type I hypersensitivity to airborne allergens in some patients.

GENETICS
The genetic basis of equine AD is largely unknown. Based on anecdotal reports and one study, Arabians seem to be predisposed, but the number of affected horses was small and no further genetic studies were reported.

INCIDENCE/PREVALENCE
After IH, AD it is the second most common hypersensitivity in the horse.

GEOGRAPHIC DISTRIBUTION
Worldwide

SIGNALMENT
• No age or gender predisposition has been identified
• In most animals, the first clinical sign is pruritus, often affecting the head and legs
• Initial pruritus may only be seasonal
• With time, pruritus becomes more severe, more generalized, and year round

SIGNS
• AD may present as a pruritus with no primary lesions or perhaps mild erythema, or with pruritus leading to secondary lesions such as alopecia, excoriations, and crusting
• It may also present as urticaria
• Secondary surface infections may cause a bacterial folliculitis, which may be clinically mistaken for dermatophytosis

CAUSES
• The most common environmental allergens causing equine AD are storage mites, mold spores, and pollens
• Depending on the geographic location and the exact type of allergen, mold spores and pollens may have a strict seasonal occurrence or may be perennial
• Many horses have concurrent IH

RISK FACTORS
Concurrent pruritic dermatosis, such as IH or ectoparasitic disease (summation effect).

 DIAGNOSIS

DIFFERENTIAL DIAGNOSIS
The list of differential diagnoses varies with the predominant site of pruritus (Table 1. As there is no reliable test differentiating AD from other hypersensitivities, ectoparasites, or other differential diagnoses, those diseases must be ruled out before AD can be confirmed.

CBC/BIOCHEMISTRY/URINALYSIS
Hemogram may reveal an eosinophilia but this is nonspecific for AD as ecto- and endoparasite burdens or IH may show this change.

OTHER LABORATORY TESTS
• A number of tests are used to identify the offending allergens in AD
• An ELISA that uses the Fc-epsilon receptor on the immunoglobulin IgE as the detection platform to identify serum IgE compared better in one study than a radioallergosorbent test and a polyclonal antibody-based ELISA

Table 1

Differential diagnoses for AD	
Body location	*Differential diagnoses*
Face	CAFR and IH, trombiculosis, *Dermanyssus gallinae*
Ears	CAFR and IH, *Psoroptes*
Neck	CAFR and IH
Mane	CAFR and IH, pediculosis, *Psoroptes*
Legs, pastern	CAFR, IH, and contact hypersensitivity, trombiculosis, *Dermanyssus gallinae*, *Chorioptes*
Dorsum	CAFR and IH, pediculosis
Ventrum	CAFR and IH, contact hypersensitivity, trombiculosis, *Dermanyssus gallinae*

• Histamine-releasing assays may be useful but are not commercially available
• None of these tests reliably differentiates AD from other skin disease and, thus, cannot be used to establish a diagnosis
• These tests serve as a guide to choosing offending allergens used in ASIT, together with the history of the patient including possible seasonality and/or specific locations

IMAGING
• Skin—N/A
• Respiratory signs—thoracic radiographs

OTHER DIAGNOSTIC PROCEDURES
• Intradermal skin tests detect the level of allergen-specific IgE in the skin directed to a panel of allergens that are region specific and thought to be clinically relevant
• Knowledge of predominant allergens and their seasonality in the area of one's practice is essential when interpreting results of allergy tests
• False-positive reactions or results that indicate subclinical sensitization may occur with both serum and intradermal testing in the horse. Several studies with control groups of healthy nonallergic horses had immediate or late-phase IDT reactions, although horses with AD, urticaria, and severe asthma showed a higher number of positive reactions. As such, IDT results cannot differentiate a hypersensitivity from another pruritic skin disease, but rather act only as a guide to choose offending allergens for ASIT
• Surface cytology from erosions or ulcers shows a neutrophilic exudate with intra- and/or extracellular cocci representative of a secondary bacterial folliculitis
• Perform skin scrapings to rule out ectoparasites
• Perform dermatophyte cultures to help rule out secondary dermatophytosis

PATHOLOGIC FINDINGS
Skin biopsies submitted for histopathology from horses with AD typically reveal edema with a superficial to deep, perivascular to interstitial, eosinophilic dermatitis and possible epidermitis pointing to hypersensitivities or ectoparasites and are not diagnostic for environmental allergy. Biopsies may be useful to rule out differential diagnoses.

 TREATMENT

APPROPRIATE HEALTH CARE
• Identification and avoidance of the offending allergen is the best strategy for horses with AD
• In rare cases, changing the type of stabling, paddock, or feeding habits will lead to clinical remission

- In the majority of cases, the etiologic allergens will either be ubiquitous or not identified and therefore unavoidable

NURSING CARE
N/A

ACTIVITY
- Horses with mild AD may be worked normally with appropriate symptomatic therapy. Severely pruritic horses may not be able to perform
- Use of some antipruritic medications are illegal in competing horses

DIET
A diet high in polyunsaturated fatty acids or supplementation of such fatty acids as cold-pressed linseed or flax seed oil has been recommended. One small randomized, placebo-controlled, double-blind cross-over trial showed a reduction in the intradermal skin test response to *Culicoides* in AD horses after 42 days of supplementation with flaxseed.

CLIENT EDUCATION
- Clients rarely appreciate learning that their horse has a chronic skin disease that requires ongoing, long-term management. The need for a thorough workup to confirm a diagnosis of AD (by exclusion) is step 1. Client acceptance of long-term therapy is step 2
- Owners need to decide if they will limit treatment to symptomatic therapy or if they will choose ASIT, which is the only specific treatment available and currently the only chance of "cure"
- As they are active participants in the treatment regime, owners also need to understand how to assess response to therapy, be aware of signs of adverse effects, and when to consult the veterinarian for a needed change in treatment

SURGICAL CONSIDERATIONS
N/A

MEDICATIONS
DRUG(S) OF CHOICE
- Treatment of choice for horses with AD is ASIT. ASIT is an extract containing offending allergens that is given subcutaneously at regular intervals
- Base the selection of allergens for inclusion in ASIT on test results, the history of the patient, and local exposure to regional allergens
- Tailor the amount and the frequency of administration of ASIT to the patient's response. For example, pruritus directly after the injection prompts a decrease in the amount or strength of ASIT, whereas increased pruritus at the end of the treatment interval before the next injection is due suggests a need to increase ASIT frequency of administration

CONTRAINDICATIONS
None

PRECAUTIONS
One possible (albeit very rare) adverse effect of ASIT is anaphylaxis. This can have particularly dramatic consequences in horses with concurrent severe asthma. In such patients, injection of the allergen extract should be preceded by 2 h by administration of an antihistamine (see Alternative Drugs) and epinephrine should be available. Monitor the horse closely for the first hour after immunotherapy injection.

POSSIBLE INTERACTIONS
None

ALTERNATIVE DRUGS
- There are a number of drugs used for symptomatic therapy, as an alternative or concurrent treatment to ASIT
- The most frequently used drugs for allergic horses are glucocorticoids. They inhibit a wide array of inflammatory mediators and cells and thus have a high efficacy in the treatment of equine pruritus. Prednisolone is preferred. It is initially given at 0.5–1 mg/kg/day and tapered after 7–14 days to the lowest possible dose every 48 h. Recent well-conducted studies have not found an association between prednisolone administration and laminitis. An alternative to prednisolone is dexamethasone, which is given initially at 0.05–0.1 mg/kg/day for a few days and then tapered to 0.01 mg/kg every third day or less, if possible
- Antihistamines are used for long- or short-term control of pruritus
- Pharmacokinetic data for many antihistamines in the horse are unknown
- Antihistamines used in the horse and their doses are listed in Table 2 Assess efficacy after 2 weeks of therapy
- Polyunsaturated omega 3 and 6 fatty acids act most likely through their influence on the immune response as well as the epidermal barrier. Their effect on horses with AD is not as clear as the one seen on canine AD. Studies have shown variable results with commercial

Table 2

Antihistamines and their dose recommended for equine dermatitis	
Antihistamine	*Dose*
Cetirizine	0.2–0.4 mg/kg every 12 h
Hydroxyzine	1 mg/kg every 8–12 h
Amitriptyline	1 mg/kg every 12 h
Chlorpheniramine (chlorphenamine)	0.25 mg/kg every 12 h
Diphenhydramine	1 mg/kg every 8–12 h
Doxepin	0.5 mg/kg every 12 h

products, flax seed, or linseed oil. If fatty acid supplementation is beneficial, improvement may occur within 4–8 weeks after commencement

FOLLOW-UP
PATIENT MONITORING
Severity of patient's disease will dictate the need for monitoring. Patients with severe uncontrolled pruritus should be assessed frequently to ensure secondary infections are managed and controlled.

PREVENTION/AVOIDANCE
- Prevention may be possible if the horse is relocated to a different ecologically diverse geographic location
- Avoidance of allergens is not always possible or practical, especially as many patients have multiple allergens contributing to their disease

POSSIBLE COMPLICATIONS
- Change in allergen exposure or load precipitating disease flare or recurrence of previously controlled AD
- Secondary bacterial infections
- Adverse effects to symptomatic medications

EXPECTED COURSE AND PROGNOSIS
AD is a chronic skin disease and spontaneous remission is rare. Therapies should be continued long term. Prognosis is good to fair with appropriate management.

MISCELLANEOUS
ASSOCIATED CONDITIONS
- Severe equine asthma
- Allergic conjunctivitis
- IH

AGE-RELATED FACTORS
Severity worsens with age.

ZOONOTIC POTENTIAL
N/A

PREGNANCY/FERTILITY/BREEDING
Long-term use of corticosteroids is contraindicated during pregnancy.

SYNONYMS
Equine atopy.

SEE ALSO
- Ectoparasites
- Heaves (severe equine asthma, RAO)
- Insect hypersensitivity
- Urticaria

ABBREVIATIONS
- AD = atopic dermatitis
- ASIT = allergen-specific immunotherapy
- CAFR = cutaneous adverse food reaction
- ELISA = enzyme-linked immunosorbent assay
- IDT = intradermal dilutional test

(CONTINUED)

- Ig = immunoglobulin
- IH = insect bite hypersensitivity
- IL = interleukin
- Th2 = T-helper cell 2

Suggested Reading

Fadok VA. Update on equine allergies. Vet Clin North Am Equine Pract 2013;29:541–550.

Hallamaa R, Batchu K. Phospholipid analysis in sera of horses with allergic dermatitis and in matched healthy controls. Lipids Health Dis 2016;15:45.

Hamza E, Mirkovitch J, Steinbach F, Marti E. Regulatory T cells in early life: comparative study of CD4+CD25high T cells from foals and adult horses. PLoS One 2015;10:e0120661.

Loewenstein C, Mueller RS. A review of allergen-specific immunotherapy in human and veterinary medicine. Vet Dermatol 2009;20:84–98.

Lorch G, Hillier A, Kwochka KW, et al. Comparison of immediate intradermal test reactivity with serum IgE quantitation by use of a radioallergosorbent test and two ELISA in horses with and without atopy. J Am Vet Med Assoc 2001;218:1314–1322.

Lorch G, Hillier A, Kwochka KW, et al. Results of intradermal tests in horses without atopy and horses with atopic dermatitis or recurrent urticaria. Am J Vet Res 2001;62:1051–1059.

Marsella R. Equine allergy therapy: update on the treatment of environmental, insect bite hypersensitivity, and food allergies. Vet Clin North Am Equine Pract 2013;29:551–557.

Morgan EE, Miller Jr WH, Wagner B. A comparison of intradermal testing and detection of allergen-specific immunoglobulin E in serum by enzyme-linked immunosorbent assay in horses affected with skin hypersensitivity. Vet Immunol Immunopathol 2007;120:160–167.

O'Neill W, McKee S, Clarke AF. Flaxseed (*Linum usitatissimum*) supplementation associated with reduced skin test lesional area in horses with *Culicoides* hypersensitivity. Can J Vet Res 2002;66:272–277.

Petersen A, Schott 2nd HC. Effects of dexamethasone and hydroxyzine treatment on intradermal testing and allergen-specific IgE serum testing results in horses. Vet Dermatol 2009;20:615–622.

Scott DW, Miller Jr WH, eds. Equine Dermatology, 2e. Maryland Heights, MO: Elsevier Saunders, 2011.

Stepnik CT, Outerbridge CA, White SD, Kass PH. Equine atopic skin disease and response to allergen-specific immunotherapy: a retrospective study at the University of California-Davis (1991–2008). Vet Dermatol 2012;23:29–35.

Author Ralf Mueller
Consulting Editor Gwendolen Lorch
Acknowledgment The author acknowledges the prior contribution of Gwendolen Lorch.

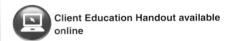 **Client Education Handout available online**

ATRIAL FIBRILLATION

BASICS

DEFINITION
• An irregularly irregular cardiac rhythm, with variable intensity heart sounds and pulses and inconsistent diastolic intervals
• Can be paroxysmal (resolving spontaneously within 48 h of onset), persistent, or permanent

PATHOPHYSIOLOGY
• A critical atrial mass must be present for AF to occur
• Predisposing factors—large atrial mass, atrial remodeling and fibrosis, high vagal tone, shortened and nonhomogeneous effective refractory period, potassium depletion, atrial premature complexes, bradycardia, predisposing arrhythmias (atrial tachycardia or atrial flutter), and rapid atrial pacing
• Produces no change in cardiac output at rest in the absence of significant underlying cardiac disease
• During high-intensity exercise, produces a significant increase in exercising HR (often 40–60 bpm higher than when in NSR) and subsequent fall in cardiac output and exercise capacity
• Present in many horses with CHF but is not the cause of CHF

SYSTEMS AFFECTED
Cardiovascular

SIGNALMENT
Higher incidence in Standardbred, draft, and Warmblood horses.

SIGNS
General Comments
Exercise intolerance in high performance animals; often an incidental finding in horses performing only light work.

Historical Findings
• Exercise intolerance
• Exercise-induced pulmonary hemorrhage—often profuse
• Weakness or collapse

Physical Examination Findings
• Irregularly irregular heart rhythm
• Variable intensity heart sounds and arterial pulses

• Absent fourth heart sound
• Cardiac murmurs with predisposing cardiac disease

CAUSES
• Normal horses have sufficient atrial mass and high vagal tone to develop AF without evident underlying heart disease—"lone" AF
• Diseases causing atrial enlargement further predispose horses to AF

RISK FACTORS
• AV valve insufficiency
• CHF
• Electrolyte disturbances

DIAGNOSIS

DIFFERENTIAL DIAGNOSIS
• Second-degree AV block—regular rhythm is interrupted by pauses containing fourth heart sound
• Atrial tachycardia with second-degree AV block—rhythm usually is regularly irregular; fourth heart sounds are present
• Atrial flutter—rhythm usually irregularly irregular; need ECG to differentiate
• NSR with multifocal ventricular premature complexes—need ECG to differentiate

CBC/BIOCHEMISTRY/URINALYSIS
Low plasma potassium or urinary fractional excretion of potassium may be present.

OTHER LABORATORY TESTS
Elevated cardiac troponin I or cardiac troponin T possible but usually within the normal range.

IMAGING
ECG
• No P waves, replaced by baseline "f" waves (Figure 1)
• The "f" waves may be coarse or fine and may occur 300–500 times per minute
• Irregular R–R interval
• Some variation in the amplitude of QRS and T complexes usually is present, but these complexes are otherwise normal in appearance

Echocardiography
• Many have little or no discernible underlying cardiac disease; therefore, the echocardiogram is normal

• Some have low shortening fraction (24–32%). This should return to normal within several days of conversion to normal NSR
• Mild left atrial enlargement occasionally occurs with permanent AF
• Atrial enlargement due to AV valve insufficiency, underlying myocardial disease, or congenital defects may be present

OTHER DIAGNOSTIC PROCEDURES
Continuous 24 h Holter Monitoring
• Use with suspected paroxysmal AF to identify underlying arrhythmias
• Use with persistent AF to determine if other concurrent arrhythmias are present

Exercise ECG
Use to detect exercise-induced arrhythmias and conduction abnormalities and to determine horse and rider safety and exercise limitations if the AF is not or cannot be converted.

PATHOLOGIC FINDINGS
• Grossly and histopathologically normal heart in horses with no underlying cardiac disease
• Focal or diffuse atrial fibrosis may be present in horses with longstanding AF
• Myocarditis, myocardial necrosis, and fatty infiltration have been documented in affected horses
• Both atrial and ventricular enlargement in horses with significant AV valvular disease

TREATMENT

AIMS
• Restoration of NSR and athletic performance in horses with no, minimal, or mild underlying heart disease
• Assessment of rider/driver/handler safety if cardioversion is not successful or not desired; rate control if indicated
• Palliative care for horses with AF in conjunction with CHF

APPROPRIATE HEALTH CARE
• Monitor horses for 24–48 h to determine if the condition will spontaneously resolve (i.e. paroxysmal)
• In horses with AF and CHF, institute treatment for CHF—using digoxin

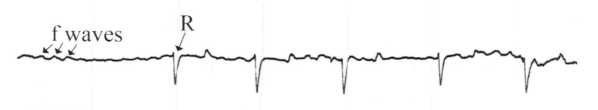

Figure 1.

Base–apex lead 25 mm/s, 5 mm = 1 mV.

(CONTINUED)

(0.0022 mg/kg IV every 12 h or 0.011 mg/kg PO every 12 h), furosemide (1–2 mg/kg IV every 8 h, not PO), or torsemide (0.5–1 mg/kg PO every 12 h) and ACE inhibitor (benazepril at 1 mg/kg PO every 12 h), if indicated
• If AF is persistent, CHF is not present, and exercise intolerance is present, pharmacologic cardioversion or TVEC should be considered

NURSING CARE
• Perform continuous ECG throughout attempted conversion to NSR
• Keep horses quiet during pharmacologic cardioversion

ACTIVITY
• Horses with AF should not perform high-intensity exercise
• Horses with AF can usually perform successfully in lower level athletic work, as broodmares, and as breeding stallions
• An exercising ECG is indicated to ensure safety of horse and rider for intended use if cardioversion is not successful or not elected

DIET
• Oral potassium supplementation may be indicated with low plasma potassium, or low urinary fractional excretion of potassium or with excessive sweating
• Potassium chloride salt can be added to the feed (1 tablespoon every 12 h, gradually increasing to 28 g (1 oz) every 12 h)

CLIENT EDUCATION
• Discuss treatment-associated risks with owners—see Possible Complications
• Discuss predisposing factors to minimize the likelihood of recurrence

SURGICAL CONSIDERATIONS
• TVEC under general anesthesia is usually successful (success rate similar to quinidine)
• This utilizes a biphasic current delivered between electrodes placed in the right atrium and left pulmonary artery using pressure waveforms, echocardiography, and radiography or robotic fluoroscopy to guide and confirm electrode placement

 MEDICATIONS

DRUG(S) OF CHOICE
The drug of choice for conversion is quinidine sulfate or gluconate.

Quinidine Gluconate
• Indicated with AF of duration ≤2 weeks and no underlying cardiac disease
• Administered in boluses of 0.5–1 mg/kg every 5–10 min to a total dose of 12 mg/kg

Quinidine Sulfate
• Indicated in horses with persistent AF
• Administered via nasogastric intubation at 22 mg/kg every 2 h to a total of 4–6 treatments, then every 6 h until the horse

shows signs of toxicity or has converted to NSR

CONTRAINDICATIONS
• Do not administer quinidine sulfate or gluconate to horses with AF and CHF
• Horses with a resting HR of >60 bpm and/or grade 3/6 or louder systolic murmurs are likely to have CHF
• TVEC may be preferable in horses with wide QRS morphology with increased ventricular response rate

PRECAUTIONS
Quinidine is associated with the following complications.

Cardiovascular
• Prolonged QRS duration—indicates quinidine toxicity
• Prolonged QT interval—increases risk of ventricular arrhythmias
• Rapid supraventricular tachycardia—treat aggressively with digoxin to slow HR
  ○ Digoxin is recommended in conjunction with quinidine in horses with myocardial dysfunction or rapid HR during quinidine treatment
  ○ If HR exceeds 100 bpm, consider digoxin—0.011 mg/kg PO or 0.0022 mg/kg IV
  ○ If HR exceeds 150 bpm, consider digoxin (0.0022 mg/kg IV) and sodium bicarbonate (1 mEq/kg IV)
  ○ Detomidine or diltiazem may also be used to control rate with close monitoring of blood pressure
  ○ If a horse receiving quinidine only on day 1 does not convert, consider adding digoxin orally on day 2
  ○ Base subsequent digoxin administration during quinidine treatment on serum digoxin concentration and need to control HR or to improve myocardial contractility
• Ventricular arrhythmias do not require treatment if ventricular rhythm is slow (<120 bpm), uniform, and no R-on-T is detected
  ○ If treatment indicated use magnesium sulfate—2–5 mg/kg bolus IV every 5 min to 50 mg/kg total
• Hypotension—monitor and treat, if severe, with IV fluids to effect and, if necessary, phenylephrine (0.1–0.2 µg/kg/min IV to effect)
• Sudden death—try to prevent with continuous ECG monitoring and treatment of any concerning arrhythmias that occur

Gastrointestinal
• Flatulence—resolves on return of quinidine plasma concentrations to negligible levels
• Oral ulcerations—prevent by administering quinidine via nasogastric tube
• Diarrhea—resolves on return of quinidine plasma concentrations to negligible levels
• Colic—associated with increasing number of doses; treat with analgesics as needed

Respiratory
Upper respiratory tract obstruction—indicates quinidine toxicity; treat with passage of a nasotracheal tube to relieve the upper airway obstruction; administer corticosteroids and antihistamines; emergency tracheotomy, if necessary.

Dermatologic
Urticaria—treat with corticosteroids and antihistamines.

Reproductive
Paraphimosis—resolves on return of plasma quinidine concentration to negligible levels.

Musculoskeletal
Laminitis—if the horse is uncomfortable, administer analgesics.

Neurologic
• Indicates quinidine toxicity
• Ataxia—resolves on return of plasma quinidine concentration to negligible levels
• Convulsions—administer anticonvulsants
• Bizarre behavior—resolves on return of plasma quinidine concentration to negligible levels

PATIENT MONITORING DURING TREATMENT WITH QUINIDINE
• Perform continuous ECG during treatment, because antiarrhythmic drugs are also arrhythmogenic
• Measure QRS and QT duration before each dose; discontinue treatment if QRS or QT duration ≥25% of the pretreatment value
• Discontinue treatment if rapid supraventricular tachycardia, ventricular arrhythmias, diarrhea, colic, ataxia, convulsions, bizarre behavior, urticaria, upper respiratory tract obstruction, or laminitis occurs

POSSIBLE INTERACTIONS
Quinidine results in increased steady-state digoxin concentration, causing potential digoxin toxicity.

ALTERNATIVE DRUGS
• IV amiodarone has been successful but has a lower cardioversion rate
• Flecainide has been associated with fatal ventricular arrhythmias and is not recommended

 FOLLOW-UP

PATIENT MONITORING FOLLOWING CONVERSION
• Following conversion, perform 24 h Holter ECG. If atrial ectopy is found, rest and corticosteroid therapy may be indicated
• Evaluate left atrial contractile function; if absent or decreased, rest for 4 weeks and reevaluate
• Regularly monitor cardiac rhythm; any irregularities or poor performance should prompt reexamination

ATRIAL FIBRILLATION   (CONTINUED)

- If in permanent AF, informed adult rider should monitor exercising HR with HR monitor
- Retire horse if exercising HR >220 bpm or ventricular arrhythmias or conduction abnormalities are induced by exercise or sympathetic nervous system stimulation

PREVENTION/AVOIDANCE
- Discontinue administration of furosemide and bicarbonate milkshakes
- Administer potassium or other electrolyte supplementation, if indicated
- Consider administration of ACE inhibitor to minimize atrial remodeling and fibrosis
- Consider administration of vitamin C
- Avoid thyroid hormone supplementation
- See chapter Supraventricular arrhythmias

POSSIBLE COMPLICATIONS
- If AF is not or cannot be treated, clinical signs will persist
- Some horses with AF also have exercise-induced aberrant conduction, ventricular arrhythmias or R-on-T complexes; if AF is not or cannot be converted and the horse is to continue to be used for ridden exercise, exercising ECG is indicated to ensure horse and rider safety—see chapter Ventricular arrhythmias

EXPECTED COURSE AND PROGNOSIS
- Most horses with little or no underlying cardiac disease convert to NSR with quinidine or TVEC cardioversion
- Recurrences occur in ≅15% of horses with a suspected duration of ≤4 months
- Recurrences occur in ≅45% of horses with a duration of AF of >4 months
- Recurrence is most likely during the first year after conversion but can occur at any time
- Recurrence likely in horses with left atrial enlargement or mitral regurgitation
- Prognosis for return to the previous level of athletic performance is excellent in converted horses without significant underlying cardiovascular disease

- Horses with permanent AF that do not convert to NSR with treatment or that are not candidates for conversion usually have a normal life expectancy and can be safely used for lower level athletic performance, as long as their exercising HR is <220 bpm and there is no aberrant conduction, ventricular arrhythmias, or R-on-T complexes
- With significant valvular insufficiency, severity of the valvular heart disease and its progression determine the horse's useful performance life and life expectancy
- Horses with CHF usually have severe underlying valvular heart or myocardial disease and have a guarded to grave prognosis for life
- Most affected horses treated for CHF respond to the supportive therapy and improve for a short time but are euthanized within 2–6 months of initiating treatment

 MISCELLANEOUS

ASSOCIATED CONDITIONS
Any cardiac disease resulting in atrial enlargement predisposes to AF.

AGE-RELATED FACTORS
Older horses are more likely to have significant underlying cardiac disease, with valvular insufficiency and atrial enlargement and are not usually candidates for conversion.

PREGNANCY/FERTILITY/BREEDING
- Affected pregnant mares without underlying cardiac disease and CHF should not experience any problems
- Affected pregnant mares with CHF—treat for the underlying cardiac disease with digoxin and furosemide. Although not studied in the horse, ACE inhibitors are contraindicated in pregnant mares due to the risk of birth defects documented in other species

SYNONYMS
A fib, AF

SEE ALSO
- Mitral regurgitation
- Myocardial disease
- Supraventricular arrhythmias
- Tricuspid regurgitation
- Ventricular arrhythmias

ABBREVIATIONS
- ACE = angiotensin-converting enzyme
- AF = atrial fibrillation
- AV = atrioventricular
- CHF = congestive heart failure
- HR = heart rate
- NSR = normal sinus rhythm
- TVEC = transvenous electrical cardioversion

Suggested Reading
De Clercq D, van Loon G, Baert K, et al. Effects of an adapted intravenous amiodarone treatment protocol in horses with atrial fibrillation. Equine Vet J 2007;39:344–349.
Decloedt A, Schwarzwald CC, De Clercq D, et al. Risk factors for recurrence of atrial fibrillation in horses after cardioversion to sinus rhythm. J Vet Intern Med 2015;29:946–953.
McGurrin MK, Physick-Sheard PW, Kenney DG, et al. Transvenous electrical cardioversion of equine atrial fibrillation: technical considerations. J Vet Intern Med 2005;19:695–702.
Reef VB, Levitan CW, Spencer PA. Factors affecting prognosis and conversion in equine atrial fibrillation. J Vet Intern Med 1988;2:1–6.
Reef VB, Reimer JM, Spencer PA. Treatment of equine atrial fibrillation: new perspectives. J Vet Intern Med 1995;9:57–67.
van Loon G, Blissitt KJ, Keen JA, et al. Use of intravenous flecainide in horses with naturally-occurring atrial fibrillation. Equine Vet J 2004;36:609–614.

Author Virginia B. Reef
Consulting Editor Celia M. Marr and Virginia B. Reef

BASICS

DEFINITION
• A congenital defect (i.e. hole) in the interatrial septum that creates a communication between the right and left atria
• Can be located in the atrial septum immediately adjacent to the ventricular septum (i.e. atrium primum defect), in the area of the foramen ovale (i.e. atrium secundum defect), or in the most basilar portion of the interatrial septum (i.e. sinus venosus-type defect)
• ASD can occur in isolation or in conjunction with other cardiac anomalies in complex congenital cardiac disease
• The atrial septum forms in the fetus from the septum primum and the septum secundum. The slit-like communication between these septa (i.e. the foramen ovale) allows passage of blood from right to the left atrium in the fetus
• The foramen ovale is functionally closed in normal neonates within 24–48 h of birth, but anatomic closure may not be complete until 9 weeks

PATHOPHYSIOLOGY
• A patent foramen ovale occurs when the foramen ovale fails to close
• Failed formation of 1 of the 2 septa results in the other forms of ASD
• Blood shunts from the higher pressure left atrium to the lower pressure right atrium in foals with ASD, creating a left atrial, right atrial, and right ventricular volume overload
• Size of the ASD determines severity of the volume overload. In horses with a large ASD, the right and left atrial and right ventricular volume overload is severe
• Over time, stretching of the tricuspid annulus occurs, and tricuspid regurgitation develops. As the tricuspid regurgitation becomes more severe, increases in right atrial pressure result in increased hepatic venous pressure and development of clinical signs of right-sided CHF

SYSTEMS AFFECTED
Cardiovascular

GENETICS
• Not yet determined in horses
• Although heritable in other species, it is rare in horses

INCIDENCE/PREVALENCE
These defects are uncommon as isolated congenital defects and more frequently occur in conjunction with complex congenital heart disease, particularly tricuspid and pulmonic atresia.

SIGNALMENT
Most frequently diagnosed in neonates, foals, and young horses, but may be diagnosed at any age.

SIGNS
General Comments
May be detected as an incidental finding, but usually is part of a more complex, congenital cardiac disorder.

Historical Findings
• Exercise intolerance—medium-sized to large ASDs
• CHF—large ASDs

Physical Examination Findings
• No murmur may be present, or a coarse, band- or ejection-shaped, holosystolic murmur with point of maximal intensity in the pulmonic valve area may be detected
• Premature beats or an irregularly irregular heart rhythm of AF may be present with larger ASDs

CAUSES
• Failed closure of the foramen ovale
• Congenital malformation of the interatrial septum

RISK FACTORS
• Premature foal
• Neonatal pulmonary hypertension
• Neonatal respiratory distress syndrome

DIAGNOSIS

DIFFERENTIAL DIAGNOSIS
• Physiologic flow murmur—differentiate echocardiographically
• Pulmonic stenosis (rare)—murmur usually louder; differentiate echocardiographically
• Aortic stenosis (rare)—murmur usually louder; weak arterial pulses; differentiate echocardiographically
• Tricuspid atresia—murmur usually louder; foal is unthrifty, tachycardic, and hypoxemic; differentiate echocardiographically
• Pulmonic atresia—murmur usually louder; may have a continuous machinery murmur; foal is unthrifty, tachycardic, and hypoxemic; differentiate echocardiographically

CBC/BIOCHEMISTRY/URINALYSIS
N/A

OTHER LABORATORY TESTS
N/A

IMAGING
ECG
• Atrial premature depolarizations or AF may be present in horses with right and left atrial enlargement
• Persistent AF has been reported in some affected foals and horses

Echocardiography
• Can determine location of the ASD
• Atrial septal dropout is detected at the ASD location and should be confirmed by visualization in 2 mutually perpendicular planes

• The left and right atria and right ventricle are enlarged, dilated, and have a rounded appearance
• Paradoxical septal motion is detected with a severe right ventricular volume overload
• Pulmonary artery dilatation is seen in horses with a large shunt
• Interrogate the entire atrial septum with pulsed-wave or color-flow Doppler with suspected ASD
• Contrast or color-flow Doppler reveals the shunt from the left to the right atrium through the ASD
• A small amount of positive contrast may be seen in the left atrium in horses with normal pulmonary arterial pressures or with the Valsalva maneuver during contrast echocardiography
• A jet of tricuspid regurgitation may be present in horses with a large ASD and marked right atrial and ventricular volume overload

Thoracic Radiography
Increased pulmonary vascularity and cardiac enlargement may be detected in horses with large shunts.

OTHER DIAGNOSTIC PROCEDURES
Cardiac Catheterization
• Right-sided catheterization can be performed to directly measure right atrial, right ventricular, and pulmonary arterial pressures and to sample blood for oxygen content
• Elevated right atrial, right ventricular, and pulmonary arterial pressures and increased oxygen saturation of right ventricular and pulmonary arterial blood have been seen in horses with larger ASDs

Continuous 24 h Holter Monitoring
Use in identifying intermittent atrial premature depolarizations.

PATHOLOGIC FINDINGS
• Defect in the atrial septum
• Jet lesions along the defect margins and on the adjacent right atrial endocardium
• Left atrial, right atrial, and right ventricular enlargement and thinning of the left atrial, right atrial, and right ventricular free wall in horses with a significant shunt
• Pulmonary artery dilatation in horses with a large shunt or that have developed pulmonary hypertension
• With CHF, ventral and peripheral edema, pleural effusion, pericardial effusion, chronic hepatic congestion, and, occasionally, ascites may be detected

TREATMENT

AIMS
• Management by intermittent monitoring in horses with small ASDs

• Palliative care in horses with large ASDs and those with complex congenital cardiac defects

APPROPRIATE HEALTH CARE
• Most affected horses require no treatment and can be monitored on an outpatient basis
• Monitor horses with large shunts on an annual basis
• Affected horses with CHF can be treated for CHF with positive inotropic drugs, vasodilators, and diuretics. Consider humane destruction if CHF develops, however, because only short-term, symptomatic improvement can be expected

NURSING CARE
N/A

ACTIVITY
• Affected horses are safe to continue in full athletic work until significant tricuspid regurgitation or AF develops
• Horses with small defects can be in unrestricted activity and may be able to compete reasonably successfully in upper level athletic competition
• Monitor horses with hemodynamically significant defects echocardiographically on an annual basis to ensure they are safe to ride and compete. These horses can be used for lower level athletic competition but are unlikely to compete at the upper levels of athletic performance
• Affected horses that develop AF need a complete cardiovascular examination to determine if they are safe to use for lower level athletic performance
• Horses with significant pulmonary artery dilatation no longer are safe to ride

DIET
N/A

CLIENT EDUCATION
• Regularly monitor cardiac rhythm; any irregularities of the rhythm, other than second-degree atrioventricular block, should prompt ECG
• Carefully monitor for exercise intolerance, respiratory distress, prolonged recovery after exercise, increased resting respiratory or heart rate, cough, generalized venous distention, jugular pulses, or ventral edema; if detected, obtain a cardiac reexamination

SURGICAL CONSIDERATIONS
• Closure of the ASD would be possible with a transvenous umbrella catheter if the diameter of the umbrella was large enough to close the defect
• Surgical closure is not financially feasible or practical for obtaining equine athletes at this time

MEDICATIONS
DRUG(S) OF CHOICE
N/A

CONTRAINDICATIONS
N/A

PRECAUTIONS
N/A

POSSIBLE INTERACTIONS
N/A

ALTERNATIVE DRUGS
N/A

FOLLOW-UP
PATIENT MONITORING
Frequently monitor cardiac rate, rhythm, and respiratory rate and effort.

PREVENTION/AVOIDANCE
N/A

POSSIBLE COMPLICATIONS
Large ASD—AF; CHF.

EXPECTED COURSE AND PROGNOSIS
• Horses with small defects should have a normal performance life and life expectancy
• Horses with moderate defects also have a normal life expectancy. These horses usually perform successfully only at lower levels of athletic competition, and they may develop AF
• Horses with large defects have a guarded prognosis, because they may have a shortened life expectancy and performance life, even at the lower levels of athletic competition
• Affected horses with CHF usually have a guarded to grave prognosis for life. Most such horses being treated for CHF should respond to the supportive therapy and transiently improve; however, once CHF develops, euthanasia is recommended

MISCELLANEOUS
ASSOCIATED CONDITIONS
• Complex congenital cardiac disease, particularly tricuspid and pulmonic atresia, is likely
• Tricuspid regurgitation can develop in horses with significant left atrial, right atrial, and right ventricular volume overload

secondary to stretching of the tricuspid annulus
• Pulmonic regurgitation can develop in horses with isolated defects
• Pulmonic valve leaflets may no longer coapt with stretching of the pulmonary artery from the volume overload

AGE-RELATED FACTORS
Young horses are more likely to be diagnosed.

ZOONOTIC POTENTIAL
N/A

PREGNANCY/FERTILITY/BREEDING
Breeding affected horses is discouraged. The condition is rare, however, and the heritable nature of this defect in horses is not known.

SYNONYMS
N/A

SEE ALSO
• Atrial fibrillation
• Supraventricular arrhythmias

ABBREVIATIONS
• AF = atrial fibrillation
• ASD = atrial septal defect
• CHF = congestive heart failure

Suggested Reading
Physick-Sheard PW, Maxie MG, Palmer NC, Gaul C. Atrial septal defect of the persistent ostium primum type with hypoplastic right ventricle in a Welsh Pony foal. Can J Comp Med 1985;49:429–433.
Reef VB. Cardiovascular disease in the equine neonate. Vet Clin North Am Equine Pract 1985;1:117–129.
Reef VB. Echocardiographic findings in horses with congenital cardiac disease. Compend Contin Educ Pract Vet 1991;13:109–117.
Reef VB. Cardiovascular ultrasonography. In: Reef VB, ed. Equine Diagnostic Ultrasound. Philadelphia, PA: WB Saunders, 1998:215–272.
Reppas GP, Canfield PJ, Hartley WJ, et al. Multiple congenital cardiac anomalies and idiopathic thoracic aortitis in a horse. Vet Rec 1996;138:14–16.
Taylor FG, Wooton PR, Hillyer MH, et al. Atrial septal defect and atrial fibrillation in a foal. Vet Rec 1991;128:80–81.

Author Virginia B. Reef
Consulting Editors Celia M. Marr and Virginia B. Reef

BASICS

OVERVIEW
• A form of severe nonexertional rhabdomyolysis due to eating plant material containing toxin hypoglycin A; aka "seasonal pasture myopathy"
• Horses ingest toxin-containing seeds from box elder (*Acer negundo*, midwest USA and Canada) or sycamore maple (*Acer pseudoplatanus*, UK and northern Europe)
• Metabolized hypoglycin A inhibits acyl-coenzyme A dehydrogenase, resulting in massive aerobic metabolism disruption and severe type I muscle fiber damage
• Necrosis of skeletal, respiratory, and cardiac muscles results in myoglobinuria, weakness, recumbency, respiratory difficulty, renal damage, and death in a high proportion of affected horses

SIGNALMENT
• Typically ≤3 years of age
• Any breed or gender

SIGNS
• Weakness, stiffness, rapid progression to recumbency and death in 72 h
• Discolored (red/brown) urine
• Tachycardia, respiratory difficulty
• ± Bright and appetent while recumbent
• ± Subclinical disease in pasture mates

CAUSES AND RISK FACTORS
• Consumption of seeds containing hypoglycin A
• >12 h of pasture access
• Young age, dietary indiscretion
• Competitive feeding situations
• Lack of supplemental feeding, particularly during cold or inclement weather
• Overgrazed pastures

DIAGNOSIS

DIFFERENTIAL DIAGNOSIS
Conditions causing weakness, stiffness, recumbency, and/or discolored urine such as laminitis, tetanus, colic, viral encephalitides, acute exertional rhabdomyolysis, selenium deficiency, red maple (*Acer rubrum*) toxicity, and other disorders causing intravascular hemolysis/methemoglobinemia.

CBC/BIOCHEMISTRY/URINALYSIS
• Elevated serum creatine kinase (>100 000 U/L in many), aspartate aminotransferase, and lactate dehydrogenase
• Hypochloremia, hypocalcemia, hyponatremia, hyperkalemia
• Azotemia
• Hyperglycemia, hyperlipemia, hyperlactatemia
• Myoglobinuria

OTHER LABORATORY TESTS
• Cardiac troponin I or T
• Methylenecyclopropylacetic acid conjugates (hypoglycin A metabolite) in serum or urine

IMAGING
Echocardiography (in survivors).

OTHER DIAGNOSTIC PROCEDURES
Muscle biopsy—excessive lipid accumulation in type I skeletal muscle fibers.

PATHOLOGIC FINDINGS
• Massive skeletal muscle necrosis
• Cardiac muscle necrosis in ~50% of cases
• Acute tubular necrosis ± pigmenturia

TREATMENT

• Reduce discomfort, prevent further muscle necrosis, restore fluid volume and acid–base and electrolyte status, reverse shock, and prevent renal damage
• Prompt, intensive supportive care. Hospitalization to provide appropriate fluid therapy and to manage recumbency
• IV or oral fluid therapy with balanced electrolyte solutions until myoglobinuria resolves
• Deep bedding, head and eye protection, and limb wraps are indicated for recumbent horses
• ± Slinging

MEDICATIONS

DRUG(S) OF CHOICE
• Analgesics—butorphanol (0.01–0.04 mg/kg IM or IV; or as a CRI at 23.7 µg/kg/h after a loading dose of 17.8 µg/kg IV); lidocaine (CRI at 30–50 µg/kg/min after a loading dose of 1.3 mg/kg IV slowly); and flunixin meglumine (0.5–1.1 mg/kg IV or PO)
• Antioxidant drugs—DMSO (1 g/kg IV or PO as a 10% solution), vitamin C (30 mg/kg IV diluted in fluids), vitamin E (2000–5000 IU PO every 24 h)
• Muscle relaxants—methocarbamol (5–22 mg/kg IV slowly, every 6–12 h) and dantrolene (4–6 mg/kg PO every 12 h). Dantrolene prevents additional muscle necrosis and may speed return of function, but is poorly absorbed in horses that have not eaten within 4 h prior to administration
• Insulin (0.2–0.4 U/kg insulin glargine IV or SC every 24 h) for hyperlipemia

CONTRAINDICATIONS/POSSIBLE INTERACTIONS
• Avoid NSAIDs in horses with azotemia, myoglobinuria, or profound shock
• Avoid dantrolene in horses with hyperkalemia

FOLLOW-UP

PATIENT MONITORING
Close monitoring of clinical and clinicopathologic variables is essential in affected horses, including serial monitoring of serum muscle enzymes, cardiac troponin, creatinine, and other relevant variables.

PREVENTION/AVOIDANCE
• Prevent access to causative tree species via fencing or tree removal
• Provide supplemental feeding during inclement weather or remove horses from pasture

POSSIBLE COMPLICATIONS
• Acute or chronic renal insufficiency secondary to myoglobinuria
• Acute or chronic cardiac dysfunction
• Atrophy of skeletal musculature

EXPECTED COURSE AND PROGNOSIS
• Guarded to grave prognosis with a 75–80% fatality rate. Surviving horses can have chronic complications
• Survivors require months of rest. Reevaluation including assessment of cardiac function is recommended before return to exercise

MISCELLANEOUS

ASSOCIATED CONDITIONS
• Heart failure
• Renal insufficiency

AGE-RELATED FACTORS
Highest prevalence in young horses.

PREGNANCY/FERTILITY/BREEDING
N/A

SEE ALSO
Exertional rhabdomyolysis syndrome

ABBREVIATIONS
• CRI = constant rate infusion
• DMSO = dimethyl sulfoxide
• NSAID = nonsteroidal anti-inflammatory drug

Suggested Reading
Valberg SJ, Sponseller BT, Hegeman AD, et al. Seasonal pasture myopathy/atypical myopathy in North America associated with ingestion of hypoglycin A within seeds of the box elder tree. Equine Vet J 2013;45:419–426.

Author Erica C. McKenzie
Consulting Editor Elizabeth J. Davidson

AURAL PLAQUES

BASICS

OVERVIEW
Aural plaques are whitish plaques on the inner pinnal surface of horses that are caused by EcPV.

SIGNALMENT
• Common in all sexes and breeds but rarely observed in horses <1 year old
• Incidence ranges from 14.8% of Brazilian horses to 20–24% of horses in the USA
• 85% of Brazilian farms had at least one horse affected

SIGNS
• Depigmented, well-demarcated papules and plaques covered with keratin deposits located on the concave pinnal surface. Lesions are single, multiple, or coalescing and may affect 1 or both pinna
• Horses can be asymptomatic or may resent bridling or handling of the ears
• Symptoms may be aggravated by biting flies

CAUSES AND RISK FACTORS
• Lesions contain EcPV, with EcPV types 3, 4, 5, and/or 6 consistently identified in biopsies
• Abrasions and biting flies, particularly black flies, are likely involved in viral transmission
• Ear grooming is associated with an 8.6-fold increased risk of coalescing (severe) lesions
• Increased horse density

DIAGNOSIS

DIFFERENTIAL DIAGNOSIS
Sarcoids—more often on the external surface of the pinna or at the margins of the ear. May coexist with aural plaques.

CBC/BIOCHEMISTRY/URINALYSIS
N/A

OTHER LABORATORY TESTS
N/A

IMAGING
N/A

OTHER DIAGNOSTIC PROCEDURES
Diagnosis is based on classic appearance and can be confirmed by biopsy.

TREATMENT
• Aural plaques are not known to resolve without treatment. Horses without ear sensitivity do not require treatment

• CO$_2$ laser ablation has been used but long-term efficacy is unknown
• Ear handling and ear clipping should be minimized in affected horses that are not being treated
• Ears should be protected from biting flies to avoid aggravation of the condition

MEDICATIONS

DRUG(S) OF CHOICE
• Topical imiquimod, an immune response modifier with antiviral activity, is the only drug shown to be consistently effective
• Imiquimod 5% cream resolves the plaques in 87–88% of horses and clears the infection with EcPV in 71% of ears biopsied
• Each lesion must be treated. Imiquimod is applied topically as a thin layer 2 or 3 times per week at least every other week until resolution, typically 3–4 months of every other week therapy (9–48 treatments). Alternatively, horses may be treated every 48 h for faster resolution (8–30 applications). A strong local inflammatory response is consistently observed with imiquimod due to its mechanism of action. The exudate and inflammation can make it difficult to handle and clean the ears prior to the next treatment. Sedation is often needed, particularly for the second or third treatment weeks. Inflammation generally resolves 7 days after the last treatment. Owners should be warned of the reaction and temporarily increased sensitivity due to local inflammation

CONTRAINDICATIONS/POSSIBLE INTERACTIONS
Imiquimod can cause inflammation of normal skin. No need to wash off the imiquimod until the next treatment is due.

FOLLOW-UP

PATIENT MONITORING
• Monitor for appropriate cleaning, application of imiquimod, and for complete resolution
• Clients may have difficulty cleaning the area sufficiently prior to treatment, resulting in poor contact of the drug with the plaques. Sedation is required for subsequent treatment if the repeated treatment occurs before 7 days after the last application. Inflammation caused by imiquimod can make it difficult to determine if the plaque resolution has occurred. Discontinuation of treatment for

1–2 weeks allows for better evaluation. Reevaluation at 1 month post treatment is strongly recommended. Assume any whitish areas are residual plaques. Recurrence is possible but infrequent within the subsequent 2 years if the plaques were resolved and flies controlled

PREVENTION/AVOIDANCE
• Not possible
• Use of fly repellents with permethrin/pyrethrin (for quick insect knockdown) and piperonyl butoxide (as a pesticide synergist) with fly masks that provide ear coverage may help prevent development

POSSIBLE COMPLICATIONS
• Ear sensitivity and pain
• Imiquimod can cause erosions or ulcers, particularly if applied in a thick layer. Erosions are more common in the first month of treatment. The severity of the reaction decreases as the plaques resolve

EXPECTED COURSE AND PROGNOSIS
• Aural plaques persist without treatment
• Post-treatment skin depigmentation may occur
• Ear sensitivity and head shyness improves after resolution of plaques despite the inflammation and challenges with ear handling during treatment

MISCELLANEOUS

ASSOCIATED CONDITIONS
None known.

AGE-RELATED FACTORS
None known.

ZOONOTIC POTENTIAL
None

SEE ALSO
• Papillomatosis
• Sarcoid

ABBREVIATIONS
EcPV = *Equus caballus* papillomavirus

Internet Resources
University of Minnesota, Veterinarian instructions for Aldara. http://www.vetmed.umn.edu/centers-programs/clinical-investigation-center/completed-clinical-studies/veterinarian-instructions-aldara

Author Erin Malone
Consulting Editor Gwendolen Lorch
Acknowledgment The author and editor acknowledge the prior contribution of Sheila Torres.

BASICS

DEFINITION
• Azotemia—the accumulation of nitrogenous waste (e.g. urea, Cr, other nitrogenous substance) in blood, plasma, or serum.
• Uremia—the clinical manifestation of azotemia; a multisystem disorder resulting from the effects of uremic toxins on cellular metabolism and function. Cr and BUN typically are measured in serum and used as indices of azotemia

PATHOPHYSIOLOGY
• BUN concentration is determined by the rate of urea synthesis by hepatocytes and rate of clearance by the kidneys. • Increased protein catabolism results in elevated BUN concentration. • Decreased GFR may result from decreased renal perfusion, renal disease, or urinary obstruction. • Azotemia results from resorption of urine following urinary tract rupture. • Cr is a result of muscle creatine metabolism. • Renal excretion of Cr is dependent on GFR. • Cr is not resorbed by renal tubules. • Low BUN concentration may result after prolonged diuresis or as a result of impaired liver function

SYSTEMS AFFECTED
• Depend on the underlying causes.
• Generalized effects—depression, weight loss, edema, dehydration. • Gastrointestinal tract—anorexia, uremic stomatitis, uriniferous breath, excessive dental tartar, oral/gastric ulceration, protein losing enteropathy, diarrhea.
• Neuromuscular—lethargy, gait imbalance, behavioral changes, seizures.
• Endocrine/metabolic—renal secondary hyperparathyroidism, inadequate production of erythropoietin and 1,25-dihydroxycholecalciferol (calcitriol).
• Cardiovascular—hypertension, heart murmur, cardiac dysrhythmia.
• Hemolymphatic—anemia

GENETICS
Healthy, heavily muscled Quarter Horses might have serum Cr concentrations >2.0 mg/dL.

INCIDENCE/PREVALENCE
N/A

GEOGRAPHIC DISTRIBUTION
N/A

SIGNALMENT
• Neonatal male foals (ruptured bladder at parturition). • Any breed, age, or sex

SIGNS
General Comments
Unless the animal is uremic, clinical findings are limited to the process causing azotemia such as dehydration, urinary outflow tract obstruction, urinary outflow tract, or rupture.

Historical Findings
• Polyuria/polydipsia. • Weight loss.
• Anorexia. • Abnormal urination. • Lethargy.
• Uriniferous breath. • Poor performance.
• Lumbar pain. • Colic. • Poor hair coat.
• Prolonged posturing to urinate. • Stranguria

Physical Examination Findings
• Fever. • Anorexia. • Obtundation. • Poor body condition. • Ventral edema. • Oral ulceration. • Excessive dental tartar. • Scleral injection. • Colic. • Distended abdomen.
• Urine scald. • Dysuria. • Hematuria.
• Halitosis

CAUSES
Prerenal Azotemia
• Renal hypoperfusion caused by decreased circulating volume or decreased blood pressure. • Increased protein catabolism

Renal Azotemia
• AKI or CRF—primary renal dysfunction affecting glomeruli, renal tubules, renal interstitium, or renal vasculature ○ Prolonged dehydration. ○ Polycystic kidney disease.
○ Pigment nephropathy (e.g. hemoglobin, myoglobin). ○ Nephrotoxic drugs (e.g. NSAIDs, aminoglycoside, tetracycline, polymyxin B). ○ Toxicities (e.g. cantharidin, red maple leaf, vitamin K3). ○ Leptospirosis.
○ Neoplasia

Postrenal Azotemia
• Obstruction of the urinary tract (e.g. urolithiasis). • Rupture of urinary tract

RISK FACTORS
• Prolonged exposure to nephrotoxic drugs, especially with concurrent dehydration.
• Rhabdomyolysis

DIAGNOSIS

DIFFERENTIAL DIAGNOSIS
Elevated serum Cr concentration can be seen in healthy, heavily muscled horses.

CBC/BIOCHEMISTRY/URINALYSIS
CBC
Nonregenerative anemia caused by decreased erythropoietin production can occur with CRF.

Biochemistry
• Elevations in serum Cr and BUN concentrations indicate azotemia. In horses, BUN:Cr ratio is unreliable in differentiating AKI and CRF. • Hyponatremia and hypochloremia are common in horses with renal disease and can occur with third-compartment spacing of urine.
• Hyperkalemia is a common finding in AKI and uroperitoneum. • Hypercalcemia and hypophosphatemia are often found with CRF; hypocalcemia and hyperphosphatemia can be found with AKI. • Hypercalcemia in renal failure depends upon dietary content and intake of calcium

Urinalysis
• USG >1.020 and urine osmolality >500 mOsm/kg are consistent with prerenal azotemia. • Fluid therapy and some medications (e.g. furosemide, α_2-receptor agonists, corticosteroids) may render the USG value inconclusive. • Dehydrated horses with primary renal disease usually lose the ability to concentrate urine; USG and osmolality are <1.020 and <500 mOsm/kg, respectively

OTHER LABORATORY TESTS
• Blood gas analysis—metabolic acidosis might be present with uremia. • Urine PCR for *Leptospira* sp.

IMAGING
Ultrasonography
• The urinary tract can be examined either transrectally or transabdominally. • Bladder ultrasonography is best performed transrectally using a 5 MHz probe.
• Transabdominal ultrasonography of the kidneys is best performed with a 2.5–3 MHz probe. • Assess the size and shape of both kidneys and architecture and echogenicity of the parenchyma. • The renal medulla is more echoluent than the renal cortex. • The renal pelvis varies in echogenicity. • With AKI, kidneys may be normal, enlarged, or hydronephrotic, and parenchymal abnormalities are often not detected. • With CRF, kidneys are usually smaller and more echogenic than normal. • Cystic or mineralized areas are more often associated with CRF or congenital anomalies. • Acoustic shadowing represents calculi formation

Renal Scintigraphy
May be used to document renal function but is not commonly performed.

OTHER DIAGNOSTIC PROCEDURES
Urine GGT:Cr Ratio
• Reflects GGT leakage from damaged renal tubular epithelium compared with the normal excretion of Cr. • Calculated as (urine GGT/urine Cr) × 100. • A ratio of >25 suggests proximal tubular damage; this elevation may occur before azotemia develops.
• Finding an elevated ratio depends on having enough remaining tubules that can leak GGT; severe renal fibrosis may yield normal values

Fractional Excretion of Electrolytes
• Measurement of electrolytes in serum and urine can be compared to assess renal damage.
• Calculated as (urine [electrolyte] × serum Cr/serum [electrolyte] × urine Cr). • Reported reference intervals for sodium fractional excretion range from 0.01 to 0.70. • Poor indicator of renal function

Rectal Examination
• Bladder—determine size, wall thickness, and presence of calculi or mural mass. • Left kidney—determine size and texture.
• Ureter—usually not detectable upon palpation, may be enlarged in association with pyelonephritis or ureterolithiasis

Ultrasonography-Guided Renal Biopsy
Can be used to confirm the diagnosis of primary renal disease, differentiate AKI from CRF, and identify a specific cause.

Urethrocystoscopy
• To evaluate abnormal urination. • In adult males, a flexible endoscope with an outside diameter of <12 mm and a length of ≥1 m is adequate to evaluate the urethra and urinary bladder. • Normal urethral mucosa is pale pink, with longitudinal folds. • If the urethra is dilated with air (e.g. to aid passage of the endoscope), the mucosa may appear reddened, and a prominent vascular pattern may appear. • The ischial arch and colliculus seminalis are the most common sites of posturination or postbreeding hemorrhage in geldings and stallions. • In the dorsal aspect of the bladder trigone, the ureteral openings can be visualized to determine the source of hematuria or pyuria. • Biopsy of a bladder mass or collection of a sterile urine sample can be obtained

PATHOLOGIC FINDINGS
Dependent on the underlying cause.

TREATMENT

Prerenal Azotemia
Correct the underlying cause of renal hypoperfusion and/or correct the dehydration.

Renal Azotemia
• Dependent on the underlying cause.
• Supportive care to alleviate clinical signs of uremia; correct fluid, electrolyte, and acid–base abnormalities

Postrenal Azotemia
• Eliminate urinary obstruction or correct cause of urine leakage ○ Surgical intervention often is required, but correction of any metabolic derangements is paramount

MEDICATIONS

DRUG(S) OF CHOICE
Dependent on the underlying cause.

Fluids
• IV fluid therapy is indicated for most azotemic patients. • Commonly used fluids—0.9% saline, Plasmalyte, lactated Ringer's solution. • Base the amount of fluid administration on dehydration or volume deficit. • Correction of the fluid deficit can occur during the first 6 h without untoward effects, except in patients with hypoproteinemia/hypoalbuminemia and with signs of cardiac disease

CONTRAINDICATIONS
• Use nephrotoxic drugs (e.g. NSAIDs, aminoglycosides) with caution in patients with azotemia. • K⁺-containing IV fluid solutions (e.g. Plasmalyte, lactated Ringer's solution) in the presence of hyperkalemia

PRECAUTIONS
• Use caution when administering fluids to horses with AKI and CRF because they may develop significant peripheral and pulmonary edema. • Use IV fluids cautiously in oliguric or anuric patients to minimize overhydration. • Use NSAIDs and corticosteroids with caution. Although they can limit renal inflammation, they can also nonselectively block vasodilatory mediators of renal blood flow under conditions of renal hypoperfusion and are not recommended for CRF. • Horses should be well hydrated when using NSAIDs and aminoglycosides

POSSIBLE INTERACTIONS
Be aware of additive effects of nephrotoxic drugs.

ALTERNATIVE DRUGS
N/A

FOLLOW-UP

PATIENT MONITORING
• Serum Cr, BUN and electrolyte concentrations within 24 h after initiating fluid therapy, hydration status, and urine outflow. • Monitoring body weight of foals and adult horses may be helpful. • With severe electrolyte or acid-base derangements, more frequent monitoring may be required

POSSIBLE COMPLICATIONS
• Failure to promptly correct prerenal azotemia caused by renal hypoperfusion may result in AKI. • Failure to correct renal azotemia may result in uremia. • Failure to correct postrenal azotemia may result in renal damage or death caused by hyperkalemia and uremia

EXPECTED COURSE AND PROGNOSIS
• Dependent on the underlying cause. • With CRF, serum Cr concentrations >5 mg/dL indicates a marked decline in GFR. A grave prognosis is associated with serum Cr concentrations >10 mg/dL

MISCELLANEOUS

ASSOCIATED CONDITIONS
Dependent on the underlying cause.

AGE-RELATED FACTORS
• AKI may occur at any age, but older horses may be at higher risk for azotemia regardless of the cause. • Ruptured bladder is more common in male neonatal foals

PREGNANCY/FERTILITY/BREEDING
The ability of a mare to maintain a viable pregnancy decreases as renal function decreases.

SYNONYMS
Acute renal failure

SEE ALSO
• Acidosis, metabolic
• Acute kidney injury (AKI) and acute renal failure (ARF)
• Chronic kidney disease
• Potassium, hyperkalemia
• Urolithiasis
• Uroperitoneum, neonate

ABBREVIATIONS
• AKI = acute kidney injury. • BUN = blood urea nitrogen. • Cr = creatinine.
• CRF = chronic renal failure. • GFR = glomerular filtration rate. • GGT = γ-glutamyltransferase.
• NSAID = nonsteroidal anti-inflammatory drug. • PCR = polymerase chain reaction.
• USG = urine specific gravity

Suggested Reading
Van Metre DC, Soto DR. Diseases of the renal system. In: Smith B, ed. Large Animal Internal Medicine, 5e. St. Louis, MO: Elsevier Mosby, 2015:873–895.

Author Sandra D. Taylor
Consulting Editor Sandra D. Taylor
Acknowledgment The author/editor acknowledges the prior contribution of Terry C. Gerros.

BASICS

OVERVIEW
• Broad term to describe pain in the thoracolumbar spine and/or its associated ligaments and muscles
• Cause for poor performance, altered gait, and undesirable behavior in the ridden horse

SIGNALMENT
• Middle-aged performance horses
• Jumping, racing, and dressage horses

SIGNS

Historical Findings
• Decrease or change in performance
• Previous trauma such as a fall or starting gate "incident"
• Resentment to grooming, saddling, or ridden ("cold backed")
• Ill-defined gait alternations when ridden (rearing, bucking, lack of impulsion, stiff gait)

Physical Examination Findings
• Back muscle atrophy
• Kyphosis ("roached back")
• Lordosis
• Scoliosis
• Resentment, muscle spasm, fasciculation when palpate back

CAUSES AND RISK FACTORS
• Spinal malformations
• Short-backed or long-backed conformation
• Poor or improper training methods
• Chronic coexisting hindlimb lameness
• Poorly fitting saddle
• Sports that require jumping
• Specific diseases that cause primary back pain
  ○ Impingement (overriding) of dorsal spinous processes ("kissing spines")
  ○ Fractured withers
  ○ Vertebral bone fractures, spondylosis, or discospondylosis
  ○ Osteoarthritis of thoracolumbar spine
  ○ Supraspinous desmitis

DIAGNOSIS

DIFFERENTIAL DIAGNOSIS
• Lameness, especially hindlimb
• Exertional rhabdomyolysis—elevated muscle enzymes, muscle biopsy
• Polysaccharide storage myopathy—muscle biopsy
• EPM—neurologic deficits, elevated titer in CSF, serology
• HYPP—DNA testing

CBC/BIOCHEMISTRY/URINALYSIS
± Mild elevation in serum creatine kinase, aspartate aminotransferase, lactate dehydrogenase.

OTHER LABORATORY TESTS
Serology and CSF for EPM.

IMAGING
• Radiography—overriding dorsal spinous processes, spondylosis, vertebral fracture
• Nuclear scintigraphy—increased radiopharmaceutical uptake in thoracolumbar spine and/or back muscles
• US—supraspinous desmitis, calcification, or acute epaxial muscle injury

OTHER DIAGNOSTIC PROCEDURES
• Diagnostic analgesia—local infiltration between dorsal spinous processes or back muscles
• Neurologic examination, CSF analysis
• Muscle biopsy
• DNA analysis for HYPP

TREATMENT
• Appropriate treatment for primary lameness
• Training management—progressive warmup exercise without rider
• Replace poorly fitting saddle
• Extracorporeal shock wave therapy—3 treatments at 3 week intervals at site of injury
• Surgery—resection of affected dorsal spinous processes, interspinous desmotomy
• For vertebral body fracture—stall rest for 2 months followed by small paddock turnout for 2 months
• Additional treatments:
  ○ Acupuncture
  ○ Physical therapy (massage)
  ○ Therapeutic US
  ○ Laser therapy
  ○ Magnetic blanket

MEDICATIONS

DRUG(S) OF CHOICE
• NSAIDs—phenylbutazone (2.2–4.4 mg/kg every 12–24 h)
• Perispinal injections—local infiltration of corticosteroids (40–60 mg of methylprednisolone acetate per site) ± Sarapin
• Intra-articular methylprednisolone acetate (20–40 mg) in vertebral facet or sacroiliac joints. US guidance ensures accurate placement
• Methocarbamol (10 mg/kg IV or 40–60 mg/kg PO daily)
• Mesotherapy—intradermal injections corresponding to the sites of pain. After treatment, exercise is restricted and gradually increased

CONTRAINDICATIONS/POSSIBLE INTERACTIONS
Gastrointestinal sensitivity with phenylbutazone.

FOLLOW-UP

PATIENT MONITORING
Periodic lameness and behavior evaluation.

PREVENTION/AVOIDANCE
• Avoid poorly fitting tack
• Institute proper training and treatment once diagnosed; frequent treatments are often necessary

POSSIBLE COMPLICATIONS
• Failure of accurate diagnosis and treatment
• Infection after injection(s)

EXPECTED COURSE AND PROGNOSIS
• For acute epaxial muscle injury, early diagnosis and treatment is usually successful
• For most other back pain, accurate diagnosis is difficult and selecting appropriate treatment is challenging. Prognosis is variable and determined by response to therapy
• Vertebral body fracture can be successfully treated with early diagnosis and rest

MISCELLANEOUS

ASSOCIATED CONDITIONS
Distal tarsitis, bilateral stifle disease.

AGE-RELATED FACTORS
None

SEE ALSO
• Distal tarsitis
• Equine protozoal myeloencephalitis (EPM)
• Exertional rhabdomyolysis syndrome
• Hyperkalemic periodic paralysis
• Polysaccharide storage myopathy

ABBREVIATIONS
• CSF = cerebrospinal fluid
• EPM = equine protozoal myeloencephalitis
• HYPP = hyperkalemic periodic paralysis
• NSAID = nonsteroidal anti-inflammatory drug
• US = ultrasonography, ultrasound

Suggested Reading
Denoix JM, Dyson SJ. Thoracolumbar spine. In: Ross MW, Dyson SJ, eds. Diagnosis and Management of Lameness in the Horse. St. Louis, MO: Elsevier Saunders, 2011:592–605.

Author Elizabeth J. Davidson
Consulting Editor Elizabeth J. Davidson
Acknowledgment The author/editor acknowledges the prior contribution of Benson B. Martin Jr.

BACTEREMIA/SEPSIS

B

BASICS

DEFINITION
- *Bacteremia*—the presence of viable bacteria in the circulating blood
- Sepsis—systemic disease caused by circulating microorganisms, including viral and fungal microorganisms, and their products
- *Endotoxemia*—the presence of endotoxin (lipopolysaccharide) within the circulating blood; implies the presence of associated clinical signs

PATHOPHYSIOLOGY
- Bacteremia—bacteria must gain access to the circulation via a breach of normal protective mechanisms. Occurs most commonly in the neonate. Portals of entry include respiratory and GI tracts, placenta, umbilicus, and surgical and traumatic wounds. In healthy animals, normal defense mechanisms rapidly clear circulating bacteria from the bloodstream
- Sepsis—normal defense mechanisms are overwhelmed, allowing the establishment of localized or generalized infection. The immunity is less effective in the neonate than in the adult, increasing the risk of sepsis
- Pathogens in neonatal sepsis—majority are Gram-negative bacteria (*Escherichia coli*), Gram-positive bacteria are rapidly increasing, viral, fungal, and protozoal pathogens
- Adult sepsis associated with enterocolitis—compromised GI barrier provides a route for entry of bacteria and fungi
- Endotoxemia—LPS from the bacteria cell wall of Gram-negative pathogens. Recognized as a sequela to Gram-negative neonatal sepsis. Associated with enterocolitis and pleuropneumonia in adults
- Circulating LPS interacts with immune cells to initiate production of a cascade of soluble immune mediators to produce a wide variety of systemic effects. Imbalance in the production of immune mediators can result in SIRS and severe sepsis/septic shock.

SYSTEMS AFFECTED
- All body systems can be affected
- Cardiovascular—hyperdynamic responses in early septic shock, systemic hypoperfusion, and cardiac depression in later stages

SIGNALMENT
- Foals generally within the first 3 days of age, although may occur at almost any age
- Adult horses of any age, sex, or breed

SIGNS

General Comments
A large variety of clinical signs are associated with infection, and specific signs depend on the stage of the disease process and the organ systems involved.

Historical Findings
- Foals with sepsis may have a history of perinatal problems, dystocia, premature/dysmature/postmature birth, previous abnormal siblings, etc. Failure of transfer of passive immunity is commonly reported. Poor management and poor environmental conditions may be present
- Affected adults may have concurrent immunosuppression or other disease processes

Physical Examination Findings
- Early signs—nonspecific, vague, or nonexistent. Easily attributable to other disease processes. Signs include lethargy, scleral injection, petechiation, mucous membrane injection, loss of suck reflex in foals, increased lethargy, or sleepiness
- Fever is present inconsistently
- Diarrhea may be the earliest localizing sign in septic foals
- Other signs—seizures, colic, respiratory distress, uveitis, subcutaneous abscesses, lameness, gait abnormality, joint distention, and periarticular edema
- Early SIRS/sepsis—normal blood pressures and blood pressure gradient, variable fever, injected mucous membranes, normal to brisk capillary refill time, tachycardia, agitation, and depression
- Late-stage septic shock is characterized by hypoperfusion and cool distal limbs and extremities, depression, unresponsiveness, hypotension, hypothermia, and gray mucous membranes with delayed capillary refill time

DIAGNOSIS

DIFFERENTIAL DIAGNOSIS

Foals
Hypoxic ischemic asphyxial syndromes, inflammatory perinatal insult, prematurity, and viral sepsis.

Adults
Early sepsis can be confused with almost any disease process. Late-stage septic shock is difficult to misdiagnose. Major differentials—hypovolemia (e.g. blood loss) and cardiogenic shock.

CBC/BIOCHEMISTRY/URINALYSIS

CBC
- Leukocytosis or leukopenia
- Increased band neutrophils
- Neutropenia
- Thrombocytopenia with associated DIC
- Fibrinogen normal, increased, or decreased (DIC), depending on stage of disease
- Serum amyloid A increased

Biochemistry
- Hypoglycemia in foals and some adult horses
- Metabolic acidosis and increased L-lactate concentrations with advancing hypoperfusion

- Increased creatinine and serum urea nitrogen concentrations with dehydration and AKI secondary to renal hypoperfusion in late stages
- Endstage sepsis is associated with multisystem organ failure

Urinalysis
- Increased protein and cells, altered fractional excretions of sodium and potassium, and isosthenuria or hyposthenuria with AKI
- Urinary parameters may not be valid in animals on IV fluid therapy

OTHER LABORATORY TESTS

Arterial Blood Gas Analysis
Hypoxemia, hypercapnia, and/or acidosis (mixed respiratory and metabolic), particularly in animals with acute respiratory distress syndrome and/or pulmonary edema.

IMAGING
- Depends on predisposing or associated condition
- Cardiac ultrasonography—increases in fractional shortening and decreased end-systolic volume (early stages), decreased cardiac contractility and ejection fractions (late stages)

OTHER DIAGNOSTIC PROCEDURES
- Blood culture required for definitive diagnosis
- Loss of normal barriers for bacterial translocation may result in isolation of microbes not causing primary disease
- Culture from localized infection
- Serial fecal cultures/PCR in cases of suspected salmonellosis, clostridiosis
- Clostridial toxin determination from feces

PATHOLOGIC FINDINGS
- Pathology is associated with affected organ systems
- Findings associated with DIC include jugular thrombosis, pulmonary thromboembolism, general or localized petechiae and ecchymoses, spontaneous hemorrhage, hemorrhage associated with venipuncture, and laminitis
- Severe sepsis/septic shock and endstage multiorgan failure findings may include pulmonary edema, tubular and interstitial nephritis, hepatic lipidosis, hepatic necrosis, myocardial necrosis, and/or GI mucosal abnormalities

TREATMENT

APPROPRIATE HEALTH CARE
Septic neonates and adults without evidence of septic shock may be treated at the farm. Referral to a facility where advanced 24 h care can be more readily provided when evidence of early or late septic shock.

(CONTINUED)   **BACTEREMIA/SEPSIS**

B

NURSING CARE
Septic shock—intensive nursing care including continuous IV fluid therapy, nutritional support, intranasal oxygen supplementation, frequent turning of recumbent foals to prevent decubital sores and lung atelectasis, heat lamps and warming blankets to prevent hypothermia.

ACTIVITY
Restricted

DIET
• Patients are frequently anorexic
• GI function often compromised and rest is required
• Parenteral nutrition considered for all foals and in adults (when finances are not a primary concern)
• Do not feed enterally foals with evidence of GI discomfort and/or bloat, foals and adults with hypothermia

CLIENT EDUCATION
Foals and adults that do not have serious additional disease beyond localized or mild sepsis frequently respond to treatment and survive. Survival decreases with the onset of severe sepsis. Foals and adults with hypotensive septic shock have a guarded to grave prognosis, even with intensive care.

SURGICAL CONSIDERATIONS
• Drained localized abscesses
• Remove infected umbilical remnants if medical therapy proves ineffective and if patient is stable enough to warrant general anesthesia
• Infected joints—lavage and/or arthroscopy for debridement, local antimicrobial therapies such as joint injection or regional limb perfusion

MEDICATIONS
DRUG(S) AND FLUIDS
• Broad-spectrum antimicrobial therapy—culture is pending or results are negative. Antimicrobial therapy should then be based on culture and sensitivity
• Equine plasma—foals with failure of passive transfer of maternal antibody
• Plasma and/or whole blood are ideal volume expander fluids

• Hyperimmune antiendotoxin plasma (J-5) therapy and/or polymyxin B (for a maximum of 3 days; monitor renal function closely)
• IV fluids—adults and foals with dehydration and either early or late septic shock
• Crystalloids—initial shock boluses of 20 mL/kg over 20 min; reassess patient and give additional boluses as necessary
• Hypotensive septic shock—may require pressor agents via constant rate of infusion with concurrent blood pressure and cardiac rate and rhythm monitoring
• NSAIDs (flunixin meglumine 1.0–0.25 mg/kg TID IV to adult horses) to aid in combating endotoxemia; use judiciously in foals due to complications of GI ulceration and renal dysfunction
• IV DMSO (controversial) 0.25–1.0 g/kg SID or BID as an anti-inflammatory agent and for diuresis
• Short-acting corticosteroid therapy (controversial) dexamethasone 0.01–0.1 mg/kg IV SID with septic shock

CONTRAINDICATIONS, PRECAUTIONS, POSSIBLE INTERACTIONS, ALTERNATIVE DRUGS
• Corticosteroids—associated with laminitis in the adult horse
• Pressor agents—cardiac dysrhythmias or decreased renal perfusion at certain dosages
• Aminoglycoside antimicrobials, oxytetracycline, and polymyxin B—AKI

FOLLOW-UP
PATIENT MONITORING
• All interventions should be monitored carefully for any change in the patient's condition
• Electrolyte and creatinine values daily if animals are on IV fluids. Any decrease in urinary output is suggestive of poor renal perfusion and possible renal failure
• Blood glucose twice daily if possible, particularly in septic shock
• Frequent arterial blood gas determinations in cases of septic shock
• Arterial blood pressure, heart rate, and rhythm

• Serial white blood cell counts, fibrinogen
• Antimicrobial treatment should continue until clinical signs are resolved and white blood count and fibrinogen concentration are within normal range

PREVENTION/AVOIDANCE
• Treat by prevention
• Early ingestion of good-quality colostrum by neonates and good management practices

MISCELLANEOUS
ABBREVIATIONS
• AKI = acute kidney injury
• DIC = disseminated intravascular coagulopathy
• DMSO = dimethylsulfoxide
• GI = gastrointestinal
• LPS = lipopolysaccharide
• NSAID = nonsteroidal anti-inflammatory drug
• PCR = polymerase chain reaction
• SIRS = systemic inflammatory response syndrome

Suggested Reading
Giguère S, Weber EJ, Sanchez LC. Factors associated with outcome and gradual improvement in survival over time in 1065 equine neonates admitted to an intensive care unit. Equine Vet J 2017;49:45–50.
Holcombe SJ, Jacobs CC, Cook VL, et al. Duration of in vivo endotoxin tolerance in horses. Vet Immunol Immunopathol 2016;173:10–16.
Moore JN, Vandenplas ML. Is it the systemic inflammatory response syndrome or endotoxemia in horses with colic? Vet Clin North Am Equine Pract 2014;30:337–351.
Wilkins PA. Prognostic indicators for survival and athletic outcome in critically ill neonatal foals. Vet Clin North Am Equine Pract 2015;31:615–628.
Wong DM, Wilkins PA. Defining the systemic inflammatory response syndrome in equine neonates. Vet Clin North Am Equine Pract 2015;31:463–481.

Author Pamela A. Wilkins
Consulting Editor Ashley G. Boyle

BACTERIAL DERMATITIS—METHICILLIN-RESISTANT STAPHYLOCOCCI

B

BASICS

DEFINITION
• Staphylococci are Gram-positive, opportunistic pathogens that can cause a variety of infections, including skin and soft tissue infections
• Methicillin (meticillin) resistance is conferred predominantly by the *mecA* gene, which encodes an PBP2a that confers resistance to almost all beta-lactam antimicrobials (penicillin, cephalosporins, carbapenems). MRS are also often resistant to many other drug classes
• MRSA is a potential zoonotic pathogen
• Staphylococci (including MRS) are commensal organisms and are often found as mucosal colonizers and on the skin
• There are two main classifications of staphylococci—coagulase positive and coagulase negative:
  ○ Coagulase-positive staphylococci are the most common causes of disease. *S. aureus* is the main coagulase-positive *Staphylococcus* in horses. *S. pseudintermedius* is a common canine pathogen that has sporadically been identified in horses
  ○ Coagulase-negative species are generally less pathogenic and are most often identified as contaminants or commensals
  ○ Any *Staphylococcus* can acquire methicillin resistance genes. Methicillin resistance does not make a *Staphylococcus* more virulent, but it complicates treatment when infections develop
• MRS cause infections at various body sites. Dermatitis may occur alone or associated with infections at other sites

GENETICS
No genetic predisposition has been identified.

INCIDENCE/PREVALENCE
• The incidence of staphylococcal dermatitis is unclear but is likely low
• MRSA colonization can be found in the nares of 0–2% of healthy horses in most regions, with higher prevalences sporadically identified. MR-CoNS colonization is much more common, ranging from 30% to 60%, and high rates of skin carriage or colonization are likely
• Staphylococcal skin diseases are virtually always secondary to an inciting cause that damages the skin barrier or host immune response. Infections more common in the spring and summer in most regions, likely because of factors such as heavy riding/training, higher temperature, higher humidity, increased time outdoors and in rainy conditions, increased biting insect populations and shedding

GEOGRAPHIC DISTRIBUTION
MRSA infections have been reported in many countries in North America, Europe, and Asia. It is likely that MRSA is distributed in the horse population worldwide. MR-CoNS are ubiquitous.

SIGNALMENT
There are no breed, age, or sex predilections.

SIGNS
Infections caused by MRS are not clinically discernable from those caused by susceptible strains. Clinical signs vary with the type of disease, and details are provided under specific topics.

CAUSES
Causes of specific staphylococcal dermatologic diseases are covered elsewhere. There should be no difference for infections caused by MRS.

RISK FACTORS
Risk factors for methicillin-resistant staphylococcal dermatitis have not been reported. A history of MRSA infection or colonization on the farm should increase suspicion. Prior antimicrobial therapy and hospitalization are associated with a higher risk of colonization by MRSA. Infections often occur in the absence of identifiable risk factors.

DIAGNOSIS

DIFFERENTIAL DIAGNOSIS
Differential diagnoses vary with the type of dermatologic disease and are covered elsewhere.

CBC/BIOCHEMISTRY/URINALYSIS
These may be indicated to identify an underlying disease (e.g. hyperadrenocorticism).

OTHER LABORATORY TESTS
• Cytologic examination—an abundance of neutrophils and clusters of intra- and extracellular cocci is suggestive of staphylococcal infection, but cannot identify MRS
• Identification of MRS involves isolation of the *Staphylococcus* spp. and identification of oxacillin or cefoxitin resistance, detection of *mecA* by PCR, and/or identification of PBP2a
• Interpretation of cultures of superficial skin surfaces can be difficult because staphylococci, particularly coagulase-negative species, are common on normal skin. Sampling should be done to limit the likelihood of contamination (e.g. sampling of intact pustules vs. superficial swabs of affected skin surfaces). Isolation of MRS, particularly MR-CoNS, from skin does not necessarily imply relevance

IMAGING
N/A

OTHER DIAGNOSTIC PROCEDURES
None

PATHOLOGIC FINDINGS
N/A

TREATMENT

AIMS
Aims of treatment are to eliminate the clinical signs of infection and to limit the risk of transmission to other horses or humans. Addressing underlying risk factors is critical. Elimination of MRS from the body, at either the site of infection or colonization sites (e.g. nose, pharynx) would be desirable but is not the goal, because colonization with MRS after a successful clinical response is not uncommon.

APPROPRIATE HEALTH CARE
Most cases can be managed on the farm or as outpatients. The main reasons for hospitalization would be severe infection and an inability of the owner to properly treat the horse.

NURSING CARE
Nursing care is dependent on the specific staphylococcal disease. Infection control precautions should be instituted as described below.

ACTIVITY
Medically, there is no reason to limit activity. The main reason to limit activity is for infection control. MRSA is transmissible to other horses and humans, and infected horses should be isolated. There is less concern with other MRS.

DIET
There are no specific requirements.

CLIENT EDUCATION
• *MRSA is a zoonotic disease* and clients should be counseled on the risk of transmission
• Barrier precautions (gloves, protective outerwear) should be used when handling affected horses
• Hand hygiene (handwashing, use of alcohol-based hand rub) should be performed when in contact with the horse or its environment. The affected horse should be isolated from other horses until clinical signs have resolved. Some risk is still present after clinical cure because of the potential for post-treatment colonization, and the infection control approach is a case-by-case basis, considering the risk status of other horses and people on the farm, whether MRSA likely originated on the farm, the ability to use isolation measures on the farm, and the intended use

SURGICAL CONSIDERATIONS
N/A

(CONTINUED)   BACTERIAL DERMATITIS—METHICILLIN-RESISTANT STAPHYLOCOCCI

MEDICATIONS

DRUG(S) OF CHOICE
• Dermatitis caused by MRS should be approached identically to disease caused by susceptible staphylococci, with the exception of the chosen antimicrobial
• Topical therapy (e.g. chlorhexidine bathing) can be effective as the sole treatment of superficial disease. Shampooing affected areas 3 or 4 times per week is commonly used in dogs and would likely be similarly effective in horses. Topical antimicrobials include mupirocin and fusidic acid, although resistance to these drugs has emerged and there are public health concerns about use of these drugs in horses
• With deeper involvement, poor response to topical therapy, or when proper topical therapy is not possible, systemic antimicrobials are indicated. Antimicrobials should be selected based on culture and susceptibility testing. MRS should be considered resistant to all beta-lactam antimicrobials, regardless of in vitro results. Fluoroquinolones should be avoided if possible because resistance can develop quickly and clinical response may be unpredictable. MRS may be susceptible to rifampin (rifampicin), but this drug should always be used with another antimicrobial to which the isolate is susceptible
• For superficial infections, 2–4 weeks should be adequate, with shorter durations possible in some cases, particularly when topical therapy can also be used and when an underlying problem can be corrected (e.g. irritation from tack) or is not persistent (e.g. surgical wound)
• For deep infections, it is important that treatment duration is adequate; 10–12 weeks of therapy (or more) may be required in some cases

CONTRAINDICATIONS
None

PRECAUTIONS
Horses should be prevented from licking sites where topical antimicrobials have been applied, as that might reduce efficacy or pose a risk for antimicrobial-associated diarrhea.

POSSIBLE INTERACTIONS
N/A

ALTERNATIVE DRUGS
There are ethical concerns about the use of drugs that are important in human medicine such as vancomycin and linezolid, and there is minimal pharmacokinetic and safety information available for horses. Use of these drugs should be discouraged.

FOLLOW-UP

PATIENT MONITORING
• Clinical response should be monitored. If there is poor initial response, the diagnosis should be reconsidered
• Culture of the affected site after clinical cure is not recommended because the presence of MRS after clinical cure is not uncommon
• Post-treatment testing for MRSA colonization (e.g. nasal swab culture) can be indicated as part of the infection control response in some situations

PREVENTION/AVOIDANCE
Prudent antimicrobial use is important to decrease the prevalence of MRSA in the population and to reduce the chance of a horse acquiring MRSA. The same probably applies to many other MRS, although it is likely that MR-CoNS are part of the normal microbiota and there are no effective means of eliminating normal commensals. Application of general infection control practices may be useful for restricting the spread and impact of MRS infections.

POSSIBLE COMPLICATIONS
Systemic manifestations secondary to dermatitis are rare.

EXPECTED COURSE AND PROGNOSIS
The prognosis is more dependent on the type of disease than the pathogen involved and is good as long as an appropriate antimicrobial can be identified and administered.

MISCELLANEOUS

ASSOCIATED CONDITIONS
None

AGE-RELATED FACTORS
None

ZOONOTIC POTENTIAL
MRSA is a zoonotic pathogen, and transmission from colonized and infected horses to humans has been documented. Infection control precautions should be implemented to limit contact with infected horses. These include the use of barrier precautions (gloves, dedicated outerwear) whenever the horse or its environment is contacted, restricted contact, and careful attention to hand hygiene. People at higher risk for developing an MRSA infection, such as immunocompromised individuals, should not have contact with infected or colonized horses. The risk with other MRS is unclear and is likely minimal; however, it is sensible to implement the same precautions with any multidrug-resistant infection.

PREGNANCY/FERTILITY/BREEDING
There are no additional concerns.

SYNONYMS
N/A

SEE ALSO
Bacteremia/sepsis

ABBREVIATIONS
• MR-CoNS = methicillin-resistant coagulase-negative staphylococci
• MRS = methicillin-resistant staphylococci
• MRSA = methicillin-resistant *Staphylococcus aureus*
• PBP2a = penicillin binding protein 2a
• PCR = polymerase chain reaction

Suggested Reading
Bergström K, Bengtsson B, Nyman A, et al. Longitudinal study of horses for carriage of methicillin-resistant *Staphylococcus aureus* following wound infections. Vet Microbiol 2013;163:388–391.

Author J. Scott Weese
Consulting Editor Gwendolen Lorch

BILE ACIDS

BASICS

OVERVIEW
- BAs are cholesterol derivatives made by the liver and secreted via the biliary tree into the small intestine, where they emulsify dietary lipid and enhance its digestion by pancreatic lipases
- Primary functions of BAs:
  - Facilitate cholesterol excretion
  - Stimulate hepatic bile flow
  - Enhance dietary lipid absorption
- During digestion, primary BAs are dehydroxylated by enteric bacteria to secondary BAs
- BAs are reabsorbed from the gastrointestinal tract in the ileum; they are transported back to the liver via portal circulation, where they are extracted by the liver, conjugated, and resecreted. Approximately 90% of the BA pool is concentrated in the enterohepatic circulation, and may be recycled 10–40 times/day
- Under physiologic conditions, equilibrium exists between intestinal absorption, hepatic uptake from the portal circulation, and hepatic secretion of BAs; this is represented and quantified as the SBAs
- Assessment of SBAs in the horse can be performed at any time, as the horse does not store BAs in a gallbladder between meals. Further, SBA concentrations do not display diurnal variation in this species
- Reference range < 12 μmol/L
- Elevated SBA concentration is a sensitive and specific marker of hepatic disease; however, the nature of the lesion cannot be determined by this parameter alone
- The primary BAs are taurocholic, taurochenodeoxycholic, and glycochenodeoxycholic acid; the majority of BAs are conjugated with taurine. Conjugation is required for secretion
- Three general mechanisms increase SBAs:
  - Failure of hepatocytes to extract BAs from portal blood
  - Biliary stasis
  - Portosystemic shunting

SIGNALMENT
Any breed, age, or sex.

SIGNS
- BA accumulation in the skin has been suggested to induce pruritus
- Signs of hepatic dysfunction
  - Icterus
  - Anorexia, weight loss
  - Depression
  - Edema
  - Hepatic encephalopathy
  - Photosensitization
  - Colic
  - Diarrhea
  - Hemolysis (rare, but significant)
  - Hemorrhagic diathesis (rare)

CAUSES AND RISK FACTORS
- Acute disease
  - Theiler's disease
  - Hepatic lipidosis
  - Tyzzer's disease
  - Cholangiohepatitis
  - Biliary obstruction
    - Cholelithiasis/choledocholithiasis
    - Colon displacement
- Parasitic hepatitis
- Toxic hepatopathy (iron, drugs, plants, mycotoxins)
- Viral hepatitis (equine infectious anemia, equine viral arteritis, equine herpesvirus 1)
- Chronic disease
  - Pyrrolizidine alkaloid toxicity
  - Chronic active hepatitis
  - Cholelithiasis
  - Neoplasia
  - Hepatic abscess
- Congenital disease
  - Portosystemic shunt

DIAGNOSIS

CBC/BIOCHEMISTRY/URINALYSIS
- CBC—may suggest inflammation (leukocytosis, neutrophilia) or anemia of chronic disease
- Biochemistry—increased γ-glutamyltransferase, aspartate aminotransferase, sorbitol dehydrogenase, alkaline phosphatase, bilirubin; decreased albumin, blood urea nitrogen, glucose

OTHER LABORATORY TESTS
- Blood ammonia concentration
- Plasma fibrinogen concentration

IMAGING
- Hepatic ultrasonography
  - Hyperechogenicity noted in cases of hepatic fibrosis, hepatic lipidosis
  - Nodules
  - Biliary dilatation
  - Choleliths
  - Hepatomegaly

OTHER DIAGNOSTIC PROCEDURES
- Biopsy to characterize hepatic lesions and formulate prognosis (acute hepatitis vs. hepatic fibrosis)
- Coagulation profile prior to collecting biopsy, but coagulopathy does not predict risk of biopsy complication

TREATMENT
- Treatment of underlying cause
- Supportive care, as initial inciting insult may no longer be present (e.g. pyrrolizidine alkaloid hepatotoxicity)
- Low-protein, highly soluble carbohydrate diet with low aromatic amino acid to branched-chain amino acid ratio

MEDICATIONS

DRUG(S) OF CHOICE
Dependent on the underlying cause.

CONTRAINDICATIONS/POSSIBLE INTERACTIONS
Dependent on the underlying cause.

FOLLOW-UP

PATIENT MONITORING
Serial monitoring of biochemistry and SBAs.

PREVENTION/AVOIDANCE
- Use caution in the administration of equine-origin biologics (e.g. plasma, tetanus anti-toxin) to adult horses
- Avoid exposure to hepatotoxic plants and medications

POSSIBLE COMPLICATIONS
- Coagulopathy and hemorrhagic diathesis with severe hepatic failure
- Self-trauma in patients with hepatic encephalopathy

EXPECTED COURSE AND PROGNOSIS
- Dependent on the underlying cause, but most etiologies carry a prognosis that is guarded to poor
- SBA concentration >50 μmol/L has been associated with a poor prognosis in horses with pyrrolizidine alkaloid toxicosis, and SBA concentration >20 μmol/L has been associated with nonsurvival (short and long term) in equine liver disease

MISCELLANEOUS

AGE-RELATED FACTORS
The SBA concentration of neonatal foals is substantially higher than that observed in adult horses.

SEE ALSO
- Acute hepatitis in adult horses (Theiler disease)
- Cholelithiasis
- Hepatic encephalopathy
- Photosensitization
- Pyrrolizidine alkaloid toxicosis
- Tyzzer disease (*Clostridium piliforme*)

ABBREVIATIONS
- BA = bile acid
- SBA = serum bile acid

Suggested Reading
Dunkel B, Jones SA, Pinilla MJ, Foote AK. Serum bile acid concentrations, histopathological features, and short- and long-term survival in horses with hepatic disease. J Vet Intern Med 2015;29(2):644–650.

Author Teresa A. Burns
Consulting Editor Sandra D. Taylor

BILIRUBIN (HYPERBILIRUBINEMIA)

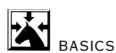

BASICS

DEFINITION
Hyperbilirubinemia is increased bilirubin in the blood.

PATHOPHYSIOLOGY
• Most bilirubin in the blood of healthy horses originates from the breakdown of hemoglobin by macrophages that have phagocytized aged or damaged erythrocytes
• Macrophages release water-insoluble, unconjugated (indirect) bilirubin into blood where it binds to albumin. This form of bilirubin does not pass through glomeruli into urine. It enters hepatocytes by a carrier-mediated process. A small amount is refluxed into blood; most is conjugated to a water-soluble form that is excreted into the biliary system. Little conjugated (direct) bilirubin is regurgitated back into systemic circulation
• Conjugated bilirubin is filtered by glomeruli and bilirubinuria can occur with hyperbilirubinemia
• Normal horses have higher blood concentrations of bilirubin than many other species
• Hyperbilirubinemia occurs with decreased food intake, hemolytic anemia, hepatocellular disease, and cholestatic disorders

SYSTEMS AFFECTED
Skin
• Icterus (yellow discoloration of skin, sclera, or mucous membranes) may be detected when total bilirubin concentrations >2–3 mg/dL. Hyperbilirubinemia can be present without visible icterus
• Slight yellow discoloration of sclera or mucous membranes occurs in 10–15% of normal horses

Renal/Urologic
Dark-colored urine occurs with bilirubinuria.

GENETICS
N/A

INCIDENCE/PREVALENCE
N/A

GEOGRAPHIC DISTRIBUTION
N/A

SIGNALMENT
• All ages and breeds are affected
• Newborns are at risk for neonatal isoerythrolysis

SIGNS
Historical Findings
• Anorexia
• Depression
• Lethargy
• Weakness
• Icterus

Physical Examination Findings
• Hemolytic anemia—pale mucous membranes, tachycardia, and tachypnea
• Hepatocellular or cholestatic disorders—weight loss, behavioral changes, colic, fever, diarrhea, ascites, edema, hemorrhagic diathesis, photosensitization

CAUSES
Prehepatic (Hemolytic) Hyperbilirubinemia
• Hemolytic disorders cause elevated total bilirubin (primarily unconjugated) when production overwhelms the ability of hepatocytes to uptake, conjugate, and excrete bilirubin
• Conjugated bilirubin may increase due to increased hepatic production or concurrent hepatobiliary disease
• Causes for hemolysis include immune-mediated disorders (e.g. neonatal isoerythrolysis, idiopathic, or secondary to drug therapy, infection, neoplasia), infectious diseases (e.g. piroplasmosis, equine infectious anemia), oxidant damage (e.g. red maple leaf intoxication), fragmentation (e.g. disseminated intravascular coagulation), administration of hypotonic fluids and severe hepatic failure

Fasting Hyperbilirubinemia
• Unconjugated bilirubin predominates with minimal increases in conjugated bilirubin
• Elevated bilirubin in the blood occurs within 12–15 h of onset of anorexia or fasting
• Bilirubinemia plateaus after 2–3 days and is usually <8 mg/dL but may be as high as 12 mg/dL
• The mechanism likely involves impaired bilirubin uptake by hepatocytes
• Values normalize once food intake resumes

Hepatic Hyperbilirubinemia
• Hepatocellular disorders increase bilirubin by impairing bilirubin uptake, conjugation, or excretion into biliary canaliculi
• Unconjugated bilirubin predominates

Cholestatic Hyperbilirubinemia
• Decreased bilirubin excretion occurs with obstruction of bile flow due to hepatocyte swelling, periportal compression of bile ducts, or extrahepatic blockage of bile ducts
• Endotoxemia/sepsis may cause functional cholestasis
• Suspect cholestatic disease when conjugated bilirubin comprises >25% of total bilirubin; conjugated bilirubin rarely exceeds 30–40% of total bilirubin

RISK FACTORS
• Hyperbilirubinemia is common with anorexia
• Mild hyperbilirubinemia may occur for several days after prolonged exercise
• Administration of equine biologics (e.g. plasma, tetanus anti-toxin) is associated with Theiler's disease

DIAGNOSIS

DIFFERENTIAL DIAGNOSIS
N/A

CBC/BIOCHEMISTRY/URINALYSIS
• Total and conjugated bilirubin are measured in serum or heparinized plasma. Unconjugated bilirubin is calculated
• Exposure to sunlight or fluorescent lighting may decrease bilirubin concentration
• Separate serum/plasma from cells as soon as possible and protect from light
• Hemolysis, lipemia, or some drugs may alter bilirubin measurement depending on the methodology used

Prehepatic Hyperbilirubinemia
• Moderate to severe decreases in RBC count, hematocrit, and hemoglobin
• Hemoglobinemia and hemoglobinuria occur if hemolysis is intravascular
• Total protein and albumin concentrations are usually normal
• Blood smear may reveal morphologic changes supporting hemolysis (e.g. agglutination, spherocytes, Heinz bodies, eccentrocytes, schistocytes, pyknocytes) or organisms
• Neutrophilia with a left shift may be present
• The activity of liver enzymes (e.g. AST, SDH) may be normal to slightly elevated due to hypoxia

Fasting Hyperbilirubinemia
• RBC count, hematocrit, and hemoglobin are normal to slightly decreased if anemia is not part of the disorder causing anorexia
• Liver enzyme activities are normal if hepatobiliary disease is absent

Hepatic Hyperbilirubinemia
• RBC count, hematocrit, and hemoglobin concentration are normal to slightly decreased
• Albumin concentration usually is normal in acute and decreased in chronic hepatocellular disease with loss of function
• Globulin concentrations are normal to increased
• Liver enzyme (e.g. AST, SDH, ALP, GGT) activities are significantly increased; the degree of elevation lessens with chronicity
• With impairment of hepatic function, BUN, glucose, and cholesterol concentrations may decrease. Bile acids and ammonia concentrations increase
• Elevated triglyceride concentrations occur with hyperlipemia and hepatic lipidosis

Cholestatic Hyperbilirubinemia
• RBC count, hematocrit, and hemoglobin are normal to slightly decreased
• Total protein, albumin, BUN, and glucose concentrations usually are normal
• Activities of enzymes indicative of hepatocellular damage (e.g. AST, SDH) may increase if there is concurrent hepatocyte

BILIRUBIN (HYPERBILIRUBINEMIA) (CONTINUED)

B

damage; those indicative of cholestasis (e.g. ALP, GGT) are moderately to markedly increased
• Serum bile acids are elevated
• Bilirubinuria is detected

OTHER LABORATORY TESTS
• Prehepatic hyperbilirubinemia—consider Coggins test, Coombs test, osmotic fragility, serology, or PCR testing to determine the cause of anemia
• Hepatic hyperbilirubinemia—measure clotting times (prothrombin time, activated partial thromboplastin time) in horses with hemorrhagic diathesis or before surgery to assess risk of hemorrhage

IMAGING
Ultrasonography is useful to evaluate liver size, changes in hepatic parenchyma, and biliary patency.

OTHER DIAGNOSTIC PROCEDURES
Hepatic biopsy for histopathology and bacterial culture may identify the cause of hepatic disease.

PATHOLOGIC FINDINGS
• Hepatic disorders associated with hyperbilirubinemia include Theiler's disease, infectious hepatitis, toxic hepatopathies, chronic active hepatitis, amyloidosis, neoplasia, and hepatic lipidosis
• Cholestatic disorders associated with hyperbilirubinemia include cholangitis, cholelithiasis, hepatitis, neoplasia, fibrosis, large colon displacement, and biliary hyperplasia

TREATMENT
• Prehepatic hyperbilirubinemia—eliminate the inciting cause of erythrocyte destruction
• Fasting hyperbilirubinemia—correct the underlying cause for decreased food intake
• Hepatic or cholestatic hyperbilirubinemia—eliminate the underlying cause and provide supportive care until the liver regenerates

APPROPRIATE HEALTH CARE
• Medical management is appropriate for most horses
• Surgery is required in some cases of biliary obstruction

NURSING CARE
• IV fluid therapy may be required to maintain hydration, tissue perfusion, and electrolyte balance
• Compatible whole-blood or packed RBC transfusion is rarely required to restore erythrocyte mass in severely anemic horses

ACTIVITY
Restrict activity until underlying abnormalities are corrected.

DIET
• Fasting hyperbilirubinemia—offer a high-quality diet; icterus will resolve when food intake resumes
• Decreased hepatic function—provide a balanced, high-carbohydrate, low-protein diet; oat or grass hay is recommended

CLIENT EDUCATION
N/A

SURGICAL CONSIDERATIONS
N/A

MEDICATIONS
DRUG(S) OF CHOICE
Prehepatic Hyperbilirubinemia
• Discontinue any current drugs if suspect drug-induced IMHA
• Treatment of IMHA includes immunosuppressive doses of corticosteroids (dexamethasone 0.1–0.2 mg/kg IM or IV SID), decreasing gradually once hematocrit stabilizes

Hepatic or Cholestatic Hyperbilirubinemia
• Bacterial hepatitis or cholangitis are best treated with antibiotics determined by culture and sensitivity results
• Chronic active (nonsuppurative) hepatitis with a suspected immune-mediated origin may respond to dexamethasone (0.05–0.1 mg/kg) or prednisolone (1 mg/kg) daily for 4–7 days, then gradually decrease over several days
• Hepatic encephalopathy—neomycin (10–100 mg/kg PO every 6 h for 1 day); lactulose (333 mg/kg PO every 8 h)

CONTRAINDICATIONS
Hepatic or cholestatic hyperbilirubinemia:
• Avoid drugs known to be hepatotoxic
• Drugs associated with hepatocellular diseases include phenothiazine and erythromycin
• Drugs associated with idiosyncratic hepatotoxicity include aspirin, diazepam, halothane, isoniazid, nitrofurantoin, phenobarbital, phenytoin, rifampin (rifampicin), and sulfonamides

PRECAUTIONS
Hepatic or cholestatic hyperbilirubinemia:
• Use drugs cautiously because many require biotransformation or excretion in the liver and dosages may need to be altered
• Avoid analgesics, anesthetics, and barbiturates if possible

POSSIBLE INTERACTIONS
N/A

ALTERNATIVE DRUGS
N/A

FOLLOW-UP
PATIENT MONITORING
• Hemolytic hyperbilirubinemia—serial CBCs as indicated by the underlying disease process
• Hepatic or cholestatic hyperbilirubinemia—regular measurement of liver enzyme activities, albumin, and bilirubin

PREVENTION/AVOIDANCE
Dependent on the underlying cause.

POSSIBLE COMPLICATIONS
Dependent on the underlying cause.

EXPECTED COURSE AND PROGNOSIS
Dependent on the underlying cause.

MISCELLANEOUS
ASSOCIATED CONDITIONS
N/A

AGE-RELATED FACTORS
Bilirubin often is elevated in neonates because of decreased hepatic function and increased turnover of fetal hemoglobin; values usually decrease to adult concentrations within 1–2 weeks of birth.

ZOONOTIC POTENTIAL
N/A

PREGNANCY/FERTILITY/BREEDING
N/A

SYNONYMS
• Icterus
• Jaundice

SEE ALSO
• Anemia
• Bile acids

ABBREVIATIONS
• ALP = alkaline phosphatase
• AST = aspartate aminotransferase
• BUN = blood urea nitrogen
• GGT = γ-glutamyltransferase
• IMHA = immune-mediated hemolytic anemia
• PCR = polymerase chain reaction
• RBC = red blood cell
• SDH = sorbitol dehydrogenase

Suggested Reading
Carlson KL. Hepatic diseases in the horse. In: Sprayberry KA, Robinson NE, eds. Robinson's Current Therapy in Equine Medicine, 7e. Philadelphia, PA: WB Saunders, 2015:287–293.
Peek SF. Hemolytic disorders. In: Sprayberry KA, Robinson NE, eds. Robinson's Current Therapy in Equine Medicine, 7e. ST. Louis, MO: WB Saunders, 2015:492–495.

Author Jennifer S. Thomas
Consulting Editor Sandra D. Taylor

BIOSECURITY, DISINFECTANTS IN THE BREEDING SHED

BASICS

DEFINITION
Biosecurity:
- All actions taken to reduce the risk of introduction and spread of infectious diseases
- Breeding shed biosecurity typically concentrates on venereally transmitted diseases; outbreaks of any contagious disease have significant impacts on horse health
- Equine herpesvirus myeloencephalopathy outbreaks affecting equine facilities have increased biosecurity awareness
- Must address contagious diseases beyond those that affect the reproductive tracts of mares and stallions

BIOSECURITY PRINCIPLES
Biosecurity protocols should be tailored to the individual facility:
- Owners, managers, and veterinarians must know and abide by all current requirements for CEM testing and EAV testing and vaccination
- Examine all horses arriving for signs of disease, includes leased teaser stallions, nurse mares
- Group farm horses by use and age
- Separate resident horses from transient horses (layovers, show horses, and pleasure horses)
- When possible, personnel routinely working with pregnant mares and foals (high-risk populations) should not work with other horses
- New arrivals must be accompanied by a certificate of veterinary inspection, negative equine infectious anemia test, and complete history of vaccination and deworming
- Minimum 2 week quarantine to monitor horses (BID rectal temperature) from low-risk premises, including comprehensive vaccinations and biosecurity protocols; no active infectious disease issues, vaccination and deworming updates, and health assessments
- Minimum 21–28 days quarantine if unknown health history and vaccinations. Allow no nose-to-nose contact over fence lines with resident horses. Use separate equipment (rakes, shovels, buckets, grooming equipment, etc.) not shared with resident horse population

PATHOGENS
- Equine venereal disease outbreaks are primarily caused by *Taylorella equigenitalis*, EAV, and EHV-3
- *T. equigenitalis*—Gram-negative coccobacillus; causes CEM
  - Transmission—venereal contact, contaminated semen, contaminated fomites including phantoms (stallion to stallion)
- EAV—lipid-enveloped RNA virus, family Arteriviridae

- Transmission—respiratory secretions, aerosolization of virus-contaminated materials, and coitus
- EHV-3 causes equine coital exanthema; highly contagious via natural cover, artificial insemination, nose-to-nose contact, contaminated fomites
- Dourine is a trypanosomal disease (*Trypanosoma equiperdum*)
  - Transmission—only by coitus
  - Eradicated from North America, most of Europe; exists in other areas of the world
- Veterinarians—must be aware of local, state, and national reporting requirements
- Other bacterial infections, e.g. *Pseudomonas aeruginosa* and *Klebsiella pneumoniae*, can be transmitted by coitus, artificial insemination, contaminated breeding equipment, fomites
- *T. equigenitalis*, EAV, and EHV—easily killed by thorough cleaning with detergent and commonly used disinfectants in the breeding shed
- Transmission (viral and bacterial pathogens) can occur any time horses are co-mingled or equipment is shared
  - Of significant importance are EHVs, equine influenza virus, EAV, *Streptococcus equi*, and other respiratory pathogens
  - Nose-to-nose contact, nasal contact of contaminated surfaces (stalls, stocks, phantoms), and shared equipment can all result in pathogen spread
  - *Salmonella* spp. and other pathogens can be spread by the fecal–oral route
  - Breeding shed biosecurity requires overall farm biosecurity measures

CLEANING AND DISINFECTION
- Specific breeding equipment (artificial vaginas, wash buckets, etc.) is addressed elsewhere
- Must keep clean and disinfected—the breeding shed, to include teasing stalls, mare stocks, aisle ways
- Teasing stalls or stocks permit teaser stallions contact with mares to confirm receptivity. Nose-to-nose contact between the two should be avoided

STALLS, STOCKS, TEASING CHUTES
- Ideal surfaces are made of nonporous material, easily cleaned with detergents, rinsed, and then sprayed with an appropriate disinfectant
- Raw wood/dirt floors—virtually impossible to adequately clean and disinfect
  - Wood surfaces (including stocks) can be cleaned and sealed with several coats of paint or polyurethane wood sealant to make a cleanable surface
  - Concrete block stalls—porous until painted
  - Any surface contaminated with bodily fluids and nasal secretions should be scrubbed with detergent and rinsed with potable water
  - Avoid pressure washers—can aerosolize pathogens

- Garden hose nozzles (<0.8 MPa (120 psi) water pressure) can be used
- Mares brought only for live cover—house temporarily in stalls to be teased by stallions
  - Remove manure in between mares
  - Remove bedding soiled with urine and vaginal discharges; clean surfaces with detergent before the stall is used again
  - Leptospires are shed in urine; vaginal discharges can be source of pathogens. If stall floors are dirt, packed clay, or sand, wet areas can thoroughly be sprinkled with barn lime to discourage pathogen retention

PHANTOMS
- Routinely used to collect semen, constructed of a variety of materials
- To significantly reduce the risk of venereal transmission, phantoms, regardless of surface material, can be wrapped in disposable plastic (available in 50 cm (20 inch) wide rolls, discount warehouses/online)
  - Wrapping includes any padded area for the stallions' front legs, and bite bars, with sufficient overlap of layers to prevent it from being dislodged during collection
  - Afterwards, workers wearing disposable gloves tear the plastic, carefully fold the edges towards the top to contain any bodily fluids before throwing the material away, followed by discarding their own gloves
  - Care must be taken to minimize the spread of any bodily fluids back onto the phantom or onto the floor while disposing of the plastic
- Any areas of the phantom visibly contaminated or dirty should be washed with detergent, rinsed with potable water, and allowed to dry
- After every use (whether washed or not), the entire phantom should be sprayed with 70% isopropyl or ethyl alcohol and allowed to dry. Workers should then don new disposable gloves and completely wrap the phantom with plastic wrap before the next stallion is collected
- Covering only parts of the phantom in contact with the penis is inadequate; nasal secretions can spread respiratory pathogens
- If covered with a washable, nonporous fabric, at the very least, wrap the phantom closest to the hind limbs of the stallion in disposable plastic. After use, discard the plastic, wash the entire phantom, rinse. When dry, spray with alcohol; allow to dry
- If fleece padding is used to protect the stallion's medial carpi, plastic wrap can also protect this material
- Alternatively, individual fleece can be used for each stallion and routinely washed with detergent

BREEDING SHED FLOORS
- Floors of dirt, sand, shredded rubber, and other loose material cannot be cleaned and disinfected, but provide traction and cushion to horses

B

• Can reduce dust by wetting down with water prior to using the breeding shed
• Textured rubber mats with sealed seams provide a cleanable surface
• Keep the breeding shed floor clean and free of organic matter

MISCELLANEOUS BREEDING SHED EQUIPMENT
• Leather shrouds (bite covers) to protect mares' necks from stallions' teeth, should be cleaned with detergent and water in between uses; could be contaminated with nasal secretions
• Leather aprons used to prevent the teaser stallion from accidental penetrating a mare should be dedicated to one stallion; thoroughly clean after each use
  ◦ An apron used by several stallions must be cleaned with soap and water, rinsed, sprayed with 2% chlorhexidine solution and allowed to dry before reuse
  ◦ Leather is a porous material and cannot completely be disinfected

HAND HYGIENE
• After completing one mating or semen collection, discard any disposable gloves in a proper receptacle
• Thoroughly wash hands with liquid soap and water; dry with disposable paper towels
• Antimicrobial hand soap is unnecessary and recommended only during disease outbreak situations
• Avoid bar soap, it can harbor pathogens
• Disposable gloves do not guarantee that glove tears do not occur, inadvertently contaminating hands
• Proper handwashing is critical for biosecurity

DISINFECTANT CHOICES
For stall surfaces, stocks, padded breeding chutes, and barn aisle ways:
• Commonly used horse barn disinfectants include peroxygenase compounds, phenolics, and quaternary ammonium compounds

• Bleach is quickly inactivated by any organic matter; use only on hard, nonporous materials that are thoroughly precleaned
• Ethyl or isopropyl alcohol (70%) are disinfectants used on cleaned phantoms, but are not routine stall disinfectants. Phantom disinfectants readily evaporate and leave no chemical residue that could irritate stallions
• Remove organic matter by thorough scrubbing with detergent and water to remove >90% of bacteria and inactivate lipid-enveloped viruses on barn surfaces
• Avoid power washing. Any disinfectant will be compromised by organic matter; cleaning cannot be overemphasized
• Some detergents (cationic, anionic, or nonionic) can inactivate certain disinfectants and must be considered in the choice of cleaning products and disinfectants
• No disinfectant is effective against all known equine pathogens and also safe. No product is currently available that cleans and disinfects in one step. Active ingredients and directions for use must be understood by all farm employees as misuse can cause significant injury. Never mix different disinfectants together
• Manufacturers of disinfectants approved by the United States Environmental Protection Agency provide label instructions that must be followed. Recommended personal protective equipment (glove type, eye protection, etc.), dilution and application instructions, and surface contact time should strictly be followed. Thorough knowledge of Material Safety Data Sheet information is also necessary

 MISCELLANEOUS

ASSOCIATED CONDITIONS
N/A

AGE-RELATED FACTORS
N/A

ZOONOTIC POTENTIAL
No known zoonotic potential for EHV, EAV, *T. equigenitalis*, or *Trypanosoma equiperdum*.

PREGNANCY/FERTILITY/BREEDING
N/A

SYNONYMS
N/A

SEE ALSO
• Contagious equine metritis (CEM)
• Dourine
• Equine herpesvirus myeloencephalopathy
• Viral arteritis (EVA)

ABBREVIATIONS
• CEM = contagious equine metritis
• EAV = equine arteritis virus
• EHV = equine herpesvirus
• EVA = equine viral arteritis

Internet Resources
The Center for Food Security and Public Health. http://www.cfsph.iastate.edu
Equine Disease Communication Center. http://www.equinediseasecc.org

Suggested Reading
Burgess BA, Traub-Dargatz JL. Biosecurity and control of infectious disease outbreaks. In: Sellon DC, Long MT, eds. Equine Infectious Diseases, 2e. St. Louis, MO: Elsevier, 2014:530–543.
Timoney PJ. Horse species symposium: contagious equine metritis: an insidious threat to the horse breeding industry in the United States. J Anim Sci 2011;89:1552–1560.

Author Roberta M. Dwyer
Consulting Editor Carla L. Carleton

BLOOD AND PLASMA TRANSFUSION REACTIONS

BASICS

DEFINITION
• Blood and/or blood components can be administered as biological therapeutic agents
• A TR is an adverse clinical consequence or reaction to the administration of blood or blood component
• Administration of nonideal BP may induce a TR due to the additional unnecessary components (usually plasma) of the BP

PATHOPHYSIOLOGY
• TRs can be immune-mediated or nonimmune mediated; may or may not involve hemolysis of recipient or donor RBCs; can occur immediately or be delayed hours to days after administration; and may involve the transmission of an infectious agent
• Different methods of processing whole blood into components achieve different levels of purity and can affect the incidence of TR
• Improper methods and techniques of collection, processing, storage, or administration of the BP can induce a TR

Immune-Mediated Reactions
• Sourced from other horses, BPs contain antigens that can be recognized by the recipient as foreign (alloantigens) and induce an immune-mediated reaction in the recipient
• Autologous alloantibodies to RBC surface antigens do not naturally occur in horses, thus hemolytic reactions are uncommon during first blood transfusions; alloantibodies to RBC antigens develop within 3–10 days of exposure (original transfusion) and therefore caution is indicated with subsequent transfusions
• Immune-mediated TRs can be induced by administered RBCs, WBCs, plasma proteins, or platelets interacting with the recipient's immune system
• Common immune-mediated reactions include hemolysis (acute or delayed), febrile nonhemolytic TR, allergic reactions ranging from mild urticaria to severe anaphylaxis, thrombocytopenia, transfusion-related acute lung injury, and post-transfusion purpura
• Anaphylaxis represents the most severe form of allergic transfusion reaction and can occur following administration of very small volumes of BP (a few mL)

Nonimmune-Mediated Reactions
• Common nonimmune-mediated reactions include circulatory volume overload; hypocalcemia, e.g. citrate toxicity; coagulopathy, e.g. excess anticoagulant administration; transmission of blood-borne infectious agents; hemosiderosis and hemoglobinemia; and hyperkalemia, e.g. administration of hemolyzed RBCs
• Blood-borne infectious agents transmissible by plasma include Theiler disease-associated virus (serum hepatitis) and equine infectious

anemia virus and in whole blood include *Babesia* spp. and *Anaplasma phagocytophilum*
• Hepatic failure is a complication in foals receiving blood transfusion(s) especially those receiving >4 L of blood; deferoxamine enhances urinary iron elimination and decreases hepatic iron accumulation, reducing the risk of hepatic failure in these foals

SYSTEMS AFFECTED
• Hemic/lymphatic/immune
• Other systems depending on TR

GENETICS
Differences in inherited blood types, WBC and platelet antigens, and protein polymorphism contribute to incidence.

INCIDENCE/PREVALENCE
• Plasma—horses <7 days of age 9.7%; horses >7 days of age and adults <2% (commercial, plasmapheresis) and 10% (inhouse, gravity sedimentation)
• Whole blood—adult horses 16%

GEOGRAPHIC DISTRIBUTION
N/A

SIGNALMENT
Foals <7 days at higher risk of plasma-induced TR.

SIGNS
General Comments
Variable signs dependent on cause.

Historical Findings
• Previous transfusion of blood or BP
• Transfusion of old, damaged, or hemolyzed blood or BP
• Improper aseptic technique for collection or administration of blood or BP
• Improper storage or handling of blood, BP, or transfusion supplies and equipment

Physical Examination Findings
Immune-Mediated Reactions
• Acute hemolysis and delayed immune-mediated hemolysis; fever, restlessness, tachycardia, tachypnea
• Febrile nonhemolytic TR—increase in body temperature >1°C during transfusion with or without malaise, signs of abdominal pain, tachycardia, and tachypnea
• Allergic reaction—piloerection, pruritus, urticaria, tachycardia, tachypnea, dyspnea, nasal and/or pulmonary edema, signs of abdominal pain, muscle fasciculations
• Anaphylaxis—signs of abdominal pain, diarrhea, tachycardia, tachypnea, dyspnea, nasal and/or pulmonary edema, hypotension, shock, cardiac dysrhythmias, loss of consciousness, cardiac arrest, death, fever often absent
Nonimmune-Mediated Reactions
• Contaminated transfusion—fever, tachycardia, tachypnea
• Circulatory volume expansion— hypertension, jugular vein distention, pulmonary edema, cardiac dysfunction, dyspnea, tachypnea

• Hypocalcemia—cardiac dysrhythmias, ileus, signs of abdominal pain, synchronous diaphragmatic flutter ("thumps"), tachycardia (bradycardia if severe hypocalcemia), tachypnea, muscle fasciculations, trismus

CAUSES
Immune-Mediated Reactions
• Hemolytic TRs involve either antibodies directed against recipient RBCs present in administered plasma or preexisting or acquired antibodies in the recipient's own plasma directed against transfused RBCs (inducing immediate or delayed TR respectively)
• Antibodies binding RBC surface alloantigens cause complement activation, RBC lysis, and cytokine release
• Febrile, nonhemolytic TRs are likely associated with leukocyte-derived cytokines and/or circulating antileukocyte antibodies in the recipient; most common TR
• Allergic/anaphylactic reaction is an IgE-mediated (type 1) hypersensitivity reaction due to interaction of a donor antigen with recipient IgE antibodies results in mast cell degranulation, histamine release, and complement activation
Nonimmune-Mediated Reactions
• Related to the physical volume of the administered BP into the vascular space if the recipient's circulating volume is not reduced, degradation of RBCs or WBCs in the BP, contamination of the BP at the time of collection (infectious agents), or the effect of the anticoagulant
• Pyrogens and proinflammatory substances can accumulate during storage or can be released by degradation of leukocytes during storage

RISK FACTORS
See Historical Findings.

DIAGNOSIS

DIFFERENTIAL DIAGNOSIS
• Hemolysis—exclude other causes including electrolyte concentration of administered IV and/or any additives to IV fluids
• Fever, respiratory distress, hypotension or shock—exclude other causes of systemic inflammation or anaphylaxis (concurrently administered medications)
• Signs of abdominal pain—exclude primary gastrointestinal lesion
• Urticaria—exclude adverse drug reaction to concurrently administered medication

CBC/BIOCHEMISTRY/URINALYSIS
• Hemoglobinemia, hemoglobinuria, hyperbilirubinemia, bilirubinuria, anemia that may be progressive/persistent anemia for 3–5 days post transfusion

BLOOD AND PLASMA TRANSFUSION REACTIONS (CONTINUED)

- Spherocytes identified on blood smear evaluation confirm immune-mediated hemolysis
- Evidence of secondary organ dysfunction

OTHER LABORATORY TESTS
Cross-match (major and minor) not 100% sensitive for the detection of an impending TR.

IMAGING
N/A

OTHER DIAGNOSTIC PROCEDURES
- Culture of transfused blood or blood culture from recipient with suspected sepsis
- Blood pressure and central venous pressure for circulatory volume overload

PATHOLOGIC FINDINGS
No pathognomonic findings.

TREATMENT

APPROPRIATE HEALTH CARE
- Initial management of mild reactions includes slowing rate of transfusion or temporarily discontinuing until TR is controlled
- Severe reaction or anaphylaxis should prompt immediate cessation of transfusion
- Acute hemolytic reactions may require blood transfusions from alternate, compatible donors if available or plasma transfusion from a different donor/batch of plasma
- Monitor heart and respiratory rate and determine blood pressure

NURSING CARE
- Manage hypotension with IV crystalloid fluid therapy
- Low-volume resuscitation with hypertonic solutions or colloids can be used for hypotensive shock

ACTIVITY
Minimizing exertion during a TR reduces the likelihood of collapse from hypotension.

DIET
N/A

CLIENT EDUCATION
N/A

SURGICAL CONSIDERATIONS
N/A

MEDICATIONS

DRUG(S) OF CHOICE
- Mild reactions—antihistamine, e.g. diphenhydramine (0.5–2.0 mg/kg IV or IM) or hydroxyzine (0.5–1.0 mg/kg IM); NSAID,

e.g. flunixin meglumine (0.25–1.1 mg/kg IV or PO; if administering PO increase dose by 30% to account for bioavailability)
- Moderate to severe reaction—corticosteroids, e.g. prednisolone sodium succinate (1 mg/kg IV) or dexamethasone (0.05–0.1 mg/kg IV)
- Anaphylaxis—corticosteroid together with epinephrine (0.01–0.02 mg/kg IV or IM (1:10 000 dilution = 0.1 mg/mL))
- Appropriate antimicrobial therapy in cases of sepsis
- If volume overload with pulmonary edema is suspected, diuretics (furosemide 1 mg/kg IV every 1–12 h or CRI of 0.12 mg/kg/h after loading dose of 0.12 mg/kg) and intranasal oxygen (15 L/min)
- Deferoxamine 14 mg/kg SC BID, 14 days if transfusion-induced iron overload

CONTRAINDICATIONS
N/A

PRECAUTIONS
Agitation and excitement reported following antihistamine administration.

POSSIBLE INTERACTIONS
N/A

ALTERNATIVE DRUGS
N/A

FOLLOW-UP

PATIENT MONITORING
Physical examination, including heart rate, respiratory rate, and rectal temperature, every 5 min for the first 15 min and then every 15 min during infusion.

PREVENTION/AVOIDANCE
- Pretransfusion testing with major and minor cross-match reduces, but does not eliminate, possibility of hemolytic TR
- Administer BP using an administration set with an inline filter through an aseptically inserted venous catheter with correct and aseptic handling of BP, transfusion supplies, and equipment
- Commence administration of biologic product slowly (0.1 mL/kg/h); if no reaction observed during the first 15 min increase rate of administration without exceeding 10–20 mL/kg/h
- Select healthy blood donors free from infectious agents and/or registered BPs
- Collect, store, and administer blood or BPs appropriately

POSSIBLE COMPLICATIONS
- Delayed hemolysis indicates alloantibodies have been induced and future hemolysis TR probable; cross-match indicated

- Secondary organ failure can result from impaired oxygen delivery and/or toxic effects of hemolytic products (e.g. pigment nephropathy, renal failure, disseminated intravascular coagulopathy)
- Volume overload can lead to cardiac failure

EXPECTED COURSE AND PROGNOSIS
- Most TRs follow an acute course
- Prognosis is good if mild or moderate, but guarded if marked, anaphylactic reaction occurs, the animal is severely ill, or TR not recognized

MISCELLANEOUS

ASSOCIATED CONDITIONS
N/A

AGE-RELATED FACTORS
See Signalment.

ZOONOTIC POTENTIAL
None

PREGNANCY/FERTILITY/BREEDING
An acute, severe, TR with resultant hypotension and tissue ischemia in a pregnant mare may result in death/abortion of a fetus.

SYNONYMS
None

SEE ALSO
- Anaphylaxis
- Anemia, immune mediated
- Hemorrhage, acute
- Hemorrhage, chronic
- Neonatal isoerythrolysis
- Thrombocytopenia

ABBREVIATIONS
- BP = blood product
- CRI = constant rate infusion
- IgE = immunoglobulin E
- NSAID = nonsteroidal anti-inflammatory drug
- RBC = red blood cell
- TR = transfusion reaction
- WBC = white blood cell

Suggested Reading
Hart KA. Pathogenesis, management and prevention of blood transfusion reactions in horses. Equine Vet Educ 2011;23:343–345.
Author Jamie G. Wearn
Consulting Editors David Hodgson, Harold C. McKenzie, and Jennifer L. Hodgson.
Acknowledgment The author and editors acknowledge the prior contribution of Jane Wardrop and Jennifer L. Hodgson.

BASICS

DEFINITION
- A diagnostic procedure used to identify pathogenic organisms in the bloodstream
- A positive blood culture is one in which organisms are recovered from the sample. Organisms must be interpreted as pathogens or contaminants based on their identification and the patient's clinical signs
- A negative blood culture does not rule out microbial infection
- Bacterial aerobic and/or anaerobic culture, and/or fungal culture may be requested. Bacterial aerobic culture is often the most rewarding
- Prior to collecting the blood sample, skin must be surgically prepared to avoid contamination of the sample by normal skin flora. Samples are collected prior to administration of antibiotics, or after a 24 h antibiotic discontinuation, to optimize the recovery of organisms
- It is recommended that multiple, usually three, samples be collected either from different sites or from the same site with at least 20 min between each sample
- Samples should not be collected via indwelling catheters
- Samples must be immediately transferred into blood culture-appropriate containers (e.g. Isolator™ tubes, blood culture bottles), with the total volume to be collected depending on the container used
- The testing laboratory should be contacted for specific instructions prior to sample collection

PATHOPHYSIOLOGY
A positive culture occurs when microorganisms are present in the systemic circulation due to a generalized infection or during a transient bacterial shower, such as following a dental procedure or occasionally in healthy neonatal foals. A positive culture due to contamination by normal skin flora may also occur if the skin is not properly prepared prior to sample collection.

SYSTEMS AFFECTED
- Hemolymphatic—assuming that contamination from skin has not occurred, microorganisms must be present in circulation for a blood culture to be positive
- Adults—commonly associated with GI disease including ischemic necrosis, colitis, and proximal enteritis. May also be secondary to respiratory (pleuropneumonia), muscular (clostridial myositis), or reproductive (metritis) infections. Septicemia (SIRS caused by blood infection) can lead to multiorgan dysfunction and failure
- Foals—often no primary site of infection is detectable. Can be secondary to bacterial translocation from the GI tract or umbilicus

GENETICS
Genetic factors may increase susceptibility to infectious disease, e.g. DNA-dependent protein kinase deficiency causing SCID in Arabian horses.

INCIDENCE/PREVALENCE
- Positive blood culture in adult horses is uncommon
- False-negative blood culture results can occur despite current bacteremia due to the dilutional effect of the blood volume

GEOGRAPHIC DISTRIBUTION
N/A

SIGNALMENT
- Any breed, age, or sex
- Positive cultures are most common in neonatal foals with septicemia

SIGNS

Historical Findings
- Recent dental float in a horse with PPID
- Neonatal foal that failed to nurse within 8–12 h or did not receive adequate colostrum from the dam

Physical Examination Findings
- Signs may be referable to a primary site of infection
- Absence of pyrexia does not rule out septicemia
- Adults—signs may include fever, anorexia, depression, tachycardia, tachypnea, and mucous membrane hyperemia. Dehydration and hypovolemic shock may be present
- Foals—signs may include recumbency, poor suckle reflex, weakness, diarrhea, colic, and increased or decreased heart rate, respiratory rate, and temperature

CAUSES
With the exception of transient bacteremia, the blood is normally a sterile site, so any organisms present in the blood raise concern.

Adults
Bacteremia involving *Streptococcus* spp., *Actinobacillus* spp., and *Pseudomonas aeruginosa*, among others, has been reported.

Neonatal Septicemia
- Gram-negative bacteria (most common)—*Escherichia coli, Actinobacillus* spp., *Klebsiella* spp., *Salmonella* spp., *Enterobacter* spp.
- Gram-positive bacteria—*Enterococcus* spp., *Streptococcus* spp., *Staphylococcus* spp., and the anaerobic *Clostridium* spp.
- Fungi—*Candida* spp.

RISK FACTORS

Adults
- Venous catheterization (thrombophlebitis)
- Immunosuppression (PPID, prolonged illness, stress, exogenous corticosteroids)
- Local infection or abscess, such as pulmonary infection, penetrating wound, castration or other surgical site infection, septic arthritis, or synovitis

Neonates
- Maternal illness or placentitis
- FPT
- Heavy exposure to environmental pathogens
- Omphalophlebitis
- SCID

DIAGNOSIS

DIFFERENTIAL DIAGNOSIS
- Signs of SIRS without bacteremia (e.g. trauma, burns, acidosis) may mimic signs of septicemia
- Sample contamination due to poor collection technique

CBC/BIOCHEMISTRY/URINALYSIS
Abnormalities vary depending on organ system involved, but may include the following:

CBC
- Leukopenia or leukocytosis, degenerative left shift, toxic changes to neutrophils, elevated plasma fibrinogen concentration
- Elevated packed cell volume and total protein with dehydration and hypovolemic shock

Biochemistry
- Hyperproteinemia in adults due to dehydration
- Hypoproteinemia may reflect FPT in foals
- Hypoalbuminemia if septicemia caused by colitis, pleuropneumonia, or metritis
- Hyperglobulinemia if chronic antigenic stimulation
- Hypoglycemia is common in foals with septicemia

OTHER LABORATORY TESTS
- Abnormalities that may be present in abdominal, pleural, synovial, or cerebrospinal fluid if these are sites of primary infection—increased protein, increased total nucleated cell count with degenerative changes in cell morphology and intracellular bacteria
- Blood lactate concentration may be elevated
- Low serum immunoglobulin concentrations in neonates might indicate septicemia secondary to FPT
- Arterial blood gas analysis may reveal metabolic acidosis and hypoxemia
- Abnormalities in the clotting profile—increased prothrombin time, activated partial thromboplastin time, fibrin degradation products or D-dimer test; thrombocytopenia may occur in association with DIC in severely affected patients

IMAGING
Dependent on the underlying cause.

OTHER DIAGNOSTIC PROCEDURES
- If a focus of infection is identified, culture and/or biopsy of a sample collected from that area is indicated

BLOOD CULTURE (CONTINUED)

B

• Endoscopy, thoracoscopy, laparoscopy may be indicated

PATHOLOGIC FINDINGS
Dependent on the underlying cause.

TREATMENT

APPROPRIATE HEALTH CARE
Hospitalization with inpatient medical management.

NURSING CARE
N/A

ACTIVITY
N/A

DIET
Anorexia occurs in many patients with septicemia. Therefore, monitor nutritional intake and supplement with nasogastric feeding or total or partial parenteral nutrition where appropriate.

CLIENT EDUCATION
• Endocarditis or primary internal abscessation may be difficult to treat successfully. Treatment may be prolonged and costly
• Neonates with septicemia carry a poor prognosis without intensive care

SURGICAL CONSIDERATIONS
• Surgical drainage or resection of an infected focus should be performed when possible
• Surgical lavage and debridement of infected synovial structures or osteomyelitic lesions
• Consider surgical excision with acquired patent urachus or omphalophlebitis if not responding to medical therapy

MEDICATIONS

DRUG(S) OF CHOICE
• Fluid therapy
• Appropriate antimicrobial therapy (broad spectrum initially, then according to antimicrobial susceptibility testing results)
• Parenteral antimicrobials should be continued for 24–48 h beyond the resolution of clinical signs and normalization of clinicopathologic abnormalities
• Combination therapy with a beta-lactam and an aminoglycoside is a common approach. Third-generation cephalosporins present an alternative
• Peak and trough concentration therapeutic drug monitoring is recommended for aminoglycoside therapy
• NSAID therapy is useful in addressing SIRS and pain

CONTRAINDICATIONS
Fluoroquinolones and tetracyclines in foals.

PRECAUTIONS
• Ensure pathogen is sensitive to selected antimicrobial and that the antimicrobial has suitable penetration and action in vivo
• Reevaluate antimicrobials if inadequate response to therapy
• Use caution with NSAIDs in dehydrated patients or those with SIRS-associated hypotension to decrease risk of nephrotoxicity
• Antibiotic administration can cause colitis in adult horses

POSSIBLE INTERACTIONS
N/A

ALTERNATIVE DRUGS
Probiotics may be useful in decreasing the risk of antibiotic-associated diarrhea, but evidence is primarily anecdotal to date.

FOLLOW-UP

PATIENT MONITORING
• Appropriate monitoring within intensive care facility is required
• Follow-up ultrasonography, radiography, or echocardiography allows assessment of changes at primary and secondary sites of infection
• Repeat sampling and culture of primary sites of infection where appropriate

PREVENTION/AVOIDANCE
Adults
Proper management of infectious diseases may reduce the chance of septicemia developing.

Foals
• Measure serum or plasma immunoglobulin concentration in neonates at 12–24 h of age to detect FPT
• Observe foaling in a clean environment and ensure successful nursing

POSSIBLE COMPLICATIONS
• Laminitis
• Multiorgan dysfunction syndrome
• DIC
• Valvular endocarditis
• Meningitis

EXPECTED COURSE AND PROGNOSIS
• Outcomes of adult sepsis depend on the primary infection and severity
• Survival rate of septic neonatal foals is approximately 65–70% with intensive care. Secondary joint infection decreases the odds of successful performance as adults

MISCELLANEOUS

ASSOCIATED CONDITIONS
See Possible Complications.

AGE-RELATED FACTORS
• Young horses (6 months to 3 years) are generally more susceptible to novel viral infections that can predispose to colitis and pleuropneumonia
• PPID in older horses (>15 years) can cause immunosuppression
• Risk of FPT in neonates

ZOONOTIC POTENTIAL
Dependent on the underlying cause.

PREGNANCY/FERTILITY/BREEDING
• Ascending placentitis may result in abortion or neonatal septicemia
• Bacterial metritis can cause infertility

SYNONYMS
N/A

SEE ALSO
• Bacteremia/sepsis
• Endocarditis, infective
• Endotoxemia
• Failure of transfer of passive immunity (FTPI)
• Fever
• High-risk pregnancy
• Immunosuppression
• Omphalophlebitis
• Septicemia, neonate
• Thrombophlebitis

ABBREVIATIONS
• DIC = disseminated intravascular coagulopathy
• FTPI = failure of transfer of passive immunity
• GI = gastrointestinal
• NSAID = nonsteroidal anti-inflammatory drug
• PPID = pituitary pars intermedia dysfunction
• SCID = severe combined immunodeficiency
• SIRS = systemic inflammatory response syndrome

Suggested Reading
Kirn TJ, Weinstein MP. Update on blood cultures: how to obtain, process, report, and interpret. Clin Microbiol Infect 2013;19:513–520.
Roy MF. Sepsis in adults and foals. Vet Clin Equine 2004;20:41–61.
Taylor S. A review of equine sepsis. Equine Vet Educ 2015;27:99–109.
Theelen MJP, Wilson WD, Edman JM, et al. Temporal trends in prevalence of bacteria isolated from foals with sepsis: 1979-2010. Equine Vet J 2013;46:169–173.

Author G. Kenitra Hendrix
Consulting Editor Sandra D. Taylor
Acknowledgment The author and editor acknowledge the prior contributions of Jill E. Parker and Laura C. Fennell.

B

BASICS

OVERVIEW
• Cyanobacterial proliferations may occur in fresh and salt water
• BGA toxin can lead to an acute intoxication affecting the liver and the central nervous system
• Microcystins are hepatotoxic BGA toxins
• Microcystins have also been detected in dietary supplements used in animals
• Anatoxins, including anatoxin-a and anatoxin-a$_s$, are neurotoxic BGA toxins
• Cyanotoxin poisoning has occurred in animals and humans, with a presumptive iatrogenic case reported in a horse

SIGNALMENT
N/A

SIGNS
Microcystin
• Acute hepatotoxicosis—anorexia, depression, diarrhea, colic, weakness, pale mucous membranes and shock
• Progression of disease is rapid and death generally occurs within several hours of exposure
• Animals that survive the acute intoxication may develop hepatogenous photosensitization

Anatoxin-a
• Rapid onset of rigidity and muscle tremors, followed by paralysis, cyanosis, and death as a result of potent nicotinic cholinergic stimulation
• Progression is very rapid and death usually occurs within minutes to a few hours of exposure

Anatoxin-a$_s$
• Rapid onset of excessive salivation, lacrimation, diarrhea, and urination is associated with muscarinic overstimulation
• Clinical signs of nicotinic overstimulation include tremors, incoordination, and convulsions
• Respiratory arrest and recumbency may be seen prior to death
• Progression is very rapid and animals may die within 30 min of exposure

CAUSES AND RISK FACTORS
• BGA blooms are increased with high water temperature and elevated nutrient concentrations. Steady winds that propel toxic blooms to shore allow for ingestion by drinking animals
• Dietary supplements containing the BGA *Spirulina platensis* and *Aphanizomenon flos aquae* can be contaminated with microcystins

DIAGNOSIS

DIFFERENTIAL DIAGNOSIS
• Microcystin toxicosis—other causes of acute liver failure
• Anatoxin-a—cyanide, yew, oleander, poison hemlock, insecticides, ionophore antibiotics, intestinal compromise (e.g. torsion)
• Anatoxin-a$_s$—organophosphorus and carbamate insecticides, slaframine

CBC/BIOCHEMISTRY/URINALYSIS
• Microcystins—increases in serum aspartate aminotransferase, sorbitol dehydrogenase, and bile acids, direct and total bilirubin, ammonia, hyperkalemia, hypoglycemia, bilirubinuria
• Anatoxin-a and anatoxin-a$_s$—no significant findings

OTHER LABORATORY TESTS
Anatoxin-a$_s$—depressed blood cholinesterase activity.

DIAGNOSTIC PROCEDURES
• Identification of the algae in the suspect water source or stomach contents. However, morphological identification alone cannot predict the hazard level
• Detection of microcystins in gastric contents is confirmatory
• Mouse bioassay (IP injection of algal bloom extract) was used in the past to determine the toxicity of algal blooms

PATHOLOGIC FINDINGS
Detection of algal bloom material in GI tract and/or on legs or muzzle.

Microcystin
• Liver enlargement and soft, friable appearance; histologic lesions include progressive centrilobular hepatocyte necrosis and intrahepatic hemorrhage
• Alzheimer type II cells present with hepatoencephalopathy

Anatoxin-a and Anatoxin-a$_s$
No lesions are found.

TREATMENT

• Often unsuccessful because of the rapid onset of clinical signs and death
• GI decontamination with activated charcoal can be attempted but efficacy is questionable
• Microcystin toxicosis—provide supportive therapy to treat hypovolemia, electrolyte imbalances, hyperammonemia; protect from sun exposure if hepatogenous photosensitization is present
• Anatoxin-a toxicosis—general supportive care and specific measures to control seizures
• Anatoxin-a$_s$ toxicosis—atropine should be given at a test dose to determine its efficacy in

animals with life-threatening clinical signs. Can then be given repeatedly until cessation of salivation

MEDICATIONS

DRUG(S) OF CHOICE
• AC (1–4 g/kg in water slurry (1 g of AC in 5 mL of water) PO)
• Diazepam (adults 25–50 mg IV, repeat in 30 min if necessary; foal 0.05–0.4 mg/kg IV, repeat in 30 min if necessary) for seizure control
• Lactulose (0.5 mL/kg via nasogastric tube every 6 h)
• Atropine (given to effect, IV) in anatoxin-a$_s$ intoxication

CONTRAINDICATIONS/POSSIBLE INTERACTIONS
Atropine administration can lead to severe colic signs.

FOLLOW-UP

PATIENT MONITORING
Microcystin toxicosis—monitor liver function, coagulation status, and risk of photosensitization.

PREVENTION/AVOIDANCE
• Denied access to water with visible algal blooms
• Reduce fertilizer application and run-off in fields surrounding ponds used for drinking water
• Use algicides for chemical control of algal blooms

EXPECTED COURSE AND PROGNOSIS
• Animals poisoned with BGA toxins are often found dead
• Animals that survive acute microcystin poisoning may suffer from photosensitization

MISCELLANEOUS

ABBREVIATIONS
• AC = activated charcoal
• BGA = blue-green algae
• GI = gastrointestinal

Suggested Reading
Puschner B, Roegner AF. Cyanobacterial (blue-green algae) toxins. In: Gupta RC, ed. Veterinary Toxicology: Basic and Clinical Principles, 2e. San Diego, CA: Elsevier, 2012:953–965.

Author Birgit Puschner
Consulting Editors Wilson K. Rumbeiha and Steve Ensley

BORDETELLA BRONCHISEPTICA

B

BASICS

OVERVIEW
- Respiratory pathogen in dogs, rabbits, rodents, cats, and guinea pigs
- Role as an opportunistic pathogen is debated
- Isolated from nasal swabs in some normal horses, tracheal cultures of horses with pneumonia, and a guttural pouch
- Has been associated with abortion and infertility in mares

SIGNS

Respiratory
- Lethargy, nasal discharge, cough, lymphadenopathy, pyrexia, and weight loss
- Thoracic auscultation may reveal intermittent crackles and wheezes

Reproductive
Abortion, increased uterine fluid, increased uterine wall thickness, hyperemic vaginal wall.

CAUSES AND RISK FACTORS
- Small, Gram-negative aerobic rod that requires minimal nutrition
- Grows slowly. Poor competitor in host environments. Proliferates when other microorganisms have been eliminated (i.e., prior antibiotic administration). Prior antibiotic administration
- The pathogenicity is mediated by specific adhesins and toxins. Fimbriae and filamentous hemagglutinin allow for mucociliary adherence as well as suppression of inflammation and prolonged colonization. Damage of the respiratory epithelium leads to increased mucus secretion and reduced mucociliary clearance. The extent of epithelial damage by toxins may prolong therapy needed for resolution
- Factors that disrupt host airway defense mechanisms, such as travel, recent viral infections, anesthesia, and inadequate ventilation

DIAGNOSIS

DIFFERENTIAL DIAGNOSIS
- Other infectious causes of lower or upper airway disease
- Nasopharyngeal swabs can be submitted for PCR to look for viral causes of respiratory disease, such as equine influenza virus and equine herpesvirus 1 and 4
- Noninfectious causes of lower airway disease
- Laryngeal and guttural pouch diseases
- Other infectious causes of infertility and abortion

CBC/BIOCHEMISTRY/URINALYSIS
Respiratory infection may be associated with leukocytosis, elevated fibrinogen, and increased SAA.

OTHER LABORATORY TESTS
- Tracheobronchial aspirate cytology—neutrophilic inflammation, intracellular and extracellular bacteria. Gram stain—pink rods
- Real-time PCR assay available, aerobic culture is most commonly used for definitive diagnosis and susceptibility pattern evaluation
- Uterine swab for culture and cytology

IMAGING
- Thoracic US and radiography
- Transrectal uterine US—the combined uterine placental thickness, placental attachment during pregnancy

OTHER DIAGNOSTIC PROCEDURES

Endoscopy
Evaluate upper respiratory tract and tracheal mucosa.

Uterine biopsy
Evaluation of the endometrium and prognosticate the ability of a mare to carry a foal to term.

TREATMENT
Will depend on the severity of lung and pleural involvement; rest for several weeks following resolution of the clinical signs.

MEDICATIONS
- Antimicrobial therapy should be based on susceptibility results due to variation in *B. bronchiseptica* susceptibility patterns
- Decreased susceptibility has been reported for some beta-lactam antibiotics (penicillins and cephalosporins), due to production of beta-lactamases or low membrane permeability to cephalosporins
- Most reported isolates are sensitive to gentamicin (6.6 mg/kg IV every 24 h), oxytetracycline (6.6 mg/kg IV every 12 h), and trimethoprim–sulfamethoxazole (30 mg/kg PO every 12 h). Isolates with increased minimum inhibitory concentration values of trimethoprim-sulfamethoxazole and tetracycline have been reported. Therapy should continue until clinical signs resolve and should provide coverage for any other pathogenic bacteria isolated
- Therapy for endometritis with antibiotics should be based on susceptibility

FOLLOW-UP

PATIENT MONITORING
- Thoracic auscultation, rectal temperature, white blood cell count, plasma fibrinogen, SAA, thoracic radiographic, and US findings
- Repeat tracheobronchial aspirates are used to ensure resolution of neutrophilic inflammation on cytology

POSSIBLE COMPLICATIONS
Chronic pneumonia, lung abscessation, pleuritis, pleuropneumonia.

EXPECTED COURSE AND PROGNOSIS
- Resolution within 2 weeks with effective antimicrobial therapy
- Relapses and recurrent infections have been reported and may require additional therapy
- Coinfections—treatment should be extended, complications more likely
- *B. bronchiseptica* isolated from the endometrium resolved after 5 days of antibiotics

MISCELLANEOUS

SEE ALSO
- Aspiration pneumonia
- Cough, acute/chronic
- Expiratory dyspnea
- Fungal pneumonia
- Pleuropneumonia
- Pneumonia, neonate

ABBREVIATIONS
- PCR = polymerase chain reaction
- SAA = serum amyloid A
- US = ultrasonography, ultrasound

Suggested reading
Garcia-Cantu MC, Hartmann FA, Brown CM, Darien BJ. *Bordetella bronchiseptica* and equine respiratory infections: a review of 30 cases. Equine Vet Educ 2000;12:45–50.
Prüller S, Rensch U, Meemken D, et al. Antimicrobial susceptibility of *Bordetella bronchiseptica* isolates from swine and companion animals and detection of resistance genes. PLoS One 2015;10(8):e0135703.

Authors Benjamin J. Darien and Sarah M. Raabis
Consulting Editor Ashley G. Boyle
Acknowledgment The authors and editor acknowledge the prior contribution of Jane E. Axon.

BASICS

DEFINITION
Gradually progressive, symmetric muscular weakness in horses characterized by flaccid paralysis and dysphagia.

PATHOPHYSIOLOGY
• Systemic absorption of the *Clostridium botulinum* neurotoxin inhibits acetylcholine release at the neuromuscular junction, leading to flaccid paralysis
• After toxin absorption from the digestive tract or infected wounds, botulinum toxin circulates in the bloodstream and, subsequently, is bound by specific endopeptidase receptors on motor end plates. Once attached to the receptor, the toxin is translocated within the cell and bound to acetylcholine vesicles, preventing electrical signals from reaching the myoneural junctions
• With relatively small doses of toxin, clinical signs may not become apparent for ≥10 days after ingestion. However, horses may become recumbent and die within 8 h with massive doses
• Botulism spores are relatively ubiquitous in the environment. Ingestion rarely leads to clinical botulism, however, because the spores do not elaborate toxin unless present in an anaerobic environment with a high pH and appropriate nutrients
• Botulism spores are pH sensitive and do not form toxin at pH < 4.5
• Three forms of the disease are recognized in horses. The most common in adult horses is ingestion of the preformed toxin. Young foals develop toxicoinfectious botulism through ingestion of spores and subsequent sporulation with toxin formation in the gut. Toxin elaboration can also occur in wounds such as castration sites and deep penetrating wounds, including deep IM injections (wound botulism)

SYSTEMS AFFECTED
Neuromuscular
• Progressive muscular weakness over several hours to days frequently manifests as trembling of the larger muscle groups, especially triceps and gluteals
• As clinical signs progress, affected horses lie down more frequently than normal and may become unable to stand. They may struggle to stand, get up and stand for several minutes, then lie down, at first in sternal recumbency, then later lateral recumbency
• Slow chewing and dysphagia may be seen in adult horses. Drooling and feed at the nostrils may also be noted due to difficulty swallowing
• Affected foals attempt to suckle the mare, but milk drools from the foal's mouth

GI
Colic may be the primary sign prior to showing weakness. Intestinal ileus is common.

Respiratory
Respiratory distress during the terminal phases of botulism. Secondary aspiration pneumonia possible.

Ophthalmic
Moderate mydriasis with intact pupillary light reflex.

Renal/Urologic
• Horses that remain standing can void the bladder, which helps to differentiate botulism from herpesvirus infections
• Down horses will retain urine in the bladder, requiring periodic catheterization

Cardiovascular
Tachycardia and cardiac arrhythmia may be present independently of stress or dehydration.

INCIDENCE/PREVALENCE
Type B
• More than 85% of equine botulism cases in the USA
• Most frequently occurs in the mid-Atlantic region in North America
• May occurs as an individual or multiple cases
• Several cases occurring over a few days suggests a point source of toxin such as silage (haylage) or spoiled hay from large hay bales

Type A
Typically occurs in the western USA, especially in Idaho, Utah, and California.

Type C
• May occur when a decomposing carcass contaminates feed materials
• More common in Arizona and New Mexico

SIGNALMENT
Mean Age and Range
• Foals—peak occurrence between 6 days and 6 weeks of age
• Adults—any age

SIGNS
Historical Findings
• Generalized muscle weakness or dysphagia typically is the first clinical sign detected
• Astute owners also may detect mild depression, decreased exercise tolerance, and reluctance to eat hay or grain

Physical Examination Findings
• Generalized muscle weakness, with early signs being toe-dragging, decreased tail tone, eyelid tone, and tongue tone
• A "grain test" can be used to assess for early dysphagia. Most normal horses should be able to consume 225 mL (8 oz) of grain within 2 min
• As the disease progresses, dysphagia becomes more obvious, and muscular weakness may progress to the point of recumbency and respiratory paralysis
• Vital signs are normal during the early stages of disease. Once the horse is recumbent, however, both the heart and respiratory rate

increase in proportion to the intensity of the struggle to rise
• Borborygmus sounds are typically reduced

CAUSES
• The source of toxin in most cases of individual equine botulism is rarely determined but most likely is ingestion of a small amount of preformed toxin in roughage (typically hay). It is often impossible to subsequently identify toxin in roughage samples, because the offending material has been consumed
• In herd outbreaks, the point source is most often hay in plastic bags or round bales
• Rarely has commercial grain been associated with equine botulism
• Roughage contaminated with a carcass typically results in type C botulism
• Wound botulism may develop secondary to infected castration sites, clamped umbilical hernias, and deep IM injections with counterirritants—iodine preparations

RISK FACTORS
• Feed sources—silage or fermented forages
• Foals from unvaccinated mares in endemic areas are at risk of toxicoinfectious botulism

DIAGNOSIS

DIFFERENTIAL DIAGNOSIS
• Equine herpes myeloencephalopathy, atypical myopathy, hyperkalemic periodic paralysis, equine motor neuron disease, West Nile virus
• Toxins—ionophores, organophosphates
• Equine protozoal myelitis and guttural pouch mycosis (dysphagia)
• Neonatal foals—generalized weakness due to sepsis or white muscle disease

CBC/BIOCHEMISTRY/URINALYSIS
Until affected horses are recumbent, CBC and biochemistry profiles are within normal limits.

OTHER LABORATORY TESTS
• An arterial blood gas is needed to diagnose hypercapnia and hypoxemia, and can help determine the need for mechanical ventilation in foals
• Electromyography is not often used but should show abundant small amplitude action potentials in the face of flaccid paralysis

DIAGNOSTIC PROCEDURES
• Identification of toxin or spores in feed materials or GI contents via mouse bioassay has been considered the gold standard for testing, but these tests may take as long as 2–4 weeks to complete. In addition horses appear to be more sensitive to the toxin than mice, and levels detrimental to horses may not harm mice
• PCR for detection of botulism neurotoxin in feces, GI content, or feed has been shown to be sensitive and specific, and provides more

BOTULISM (CONTINUED)

rapid and cost-effective testing than the mouse bioassay
• Diagnosis is most often based on clinical signs and ruling out other causes of dysphagia or weakness. Treatment with antitoxin should not be delayed in suspected cases of botulism

PATHOLOGIC FINDINGS
Lack of gross and histologic lesions typifies horses with botulism.

TREATMENT
APPROPRIATE HEALTH CARE
Confine affected horses to a box stall with no additional physical activity. Inpatient hospitalization is recommended.

NURSING CARE
• Provide soups made with pelleted complete feed in a low ridge bucket placed on the ground if horses are not recumbent
• Enteral fluid therapy may be required in horses with complete dysphagia
• Enteral nutrition can be provided via nasogastric feeding tube. Powdered or blenderized pelleted complete feeds can be used
• Neonates should be fed mare's milk every 2 h
• For horses that are unable to sit sternal, IV fluids and parenteral nutrition may be used to reduce the risk of aspiration
• Recumbent horses require an immense amount of nursing care to minimize decubital sores and other complications
• Recumbent horses, especially males, may need to have their bladder catheterized periodically
• Mechanical ventilation should be used in foals with signs of respiratory fatigue or failure

ACTIVITY
• Restriction of any muscular activity of affected horses is critical
• Assistance manually or with a sling to rise from recumbency or turn to opposite recumbency 4 times/day. Maintain recumbent horses in sternal position if possible
• Slings should be used with caution as the stress of slinging may hasten death
• Horses that struggle excessively when down or remain down for more than 24 h have very poor prognosis for survival

CLIENT EDUCATION
• Once botulism has occurred on a farm, annual vaccination of all horses on the farm is strongly recommended every year
• Vaccination of horses prior to feeding with silage (haylage) is advised in high-risk regions.

• After the occurrence of botulism in one horse, owners should be very diligent for signs in other horses

MEDICATIONS
DRUG(S) OF CHOICE
• Multivalent botulinum antitoxin administered soon after the onset of clinical signs is *critical.* Monovalent (type B) antitoxin is also commercially available and is appropriate for treating horses in the eastern USA and Canada
• Antitoxin will not reverse clinical signs at it will not neutralize unbound toxin. Antitoxin should stop progression of the disease and allow patients to improve by growing more motor end plates at the myoneural junctions
• Crystalline penicillin or metronidazole may be used in cases of wound botulism. Broad-spectrum antimicrobials are indicated for treatment of aspiration pneumonia when present
• Laxatives such as mineral oil may be needed to treat horses with GI ileus

CONTRAINDICATIONS
• *Aminoglycosides, procaine penicillin, and tetracycline are contraindicated due to their interference at the neuromuscular junction.*
• Penicillins and metronidazole, although useful for treatment of the botulism organisms, may also contribute to a reduction in normal GI flora and subsequent overgrowth of *C. botulinum*

FOLLOW-UP
PATIENT MONITORING
• Monitor hydration status and ventilation. Respiratory fatigue and aspiration pneumonia can rapidly lead to respiratory distress
• Mild improvement in strength and swallowing function may be seen as early as 1 week, but full recovery is not expected for at least 1 month

PREVENTION/AVOIDANCE
• 3 doses of monovalent type B botulinum toxoid ≅4 weeks apart are recommended to provide the most complete protection
• Annual revaccination with a single dose of toxoid is adequate to maintain effective protection
• Adequately vaccinated mares provide passive protection to newborn foals for several weeks if colostrum ingestion is adequate. Mares should be vaccinated 4–6 weeks before foaling
• Foals of unvaccinated mares can be vaccinated within the first 2–3 weeks of life

POSSIBLE COMPLICATIONS
• Aspiration pneumonia secondary to dysphagia is a concern, but many horses recover without intensive antibiotic therapy
• Ventilatory failure will lead to death in adults, and requires mechanical ventilation in foals
• Massive decubital sores may result from recumbency in adults with botulism

EXPECTED COURSE AND PROGNOSIS
• The more rapid the onset of clinical signs, the poorer is the prognosis for survival
• Overall survival rate in adults is approximately 50%, with poor chance of survival in horses that lost the ability to stand
• Once given the antitoxin, horses remain stable for 2–4 days and then gradually improve during the next 5–10 days as they regain their ability to swallow both water and roughage. Muscle strength gradually returns during the next 30 days. Weak tongues may persist for several weeks, but affected horses seem to eat and swallow normally
• Foals are reported to have a better prognosis (>96% for treated foals), although 30% required mechanical ventilation

MISCELLANEOUS
SYNONYMS
• Forage poisoning in adults
• Shaker foal syndrome

ABBREVIATIONS
• GI = gastrointestinal
• PCR = polymerase chain reaction

Suggested Reading
Johnson AL, McAdama-Gallagher SC, Aceto H. Outcome of adult horses with botulism treated at a veterinary hospital: 92 cases (1989-2013). J Vet Intern Med 2015;29:311–319.
Johnson AL, McAdama-Gallagher SC, Aceto H. Accuracy of a mouse bioassay for the diagnosis of botulism in horses. J Vet Intern Med 2016;30:1293–1299.
Stratford CH, Mayhew IG, Hudson NPH. Equine botulism: a clinical approach to diagnosis and management. Equine Vet Educ 2014;26:441–448.
Wilkins PA, Palmer JE. Botulism in foals less than 6 months of age: 30 cases (1989–2002). J Vet Intern Med 2003;17:702–707.

Author Margaret C. Mudge
Consulting Editor Caroline N. Hahn

BASICS

OVERVIEW
• Any cardiac arrhythmia associated with a slow heart rate
• Physiologic—first- and second-degree AVB, sinus arrhythmia, and sinus blocks and pauses
• Pathologic—atrial standstill and advanced second- and third-degree AVB

SIGNALMENT
N/A

SIGNS
• A slow regularly irregular rhythm
• Physiologic—no clinical signs, easily abolished by exercise or excitement
• With second- and third-degree AVB, audible fourth (atrial) heart sounds heard during the pauses
• Pathologic—weakness and syncope

CAUSES AND RISK FACTORS
• Physiologic—a common normal mechanism to modify heart rate and blood pressure
• Pathologic—uncommon but can occur with potassium disturbances and myocardial pathology
• Profound hyperkalemia is associated with sinus bradycardia, atrial standstill, and third-degree AVB and can be seen with renal failure and in foals with uroperitoneum
• Advanced second-degree AVB can also occur with α_2-adrenergic sedative drugs and with halothane
• Pathologic bradyarrhythmias occur as a terminal event

DIAGNOSIS

DIFFERENTIAL DIAGNOSIS
• Sinus bradycardia
• AVB
• AF with a slow heart rate

CBC/BIOCHEMISTRY/URINALYSIS
• Hyperkalemia may be present.
• Cardiac troponin I or T may be increased with myocardial pathology

IMAGING
• ECG to characterize the bradyarrhythmia and to identify AF
• With AVB, there is prolongation of the PR interval (first degree), intermittent P waves without a following QRS complex (second degree), or complete dissociation of the P and QRS complexes (third degree)
• With atrial standstill, P waves are absent
• With sinus bradycardias, every P is followed by a QRS complex, but there is intermittent waxing and waning of the P–P interval and

the R–R interval; with sinus pauses, there is a prolonged P–P interval; and with sinus blocks, the P–P interval is intermittently prolonged to more than two normal cardiac cycles
• Echocardiography to identify underlying heart disease with pathologic bradyarrhythmias

TREATMENT

• Physiologic—no treatment. An exercising ECG documents the disappearance of the arrhythmia
• Pathologic—identify predisposing causes (drugs or hyperkalemia) and remove them if possible
• With uroperitoneum, abdominal drainage is indicated, but the foal's electrolyte status must be stabilized before general anesthesia and surgery
• With pathologic bradyarrhythmias secondary to myocardial pathology, anti-inflammatory medications may be appropriate
• Some cases of third-degree AVB have successfully been treated by placement of transvenous pacemakers

MEDICATIONS

DRUG(S) OF CHOICE
For treatment of hyperkalemia consider the following drugs:
• If symptomatic (bradycardia, muscle weakness) or serum potassium concentration >7.0 mmol/L
  ○ Calcium borogluconate 23% 0.2–0.4 mL/kg IV
  ○ Dextrose 0.5 g/kg with soluble insulin 0.1 unit/kg in 500 mL saline as IV infusion over 30–45 min
  ○ Sodium bicarbonate 1 mEq/kg IV over 15 min, can be repeated
• If not symptomatic and <7.0 mmol/L
  ○ Diurese with at least 5 mL/kg/h lactated Ringer's solution
  ○ Furosemide 1 mg/kg IV if horse well perfused
• For treatment of myocardial pathology, corticosteroids such as prednisolone 1 mg/kg PO every 48 h or dexamethasone 0.05–0.1 mg/kg IV or 0.1 mg/kg PO every 24 h for 3 or 4 days and then continued every 3–4 days in decreasing dosages are recommended
• Where life-threatening bradyarrhythmias are observed during cardiopulmonary resuscitation, atropine or glycopyrrolate

(glycopyrronium) can be administered at 0.005–0.01 mg/kg IV

CONTRAINDICATIONS/POSSIBLE INTERACTIONS
• Care should be taken that discontinuation of dextrose infusions does not lead to hypoglycemia, particularly when insulin has been administered concurrently
• High-dose corticosteroid therapy has been associated with laminitis, particularly when other laminitis risk factors are present

FOLLOW-UP

PATIENT MONITORING
Horses with pathologic bradyarrhythmias should have their ECG monitored frequently until the arrhythmia resolves.

POSSIBLE COMPLICATIONS
Pathologic bradyarrhythmias can be fatal.

EXPECTED COURSE AND PROGNOSIS
The clinical course and prognosis are generally determined by the underlying cause.

MISCELLANEOUS

ASSOCIATED CONDITIONS
• Uroperitoneum
• Renal failure
• Myocardial disease

AGE-RELATED FACTORS
More common in foals with uroperitoneum

PREGNANCY/FERTILITY/BREEDING
Third-degree AVB will lead to a profound decrease in cardiac output and compromise blood supply to the fetus. A transvenous pacing device should be considered in pregnant mares.

SEE ALSO
• Atrial fibrillation
• Myocardial disease

ABBREVIATIONS
• AF = atrial fibrillation
• AVB = atrioventricular block

Suggested Reading
Reef VB, Bonagura J, Buhl R, et al. Recommendations for management of equine athletes with cardiovascular abnormalities. J Vet Intern Med 2014;28:749–761.

Author Virginia B. Reef
Consulting Editor Celia M. Marr and Virginia B. Reef
Acknowledgment The author acknowledges the prior contribution of Celia M. Marr.

BROAD LIGAMENT HEMATOMA

B

BASICS

DEFINITION
• A rupture of the utero-ovarian, middle uterine, or external iliac arteries near the time of parturition. • Hemorrhage from the arteries can accumulate in the abdomen or into the broad ligament, forming a hematoma

PATHOPHYSIOLOGY
• With aging, the utero-ovarian and middle uterine artery walls undergo degenerative processes believed to result in loss of elasticity. • Secondary to the increased size or stretching, the arteries are more prone to rupture. • Preexisting damage to the intima and underlying media of the external iliac arteries (e.g. parasites) may predispose them to rupture

SYSTEMS AFFECTED
• Reproductive. • Cardiovascular

GENETICS
Unknown

INCIDENCE/PREVALENCE
Unknown

SIGNALMENT
• Pregnancy. • Most common in mares >12 years of age. • Any breed

SIGNS
General Comments
• Broad ligament hematoma—the hemorrhage contained between layers of the broad ligament; usually not fatal. • Intraperitoneal hemorrhage (i.e. free blood into the abdomen) is a fatal sign
Historical Findings
• No cardinal, characteristic signs before artery rupture. • Pale mucous membranes, tachycardia. • After rupture and with accumulation of hemorrhage, mares may become shocky or show colic from pain associated with stretching of the mesometrium, the portion of the broad ligament attached to the uterus
Physical Examination Findings
• Clinical signs suggestive of hemorrhagic shock (tachycardia, delayed CRT, sweating, etc.). • May appear anxious. • TRP may reveal an enlarged broad ligament—unilateral is most common, but bilateral may occur

CAUSES
Degeneration of arterial vessel walls related to age.

RISK FACTORS
Risk factors include pregnancy and aging.

DIAGNOSIS

DIFFERENTIAL DIAGNOSIS
• Colic from other causes. • Ilial fractures and pelvic abscesses

CBC/BIOCHEMISTRY/URINALYSIS
Varying degrees of anemia after 24 h of hematoma formation.

IMAGING
US imaging is useful to differentiate hemorrhage from purulent material.

OTHER DIAGNOSTIC PROCEDURES
• TRP is the preferred diagnostic method to confirm the condition, but it must be gentle and brief; identify the broad ligament enlargement, but do not disrupt the integrity of the myometrial walls that are containing the hemorrhage (avoid rough handling, leading to broad ligament rupture—losing the *field of containment*). • US imaging of contents captured within the mesometrium may be useful. Hemorrhage becomes increasingly hyperechoic as the clot consolidates and contracts.

PATHOLOGIC FINDINGS
• Acute hemorrhagic enlargement in the broad ligaments/mesometrium during the peripartal period. • Free hemorrhage in the abdomen

TREATMENT

APPROPRIATE HEALTH CARE
• Avoid moving the mare until she is medically stable, and the hematoma clots, contracts, and begins noticeably to reduce in size. • Prevent the mare from rolling, running, or becoming excited

NURSING CARE
Maintain a quiet environment.

ACTIVITY
Restrict activity as much as possible, including hand-walking, if necessary.

CLIENT EDUCATION
• Possibility of occurrence increases with age. • Consider the possibility of arterial rupture before breeding an old mare

SURGICAL CONSIDERATIONS
Attempts to ligate the damaged vessel may lead to further hemorrhage.

MEDICATIONS

CONTRAINDICATIONS
• Agents to enhance clotting have little or no value. • Oxytocin administration

PRECAUTIONS
• If broad ligament hemorrhage began prepartum, be careful when extracting a fetus if the mare is in dystocia. • Avoid transport to a veterinary hospital as it may result in fatal bleeding

FOLLOW-UP

PATIENT MONITORING
• Monitor packed cell volume, total solids, capillary refill time, and color of mucous membranes if broad ligament hematoma is diagnosed. • Avoid TRPs once a hematoma has been confirmed

POSSIBLE COMPLICATIONS
• Death. • Abscess formation in the hematoma

EXPECTED COURSE AND PROGNOSIS
• Best outcome—slow regression of a hematoma, the broad ligament is unlikely to return entirely to its pre-hematoma size and shape. • Once affected, mares are at increased risk of future rupture

MISCELLANEOUS

ASSOCIATED CONDITIONS
• Abscess formation. • Dystocia

PREGNANCY/FERTILITY/BREEDING
Occurs either at or near term during an otherwise normal pregnancy.

SYNONYMS
Mesometrial hematoma

SEE ALSO
Dystocia

ABBREVIATIONS
TRP = transrectal palpation
US = ultrasonography, ultrasound

Suggested Reading
Dascanio JJ. Abdominocentesis in the postpartum mare. In: Dascanio JJ, McCue P, eds. Equine Reproductive Procedures. Ames, IA: Wiley Blackwell, 2014:312–313.
Oikawa M, Nambo Y, Miyamoto M, et al. Postpartum massive hematoma within the broad ligament of the uterus in a broodmare possibly caused by rupture of the uterine artery (case report). J Equine Sci 2009;20(3):41–46.
Ueno T, Nambo Y, Tajima Y, Umemura T. Pathology of lethal peripartum broad ligament haematoma in 31 Thoroughbred mares. Equine Vet J 2010;42(6):529–533.

Author Carla L. Carleton
Consulting Editor Carla L. Carleton
Acknowledgment The author and editor acknowledges the prior contribution of Walter R. Threlfall.

BASICS

OVERVIEW
• Chronic bacterial zoonosis caused by *Brucella abortus*, and more rarely *Brucella suis*
• Predilection of the organism for synovial structures results in supraspinous bursitis (fistulous withers)
• Usually acquired from infected cattle and occasionally pigs
• Difficult to treat

SIGNS
• Most seropositive horses are asymptomatic
• Supraspinous bursitis is marked by painful swelling over the withers, which may open and drain purulent material
• Supra-atlantal bursitis (poll evil), abscess localized in tendons, bursae, and joints may also occur
• Osteomyelitis and osteoarthritis—hocks, pasterns, fistula in ribs
• Generalized illness marked by fever, stiffness, poor appetite, and lethargy may occur
• Occasionally, widespread infection with sepsis is observed
• Reproductive disorders are rare

CAUSES AND RISK FACTORS
• Rearing horses among cattle and pigs. Transmission among horses is very unlikely
• Infection occurs mainly by the oral route, through ingestion of contaminated food and water. *Brucella* spp. can survive in the environment for weeks, so horses grazing on pastures recently occupied by infected cattle are at risk
• Bacteria colonize initially the oronasal mucosa, reach regional lymph nodes, and begin replication within phagocytes, leading to granuloma formation. Infection can also occur through skin, air, venereal, conjunctival, and transcutaneous routes
• Horses are accidental or terminal hosts

DIAGNOSIS

DIFFERENTIAL DIAGNOSIS
Clinical signs are not specific. Other microorganisms may also cause fistulous withers, supraspinous bursitis or joint infections. Failure to identify *Brucella* spp. does not rule out infection. Antimicrobial treatment can reduce culture sensitivity. Reproductive failure and abortion can be confirmed by history, culture, PCR, and histopathology of placental and fetal tissues.

LABORATORY TESTS
Horse anti-*Brucella* antibodies can be detected by plate agglutination test, standard tube test, 2-mercaptoethanol, and complement fixation test. Rising titer in paired sera 2 weeks apart is diagnostic. Titer ≥100, with history of exposure to infected cattle and typical clinical signs, is usually diagnostic. Retest acute cases after 2 weeks before ruling out brucellosis.

IMAGING
• Dorsal spinous processes—radiographs help differentiate fractures versus osteomyelitis
• Contrast radiography and ultrasonography to determine location of fluid pockets and fistulous tracts

OTHER DIAGNOSTIC PROCEDURES
Culture and PCR. *Brucella* spp. is hard to isolate and requires biosafety level 3 procedures. Secondary pathogens are usually isolated.

PATHOLOGIC FINDINGS
• Affected bursae have a thickened capsule and clear fluid unless fistulated, when exudate is usually purulent
• Osteomyelitis of the dorsal spinous processes possible

TREATMENT

• Notify state regulatory authorities. Treatment in horses is not usually recommended, and sometimes forbidden. When done, it is based on clinical manifestations
• Animals should be isolated. Use personal protection equipment (gloves, long sleeve coats, glasses, N95 masks)
• Lavage fistulous tracts with an antiseptic solution (0.1% povidone iodine or 10–50% DMSO solution)
• Hydrotherapy
• No riding
• Surgical curettage of the affected soft tissue and bone is indicated in cases that do not respond to antibiotic treatment. Patients may require more than 1 surgery
• Treatment is usually required for 3–4 months, with risks of permanent chronic infection

MEDICATIONS

DRUG(S) OF CHOICE
• Tetracyclines, chloramphenicol, streptomycin, and some sulfonamides. Success rates are variable

• Flunixin meglumine (1 mg/kg every 12 h) or phenylbutazone (2–4 mg/kg PO or IV every 12 h) reduce fever and inflammation
• *B. abortus* S19 vaccination was described. This extralabel use of vaccine may cause serious adverse effects, such as fever, inflammation, and death

CONTRAINDICATIONS/POSSIBLE INTERACTIONS
Informed consent should be obtained before treatment with S19, dexamethasone (0.25 mg/kg IV), aspirin (35 mg/kg PO), or flunixin meglumine (1.1 mg/kg).

FOLLOW-UP

In *Brucella*-free or low-prevalence areas, infection in horses is low.

MISCELLANEOUS

ZOONOTIC POTENTIAL
Direct contact with infected material, ingestion, or inhalation, or by inoculation with live vaccine. Drainage of abscesses exposes humans to high risk of infection, as well as administration of S19. Use of antimicrobials for treatment of equine brucellosis can lead to serious public health risk due to appearance of resistant strains.

SYNONYMS
• Bang disease
• Undulant fever

SEE ALSO
• Back pain
• Chronic weight loss
• Fever
• Osteoarthritis

ABBREVIATIONS
• DMSO = dimethyl sulfoxide
• PCR = polymerase chain reaction

Suggested Reading
Hawkins JF, Fessler JF. Treatment of supraspinous bursitis by use of debridement in standing horses: 10 cases (1968–1999). J Am Vet Med Assoc 2000;217: 74–78.

Authors Elaine M.S. Dorneles and Andrey P. Lage
Consulting Editor Ashley G. Boyle
Acknowledgment The authors and editor acknowledge the prior contribution of Laura K. Reilly.

BRUXISM

B

BASICS

DEFINITION
Bruxism is the medical term characterizing rhythmic or spasmodic nonfunctional motor activity such as gnashing, grinding, or clenching of the teeth. Bruxism may occur intermittently or, in more severe cases, may become incessant. It has a multifactorial etiology.

PATHOPHYSIOLOGY
Bruxism in animals develops secondary to diseases, medications, and/or toxins. The biomechanics of mandibular movement is a function of the neurologic input from cortical and stomatognathic sources acting to initiate or restrict muscular contracture. During bruxism the neuromuscular protecting mechanisms, which are present during normal functional activities, are absent or reflex thresholds are raised, resulting in less influence over masticatory muscle activity. Bruxism may be seen in a variety of clinical disorders:
• Foals—intermittent bruxism may occur with any painful condition. It is most commonly associated with gastroduodenal ulceration, gastritis, and esophagitis. In cases when gastric outflow is inhibited by stricture of the pylorus or duodenum subsequent gastroesophageal reflux results in corrosive esophagitis
• Adults—bruxism in adults is often associated with pharyngeal pain or pain at the esophagus in the area of the palatopharyngeal arch. This area can be irritated by nasogastric intubation and indwelling nasogastric tubes. However, bruxism may occur in response to almost any painful condition. It is also observed with esophagitis and gastric ulceration
• Inappropriate horse tack and stringent training methods may also cause bruxism. Occasionally, bruxism may become a vice, which can express itself without a specific provocation or the act of bruxism can be triggered by specific activities related to management and/or training
• Bruxism is often associated with neurologic disorders. Disturbances in brain neurotransmission, especially the central dopaminergic system, have been strongly associated with the etiopathogenesis of bruxism

SYSTEMS AFFECTED
Most often the stomatognathic system, GI tract.

SIGNALMENT
No age, breed, or sex predilection.

SIGNS
Bruxism is a nonspecific clinical sign. It is usually a sign of discomfort or pain, or

occasionally indicates frustration or neurologic disease. Bruxism can therefore be present with a variety of other clinical signs associated with the primary disease.

Historical Findings
These are generally associated with primary disease. The health status of other horses on the premises should be checked. A history of recent nasogastric intubation or indwelling nasogastric tube may indicate traumatic causes for bruxism. Signs such as recent or ongoing colic, appetite, feces consistency, and attitude should be evaluated.

Physical Examination Findings
When associated with pharyngeal pain, mild dysphagia may be present, which is frequently characterized by salivation or by holding saliva in the mouth for prolonged periods. With gastric ulceration, foals may exhibit poor appetite, intermittent nursing (may nurse for a short period and then act mildly uncomfortable), episodes of mild colic, diarrhea, pot-bellied appearance, salivation, or dorsal recumbency. Salivation and bruxism are usually indicative of severe glandular or duodenal ulcers with concurrent gastroesophageal reflux and delayed gastric emptying. Adults with gastric ulceration may also exhibit poor appetite, lethargy, poor body condition, rough hair coat, and low-grade colic. In cases of esophageal rupture bruxism may be accompanied by severe ptyalism.

CAUSES
Trauma from nasogastric intubation, irritation from indwelling nasogastric tubes, gastroduodenal ulceration, reflux esophagitis, neurologic diseases (i.e. Borna disease, rabies), dental problems, any painful condition.

RISK FACTORS
Passage of nasogastric tube, indwelling nasogastric tube, inappropriate horse tack, stringent training methods, any painful disease.

DIAGNOSIS

DIFFERENTIAL DIAGNOSIS
• Traumatic pharyngitis/esophagitis
• Gastritis/esophagitis
• Gastroduodenal ulceration
• Reflux esophagitis
• Gastric impaction
• Small intestine obstruction
• Borna disease
• Rabies
• Equine protozoal myeloencephalitis
• Head trauma
• Bacterial meningitis
• Foreign body or mass of the oral cavity, pharynx, esophagus, or stomach
• Severe inflammatory condition of the oral cavity, pharynx, esophagus, or stomach

CBC/BIOCHEMISTRY/URINALYSIS
These parameters are useful for identifying the primary cause for bruxism.

OTHER LABORATORY TESTS
N/A

DIAGNOSTIC PROCEDURES
Endoscopic Examination
Endoscopy is of value in determining if bruxism is a response to traumatic pharyngitis or esophagitis, reflux esophagitis, esophageal rupture, and/or gastroduodenal ulceration. Pharyngitis might be obvious; however, in some cases the lesion is in or behind the palatopharyngeal arch and difficult to visualize.

TREATMENT
• Treatment of primary disease is indicated
• Bruxism may be the sequela of serious medical conditions that require inpatient monitoring and care. If the patient is not drinking or is losing fluids through salivation, appropriate IV fluid therapy should be administered

MEDICATIONS
DRUG(S) OF CHOICE
• Patients with painful conditions may benefit from administration of NSAIDs for pain control. In general, flunixin meglumine and ketoprofen are preferred for treatment of visceral pain, whereas phenylbutazone is preferred for musculoskeletal pain. Flunixin meglumine is administered at 1.1 mg/kg (IV or PO), ketoprofen at 2.2 mg/kg (IV), and phenylbutazone at 2.2–4.4 mg/kg. Other NSAIDs are less often prescribed (vedaprofen, meloxicam). NSAIDs should not be used before GI mucosal erosions are excluded as a cause for bruxism
• Gastric ulceration is most often treated with PPIs (omeprazole) or histamine H_2 receptor antagonists. Omeprazole is administered at 1–4 mg/kg PO once daily. Omeprazole has a time- and dose-related effect on healing of gastric ulcers. Therefore, higher doses result in more rapid and complete healing. However, lower doses are frequently effective in relieving clinical signs and promoting healing. Omeprazole requires 3–5 days of treatment for maximum antisecretory effect to occur, and prolonged treatment to achieve satisfactory ulcer healing. Cimetidine is administered at 20–25 mg/kg PO or at 4–6 mg/kg IV every 6–8 h. Ranitidine is administered at 6–8 mg/kg PO or 1.5–2.0 mg/kg IV every 6–8 h
• The use of mucosal protectants, especially in foals, is warranted. Sucralfate is administered

(CONTINUED)

at 10–20 mg/kg PO every 6–8 h, and 20–40 mg/kg PO every 8 h in foals and adults, respectively. Sucralfate is likely to be ineffective in the treatment of equine squamous gastric disease but could possibly be effective in equine glandular gastric disease

PRECAUTIONS
Indiscriminate treatment with NSAIDs may initiate or worsen gastroduodenal ulceration and can result in toxicosis if administered in excessive doses or to dehydrated animals. NSAIDs also prolong mucosal healing. Between ketoprofen, flunixin meglumine, and phenylbutazone, the last has the greatest potential for toxicity. When frequent dosing is necessary, ketoprofen has been shown to have less potential for toxicosis than flunixin meglumine or phenylbutazone.

POSSIBLE INTERACTIONS
Cimetidine and, to a lesser extent, omeprazole are hepatic cytochrome P450 inhibitors and might slow the metabolism of concurrently administered compounds that require this enzyme for metabolism and elimination. Treatment with PPIs and/or sucralfate may also have a negative impact on other medications.

ALTERNATIVE DRUGS
Butorphanol, xylazine, and detomidine may also be used for short-term relief of pain. For gastric ulceration, antacid compounds buffer gastric acid. They are impractical to use in most instances, and must be administered 4–6 times daily at approximately 250 mL/450 kg horse. Spasmolytic drugs (hyoscine *N*-butylbromide) alone or in combination with metamizole (dipyrone) can indirectly provide analgesia by reducing spasms of the intestine. Lidocaine is also

effective in treating pain (1.3 mg/kg IV as a bolus followed by a 0.05 mg/kg/min infusion for 24–72 h). Side effects of all pain relief drugs should be carefully considered.

FOLLOW-UP

PATIENT MONITORING
Patients exhibiting bruxism often have serious medical problems and should be thoroughly evaluated. Foals exhibiting bruxism should be monitored carefully for development of gastroesophageal reflux and diminished gastric emptying.

POSSIBLE COMPLICATIONS
There are no significant complications associated with the bruxism itself. Bruxism results in sustained muscle contraction for long periods, which, unlike functional activity, can result in fatigue, pain, and spasms of masticatory muscles. Most complications are associated with the primary disease.

MISCELLANEOUS

ASSOCIATED CONDITIONS
Usually associated with primary disease.

AGE-RELATED FACTORS
N/A

ZOONOTIC POTENTIAL
In endemic areas, rabies should be considered in patients showing neurologic signs of undetermined etiology.

PREGNANCY/FERTILITY/BREEDING
N/A

SYNONYMS
• Odontoprisis
• Teeth grinding

SEE ALSO
• Gastric ulcers and erosions (equine gastric ulcer syndrome, EGUS)
• Regurgitation/vomiting/dysphagia

ABBREVIATIONS
• GI = gastrointestinal
• NSAID = nonsteroidal anti-inflammatory drug
• PPI = proton pump inhibitor

Suggested Reading
Dauphin G, Legay V, Pitel PH, Zientara S. Borna disease: current knowledge and virus detection in France. Vet Res 2002;33:127–138.
Ella B, Ghorayeb I, Burbaud P, Guehl D. Bruxism in movement disorders: a comprehensive review. J Prosthodont 2017;26(7):599–605.
Falisi G, Rastelli C, Panti F, et al. Psychotropic drugs and bruxism. Expert Opin Drug Saf 2014;13:1319–1326.
Hardy J, Stewart RH, Beard WL, Yvorchuk-St-Jean K. Complications of nasogastric intubation in horses: nine cases (1987–1989). J Am Vet Med Assoc 1992;201:483–486.
Murali RV, Rangarajan P, Mounissamy A. Bruxism: conceptual discussion and review. J Pharm Bioallied Sci 2015;7:S265–270.
Sykes BW, Hewetson M, Hepburn RJ, et al. European College of Equine Internal Medicine consensus statement—equine gastric ulcer syndrome in adult horses. J Vet Intern Med 2015;29:1288–1299.

Author Modest Vengust
Consulting Editors Henry Stämpfli and Olimpo Oliver-Espinosa

BURDOCK PAPPUS BRISTLE KERATOPATHY

BASICS

DEFINITION
• Burdock pappus (*Arctium* spp.) bristles are common conjunctival foreign bodies in the northeastern USA that can lead to chronic, nonhealing lesions of the cornea
• The burdock plant releases tiny, sharply pointed bristles that attach to skin and mucous membranes. They can cause dermal irritation, respiratory disease, and ocular disease in many species including horses and humans. When the bristles lodge in the conjunctiva, they contact the cornea causing irritation and corneal ulceration. The bristles may release irritating substances
• Systems affected—ophthalmic

GENETICS
No breed predilections for this conjunctival foreign body.

INCIDENCE/PREVALENCE
Common condition in the northeastern USA.

GEOGRAPHIC DISTRIBUTION
More common in the northeastern USA; however, the plant has been found in all of the contiguous United States except Florida.

SIGNALMENT
No age or sex predilection.

SIGNS
• History of unilateral ocular signs including photophobia, blepharospasm, lacrimation, discharge characterized as either serous or mucopurulent, and fluorescein retention on the cornea
• Most ulcers are near the nasal limbus, near the nictitans
• The corneal erosions or ulcerations persist despite topical medical therapy

CAUSES
Burdock pappus bristles are a common source of small conjunctival foreign bodies. The bristles may release irritating substances.

DIAGNOSIS

DIFFERENTIAL DIAGNOSIS
• Lid abnormalities such as distichiasis, trichiasis, and entropion; neuroparalytic and neurotrophic keratitis
• Corneal dystrophies; indolent corneal ulcers, eosinophilic keratitis, and corneal foreign bodies
• Inappropriate topical corticosteroid therapy causing delayed corneal healing

CBC/BIOCHEMISTRY/URINALYSIS
N/A

OTHER LABORATORY TESTS
Rule out infectious causes (bacterial or fungal) with corneal scrapings for cytology, aerobic bacterial, and fungal culture of the wound bed.

IMAGING
N/A

OTHER DIAGNOSTIC PROCEDURES
N/A

PATHOLOGIC FINDINGS
N/A

TREATMENT

APPROPRIATE HEALTH CARE
• Find the bristle. Apply topical anesthetic. Retropulse the eye using gentle, transpalpebral pressure on the globe. Delicately evert the third eyelid and investigate the posterior face using a focal light source
• Conjunctivectomy of the bristle foreign body and surrounding tissue under sedation, topical anesthesia, and auriculopalpebral nerve block
• Debridement of the conjunctiva behind the nictitans is often necessary

NURSING CARE
Topical antibiotic therapy 4–6 times a day until resolution of the corneal ulcer is recommended.

ACTIVITY
The patient's activity should be restricted to stall rest or small paddock turnout until resolution of the keratitis.

DIET
N/A

CLIENT EDUCATION
• Patients should become progressively more comfortable after removal of the foreign body. If worsening is noted, reexamination is warranted
• If there is evidence of self-trauma when ocular disease is present, a protective hood covering the affected eye should be placed on the horse

SURGICAL CONSIDERATIONS
N/A

MEDICATIONS

DRUG(S) OF CHOICE
After conjunctivectomy—follow-up therapy with topical antibiotics 4–6 times daily (e.g. neomycin–polymyxin B–bacitracin ointment, erythromycin ointment), topical 1% atropine SID to TID, and 1–2 g phenylbutazone BID PO.

CONTRAINDICATIONS, POSSIBLE INTERACTIONS
• Horses receiving topical atropine should be monitored for colic
• Secondary infection can result in a rapidly worsening condition. See chapter Corneal ulceration for further information

FOLLOW-UP

PATIENT MONITORING
Recheck in 5–7 days to monitor epithelialization of the ulcer, improvement in patient comfort, and decrease in keratitis/conjunctivitis.

PREVENTION/AVOIDANCE
Ubiquitous in the environment due to airborne dispersion, contact with the bristles may be difficult to avoid in certain areas. However, they should be removed if identified in pasture.

POSSIBLE COMPLICATIONS
Secondary bacterial infection.

EXPECTED COURSE AND PROGNOSIS
After removal of the bristle, healing of the corneal defect occurs within 3–14 days.

MISCELLANEOUS

ASSOCIATED CONDITIONS
Secondary bacterial infection.

AGE-RELATED FACTORS
N/A

ZOONOTIC POTENTIAL
None

PREGNANCY/FERTILITY/BREEDING
N/A

SEE ALSO
• Calcific band keratopathy
• Corneal/scleral lacerations
• Corneal ulceration
• Eosinophilic keratitis
• Superficial nonhealing ulcers

Suggested Reading
Brooks DE. Ophthalmology for the Equine Practitioner, 2e. Jackson, WY: Teton NewMedia, 2009.
Gilger BC. Equine ophthalmology. In: Gelatt KN, ed. Veterinary Ophthalmology, 5e. Ames, IA: Wiley, 2013:1560–1609.
Gilger BC. Equine Ophthalmology, 3e. Ames, IA: Wiley, 2017.

Author Caroline Monk
Consulting Editor Caryn E. Plummer
Acknowledgment The author and editor acknowledge the prior contribution of Andras M. Komaromy and Dennis E. Brooks.

CALCIFIC BAND KERATOPATHY

BASICS

OVERVIEW
Calcific band keratopathy consists of depositions of calcium (hydroxyapatite) in or adjacent to the basement membrane of the corneal epithelium and anterior stroma and is a possible complication of chronic uveitis. The ophthalmic system is affected.

SIGNALMENT
All ages and breeds affected.

SIGNS
• In addition to signs of chronic uveitis (e.g. synechiae, miosis, aqueous flare), variably dense, white, dystrophic bands or chalky plaques are noted in the interpalpebral region of the central cornea. These areas are often associated with scattered areas of fluorescein retention, usually the result of the lesions elevating the overlying epithelium
• Calcium deposited at the level of the corneal epithelial basement membrane may accumulate and disrupt the epithelium to result in painful ulcers and a secondary reflex uveitis

CAUSES AND RISK FACTORS
The exact pathogenesis of calcium band keratopathy is unknown. It is an occasional complication of chronic cases of uveitis and has been noted following the chronic application of topical corticosteroids or phosphate-containing solutions (usually as a therapy for uveitis). Alterations of pH in the superficial cornea of the interpalpebral space and evaporation of tears in the same region have been postulated as contributing factors for the development of this condition.

DIAGNOSIS

DIFFERENTIAL DIAGNOSIS
Lid abnormalities such as distichiasis, trichiasis, and entropion resulting in keratitis and corneal injury; bacterial or fungal keratitis; eosinophilic keratitis; corneal lipid degeneration; neuroparalytic and neurotrophic keratitis; keratoconjunctivitis sicca; corneal dystrophies; corneal foreign bodies; and chronic epithelial erosion (indolent ulceration).

CBC/BIOCHEMISTRY/URINALYSIS
N/A

OTHER LABORATORY TESTS, DIAGNOSTIC PROCEDURES
• Rule out infectious causes (bacterial or fungal) with corneal scrapings for cytology and culture. Scraping procedure causes audible and tactile evidence of mineralization
• The dull, gritty appearance and character of corneal calcium are helpful in the diagnosis
• Biopsy sample can be taken to histologically support the diagnosis of calcific band keratopathy. Von Kossa and alizarin red stains can detect the presence of calcium

IMAGING
N/A

PATHOLOGIC FINDINGS
• Special stains (e.g. Kossa's method or alizarin red) confirm the presence of calcium deposits at the level of the lamina propria of the epithelium and underlying superficial stroma
• Vascularization is often noted, and an associated lymphocytic and neutrophilic cellular reaction is frequently present around the calcium deposits

TREATMENT
• Superficial keratectomy is recommended. If calcific deposits are not removed, affected eyes remain painful despite medical treatment because of persistent or recurrent ulceration. Debridement with a diamond burr or application of topical EDTA during debridement may be effective in removing some superficial mineral
• Inappropriate topical corticosteroid therapy may cause delayed corneal healing

MEDICATIONS

DRUG(S) OF CHOICE
• Topically administered calcium-chelating drugs (dipotassium EDTA 13.8%; Sequester-Sol) to dissolve the calcium deposits are usually only helpful if the corneal epithelium is absent or compromised
• Topical antibiotic (e.g. chloramphenicol, bacitracin–neomycin–polymyxin B), atropine (1%), and systemic nonsteroidal anti-inflammatory drugs (e.g. flunixin meglumine 0.25–1 mg/kg BID PO, IM, IV) should be used to protect any ulcerations and treat any resultant uveitis until the keratectomy site heals

CONTRAINDICATIONS/POSSIBLE INTERACTIONS
Risk of opportunistic infections due to topical corticosteroids for treatment of uveitis. The rate of post-keratectomy infections can be high, usually owing to a compromised cornea from chronic uveitis or prior use of topical corticosteroids.

FOLLOW-UP

EXPECTED COURSE AND PROGNOSIS
• Healing of keratectomy sites can occur with slight to severe scarring
• Recurrence of calcium band keratopathy is possible with continued episodes of uveitis
• The prognosis for vision is guarded because of subsequent corneal scarring and further uveitis episodes
• Horses with dystrophic calcification due to severe corneal injury or infection in areas other than the interpalpebral fissure usually fare better than those with palpebral fissure lesions

MISCELLANEOUS

ASSOCIATED CONDITIONS
Complication of uveitis.

SEE ALSO
• Burdock pappus bristle keratopathy
• Corneal/scleral lacerations
• Corneal ulceration
• Eosinophilic keratitis
• Equine recurrent uveitis
• Glaucoma
• Ulcerative keratomycosis
• Viral (herpes) keratitis (putative)

Suggested Reading
Brooks DE. Ophthalmology for the Equine Practitioner, 2e. Jackson, WY: Teton NewMedia, 2008.
Brooks DE, Matthews AG. Equine ophthalmology. In: Gelatt KN, ed. Veterinary Ophthalmology, 4e. Ames, IA: Blackwell, 2007:1165–1274.
Gilger BC, ed. Equine Ophthalmology, 3e. Ames, IA: Wiley, 2017.

Author Caryn E. Plummer
Consulting Editor Caryn E. Plummer

CALCIUM, HYPERCALCEMIA

BASICS

DEFINITION
Serum total calcium concentration greater than the reference interval.

PATHOPHYSIOLOGY
• PTH, calcitonin, and vitamin D act in conjunction with the intestine, bone, kidneys, and parathyroid glands to maintain calcium homeostasis. The calcium-sensing receptor, found in cell types that secrete calciotropic hormones, is central to calcium regulation and detects changes in ionized calcium.
• Calcium absorption occurs primarily in the proximal small intestine. Serum calcium concentration is more dependent on the amount of dietary calcium and less dependent on vitamin D. • The kidney is important in calcium regulation; horses excrete a larger proportion of absorbed calcium in the urine than other mammals do. Calcium is also eliminated through sweat, milk, and feces.
• Disturbances in calcium homeostasis leading to hypercalcemia occur with organ dysfunction, abnormalities in hormonal balance and control, administration of vitamin D products or ingestion of plants containing vitamin D-like compounds, or production of a parathyroid hormone analog in certain malignancies. • With CRF, ability of the kidney to excrete calcium is compromised, causing hypercalcemia especially in horses on a high calcium diet.
• Hypercalcemia of malignancy is associated with certain types of neoplasia. Tumor cells produce and secrete PTHrP or related products, causing increased osteoclastic bone resorption and renal resorption of calcium.
• Hypercalcemic states can lead to widespread soft tissue mineralization

SYSTEMS AFFECTED
General Comments
Although uncommon, metastatic calcification may develop with hyperphosphatemia and concurrent hypercalcemia (hypervitaminosis D) when the calcium x phosphorus product (in mg/dL) is greater than 70. Vasculature of lungs, pleura, kidneys, endocardium, and stomach are prone.

Cardiovascular
ECG changes associated with increased serum calcium progress from bradycardia to tachycardia to ventricular fibrillation.

Endocrine/Metabolic
Hypercalcemia stimulates calcitonin release from thyroid C-cells, which acts by decreasing osteoclastic bone resorption as a compensatory mechanism to decrease plasma calcium concentration.

GI
Possible decreased contractility of GI smooth muscle. Constipation may occur.

Renal
Soft tissue mineralization may occur with concurrent hypercalcemia and hyperphosphatemia.

GENETICS
N/A

INCIDENCE/PREVALENCE
N/A

GEOGRAPHIC DISTRIBUTION
N/A

SIGNALMENT
Renal Disease
Dependent on the underlying cause.

Hypercalcemia of Malignancy
• Lymphoma is a common neoplasm in horses. • Horses with lymphoma are typically young to middle-aged (5–10 years). • SCC generally occurs in older animals. • Cutaneous SCC more commonly occurs on nonpigmented areas, so Appaloosas, Paints, and some draft breeds are predisposed

SIGNS
General Comments
Dependent on the underlying cause.

Historical Findings
• With renal disease/failure, poor performance and/or weight loss, mild colic signs or abnormal urination may be noted. Recent or long-term nephrotoxic medications (e.g. NSAIDs, aminoglycosides) may be included in the history. • With lymphoma, weight loss, lethargy, edema, recurrent fever, and/or lymphadenopathy may be present. • With gastric SCC, horses may exhibit signs of esophageal obstruction (e.g. dysphagia, ptyalism, choke), and/or have a prolonged history of halitosis, anorexia and weight loss. Intraabdominal SCC may cause chronic weight loss and intermittent colic. • Horses with hypervitaminosis D may exhibit limb stiffness and painful flexor tendons and suspensory ligaments. • Primary hyperparathyroidism is rare; history may include anorexia, weight loss, or changes in facial bone structure

Physical Examination Findings
Renal Disease
• Ventral edema—frequently seen with glomerulonephritis. • Oral ulcerations. • Hematuria or PU/PD. • On rectal palpation, some horses with AKI may have enlarged painful kidneys; horses with CRF may have small kidneys with irregular surface
Neoplasia
• Cutaneous SCC—proliferative/erosive masses or nonhealing wounds in the periorbital region, genitalia, lips, nose, or anus; during late/advanced stages, signs might be referable to location of metastasis.
• Abdominal mass might be palpated per rectum in cases of metastatic SCC or GI lymphoma. • Gastric SCC—weight loss, halitosis. • Lymphoma: dependent on

location of tumor (e.g. cutaneous GI, mediastinal or multicentric)
Primary Hyperparathyroidism
Bone remodeling (osteodystrophy of facial bones).

CAUSES
Renal Disease
• Hyper-, hypo-, or normocalcemia occurs with AKI. • Hypercalcemia in AKI or CRF is more apt to develop in horses fed high-calcium rations. • AKI may progress to CRF. Causes—glomerulonephritis from immune complex deposition (e.g. streptococcal infection, equine infectious anemia), nephrotoxins (e.g. aminoglycosides, NSAIDs, vitamin K3, heavy metals [especially mercury], hemoglobin, myoglobin), chronic urinary tract obstruction, interstitial nephritis, amyloidosis, pyelonephritis, nephrolithiasis and ureterolithiasis, and congenital abnormalities (e.g. renal hypoplasia or polycystic kidneys)

Neoplasia
• The most common paraneoplastic finding in horses is hypercalcemia. • Tumors associated with hypercalcemia—lymphoma, SCC, multiple myeloma, adrenocortical carcinoma, malignant mesenchymoma of the ovary, and ameloblastoma

Hypervitaminosis D
Hypercalcemia from increased GI absorption and bone resorption is associated with ingestion of plants containing vitamin D-like substances (*Solanum* spp., *Cestrum diurnum, Trisetum flavescens*) or administration of vitamin D.

Exercise
Because calcium is present in sweat, plasma concentrations may be reduced with large volumes of sweat loss.

Primary Hyperparathyroidism (Rare)
Parathyroid adenoma, parathyroid hyperplasia, carcinoma.

Neonatal Hypercalcemia and Asphyxia (Rare)
Asphyxia; may be associated with placental insufficiency and excessive PTHrP.

Granulomatous Disease (Rare)
Hypercalcemia due to unregulated production of calcitriol by macrophages may be seen in horses with idiopathic systemic granulomatous disease.

RISK FACTORS
See Signalment and Causes.

DIAGNOSIS

DIFFERENTIAL DIAGNOSIS
See Causes.

CBC/BIOCHEMISTRY/URINALYSIS

• Azotemia (increased serum Cr and urea nitrogen concentrations) and isosthenuria (USG 1.008–1.015) support the diagnosis of renal disease, but other causes of azotemia with concurrent PU/PD must be ruled out.
• Hypophosphatemia, mild hyponatremia and hypochloremia, and normo- or hyperkalemia can be present. • Moderate to marked proteinuria is common with glomerulonephritis. • Suspect urinary tract infection with moderate to many leukocytes in urine sediment. • Hypercalcemia without concurrent azotemia or isosthenuria implies causes other than renal; suspect neoplasia.
• Consider vitamin D intoxication with concurrent hypercalcemia and hyperphosphatemia. Hyperphosphatemia is the earliest abnormality and may be more reliable for indicating hypervitaminosis D in oversupplementation than hypercalcemia. Hyperphosphatemia may be absent in plant intoxication. USG may be low

OTHER LABORATORY TESTS

• Measurement of ionized calcium concentration by ion-selective electrodes requires special sample handling (collected in anaerobic conditions and analyzed promptly) and is becoming more readily available.
• With suspected primary hyperparathyroidism, measurement of PTH is indicated

IMAGING

Ultrasonography of kidneys during CRF may reveal increased echogenicity (i.e. fibrosis) and is useful in assessing abnormalities (e.g. polycystic kidneys).

OTHER DIAGNOSTIC PROCEDURES

• Fine needle aspiration or tissue biopsy of masses (endoscopic or ultrasonography guided) are indicated for establishing the diagnosis of neoplasia. • Abdominal or thoracic fluid cytology may reveal neoplastic cells. • Renal biopsy sometimes is useful in determining the cause of renal disease

PATHOLOGIC FINDINGS

Dependent on the underlying cause.

TREATMENT

DIET

Renal disease—salt restriction is indicated if ventral edema develops, and a diet of high-quality carbohydrates (e.g. corn, oats), roughage (e.g. grass hay), and free access to fresh water is recommended. Avoid feeds high in protein or calcium.

SURGICAL CONSIDERATIONS

Surgical excision, local chemotherapy, radiotherapy, cryosurgery, or hyperthermia are options with some localized tumors.

MEDICATIONS

DRUG(S) OF CHOICE

AKI (Hypercalcemia Less Likely)
• IV fluid therapy/diuresis. • Discontinue nephrotoxic drugs

CRF
• Good nutritional support and free access to fresh water, fluids and electrolytes, salt blocks if edema is absent (restrict if hypertension or edema develops), and vitamin B complex.
• Anabolic steroids may help to prevent muscle wasting. • With severe hypercalcemia, administration of physiologic saline with loop diuretics (e.g. furosemide) will promote urinary calcium excretion

Hypervitaminosis D
Removal of the source of vitamin D, fluid diuresis, corticosteroid administration, and low calcium and phosphorus feeds.

CONTRAINDICATIONS

• Do not feed hypercalcemic horses legume hays or high-calcium rations. • Fluid therapy for hypercalcemic horses should be devoid of calcium. • Thiazide diuretics promote renal resorption of calcium. • Avoid aminoglycoside antibiotics and NSAIDs if possible

PRECAUTIONS
N/A

POSSIBLE INTERACTIONS
N/A

ALTERNATIVE DRUGS
N/A

FOLLOW-UP

PATIENT MONITORING
Renal disease—serial biochemistries.

PREVENTION/AVOIDANCE
• Judicious use of nephrotoxic drugs.
• Ultraviolet-blocking fly masks in horses with nonpigmented facial skin

POSSIBLE COMPLICATIONS
Soft tissue mineralization.

EXPECTED COURSE AND PROGNOSIS
• Supportive therapy may prolong life substantially in polyuric (urine output > 18 mL urine/kg/day), stabilized patients. • With CRF, serum Cr concentration > 5 mg/dL indicates a marked decline in glomerular filtration rate. A grave prognosis is associated with serum Cr concentrations > 10 mg/dL. • Unless cutaneous or localized, neoplasia carries a guarded to poor prognosis. • Removal of vitamin D sources may result in recovery of hypervitaminosis D with time, but with soft tissue mineralization in the heart or kidney, the prognosis is poor

MISCELLANEOUS

ASSOCIATED CONDITIONS
N/A

AGE-RELATED FACTORS
N/A

ZOONOTIC POTENTIAL
N/A

PREGNANCY/FERTILITY/BREEDING
Increased calcium concentration in mammary secretions is a good indicator of impending parturition.

SYNONYMS
• Hypercalcemia of malignancy—humoral hypercalcemia of malignancy, pseudohyperparathyroidism
• Metastatic calcification—soft tissue mineralization

SEE ALSO
• Gastric neoplasia
• Lymphosarcoma
• Phosphorus, hyperphosphatemia
• Phosphorus, hypophosphatemia
• Primary hyperparathyroidism

ABBREVIATIONS
• AKI = acute kidney injury
• Cr = creatinine
• CRF = chronic renal failure
• GI = gastrointestinal
• NSAID = nonsteroidal anti-inflammatory drug
• PTH = parathyroid hormone
• PTHrP = parathyroid hormone-related peptide
• PU/PD = polyuria/polydipsia
• SCC = squamous cell carcinoma
• USG = urine specific gravity

Suggested Reading
Aguilera-Tejero E. Calcium homeostasis and derangements. In: Fielding CL, Magdesian KG, eds. Equine Fluid Therapy. Ames, IA: Wiley, 2015:55–75.
Toribio RE. Parathyroid gland, calcium and phosphorus regulation. In: Smith BP, ed. Large Animal Internal Medicine, 5e. St. Louis, MO: Elsevier Mosby, 2015:1244–1252.

Author Karen E. Russell
Consulting Editor Sandra D. Taylor

CALCIUM, HYPOCALCEMIA

 BASICS

DEFINITION
Total serum calcium concentration less than the reference interval.

PATHOPHYSIOLOGY
• Calcium, a major component of bone, also is necessary for blood coagulation, muscle contraction and neuromuscular excitability, hormone secretion, and enzyme activation
• Fractions of total serum calcium concentration occur as protein bound (50%), ionized (40%), or complexed with other anions (10%)
• Ionized calcium is the physiologically active fraction
• Of the protein-bound fraction, ≅50% is complexed with albumin. Serum albumin has a direct effect on total serum calcium concentration. Ionized calcium usually is not affected by albumin concentrations
• Acidosis increases ionized calcium by decreasing protein binding. Total calcium concentration usually remains within the reference interval
• Hypocalcemia can be seen with dietary deficiency or imbalance, sepsis, GI disease, hypocalcemic tetany (e.g. lactation, transport, idiopathic, eclampsia), hypoalbuminemia or hypoproteinemia, toxicosis (cantharidin [blister beetle], oxalate), administration of certain drugs (tetracycline, furosemide, bicarbonate), excessive sweating, rhabdomyolysis, renal disease, or pancreatic disease

SYSTEMS AFFECTED
Musculoskeletal
• In response to hypocalcemia, calcium is mobilized from bone to maintain other metabolic functions
• Consequences include too little or abnormal bone formation, bone demineralization, and a skeleton more prone to injury

Neuromuscular
• Most acute cases manifest as tetany rather than paresis
• Hypocalcemia may lead to increased neuroexcitability and seizures

GI
Decreased contractility may lead to hypomotility and ileus.

Reproductive
Retained placenta and acute endometritis are seen in mares with hypocalcemia and may occur as a result of decreased uterine tone and contractility, possibly resulting from a mechanism similar to that seen with ileus.

Cardiovascular
SDF (i.e. contraction of one or both flanks coincident with heartbeat) is thought to result from altered membrane potential of the phrenic nerve and its discharge in response to electrical impulses generated during myocardial depolarization.

GENETICS
N/A

INCIDENCE/PREVALENCE
N/A

GEOGRAPHIC DISTRIBUTION
N/A

SIGNALMENT
• Lactation tetany most frequently occurs in mares ≅10 days post foaling or 1–2 days post weaning
• Draft breeds are more susceptible

SIGNS
Historical Findings
Owners may describe lethargy, colic, anorexia, or depression after ingestion of alfalfa; lameness, swollen painful joints, or poor growth; diets of high grain content and low-quality roughage or bran supplement added to grain.

Physical Examination Findings
• Tetany, increased muscle tone or weakness, stiffness, muscle fasciculations, SDF, tachypnea, cardiac arrhythmias, ileus, colic, hyperthermia, sweating, excitation
• In severe cases, incoordination, recumbency, convulsions, death
Dietary Calcium Deficiency or Imbalance
• Early signs include intermittent shifting-leg lameness, generalized joint tenderness, stilted gait
• As the disease progresses, abnormal bone formation and enlarged facial bones (e.g. NHP, bighead disease)
Cantharidin Toxicosis
• Colic
• GI or urinary tract irritation
• Elevated respiratory and heart rates
• Diarrhea
• Fever
• Sweating
• Shock

CAUSES
Hypoalbuminemia or Hypoproteinemia
• The protein-bound fraction of calcium is directly affected by serum protein concentration; low serum protein concentrations may mask hypercalcemia
• Correction formulas determined for dogs have not been validated in horses

Dietary Calcium Deficiency or Imbalance
• Occurs from lack of dietary calcium, or factors limiting calcium utilization—excess phosphorus (in the form of inorganic phosphorus, phytate phosphate); oxalic acid
• In young animals, skeletal mass does not keep up with increasing body size; the skeleton is more prone to injury
• NHP occurs from low calcium and excess phosphorus intake. Parathyroid hormone increases as compensatory mechanism
• Rickets occurs from combined calcium and vitamin D deficiency
• Growing animals with vitamin D deficiency may be hypocalcemic, hypophosphatemic, and have elevated ALP. Vitamin D deficiency causes defective mineralization of new bone, resulting in painful swelling of the physis and metaphysis of long bones and costochondral junctions, bowed limbs, and stiff gait
• Natural cases of rickets in foals are not well documented

Cantharidin Toxicosis
Ingestion of alfalfa hay or alfalfa-containing products contaminated with blister beetles (*Epicauta* spp.).

Hypocalcemic Tetany (Lactation, Transport)
• Lactation tetany occurs ≅10 days post foaling or 1–2 days post weaning
• Draft mares, mares that produce large amounts of milk, and mares on pasture only or on a marginal plane of nutrition are at greatest risk
• Prolonged transportation or strenuous activity can predispose to hypocalcemia and tetany
• Concurrent hypomagnesemia is common in hypocalcemic tetany

Sepsis and GI Disease
• Sepsis and GI disease are common causes of hypocalcemia
• Endotoxemia may be the underlying stimulus that triggers several mechanisms leading to hypocalcemia
• Plasma calcium concentrations may decline during the postoperative period after abdominal surgery and while receiving IV fluid therapy
• Hypocalcemia may contribute to ileus

Excessive Sweating and Exertional Rhabdomyolysis
• Horses lose calcium, chloride, and potassium in sweat
• Endurance horses are especially prone to electrolyte imbalances and acid–base disturbances (e.g. alkalosis) after prolonged activity, and may develop SDF. In addition to calcium loss in sweat, the ionized calcium fraction is further reduced in alkalosis
• Hypocalcemia has been reported in neonatal foals with severe rhabdomyolysis. The pathogenesis of hypocalcemia in exertional rhabdomyolysis is not understood

Renal Disease
Horses with acute kidney injury may be hypo-, hyper-, or normocalcemic. Although hypercalcemia is more common, some horses in chronic renal failure may have normocalcemia early in the disease process or if not on an alfalfa or high calcium diet.

Oxalate Toxicity
Several plant species contain oxalates, which, in excess, reduce calcium absorption.

C

Drug Induced
- Oxytetracycline—acute signs of hypocalcemia may occur immediately following drug administration
- Furosemide—promotes diuresis and inhibits calcium reabsorption at the level of the distal tubules in the kidney; horses may not exhibit clinical signs

RISK FACTORS
See Causes.

DIAGNOSIS
DIFFERENTIAL DIAGNOSIS
Tetany/Stiffness
- Tetanus—normal serum calcium concentration, history of wound, does not exhibit SDF, does not respond to treatment with calcium, hyperresponsive to sound, and prolapse of the third eyelid
- Strychnine—normal serum calcium concentration
- Exertional rhabdomyolysis, myositis—marked increases in creatine kinase and aspartate aminotransferase activity; myoglobinuria
- Laminitis—lameness, bounding digital pulses, and characteristic stance

SDF
Asynchronous diaphragmatic flutter (hiccups).

CBC/BIOCHEMISTRY/URINALYSIS
- General—concurrent hypomagnesemia commonly is seen during many conditions associated with hypocalcemia
- Cantharidin toxicosis—hypomagnesemia, hematuria, and normal to isosthenuric urine specific gravity
- Excessive exercise, endurance events—SDF—hypocalcemia, hypokalemia, hypochloremia, and alkalosis
- NHP—normal renal function; depending on stage of disease, hypocalcemia, hyperphosphatemia, and elevated ALP concentration
- Pancreatic disease—increased amylase, lipase, γ-glutamyltransferase, and peritoneal amylase

OTHER LABORATORY TESTS
- Measurement of ionized calcium concentration by ion-selective electrodes requires special sample handling and may not be readily available
- Dietary deficiency or imbalance—inspection of feed, chemical analysis for calcium and phosphorus
- NHP—increased urinary phosphorus and decreased urinary calcium concentrations
- Cantharidin toxicosis—presence of blister beetles in hay; determination of cantharidin

in urine or stomach contents is definitive; loss of activity of toxic principal in urine occurs ≅5 days after consumption; urine collected early is most diagnostic

IMAGING
Conventional radiology has little benefit in detecting loss of skeletal mineralization until losses exceed 30%.

OTHER DIAGNOSTIC PROCEDURES
N/A

PATHOLOGIC FINDINGS
Dependent on the underlying cause.

TREATMENT
- General—symptomatic to control pain with analgesics, maintain hydration with fluids, broad-spectrum antibiotics for suspected bacterial infections, supplementation with high-calcium feeds (e.g. alfalfa, legume hays)
- NHP—correct dietary deficiency or imbalance by supplying the deficient nutrient
- Cantharidin toxicosis—no antidote available, remove contaminated feed, supportive therapy (e.g. activated charcoal, evacuate GI tract, diuretics)
- Sources of calcium include alfalfa or legume hay, molasses, limestone, bonemeal, or dicalcium phosphate
- Dietary calcium–phosphorus ratio should not exceed 1.5–2:1

MEDICATIONS
DRUG(S) OF CHOICE
IV calcium solutions—20% calcium borogluconate diluted with saline, dextrose, or lactated Ringer's solution.

CONTRAINDICATIONS
N/A

PRECAUTIONS
- Calcium is cardiotoxic. Administer solutions containing calcium slowly, with constant monitoring of heart rate and rhythm. Stop treatment at once if dysrhythmia or bradycardia develops
- Rapid IV administration of tetracycline, which chelates calcium, can lead to cardiac arrhythmias, collapse, and death
- Furosemide administration promotes urinary calcium and magnesium excretion
- Excessive bicarbonate administration causes alkalosis, which decreases calcium

POSSIBLE INTERACTIONS
N/A

ALTERNATIVE DRUGS
N/A

FOLLOW-UP
PATIENT MONITORING
With hypocalcemic tetany, recovery may take several days and relapses can occur.

PREVENTION/AVOIDANCE
See Causes.

POSSIBLE COMPLICATIONS
N/A

EXPECTED COURSE AND PROGNOSIS
Dependent on the underlying cause.

MISCELLANEOUS
ASSOCIATED CONDITIONS
SDF—oral administration of large quantities of sodium bicarbonate to hypochloremic and volume-depleted horses, salmonellosis, severe diarrhea, laminitis, abdominal disorders, postoperative rhabdomyolysis, myositis, uterine torsion, lactation tetany, overexertion, cantharidin toxicosis, thoracic hematoma, and trauma.

AGE-RELATED FACTORS
N/A

PREGNANCY/FERTILITY/BREEDING
See Hypocalcemic Tetany (Lactation, Transport).

SYNONYMS
- NHP—bighead disease, bran disease, osteodystrophia fibrosa, and Miller disease
- SDF—thumps

SEE ALSO
- Calcium, hypercalcemia
- Cantharidin toxicosis
- Metabolic Disorders in Endurance Horses
- Phosphorous, hyperphosphatemia
- Phosphorus, hypophosphatemia

ABBREVIATIONS
- ALP = alkaline phosphatase
- GI = gastrointestinal
- NHP = nutritional secondary hyperparathyroidism
- SDF = synchronous diaphragmatic flutter

Suggested Reading
Aguilera-Tejero E. Calcium homeostasis and derangements. In: Fielding CL, Magdesian KG, eds. Equine Fluid Therapy. Ames, IA: Wiley, 2015:55–75.
Toribio RE. Parathyroid gland, calcium and phosphorus regulation. In: Smith BP, ed. Large Animal Internal Medicine, 5e. St. Louis, MO: Elsevier Mosby, 2015:1244–1252.

Author Karen E. Russell
Consulting Editor Sandra D. Taylor

CANTHARIDIN TOXICOSIS

C

BASICS

OVERVIEW
• Cantharidin is the toxic compound found in blister beetles (primarily *Epicauta* spp. but also *Pyrota* spp.)
• Toxicosis results from ingestion of baled alfalfa hay, or other alfalfa feeds, containing dead blister beetles
• Cantharidin is rapidly absorbed from the GI tract and is excreted unchanged in the urine
• The vesicant properties of cantharidin cause irritation, vesicle formation, ulceration, or erosions throughout the GI tract and bladder
• Colic and/or sudden death
• Hypocalcemia, hypomagnesemia, renal failure, cardiac abnormalities
• Large swarms of blister beetles concentrate in alfalfa fields from the southern USA

SIGNALMENT
• All ages affected
• No genetic or sex predisposition

SIGNS
• Typically several horses are affected within minutes to hours after feeding
• Severity depends on the amount of cantharidin ingested
• High doses = sudden death within hours; lower doses = symptoms that last for days
• Restlessness, irritability
• Sweating, fever
• Colic, pawing the ground
• Muscle fasciculations
• Diaphragmatic flutter
• Anorexia, loose stools, oral lesions
• Playing in water without drinking
• Congested mucous membranes, increased capillary refill times
• Tachycardia, tachypnea
• Stranguria, hematuria
• Aggressive behavior
• Seizures before death

CAUSES AND RISK FACTORS
• Feeding of baled alfalfa that has been crimped or alfalfa cubes/pellets increases risk
• Large swarms of beetles within fields among mature alfalfa or flowering plants
• Malicious poisoning has occurred

DIAGNOSIS

DIFFERENTIAL DIAGNOSIS
• Colic from a variety of other causes
• Ionophore toxicosis
• History of feeding alfalfa or alfalfa products, hypocalcemia with or without concurrent hypomagnesemia, and discovery of beetles in hay or GI contents

CBC/BIOCHEMISTRY/URINALYSIS
• Hypocalcemia
• Hypomagnesemia

• Hyposthenuria with possible hematuria
• Hyperproteinemia and increased packed cell volume due to dehydration
• Leukocytosis may be observed in cases of bacterial infection-compromised GI epithelium

OTHER LABORATORY TESTS
N/A

IMAGING
N/A

OTHER DIAGNOSTIC PROCEDURES
• Analysis of urine or intestinal contents by HPLC or GC-MS
• Any level of cantharidin detected is considered clinically significant
• Urine (500 mL) is the specimen of choice for cantharidin analysis
• Intestinal contents (500 mL) can also be tested
• Analysis for cantharidin should be done early on since it is rapidly excreted through the urine unchanged
• Liver, kidney, and serum can be used but are not the specimens of choice

PATHOLOGIC FINDINGS
• Large doses can result in sudden death without gross lesions
• Gross lesions may include ulceration of the oral mucosa and lips but are most common in the terminal esophagus, stomach, and the intestines, which may consist of areas of ulceration or erosion that may (or may not) be hemorrhagic
• Hyperemic areas of the mucosal lining of the entire GI tract and urinary bladder have been noted
• White streaks on the heart may be seen grossly
• Microscopic lesions include acantholysis of the mucosa of the GI tract, epithelium of the urinary tract, and endothelium of vessels. Myocarditis, renal tubular nephrosis, and degenerative changes in the kidneys and GI tract can also be seen

TREATMENT

• Cantharidin toxicosis is an emergency and requires in-hospital treatment
• Focus treatment on enhancing fecal and urinary elimination of cantharidin, correcting dehydration, managing serum calcium and magnesium abnormalities, and controlling pain
• Intensive supportive treatment may be required for 3–10 days, depending on the severity of illness
• Initiate fluid therapy to adequately rehydrate the horse, decrease serum cantharidin levels, and aid in toxin excretion via the kidneys
• Monitor serum calcium frequently
• Stall rest for 5–10 days

MEDICATIONS

DRUG(S) OF CHOICE
• Administer AC (1–4 g/kg as an aqueous slurry) via nasogastric tube, then mineral oil (2–4 L) 2–3 h later to prevent occupation of adsorptive sites on the AC
• Repeated doses of mineral oil recommended
• Adult horses may receive 500 mL of a commercial calcium-containing fluid (not exceeding 23 g of calcium compound per 100 mL) if administered slowly. Dilute commercial calcium preparations in isotonic fluids to decrease the chance of adverse cardiac responses and to allow more rapid administration. Dilute calcium in a ratio of 1:4 with saline or dextrose if frequent administration is required to control synchronous diaphragmatic flutter or muscle fasciculations
• Hypomagnesemia may require addition of magnesium as well as calcium to the isotonic fluids
• Prednisolone sodium succinate (50–100 mg as an initial dose) may be administered IV over 1 min for severe shock
• Consider sucralfate (1 g per 45 kg PO every 6–8 h) in horses exhibiting clinical signs of gastritis—water playing
• Commonly prescribed analgesics (e.g. flunixin meglumine) may not provide adequate pain relief. Therefore, administer α₂-adrenergic agonists (e.g. detomidine 20–40 µg/kg IV or butorphanol tartrate 0.02–0.1 mg/kg IV every 3–4 h, not to exceed 48 h). Detomidine at 40 µg/kg dose should provide analgesia for 45–75 min
• Xylazine (1.1 mg/kg IV) is also an α₂-adrenergic agonist and may be substituted for detomidine for analgesia
• Use broad-spectrum antibiotic therapy if septic complications from GI mucosal ulceration are likely

CONTRAINDICATIONS/POSSIBLE INTERACTIONS
• Do not include calcium in fluids containing sodium bicarbonate because of possible precipitation of calcium
• Aminoglycoside antibiotics are potentially nephrotoxic and should be avoided
• Nonsteroidal anti-inflammatory drugs should be used with caution because of potential GI and renal complications
• Diuretics—furosemide
• Acepromazine maleate—may potentiate shock
• Do not administer detomidine concurrently with potentiated sulfonamides (e.g. trimethoprim–sulfa combinations) because fatal dysrhythmias can result
• Use caution with corticosteroids—they are reported to cause laminitis

(CONTINUED) **CANTHARIDIN TOXICOSIS**

 FOLLOW-UP

PATIENT MONITORING
Monitor hydration status, electrolytes, and response to analgesics.

PREVENTION/AVOIDANCE
• Do not feed contaminated alfalfa
• Owners should inspect hay for beetles when feeding. Inspection can be aided by feeding small individual flakes instead of large bales. This may not be possible for hay cubes
• Cut hay before the bloom stage so plants do not attract adult blister beetles. First cutting and late cuttings are often safer because they are before and after peak beetle activity, respectively
• Avoid driving equipment over and crushing standing or cut hay

POSSIBLE COMPLICATIONS
• Complications are unusual, but laminitis has been reported

• Any time the heart is damaged, there could be the possibility of sudden death

EXPECTED COURSE AND PROGNOSIS
• Prognosis ranges from poor to excellent and depends on the amount of cantharidin ingested, early recognition of intoxication, and aggressiveness of therapy
• A more favorable prognosis may be given if the animal survives for 2–3 days after toxin exposure

 MISCELLANEOUS

PREGNANCY/FERTILITY/BREEDING
Use corticosteroids with caution in pregnant mares.

SYNONYMS
• Blister beetle poisoning
• Equine cantharidiasis

ABBREVIATIONS
• AC = activated charcoal
• GC-MS = gas chromatography mass spectrometry
• GI = gastrointestinal
• HPLC = high-pressure liquid chromatography

Suggested Reading
Gwaltney-Brant SH, Dunayer EK, Youssef HY. Terrestrial zootoxins. In: Gupta RC, ed. Veterinary Toxicology: Basic and Clinical Principles. San Diego, CA: Elsevier, 2012:969–992.
Stair EL, Plumlee KH. Insects. In: Plumlee KH, ed. Clinical Veterinary Toxicology. St. Louis, MO: Mosby, 2004:101–103.

Author Scott L. Radke
Consulting Editors Wilson K. Rumbeiha and Steve Ensley
Acknowledgment The editors acknowledge the prior contribution of Sandra E. Morgan.

CARDIOTOXIC PLANTS

BASICS

DEFINITION
• Major toxins are cardiac glycosides found in a number of unrelated plants, e.g. oleander (*Nerium oleander*), summer pheasant's eye (*Adonis aestivalis*), foxglove (*Digitalis purpurea*), lily of the valley (*Convallaria majalis*), dogbane (*Apocynum* spp.), and some species of milkweed (*Asclepias* spp.)
• Oleander most common
• Other cardiotoxic plants that have poisoned horses include yew (*Taxus* spp.), grayanotoxin-containing plants (*Rhododendron* spp., *Kalmia* spp., and *Pieris japonica*), avocado (*Persea* spp.), death camas (*Zigadenus* spp.), and cheeseweed mallow (*Malva parviflora*)

PATHOPHYSIOLOGY
• Acute intoxications and are rapidly absorbed from the GI tract
• Cardiac glycosides have positive inotropic effect due to increased intracellular Ca^{2+}. Also, direct effects on the sympathetic nervous system
• Yews contain taxine alkaloids (major alkaloids are taxine A and taxine B) that are rapidly absorbed, metabolized, conjugated in the liver, and eliminated in urine as conjugated benzoic acid (hippuric acid). Increase cytoplasmic calcium, resulting in the depression of cardiac depolarization and conduction. Yews also contain nitriles (cyanogenic glycoside esters), ephedrine, and irritant oils that may cause colic and diarrhea
• Grayanotoxins are diterpenes that exert toxicity by maintaining cells in a state of depolarization. The membrane effects caused by grayanotoxins account for the observed responses of skeletal and myocardial muscle, nerves, and the central nervous system
• The toxic compound in avocado is persin, but the exact mechanism of action remains unclear
• Death camas contains steroidal alkaloids such as zygacine and zygadenine. The alkaloids decrease blood pressure, slow the heart rate, and lead to respiratory depression
• Cyclopropene fatty acids present in cheeseweed mallow are suspected to impair beta-oxidation, leading to acute myopathy and cardiomyopathy

SYSTEMS AFFECTED
• Cardiovascular
• GI

INCIDENCE/PREVALENCE
• Ingestion of dried oleander clippings or oleander-contaminated hay is a common cause of toxicity
• Yew, death camas, and avocado poisoning are relatively uncommon
• Grayanotoxin and cheeseweed mallow poisonings are uncommon in horses

GEOGRAPHIC DISTRIBUTION
• Cardiotoxic plants have specific distributions in the USA
• Oleander—southern USA; summer pheasant's eye limited to northern California
• Grayanotoxins are widely distributed in the USA
• Avocado is extensively cultivated in California and Florida
• Death camas species are most abundant in the spring
• Cheeseweed mallow is a common weed found in pastures in the USA

SIGNALMENT
No breed, age, or sex predilections.

SIGNS
• Acute death common
• Colic often seen within hours of exposure
• Progression is rapid and animals develop weakness, tremors, excessive salivation, incoordination, dyspnea, and sometimes convulsions
• Irregular fast pulse with tachycardia, ventricular arrhythmias, or gallop rhythms are common
• *Adonis* spp. poisoning in horses leads to GI stasis, anorexia, dyspnea, and cardiac arrhythmias
• Horses exposed to avocado develop subcutaneous edema of the head and chest, submandibular edema, respiratory dyspnea, and cardiac arrhythmias
• *Taxus* poisoning—incoordination, nervousness, difficulty in breathing, bradycardia, diarrhea, and convulsions, but sudden death is often all that is seen
• Grayanotoxin poisoning—depression, severe salivation, and abdominal pain. In severe cases, the animals may become laterally recumbent and develop seizures, tachycardia, tachypnea, and pyrexia
• Cheeseweed mallow poisoning—diffuse sweating, muscle fasciculations, and tachycardia

CAUSES
• Oleander and yew—most common cause of acute poisoning with cardiogenic plants
• All parts of oleander are toxic, whether fresh or dried; 5–10 leaves can cause illness and death in an adult horse
• All parts of the yew, green or dried, with the exception of the red fleshy part surrounding the seed (aril portion) are toxic. Ingestion of yew clippings is most often the cause of poisonings
• Grayanotoxin poisoning usually occurs when animals are offered plant trimmings or stray into wooded areas where little else is available to eat. The leaves of the plants are considered the greatest risk
• Avocado leaves are especially toxic, but ingestion of fruit and seeds can also result in poisoning
• Death camas leaves during the early stages of growth pose the greatest risk for poisoning.

Seeds and fruits as well as the dried plant in hay are also toxic
• Compounds responsible for cheeseweed mallow poisoning are suspected to be cyclopropene fatty acids that have highest concentrations in seeds

RISK FACTORS
• Fresh plant material is often considered to be of low palatability, so animals are most likely to ingest dried plant material
• Contamination of hay or hay cubes with oleander is of great risk
• The Guatemalan race of avocados and its hybrid ("Fuerte") are reportedly toxic, while the Mexican race has low toxicity

DIAGNOSIS

DIFFERENTIAL DIAGNOSIS
• Ionophore antibiotics—detection in the feed, histologic lesions
• Cyanide poisoning—mucous membranes are initially bright cherry red; evidence of exposure to cyanogenic plants, chemical analysis for cyanide in GI contents, liver, or muscle
• Organophosphorus or carbamate insecticide exposure—commonly associated with GI and neurologic signs, evaluation of cholinesterase activity, detection in GI contents
• Exposure to neurotoxic plants, such as poison hemlock, water hemlock, tree tobacco, lupine—chemical analysis for plant toxins in GI contents, history of presence of plants in the environment
• Exposure to star of Bethlehem—severe diarrhea
• Myocarditis—murmurs are usually present; differentiate echocardiographically
• Endocarditis—fever; differentiate echocardiographically
• Intestinal compromise—physical examination

CBC/BIOCHEMISTRY/URINALYSIS
• Serum chemistry changes are limited
• Myocardial damage may result in hyperkalemia, elevated lactate dehydrogenase, creatine kinase, and aspartate aminotransferase activities, and elevated cardiac troponin I

OTHER LABORATORY TESTS
• Analytic detection of cardiotoxins in serum, stomach, cecal, or colon contents, and liver
• Visual and microscopic examination of stomach or intestinal contents for plant fragments
• Acyl carnitine profiles are altered after cheeseweed mallow exposure

DIAGNOSTIC PROCEDURES
ECG disturbances are supportive—atrioventricular conduction blocks and ventricular arrhythmias.

(CONTINUED)   **CARDIOTOXIC PLANTS**

PATHOLOGIC FINDINGS
- In peracute cases, no lesions are found
- Postmortem lesions are generally nonspecific in animals that die
- Oleander poisoning—fluid in the pericardium and body cavities, endocardial hemorrhages, and multifocal myocardial degeneration and necrosis. Mural thrombi and subepicardial hemorrhage can be seen
- *Taxus* poisoning—mild to moderate endocardial hemorrhages in both ventricles. Histologically, acute multifocal contraction band necrosis of the ventricular wall and the papillary muscles and occasional neutrophilic and lymphocytic infiltrates in the interstitium of the myocardium are noted
- No or very few lesions with yew, grayanotoxin, or death camas poisoning
- Avocado poisoning—fluid accumulation in the pericardial sac and in the thoracic and abdominal cavities
- Cheeseweed mallow poisoning results in myocardial necrosis in atrial and ventricular walls. Skeletal muscle necrosis may also be seen

TREATMENT
AIMS
- Prevent further exposure to cardiotoxic plant
- Decontamination
- Provide supportive therapy

APPROPRIATE HEALTH CARE
- Immediate removal of the toxic plant material to prevent further exposure. Provide the animals with good quality feed
- Adsorption of toxins with AC has been suggested. Multidose AC is beneficial in oleander intoxications
- Treatment of animals exposed to cardiotoxic plants is primarily supportive and symptomatic. Supportive therapy should include administration of IV fluids, antiarrhythmics, and antibiotics if indicated
- Avoid stress
- If edema is present in avocado poisoning, administration of diuretics is recommended
- Atropine should be considered in cases of severe bradycardia

NURSING CARE
- Decontamination procedures include administration of AC (1–4 g/kg PO in a watery slurry (1 g of AC in 5 mL of water)) via stomach tube

- Correct electrolyte losses according to clinical chemistry findings. Recommended IV fluid in oleander poisoning is 0.9% NaCl with 2.5% dextrose as a constant rate infusion of 3 mg/kg/h

ACTIVITY
Keep the animal quiet.

DIET
Provide high-quality diet free of toxic plants.

CLIENT EDUCATION
- Recognize cardiotoxic plants of concern in the geographic location and prevent access by the horse
- Provide adequate forage to limit ingestion of toxic plants

SURGICAL CONSIDERATIONS
N/A

MEDICATIONS
DRUG(S) OF CHOICE
- Antiarrhythmics (guided by ECG monitoring)
- Atropine (0.01–0.02 mg/kg IV) to treat bradyarrhythmias
- AC

CONTRAINDICATIONS
- Do not administer potassium in fluids if hyperkalemia is present
- Avoid calcium-containing solutions and quinidine

ALTERNATIVE DRUGS
Anticardiac glycoside Fab antibodies have been used in humans and small animals, but their efficacy is unknown in poisoned horses.

FOLLOW-UP
PATIENT MONITORING
Monitor progression of clinical signs and evaluate ECG.

PREVENTION/AVOIDANCE
- Horses should be denied access to landscaped yards and discarded clippings
- Suspect forage should be inspected for the presence of cardiotoxic plants before allowing access
- Hay should be inspected carefully for weeds, as many cardiotoxic plants remain toxic when dried (oleander, death camas, yew)

POSSIBLE COMPLICATIONS
N/A

EXPECTED COURSE AND PROGNOSIS
- Animals poisoned with cardiotoxic plants are often found dead
- Cardiotoxic plant exposure progresses so rapidly that treatment is often too late. In oleander and yew intoxications, the prognosis is poor
- If treatment is initiated promptly after the onset of clinical signs, the prognosis is fair
- Animals that survive the acute poisoning may suffer from myocardial damage and may be more prone to stress

MISCELLANEOUS
ASSOCIATED CONDITIONS
N/A

AGE-RELATED FACTORS
N/A

ZOONOTIC POTENTIAL
N/A

PREGNANCY/FERTILITY/BREEDING
N/A

ABBREVIATIONS
- AC = activated charcoal
- GI = gastrointestinal

Suggested Reading
Bauquier J, Stent A, Gibney J, et al. Evidence for marsh mallow (*Malva parviflora*) toxicosis causing myocardial disease and myopathy in four horses. Equine Vet J 2017;49(3):307–313.
Casteel SW. Taxine alkaloids. In: Plumlee KH, ed. Clinical Veterinary Toxicology. St. Louis, MO: Mosby, 2004:379–381.
Galey FG. Cardiac glycosides. In: Plumlee KH, ed. Clinical Veterinary Toxicology. St. Louis, MO: Mosby, 2004:386–388.
Puschner B. Grayanotoxins. In: Plumlee KH, ed. Clinical Veterinary Toxicology. St. Louis, MO: Mosby, 2004:412–415.
Tiwary AK, Puschner B, Kinde H, et al. Diagnosis of Taxus (yew) poisoning in a horse. J Vet Diagn Invest 2005;17:252–255.

Author Birgit Puschner
Consulting Editors Wilson K. Rumbeiha and Steve Ensley

CASTRATION, HENDERSON CASTRATION INSTRUMENT

BASICS

OVERVIEW
• Common technique for the elective surgical removal of the testes in equids
• Organ systems affected—reproductive

SIGNALMENT
Intact male equids of any age.

SIGNS
Normal testis size, shape, and consistency.

CAUSES AND RISK FACTORS
N/A

DIAGNOSIS

DIFFERENTIAL DIAGNOSIS
N/A

CBC/BIOCHEMISTRY/URINALYSIS
Laboratory parameters should be normal prior to routine castration.

OTHER LABORATORY TESTS
N/A

IMAGING
N/A

OTHER DIAGNOSTIC PROCEDURES
N/A

PATHOLOGIC FINDINGS
N/A

TREATMENT
• The castration uses a closed technique under general anesthesia
• The patient is placed in lateral recumbency with the upper rear limb pulled lateral/caudal to expose the testes
• The patient is scrubbed and prepared for surgery as described for routine castration
• The testes are exposed following a scrotal skin incision over each testis or by removing a 3 cm strip of the median raphe of the scrotum
• The fascia is stripped away from the exteriorized testicle, exposing the spermatic cord as far proximal as possible
• The Henderson instrument is inserted into a 14.4 V cordless hand drill with a 0.95 cm (0.375 inch) removable chuck
• The drill is placed in a sterile shroud
• The pliers of the instrument are placed on the spermatic cord just proximal to the testis
• The drill is powered to rotate the instrument in a slow clockwise direction. Allow the tip of the instrument to be drawn into the incision, approximately 2 cm, as it starts to rotate. As the spermatic cord twists, do not allow the

instrument to go any farther into the incision. The rotation can moderately be increased, as the cord starts to elongate just before it severs. Once the cord fatigues, more tension can be placed on the cord to complete its separation and removal of the testis. A tightly coiled cord is left behind, which achieves hemostasis
• The instrument is removed and the operation is repeated on the other side. The incision site is inspected for bleeders. Excess fascia and/or fat is removed. The incision is left open and sprayed with a topical antiseptic/spray bandage. The horse is allowed to stand and is put into a stall to complete anesthetic recovery

MEDICATIONS

DRUG(S) OF CHOICE
Anesthesia
• Preoperative sedation with xylazine (1.0–1.1 mg/kg IV)
• Butorphanol (0.01–0.02 mg/kg IV) may be combined with xylazine to further sedation and analgesia
• Induction with ketamine hydrochloride (2.2 mg/kg IV) combined with diazepam (0.03–0.06 mg/kg IV)
• Anti-inflammatory therapy to help control swelling and pain postoperatively—phenylbutazone (2–4 mg/kg PO or IV) or flunixin meglumine (1 mg/kg) or ketoprofen (0.5 mg/kg)
• Antibiotic therapy is not needed in a routine, uncomplicated castration
• Tetanus toxoid prophylaxis

CONTRAINDICATIONS/POSSIBLE INTERACTIONS
N/A

FOLLOW-UP
N/A

PATIENT MONITORING
• The patient should be confined to the stall until complete recovery from anesthesia
• The surgical site should be monitored daily for hemorrhage, evisceration, excessive swelling, and/or infection
• Forced exercise twice daily for a minimum of 20 min for the first 10–12 days to help reduce swelling and improve drainage
• Cold water therapy for 15–20 min daily for 3–5 days

PREVENTION/AVOIDANCE
N/A

POSSIBLE COMPLICATIONS
• Hemorrhage—excessive hemorrhage may occur if too much tension is put on the spermatic cord before it fatigues and fractures
• Treatment for excessive hemorrhage should include identification and ligation of blood vessels
• Excessive preputial/scrotal swelling results from poor drainage from the scrotum:
  ○ Tranquilization, surgical scrub, and manually opening the surgical site will allow drainage
• Excessive preputial/scrotal swelling may also result from infection. If infected—antibiotics, anti-inflammatory therapy, and drainage of the site are indicated
• Evisceration of the abdominal contents is an uncommon occurrence, which can be fatal if not treated. The horse should be anesthetized, the intestinal contents cleaned, and viable intestine replaced. The superficial ring should be sutured closed
• Some males may continue to display male-like behavior despite castration. This is a learned behavior and is not associated with testosterone production

EXPECTED COURSE AND PROGNOSIS
N/A

MISCELLANEOUS

ASSOCIATED CONDITIONS
A simplified version of the technique, "Equitwister," has been described.

AGE-RELATED FACTORS
N/A

ZOONOTIC POTENTIAL
N/A

PREGNANCY/FERTILITY/BREEDING
N/A

SEE ALSO
Castration, routine

Internet Resources
1 The Horse. The Equitwister: a simplified way to castrate working equids. http://www.thehorse.com/articles/37413/the-equitwister-a-simplified-way-to-castrate-working-equids

Suggested Reading
Reilly MT, Cimetti LJ. How to use the Henderson castration instrument and minimize castration complications. Proceedings of the 51st American Association of Equine Practitioners (AAEP), Seattle (3–7 December 2005). Lexington, KY: AAEP, 2005.

Author Ahmed Tibary
Consulting Editor Carla L. Carleton

BASICS

OVERVIEW
Routine surgical removal of the testes is the most common surgical technique in the male equid for sterilization; eliminates male behavior.

SIGNALMENT
Intact male horse.

SIGNS
Performed on male with normal descended testes.

CAUSES AND RISK FACTORS
Mules and males not intended for breeding.

DIAGNOSIS
N/A

DIFFERENTIAL DIAGNOSIS
N/A

CBC/BIOCHEMISTRY/URINALYSIS
Laboratory parameters should be normal prior to routine castration.

OTHER LABORATORY TESTS
N/A

IMAGING
N/A

OTHER DIAGNOSTIC PROCEDURES
N/A

PATHOLOGIC FINDINGS
N/A

TREATMENT
• Castration can be performed standing using local anesthesia or in lateral recumbency under general anesthesia
• Standing castration—advantage that recovery is faster and with less risk of injury during anesthetic recovery
• Castration using general anesthesia, placing the animal in lateral recumbency, allows for greater safety for the surgeon, better exposure to the surgical site, and much better analgesia
• Closed technique (vaginal tunic is not incised) versus open technique (vaginal tunic is opened and the testes are completely exposed)—can be standing or under general anesthesia
• Three 30 s scrubs of the scrotal area using povidone–iodine (Betadine) and/or chlorhexidine scrub; 2–3 mL of lidocaine is injected into each testis or spermatic cord, to achieve further analgesia before the last scrub

• 2 incisions are made over the testes, 1 cm from the midline of the scrotum, and a 3–4 cm strip of skin is removed, exposing the testes
• The fascia is stripped away from 1 exteriorized testicle to expose the spermatic cord to the inguinal ring
• *Closed technique*—the emasculators are placed as close to the body wall as possible to remove as much of the cord as possible
• *Open technique*—the tunic over the testis is excised and the testis is exposed. The emasculators are placed closed to the body wall on the artery, vein, and nerve of the exposed cord and are emasculated followed by the exposed tunic, which is emasculated close to the body wall
• The other testis is removed using either the closed or open technique
• In large stallions, the mesorchium should be separated above the epididymis and the cord separated into the neurovascular and musculofibrous (cremaster muscle, vaginal tunic, and ductus deferens) portions before emasculation
• Following emasculation, maintain hold on one side of the stump to keep it in view and observe it for any bleeding. If there is no bleeding from the site, the incision is inspected to ensure that it is open and will drain readily (to avoid serum accumulation)
• Remove any loose tags of fascia or fat that protrude from the incision
• Spray the area with an antiseptic solution and fly spray

MEDICATIONS

DRUG(S) OF CHOICE
General Anesthesia
• Preoperative sedation with xylazine (1.0–1.1 mg/kg IV) with or without butorphanol (0.01–0.02 mg/kg IV)
• Induction with ketamine hydrochloride (2.2 mg/kg IV) combined with diazepam (0.03–0.06 mg/kg IV)
• Anti-inflammatory therapy—phenylbutazone (2–4 mg/kg PO or IV)
• Antibiotic therapy is not needed for a routine, uncomplicated castration
• Tetanus toxoid ± antitoxin depending on vaccination history

FOLLOW-UP

PATIENT MONITORING
• Minimum of 20 min of moderate, daily forced exercise BID is essential

• The surgical site should be monitored daily for hemorrhage, evisceration, excessive swelling, and/or infection
• Cold water therapy/hydrotherapy for 15–20 min daily for 3–5 days

POSSIBLE COMPLICATIONS
• Minor hemorrhage occurs through the skin, which should stop within 30 min
• Treatment for excessive hemorrhage is identification and ligation of bleeding vessels
• Excessive preputial/scrotal swelling results from poor drainage from the scrotum
  ○ Tranquilization, surgical scrub, and manually opening (stretching) the surgical site will facilitate drainage
  ○ Moderate forced exercise is the best means to ensure the surgical site will remain open and draining
  ○ Excessive preputial/scrotal swelling may also result from infection. If infected, antibiotics, anti-inflammatory therapy, and drainage of the site are indicated
• Evisceration of the abdominal contents is an uncommon occurrence, which can be fatal if left untreated. The horse should be anesthetized and the intestinal contents cleaned and viable intestine replaced. The superficial inguinal ring should be sutured closed
• Masculine behavior following castration is a reflection of learned behavior

MISCELLANEOUS

ASSOCIATED CONDITIONS
N/A

AGE-RELATED FACTORS
Castration of prepubertal horses may result in a taller animal when mature.

ZOONOTIC POTENTIAL
N/A

PREGNANCY/FERTILITY/BREEDING
N/A

SEE ALSO
Castration, Henderson castration instrument

Suggested Reading
Kilcoyne I. Equine castration: a review of techniques, complications and their management. Equine Vet Educ 2013;25:479–482.

Author Ahmed Tibary
Consulting Editor Carla L. Carleton
Acknowledgment The author and editor acknowledge the prior contribution of Alfred B. Caudle.

CENTAUREA AND ACROPTILON TOXICOSIS

BASICS

OVERVIEW
• *Centaurea solstitialis* (yellow star thistle) is an annual weed found commonly in the northwestern USA. The plant is about 1 m in height. The flower is yellow with a composite head and sharp thorns around the flower head
• *Acroptilon repens*, with synonyms *Centaurea repens* and *Rhaponticum repens* (Russian knapweed), is a perennial weed found mainly in western USA; it can appear in eastern USA as well. The plant is about 1 m in height and has a cone-shaped flowering head that is pinkish-purple with spreading rhizomes, which make control difficult. In general, it is not readily grazed
• Ingestion of either plant can result in ENE, or "chewing disease," characterized by the abrupt appearance of difficulties in eating and drinking. Typically, affected animals lose condition and die

SIGNALMENT
There is no breed, age, or sex predilection.

SIGNS
• Depression/drowsiness
• Difficulty eating and drinking
• Aimless walking with head low
• Head pressing
• Abnormal gait or incoordination
• Hypertonicity of facial and lip muscles
• Tongue lolling
• Loss of body condition
• Dehydration
• Death

CAUSES AND RISK FACTORS
• The toxic principal has not been conclusively identified, although it is suspected to be repin, a sesquiterpene lactone
• Toxicosis is usually chronic rather than acute, requiring plant consumption for at least 2–3 weeks

• A lethal dose of fresh plant material has been given as 2.3–2.6 kg/100 kg body weight for *C. solstitialis* and 1.8–2.5 kg/100 kg body weight for *A. repens*. Often clinical signs will appear suddenly after prolonged ingestion of the plant. Dried plants can also be toxic

DIAGNOSIS

DIFFERENTIAL DIAGNOSIS
• Teeth or mouth abnormalities
• Other chronic disease processes

CBC/BIOCHEMISTRY/URINALYSIS
N/A

OTHER LABORATORY TESTS
N/A

IMAGING
MRI can be used to identify brain lesions.

OTHER DIAGNOSTIC PROCEDURES
• Positive identification of plants
• Evidence of consumption of *C. solstitialis* or *A. repens*
• Plant particles in the stomach can be submitted for feed microscopy

PATHOLOGIC FINDINGS
ENE—foci of necrotic tissue found in the brain, specifically in the globus pallidus and substantia nigra. Several aspects of ENE have been likened to human Parkinson disease.

TREATMENT
• Removal from pasture or source of plants
• Supportive care

MEDICATIONS

DRUG(S) OF CHOICE
N/A

CONTRAINDICATIONS/POSSIBLE INTERACTIONS
N/A

FOLLOW-UP
Remove any nonaffected animals from suspect source.

MISCELLANEOUS

ABBREVIATIONS
• ENE = equine nigropallidal encephalomalacia
• MRI = magnetic resonance imaging

Suggested Reading
Burrows GE, Tyrl RJ. Toxic Plants of North America. Ames, IA: Iowa State University Press, 2001:156–160.
Chang HT, Rumbeiha WK, Patterson JS, et al. Toxic equine parkinsonism: an immunohistochemical study of 10 horses with nigropallidal encephalomalacia. Vet Pathol 2012;49(2):398–402.
Sanders SG, Tucker RL, Bagley RS, Gavin PR. Magnetic resonance imaging features of equine nigropallidal encephalomalacia. Vet Radiol Ultrasound 2001;42(4):291–296.

Author Larry J. Thompson
Consulting Editors Wilson K. Rumbeiha and Steve Ensley

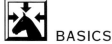

BASICS

OVERVIEW
• A genetic neurologic disease due to neonatal apoptosis of cerebellar Purkinje cells
• The cerebellum processes peripheral proprioceptive input and coordinates the quality of motor activity through its efferent pathways; simplistically, it "tones down" somatic upper motor neurons in the brainstem
• Cerebellar abiotrophy may be an inherited metabolic defect of cortical cerebellar neurons in some breeds, particularly Arabians of Polish, Egyptian, and Spanish types
• The result is formation and then premature death of these neurons during late fetal or early postnatal life, resulting in a cerebellum that may be normal at birth and degenerates thereafter
• Gene mapping of affected Arabian foals has indicated an autosomal recessive single nucleotide polymorphism with variable expression that results in the downregulation of the gene *MUTYH*, involved in the repair of DNA

SIGNALMENT
• Cerebellar abiotrophy occurs in lines of Arabian horses and has occasionally been noted in breeds descended from Arabian horses and Oldenburg, Gotland, and Eriskay foals
• Foals may be affected at birth, but often disease is not evident until a few weeks or months of age

SIGNS

Historical Findings
• Foals appear normal at birth as these clinical syndromes, for the most part, are not congenital

• Affected animals also have a normal gait for a period postnatally, then demonstrate a syndrome related to progressive cerebellar degeneration

Physical Examination Findings
• Head tremor is a characteristic finding in affected horses. It manifests when the horse is heating or with other voluntary movements of the head (intention tremor)
• A basewide stance and hypermetric or hypometric ataxia may be prominent; some affected animals show hypometric gait at a walk, which becomes hypermetric at faster gaits
• There is no weakness. Intention tremor, an absent menace response with intact vision and pupillary light reflexes, is also evident

DIAGNOSIS

• Signalment and clinical signs are characteristic
• A genetic screening test is available. Necropsy will be definitive

DIFFERENTIAL DIAGNOSIS
Cerebellar hypoplasia, i.e. a cerebellum that is small at birth with no further signs of degeneration, is extremely rare in horses. Cerebellar dysfunction due to a structural lesion is also very unusual in horses.

CBC/BIOCHEMISTRY/URINALYSIS
No specific abnormalities.

IMAGING
A small cerebellum is evident on morphometric MRI.

PATHOLOGIC FINDINGS
On gross postmortem examination, the cerebellum weighs less than 10% of the whole brain weight. Histologically, evidence of

degenerative Purkinje and granular cells and swollen Purkinje axons ("torpedoes") may be prominent.

FOLLOW-UP

EXPECTED COURSE AND PROGNOSIS
Poor; this is a progressive condition. Rarely, mildly affected horses may not show increasing signs.

MISCELLANEOUS

ABBREVIATIONS
MRI = magnetic resonance imaging

Suggested Reading
Brault LS, Famula TR, Penedo MC. Inheritance of cerebellar abiotrophy in Arabians. Am J Vet Res 2011;72:940–944.
Cavalleri JM, Metzger J, Hellige M, et al. Morphometric magnetic resonance imaging and genetic testing in cerebellar abiotrophy in Arabian horses. BMC Vet Res 2013;9:105.
MacKay RJ. Neurodegenerative disorders. In: Furr M, Reed S, eds. Equine Neurology, 2e. New York, NY: Wiley Blackwell, 2016:328–342.
Mayhew IG. Large Animal Neurology, 2e. Oxford, UK: Wiley Blackwell, 2008.
Author Caroline N. Hahn
Consulting Editor Caroline N. Hahn

CERVICAL LESIONS

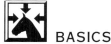

BASICS

DEFINITION
• Inflammation, lacerations, adhesions, and inability to dilate during estrus
• Congenital abnormalities and neoplasia of the cervix uncommon

PATHOPHYSIOLOGY
• The mare's cervix is a tubular structure 5.0–7.5 cm long and 3.5–4.0 cm in diameter, which protects the uterus from the external environment and contamination
• The cervix is formed by an inner circular smooth muscle layer, rich in collagen elastic fibers, and an outer longitudinal smooth muscle layer connecting the vagina with the uterus
• The cervix opens/relaxes depending on hormonal influence and the stage of estrus
• Impaired normal cervical function and competency may lead to infertility, chronic uterine infections, and possible pregnancy loss

SYSTEMS AFFECTED
Reproductive

GENETICS
N/A

INCIDENCE/PREVALENCE
Lacerations are more common in old and/or pluriparous mares. Lack of cervical relaxation is more common in old maiden mares and mares with fibrosis due to extensive cervical manipulation.

SIGNALMENT
• Old (mean age 11–13 years), pluriparous mares (mean parity before surgery 6.2 years) after either normal parturition or dystocia. These mares are more predisposed to cervicitis caused by pneumovagina, urovagina, delayed uterine clearance, and endometritis
• Young or old, maiden mares

SIGNS

Historical Findings
• Infertility
• Poor uterine drainage
• Chronic or recurrent endometritis
• Pyometra
• Pregnancy loss

Physical Examination Findings
• Poor perineal conformation
• Pneumovagina, urovagina, exudate coming through the cervix; cervical and vaginal mucosal irritation; cervical lacerations or mucosal roughness; adhesions between the cervix and vaginal fornix or in the cervical lumen
• Manual examination of the cervix:
  ○ During diestrus—to evaluate cervical closure and tone, the presence and extent of lacerations or adhesions
  ○ During estrus—extent of cervical dilation, assess cervical patency, ability to relax, the presence of intraluminal adhesions
• Ultrasonography of the uterus—presence of intrauterine fluid before or after breeding, quantity, and flocculence

CAUSES

Infectious
• Poor perineal conformation
• Severe acute cervicitis after inoculation/infection with *Taylorella equigenitalis* (contagious equine metritis)
• See also chapters Endometritis and Placentitis

Noninfectious
Cervical Trauma
Parturition, manipulation, and traction; extended fetal pressure against the cervical walls; and use of a fetotome can cause bruising of the cervix.
Two Types of Lacerations
• Overstretching or partial-thickness laceration of the muscular layer with intact mucosa
• Full-thickness laceration occurring during normal, prolonged parturition or dystocia, most frequently occurring in the vaginal portion of the cervix but may extend toward the uterus as far as, and including, the internal cervical os*Adhesions*
• Sequela of cervical trauma during parturition or originating from the use of irritating solutions for uterine therapy, pyometra, and, rarely, chronic endometritis
• Can obliterate the cervical lumen and prevent it from opening and closing properly
Cervicitis
• Iatrogenic, e.g. chemical substances placed in the uterus
• Secondary to trauma, e.g. parturition, dystocia, obstetric manipulation
Idiopathic
• Maiden mares (young or old) with impaired cervical relaxation during estrus with no associated fibrosis or adhesions
• Older mares that have undergone numerous embryo transfer flushes or cervical manipulation can develop a fibrotic cervix or adhesions preventing cervical relaxation
• Maiden mares that conceive will dilate their cervix normally at parturition while a fibrotic cervix is at greater risk of tearing
Neoplasia
Very rare.
Developmental Abnormalities
Rare
Congenital Incompetency
Cervical aplasia, hypoplasia, and double cervix.

RISK FACTORS
• Pluriparous and old mares
• Prolonged natural or assisted parturition
• >2 or 3 cuts with the fetotome

• Maiden mares
• Aggressive uterine therapy
• Concurrent acute and chronic endometritis
• Pyometra

DIAGNOSIS

DIFFERENTIAL DIAGNOSIS
Other causes of vaginal discharge:
• Urovagina/uterus
• Endometritis
• Pyometra
• Placentitis
• Cystitis/urolithiasis

CBC/BIOCHEMISTRY/URINALYSIS
N/A

OTHER LABORATORY TESTS
N/A

IMAGING
Transrectal ultrasonography—fluid accumulation in the uterine lumen caused by a tight cervix, e.g. while still in estrus after breeding or adhesions. If cervix is incomplete owing to a laceration the accumulation of fluid may be due to inflammation and endometritis. Length and width of the cervix can be determined as well as defects of or within the cervix.

OTHER DIAGNOSTIC PROCEDURES
Cervical Examination
• The cervix is examined by TRP, direct visualization with a speculum, and direct vaginal/digital palpation. The last is recommended over speculum examination
• TRP—determines the size, tone, length, and degree of relaxation
• Vaginoscopy—provides information regarding cervical and vaginal color, e.g. hyperemia; presence of edema, secretions, e.g. pus, urine; cysts, varicose veins, or adhesions between the cervical os and vagina
• Digital palpation of the cervix is essential to evaluate lacerations or intraluminal adhesions. It is performed by placing the index finger into the cervical lumen and the thumb on the vaginal side of the cervix, then feeling carefully around its full perimeter for defects and throughout the lumen to the internal os
• During the noncycling phase of the year, place mare on exogenous progesterone for 7 days to evaluate cervical tone, competency, and its ability to close
• Only major defects can be detected immediately postpartum. Evaluate 6 days post ovulation after foal heat for maximal closure and competency. If the cervix has a questionable defect or closure an additional 7 days of exogenous progesterone can aid in diagnosis

PATHOLOGIC FINDINGS
N/A

(CONTINUED)

TREATMENT

APPROPRIATE HEALTH CARE

• Treatment of choice for cervical lacerations depends on the severity (thickness) and extent (length) of the lesion
• Mucosal and submucosal lacerations (up to two-thirds thickness of the wall) can be treated daily with antimicrobial/steroidal anti-inflammatory ointment to avoid cervical adhesions while healing
• Begin treatment of cervical lacerations immediately postpartum to prevent adhesions and infection
• Cervical lacerations of the external os or up to one-third of the length of the cervix may be managed using exogenous progesterone supplementation during diestrus (starting day 6 post ovulation) as long as persistent endometritis does not exist, and pregnancy can be achieved
• Cervical defects more than one-third of the length should be surgically corrected. Healing occurs with fibrous tissue, which lacks the ability to relax or soften as occurs with normal cervical smooth muscle
• Potential postsurgical problems—incomplete cervical dilation/relaxation, retention of intraluminal fluid, adhesions, pyometra, recurrent cervical lacerations during parturition that require repair

Treatment for adhesions
• Recently formed adhesions are debrided daily (manual), and antibiotic/steroid ointment is applied BID
• Cervical adhesions may be bypassed manually by artificial insemination or reduced surgically, recognizing that lack of cervical relaxation affects uterine clearance

Treatment for lack of cervical dilation
• Postbreeding treatment for delayed uterine clearance.
• Manual dilation of the cervix
• Prostaglandin E_1 (misoprostol) placed on/in the cervix
• N-butylscopolammonium bromide (hyoscine butylbromide; Buscopan) cream on/in the cervix. Topical creams relax the muscular cervix better than a fibrotic cervix
• A cervical wedge resection can be performed on the old fibrotic cervix that does not dilate. However, since closure is then incomplete, assisted reproductive techniques, e.g. embryo transfer, are necessary to establish pregnancy

NURSING CARE
• When using antiseptics or nonbuffered antibiotics, check for signs of acute mucosal irritation before administering subsequent treatments
• Following cervical surgical repair—palpation of the cervical canal is necessary to prevent adhesion formation

ACTIVITY
N/A

DIET
N/A

CLIENT EDUCATION
• Routine postpartum evaluation of the reproductive tract of the mare, especially when there is a history of assisted, prolonged manipulation or unassisted, traumatic parturition
• Early identification and treatment of traumatic injuries avoids loss of time during the breeding season; decreases the risk for infertility
• Lack of cervical relaxation necessitates treatment for poor uterine clearance

SURGICAL CONSIDERATIONS
• Cervical repair may be warranted for small cervical lacerations if coupled with a history of infertility and chronic endometritis
• Surgery can be performed standing under epidural anesthesia; if the cervical lesion is extensive or difficult to visualize (usually ventral lesions) general anesthesia and hoisting the pelvic limbs to achieve a Trendelenburg position may be necessary:
• Cervical adhesions should be identified by palpation per vagina and reduced by sharp or blunt dissection depending on the extent of external versus internal cervical involvement
   ○ Excess scar tissue may be trimmed
   ○ Before and after surgery—mares are usually administered broad-spectrum antibiotics and anti-inflammatories
• With a successful surgical repair, prognosis is fair to good for delivering a term foal
• Anatomic defects resulting in cervicitis, such as pneumovagina and urovagina, can be surgically corrected by a Caslick vulvoplasty or a Pouret or Gadd procedure
• Perform endometrial biopsy before surgery to evaluate the endometrium (biopsy category). Unnecessary repair and expense can be avoided if it is found that surgery cannot improve the mare's ability to carry a fetus to term

MEDICATIONS

DRUG(S) OF CHOICE
• Progestin supplementation (altrenogest)
   ○ Double dose (0.088 mg/kg PO daily) during surgery
• Systemic and oral antibiotics
   ○ See chapter Endometritis
• NSAIDs
   ○ Flunixin meglumine—anti-inflammatory dose 1 mg/kg IV or IM BID
   ○ Phenylbutazone—2.2–4.4 mg/kg IV or PO BID
• Prostaglandin E_1 for cervical relaxation—misoprostol 2000 µg/3 mL tube

intracervically 4 h before breeding. Cervix will be dilated for 8 h
• Less effective in older mares with previous cervical trauma
• Frequent application produces irritation
• N-butylscopolammonium bromide (Buscopan) cream aids in normal cervical relaxation more than with a fibrotic cervix
• Local therapy
   ○ Anti-inflammatory, antibiotic, and antifungal cream (Panalog or Animax). Frequency of application is based on severity of lesion or adhesions

CONTRAINDICATIONS
See chapter Endometritis.

PRECAUTIONS
• Certain antiseptics and nonbuffered antibiotics should be used with caution to treat infections of the vagina and uterus since some can cause inflammation and adhesions
• Minimize forced extraction during dystocia, use ample lubrication, and consider cesarean section in cases with intractable cervical induration, poor dilation of the birth canal, as well as with large, deformed, or contracted foals

FOLLOW-UP

PATIENT MONITORING
• Palpation of the cervix and application of sterile lube, an antiadhesion cream, or steroid/antibiotic cream—commence 5–7 days post surgery, continue every 3–4 days for approximately 21 days so that adhesions and stricture of the cervical canal may be prevented
• Sexual rest for 4–6 weeks
• If live cover is necessary, i.e. Thoroughbreds, the use of a stallion roll is advised to limit full intromission during cover

PREVENTION/AVOIDANCE
• Unnecessary manipulation during parturition
• Use of irritants
• Check for normalcy of anatomic barriers that protect the genital tract (perineum, vulva, vestibulovaginal sphincter, and cervix); repair any defects

POSSIBLE COMPLICATIONS
• The scar/site of repair lacks the elasticity of normal cervical tissue. A high percentage will tear again at the next foaling and require annual surgical repair after foaling
• Cervical repair usually prevents complete relaxation during estrus; treatment for delayed or poor uterine clearance may be necessary
• The decision to perform subsequent surgeries is based on the degree of cervical damage after the most recent foaling, assessment of surgical cost, and breeding/treatment expenses versus the potential value of an additional foal

CERVICAL LESIONS

• Lack of cervical dilation or continued/reformed adhesions lead to poor uterine clearance, potentially producing chronic retention of intraluminal fluid, chronic endometritis, and pyometra

EXPECTED COURSE AND PROGNOSIS
• Fair to good for maintenance of pregnancy after successful repair of cervical lacerations
• Guarded prognosis if repair was extensive or unsuccessful

MISCELLANEOUS

ASSOCIATED CONDITIONS
N/A

AGE-RELATED FACTORS
Most common in old, pluriparous mares and young or old maiden mares.

ZOONOTIC POTENTIAL
N/A

PREGNANCY/FERTILITY/BREEDING
See Expected Course and Prognosis.

SEE ALSO
• Artificial insemination
• Delayed uterine involution
• Dystocia
• Endometritis
• Pyometra

ABBREVIATIONS
• NSAID = non-steroidal anti-inflammatory drug
• TRP = transrectal palpation

Suggested Reading
Blanchard TL, Varner D, Schumacher J. Surgery of the mare reproductive tract. In: Manual of Equine Reproduction. St. Louis, MO: Mosby, 1998:165–167.
Makloski-Cohorn CL. Post-operative fertility in mares with cervical defects. Masters thesis. Oklahoma State University, 2009.
O'Leary JM, Rodgerson DH. Foaling rates after surgical repair of ventral cervical lacerations using a Trendelenburg position in 18 anesthetized mares. Vet Surg 2013;42:716–720.
Sertich PL. Cervical problems in the mare. In: McKinnon AO, Voss JL, eds. Equine Reproduction. Philadelphia, PA: Lea & Febiger, 1993:404–407.

Author Karen Wolfsdorf
Consulting Editor Carla L. Carleton
Acknowledgment The author and editor acknowledge the prior contribution of Maria E. Cadario.

CERVICAL VERTEBRAL MALFORMATION

BASICS

OVERVIEW
CVM causes ataxia owing to spinal cord compression. It is the most common cause of ataxia in horses in Europe and Australasia and is an important differential diagnosis in regions affected by inflammatory diseases such as EPM and WNV.

SIGNALMENT
• CVM is reported to be due to either developmental bone disease (type 1 CVM) or secondary to osteoarthritis of the caudal cervical intervertebral joints (type 2 CVM), associated with older horses
• There can be an overlap of these classifications. Affected horses are often large-framed, fast-growing horses
• There likely is a genetic predisposition for the disease. Breeding trials involving both affected males and females have been unable to produce CVM cases but offspring did have a higher prevalence of osteochondritis dissecans lesions in other joints

SIGNS
• Signs can be acute and include progressive paresis and ataxia
• Because of the anatomy of the spinal cord initially signs will only be evident in the pelvic limbs, but eventually the thoracic limbs will be involved as well
• The neurologic signs are due to proprioceptive and upper motor neuron deficits and are characterized by bilaterally symmetric knuckling of the fetlocks, toe dragging, swaying of the body when moving, dysmetria, a "floating" thoracic limb gait, circumduction of the outside pelvic limb when tightly circled, and the horse stepping on its own feet

CAUSES AND RISK FACTORS
• Type 1 CVM is likely a manifestation of DOD; cases have an increased incidence of DOD and osteochondrosis in other joints
• Type 2 CVM is associated with significant arthropathies of the caudal cervical articular processes. External trauma and exercise are likely involved in the pathogenesis

DIAGNOSIS

DIFFERENTIAL DIAGNOSIS
• Cervical fractures—history and/or evidence of trauma. Cervical radiographs

• EPM—CSF and serum antibody titers
• Equine degenerative myeloencephalopathy—young animals with history of low vitamin E status
• Equine herpesvirus 1—history of respiratory illness in other horses, cauda equina signs, viral identification using PCR or culture, CSF titers, CSF xanthochromia, rapidly progressive disease

IMAGING
Standing plain film lateral cervical radiographs.

Type 1 CVM
• Obvious vertebral malformation and malarticulation of the cervical vertebrae is common
• Diagnosis is made by demonstrating a decreased diameter of the vertebral canal on lateral cervical radiographs
• Myelography may contribute additional information and probably should be performed if the horse is going to surgery; however, it is rarely necessary in order to make the diagnosis

Type 2 CVM
• The spinal cord in type 2 CVM is compressed secondary to osteoarthritis of the caudal (C6–T1) cervical vertebrae
• Diagnosis made by showing enlarged and remodeled intervertebral joints of the caudal cervical vertebrae on radiographs, although the specificity of the technique is low due to many normal older horses having similar radiographic changes

TREATMENT

• Conservative therapy—horses that are overtly ataxic will never recover completely but will become stronger with time. Owners must be counseled about the risk of injury to the handler even if the horse is retired to pasture. In very young animals with radiographic signs of CVM severe, long-term dietary restriction may be helpful; however, it is not recommended to attempt to ride any horses that have clinical signs so a neurologic examination must be passed before training could commence
• Surgical—ventral cervical vertebral stabilization. This procedure uses a stainless-steel basket filled with cancellous bone graft to fuse the vertebrae. This has proved successful for both forms of CVM. The procedure is most successful in younger

and mildly affected horses. Horses can take up to a full year to show improvement of neurologic deficits; some never fully recover but still become athletes. Owners should be aware that this is a long-term commitment and there are still liability issues involved if the horse is put into training

MEDICATIONS
None indicated; corticosteroids give no long-term benefit.

FOLLOW-UP

PREVENTION/AVOIDANCE
Avoid overfeeding rapidly growing foals.

POSSIBLE COMPLICATIONS
Falling on rider and handler is a serious risk.

EXPECTED COURSE AND PROGNOSIS
• Once clinical signs are seen, prognosis for performance is grave unless surgery is undertaken
• Mildly affected horses may be kept as pets as they may not progress; breeding type 1 CVM horses is strongly discouraged

MISCELLANEOUS

SEE ALSO
• Degenerative myeloencephalopathy
• Equine herpesvirus myeloencephalopathy
• Equine protozoal myeloencephalitis (EPM)
• Neuroaxonal dystrophy/equine

ABBREVIATIONS
• CSF = cerebrospinal fluid
• CVM (some use CSM) = cervical vertebral malformation
• DOD = developmental orthopedic disease
• EPM = equine protozoal myeloencephalitis
• PCR = polymerase chain reaction
• WNV = West Nile virus

Suggested Reading
Mayhew IG. Large Animal Neurology, 2e. Oxford, UK: Wiley Blackwell, 2008.

Author Caroline N. Hahn
Consulting Editor Caroline N. Hahn

C

CESTRUM DIURNUM TOXICOSIS

BASICS

OVERVIEW
• *Cestrum diurnum* (day-blooming jessamine or jasmine) is a large shrub with alternate, simple leaves that have smooth margins and are lanceolate or elliptic in shape
• The fragrant and showy blooms are ≅2.5 cm in length and are 5-part flowers that appear in the axillary clusters. The flowers are white and sweet scented in the day
• The fruit is a small berry that is spheric and black when mature
• The plant, introduced into the USA from the West Indies, prefers warmer areas, and is used ornamentally in the south. It also may be found wild in the Florida Keys and in south Texas
• The plant is a member of the Solanaceae family and contains several toxins. The unripe berry contains solanine, a GI irritant, and a cholinesterase-inhibiting glycoalkaloid. The ripe berry contains tropane alkaloids. Traces of saponins and nicotine are found as well
• The agent of greatest concern is 1,25-dihydroxycholecalciferol. The glycoside is hydrolyzed to yield the active vitamin D3. There are about 30 000 IU of D3 equivalents/kg of plant. The resultant effects are increased calcium absorption and increased calcium-binding protein
• Ingestion of the plant results in hypercalcemia secondary to excessive calcium absorption and metastatic tissue calcification

SIGNALMENT
N/A

SIGNS
• Progressive weight loss and lameness, increasing in severity during a 2–6 month period
• Affected horses become stiff, are reluctant to move, and develop a short, choppy gait
• Reluctance to move is especially evident when turning
• Flexor and suspensory ligaments sensitive to palpation
• Slight to moderate kyphosis
• Elevated pulse and respiratory rates

CAUSES AND RISK FACTORS
N/A

DIAGNOSIS

DIFFERENTIAL DIAGNOSIS
Vitamin D intoxication from other sources—historical or laboratory evidence of vitamin D oversupplementation; evidence of plant ingestion; some rodenticides contain cholecalciferol and are capable of causing similar clinical signs.

CBC/BIOCHEMISTRY/URINALYSIS
• Hypercalcemia
• Serum phosphorus remains within normal limits

OTHER LABORATORY TESTS
N/A

IMAGING
Evidence of tissue calcification.

OTHER DIAGNOSTIC PROCEDURES
N/A

PATHOLOGIC FINDINGS
Gross
• Hypervitaminosis D results in widespread soft tissue mineralization (i.e. calcification), especially in arteries, ligaments, and tendons
• Forelimb flexor tendons are more severely affected than those of the pelvic limb; however, all suspensory ligaments are calcified
• Calcification occurs in the kidneys, lungs, large blood vessels, and GI tract but is not a consistent finding
• Heart calcification can occur, with the most severely calcified portion of the heart being the left atrium
• Generalized osteoporosis and emaciation

Histopathologic
Hyperplasia of the parathyroid chief cells (i.e. C cells).

TREATMENT
• No documented efficacious treatment
• Pain relief
• Promote diuresis and calciuresis with normal saline

MEDICATIONS

DRUG(S) OF CHOICE
• Promote diuresis and calciuresis with furosemide (1 mg/kg IV initial dose; if no increase in urine output is noted within 1 h, the dose can be increased to 5–10 mg/kg IV; 1–3 mg/kg IV BID–QID). However, care should be taken to ensure that the horse does not become dehydrated. Preferable means of inducing diuresis is administration of isotonic, calcium-free fluids
• Corticosteroids decrease bone release and intestinal absorption of calcium and promote calciuresis

• Salmon calcitonin prevents mobilization of calcium from bones (dosage not well established)
• Pamidronate disodium (pamidronic acid) also prevents demineralization of bones

CONTRAINDICATIONS/POSSIBLE INTERACTIONS
N/A

FOLLOW-UP

PATIENT MONITORING
Monitor serum calcium concentrations.

PREVENTION/AVOIDANCE
• Prevent access to the plant
• When preventing access is impossible, remove the plant itself, because the dead leaves remain toxic

POSSIBLE COMPLICATIONS
N/A

EXPECTED COURSE AND PROGNOSIS
N/A

MISCELLANEOUS

ASSOCIATED CONDITIONS
N/A

AGE-RELATED FACTORS
N/A

ZOONOTIC POTENTIAL
N/A

PREGNANCY/FERTILITY/BREEDING
N/A

ABBREVIATIONS
GI = gastrointestinal

Suggested Reading
Burrow GE, Tyrl RJ. Toxic Plants of North America. Ames, IA: Iowa State University Press, 2001: 1111–1113.
Krook L, Wasserman RH, Shively JN, et al. Hypercalcemia and calcinosis in Florida horses: implication of the shrub, *Cestrum diurnum*, as the causative agent. Cornell Vet 1975;65:26–56.

Author Tam Garland
Consulting Editors Wilson K. Rumbeiha and Steve Ensley

Client Education Handout available online

BASICS

DEFINITION
Serum chloride concentration greater than the reference range.

PATHOPHYSIOLOGY
- Chloride is the major anion in the extracellular fluid
- Serum chloride concentrations may increase and decrease in proportion to changes in serum sodium concentrations; these proportional increases and decreases relate to changes in body water and sodium homeostasis
- Changes in serum chloride concentrations not proportional to those in serum sodium concentrations usually relate to acid–base abnormalities
- Serum chloride concentrations tend to vary inversely with serum bicarbonate concentrations
- Metabolic acidosis with a normal or low AG may be accompanied by hyperchloremia; in metabolic acidosis with a high AG, serum chloride concentration is normal or low
- Hyperchloremia may also occur when the serum bicarbonate concentration decreases in compensation for respiratory alkalosis

SIGNALMENT
N/A

SIGNS
- Dependent on the underlying cause
- Neuromuscular—severe hypernatremia and hyperchloremia, resulting in marked hyperosmolality, may cause neurologic abnormalities because of water loss from neurons

CAUSES
Chloride Increased Proportionately to Sodium
- High total body chloride—excessive NaCl intake (i.e. salt poisoning) with water restriction (rare)
- Iatrogenic causes—administration of excessive hypertonic NaCl
- Normal total body chloride with excessive free water loss—inadequate water intake, early stages of diarrhea, central or nephrogenic diabetes insipidus, prolonged hyperventilation

Chloride Increased Disproportionately to Sodium
- Metabolic acidosis with a low or normal AG—RTA, an uncommon disorder in horses, results in striking hyperchloremia, hypobicarbonatemia (especially with proximal type II RTA) and metabolic acidosis
- Compensated respiratory alkalosis—decreased bicarbonate as a compensatory response results in increased chloride

- Acetazolamide treatment for hyperkalemic periodic paralysis

RISK FACTORS
- Inadequate water intake
- Psychogenic disorders leading to excessive consumption of salt/mineral block supplements

 DIAGNOSIS

DIFFERENTIAL DIAGNOSIS
- History or physical examination to detect decreased water intake or excessive water loss resulting in dehydration
- Diseases resulting in metabolic acidosis with a normal or low AG—RTA (uncommon) or renal failure

CBC/BIOCHEMISTRY/URINALYSIS
Serum electrolyte analysis.

OTHER LABORATORY TESTS
- Blood gas analysis is indicated when increases in chloride concentration are disproportionate to sodium concentration
- Evaluate for primary metabolic (e.g. hypobicarbonatemia) or compensated respiratory alkalosis (decreased PCO_2)
- Urinalysis including pH determination, especially when RTA is suspected
- Determine serum potassium and bicarbonate concentrations to calculate AG

IMAGING
If neurologic signs are present, MRI may show CNS edema formation.

OTHER DIAGNOSTIC PROCEDURES
N/A

PATHOLOGIC FINDINGS
N/A

 TREATMENT
Treat the underlying cause.

 MEDICATIONS

DRUG(S) OF CHOICE
- Treat the primary cause
- Change fluid therapy regimens in cases of iatrogenic causes of hyperosmolar fluid administration
- If sodium and chloride increases are proportional, ensure adequate water availability
- If hypernatremia and hyperchloremia are longstanding, correction should be gradual to avoid neurologic damage

- If chloride is increased disproportionately to sodium, evaluate and treat the acid–base imbalance

CONTRAINDICATIONS
N/A

POSSIBLE INTERACTIONS
N/A

 FOLLOW-UP

PATIENT MONITORING
Serum electrolyte concentrations and acid–base status to monitor response to fluid therapy.

PREVENTION/AVOIDANCE
Ensure a clean fresh water supply at all time.

POSSIBLE COMPLICATIONS
- Dependent on the underlying cause
- Hypernatremia—seizures, convulsions, and permanent neurologic damage are possible in severe cases
- Rapid replacement of the fluid deficit with water in markedly hyperosmotic animals may result in cerebral edema and neurologic abnormalities. Reducing hypertonicity of tissues with relatively hypotonic solutions should be performed slowly to prevent edema formation

EXPECTED COURSE AND PROGNOSIS
- Dependent on the underlying cause
- Poor if neurologic dysfunction is evident and worsens during treatment. This suggests cerebral edema

 MISCELLANEOUS

SEE ALSO
- Acidosis, metabolic
- Sodium, hypernatremia

ABBREVIATIONS
- AG = anion gap
- CNS = central nervous system
- MRI = magnetic resonance imaging
- PCO_2 = partial pressure of carbon dioxide
- RTA = renal tubular acidosis

Suggested Reading
Magdesian KG. Critical care and fluid therapy. In: Smith BP, ed. Large Animal Internal Medicine, 5e. St. Louis, MO: Elsevier Mosby, 2015:1369–1387.

Author Samuel D.A. Hurcombe
Consulting Editor Sandra D. Taylor

CHLORIDE, HYPOCHLOREMIA

BASICS

DEFINITION
Serum chloride concentration less than the reference range.

PATHOPHYSIOLOGY
• Chloride is a major anion in the extracellular fluid
• Serum chloride concentrations may increase and decrease in proportion to changes in serum sodium concentrations
• Alterations in serum chloride concentrations not proportional to changes in serum sodium concentrations usually relate to acid–base abnormalities
• Serum chloride concentrations tend to vary inversely with serum bicarbonate concentrations

SIGNALMENT
N/A

SIGNS
• Dependent on the underlying cause
• If severe and acute hyponatremia, lethargy, blindness, seizures, tremors, and abnormal gait are possible
• If related to an acid–base abnormality, the respiratory rate may be affected. If there is alkalemia, this may cause ionized hypocalcemia and synchronous diaphragmatic flutter

CAUSES

Proportionate Decreases in Sodium and Chloride
• Third spacing—when fluid accumulates in body spaces (e.g. abdominal and thoracic cavities, GI tract); ruptured urinary bladder in foals, abdominal effusions associated with colic, colitis, and peritonitis
• Iatrogenic—orally administered hypotonic fluids or excessive IV administration of 5% dextrose solution
• Inappropriate water retention caused by heart failure, hepatic fibrosis, severe hypoproteinemia, or syndrome of inappropriate antidiuretic hormone secretion

Disproportionate Decreases in Sodium and Chloride
• Renal disease
• Diarrhea and diseases causing fluid sequestration in the GI tract
• Prolonged diuresis or glucosuria may result in medullary washout and subsequent hyponatremia, hypochloremia, and metabolic alkalosis
• Adrenal insufficiency
• Primary metabolic alkalosis—serum chloride concentration decreases in compensation for increased serum bicarbonate concentration. Metabolic alkalosis may result from excessive sweating. Equine sweat contains a proportionally higher concentration of chloride than sodium;

enhanced renal bicarbonate reabsorption occurs in compensation for chloride loss
• Compensatory response to respiratory acidosis—serum bicarbonate concentration increases in compensation for respiratory acidosis; serum chloride concentration decreases to maintain electroneutrality
• Metabolic acidosis with increased AG is often associated with colic because of increased concentrations of other anions (e.g. L-lactate) that maintain electroneutrality
• Furosemide—results in disproportionate loss of chloride in the thick ascending loop of Henle

RISK FACTORS
See Causes.

DIAGNOSIS

DIFFERENTIAL DIAGNOSIS

Proportionate Decreases in Sodium and Chloride
• Ascites suggests third spacing. In foals, consider ruptured urinary bladder. In adults, consider peritonitis, heart failure, and other causes of ascites
• Thoracic effusion suggests third spacing. Consider pleuritis, neoplasia, and other causes of thoracic effusions
• Diarrhea suggests GI loss
• Polyuria/polydipsia indicates the need for renal function assessment

Disproportionate Decreases in Chloride Compared with Sodium
• Normal or low AG—consider excessive sweating as a cause of metabolic alkalosis; evaluate respiratory and neurologic systems for possible causes of respiratory acidosis
• Increased AG—consider colic and other causes of increased lactate, phosphate, sulfate, or protein

CBC/BIOCHEMISTRY/URINALYSIS
• Concurrent hyponatremia—consider diseases resulting in loss of sodium and chloride
• Decreased serum potassium concentration—GI fluid loss or anorexia
• Increased potassium concentration—renal disease or uroperitoneum
• Increased bicarbonate concentration—metabolic alkalosis or compensation for respiratory acidosis
• Decreased bicarbonate concentration and increased AG—increased concentrations of ions other than bicarbonate or chloride
• Azotemia—dehydration, renal failure, or uroperitoneum

OTHER LABORATORY TESTS
• Urinary fractional excretion $([Na_u^+/Na_s^+]/[Cr_u/Cr_s])$; increased fractional excretion accompanying hypochloremia suggests renal disease or furosemide treatment

• Blood gas analysis if the decrease in chloride is disproportionate to sodium
• Abdominal or thoracic fluid examination

IMAGING
Ultrasonography to evaluate GI distention/dilatation or third spacing.

PATHOLOGIC FINDINGS
N/A

OTHER DIAGNOSTIC PROCEDURES
N/A

TREATMENT
Treat the underlying cause.

MEDICATIONS

DRUG(S) OF CHOICE
• If sodium and chloride decreases are proportional, see the discussion of treatment in chapter Sodium, hyponatremia
• If chloride is decreased disproportionately compared with sodium, address acid–base imbalance

CONTRAINDICATIONS
N/A

POSSIBLE INTERACTIONS
N/A

FOLLOW-UP

PATIENT MONITORING
Serum electrolyte concentrations and acid–base status.

EXPECTED COURSE AND PROGNOSIS
Dependent on the underlying cause.

✓ MISCELLANEOUS

SEE ALSO
• Sodium, hyponatremia
• Uroperitoneum, neonate

ABBREVIATIONS
• AG = anion gap
• GI = gastrointestinal

Suggested Reading
Groover ES, Woolums AR, Cole DJ, LeRoy BE. Risk factors associated with renal insufficiency in horses with primary gastrointestinal disease: 26 cases (2000-2003). J Am Vet Med Assoc 2006;228:572–577.

Author Samuel D.A. Hurcombe
Consulting Editor Sandra D. Taylor

BASICS

OVERVIEW
- Refers to calculi in the biliary tree
- Relatively uncommon
- The pathogenesis possibly involves retrograde bacterial infection from the small intestine. Ascending infection is thought to initiate a cholangitis/cholangiohepatitis, which may be a predisposing factor in cholelith formation
- Plant material has occasionally been found in choleliths, further supporting retrograde invasion of bacteria and even ingesta from the duodenum as a predisposing factor of disease
- Deconjugation of bilirubin diglucuronide by bacterial β-glucuronidase occurs with subsequent precipitation of calcium bilirubinate, and cementation by anionic glycoproteins is thought to result in the formation of calculi

SIGNALMENT
- Most affected horses are 5–15 years old; cases of cholelithiasis have been reported in horses as young as 3 years
- No breed or sex predilections
- No reported geographic distribution

SIGNS
- Intermittent colic
- Icterus
- Fever
- Depression
- Weight loss
- Hepatic encephalopathy
- Photosensitization

CAUSES AND RISK FACTORS
- The condition is sporadic
- No clearly established risk factors have been identified

DIAGNOSIS

DIFFERENTIAL DIAGNOSIS
- Other causes of chronic liver disease can be differentiated with US and biopsy
- Mild, recurrent colic may be caused by gastrointestinal problems; however, most of these conditions are not accompanied by changes in serum liver enzymes or icterus. Right dorsal displacement of the large colon can result in mild colic, icterus, and increases in serum GGT and conjugated bilirubin

CBC/BIOCHEMISTRY/URINALYSIS
- Markedly elevated hepatobiliary enzymes GGT (commonly 7–20 times normal),

alkaline phosphatase, and bilirubin; mild to moderate increases in hepatocellular enzymes sorbitol dehydrogenase, glutamate dehydrogenase, and aspartate aminotransferase (2–4 times normal). Significantly elevated serum bile acids
- Increase in the conjugated bilirubin fraction to >25% of the total bilirubin is common, but in approximately one-third of cases the conjugated/total bilirubin is <25%
- CBC—neutrophilia
- Fibrinogen and globulin—elevated (except in cases of common variable immunodeficiency)

OTHER LABORATORY TESTS
Prothrombin time and activated partial thromboplastin time—may be prolonged.

IMAGING
- US reveals increased hepatic echogenicity, hepatomegaly, distended bile ducts, and occasionally calculi are visualized. Choleliths seen in 50–75% of cases
- Duodenoscopy may reveal a "bulge" at the level of the major duodenal papilla if obstruction is in the common bile duct

OTHER DIAGNOSTIC PROCEDURES
Liver biopsy and aerobic and anaerobic bacterial culture of biopsy sample. Positive cultures are obtained in approximately 50% of cases.

PATHOLOGIC FINDINGS
Hepatomegaly, periportal fibrosis, dilation of bile ducts, and inflammation. Concentric fibrosis is present around ducts in some cases with obstructing stones.

TREATMENT
- Medical therapy
- Choledocholithotomy or choledocholithotripsy should be considered in cases unresponsive to medical therapy

MEDICATIONS

DRUG(S) OF CHOICE
- Long-term antibiotic therapy ideally based on culture and sensitivity results from liver biopsy
- Gram-negative enteric and mixed anaerobic bacteria are the most frequently isolated; antibiotics with good Gram-negative activity (enrofloxacin, third-generation cephalosporins, aminoglycosides, trimethoprim–sulfamethoxazole) and

antimicrobials effective against enteric anaerobes (penicillin, metronidazole, chloramphenicol) should be selected
- Ursodiol (ursodeoxycholic acid)—anti-inflammatory and choleretic agent
- DMSO—solubilize calcium bilirubinate
- IV fluids and anti-inflammatories

FOLLOW-UP

PATIENT MONITORING
- Sequential US
- Continue antimicrobial therapy until clinical and biochemical recovery has occurred

EXPECTED COURSE AND PROGNOSIS
- Prognosis depends on severity
- Surgical intervention is not easy due to difficulty accessing the biliary tree

MISCELLANEOUS

SEE ALSO
- Icterus (prehepatic, hepatic, posthepatic)

ABBREVIATIONS
- DMSO = dimethylsulfoxide
- GGT = γ-glutamyltransferase
- US = ultrasonography, ultrasound

Suggested Reading
Divers TJ. The equine liver in health and disease. Proc Am Assoc Equine Pract 2015;61:66–103.
Johnson JK, Divers TJ, Reef VB, et al. Cholelithiasis in horses: ten cases (1982–1986). J Am Vet Med Assoc 1989;194:405–409.
Peek SF, Divers TJ. Medical treatment of cholangiohepatitis and cholelithiasis in mature horses: 9 cases (1981–1998). Equine Vet J 2000;32:301–306.

Authors Kathleen R. Mullen and Thomas J. Divers
Consulting Editors Michel Lévy and Heidi Banse

Acknowledgment The authors and editors acknowledge the prior contribution of Christopher M. Brown.

Client Education Handout available online

CHORIORETINITIS

BASICS

OVERVIEW
• The choroid and retina are closely related anatomically and physiologically. The choroid is the primary supply of blood to the retina. Chorioretinitis is inflammation of the choroid and retina
• Systems affected—ophthalmic

SIGNALMENT
N/A

SIGNS
• Chorioretinitis manifests in equine eyes as "bullet-hole" retinal lesions, diffuse chorioretinal lesions, horizontal band lesions of the non-tapetal retina, and peripapillary chorioretinal lesions. Lesions near the optic disc are more likely to affect vision than peripheral retinal lesions
• Focal chorioretinopathy, or "bullet-hole" lesions, are focal or multifocal circular scars of the peripapillary and non-tapetal regions. They consist of a depigmented periphery and a hyperpigmented central area. Acute lesions, which are uncommon, appear as white or gray exudative lesions. It has been suggested that vision may be impaired if there are more than 10–20 bullet-hole lesions. However, a recent study showed that even horses with over 100 lesions per eye have not demonstrated visual impairment or changes to their retinal function, evaluated by electroretinography
• EHV-1 may be associated with "bullet-hole" lesions in horses. This type of lesion is nonprogressive, can be seen in all age groups, and is considered an incidental finding
• Diffuse chorioretinal lesions are vermiform, circular, or band-shaped lesions that are hyperreflective in the tapetal retina, and large depigmented areas in the non-tapetal retina. These lesions are uncommon. They represent prior widespread inflammatory or infarctive disease with subsequent retinal degeneration. Optic nerve atrophy may accompany these lesions, and vision is markedly reduced
• Peripapillary chorioretinitis occurs adjacent to the optic disc. Fluffy, raised exudates are found in the active stage. Vasculitis can be observed in some cases with white or pale exudates surrounding affected retinal vessels. In the chronic stage, scar tissue develops, often, but not necessarily, in a butterfly shape around the papilla. "Butterfly lesions" may be associated with ERU, especially with concurrent signs of anterior uveitis, but, unlike previously thought, they are not pathognomonic for ERU

CAUSES AND RISK FACTORS
• Lesions can be caused by infectious agents (e.g. leptospirosis, EHV-1, *Onchocerca cervicalis* microfilaria), idiopathic or immune-mediated uveitis, trauma, or vascular disease
• Foals born to mares with respiratory disease can have chorioretinitis

DIAGNOSIS

DIFFERENTIAL DIAGNOSIS
Usually, chorioretinitis does not recur, unless it is part of the ERU syndrome.

CBC/BIOCHEMISTRY/URINALYSIS
Possible signs of systemic disease, such as infection or an immune-mediated disorder.

OTHER LABORATORY TESTS
Rule out infectious causes of chorioretinitis by serologically testing for infectious agents.

IMAGING
N/A

OTHER DIAGNOSTIC PROCEDURES
Maze testing will help to assess visual impairment, and electroretinography will help to assess functionality of the retina.

PATHOLOGIC FINDINGS
The type of cellular reaction depends on underlying cause.

TREATMENT
• Remove underlying cause if known
• Observed changes cannot be reversed
• Goal of treatment is to stop the progression of an active disease process
• Chronic, inactive lesions do not require treatment

MEDICATIONS

DRUG(S) OF CHOICE
• Systemic medication according to the underlying cause
• In addition, if lesions appear active, systemic nonsteroidal drugs such as flunixin meglumine (0.25–1.0 mg/kg BID PO) or phenylbutazone (1 g BID IV or PO)
• Topical medication is only indicated if anterior uveitis is also present: prednisolone acetate (1%) or topical NSAIDs (e.g.

diclofenac or flurbiprofen) at least 4–6 times a day, and atropine (1%) SID–QID

CONTRAINDICATIONS/POSSIBLE INTERACTIONS
• Topical steroids should be avoided if a corneal defect is present
• Horses receiving topical atropine should be monitored for colic

FOLLOW-UP

EXPECTED COURSE AND PROGNOSIS
The goal of the treatment for active chorioretinitis is to preserve the present status, i.e. to prevent progression of the disease.

MISCELLANEOUS

ASSOCIATED CONDITIONS
Possible signs of systemic infection.

AGE-RELATED FACTORS
N/A

ZOONOTIC POTENTIAL
Dependent on the underlying cause.

PREGNANCY/FERTILITY/BREEDING
Some infectious agents causing chorioretinitis can threaten pregnancy (e.g. *Leptospira*).

SEE ALSO
• Equine recurrent uveitis
• Ischemic optic neuropathy

ABBREVIATIONS
• EHV-1 = equine herpesvirus 1
• ERU = equine recurrent uveitis
• NSAID = nonsteroidal anti-inflammatory drug

Suggested Reading
Brooks DE. Ophthalmology for the Equine Practitioner, 2e. Jackson, WY: Teton NewMedia, 2008.
Gilger BC. Equine ophthalmology. In: Gelatt KN, Gilger BC, Kern TJ, eds. Veterinary Ophthalmology, 5e. Ames, IA: Wiley Blackwell, 2013:1560–1609.
Gilger BC. Equine Ophthalmology, 3e. Philadelphia, PA: WB Saunders, 2017.
Author Gil Ben-Shlomo
Consulting Editor Caryn E. Plummer
Acknowledgment The author and editor acknowledge the prior contribution of Andras M. Komaromy and Dennis E. Brooks.

C

BASICS

DEFINITION
Chronic diarrhea is defined as increased water content of feces of >2 weeks' duration. It can be constant or intermittent.

PATHOPHYSIOLOGY
Pathophysiology depends on the underlying cause, all leading to disturbances in large intestinal function. Homeostasis between fluid absorption, fluid secretion, motility, and permeability is disturbed. The dysbiosis (abnormal bacterial flora) contributes to altered function of the GI tract.

SYSTEMS AFFECTED
• GI—the main clinical sign is diarrhea. Recurrent colic also occurs.
• Cardiovascular—dehydration and endotoxemia are rarely features of chronic diarrhea. • Musculoskeletal—weight loss is common. Ventral edema can develop.
• Renal/urologic—renal insufficiency can occur if dehydration is present

GENETICS
None

INCIDENCE/PREVALENCE
Sporadic condition.

GEOGRAPHIC DISTRIBUTION
Worldwide

SIGNALMENT
There is no reported breed, age, or sex predilection. Foals may also be affected.

SIGNS
Historical Findings
Colic, abnormal fecal consistency, and weight loss are commonly reported. These signs may be intermittent or constant and vary in severity from mild to severe. There might be a history of antimicrobial use or management changes in the recent past.

Physical Examination Findings
• Horses can be lethargic and show varying degrees of anorexia. • Diarrhea varies from cowpat to watery and is often malodorous and sometimes contains abnormal contents such as blood. Fecal appearance might be normal if the condition is intermittent. • Signs of colic and abdominal discomfort may be present. Abdominal wall tension may be increased and GI sounds are often hypermotile. • Affected horses often have decreased body condition scores, muscle wasting, and poor hair coat. Fecal staining of the hindlimbs and tail is often present and can lead to hindlimb dermatitis. • Cardiovascular parameters are usually normal. • Ventral pitting edema can occur due to hypoproteinemia

CAUSES
There are many causes; in up to 50% of cases a cause cannot be established. • Dietary ○ Incorrect amount or type of feed.

○ Contaminated/spoiled feed. ○ Poor quality feed. • Dental abnormalities. • GI diseases ○ Peritonitis. ○ Abdominal abscess. ○ IBD. ○ GI neoplasia. ○ Sand impaction. ○ Chronic impaction. ○ Chronic salmonellosis. ○ GI parasitic disease. ○ Right dorsal colitis. ○ Horses <1 year of age—EPE. ○ Foals—gastric ulcers. • Chronic cardiac, liver, or renal disease

RISK FACTORS
Antimicrobial use, transportation, dietary changes, surgery, and other GI disorders have been shown to cause dysbiosis. Other risk factors depend on the underlying disease.

DIAGNOSIS

DIFFERENTIAL DIAGNOSIS
Chronic cardiac, liver, or renal diseases.

CBC/BIOCHEMISTRY/URINALYSIS
CBC
Elevated packed cell volume from dehydration can occur. White blood cell count (leukopenia with neutropenia and a left shift or leukocytosis and neutrophilia) are rare.

Biochemistry
• Serum electrolyte concentrations are usually decreased. • Hypoproteinemia is common and is usually characterized by hypoalbuminemia. Globulin levels vary from low to high, depending on whether losses in the intestinal lumen occur or the production is increased (lymphoma, abscess, chronic infection). • Prerenal azotemia can be present if the animal is dehydrated and can result in renal insufficiency if untreated. • Acute-phase proteins (amyloid A, fibrinogen) can be elevated. Other abnormalities depend on the underlying disease

Urinalysis
Hypersthenuria can be present if the animal is dehydrated or decreased if renal disease is present.

OTHER LABORATORY TESTS
Abdominocentesis
Can be normal or show increased protein concentration and cell count in peritonitis, lymphoma, or abdominal abscesses. With neoplasia, cytologically abnormal cells can sometimes be found.

Glucose/Xylose Absorption Test
Evaluates the capacity of the intestine to absorb glucose (and indirectly other nutrients). It is commonly abnormal in IBD, neoplasia, and EPE.

IMAGING
Abdominal Ultrasonography
Thickened small intestinal walls are suggestive of IBD, EPE, or lymphoma. Thickened large intestinal walls are suggestive of right dorsal colitis, neoplasia, or wall edema due to

hypoproteinemia. Intestinal contents are often "fluidy." Increased abdominal fluid is sometimes present. Masses suggestive of intra-abdominal tumors, abscesses, or enlarged lymph nodes can sometimes be imaged in the abdomen or the intestinal wall. The liver and spleen should be thoroughly evaluated for signs of disease.

Thoracic Ultrasonography and Radiographs
Can be performed to evaluate signs of thoracic lesions if a neoplastic lesion is suspected.

Echocardiography
If chronic cardiac disease is suspected.

OTHER DIAGNOSTIC PROCEDURES
Rectal Examination
Evaluate the walls of the intestine and check for masses suggestive of neoplasia, abscess, or enlarged lymph nodes. Chronic impactions can also be felt.

Nasogastric Intubation
To check for reflux if signs of colic are present and a GI lesion cannot be ruled out.

Fecal Sand Sedimentation
If positive, chronic sand impaction should be suspected. Fecal flotation and fecal egg count for parasites.

Fecal Culture
Salmonella culture. If EPE is suspected fecal and serum samples should be sent for testing. Bacteriologic evaluation of fecal samples is not diagnostic for dysbiosis. There is no available diagnostic test for dysbiosis.

Gastroscopy
Gastric ulcers and pyloric stenosis (particularly in foals), gastric neoplasia, and evaluate the duodenum. A duodenal and/or rectal biopsy can be submitted for histologic evaluation to test for IBD and lymphoma.

Laparoscopy or Exploratory Laparotomy
Full-thickness intestinal biopsies as a last test if no causes can be found with other diagnostics.

PATHOLOGIC FINDINGS
Dependent on the underlying cause. Large intestinal walls are often edematous and intestinal contents are excessively liquid.

TREATMENT

APPROPRIATE HEALTH CARE
Depending on underlying cause, some horses can be managed on the farm. As diagnostics often require specialized equipment referral to a hospital may be indicated.

NURSING CARE
• IV fluid therapy using a balanced electrolyte solution should be instituted if dehydration is present. The rate of fluid administration depends on the degree of dehydration and the fluid loss through diarrhea. In severely

hypokalemic horses, 20–40 mEq/L of KCl can be added to lactated Ringer's solution. IV administration of KCl should not exceed 0.5 mEq/kg/h. • Hindlimbs and tail should be cleaned daily. Petroleum jelly can be applied to prevent dermatitis. • Physical therapy (cold hosing) and bandaging of the lower limbs should be applied to decrease edema formation. • Fecal microbial transplantation (transfer of feces from a healthy horse via nasogastric tube) can be performed in an attempt to restore the GI microbiota

ACTIVITY
Depending on the underlying condition, work has to be reduced or stopped. Diarrheic horses should be considered infectious until infectious causes have been ruled out.

DIET
• Provide free-choice good quality hay. Hay can be fed from a hay net to prevent head edema if hypoproteinemia is present. • Fecal consistency may normalize in some horses by replacing hay with pelleted or cube hay. • Higher energy feeds should be avoided unless indicated based on underlying disease. • Anorexic animals may benefit from forced enteral feeding or parenteral nutrition. • Free-choice water and a salt block should be offered at all times to allow the horse to compensate for fecal fluid losses. • A balanced oral electrolyte solution (35 g KCl and 70 g NaCl in 10 L of water) can be offered in addition to water to compensate for electrolyte losses. • Additional dietary recommendations depend on underlying disease

CLIENT EDUCATION
Salmonellosis is a potential cause of chronic diarrhea that may be zoonotic. Diagnosis can be challenging and costly.

MEDICATIONS
DRUG(S) OF CHOICE
Medication depends on the underlying cause. The following applies to chronic diarrhea in which no cause can be found.

Antimicrobials
The use of antimicrobial drugs in chronic diarrhea is contraindicated unless a specific infectious cause can be determined. Antimicrobials will further disrupt the colonic microbiota.

NSAIDs
Flunixin meglumine can be given (1.1 mg/kg every 12 h IV) to control signs of colic, unless right dorsal colitis is the cause.

Antidiarrhea Drugs
Di-tri-octahedral smectite (500 kg horse: 2–3 mg/kg loading dose followed by 1 mg/kg every 6–12 h PO).

CONTRAINDICATIONS
• Metronidazole to alter the colonic microbiota is questionable. • There is no evidence for iodochlorhydroxyquin (clioquinol) to modify the microbiota. • Probiotics have questionable efficacy in horses

PRECAUTIONS
• Di-tri-octahedral smectite can cause impaction if administered beyond resolution of diarrhea. • At a dose of 1.1 mg/kg, flunixin meglumine may be nephrotoxic in dehydrated animals

ALTERNATIVE DRUGS
• Any licensed NSAID can be used instead of flunixin meglumine. • Bismuth subsalicylate, up to 4 L/500 kg every 12 h PO or activated charcoal (1 g/kg every 24 h PO) instead of di-tri-octahedral smectite

FOLLOW-UP
PATIENT MONITORING
Depending on disease and chosen treatment, monitoring may be frequent or periodic until resolution of clinical signs.

PREVENTION/AVOIDANCE
Feed, particularly hay, should be of good quality. Risk factors should be avoided if possible.

POSSIBLE COMPLICATIONS
Chronic diarrhea can be an intermittent disease and might recur. Often it is not possible to determine the exact cause or cure the horse. Complications include hindlimb dermatitis.

EXPECTED COURSE AND PROGNOSIS
The course and prognosis depend on the underlying disease. In cases where a cause cannot be found, response to therapy and management changes has to be monitored. If diarrhea resolves, it might recur. Prognosis for survival is good, even if diarrhea cannot be resolved; however the prognosis for use might be guarded depending on the severity.

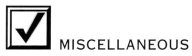

MISCELLANEOUS
ASSOCIATED CONDITIONS
• Hindlimb dermatitis. • Weight loss. • Chronic or recurrent colic

AGE-RELATED FACTORS
None

ZOONOTIC POTENTIAL
Salmonellosis

PREGNANCY/FERTILITY/BREEDING
N/A

SYNONYMS
N/A

SEE ALSO
• Acute kidney injury (AKI) and acute renal failure (ARF)
• Gastric ulcers and erosions (equine gastric ulcer syndrome, EGUS)
• Gastric ulcers, neonate
• *Lawsonia intracellularis* infections in foals
• Lymphosarcoma
• Peritonitis
• Probiotics in foals and horses
• Right dorsal colitis
• Salmonellosis
• Sand impaction and enteropathy

ABBREVIATIONS
• EPE = equine proliferative enteropathy
• GI = gastrointestinal
• IBD = inflammatory bowel disease
• NSAID = nonsteroidal anti-inflammatory drug

Suggested Reading
Mullen KR, Yasuda K, Divers TJ, Weese JS. Equine faecal microbiota transplant: current knowledge, proposed guidelines and future directions. Equine Vet Educ 2018;30:151–160.
Schoster AS, Weese JS, Guardabassi LG. Probiotic use in horses—what is the evidence for their clinical efficacy. J Vet Intern Med 2014;28:1640–1652.
Staempfli HR, Oliver OE. Chronic diarrhea and weight loss in three horses. Vet Clin North Am Equine Pract 2006;22:27–35.

Author Angelika Schoster
Consulting Editors Henry Stämpfli and Olimpo Oliver-Espinosa

 Client Education Handout available online

BASICS

DEFINITION
Substantial and permanent decrease in GFR.

PATHOPHYSIOLOGY
- Usually a consequence of GN or CIN
- Impaired urine-concentrating ability (i.e. isosthenuria) occurs when more than two-thirds of nephron function is lost
- Azotemia develops after loss of more than three-fourths of nephron function
- Disturbances in fluid, electrolyte, and acid–base homeostasis are less severe than with AKI/ARF, but the loss of renal function is irreversible

SYSTEMS AFFECTED
- Renal/urologic—failure
- Endocrine/metabolic—disturbances in electrolyte and acid–base homeostasis; decreased erythropoietin production
- GI—inappetence, possible diarrhea, and increased risk of ulcers
- Nervous/neuromuscular—occasional ataxia or dementia in severe CKD; tremors or muscle fasciculations may accompany metabolic disturbances
- Hemic/lymphatic/immune—platelet dysfunction, increased susceptibility to infection, anemia

GENETICS
N/A

INCIDENCE/PREVALENCE
Reported to be 0.12%.

GEOGRAPHIC DISTRIBUTION
N/A

SIGNALMENT
Breed Predilections
- May be more common in Clydesdales
- A heritable form of PKD may occur in Arabians and Paints

Mean Age and Range
Older horses (>15 years) are at greater risk (prevalence 0.5%); however, this may reflect more extensive investigation of valuable animals.

SIGNS
Historical Findings
- Insidious-onset lethargy, partial anorexia, and weight loss
- Ventral edema and mild polyuria and polydipsia (with clear-appearing urine)
- At an earlier stage, decreased performance

Physical Examination Findings
- Weight loss, poor hair coat, mild lethargy, reduced appetite, edema, excessive dental tartar, and uremic odor in the oral cavity may be found
- Affected horses usually are not dehydrated
- Voided urine usually is clear and pale yellow
- Rectal examination may reveal a small, firm left kidney with an irregular surface and,

rarely, ureteral distention due to obstruction with uroliths
- With endstage disease, anuria may develop with anorexia, and more marked lethargy may be accompanied by ataxia, hypermetria, and mental obtundation

CAUSES
- Immune-mediated GN initiated by chronic infections (e.g. equine infectious anemia, streptococcal diseases) or autoimmune disease
- CIN encompasses all non-GN causes and may be a sequela to ischemic or nephrotoxic AKI/ARF
- Less commonly, ascending infections may lead to bilateral pyelonephritis and nephrolithiasis and/or ureterolithiasis
- Long-term use of NSAIDs with medullary necrosis and nephrolithiasis
- Amyloidosis and renal neoplasia—rare
- In horses <5 years of age and with no history of medical problems, anomalies of development—renal hypoplasia or dysplasia; PKD

RISK FACTORS
- Previous episodes of AKI/ARF or UTI
- Prior medical or surgical diseases, especially when treatment included aminoglycoside antibiotics and NSAIDs
- Long-term use of NSAIDs
- CKD may develop months to years after nephrotoxin-induced AKI

DIAGNOSIS

DIFFERENTIAL DIAGNOSIS
- All disorders that may lead to lethargy, partial anorexia, and weight loss
- AKI/ARF—supported by an underlying disease process producing renal ischemia or recent/concurrent exposure to nephrotoxic agents
- Postrenal failure—supported by stranguria, anuria, or uroperitoneum

CBC/BIOCHEMISTRY/URINALYSIS
- Normal to low packed cell volume (attributed to decreased serum erythropoietin concentration and shortened RBC life span), platelets normal to decreased
- Increased BUN (100–250 mg/dL; 36–89 mmol/L) and Cr (2.0–20 mg/dL; 177–1768 μmol/L); BUN:Cr ratio usually >10; Cr usually >5.0 mg/dL (440 μmol/L) with horses presented for chronic ill thrift
- Variable hyponatremia, hypochloremia, and hyperkalemia—less severe than with AKI/ARF
- Hypercalcemia and hypophosphatemia are unique to horses
- Mild to moderate hypoalbuminemia, hypertriglyceridemia, and hypercholesterolemia
- Mild to moderate metabolic acidosis may accompany endstage disease

- USG—isosthenuria (1.008–1.014) is a hallmark feature
- GN—moderate to marked proteinuria that may increase USG to 1.020
- Urine sediment is relatively devoid of crystals, but otherwise may be unremarkable. Increased RBCs support lithiasis or neoplasia, and increased leukocytes support UTI

OTHER LABORATORY TESTS
- Increased fractional clearances of sodium and chloride with advanced disease
- Increased urine protein–urine creatinine ratio (>2:1) supports GN
- Quantitative urine culture and antimicrobial sensitivity even in the absence of pyuria
- Coagulation panel when performing renal biopsy or investigating GN (decreased antithrombin III)

IMAGING
Transabdominal and Transrectal Ultrasonography
- Kidneys may be small (diameter <6 cm; length <12 cm), with irregular surfaces
- Increased parenchymal echogenicity (similar to that of the spleen), loss of detail of corticomedullary junction
- Nephrolithiasis/ureterolithiasis and variable hydronephrosis may be detected
- Multiple cystic structures may be found with PKD or pyelonephritis

Urethroscopy/Cystoscopy
- Useful with suspected obstructive disease or pyelonephritis
- Urine samples may be collected from each ureter by catheterization

OTHER DIAGNOSTIC PROCEDURES
GFR
Measuring changes in GFR, by plotting the inverse of Cr over time, may be the most accurate way to follow the progressive decrease in renal function.

Biopsy
- Percutaneous renal biopsy with routine histopathology, immunohistochemistry, and electron microscopy of the sample may provide information regarding cause (GN versus CIN) but rarely affects prognosis or progression of CKD
- Pursue biopsy with caution, because life-threatening hemorrhage can be a complication

Blood Pressure
Serial measurement of blood pressure may reveal persistent hypertension and support for use of antihypertensive medications, especially in cases of GN with proteinuria.

PATHOLOGIC FINDINGS
Gross
- Firm, shrunken, pale kidneys, with irregular surfaces and narrowed cortices
- Renal capsule is often adhered to underlying parenchyma

CHRONIC KIDNEY DISEASE   (CONTINUED)

• See chapters Urolithiasis and Urinary tract infection (UTI)
• Enlarged kidneys with multiple cysts are found with PKD

Histopathologic
• Variable glomerular, tubular, and interstitial changes
• Endstage CKD may preclude categorization of the initiating cause

TREATMENT

APPROPRIATE HEALTH CARE
Inpatient/outpatient medical management.

NURSING CARE

Fluid Therapy
• With stable CKD short-term diuresis with IV fluid therapy is rarely beneficial and may carry an increased risk of thrombophlebitis
• IV fluid therapy can be pursued to rule out AKI/ARF or acute-on-chronic disease—5% dextrose or isotonic (0.9%) saline at 1.5–2-fold the maintenance rate for 24–48 h with daily assessment of changes in body weight, BUN and Cr, serum electrolyte concentrations, and USG
• Increased urine output and decreased azotemia should occur in patients with AKI/ARF or acute-on-chronic disease
• Horses with more severe CKD typically gain weight and develop edema, with little decrease in magnitude of azotemia

Oral Electrolyte Supplementation
With serum bicarbonate <20 mEq/L, 30 g of sodium bicarbonate may be administered once or twice daily.

ACTIVITY
When clinical signs are mild and the horse's attitude is good, light exercise can be continued.

DIET
• Access to fresh water at all times
• The ideal diet provides adequate caloric intake without excessive protein intake
• Offering a variety of concentrate feeds, bran mash, and access to good quality pasture is the recommended diet. Grass hay is preferred to alfalfa owing to the higher protein and calcium content of the latter; however, if appetite for grass hay is poor, feed alfalfa
• Supplementation with fat effectively increases caloric intake
• Supplement omega-3 fatty acids (flax seed, fresh grass pasture) and antioxidants (vitamins C and E)

SURGICAL CONSIDERATIONS
Surgery is only required for acute-on-chronic disease due to obstructive urolithiasis.

MEDICATIONS

DRUG(S) OF CHOICE
• Corticosteroids may be used with caution in patients with GN and proteinuria
• Angiotensin-converting enzyme inhibitors (benazepril 0.5 mg/kg PO every 24 h) may be helpful in patients with hypertension, proteinuria, and edema

CONTRAINDICATIONS
• NSAIDs may exacerbate renal hypoperfusion and the decline in GFR
• Avoid all nephrotoxic medications unless specifically indicated for a concurrent disease process, and then modify dosage accordingly

PRECAUTIONS
Discontinue oral electrolyte supplementation if it produces or exacerbates edema.

POSSIBLE INTERACTIONS
N/A

FOLLOW-UP

PATIENT MONITORING
• Monitor response to fluid therapy closely—as little as 40 mL/kg of IV fluids (20 L to a 500 kg horse) may produce pulmonary edema in oliguric/anuric patients
• Assess clinical status (emphasizing attitude and appetite), edema formation, body weight, and magnitude of azotemia at least monthly during the initial few months of supportive care and every 2–3 months thereafter
• Assess electrolyte and acid–basis status whenever changes in clinical status are noted

PREVENTION/AVOIDANCE
• Anticipate compromised renal function in patients with other diseases or prolonged anesthesia and surgery; minimize dehydration and potential renal damage
• Ensure adequate hydration status in patients receiving nephrotoxic medications
• Avoid use of NSAIDs unless necessary

POSSIBLE COMPLICATIONS
• Pulmonary and peripheral edema with fluid therapy
• Increased risk of thrombophlebitis with IV fluid therapy
• Oral and GI ulceration or GI bleeding
• Signs of neurologic impairment—ataxia, mental obtundation

EXPECTED COURSE AND PROGNOSIS
• Issue a poor prognosis and consider euthanasia for horses that are emaciated, anuric, or have Cr >10 mg/dL (850 µmol/L) at initial evaluation

• Issue a guarded prognosis for short-term survival for horses with Cr of 5–10 mg/dL (440–850 µmol/L) at initial evaluation
• Issue a fair prognosis for short-term survival for horses with Cr <5 mg/dL (440 µmol/L) that are in good body condition at initial evaluation
• Horses with GN typically have a poorer prognosis and more rapid decline in renal function than horses with CIN

MISCELLANEOUS

ASSOCIATED CONDITIONS
Hypertension

AGE-RELATED FACTORS
In horses <5 years of age, CKD may be due to a developmental anomaly—renal hypoplasia or dysplasia.

PREGNANCY/FERTILITY/BREEDING
Pregnant mares may be at increased risk of UTI. Mares with CKD have successfully carried foals to term but the prognosis for a viable foal is guarded.

SYNONYMS
• Chronic renal failure
• Kidney failure

SEE ALSO
• Acute kidney injury (AKI) and acute renal failure (ARF)
• Urinary tract infection (UTI)
• Urolithiasis

ABBREVIATIONS
• AKI = acute kidney injury
• ARF = acute renal failure
• BUN = blood urea nitrogen
• CIN = chronic interstitial nephritis
• CKD = chronic kidney disease
• Cr = creatinine
• GFR = glomerular filtration rate
• GI = gastrointestinal
• GN = glomerulonephritis
• NSAID = nonsteroidal anti-inflammatory drug
• PKD = polycystic kidney disease
• RBC = red blood cell
• USG = urinary specific gravity
• UTI = urinary tract infection

Suggested Reading
McLeland S. Diseases of the equine urinary system. Vet Clin North Am Equine Pract 2015;31(2):377–387.

Author Harold C. Schott II
Consulting Editor Valérie Picandet

CHRONIC PROGRESSIVE LYMPHEDEMA

BASICS

OVERVIEW
• CPL is a disorder characterized by lymphedema of the lower extremities, leading to recurrent infections and severe fibrosis
• Affected organ systems are hemic/lymphatic/immune and skin/exocrine. Exact pathogenesis is unknown
• Elastin within the skin and around lymphatic vessels of the skin and subcutis is altered with increased levels of circulating anti-elastin antibodies
• Ineffective lower extremity lymph drainage leads to lymph stasis, which induces diffuse nodular fibrosis and ischemia of the skin and subcutaneous tissues
• Heavy feathering and decreased skin barrier function due to LE and ischemia foster recurrent bacterial and parasitic dermatitis

SIGNALMENT
• Draft horses with heavy feathering are affected—Shires, Clydesdales, Belgian draft horses, Friesians, Gypsy Vanners, some German draft breeds, and English Cobbs. Certain familial lines of draft horse breeds are more affected
• The high incidence of CPL in certain breeds suggests a genetic component. Evaluation of *FOXC2* (LE–distichiasis syndrome) and *ATP2A2* (Darier–White disease) genes revealed no association with CPL. Other candidate genes are *ubiquitin protein ligase E3A*, *CD109*, *transforming growth factor*-β and *myotubularin-related protein 6*

SIGNS
• Develops as early as 2–4 years of age and progresses throughout life
• Often more pronounced in the hind legs
• Starts in the fetlock and pastern and expands proximally
• Mild and/or early CPL—often not diagnosed under heavy feathering
  ◦ After clipping mild pitting edema is appreciated resulting in lack of distinction of tendons and metatarsus/metacarpus and fetlock
  ◦ There is mild rippling of skin surface of pastern and fetlock
  ◦ Scaling
  ◦ *Chorioptes* infestation results in pruritus and stomping
  ◦ Oozing and crusting due to secondary infections
• Severe/chronic CPL—lesions progress to carpus and tarsus
  ◦ Leg swelling is firm from fibrosis of the CPL
  ◦ Numerous firm folds and nodules can be palpated
  ◦ Skin surface is extremely scaly, moist, and often greasy
  ◦ Erosions and ulcers occur due to self-trauma (pruritus and interference of movement)
  ◦ Persistent infections affect deeper tissues and induce lymphangitis and swelling of the entire leg
  ◦ Coronary band is markedly hyperkeratotic and hyperplastic
  ◦ Hoof quality is poor; may be brittle and chipped with splits and cracks
  ◦ Repeated bouts of thrush and deep hoof abscesses are common
  ◦ Chestnuts and ergots tend to be misshapen and hyperkeratotic

CAUSES AND RISK FACTORS
• Heavy long feathering in association with wet and muddy environment
• Lack of movement increases the LE

DIAGNOSIS

Clinical presentation and history are characteristic. Thorough palpation of lower legs is necessary to identify early pitting edema.

DIFFERENTIAL DIAGNOSIS
Pastern dermatitis in draft horses, in particular if several legs are affected, raises the concern for CPL.

CBC/BIOCHEMISTRY/URINALYSIS
N/A

OTHER LABORATORY TESTS
Skin scrapings and bacterial culture assist in identification of chorioptic mites or secondary pyoderma, respectively.

IMAGING
Lymphangiography illustrates dilated, tortuous lymphatic vessels in the distal legs and confirms the diagnosis.

OTHER DIAGNOSTIC PROCEDURES
N/A

TREATMENT
• No curative treatment exists. Early recognition and careful management can drastically improve the condition and slow progression of the disease
• Clipping of feathers is imperative for successful long-term management
• Legs need to be kept clean and dry

Activity
• Exercise increases circulation, lymph drainage, and lymph flow. Light exercise can be performed with the horse wearing compression bandages that constitute part of combined decongestive therapy
• Cold water rinses are recommended on limbs with clipped feathers after exercise. Skin needs to be dried after rinsing
• Routine hoof care is important to avoid thrush
• Combined decongestive therapy—includes daily manual lymph drainage massage by a trained person and compression bandaging using specialized short-stretch bandages in phases 1 and 2. Horses can be walked with the bandages

Client Education
Owners must commit to life-long management.

SURGICAL CONSIDERATIONS
Surgical debulking of nodules or epidermal shaving with subsequent compression bandaging has been suggested. However, intervention will disrupt the lymphatic vascular bed and enhance LE, unless stringent compression treatment is used.

MEDICATIONS

DRUG(S) OF CHOICE
Treatment of *Chorioptes* is crucial (fipronil or lime sulfur sprays; ivermectin; moxidectin). Bacterial infections need to be treated.

FOLLOW-UP

POSSIBLE COMPLICATIONS
Permanent lameness and a poor quality of life.

EXPECTED COURSE AND PROGNOSIS
CPL can lead to premature euthanasia.

MISCELLANEOUS

AGE-RELATED FACTORS
Progression with age.

ABBREVIATIONS
• CPL = chronic progressive lymphedema
• LE = lymphedema

Suggested Reading
Affolter VK. Chronic progressive lymphedema in draft horses. Vet Clin North Am Equine Pract 2013;29(3):589–605.

Author Verena K. Affolter
Consulting Editor Gwendolen Lorch

C

CHRONIC WEIGHT LOSS

BASICS

DEFINITION
Can be defined as loss of body weight over time (>4–5 weeks) due to decreased fat and muscle mass or loss of GI content and total body water, or a combination of these factors.

PATHOPHYSIOLOGY
Weight loss can result from many causes— lack of adequate food and/or water, poor quality food, inability to prehend or swallow, maldigestion or malabsorption of food, increased loss of nutrients once absorbed, and increased catabolism. Inadequate caloric intake is likely the most common cause of weight loss, and may also be due to specific nutrient deficiencies, chronic liver disease, neoplasia, malabsorption, and chronic infections. The pathophysiologic events leading to weight loss are manifold and depend on underlying causes. For details, see specific problems.

SYSTEMS AFFECTED
GI
• Dental diseases. • Parasitism. • Oral ulcerations. • Tongue paralysis. • Pharyngeal paresis or paralysis. • Retropharyngeal masses. • Esophageal strictures. • Gastric ulceration. • Intestinal malabsorption. • Maldigestion. • Intestinal infections and noninfectious inflammatory, infiltrative, and neoplastic disorders. • Intestinal motility disturbances. • Intra-abdominal abscesses. • Chronic grass sickness. • Sand enteropathy

Endocrine/Metabolic
• Pituitary adenoma of the pars intermedia in the horse due to increased metabolic rate, including muscle wasting induced by hyperadrenocorticism. • Diabetes mellitus due to endocrine pancreatic insufficiency. • Nutritional secondary hyperparathyroidism

Hemic/Lymphatic/Immune
• Lymphoma, leading to cancer cachexia. • Inflammatory bowel disease leading to malabsorption. • EIA. • Chronic piroplasmosis

Hepatobiliary
• Chronic hepatic failure. • Cholangiohepatitis. • Hepatic abscess

Cardiovascular
• Congestive heart failure, leading to decreased liver and GI function. • Valvular endocarditis due to occult infections

Renal/Urologic
Chronic renal failure.

Neuromuscular
Equine motor neuron disease and associated muscle wasting.

Behavioral
• Cribbing. • Oral stereotypy

Respiratory
• Heaves. • Chronic pleuropneumonia. • Lung abscesses

Skin/Exocrine
• Pemphigus foliaceus. • Pythiosis

Musculoskeletal
Chronic painful lameness (e.g. severe laminitis).

Nervous
Neurologic conditions that impair prehension, chewing, and swallowing.

SIGNALMENT
Varies according to the underlying cause of weight loss.

SIGNS
Signs vary according to the primary condition, but, commonly, decrease in body condition and reduced appetite are observed.

CAUSES
See Systems Affected.
The most common causes (Consultant®, Maurice White, Cornell University, 2016) include occult infections, malabsorption syndromes, chronic renal failure, liver failure, parasitism, chronic viral infections (EIA), and endocrinopathies.

RISK FACTORS
Any condition leading to catabolic situations.

DIAGNOSIS

CBC/BIOCHEMISTRY/URINALYSIS
A minimal database includes CBC, serum biochemical profile, and fibrinogen. CBC findings may be nonspecific, but total protein might be increased (e.g. due to hyperglobulinemia in occult infections) or decreased (e.g. due to protein-losing enteropathies). Anemia of chronic disease might be present. There might be leukocytosis. Biochemistry should help to differentiate between specific organ failure problems such as hepatic or renal diseases. Serum electrophoresis might assist in characterizing dysproteinemias and in separating conditions such as occult infections from neoplasia or parasitism.

OTHER LABORATORY TESTS
Hyperfibrinogenemia in inflammatory or neoplastic disease.

DIAGNOSTIC PROCEDURES
• Abdominocentesis can be useful in identifying the abdomen to be the site of occult infections. • Ultrasonography is used to detect abscesses (abdominal, pleural, wall

thickening of jejunum and colon, etc.). • In individual cases, exploratory laparotomy/ laparoscopy might be required. • Glucose and xylose absorption tests when small intestine malabsorption is suspected. • When stomach ulcers are suspected, gastroscopy should be performed. • Echocardiography in cases of congestive heart failure

TREATMENT
See specific conditions.

MEDICATIONS

DRUG(S) OF CHOICE
See specific conditions.

FOLLOW-UP
Reports of case studies indicate a survival probability of around 70%.

PATIENT MONITORING
Monitor feed intake and body weight of the animal.

POSSIBLE COMPLICATIONS
Secondary infections due to the debilitated immune system of the horse.

MISCELLANEOUS

AGE-RELATED FACTORS
Poor dentition might be a major factor in weight loss in geriatric horses.

ZOONOTIC POTENTIAL
Chronic salmonellosis.

ABBREVIATIONS
• EIA = equine infectious anemia.
• GI = gastrointestinal

Suggested Reading
Metcalfe LVA, More SJ, Duggan V, Katz LM. A retrospective study of horses investigated for weight loss despite a good appetite (2002–2011). Equine Vet J 2013;45:340–345.
Stämpfli H, Oliver OE. Chronic diarrhea and weight loss in three horses. Vet Clin North Am Equine Pract 2006;22:e27–e35.

Author Olimpo Oliver-Espinosa
Consulting Editors Henry Stämpfli and Olimpo Oliver-Espinosa

BASICS

OVERVIEW
• Cleft palate (palatoschisis) is a rare defect of the secondary (hard and soft) palates
• Congenital clefts result from an interruption of the midline closure of the embryonic palatine folds. Closure of the palate proceeds from rostral to caudal, so either the soft palate or both soft and hard palate may be affected
• Acquired clefts result from trauma during surgery and may involve the hard or soft palate

SIGNALMENT
• Congenital cleft palate is seen in horses of any breed and gender, with a reported frequency of 4% of all congenital abnormalities. Age of presentation is often dependent on the severity of the cleft
• Acquired clefts occur in horses of any age that have a history of recent surgery

SIGNS
• Milk draining from a foal's nose after nursing
• Water- or food-stained discharge from the nares of adult horses
• Coughing
• Signs of aspiration pneumonia—fever, lethargy, increased respiratory rate, abnormal lung sounds
• Chronic clefts—stunted due to lack of adequate nutritional intake and persistent respiratory disease
• Horses >1 year of age may present for abnormal respiratory noise

CAUSES AND RISK FACTORS
• Congenital—toxins, nutritional deficiencies, infection, hormonal and environmental factors, and metabolic abnormalities at the time of palate fusion (around the 47th day of gestation)
• Acquired—iatrogenic trauma to the palate during pharyngeal or oral surgery

DIAGNOSIS

DIFFERENTIAL DIAGNOSIS
• Esophageal obstruction
• Dysphagia
• Pneumonia

CBC/BIOCHEMISTRY/URINALYSIS
CBC and fibrinogen—leukocytosis and hyperfibrinogenemia secondary to aspiration pneumonia.

OTHER LABORATORY TESTS
• Immunglobulin G assessed in all neonatal foals
• Blood cultures indicated in foals with pneumonia or failure of transfer of passive immunity

IMAGING
• Thoracic radiographs can determine the extent of aspiration pneumonia
• Thoracic ultrasonography will provide information regarding the pleural surface

OTHER DIAGNOSTIC PROCEDURES
Endoscopy (nasal or oral) is essential to determine the extent and prognosis.

TREATMENT
• Primary surgical closure of the cleft—transhyoid pharyngotomy for caudal clefts of the soft palate or a mandibular symphysiotomy for extensive soft palate defects or concurrent hard palate clefts
• Extensive nursing care is required in neonates after surgery
• Severity of aspiration pneumonia may increase anesthetic risk
• Small defects at the caudal edge of the soft palate without signs of a respiratory infection may not require surgical repair
• A laryngeal tie-forward has been described to treat dysphagia and respiratory infections for small, caudal defects in horses >1 year of age

MEDICATIONS

DRUG(S) OF CHOICE
• Prompt administration of broad-spectrum antibiotics is indicated for respiratory infections
• Antimicrobial combinations include sodium or potassium penicillin (22 000–44 000 U/kg IV every 6 h), an aminoglycoside (gentamicin in adults (6.6 mg/kg IV every 24 h) or amikacin in foals (25 mg/kg IV every 24 h)), and metronidazole (15–25 mg/kg PO every 8 h)
• NSAIDS—for endotoxemia and inflammation (flunixin meglumine (1.1 mg/kg IV/PO every 12 h) or ketoprofen (1.1–2.2 IV every 12 h))

CONTRAINDICATIONS/POSSIBLE INTERACTIONS
Aminoglycosides and NSAIDS have negative renal and gastrointestinal side effects, especially in dehydrated patients.

FOLLOW-UP

PATIENT MONITORING
• Evaluate the suture line by endoscopy no earlier than 1 week after surgery to prevent dehiscence
• Monitor clinical signs of pneumonia, including temperature, respiratory rate, and effort
• Follow progress of pneumonia by radiography for pulmonary lesions or ultrasonography for pleural lesions
• Patients with extensive repairs, especially those involving the hard palate, should be fed via nasogastric tube to reduce the risk of dehiscence of the suture line

PREVENTION/AVOIDANCE
Owners are recommended not to breed animals with cleft palates, although inheritance is unknown.

POSSIBLE COMPLICATIONS
• Dehiscence
• Incisional infection
• Persistent soft palate displacement
• Oronasal fistula
• Pneumonia
• Chronic nasal discharge

EXPECTED COURSE AND PROGNOSIS
• Successful repair occurs in 50–60% of patients with midline clefts and minimal tissue loss
• Clefts involving both hard and soft palate, >20% of the soft palate alone, or asymmetrical clefts have a poor prognosis
• Prognosis is reduced by concurrent respiratory disease
• Guarded prognosis for future athleticism—may also have persistent respiratory insufficiency after resolution of pneumonia

MISCELLANEOUS

ASSOCIATED CONDITIONS
• Aspiration pneumonia
• Esophageal obstruction (choke)
• Exercise intolerance
• Pneumonia, neonate

SEE ALSO
Pneumonia, neonate

ABBREVIATIONS
NSAID = nonsteroidal anti-inflammatory drug

Suggested Reading
Tate LP. Surgical repair of cleft palate. In: Hawkins J, ed. Advances in Equine Upper Respiratory Surgery. Hoboken, NJ: Wiley, 2015:195–206.

Author Amelia S. Munsterman
Consulting Editor Margaret C. Mudge

C

CLITORAL ENLARGEMENT

BASICS

OVERVIEW
• The clitoris appears larger than normal and may to protrude through the vulvar lips at the ventral commissure
• It develops from the embryonic genital tubercle in the absence of testicular testosterone production, or the conversion of testosterone by 5α-reductase to the active form, dihydrotestosterone
• The clitoris is the female homolog of the penis
• Anatomy
  ◦ Corpus cavernosum clitoris—erectile tissue
  ◦ Corpus clitoris (body of the clitoris)—5 cm in length
  ◦ Crura—attached to the ischial arch
  ◦ Glans clitoris—2.5 cm in diameter; situated in the fossa at the ventral commissure of the vulva; well-developed median sinus and lateral sinuses may be present
• Systems affected—reproductive
• May be associated with sex chromosome abnormalities

SIGNALMENT
• Females
• Congenital
• Concurrent ovarian neoplasia—GTCT
• Iatrogenic drug administration—anabolic steroid, progestin
• Intersex condition

SIGNS
• Historical—known drug administration; female offspring of treated mare
• Enlargement of the glans clitoris beyond the expected norm
• May be visible externally as swelling of the ventral vulvar commissure
• May protrude from the clitoral fossa between labia
• May be associated with abnormal cyclicity
• May be associated with other structural genital anomalies, internal and/or external
• May be associated with stallion-like behavior and conformation

CAUSES AND RISK FACTORS
• Administration of anabolic steroids
• Progestin (altrenogest) usage for estrus control, behavior modification, and pregnancy maintenance; female progeny have associated altered gonadotropin secretion and increased clitoral size to 21 months of age; no effect on reproductive function
• Aberrant endogenous sex-steroid production—granulosa cell tumor in dam during gestation alters fetal development
• Hormonally active ovarian neoplasm in a postpubertal female—GTCT

• Mixoploidy or sex chromosome aberration—presence of testis-determining factor

DIAGNOSIS

DIFFERENTIAL DIAGNOSIS
• Intersex conditions
• Pseudohermaphrodite—may be associated with clitoral enlargement
• Hypospadias penis
• Hypoplastic penis with incomplete closure of embryonic urethral folds
• Associated with prominent perineal median raphe, ventrally displaced vulva, and caudad direction of penis
• Most common presentation—64,XX male

CBC/BIOCHEMISTRY/URINALYSIS
N/A

OTHER LABORATORY TESTS
Hormonal Assay
• Testosterone/hCG challenge—baseline blood sample; administer 3000 IU hCG IV, with additional blood samples collected at 3 and 24 h; increased testosterone indicates testicular tissue is present, i.e. Leydig cell production
• Estrone sulfate—produced by Sertoli cells in the testicle; couple with hCG challenge to improve diagnostic accuracy
• Investigate (rule out presence of) a GTCT by measurement of inhibin (sensitivity 80%), anti-Müllerian hormone (98%), and testosterone (48%)

Immunology
• Test for presence of 5α-reductase or cytosolic receptor
• Use labial skin only, as the receptors are site specific

IMAGING
• Ultrasonography coupled with transrectal palpation of internal genitalia for ovarian pathology or internal genital anomaly
• Note there is no pathognomonic appearance of a GTCT

OTHER DIAGNOSTIC PROCEDURES
N/A

PATHOLOGIC FINDINGS
N/A

TREATMENT
N/A

MEDICATIONS

DRUG(S) OF CHOICE
N/A

CONTRAINDICATIONS/POSSIBLE INTERACTIONS
N/A

FOLLOW-UP

PATIENT MONITORING
N/A

PREVENTION/AVOIDANCE
• Rational causative drug use
• If genetic, analysis of pedigree
• If heritable, elimination of parent stock from breeding pool

POSSIBLE COMPLICATIONS
N/A

EXPECTED COURSE AND PROGNOSIS
N/A

MISCELLANEOUS

ASSOCIATED CONDITIONS
Intersex conditions.

AGE-RELATED FACTORS
Congenital

ZOONOTIC POTENTIAL
N/A

PREGNANCY/FERTILITY/BREEDING
Associated abnormalities may preclude fertility.

SEE ALSO
Disorders of sexual development

ABBREVIATIONS
• GTCT = granulosa–theca cell tumor
• hCG = human chorionic gonadotropin

Suggested Reading
Ball BA, Almeida J, Conley AJ. Determination of serum anti-Müllerian hormone concentrations for the diagnosis of granulosa-cell tumours in mares. Equine Vet J 2013;45:199–203.
Christensen BW, Meyer-Wallen VN. Sex determination and differentiation. In: McKinnon AO, Squires EL, Vaala WE, Varner DD, eds. Equine Reproduction, 2e. Ames, IA: Wiley Blackwell, 2011:2211–2221.
Lear TL, Villagomez AF. Cytogenetic evaluation of mares and foals. In: McKinnon AO, Squires EL, Vaala WE, Varner DD, eds. Equine Reproduction, 2e. Ames, IA: Wiley Blackwell, 2011:1951–1962.

Author Peter R. Morresey
Consulting Editor Carla L. Carleton

BASICS

DEFINITION
Clostridial myositis is an infection of muscle by *Clostridium* spp. most frequently associated with IM injection. The infection may remain localized and form a focal abscess or migrate along fascial planes, resulting in diffuse necrotizing cellulitis.

PATHOPHYSIOLOGY
The frequent temporal association between IM injections and clostridial myositis suggests entry of the organism at the time of injection. However, injection of irritating substances may produce local tissue necrosis and an anaerobic environment ideal for proliferation of spores that may already be present in muscle. Because of the ubiquitous nature of clostridial organisms both in the environment and as commensals in the horse, they may contaminate wounds and surgical sites. The release of potent clostridial exotoxins leads to local tissue necrosis, systemic toxemia, and organ dysfunction. In this most severe form, the term "malignant edema" is used to reflect the systemic involvement and high mortality.

SYSTEMS AFFECTED
Musculoskeletal
This is the primary system affected. Necrotizing toxins released by the organism lead to local soft tissue necrosis. Osteitis of cervical vertebrae in close proximity to the infection may occur.

Cardiovascular/Hemic
Exotoxins absorbed from the site of infection may induce intra- or extravascular hemolysis and increased capillary permeability. Transient hypertrophic cardiomyopathy has been documented.

Renal/Hepatobiliary
Toxemia can lead to multiple organ dysfunction.

GENETICS
N/A

INCIDENCE/PREVALENCE
Some geographic areas may have a greater incidence owing to higher environmental contamination by clostridial organisms.

SIGNALMENT
Clostridial myositis occurs in horses of any breed or age.

SIGNS
Historical Findings
IM injection with a non-antibiotic medication is the most common cause of clostridial myositis, and thus owners should be questioned about recent medications, treatments, or illnesses. Depending on the site of infection, horses may be stiff and reluctant to walk, lame, or unwilling to raise or lower the head to eat. Pain and systemic toxemia

may lead to anorexia and tachypnea. Vague signs of discomfort are easily mistaken for colic.

Physical Examination Findings
If myonecrosis is related to IM injection, common sites of injection should be palpated for heat, pain, swelling, and crepitus. Small puncture wounds are occasionally only visible once the hair over the affected area is clipped. Swellings are initially warm and painful and later become cool, firm, and necrotic. Muscle pain may cause a lame or stiff gait, reluctance to walk, depression, anorexia, tachypnea, and tachycardia. Dehydration, depression, delayed CRT, poor peripheral pulses, and cool extremities suggest systemic toxemia and inadequate peripheral perfusion and shock. Oral mucous membranes may be dark red to blue. Fever is common.

CAUSES
Clostridial myositis is most often associated with *Clostridium perfringens* (type A) and *Clostridium septicum*, but *Clostridium chauvoei, Clostridium novyi, Clostridium fallax,* and *Clostridium sordellii* have also been reported.

RISK FACTORS
Although any IM injection could potentially result in a clostridial infection, medications that are irritating and result in tissue necrosis are frequently associated with this syndrome. Flunixin meglumine is most commonly implicated; however, IM injection of other medications such as xylazine, ivermectin, vitamin B complex, antihistamines, phenylbutazone, dipyrone (metamizole), synthetic prostaglandins, and vaccines have also been associated with clostridial myositis.

DIAGNOSIS

DIFFERENTIAL DIAGNOSIS
When clostridial myositis is secondary to an injection, the diagnosis can be complicated by previous medical problems. Pain associated with myonecrosis may be confused with colic, exertional myopathy, laminitis, or abscesses from other causes. Severe pain, fever, toxemia, and shock rarely result from an abscess due to other less virulent organisms.

CBC/BIOCHEMISTRY/URINALYSIS
If clostridial infection is localized into an abscess, a CBC may reveal only a modest leukocytosis with left shift and neutrophilia. Hyperfibrinogenemia may be present if infection is present for more than a few days. When severe systemic toxemia develops, anemia, leukopenia, thrombocytopenia, and intra-/extravascular hemolysis can occur. If IMHA is present, spontaneous autoagglutination may be seen. Increases in muscle enzymes creatine kinase and aspartate aminotransferase may be mild compared with

the apparent severity of toxemia perhaps due to the focal nature of the disease, destruction of enzyme, or lack of enzyme absorption into the systemic circulation. Dehydration and shock may result in azotemia and hemoconcentration. Increases in hepatic enzymes, total bilirubin, and bile acids may occur. Hemoglobinuria/myoglobinuria may be present. Urinalysis results should be evaluated with the serum chemistry to measure renal insult.

OTHER LABORATORY TESTS
Clostridial toxins may result in DIC and alterations in clotting factors. Elevation in cardiac troponin I may suggest myocardial injury and should be paired with echocardiography. A direct Coombs test may be positive in cases developing IMHA.

IMAGING
Ultrasonography may reveal an encapsulated abscess or diffuse tissue edema, necrosis, cellulitis, and echogenic foci of emphysema. Differentiation between focal abscesses and diffuse cellulitis aids in defining areas for treatment. Abscesses should be lanced and lavaged. Fasciotomy/myotomy is appropriate if diffuse cellulitis and myonecrosis are present.

OTHER DIAGNOSTIC PROCEDURES
A tentative diagnosis can be made based on a history of IM injection or wound and a rapid onset of clinical signs. Diagnosis can be confirmed by aspiration of purulent or serosanguineous material for anaerobic culture, cytology, or fluorescent antibody identification. Care should be taken to properly prepare sites for aspiration to avoid contamination with surface organisms. Samples should be collected and placed in a medium designed for transportation of anaerobic specimens and submitted to a laboratory as soon as possible. Muscle biopsies frequently reveal characteristic Gram-positive rods.

PATHOLOGIC FINDINGS
Systemic toxemia results in the degeneration of parenchymatous tissues. Malodorous serosanguineous fluid and emphysema are present in dark-colored necrotic muscle.

TREATMENT

APPROPRIATE HEALTH CARE
Treatment options are dictated by the severity of the disease. Focal encapsulated abscesses may be managed in the field; however, referral should be considered for horses with signs of systemic toxemia (tachycardia, increased CRT, abnormal mucous membrane color, poor peripheral pulses, or cool extremities).

NURSING CARE
Oral or parenteral fluids are indicated if dehydration is present and balanced polyionic

CLOSTRIDIAL MYOSITIS (CONTINUED)

fluids (lactated or acetated Ringer's solution) should be administered IV if there are signs of shock. Hot-packing may aid in drainage of abscesses, whereas later in the course of the disease cold hydrotherapy may decrease the activity of inflammatory mediators. Feed and water should be provided at head level for horses with neck pain associated with infection of cervical musculature.

ACTIVITY
Activity should be limited to decrease movement of bacteria along fascial planes.

DIET
N/A

CLIENT EDUCATION
Clients should be educated on which medications are appropriately given IM. Alternate routes of administration for certain medications, such as orally for flunixin meglumine, should be emphasized.

SURGICAL CONSIDERATIONS
Focal abscesses may be drained by incision, lavage, and placement of a drain. Diffuse cellulitis and tissue edema are important to identify echographically because medical management may be more appropriate for this type of infection. Depending on the severity of the disease, fenestration of infected tissue with vertical incisions is helpful in reducing an anaerobic environment. Incisions are made through skin and necrotic muscle so as to aerate tissues and reduce pressure associated with severe edema. Minimal sedation and hemostasis are frequently necessary owing to the necrotic nature of the tissue incised.

MEDICATIONS

DRUG(S) OF CHOICE
• Horses with severe systemic signs are initially given potassium or sodium penicillin (44 000 IU/kg IV) every 2–4 h until stabilized and then 4 times daily. Focal abscesses can be managed with drainage and penicillin (22 000 IU/kg IM every 12 h)
• Metronidazole (15–25 mg/kg PO every 6 h) is also effective against *Clostridium* spp. and can be given orally or rectally

• Oxytetracycline (6.6 mg/kg IV every 24 h) has also been successfully paired with metronidazole
• Analgesics and anti-inflammatory medications (flunixin meglumine 1.1 mg/kg IV every 12 h) are indicated

CONTRAINDICATIONS
N/A

PRECAUTIONS
Hydration and renal function should be monitored when using nonsteroidal anti-inflammatory medications in horses with severe systemic disease.

POSSIBLE INTERACTIONS
N/A

ALTERNATIVE DRUGS
• Chloramphenicol (50 mg/kg PO every 6) also has activity against anaerobic bacteria; however, owing to the potential for irreversible aplastic anemia in people, its use should be avoided if possible
• Trimethoprim-potentiated sulfonamides are efficacious in vitro but have questionable in vivo efficacy
• Rifampin (rifampicin) is effective against most *Clostridium* spp.; however, it is generally used in combination with other antimicrobials owing to the development of resistance

FOLLOW-UP

PATIENT MONITORING
N/A

PREVENTION/AVOIDANCE
Avoiding IM injection of irritating or frequently implicated medications may reduce the incidence of *Clostridium* myositis.

POSSIBLE COMPLICATIONS
Severe toxemia may lead to shock, renal insufficiency, hepatobiliary insult, laminitis, intravascular hemolysis, cardiomyopathy, DIC, collapse, or death.

EXPECTED COURSE AND PROGNOSIS
Small, focal abscesses may respond well to drainage and systemic antimicrobials. Horses with diffuse myositis, toxemia, and shock

have a guarded to poor prognosis in spite of aggressive therapy. *C. septicum* and *C. chauvoei* infections are usually fatal; however, *C. perfringens* infections have a better prognosis.

MISCELLANEOUS

ASSOCIATED CONDITIONS
N/A

AGE-RELATED FACTORS
N/A

ZOONOTIC POTENTIAL
C. perfringens is the most common cause of malignant edema in people.

PREGNANCY/FERTILITY/BREEDING
N/A

SYNONYMS
• Clostridial cellulitis
• Clostridial myonecrosis
• Malignant edema

SEE ALSO
• Botulism
• *Clostridium difficile* infection
• Tetanus
• Tyzzer disease (*Clostridium piliforme*)

ABBREVIATIONS
• CRT = capillary refill time
• DIC = disseminated intravascular coagulation
• IMHA = immune-mediated hemolytic anemia

Suggested Reading
Peek SF, Semrad AD, Perkins GA. Clostridial myonecrosis in horses (37 cases 1985–2000). Equine Vet J 2003;35(1):86–92.
Rebhun WC, Shin SJ, King JM, et al. Malignant edema in horses. J Am Vet Med Assoc 1985;187:732–736.

Author Liz Arbittier
Consulting Editor Ashley G. Boyle
Acknowledgment The author and editor acknowledge the prior contribution of Kerry E. Beckman.

CLOSTRIDIUM DIFFICILE INFECTION

BASICS

DEFINITION
CDI is an inflammation of the small intestine, cecum, and large colon commonly resulting in diarrhea and varying degrees of toxemia.

PATHOPHYSIOLOGY
Clostridium difficile is a Gram-positive spore-forming bacterium found in a small percentage of healthy adult horses, and a larger percentage of young healthy foals. It is acquired through ingestion of spores. The disease is hypothesized to occur from a disruption of the normal resident GI microbiota, often as a result of antimicrobial exposure. *C. difficile* produces 2 major toxins (A and B), a cytotoxin and an enterotoxin, that work synergistically. However, strains that only produce toxin B are capable of inducing disease. These toxins cause clinical signs by their direct toxic effects on the colon and through proinflammatory effects on neutrophils. The net result are varying degrees of fluid secretion, mucosal damage, and intestinal inflammation. Some strains of *C. difficile* also produce a binary toxin, but its role in equine enterocolitis is unknown.

SYSTEMS AFFECTED
GI
C. difficile can cause soft–loose to profuse and watery diarrhea, mild to severe colic, and, occasionally, fever.

Cardiovascular
Dehydration and cardiovascular shock can ensue.

Musculoskeletal
Peripheral edema and laminitis.

INCIDENCE/PREVALENCE
It is usually sporadic, but outbreaks have been reported and are most common in foals on breeding farms.

SIGNALMENT
There is no reported breed, age, or sex predilection.

SIGNS
Historical Findings
Depression, anorexia, diarrhea, colic, and/or pyrexia. Recent or current antibiotic use.

Physical Examination Findings
• Diarrhea in most cases that may be associated with dehydration, and tachycardia
• Rectal temperature may be subnormal, normal, or increased
• Signs of endotoxemia and peripheral edema may be present
• Colic may result from inflammation, fluid, and gas distention of the GI tract

CAUSES
Infectious
The proliferation of the toxigenic *C. difficile* and the production of its exotoxins.

RISK FACTORS
• Not clearly established; however, antibiotics and hospitalization have been associated with both colonization and disease
• Reported in mares whose foals were being treated with erythromycin succinate
• Hospitalization, as in humans, but equine hospital outbreaks are very rare
• Other stressors, such as surgery and transportation, may play a role in sporadic cases

DIAGNOSIS

DIFFERENTIAL DIAGNOSIS
• Salmonellosis
• Potomac horse fever
• *Clostridium perfringens* enterocolitis
• Cyathostomiasis
• NSAID-induced colitis
• Cantharidin toxicosis
• Chronic sand impaction
• Idiopathic colitis

CBC/BIOCHEMISTRY/URINALYSIS
CBC
The packed cell volume is often elevated. Total protein levels are variable and may be increased due to hemoconcentration or decreased due to protein loss. Leukopenia with neutropenia with left shift is often present. Neutrophils may be degenerate. A leukocytosis develops at later stages of the disease.

Biochemistry
Hyponatremia and hypochloremia are characteristic. Hypokalemia is sometimes present, but hyperkalemia in response to a metabolic acidosis can occur. Hypocalcemia and hypoalbuminemia are also common. Prerenal azotemia is common in dehydrated animals.

OTHER LABORATORY TESTS
• Culture of this organism is difficult, and is not diagnostic
• The clinical standard for diagnosis is detection of *C. difficile* toxins A or B in feces using enzyme immunoassays, and some commercial assays have good sensitivity and specificity. Tests that only detect toxin A can be used but because strains that only produce toxin B can cause disease in horses, false-negative cases can occur
• Antigen testing of feces via immunoassay can be used as a screening test. Antigen-negative results have a high negative predictive value, but antigen-positive samples should be tested further to determine whether toxins are present
• PCR is commonly used to detect toxin genes in fecal samples of human patients and in horses. While potentially highly sensitive and specific, the same concerns exist as for culture, as positive results will be obtained

from horses that are colonized with strains containing toxin genes in the absence of production of toxins
• Bacterial culture for *Salmonella* spp. should also be performed because it is a major differential diagnosis, and co-infection can occur

IMAGING
The large colon contents may appear hypoechoic with increased motility and the intestinal wall may be thickened.

OTHER DIAGNOSTIC PROCEDURES
Palpation per rectum to rule out another GI lesion.

PATHOLOGIC FINDINGS
Gross abnormalities include fluid intestinal contents, and multifocal hemorrhagic or diffusely darker appearance of the serosal surface of the small and large intestines. More severe cases may have marked intestinal edema and hemorrhage, with petechiae and ecchymoses throughout. Histologically, depending on the severity, the small and large intestine may have mucosal necrosis, mucosal and/or submucosal thrombosis, hemorrhage, edema, congestion, neutrophilic infiltration, fibrinonecrotic pseudomembranes, and occasionally numerous Gram-positive rods on the superficial mucosa can be present.

TREATMENT

APPROPRIATE HEALTH CARE
Best managed intensively owing to the frequent need for aggressive fluid therapy and the high risk of secondary problems. If the diarrhea is not severe and adequate hydration can be maintained, treatment on farm could be attempted.

NURSING CARE
IV fluid therapy with balanced polyionic electrolyte solution is the most important supportive treatment. Sodium bicarbonate may be required to correct a severe metabolic acidosis. In severely hypokalemic horses, 20–40 mEq/L of potassium chloride can be added to the IV fluids. IV administration of KCl should not exceed 0.5 mEq/kg/h. Oral supplementation with KCl (50 g every 6 or 8 h) is also effective to correct hypokalemia. An oral electrolyte solution along with clean, fresh drinking water should be provided. Hypertonic saline (4–6 mL/kg IV of 5–7.5% NaCl) may be indicated in severely dehydrated animals. Feet should be iced for 72 h continuously in an attempt to prevent laminitis.

ACTIVITY
Animals should be handled accordingly and an isolated area should be used and disinfected appropriately because diarrheic horses are potentially infectious.

CLOSTRIDIUM DIFFICILE INFECTION   (CONTINUED)

DIET
Free-choice hay, preferably in a hay net, because hypoproteinemic horses eating off the ground may develop severe facial edema. Large amounts of grain should be avoided due to the risk of further GI flora disruption. Owing to the severe catabolic state that occurs in colitis, forced enteral feeding or partial or total parenteral nutrition may be required.

CLIENT EDUCATION
Clients should be made aware of the potential for mortality and the serious risk of secondary problems such as laminitis and jugular vein thrombosis. They should also be warned that the horse should be considered infectious, and appropriate sanitation of contaminated areas should be recommended.

SURGICAL CONSIDERATIONS
N/A

MEDICATIONS

DRUG(S) OF CHOICE
• Metronidazole—15–25 mg/kg PO every 6–8 h
• Flunixin meglumine—0.25–0.5 mg/kg every 8 h IV for its purported antiendotoxic effects; 1.1 mg/kg for analgesia
• Fresh-frozen plasma—<40 g/L (4.0 g/dL); although not proved to be of added benefit in cases of colitis
• KCL—25–50 g PO every 12–24 h. Oral administration of KCl once or twice a day is an easy and cost-effective route of supplementation
• Laminitis treatment—see chapter Laminitis

CONTRAINDICATIONS
Metronidazole may be teratogenic and is therefore contraindicated in pregnant mares.

PRECAUTIONS
Flunixin meglumine may be nephrotoxic in dehydrated animals. It may mask severe pain that indicates a surgical lesion, and should be used judiciously when the diagnosis is still in question.

POSSIBLE INTERACTIONS
Cimetidine should not be used concurrently with metronidazole because there is interaction through hepatic inhibition.

ALTERNATIVE DRUGS
N/A

FOLLOW-UP

PATIENT MONITORING
Frequent monitoring of hydration status, character and volume of diarrhea, and for presence of edema, and observe for signs of colic and laminitis.

PREVENTION/AVOIDANCE
Antibiotics should be used judiciously to decrease the risk of disruption of the GI microflora.

POSSIBLE COMPLICATIONS
• Endotoxemia
• Laminitis
• Jugular vein thrombosis
• Renal failure

EXPECTED COURSE AND PROGNOSIS
Mortality rates range from 10% to 40%; however, referral hospital-based studies are a biased population and the overall mortality rate is likely lower. Death can occur from the primary GI disease; however, euthanasia is often opted for due to cost of treatment, poor response to initial treatment, or development of severe laminitis. The prognosis is good when the diarrhea resolves shortly after presentation and no signs of laminitis occur.

MISCELLANEOUS

ASSOCIATED CONDITIONS
• Laminitis
• Venous thrombosis

AGE-RELATED FACTORS
N/A

ZOONOTIC POTENTIAL
Some *C. difficile* strains found in horses are also found in people with CDI. While it is unknown whether horse–human transmission occurs, it is advisable to treat all affected horses as zoonotic risks.

PREGNANCY/FERTILITY/BREEDING
Metronidazole should not be administered to pregnant mares. An increased risk of abortion may be present due to endotoxemia and hypovolemic shock.

SYNONYMS
• *C. difficile*-associated diarrhea
• *C. difficile* enterocolitis

SEE ALSO
Laminitis

ABBREVIATIONS
• CDI = *Clostridium difficile* infection
• GI = gastrointestinal
• NSAID = nonsteroidal anti-inflammatory drug
• PCR = polymerase chain reaction

Suggested Reading
Baverud V, Gustafsson A, Franklin A, et al. *Clostridium difficile* associated with acute colitis in mature horses treated with antibiotics. Equine Vet J 1997;29:279–284.
Weese JS, Toxopeus L, Arroyo L. *Clostridium difficile* associated diarrhoea in horses within the community: predictors, clinical presentation and outcome. Equine Vet J 2006;38:185–188.

Authors Luis G. Arroyo and J. Scott Weese
Consulting Editors Henry Stämpfli and Olimpo Oliver-Espinosa

COAGULATION DEFECTS, ACQUIRED

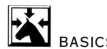

BASICS

DEFINITION
• Results in hemostatic dysfunction and subsequent bleeding tendencies
• They may be classified as:
  ◦ Disorders that impair fibrin clot formation, known as coagulation defects
  ◦ Disorders that impair platelet plug formation due to platelet function deficiencies (e.g. idiopathic thrombocytopenia, thrombasthenia, antiplatelet drug administration) or endothelial damage (e.g. vasculitis)
  ◦ Disorders in which primary hemostasis and coagulation factor pathways are inadequate due to a consumptive coagulopathy (e.g. DIC)

PATHOPHYSIOLOGY
• Vitamin K is essential for hepatic synthesis of several coagulation factors (II, VII, IX, and X) and protein C
• Vitamin K deficiency results in a gradual decrease of circulating coagulation factors, causing progressive coagulation impairment and unexpected bleeding
• The rate of decrease in coagulation factor concentrations depends on their half-lives. Factor VII has the shortest half-life (<6–7 h) and its concentration decreases rapidly, affecting the extrinsic coagulation pathway and prolonging PT. As the condition progresses, concentrations of other coagulation factors decrease, affecting also the intrinsic pathway and prolonging aPTT
• In cases of hepatic failure, a coagulation defect occurs as a result of a decrease in coagulation factor synthesis, especially fibrinogen and the vitamin K-dependent factors
• An acquired coagulation factor VIII (hemophilia A) deficiency was recently reported in a mare with hematomas, hemoabdomen, and blood loss anemia. The development of anti-factor VIII antibodies was considered idiopathic. The mare responded to transfusions of fresh whole blood and plasma and immunosuppressive treatment

SYSTEMS AFFECTED
• Hemic/lymphatic/immune—coagulation deficiencies are associated with prolonged bleeding after wounds/trauma or spontaneous hemorrhages
• Other systems may be affected, depending on the sites of hemorrhage. The most frequently affected systems are the musculoskeletal, respiratory, and GI systems

INCIDENCE/PREVALENCE
• Vitamin K deficiency in horses is very rare. However, toxicosis caused by ingestion of moldy sweet clover (*Melilotus officinalis*) hay has been reported

• Anticoagulant toxicosis is rare now because warfarin administration is currently not recommended in horses, and heparin administration is restricted to patients receiving critical care
• Abnormal coagulation is common in horses (up to 50%) with hepatic disease

SIGNS

General Comments
• Historical findings depend on etiology
• Clinical signs of acquired coagulation defects are similar to those of the hemorrhagic form of DIC, but must be differentiated in order to institute appropriate therapy

Historical Findings
• Excessive hemorrhage after minor trauma or surgery
• Unexplained epistaxis or other mucosal bleeding
• Previous exposure to moldy sweet clover hay or rodenticides
• Previous anticoagulant administration

Physical Examination Findings
• Characterized by spontaneous bleeding from body orifices or into body cavities and hematoma formation
• The most common signs associated with spontaneous hemorrhage include SC or IM hematomas, hemarthrosis, epistaxis, hematuria, melena, and ecchymoses in mucous membranes
• Prolonged bleeding from wounds or after minor surgical procedures possible
• Usually, there are no petechial hemorrhages in mucous membranes. This may be used to distinguish this condition from a primary hemostatic deficiency (e.g. platelet disorder) and DIC. In cases of DIC, other clinical signs associated with the underlying disease are also observed

CAUSES
• The most common causes of vitamin K deficiency are:
  ◦ Ingestion of moldy sweet clover (*Melilotus* spp.); fresh, in hay or in silage
  ◦ Ingestion of plants containing coumarine glycosides—ferns, some pines, and the Mediterranean plant *Ferula communis*
  ◦ Accidental ingestion of rodenticides containing first- or second-generation anticoagulants
  ◦ Chronic intestinal malabsorption problems that decrease vitamin K absorption
  ◦ Hepatic failure
• Anticoagulants used in equine medicine that may cause a coagulation deficiency disorder are:
  ◦ Warfarin, which has previously been advocated as an oral anticoagulant for use in horses (no longer recommended)
  ◦ Heparin (unfractionated and LMWH), which is recommended for treatment of endotoxemia

RISK FACTORS
Administration of warfarin together with other albumin-binding drugs, such as phenylbutazone, or any condition that causes hypoalbuminemia, may increase the risk of warfarin toxicosis.

DIAGNOSIS

DIFFERENTIAL DIAGNOSIS
• Other causes of spontaneous hemorrhage and/or ecchymosis
• DIC (hemorrhagic form) can be difficult to distinguish from an acquired coagulation defect. Clinical signs, identification of an underlying disease consistent with DIC, and plasma D-dimer concentrations may assist differentiation
• Inherited coagulation deficiencies (e.g. hemophilia A) can also be difficult to distinguish from an acquired coagulation defect
• Platelet disorders (i.e. thrombocytopenia) can be differentiated by platelet counts or tests of platelet function
• Vasculitis can be differentiated by histopathology and identification of the underlying cause of vasculitis

CBC/BIOCHEMISTRY/URINALYSIS
• Platelet count usually remains within the normal range. Thrombocytopenia is rarely observed, in contrast to DIC
• Urinalysis may show hematuria
• In cases of hepatic failure, liver enzymes (i.e. sorbitol dehydrogenase, glutamate dehydrogenase, γ-glutamyltransferase) are markedly elevated

OTHER LABORATORY TESTS
• PT and aPTT are prolonged (>15 and 65 s, respectively). In the initial stages of vitamin K deficiency, regardless of its cause, PT values are prolonged first and aPTT may remain within normal limits. In more chronic cases, PT and aPTT are markedly prolonged. Ongoing monitoring is recommended to assess clinical progression
• ACT (a simple variation of aPTT) is also prolonged. While ACT is simpler to perform, PT and aPTT are usually more reliable
• Plasma D-dimer concentration is commonly normal (0–500 ng/mL), although body cavity hemorrhages and hematomas may produce a mild increase (normally <1000 ng/mL). Increases in D-dimer concentration >2000 ng/mL are commonly observed in horses with DIC but rare in vitamin K deficiency
• Thrombin time and aPTT are specifically recommended to detect overdoses of unfractionated heparin as these are markedly prolonged in heparin toxicosis. However, an overdose of LMWH must be confirmed by measuring plasma anti-factor Xa activity and

aPTT, which are above therapeutic limits and markedly prolonged, respectively

IMAGING
Ultrasonography and radiography may be used to diagnose and monitor the progression of body cavity hemorrhages and other sites of hemorrhage.

OTHER DIAGNOSTIC PROCEDURES
Cytology of collected fluid can confirm the presence of body cavity hemorrhages, hemarthroses, or hematomas.

PATHOLOGIC FINDINGS
Hemorrhages and hematomas in a variety of tissues, especially the respiratory and GI tracts.

TREATMENT

AIMS
• In vitamin K deficiency (i.e. rodenticide toxicities) treatment consists of removal of the source of the toxin, vitamin K administration, and restoration of coagulation factor synthesis
• The aim of this treatment differs from the aims of treatment for hemorrhagic DIC, and it is important to differentiate if the coagulation defect is due to vitamin K deficiency or DIC prior to treatment
• In hepatic failure the aim of treatment is to replace the deficient coagulation factors and to treat the underlying cause of liver failure

APPROPRIATE HEALTH CARE
• Should be managed as inpatients due to the need for close monitoring of clotting times and for control of bleeding complications
• Patients with profuse bleeding should be managed as a life-threatening emergency

NURSING CARE
• Fresh (frozen) plasma transfusion in cases of severe bleeding in order to replace plasma clotting factors
• Minimize trauma and venipunctures in these patients

ACTIVITY
Minimize exercise and trauma while clotting times (PT and aPTT) remain prolonged.

DIET
Green leafy feeds, including hay and fresh pasture, are high in vitamin K1. Thus, good quality alfalfa hay is recommended.

MEDICATIONS

DRUG(S) OF CHOICE
• Vitamin K deficiency should be treated with vitamin K1 (0.5–1 mg/kg SC every 6 h) until PT values return to normal. In horses intoxicated with brodifacoum, several weeks of vitamin K1 therapy (2.5 mg/kg SC or PO every 12 h) may be required due to the long half-life of this toxin
• Antifibrinolytic drugs, such as aminocaproic acid (20–40 mg/kg IV diluted in saline and given over 30–60 min), may be used in order to reduce bleeding until coagulation factors are restored
• In heparin toxicosis, heparin antagonists such as protamine sulfate (1 mg for every 100 U of heparin administered) may have significant side effects and are not recommended

CONTRAINDICATIONS
• Administration of other anticoagulants and/or antiplatelet drugs may worsen the coagulation defect
• Parenterally administered vitamin K3 is nephrotoxic to horses and may produce signs of colic and acute renal failure

POSSIBLE INTERACTIONS
Other drugs may interfere with vitamin K1 binding and should be avoided—phenylbutazone, heparin, phenytoin, salicylates, quinidine, potentiated sulfonamides, and steroid hormones.

FOLLOW-UP

PATIENT MONITORING
• Monitor PT and aPTT until normalization
• Plasma D-dimer concentration and platelet count may also be monitored

PREVENTION/AVOIDANCE
Warfarin administration is not recommended.

POSSIBLE COMPLICATIONS
Tissue hemorrhages may be complicated by secondary infections.

EXPECTED COURSE AND PROGNOSIS
• Vitamin K deficiencies have a good prognosis and rapid resolution when diagnosed and treated early

• Coagulation defects due to hepatic failure have a guarded prognosis

MISCELLANEOUS

PREGNANCY/FERTILITY/BREEDING
Rodenticides may cross the placenta, causing fetal coagulation defects.

SYNONYMS
Hypocoagulable disorders.

SEE ALSO
• Anticoagulant rodenticide toxicosis
• Coagulation defects, inherited
• Dicoumarol (moldy sweet clover) toxicosis
• Disseminated intravascular coagulation
• Hemorrhage, acute
• Petechiae, ecchymoses, and hematomas
• Purpura haemorrhagica
• Thrombocytopenia

ABBREVIATIONS
• ACT = activated clotting time
• aPTT = activated partial thromboplastin time
• DIC = disseminated intravascular coagulation
• GI = gastrointestinal
• LMWH = low-molecular-weight heparin
• PT = prothrombin time

Suggested Reading
Monreal L. Monitoring the coagulation system. In: Corley K, Stephan J, eds. The Equine Hospital Manual. Oxford, UK: Blackwell, 2008:401–408.
Sellon DC. Disorders of the hematopoietic system. In: Reed SM, Bayly WM, Sellon DC, eds. Equine Internal Medicine, 2e. St. Louis, MO: WB Saunders, 2004:721–768.

Author Eduard Jose-Cunilleras
Consulting Editors David Hodgson, Harold C. McKenzie, and Jennifer L. Hodgson
Acknowledgment The author and editors acknowledge the prior contribution of Luis Monreal.

BASICS

OVERVIEW

• Several rare inherited coagulation deficiencies occur in horses:
  ○ vWD (vWF deficiency)—vWF is involved in platelet adhesion, and this defect results in abnormal platelet adhesion and platelet plug formation
  ○ Glanzmann thrombasthenia is a deficiency/dysfunction of the platelet glycoprotein IIb/IIIa complex, critical to platelet adhesion and aggregation
  ○ Hemophilia A (factor VIII deficiency) results in a defect in the intrinsic coagulation pathway, with deficient clot formation
  ○ Prekallikrein deficiency leads to defective initiation of the intrinsic coagulation pathway as this glycoprotein stimulates activation of factor XII
  ○ Protein C deficiency results in a hypercoagulable state and thrombotic events, as protein C is a critical coagulation inhibitor

SIGNALMENT

• Most disorders are inherited in an autosomal recessive pattern and occur in young purebred horses
• Hemophilia A is most common, and has been diagnosed in Thoroughbred, Standardbred, Quarter Horse, Tennessee Walking Horse, and Arabian colts. It is an X-linked recessive chromosomal abnormality usually evident in colts <6 months of age (up to 3 years)
• Prekallikrein deficiency has been reported in families of American Miniature and Belgian horses, affecting males and females. Horses with signs are homozygous, while heterozygous horses are asymptomatic
• vWF deficiency has been reported in young Quarter Horses and Thoroughbreds
• Glanzmann thrombasthenia has been reported in young and adult horses (Thoroughbred cross; Quarter Horse; Peruvian Paso; Oldenburg)
• Protein C deficiency has been diagnosed in a Thoroughbred colt

SIGNS

There are 3 clinical forms:
• When the defect affects platelet function or primary hemostasis (e.g. vWF deficiency, Glanzmann thrombasthenia), signs are spontaneous epistaxis or bleeding involving mucosal surfaces and prolonged bleeding after trauma/surgery. Petechiae may be observed
• When the defect affects clot formation or secondary hemostasis (e.g. hemophilia A),

signs are a bleeding tendency with spontaneous hemorrhages or prolonged bleeding after trauma/surgery. Bleeding into body cavities, joints, muscles, and subcutaneously is common
• When the defect is related to a coagulation inhibitor defect (e.g. protein C deficiency), signs are related to the subsequent hypercoagulable state (thrombosis)

DIAGNOSIS

DIFFERENTIAL DIAGNOSIS

• Disseminated intravascular coagulation (hemorrhagic form)—clinical signs and plasma D-dimer concentrations may aid differentiation
• Acquired coagulation defects can be difficult to distinguish from inherited defects
• Platelet disorders (e.g. thrombocytopenia) can be differentiated by platelet counts or tests of platelet function

CBC/BIOCHEMISTRY/URINALYSIS

• Few or no changes in CBC, serum biochemistry, and urinalysis
• Most affected animals have normal platelet counts, but mild thrombocytopenia may be noted if profuse bleeding has occurred

OTHER LABORATORY TESTS

• vWD—prolonged TBT, normal to prolonged aPTT, and decreased plasma vWF antigen concentration
• Glanzmann thrombasthenia—prolonged TBT but normal platelet count, PT, aPTT, and vWF antigen concentration. Platelet aggregation responses are markedly impaired
• Hemophilia A—prolonged aPTT, normal PT, and reduced plasma factor VIII activity
• Prekallikrein deficiency—prolonged aPTT, normal PT, and reduced plasma prekallikrein activity
• Protein C deficiency—reduced plasma protein C activity and/or antigen concentration

IMAGING

Ultrasonography for suspected hematomas, hemothorax, or hemoperitoneum.

OTHER DIAGNOSTIC PROCEDURES

Cytology can confirm the presence of internal hemorrhage.

TREATMENT

Potential treatments focus on restoration of the deficient factor by means of whole blood or plasma transfusions. Owners should be informed that these diseases have no cure.

MEDICATIONS

CONTRAINDICATIONS/POSSIBLE INTERACTIONS

Other treatments affecting platelet function (e.g. colloids) or coagulation (e.g. heparin) may exacerbate bleeding tendency.

FOLLOW-UP

PATIENT MONITORING

Continuous monitoring is indicated due to the risk of recurrent hemorrhage.

PREVENTION/AVOIDANCE

• Affected animals and their parents should not be used for breeding
• Preoperative blood transfusions may be necessary to reduce intrasurgical and postsurgical risk of bleeding

EXPECTED COURSE AND PROGNOSIS

There is no cure.

MISCELLANEOUS

PREGNANCY/FERTILITY/BREEDING

N/A

SEE ALSO

• Coagulation defects, acquired
• Hemorrhage, acute
• Hemorrhage, chronic

ABBREVIATIONS

• aPTT = activated partial thromboplastin time
• PT = prothrombin time
• TBT = template bleeding time
• vWD = von Willebrand disease
• vWF = von Willebrand factor

Suggested Reading
Zimmel DN. Hemostatic disorders. In: Robinson NE, ed. Current Therapy in Equine Medicine, 5e. Philadelphia, PA: Saunders, 2003:351–354.

Author Eduard Jose-Cunilleras
Consulting Editors David Hodgson, Harold C. McKenzie, and Jennifer L. Hodgson
Acknowledgment The author and editors acknowledge the prior contribution of Luis Monreal.

COCCIDIOIDOMYCOSIS

BASICS

OVERVIEW
• *Coccidioides immitis* and *Coccidioides posadasii* are saprophytic soil fungi endemic to the southwestern USA, including parts of California, Arizona, New Mexico, Texas, Nevada, and Utah
• Animals and humans become infected when they inhale arthroconidia released into the air from growing mycelia, after which the arthroconidia enlarge to form a spherule that can then rupture to release endospores. The endospores can mature into additional endosporulating spherules, leading to rapid proliferation of infective units within the affected host
• Because of the respiratory route of exposure, the organism commonly causes localized respiratory tract infections but can spread by blood and lymph to other organs such as bone, skin, and abdominal viscera
• There are multiple specific forms of disease, including interstitial pneumonia, osteomyelitis, mastitis, abortion, and disseminated and cutaneous forms. Prognosis and diagnosis vary greatly depending on the form
• Serologic survey data show that 4.1% of horses in endemic areas carry a low positive IgG titer to *C. immitis*, all of which were asymptomatic and showed spontaneous resolution of their positive titers over a 2–6 month period, suggesting that exposure does not always result in clinical infection

SIGNALMENT
All age groups are susceptible to the illness.

SIGNS
• Presenting signs vary with disease form, but commonly include fever, chronic weight loss, present or historical respiratory signs, and an inflammatory leukogram
• Abortion, cutaneous lesions, and localized infections such as mastitis can also be seen

CAUSES AND RISK FACTORS
Residing in the endemic area is the main risk factor for disease.

DIAGNOSIS

DIFFERENTIAL DIAGNOSIS
Other systemic diseases causing fever, lethargy, an inflammatory leukogram, and pyogranulomatous lesions including infections with *Streptococcus equi* ssp. *equi*, *Rhodococcus equi*, and *Corynebacterium pseudotuberculosis*.

CBC/BIOCHEMISTRY/URINALYSIS
Typically include hyperfibrinogenemia, leukocytosis, mature neutrophilia, and hyperglobulinemia.

IMAGING
• Thoracic ultrasonography will often reveal pleural roughening, demonstrated as a comet-tail artifact, areas of pulmonary consolidation, and possible pleural effusion. Abdominal ultrasonography may detect a localized internal abscess or increased abdominal fluid
• Thoracic radiographs will often show a diffuse/interstitial miliary pattern consistent with granulomatous pneumonia

OTHER DIAGNOSTIC PROCEDURES
• With respiratory signs, a transtracheal wash is the diagnostic procedure of choice, as it may yield the organism on microbiologic culture as well as confirm suppurative inflammation on cytology
• Serology is also a key diagnostic test, as horses develop an initial IgM antibody response acutely following infection by the organism, followed shortly after by an IgG antibody response
• Magnitude of serologic titer has been statistically correlated with various forms of disease and may aid greatly in the decision to treat and prognosis for survival

PATHOLOGIC FINDINGS
Isolated or disseminated granulomatous lesions are the hallmark of the disease.

TREATMENT

Commonly accepted that prognosis is poor once the animal shows clinical disease. However, recent successful cases reported may prove that the pulmonary form of disease, especially if caught early before dissemination has occurred, may respond well to antifungal treatment.

MEDICATIONS

DRUG(S) OF CHOICE
• Horses with persistent elevated rectal temperature, anorexia, and lethargy can be treated with NSAIDs such as flunixin meglumine (0.5–1.1 mg/kg every 12–24 h IV or PO) or phenylbutazone (2–4 mg/kg every 12–24 h IV or PO) for 5–7 days, as long as their hydration status is believed normal
• Antifungal treatment using fluconazole at 14 mg/kg loading dose followed by 5 mg/kg PO every 24 h has been shown effective in pulmonary cases. Treatment duration may be several months and needs to be determined based on response to treatment, resolution of bloodwork abnormalities, and waning of serologic titer

FOLLOW-UP

PREVENTION/AVOIDANCE
• Environmental exposure can be difficult to prevent or avoid if living in an endemic area
• Precautions need to be taken to prevent secondary exposure from an animal with external infection or an infected carcass

MISCELLANEOUS

ABBREVIATIONS
• Ig = immunoglobulin
• NSAID = nonsteroidal anti-inflammatory drug

Suggested Reading
Higgins JC, Leith GS, Voss ED, Pappagianis D. Seroprevalence of antibodies against *Coccidioides immitis* in healthy horses. J Am Vet Med Assoc 2005;226:1888–1892.
Higgins JC, Leith GS, Pappagianis D, Pusterla N. Treatment of *Coccidioides immitis* pneumonia in two horses with fluconazole. Vet Rec 2006;159:349–351.
Higgins JC, Pusterla N, Pappagianis D. Comparison of *Coccidioides immitis* serological antibody titres between forms of clinical coccidioidomycosis in horses. Vet J 2007;173:118–123.

Author Jill C. Higgins
Consulting Editor Ashley G. Boyle

Client Education Handout available online

BASICS

OVERVIEW
Equine coccidiosis is a protozoal infection of the intestinal tract that is mainly associated with *Eimeria leuckarti*; however, *Eimeria uniungulsti* and *Eimeria solipedum* have also been reported worldwide. The pathogenic capacity of equine species of coccidia have not been clearly demonstrated; nevertheless, it has been determined that these protozoa affect epithelial cells of the small intestine, where they undergo development in cells displaced into the lamina propria and cause an increase in cell lifespan from a normal duration of 3–5 days to 28 days. Oocysts of *E. leuckarti* have been identified in the feces of normal horses and horses with diarrhea. The prepatent period is normally between 16 and 36 days. The meronts (schizonts) develop in the jejunum and ileum, mainly in the lacteals of these intestinal sections. This infestation has a worldwide distribution and has been reported on 5 continents. International reports indicated a prevalence of 0.6–2.6% mainly in foals. However, recent studies in Kentucky have shown prevalences of *E. leuckarti* oocysts of between 28% and 41.6% in foals and of between 86% and 100% of the farms studied.

SIGNALMENT
Detection of the causative organism is more prevalent in foals but it also occurs in adult horses. The organism is also a parasite of donkeys.

SIGNS
Because there are so many doubts about the pathogenic properties of the etiologic agent of equine coccidiosis, its presence is often considered an incidental finding. Signs associated with this infestation are profuse diarrhea despite not being observed frequently, massive intestinal hemorrhage, chronic diarrhea, jejunitis, and cecocolic intussusception; in some cases it has also been associated with weight loss and hair matting.

CAUSES AND RISK FACTORS
The causative organisms of equine coccidiosis are *E. leuckarti*, *E. uniungulsti*, and *E. solipedum*. Despite reports that *E. leuckarti* is more frequently seen in young animals, it has been suggested that age should not be considered a risk factor in this infection.

DIAGNOSIS

By identification of oocyst in feces. These oocysts are ovoidal, dark brown in color, 70–84 μm in length by 47–57 μm in width, and they have a 2-layer external wall (6–7.3 μm); they also have a micropyle at the narrower pole of the oocyst without a polar cap.

DIFFERENTIAL DIAGNOSIS
The finding of oocysts in the feces of any horse with diarrhea should not be taken as evidence of cause and effect. A thorough investigation for other causes of diarrhea (e.g. salmonellosis, Potomac horse fever, cyathostomiasis) should be undertaken.

CBC/BIOCHEMISTRY/URINALYSIS
N/A

OTHER LABORATORY TESTS
Fecal flotation is the main diagnostic test. Saturated sodium nitrate gives better concentration of oocysts of *E. leuckarti*; however, it has been shown recently that a sedimentation–flotation technique has been more sensitive for diagnosis of *E. leuckarti* infection.

TREATMENT

There is no therapeutic regimen reported for equine coccidial infestation.

Suggested Reading
De Souza PNB, Bomfimb TCB, Huber F, et al. Natural infection by *Cryptosporidium* sp, *Giardia* sp and *Eimeria leuckarti* in three groups of equines with different handlings in Rio de Janeiro, Brazil. Vet Parasitol 2009;160:327–333.
Dos Santos CS, Pereira B, Teixeira VL, Gomes CW. *Eimeria leuckarti* Flesch, 1883 (Apicomplexa: Eimeriidae) from horse foals in Rio de Janeiro. Coccidia 2014;2:40–44.
Gundłach JL, Sadzikowski AB, Studzińska MB. Protozoal invasions of horses. Ann Univ Mariae Curie Sklodowska (Vet) 2006;61:31–44.
Hirayama K, Okamoto M, Sako T, et al. Eimeria organisms develop in the epithelial cells of equine small intestine. Vet Pathol 2002;39:505–508.
Lyons ET, Tolliver SC. Prevalence of parasite eggs (*Strongyloides westeri*, *Parascaris equorum*, and strongyles) and oocysts (*Emeria leuckarti*) in the feces of Thoroughbred foals on 14 farms in central Kentucky in 2003. Parasitol Res 2004;94:400–404.
Lyons ET, Drudge JH, Tolliver SC. Natural infection with *Eimeria leuckarti*: prevalence of oocysts in feces of horse foals on several farms in Kentucky during 1986. Am J Vet Res 1988;49:96–98.
Lyons ET, Tolliver SC, Collin SS. Field studies on endoparasites of Thoroughbred foals on seven farms in central Kentucky in 2004. Parasitol Res 2006;98:496–500.
Studzińska MB, Tomczuk K, Sadzikowski AB. Prevalence of *Eimeria leuckarti* in young horses and usefulness of some coproscopical methods for its detection. Bull Vet Inst Pulawy 2008;52:541–544.
Sudan V, Sharma RL, Gupta SR, Borah MK. Successful therapeutic management of concurrent subclinical *Eimeria leuckarti* and *Babesia* (*Theileria*) *equi* infection in a mare. J Parasit Dis 2013;37:177–180.
Uslu U, Guçlu F. Prevalence of endoparasites in horses and donkeys in Turkey. Bull Vet Inst Pulawy 2007;51:237–240.

Authors Rubiela Castañeda-Salazar and Olimpo Oliver-Espinosa
Consulting Editors Henry Stämpfli and Olimpo Oliver-Espinosa

COLIC, CHRONIC/RECURRENT

BASICS

DEFINITION
• Chronic colic originating usually, but not exclusively, from the GI tract and that has been present constantly or intermittently for >3 days. It may also originate from other abdominal organs such as liver, spleen, kidney, uterus, and peritoneum
• *Chronic abdominal pain* refers to continuous or intermittent signs of abdominal pain of >3 days' duration
• *Recurrent abdominal pain* refers to several episodes of transient or prolonged abdominal pain separated by a period of a few days or weeks in which the horse is usually normal

PATHOPHYSIOLOGY
Pain from within the intestinal tract may result from intramural tension, tension on a mesentery, inflammation, spasm associated with hypermotility, or a combination of those. Most cases of chronic colic usually exclude strangulating obstructive events.

SYSTEMS AFFECTED
• GI
• Cardiovascular—may be affected as a result of progressive dehydration, toxemia
• Other systems such as urinary, reproductive, or hepatic may be involved

SIGNALMENT
Non-specific. Previous abdominal surgery results in a risk of adhesions leading to chronic colic.

SIGNS

General Comments
Signs of abdominal pain are usually mild to moderate.

Historical Findings
• There may be a recent history of change in diet or exercise regimen, lack of access to drinking water, deworming, weight loss, previous infection, or abdominal surgery
• A change in attitude (depression), appetite, and fecal output may be noticed

Physical Examination Findings
Vital signs are usually normal to moderately affected. The following signs might be observed:
• General findings—none to moderate abdominal distention; weight loss
• Cardiovascular findings—normal to mild changes in color of the mucous membrane, increase in capillary refill time, normal to moderate increase in heart rate, and dehydration may occur with time. May have signs of endotoxemia such as hyperemic mucous membranes and increase in heart rate
• GI findings—normal, decreased, or increased gut motility; abnormal sounds may be heard in sand impactions; may have a

gas-filled viscus on percussion; may have presence of gastric reflux on passage of the nasogastric tube. Feces are normal, reduced, or absent, or there may be diarrhea
• Abnormalities on rectal examination—distention of a viscus by gas, liquid, or food; displacement of a viscus; abnormal intestinal diameter or wall thickness; uterine or renal abnormalities; palpation of a mass. May have a painful response on palpation of a specific area

CAUSES
The most common cause of chronic colic located at the GI level is large colon impaction, but there are others causes, such as chronic peritonitis, enteritis/colitis, colonic displacement, parasite infestation, ulceration, and intussusception. For recurrent abdominal pain, the most common cause is spasmodic colic but also includes processes such as chronic ulceration, non-total disturbance of the intestinal lumen due to adhesions, stricture, intussusception, enteroliths, intra-abdominal masses such as abscesses and neoplasms, and sand impactions.

GI
• Gastric—gastric ulcer, gastric neoplasia
• Small intestine—duodenal ulcer, duodenojejunal enteritis, chronic inflammatory bowel disease, adhesions, stricture, intussusception, neoplasia, impaction, muscular hypertrophy, etc.
• Large intestine, cecum, and small colon—impaction, adhesions, ulceration, spasmodic colic, enteroliths, fecalith, sand impaction, neoplasia, chronic inflammatory bowel disease, displacement

Reproductive
• Ovarian tumor
• Uterine torsion
• Late stage of pregnancy

Renal/Urologic
• Renal/ureteral/bladder/urethral calculi
• Pyelonephritis
• Cystitis
• Renal inflammatory process

Hepatobiliary
• Hepatitis
• Hepatobiliary calculi
• Abscesses

Other Systems Affected
• Peritonitis
• Mesenteric abscesses
• Abdominal neoplasia (e.g. lymphosarcoma)

RISK FACTORS
Previous surgery, diet, environment, excessive use of NSAIDs, *Anoplocephala* infestation, larval cyathostomiasis, strongylosis, no access to water, sudden change in exercise, history of deworming, pregnancy. Horses with severe dental disease may fail to masticate coarse herbage and be prone to impactions.

DIAGNOSIS

DIFFERENTIAL DIAGNOSIS
Other causes of pain that might resemble pain originating from the abdominal cavity include myositis, pleuropneumonia, and neurologic and musculoskeletal injury.

CBC/BIOCHEMISTRY/URINALYSIS
• Packed cell volume and total protein might be increased due to dehydration
• Hypoproteinemia is seen in conditions such as chronic ulceration, intussusception, neoplasia, parasitism, infectious disease, and chronic inflammatory bowel disease. Total globulin concentration may be increased in chronic inflammatory processes and strongyle parasitism
• The fibrinogen concentration is increased in the presence of inflammation
• Leukocytosis in chronic inflammatory processes
• Anemia may result from chronic inflammatory processes or chronic bleeding
• Hypochloremia, hyponatremia, and low bicarbonate concentrations seen in colitis
• Presence of azotemia occurs in severely dehydrated horses or in cases of renal disease. Liver enzymes may also be increased if hepatic disease is present

OTHER LABORATORY TESTS
• Abdominal paracentesis—cytology of the abdominal fluid may be normal or may reveal the presence of an inflammatory process. The presence of abnormal or mitotic cells may suggest lymphosarcoma. Bacteriology of abdominal fluid in cases of peritonitis may be helpful in isolating an agent and appropriately choosing antibiotic therapy
• Melena in feces—ulcerative disease, intussusceptions of the small intestine
• Fecal analysis for the presence of parasite eggs and sand
• Fecal bacteriology might help to identify the cause of inflammatory abdominal pain (*Salmonella* spp., *Clostridia* spp.)
• Urinalysis—change in specific gravity or an increase in leukocyte content, red blood cells, and pH may be noticed if renal disease is present

IMAGING
• Radiographs—may be useful in identification of sand impaction or enteroliths
• Ultrasonography—evaluation of abdominal fluid, wall thickness and diameter of small intestine, nephrosplenic space, and motility and wall thickness of the large intestine; and abnormal findings such as intussusception, abscess, or adhesions. Also useful in evaluating the kidneys, liver, spleen, and uterus

• Gastroscopy—evaluation of the glandular and nonglandular part of the stomach for ulcer or impaction
• Cystoscopy—evaluation of the urethra, bladder, and opening of the ureters for inflammation, urolithiasis
• Laparoscopy—visualization of abdominal viscera

OTHER DIAGNOSTIC PROCEDURES
• Biopsy—intestinal, liver, or renal biopsy for histology
• Histology—biopsy of kidney or liver if these are suspected to be the origin of the problem; intestinal biopsy
• Exploratory laparotomy or laparoscopy—to identify the origin of the problem if it has not been determined by other tests

TREATMENT
The treatment depends on the source of the problem. The treatment may be supportive or curative, medical, or surgical. Moderate or severe cases of cecal impaction are an indication to perform exploratory laparotomy to prevent cecal rupture.

MEDICATIONS
DRUG(S) OF CHOICE
Analgesics
Analgesics control the abdominal pain, and include:
• NSAIDs—flunixin meglumine, dipyrone (metamizole), ketoprofen
• α_2-Blockers, such as xylazine, detomidine, or romifidine, can also be given in more severe cases
• Although usually not needed unless signs of pain are severe, narcotic analgesics such as butorphanol can be given alone or in conjunction with an α_2-blocker

Spasmolytics
N-butylscopolammonium bromide (hyoscine butylbromide; Buscopan).

Laxatives
To soften ingesta; mainly used for impaction:
• Mineral oil—10 mL/kg via nasogastric tube
• Osmotic laxative—diluted magnesium sulfate in 4 L warm water via nasogastric tube
• Dioctyl sodium succinate (docusate sodium)
• IV balanced electrolytes solution

Fluids
• Parenteral—in cases of dehydration or moderate to severe impaction, IV fluid therapy should be initiated with a balanced electrolyte solution (lactated Ringer's solution). Unbalanced electrolytes should be corrected, especially hypokalemia and hypocalcemia, which are important for intestinal motility
• Orally—in cases of impaction where good GI motility is present, 5 L of water every 2 h can be given by nasogastric tube (check for gastric reflux prior to giving water)

Antibiotic Therapy
Antibiotic therapy should be started if peritonitis or infectious disease is suspected, or if surgery is performed. Usually, broad-spectrum antibiotics such as a combination of penicillin (20 000 IU/kg IV QID) and gentamicin (6.6 mg/kg IV SID) or trimethoprim–sulfamethoxazole (30 mg/kg IV BID) are given. Surgical exploration may be necessary to determine the cause of chronic or recurrent signs of abdominal discomfort.

PRECAUTIONS
• Repeated use of α_2-blockers and butorphanol may cause ileus
• Repeat doses of NSAIDs, especially in cases of dehydration, can result in gastric or large colon ulceration as well as renal damage

POSSIBLE INTERACTIONS
N/A

ALTERNATIVE DRUGS
N/A

FOLLOW-UP
PATIENT MONITORING
The heart rate and cardiovascular status of the horse should be monitored closely to detect any deterioration.

POSSIBLE COMPLICATIONS
Chronic signs of pain nonresponsive to medical treatment, intestinal rupture secondary to intestinal necrosis due to an enterolith, and severe impaction are indications for an exploratory laparotomy.

MISCELLANEOUS
ZOONOTIC POTENTIAL
N/A

PREGNANCY/FERTILITY/BREEDING
Late stage of pregnancy can result in intermittent mild signs of abdominal discomfort.

SYNONYMS
Chronic/recurrent colic

ABBREVIATIONS
• GI = gastrointestinal
• NSAID = nonsteroidal anti-inflammatory drug

Suggested Reading
Hackett ES. Specific causes of colic. In: Southwood LL, ed. Practical Guide to Equine Colic. Ames, IA: Wiley Blackwell, 2013:204–230.
Hillyer MH, Mair TS. Chronic colic in the mature horse: a retrospective review of 106 cases. Equine Vet J 1997;29:415–420.
Hillyer MH, Mair TS. Recurrent colic in the mature horse: a retrospective review of 58 cases. Equine Vet J 1997;29:421–424.
Mair T, Divers T, Ducharme N. Manual of Equine Gastroenterology. Philadelphia, PA: WB Saunders, 2002:101–141.
Mair T, Divers T, Ducharme N. Manual of Equine Gastroenterology. Philadelphia, PA: WB Saunders, 2002:427–442.
Southwood LL. Gastrointestinal parasitology and anthelmintics. In: Southwood LL, ed. Practical Guide to Equine Colic. Ames, IA: Wiley Blackwell, 2013:316–324.

Author Nathalie Coté
Consulting Editor Henry Stämpfli and Olimpo Oliver-Espinosa

COLIC IN FOALS

C

BASICS

DEFINITION
Colic refers to abdominal pain, most commonly due to a GI disorder.

PATHOPHYSIOLOGY
• Obstructive GI conditions, such as meconium impaction, cause gas and fluid distention proximal to the obstruction, and subsequent abdominal distention and associated pain due to stimulation of intestinal wall stretch receptors within the GI tract. Prolonged/severe distention or direct compression by an intraluminal mass (e.g. impaction) can lead to reduced intestinal wall perfusion and ischemic injury, leading to secondary reperfusion injury when blood flow is reinstituted
• Enteritis and enterocolitis (see chapter Diarrhea, neonate) can be caused by a variety of bacterial and viral organisms. Small intestine and colon can become distended with fluid and gas secondary to enterocolitis and may also have spasmodic contractions, leading to colic pain
• Strangulating lesions of the small or large intestine (such as small intestinal volvulus) generally cause acute, severe pain, and rapid hemodynamic deterioration
• Duodenal stricture or obstruction can occur secondary to gastroduodenal ulceration, usually in foals 1–4 months of age
• Damage to the intestinal wall secondary to enterocolitis, obstruction, or strangulation can lead to bacterial translocation and subsequent endotoxemia. Endotoxin is responsible for many of the clinical signs (fever, tachycardia, leukopenia, injected mucous membranes)
• Adhesions are a relatively common complication of abdominal surgery in neonatal foals. They form as fibrin adheres to areas of serosal injury

SYSTEMS AFFECTED
• GI
• Cardiovascular—decreased fluid intake, third spacing of fluid in the intestinal lumen, abdominal effusion, and losses via reflux or diarrhea can lead to hypovolemia, hypovolemic shock, and dehydration. Endotoxemia will compound the effects on the cardiovascular system and may lead to decompensated shock

GENETICS
• Generalized abdominal pain or colic does not have a genetic predisposition
• Specific causes of colic, such as lethal white syndrome, do have a genetic basis

INCIDENCE/PREVALENCE
The incidence of colic in foals appears to be lower than that in adult horses; however, there are causes of colic that are specific to or more common in foals.

GEOGRAPHIC DISTRIBUTION
No specific geographic distribution, although sand colic is more prevalent in coastal areas or local turnout areas with high levels of sand.

SIGNALMENT
• Miniature horses have a higher incidence of fecalith formation
• Overo-overo cross Paint foals are at risk of intestinal aganglionosis (LWFS)
• Foals 24–48 h of age are most commonly affected by meconium impaction and enterocolitis. Less commonly, atresia coli, LWFS, GI ulceration, and congenital inguinal hernias are causes of neonatal colic
• Foals 2–5 days of age—enterocolitis, ruptured bladder, atresia coli, atresia ani, gastric ulcers
• Foals 5 days to 6 months of age—enterocolitis, gastric ulcers, duodenal ulcers and stenosis, small intestinal volvulus, intussusception, hernias (inguinal, scrotal, diaphragmatic), phytobezoar, drug-induced colic (antimicrobial-associated enterocolitis, NSAID-associated GI ulcerative disease), abscessation, and ascarid impaction
• Colts are at risk of inguinal hernias and appear to be at higher risk of ruptured bladder and meconium impaction

SIGNS
Signs of colic in neonatal foals can be inconsistent, and may be complicated by concurrent disease states (e.g. septicemia). Foals may be depressed and anorexic rather than displaying "classic" colic signs such as pawing or rolling.

Historical Findings
• Not nursing well—foal may have dried milk on its head, and mare's udder will be full
• Decreased fecal passage
• Persistent posturing to urinate/defecate
• Poor weight gain, unthrifty appearance
• Previous gastric ulceration can predispose to gastric outflow obstruction in older foals

Physical Examination Findings
• Depression, lethargy
• Abdominal distention
• Reduced nursing
• Tachycardia, tachypnea
• Tail flagging, straining/tenesmus
• Decreased or increased borborygmi
• Rolling, lying on back, restlessness, persistent recumbency, stretching out of limbs
• Signs of self-trauma (e.g. abrasions over the eyes) indicate colic pain prior to presentation

CAUSES
• Bacterial—septicemia can lead to enterocolitis. Other common causes of enterocolitis in foals include *Clostridium difficile* and/or *perfringens*, rotavirus, corona virus, *Escherichia coli*, *Actinobacillus equuli*, and *Salmonella* spp.
• Congenital—intestinal atresia, LWFS, and hernia are congenital problems in foals

• Intussusceptions are associated with tapeworm infestations in older foals and adults; this is not a common cause of colic in neonates, but may be related to altered peristalsis
• Small intestinal volvulus can occur secondary to enteritis or may be idiopathic—progressive fluid distention and altered motility may contribute to volvulus at the base of the mesentery
• Diaphragmatic hernias are uncommon in neonatal foals but may be congenital or traumatic in origin

RISK FACTORS
• FTPI places foals at higher risk of septicemia (and therefore enterocolitis) and might predispose to meconium retention
• NSAIDs and stress contribute to formation of gastric and duodenal ulcers in foals
• Neonatal maladjustment syndrome can result in localized ischemic perfusion injury to the intestinal mucosa, resulting in generalized small intestine ileus, mucosal injury, and bacterial translocation

DIAGNOSIS

DIFFERENTIAL DIAGNOSIS
• Simple obstruction—should not have significant metabolic deterioration in the acute stages; if foal is <48 h of age, suspect meconium impaction
• Strangulating obstruction—small intestinal volvulus, large intestinal volvulus, strangulating hernia; rapid deterioration, pain refractory to analgesics, usually have pronounced abdominal distention
• Enterocolitis—reflux or diarrhea present; fluid-filled bowel on US and thickened intestinal wall; suspect in leukopenic or septicemic foals
• Uroperitoneum—abdominal fluid and serum electrolytes and creatinine are usually diagnostic
• Diaphragmatic hernia—thoracic/abdominal radiography and US are most useful

CBC/BIOCHEMISTRY/URINALYSIS
• Dehydration, hypovolemia, and hypoglycemia are common in neonatal foals that have not been nursing
• Leukopenia (especially with enterocolitis/septicemia) and leukocytosis are commonly seen with GI inflammation
• Electrolyte disturbances are seen with uroperitoneum (hyperkalemia, hyponatremia, hypochloremia)
• Azotemia (prerenal or postrenal) with dehydration or uroabdomen

OTHER LABORATORY TESTS
Immunoglobulin G will be low (<800 mg/dL) if there is FTPI.

(CONTINUED)   **COLIC IN FOALS**

C

IMAGING
- Abdominal radiography
  ◦ Gas dilation of large and small intestine is visible. Radiodense fecaliths, impactions, and foreign material (sand) may be visualized. Standing or lateral views are usually adequate, although a dorsoventral view can be obtained, if needed
  ◦ Contrast radiography (upper GI) is useful for identifying gastric outflow obstruction; barium enemas can help in diagnosis of meconium impaction and atresia coli
- Abdominal US—evaluation of the small intestine is best performed with US; distention, wall thickness, and motility can be assessed. Free abdominal fluid may be seen on US, and the integrity of the bladder and urachus can also be assessed

OTHER DIAGNOSTIC PROCEDURES
- Abdominocentesis—indicated if there is excessive free fluid, or if information from abdominal fluid will change the treatment or surgical decision. Use a 20-gauge needle or teat cannula. Normal values: WBCs <5000/μL, TP <2.5 g/dL. TP can increase with enteritis; WBCs, TP, and lactate may increase with ischemic lesions. Caution should be used when there is significant abdominal distention—bowel in foals is very friable, and there is a risk of intestinal perforation and laceration
- Measure abdominal circumference to monitor for increasing abdominal distention
- Digital rectal examination—use a well-lubricated finger; may detect firm meconium
- Nasogastric reflux—net reflux >500 mL (usually >2 L) may indicate small intestinal ileus, enteritis, or pyloric outflow obstruction. Normal gastric emptying time for liquids is approximately 30 min. Relief of pain after refluxing is suggestive of enteritis or a gastric outflow obstruction
- Gastroduodenal endoscopy—identify gastric ulcers and duodenal ulceration/stricture

TREATMENT
AIMS
- Pain management—may be needed for short-term management of acute colic. Repeated administration of analgesics, antispasmodics, or sedation should always be accompanied by reassessment of the foal's status (possible need for changes in treatment or a decision for surgery)
- Treat underlying conditions—septicemia, neonatal maladjustment syndrome
- Antimicrobials for perioperative coverage or for treatment of enterocolitis
- Supportive care—rehydration, treatment of hypotension and acidosis; correct electrolyte imbalances

- Decision for surgery is based on the severity of pain, lack of response to analgesics, increasing abdominal distention, evidence of strangulation, or deterioration of condition despite medical treatment
- Ulcer prophylaxis or treatment of existing ulcers. Septicemic neonates usually have alkaline gastric pH, and treatment with PPIs or H_2 blockers may be contraindicated in this group. Use of prophylactic PPIs has been shown to increase the risk of *Salmonella* spp. in septicemic neonates

APPROPRIATE HEALTH CARE
If colic is persistent (unresponsive to initial medications), the foal should be referred for inpatient medical evaluation, treatment, possibly for emergency medical stabilization, and, if required, for emergency surgery.

NURSING CARE
- Fluid therapy—balanced electrolyte replacement fluids (Plasma-Lyte 148 or lactated Ringer's solution) for rehydration, unless hyperkalemia is present (0.9% saline). Hypertonic solutions should not be used
- Gastric decompression (reflux) via a nasogastric tube for cases of enteritis or gastric outflow obstruction
- Broad-spectrum antimicrobial coverage for primary septicemia and secondary bacterial translocation

ACTIVITY
- The foal may be confined to a stall or small pen/cage while IV fluids are administered and the foal is observed closely for changes in clinical condition
- If abdominal surgery is performed, the foal should be restricted to a stall for 3–4 weeks, and a small paddock for an additional 4 weeks to allow for healing of the ventral midline incision

DIET
Partial or complete parenteral nutrition is indicated if enteral feeding cannot be tolerated (due to obstruction, ileus, or enterocolitis).

CLIENT EDUCATION
- Discuss the importance of adequate colostrum intake if FTPI is an underlying risk factor
- If there is a congenital problem (LWFS), discourage rebreeding the same mare and stallion and recommend genetic testing

SURGICAL CONSIDERATIONS
- Surgery may be indicated if the foal is persistently painful and refractory to analgesics, has progressive abdominal distention, has evidence of sepsis or ischemia on abdominocentesis, has uroabdomen, or has evidence of complete obstruction on abdominal radiographs or US
- The foal must be stabilized prior to surgery, especially if there are significant electrolyte or acid–base derangements, as these metabolic

abnormalities increase the risk of arrhythmia and anesthetic complications
- Abdominal adhesions are a frequent and serious consequence of abdominal surgery in foals. Precautions such as gentle tissue handling, administration of NSAIDs and broad-spectrum antimicrobial drugs, lubrication of serosal surfaces with sodium carboxymethylcellulose, lavage, hyaluronic acid, and omentectomy should be taken to help reduce the chance of significant postoperative adhesions

MEDICATIONS
DRUG(S) OF CHOICE
Pain Management
- α_2-Agonist, e.g. xylazine (0.4–1.0 mg/kg IV)
- Butorphanol (0.04–0.1 mg/kg IV)
- NSAIDs, e.g. flunixin meglumine (0.5–1.1 mg/kg IV every 12 h)
- Butylscopolamine (0.1–0.2 mg/kg IV every 12 h)

Antimicrobials
- Penicillin (22 000 IU/kg IV every 6 h)
- Amikacin (25 mg/kg IV every 24 h)

Ulcer Prophylaxis
See chapter Gastric ulcers, neonate

CONTRAINDICATIONS
Enrofloxacin should not be used in foals.

PRECAUTIONS
- NSAIDs increase the risk of gastric ulceration and can also mask a more serious underlying condition
- Aminoglycosides should not be used in dehydrated or azotemic foals

ALTERNATIVE DRUGS
Cephalosporins can be used as a broad-spectrum antimicrobial (ceftiofur 5–10 mg/kg IV every 6–12 h).

FOLLOW-UP
PATIENT MONITORING
- The neonatal foal with colic should be monitored closely for dehydration, hypoglycemia, and changes in cardiovascular status
- Measure abdominal circumference and monitor for fecal passage to assess for resolution of impaction and gas distention

PREVENTION/AVOIDANCE
Adequate colostrum intake should reduce the risk of meconium impaction and may reduce the risk of infectious enterocolitis.

POSSIBLE COMPLICATIONS
- In foals <7 days of age, concurrent diseases such as septicemia, neonatal maladjustment

syndrome, and prematurity are common (colic is usually secondary)
• Recurrence of colic is possible in cases of enterocolitis
• Adhesions are a common complication of colic surgery in foals, with as many as 30% developing clinically significant intestinal adhesions

EXPECTED COURSE AND PROGNOSIS
• Simple obstruction, such as meconium impaction, has an excellent prognosis. Other medical colic will often resolve within 24–48 h of treatment, although colic complicated by debilitating diseases such as sepsis has a more guarded prognosis
• Short-term survival has been reported to be 61–65% for foals with colic surgery
• Long-term survival in surgically treated foals is approximately 35–45%, with poorer prognosis for foals <14 days of age and for foals with strangulating GI lesions
• Atresia coli, LWFS, and gastroduodenal rupture have a grave prognosis

MISCELLANEOUS

ASSOCIATED CONDITIONS
Septicemia

AGE-RELATED FACTORS
Specific types of colic (e.g. meconium impaction, ruptured bladder) in foals are age related.

SEE ALSO
• Diarrhea, neonate
• Lethal white foal syndrome
• Meconium retention

ABBREVIATIONS
• FTPI = failure of transfer of passive immunity
• GI = gastrointestinal
• LWFS = lethal white foal syndrome
• NSAID = nonsteroidal anti-inflammatory drug
• PPI = proton pump inhibitor
• TP = total protein
• US = ultrasonography, ultrasound
• WBC = white blood cell

Suggested Reading
Furr M. Diagnosis of colic in the foal. In: Blikslager AT, White NA, Moore JN, Mair TS, eds. The Equine Acute Abdomen, 3e. Hoboken, NJ: John Wiley & Sons, Inc, 2017:413–417.
Mackinnon MC, Southwood LL, Burke MJ, Palmer JE. Colic in equine neonates: 137 cases (2000–2010). J Am Vet Med Assoc 2013;243(11):1586–1595.
Vatistas NJ, Snyder JR, Wilson WD, et al. Surgical treatment for colic in the foal (67 cases): 1980–1992. Equine Vet J 1996;28:139–145.

Author Eric L. Schroeder
Consulting Editor Margaret C. Mudge
Acknowledgment The author acknowledges the prior contribution of Margaret C. Mudge.

COMPLEX CONGENITAL CARDIAC DISEASE

BASICS

DEFINITION
• The term complex congenital cardiac disease encompasses numerous defects or anomalies of the heart, which form during embryogenesis and are therefore present from birth
• Congenital cardiac defects can be classified as hypoplasia, obstruction defects, septal defects, and cyanotic defects
• To be described as complex, more than 1 specific defect is present, although frequently these include patent ductus arteriosus and/or ventricular or atrial septal defect, which can also occur singly (see chapters Atrial septal defect and Ventricular septal defect (VSD))

PATHOPHYSIOLOGY
• In the embryo, formation of the heart begins with a straight tube of mesenchymal cells. This forms segments (atria, primitive ventricle, bulbus cordis, conus, and truncus) and then, through cardiac looping, the bulbus cordis migrates relative to the ventricle to take up positions that enable the formation of the right and left ventricles
• Septation of the right and left atria involves ingrowths of the septum and the septum secundum. Simultaneously, the atrioventricular canals remodel to align with their respective ventricles and ventricular septation begins. Failure at this stage can lead to a common ventricle or, more commonly, a range of ventricular septal defects
• The formation of the aortic and pulmonary trunks is achieved by truncoconal septation and spiraling of the conus. Abnormalities at this stage can lead to a wide range of malformations, of which the most commonly reported in the horse is tetralogy of Fallot
• Hypoplasia results in failure of formation of 1 of the ventricles
• Obstruction defects occur when heart valves, arteries, or veins are blocked; pulmonic stenosis is the most commonly reported form in horses
• Septal defects can involve the atrial and/or the ventricular septum
• Cyanotic defects arise when the defects lead to right-to-left shunting of blood such than unoxygenated blood reaches the systemic circulation. Examples include tetralogy of Fallot, tricuspid atresia, persistent truncus arteriosus, and transposition of the great vessels

SYSTEMS AFFECTED
Cardiovascular

GENETICS
• Not yet determined in horses
• Complex congenital cardiac diseases are heritable in other species

INCIDENCE/PREVALENCE
Congenital cardiac defects accounted for 3.5% of all congenital defects in 1 pathologic survey, and 1 report estimated that they occur in around 1–5 in 1000 births.

SIGNALMENT
• Arabian horses appear to be predisposed to complex congenital cardiac defects
• Murmurs usually are detectable at birth
• Diagnosed most frequently in neonates, foals, and young horses but can be found at any age

SIGNS
General Comments
Complex cardiac disease is more likely to present with signs of severe cardiac compromise than single (or simple) defects.

Historical Findings
Depending on the specific defect and its severity, affected foals will present with lethargy, exercise intolerance, and failure to grow at expected rates.

Physical Examination Findings
• Cardiac murmurs are generally loud (grade ≥4/6), and often have a precordial thrill. The point(s) of maximal intensity will depend on the specific defect and the structures involved
• Tetralogy of Fallot produces murmurs on both sides of the chest but typically the loudest murmur is over the pulmonic valve on the left side
• Tricuspid atresia creates its loudest murmur over the tricuspid valve area on the right side
• Many complex cardiac defects are associated with cyanosis and affected foals have bluish mucous membranes

CAUSES
Failure of development at 1 or more stages of cardiac embryogenesis. In humans, both genetic and environmental factors (e.g. maternal illness, infection, and drugs) are associated with congenital cardiac defects but these factors have not been identified in horses.

RISK FACTORS
Arabian breed.

DIAGNOSIS

DIFFERENTIAL DIAGNOSIS
Loud murmurs and signs of cardiac compromise in young horses can also be associated with infective endocarditis. Differentiate echocardiographically.

CBC/BIOCHEMISTRY/URINALYSIS
Arterial blood gas analysis may show hypoxia in cyanotic disorders. The red blood cell count and packed cell volume may increase in response to chronic hypoxia.

OTHER LABORATORY TESTS
N/A

IMAGING
Echocardiography
Using 2-dimensional Doppler and contrast echocardiography, a segmental approach is useful:
Step 1. Assess the atrial arrangement—the right side has a triangular appendage and the left side is tubular and narrow based
Step 2. Assess the ventricular arrangement—the right ventricle has coarse apical trabeculations, a moderator band, and septomarginal trabeculations, and the atrioventricular valve is attached directly to the septum; the left ventricle has fine trabeculations and a smooth upper part of the septum without attachment of the atrioventricular valve. The ventricular morphology can be indeterminate or hypoplastic
Step 3. Assess atrioventricular connections—determine if there are 2 atria, and that these are connected to the appropriate ventricle
Step 4. Assess atrioventricular valves—evaluate the number of cusps, their shape, connections, and presence of regurgitation and stenosis
Step 5. Assess ventriculoarterial connections—coronary arteries originate from the aorta, and the main pulmonary artery from 2 branches. Check great vessels are connected to the appropriate ventricle and look for atresia
Step 6. Assess arterial valves—evaluate the number of cusps, their shape, connections, and presence of regurgitation and stenosis
Step 7. Associated malformations—a range of specific lesions should be evaluated:
a. Shunts
b. Outflow tract obstructions
c. Coronary abnormalities
d. Anomalies of systemic and pulmonary venous connections
e. Abnormalities of the aorta and aortic arch

Thoracic Radiography
• Increased pulmonary vascularity and cardiac enlargement may be detected
• Pulmonary edema may be detected in foals or horses with congestive heart failure
• Contrast angiography can help delineate specific defects such as common truncus arteriosus or anomalies of the great vessels

OTHER DIAGNOSTIC PROCEDURES
Cardiac Catheterization
Right-sided cardiac catheterization to directly measure pulmonary arterial and capillary wedge pressures and to sample blood for oxygen content. Abnormalities detected will vary depending on the specific defect(s) that are present.

PATHOLOGIC FINDINGS
Specific pathologic findings will reflect the defect(s) that are present. In addition, there may be pathologic changes associated with

COMPLEX CONGENITAL CARDIAC DISEASE   (CONTINUED)

right heart failure, such as peripheral edema, hepatic congestion, and ascites, and/or left heart failure, such as pulmonary edema.

TREATMENT

Treatment of complex congenital cardiac defects has not been attempted in horses.

ACTIVITY

Horses with complex congenital cardiac disease should not be used for any form of work.

MEDICATIONS

DRUG(S) OF CHOICE
N/A

CONTRAINDICATIONS
N/A

ALTERNATIVE DRUGS
N/A

FOLLOW-UP

PATIENT MONITORING
Frequently monitor the horse's cardiac rate, rhythm, respiratory rate, and effort.

PREVENTION/AVOIDANCE
N/A

POSSIBLE COMPLICATIONS
Congestive heart failure.

EXPECTED COURSE AND PROGNOSIS
• Some mildly affected cases may be able to live relatively comfortably with a nonathletic lifestyle of variable periods
• Horses with associated congestive heart failure usually have a guarded to grave prognosis for life

MISCELLANEOUS

AGE-RELATED FACTORS
Young horses are more likely to be diagnosed with this defect.

ZOONOTIC POTENTIAL
N/A

PREGNANCY/FERTILITY/BREEDING
Breeding affected horses should be discouraged even though the condition is rare and the heritable nature of this defect is not known.

SYNONYMS
NA

Suggested Reading
Buergelt CD. Equine cardiovascular pathology: an overview. Anim Health Res Rev 2003;4:109–129.

Crowe MW, Swerczek TW. Equine congenital defects. Am J Vet Res 1984;46:353–358.

Marr CM. Cardiac murmurs: congenital heart disease. In: Marr CM, Bowen M, eds. Cardiology of the Horse, 2e. Edinburgh, UK: Saunders Elsevier, 2010:187–197.

Marr CM. The equine neonatal cardiovascular system in health and disease. Vet Clin North Am Equine Pract 2015;31:545–565.

Schwarzwald CC. Sequential segmental analysis—a systemic approach to the diagnosis of congenital cardiac defects. Equine Vet Educ 2008;20:305–309.

Author Celia M. Marr
Consulting Editors Celia M. Marr and Virginia B. Reef

BASICS

DEFINITION
Maternal structural or functional defects that prevent:
- The fertilized ovum from normal embryonic development
- Transport of the embryo into the uterus by day 6 after ovulation
- Embryonic survival until pregnancy is diagnosed by transrectal US ≥14 days after ovulation

PATHOPHYSIOLOGY
The *normal* rate of conception failure is ≈ 30% for young mares (based on day 14–16 US) but approaches 50–70% in older, subfertile mares.
Some of the specific causes of failure of conception are as follows:
- Defective embryos
  ○ Old mares
  ○ Seasonal effects
  ○ Transferred embryos from older mares or embryos generated by IVF or other reproductive technologies
- Unsuitable/hostile uterine environment
  ○ Endometritis can result in early CL regression and failure of maternal recognition of pregnancy
  ○ Endometrial periglandular fibrosis
  ○ Lymphatic cysts of sufficient size to impede embryonic mobility and failure of maternal recognition of pregnancy
  ○ Inadequate secretion of histotrophs
- Xenobiotics
  ○ Equine fescue toxicosis and ergotism
  ○ Phytoestrogens, anecdotal
- Oviductal disease
  ○ Unsuitable/hostile environment for embryonic development
  ○ Oviductal blockage
- Endocrine disorders
  ○ Hypothyroidism—anecdotal
  ○ Luteal insufficiency—anecdotal
  ○ Endocrine disorders, such as PPID and EMS/IR
- Maternal disease
  ○ Fever
  ○ Pain, such as that associated with severe laminitis—anecdotal
Depending on the specific infectious cause, the pathophysiologic mechanisms for conception failure can involve 1 or more of the following:
- Defective embryo which cannot continue to develop
- Unsuitable oviductal or uterine environment that prevents fertilization and/or embryonic development
- Oviductal blockage or impaired function
- Failure of maternal recognition of pregnancy
- Early CL regression
- Luteal insufficiency—anecdotal

SYSTEMS AFFECTED
Reproductive

SIGNS

Historical Findings
1 or more of the following:
- After appropriately timed breeding with semen of normal fertility:
  ○ Failure of pregnancy diagnosed by transrectal US at >14 days after ovulation
  ○ Failure of pregnancy diagnosed by TRP at >25 days after ovulation
  ○ Return, possibly early, to estrus
- History of PMIE
- Previous exposure to endophyte-infected fescue or ergotized grasses and grains
- Geographic location, especially in relation to endophyte-infected fescue pastures/hay and/or ergotized grasses or grains
- *Recent* systemic disease

Physical Examination Findings
- Nonpregnant uterus, possibly with edema of endometrial folds or accumulation of intrauterine (luminal) fluid
- Absence of a CL
- Mucoid or mucopurulent vulvar discharge

RISK FACTORS
- Older mares >15 years of age, especially those with moderate/severe endometritis, periglandular fibrosis, and/or lymphatic cysts
- Anatomical defects predisposing the genital tract to endometritis
- Seasonal effects
- Foal heat breeding—anecdotal and somewhat controversial
- Inadequate nutrition
- Exposure to xenobiotics—fescue toxicosis and ergotism
- Some heterospecific matings, e.g. stallion crossed with jenny
- Susceptibility to PMIE
- Geographic location, especially in relation to endophyte-infected fescue pastures/hay and/or ergotized grasses or grains
- Preexisting PPID and EMS/IR
- Severe laminitis
- Transfer of embryos from older mares or those generated using IVF or other reproductive technologies

DIAGNOSIS

DIFFERENTIAL DIAGNOSIS

Mistiming of Insemination or Breeding
- Monitor follicular development and ovulation by TRP or US
- Appropriate timing of insemination or breeding
- Ovulation induction to complement timing of insemination or breeding

EED
Transrectal US detects pregnancy at >14 days, but the pregnancy is absent on subsequent examination at <40 days of gestation.

Pregnancy Undetected by Transrectal US
Careful, systematic visualization of the horns, uterine body, including near cervix; a slow sweep, twice over the entire tract, to avoid missing an early vesicle (yolk sac) of pregnancy.

Ovulation Failure
- TRP or US (preferred) to confirm ovulation and presence of a CL
- Serum P_4 level 6–7 days after ovulation or at end of estrus

Poor Semen Quality
Monitoring/examination of ejaculate for adequate number of spermatozoa with progressive motility and normal morphology.

Ejaculation Failure
- Observation of flagging of stallion's tail
- Palpation of ventral penile surface during live cover or collection of semen in an artificial vagina to confirm ejaculation was complete—6–10 pulses of the urethra
- Examination of dismount semen sample for motile spermatozoa

Mishandling of Semen
Systematic review of all semen-handling procedures and equipment/supplies coming into contact with semen.

Impaired Spermatozoal Transport
- Transrectal US to ensure absence of intrauterine fluid at insemination or breeding
- Vaginal speculum and digital cervical examination to ensure cervical patency/rule out urovagina

DIAGNOSTIC PROCEDURES
- CBC and serum biochemistry for inflammatory or stress leukocyte response, and/or other organ system involvement. Not indicated unless the mare has recently been ill
- ELISA or radioimmunoassay analyses for maternal P_4 useful at <80 days of gestation (normal levels vary from >1 to >4 ng/mL, depending on reference laboratory). Maternal estrogen concentrations can reflect fetal estrogen production and viability, especially conjugated estrogens, e.g. estrone sulfate
- Anecdotal reports of lower triiodothyronine/thyroxine levels in mares with a history of conception failure, EED, or abortion (somewhat controversial)
- Specialized testing for PPID or EMS/IR
- Cytogenetic studies to detect chromosomal abnormalities
- Endometrial biopsy procedures to assess endometrial inflammation and/or fibrosis
- Vaginal speculum examination and hysteroscopy if structural abnormalities suspected in the cervix or uterus
- Feed or environmental analyses for specific xenobiotics, including ergopeptine alkaloids, phytoestrogens, heavy metals
- Transrectal US is essential to confirm ovulation and early pregnancy, and to detect intrauterine fluid and lymphatic cysts

C

• A thorough reproductive evaluation prebreeding for individuals predisposed to conception failure, e.g. barren, old mares with a history of conception failure and/or endometritis
• Transrectal US, vaginal speculum, endometrial cytology/culture, and endometrial biopsy to detect anatomic defects, endometritis, or fibrosis
• Transrectal US, if performed earlier than normal, at 10 days post ovulation, may determine the presence of an embryo; however, there can be confusion between embryonic vesicles and lymphatic cysts
• Embryo recovery, procedures as for ET, to detect embryonic transport into the oviduct or into the uterus (flushing procedure might be therapeutic as well)
• Hysteroscopy of uterine lumen and uterotubal junctions
• Oviductal patency can be assessed using a variety of procedures
• Laparoscopy can be used to evaluate normal structure and function and ovarian–oviductal interactions

PATHOLOGIC FINDINGS
An endometrial biopsy can demonstrate the presence of moderate to severe chronic endometritis, endometrial periglandular fibrosis, and/or lymphatic lacunae.

TREATMENT
APPROPRIATE HEALTH CARE
• Treat preexisting endometritis before insemination or breeding of mares during physiologic breeding season
• Mares should have adequate body condition
• Inseminate or breed foal heat mares if ovulation occurs >9–10 days postpartum and no intrauterine fluid is present
• Uterine lavage 4–8 h post mating with administration of oxytocin and/or cloprostenol to treat PMIE
• Progestin supplementation—somewhat controversial
• Anecdotal reports of oviductal flushing to resolve oviductal occlusion
• Depending on breed restrictions, various forms of advanced reproductive technologies (e.g. zygote or embryo retrieval from the oviduct or uterus for ET and oocyte retrieval and successful IVF with subsequent ET)
• Primary, age-related (most are from aged mares) embryonic defects are refractory to treatment
• Most cases of conception failure can be handled in an ambulatory situation
• Increased frequency of US monitoring of follicular development and ovulation to permit insemination closer to ovulation, as well as more technical diagnostic procedures, may need to be performed in a hospital setting. Adequate restraint and optimal

lighting might not be available in the field to permit quality US examination

NURSING CARE
• Generally requires none
• Minimal nursing care might be necessary after more invasive diagnostic and therapeutic procedures

ACTIVITY
• Generally no restriction of broodmare activity, unless contraindicated by concurrent maternal disease or diagnostic or therapeutic procedures
• Preference may be to restrict activity of mares in competition because of the impact of stress on cyclicity and ovulation

DIET
Generally no restriction, unless indicated by concurrent maternal disease (e.g. EMS) or nutritional problems (e.g. under- or overnourished).

CLIENT EDUCATION
• Emphasize the *aged* mare's susceptibility to conception failure and her refractoriness to treatment
• Discuss susceptibility of mares with preexisting systemic disease (e.g. PPID and EMS/IR) to EED
• Inform clients regarding
  ○ the cause, diagnosis, and treatment of endometritis
  ○ the seasonal aspects and nutritional requirements of conception
  ○ the role that endophyte-infected fescue and certain heterospecific breedings might play in conception failure

SURGICAL CONSIDERATIONS
• Indicated for repair of anatomical defects predisposing mares to endometritis
• Certain diagnostic and therapeutic procedures discussed above might also involve some surgical intervention

MEDICATIONS
DRUG(S) OF CHOICE
Altrenogest
• Mares with a history of conception failure or moderate to severe endometritis (i.e. no active, infectious component) or fibrosis can be administered altrenogest (0.044–0.088 mg/kg PO once a day) beginning 2–3 days after ovulation or at diagnosis of pregnancy and continued until at least 90–100 days of gestation (taper daily dose over a 14 day period at the end of treatment)
• Altrenogest administration can be started later during gestation, continued longer, or used for only short periods of time, depending on serum P_4 levels during the first 80 days of gestation (>1 to >4 ng/mL depending on

reference laboratory), clinical circumstances, risk factors, and clinician preference
• If used near term, altrenogest frequently is discontinued 7–14 days before the expected foaling date, depending on the case, unless otherwise indicated by assessment of fetal maturity/viability or by questions regarding the accuracy of gestational length

Oxytocin
IM administration of 10–20 IU, 4–8 hours post mating for PMIE.

Cloprostenol
IM administration of 250 μg 12–24 hours post mating for PMIE.

PRECAUTIONS, POSSIBLE INTERACTIONS
• Use altrenogest only to prevent conception failure of noninfectious endometritis
• Care should be taken in the administration of cloprostenol or other prostaglandins following ovulation to prevent interference with CL formation and function
• Iatrogenic administration of oxytocin and cloprostenol to pregnant mares. Use transrectal US to diagnose pregnancy at ≥14–16 days after ovulation to identify intrauterine fluid or pyometra early in the disease course for appropriate treatment
• If pregnancy is diagnosed, frequent monitoring (weekly initially) may be indicated to detect EED
• Altrenogest is absorbed through the skin, so persons handling this preparation should wear gloves and wash their hands
• Cloprostenol can be absorbed through the skin, so persons handling this preparation should wear gloves and wash their hands after treating mares
• Although supplemental progestins are commonly used to treat cases of conception failure, their efficacy is controversial
• Primary, age-related, embryonic defects do not respond to supplemental progestins

ALTERNATIVE DRUGS
• Injectable P_4 (150–500 mg/day, oil base) can be administered IM, once daily instead of the oral formulation. Variations, contraindications, and precautions are similar to those associated with altrenogest
• Other injectable and implantable progestin preparations are available commercially for use in other species. Any use in horses of these products is off-label, and no scientific data are available regarding their efficacy
• Newer, repository forms of P_4 are occasionally introduced; however, some evidence of efficacy should be provided prior to use
• Other prostaglandin products (e.g. prostaglandin $F_{2\alpha}$) have been used to prevent PMIE, but their efficacy has been suggested to be less than that of cloprostenol, with a greater risk for interference with subsequent CL formation and function

• Thyroxine supplementation has been successful (anecdotally) for treating mares with histories of subfertility—controversial/considered deleterious by some clinicians
• Appropriate medications for any other systemic diseases

 FOLLOW-UP

PATIENT MONITORING
• Accurate teasing records
• Reexamination of mares treated for endometritis before breeding
• Early examination for pregnancy by transrectal US
• Monitor embryonic and fetal development with transrectal or transabdominal US

PREVENTION/AVOIDANCE
• Recognition of at-risk mares
• Management of endometritis before breeding
• Removal of mares from fescue-infected pasture and ergotized grasses and grains after breeding and during early gestation
• Prudent use of medications in bred mares
• Exposure to known toxicants

POSSIBLE COMPLICATIONS
• Later EED
• High-risk pregnancy
• Abortion—infectious or noninfectious, depending on the circumstances

EXPECTED COURSE AND PROGNOSIS
• Young mares with resolved cases of endometritis can have a fair to good prognosis for conception and completion of pregnancy
• Older mares (>15 years of age) with a history of preexisting systemic disease, chronic, moderate to severe endometritis, endometrial periglandular fibrosis, and/or lymphatic cysts, as well as conception failure and/or EED generally have a guarded to poor prognosis for conception success, safe completion of pregnancy, and delivery of a healthy foal

 MISCELLANEOUS

SYNONYMS
• EED
• Infertility
• Subfertility

SEE ALSO
• Abortion, spontaneous, infectious
• Abortion, spontaneous, noninfectious
• Early embryonic death
• Embryo transfer
• Endometrial biopsy
• Endometritis
• Ovulation failure

ABBREVIATIONS
• CL = corpus luteum
• EED = early embryonic death
• ELISA = enzyme-linked immunosorbent assay
• EMS = equine metabolic syndrome
• ET = embryo transfer
• IR = insulin resistance
• IVF = in vitro fertilization
• P_4 = progesterone
• PMIE = post-mating-induced endometritis
• PPID = pituitary pars intermedia dysfunction
• TRP = transrectal palpation
• US = ultrasonography, ultrasound

Suggested Reading
Ball BA. Embryonic loss. In: McKinnon AO, Squires EL, Vaala WE, Varner DD, eds. Equine Reproduction, 2e. Ames, IA: Wiley Blackwell, 2011:2327–2338.

Author Tim J. Evans
Consulting Editor Carla L. Carleton

CONGENITAL CARDIAC ABNORMALITIES

C

BASICS

DEFINITION
Congenital cardiac abnormalities include any structural cardiac malformation present from birth, usually due to either a failure in embryologic development or a persistence of fetal circulation.

PATHOPHYSIOLOGY
• VSD is the most common defect in foals and occurs when there is incomplete development of the ventricular septum during embryonic development
• A high (paramembranous) defect in the ventricular septum, within the left ventricular outflow tract, is most common; a subpulmonic defect (less common) communicates below the pulmonary valve. Muscular VSDs occur in any portion of the muscular septum
• ASDs—can involve various portions of the atrial septum due to failure of ingrowth from several areas, most often as part of complex congenital defects. Requires differentiation from PFO
• PDA—ductus arteriosus shunts blood from the pulmonary artery to the descending aorta in the fetal circulation; it can remain patent as a single defect or, more commonly, as part of a complex congenital cardiac abnormality. The ductus arteriosus normally closes in response to changes in pressure gradients at birth, inhibition of prostaglandins, and increased local oxygen tension
• PFO—the foramen ovale shunts blood from the right atrium to the left atrium to bypass the lungs in the fetal circulation. The foramen ovale normally closes when the lungs expand (pulmonary vascular resistance falls). This opening can remain patent if pulmonary hypertension is present. In normal foals functional closure occurs in the first 24–48 h of life
• Truncus arteriosus—normally partitions into aorta and pulmonary artery in the fetus. If there is failure to partition, communication occurs across a large VSD
• Tricuspid atresia—absence of the right atrioventricular orifice, preventing flow of blood from right atrium to right ventricle. Blood must be shunted across an ASD or PFO
• Pulmonary atresia with VSD—the right ventricular outflow does not connect with the pulmonary artery. A large malalignment VSD is usually present, and the fetal truncus arteriosus is unequally partitioned, causing marked dilation of the aorta and severe atresia or hypoplasia of the pulmonary trunk
• TOF includes VSD, right ventricular outflow obstruction, overriding aorta, and right ventricular hypertrophy. TOF is the most common cause of right-to-left shunt. Pentalogy of Fallot includes ASD in addition to the above abnormalities
• Left-to-right shunting occurs with ASD, VSD, and PDA. Blood shunted from the left ventricle to the right heart will increase volume in the pulmonary artery, and will therefore increase venous return to the left atrium and left ventricle, eventually causing left ventricular hypertrophy and dilation. Larger shunts will result in left-sided heart failure and significant pulmonary hypertension. VSDs that allow pressures to equilibrate between left and right ventricles can lead to biventricular hypertrophy
• Right-to-left shunting can occur in tricuspid valve atresia and ASD or pulmonary valve atresia and VSD, or in chronic pulmonary vascular disease

SYSTEMS AFFECTED
• Cardiovascular
• Respiratory

GENETICS
There is thought to be a genetic predisposition to congenital cardiac abnormalities, although the specific genetic factors are unknown at this time.

INCIDENCE/PREVALENCE
• 0.7–0.8% of foals and fetuses that undergo postmortem examination have congenital cardiac abnormalities
• 3.5% of congenital defects in foals were heart defects

GEOGRAPHIC DISTRIBUTION
N/A

SIGNALMENT
• Defects are present from birth; however, the time to recognition of the problem will vary depending on the severity of clinical signs. Cardiac anomalies are most often recognized in the first weeks to months after birth
• Congenital cardiac defects appear to be more common in Arabians, Standardbreds, Welsh Mountain ponies, and possibly Morgan foals
• VSD appears to have a genetic link in the Arabian breed. Standardbred and Quarter Horse breeds may also be more commonly affected with VSD
• No sex predilection

SIGNS
Commonly, left-to-right shunts secondary to congenital cardiac anomalies will result in left-sided or biventricular heart failure, leading to signs of exercise intolerance, respiratory distress, and jugular venous distention.

Historical Findings
• Premature foals may be at higher risk of left-to-right shunts at the foramen ovale
• Exercise intolerance
• Stunted growth

Physical Examination Findings
• Heart murmur—usually grade 3/6 or higher, but absence of a murmur does not rule out congenital cardiac anomaly
  ○ VSD—holosystolic, auscultated on both sides, but point of maximal intensity usually on right; louder murmur generally correlates with smaller defect
  ○ PDA—continuous machinery murmur, usually loudest on left; heard in most foals for the first 15 min of life; can be heard in normal foals for up to the first 3 days of life
  ○ TOF—loud, left-sided systolic murmur; may have a palpable thrill
• Lethargy, weakness
• Cyanotic mucous membranes at rest or with exercise (most common with right-to-left shunting)
• Tachypnea/dyspnea; may have harsh lung sounds
• Jugular venous distention
• Bounding pulses

CAUSES
• Teratogenic exposure, viral infection, or hypoxic damage early in pregnancy are suspected causes of congenital cardiac abnormalities
• Breed is likely a risk factor
• Prematurity may also be associated with failure to revert from fetal circulation

RISK FACTORS
See Causes.

DIAGNOSIS

DIFFERENTIAL DIAGNOSIS
• Pneumonia—thoracic radiographs and 2D echocardiography should elucidate the cause of respiratory compromise
• Physiologic cardiac murmur—usually left-sided, systolic; no echocardiography abnormalities, and foal should not show clinical signs of cardiac disease
• Anemia—lethargy and weakness

CBC/BIOCHEMISTRY/URINALYSIS
Polycythemia may be seen in response to chronic hypoxemia.

OTHER LABORATORY TESTS
Blood gas analysis—arterial hypoxemia, usually minimally responsive to oxygen supplementation, especially with right-to-left shunts. Arterial CO_2 is normal or reduced.

IMAGING
• Echocardiography—2D views can often confirm the defect, although Doppler studies are often needed to find VSDs in atypical locations and to estimate the pressure difference across the ventricles. Contrast echocardiography using agitated normal

saline solution administered through the jugular vein ("bubble study") allows identification of right-to-left shunting
• Radiography—cardiomegaly, pulmonary edema, and overcirculation of the pulmonary vasculature may be detected

OTHER DIAGNOSTIC PROCEDURES
ECG should be used to detect arrhythmias. Cardiac catheterization can be performed to measure pulmonary artery and pulmonary capillary wedge pressures

PATHOLOGIC FINDINGS
Cardiac malformations are detected on gross examination at necropsy.

TREATMENT

APPROPRIATE HEALTH CARE
There are no current surgical recommendations for horses with cardiac defects. Although PDA and VSD have been successfully treated surgically in dogs, there are no surgical procedures currently described for use in foals. Medical management may be used for horses with CHF or acute decompensation.

NURSING CARE
Supportive care with optimization of perfusion, oxygenation, and appropriate exercise restriction constitute care.

ACTIVITY
Foals with significant shunts or complex cardiac defects are usually exercise intolerant and can become cyanotic when exercised.

DIET
N/A

CLIENT EDUCATION
Breeding of affected animals should be discouraged.

MEDICATIONS

DRUG(S) OF CHOICE
• Digoxin (0.011 mg/kg PO once daily and 0.0022 mg/kg IV every 12 h) to improve myocardial function and control tachycardia. Digoxin levels should be monitored to avoid toxic levels
• Furosemide (1–2 mg/kg IV or IM PRN) to treat pulmonary edema. Monitor serum electrolyte concentrations and acid–base status with prolonged therapy

CONTRAINDICATIONS
Digoxin and furosemide should not be used in dehydrated patients. Acid–base or electrolyte abnormalities may increase the toxicity of digoxin in individual patients. Digoxin should not be used in horses with existing ventricular arrhythmias. Furosemide may cause electrolyte and acid–base abnormalities with prolonged therapy.

PRECAUTIONS
N/A

POSSIBLE INTERACTIONS
Free serum concentrations of digoxin may be increased if quinidine is given concurrently.

ALTERNATIVE DRUGS
N/A

FOLLOW-UP

PATIENT MONITORING
• Horses with small VSDs can have successful athletic careers but should be monitored for development of CHF and atrial fibrillation (exercise intolerance, coughing, dyspnea, lethargy)
• Repeat echocardiography (recommended yearly) is useful for evaluating development of ventricular enlargement or hypertrophy as well as valvular insufficiency
• Perform exercise ECG in horses with moderate to large VSDs, as part of a prepurchase examination, or when presenting with exercise intolerance

PREVENTION/AVOIDANCE
Horses with congenital cardiac anomalies should not be used for breeding, as the defects may be heritable.

POSSIBLE COMPLICATIONS
CHF

EXPECTED COURSE AND PROGNOSIS
• The prognosis with a VSD is dependent on the size of the defect, size of the cardiac chambers, maximal shunt velocity, and presence of significant aortic or mitral regurgitation, pulmonary hypertension, or CHF. Horses with membranous VSDs that measure <2.5 cm at the largest diameter or a VSD-to-aortic root diameter <0.4 (and that have a higher peak velocity of shunt flow >4.5 m/s) tend to have a good athletic prognosis. Horses with moderate defects may only be normal at rest
• Horses with large VSDs or with multiple congenital cardiac defects may be small and stunted and are likely to develop signs of CHF

MISCELLANEOUS

ASSOCIATED CONDITIONS
N/A

AGE-RELATED FACTORS
N/A

ZOONOTIC POTENTIAL
N/A

PREGNANCY/FERTILITY/BREEDING
Mares with significant shunting of blood due to congenital cardiac defects may develop signs of CHF during late-term pregnancy due to increased demand for cardiac output.

SEE ALSO
• Atrial septal defect
• Complex congenital cardiac disease
• Patent ductus arteriosus
• Ventricular septal defect (VSD)

ABBREVIATIONS
• 2D = two-dimensional
• ASD = atrial septal defect
• CHF = congestive heart failure
• PDA = patent ductus arteriosus
• PFO = patent foramen ovale
• TOF = tetralogy of Fallot
• VSD = ventricular septal defect

Suggested Reading
Bonagura JD, Reef VB. Disorders of the cardiovascular system. In: Reed SM, Bayly WM, Sellon DC, eds. Equine Internal Medicine, 2e. St. Louis, MO: WB Saunders, 2004:355–459.
Chope K. Cardiac disorders. In: Paradis MR, ed. Equine Neonatal Medicine: A Case-Based Approach. Philadelphia, PA: Saunders, 2006:247–258.
Marr CM, Bowen M. Cardiology of the Horse, 2e. Edinburgh, UK: Saunders Elsevier, 2010.
Reef VB. Evaluation of ventricular septal defects in horses using two-dimensional and doppler echocardiography. Equine Vet J Suppl 1995;19:86–95.
Reef VB, Bonagura R, Buhl MKJ, et al. Recommendations for management of equine athletes with cardiovascular abnormalities. J Vet Intern Med 2014;28:749–761.

Author Laura K. Dunbar
Consulting Editor Margaret C. Mudge
Acknowledgment The author acknowledges the prior contribution of Margaret C. Mudge.

Client Education Handout available online

CONIUM MACULATUM (POISON HEMLOCK) TOXICOSIS

C

 BASICS

OVERVIEW
- A potent toxic plant causing neurotoxicity and rapid death in horses
- *Conium maculatum* (poison hemlock) is also known as spotted hemlock, European hemlock, Nebraska fern, and California fern
- The plant is a biennial herb with a fern-like appearance growing up to 3 m (10 feet) in height, with a smooth, hollow, purple-spotted stem and a stout, white to pale yellow taproot
- The lacy, triangular leaves resemble those of carrots and have a musky odor, like that of a parsnip, when crushed
- Small, white flowers cluster in flat-topped umbels 4–6 cm across
- Grayish, round, tiny fruit with flattened ridges are produced during the second year
- The plant commonly grows in disturbed soil along roadsides, field edges, railroad tracks, and stream banks throughout North America, with the exception of the southwestern deserts
- The whole green plant is toxic at levels of ≅1% of body weight; 2–2.5 kg (4–5 lb) of fresh leaves are lethal for horses
- The plant contains numerous piperidine alkaloids, with the most toxic being *N*-methyl coniine and γ-coniceine; coniine acts similarly to nicotine, first causing stimulation and then depression of the central nervous system

SIGNALMENT
Horses readily eat the plant even if other forage is present.

SIGNS
- The clinical course is rapid, and horses may be found dead or die within a few hours
- Initial signs include mydriasis, salivation, hypotension, colic, and diarrhea
- Neurologic signs develop rapidly and include apprehension, muscle tremors, muscular weakness, incoordination, recumbency, paralysis, and coma
- Horses may become recumbent and comatose and remain that way for hours to days before either recovering or dying from respiratory depression
- Death results from respiratory failure

CAUSES AND RISK FACTORS
- The plant appears during the early spring, and most toxicoses occur at this time, when the plant is most palatable
- The level of *N*-methyl coniine increases as the plant matures; the root becomes toxic only later in the year
- The highest alkaloid concentration is in the seeds
- Drying seems to reduce, but not eliminate, the toxicity

 DIAGNOSIS

DIFFERENTIAL DIAGNOSIS
Other causes of sudden death in horses—lightning strike, red maple toxicosis, yew toxicosis, cyanogenic glycoside-containing plant toxicosis, cardiac glycoside toxicosis, ionophore toxicosis, cardiac dysfunction/arrhythmia, aortic aneurysm/rupture, blister beetle toxicosis.

CBC/BIOCHEMISTRY/URINALYSIS
N/A

OTHER LABORATORY TESTS
Chemical analysis for coniine in stomach contents and urine is available.

IMAGING
N/A

OTHER DIAGNOSTIC PROCEDURES
N/A

PATHOLOGIC FINDINGS
- Plant material in stomach; stomach contents, urine, and exhaled air may have a characteristic mousy odor
- Nonspecific lesions at necropsy include diffuse congestion of the lungs, liver, and myocardium

 TREATMENT

- General supportive treatment
- Early gastrointestinal decontamination may be useful
- Maintain body fluid and electrolyte balance
- Respiratory support by mechanical ventilation may be helpful
- Adequate nursing care of recumbent animals

 MEDICATIONS

DRUG(S) OF CHOICE
- AC (1–4 g/kg PO in water slurry (1 g of AC in 5 mL of water))
- 1 dose of a cathartic PO with AC if no diarrhea or ileus—70% sorbitol (3 mL/kg) or sodium or magnesium sulfate (250–500 mg/kg)

CONTRAINDICATIONS/POSSIBLE INTERACTIONS
N/A

 FOLLOW-UP

PATIENT MONITORING
Monitor respiration in recumbent animals.

PREVENTION/AVOIDANCE
- Remove poison hemlock from areas accessible to horses. Treatment with herbicides may be attempted, but ensure that all plants are dead before reintroducing horses because herbicide-treated plants may be more palatable
- Do not feed hay that contains poison hemlock. Seeds may contaminate grains, making these feeds unsafe for consumption

POSSIBLE COMPLICATIONS
N/A

EXPECTED COURSE AND PROGNOSIS
- Very guarded early prognosis
- Clinical course may last several hours to 1–2 days
- Onset of signs occurs within ≅2 h of ingestion
- In severe cases, death occurs within 5–10 h of the onset of signs
- Because both the quantity of alkaloid in the plant and the quantity of plant consumed vary, not all horses that eat poison hemlock die

 MISCELLANEOUS

ASSOCIATED CONDITIONS
N/A

AGE-RELATED FACTORS
N/A

ZOONOTIC POTENTIAL
N/A

PREGNANCY/FERTILITY/BREEDING
Poison hemlock has teratogenic effects in cattle and pigs; however, teratogenicity has not been reported in horses.

SEE ALSO
N/A

ABBREVIATIONS
AC = activated charcoal

Suggested Reading
Burrows GM, Tyrl RJ. Toxic Plants of North America, 2e. Ames, IA: Wiley Blackwell, 2013:66–70.
Lopez TA, Cid MS, Bianchini ML. Biochemistry of hemlock (*Conium maculatum* L.) alkaloids and their acute and chronic toxicity in livestock. A review. Toxicon 1999;37:841–865.
Vetter J. Poison hemlock (*Conium maculatum* L.). Food Chem Toxicol 2004;42:1373–1382.

Author Sharon Gwaltney-Brant
Consulting Editors Wilson K. Rumbeiha and Steve Ensley
Acknowledgment The author and editors acknowledge the prior contribution of Anita M. Kore.

BASICS

DEFINITION
Conjunctivitis is inflammation of the mucous membrane that covers the posterior aspects of the eyelids and nictitating membrane (palpebral conjunctiva) and the superficial surface of the sclera (bulbar conjunctiva). It may be infectious or noninfectious.

PATHOPHYSIOLOGY
• Conjunctivitis is a nonspecific finding
• Infectious and noninfectious diseases of the lids, cornea, sclera, anterior uvea, nasolacrimal system, and orbit as well as systemic diseases can result in conjunctivitis
• Conjunctiva is a mucous membrane so it can also reflect systemic dysfunction through changes in color and in vascular appearance, as in anemia and jaundice
• Environmental allergies or irritants may cause conjunctivitis
• Habronemiasis is a parasitic conjunctivitis caused by aberrant migration of *Habronema* larvae. Habronemiasis may occur concurrently with SCC, which makes histologic examination of affected tissues crucial
• Onchocerciasis can cause conjunctivitis, keratitis, and keratouveitis. The causative agent is *Onchocerca cervicalis* and the insect vector is the female *Culicoides*. Migrating larvae may invade the conjunctiva, cornea, and anterior uvea resulting in inflammation
• The development of SCC has been associated with cell damage caused by the UV component of solar radiation. Animals with higher levels of exposure to sunlight or that live in high altitudes are more prone

SYSTEMS AFFECTED
Ophthalmic

GENETICS
No proven genetic basis for conjunctivitis. However, breed predilection for ocular SCC suggests genetic influence.

INCIDENCE/PREVALENCE
Common

GEOGRAPHIC DISTRIBUTION
None identified for conjunctivitis specifically. However, animals with higher levels of exposure to UV light are more prone to development of SCC.

SIGNALMENT
• Neonates—conjunctivitis may be associated with neonatal maladjustment syndrome, septicemia, uveitis immune-mediated hemolytic anemia, and environmental irritants; subconjunctival or episcleral hemorrhages may occur secondary to birth trauma or neonatal maladjustment syndrome. Conjunctivitis secondary to pneumonia is seen most commonly in 1–6 month old foals

• Adults—ocular SCC prevalence increases with age

SIGNS
• Conjunctivitis—conjunctival hyperemia, chemosis, and ocular discharge vary with type of disease
• Onchocerciasis—limbal conjunctival thickening and depigmentation, corneal edema, vascularization, stromal cellular infiltrate
• SCC has 2 characteristic appearances—proliferative mass which may or may not be ulcerated, or diffuse thickening and ulceration of tissue. May resemble granulation tissue or just an area of increased redness in the conjunctiva
• Habronemiasis—appearance ranges from granulomas, nodules, to small raised caseated plaques on the conjunctiva
• Dermoid—pigmented mass involving the limbus and varying degrees of the cornea

CAUSES OF CONJUNCTIVITIS
• Infectious
  ○ Parasitic—*Habronema megastoma, H. muscae, Draschia megastoma, Onchocerca cervicalis, Thelazia lacrimalis, Trypanosoma* spp.
  ○ Viral—adenovirus, equine herpesvirus types 1, 2, 4, and 5, equine infectious anemia, equine viral arteritis, influenza
  ○ Bacterial—*Moraxella equi, Streptococcus equi* ssp. *equi, Rhodococcus equi, Actinobacillus* spp., leptospirosis
  ○ Mycotic—*Aspergillus* spp., *Fusarium*
  ○ Protozoal—equine protozoal myeloencephalitis
• Neoplastic—SCC, lymphoma, papilloma, hemangioma, hemangiosarcoma, mastocytoma, melanoma, multiple myeloma, etc.
• Secondary to other ocular/adnexal disease—ulcerative keratitis, corneal stromal abscess, anterior uveitis, equine recurrent uveitis, obstructed nasolacrimal duct
• Secondary to trauma—orbital fractures, scleral perforation
• Secondary to environmental causes—foreign bodies and debris, allergic reactions to dust, environmental pollutants
• Secondary to systemic disease—polyneuritis equi, vestibular disease syndrome, African horse sickness, epizootic lymphangitis, neonatal maladjustment syndrome

RISK FACTORS
• Recumbent foals are at risk for conjunctivitis secondary to environmental irritants
• White, chestnut, and palomino coat color predispose to ocular SCC
• Lightly pigmented animals and those residing in areas with high UV indices are at the greatest risk
• Warm weather and climates with heavy fly populations are risk factors for habronemiasis and other parasitic infections

DIAGNOSIS

C

DIFFERENTIAL DIAGNOSIS
• Conjunctivitis is a nonspecific sign, reflecting the eye's limited mechanisms of response to injury. It is critical to differentiate primary conjunctivitis from conjunctivitis associated with ocular or systemic disease
• Nodular/mass lesions of conjunctiva—habronemiasis, SCC, mastocytoma, hemangioma, hemangiosarcoma, papilloma, and other neoplastic infiltrates, fungal granulomas, nodular necrobiosis, pseudotumors, dermoids, foreign body reaction

CBC/BIOCHEMISTRY/URINALYSIS
N/A

OTHER LABORATORY TESTS
• Cytology to identify mycotic, bacterial causes of conjunctivitis
• Culture and sensitivity of mucopurulent discharge may be considered if a primary bacterial cause is suspected (uncommon in horses)
• Habronemiasis—conjunctival scraping reveals eosinophils, mast cells, neutrophils, plasma cells, rarely larvae
• Biopsy and histopathology should be performed for mass lesions

IMAGING
N/A

OTHER DIAGNOSTIC PROCEDURES
Complete ophthalmic examination is indicated to identify adnexal and ocular causes of conjunctivitis, including a thorough adnexal examination, fluorescein staining, and examination for signs of anterior uveitis.

Conjunctival Biopsy
• Onchocerciasis—microfilariae, eosinophils, lymphocytes
• Habronemiasis—eosinophils, mast cells, neutrophils, plasma cells, rarely larvae
• SCC—epithelial cells with neoplastic characteristics
• Lymphoma—large population monomorphic lymphocytes with neoplastic characteristics

TREATMENT

APPROPRIATE HEALTH CARE
• Most horses with simple conjunctivitis associated with parasitic, bacterial, viral, and environmental causes can be treated on an outpatient basis
• Treatment of some systemic and ocular diseases associated with complicated conjunctivitis may require hospitalization

NURSING CARE
Ensure topical medications can be administered appropriately.

ACTIVITY
• Restriction of activity may be required in cases where conjunctival disease is associated with systemic illness
• If environmental irritation is suspected, then exposure to the inciting substance should be restricted or eliminated
• Animals with ocular involvement/disease should not be ridden if visual status is compromised

DIET
No change in diet is necessary. Hay should be fed at ground level rather than elevated hay racks or bags to avoid further irritation of the conjunctiva by dust and debris.

CLIENT EDUCATION
If there is evidence of self-trauma, a protective hood covering the affected eye should be placed on the horse. The client should be instructed to contact the veterinarian if the condition worsens in any way or shows little to no signs of improvement.

SURGICAL CONSIDERATIONS
• Treatment of conjunctival neoplasia may involve local resection, with adjunctive beta-irradiation, cryotherapy, radiofrequency hyperthermia, or topical chemotherapy
• Small lacerations of the conjunctiva will heal without primary closure. Large lacerations should be sutured with fine absorbable suture
• Conjunctival foreign bodies and debris can usually be removed with topical anesthesia and liberal flushing of conjunctival fornices

MEDICATIONS

DRUG(S) OF CHOICE
• Parasitic conjunctivitis—habronemiasis: topical 0.03% echothiophate iodide (ecotiopate iodide; phospholine iodide) and neomycin/polymyxin B with dexamethasone every 12 h. Multifocal lesions will require oral ivermectin. Intralesional triamcinolone may reduce size of granulomas, but this long-acting steroid must be used with extreme caution and not at all if the cornea is compromised in any way. Onchocerciasis—systemic ivermectin with topical anti-inflammatories. Thelazia—topical phospholine iodide, flush conjunctival fornix

• Conjunctival lacerations—treat with prophylactic broad-spectrum antibiotic topically
• Allergic conjunctivitis—topical corticosteroid, reduce/eliminate exposure to inciting cause if possible, lubricating ophthalmic ointment before turnout
• Other systemic medication as indicated by concurrent systemic disease

CONTRAINDICATIONS
N/A

PRECAUTIONS
N/A

POSSIBLE INTERACTIONS
N/A

FOLLOW-UP

PATIENT MONITORING
The patient should be rechecked soon after beginning therapy (3–4 days), with specific time frame determined by disease and severity. Subsequent rechecks are dictated by the specific diagnosis, the severity, and response to treatment.

PREVENTION/AVOIDANCE
• Fly control in barns and pastures, fly hoods, and frequent periocular administration of insect repellent can help prevent the development of habronemiasis
• A preventative health program including regular deworming with avermectins will help prevent habronemiasis and onchocerciasis
• The incidence of allergic/environmental conjunctivitis can be reduced/prevented by avoidance of the inciting agent
• Treat any underlying ocular or systemic disease that may promote the conjunctival disease
• Limit solar exposure in lightly pigmented animals to decrease the incidence of SCC

POSSIBLE COMPLICATIONS
Possible complications of treatment include depigmentation in region of treatment, recurrence, and metastatic spread (if neoplastic).

EXPECTED COURSE AND PROGNOSIS
• Infectious conjunctivitis usually responds to appropriate treatment
• Failure to respond or recurrence suggests an unidentified underlying cause (i.e. recurrent bacterial conjunctivitis associated with an unrecognized foreign body)

• Course and prognosis of conjunctival neoplasia depend on the specific type of neoplasia and the extent of invasion of surrounding tissues
• Viral conjunctivitis may be recurrent
• Allergic conjunctivitis is often difficult to eliminate completely owing to the nature of the horse's environment
• Many systemic diseases that have conjunctivitis as a clinical sign can have serious and life-threatening consequences

MISCELLANEOUS

ASSOCIATED CONDITIONS
N/A

AGE-RELATED FACTORS
N/A

ZOONOTIC POTENTIAL
N/A

PREGNANCY/FERTILITY/BREEDING
Systemic absorption of topically applied medication is possible. Benefits of treatment should be considered against any risks posed to the fetus.

SYNONYMS
N/A

SEE ALSO
• Corneal ulceration
• Equine recurrent uveitis
• Eyelid diseases
• Ocular/adnexal squamous cell carcinoma
• Ocular problems in the neonate
• Ulcerative keratomycosis

ABBREVIATIONS
SCC = squamous cell carcinoma

Suggested Reading
Brooks DE. Ophthalmology for the Equine Practitioner, 2e. Jackson, WY: Teton NewMedia, 2008.
Gilger BC. Equine ophthalmology. In: Gelatt KN, ed. Veterinary Ophthalmology, 5e. Ames, IA: Wiley, 2013:1560–1609.
Gilger BC. Equine Ophthalmology, 3e. Philadelphia, PA: WB Saunders, 2017.
Author Caroline Monk
Consulting Editor Caryn E. Plummer
Acknowledgment The author acknowledges the prior contribution of Caryn E. Plummer.

CONTAGIOUS EQUINE METRITIS (CEM)

BASICS

DEFINITION
• Genital infection of stallions and mares caused by *Taylorella equigenitalis*
• A reportable, highly contagious, nonlife-threatening disease
• Transmitted primarily by coitus but also by contaminated equipment
• Stallions are asymptomatic carriers
• Clinical signs only in mares; range from none to acute endometritis
• Abortion may occur in mid- to late gestation
• Regulations for interstate shipment (USA) of semen and embryos lack uniformity

PATHOPHYSIOLOGY
Stallions
• The organism is harbored in various external regions of the genital tract including fossa glandis, urethral sinus, smegma, terminal urethra, preputial surface, and pre-ejaculatory fluid
• Indirect transmission can occur by not following appropriate sanitary protocols when handling stallion external genitalia

Mares
• Up to 30–40% of mares bred by an infected stallion develop the disease:
  ○ A mare may also be exposed by breeding with fresh-cooled or extended semen from a carrier stallion
  ○ Indirect transmission can occur by inadequate sanitary protocols when handling stallions and mares, fomite spread, and contaminated equipment, including speculums, tail wraps, and obstetric equipment
• Clinical signs range from none to acute endometritis. Acute infection may remain asymptomatic, allowing the organism to persist for prolonged periods within a population of horses
• The organism initially is found in the endometrium and cervix and less frequently in the vagina, vulva, clitoris, and oviducts
• From 3 weeks to 4 months following exposure, the organism occasionally can be recovered from the ovarian surface, oviduct, uterus, cervix, and vagina
• The organism is more reliably isolated from the clitoral fossa and sinuses as it can persist in these sites
• Mares may be mechanical carriers via smegma of the clitoral fossa
• The organism may be harbored throughout pregnancy. It is subsequently also recoverable from placentae of positive mares and genitalia of colts and fillies
• Acquired in utero, at parturition, or via contact with bedding or pasture contaminated with infected fluids

SYSTEMS AFFECTED
Reproductive

GENETICS
N/A

INCIDENCE/PREVALENCE
Transmission is dependent on carrier stallion live cover or shipped semen, or the use of contaminated equipment.

SIGNALMENT
Breeding-age mares and stallions from countries identified as CEM affected.

SIGNS
Stallions
• Inapparent infection, retained locally on external genitalia, no systemic antibody response is detectable
• 1 report (necropsy) of infection involving testes and accessory sex glands

Mares
• Within 2–7 days (experimental) or up to 13 days (field challenge) of infection, mares develop varying amount of odorless, grayish, mucopurulent discharge
• Intrauterine fluid accumulation often present with transrectal ultrasonography
• Diffuse endometritis and cervicitis—severe and plasmacytic by 14 days; declines and persists as mild, diffuse, and multifocal for as long as 2 weeks
• Shortened diestrus because of premature luteolysis
• Temporary infertility
  ○ Short-term infertility differential diagnosis should consider CEM even in the absence of inflammation or vaginal discharge
  ○ Pregnancy may successfully be maintained in the presence of infection
  ○ Abortion may occur in mid- to late gestation
• No systemic involvement
• Reexposure experimentally associated with no to minimal signs of disease

CAUSES
• 2 strains of *T. equigenitalis* based on sensitivity to streptomycin (majority of strains are sensitive)
• *Taylorella asinigenitalis* resembles *T. equigenitalis*
  ○ Has been isolated from donkey jacks at routine testing for CEM
  ○ There is cross-reactivity with the CF utilized to identify mares recently infected with *T. equigenitalis*

RISK FACTORS
• Carrier stallion
• Contaminated equipment
• No lifelong immunity
• Previous exposure does not afford absolute protection against subsequent challenge

DIAGNOSIS

DIFFERENTIAL DIAGNOSIS
• Bacterial and fungal endometritis

• Pyometra
• Vaginitis
• Urinary tract infection
• Urine pooling
• Neoplasia of the uterus or vagina
• Persistent hymen

CBC/BIOCHEMISTRY/URINALYSIS
Unremarkable

OTHER LABORATORY TESTS
• Speculum examination
• Collection of cervical discharge
• Isolation of organism

IMAGING
Ultrasonography—intrauterine fluid suggestive of endometritis.

OTHER DIAGNOSTIC PROCEDURES
Serology
• Detectable antibody in acute cases
  ○ Mares only CF positive 21–45 days post infection
• No value in stallions, because contamination is surface only

Bacterial Cultures
• Stallions—urethral fossa and urethral sinus, distal urethra, penile skin, and preputial folds
• Mares—clitoral sinus and fossa; endometrium, vaginal fluid, and cervix of estrus mare
• Exacting culture requirements for *T. equigenitalis*
  ○ Immediately place swabs in Amies charcoal medium
  ○ Keep at 4°C for transport. Do not freeze.
• Plate samples within 48 h of collection in chocolate agar at 5% CO_2
• Colonies usually form in 2–3 days; a recent streptomycin-sensitive strain may take as long as 6 days
• Reportable disease that requires a federally approved laboratory for identification

Cytology (Mares)
• Presence of polymorphonuclear cells indicative of endometritis
• Presence of morphologically suggestive bacteria
  ○ Free or phagocytized Gram-negative coccobacilli seen individually or in pairs, arranged end to end

Test Breeding (Stallions)
• Breed to 2 known CEM-negative mares following 3 negative stallion cultures over 1 week
• Post breeding, mares assessed by repeated PCR and culture; seroconversion (CF antibodies) between 21 and 45 days
• Does not consistently lead to colonization and seroconversion of test mares; therefore test breed in conjunction with direct assessment of stallion

PCR
• Rapid and cost-effective test for mares and stallions
• Not sufficiently validated for screening of cooled or frozen semen, and embryos

CONTAGIOUS EQUINE METRITIS (CEM)

• Experimentally can discriminate between *T. equigenitalis* and *T. asinigenitalis*
• Used in conjunction with culture, more effective technique than culture alone

PATHOLOGIC FINDINGS
N/A

TREATMENT

APPROPRIATE HEALTH CARE
Under federal supervision at approved quarantine station.

Stallions
• Completely extrude and wash penis in chlorhexidine 4% scrub
• Remove all smegma, especially from the urethral fossa and skin folds of prepuce
• Dry all structures completely
• Nitrofurazone 0.2% or silver sulfadiazine 1% dressing is applied liberally
• Repeat above procedure daily for 5 days

Mares
• Acute endometritis:
  ◦ Intrauterine antibiotics—crystalline penicillin ($5-10 \times 10^6$ IU for 5–7 days), ampicillin (2 g in 60 mL normal saline for 3–5 days)
  ◦ Systemic antimicrobials—trimethoprim–sulfamethoxazole (30 mg/kg PO for 5 days)
• Clitoral carriers:
  ◦ Cleansing of the clitoral fossa and sinuses with chlorhexidine scrub to remove all smegma
  ◦ Pack with nitrofurazone 0.2% or 1% silver sulfadiazine ointment
  ◦ Repeat daily for 5 days
• May be beneficial to combine above protocols to prevent colonization of clitoris during treatment
• Several treatment cycles may be necessary to eliminate infection/carrier state
Retest all treated mares and stallions no less than 21 days following above protocols to ensure freedom from colonization with *T. equigenitalis.*

SURGICAL CONSIDERATIONS
Mares—clitoral sinusectomy or clitorectomy for intractable cases.

MEDICATIONS

DRUG(S) OF CHOICE
See Treatment.

CONTRAINDICATIONS
N/A

PRECAUTIONS
• Mucosal irritation from drugs
• Concurrent systemic antimicrobial treatment of mares and stallions may reduce bacterial load and therefore diminish chance of successful culture in carrier animals

FOLLOW-UP

PATIENT MONITORING

Culture (Timing)
• Swabs—at least 7 days after the last day of treatment with systemic antimicrobials, or 21 days following topical antimicrobials, must elapse before testing
• Use most current protocol as dictated by the country regulations. In USA (USDA/APHIS):
  ◦ Mares—3 consecutive estrus periods
  ◦ Stallions—every 2 days for 3 sets

Culture (Locations)
• Mares—swab the clitoris and endometrium at estrus before breeding; swab during abnormal estrous intervals
• Stallions—swabs from teaser and breeding stallions before season begins, as described in Bacterial Cultures

Culture (Equipment)
Disposable gloves, sleeves, and speculum. Clean disposable tail wrap.

PREVENTION/AVOIDANCE
• All horses older than 2 years entering the USA from CEM-affected countries must follow treatment and testing protocol
• Mares—culture 3 times in 7 days, then treat for 5 days; if 3 negative cultures are obtained, the mare is released
• Stallions require a set of negative cultures followed by negative test breeding to 2 known CEM-negative mares; if positive, treat, then repeat cycle until 3 consecutive, negative culture results and negative test breeding results are obtained
• Use artificial insemination when feasible or permitted by breed society regulations

EXPECTED COURSE AND PROGNOSIS
Recovery with treatment.

MISCELLANEOUS

SYNONYMS
Formerly *Haemophilus equigenitalis.*

SEE ALSO
N/A

ABBREVIATIONS
• CEM = contagious equine metritis
• CF = complement fixation test
• PCR = polymerase chain reaction
• USDA/APHIS = United States Department of Agriculture/Animal and Plant Health Inspection Service

Suggested Reading
Baverud V, Nystrom C, Johansson KE. Isolation and identification of *Taylorella asinigenitalis* from the genital tract of a stallion, first case of a natural infection. Vet Microbiol 2006;116:294–300.
Carleton CL, Donahue JM, Marteniuk JV, et al. Bacterial and fungal microflora on the external genitalia of male donkeys (*Equus asinus*). Anim Reprod Sci 2015;153:62–68.
Dennis S, Pearson LK, Campbell AJ, Tibary A. Interstate equine semen and embryo shipment regulations in the United States and their implications on control of disease transmission. J Equine Vet Sci 2014;34(7):897–902.
Klein C, Donahue JM, Sells SF, et al. Effect of antimicrobial-containing semen extender on risk of dissemination of contagious equine metritis. J Am Vet Med Assoc 2012;241(7):916–921.
Schulman ML, May CE, Keys B, Guthrie AJ. Contagious equine metritis: artificial reproduction changes the epidemiologic paradigm. Vet Microbiol 2013;167(1):2–8.
Timoney PJ, Kristula MA, Ford ES, et al. Contagious equine metritis: efficacy of US post-entry testing protocols for identifying carrier stallions and mares. J Equine Vet Sci 2016;39:S60.
Wakeley PR, Errington J, Hannon S, et al. Development of a real time PCR for the detection of *Taylorella equigenitalis* directly from genital swabs and discrimination from *Taylorella asinigenitalis*. Vet Microbiol 2006;118:247–254.
Watson ED. Swabbing protocols in screening for contagious equine metritis. Vet Rec 1997;140:268–271.
Wood JL, Kelly L, Cardwell JM, Park AW. Quantitative assessment of the risks of reducing the routine swabbing requirements for the detection of *Taylorella equigenitalis*. Vet Rec 2005;157:41–46.

Author Peter R. Morresey
Consulting Editor Carla L. Carleton

C

BASICS

OVERVIEW
• Ocular trauma may have possible effects on any ocular structure such that ocular injury can have a variety of manifestations
• Blunt injuries carry a worse prognosis than injury from sharp objects as blunt forces are transmitted and often reverberate throughout the eye. Sharp, penetrating injuries generally have the forces localized to the site of impact

SIGNALMENT
Any age and breed of horse may suffer corneal laceration.

SIGNS
• The eye may be cloudy, red, and painful. Blepharospasm and lacrimation are present with focal or generalized corneal edema. Slight ventral deviation of the eyelashes of the upper eyelid may be a subtle sign of corneal ulceration
• Full-thickness corneal/scleral perforations are usually associated with iris prolapse, shallow anterior chamber, and hyphema. If the corneal lesion extends to the limbus, the sclera should also be carefully checked for perforation. Scleral wounds can be obscured by conjunctival chemosis and hemorrhage

CAUSES AND RISK FACTORS
Trauma from nails, buckets, light fixtures, vegetative material, and tree branches can result in corneal/scleral lacerations.

DIAGNOSIS

DIFFERENTIAL DIAGNOSIS
Ocular pain may also be found with corneal ulcers, uveitis, conjunctivitis, glaucoma, blepharitis, and dacryocystitis.

CBC/BIOCHEMISTRY/URINALYSIS
N/A

OTHER LABORATORY TESTS
N/A

IMAGING
N/A

OTHER DIAGNOSTIC PROCEDURES
Fluorescein dye staining of the cornea will reveal the laceration. Fluorescein dye may enter the anterior chamber. Seidel's test may reveal leakage of aqueous humor from the anterior chamber through the corneal laceration.

PATHOLOGIC FINDINGS
N/A

TREATMENT
• Medical therapy should be sufficient for superficial, nonperforating lacerations. Deep or irregular corneal lacerations require surgical repair and more aggressive therapy for iridocyclitis. Direct corneal suturing and conjunctival flaps are indicated to more rapidly restore corneal integrity
• Both small and large full-thickness corneal perforations should be surgically repaired. Complications include infection, iris prolapse, anterior synechiae, cataract formation, and persistent iridocyclitis. Both small and large corneal or scleral full-thickness defects can result in phthisis bulbi if left untreated
• An eye with a traumatic corneal perforation that defies repair, extensive extrusion of intraocular contents, severe intraocular hemorrhage, or evidence of infection should be enucleated

MEDICATIONS

DRUG(S) OF CHOICE
Medical therapy alone should be sufficient for superficial, nonperforating lacerations. Topically applied antibiotics (chloramphenicol, bacitracin–neomycin–polymyxin B, gentamicin; every 2–6 h), atropine (1%; QID), and serum (every 1–6 h) are recommended. Systemic NSAIDs (phenylbutazone 2 mg/kg BID PO; flunixin meglumine 1 mg/kg BID PO, IM, IV) and broad-spectrum parenteral antibiotics are also indicated for full-thickness lesions.

CONTRAINDICATIONS/POSSIBLE INTERACTIONS
Horses receiving topically administered atropine should be monitored for signs of colic.

FOLLOW-UP

PATIENT MONITORING
• The horse should be protected from self-trauma with hard- or soft-cup hoods
• Horses with corneal lacerations and secondary uveitis should be stall rested until the condition is healed. Intraocular hemorrhage and increased severity of uveitis are sequelae to overexertion
• Diet should be consistent with the training and activity level of the horse

PREVENTION/AVOIDANCE
N/A

POSSIBLE COMPLICATIONS
• Failure to detect a scleral tear will result in chronic hypotony and globe atrophy (phthisis bulbi)
• The eye of the horse does not tolerate much damage to its vasculature. Severe intraocular hemorrhage usually results in phthisis bulbi
• Injury to the lens, iris, and retina can accompany blunt or sharp corneal/scleral trauma
• Septic intrusion into the globe results in painful endophthalmitis. Such infection can spread to surrounding soft tissues and necessitates enucleation

EXPECTED COURSE AND PROGNOSIS
• Small corneal lacerations can heal quickly if surgical and medical therapy is prompt. Larger lesions are associated with more uveitis and will be slower to heal
• If the horse has a dazzle reflex in the damaged eye and a consensual pupillary light reflex in the fellow eye, then repair should be attempted

MISCELLANEOUS

ASSOCIATED CONDITIONS
Corneal lacerations in the horse are always accompanied by varying degrees of iridocyclitis.

AGE-RELATED FACTORS
N/A

ZOONOTIC POTENTIAL
N/A

PREGNANCY/FERTILITY/BREEDING
N/A

SEE ALSO
Iris prolapse

ABBREVIATIONS
NSAID = nonsteroidal anti-inflammatory drug

Suggested Reading
Brooks DE. Ophthalmology for the Equine Practitioner, 2e. Jackson, WY: Teton NewMedia, 2008.
Brooks DE, Matthews AG. Equine ophthalmology. In: Gelatt KN, ed. Veterinary Ophthalmology, 4e. Ames, IA: Blackwell, 2007:1165–1274.
Gilger BC, ed. Equine Ophthalmology, 3e. Philadelphia, PA: WB Saunders, 2017.

Author Caryn E. Plummer
Consulting Editor Caryn E. Plummer
Acknowledgment The author/editor acknowledges the prior contribution of Dennis E. Brooks.

CORNEAL STROMAL ABSCESSES

BASICS

OVERVIEW
A corneal abscess may develop after epithelial cells adjacent to a small defect migrate over the wound to seal infectious agents or foreign bodies in the stroma. This re-epithelialization forms a barrier that protects the bacteria or fungi from topical antimicrobial medications.

SIGNALMENT
All ages and breeds of horses are at risk.

SIGNS
• The eye may be cloudy and red. Blepharospasm and epiphora are usually present. Slight downward deviation of the upper eyelashes may be a subtle sign of ocular pain
• The diagnosis of stromal abscess is based on the presence of a focal, yellow-white infiltrate within the cornea. A mild to fulminating iridocyclitis occurs secondary to what appears initially to be a relatively benign corneal disease, causing severe pain and potentially blinding sequelae. Corneal vascularization is variable at presentation
• Initial clinical signs suggestive of minor corneal trauma. Fluorescein dye retention may be present initially and treatment for corneal ulceration results in re-epithelialization. Days to weeks later, the iridocyclitis worsens and a corneal abscess is visible

CAUSES AND RISK FACTORS
Corneal stromal abscesses can be sterile or caused by bacteria or fungi.

DIAGNOSIS

DIFFERENTIAL DIAGNOSIS
• Ocular pain may be caused by corneal ulcers, anterior uveitis, or equine recurrent uveitis
• A history of trauma or corneal ulceration and a yellow-white cellular stromal infiltrate will facilitate diagnosis of stromal abscess

DIAGNOSTIC PROCEDURES
• Cytologic, microbiologic, and histologic specimens may fail to yield an etiology. It may be that toxins released by dying bacteria and fungi and degenerating leukocytes continue the stimulus for keratitis and anterior uveitis

• Keratectomy specimens may be the only way to obtain an etiologic diagnosis

TREATMENT
• Many stromal abscesses initially respond positively with improving uveitis to topical mydriatics/cycloplegics and topical antimicrobials and systemic NSAIDs
• Scraping over the stromal abscess may aid drug penetration in the early stages but it may damage the superficial cornea, which may limit surgical options
• The use of systemic NSAIDs should be carefully adjusted to allow the control of anterior uveitis without significantly inhibiting necessary corneal vascularization
• Deep corneal abscesses respond poorly to medical therapy. Most stromal abscesses involving Descemet's membrane are fungal infections. Deep lamellar and penetrating keratoplasties are utilized in eyes with deep abscesses, and eyes with rupture of the abscess into the anterior chamber. This aggressive surgical therapy can be very successful and is done to eliminate antigenic stimulation from the sequestered organisms and to remove the necrotic debris, metabolites, and toxins
• Horses that undergo surgery early in the course of this disease tend to have a more rapid recovery than those in which surgery is delayed. If a positive response to medical therapy is not seen quickly, especially when the stromal abscesses are deep or severe uveitis is present, surgery should be considered
• The decision to perform surgery is based on continued progression of anterior uveitis despite medical therapy or relapses of uveitis when treatment is tapered, or imminent or preexistent rupture of the abscess into the anterior chamber
• Corneal transplantation is an effective treatment

MEDICATIONS

DRUG(S) OF CHOICE
Topically applied antibiotics and antifungals (natamycin, miconazole, voriconazole every 4–6 h), atropine (1%; QID) are recommended. Systemic NSAIDs (flunixin meglumine 1 mg/kg BID PO, IM, IV) are also indicated. In some cases where surgical removal of the abscess is not possible, an intracorneal injection of voriconazole may improve healing.

FOLLOW-UP

PATIENT MONITORING
• Ocular pain should diminish with resolution of the abscess. Self-trauma can be minimized with hard- or soft-cup face-masks or hoods
• Topical atropine may alter gastrointestinal motility and horses should be monitored for colic
• Horses should be stall rested until the condition is healed
• Diet should be consistent with the activity and training level of the horse

POSSIBLE COMPLICATIONS
Endophthalmitis, persistent uveitis, synechiae, and cataract are complications of stromal abscesses.

EXPECTED COURSE AND PROGNOSIS
• Most stromal abscesses do not completely heal until they become vascularized
• Enucleation of painful blind eyes is necessary in some cases

MISCELLANEOUS

ABBREVIATIONS
NSAID = nonsteroidal anti-inflammatory drug

Suggested Reading
Brooks DE. Ophthalmology for the Equine Practitioner, 2e. Jackson, WY: Teton NewMedia, 2008.
Brooks DE, Matthews AG. Equine ophthalmology. In: Gelatt KN, ed. Veterinary Ophthalmology, 4e. Ames, IA: Blackwell, 2007:1165–1274.
Gilger BC, ed. Equine Ophthalmology, 3e. Philadelphia, PA: WB Saunders, 2017.

Author Caryn E. Plummer
Consulting Editor Caryn E. Plummer
Acknowledgment The author/editor acknowledges the prior contribution of Dennis E. Brooks.

CORNEAL ULCERATION

BASICS

DEFINITION
- Corneal ulceration is a sight-threatening disease requiring early clinical diagnosis, laboratory confirmation, and appropriate medical and surgical therapy
- Ulcers can range from simple, superficial breaks or abrasions in the corneal epithelium to full-thickness corneal perforations with iris prolapse
- Prompt therapy is necessary to prevent progression and sight- and globe-threatening complications

PATHOPHYSIOLOGY
- The thickness of the equine cornea is 0.9–1.2 mm
- The normal equine corneal epithelium is 8–10 cell layers thick but increases to 10–15 cell layers following corneal injury. The epithelial basement membrane is not completely formed 6 weeks following corneal injury, in spite of the epithelium completely covering the ulcer site. Healing time of a 7 mm diameter, midstromal depth corneal trephine wound was nearly 12 days in noninfected wounds
- Bacterial and fungal organisms normally found in the horse conjunctival flora are potential ocular pathogens. *Staphylococcus, Streptococcus, Pseudomonas, Aspergillus*, and *Fusarium* spp. are commonly isolated from equine corneal ulcers
- A defect in the tear film or corneal epithelium allows bacteria or fungi to adhere to the cornea and to initiate infection
- Tear film neutrophils and some bacteria and fungi are associated with highly destructive protease and collagenase enzymes that can result in rapid corneal stromal degradation and corneal thinning in the horse. Excessive protease activity is termed "melting" and results in a gelatinous appearance of the stroma. Severely affected corneas are at great risk of perforation
- Horse corneas demonstrate a strong fibrovascular healing response

SYSTEMS AFFECTED
Ophthalmic

INCIDENCE/PREVALENCE
Common and may be associated with bacterial and fungal infection.

SIGNALMENT
All ages and breeds.

SIGNS
- The eye may be cloudy, red, and painful
- Blepharospasm and epiphora
- A corneal defect may be obvious or may require the application of topical fluorescein to highlight its margins
- Corneal edema may surround the ulcer or involve the entire cornea

- White- to cream-colored infiltrate may be present in the stroma in or around a corneal ulcer and is usually indicative of the presence of an infectious agent
- Signs of anterior uveitis are found to some extent with every corneal ulcer and include miosis, aqueous flare, fibrin, hyphema, or hypopyon

CAUSES
- Trauma
- Infection should be considered possible in every corneal ulcer in the horse. Infectious keratitis develops in eyes with traumatic corneal abrasions, and eyes with epithelial defects due to chronic edema, keratoconjunctivitis sicca, exposure keratitis, neurotrophic keratitis, and neuroparalytic keratitis. Immunosuppressive conditions and topical steroids predispose to the development of corneal infections. Fungal involvement should be suspected if there is a history of corneal injury with vegetative material, or if a corneal ulcer has received prolonged antibiotic and/or corticosteroid therapy with minimal or no improvement
- Foreign bodies, chemical burns, and immune mechanisms may also cause corneal ulceration
- Persistent superficial ulcers may become indolent due to hyaline membrane formation on the ulcer bed

RISK FACTORS
- The prominent eye of the horse may predispose to injury
- Tear film proteases are elevated in both eyes of a horse with an ulcer in 1 eye
- Healing of ulcers does not occur until tear film proteases are reduced to baseline levels

DIAGNOSIS

DIFFERENTIAL DIAGNOSIS
- Fluorescein dye (undiluted) retention is diagnostic of a corneal ulcer
- Uveitis, blepharitis, conjunctivitis, glaucoma, and dacryocystitis must be considered in the differential for a painful eye

LABORATORY TESTS
- Microbial culture and susceptibility for bacteria and fungi are recommended with rapidly progressive and deep corneal ulcers
- Corneal cultures should be obtained first, followed by corneal scrapings for cytology
- Mixed bacterial and fungal infections can be present
- Vigorous corneal scrapings, at the edge and base of the lesion, to detect bacteria and deep hyphal elements can be obtained following application of a topical anesthetic with the handle end of a sterile scalpel blade or a cytology brush. Superficial swabbing may not always yield organisms. Stain cytologic

specimens with Gram, Giemsa, or Wright's stain

DIAGNOSTIC PROCEDURES
- All corneal injuries should be fluorescein stained to detect corneal ulcers. Small corneal abrasions are detected through the use of oblique transillumination and fluorescein dye retention
- A "crater-like" defect that retains fluorescein dye at its periphery and is clear in the center is a descemetocele, and indicates the globe is at high risk of rupture. Descemet's membrane in the horse is 21 μm thick

PATHOLOGIC FINDINGS
- Many early cases present initially as minor corneal epithelial ulcers or infiltrates, with blepharospasm, epiphora, and photophobia
- At first, anterior uveitis and corneal vascularization may not be clinically pronounced
- Superficial and deep corneal vascularization and painful uveitis may occur
- Extensive stromal lesions, vascularization, conjunctival injection, and corneal edema may then become evident
- Corneal collagen breakdown or "melting" appears as a gelatinous, gray opacity in the margins and/or central regions of an ulcer. Melting corneal collagen may appear to drip off the surface of the eye
- Cellular infiltrate may develop rapidly and appears as white-to-yellow corneal opacities
- A descemetocele can be recognized as a clearing at the bottom of a deep ulcer. It does not retain fluorescein dye, whereas deep ulcers (with some remaining corneal collagen) retain fluorescein
- Deep penetration of the stroma to Descemet's membrane with perforation of the cornea is a possible sequela to all corneal ulcers in horses

TREATMENT

APPROPRIATE HEALTH CARE
- Corneal ulceration should always be considered an emergency
- The horse cornea can rapidly deteriorate if ulcerated and is prone to infection
- Subpalpebral lavage treatment systems are used to treat a fractious horse or for frequent therapy

ACTIVITY
Horses should be stall rested until the condition is healed.

CLIENT EDUCATION
- A slowly progressive, indolent course often belies the seriousness of the ulcer
- Corneal ulcers in horses may rapidly progress to descemetoceles or perforations
- Corneal ulcers in horses are often very slow to heal

CORNEAL ULCERATION   (CONTINUED)

- Anterior uveitis may be difficult to control
- Scarring and vascularization of the cornea are common to the horse following ulceration

SURGICAL CONSIDERATIONS
- Surgical placement of a conjunctival flap, corneoconjunctival transposition, or corneal transplantation may be indicated for rapidly progressive and deep corneal ulcers
- Removing necrotic tissue by keratectomy speeds healing, minimizes scarring, and decreases the stimulus for iridocyclitis
- Conjunctival grafts or flaps are used for the clinical management of deep, melting, and large corneal ulcers, descemetoceles, and for perforated corneal ulcers with and without iris prolapse
- Amniotic membrane grafts or synthetic collagen grafts are used to facilitate healing and decrease scar tissue development in large or melting corneal ulcers
- Panophthalmitis following perforation through a corneal stromal ulcer has a grave prognosis and enucleation may be considered
- Persistent ulcers may need surgical debridement with a diamond burr or a superficial keratectomy to remove the hyaline membrane slowing healing

MEDICATIONS
DRUG(S) OF CHOICE
- Topically applied antibiotics, such as neomycin–polymyxin B–bacitracin, gramicidin, chloramphenicol, gentamicin, ofloxacin, ciprofloxacin, or tobramycin ophthalmic solutions, may be used for bacterial ulcers. Amikacin (10 mg/mL) may also be used topically. Frequency of medication varies from every 1 h to every 8 h
- Topical 1% atropine (every 4 h, then decrease the frequency of administration as soon as the pupil dilates) to stabilize the blood–aqueous barrier, to minimize pain from ciliary muscle spasm, and to cause pupillary dilatation

- Topically administered autogenous serum is used in ulcers with evidence of collagenolysis, infection, or chronicity. The serum can be administered topically as often as possible. Acetylcysteine (5%) or sodium EDTA (0.2–1.0%) can also be administered until stromal liquefaction diminishes. Multiple anticollagenase medications may be needed to arrest melting in some horse eyes
- Systemic and topically administered NSAIDs such as phenylbutazone (1 g BID PO) or flunixin meglumine (1 mg/kg BID IV, IM, or PO) to reduce uveal exudation and relieve ocular discomfort

CONTRAINDICATIONS
Topical corticosteroids may encourage growth of bacterial and fungal opportunists and also impair collagen production and epithelial migration and adhesion.

PRECAUTIONS
Horses receiving topically administered atropine should be monitored for signs of colic.

ALTERNATIVE DRUGS
Topical autogenous serum can reduce tear film and corneal protease activity in corneal ulcers. It can be stored at room temperature; however, refrigeration is recommended. Replace the serum with fresh every 8 days.

FOLLOW-UP
PATIENT MONITORING
- The clarity of the cornea, the depth and size of the ulcer, the degree of corneal vascularization, the amount of tearing, the pupil size, and intensity of the anterior uveitis should be monitored. Serial fluorescein staining of the ulcer is indicated to assess re-epithelialization
- As the cornea heals, the stimulus for the uveitis will diminish, and the pupil will dilate with less frequent atropine administration
- Self-trauma should be reduced with hard- or soft-cup hoods

PREVENTION/AVOIDANCE
Corneal ulcers in horses should be aggressively treated no matter how small or superficial they may be. Progression is common and consequences can be severe.

POSSIBLE COMPLICATIONS
Globe rupture, phthisis bulbi, and blindness are possible sequelae.

EXPECTED COURSE AND PROGNOSIS
- Corneal ulcer often heals slowly and with scarring. There is a strong tendency to vascularize
- If the replication and spread of bacteria are not halted, the process of stromal degradation and "melting" ultimately leads to total loss of stromal tissue and corneal perforation
- Conjunctival flaps or corneal grafts may be necessary to save the globe and vision but are associated with scarring of the ulcer site

MISCELLANEOUS
ASSOCIATED CONDITIONS
- Corneal infection and iridocyclitis are always major concerns for even the slightest corneal ulcerations
- Iridocyclitis or uveitis is present in all types of corneal ulcers and must be treated in order to preserve vision

ABBREVIATIONS
NSAID = nonsteroidal anti-inflammatory drug

Suggested Reading
Brooks DE. Ophthalmology for the Equine Practitioner, 2e. Jackson, WY: Teton NewMedia, 2008.
Gilger BC, ed. Equine Ophthalmology, 3e. Philadelphia, PA: WB Saunders, 2017.

Author Caryn E. Plummer
Consulting Editor Caryn E. Plummer
Acknowledgment The author/editor acknowledges the prior contribution of Dennis E. Brooks.

C

BASICS

DEFINITION
Causes in order of frequency—(1) external abscesses, (2) internal infection, (3) ulcerative lymphangitis.

PATHOPHYSIOLOGY
• Soil-borne, Gram-positive, pleomorphic, intracellular facultative anaerobic rod
• Likely transmitted by mechanical vectors (flies), horse-to-horse contact, and contaminated soil
• Portals of entry—traumatized mucous membranes or skin, including insect-induced ventral midline dermatitis
• Incubation time 3–4 weeks
• Exotoxin phospholipase D increases vascular permeability to promote spread of infection through tissue and lymphatics and causes local edema and pain. Internal abscesses result from hematogenous or lymphatic spread
• Most immunocompetent horses mount a strong immune response and have a single bout of infection

SYSTEMS AFFECTED
External Abscesses
• Skin
• Lymphatic
• Musculoskeletal

Internal Infection
• Hepatobiliary
• Renal
• Respiratory
• Other (nervous, reproductive)

Ulcerative Lymphangitis
• Musculoskeletal
• Lymphatic

INCIDENCE/PREVALENCE
Endemic farms—sporadic. Naive populations—higher incidence. Mortality rate—<1% for external abscesses, 30–40% for internal infection.

GEOGRAPHIC DISTRIBUTION
Most common—southwestern USA; seen throughout North America.

SIGNALMENT
All ages affected. Foals <6 months old are rarely affected, suggesting passive transfer of immunity when born to mares in endemic areas. No sex predilection.

SIGNS
External Abscesses
• Historic cases on the property
• Edema of pectorals, axillae, ventrum, or inguinal area
• Progress to larger localized, painful and firm swellings in which small, multifocal abscesses develop
• Mature abscesses may have a palpable soft depression (Web Figure 1)

• Purulent material—thick, non-odorous, and tan
• Limb edema or lameness (triceps or inguinal areas)
• Variable signs of systemic inflammation/discomfort (fever, lethargy, anorexia, tachycardia)

Internal Infection
• History of external abscess weeks prior
• Anorexia
• Lethargy
• Weight loss
• Fever
• Dependent edema
• Tachycardia
• Tachypnea, nasal discharge (respiratory disease)
• Abdominal discomfort
• Abnormal urination (urinary tract disease)

Ulcerative Lymphangitis
• Limb edema (cellulitis/lymphangitis)
• Multiple draining lesions
• Lameness
• Variable signs of systemic inflammation/discomfort

Other
• Lameness (osteomyelitis, septic arthritis, or tenosynovitis)
• Neurologic signs (meningitis)
• Stridor (arytenoid chondritis)
• Nasal discharge (sinusitis, guttural pouch empyema)
• Vaginal discharge, abortion (metritis, placentitis)

CAUSES
• *Corynebacterium pseudotuberculosis* biovar *equi* (nitrate reductase positive)
• Biovar *ovis* (nitrate negative) causes caseous lymphadenitis in small ruminants
• Natural cross-species transmission does not occur

RISK FACTORS
• Endemic disease
• High ambient temperatures or drought. Most cases are diagnosed in summer and fall. Increased insect vectors after a wet, mild winter
• Poor vector control
• Immunocompromised horses

DIAGNOSIS

DIFFERENTIAL DIAGNOSIS
External Abscesses
• Other bacterial infections (e.g. *Streptococcus equi* ssp. *equi* and *S. equi* ssp. *zooepidemicus*)
• Hematoma/seroma
• Neoplasia
• Other causes for ventral edema (e.g. hypersensitivity, hypoproteinemia, vasculitis)
• Other causes for lameness

Internal Infection
• Other infectious organisms (e.g. *S. equi* ssp. *equi* and *S. equi* ssp. *zooepidemicus*, *Coccidioides immitis*)
• Foreign body
• Hepatopathy, splenitis, pyelonephritis, peritonitis, respiratory disease of other etiologies
• Neoplasia

Ulcerative Lymphangitis
• Other infectious causes of cellulitis/lymphangitis
• Immune-mediated vasculitis
• Exotic infectious disease (e.g. *Burkholderia mallei*, *Histoplasma capsulatum* var. *farciminosum*)
• Other—osteomyelitis, septic arthritis, meningitis, upper airway disease of other etiologies

CBC/BIOCHEMISTRY/URINALYSIS
• Anemia of chronic inflammation
• Leukocytosis with neutrophilia
• Hyperfibrinogenemia
• Hyperglobulinemia
• Biochemical abnormalities relate to the organs affected and systemic illness
• Pyuria—renal abscess

OTHER LABORATORY TESTS
• Gram stain—Gram-positive, pleomorphic rods
• Bacterial culture
• PCR—may be more sensitive in cases that are culture negative (e.g. previous treatment with antimicrobials, low quantities of bacteria)
• Synergistic hemolysin inhibition test—measures immunoglobulin G to exotoxin. Titers—negative ≤16, exposure or acute infection = 16–128, internal infection ≥512 provided no concurrent external abscess. Exposure, active disease, and recovery titers overlap. May stay increased after infection for months

IMAGING
Ultrasonography
• Early external infection—diffuse edema. Mature abscesses have thick capsules with heterogeneous contents and variable loculations
• Internal infection—thoracic: consolidation, pleural changes/effusion; abdominal: increased peritoneal fluid, abnormalities in the viscera or lymph nodes
• Abscesses are singular or multifocal within organ parenchyma, often thinly encapsulated with hypoechoic contents, and the organ may be enlarged

Radiography
• Thoracic radiographs—diffuse or patchy interstitial and/or alveolar patterns with pneumonia
• Limb radiographs—rule out other causes of lameness or osteomyelitis

CORYNEBACTERIUM PSEUDOTUBERCULOSIS (CONTINUED)

OTHER DIAGNOSTIC PROCEDURES
Abdominocentesis—peritonitis. Transtracheal wash—septic bronchopneumonia; culture and antimicrobial sensitivity. Endoscopy—guttural pouch or laryngeal involvement. Blood culture—in severe sepsis.

PATHOLOGIC FINDINGS
Abscesses are encapsulated with purulent contents and may distort surrounding tissues.

TREATMENT

APPROPRIATE HEALTH CARE
• Most noncomplicated external abscesses or ulcerative lymphangitis can be dealt with in the field or as an outpatient
• Biosecurity to prevent spread of exudate is advised for draining external abscesses

NURSING CARE
• External abscesses—hot packs/poultices encourage abscess maturation. Mature abscesses may rupture spontaneously or be surgically lanced and lavaged with saline and/or antiseptic solutions
• Internal infection—supportive care
• Ulcerative lymphangitis—topical antimicrobials and frequent bandage changes to provide wound coverage and compression. Free-choice exercise and hand-walking
• Application of insect repellent to prevent vectoring of infectious material

CLIENT EDUCATION
• Nondraining lesions—not directly infectious
• Draining lesions—confine to a single area; exudate carries high bacterial load and should be collected, disinfected, and disposed of in a closed system

SURGICAL CONSIDERATIONS
• Mature external abscesses can be lanced at a dependent site, with or without ultrasonography guidance. Lancing immature abscesses may increase tissue inflammation
• Abscesses deep to large muscle groups (e.g. triceps)—drainage through insertion of a chest tube
• Septic peritonitis may require an abdominal drain and lavage

MEDICATIONS

DRUG(S) OF CHOICE
• Uncomplicated external abscesses—antimicrobials often not indicated
• Horses with external abscesses and concurrent systemic illness, recurrent infections, or poor immunity and horses with internal infection or ulcerative lymphangitis require antimicrobials until evidence of infection has completely resolved
• Susceptible in vitro to many antimicrobials and does not appear to be developing widespread resistance
• Effectiveness in vivo depends on penetration through the abscess capsule, activity in exudate, intracellular bacterial location, and drug bioavailability
• External abscesses—trimethoprim–sulfamethoxazole (30 mg/kg PO every 12 h), trimethoprim–sulfadiazine (24 mg/kg PO every 12 h), or minocycline (4 mg/kg PO every 12 h). Sulfas and beta-lactams may be inactivated in presence of large, acidic abscess
• Internal abscesses—minocycline (4 mg/kg PO every 12 h), doxycycline (10 mg/kg PO every 12 h), enrofloxacin (7.5 mg/kg PO every 24 h), trimethoprim–sulfas (doses above), and potassium penicillin (20 000–40 000 IU/kg IV every 4–6 h). Rifampin (rifampicin) (5 mg/kg PO every 12 h) is highly effective when added to another antimicrobial (e.g. trimethoprim–sulfa). Ceftiofur is less effective due to a high minimum inhibitory concentration
• Ulcerative lymphangitis—treat aggressively with long-term antimicrobials
• NSAIDs—control discomfort and inflammation

CONTRAINDICATIONS
• Enrofloxacin—contraindicated in growing horses
• Chloramphenicol and doxycycline have variable bioavailability in horses and may be less effective in vivo

ALTERNATIVE DRUGS
Immunostimulants—not critically evaluated or currently recommended.

FOLLOW-UP

PREVENTION/AVOIDANCE
Insect Vector Control
• Prompt disposal of organic debris, fly repellent systems, fly predators, or feed-through insect growth regulators
• Apply topical insect repellents (particularly ventral midline and wounds)
Biosecurity
• Disposable gloves and handwashing
• Isolate horses with draining external abscesses
• Collect, disinfect, and dispose of exudate
• Conditionally licensed bacterin vaccine available (Boehringer Ingelheim International GmbH)

POSSIBLE COMPLICATIONS
Disseminated disease and purpura haemorrhagica

EXPECTED COURSE AND PROGNOSIS
• External abscesses—simple abscesses: 14–30 days to fully resolve; additional abscesses may develop from lymphatic spread. Prognosis: good
• Internal infection—>30 days, often 90–120 days. Prognosis: fair to good if treated
• Serially monitor leukogram, globulins and ultrasound findings
• Ulcerative lymphangitis—≥30 days. Prognosis: good

MISCELLANEOUS

ZOONOTIC POTENTIAL
Rarely occurs; 1 reported student developed pneumonia after exposure to an infected horse, likely from bacterial inhalation in a contaminated environment.

PREGNANCY/FERTILITY/BREEDING
Abortion from placentitis or fetal infection may occur.

SYNONYMS
• Pigeon fever
• Dryland distemper

ABBREVIATIONS
• NSAID = nonsteroidal anti-inflammatory drug
• PCR = polymerase chain reaction

Internet Resources
Center for Equine Health, University of California, Davis. http://viewer.zmags.com/publication/67e69b2d#/67e69b2d/1

Suggested Reading
Pratt SM, Spier SJ, Carroll SP, et al. Evaluation of clinical characteristics, diagnostic test results, and outcome in horses with internal infection caused by *Corynebacterium pseudotuberculosis*: 30 Cases (1995–2003). J Am Vet Med Assoc 2005;227:441–448.

Authors Sharon J. Spier and Emily H. Berryhill
Consulting Editor Ashley G. Boyle
Acknowledgment The authors and editor acknowledge the prior contribution of Mathilde Leclère.

Client Education Handout available online

BASICS

DEFINITION
A sudden, forceful, noisy expulsion of air through the glottis to clear mucus and particles from the tracheobronchial tree and glottis.

PATHOPHYSIOLOGY
• This reflex is a protective respiratory defense mechanism that, together with the mucociliary escalator, clears undesired material from the tracheobronchial tree proximal to the level of segmental bronchi
• Initiated by stimulation of irritant receptors that ramify between epithelial cells from the level of the larynx down to the distal bronchioles and by receptors located in the lung parenchyma and pleura
• Receptors are stimulated by mechanical deformation, chemically inert dust particles, foreign bodies, pollutant gases, exposure to cold or hot air, inflammatory conditions, excessive mucus or exudates, and chemical mediators such as histamine
• Most of the afferent impulses travel in the vagus nerve, but also in the glossopharyngeal, trigeminal, and phrenic nerves, to cough centers in the medulla oblongata

SYSTEMS AFFECTED
• Respiratory
• Musculoskeletal
• Cardiovascular
• Nervous

INCIDENCE/PREVALENCE
• Mostly unknown
• Among horses without acute respiratory infection, prevalence of cough at rest or during exercise is reported to vary between 10% and 50 %, depending on the study population

GEOGRAPHIC INCIDENCE
Worldwide

SIGNALMENT
• All ages, breeds, and sexes
• Cough resulting from viral or bacterial infections is more common in weanlings and yearlings while cough associated with equine asthma or other chronic conditions is observed in more mature horses

SIGNS
Historical Findings
• Season and activity
  ○ Cough associated with equine asthma typically has a higher incidence when horses are confined indoors, except for the summer form of equine asthma (summer pasture-associated equine asthma)
• Housing and feeding practices
  ○ Cough associated with equine asthma is exacerbated by exposure to hay and straw and poor ventilation; however, cough from other causes can also be exacerbated by inhaled irritants
  ○ Silicosis typically occurs in horses fed on the ground or grazed in dusty paddocks in areas such as the Monterey Peninsula of California, which have exposed cristobalite silica shale
• Speed of onset, contagiousness, duration
  ○ Sudden onset and rapid spread are characteristics of viral infections
  ○ Cough associated with lungworms also typically has a sudden onset and may affect multiple horses, but it tends to become chronic, while viral infections typically do not
  ○ Cough associated with foreign body or food aspiration into the tracheobronchial tree is sudden in onset but does not spread to affect other horses
  ○ Gradual onset and chronic course are typical for equine asthma, interstitial pneumonia, fungal pneumonia, and thoracic neoplasia
  ○ Exercise frequently precipitates cough caused by many conditions, particularly those associated with airway irritation or fluid accumulation in airways

Physical Examination Findings
• Fever—usually indicates an infectious cause. Low-grade fever can be present with neoplasia (e.g. lymphoma)
• No fever—typically found in equine asthma, upper airway abnormalities (other than retropharyngeal abscess), parasitic pneumonia, exercise-induced pulmonary hemorrhage, and some neoplasia (e.g. bronchial carcinoma)
• Food return via the nose—typically indicates esophageal obstruction, aspiration of food secondary to anatomic or neurologic derangement in the upper airway, severe pharyngeal inflammation, or cleft palate
• Pleurodynia—typically occurs with pleuropneumonia, less commonly with noninfectious pleural inflammation
• Nasal discharge—reflects disease characterized by exudation or drainage of mucus or purulent exudate from the lower airways, nasopharynx, guttural pouches, nasal passages, or paranasal sinuses
• Harsh, persistent cough suggests involvement of the major airways or exudate in the large airways secondary to pulmonary disease
• Soft, infrequent cough often reflects equine asthma, interstitial lung disease, or pulmonary edema secondary to cardiac failure

CAUSES
Most coughs are initiated by stimulation of receptors in the trachea and bronchi; therefore, cough is more likely to originate from diseases involving the lower respiratory tract.

Lower Respiratory Tract Diseases
• Bronchial—inflammation, infection, allergy/hypersensitivity, foreign body, and tumor
• Pulmonary—inflammation, infection, aspiration pneumonia, pulmonary edema, tumor, acute bronchointerstitial pneumonia, pneumoconiosis, and granulomatous pneumonia
• Pulmonary vascular—thrombosis/embolism, congestive cardiac failure, and pulmonary hypertension
• Pleural—inflammation, infection, hernia, and tumor

Upper Respiratory Tract Diseases
• Nasopharyngeal—pharyngitis, nasopharyngeal foreign body, cyst, or tumor; strangles, cleft palate, dorsal displacement of the soft palate, guttural pouch empyema, tympany, or mycosis (secondary to aspiration)
• Laryngeal—hemiplegia with dynamic collapse, inflammation/chondritis, epiglottic entrapment or ulcer, foreign body, tumors, previous laryngeal surgery
• Tracheal—inflammation, foreign body, smoke or chemical irritation, collapse, and tumor
• Dysphagia from any cause resulting in food aspiration

RISK FACTORS
See the individual conditions causing cough.

DIAGNOSIS

DIFFERENTIAL DIAGNOSIS
Differentiating Similar Signs
Cough is not easily confused with other signs.

Differentiating Causes
See Historical Findings, Physical Examination Findings, and Risk Factors.

CBC/BIOCHEMISTRY/URINALYSIS
• Neutrophilia, hyperfibrinogenemia, and elevated serum globulin concentration are common in bacterial infections and some malignant tumors
• Lymphopenia and lymphocytosis are common in viral infections
• Eosinophilia is a common finding in lungworm infection and some horses with granulomatous interstitial lung disease

IMAGING
• Thoracic radiography for differentiating types of lower respiratory tract disorders (consolidation, mass lesions, infiltrative interstitial disease, and pleural effusion)
• Thoracic ultrasonography in patients with superficial pulmonary consolidation, pleural disease, or mediastinal mass
• Radiography of the upper airways and proximal esophagus
• Echocardiography if primary cardiac disease or right heart disease secondary to a pulmonary condition is suspected

COUGH, ACUTE/CHRONIC   (CONTINUED)

OTHER DIAGNOSTIC PROCEDURES
- Arterial blood gases in patients with signs of respiratory distress
- Visual inspection of the upper airways, guttural pouches, trachea, and bronchi with endoscopy. If indicated, the pleural space can be visualized by thoracoscopy
- Biopsy specimens of lesions or airway walls can be collected via endoscopy, transcutaneous lung biopsy, or thoracoscopy
- Collection of nasopharyngeal swabs or washes from horses with acute-onset cough and fever help to establish the diagnosis of acute viral infection and strangles (for culture and PCR)
- Transtracheal or transendoscopic aspiration with cytology and culture for evaluation of infectious (and some inflammatory) lower respiratory tract disorders
- Bronchoalveolar lavage with cytology for evaluation of lower respiratory tract disorders (equine asthma, silicosis, and granulomatous lung disease)
- Thoracocentesis with cytologic evaluation and culture of aspirated fluid
- Direct and flotation fecal tests (e.g. Baermann) to detect ova or larvae of respiratory parasites and ascarids. Testing of donkeys or mules co-grazed with affected horses
- Echocardiography and ECG in patients with suspected cardiac disease

TREATMENT

AIMS
- Based on the underlying cause
- Regardless of the cause, decrease stimulation of irritant receptors

APPROPRIATE HEALTH CARE
Horses presented with cough usually are evaluated as outpatients but the presence of respiratory distress, pleural effusion, congestive cardiac failure, or other features of a serious disease process are indications for hospitalization.

NURSING CARE
Horses with suspected viral respiratory disease and contacts in the same airspace should be isolated as a group. Do not allow other horses to enter the same airspace occupied by sick horses.

ACTIVITY
Exercise restriction is best until a cause for the cough is established and corrected, especially when activity aggravates the cough.

HOUSING AND DIET
Regardless of the cause, decrease inhalation of dust, cold air, or noxious gas. For pharyngeal conditions, soft and moist diet can decrease mechanical irritation of the nasopharynx.

CLIENT EDUCATION
Inform owners that a wide variety of conditions can be responsible for the cough and that an extensive workup may be required to define and treat the underlying cause.

MEDICATIONS

DRUG(S) OF CHOICE
Treatment is directed at the underlying cause rather than at attempting symptomatic relief by using cough suppressants.

CONTRAINDICATIONS
- In general, avoid using corticosteroids unless an allergic-type disease or airway hyperreactivity is suspected, and evidence of infection or parasitic infestation is lacking
- Foals with acute respiratory distress syndrome (i.e. acute bronchointerstitial pneumonia) may benefit from corticosteroids even when an underlying infectious cause is present
- Do not use cough suppressants in patients with heart disease or when a respiratory infection is present (unless infection is under control and cough is causing significant discomfort)

PRECAUTIONS
- Cough suppressants—indiscriminate use may obscure warning signs of serious pulmonary or cardiac disorders
- Bronchodilator therapy may exacerbate hypoxemia in patients with ventilation–perfusion mismatch
- NSAIDs may mask fever and pleurodynia

FOLLOW-UP

PATIENT MONITORING
Cough may persist for several weeks after resolution of other signs in horses with

infectious respiratory disease because restoration of normal structure and function in the respiratory mucosa takes several weeks.

PREVENTION/AVOIDANCE
Contingent on diagnosis.

POSSIBLE COMPLICATIONS
Some diseases that cause cough also can induce prolonged or permanent respiratory dysfunction and even death.

EXPECTED COURSE AND PROGNOSIS
Contingent on diagnosis.

MISCELLANEOUS

AGE-RELATED FACTORS
See Historical Findings.

SEE ALSO
- Acute respiratory distress
- Purulent nasal discharge

ABBREVIATIONS
- NSAID = nonsteroidal anti-inflammatory drug
- PCR = polymerase chain reaction

Suggested Reading
Kohn CW. Cough. In: Reed SM, Bayly WM, Sellon DC, eds. Equine Internal Medicine, 3e. St. Louis, MO: WB Saunders, 2010:122–126.
Korpas J, Tomori Z. Cough and other respiratory reflexes. Prog Respir Res 1979;12:15–18.
Korpas J, Widdicombe JG. Aspects of the cough reflex. Respir Med 1991;85(Suppl. A):3–5.
Wasko AJ, Barkema HW, Nicol J, et al. Evaluation of a risk-screening questionnaire to detect equine lung inflammation: results of a large field study. Equine Vet J 2011;43:145–152.
Wilson WD, Lofstedt J, Lakritz J. Cough. In: Smith BP, ed. Large Animal Internal Medicine, 5e. St. Louis, MO: Elsevier Mosby, 2015:40–48.

Authors Mathilde Leclère and W. David Wilson
Consulting Editors Mathilde Leclère and Daniel Jean

BASICS

DEFINITION
The cytoplasmic enzyme responsible for the reversible conversion of creatine phosphate and adenosine diphosphate (ADP) to creatine and adenosine triphosphate (ATP), which is used for muscle contraction. Provides the sole source for energy in muscle at the initiation of exercise.

PATHOPHYSIOLOGY
• Skeletal muscle, myocardium, and brain isoenzymes, with virtually no exchange between cerebrospinal fluid and blood. Significant increases in serum CK values are attributed to skeletal or cardiac muscle injury
• Analysis of individual isoenzymes is generally not performed in the clinical setting. Use of serum CK activity to detect cardiac disease in horses is not recommended
• Serum half-life of CK activity is <2 h in horses
• After injury, serum activity typically peaks within 12 h and returns to normal in 2–3 days (or, sometimes, as long as 7 days), provided the damage is not active and persistent
• The severity of the increase directly reflects the severity of active muscle injury

SYSTEMS AFFECTED
• Increased serum activity is typically a result of skeletal muscle injury, and not a primary cause of disease
• Dependent on the underlying cause

GENETICS
The following breed predispositions have been identified:
• PSSM type 1—Quarter Horses, Paints, and draft horses
• PSSM type 2—Quarter Horses and Warmbloods
• Malignant hyperthermia—Quarter Horses
• HYPP—Quarter Horses

INCIDENCE/PREVALENCE
N/A

GEOGRAPHIC DISTRIBUTION
• Box elder trees are widespread throughout the USA but are more common in central and eastern USA
• White snakeroot is native to central and eastern USA

SIGNALMENT
• See Genetics
• Any breed, age, or sex
• NMD (vitamin E/selenium deficiency) typically occurs in foals

SIGNS
Historical Findings
• Recent exercise, especially if sporadic
• Exercise intolerance
• Recent surgery or lameness (recumbency)

Physical Examination Findings
• Palpably firm, painful muscles, stiff gait, reluctance to move (exertional rhabdomyolysis)
• Dark red or brown urine (myoglobinuria secondary to myonecrosis)
• Toxic myopathies—trembling, dysphagia, respiratory distress, difficulty elevating head, arrhythmias, sudden death

CAUSES
• Exertional rhabdomyolysis (i.e. azoturia, Monday morning disease, set-fast, tying-up)
• Trauma—prolonged recumbency, parturition, surgery, blunt trauma
• Exercise/endurance event
• Heat stroke
• Clostridial myositis
• PSSM
• NMD
• Immune-mediated myositis
• Malignant hyperthermia
• Toxins—SPM (box elder seeds), white snakeroot (tremetol), ionophores (monensin)
• HYPP (rarely causes increase in CK)

RISK FACTORS
• Improper conditioning
• Heavy training after prolonged rest
• Prolonged recumbency from any cause
• Monensin administration
• Trauma
• IM injection
• Seizures
• General anesthesia
• Feed and water restriction prior to transport
• Exposure to box elder seeds or white snakeroot
• Trailering

 DIAGNOSIS

DIFFERENTIAL DIAGNOSIS
• Acute gastrointestinal disease (trembling, sweating, colic)
• Laminitis (reluctance to move, stiffness)
• Equine motor neuron disease (muscle trembling, recumbency)
• Tetanus (third eyelid prolapse and stiffness might resemble HYPP episode)
• Hemolysis, severe dehydration, liver disease, red maple leaf toxicity (dark urine)

LABORATORY FINDINGS
Drugs That May Alter Laboratory Results
N/A

Disorders or Problems That May Alter Laboratory Results
• Improper sample handling (consult with laboratory); gross hemolysis
• Very high serum CK activity itself can alter reported values because serum contains inhibitors of CK activity. Sample dilution may be necessary to bring extremely high values into the range of linearity for the instrument, but the resultant reduction in serum volume fraction reduces the inhibitor concentrations, resulting in higher CK values. This becomes important when CK values are monitored over time, because the actual value obtained from a diluted sample may not be accurate

Valid if Run in a Human Laboratory?
Yes

CBC/BIOCHEMISTRY/URINALYSIS
• Increased plasma fibrinogen concentration (with or without inflammatory leukogram) may be present with infectious causes, and physiologic leukocytosis may be present in horses that are excited, nervous, or in pain from myonecrosis
• Initially, serum CK activity increases (peaks in 5–12 h), and if muscle damage is not continuous returns to baseline (usually by 2–3 days)
• Increased serum AST activity, depending on the time course. AST may take several days to peak, has a more modest increase, and takes longer to return to baseline (may take several weeks)
• If CK remains increased, myonecrosis is ongoing; if AST remains increased but CK is falling, myonecrosis is not likely to be progressing
• The degree of increase in CK activity may be helpful
• Modest increases (<1000 IU/L), usually in the absence of increased AST, occur in normal horses from training, transport, or exercise
• Endurance events may increase CK values to >1000 IU/L, but activities generally return to baseline within 24–48 h
• IM injections result in relatively mild to moderate increases in CK activity
• PSSM, exertional rhabdomyolysis, immune-mediated myositis, and NMD generally have severe elevations in CK activity (thousands or may exceed 100,000 IU/L)
• In milder forms of chronic exertional rhabdomyolysis, CK may be <1500–10,000 IU/L
• HYPP results in normal to mildly increased serum CK activity, even during an episode
• Moderate to severe myonecrosis results in myoglobinuria, regardless of the cause, but the absence of myoglobinuria does not rule out mild forms of chronic exertional rhabdomyolysis

OTHER LABORATORY TESTS
• Vitamin E/selenium determinations when indicated
• Serum and urine acylcarnitines for SPM
• Urine tremetone/tremetol for white snakeroot

IMAGING
N/A

OTHER DIAGNOSTIC PROCEDURES
• Biopsy for histopathology or muscle function tests to identify subtle cases of chronic exertional rhabdomyolysis or PSSM. The laboratory must specialize in muscle

C

CREATINE KINASE (CK)

evaluation and be consulted before sample collection
• Electromyography to rule out neuromuscular disease; also helpful in HYPP
• Genetic tests for PSSM and malignant hyperthermia
• Plant identification if suspect toxicity

PATHOLOGIC FINDINGS
Local or diffuse skeletal and/or cardiac muscle necrosis, depending on the underlying cause.

TREATMENT
ACTIVITY
• During an episode, minimize movement initially, but gradually resume activity when the horse is no longer reluctant to move
• Regular exercise decreases incidence of exertional rhabdomyolysis

DIET
• Horses with dysphagia from toxin exposure should be provided with parenteral nutrition or enteral feeding through a stomach tube
• Horses with PSSM and HYPP should adhere to a strict diet (refer to See Also)

CLIENT EDUCATION
See Activity and Diet.

MEDICATIONS
DRUG(S) OF CHOICE
• IV fluid therapy with balanced electrolytes is indicated in moderate to severe cases, especially if myoglobinuria or sweating is present
• Continue IV fluids at least until hydration is restored and urine appears normal
• NSAID administration for acute, severe myonecrosis to decrease inflammation and pain (see Precautions)
• Corticosteroids for immune-mediated myositis
• Acepromazine at low doses for vasodilation and anxiety relief
• Opiates with or without α-agonists to decrease pain
• Dantrolene sodium (recommended dosage varies by author—2 or 10 mg/kg as a loading

dose; alternatively 2.5 mg/kg every 1 h) diluted in normal saline and administered by stomach tube to reduce calcium release from sarcoplasmic reticulum
• Diazepam or phenobarbital for seizures

CONTRAINDICATIONS
Diuretics

PRECAUTIONS
• Use caution with nephrotoxic drugs (e.g. NSAIDs, aminoglycosides, tetracyclines) if myoglobinuria is present
• If phenobarbital is used, titrate the dose to the patient

POSSIBLE INTERACTIONS
N/A

ALTERNATIVE DRUGS
N/A

FOLLOW-UP
PATIENT MONITORING
• Serum CK and AST measurements 24–48 h after initial sampling, because persistent increases indicate ongoing muscle damage. Reassess if parameters have not normalized
• Blood urea nitrogen, creatinine, and electrolyte determinations at similar timepoints to monitor renal and electrolyte status, as well as response to therapy in cases of moderate to severe myonecrosis

PREVENTION/AVOIDANCE
Dependent on the underlying cause.

POSSIBLE COMPLICATIONS
Myoglobin released from damaged muscles can cause irreversible renal failure (pigment nephropathy) without aggressive supportive care/diuresis.

EXPECTED COURSE AND PROGNOSIS
Dependent on the underlying cause.

MISCELLANEOUS
ASSOCIATED CONDITIONS
Pigment nephropathy.

AGE-RELATED FACTORS
N/A

ZOONOTIC POTENTIAL
N/A

PREGNANCY/FERTILITY/BREEDING
N/A

SYNONYMS
• Creatine phosphokinase
• Seasonal pasture myopathy/atypical myopathy

SEE ALSO
• Seasonal Pasture Myopathy/Atypical Myopathy
• Exertional rhabdomyolysis syndrome
• Monensin toxicosis
• Nutritional myodegeneration
• Pigmenturia (hematuria, hemoglobinuria, and myoglobinuria)
• Polysaccharide storage myopathy

ABBREVIATIONS
• AST = aspartate aminotransferase
• CK = creatine kinase
• HYPP = hyperkalemic periodic paralysis
• NMD = nutritional myodegeneration
• NSAID = nonsteroidal anti-inflammatory drug
• PSSM = polysaccharide storage myopathy
• SPM = seasonal pasture myopathy

Suggested Reading
Aleman M. A review of equine muscle disorders. Neuromuscul Disord 2008;18:277–287.
Billings A. Skeletal muscle. In: Walton RM, ed. Equine Clinical Pathology. Ames, IA: Wiley Blackwell, 2014:153–180.
Hall RL, Bender HS. Muscle. In: Latimer KS, ed. Duncan & Prasse's Veterinary Laboratory Medicine Clinical Pathology, 5e. Hoboken, NJ: Wiley Blackwell, 2011:283–294.

Author Katie M. Boes
Consulting Editor Sandra D. Taylor
Acknowledgment The author and editor acknowledge the prior contribution of Ellen W. Evans and Elizabeth A. Walmsley.

BASICS

DEFINITION
- Failure of 1 or both testes to descend completely into the scrotal sac
- Affected males are referred to as rigs, ridglings, originals, or, if the testis is located in the inguinal canal, high flankers
- Complete abdominal cryptorchid—when the testis and entire epididymis are contained within the abdomen
- Incomplete abdominal cryptorchid—when the testis and most of the epididymis are intra-abdominal but the ductus deferens and cauda epididymis (i.e. tail) are located in the inguinal canal
- Inguinal cryptorchid—when the testis is located in the inguinal canal
- Ectopic cryptorchid—when the testis is subcutaneous and cannot be displaced manually into the scrotum

PATHOPHYSIOLOGY
- Embryologically, testes develop adjacent to the kidneys and are situated in the dorsal abdomen. Both testes descend ventrally through the abdominal cavity and inguinal canals into the scrotum sometime during the last 30 days of gestation or first 10 days after birth
- Failure of the testes to descend may result from abnormal development or function of the gubernaculum, failure of the fetal testis to regress in size and allow it to pass through the vaginal ring into the inguinal, or insufficient intra-abdominal pressure
- Cryptorchidism has been associated with failure to produce insulin-like peptide 3, testosterone, and/or their respective receptors
- Cryptorchidism is commonly unilateral, although up to 15% of cases are bilateral. The ratio of inguinal to abdominal testis retention varies from one study to another and may reflect differences in horse populations. Some studies report a higher incidence of abdominally retained left testes
- Spermatogenesis is arrested at the spermatogonia stage in the abdominally retained testis. If testes are retained in the inguinal canal, development may proceed to the primary spermatocyte stage
- Unilateral cryptorchids have normal fertility while bilateral cryptorchid stallions are sterile
- Cryptorchidism has been associated with increased incidence of testicular tumors

SYSTEMS AFFECTED
Reproductive

GENETICS
- Cryptorchidism is suspected to be a heritable condition in some breeds, but scientific evidence on the mode of heritability is lacking
- Heritability of cryptorchidism was estimated to be 0.12–0.35 in Icelandic horses

INCIDENCE/PREVALENCE
- Prevalence in horses has been estimated to be 2–8%
- Higher incidence/risk—Friesian, Quarter Horse, Percheron, Saddlebred, Icelandic, and pony breeds
- Lower incidence/risk—Thoroughbreds, Standardbreds, Morgans, and Tennessee Walking Horses

SIGNALMENT
- All breeds
- Absence of a palpable testis in the scrotal sac by 1 month of age is presumptive evidence of cryptorchidism. After 12 months, inguinal retained testes rarely enter the scrotum but, reportedly, have entered in horses as old as 2–3 years of age
- Unilateral is ≅10-fold more prevalent than bilateral
- The left testis is retained slightly more often than the right in horses
- Left testes more often are intra-abdominal; right testes are equally likely to be inguinal or abdominal

SIGNS

Historical Findings
- Stallion-like behavior in presumed geldings
- Rarely associated with pain or other signs of disease
- Isolated reports of torsion of the retained testis and of intestinal strangulation in association with a retained testis

Physical Examination Findings
Undescended testes are smaller and softer than scrotal testes.

CAUSES
- Cause unknown
- Genetic research suggests a complex mechanism of inheritance involving several genes. The decreasing incidence of cryptorchidism in certain lines of horses suggests that *selective breeding* influences the incidence
- Both autosomal dominant and autosomal recessive modes of inheritance have been proposed
- In addition to genetics, other factors implicated in abnormal testicular descent include inadequate gonadotropic stimulation, intrinsically defective testes, and mechanical impediment of descent, all of which may, in turn, have a genetic basis
- Cryptorchidism has been associated with intersexuality and abnormal karyotypes

RISK FACTORS
See Causes.

DIAGNOSIS

- Complete history
- Behavioral observation

- Often diagnostic to conduct a thorough visual examination and to palpate the scrotum and external inguinal region
- External deep inguinal palpation and transrectal palpation often require tranquilization or sedation

DIFFERENTIAL DIAGNOSIS
- Bilateral cryptorchid stallion
- Cryptorchid hemicastrate
- Gelding
- True anorchidism, in which neither testis develops, is extremely rare
- Monorchid animals, having failed to develop a second testis, have been described in isolated reports

CBC/BIOCHEMISTRY/URINALYSIS
N/A

OTHER LABORATORY TESTS

hCG Stimulation Test
- Administer hCG (6000–12 000 IU IV) and collect blood samples as follows—baseline (preadministration) and after 2 h
- Stallions and cryptorchids show a 2–3-fold increase in serum testosterone levels
- Geldings show no change in testosterone levels
- Very high specificity in unilaterally castrated horses (97%)

Serum Conjugated Estrogen Concentration
- Estrone sulfate
- Stallions and cryptorchids, >400 pg/mL
- Geldings, <50 pg/mL
- Not reliable in horses <3 years and in donkeys of any age; donkeys have no detectable conjugated estrogens

Serum Testosterone Concentration
- Stallion and cryptorchids, >100 pg/mL
- Geldings, <40 pg/mL
- Unreliable in horses <18 months of age
- Less reliable than hCG stimulation test and conjugated estrogen determination because of wide seasonal variation in basal concentrations (inconclusive results 14%)

Serum Inhibin Concentration
- Stallions, 1–3 ng/mL
- Gelding, negligible

Serum AMH concentration
Serum AMH is higher in cryptorchid stallions than in geldings.

IMAGING
- Parenchyma of a cryptorchid testis is less echogenic and smaller than that of a normal descended testis
- Percutaneous transinguinal US is highly effective for inguinal testes and has a sensitivity of 98% and a specificity of 97%
- Transrectal US has a very high sensitivity and specificity for the identification of abdominally retained testes

OTHER DIAGNOSTIC PROCEDURES
Less invasive procedures usually are sufficient to diagnose the problem and often are used in

CRYPTORCHIDISM

conjunction with laparoscopic cryptorchidectomy.

PATHOLOGIC FINDINGS
• Cryptorchid testes are often small and soft
• Seminiferous tubules are poorly developed (round with no lumen) and spermatogenesis is arrested
• Elevated body temperature may induce interstitial cell hyperplasia
• Testicular neoplasia is possible

TREATMENT

APPROPRIATE HEALTH CARE
Surgical removal of the retained testis.

NURSING CARE
N/A

ACTIVITY
N/A

DIET
N/A

CLIENT EDUCATION
Recommend castration of the cryptorchid individual.

SURGICAL CONSIDERATIONS
• Cryptorchidectomy via standard or laparoscopic approaches
• Standard approaches—inguinal, parainguinal, paramedian, suprapubic, and flank; choice is dictated by the location of the testis
• Laparoscopy can be performed with the horse standing or in dorsal recumbency. Remove the retained testis before the descended testis
• Another, less reliable technique involves laparoscopic cautery and transection of the spermatic cord to induce avascular necrosis of the testis. Revascularization can occur, with subsequent production of testosterone

MEDICATIONS

DRUG(S) OF CHOICE
N/A

CONTRAINDICATIONS
N/A

PRECAUTIONS
N/A

POSSIBLE INTERACTIONS
N/A

ALTERNATIVE DRUGS
N/A

FOLLOW-UP

PATIENT MONITORING
• Cessation of stallion-like behavior occurs concomitant with decreasing androgen levels
• Some stallions castrated at an older age or, after having bred mares, retain stallion-like behavior even after removal of all testicular tissue

POSSIBLE COMPLICATIONS
• Complications are uncommon, usually those associated with cryptorchidectomy
• Possible sequelae—infection, hemorrhage, adhesion formation, eventration, and incomplete castration

MISCELLANEOUS

ASSOCIATED CONDITIONS
Testicular cysts and neoplasia (e.g. teratoma, interstitial cell tumor, seminoma, Sertoli cell tumor) have been reported.

AGE-RELATED FACTORS
Endocrine assay is not reliable as a diagnostic tool in prepubertal males.

ZOONOTIC POTENTIAL
N/A

PREGNANCY/FERTILITY/BREEDING
N/A

SYNONYMS
Lay terms include rigs, ridglings, originals, or, if the retained testis is inguinal, high flanker.

SEE ALSO
• Aggression
• Stallion sexual behavior problems

ABBREVIATIONS
• AMH = anti-Müllerian hormone
• hCG = human chorionic gonadotropin
• US = ultrasonography, ultrasound

Suggested Reading
Claes A, Ball BA, Corbins CJ, Conley AJ. Anti-Mullerian hormone as a diagnostic marker for equine cryptorchidism in three cases with equivocal testosterone concentrations. J Equine Vet Sci 2014;34:442–445.
Coomer RPC, Gorvy DA, McKane SA, Wilderjans H. Inguinal percutaneous ultrasound to locate cryptorchid testes. Equine Vet Educ 2016;28:150–154.
Eriksson S, Jaderkvist K, Dalin A, et al. Prevalence and genetic parameters for cryptorchidism in Swedish-born Icelandic horses. Livest Sci 2015;180:1–5.
Mueller POE, Parks H. Cryptorchidism in horses. Equine Vet Educ 1999;11:77–86.
Schurink A, de Jong A, de Nooij HR, et al. Genetic parameters of cryptorchidism and testis size in Friesian colts. Livest Sci 2016;190:136–140.

Author Ahmed Tibary
Consulting Editor Carla L. Carleton
Acknowledgment The author and editor acknowledge the prior contribution of Jane A. Barber and Philip Prater.

BASICS

OVERVIEW
• Cryptosporidiosis is a zoonosis affecting a variety of species of animals including humans. Cryptosporidia are now recognized to be a major waterborne parasite worldwide
• *Cryptosporidium* is an apicomplexan parasite in the order *Eucoccidiorida*
• Reported prevalence in nondiarrheic horses ranges from 0% to 23% with a peak reported at 5–8 weeks of age
• Little is known about the specific pathogenicity
• The syndrome has a range of presentations from asymptomatic shedding of oocysts in feces to severe disease
• In foals pathogenicity is not clear and cryptosporidia-associated diarrhea in foals has mostly been described in immunodeficient foals
• Horse infection is by ingestion of *Cryptosporidium* oocytes
• In most species cryptosporidia infect ileal and proximal colonic epithelial cells, often resulting in impaired absorption and increased secretion (clinically observed mostly as diarrhea)
• Cryptosporidia life cycle has 6 phases, which are completed within same host and may result in persistent chronic infection (auto-reinfection)
• In a few genotyping studies in foals *C. parvum* was the most common strain
• In several species cryptosporidiosis is an emerging disease, but the reason for this is unclear

• It is not a very significant pathogen and seems to be associated with co-infections in foals with diarrhea

SIGNALMENT
• Clinically affected foals are often immunocompromised regardless of breed and sex. Common in foals with severe combined immunodeficiency
• Malodorous diarrhea; mild depression, thin body condition, no overt clinical signs

CAUSES AND RISK FACTORS
• *C. parvum*—horse-adapted cryptosporidium (rare); overcrowding; part of the foal diarrhea complex
• Infection via fecal–oral route (zoonosis); incubation period not very well established in foals (in humans, variable: 1–12 days, with an average of 7 days)
• Poor hygiene management

DIAGNOSIS

Sucrose wet mount demonstrating organisms in feces with light microscopy. Acid-fast staining. DNA of organisms in feces using PCR.

DIFFERENTIAL DIAGNOSIS
• Foal diarrhea associated with other organisms of the foal diarrhea complex
• Transient lactose intolerance

CBC/BIOCHEMISTRY/URINALYSIS
CBC unspecific or normal. Low serum albumin and total protein possible with severe cases.

OTHER LABORATORY TESTS
N/A

TREATMENT

Supportive to correct dehydration, acid–base disorders and electrolyte imbalances, and energy demands. If animals are severely catabolic parenteral or oral nutritional support is indicated. No specific effective anti-protozoal treatment is currently available for horses.

MISCELLANEOUS

SEE ALSO
Diarrhea, neonate

ABBREVIATIONS
PCR = polymerase chain reaction

Suggested Reading
Burton AJ, Nydam DV, Dearen TK, et al. The prevalence of *Cryptosporidium*, and identification of the *Cryptosporidium* horse genotype in foals in New York State. Vet Parasitol 2010;174(1-2):139–144.
Slovis NM, Elam J, Estrada M, Leutenegger CM. Infectious agents associated with diarrhoea in neonatal foals in central Kentucky: a comprehensive molecular study. Equine Vet J 2014;46(3):311–316.
Author Henry Stämpfli
Consulting Editors Henry Stämpfli and Olimpo Oliver-Espinosa

C

CUTANEOUS PHOTOSENSITIZATION

BASICS

DEFINITION
Photosensitization is an uncommon cause of mild to severe dermatitis that occurs when the skin becomes sensitized by contact or ingestion of a photodynamic agent with subsequent exposure to ultraviolet light. The spectrum of disease ranges from a simple annoyance from pasture plant contact to a life-threatening crisis of hepatogenous origin.

PATHOPHYSIOLOGY
• Photodynamic agents responsible for photosensitization are phototoxic or photo-allergic (requiring prior sensitization). Both types of compounds can reach the skin via the bloodstream or by direct contact. Photodynamic agents are activated when exposed to UV or visible light, producing reactive oxygen intermediates which cause damage to superficial blood vessels and the epidermis
• The recognized types of photosensitization in horses include primary photosensitivity (type 1 photosensitivity), hepatogenous photosensitivity (type 2 photosensitivity), and photosensitivity of unknown etiology
• Primary photosensitization occurs from ingestion of a photodynamic agent that is absorbed directly from the digestive tract and reaches the skin via the circulation. This results from ingestion of plants such as St. John's wort, buckwheat, spring parsley, and *Ammi* spp.
• Hepatogenous photosensitization is the most common type of photosensitization affecting horses and occurs secondary to hepatic injury from increases in phylloerythrin in the skin. Compromised hepatic function results in a decreased capacity to excrete phylloerythrin, resulting in accumulation. As phylloerythrin is a photodynamic agent, elevated cutaneous levels causes photosensitivity. Hepatogenous photosensitization occurs from any disease that results in severe liver damage and cholestasis. Examples include pyrrolizidine alkaloid PA toxicity, cholelithiasis, bacterial cholangitis, and ingestion of toxic plants and mycotoxins
• Contact photosensitization can occur in horses grazing pastures containing various legumes (e.g. clover, alfalfa)
• Drugs and chemicals can result in primary photosensitization through a variety of mechanisms (e.g. fly sprays, antimicrobial shampoos and tetracycline antibiotics)

SYSTEMS AFFECTED
• Skin—light-/white-skinned/-haired areas are most susceptible to UV ray exposure, thus are the most commonly affected areas of skin. Lesions may extend into dark-haired areas. Erythema and edema may be followed by vesicles, bullae, ulcers, oozing, crusting, scaling, and hair loss. Secondary bacterial infections are common
• Hepatobiliary—hepatogenous photosensitivity is the most common type of photosensitization affecting horses and occurs secondary to hepatic injury, resulting in the elevation of phylloerythrin levels within the skin

GENETICS
There is no genetic predisposition, although white-skinned/-haired horse breeds are more susceptible.

INCIDENCE/PREVALENCE
Uncommon

GEOGRAPHIC DISTRIBUTION
Possibly increased in geographic areas closer to the equator.

SIGNALMENT
Breed Predilections
Any breeds with white-/light-skinned/-haired areas.

Mean Age and Range
Adult horses

Predominant Sex
None

SIGNS
General Comments
• Signs begin soon after exposure to sunlight and include erythema, edema, exudation, crust formation, and skin necrosis in poorly haired, white/unpigmented areas that include the muzzle, eyelids, face, ears, vulva, perineum, sheath, and occasionally coronary bands
• Pigmented skin and more heavily haired areas are generally protected
• Initial signs are erythema and edema ± severe pruritus
• Serum transudation, erosion, or ulceration may occur, commonly resulting in a secondary bacterial invasion
• Extensive necrosis can lead to the sloughing of affected tissues
• Icterus is often present in cases of hepatogenous photosensitization
• Hemolysis may occur due to increased red blood cell fragility secondary to toxic and septic dermatitis and vasculitis

Historical Findings
Owner reports clinical signs of dermatitis or other signs such as lethargy, anorexia, mild colic, jaundice.

Physical Examination Findings
• Dermatitis as above
• Icterus, poor body condition, anorexia, somnolence, and intermittent mild colic with hepatic involvement may occur
• Neurologic abnormalities are typically associated with advanced liver dysfunction and range from subtle behavioral abnormalities to stupor, head pressing, and coma

• Other signs of liver disease include colitis, polydipsia, and cranial nerve abnormalities

CAUSES
• Primary photosensitization—St. John's wort (*Hypericum perforatum*), buckwheat (*Fagopyrum* spp.), spring parsley (*Cymopterus watsoni*), *Ammi* spp., and alsike clover (*Trifolium hybridum*) can cause the primary or secondary hepatogenous form
• Secondary photosensitization/hepatogenous—PA toxicity (e.g. *Senecio* spp., *Crotalaria* spp.). Toxicity associated with kleingrass, alsike clover, *Nolina texana*, *Agave lechuguilla*, *Phyllanthus abnormis*, *Lantana camara*, xanthium, and fumonisins; mycotoxicosis, cholestatic hepatopathy, serum hepatitis (Theiler disease)

RISK FACTORS
White-/light-pigmented/-haired skin; preexisting hepatopathy.

DIAGNOSIS

DIFFERENTIAL DIAGNOSIS
Any dermatitis that is limited to the unpigmented areas of the horse's body; sunburn, contact dermatitis, dermatophilosis, photoactivated vasculitis, bacterial, fungal, or parasitic infections, pemphigus foliaceus, immune-mediated vasculitis, purpura haemorrhagica, drug reaction.

CBC/BIOCHEMISTRY/URINALYSIS
• Primary photosensitization—neutrophilia, hyperglobulinemia, hypoalbuminemia
• Secondary photosensitization—elevated serum GGT, sorbitol dehydrogenase, aspartate aminotransferase; hypoglycemia and decreased albumin and blood urea nitrogen. Clotting factors may be abnormal. Serum globulins may be increased. Bile acids are often elevated, indicating abnormal liver function
• If endotoxemia is involved, there may be neutrophilia or neutropenia with a left shift. With chronicity, there may be nonregenerative anemia and hyperfibrinogenemia
• Horses with subclinical PA toxicity may have elevated GGT, so it may be beneficial to serially monitor GGT in horses on the same property where there is a known case of this toxicity

OTHER LABORATORY TESTS
A percutaneous liver biopsy can help to determine a definitive diagnosis and prognosis. Evaluation of a clotting profile (prothrombin time and activated partial thromboplastin time) should be performed prior to percutaneous biopsy. Biopsy samples should be submitted for both microscopic examination and culture.

(CONTINUED)

IMAGING
Transabdominal ultrasonography enables evaluation of liver size, architecture, determination of the presence of masses or choleliths, and evaluation of blood vessels and the biliary tree.

OTHER DIAGNOSTIC PROCEDURES
History, physical examination, bloodwork, skin biopsy, liver biopsy.

PATHOLOGIC FINDINGS
Skin—superficial dermal blood vessel degeneration and thrombosis, perivascular inflammation. Chronic lesions show a lymphocytic perivascular dermatitis, epidermal hyperplasia, and hyperkeratosis, with serous crust formation. Apoptotic keratinocytes, "sunburn cells," may be present.

TREATMENT

APPROPRIATE HEALTH CARE
• Early treatment will provide the most positive outcome
• Prevent further damage by placing the animal in a darkened stall away from direct sunlight, by removing the source of the photodynamic agent, and by symptomatically treating affected areas
• The lesions should be thoroughly and gently cleansed. Mild antiseptics can be applied depending on the stage of damage. Protective ointments (i.e. silver sulfadiazine, nitrofurazone) are helpful
• Corticosteroids can be given to reduce inflammation and pruritus
• Antibiotics may be necessary if a secondary bacterial infection has developed
• If liver disease is present, it must be immediately addressed

NURSING CARE
• Cold hydrotherapy is helpful in removing skin surface debris and will decrease inflammation and prevent myiasis
• Affected areas should be dried before bandaging is applied. Bandaging with clean nonstick materials (i.e. Adaptic™) and sheet cotton covered with firm pressure but not constricting elastic wrapping tape (7.5 cm (3 inches) or greater width) should be considered for affected legs that have swelling and exudate
• Horses with severe dermatitis and cellulitis will have swelling and heat in affected areas

ACTIVITY
Stall rest and hand-walking as the patient tolerates; no forced exercise; protect from sunlight.

DIET
Provide a good plane of nutrition, including high quality hay and concentrate as needed. Horses with hepatic disease require a low-protein diet, grass hays (oat hay is recommended if available), and beet pulp rather than high protein grains.

CLIENT EDUCATION
Clients can provide nursing care.

SURGICAL CONSIDERATIONS
Surgical debridement is indicated in cases with tissue necrosis.

MEDICATIONS

DRUG(S) OF CHOICE
• Systemic antimicrobial therapy may be indicated; beta-lactam antimicrobials are indicated due to the risk of clostridial diseases and other anaerobic bacterial infections. Standard dosing of ceftiofur sodium (2.2 mg/kg IV or IM every 6–8 h) or procaine penicillin G (22 000 IU/kg IM every 24 h) or penicillin G potassium (22 000 IU/kg IV every 6 h) combined with an aminoglycoside and oral metronidazole (20–25 mg/kg PO) is recommended
• Treatment for cellulitis should continue for 10–14 days or possibly longer
• Seriously affected animals may require fluid therapy and systemic antibiotics
• Supplementation with B vitamins is helpful and can be administered in IV fluids or IM
• Pentoxifylline may be helpful in cases involving vasculitis

CONTRAINDICATIONS, PRECAUTIONS, POSSIBLE INTERACTIONS
Avoid drugs that may exacerbate hepatopathy such as halothane, isoflurane, phenobarbital, copper disodium edetate, and high doses of ivermectin, isoniazid, nitrofurans, aspirin, dantrolene, macrolide antibiotics such as erythromycin, rifampin (rifampicin), anabolic steroids, phenothiazine tranquilizers, and diazepam.

ALTERNATIVE DRUGS
Topical natural aids for healing may include manuka honey, or botanical salves may accelerate healing.

FOLLOW-UP

PATIENT MONITORING
Serial GGT levels of herd mates in horses with PA toxicity; monitor patient hepatic enzymes and hemogram.

PREVENTION/AVOIDANCE
Avoid photosensitizing and hepatotoxic agents.

POSSIBLE COMPLICATIONS
Secondary bacterial infections; hepatoencephalopathy.

EXPECTED COURSE AND PROGNOSIS
Early recognition, supportive care, and treatment, while removing the cause of photosensitization will provide a fair prognosis for full recovery.

MISCELLANEOUS

ASSOCIATED CONDITIONS
Hepatopathy

AGE-RELATED FACTORS
Older horses may be more susceptible.

ZOONOTIC POTENTIAL
NA

PREGNANCY/FERTILITY/BREEDING
Breeding may resume once the patient has recovered.

SYNONYMS
• Photoallergy
• Sun poisoning

SEE ALSO
• Pyrrolizidine alkaloid toxicosis
• Toxic hepatopathy

ABBREVIATIONS
• GGT = γ-glutamyltransferase
• PA = pyrrolizidine alkaloid
• UV = ultraviolet

Suggested Reading
Knottenbelt DC. The approach to the equine dermatology case in practice. Vet Clin North Am Equine Pract 2012;28:131–153.

Author Rebecca S. McConnico
Consulting Editor Gwendolen Lorch

Client Education Handout available online

CYANIDE TOXICOSIS

C

BASICS

OVERVIEW

• The ingestion of plants containing cyanogenic glycosides can result in cyanide toxicosis. Although 55 cyanogenic glycosides have been reported (amygdalin, prunasin, and dhurrin, among others) in over 1000 different species of plants, the most important sources for animals have been the following genera: *Prunus, Sorghum, Triglochin, Pyrus, Suckleya,* and *Amelanchier*. Damage to the plant (including wilting and mastication) results in enzymatic degradation of the glycoside and release of cyanide
• Cyanide ion has great affinity for the iron of cytochrome c oxidase and will inhibit electron transport and cellular respiration
• The blood can carry oxygen but oxygen cannot be utilized by the cells, resulting in tissue anoxia

SIGNALMENT

No breed, size, sex, or age predilection.

SIGNS

• Onset usually rapid (20–120 min) after large ingestion
• Tachypnea
• Dyspnea
• Weakness
• Tachycardia
• Bright red mucous membranes
• Recumbency
• Terminal seizure-like activity
• Death

CAUSES AND RISK FACTORS

• Ingestion of large amounts of (usually wilted) plant material containing high concentrations of cyanogenic glycosides
• Typical scenario is ingestion of fresh but wilted cherry leaves from branches broken off during storms
• Reports indicate 100 g of wild black cherry leaves can be fatal to a 45 kg animal
• Cyanide is volatile and dried cherry leaves or hay made from *Sorghum* spp. are generally safe

DIAGNOSIS

DIFFERENTIAL DIAGNOSIS

CO poisoning—measurement of carboxyhemoglobin in blood, CO measurement in environment, identified source for CO production.

CBC/BIOCHEMISTRY/URINALYSIS

N/A

OTHER LABORATORY TESTS

• Cyanide analysis of blood, suspect material, or stomach contents
• Place samples in airtight container and freeze immediately
• Identification of suspect plant material in ingesta

IMAGING

N/A

OTHER DIAGNOSTIC PROCEDURES

N/A

PATHOLOGIC FINDINGS

• Blood is bright red
• Tracheal or pulmonary congestion or hemorrhage
• Other nonspecific agonal changes may be present

TREATMENT

• Supportive care
• Supplemental oxygen administration

MEDICATIONS

DRUG(S) OF CHOICE

• Treatment must be administered soon after clinical signs are exhibited to be effective
• Sodium nitrite is used to induce a methemoglobinemia, causing cyanide to dissociate from cytochrome c oxidase and react with methemoglobin to form cyanmethemoglobin. Sodium thiosulfate will convert cyanide (by the enzyme rhodanese) to thiocyanate, which is excreted
• Sodium nitrite 10–20 mg/kg as a 20% solution
• Sodium thiosulfate 30–40 mg/kg as a 20% solution
• Can be administered IV as a mixture of 1 mL of 20% sodium nitrite and 3 mL of 20% sodium thiosulfate at 4 mL per 45 kg of body weight. AC may help bind cyanide remaining in the GI tract
• Oral sodium thiosulfate (up to 20 g in solution) might detoxify cyanide in the GI tract

CONTRAINDICATIONS/POSSIBLE INTERACTIONS

N/A

FOLLOW-UP

PATIENT MONITORING

N/A

PREVENTION/AVOIDANCE

Avoid additional exposure to cyanide-containing plants.

POSSIBLE COMPLICATIONS

N/A

EXPECTED COURSE AND PROGNOSIS

Death or recovery occurs rapidly.

MISCELLANEOUS

ASSOCIATED CONDITIONS

• *Sorghum* cystitis–ataxia syndrome has been reported in horses following exclusive, long-term grazing on *Sorghum* pastures
• Syndrome is characterized by hindlimb ataxia, urinary incontinence, and subsequent skin irritation or scalding and cystitis
• The lumbar and sacral segments of the spinal cord may have focal axonal degeneration and demyelination
• Probably caused by thiocyanates formed from high, sublethal cyanide ingestion

AGE-RELATED FACTORS

N/A

ZOONOTIC POTENTIAL

N/A

PREGNANCY/FERTILITY/BREEDING

N/A

ABBREVIATIONS

• AC = activated charcoal
• GI = gastrointestinal

Suggested Reading
Cheeke PR. Natural Toxicants in Feeds, Forages, and Poisonous Plants. Danville, IL: Interstate Publishers Inc., 1998.
Cope R. Overview of cyanide poisoning. In: Aiello SE, Moses MA, eds. Merck Veterinary Manual, 11e. Kenilworth, NJ: Merck Sharp & Dohme Corp., 2016.
Author Larry J. Thompson
Consulting Editors Wilson K. Rumbeiha and Steve Ensley

BASICS

DEFINITION
Cyathostomins, also termed small strongyles or small red worms, are considered the most prevalent and important equine intestinal parasite. The increasing prevalence of cyathostomins, widespread anthelmintic resistance, and difficulty preventing and treating larval cyathostominosis pose significant challenges for veterinarians.

PATHOPHYSIOLOGY
Cyathostomins comprise over 50 species of small strongyles. Their life cycle is direct and does not involve an intermediate host or extraintestinal migration. The minimum prepatent period is 5 weeks. Adult cyathostomins, located predominantly in the colon and cecum, produce large numbers of eggs, which account for almost all of the strongyle eggs in equine feces. Eggs hatch and develop on pasture, through L_1 and L_2 stages to the infective L_3 stage. L_3 acquire a protective sheath which facilitates prolonged survival on pasture, even in freezing conditions, although survival is reduced by hot and dry weather. Ingested L_3 penetrate the mucosa and submucosa of the cecum and colon. A small proportion of L_3 develop into L_4 without interruption, while it is thought that, in some individuals, up to 90% undergo prolonged periods (measured up to 3 years) of inhibited development as encysted early L_3. In temperate climates most larvae undergo inhibition in winter, while in tropical climates this may occur in summer. Clinical disease, termed acute larval cyathostominosis, results from en masse ingress or emergence of large numbers (millions) of previously encysted larvae as L_4, typically in the fall, winter, or early spring. The host inflammatory response to migrating larvae causes colitis and typhlitis. Water, electrolytes, and proteins leak into the intestinal lumen, and luminal endotoxins are absorbed systemically. Hypoproteinemia may cause peripheral and intestinal edema. Dysmotility and inflammation of the large intestine may cause severe colic. Death may result from hypovolemic and endotoxic shock. Luminal adult cyathostomins (6–20 mm long) may cause catarrhal colitis, with resultant lethargy, weight loss, and diarrhea, but typically only in young naive horses that have heavy burdens. Cyathostomins may also cause nonspecific colic, nonstrangulated intestinal infarction, granulomatous colitis, cecal tympany, and cecocolic or cecocecal intussusceptions.

SIGNALMENT
All ages can be infested, although young (<5 years old) and geriatric horses are more susceptible. Larval cyathostominosis is more common in young horses.

SIGNS
• Acute larval cyathostominosis may cause acute-onset diarrhea, anorexia, lethargy, dramatic weight loss, weakness, pyrexia, colic, peripheral edema, dehydration, and signs of endotoxemia
• High burdens of adult cyathostomins may cause ill thrift

RISK FACTORS
• Risk factors for cyathostomin infestation include age, season, time since last deworming, and high pasture larval burdens. The latter reflect inadequate parasite control measures, including high stocking density, overgrazing of pastures, inappropriate use of anthelmintics, and failure to remove feces from pastures
• Anthelmintic treatment may precipitate acute larval cyathostominosis

DIAGNOSIS

DIFFERENTIAL DIAGNOSIS
Other causes of diarrhea including *Clostridium difficile*, *Clostridium perfringens*, salmonellosis, and proliferative enteropathy should be considered.

CBC/BIOCHEMISTRY/URINALYSIS
While hypoalbuminemia, hyperglobulinemia, particularly involving the β-globulin fraction, increased acute phase proteins, increased serum alkaline phosphatase, neutrophilia, and microcytic anemia are common, none of these findings is specific for cyathostominosis. Systemic eosinophilia is uncommon.

OTHER LABORATORY TESTS
Histologic examination of rectal mucosal biopsies or biopsies of the large intestine and cecum may identify larvae and/or the associated inflammatory response. Abdominocentesis and fecal culture may aid evaluation of other differential diagnoses.

IMAGING
Abdominal ultrasonography may identify mural edema and thickening of the colon and cecum, liquid colonic and cecal contents, and possibly ascites.

OTHER DIAGNOSTIC PROCEDURES
A high suspicion of larval cyathostominosis may be obtained from typical clinical signs, signalment, and history. Confirmation is made by gross observation of large numbers of small red L_4 and L_5 larvae in feces or on the sleeve used to perform a per rectum examination. To aid detection of larvae, feces can be diluted (1:10 in water) and examined under a microscope × 10. Fecal egg counting is unreliable for diagnosis of larval cyathostominosis; indeed counts are often negative because the infestation may comprise primarily immature larvae.
Large burdens of adult parasites in horses with ill thrift may be evidenced by a high fecal strongyle egg count. Fecal strongyle egg counts are also an essential component of a targeted worming program.

PATHOLOGIC FINDINGS
• Acute larval cyathostominosis induces acute typhlitis and colitis with mucosal hyperemia, edema, hemorrhage, congestion, ulceration, and necrosis. Transillumination of the mucosa from the serosal surface may aid visualization of cyathostomin larvae, which appear as small (1–2 mm), gray to red mucosal nodules. Histologic examination reveals large numbers of mucosal and submucosal cyathostomin larvae, edema, and infiltration with lymphocytes, eosinophils, plasma cells, and macrophages. Adult worms may be present within the lumen
• Chronic cases may have only mucosal thickening

TREATMENT

• For routine control of adult cyathostomins, anthelmintic treatment is generally recommended when fecal strongyle egg cell counts exceed 200 eggs per gram. An effective anthelmintic must be used. In developed regions, benzimidazole resistance is widespread and pyrantel resistance is present on many premises. Suspected moxidectin-resistant cyathostomins have been reported in donkeys, and shortening of the egg reappearance times after ivermectin and moxidectin administration has been documented in horses in several regions. Moxidectin is the treatment of choice for eliminating encysted larvae when dosing horses in fall and winter. Horses should receive the correct dose of anthelmintic, ideally based on an objective assessment of body weight
• Acute larval cyathostominosis requires intensive treatment. Moxidectin should be administered since this is the only anthelmintic with good efficacy against larvae. Care should be taken when calculating the dose as moxidectin can be toxic at twice the recommended dose, especially in thin horses. Glucocorticoids (prednisolone at 1 mg/kg PO SID or dexamethasone 0.1 mg/kg IV SID) may attenuate intestinal inflammation and reduce the associated morbidities. Supportive therapy includes correction of fluid, electrolyte and acid–base abnormalities, oncotic support (plasma, synthetic colloids), and analgesia.

MEDICATIONS

DRUG(S) OF CHOICE
• Moxidectin 0.4 mg/kg PO has licensed efficacy against all stages of cyathostomins,

C

and in drug-sensitive populations suppresses fecal egg counts for approximately 3 months following treatment. A single dose of moxidectin 0.4 mg/kg PO is indicated for acute larval cyathostominosis
• Ivermectin 0.2 mg/kg PO has licensed efficacy against adult stages, luminal larval stages, and developing stages of larvae in mucosa, but variable low efficacy has been observed against inhibited stages
• Oxfendazole 10 mg/kg PO or fenbendazole 5 mg/kg PO will control benzimidazole-susceptible strains of adults and developing larvae, but should be avoided on premises which have benzimidazole resistance. Administration of fenbendazole for 5 consecutive days is no longer indicated for acute larval cyathostominosis or larvicidal treatments in the fall/winter in temperate regions
• Pyrantel embonate 19 mg/kg PO kills adults but not inhibited larvae. It can be used as an alternative to moxidectin for routine strategic deworming of horses during spring and summer, but should be avoided where resistance occurs

FOLLOW-UP

PREVENTION/AVOIDANCE
• An integrated parasite control program, ideally designed by a veterinarian, which is tailored to the needs of individual premises, should be implemented. The key objective is to reduce the number of infective larvae on the pasture. All horses on the premises should be included in the program

• Strategic targeted deworming should be practiced to reduce anthelmintic use and consequently minimize development of anthelmintic resistance. Repeated interval dosing throughout the life of each horse should be avoided. Since most adult horses have some immunity against cyathostomins, only a small portion (~20%) of the herd harbors significant numbers of egg-producing adults, thereby contributing to the bulk of the pasture larval burden. These animals are identified by performing frequent fecal strongyle egg counts on all horses throughout the grazing season. The frequency of testing is dependent on the anthelmintics that are used for treatment and testing after treatment should occur at or soon after the expected egg reappearance period (this information is available on datasheets). An effective anthelmintic is then administered only to those with >200 eggs per gram. Moxidectin is commonly administered to all horses in fall/winter to reduce the cyathostomin burden, including inhibited larvae, and to eliminate large strongyles from horses that had not received an anthelmintic earlier in the grazing season. The efficacy of particular anthelmintics on premises should be assessed annually, ideally in summer, by undertaking a fecal egg count reduction test
• Anthelmintic treatment is only an adjunct to good pasture management. Pasture parasite burden can be reduced by removing feces from pastures twice weekly, avoidance of overstocking, rotating pastures, and grazing horse pastures with ruminants. Harrowing pasture can reduce pasture larval burden but only in dry weather; harrowing in wet weather is detrimental because it disperses infective

larvae away from fecal-contaminated zones. New arrivals should be quarantined and dewormed with moxidectin/praziquantel before being admitted to the herd

EXPECTED COURSE AND PROGNOSIS
Larval cyathostominosis has a guarded prognosis, with up to 50% of affected horses dying despite appropriate intensive treatment. For survivors, return to normal intestinal function may be slow.

MISCELLANEOUS

SEE ALSO
• Chronic diarrhea
• Protein, hypoproteinemia
• Protein-losing enteropathy (PLE)

Suggested Reading
Lester HE, Matthews JB. Control of equine nematodes: making the most of faecal egg counts. In Pract 2015;37:540–544.
Matthews JB. Anthelmintic resistance in equine nematodes. Int J Parasitol Drugs Drug Resist 2014;4:310–315.
Nielsen MK, von Samson-Himmelstjerna G, Pfister K, et al. The appropriate anti-parasitic treatment; coping with emerging threats from old adversaries. Equine Vet J 2016;48:374–375.

Author Bruce McGorum
Consulting Editors Henry Stämpfli and Olimpo Oliver-Espinosa

Client Education Handout available online

CYTOLOGY OF BRONCHOALVEOLAR LAVAGE (BAL) FLUID

BASICS

OVERVIEW
- Material is collected from the small airways and alveoli by flushing with sterile saline, lactated Ringer's solution, or phosphate-buffered saline and suctioning back through an endoscope or cuffed BAL tube, which has been placed in a bronchus
- Fluid is collected into sterile nonadherent tubes for cytology and bacterial culture. Samples should be kept on ice until analysis. If the analysis is delayed for more than a few hours, samples should be kept in EDTA tubes or in fixatives for cytology
- Cytocentrifuged slides are preferred but sediment preparations and direct smears are adequate alternatives. Slides are preferable stained with automated Romanowsky, May–Grünwald–Giemsa, and toluidine blue stains to visualize mast cells
- Total nucleated cells may be counted but this is not routine because standardizing the amount of saline recovered is difficult
- Total protein of fluid is low and not routinely measured
- BAL fluid from normal horses contains predominantly macrophages and lymphocytes, with small numbers of columnar epithelial cells, neutrophils, mast cells, and occasionally eosinophils. A differential cell count should be performed on 400 cells
- Most samples contain a small amount of mucus
- Presence of squamous epithelial cells indicates contamination from oropharynx

Pathophysiology
- Material present in fluid from a BAL represents the region of lungs being sampled
- Abnormalities include increased inflammatory cells, organisms, evidence of hemorrhage, increased mucus and goblet cells, and pollens/particulates that pass the mucociliary clearance apparatus
- Chronic inflammation causes increased mucus
- Neoplastic cells from lung tumors typically are not found in BAL samples
- May not be diagnostic for focal lung lesions, mild diffuse disease, or severe, chronic airway disease that prevents lavage fluid from reaching affected alveoli

CAUSES OF ABNORMAL CYTOLOGY
- Acute or chronic inflammation
- Equine asthma (IAD, heaves)
- EIPH
- Parasitic inflammation
- Idiopathic eosinophilic inflammation
- Neoplasia
- EMPF

DIAGNOSIS

DIFFERENTIAL DIAGNOSIS

Acute or Chronic Inflammation
- Acute pulmonary inflammation is associated with increased neutrophils, which may be degenerative, especially when bacteria are present (e.g. pneumonia, pleuropneumonia)
- If bacteria are primarily extracellular, examine samples for oropharyngeal contamination
- Fungal elements are usually associated with increased macrophage and neutrophil numbers. They reflect their presence in the environment and a decrease in mucociliary clearance. It does not allow for a diagnosis of fungal pneumonia
- *Pneumocystis jiroveci* (previously *carinii*) may be observed in immunosuppressed horses and more easily identified using Gömöri methenamine silver stains and other silver stains

Mild to Moderate Equine Asthma (IAD)
Characterized by increased neutrophils (>5–10%), mast cells (>2%), or eosinophils (>1%). Increases in one or more granulocyte populations may be present. Normal values may vary depending on the technique used for BAL fluid collection.

Severe Equine Asthma (Recurrent Airway Obstruction, Heaves)
- BAL samples contain an increased percentage of neutrophils (usually >20–25%) with an increased amount of mucus or goblet cells
- Eosinophil and mast cell numbers are rarely increased

EIPH
- A few RBCs may be seen if mild trauma occurs during sampling
- Phagocytized RBCs or macrophages containing breakdown products of hemoglobin suggest pulmonary hemorrhage before sampling. These may be present for 3 weeks following intrapulmonary bleeding

Parasitic Inflammation
Infection with the lungworm *Dictyocaulus arnfieldi* is associated with large numbers of eosinophils and macrophages; larvae are not usually seen.

Idiopathic Eosinophilic Pneumonia
Increased numbers of eosinophils are usually present.

Neoplasia
BAL fluid analysis is not typically useful in the diagnosis of pulmonary neoplasia.

LABORATORY TESTS
- Bacterial or fungal cultures of BAL fluid are usually not recommended because of contamination of the upper airways during sampling
- Baermann funnel fecal examination (lungworms)
- PCR of BAL for equine herpesvirus 5 (EMPF)

TREATMENT
Dependent on the underlying cause.

FOLLOW-UP

PATIENT MONITORING
Within 48 h of BAL, a significant influx of neutrophils occurs into the lung; recognize this effect if repeated BALs are analyzed.

MISCELLANEOUS

SEE ALSO
- Cytology of tracheal aspiration (TA) fluid
- Equine asthma
- Exercise-induced pulmonary hemorrhage (EIPH)
- Heaves (severe equine asthma, RAO)
- Inflammatory airway diseases—IAD in performance horses (mild and moderate equine asthma)
- Lungworm—parasitic bronchitis and pneumonia
- Summer pasture-associated equine asthma (pasture asthma)

ABBREVIATIONS
- BAL = bronchoalveolar lavage
- EIPH = exercise-induced pulmonary hemorrhage
- EMPF = equine multinodular pulmonary fibrosis
- IAD = inflammatory airway disease
- PCR = polymerase chain reaction
- RBC = red blood cell

Suggested Recading
Couetil LL, Cardwell JM, Gerber V, et al. Inflammatory airway disease of horses—revised consensus statement. J Vet Intern Med 2016;30:503–515.

Author Susan J. Tornquist
Consulting Editor Sandra D. Taylor

CYTOLOGY OF PLEURAL FLUID

BASICS

OVERVIEW
- Fluid collected from the pleural space by aspiration between the intercostal spaces. Samples are collected aseptically into a sterile tube for bacterial culture and into EDTA for cell count, cytology, and protein determination
- Normal equine pleural fluid is clear and light yellow, with a protein content <2.5 g/dL and a nucleated cell count of <10,000 cells/μL. Few nondegenerative neutrophils and large mononuclear cells, including mesothelial cells and macrophages, constitute most of the cells. Small numbers of RBCs may reflect minor hemorrhage secondary to sampling
- Measurement of glucose, lactate, and pH may help in identifying bacterial pleuropneumonia, which typically yields fluid values with a glucose of <40 mg/dL, a high lactate, and a low pH.

Pathophysiology
- Pleural fluid normally is a dialysate of the plasma, present in a small volume, and drained from the pleural cavity via lymphatic vessels
- An increased volume of fluid constitutes an effusion, the character of which reflects the initiating process—inflammation, neoplasia, decreased oncotic pressure, or hemorrhage

Systems Affected
- Respiratory
- Cardiovascular
- Hemic/lymphatic
- Hepatobiliary

SIGNALMENT
Any breed, age, or sex.

SIGNS
- Dyspnea
- Depression
- Weight loss
- Fever
- Cough
- Nasal discharge
- Reduced lung sounds
- Exercise intolerance
- Ventral edema

CAUSES AND RISK FACTORS
- Pleuritis—inflammation caused by pleuropneumonia, ruptured abscess, external trauma, foreign bodies, or primary pleuritis
- Neoplasia including lymphoma, metastatic SCC, metastatic adenocarcinoma, melanoma, or mesothelioma
- Hemorrhage
- Decreased oncotic pressure—hypoalbuminemia
- Increased hydrostatic pressure—congestive heart failure

DIAGNOSIS

DIFFERENTIAL DIAGNOSIS

Pleuritis
- Inflammation results in fluid with an increased cell count and protein content. This commonly is associated with pneumonia or lung abscessation and often is bacterial
- A predominantly neutrophilic response is seen in acute inflammation
- If bacteria are present, neutrophils may appear degenerative, and bacteria may be seen intracellularly. Culture is suggested when neutrophils are increased
- As inflammation becomes chronic, the proportion of large mononuclear cells increases, and these cells may appear vacuolated or actively phagocytic

Neoplasia
- If cells from an intrathoracic tumor are shed into the pleural fluid, a diagnosis of neoplasia may be made by cytologic examination
- The most common tumor causing pleural effusion is lymphoma, often characterized by large lymphocytes with prominent nucleoli and deeply basophilic cytoplasm. Lymphoma that is not lymphoblastic is hard to diagnose because neoplastic lymphocytes may appear morphologically normal
- Primary mesothelioma, metastatic gastric SCC, melanoma, and adenocarcinoma may exfoliate cells into the fluid

Hemorrhage
- Most hemorrhage in fluid samples is mild and iatrogenic
- Hemorrhage into the thorax before sampling may cause hemolysis and phagocytosis of RBCs; RBC breakdown products may be seen

Decreased Oncotic Pressure
Hypoalbuminemia may cause a cytologically normal transudate because of reduced oncotic pressure in the plasma.

Increased Hydrostatic Pressure
Effusions that result from heart failure (increased hydrostatic pressure) usually have higher cell counts (normal distribution of cells) and protein content than a pure transudate.

CBC/BIOCHEMISTRY/URINALYSIS
- Inflammation may be associated with leukocytosis, left shift, toxic changes in neutrophils, and hyperfibrinogenemia
- Hypoalbuminemia may support the diagnosis of a transudate

OTHER LABORATORY TESTS
- If bacterial pleuropneumonia or abscessation is suspected, aerobic and anaerobic culture of pleural fluid is recommended
- Cytologic analysis
- Fluid glucose, lactate, and pH

IMAGING
Radiography and ultrasonography may help to localize pleural fluid and to characterize pathologic processes.

OTHER DIAGNOSTIC PROCEDURES
Tracheal aspiration (cytology, aerobic and anaerobic culture) may help in establishing the diagnosis of pleuropneumonia, lung abscessation, or neoplasia.

TREATMENT
Dependent on the underlying cause.

FOLLOW-UP

PATIENT MONITORING
Following sampling, patients should be monitored for local hemorrhage, cellulitis, emphysema, or abscess at the site.

POSSIBLE COMPLICATIONS
- Hemorrhage, epistaxis
- Pneumothorax if air is allowed to enter the thoracic cavity

EXPECTED COURSE AND PROGNOSIS
Dependent on the underlying cause.

MISCELLANEOUS

ZOONOTIC POTENTIAL
(*Coccidioides immitis*) can cause pneumonia in horses and is zoonotic (Valley Fever). Primarily in southwestern USA.

SEE ALSO
- Pleuropneumonia
- Tumors of the respiratory system

ABBREVIATIONS
- RBC = red blood cell
- SCC = squamous cell carcinoma

Suggested Reading
Arroyo MG, Slovis NM, Moore GE, Taylor SD. Factors associated with survival in 97 horses with septic pleuropneumonia. J Vet Intern Med 2017;31(3):894–900.
Hewson J, Arroyo LG. Respiratory diseases: diagnostic approaches in the horse. Vet Clin North Am Equine Pract 2015;31(2):307–336.

Author Susan J. Tornquist
Consulting Editor Sandra D. Taylor

CYTOLOGY OF TRACHEAL ASPIRATION (TA) FLUID

BASICS

DEFINITION
• TA of fluid may be performed by two commonly used methods
• In the percutaneous technique, fluid is aspirated from the tracheal lumen using sterile polyethylene tubing, a catheter inserted through a cannula, or a large-bore needle inserted between the sterilely prepared tracheal rings. The site is infiltrated with 2% lidocaine and a small skin incision made prior to passing the needle or cannula. With this method, a sterile sample from the airways is more easily obtained, but complications can occur
• Another method for obtaining samples is via passage of an endoscope through the nostrils and pharynx into the trachea. A catheter is then advanced through the endoscope biopsy channel beyond the tip of the endoscope and into the trachea. This method is less invasive than the percutaneous technique, but the sample is more likely to be contaminated as the endoscope passes through the nares and pharynx. The use of dedicated double lumen catheters decreases the level of contamination
• With either method, sterile saline (10–60 mL) or lactated Ringer's solution is instilled and immediately recovered by applying suction with a syringe. If the attempt to recover fluid is not successful, the tubing or catheter may be moved a few centimeters in either direction, and additional fluid may be injected
• The sample is aliquoted into a sterile tube for culture and into a tube containing EDTA for cytology
• Direct smears, sediment preparations, or cytocentrifuged slides are made for cytologic examination. Making slides soon after collection of fluid avoids artifactual changes in cells and limits the confounding overgrowth of bacteria that can occur when there is contamination of the sample
• Most commonly, air-dried slides are stained with Wright's or Diff-Quik. Diff-Quik is a non-metachromatic stain and it may fail to stain mast cell granules, making identification of mast cells problematic
• Cell counts are not typically performed because the amount of fluid infused and recovered is variable and the presence of mucus can lead to irregular distribution of cells
• Protein content is not commonly determined because wash fluids usually are low in protein
• In aspirates from normal horses, columnar epithelial cells, which may appear ciliated or nonciliated, are the most common cell type. Macrophages are also present in moderate numbers, along with small numbers of nondegenerative neutrophils and occasional eosinophils and lymphocytes. Multinucleated macrophages may be seen in low numbers
• Mucus is present in many samples and appears as strands of purple fibrillar material. NETs have a similar appearance and are generally confused with mucus in the presence of activated neutrophils
• Squamous epithelial cells, organisms, and debris from the oropharynx or skin may be present and indicate contamination

PATHOPHYSIOLOGY
• Samples from normal horses have a wide range of cell types and generally do not contain the same cell types as those obtained using BAL. This reflects differences in cell populations in the trachea compared with those lining alveolar spaces. Tracheal aspirates contain cells from all areas of the lung and may be useful in detecting focal lung lesions
• Acute inflammation of the respiratory tract often causes migration of inflammatory cells to the trachea
• Other conditions (e.g. severe equine asthma) may not be diagnosed as readily by TA as by BAL
• Chronic inflammation or irritation causes increased mucus production by epithelial cells of the airways. This is a feature of equine asthma. The presence or amount of mucus may or may not be associated with increased numbers or percentages of neutrophils in these conditions
• With suspected septic conditions, sterile collection of material by TA is preferred over BAL; however, bacteria in the trachea without cytologic evidence of neutrophilic inflammation suggests nonpathogenic colonization of the trachea

SYSTEMS AFFECTED
• Respiratory
• Hemic/lymphatic

GENETICS
N/A

INCIDENCE/PREVALENCE
N/A

GEOGRAPHIC DISTRIBUTION
N/A

SIGNALMENT
• Any breed, age, or sex
• Foals 1–6 months of age are susceptible to pneumonia caused by *Rhodococcus equi*

SIGNS
• Coughing
• Dyspnea
• Exercise intolerance
• Nasal discharge
• Fever

CAUSES
• Pneumonia
• Equine asthma
• EIPH
• Parasitic inflammation (lungworms)

• Idiopathic eosinophilic pneumonia
• Neoplasia

RISK FACTORS
• History of *R. equi* previously on premises; see Signalment
• Young performance horses (e.g. racehorses) are at higher risk for developing upper respiratory tract viral infections, secondary bacterial pleuropneumonia, mild and moderate equine asthma (inflammatory airway disease), and EIPH
• Long-distance transportation
• Proximity to donkeys (lungworms)

DIAGNOSIS

DIFFERENTIAL DIAGNOSIS

Acute or Chronic Inflammation
• Acute pulmonary inflammation is characterized by increased neutrophil numbers (generally >20%). This is most often associated with increased mucus and NET production
• Bacterial infection often causes neutrophil degeneration
• Bacteria may be present intracellularly or extracellularly. If primarily extracellular and increased numbers of degenerative neutrophils are not seen, examine cytologic samples for signs of oropharyngeal contamination, which may lead to a false diagnosis of pneumonia
• As inflammation becomes more chronic, macrophage numbers typically increase, and neutrophils may decrease but still be present in increased numbers
• Fungal elements may be observed, and are generally indicative of environmental conditions and decreased mucociliary clearance rather than fungal pneumonia
• Viral infection of the lungs does not produce a typical inflammatory pattern
• *Pneumocystis jirovecii* (previously *carinii*) may be observed in immunosuppressed horses

Equine Asthma of All Severities
• The number and percentage of neutrophils or eosinophils may be increased in equine asthma. However, tracheal wash cytology is not considered an alternative to BAL fluid cytology for this condition
• Evidence of increased mucus, Curschmann's spirals (i.e. casts of inspissated mucus from small airways), or increased goblet cells (i.e. columnar epithelial cells with distinct, round, purple granules of mucus in the cytoplasm) are usually present in severe equine asthma
• Severity of clinical signs and airway obstruction is not correlated with cytologic findings in many cases

EIPH
• Few to moderate numbers of intact RBCs because of mild hemorrhage during TA are common

CYTOLOGY OF TRACHEAL ASPIRATION (TA) FLUID   (CONTINUED)

• Phagocytized RBCs or macrophages containing breakdown products of hemoglobin (e.g. hemosiderin) are consistent with pulmonary hemorrhage prior to sampling

Parasitic Inflammation
• Infection with the lungworm, *Dictyocaulus arnfieldi,* most often results in large numbers of eosinophils and macrophages in the sample
• Larvae have been found in unfixed, unstained sediment of tracheal fluid

Idiopathic Eosinophilic Pneumonia
• Respiratory allergic reactions typically are associated with increased numbers of eosinophils
• Mast cells, neutrophils, and lymphocytes also may be present

Neoplasia
TA is not usually considered a useful technique for the diagnosis of equine pulmonary neoplasia.

CBC/BIOCHEMISTRY/URINALYSIS
Inflammatory respiratory disease may be associated with neutrophilia, left shift, and hyperfibrinogenemia; however, these findings are neither consistent nor specific for respiratory disease.

OTHER LABORATORY TESTS
• Bacterial or fungal culture of aspirated fluid
• Baermann funnel technique to detect lungworm larvae in feces may be indicated with marked eosinophilic inflammation and appropriate history
• PCR, virus isolation, ELISA, or fluorescent antibody staining for infectious agents may be performed

IMAGING
Radiology and ultrasonography may be useful in localizing and characterizing lung lesions. CT may be useful in identifying lesions in some cases.

OTHER DIAGNOSTIC PROCEDURES
BAL
• More accurate in assessing lower airway disease, whereas TA allows assessment of overall lung and airway conditions

• Upper airway endoscopy
• Lung biopsy
• Bronchoscopy
• Pleuroscopy
• Pulmonary function testing

PATHOLOGIC FINDINGS
Dependent on the underlying cause.

TREATMENT
Directed at the underlying cause.

FOLLOW-UP
PATIENT MONITORING
Following transcutaneous TA, patients should be monitored for local hemorrhage, cellulitis, emphysema, or abscess at the site.

PREVENTION/AVOIDANCE
N/A

POSSIBLE COMPLICATIONS
• With transcutaneous TA, uncommon complications include infection, hemorrhage, or emphysema. Rarely, the catheter may snap inside the trachea; the catheter is usually coughed up
• With the endoscopic procedure, epistaxis may occur. The endoscope should always be thoroughly disinfected between patients

EXPECTED COURSE AND PROGNOSIS
Dependent on the underlying cause.

MISCELLANEOUS
ASSOCIATED CONDITIONS
N/A

AGE-RELATED FACTORS
• Foals normally may have increased neutrophils in TA fluid numbers
• Pneumonia in foals 1–6 months of age

ZOONOTIC POTENTIAL
Coccidioidomycosis (*Coccidioides immitis*) can cause pneumonia in horses and is zoonotic (Valley Fever). Primarily in southwestern USA.

PREGNANCY/FERTILITY/BREEDING
N/A

SYNONYMS
• Tracheal wash
• Transtracheal wash

SEE ALSO
• Aspiration pneumonia
• Cytology of bronchoalveolar lavage (BAL) fluid
• Exercise-induced pulmonary hemorrhage (EIPH)
• Pleuropneumonia
• *Rhodococcus equi (Prescottella equi)*

ABBREVIATIONS
• BAL = bronchoalveolar lavage
• CT = computed tomography
• EIPH = exercise-induced pulmonary hemorrhage
• ELISA = enzyme-linked immunofluorescence assay
• NET = neutrophil extracellular trap
• PCR = polymerase chain reaction
• TA = tracheal aspiration

Suggested Reading
Couetil LL, Cardwell JM, Gerber V, et al. Inflammatory airway disease of horses—revised consensus statement. J Vet Intern Med 2016;30:503–515.
Holcombe SJ, Robinson NE, Derksen FJ, et al. Effect of tracheal mucus and tracheal cytology on racing performance in thoroughbred racehorses. Equine Vet J 2006;38:300–304.
Robinson NE, Berney C, Eberhart S. Coughing, mucus accumulation, airway obstruction, and airway inflammation in control horses and horses affected with recurrent airway obstruction. Am J Vet Res 2003;64:550–557.

Author Susan J. Tornquist
Consulting Editor Sandra D. Taylor

BASICS

DEFINITION
The nasolacrimal system has both secretory and drainage components. Drainage of ocular secretions occurs through the puncta of the upper and lower eyelids into the nasolacrimal canaliculi, and subsequently the nasolacrimal sac, a dilation smaller than in most other species. The sac drains to the nasolacrimal duct in the lacrimal canal of the lacrimal and maxillary bones, then opens into the ventrolateral nasal cavity. Dacryocystitis is inflammation of the lacrimal sac and/or NLD. It is seen frequently in horses.

PATHOPHYSIOLOGY
• Dacryocystitis may develop as a primary problem or secondary to duct obstruction
• Usually dacryocystitis occurs as the result of obstruction of the NLD by accumulation of material, followed by secondary retention of tears in the duct and bacterial proliferation in the stagnant tears
• Congenital abnormalities—eyelid punctal atresia, nasolacrimal duct agenesis or incomplete formation of the duct, nasal punctal atresia, and imperforate nasal puncta
• Acquired abnormalities—fractures and other traumatic insults, inflammation, strictures, accumulation of environmental debris or foreign bodies, neoplasia, granulomas, sinusitis, upper arcade dental disease, idiopathic

SYSTEMS AFFECTED
Ophthalmic

GENETICS
There are no breed predilections for or known genetic influence on development of dacryocystitis.

INCIDENCE/PREVALENCE
Common

GEOGRAPHIC DISTRIBUTION
None identified.

SIGNALMENT
• Dacryocystitis associated with a congenital abnormality of the nasolacrimal system is usually seen within the first 2–6 months of life, but occasionally not until 1–2 years of age, especially if the animal has been turned out after weaning
• Acquired obstruction may occur at any point during an animal's life; however, for those induced by neoplastic causes, the incidence increases with age
• No proven sex predilection

SIGNS
• Thick mucopurulent discharge at the medial canthus, reflux exudation upon manipulation of the medial eyelid, mild conjunctival hyperemia

• May be unilateral or bilateral when associated with congenital causes; acquired obstructions are usually unilateral
• Atresia of the nasal puncta is most commonly unilateral
• Globe and conjunctiva are usually not involved, unless chronic dacryocystitis has resulted in blepharoconjunctivitis or keratoconjunctivitis

CAUSES
Congenital Obstruction
• Nasal puncta atresia
• Nasolacrimal duct agenesis
• Eyelid puncta atresia

Acquired Obstruction
• Traumatic disruption
• Foreign body
• Neoplasia (especially SCC)
• Granuloma (habronemiasis)
• Sinusitis, rhinitis
• Periodontitis
• Fibrosis secondary to chronic inflammation
• *Thelazia lacrymalis*

RISK FACTORS
• White, chestnut, and palomino coat color and light periocular skin pigmentation predispose to ocular SCC
• Warm weather and climates with a heavy fly population are a risk factor for habronemiasis and other parasitic causes

DIAGNOSIS

DIFFERENTIAL DIAGNOSIS
One must differentiate dacryocystitis from other causes of mucopurulent ocular discharge, including bacterial or parasitic conjunctivitis, neoplasia of eyelid or conjunctiva, secondary infection following ocular or eyelid injury, ocular foreign body.

CBC/BIOCHEMISTRY/URINALYSIS
Results usually normal.

OTHER LABORATORY TESTS
• Aerobic and anaerobic bacterial culture and sensitivity of material flushed from puncta
• Habronemiasis—scraping of the granuloma reveals eosinophils, mast cells, neutrophils, plasma cells, occasionally larvae
• Biopsy and histopathology of mass lesions are necessary for proper diagnosis

IMAGING
• Skull radiographs if fracture suspected from history or physical examination
• Contrast dacryocystorhinography assists in identifying cause and location of obstruction. It involves instillation of 4–6 mL of radiopaque solution into the puncta, followed by radiography or CT. General anesthesia is necessary for this latter diagnostic technique
• Rhinoscopy is indicated if sinusitis/rhinitis suspected

• Microvideoendoscopy may be used to directly visualize NLD lesions

OTHER DIAGNOSTIC PROCEDURES
• Complete ophthalmic examination is indicated to identify any primary ocular problem causing mucopurulent discharge or secondary ocular involvement
• Patency of the duct may be assessed initially by the Jones dye test. Fluorescein dye is instilled into the eye, and the nasal puncta is observed for appearance of fluorescein within 5 min. Attempt should be made to flush the duct with saline or irrigating solution from patent nasal puncta. Topical anesthetic should be applied to both nasal mucosa and conjunctiva
• Cannulation of the nasolacrimal duct is performed using a 5 French urinary catheter or polyethylene tubing (size 160), inserted through the nasal or eyelid puncta. Catheter may hit a blind end several centimeters from the nasal punctal opening where the duct is pressed laterally by a cartilaginous plate in the alar fold, and should be directed laterally
• Dental and oral examination, and potentially dental radiography, should be performed if dental disease is suspected as inciting cause of dacryocystitis

PATHOLOGIC FINDINGS
• Habronemiasis—eosinophils, mast cells, neutrophils, plasma cells, rarely larvae
• SCC—epithelial cells with neoplastic characteristics
• Other histopathologic findings possible depending on the type of neoplasia present

TREATMENT

APPROPRIATE HEALTH CARE
Patients that require surgical intervention to reestablish patency of the duct would be hospitalized on a short-term basis. Those in which patency is reestablished with simple irrigation or cannulation can be treated on an outpatient basis.

NURSING CARE
Ensure that topical medications can be administered appropriately prior to dispensing.

ACTIVITY
Restriction of activity may be required for a short time following surgical procedures.

DIET
No change in diet is necessary. Hay should be fed at ground level rather than from elevated hayracks or bags if ocular disease is present.

CLIENT EDUCATION
Clients should be informed of the potential for recurrence in cases of acquired obstruction or when a cause is unidentified.

SURGICAL CONSIDERATIONS
• Uncomplicated obstructions may be relieved by simply flushing the NLD and then applying topical broad-spectrum antibiotics and possibly anti-inflammatory agents
• Nasolacrimal duct agenesis accompanied by nasal or eyelid punctal atresia necessitates surgical creation of a proximal or distal opening. If the duct is present, flushing of the nasolacrimal system results in dilation of tissue overlying the site of the atretic or imperforate puncta. An incision through overlying tissue will establish patency, and a 5 French catheter placed in the nasolacrimal duct will allow epithelialization of the new puncta. Severe hemorrhage may occur following incision over the atretic nasal puncta. The ends of the catheter/stent are sutured to the skin of the muzzle and near the medial canthus, and the catheter/stent is left in place for 2–3 weeks and sometimes longer
• Acquired obstructions are treated by removal of the inciting cause when possible, irrigating the duct, and catheterization of the duct for 2–3 weeks. The indwelling stent is sutured to skin as described for congenital lesions
• Conjunctivorhinostomy involves creation of a mucous membrane-lined fistula between the ventromedial conjunctival surface and nasal cavity. This procedure is indicated for nasolacrimal duct obstruction that cannot be relieved with flushing or cannulation. Alternatively, canaliculorhinostomy involves creating a pathway from the canaliculi to the nasal cavity. Conjunctivosinostomy creates a connection between the conjunctiva and the maxillary sinus. All of these procedures must be performed under general anesthesia and involve drilling a hole through the lacrimal bone into the nasal cavity or the sinus and placing a stent until the connection is permanent and the incisions heal

MEDICATIONS
DRUG(S) OF CHOICE
• Topical triple antibiotic solution (neomycin–polymyxin B–bacitracin) placed in the eye 3 or 4 times daily until the catheter is removed or until culture results specify the need to change antimicrobial agents
• Topical corticosteroids (1% prednisolone acetate or 0.1% dexamethasone) are recommended to decrease swelling in the NLD as long as there are no ocular surface problems (corneal ulceration) that would make their use contraindicated
• Systemic antibiotics (trimethoprim–sulfonamide or ceftiofur) are absolutely critical for 7–10 days if surgical establishment of the NDL has been performed. An appropriate antibiotic solution should be flushed through the indwelling stent on a daily or every other day basis

CONTRAINDICATIONS
N/A

PRECAUTIONS
N/A

POSSIBLE INTERACTIONS
N/A

ALTERNATIVE DRUGS
N/A

FOLLOW-UP
PATIENT MONITORING
The patient should be rechecked soon after the initial procedure to establish patency (7–10 days), with the specific time frame determined by severity. Subsequent rechecks are dictated by severity of disease and response to treatment.

PREVENTION/AVOIDANCE
Fly control in barns and pastures, fly hoods, frequent periocular administration of insect repellent, and regular deworming with avermectins, decreasing environmental dust, debris, and other material that may accumulate in the NLD, and decreasing the amount or exposure to allergens may prevent the development of or decrease the incidence or severity of NLD obstructions and dacryocystitis.

POSSIBLE COMPLICATIONS
Potential complications vary with the inciting cause. They include recurrence of the dacryocystitis and failure to maintain patency of the duct.

EXPECTED COURSE AND PROGNOSIS
• The prognosis for NLD obstructions and dacryocystitis is good, but depends upon the location, extent, and cause of the obstruction
• Acquired obstructions resulting in dacryocystitis are more difficult to treat than congenital abnormalities
• Foreign body and periodontal causes have the best response to therapy of acquired obstructions
• Cannulation of the duct may be impossible in cases of neoplasia and maxillary fractures, and permanent correction of the obstruction and subsequent dacryocystitis may not be possible

MISCELLANEOUS
ASSOCIATED CONDITIONS
N/A

AGE-RELATED FACTORS
N/A

ZOONOTIC POTENTIAL
N/A

PREGNANCY/FERTILITY/BREEDING
Systemic absorption of topically applied medication is possible. Benefits of treatment should be considered against any risks posed to the fetus.

SEE ALSO
• Ocular/adnexal squamous cell carcinoma
• Ocular problems in the neonate

ABBREVIATIONS
• CT = computed tomography
• NLD = nasolacrimal duct
• SCC = squamous cell carcinoma

Suggested Reading
Brooks DE. Ophthalmology for the Equine Practitioner, 2e. Jackson, WY: Teton NewMedia, 2008.
Gilger BC. Equine ophthalmology. In: Gelatt KN, Gilger BC, Kern TJ, eds. Veterinary Ophthalmology, 5e. Ames, IA: Wiley Blackwell, 2013:1560–1609.
Gilger BC. Equine Ophthalmology, 3e. Philadelphia, PA: WB Saunders, 2017.

Author Caroline Monk
Consulting Editor Caryn E. Plummer
Acknowledgment The author acknowledges the prior contribution of Caryn E. Plummer.

DELAYED UTERINE INVOLUTION

BASICS

DEFINITION
• Involution is normally complete by 13–25 days, with the exception of normal size, which may require as long as 35 days. • Delayed uterine involution may be the result of size, tone, endometrial regeneration, or elimination of bacteria from the uterine lumen

PATHOPHYSIOLOGY
• Placentation in the equine is diffuse allantochorial microcotyledonary, which allows rapid uterine involution. • Microcaruncular involution is complete by day 9 postpartum and complete histologic repair is observed by day 14. • DUC may follow dystocia or RFM and is characterized by compromised ability to eliminate postpartum debris and bacteria from the uterus. • DUC origin can be: ○ Mechanical, e.g. decreased muscular contractions, decreased exercise. ○ Inflammatory, e.g. neutrophil influx. ○ Immunologic

SYSTEMS AFFECTED
Reproductive

SIGNALMENT
• Any mare. • More prevalent in old mares. • Draft breeds are predisposed

SIGNS
General Comments
Rapid uterine involution is necessary in mares because foal heat and rebreeding can occur within 5–18 days postpartum.

Historical Findings
Suspected if failure to conceive when bred during an early foal heat.

Physical Examination Findings
Increased uterine size, intrauterine fluid, or abnormal vaginal discharge.

CAUSES
• Anatomic defects. • Poor uterine contraction. • Poor uterine clearance

RISK FACTORS
• Old mares. • Dystocia and RFM. • Contaminated uterus at parturition

DIAGNOSIS

DIFFERENTIAL DIAGNOSIS
• Metritis. • Delayed uterine involution may accompany metritis

CBC/BIOCHEMISTRY/URINALYSIS
N/A

OTHER LABORATORY TESTS
Endometrial cytology—presence of neutrophils.

IMAGING
US
• Fluid within the postpartum uterine lumen. • Decreased uterine tone and/or increased uterine size

OTHER DIAGNOSTIC PROCEDURES
Endometrial bacteriology.

PATHOLOGIC FINDINGS
Indicators of delayed uterine involution, 12–15 days postpartum.

Uterus
• Intraluminal fluid. • Decreased tone. • Endometrial cytology, increased number of leukocytes

Vulva/Vulvar
Discharge persists.

TREATMENT

APPROPRIATE HEALTH CARE
• May accompany uterine infections or inflammation. • Systemic antibiotics are not indicated. • Local, intrauterine instillation of antibiotics may be contraindicated

ACTIVITY
Normal activity.

CLIENT EDUCATION
• Not all mares are ready to be bred at foal heat. • All mares should undergo a postpartum examination even if foaling appeared to be normal. • Decision for foal heat breeding should be based on serial TRP

MEDICATIONS

DRUG(S) OF CHOICE
• Oxytocin (10 IU IV or 20 IU IM every 2 h for the first 24 h postpartum) and prostaglandin $F_{2\alpha}$ (10 mg IM) or a prostaglandin analog (cloprostenol 250 µg IM) have been used to promote uterine involution, but their efficacy is not known. • Uterine flushes when indicated (i.e. presence of a large amount of intrauterine debris). • Antibiotics—*only* if a bacterial pathogen is confirmed present

PRECAUTIONS
Do not overtreat delayed uterine involution with unnecessary antibiotics or other local or systemic medications.

FOLLOW-UP

PATIENT MONITORING
Examination of the uterus to determine return to normal is essential after therapy—TRP; ultrasonography.

PREVENTION/AVOIDANCE
• Light exercise during late gestation and postpartum. • Barn hygiene—mare's stall should be bedded with clean straw for foaling and during the first several days postpartum

POSSIBLE COMPLICATIONS
• Failure to conceive. • Early embryonic death

EXPECTED COURSE AND PROGNOSIS
• Majority of mares return to normal without treatment. • In some cases, involution remains incomplete and may prevent conception or pregnancy maintenance

MISCELLANEOUS

ASSOCIATED CONDITIONS
May or may not be coupled with a uterine infection.

SEE ALSO
• Dystocia
• Postpartum metritis
• Retained fetal membranes
• Vaginitis and vaginal discharge
• Vulvar conformation

ABBREVIATIONS
• DUC = delayed uterine clearance.
• RFM = retained fetal membranes.
• TRP = transrectal palpation

Suggested Reading
Carluccio A, Contri A, Tosi U, et al. Survival rate and short-term fertility rate associated with the use of fetotomy for resolution of dystocia in mares: 72 cases (1991-2005). J Am Vet Med Assoc 2007;230:1502–1505.
McKinnon AO, Squires EL, Harrison LA, et al. Ultrasonographic studies on the reproductive tract of mares after parturition: effect of involution and uterine fluid on pregnancy rates in mares with normal and delayed first postpartum ovulatory cycles. J Am Vet Med Assoc 1988;192:350–353.
Steiger K, Kersten F, Aupperle H, et al. Puerperal involution in the mare—morphological studies in correlation with course of birth. Theriogenology 2002;58:783–786.
Stewart DR, Kindahl H, Stabenfeldt GH, Hughes JP. Concentrations of 15-keto-13,14-dihydroprostaglandin $PGF_2\alpha$ in the mare during spontaneous and oxytocin induced foaling. Equine Vet J 1984;16:270–274.

Author Ahmed Tibary
Consulting Editor Carla L. Carleton
Acknowledgment The author and editor acknowledge the prior contribution of Walter R. Threlfall.

D

DERMATOMYCOSES, SUBCUTANEOUS (SC)

BASICS

DEFINITION
SC fungal infections are generally secondary to wound inoculations, have invaded the viable tissues of the skin, and are subdivided into the following categories:
- Phaeohyphomycoses and eumycotic mycetomas—nodular, slowly extensive mycoses due to dematiaceous pigmented fungi (melanin pigments). With mycetomas, the lesions contain fungal grains that can be either pigmented or nonpigmented and the disease is rarely invasive
- Sporotrichosis—slowly extensive SC infection due to the yeast phase of *Sporothrix schenckii*; slowly invasive
- Oomycosis—pythiosis: SC and extensive infection due to *Pythium insidiosum,* rapidly invasive (not true fungi)
- Zygomycoses—deep, rapidly invasive infections from 2 orders in the Zygomycetes class (Entomophthorales and Mucorales), rapidly invasive

PATHOPHYSIOLOGY
- Phaeohyphomycoses and eumycotic mycetomas—most dematiaceous fungi exist on soil and plants. After inoculating a wound, the fungus induces chronic inflammation
- Sporotrichosis—infection from wounds. The mold form is normally present in soil, plants, wood, and water. After inoculation, the fungus changes to a yeast phase that slowly proliferates and extends to lymphatic vessels and lymph nodes
- Pythiosis—*P. insidiosum* develops on aquatic plants. Motile spores in water are attracted by damaged skin tissue and germinate on the surface of the skin. SC invasion results in proliferative necrotic extensive lesions
- Zygomycoses—after inoculation, the fungi develop in the dermis, resulting in a pyogranulomatous inflammation with tropism for blood vessels

SYSTEMS AFFECTED
- Skin—all
- Phaeohyphomycoses and eumycotic mycetomas—regional lymphatic
- Sporotrichosis—regional lymphatic
- Pythiosis—secondarily systemic
- Zygomycoses—occasionally rhinofacial, nasopharyngeal

INCIDENCE/PREVALENCE
- Dependent on geographic distribution
- Phaeohyphomycoses—rare in USA. Eumycotic mycetomas—most commonly reported fungus in the USA being *Pseudallescheria boydii*; account for approximately 9.5% of cases of equine non-neoplastic nodular lesions submitted for histopathology in the Pacific northwest of the USA
- Sporotrichosis—worldwide and areas of high humidity and mild temperatures

- Pythiosis—most cases are seen during the summer and fall. The environmental factors of water, decaying vegetation, and temperatures between 30°C and 40°C are the most influential factors governing the occurrence
- Zygomycoses—found in soil and decaying vegetation. Cases occur throughout the year

GEOGRAPHIC DISTRIBUTION
- Eumycotic mycetomas—found most frequently near the Tropic of Cancer, including Africa, North, South, and Central America, India, and southern Asia, and less commonly in the USA and Europe
- Sporotrichosis—most common in warm countries, endemic in Spain and Italy
- Pythiosis—in tropical and subtropical areas of the world (e.g. Thailand, Japan, Indonesia, Burma, New Guinea, Colombia, Costa Rica, Brazil, and Australia). In the USA, cases are mainly seen in the Gulf Coast region and other southern states; however, it has also been documented in Oklahoma, Arkansas, Missouri, Kentucky, Tennessee, North and South Carolina, Virginia, New Jersey, and southern Indiana
- Zygomycoses—*Rhizopus, Mucor, Absidia* (Mucorales) have a worldwide distribution. The 2 major species of Entomophthorales are *Basidiobolus ranarum* (Americas, Australia, Asia, and tropical Africa) and *Conidiobolus coronatus* (tropical Africa and southeast Asia). In the USA, states along the Gulf of Mexico

SIGNALMENT
- Cutaneous granulomas most common in young (mean age 6 ± 4.2 years), with no breed or sex bias
- Pythiosis—commonly affected horses have had prolonged contact with water in lakes, ponds, swamps, and flooded areas. The horse is the most susceptible species

SIGNS
Phaeohyphomycosis
- Firm, single or multiple well-circumscribed dermal nodules (1–10 cm) on the face and legs but can be widely scattered
- Lesions initially haired but become alopecic, eroded, ulcerated, and drain
- Papular satellites possible
- Grossly pigmented, nonpruritic, and nonpainful

Eumycotic Mycetomas
- SC lesions occur anywhere; however, single or multiple nodules on the head including lips and ears and neck are the most common involved sites
- As lesions progress, they become firm, alopecic, ulcerative plaques or nodules that may drain serous, purulent, or hemorrhagic discharge that may contain black or white grains. Average size 7 mm
- On the cut surface, suppurative exudate contains generally brown to black (rarely white to yellow) tissue grains (1–2 mm in size)

- Mycetomas discharge tissue grains in contrast to phaeohyphomycoses, which do not

Sporotrichosis
- Cutaneolymphatic form most common. Firm dermal to SC nodules (1–5 cm) common on the distal extremity but can be found on the chest, proximal foreleg, shoulder, and perineal region
- Nodules linearly disposed along lymphatics and lymph nodes draining the area of the lesion
- Lymphangitis with enlarged thickened "corded" vessels
- Possible secondary fistulation with hemorrhagic rust to brown thin seropurulent fluid
- Usually nonpruritic, nonpainful
- Primary cutaneous form occurs but is uncommon

Pythiosis
- Disease affects ventral part of the body including the legs, chest, and ventrum. Occasionally nasal
- Progressive development of cutaneous or SC nodular tumor-like, ulcerative lesion; thick, sticky material exudes from the wound
- Rapidly enlarging; may reach 50 cm in diameter
- Pruritus frequent, sometimes intense
- Visible hard, gritty, yellowish to gray coral-like masses named "kunkers" (rice grain to several centimeters) which are composed of fungal hyphae, host exudates, and protein
- Possible extension (bones, joints, lungs, digestive tract)

Zygomycoses
- *Basidiobolus* infects the lateral aspects of the head, neck, and body; lesions are usually single nodular eroded to ulcerative granulomas that may demonstrate moderate to severe pruritus
- Fistulous tracts discharge a serosanguineous exudate from the lesions, which are frequently traumatized and can contain small, gritty, yellow-white coral-shaped bodies (0.7–1.7 mm)
- *Conidiobolus* affects almost exclusively the mucosa of the nose and mouth
- Ulcerative firm, single or multiple to coalescing lesions that may have a cobblestone appearance and may cause mechanical blockage, resulting in dyspnea and nasal discharge
- Vascular invasion and hematogenous spread more common with mucormycosis than entomophthoromycosis

CAUSES
- Phaeohyphomycoses—*Drechslera spinferum, Alternaria alternata, Exserohilum rostratum, Cladosporium* spp.
- Eumycotic mycetomas—*Curvularia* spp., *Madurella* (black grained mycetomas), *Scedosporium/Pseudallescheria* complex,

Phialophora, and *Aspergillus versicolor* (white grained mycetomas), *Alternaria* spp.
• Sporotrichosis—*Sporothrix schenckii* complex
• Pythiosis—*P. insidiosum*
• Zygomycoses—2 orders:
• Mucorales (genera include *Rhizopus, Mucor* spp., *Absidia*, and *Mortierella*)
• Entomophthorales (genera include *Conidiobolus* spp. and *Basidiobolus*)

DIAGNOSIS

DIFFERENTIAL DIAGNOSIS
• Phaeohyphomycoses and eumycotic mycetomas—neoplasia (sarcoid, squamous cell carcinoma, cutaneous lymphoma, melanoma), granulomas (foreign bodies, eosinophilic, bacterial), sporotrichosis, insect bite reactions, histoplasmosis, and molluscum contagiosum
• Sporotrichosis—cutaneous habronemiasis, foreign body and infectious granulomas, sarcoids, neoplasia, ulcerative, and histoplasmosis
• Pythiosis and zygomycoses—as for sporotrichosis and extreme granulation tissue

CBC/BIOCHEMISTRY/URINALYSIS
Pythiosis—anemia and hypoproteinemia.

OTHER LABORATORY TESTS
• Sporotrichosis—mold phase growth at 27°C or yeast growth on blood agar CO_2 enriched at 37°C
• Direct fluorescent antibody tests on biopsy specimen are performed at specialized laboratories like the Centers for Disease Control and Prevention, Atlanta, GA
• PCR from skin biopsy for identification of *chitin synthase 1* gene
• Pythiosis—serology (ELISA, Western blot) and molecular tests (PCR) conducted by Pan American Veterinary Labs, Hutto, TX (www.pavlab.com): accurate and rapid diagnosis

DIAGNOSTIC PROCEDURES
• Definitive diagnosis for all SC mycoses is by demonstration of the organism via cytologic examination of exudate, culture of tissue or exudates, and/or histopathology
• Pythiosis—tissue samples should be submitted via overnight shipping at room temperature. Procedures for determination of the agent include: (1) wet mount examination in 10% KOH followed by culturing, (2) detection of anti-*P. insidiosum* antibodies using serological assays, and (3) detection of DNA of the agent in the infected tissue by PCR and sequencing

PATHOLOGIC FINDINGS
• Phaeohyphomycoses and eumycotic mycetomas—granuloma with central core of cellular debris and neutrophils surrounded by lymphocytes and epithelioid macrophages,

organisms with septate and branched hyphae, thick walled, pigmented, or not hyphae or yeast-like elements (organized in grains in mycetomas)
• Sporotrichosis—special stains are required (periodic acid–Schiff or GMS) as yeast are difficult to detect. Typically elongated yeasts in a granulomatous reaction with multinucleated giant cells
• Pythiosis—pyogranulomatous dermatitis and panniculitis with eosinophils. Wide and irregular hyphae (special stains), frequently surrounded by eosinophilic Splendore–Hoeppli reaction and kunkers
• Zygomycoses—in excised tissues, a thickened fibrotic dermis has scattered, red to creamy white areas with a central core of necrotic tissue, which often contains hyphal forms surrounded by eosinophilic infiltrate of the Splendore–Hoeppli phenomenon. Tissue sections stained with GMS reveal large, branching, sometimes septate, 4–20 μm hyphae

TREATMENT

AIMS
Attempt to reduce fungal burden via both medical and surgical management.

APPROPRIATE HEALTH CARE
• The treatment of choice is aggressive surgical excision of all infected tissue (at least 2–3 cm of apparent healthy margins)
• Chronic disease may not allow complete surgical excision
• Medical management may reduce nonresectable lesions to the point that they become resectable

CLIENT EDUCATION
• All SC dermatomycoses carry a fair to guarded prognosis if complete surgical excision cannot be achieved
• Treatment duration is a least 3 weeks but often much longer
• Treatment is expensive

SURGICAL CONSIDERATIONS
• Wide surgical excision should be performed for all SC mycoses
• Phaeohyphomycoses—the only effective treatment
• Eumycotic mycetomas—recurrence is common if incomplete excision
• Sporotrichosis—effective in limiting the disease
• Pythiosis—only possible in early cases
• Zygomycoses—early removal effective

MEDICATIONS

DRUG(S) OF CHOICE
• Phaeohyphomycoses—fluconazole loading dose of 14 mg/kg given once followed by

5 mg/kg PO every 24 h concurrently with inorganic potassium iodide at 10–15 g every 24 h (for horses), 5–10 g every 24 h for ponies for 30 days or 1 month beyond clinical cure
• Sporotrichosis—ethylene diamine dihydroiodide, drug of choice administered as a feed additive at a dosage of 1–2 mg/kg every 12–24 h × 1 week; then reduce to 0.5–1.0 mg/kg every 24 h for the remainder of the treatment. Continue treatment at least 1 month past clinical cure
• Alternative systemic antimycotic therapy; sodium iodine therapy (125 mL of 20% solution IV slowly for 3 days) then 30 g/horse daily IM injection for 30 days
• Zygomycoses and pythiosis—amphotericin B given systemically after surgical excision must be dissolved in 5% dextrose and water. Initial daily dose is 0.3 mg/kg. Every third day the dose is increased by 0.1 mg/kg until a maximum dose of 0.8–0.9 mg/kg/day is reached. Lesions of the extremities should receive surgical excision of exuberant granulation tissue followed by IV regional limb profusion of 50 mg amphotericin B (10 mL) in a 10% solution of medical grade dimethylsulfoxide (6 mL) and lactated Ringer's solution (44 mL)

CONTRAINDICATIONS
Use of azoles in horses with compromised hepatic function warrants careful monitoring of liver function during treatment or avoiding use of the drug if further hepatic compromise is considered to have serious clinical consequences.

PRECAUTIONS
• Tolerance to iodides is variable and some horses show signs of iodism. Stop treatment for at least 1 week; then reinstitute at 75% of dosage responsible for toxic signs
• Baseline biochemical profile should be performed to evaluate liver enzymes before administration of azoles
• Ketoconazole is not recommended in the horse due to poor bioavailability

ALTERNATIVE DRUGS
Pythiosis—immunotherapy with USDA licensed *P. insidiosum* vaccine has been reported to be effective in control or resolution of the disease in > 85% of affected horses. Can be combined with concurrent therapies.

FOLLOW-UP

PATIENT MONITORING
• Reevaluate every 2–3 weeks for clinical signs and side effects associated with treatments
• Pythiosis—ELISA serology can be used to monitor response to therapy; serology should be checked 2–3 months after surgery or every 3 months during medical therapy

DERMATOMYCOSES, SUBCUTANEOUS (SC)   (CONTINUED)

POSSIBLE COMPLICATIONS
• Phaeohyphomycoses and eumycotic mycetomas—osteomyelitits, arthritis, myositis
• Pythiosis—acute abdomen and death from gastrointestinal thrombosis and perforation

EXPECTED COURSE AND PROGNOSIS
• Unresponsive to therapy—not unexpected; consider alternative treatment or combined treatment regimens (supersaturated potassium iodide, amphotericin B, and itraconazole)
• Phaeohyphomycoses—wide surgical excision may be curative; horses with multiple lesions may heal spontaneously within 3 months after the diagnosis
• Eumycotic mycetomas—some response to aggressive surgical removal of affected nodules, but recurrence is common. May stay localized for years and not invade muscle or bone
• Pythiosis—prognosis varies with treatment response

• Zygomycoses—chronic lesions have a poorer prognosis

MISCELLANEOUS

ZOONOTIC POTENTIAL
Sporotrichosis—humans are susceptible to sporotrichosis; however, there are no reports of transmission from an infected horse.

PREGNANCY/FERTILITY/BREEDING
• Systemic iodides may cause abortion
• Azoles antifungals are tetratogenic and should not be used in pregnant mares

SYNONYMS
• Phaeohyphomycoses and mycetomas—chromomycosis, pseudomycetoma (dermatophytic mycetoma)
• Pythiosis—swamp cancer, phycomycosis, hyphomycosis, Florida horse leeches

• Zygomycoses—mucormycosis, entomophoromycosis, basidiobolomycosis, and conidiobolomycosis

ABBREVIATIONS
• ELISA = enzyme-linked immunosorbent assay
• GMS = Gömöri methenamine silver stain
• PCR = polymerase chain reaction
• USDA = United States Department of Agriculture

Suggested Reading
Renata GS, Cravalho MB, Freitas SH, et al. Evaluation of intravenous regional perfusion with amphotericin B and dimethylsulfoxide to treat horses for pythiosis of a limb. BMC Vet Res 2015;11:152.

Author Gwendolen Lorch
Consulting Editor Gwendolen Lorch
Acknowledgment The author/editor acknowledges the prior contribution of Patrick Bourdeau.

BASICS

DEFINITION
• Superficial cutaneous fungal infections develop in the stratum corneum, hair, and hoof. They include dermatophytoses and yeast dermatoses
• Dermatophytoses are generally highly contagious dermatoses due to keratinophilic fungi of the *Microsporum* and *Trichophyton* genera
• Yeast—superficial fungal dermatoses. Most important yeasts are *Malassezia* and *Candida albicans*

PATHOPHYSIOLOGY
• Dermatophytoses—2 zoophilic species identified specifically in horses: *Trichophyton equinum* and *Microsporum equinum*
• Transmission by contact with clinically infected or asymptomatic carrier horses, other animal species, insect bites, or fomites. Dermatophyte spores have a very long resistance in the environment (months to years)
• The spores remain quiescent until local conditions stimulate arthroconidia to germinate and invade the stratum corneum and hair follicles. Protease production digests keratin and initiates skin and hair damage
• Yeast—(*Malassezia* spp.) is a lipophilic yeast present on the skin of most horses. Proliferation may induce inflammation

SYSTEMS AFFECTED
Skin/exocrine

GENETICS
N/A

INCIDENCE/PREVALENCE
Dermatophytoses—1 of the 10 most frequent skin conditions in horses. Higher incidence on training farms than breeding farms.

GEOGRAPHIC DISTRIBUTION
• Dermatophytoses—worldwide
• Yeast—presumably worldwide

SIGNALMENT
• Dermatophytes—any age. More frequent in young horses
• Yeast—no breed predilection. *Malassezia* (intermammary fossa) possibly more frequent in mares. Nonseasonal

SIGNS

Dermatophytes
• Clinical disease is usually evident within 1–6 weeks after exposure and clinical signs are highly variable
• Evolution influenced by host (age, immune status), fungus, and time. More inflammation is frequent with *Trichophyton* sp. Papules, tufted hairs, or urticaria-like lesions at early stage
• Annular alopecia (1–10 cm in diameter) and scaling with an erythematous margin. Become

polycyclic by coalescence or grow centripetally. New hair growth may occur in the center of the lesion but active disease continues to occur at the periphery
• May have single or multiple lesions in a cluster or generalized
• Moderate erythema (visible on white horses)
• Crusts occasionally thick. Infrequently multiple papular forms (miliary). Subcutaneous forms (mycetomas) are rare in horses
• Pruritus usually minimal, except with *Trichophyton bullosum*

Physical Examination Findings
• Frequently starts on areas exposed to trauma or are in contact with saddles, bridles, and harness
• Most lesions are located on the face, neck, dorsolateral thorax, forelimbs, and girth
• More or less rapidly extensive
• Individual lesions spontaneously cure with regrowth of hair from the center (occasionally darker in color)
• Mane and tail generally spared

Yeast
• *Malassezia*—intertrigo (axillae, groin, mammary gland, prepubital fossa); odor; greasiness and sticky brownish material
• *Candida*—acute inflammation, erythema, pustular, erosion, exudates (occasionally whitish) mainly periorificial, vulvovaginal, perineal, or intertriginous areas, occasionally pruritic (even painful if *Candida*). Nodular cutaneous candidiasis represented as firm, painful nodules covered by a normal hair coat has been reported

CAUSES
• Yeast—immunosuppressive diseases (viral infections, neoplasia) or immunosuppressive drug therapy may predispose to candidiasis
• Vulvovaginal candidiasis was reported in Thoroughbred mares following oral administration of a synthetic progestogen
• Defects in cornification and hypersensitivity

RISK FACTORS

Dermatophytes
• Contaminated barns and confined animals
• Young age (<3 years) and high humidity
• Recent introduction of new horses or other animals

Yeast
Candidosis precipitated by antibiotic treatments.

DIAGNOSIS

DIFFERENTIAL DIAGNOSIS

Dermatophytoses
• Bacterial folliculitis (mainly staphylococcal)—similar to identical annular lesions; same predisposed body locations, more frequent during hot periods

• Dermatophilosis (folliculitis with thick crusts and alopecia)
• Urticaria (atopy, food, drug intolerances), rapid onset, alopecia is rare
• Alopecia areata (minimal reaction of skin)
• Pemphigus foliaceus (crusts, frequently perioral)
• Eosinophilic folliculitis
• Any nodular lesions (bacterial, fungal, foreign body granulomas, neoplasms) in cases of dermatophytic mycetoma

Yeast
• Other causes of greasiness, intertrigo, or periorificial inflammation
• Other rare fungal superficial dermatoses (*Alternaria, Geotrichum*)
• Mucocutaneous candidiasis differentials include systemic lupus erythematosus, pemphigus vulgaris, erythema multiforme, drug eruptions, and vasculitis
• Nodular forms of candidiasis include infectious and sterile granulomatous disorders

CBC/BIOCHEMISTRY/URINALYSIS
Not indicated unless suspect systemic disease that is causing immunosuppression.

OTHER LABORATORY TESTS

Dermatophytes—Fungal Culture
• Gold standard to identify the dermatophyte and possible origin
• Selective dermatophyte test media are required to prevent overgrowth of commensal fungi
• Wipe the lesion with 70% alcohol, allow to dry, and then pluck the lesional hair with sterile hemostats
• May need to include inoculation of crusts

Yeast—Fungal Culture
• Necessary to identify *C. albicans*. Pathogenic when isolated from skin
• *Malassezia pachydermatis* is the only species that develops on routine medium agar at 30°C

IMAGING
N/A

OTHER DIAGNOSTIC PROCEDURES

Dermatophytoses—Scrapings and Trichoscopy
Direct microscopic examination of infected hairs—broken, embedded in crusts, thickened, and fibrous; may contain hyphae, with surrounding arthrospores.

Yeast—Cytology on Direct Smears
Abundance of narrow (*Candida*) or wide (*Malassezia*) based budding yeasts. Occasionally hyphae (*C. albicans*).

Cytology
• Abundant neutrophils, acantholytic cells (confusion with pemphigus); occasionally arthrospores (confusion with yeasts)
• Rarely concurrent bacterial folliculitis

DERMATOMYCOSES, SUPERFICIAL (CONTINUED)

TREATMENT

AIMS

Dermatophytoses
- Although considered self-limiting, the infection may last for months and horses remain carriers and sources
- The aim is to shorten the evolution, reduce lesions, and limit the risk of contamination
- Topical therapy applied to the entire body is mandatory. Other mandatory therapy includes clipping and destruction of infected hairs

Yeast
- Correction of the predisposing causes is fundamental
- Excessive moisture must be avoided

APPROPRIATE HEALTH CARE
Outpatient medical management is appropriate.

NURSING CARE
N/A

ACTIVITY
Dermatophytes—identification and isolation of infected horses are important to limit the contagion.

DIET
N/A

CLIENT EDUCATION

Dermatophytoses
- Inform clients that the disease is contagious to other horses and eventually humans. Other hosts may be of concern
- The disinfection of all materials and housing is imperative for clinical success
- The appropriate application of topical treatment is crucial for cure

SURGICAL CONSIDERATIONS
N/A except for mycetomas (wide excision).

MEDICATIONS

DRUG(S) OF CHOICE

Dermatophytoses
Topical
- Lotions or rinses are preferred to creams. Miconazole 1–2%, terbinafine 1%, or natamycin can be used for smaller, localized lesions but are not practical for treatment of generalized disease
- Lime sulfur 2%, enilconazole 0.2% (Imaverol), ketoconazole 1–2%, miconazole 2%, chlorhexidine 2–4%, and combinations of miconazole/ketoconazole with chlorhexidine. Applied at least 2 or 3 times weekly for initial therapy
- Every case should receive topical therapy
Systemic
- Griseofulvin (Fulvicin) powder. Labeled for use in horses in many countries. Proposed

dosages highly variable. Most have found no evidence that oral griseofulvin powder at the labeled dose is efficacious in horses. However, 100 mg/kg/day for 10 days was reported to be effective in a small number of horses. Superiority of benefit remains controversial especially compared with topical therapy
- Equine pharmacokinetics of terbinafine at 20 mg/kg have been determined with clinical trials demonstrating efficacy still needed

Yeast
Topical
Apply 2 or 3 times a week for at least 3 weeks.
Shampoos
- Chlorhexidine (2–4%) or preferably combined with miconazole (2%)/ketoconazole (1–2%)
- If skin is particularly greasy (*Malassezia*), use a keratolytic shampoo
- Selenium sulfide 1% or lime sulfur 2%
- For localized dermatitis, consider clipping and applying topical chlorhexidine/miconazole or azole creams, ointments, or mousses every 12 h for 3–4 weeks

CONTRAINDICATIONS
See Pregnancy/Fertility/Breeding.

PRECAUTIONS
Selenium sulfide can be irritating (rinse thoroughly).

POSSIBLE INTERACTIONS
Not reported in horses.

ALTERNATIVE DRUGS

Dermatophytoses
Essential oils have the potential to be natural fungicides. A small, randomized, open clinical trial evaluated the use of 25% tea tree oil in sweet almond oil compared with enilconazole 2% solution. Use of 25% tea tree oil mixture twice a day for 15 days was well tolerated. Horses in both groups reached clinical cure.
Oral Azoles (Fluconazole, Voriconazole, Itraconazole)
Generally cost prohibitive. Fluconazole is effective against dermatophytes and yeast dermatitis. Dose is 5 mg/kg every 24 h PO with a half-life of 38 h. Voriconazole is effective against dermatophytes. Oral absorption is 92% and half-life is 13 h. Dose is 2-4 mg/kg every 24 h or 3 mg/kg every 12 h PO.
Vaccines
- Have been developed in different species, including horses, in some countries
- Vaccination may provide a reasonable degree of protection in horses, but they are not commercially available in many regions.

Yeast
- Treatment with systemic azoles—a possible alternative but prohibitive cost
- For refractory cases, consider the use of leave-on 2% lime sulfur or enilconazole rinses applied after twice-weekly medicated shampoos

FOLLOW-UP

PATIENT MONITORING
Control at 7–10 day intervals and verify the clinical recovery.

PREVENTION/AVOIDANCE
The owner has to look carefully at other animals to detect new cases. Quarantine of new arrivals and prevent sharing of tack.

POSSIBLE COMPLICATIONS
N/A

EXPECTED COURSE AND PROGNOSIS
Dermatophytoses—with appropriate therapy, the extension is rapidly stopped and hair regrowth is noted. Complete cure in 1–4 months.

MISCELLANEOUS

ASSOCIATED CONDITIONS
Yeast—possible allergic dermatitis.

AGE-RELATED FACTORS
Any age, although young horses frequently concerned.

ZOONOTIC POTENTIAL

Dermatophytoses
Human contamination is not rare—mainly from *Trichophyton mentagrophytes*, *Trichophyton verrucosum*, or *Microsporum canis*; occasionally from *M. equinum*, *T. bullosum*; rarely from *T. equinum*.

Yeast
A minor concern, easily prevented by simple handwashing.

PREGNANCY/FERTILITY/BREEDING
The use of griseofulvin and oral azoles is contraindicated in pregnant animals.

SYNONYMS

Dermatophytoses
- Ringworm
- Microsporosis
- Trichophytosis

Yeast
- Candidosis
- Thrush

SEE ALSO
- Alopecia
- Dermatomycoses, subcutaneous (SC)
- Dermatophilosis
- Pemphigus foliaceus

Suggested Reading
Weese JS, Yu AA. Infectious folliculitis and dermatophytosis. Vet Clin North Am Equine Pract 2013;29:559–575.

Author Gwendolen Lorch
Consulting Editor Gwendolen Lorch
Acknowledgment The author/editor acknowledges the prior contribution of Patrick Bourdeau.

BASICS

OVERVIEW
Dermatophilosis is a common bacterial exudative crusting dermatitis of horses that may affect multiple horses in a barn but not necessarily all of them. It typically occurs during periods of heavy rain. Tightly adherent crusts most commonly affect the dorsum of the trunk, especially the saddle region or the dorsal surface of both hind cannon bones. It is a cause of pastern dermatitis (grease heal, scratches). This infection is easily resolved with topical and/or systemic antimicrobial therapy.

SIGNALMENT
No age, breed, or sex predilection has been recognized. Horses that are debilitated may develop a chronic infection. If a horse is kept in a wet stall or pen, chronic pastern dermatitis may ensue.

SIGNS
• Clinical lesions vary with the stage of disease. Initially, follicular and nonfollicular papules and pustules form tightly adherent crusts
• Crusts may cluster to form large coalescing crusted plaques associated with a thick yellow to light green suppurative exudate. Removal of crusts results in the distal hair ends protruding through the crust, giving a "paint brush" appearance. Moist erosive erythematosus alopecic lesions are present when the crust is removed
• Alopecia is variable. If lesions are palpated pain may be elicited
• Pastern or fetlock involvement may cause lameness and localized swelling
• Lymphadenopathy may occur

CAUSES AND RISK FACTORS
• Dermatophilosis is caused by a Gram-positive, non-acid-fast facultative anaerobic actinomycete—*Dermatophilus congolensis*
• Skin damage and moisture seem to be the 2 most important factors required for an infection to occur. Skin damage allows colonization while moisture is important to promote growth of the organism
• Biting flies and ticks may spread the disease as well as fomites. Crusts, whether on the horse or in the environment, are infectious

DIAGNOSIS

DIFFERENTIAL DIAGNOSIS
• Differential diagnoses depend on the distribution of the lesions. If the lesions are truncal, consider dermatophytosis, pemphigus foliaceus, demodicosis, staphylococcal folliculitis, and drug reactions
• If only pastern involvement, then staphylococcal folliculitis/furunculosis, dermatophytosis, *Chorioptes* infestation, trombiculosis, irritant or allergic contact dermatitis, photosensitization, and vasculitis need to be ruled out
• If limited to the white areas of the body, consider photosensitization due to liver disease, plant poisoning, or sunburn

CBC/BIOCHEMISTRY/URINALYSIS
Generally, not of value.

DIAGNOSTIC PROCEDURES
• The distribution and types of lesions present are used to establish the diagnosis
• Cytology of exudate and/or crust should be stained with a modified Wright's stain (Diff-Quik). Cytology collected by impression smears from a lesion in which the crust has been removed, and from the underside of a moist crust, is most rewarding
• *Dermatophilus* are cocci that form parallel rows within branching filaments ("railroad tracks"). Detection of the organism from chronic lesions is challenging

TREATMENT
• Be cognizant of the infectious and zoonotic potential of the crusts. Wear gloves when bathing the horse and when handling the crusts. Dispose of crusts in a trash bag; do not discarded into the environment
• *Essential* components to treatment:
  1. Keep the horse and its environment clean and dry
  2. Gentle removal of the crusts after soaking with antibacterial shampoo

MEDICATIONS

DRUG(S) OF CHOICE
• Topical therapy and establishing good management practices may be all that are needed

• Bathe with a shampoo that has antimicrobial properties every 1–2 days until the lesions are healed (typically 10–14 days). Allow shampoo contact time of 10–15 min before rinsing
• If bathing is not possible and the lesions are focal, 2–4% chlorhexidine, accelerated hydrogen peroxide, benzoyl peroxide sprays, wipes, mousses, or lotions may be used

CONTRAINDICATIONS/POSSIBLE INTERACTIONS
None

FOLLOW-UP

PATIENT MONITORING
Clinical appearance.

PREVENTION/AVOIDANCE
• Management changes—control flies, keep the environment dry
• If the horse is boarded, tell the stable manager of the diagnosis so appropriate recommendations and modifications are made
• Bacteria can survive in the environment for several years

POSSIBLE COMPLICATIONS
None

EXPECTED COURSE AND PROGNOSIS
• Many cases are self-limiting once environmental factors are corrected
• Excellent prognosis

MISCELLANEOUS

ASSOCIATED CONDITIONS
• Chronic infections may be associated with poor nutrition, heavy parasite infestation, viral diseases, or neoplasia
• In some cases, white-haired areas are more severely affected. Infection with *Dermatophilus* may result in a secondary photodermatitis

ZOONOTIC POTENTIAL
Dermatophilus congolensis is a zoonotic disease.

SEE ALSO
• Atopic dermatitis
• Bacterial dermatitis–methicillin-resistant staphylococci
• Pastern dermatitis
• Pemphigus foliaceus

Author Gwendolen Lorch
Consulting Editor Gwendolen Lorch
Acknowledgment The author/editor acknowledges the prior contribution of Paul B. Bloom.

DIAPHRAGMATIC HERNIA

BASICS

OVERVIEW
• Herniation of abdominal viscera into the thoracic cavity through a diaphragmatic defect
• Diaphragmatic hernia generally results in simple or strangulated obstruction of the herniated GI viscera and in hypoventilation

SIGNALMENT
• No sex or breed predilection
• Most frequently observed in adult horses

SIGNS
• Abdominal pain, which may vary from mild, intermittent episodes of colic to severe, intractable pain
• Alteration in respiration, which may vary from exercise intolerance, to tachypnea, to respiratory distress depending on the degree of decrease in thoracic volume
• Clinical signs suggestive of hypovolemic shock, such as blanched mucous membranes, tachycardia, and collapse, may be observed when severe hemorrhage occurs in the abdominal or thoracic cavity

CAUSES AND RISK FACTORS
• Diaphragmatic defects may be either congenital or acquired
• Congenital defect results from incomplete fusion of the pleuroperitoneal folds, causing an enlarged esophageal hiatus
• Acquired defects result from sudden increases in intrathoracic or intra-abdominal pressure. Acquired defects are usually observed after external trauma, strenuous exercise, GI distention, or pregnancy

DIAGNOSIS

DIFFERENTIAL DIAGNOSIS
• All disorders resulting in acute abdominal pain in the horse
• Pneumonia and pleuritis. Horses with diaphragmatic hernias usually are not pyrexic, are not depressed, and do not have inflammatory leukograms
• Horses with diaphragmatic hernia may be exercise intolerant

CBC/BIOCHEMISTRY/URINALYSIS
Usually normal.

OTHER LABORATORY TESTS
Blood gas analysis may reveal hypercapnia. Respiratory acidosis or uncompensated metabolic acidosis is usually observed in horses with diaphragmatic hernia. The

hypercapnia observed in horses with diaphragmatic hernia is associated with hypoventilation due to either thoracic pain and/or reduction of thoracic volume.

IMAGING
• Thoracic radiography—standing lateral thoracic radiography is used to confirm a diagnosis of diaphragmatic hernia. Radiographic signs include gas-filled loops of intestines in the thoracic cavity, increased ventral thoracic density, and absence of the cardiac shadow. The most consistent radiographic sign is loss of the diaphragmatic shadow in the area of the hernia
• Thoracic ultrasonography—reveals the presence of pleural fluid and of abdominal viscera in the thoracic cavity

OTHER DIAGNOSTIC PROCEDURES
• Auscultation of the thorax of horses with diaphragmatic hernia reveals regions of thoracic dullness or reduced cardiac sounds on the involved side of the thorax. Referred GI sounds are frequently heard over the caudoventral thorax in normal horses
• Abdominal paracentesis usually yields a normal abdominal fluid; however, in the case of an acute acquired diaphragm defect, abundant hemorrhagic fluid may be obtained
• ECG may reveal decreased amplitudes of the QRS complex

TREATMENT
• Emergency exploratory celiotomy is performed under general anesthesia with assisted positive-pressure ventilator. Surgical treatment consists of reduction of the herniated viscera, resection of devitalized intestine, and intestinal anastomosis. Repair of the diaphragmatic defect is not always possible and may require a second procedure
• In horses with acute diaphragmatic defects secondary to trauma, surgery may be delayed if the animal's condition is stable. Delay allows development of fibrosis of the edges of the defect and easier surgical closure
• Preoperative fluid volume replacement therapy is accomplished with administration of lactated Ringer's solution at a rate of 3–6 mL/kg/h

MEDICATIONS

DRUG(S) OF CHOICE
Preoperative and postoperative medications consist of systemic antibiotics (sodium

penicillin G 20 000 IU/kg IV every 6 h and gentamicin sulfate 6.6 mg/kg IV every 24 h) and NSAIDs (flunixin meglumine 1 mg/kg IV BID).

CONTRAINDICATIONS/POSSIBLE INTERACTIONS
α_2-Agonist agents, such as xylazine, detomidine, and romifidine, should be used with caution because these drugs have depressive effects in both the cardiovascular and respiratory functions.

FOLLOW-UP
• Postsurgical monitoring for the development of pneumothorax or pleural effusion
• Restrict exercise for 90 days after the surgical correction of the hernia
• Prognosis for survival of horses with diaphragmatic hernia is poor to guarded

MISCELLANEOUS

SEE ALSO
• Expiratory dyspnea
• Inspiratory dyspnea
• Pleuropneumonia
• Thoracic trauma

ABBREVIATIONS
• GI = gastrointestinal
• NSAID = nonsteroidal anti-inflammatory drug

Suggested Reading
Bristol DG. Diaphragmatic hernias in horses and cattle. Comp Cont Educ Pract 1986;8:S407–S412.
Bryant JE, Sanchez LC, Rameriz S, Bleyaert H. What is your diagnosis? Herniation of the intestines into the caudal region of the thorax. J Am Vet Med Assoc 2002;15:1461–1462.
Malone ED, Farnsworth K, Lennox T, et al. Thoracoscopic-assisted diaphragmatic hernia repair using a thoracic rib resection. Vet Surg 2001;30:175–178.

Author Ludovic P. Bouré
Consulting Editors Daniel Jean and Mathilde Leclère

BASICS

DEFINITION
• Diarrhea—increased volume and fluid content of feces, usually associated with abnormally frequent defecation
• Neonatal foal—a foal <28 days of age

PATHOPHYSIOLOGY
• Diarrhea results in loss of water and electrolytes due to increased secretion, reduced absorption, increased luminal osmolality, and altered GI transit time. Loss of disaccharidase activity (lactase) secondary to destruction of enterocytes causes maldigestion of milk sugars and subsequent osmotic diarrhea
• Bacterial toxins can cause intestinal inflammation, leading to maldigestion and malabsorption
• Small intestinal disease (enteritis), colonic disease (colitis), or a combination of both can cause diarrhea in foals
• Loss of large volumes of electrolyte-rich fluid can lead to electrolyte, fluid, and acid–base derangements
• Loss of enteric barrier function can allow absorption of enteric toxins or translocation of enteric bacteria with subsequent septicemia and multiple organ dysfunction
• Intestinal ischemia or hypoxia from hypoperfusion or acute anemia can initially result in noninfectious diarrhea that could lead to septicemia due to bacterial translocation from a breach of the intestinal barrier

SYSTEMS AFFECTED
• GI—as described earlier
• Cardiovascular—hypovolemic shock and tissue hypoperfusion; toxemia, inflammatory cytokines, electrolyte derangements, and ischemia can lead to myocardial dysfunction
• Renal—hypovolemia, reduced renal perfusion, and toxemia can cause prerenal or renal azotemia, and subsequent renal injury
• Nervous—electrolyte derangements (e.g. hyponatremia) and hypoglycemia could lead to neurologic signs, including depression and seizures; meningitis from bacterial (e.g. *Salmonella* spp., *Escherichia coli*) translocation

GENETICS
No genetic predisposition is recognized with the exception of Arabian foals with SCID.

INCIDENCE/PREVALENCE
• Common disease of foals
• 25% of foals 0–7 days of age, 40% at 8–31 days of age, and 8% at 32–180 days of age have diarrhea at some point
• Case fatality rate is low (~3%)

GEOGRAPHIC DISTRIBUTION
N/A

SIGNALMENT
Breed Predilections
N/A

Mean Age and Range
Sepsis-related diarrhea is most often seen in foals <2 weeks of age. Diarrhea due to viral infection or other causes is most commonly seen in foals <1 month of age.

Predominant Sex
None

SIGNS
Historical Findings
• Often acute onset but can become chronic. Some foals have mild diarrhea but are otherwise well
• More than 1 foal may be affected
• Determine dietary history, deworming history, history of diarrhea in neonatal foals, housing and management practices, medications administered, pregnancy history including premature lactation

Physical Examination Findings
• Early on foals are bright, alert, and responsive with normal vital signs. Depending on the etiologic agent, disease can progress rapidly to dehydration, hypovolemia, depression, and recumbency
• Consistency of diarrhea can vary from pasty to watery, and color of feces can vary from yellow to red/bloody
• Severely ill foals may show signs of colic, abdominal distention, and/or tenesmus, often before onset of diarrhea
• Rectal temperature can be normal, low, or high. Cold extremities and hypothermia are consistent with severe disease. Entropion may develop in severely dehydrated foals
• Signs of hypovolemia include depression, tachycardia, weak peripheral pulse, and cold extremities

CAUSES
Infectious and Parasitic Causes
• Most foals with diarrhea do not have a definitive diagnosis. Rule out infectious disease when there is more than 1 foal at risk
• Bacterial—e.g. *Salmonella* spp., other Gram-negative sepsis/endotoxemia, *Clostridium* (*difficile, perfringens* type C), *Rhodococcus equi* (usually >3 weeks of age)
• Viral—common: rotavirus; rare: adenovirus, coronavirus
• Protozoal—e.g. *Cryptosporidium* spp.
• Parasitic—e.g. *Strongyloides westeri* and *Parascaris equorum*

Noninfectious Causes
• Foal heat diarrhea—self-limiting in foals during the first 2 weeks of life
• Antibiotic induced
• Lactose intolerance—secondary to intestinal hypoxia or infectious diarrhea
• Cathartics—overdosing of magnesium sulfate, dioctyl sodium sulfosuccinate, mineral oil

RISK FACTORS
• Mare—short or prolonged gestation, placental disorders, dystocia, maternal diseases
• Foal—failure of transfer of passive immunity, prematurity/dysmaturity, neonatal maladjustment syndrome, hypoxia (isoerythrolysis, pneumonia)
• Environment—poor farm management, inadequate hygiene, presence of pathogenic organisms

DIAGNOSIS

DIFFERENTIAL DIAGNOSIS
• Non-diarrheal colic
• Peritonitis
• Uroperitoneum

CBC/BIOCHEMISTRY/URINALYSIS
• Mildly affected, clinically stable foals often have normal hemogram and biochemistry values
• Sick foals are often leukopenic with neutropenia
• Hypoproteinemia, depending on the cause
• Acidemia, hyperlactatemia, hyponatremia, hypochloremia, and hypoglycemia are common in symptomatic foals
• Azotemia—prerenal or renal origin
• Often foals with diarrhea have inadequate serum concentrations of IgG

OTHER LABORATORY TESTS
Infectious Causes
• Bacterial culture of feces and/or blood
• Immunoassays or molecular testing for pathogenic *Clostridium* spp. or clostridial toxins
• Immunofluorescence assay for *Cryptosporidium* spp. and *Giardia* spp.
• Immunoassay or electron microscopy for rotavirus
• Fecal floatation for nematode parasites

Noninfectious Causes
• Lactose absorption test—rarely necessary
• Test feeding of lactose-free cow's milk or oral supplementation with lactase—improvement of diarrhea in 24–48 h in lactose-intolerant foals

IMAGING
Abdominal Ultrasonography
• Distended, thickened, fluid-filled small intestines and fluid-filled large intestines
• Rule out other abdominal disease such as uroperitoneum, intussusception, and intestinal accidents

OTHER DIAGNOSTIC PROCEDURES
• Measure abdominal circumference in a systematic fashion to monitor progression of distention
• Pass nasogastric tube for evidence of reflux/ileus in colicky foals

TREATMENT

APPROPRIATE HEALTH CARE
• Foals with severe diarrhea and hypovolemia require emergency inpatient intensive care management
• Less severe cases may be treated in the field, although it should be kept in mind that neonatal foals have minimal fluid and energy reserves

NURSING CARE
• Depending on the degree of dehydration, fluids may be administered IV or PO
• IV administration of lactated Ringer's solution often is sufficient
• Isotonic 2.5% dextrose in 0.45% saline can also be used
• If acidosis does not resolve with correction of volume and electrolyte deficits, give IV or oral isotonic sodium bicarbonate (1.3%)
• Dextrose solutions (2.5–5.0%) to correct hypoglycemia
• IV plasma to correct low serum IgG concentration
• Vaseline or zinc oxide around the perineum to prevent hair loss and scalding of the skin
• Ophthalmic ointment to lubricate eyes if the foal is recumbent or develops entropion

DIET
• GI rest in foals with severe diarrhea—parenteral nutrition or enteral lactose-free cow's milk
• Return foal to nursing the mare as soon as the foal can tolerate ingestion of milk
• Some foals continue to be lactose intolerant after resolution of infectious cause of the diarrhea. Some of these foals have resolution of diarrhea when fed lactose-free cow's milk and may benefit from lactase supplementation (3000–6000 units PO every 6–8 h)

MEDICATIONS

DRUG(S) OF CHOICE
Broad-Spectrum Antimicrobial Therapy
• Penicillin (e.g. potassium penicillin (22 000 IU/kg IV every 6 h)) in combination with an aminoglycoside (e.g. amikacin (25 mg/kg IV every 24 h)), or a third-generation cephalosporin (ceftiofur sodium (4.4–8.8 mg/kg IV every 12 h)) may be indicated in foals with suspected primary or secondary bacterial enteritis or evidence of septicemia
• With suspected clostridial enteritis, metronidazole (10–15 mg/kg PO or IV every 8 h) is recommended

Intestinal Protectants
Products containing smectite, activated charcoal, or bismuth subsalicylate are often administered to foals with diarrhea. There is no objective in vivo evidence of efficacy in foals.

Antispasmodic Drugs
Use motility-altering agents with caution.

Probiotics
Probiotics are available for use in foals. Their efficacy is unproved, and in fact routine administration might be associated with increased risk of diarrhea.

CONTRAINDICATIONS
• Avoid oral antimicrobials, particularly those associated with inducing diarrhea (e.g. erythromycin)
• Avoid enteral nutrition in foals with severe diarrhea exacerbated by feeding (e.g. rotaviral diarrhea)

FOLLOW-UP

PATIENT MONITORING
• Foals can deteriorate rapidly and require intensive care
• Monitor attitude, appetite, fecal color and consistency, hydration status, and abdominal distention several times daily. Use laboratory data as clinically indicated, especially indicators of acid–base status, renal function, and serum electrolyte concentrations
• Monitor other foals for signs of diarrhea or colic

PREVENTION/AVOIDANCE
• Implement isolation protocols to control/prevent the spread of possible infectious agents
• If there is an outbreak of diarrhea due to *Salmonella* spp., institute a program of strict hygiene including washing the udder and perineum of prepartum mares immediately
• There are no vaccinations available for the common pathogens causing diarrhea in foals
• On farms that experience outbreaks of clostridial enteritis in foals, prophylaxis with metronidazole (10 mg/kg PO every 8–12 h for the first 4 days of life) might provide some protection against disease

POSSIBLE COMPLICATIONS
• Sepsis
• Intussusception
• Hypovolemic shock
• Septic peritonitis
• Septic arthritis
• Septic physitis/osteomyelitis
• Gastric ulceration

EXPECTED COURSE AND PROGNOSIS
• Prognosis for foals with rotavirus diarrhea is excellent
• Diarrhea due to *Salmonella* spp. or *Clostridium* spp. or complicated by septicemia has a guarded prognosis. Regardless of etiologic agent, severe hypothermia and cold extremities are associated with a poor outcome

MISCELLANEOUS

ASSOCIATED CONDITIONS
• Septicemia
• SCID
• Peritonitis
• Gastric ulceration

AGE-RELATED FACTORS
• Foals often develop a non-life-threatening diarrhea at 5–10 days of age (foal heat diarrhea)
• High index of suspicion for clostridial enterocolitis in foals with hemorrhagic diarrhea < 1 week of age

ZOONOTIC POTENTIAL
• *Salmonella* spp.
• *Cryptosporidium* spp.

SYNONYMS
Scours

SEE ALSO
• Colic in foals
• Fluid therapy, neonate
• Gastric ulcers, neonate

ABBREVIATIONS
• GI = gastrointestinal
• IgG = immunoglobulin G
• SCID = severe combined immunodeficiency disease

Suggested Reading
Constable PD, Hinchcliff KW, Done SH, Grunberg W. Veterinary Medicine: A Textbook of the Diseases of Cattle, Horses, Sheep, Goats and Pigs, 11e. St. Louis: Elsevier, 2017:273–276.
Magdesian KG. Neonatal foal diarrhea. Vet Clin North Am Equine Pract 2005;21:295–312.

Author Ramiro Toribio
Consulting Editor Margaret C. Mudge
Acknowledgment The author and editor acknowledge the prior contribution of Kenneth W. Hinchcliff.

DICOUMAROL (MOLDY SWEET CLOVER) TOXICOSIS

BASICS

OVERVIEW
- Sweet clover has erect stems and leaves divided into 3 segments and spikes of flowers, white or yellow, that give off a sweet odor when crushed
- Grows in moist soils throughout the USA and Canada and can reach 1.8–2.4 m (6–8 feet) high
- Sweet clover may be grown for hay or become a weed invading pastures and roadsides
- Ingestion of moldy sweet clover hay interferes with normal blood clotting in horses
- Sweet clovers (*Melilotus alba, M. officinalis*) and sweet vernal (*Anthoxanthum odoratum*) contain the nontoxic compound coumarin. When cut and baled for hay under high moisture conditions, various molds (*Penicillium* spp., *Aspergillus* spp., and others) metabolize coumarin to form dicoumarol, which leads to bleeding
- Dicoumarol in hay >20 ppm suggests potential toxicity problems; most toxicoses in livestock are reported at levels >30 ppm. Prolonged consumption of moldy hay at 10 ppm can cause clinical signs

SIGNALMENT
- All animals
- More common in cattle because horses rarely eat moldy sweet clover hay

SIGNS
- Bleeding diathesis, ranging from mild to severe
- Generally, horses show symptoms within 3–8 weeks after initial ingestion
- Hemorrhage may be internal or external—epistaxis; fecal blood
- Swellings may appear over bony protuberances of the body because of bruising and hematoma formation
- Lameness can result from hemorrhage into joint capsules and soreness may result from muscle hematomas
- Profuse hemorrhage can occur during minor surgical procedures or during parturition
- Symptoms include anemia, pale mucous membranes, weakness, abnormal heartbeat, and death
- Sudden death often is marked by massive hemorrhage into the thorax or abdominal cavity or around the brain

CAUSES AND RISK FACTORS
Dicoumarol interferes with normal blood clotting because of a reduction in the concentrations of the active forms of clotting factors II, VII, IX, and X. This results from competitive inhibition between vitamin K epoxide and dicoumarol for the enzyme vitamin K epoxide reductase, which converts inactive vitamin K epoxide back to its active vitamin K form in the body. Thus, dicoumarol causes vitamin K deficiency by inhibiting regeneration of the active form of vitamin K.

DIAGNOSIS

DIFFERENTIAL DIAGNOSIS
- Disseminated intravascular coagulation—reduced plasma concentrations of platelets and coagulant and anticoagulant proteins; increased concentrations of coagulant byproducts; petechial hemorrhages
- Severe liver disease—altered liver function tests
- Inherited deficiencies of coagulation factors—measurement of specific coagulation factors
- Immune-mediated thrombocytopenia—thrombocytopenia; petechial hemorrhages
- Anticoagulant rodenticide poisoning

CBC/BIOCHEMISTRY/URINALYSIS
Blood loss anemia.

OTHER LABORATORY TESTS
- Prolonged PT and aPTT. In horses, aPTT elevates before PT
- Chemical analysis of suspect hay for dicoumarol content
- Whole blood and/or liver tissue also may be analyzed

IMAGING
Imaging for internal bleeding.

PATHOLOGIC FINDINGS
Hemorrhages may occur in any part of the body.

TREATMENT
- Whole blood or plasma transfusions may be helpful
- Handle horses with care to avoid stress and further hemorrhaging
- Attempt correction of organ dysfunction resulting from accumulation of extravascular blood (e.g. thoracocentesis) only if life-threatening and after normal blood coagulation has been restored
- Adding alfalfa hay to the diet may help to provide a source of increased dietary vitamin K1

MEDICATIONS

DRUG(S) OF CHOICE
- Vitamin K1 (i.e. phytonadione; 1.5 mg/kg SC or IM every 12 h for up to 3 days) effectively reverses the clotting defect
- Improvement in PT after vitamin K1 therapy usually is observed within 24 h

CONTRAINDICATIONS/POSSIBLE INTERACTIONS
Do not use vitamin K3 (i.e. menadione), which is ineffective and is nephrotoxic in horses.

FOLLOW-UP

PATIENT MONITORING
Monitor for blood loss.

PREVENTION/AVOIDANCE
- Remove all moldy sweet clover hay from diet
- If hay appears moldy, or the ensilage process is in question, test hay for the presence of dicoumarol

EXPECTED COURSE AND PROGNOSIS
- Onset of clinical signs in healthy horses depends on the dicoumarol concentrations in the contaminated hay
- Prognosis is based on the severity of blood loss and damage to organ systems affected by hemorrhage

MISCELLANEOUS

PREGNANCY/FERTILITY/BREEDING
The late-term abortions observed in cattle have not been reported in horses.

SEE ALSO
Anticoagulant rodenticide toxicosis

ABBREVIATIONS
- aPTT = activated partial thromboplastin time
- PT = one-stage prothrombin time

Suggested Reading
Burrows GE, Tyrl RJ. Toxic Plants of North America, 2e. Ames, IA: Wiley Blackwell, 2013:582–586.
Knight AP. Plant Poisoning of Horses. In: Lewis LD, ed. Equine Clinical Nutrition: Feeding and Care. Baltimore, MD: Williams and Wilkins, 1995:481–482.

Author Charlotte Means
Consulting Editors Wilson K. Rumbeiha and Steve Ensley
Acknowledgment The author and editors acknowledge the prior contribution of Anita M. Kore.

DISEASES OF THE EQUINE NICTITANS

D

BASICS

DEFINITION
The nictitating membrane consists of a T-shaped cartilage with a seromucoid gland located at its base. This gland secretes a significant portion of the aqueous tear film. The nictitans is covered on both the palpebral and bulbar surfaces with conjunctiva, and diseases affecting the conjunctiva can also involve the nictitans. Movement of the nictitans distributes the tear film and protects the cornea. Protrusion of the nictitating membrane is passive in horses and occurs secondary to retraction of the globe into the orbit mediated by cranial nerve VI (abducens) contraction of the retractor bulbi muscle. Sympathetic innervation to the smooth muscles of the periorbital and Müller's muscles of the upper and lower eyelids keeps these muscles contracted for slight protrusion of the eye and an open palpebral fissure. Horner syndrome refers to sympathetic denervation, which results in passive elevation of the nictitans in addition to other clinical signs.

PATHOPHYSIOLOGY
• Protrusion of the nictitating membrane is usually a nonspecific sign of pain. Ocular diseases often result in ocular pain, enophthalmos, and secondary nictitans protrusion. Systemic disease can also cause nictitans protrusion
• Horner syndrome can be a result of central, preganglionic, or postganglionic lesions along the pathway of sympathetic innervation to the eye. Subsequent oculosympathetic paralysis is reflected in the loss of sympathetically mediated functions
• Tetanus may be a complication of elective surgery or accidental wounds. Contamination of wounds by *Clostridium tetani* and the subsequent production of a neurotoxin results in the classic "sawhorse stance" and elevated third eyelids
• HYPP attacks can involve protrusion of the third eyelid due to involuntary muscle contraction along with generalized muscle tremors and weakness

SYSTEMS AFFECTED
Ophthalmic

GENETICS
• Breed predilection for ocular SCC suggests a genetic influence
• HYPP is a dominant disorder caused by a known genetic defect for which a test is available

INCIDENCE/PREVALENCE
Common

GEOGRAPHIC DISTRIBUTION
None established.

SIGNALMENT
• No detected age distribution of Horner syndrome or protrusion of the nictitans. Ocular SCC prevalence increases with age
• There are no breed predilections for Horner syndrome
• HYPP is an inherited disease and is seen most commonly in Quarter Horses
• SCC, the most common neoplasm affecting the equine nictitans, has a high prevalence in draft horses, Appaloosas, and Paints

SIGNS
• Protrusion of the nictitating membrane, conjunctival hyperemia, chemosis, follicle development, ocular discharge
• Horner syndrome—ptosis, nictitans protrusion, slight miosis, hyperemia of nasal and conjunctival mucosa, increased temperature, and sweating of base of ear, side of face, and neck of affected side
• SCC may have different appearances—proliferative/ulcerated or thickening/ulceration of tissue
• Habronemiasis—granulomas, nodules, yellow caseous exudate, and necrotic mineralized tissue. May be ulcerated
• Tetanus causes bilateral protrusion of the nictitans, spasms of the masseter muscles, stiff gait, and increased sensitivity to external stimulation

CAUSES
Protrusion
• Ocular pain
• Horner syndrome
• Tetanus
• Enophthalmos
• Space-occupying mass in orbit
• Loss of orbital mass—starvation, dehydration
• Decreased ocular mass—microphthalmos, phthisis bulbi
• Secondary to systemic disease—hyperkalemic periodic paralysis
• Retrobulbar fat prolapse—optical illusion of protrusion
• Congenital lack of pigmentation on leading edge—optical illusion of protrusion

Change in color or texture
• Neoplasia—SCC most common
• Secondary to environmental causes—foreign bodies and debris, trauma
• Inflammation—bacterial, parasitic (habronemiasis), trauma

RISK FACTORS
• White, chestnut, and palomino coat color predisposes to SCC
• Warm weather, climates with heavy fly population are a risk factor for habronemiasis
• Deficit vaccination programs increase the risk of tetanus

DIAGNOSIS

DIFFERENTIAL DIAGNOSIS
• Ocular pain—ulcerative keratitis, corneal stromal abscess, anterior uveitis, keratomycosis, corneal laceration, conjunctivitis
• Horner syndrome—jugular vein and carotid artery injections, cervical abscesses, guttural pouch infections, neoplasia of neck and thoracic inlet, trauma to neck and thorax, mediastinal and thoracic masses
• Nodular/mass lesions of nictitans—SCC, habronemiasis, mastocytoma, hemangioma, hemangiosarcoma, papilloma, fungal granulomas, nodular necrobiosis, foreign body reaction, retrobulbar fat prolapse
• Space-occupying mass in orbit—neoplasia, abscess, hematoma, arteriovenous fistula

CBC/BIOCHEMISTRY/URINALYSIS
Results usually normal unless nictitans disease associated with systemic disease.

OTHER LABORATORY TESTS
• Habronemiasis—conjunctival scraping reveals eosinophils, mast cells, neutrophils, plasma cells, rarely larvae. Biopsy and histopathology for mass lesions
• Consider culture and susceptibility if suspect bacterial involvement
• Other specific tests as indicated when systemic disease suspected

IMAGING
N/A

OTHER DIAGNOSTIC PROCEDURES
• Complete ophthalmic examination to identify ocular causes of nictitans disease. Fluorescein stain and examination for signs of anterior uveitis (aqueous flare, miosis, hypotony). Examination behind nictitans may reveal foreign body, debris
• Pharmacologic testing to differentiate between central/preganglionic and postganglionic lesions in Horner syndrome has not been critically evaluated in horses. Topical application of 1% phenylephrine or 0.1% epinephrine—rapid mydriasis within 20 min indicates a postganglionic lesion, slow mydriasis within 30–40 min indicates a preganglionic lesion. Topical application of 0.1% pilocarpine—rapid miosis within 20 min indicates postganglionic lesion, no miosis indicates preganglionic lesion
• Testing for HYPP if history is compatible with this disease

PATHOLOGIC FINDINGS
• Habronemiasis—eosinophils, mast cells, neutrophils, plasma cells, rarely larvae
• SCC—epithelial cells with neoplastic characteristics
• Lymphoma—large population monomorphic lymphocytes with neoplastic characteristics

• Other histopathologic findings possible depending on type of neoplasia present

TREATMENT

APPROPRIATE HEALTH CARE
• Most horses with nictitans protrusion or Horner syndrome can be treated on an outpatient basis
• Treatment of some ocular (severe ulcerative keratitis, corneal stromal abscess, keratomycosis, SCC) and systemic (tetanus, severe hyperkalemic periodic paralysis) diseases associated with secondary nictitans involvement may require hospitalization

NURSING CARE
Ensure topical medications can be administered appropriately.

ACTIVITY
• If environmental irritation is suspected, then exposure to the inciting substance should be restricted or eliminated
• Animals with ocular involvement/disease should not be ridden if visual status is compromised
• Animals affected with tetanus should be kept in a quiet, dark environment

DIET
No change in diet is necessary except for HYPP. Hay should be fed at ground level rather than elevated hay racks or bags if ocular disease is present.

CLIENT EDUCATION
• If there is evidence of self-trauma when ocular disease is present, a protective hood covering the affected eye should be employed. The client should be instructed to contact the veterinarian if the condition worsens in any way
• If hyperkalemic periodic paralysis is identified, the client should be informed of the genetic basis of the disease and advised against breeding the affected animal

SURGICAL CONSIDERATIONS
• SCC is treated by surgical resection of the nictitans. Enucleation or exenteration may be necessary depending on the type of neoplasia and extent of invasion of surrounding tissue
• Foreign bodies and debris of the nictitating membrane can usually be removed with topical anesthesia and liberal flushing of conjunctival fornices

• Thorough wound lavage and debridement is necessary in cases of tetanus

MEDICATIONS

DRUG(S) OF CHOICE
• Habronemiasis—topical 0.03% echothiophate (ecothiopate) iodide (phospholine iodide) and ophthalmic neomycin/polymyxin B with dexamethasone BID. Multifocal lesions—oral avermectin. Intralesional triamcinolone (10–40 mg) may reduce size of granulomas
• Bacterial inflammation—topical broad-spectrum antibiotic initially (every 4–8 h), may change after results of bacterial culture and susceptibility
• SCC—see chapter Ocular/adnexal squamous cell carcinoma
• Other systemic medication as indicated by concurrent systemic disease

CONTRAINDICATIONS
Intralesional triamcinolone in a horse with laminitis or pituitary pars intermedia dysfunction.

FOLLOW-UP

PATIENT MONITORING
The patient should be rechecked soon after beginning therapy (3–4 days), with the specific time frame determined by disease and severity. Subsequent rechecks are dictated by severity of disease and response to treatment.

PREVENTION/AVOIDANCE
• Fly control in barns and pastures, fly hoods, frequent periocular administration of insect repellant, and regular deworming with avermectins can help prevent the development of habronemiasis
• Treat any underlying ocular or systemic disease which may be inciting the nictitans disease

POSSIBLE COMPLICATIONS
Potential complications of neoplasia of the nictitans and its treatment vary with the specific type of tumor, but include recurrence and metastasis.

EXPECTED COURSE AND PROGNOSIS
• Course and prognosis of nictitating membrane neoplasia depend on the specific

type of neoplasia and the extent of invasion of surrounding tissues
• Horner syndrome may be reversible depending on the cause. Resolution of cervical abscesses, perivenous injections, and guttural pouch disease may resolve associated Horner syndrome. Neoplastic and traumatic causes are less likely to be correctable
• Prognosis associated with nictitans protrusion secondary to systemic or ocular disease varies with the specific disease
• Tetanus is a life-threatening disease with a prolonged recovery phase and intensive supportive care

MISCELLANEOUS

AGE-RELATED FACTORS
N/A

ZOONOTIC POTENTIAL
N/A

PREGNANCY/FERTILITY/BREEDING
Systemic absorption of topically applied medication is possible. Benefits of treatment should be considered against any risks posed to the fetus.

SYNONYMS
N/A

SEE ALSO
• Conjunctival diseases
• Corneal ulceration
• Hyperkalemic periodic paralysis
• Ocular/adnexal squamous cell carcinoma
• Tetanus

ABBREVIATIONS
• HYPP = hyperkalemic periodic paralysis
• SCC = squamous cell carcinoma

Suggested Reading
Brooks DE. Ophthalmology for the Equine Practitioner, 2e. Jackson, WY: Teton NewMedia, 2008.
Gilger BC. Equine ophthalmology. In: Gelatt KN, Gilger BC, Kern TJ, eds. Veterinary Ophthalmology, 5e. Wiley Blackwell, 2013:1560–1609.
Gilger BC. Equine Ophthalmology, 3e. Ames, IA: Wiley Blackwell, 2017.

Author Caroline Monk
Consulting Editor Caryn E. Plummer
Acknowledgment The author and editor acknowledge the prior contribution of Heidi M. Denis and Dennis E. Brooks.

DISORDERS OF SEXUAL DEVELOPMENT

 BASICS

DEFINITION
- Sexual differentiation occurs sequentially at 3 levels:
  - Genetic/chromosomal
  - Gonadal
  - Phenotypic
- Errors at any level lead to varying degrees of genital ambiguity and aberrant reproductive function
  - Affected animals are known as intersexes or as particular classes of hermaphrodites
  - Hermaphrodites/intersex—both testicular and ovarian tissue is present
  - Pseudohermaphrodites—further divided into male and female pseudohermaphrodites. Genetic and gonadal sex agree, however there is ambiguous genitalia. Division is dependent on the gonadal tissue present

PATHOPHYSIOLOGY
- Genetic sex is established at fertilization
- Gonadal sex is controlled by genetic sex determination
- Phenotypic sex is governed by gonadal function and target-organ sensitivity
  - The zygote contains either an XX (female) or XY (male) complement of sex chromosomes
  - The presence of a Y chromosome dictates development of testicular tissue and a male phenotype
  - The sex-determining region of the Y chromosome is a gene (*Sry*) responsible for the initiation of testicular development, regardless of the number of X chromosomes present
  - There is no corresponding gene directing female development

Disorders of Genetic Sex
- *Sex chromosomes*
  - Abnormal number (aneuploidy)
  - Abnormal structure (deletion, duplication/insertion, reciprocal exchange, fusion, inversion)
- *Chimeras*—individual with coexisting, genetically distinct cell populations admixed in utero. Rare in horses due to separate placentation and uncommon delivery of twins. Fertilization of single ovum by multiple spermatozoa theoretically possible
- *Mosaics*—individual with coexisting, genetically distinct cell populations caused by errors in chromosomal segregation during division of a single genetic source. Nondisjunction of paired chromosomes during mitosis is implicated: abnormal sexual development occurs when sex chromosomes affected. Sexual differentiation may be ambiguous
- Normality of genetic sex development depends on chromosomal pairings during gametogenesis and fertilization

- 63,XO, monosomy X (most common). Either a normal ovum (X containing) fuses with a sperm lacking sex chromosome or an X-bearing sperm fertilizes ovum lacking X chromosome
  - Ovarian dysgenesis, infantile tubular genitalia, small stature, reduced athletic potential, lack of cervical and uterine tone, follicular activity is curtailed, with degeneration occurring during development, phenotypic female; similar to Turner syndrome in humans
- 65,XXY. Either an XY-containing sperm fuses with a normal oocyte or a Y-bearing sperm fuses with an abnormal XX oocyte
  - Hypoplastic testes, genitalia normal to hypoplastic, testes may be scrotal or retained, all infertile, phenotypic male; similar to Klinefelter syndrome in humans
- 65,XXX. Either an XX-containing sperm fuses with a normal oocyte or an X-bearing sperm fuses with an abnormal XX oocyte
  - Gonadal dysgenesis, infertility, external appearance is most often indistinguishable from a normal mare
- Numerous possible combinations (mixoploidies) are reported, as are deletions of sections (arms) of the sex chromosomes

Disorders of Gonadal Sex
- *Sex reversal syndromes*—gonadal and genetic sex may disagree because of autosomal recessive genes or translocation of TDF to X chromosomes. Karyotype is normal
- XY with no testes; instead hypoplastic ovary/streak gonad forms with degenerate follicles/oocytes; acyclic, sterile; female phenotype, therefore classified as XY female
- XX with varying degrees of testicular development, the extreme form is XX male with bilateral testicular development; otherwise, a true hermaphrodite forms with ovotestes
- True hermaphrodite with ovotestes, ambiguous genitalia; named by genetic makeup, either XX or XY
- The presence or absence of an active *Sry* gene determines the outcome of the reversal
- In the absence of testosterone or anti-Müllerian hormone, a phenotypic female develops

Disorders of Phenotypic Sex
- Phenotypic sex development involves differentiation of tubular genitalia (mesonephric and paramesonephric ducts) and external genitalia under direction of the gonad
- Male reproductive tract—gonad must produce testosterone (Leydig cells) and Müllerian-inhibitory substance (Sertoli cells) at correct time
- Degree of masculinization of external genitalia relates to the proportion of testicular tissue and hence testosterone production of the intersex gonad
- Target organ (duct system) must have cytosolic receptors for testosterone and

enzyme 5α-reductase to produce dihydrotestosterone, the androgen responsible for tubular and external genitalia differentiation
- Hypospadias—urethra opens ventrally on penis
- Epispadias—urethra opens dorsally on penis
- Hermaphrodite/intersex—genetic mosaic, both XX and XY present. Alternatively, *Sry* translocation to X chromosome. The gonad is an ovotestis, with components of both ovaries and testes. External genitalia is ambiguous
- Pseudohermaphrodite—named by the gonadal tissue present; male, testes; female, ovary. Gonadal tissue is either testicular or ovarian, there is no combination. Genetic and gonadal sex are in agreement; ambiguous external genitalia are present
- Testicular feminization—genetic and gonadal male (XY chimera, testicle) but external genitalia female; target-organ insensitivity

SYSTEMS AFFECTED
- Reproductive
- Urologic

GENETICS
See Pathophysiology.

INCIDENCE/PREVALENCE
N/A

SIGNALMENT
- Congenital disorder
- Normal external genitalia may delay detection of the problem until the affected individual enters a breeding program

SIGNS
Historical Findings
- Infertility; sterility
- Failure to display appropriate reproductive behavior with opposite sex; attraction to same sex
  - In females, apparent estrus behavior but lack of standing for mounting. Ovarian inactivity during breeding season
  - In males, normal libido, however ejaculate consistently azoospermic

Physical Examination Findings
External
- Female—normal or hypoplastic vulva; enlarged clitoris; presence of os clitoris; purulent vulvar discharge
- Male—penis, prepuce normal or hypoplastic; testes, scrotal or cryptorchid; hypospadias, epispadias (abnormal position of urinary orifice, closure of urethra)
Internal
- Abnormal gonadal position (cryptorchid), form (hypoplastic, fibrous), or type (ovotestis)
- Aberrant ductal derivatives—aplasia, hypoplasia, or cysts

CAUSES
- Congenital—heritable or spontaneous genetic abnormalities

- Genetic abnormalities—zygote fusion, abnormal sex chromosome number or structure
- Transfer of TDF to autosomal chromosome or X chromosome
- Placental admixture not reported in equines due to separate vascularity (contrast bovine freemartinism)
- Exogenous—steroid hormone use during pregnancy
- Progestins, androgens—masculinize females
- Estrogens, antiandrogens—feminize males

RISK FACTORS
N/A

DIAGNOSIS

DIFFERENTIAL DIAGNOSIS
If phenotypically normal:
- Infectious infertility
- Noninfectious infertility—female, ovarian degeneration, endometrial degeneration; male, testicular hypoplasia or degeneration

CBC/BIOCHEMISTRY/URINALYSIS
Unremarkable, unless cystitis or infection results from aberrant genital structure.

OTHER LABORATORY TESTS
Hormonal Assays
Testosterone
- Testosterone in XY mares correlates with phenotype and behavior
- hCG challenge—baseline blood sample; administer 3000 IU hCG; additional blood samples at 3 and 24 h
- An increase in testosterone indicates testicular tissue is present, Leydig cell production
Estrone Sulfate
- Source in male is the testicles, Sertoli cells
- Couple estrone sulfate test with testosterone levels (from an hCG challenge test) to improve diagnostic accuracy
Anti-Müllerian Hormone
Source in males is Sertoli cells.

Immunology
- Test for 5α-reductase or cytosolic receptor
- Use labial skin only; receptors are site specific

IMAGING
- Ultrasonography coupled with transrectal palpation; discovery of mass (neoplastic) or cyst (segmental aplasia with fluid dilations)
- Laparoscopy, laparotomy

OTHER DIAGNOSTIC PROCEDURES, PATHOLOGIC FINDINGS
- Disorders are characterized by histopathology of gonad, morphology of tubular genitalia (duct derivatives), accessory glands (male), and external genitalia (increased anogenital distance, vulval folds, blind-ended vagina)
- Karyotyping—culture of peripheral blood leukocytes and examination of metaphase spreads
  ∘ Collect whole blood in heparin or acid citrate dextrose
  ∘ Send samples unrefrigerated, by rapid courier
  ∘ Cultures require 48–72 h
- PCR
- Detection of *Sry*—whole blood in EDTA

TREATMENT

APPROPRIATE HEALTH CARE
N/A, unless resulting pathology or physical/behavioral problems develop that require gonadectomy or hysterectomy to modify behavior.

CLIENT EDUCATION
Some conditions are heritable and pedigree analysis is warranted in these cases.

SURGICAL CONSIDERATIONS
See Appropriate Health Care.

FOLLOW-UP

PATIENT MONITORING
Only if physical or behavioral complications develop.

PREVENTION/AVOIDANCE
Remove carrier animals from the breeding population; gonadectomy.

MISCELLANEOUS

ASSOCIATED CONDITIONS
If not detected early:
- Pyometra
- Cystitis
- Hematuria
- Gonadal neoplasia (intra-abdominal testis)

AGE-RELATED FACTORS
Congenital

PREGNANCY/FERTILITY/BREEDING
Fertility is rare in affected animals.

SYNONYMS
- Hermaphrodite
- Intersex
- Klinefelter syndrome, trisomy
- Mesonephric, Wolffian
- Paramesonephric, Müllerian
- Pseudohermaphrodite
- Turner syndrome, monosomy X

ABBREVIATIONS
- EDTA = ethylene diamine tetraacetic acid
- hCG = human chorionic gonadotropin
- PCR = polymerase chain reaction
- *Sry* = sex-determining region of the Y chromosome
- TDF = testis-determining factor

Suggested Reading
Bannasch D, Rinaldo C, Millon L, et al. SRY negative 64, XX intersex phenotype in an American Saddlebred horse. Equine Vet J 2007;173:437–439.
Chandley AC, Fletcher J, Rossdale PD, et al. Chromosome abnormalities as a cause of infertility in mares. J Reprod Fertil Suppl 1975;23:377–383.
Christensen BW, Meyer-Wallen VN. Sex determination and differentiation. In: McKinnon AO, Squires EL, Vaala WE, Varner DD, eds. Equine Reproduction, 2e. Ames, IA: Wiley Blackwell, 2011:2211–2221.
DeLorenzi L, Molteni L, Zannotti M, et al. X trisomy in a sterile mare. Equine Vet J 2010:469–470.
DiNapoli L, Capel B. SRY and the standoff in sex determination. Mol Endocrinol 2008;22:1–9.
Halnan CR. Equine cytogenetics—role in equine veterinary practice. Equine Vet J 1985;17:173–177.
Lear TL, Villagomez AF. Cytogenetic evaluation of mares and foals. In: McKinnon AO, Squires EL, Vaala WE, Varner DD, eds. Equine Reproduction, 2e. Ames, IA: Wiley Blackwell, 2011:1951–1962.
Meyers-Wallen VN, Hurtgen J, Schlafer D, et al. Sry XX true hermaphroditism in a Pasa Fino horse. Equine Vet J 1997;29:404–408.
Milliken JE, Paccamonti DL, Shoemaker S, Green WH. XX male pseudohermaphroditism in a horse. J Am Vet Med Assoc 1995;207:77–79.

Author Peter R. Morresey
Consulting Editor Carla L. Carleton

DISORDERS OF THE THYROID, HYPO- AND HYPERTHYROIDISM

BASICS

DEFINITION
• Once T_3 and T_4 are excreted into the circulation, >99% is bound to circulating proteins (primarily albumin)
• Protein-bound T_4 acts as a reservoir to maintain a steady supply of free T_4, which diffuses into cells, where it is deiodinated to form T_3. Similarly, the majority of circulating T_3 is protein bound, and the free T_3 is the biologically active form
• Increased amounts of T_3 and T_4 in the circulation lead to hyperthyroidism, whereas decreased amounts result in hypothyroidism. Both are pathologic conditions
• The third form of thyroid hormone in the blood is reverse T_3, which is formed from T_4 in the peripheral tissues. Concentrations of reverse T_3 decrease when there is increased production of T_3
• Goiter is an increase in thyroid size to twice its normal volume

PATHOPHYSIOLOGY
• The thyroid gland is responsible for the synthesis of the thyroid hormones T_4 and T_3. These hormones enter cells, resulting in regulation of resting metabolic rate in adult animals. In utero and in growing animals, thyroid hormones are necessary for proper bone, pulmonary, and nervous system development
• The net effect of hypothyroidism is decreased basal metabolic rate and decreased ability to respond to metabolic demands
• Horses with systemic disease can exhibit the "euthyroid sick" syndrome—circulating thyroid hormone concentrations are reduced despite the presence of a normal thyroid axis. In these instances, the decreased thyroid concentrations are a response by the diseased animal that decreases the resting metabolic rate and thus conserves energy
• Hyperthyroidism caused by either an overdose of exogenous hormone or a secreting thyroid tumor; produces an increased metabolic rate that manifests as weight loss and behavioral changes
• A wide number of factors, including, diet, fitness, disease, and drug administration, result in concentrations of thyroid hormones below the normal reference ranges. In most instances, thyroid function as measured by either the TSH or TRH response test is normal, and the horses cannot be considered hypothyroid

SYSTEMS AFFECTED
Endocrine/Metabolic
• The endocrine system is primarily affected by abnormal T_3 and T_4
• Energy metabolism is altered by hypothyroidism, and affected horses have increased serum cholesterol and metabolize lipid poorly

Musculoskeletal
• Foals affected with congenital hypothyroidism are born with underdeveloped tarsal and carpal bones, prognathism, ruptured common digital extensor tendons, and forelimb contracture
• They are often weak and need assistance to stand

Behavioral
Horses with abnormal thyroid levels may have altered behavior such as increased aggression and lethargy with hypothyroidism or nervousness and pacing with hyperthyroidism.

Cardiovascular
• Thyroidectomized horses have bradycardia, decreased cardiac output, and exercise intolerance
• Immature respiratory tract and respiratory insufficiency have been reported in hypothyroid foals

SIGNALMENT
• No sex or breed predilections for abnormal T_3/T_4 levels
• Hypothyroidism can occur at any age and exist in utero, with the foal showing characteristic signs at birth
• Iatrogenic hyperthyroidism generally occurs in adults. Thyroid tumors occur in older horses (>10 years)

SIGNS
• Hypothyroidism foals—prognathism, ruptured common digital extensor tendon, forelimb contracture, retarded ossification and crushing of the carpal and tarsal bones, weakness, and poor suckle reflex. Less common signs—goiter, angular limb deformities, respiratory distress, abdominal hernia, poor muscle development, and osteoporosis
• Hypothyroidism adults—hypothermia and bradycardia. Less common—cold intolerance, poor hair coat, and poor growth. Horses with experimentally induced hypothyroidism develop edema of the distal limbs and coarsened features
• Horses with hyperthyroidism due to a functioning tumor exhibit weight loss, pacing, and nervousness

CAUSES
• Drugs, including phenylbutazone, iodine-containing compounds, corticosteroids, and sulfa drugs, may cause low serum levels
• Ingestion of endophyte-containing fescue, high or low iodine levels, or high carbohydrate diets can decrease circulating hormone levels
• Hypothyroidism in adults is often idiopathic
• Iodine deficiency can cause hypothyroidism in horses, but this is extremely rare
• Iodine deficiency or excess in the diets of broodmares can cause hypothyroidism in their foals; ingestion of endophyte-infected fescue also can result in congenital hypothyroidism

• Training can decrease thyroid hormone levels
• In most instances, thyroid tumors are clinically silent
• Foals have increased thyroid hormone levels compared with older horses
• Very cold weather also can lead to higher thyroid hormone levels

RISK FACTORS
• Primarily dietary
• Excess or inadequate iodine or ingestion of other goitrogens can lead to hypothyroidism

DIAGNOSIS

DIFFERENTIAL DIAGNOSIS
• The primary differential diagnoses for an adult horse suspected of hypothyroidism are a pituitary tumor or insulin resistance (equine metabolic syndrome, insulin dysregulation); these horses, however, suffer from euthyroid sick syndrome. The "classic" presentation of hypothyroidism in adult horses—weight gain, laminitis, "cresty neck," and abnormal fat deposits—is now recognized as manifestations of insulin dysregulation
• Hypothyroidism can be ruled out by provocative testing with either TSH or TRH. A history of administration of a drug that decreases thyroid hormone values can explain abnormally low T_3 and T_4 levels not caused by true disease. A history of overadministration of an exogenous thyroid supplement can explain abnormally high T_3 and T_4 levels
• Differentials for foals with congenital hypothyroidism include fescue toxicosis, prematurity, angular limb deformities, and sepsis. Dietary history rules out abnormal iodine in the dam's diet. Physical examination and CBC should rule in sepsis or prematurity/dysmaturity

LABORATORY FINDINGS
Valid if Run in a Human Laboratory?
Laboratory determination of T_3, free T_3, T_4, and free T_4 is valid. Use equine reference ranges to interpret results. Free T_3 and T_4 should be determined using the equilibrium dialysis method for most accurate results.

CBC/BIOCHEMISTRY URINALYSIS
Hypothyroid horses may exhibit anemia, leukopenia, and hypercholesterolemia.

OTHER LABORATORY TESTS
To confirm the diagnosis of hypothyroidism, consider a TRH or TSH response test. TSH is currently not readily available. For a TRH stimulation test, give 1 mg TRH IV. Collect blood for T_3 and T_4 determination 0, 2, and 4 h later. One expects to see baseline T_3 and T_4 in the reference range, the T_3 to double at 2 h, and T_4 to double at 4 h.

(CONTINUED) DISORDERS OF THE THYROID, HYPO- AND HYPERTHYROIDISM

IMAGING

Ultrasonography
• Rarely useful in diagnosing hypothyroidism
• Thyroid tumor or goiter could be seen via ultrasonography

Radiography
A thyroid tumor or goiter might be seen as increased soft tissue density in the throat-latch area.

OTHER DIAGNOSTIC PROCEDURES
A fine needle aspiration or biopsy may assess the thyroid gland.

TREATMENT

APPROPRIATE HEALTH CARE
• Foals with congenital hypothyroidism may require inpatient medical management if the disease is severe
• All other horses with abnormal T_3 and T_4 levels can be treated on an outpatient basis

NURSING CARE
• Foals may need assistance if they are too weak to suckle or mechanical ventilation if they cannot ventilate on their own
• Animals with poor hair coat may need blanketing, and cold temperatures should be avoided

ACTIVITY
Limit activity in foals with musculoskeletal deformities.

DIET
• Examine the diet of any horse with hypothyroidism and the dams of foals born with hypothyroidism to ensure the proper amount of iodine is being fed
• Pregnant mares should not receive endophyte-infected fescue hay, particularly during their last months of gestation or iodine supplementation. If fescue cannot be avoided, domperidone should be given daily to counter the anti-prolactin effects of the fescue endophytes

CLIENT EDUCATION
• Prognosis for soundness is poor in most foals with congenital hypothyroidism and should be discussed with owners
• Adult horses with hypothyroidism respond well to exogenous replacement hormone, and their prognosis is generally good

• Horses with hyperthyroidism should have their dose of thyroid supplement decreased
• Animals that are euthyroid despite low blood T_3 and T_4 levels should have their primary disease treated, but do not require hormone supplementation

SURGICAL CONSIDERATIONS
If the cause of increased or decreased T_3 and T_4 concentrations is a tumor, surgical removal of the affected thyroid lobe should be curative.

MEDICATIONS

DRUG(S) OF CHOICE
For decreased T_3 and T_4 levels caused by hypothyroidism, replacement therapy with T_4 20 µg/kg maintains T_4 and T_3 levels in the normal range for 24 h; this constitutes a dose of 10 mg in a 450 kg (1000 lb) horse.

CONTRAINDICATIONS
Thyroid replacement therapies of euthyroid sick horses may cause further deterioration of the horse's condition. Thus, perform provocative testing to establish the diagnosis of hypothyroidism before beginning to treat.

PRECAUTIONS
Exogenous thyroid hormones causes downregulation and, potentially, atrophy of the thyroid gland; gradually discontinue the hormone supplement over the course of several weeks.

ALTERNATIVE DRUGS
Other sources of thyroid hormone replacement—iodinated casein (5.0 g/day) and concentrated bovine thyroid extract (10 g/day).

FOLLOW-UP

PATIENT MONITORING
• Monitor by measuring serum T_4 and T_3 levels every 30–60 days. If the serum levels are low, increase the dose of supplement until serum levels reach normal range; if the serum levels are too high or in the higher end of the normal range, decrease the dosage and retest in 30–60 days

• Reconsider the original diagnosis if the patient fails to respond after 6 weeks of therapy

POSSIBLE COMPLICATIONS
N/A

MISCELLANEOUS

ASSOCIATED CONDITIONS
• Angular limb deformities, hypognathism, weakness, and respiratory distress often are associated with congenital hypothyroidism
• Infertility and poor hair coat have been associated with hypothyroidism in adults

AGE-RELATED FACTORS
• Higher T_3 and T_4 levels are normal in neonatal foals. Levels are highest at birth (10 times adult levels), then decrease rapidly in the first weeks of life to adult levels
• Resting T_3 and T_4 levels decline gradually with age, and levels in old horses may be lower than those in younger animals

SEE ALSO
Thyroid releasing hormone (TRH) and thyroid stimulating hormone (TSH) tests

ABBREVIATIONS
• T_3 = triiodothyronine
• T_4 = thyroxine
• TRH = thyroid releasing hormone
• TSH = thyroid stimulating hormone

Suggested Reading
Allen AL, Townsend HG, Doige CE, Fretz PB. A case-control study of the congenital hypothyroidism and dysmaturity syndrome of foals. Can Vet J 1996;37:349–358.
Frank N, Sojka J, Messer NT. Equine thyroid dysfunction. Vet Clin North America Equine Pract 2002;18:305–319.
Hilderbran AC, Breuhaus BA, Refsal KR. Nonthryoidal illness syndrome in adult horses. J Vet Intern Med 2014;28:609–617.

Author Janice Kritchevsky
Consulting Editors Michel Lévy and Heidi Banse

DISSEMINATED INTRAVASCULAR COAGULATION

 BASICS

DEFINITION
• DIC is an acquired coagulation dysfunction characterized by marked activation of the coagulation system that causes excessive thrombin activation, fibrin formation, and widespread intravascular fibrin deposition
• The exaggerated activation of coagulation and subsequent deposition of microthrombi can lead to:
  ○ Ischemic lesions in organs and development of multiorgan failure
  ○ Depletion of platelets and coagulation factors (consumption coagulopathy), which may cause secondary hemorrhage
• DIC is always secondary to a severe underlying disorder. Endotoxemia secondary to GI disorders and septicemia are the main causes of DIC in adult horses and neonatal foals, respectively

PATHOPHYSIOLOGY
• Underlying diseases induce platelet activation and excessive thrombin formation, and may induce endothelial damage, inhibition of coagulation inhibitors, and defective fibrinolysis. These combine to produce uncontrolled fibrin deposition and consumptive coagulation
• 2 clinical forms of DIC can be observed:
  ○ The MOFS form occurs when activation of coagulation is severe and fibrinolytic activity is inhibited. Widespread fibrin formation and microthrombus deposition in the microcirculation produce ischemic damage to tissues, contributing to MODS and MOFS
  ○ The hemorrhagic form occurs when activation of coagulation is less severe and excess fibrin formation can be arrested by the fibrinolytic system. Increased consumption of coagulation factors and platelet depletion may cause a consumptive coagulopathy and a subsequent hypocoagulable state, resulting in bleeding diatheses
• Despite some debate there is evidence to indicate that DIC contributes to multiple organ failure

SYSTEMS AFFECTED
• Hemic/lymphatic/immune—excessive fibrin formation and deposition occurs in blood vessels
  ○ Hypercoagulation may induce vessel thrombosis after endothelial damage associated with venipunctures or catheters
• Other systems may be affected depending on the organ affected by deposition of microthrombi, and/or the sites of hemorrhage

INCIDENCE/PREVALENCE
• DIC is the most frequent hemostatic disorder of the horse. It has been reported in 55% of ischemic and 36% of severe inflammatory GI disorders
• DIC is also diagnosed in many septic newborn foals (>50%)

SIGNALMENT
N/A

SIGNS
General Comments
Clinical signs include those of the underlying disease and of DIC.

Historical Findings
Dependent upon underlying disease.

Physical Examination Findings
• In the MOFS form of DIC, horses may demonstrate clinical signs referable to the affected organ including hypotension, dyspnea, tachypnea, oliguria, colic, cardiac arrhythmias, etc.
• In the hemorrhagic form of DIC, horses may have hemorrhagic diatheses, with excessive bleeding after wound or minor trauma, petechiae, or spontaneous bleeding from mucous membranes (i.e. epistaxis, melena)
• Catheter and venipuncture site thrombosis is common

CAUSES
• Ischemic or inflammatory GI disorders
• Endotoxemia
• Neonatal septicemia
• Heat stroke
• Less common—severe hemolysis, disseminated neoplasia, and other systemic inflammatory conditions (e.g. snake bite)

RISK FACTORS
Any disease or treatment that severely activates platelets and/or coagulation pathways, inhibits the fibrinolytic system, or causes significant endothelial damage.

 DIAGNOSIS

DIFFERENTIAL DIAGNOSIS
• The MOFS form of DIC requires differentiation from other causes of hypotension, renal failure, hypoxemia, etc.
• The hemorrhagic form of DIC requires differentiation from other coagulation deficiencies (acquired or inherited)

CBC/BIOCHEMISTRY/URINALYSIS
• Thrombocytopenia (<100 000 platelets/μL) due to platelet consumption
• In cases of MODS or MOFS, plasma biochemistry abnormalities may be detected depending on organ dysfunction (e.g. increase in creatinine, blood urea nitrogen, liver enzymes, etc.)

OTHER LABORATORY TESTS
• Laboratory evidence may include:
  ○ Consumptive coagulopathy is detected by evaluating clotting times (PT and aPTT), but this is not specific for DIC. A decrease in fibrinogen concentration is also consistent with clotting factor consumption
  ○ Fibrinolytic activation increases plasma D-dimer concentration. In DIC patients concentrations may be >2000 ng/mL. This test is sensitive for DIC, but has low specificity
  ○ FDPs have also been used to assess fibrinolysis, but are less reliable and decreasingly used
  ○ Coagulation inhibitor consumption may be measured through decreases in concentrations of antithrombin activity and protein C
• No single laboratory test is sufficiently sensitive or specific, therefore a diagnosis of DIC requires a combination of laboratory findings (e.g. thrombocytopenia, prolonged clotting times, increased D-dimers, and reduced antithrombin and fibrinogen) in conjunction with appropriate clinical signs
• In the equine veterinary literature, horses are considered to have subclinical DIC if they have abnormalities in 3 of 6 traditionally available tests: (1) platelet count, (2) PT, (3) aPTT, (4) antithrombin activity, (5) fibrinogen, and (6) either D-dimers or FDPs. Horses in subclinical DIC are at risk of developing overt clinical DIC as natural coagulation inhibitors become overwhelmed

PATHOLOGIC FINDINGS
• Petechiae and ecchymoses may be seen on postmortem
• Thrombosis may be observed grossly, but microthrombosis is commonly misdiagnosed on histologic examinations when using routine stains
• Specific histochemical (PTAH) or immunohistochemical stains are required to accurately detect fibrin deposition in capillaries

 TREATMENT

AIMS
• The primary aim of treatment is to control the underlying disease causing the severe, hypercoagulable state
• The second aim is to control the hypercoagulable state (and subsequent consumptive coagulopathy)
• The mortality rate of DIC is low if patients are diagnosed and treated during the early stages of disease, but becomes high when multiorgan failure and/or bleeding diatheses are present. Thus, a key objective for management of DIC is to treat patients at risk of DIC in order to prevent hypercoagulation from developing
• Supportive therapy is required to reduce microthrombi deposition and secondary organ dysfunction and/or failure

APPROPRIATE HEALTH CARE
DIC requires emergency hospitalization and intensive care management.

NURSING CARE
• Fresh (or fresh frozen) plasma transfusion (12–20 mL/kg) is only required in cases with severe consumptive coagulopathy and bleeding diatheses. This treatment slows progression of DIC and may help improve metabolic derangements caused by some primary diseases
• Low-dose heparin therapy has also been given to patients with DIC added to the transfusion bags. However, the high cost of plasma transfusions and the poor prognosis of the hemorrhagic form of DIC makes this treatment difficult and impractical in horses
• Horses with DIC may require intensive fluid therapy to control shock, improve tissue blood supply, and reduce multiorgan failure. Crystalloid solutions (e.g. lactated Ringer's solution) are commonly used, but colloidal solutions (e.g. hetastarch) may also be indicated

ACTIVITY
Limited as required for patients in intensive care.

DIET
According to restrictions/prescriptions associated with the underlying disease.

SURGICAL CONSIDERATIONS
Only if the underlying disorder requires surgery.

MEDICATIONS

DRUG(S) OF CHOICE
• Antithrombotics (e.g. heparin) are administered in the early stages of DIC to reduce the excessive coagulation activation. They are the most effective treatment for control of this disorder, although their administration has been considered controversial
• LMWH (e.g. dalteparin, enoxaparin) are preferred as they do not produce many of the detrimental effects associated with unfractionated heparin, such as erythrocyte agglutination. The safest dose of LMWH is 50 IU/kg of dalteparin SC every 24 h (or 0.5 mg/kg of enoxaparin) over 3–4 days. If no LMWH is available, unfractionated heparin is recommended (40–100 IU/kg every 12 h)

• Unfractionated heparin administration—sodium heparin (SC or IV), calcium heparin (SC)
• The use of antiplatelet agents (e.g. aspirin) to reduce the hypercoagulable state has not been shown to be effective in horses (unlike humans or small animals)
• Clopidogrel has been demonstrated to be an effective platelet inhibitor in healthy horses, but efficacy in horses with a hypercoagulable state is unknown. Interindividual variability in the response to clopidogrel may influence clinical efficacy

CONTRAINDICATIONS
• Antifibrinolytic drugs (e.g. aminocaproic acid) should not be used in hemorrhagic patients, as it impairs fibrinolysis and worsens hypercoagulation, microthrombi deposition, and DIC
• Hypertonic saline solution should not be used to control hypotension as it may cause hemodilution of coagulation factors and increase the risk of bleeding

POSSIBLE INTERACTIONS
Colloidal solutions may be administered to patients with DIC to treat the hypoalbuminemia caused by the underlying disease (e.g. colitis). Colloidal administration may reduce platelet function and may prolong hemorrhage.

FOLLOW-UP

PATIENT MONITORING
• Repeated physical examinations, with particular attention to evidence of MODS, MOFS, bleeding, or venous thrombosis, should be performed
• PT, aPTT, D-dimer concentration, and platelet counts should be monitored to assess clinical progression and effectiveness of treatment
• In cases of MODS/MOFS, biochemical parameters indicative of tissue dysfunction should be monitored

POSSIBLE COMPLICATIONS
• MODS
• MOFS
• Shock
• Acute renal failure
• Laminitis
• Thrombophlebitis
• Fatal bleeding
• Death

EXPECTED COURSE AND PROGNOSIS
• With clinical signs of DIC, prognosis is guarded to poor. High mortality rates are due to the combination of DIC and severity of the underlying disease
• Prognosis is better if:
  ○ DIC is diagnosed early
  ○ Preventive treatment is effectively introduced

MISCELLANEOUS

ASSOCIATED CONDITIONS
• Localized or systemic ischemic or inflammatory disorders
• Heat stroke
• Others; severe hemolysis, disseminated neoplasia (i.e. melanosarcoma), etc.

SYNONYMS
Consumptive coagulopathy

SEE ALSO
• Coagulation defects, acquired
• Petechiae, ecchymoses, and hematomas
• Thrombocytopenia

ABBREVIATIONS
• aPTT = activated partial thromboplastin time
• DIC = disseminated intravascular coagulation
• FDP = fibrin(ogen) degradation product
• GI = gastrointestinal tract
• LMWH = low-molecular-weight heparin
• MODS = multiorgan dysfunction syndrome
• MOFS = multiorgan failure syndrome
• PT = prothrombin time
• PTAH = phosphotungstic acid–hematoxylin

Suggested Reading
Cesarini C, Monreal L, Armengou L, et al. Association of admission plasma D-dimer concentration with diagnosis and outcome in horses with colic. J Vet Intern Med 2010;24(6):1490–1497.
Cotovio M, Monreal L, Navarro M, et al. Detection of fibrin deposits in tissues from horses with severe gastrointestinal disorders. J Vet Intern Med 2007;21:308–313.

Author Eduard Jose-Cunilleras
Consulting Editors David Hodgson, Harold C. McKenzie, and Jennifer L. Hodgson
Acknowledgment The author and editors acknowledge the prior contribution of Luis Monreal.

DISTAL AND PROXIMAL INTERPHALANGEAL JOINT DISEASE

BASICS

OVERVIEW
- Any disease localized to DIP or PIP
- The distal limb undergoes high stresses during locomotion
- The DIP is a high-motion joint supported by collateral ligaments. Excessive or repetitive stresses such as circling, uneven ground, and/or unbalanced feet contribute to injury.
- The PIP is a low-motion joint supported by collateral, palmar, and distal sesamoidean ligaments. Sliding and rotational forces are main contributing factors
- Articular DIP/PIP diseases (osteochondrosis, fracture, luxation) may result in osteoarthritis
- DIP and PIP osteoarthritis are commonly called low ringbone and high ringbone, respectively
- Musculoskeletal—foot (DIP), pastern (PIP)

SIGNALMENT
- All breeds, sports
- Middle-aged to older horses most common

SIGNS
- Variable lameness, often chronic, progressive
- Lameness, often bilateral, although 1 limb predominates
- Lameness in any limb, forelimb more common
- Lameness worse circling or on hard ground
- Resentment of distal limb flexion
- Dorsal DIP joint distention
- Buttress foot (dorsal pastern/hoof wall distortion) in chronic DIP disease
- Firm periarticular PIP swelling in chronic disease

CAUSES AND RISK FACTORS
- Poor conformation
- Hoof imbalance
- Sports that require repetitive quick turns, abrupt stops (Western, polo, jumping)
- Osteochondrosis
- Articular phalangeal fractures

DIAGNOSIS

DIFFERENTIAL DIAGNOSIS
- Laminitis—rule out with radiography
- Other lameness causes alleviated by DIP analgesia. Palmar digital nerves lie next to DIP palmar pouch, analgesia may diffuse to palmar digital nerve. Differential includes:
  ◦ Navicular syndrome—rule out with comprehensive imaging and selective nerve blocks
  ◦ Solar pain—rule out with comprehensive imaging

CBC/CHEMISTRY/URINALYSIS
None

OTHER LABORATORY TESTS
None

IMAGING
- Radiography—± early/acute: normal. Chronic: osteophytes, loss of joint space, subchondral sclerosis.
- Ultrasonography—for DIP, ± collateral ligament desmitis. For PIP, desmitis of collateral ligaments, distal sesamoidean, or palmar pastern ligaments can contribute to disease
- Nuclear scintigraphy—± generalized increased radiopharmaceutical uptake
- MRI—± collateral ligaments desmitis, subchondral remodeling, cartilage damage, synovitis

OTHER DIAGNOSTIC PROCEDURES
- Diagnostic analgesia—DIP pain improves after palmar digital, abaxial, or IA analgesia. PIP pain improves after abaxial, palmar digital plus pastern ring block, or IA analgesia
- Diagnostic arthroscopy—limited, osseous fragment removal is challenging
- Synovial fluid analysis—rule out infectious arthritis

TREATMENT
- Rest for weeks to months
- Restore hoof balance, shorten toe, ease breakover
- IA anti-inflammatory(s)
- Reduced workload and expectations
- ± Arthroscopic osseous fragment(s) removal
- Surgical PIP arthrodesis in advanced disease
- Surgical DIP arthrodesis performed on a limited basis

MEDICATIONS

DRUG(S) OF CHOICE
- NSAIDs—phenylbutazone (2.2 mg/kg daily to every 12 h for 7–10 days)
- IA corticosteroids—methylprednisolone acetate (20–40 mg) or triamcinolone (3–6 mg)
- IA sodium hyaluronate (10–20 mg)
- Combination of IA corticosteroids and sodium hyaluronate
- Systemic chondroprotective drugs—polysulfated glycosaminoglycan (500 mg IM every 4 days for 7 treatments) or sodium hyaluronate (40 mg IV every 7 days for 3 treatments)
- Oral chondroprotective medications—glucosamine/chondroitin sulfate powder (1 scoop (3.3 g) every 12 h)

CONTRAINDICATIONS/POSSIBLE INTERACTIONS
IA corticosteroids not recommended in horses with laminitis.

FOLLOW-UP

PATIENT MONITORING
Periodic lameness and radiographic assessment are recommended. In general, DIP and PIP osteoarthritis is progressive.

PREVENTION/AVOIDANCE
Reduced workload or alterative sport may slow the progression.

POSSIBLE COMPLICATIONS
Inability to perform expected sport due to chronic lameness.

EXPECTED COURSE AND PROGNOSIS
- For PIP or DIP disease, early recognition and treatment may prolong intended use
- PIP or DIP osteoarthritis is progressive and reduced athletic soundness is expected
- In chronic or advanced PIP disease, surgical arthrodesis is indicated and many horses retain athletic ability
- Advanced DIP disease results in chronic lameness and retirement

MISCELLANEOUS

ASSOCIATED CONDITIONS
Navicular syndrome

AGE-RELATED FACTORS
Middle-aged horses most common

ZOONOTIC POTENTIALS
None

SEE ALSO
- Navicular syndrome
- Osteoarthritis

ABBREVIATIONS
- DIP = distal interphalangeal joint
- IA = intra-articular
- NSAID = nonsteroidal anti-inflammatory drug
- PIP = proximal interphalangeal joint

Suggested Reading
Dyson SJ. The distal phalanx and distal interphalangeal joint. In: Ross MW, Dyson SJ, eds. Diagnosis and Management of Lameness in the Horse, 2e. St. Louis, MO: Elsevier Saunders, 2011:349–366.
Ruggles AJ. The proximal and middle phalanges and proximal interphalangeal joint. In: Ross MW, Dyson SJ, eds. Diagnosis and Management of Lameness in the Horse, 2e. St. Louis, MO: Elsevier Saunders, 2011:387–395.

Author Elizabeth J. Davidson
Consulting Editor Elizabeth J. Davidson

BASICS

OVERVIEW
• Lower hock joint (TMT, DIT) lameness from pain/inflammation or osteochondral damage. • "Bone spavin": lay term for distal tarsal osteoarthritis. • Low-motion TMT/DIT prone to compression and rotation; excessive or repetitive forces result in inflammation and osteoarthritis. • Neonates with delayed small tarsal bone ossification may develop "juvenile bone spavin". • Musculoskeletal—hock (tarsus)

SIGNALMENT
• Any age, middle-aged most common. • Athletic horses. • Rare in ponies, donkeys, mules, draft breeds

SIGNS

Historical Findings
• Intermittent, slowly progressive hindlimb lameness. • Usually bilateral; ± unilateral hindlimb lameness. • Warm out of lameness during work. • Reduced performance—slower run times; resists stops, turns, jumps, collection, correct canter lead. • Drags hind toes

Physical Examination Findings
• Bony exostosis ± heat on medial TMT/DIT. • Worn lateral toe on hind shoe. • "Stabbing" or "stabby" hindlimb gait. • Affected limb swings toward midline. • Lameness worse after upper hindlimb flexion. • Painful to "Churchill test" (digital pressure to proximomedial second metatarsal bone while abducting limb)

CAUSES AND RISK FACTORS
• Poor conformation—sickle or cow hocks, straight hindlimb, long toe/low heel hind foot, height disparity between withers and croup. • Athletics requiring jumping, abrupt stops, or excessive hindlimb use. • Delayed small tarsal bone ossification. • Excessive exercise when young

DIAGNOSIS

DIFFERENTIAL DIAGNOSIS
• Hindlimb proximal suspensory desmitis—rule out with diagnostic analgesia ± imaging. • Stifle lameness—rule out with diagnostic analgesia ± imaging. • Tarsocrural joint pain—rule out with diagnostic analgesia ± imaging

IMAGING

Radiography
• Early disease—subtle or no lesions. • Dorsal TMT/DIT periarticular osteophytes, joint narrowing, subchondral sclerosis, ± lysis.

• Enthesophyte of dorsoproximal third metatarsal bone. • Severe—extensive bone exostosis, ankylosis.

Ultrasonography
• Medial and lateral collateral ligament desmitis. • Rule out hindlimb suspensory desmitis

Nuclear Scintigraphy
Generalized increased radiopharmaceutical uptake TMT ± DIT.

MRI
Tarsal bone edema, subchondral bone injury. Rule out proximal suspensory desmitis.

OTHER DIAGNOSTIC PROCEDURES
Diagnostic analgesia—IA TMT/DIT or regional (peroneal/tibial) analgesia; diffusion to proximal suspensory complicates interpretation.

PATHOLOGIC FINDINGS
DIT/TMT—ankylosis, bony lysis, ± cartilage erosions.

TREATMENT
• Intra-articular (IA) medication. • Rest. • Restore hoof balance, shorten hind toes. • Extracorporeal shockwave therapy. • Chemical arthrodesis with ethyl alcohol. • Surgical arthrodesis. • Cunean tenectomy

MEDICATIONS

DRUG(S) OF CHOICE
• NSAIDs—phenylbutazone (2.2 mg/kg every 12–24 h). • IA corticosteroids—methylprednisolone acetate (20–40 mg) or triamcinolone (3–6 mg). • IA sodium hyaluronate (10–20 mg). • Combination of IA corticosteroids and sodium hyaluronate. • Systemic chondroprotective drugs—polysulfated glycosaminoglycan (500 mg IM every 4 days for 7 treatments) or sodium hyaluronate (40 mg IV every 7 days for 3 treatments). • Oral chondroprotective medications—glucosamine/chondroitin sulfate powder (1 scoop (3.3 g) every 12 h). • Equithrive oral supplementation (1 scoop (1000 mb) every 12 h)

CONTRAINDICATIONS/POSSIBLE INTERACTIONS
• IA corticosteroids not recommended in horses with historical laminitis. • Chemical arthrodesis contraindicated if proximal intertarsal joint communicates with TMT/DIT or tarsal sheath. • Chemical arthrodesis—± excessive edema, swelling, necrosis, sepsis, severe postinjection pain

FOLLOW-UP

PATIENT MONITORING
• Asses lameness after IA medications. • Periodically assess lameness during athletic career. • Therapeutic trimming/shoeing every 6 weeks. • Radiographic assessment 3–4 months post chemical or surgical arthrodesis

PREVENTION/AVOIDANCE
Reduced or alterative workload.

POSSIBLE COMPLICATIONS
• Laminitis or joint sepsis secondary to IA corticosteroids. • Gastric ulceration, right dorsal colon inflammation, or kidney damage secondary to chronic NSAIDs use. • Incomplete ankylosis and continued lameness. • Persistent soft tissue swelling, skin necrosis, persistent lameness after chemical arthrodesis

EXPECTED COURSE AND PROGNOSIS
• Usually progressive but manageable with therapy. Many return to athletic use. • Distal intertarsal bone lysis has poor prognosis for athletics. • After surgical arthrodesis, 66% return to intended use but require 6–12 months for ankylosis. • Chemical arthrodesis used with caution due to possible postinjection complications

MISCELLANEOUS

ASSOCIATED CONDITIONS
• Cunean bursitis. • Proximal suspensory ligament desmitis. • Stifle disease (straight hindlimb conformation)

AGE-RELATED CONDITIONS
• Middle-aged athletic horses. • Young horses worked excessively

ABBREVIATIONS
• DIT = distal intertarsal joint
• IA = intra-articular
• MRI = magnetic resonance imaging
• NSAID = nonsteroidal anti-inflammatory drug
• TMT = tarsometatarsal joint

Suggested Reading
Jackman BR. Review of equine distal hock inflammation and arthritis. Am Assoc Equine Pract 2006;52:5–12.

Author Robin M. Dabareiner
Consulting Editor Elizabeth J. Davidson

D

DORSAL DISPLACEMENT OF THE SOFT PALATE (DDSP)

BASICS

OVERVIEW
• When the soft palate displaces dorsally, the epiglottis cannot be seen within the nasopharynx as it is in the oropharynx
• During exhalation, the caudal free margin of the soft palate billows across the rima glottis, creating an airway obstruction during exhalation
• DDSP has been estimated to affect 10% of racehorses
• This condition may be intermittent at exercise or permanent

SIGNALMENT
The most common presentation is intermittent and is seen predominantly in racehorses and to a lesser degree in sport horses.

SIGNS
• Intermittent DDSP occurs during exercise
• Usually associated with an abnormal upper respiratory noise during exhalation, often referred to as "gurgling noise"
• Approximately 10–20% of horses with DDSP do not make a noise and are referred to as "silent displacers"
• Horses with intermittent DDSP generally have a history of exercise intolerance and may make a "gurgling" noise during exhalation; concurrent with these signs is open-mouth breathing

CAUSES AND RISK FACTORS
The causes can be classified into 2 groups. (1) Intrinsic causes associated with structural abnormality such as subepiglottic cyst, subepiglottic masses, epiglottic cartilage deformity, epiglottitis, and palatal cyst or inflammation. It can also be due to decreased muscular activity of the palatinus and palatopharyngeus muscles. It may also be due to heightened sensory input of the larynx, as seen with painful conditions. (2) Extrinsic causes are those associated with factors affecting neuromuscular control of the position of the basihyoid bone and/or larynx.

DIAGNOSIS

DIFFERENTIAL DIAGNOSIS
Epiglottic entrapment.

IMAGING
Lateral radiographs of the larynx/pharynx allow identification of soft palate displacement, the length of the epiglottic cartilage, and presence of subepiglottic and palatal cysts/mass. However, these findings are more easily assessed by endoscopy.

OTHER DIAGNOSTIC PROCEDURES
• The diagnosis of intermittent DDSP is based on a history of a sudden decrease in performance in the second half of the exercise intensity or competition and generally is associated with "gurgling" expiratory respiratory noises
• Palatal instability at exercise is seen as a prodromal sign of DDSP
• Endoscopy of the upper airway at rest usually is normal but may identify structural anomalies and the presence of an ulcer on the caudal edge of the soft palate
• There is a poor correlation with the observation of DDSP at rest and during exercise
• The best diagnostic test is dynamic endoscopy (overground or treadmill)

TREATMENT

• Treatment initially is directed at modifying or eliminating factors associated with the occurrence of DDSP
• The incidence of intermittent DDSP decreases with maturity
• If upper respiratory tract inflammation was diagnosed during the examination, treatment should include judicious use of systemic anti-inflammatory medication
• Several surgical therapies and combination surgical therapies currently are performed as treatment. Certain procedures (laser or cautery-assisted treatment of the soft palate, staphylectomy, or surgical imbrication of the palate) attempt to "stiffen" the soft palate or reduce its obstructive surface (staphylectomy); there is a lack of evidence-based data in support of persistent stiffening or fibrosis being induced. Other techniques such as myectomies (sternothyroid and/or sternohyoid muscle resection) and surgical repositioning of the larynx in a dorsal and forward position (laryngeal tie-forward) are thought to optimize the position of the larynx during exercise. The latter 2 techniques (laryngeal tie-forward and sternothyroid muscles) are generally combined

MEDICATIONS

DRUG(S) OF CHOICE
A systemic and or local course of anti-inflammatory agents may be indicated to treat larynx inflammation.

CONTRAINDICATIONS/POSSIBLE INTERACTIONS
None

FOLLOW-UP

PATIENT MONITORING
Endoscopy 14–30 days after institution of medical treatment or 2–3 weeks after surgery.

POSSIBLE COMPLICATIONS
Tracheal aspiration of feed material is a possible complication after staphylectomy.

EXPECTED COURSE AND PROGNOSIS
Prognosis after surgery is approximately 60–80%.

MISCELLANEOUS

ASSOCIATED CONDITIONS
Pharyngitis

AGE-RELATED FACTORS
Higher prevalence in 2–3-year-olds.

SEE ALSO
Dynamic collapse of the upper airways

ABBREVIATIONS
DDSP = dorsal displacement of the soft palate

Suggested Reading
Barakzai SA, Johnson VS, Baird DH, et al. Assessment of the efficacy of composite surgery for the treatment of dorsal displacement of the soft palate in a group of 53 racing Thoroughbreds (1990–1996). Equine Vet J 2004;36:175–179.
Cheetham J, Piggot JH, Thorson LM, et al. Racing performance following the laryngeal tie-forward procedure: a case-controlled study. Equine Vet J 2008;40:501–507.
Ducharme NG. Pharynx. In: Auer JA, Stick JA, eds. Equine Surgery, 3e. St. Louis, MO: Saunders Elsevier, 2006:544–565.

Author Norm G. Ducharme
Consulting Editors Daniel Jean and Mathilde Leclère

DORSAL METACARPAL BONE DISEASE

BASICS

OVERVIEW
• Commonly referred to as "bucked shin complex"
• Stress-related bone injury to the dorsal aspect of MCIII resulting in dorsal metacarpal periostitis ("bucked shins") and dorsal cortical stress fracture ("saucer fracture")
• High-strain cyclic fatigue of MCIII causes decreased bone stiffness and the bone responds by adding new bone.
• Common racehorse disease in the USA and Australia
• Musculoskeletal—dorsal MCIII, occasionally MTIII

SIGNALMENT
• Young (2- and 3-year-olds) racehorses
• Thoroughbreds, Quarter Horses, Arabians, and uncommonly Standardbreds

SIGNS
• Acute soreness, tenderness, swelling of dorsal MCIII after high-speed workout ("breeze") or race
• Associated lameness, bilateral stiff or short, choppy forelimb gait
• Distinct dorsal convexity of MCIII when viewed from the lateral side
• "Saucer fractures" occur mostly in the left forelimb; focal swelling or bony knot in the dorsal or dorsolateral aspect of mid-MCIII

CAUSES AND RISK FACTORS
• Racing and race training
• Classically trained racehorses
• Racing/training on dirt tracks
• Counterclockwise racing
• Most racehorses with "saucer fracture" had previous "bucked shins"

DIAGNOSIS

DIFFERENTIAL DIAGNOSIS
• Incomplete, longitudinal MCIII cortical fracture—rule out with radiography
• Suspensory avulsion fracture—rule out with radiography, nuclear scintigraphy, ultrasonography
• Periostitis due to direct trauma

IMAGING
Radiography
• "Bucked shins"—periosteal thickening of dorsal, dorsomedial MCIII diaphysis
• "Saucer fracture"—short, oblique unicortical fracture in dorsal or dorsolateral MCIII diaphysis

Nuclear Scintigraphy
• "Bucked shins"—diffuse increased radiopharmaceutical uptake along dorsal MCIII
• "Saucer fracture"—focal increased radiopharmaceutical uptake ("hot spot") in dorsal MCIII

OTHER DIAGNOSTIC PROCEDURES
Diagnostic analgesia—generally not necessary; high palmar analgesia with dorsal proximal MCIII ring block confirms the location of the pain.

PATHOLOGIC FINDINGS
Microradiographic evaluation reveals appositional new bone formation on the dorsomedial periosteal surface of MCIII.

TREATMENT
• Cold water hosing, icing, poultice, or antiphlogistic dressing for several days
• "Bucked shins"—stall confinement and hand-walking for 2–8 weeks
• "Saucer fracture"—stall confinement and hand-walking for 4–6 weeks followed by controlled exercise (small paddock or light jogging) for another 6–8 weeks
• Surgery—osteostixis (fenestration), screw fixation, or both for "saucer fracture"
• Additional therapies:
  ○ Thermocautery ("pin firing")
  ○ Cryotherapy ("freeze firing")
  ○ Periosteal picking—percutaneous periosteum irritation with needle
  ○ Extracorporeal shockwave therapy

MEDICATIONS

DRUG(S) OF CHOICE
• NSAIDs (phenylbutazone 2.2–4.4 mg/kg every 12–24 h) for a few days
• Counterirritants ("paints" and "blisters")—topical medications

CONTRAINDICATIONS/POSSIBLE INTERACTIONS
Long-term NSAID use is contraindicated owing to resultant impaired bone healing and risk of catastrophic fracture after "saucer fracture."

FOLLOW-UP

PATIENT MONITORING
• For acute mild disease, return to soundness within several days to weeks
• For severe disease, return to soundness in months. Radiographic evaluation at monthly intervals for "saucer fracture"

PREVENTION/AVOIDANCE
• Revised training regimens to stimulate cyclic bone loading that is similar to those when racing, i.e. train at racing speeds. Horses are worked at or near racing speeds at least twice weekly, initially at very short distances and increased gradually. With each incremental increase in training speed, distance is decreased
• Avoid slow jogging and long gallops

POSSIBLE COMPLICATIONS
• Variable proportion of horses experience repeated or chronic episodes
• Prolonged or incomplete bony healing of a "saucer fracture" with conservative treatment
• Catastrophic fracture in unrecognized "saucer fracture"

EXPECTED COURSE AND PROGNOSIS
• Prognosis for most horses with "bucked shins" is very good after early recognition and strict adherence to revised training protocol
• The majority of horses with "saucer fractures" treated with osteostixis, screw fixation, or both will return to racing

MISCELLANEOUS

ASSOCIATED CONDITIONS
Most horses with "saucer fractures" had previous episode of "bucked shins."

AGE-RELATED FACTORS
Young (<4 years of age) racehorses.

ZOONOTIC POTENTIAL
None

SEE ALSO
Stress fractures

ABBREVIATIONS
• MCIII = third metacarpal bone
• MTIII = third metatarsal bone
• NSAID = nonsteroidal anti-inflammatory drug

Suggested Reading
Nunamaker DM. The bucked shin complex: etiology, pathogenesis, and conservative management. In: Ross MW, Dyson SJ, eds. Diagnosis and Management of Lameness in the Horse. St. Louis, MO: Elsevier Saunders, 2003:847–853.

Author Elizabeth J. Davidson
Consulting Editor Elizabeth J. Davidson

DOURINE

BASICS

DEFINITION
• Reported only in horses and donkeys
• Classically thought to be caused by *Trypanosoma equiperdum*; however, the position with the trypanozoon group is uncertain, with overlap noted between this and *Trypanosoma evansi* and *Trypanosoma brucei*
• Only a small number of laboratory strains of uncertain origin exist. No recent isolates have been obtained.
• Venereal-only transmission
• Tropism for genital mucosa; cannot survive outside host
• Mortality high; debilitation; predisposition to other diseases

PATHOPHYSIOLOGY
• Limited to venereal transmission; transmissible by direct contact
• Requires no vector host; low numbers of organisms in peripheral blood make biting insect transmission unlikely

SYSTEMS AFFECTED
• Gastrointestinal—weight loss; emaciation
• Cardiovascular—intense anemia, dependent edema, and urticaria
• Lymphatic—peripheral lymphadenopathy
• Nervous—meningoencephalitis, progressive weakness, paresis, and paralysis
• Musculoskeletal—progressive weakness
• Reproductive—abortion
• Ophthalmic—keratoconjunctivitis

INCIDENCE/PREVALENCE
• Enzootic; endemic in Africa, Asia, Central and South America
• Eradicated in North America
• Low prevalence in parts of Europe

SIGNALMENT
Breeding mares and stallions.

SIGNS
• Depends on strain and general health of the horse population
• 3 disease phases recognized:
  ◦ Genital—preputial and vulvar edema and tumefaction
  ◦ Cutaneous—pathognomonic widespread raised cutaneous plaques (round, ovoid, irregular) 1–10 cm in diameter; trunk, neck, chest, shoulders. Edema of mammary gland, limbs, and ventrum also reported
  ◦ Neurologic—neurologic compromise (hindquarter weakness; ataxia, hyperesthesia, and hyperalgia); lower lip droop; anemia of increasing severity during clinical course of disease (normochromic, macrocytic); emaciation, death
• Approximately 50% of affected animals die of acute disease in 6–8 weeks

Females
• Severe, edematous vulvar and perineal swelling
• Mucopurulent vulvar discharge
• Frequent, painful attempts at urination because of vaginal mucosal irritation
• Chronic cases develop urticarial subcutaneous plaques in the vulva and surrounding tissues, as well as in the neck and ventral abdomen. These may regress within hours or days to areas of depigmentation
• Abortion, if pregnant

Males
• Edema of prepuce, urethral process, penis, testes, and scrotum
• Paraphimosis may ensue
• Purulent urethral discharge
• Inguinal lymph node enlargement
• Plaques and depigmented lesions, as in females

CAUSES
• Exposure to *T. equiperdum*
• Infection occurs across intact genital mucosal barriers

RISK FACTORS
• Presence of asymptomatic carriers
• The organism periodically may be unrecoverable from the urethra or vagina
• Transmission is not certain, even from matings with animals known to be infected
• Transport of horses from areas known to be infected
• Urethral discharge from intact male
• Males may serve as noninfected mechanical carriers after breeding of infected females

DIAGNOSIS

DIFFERENTIAL DIAGNOSIS
• Equine herpesvirus 3
• Equine infectious anemia
• Equine viral arteritis
• Endometritis

CBC/BIOCHEMISTRY/URINALYSIS
• Acute infection—leukocytosis; other inflammatory changes
• Chronic, debilitating infection results in anemia and extensive multisystemic disease

OTHER LABORATORY TESTS
Cytology/Histopathology
• Causative organism in smears of body fluid or lymph node aspirates may yield organism; appears as flagellated protozoan. Mount as a wet film, appears motile with flagellar movement
• Seminal fluid, mucus from prepuce, and vaginal discharges
• Histology, immunohistochemistry, IFA

Serology
• PCR testing recently available. Species differentiation (*T. equiperdum* versus *T. evansi*) has been reported
• CF test is the most widely used and only internationally recognized test; however, developed in 1915

• Also available—agar gel immunodiffusion, IFA, and ELISA tests

DIAGNOSTIC PROCEDURES
• Diagnosis complicated by inconsistent presence of characteristic lesions, low numbers of organisms, short-lived parasitemia
• In the nervous form, the organism can be recovered from the lumbar and sacral spinal cord, sciatic and obturator nerves, and cerebrospinal fluid

PATHOLOGIC FINDINGS
Primarily emaciation with enlargement of lymph nodes, spleen, liver; periportal infiltrations in liver; and petechial hemorrhages in kidney.

TREATMENT

APPROPRIATE HEALTH CARE
• International regulations impose slaughter of CF-positive horses
• May be successful if treated early in the course of disease
• Chronic cases in particular are unresponsive to treatment

CLIENT EDUCATION
Recovered treated animals may become asymptomatic carriers.

MEDICATIONS

DRUG(S) OF CHOICE
Quinapyramine sulfate—5 mg/kg divided doses SC.

ALTERNATIVE DRUGS
• Diminazene diaceturate—7 mg/kg as 5% solution injected SC; repeat at half-dose 24 h later
• Suramin—10 mg/kg IV 2 or 3 times at weekly intervals
• 4-Melaminophenylarsine dihydrochloride—0.25–0.5 mg/kg/day for up to 6 days

FOLLOW-UP

PATIENT MONITORING
• Body weight and condition
• CBC
• Neurologic examination

PREVENTION/AVOIDANCE
• Prohibit movement of horses from infected areas
• Control breeding practices
• Eradication–serologic testing with slaughter of infected animals
• Consecutive negative tests at least 1 month apart indicate freedom from disease

(CONTINUED)

POSSIBLE COMPLICATIONS

Multisystemic nature of the disease predisposes to multisystem failure.

EXPECTED COURSE AND PROGNOSIS

• Incubation period—1 week to 3 months
• Approximately 50% of affected animals die of acute disease in 6–8 weeks
• Course of disease—usually 1–2 months but may last for 2–4 years

MISCELLANEOUS

PREGNANCY/FERTILITY/BREEDING

Abortion

ABBREVIATIONS

• CF = complement fixation
• ELISA = enzyme-linked immunosorbent assay
• IFA = immunofluorescent assay
• PCR = polymerase chain reaction

Suggested Reading

Barrowman PR. Observations on the transmission, immunology, clinical signs and chemotherapy of dourine (*Trypanosoma equiperdum* infection) in horses, with special reference to cerebrospinal fluid. Onderstepoort J Vet Res 1976;43:55–66.

Claes F, Buscher P, Touratier L, Goddeeris BM. *Trypanosoma equiperdum*—master of disguise or historical mistake? Trends Parasitol 2005;21:316–321.

Clausen PH, Chuluun S, Sodnomdarjaa R, et al. A field study to estimate the prevalence of *Trypanosoma equiperdum* in Mongolian horses. Vet Parasitol 2003;115:9–18.

Hagebock JM, Chieves L, Frerichs WM, Miller CD. Evaluation of agar gel immunodiffusion and indirect fluorescent antibody assays as supplemental tests for dourine in equids. Am J Vet Res 1993;54:1201–1208.

Hagos A, Goddeeris BM, Yilkal K, et al. Efficacy of Cymelarsan® and Diminasan® against *Trypanosoma equiperdum* infections in mice and horses. Vet Parasitol 2010;171:200–206.

Pascucci I, Di Provvido A, Cammà C, et al. Diagnosis of dourine in outbreaks in Italy. Vet Parasitol 2013;193:30–38.

Vulpiani MP, Carvelli A, Giansante D, et al. Reemergence of dourine in Italy: clinical cases in some positive horses. J Equine Vet Sci 2013;33:468–474.

Author Peter R. Morresey
Consulting Editor Carla L. Carleton

DUODENITIS–PROXIMAL JEJUNITIS (ANTERIOR ENTERITIS, PROXIMAL ENTERITIS)

BASICS

DEFINITION
DPJ is an inflammation of the proximal SI. However, this descriptive name is inaccurate because other segments of the GI tract can be affected. Ileus with SI and gastric distention occurs as a result of excessive fluid and electrolyte secretion and accumulation.

PATHOPHYSIOLOGY
• Idiopathic condition
• Lesions are more consistently found in the duodenum and proximal jejunum, but the pylorus, distal esophagus, and stomach can be affected
• Fluid and electrolyte accumulation occurs in the SI and stomach
• Signs of abdominal pain are common, likely as a result of inflammation and intestinal distention from increased secretion, decreased absorption, and poor perfusion
• The cause of the ileus is unknown, but could result from direct damage, distention, pain, toxemia, hypokalemia, and/or other electrolyte disturbances
• Net fluid movement into the SI combined with lack of aboral movement eventually results in gastric distention

SYSTEMS AFFECTED
GI
• Increased fluid secretion, decreased fluid absorption, and lack of aboral movement cause SI distention, mainly in the duodenum and proximal jejunum
• Fluid accumulation in the SI, reflux into the stomach causing gastric distention
• Signs of abdominal pain (colic)
• Some horses may develop diarrhea
• Liver enzymes can be increased, but the mechanism involved is unknown

Cardiovascular
Dehydration and hypovolemia. Cardiac arrhythmias can occur.

Musculoskeletal
• Laminitis
• Muscle mass loss can result from the severe catabolic state and restricted food intake

GENETICS
No known genetic basis.

INCIDENCE/PREVALENCE
• Anecdotally, a greater incidence in the southern USA; however, cases can occur in any region
• Can occur throughout the year; however, it is reported more often during the summer months in some areas

SIGNALMENT
• Horses >1 year are primarily affected, with a high proportion in those >9 years
• No sex predilection

SIGNS
Historical Findings
• Acute onset of colic signs
• Occasionally there is recent introduction of a high-energy diet or access to too-lush pasture

Physical Examination Findings
• Tachycardia, with 40–80 bpm
• Moderate to severe dehydration
• Animals appear more depressed than painful, especially after gastric decompression; however, some horses may be severely painful
• Fever is common
• Gastric reflux with variable volumes
• Appearance of gastric reflux varies from green to brownish-red, with or without a fetid odor
• Distended SI is usually palpable per rectum
• Clinical signs resemble those of an obstructive SI lesion. Differentiation of horses with obstructive lesions requiring surgery is critical. Horses with DPJ tend to be more depressed and to have a greater resolution of pain and lower heart rate after gastric decompression, significantly more reflux, less palpably distended SI, more GI sounds, and lower peritoneal WBC counts than horses with surgical SI lesions. None of these signs alone is diagnostic and a definitive diagnosis can be confirmed only during surgical exploration or necropsy

CAUSES
• Unknown, but infectious cause is suspected
• *Clostridium difficile* was consistently recovered from the reflux in some horses and also occasionally from the feces of affected horses. Some horses inoculated with *C. difficile* toxins developed clinical signs and lesions consistent with those found in naturally occurring disease cases
• *Clostridium perfringens* has been inconsistently recovered from reflux or feces of clinical cases
• *Salmonella* spp. and mycotoxins have been suggested as possible causes but not proven
• Intestinal dysbacteriosis is likely to occur as well and could play a role in the pathogenesis

RISK FACTORS
A recent dietary change.

DIAGNOSIS

DIFFERENTIAL DIAGNOSIS
• Any condition causing colic and gastric reflux
• Strangulating or nonstrangulating obstructive SI lesions
• Ileus
• Large colon impaction, causing SI compression

CBC/BIOCHEMISTRY/URINALYSIS
A leukocytosis may be present but is not diagnostic.

OTHER LABORATORY TESTS
• Metabolic acidosis can occur due to hypovolemia, decreased tissue perfusion, and electrolyte imbalance. Metabolic alkalosis also possible due to gastric reflux
• Abdominocentesis—increased peritoneal fluid protein level (>30 g/L, and possibly >45 g/L) with normal WBC numbers (<5–10 × 10^9 cells/L) is suggestive but is not diagnostic

IMAGING
Abdominal ultrasonography—SI distention.

PATHOLOGIC FINDINGS
Gross
• Lesions are present invariably in the duodenum, often in the jejunum, and occasionally in the pyloric region of the stomach
• Petechial and ecchymotic hemorrhages on serosal surface
• Thickened intestinal wall due to edema and inflammation
• Hyperemic mucosa

Histopathologic
• Lesions include fibrinopurulent exudation on the serosal surface, intramural hemorrhage, and hyperemia and edema of the mucosa and submucosa
• Depending on severity, there may be villous epithelial degeneration, epithelial cell sloughing, and neutrophilic infiltration
• In some cases, no gross or histologic lesions are present

TREATMENT

APPROPRIATE HEALTH CARE
Intensive treatment and monitoring required; affected horses should be managed on an inpatient basis.

NURSING CARE
• Frequent monitoring is essential, especially when the presence of a surgical lesion remains unclear
• Signs of colic and tachycardia could indicate the need for gastric decompression
• Deep bedding and prophylactic feet icing could be beneficial to laminitis

IV Fluid Therapy
• Balanced electrolyte solution
• Administer daily maintenance (30–50 mL/kg/day) plus correction of fluid deficits from dehydration and replacement of the fluid volume lost with reflux
• Monitor plasma electrolyte levels
• IV potassium supplementation— 20–40 mEq/L of KCl can be added to lactated Ringer's solution or saline. Infusion rate should not exceed 0.5 mEq/kg/h
• Hypocalcemia—slow 500 mL IV infusion of 23% calcium borogluconate

(CONTINUED) DUODENITIS–PROXIMAL JEJUNITIS (ANTERIOR ENTERITIS, PROXIMAL ENTERITIS)

Gastric Decompression
• A siphon must be established each time, because passage of a nasogastric tube does not always result in reflux. Initially, nasogastric intubation may be needed every 1–2 h
• If <5 L of fluid is obtained, the interval between refluxing can be increased
• If colic or tachycardia are observed, the stomach should be refluxed
• The tube is commonly left in place until refluxing has either ceased or decreased to 1–2 L in 4 h

ACTIVITY
If no signs of laminitis are present, it may be beneficial to walk the horse frequently for short periods of time to stimulate GI motility.

DIET
• Nothing should be given orally until the nasogastric tube is removed, after which a slow reintroduction of feed can begin
• Partial or total parenteral nutrition may be indicated

CLIENT EDUCATION
• This condition can be frustrating and expensive to treat
• Owners should be made aware that the affected horses could reflux for >1 week, and that expensive therapy (e.g. total or partial parenteral nutrition) may be indicated
• Laminitis can occur, especially in larger horses
• Reported survival rate is generally good
• Death occurs from complications (e.g. laminitis, adhesions), or horses are euthanized because of economic concerns

SURGICAL CONSIDERATIONS
• Surgical intervention is common during the early stages of this condition to differentiate from a surgical SI lesion
• Surgery may be beneficial by confirming the diagnosis and decompressing the SI, but secondary complications such as risks associated with anesthesia and adhesion formation should be considered

 MEDICATIONS

DRUG(S) OF CHOICE
• The use of antimicrobials has been suggested but their efficacy has not been proven:
  ◦ For intestinal clostridiosis, penicillin may be administered—sodium penicillin (20 000–40 000 IU/kg IV every 6 h) or metronidazole (15–25 mg/kg per rectum every 8 h)

  ◦ Broad-spectrum antibiotics may be indicated with signs of toxemia or bacteremia. Options include a penicillin–aminoglycoside combination (sodium penicillin 20 000–40 000 IU/kg IV every 6 h/gentamicin 6.6 mg/kg IV every 24 h), trimethoprim–sulfamethoxazole (24 mg/kg IV every 12 h), or ceftiofur sodium (2 mg/kg IV every 12 h)
• Low-dose flunixin meglumine 0.25–0.5 mg/kg IV every 8 h can be administered for its purported antiendotoxin as well as anti-inflammatory effects
• Once the stomach is decompressed, there usually is little need for analgesics
• Analgesics should be administered judiciously because they may mask the progression of clinical signs that might indicate a surgical lesion. If analgesia is required, flunixin meglumine 1.1 mg/kg IV every 12 h can be administered
• H_2-receptor antagonists (e.g. ranitidine 6.6 mg/kg PO every 8 h) or proton pump inhibitors (e.g. omeprazole 4 mg/kg PO every 24 h) may be indicated after refluxing has ceased because of gastric irritation from distention, the primary disease process, and prolonged nasogastric intubation
• Efficacy of prokinetic agents has not been proven

CONTRAINDICATIONS
Prokinetic agents are contraindicated in obstructive SI lesions. Consider their use once an obstructive lesion has been ruled out or when DPJ has been confirmed via exploratory laparotomy/laparoscopy.

PRECAUTIONS
• Aminoglycosides and NSAIDs are potentially nephrotoxic and should not be administered until hydration status is normal
• Antibiotics have been implicated in the development of colitis

 FOLLOW-UP

PATIENT MONITORING
During the recovery period, monitor for signs of recrudescence of disease.

PREVENTION/AVOIDANCE
Because an intestinal dysbacteriosis may be involved in pathogenesis, institute feeding changes gradually.

POSSIBLE COMPLICATIONS
• Laminitis
• Intestinal adhesions after surgical exploration

• Other less common complications—peritonitis, aspiration pneumonia, and myocardial or renal infarcts

EXPECTED COURSE AND PROGNOSIS
• Duration of reflux may be short (≤24 h) but typically lasts for 3–7 days or longer
• Survival rates range from 25% to 98%
• Prognosis is good for horses that stop refluxing within 72 h
• Death most often results from economic concerns or complications such as laminitis or adhesions

 MISCELLANEOUS

ASSOCIATED CONDITIONS
• Aspiration pneumonia
• Intestinal adhesions
• Laminitis
• Peritonitis

PREGNANCY/FERTILITY/BREEDING
Pregnant mares may be at greater risk for abortion.

SYNONYMS
• Anterior enteritis
• Gastroduodenojejunitis
• Proximal enteritis

SEE ALSO
• Acute adult abdominal pain—acute colic
• Laminitis
• Peritonitis

ABBREVIATIONS
• DPJ = duodenitis–proximal jejunitis
• GI = gastrointestinal
• NSAID = nonsteroidal anti-inflammatory drug
• SI = small intestine
• WBC = white blood cell

Suggested Reading
Arroyo LG, Stämpfli HR, Weese JS. Potential role of *Clostridium difficile* as a cause of duodenitis-proximal jejunitis in horses. J Med Microbiol 2006;55:605–608.
Cohen ND, Toby E, Roussel AJ, et al. Are feeding practices associated with duodenitis-proximal jejunitis? Equine Vet J 2006;38:526–531.
Freeman DE. Duodenitis-proximal jejunitis. Equine Vet Educ 2000;12:322–332.

Authors Luis G. Arroyo and J. Scott Weese
Consulting Editors Henry Stämpfli and Olimpo Oliver-Espinosa

DYNAMIC COLLAPSE OF THE UPPER AIRWAYS

 BASICS

DEFINITION
• This is a group of disorders that cause a transient obstruction to respiration within the pharynx, larynx, or both
• Often cyclic and synchronous with inspiration
• Results from fatigue of the musculature that normally maintains luminal patency of the pharynx and larynx

PATHOPHYSIOLOGY
• The pathophysiologies of many of the abnormalities resulting in this condition have not yet been characterized. All appear to be different forms of neuromuscular dysfunction or fatigue; however, most occur during the inspiratory phase of respiration, under the pull of high negative inspiratory pressures
• With increased respiratory effort and muscular fatigue, the condition worsens, the obstruction becomes more severe, and a vicious cycle ensues
• Airway turbulence may result in abnormal respiratory noise but is not always present

SYSTEMS AFFECTED
• Upper respiratory tract
• With severe, more chronic conditions, the cardiopulmonary system may undergo secondary changes from repeated, high negative intrathoracic pressures and hypoxia

SIGNALMENT
• Any age or breed
• More commonly diagnosed in racehorses because of the high negative inspiratory pressures created during strenuous exercise
• Thoroughbreds (2–3 years) are the largest group affected
• To date, medial deviation of the aryepiglottic folds has been most commonly identified in racehorses
• Quarter Horses with hyperkalemic periodic paralysis can have paroxysmal spasms of the pharynx and larynx during "paralytic episodes" that result in severe upper respiratory obstruction

SIGNS
• Exercise intolerance or poor performance
• Abnormal upper respiratory noise during inspiration may occur depending on the degree and type of obstruction
• Only DDSP results in expiratory noise
• Coughing
• Dysphagia

CAUSES
• Laryngeal hemiplegia most commonly affects the left arytenoid cartilage, results from idiopathic degeneration of the left recurrent laryngeal nerve, and causes a paresis of the primary abductor of the left arytenoid, the cricoarytenoideus dorsalis muscle

• Infrequently, trauma to either the left or right recurrent laryngeal nerve associated with jugular thrombophlebitis can result in laryngeal hemiplegia
• Epiglottic retroversion is presumed to be a dysfunction of the hypoepiglottic muscle on the basis of experimental reproduction of the disorder after anesthetic blockade of the nerve (i.e. the hypoglossal) that supplies the hypoepiglottic muscle
• Dorsal pharyngeal collapse can be reproduced experimentally with anesthetically induced dysfunction of the stylopharyngeus muscles
• Other forms of collapse are thought to represent either specific muscle dysfunction within the pharynx or disproportionate force between the muscle groups

RISK FACTORS
• High-speed exercise
• Hyperkalemic periodic paralysis in Quarter Horses

 DIAGNOSIS

DIFFERENTIAL DIAGNOSIS
• Laryngeal hemiplegia
• Vocal cord collapse
• Intermittent DDSP
• Pharyngeal collapse
• Epiglottic retroversion
• Medial deviation of the aryepiglottic folds
• Combinations of any of the above-mentioned distinct disorders

DIAGNOSTIC PROCEDURES
Resting Endoscopy
• Helps to evaluate any structural abnormalities predisposing to dynamic obstruction during exercise but rarely is definitive for a dynamic abnormality
• More difficult to speculate on pharyngeal than on laryngeal forms of dynamic collapse
• Assesses laryngeal and pharyngeal function during normal breathing, nasal occlusion, and swallowing
• Horses normally demonstrate some dorsal roof collapse of the pharynx and have air pass between the aryepiglottic folds and pharyngeal ostium during nasal occlusion. This is not an indication of a pharyngeal abnormality during exercise
• With prolonged nasal occlusion, 60% of horses can be made to displace their palates, but they do not experience dynamic collapse during exercise
• Horses that very readily displace their soft palate are more likely to displace it during a race
• Horses that leave their palates displaced for an extended period of time or have difficulty replacing their palates with a swallow are more likely to have a pharyngeal abnormality

during high-speed exercise. This may be a crude indication of some pharyngeal weakness
• Horses commonly demonstrate asynchrony to their arytenoid movement yet achieve full abduction of both arytenoids during nasal occlusion or after swallowing (grade 2 on a scale of 1–4). These horses do not experience dynamic collapse during exercise. Horses that cannot fully and symmetrically abduct both arytenoids after swallowing or nasal occlusion (grade 3) are considered to be impaired
• The degree of dynamic collapse depends on the degree of paresis and on the intensity of exercise. Racehorses likely undergo significant respiratory compromise with grade 3 laryngeal hemiplegia; show horses are more likely asymptomatic

Ultrasonography
Ultrasonography of the larynx can determine if there is evidence of denervation of the cricoarytenoideus lateralis that would be indicative of recurrent laryngeal neuropathy (laryngeal hemiplegia). This should not be used as the sole criterion for surgical intervention but provides strong evidence of clinically significant dysfunction in racehorses.

Endoscopy During Exercise
• Often required to determine the cause of upper respiratory collapse
• The examination can be performed over ground or on a treadmill but, regardless of the surface, the level of strenuous activity must match the performance level
• Head and neck flexion can have a significant impact on the findings and thus the position during the examination should simulate that which occurs during performance to be valid
• Other requirements to ensure a valid test:
  ○ Holter monitor to record heart rate during exercise, to determine heart rate relative to the horse's speed, and to guarantee the horse is maximally exerting itself by achieving a heart rate of ≤ 220 bpm or greater
  ○ Videoendoscope linked to a video recorder to visualize the abnormality and play back the video in slow motion if the obstruction occurs too quickly to see in real time
  ○ A physiologically fit horse exercised in tack (harness for Standardbreds) to minimize spurious results
• Because these abnormalities are dynamic, and some can be intermittent (e.g. DDSP), other factors that may affect the horse's performance should also be simulated. For example, some racehorses will only demonstrate the abnormalities during an examination if other horses are challenging them during the examination
• Measurements of upper respiratory pressures and use of flow–volume loops during treadmill exercise can document respiratory obstruction but cannot discriminate between the many different abnormalities

Analysis of Upper Respiratory Sounds
Spectrogram analysis can be used to some degree to determine if an abnormality is present and which abnormality exists.

PATHOLOGIC FINDINGS
N/A

TREATMENT

AIMS
To create a stable open airway, resistant to high negative pressures.

SURGICAL CONSIDERATIONS
• Laryngeal hemiplegia is treated with surgical laryngoplasty (i.e. tie-back procedure). The affected arytenoid is held in a fixed, partially abducted position with a nonabsorbable suture simulating the contracted cricoarytenoid muscle. An adjunctive procedure (i.e. ventriculocordectomy) also can be performed to minimize obstruction at the ventral aspect of the glottis after a tie-back. For more on this topic, see chapter Laryngeal hemiparesis/hemiplegia (recurrent laryngeal neuropathy)
• Medial deviation of the aryepiglottic folds has been treated effectively both with rest and with laser resection of the offending soft tissue; however, surgery affords a quicker return to training
• There are multiple surgical procedures to consider for intermittent DDSP, which demonstrates our inability to define the exact cause in each patient. For more on this topic, see chapter Dorsal displacement of the soft palate (DDSP)

• Rest and oral anti-inflammatory treatment has been the only mode of therapy for other forms of dynamic collapse

MEDICATIONS

DRUG(S) OF CHOICE
A 3–4 week course of an anti-inflammatory drug may be indicated during the period of rest to resolve any presumed inflammatory component causing the dysfunction.

FOLLOW-UP

PATIENT MONITORING
• Resting endoscopy is necessary several weeks after any surgical intervention, and though it will not be definitive for determining the success of the surgery it will determine the capability of the horse to resume training
• An increase in performance or diminution of noise often is the criterion used to determine a successful treatment
• Repeat exercising endoscopy is the best method to determine a successful outcome from any treatment, but only after the horse has regained fitness

POSSIBLE COMPLICATIONS
• Most common is failure to achieve primary goal
• Increasing the risk of aspiration or dysphagia is the second most common complication

EXPECTED COURSE AND PROGNOSIS
Depending on the specific cause of collapse, the prognosis ranges from guarded to good.

MISCELLANEOUS

SEE ALSO
• Arytenoid chondropathy
• Dorsal displacement of the soft palate (DDSP)
• Epiglottic entrapment
• Laryngeal hemiparesis/hemiplegia (recurrent laryngeal neuropathy)

ABBREVIATIONS
DDSP = dorsal displacement of the soft palate

Suggested Reading
Davidson EJ, Martin BB, Boston RC, Parente EJ. Exercising upper respiratory videoendoscopic evaluation of 100 nonracing performance horses with abnormal respiratory noise and/or poor performance. Equine Vet J 2011;43(1):3–8.
Garrett KS, Woodie JB, Embertson RM. Association of treadmill upper airway endoscopic evaluation with results of ultrasonography and resting upper airway endoscopic evaluation. Equine Vet J 2011;43(3):365–371.
Leutton JL, Lumsden JM. Dynamic respiratory endoscopic findings pre- and post laryngoplasty in Thoroughbred racehorses. Equine Vet J 2015;47(5):531–536.
Van Erck E. Dynamic respiratory videoendoscopy in ridden sport horses: effect of head flexion, riding and airway inflammation in 129 cases. Equine Vet J Suppl 2011;40:18–24.

Author Eric J. Parente
Consulting Editors Mathilde Leclère and Daniel Jean

DYSTOCIA

 BASICS

DEFINITION
Any difficult delivery with or without assistance.

PATHOPHYSIOLOGY
• *Hereditary*—genital tract abnormalities, twinning, ankylosis of joints, large fetal head, hydrocephalus
• *Nutrition and management*—mare's pelvic size (nutritional stunting), pelvic cavity fat, failure to observe animals near term (uterine inertia), close confinement of mares during entire gestation
• *Infectious conditions of the placenta or fetus*—can result in uterine inertia, incomplete cervical dilatation, postural abnormalities due to fetal death, loss of placental attachment sites, etc.
• *Traumatic*—abdominal wall damage can inhibit abdominal contractions; uterine torsion, pelvic fracture, etc.
• *Miscellaneous*—unexplained postural changes: posterior or transverse presentation

Primary Uterine Inertia
• Uterine overstretching (i.e. hydrops, twins) increases in older, debilitated animals
• Uterine infections
• Oxytocin—failure of its release or to effect a uterine response

Secondary Uterine Inertia
• Dystocia, uterine muscle is exhausted
• Failure of labor due to pain
• Prolonged dystocia with strong circular contractions in a fatigued uterus

Immediate Causes of Dystocia
• Most often of fetal origin
• *Maternal causes*—birth canal stenosis, small pelvis, hypoplasia, lacerations and scars of the genital tract, pelvic tumors, persistent hymen, failure of cervical dilatation, uterine inertia, abortions, twinning
• *Fetal causes*—abnormal presentation, position, posture; excessive size; anasarca, ascites, tumors, monsters; ankylosed joints, hydrocephalus, posterior or transverse presentation, wry neck

SYSTEMS AFFECTED
• Reproductive
• Others possible as condition progresses, with development of systemic illness

GENETICS
See Pathophysiology.

INCIDENCE/PREVALENCE
Dystocia rates—10%. Higher incidence—miniature horse breeds.

GEOGRAPHIC DISTRIBUTION
Wherever pregnant mares are housed.

SIGNALMENT
Any breed and ages.

SIGNS

General Comments
Dystocia is always an emergency.

Historical Findings
• Stage 2 labor >40 min or an abnormal presentation, position, and/or posture
• May include premature placental detachment with the fetus yet in utero
• Important—complete history
  ○ Mare's due date
  ○ Prior dystocia or abnormal gestations
  ○ Systemic disease during gestation
  ○ Duration active labor (stages 1 and 2)
  ○ Rupture of allantoic membrane
  ○ Rupture of amniotic membrane
  ○ Assistance given? (potential contamination)
  ○ Status of mare's mobility

Physical Examination Findings
• Do routine physical examination of the reproductive tract and fetal examination *before* deciding how to handle a dystocia
• If recumbent, unable to rise, determine:
  ○ Cause
  ○ Hydration status
  ○ In shock or into shock before procedure is complete?
  ○ CRT ± toxic mucous membranes
• TRP of genital tract performed to determine possible lacerations; uterine tone; fetal presentation, position, posture before vaginal examination
• Genital tract examination following tail wrap and meticulous perineal wash
  ○ Use liberal amounts of lubricant
  ○ Examine vulva, vagina, cervix, uterus for lacerations. Inform owner prior to palpation of the fetus or obstetric manipulation if lacerations have been identified.
• Determine fetal viability:
  ○ Gentle pressure over eyes (blink reflex?)
  ○ Place fingers in fetal mouth (suckle reflex?)
  ○ Pull on fetal limb (test—fetal retraction?)
  ○ Maximally flex limb (stimulate fetal motion, it pulls away)
  ○ Test anal sphincter, contraction?
  ○ US examination to determine presence of heart beat or blood flow
• Evaluate fetal presentation, position, posture
• Determine birth canal size, permit fetal passage?
• If fetus is dead, determine how long (may not be possible until after delivery)
  ○ Time of death classification—corneas cloudy (dead 6–12 h prior to delivery); emphysema and sloughing of hair of fetus (dead minimum 18 h prior to delivery)

CAUSES
• All posterior presentations
• All deviations from normal position (dorsosacral)
  ○ Dorsoilial
  ○ Dorsopubic
• Postural defects, flexion of the extremities (head, neck, limbs)
• Most common cause of dystocia
  ○ Carpal, shoulder, hip flexion; lateral flexion head and neck
  ○ Ankylosis of joints
  ○ Hydrocephalic fetus, anasarca

RISK FACTORS
• Major causes involve fetal malposture. It is impossible to state precisely why the fetus moves from a normal to an abnormal delivery presentation
• Increased risk in older mares and in mares with insufficient exercise

 DIAGNOSIS

DIFFERENTIAL DIAGNOSIS
• Primary prepartum colic. Similar signs, especially in early stages of dystocia. With dystocia, the mare is not only uncomfortable but is also straining. Examination of the reproductive tract (TRP and vaginal) will help to differentiate dystocia from colic
• With true breech delivery (posterior presentation, both rear legs flexed), stage 2 labor and straining may be absent

CBC/BIOCHEMISTRY/URINALYSIS
CBC—blood chemistries indicated if mare is hospitalized and results rapidly available.

IMAGING
Depending on circumstances, US may determine fetal viability.

OTHER DIAGNOSTIC PROCEDURES
• Determine mare's mucous membrane color (normal, injected, muddy) and CRT
• Mare hydration status
• Is mare ambulatory or down?
• Is she sufficiently stable to administer local anesthetics, epidurals, general anesthesia, or sedation?
• TRP is always indicated to determine if uterine lacerations are present prior to vaginal examination, fetal viability, the amount of uterine contracture around the fetus
• Vaginal examination to determine presence of uterine tears, degree of cervical relaxation and uterine contracture, fetal viability, presentation, position, posture, space between the fetus and maternal pelvis
• Field resolution is preferable when C-section is not an option and mare's straining prevents adequate room to accomplish mutation
• Heavy sedation or *light general anesthesia* of the mare:
  ○ Elevation of mare's rear quarters (suspending by her hocks; *care must be taken* to protect the hocks with padding or towels before attaching chains or straps); use a lift, front-end loader, overhead beam, etc.
  ○ Mare placed in lateral recumbency, elevate hocks no more than 45–60 cm (18–24 inches), usually sufficient
  ○ Allows weight of the fetus/fluids in the relaxed uterus to fall deeper into the

abdomen, creates additional space to accomplish mutation, subsequent extraction
○ An option whether fetus is alive or dead, especially when C-section is declined

PATHOLOGIC FINDINGS
Depends on the cause of the dystocia.

TREATMENT

APPROPRIATE HEALTH CARE
• Generally best handled on the farm
• Vaginal deliveries best accomplished shortly after a dystocia is diagnosed, whether mutation, forced extraction, or fetotomy is to be performed

NURSING CARE
• Thorough examination of the genital tract after delivery
• Broad-spectrum antibiotics placed into the uterus to reduce number of organisms introduced during mutation and extraction of the fetus. Systemic antibiotics may be necessary if systemic disease develops
• Uterine stimulants such as oxytocin can be beneficial; enhance uterine contractions and involution
• Uterine flushes or infusions may be indicated to enhance uterine contractility

ACTIVITY
Stall rest for mares undergoing C-section.

DIET
• Maintain mare's regular diet, reduce quantity fed, if indicated
• Changing diet at the time of parturition further adds to the mare's stress; should be avoided

CLIENT EDUCATION
• Mares should not be permitted to be in prolonged labor; reduces probability of neonatal survival
• As soon as possible, examine location of fetal extremities during delivery; determine if fetus is in an abnormal delivery presentation, position, or posture
• If soles of the fetus viewed at the mare's vulvar lips are *pointed down*:
  ○ Anterior presentation and dorsosacral position (=normal), or
  ○ Posterior presentation and dorsopubic position (=upside down; detorsion &/or C-section)
• Must determine if fetus's head is resting on its metacarpi (normal presentation, position, posture)

SURGICAL CONSIDERATIONS
• Decide early if a C-section is the best approach for a viable fetus:
  ○ No other correction (mutation, extraction) possible
  ○ If surgical approach can be made quickly to maintain fetal viability
• If a C-section is to be performed, timing is critical
• If fetus cannot be delivered alive, give consideration to fetotomy, especially if fetotomy will require only 1 or 2 cuts that can be done on the farm at an early stage, before the vaginal vault diameter becomes compromised (swelling, bruising)

MEDICATIONS

DRUG(S) OF CHOICE
• Epidural anesthesia may assist the delivery; reduces contractions during assisted delivery. Approximate dose—1 mL of 2% Carbocaine (mepivacaine) per 40 kg of body weight
• Xylazine (0.5–1.0 mg/kg) used for sedation alone or combined with acepromazine (0.04 mg/kg)
• General anesthetic agents for C-section or to accomplish further corrective procedures
• After delivery, administration of oxytocin at a dosage of 10–20 IU per 500 kg IM to hasten uterine contractions, involution of postpartum uterus

CONTRAINDICATIONS
Never administer oxytocin prepartum—potential to induce further uterine contracture, reducing further fetal manipulation space. Exceeding recommended doses, especially early after delivery, may result in uterine eversion (prolapse).

PRECAUTIONS
Regardless of approach, manipulate fetus carefully during delivery.

ALTERNATIVE DRUGS
• Butorphanol
• Detomidine
• Morphine

FOLLOW-UP

PATIENT MONITORING
• TRP is indicated daily or every other day to determine size and tone of the uterus
• US examination plus TRP—determine presence or absence of uterine luminal fluid

PREVENTION/AVOIDANCE
• Close observation of near-term mare to aid in early diagnosis of dystocia
• There is no method to prevent dystocia

POSSIBLE COMPLICATIONS
• After dystocia, check for lacerations—cervix, vagina, vestibule, vulva, or uterus (with resultant peritonitis)
• Uterine inflammation or infection may result from the dystocia or corrective methods used

EXPECTED COURSE AND PROGNOSIS
• Prognosis decreases with:
  ○ Duration of dystocia
  ○ Inexperienced interference
  ○ Cause of dystocia
• Mares have a grave prognosis if >24 h from onset of stage 2
• Fetuses have a guarded prognosis >40 min from onset of stage 2
• After initial examination of mare—discuss prognosis, fees, best approach to resolve dystocia with owner
• Choices of approach:
  ○ Mare standing, lateral recumbency, rear quarters elevated—assisted forced extraction, manipulation (mutation) of fetus; fetotomy
  ○ C-section
  ○ Euthanasia of mare

MISCELLANEOUS

AGE-RELATED FACTORS
Slight increase in dystocia in aged mares, may be related to decreased uterine contractions.

SYNONYMS
Difficult—foaling, labor, delivery, parturition.

ABBREVIATIONS
• CRT = capillary refill time
• C-section = Caesarean section
• TRP = transrectal palpation
• US = ultrasonography, ultrasound

Suggested Reading
McCue PM, Ferris RA. Parturition, dystocia and foal survival: a retrospective study of 1047 births. Equine Vet J 2012;44 (Suppl. 41):22–25.

Author Carla L. Carleton
Consulting Editor Carla L. Carleton
Acknowledgment The author/editor acknowledges the prior contribution of Walter R. Threlfall.

EAR TICK-ASSOCIATED MUSCLE CRAMPING

BASICS

SIGNALMENT
Horses of any age or breed.

SIGNS
• Severe and intermittent muscle cramping not associated with exercise
• Clinical signs are often misconstrued as signs of colic or mild tying up
• Focal muscle groups in various regions may have intermittent visible contraction. Intermittent prolapse of the third eyelid, sweating, pawing, muscle tremors, and muscle fasciculations may also be observed
• When muscle cramping occurs during movement, alternating limb lameness may be observed
• Percussion of muscle bodies will induce contraction of muscle groups and pain
• Muscle biopsy reveals no abnormalities except for a few necrotic muscle fibers undergoing phagocytosis
• Electromyography of 1 horse was suggestive of increased motor unit activity
• All horses had *Otobius megnini* (ear tick) infestations and had recurrence of signs until treatment was initiated for ear ticks

CAUSES AND RISK FACTORS
• The *O. megnini* ear tick is found mostly in arid regions of the western USA but may be seen in other locations
• Horses have become infected following stabling at fairground barns, older barns, and other wooden facilities
• Multiple horses were seen with the syndrome following stabling at an event in New Mexico

DIAGNOSIS

DIFFERENTIAL DIAGNOSIS
• Colic
• Myopathy
• Tetanus
• Shifting limb intermittent lameness due to muscle cramping

CBC/BIOCHEMISTRY/URINALYSIS
Concentrations of serum electrolytes and the acid–base balance are within reference limits, but activities of creatine kinase and aspartate aminotransferase are moderately high.

DIAGNOSTIC PROCEDURES
The key to diagnosis is to consider this disorder and do muscle percussion to induce cramping and look in the horse's ears for the easily seen spinose ear ticks, which are large gray ticks with prominent legs.

TREATMENT

• Treatment is removal of the ear ticks by topical administration of pyrethroid compounds or gels directly into the ear, which causes the ticks to dislodge. There is no need to manually remove the ticks
• Horses shake their heads vigorously following treatment and ear ticks can be seen flying out of the ears

MEDICATIONS

• In North America several acaricides have broad-spectrum activity against ticks
• Pyrethroids in topical form or spays have been used to kill these ear ticks with applications directly in the horse's ears
• Broad antibacterial and anti-inflammatory ointments used for canine ear infections have been applied into the horse's ears after the ticks have been removed

FOLLOW-UP

The ticks migrate from the body of the horse to the ears. It is considered appropriate to treat the body of the horse with an approved topically applied acaricide labeled for horses.

SEE ALSO
• Acute adult abdominal pain—acute colic
• Hyperkalemic periodic paralysis
• Tetanus

Suggested Reading
Madigan JE, Valberg SJ, Ragle C, Moody JL. Muscle spasms associated with ear tick (*Otobius megnini*) infestations in five horses. J Am Vet Med Assoc 1995;207(1):74–76.

Author John E. Madigan
Consulting Editor Caroline N. Hahn

EARLY EMBRYONIC DEATH

BASICS

DEFINITION
Maternal structural/functional defects preventing normal embryonic development from early pregnancy diagnosis at 14–15 days post ovulation to the beginning of the fetal stage at approximately 40 days of gestation.

PATHOPHYSIOLOGY
• Estimated to be 5–10% in younger mares; much higher in older, subfertile mares
• The causes and pathophysiology are similar to those of conception failure and include:
  ○ Embryonic defects or injury
  ○ Unsuitable uterine environment
  ○ Regression of CL secondary to endometritis
  ○ Luteal insufficiency—anecdotal
  ○ Failure of *maternal recognition of pregnancy*

SYSTEMS AFFECTED
Reproductive

SIGNS
Historical Findings
One or more of the following:
• Diagnosis of EED by transrectal US at >14 days after ovulation, following previous diagnosis of pregnancy
• Diagnosis of failure of pregnancy by TRP at >25 days after ovulation, following previous diagnosis of pregnancy
• History of PMIE
• History of abortion and/or dystocia
• Return to estrus after diagnosis of pregnancy
• Previous exposure to endophyte-infected fescue or ergotized grasses and grains
• *Recent* systemic disease

Physical Examination Findings
• Frequently, at ≤40 days after ovulation, there is no evidence by transrectal US or TRP of a previously diagnosed pregnancy
• Alternatively, at ≤40 days after ovulation, there can be evidence by transrectal US of embryonic death in a mare previously diagnosed as pregnant
• Transrectal US evidence of EED includes decreasing embryonic vesicular size, change in appearance of the fluid within the embryonic vesicle, failure to visualize the embryo proper, the absence of a heartbeat at >25 days, and/or cessation of normal embryonic growth and development, with eventual disappearance of pregnancy-associated structures
• Endometrial folds and/or intrauterine fluid might be visualized in the nonpregnant uterus
• Luteal structures may or may not be present on the ovaries, and the mare can appear to be cyclic or acyclic, depending on the circumstances
• There may or may not be a mucoid or mucopurulent vaginal discharge

RISK FACTORS
• Older mares >15 years of age, especially those with moderate/severe endometritis, endometrial periglandular fibrosis, and/or lymphatic cysts
• Anatomic defects predisposing to endometritis
• Seasonal effects
• Foal heat breeding—anecdotal and somewhat controversial
• Inadequate nutrition
• Exposure to xenobiotics—fescue toxicosis and ergotism
• Some heterospecific matings—stallion × jenny
• Susceptibility to PMIE (conception failure is more likely)
• Geographic location, especially in relation to endophyte-infected fescue pastures/hay and/or ergotized grasses or grains
• Preexisting PPID and EMS/IR
• Severe laminitis
• Transfer of embryos from older mares or those generated using IVF or other reproductive technologies

DIAGNOSIS

DIFFERENTIAL DIAGNOSIS
• Conception failure
• Misdiagnosis of pregnancy
• Pregnancies move (transuterine migration) until fixation at 16 days after ovulation; they also increase in size, and develop/exhibit heartbeats

CBC/BIOCHEMISTRY/URINALYSIS
• CBC and serum biochemistry for inflammatory response, or evidence of other organ system involvement if the mare has recently been ill
• Maternal P_4 may be useful at <80 days of gestation (>1 to >4 ng/mL, depending on the reference laboratory). Maternal estrogen concentrations can reflect fetal estrogen production and viability, especially conjugated estrogens, e.g. estrone sulfate

IMAGING
• Transrectal US should be performed every 2 weeks until at least 60 days of pregnancy in normal mares in order to detect EED
• It is necessary to follow embryonic growth and development and to distinguish the conceptus from cysts

OTHER DIAGNOSTIC PROCEDURES
• Vaginal speculum examination and hysteroscopy if structural abnormalities are suspected in the cervix or uterus
• Endometrial cytology, culture, and biopsy procedures to assess endometrial inflammation and/or fibrosis
• Feed or environmental analyses for specific xenobiotics, ergopeptine alkaloids, phytoestrogens, heavy metals, or fescue endophyte
• A thorough reproductive evaluation is indicated before breeding for individuals predisposed to EED
• Specialized testing for PPID or EMS/IR
• Cytogenetic studies to detect chromosomal abnormalities

PATHOLOGIC FINDINGS
An endometrial biopsy can demonstrate the presence of moderate to severe, chronic endometritis, endometrial periglandular fibrosis with decreased normal glandular architecture, and/or lymphatic lacunae.

TREATMENT

APPROPRIATE HEALTH CARE
• Treat preexisting endometritis before insemination or breeding of mares during physiologic breeding season
• Mares being bred should have adequate body condition
• Inseminate or breed foal heat mares if ovulation occurs >9–10 days postpartum and no intrauterine fluid is present
• Prevention of PMIE
• Depending on breed restrictions, various forms of advanced reproductive technologies (e.g. zygote, embryo) to retrieve embryos from the oviduct or uterus (days 6–8 after ovulation) for ET, and oocyte retrieval and successful IVF with subsequent ET have been used in some instances
• Most cases of EED can be handled in an ambulatory situation
• Increased frequency of US monitoring of follicular development and ovulation to permit insemination closer to ovulation, as well as more technical diagnostic procedures, may need to be performed in a hospital setting

NURSING CARE
Minimal nursing care might be necessary after more invasive diagnostic and therapeutic procedures.

ACTIVITY
• No restriction unless contraindicated by concurrent maternal disease or diagnostic or therapeutic procedures
• Preference may be to restrict activity of mares in competition because of the possible impact of stress on pregnancy maintenance, especially in mares with a history of EED

DIET
Generally no restriction, unless indicated by concurrent maternal disease (e.g. EMS) or nutritional problems, e.g. under- or overnourished.

CLIENT EDUCATION
• Emphasize the *aged* mare's susceptibility to conception failure and EED and her refractoriness to treatment

E

EARLY EMBRYONIC DEATH   (CONTINUED)

• Discuss susceptibility of mares with preexisting systemic disease (e.g. PPID and EMS/IR) to EED
• Inform clients regarding the cause, diagnosis, and treatment of endometritis; the seasonal aspects and nutritional requirements of conception; the role that endophyte-infected fescue and certain heterospecific breedings might play in conception failure

SURGICAL CONSIDERATIONS
• Indicated for repair of anatomic defects predisposing mares to endometritis
• Certain diagnostic and therapeutic procedures discussed above might also involve some surgical intervention

MEDICATIONS
DRUG(S) OF CHOICE
Altrenogest
• For mares with a history of conception failure or moderate to severe endometritis (i.e. no active, infectious component) or fibrosis—0.044–0.088 mg/kg PO once daily beginning 2–3 days after ovulation or at diagnosis of pregnancy and continued until at least 90–100 days of gestation (taper daily dose over a 14 day period at the end of treatment)
• Administration can be started later during gestation, continued longer, or used for only short periods of time, depending on serum P_4 levels during the first 80 days of gestation, clinical circumstances, and risk factors
• If used near term, altrenogest is generally discontinued 7–14 days before the expected foaling date

PRECAUTIONS, POSSIBLE INTERACTIONS
• Use altrenogest only to prevent conception failure of noninfectious endometritis
• Use transrectal US to diagnose pregnancy at ≥14–16 days after ovulation to identify intrauterine fluid or pyometra early in the disease course for appropriate treatment
• If pregnancy is diagnosed, frequent monitoring (weekly initially) may be indicated to detect EED
• Altrenogest is absorbed through the skin, so persons handling this preparation should wear gloves and wash their hands
• Although supplemental progestins are commonly used widely to treat cases of

conception failure, their efficacy is controversial
• Primary, age-related embryonic defects do not respond to supplemental progestins

ALTERNATIVE DRUGS
• Injectable P_4 (150–500 mg/day, oil base IM SID) instead of the oral formulation
• Other injectable and implantable progestin preparations are available commercially for use in other species. Any use in horses of these products is off-label, and little scientific data are available regarding their efficacy
• Newer, repository forms of P_4 are occasionally introduced; however, some evidence of efficacy should be provided prior to use
• The use of thyroxine supplementation in affected mares is controversial

FOLLOW-UP
PATIENT MONITORING
• Accurate teasing records
• Reexamination of mares treated for endometritis before breeding
• Early examination for pregnancy by transrectal US

PREVENTION/AVOIDANCE
• Recognition of at-risk mares
• Management of endometritis before breeding
• Removal of mares from fescue-infected pasture and ergotized grasses and grains after breeding and during early gestation
• Prudent use of medications in bred mares
• Avoid exposure to known toxicants

POSSIBLE COMPLICATIONS
• High-risk pregnancy
• Abortion—infectious or noninfectious

EXPECTED COURSE AND PROGNOSIS
• Young mares with resolved cases of endometritis or corrected anatomic abnormalities can have a fair to good prognosis to complete pregnancy
• Older mares (>15 years of age) with a history of preexisting systemic disease, chronic, moderate to severe endometritis, endometrial periglandular fibrosis, and/or lymphatic cysts, as well as conception failure and/or EED have a guarded to poor prognosis for conception, full-term pregnancy, and delivery of a healthy foal

MISCELLANEOUS
SYNONYMS
• Conception failure
• Infertility
• Pregnancy reabsorption
• Reabsorbed pregnancy
• Sterility
• Subfertility

SEE ALSO
• Abortion, spontaneous, infectious
• Abortion, spontaneous, noninfectious
• Conception failure in mares
• Embryo transfer
• Endometrial biopsy
• Endometritis
• Postpartum metritis
• Spermatogenesis and factors affecting sperm production

ABBREVIATIONS
• CL = corpus luteum
• EED = early embryonic death
• EMS = equine metabolic syndrome
• ET = embryo transfer
• IR = insulin resistance
• IVF = in vitro fertilization
• P_4 = progesterone
• PMIE = post-mating-induced endometritis
• PPID = pituitary pars intermedia dysfunction
• TRP = transrectal palpation
• US = ultrasonography, ultrasound

Suggested Reading
Ball BA. Embryonic loss. In: McKinnon AO, Squires EL, Vaala WE, Varner DD, eds. Equine reproduction, 2e. Ames, IA: Wiley Blackwell, 2011:2327–2338.
Canisso IF, Stewart J, Coutinho da Silva MA. Endometritis: managing persistent post-breeding endometritis. Vet Clin North Am Equine Pract 2016;32(3):465–480.
Evans TJ. Endocrine disruptive effects of ergopeptine alkaloids on pregnant mares. Vet Clin North Am Equine Pract 2011;27(1):165–173.
Ferris RA. Endometritis: diagnostic tools for infectious endometritis. Vet Clin North Am Equine Pract 2016;32(3):481–498.
Scoggin CF. Endometritis: nontraditional therapies. Vet Clin North Am Equine Pract 2016;32(3):499–511.

Author Tim J. Evans
Consulting Editor Carla L. Carleton

EASTERN (EEE), WESTERN (WEE), AND VENEZUELAN (VEE) EQUINE ENCEPHALITIDES

BASICS

DEFINITION
EEEV, WEEV, and VEEV cause encephalomyelitides in North and South America that spread from wild (sylvatic) reservoirs to horses and humans and other mammals, most often by mosquito species. Historically there have been North and South American EEEV variants; the South American EEEV is now designated as MDV. This virus causes disease outbreaks in horses.

PATHOPHYSIOLOGY
• Varying degrees of destructive encephalomyelitis associated with intraneuronal viral replication and severe infiltration of polymorphonuclear cells
• EEEV is one of the most pathogenic neurotropic viruses known
• In recent years WEEV has not caused any outbreaks; however a variant of WEEV, Highlands J virus, actively circulates in Florida
• VEEV is the only arbovirus where, in epizootics, horses are *not* dead-end hosts

SYSTEMS AFFECTED
Central nervous system, especially the cerebral cortex.

INCIDENCE/PREVALENCE
• In certain geographic locations, the annual locale incidence is consistent with spikes in activity depending on weather conditions
• Large outbreaks can occur in new locations, and are occurring more frequently in the northern USA and Canada

GEOGRAPHIC DISTRIBUTION
North and South America only.

SIGNALMENT
• There is no associated breed or sex predisposition
• Young horses may be at greater risk for development of EEE

SIGNS
Historical Findings
• For North American alphaviruses, EEEV occurs east of the Mississippi River while WEEV primarily occur in the west
• VEE cases have been reported in southern Texas and South America and occasionally in nearby locales
• Florida is also considered an at-risk state for VEE
• Significant MDV and VEEV outbreaks occur in Central and South America
• Unvaccinated horses in endemic areas are at high risk
• New arrivals of horses in endemic areas that are undervaccinated
• Even in the southeast, while EEEV can occur year-round, peak incidence is midsummer

Physical Examination Findings
• 48–96 h before onset of neurologic signs fever, inappetence, and depression can occur
• Some horses may demonstrate lameness and even abdominal pain

Neurologic Findings
• Clinical signs, which vary in severity with each virus, usually are referable to diffuse cerebral disease, but sometimes signs of spinal cord disease predominate
• Fever, prodromal malaise, colic, and anorexia may initially be evident; then there is a progressive, but often abrupt, onset of somnolence and peracute to acute diffuse brain signs
• Dementia, head pressing, ataxia, blindness, circling, and seizures often present
• Signs of spinal cord or brainstem involvement may occur first, occasionally with focal sensory, reflex, and lower motor neuron signs, particularly in the brainstem
• Gastrointestinal abnormality, severe obtundation, recumbence, and death may be noted before neurologic deficits are evident.
• Other associated signs include abortion, oral ulceration, pulmonary hemorrhage, and epistaxis

CAUSES
Etiologic Agent
• EEEV, WEEV, and VEEV are single-stranded, enveloped positive-sense RNA viruses in the family Togaviridae, genus *Alphavirus*
• They are all mosquito borne with birds the primary reservoir host for EEEV and rodents the reservoir host for endemic VEEV
• When epizootic VEEV occurs, there is virus mutation, change in the mosquito vector, and reservoir changes to equids

RISK FACTORS
Poor vaccination programs and the presence of dense populations of insects (most often mosquitoes) spreading viral particles from the sylvatic reservoirs, which often include birds, rodents, and reptiles.

DIAGNOSIS

• Immunoglobulin M capture ELISA titer ≥400 confirmatory in a clinical animal
• A 4-fold rise in titer between acute and convalescent (7–10 days later) serum samples is considered positive for the diseases, although EEEV horses rarely survive to a second test
• An increased single sample titer in an unvaccinated severely affected animal is a probable diagnosis
• Any single sample analysis must be interpreted cautiously if there is a history of vaccination against the viruses

• Vaccinal versus wild virus-induced titers historically have been used to determine EEEV exposure
• EEE-to-WEE titer ratios of 4 or more are suspicious for EEE infection
• Ratio of 8 or more is highly indicative of EEE

DIFFERENTIAL DIAGNOSIS
WNV, rabies, leukoencephalomalacia, and hepatic encephalopathy—WNV encephalomyelitis in the USA tends to result in less severe cerebral and more prominent spinal cord signs than EEEV.

CBC/BIOCHEMISTRY/URINALYSIS
Cerebrospinal fluid analysis is highly indicative—consisting of predominately polymorphonuclear cells that are nondegenerate with a corresponding increase in total protein.

PATHOLOGIC FINDINGS
• Gross necropsy findings are nonspecific but often have extremely congested meninges
• A gray discoloration with petechial hemorrhages of the brain and spinal cord is evident
• Brain swelling can be present with even some occipital–subtentorial herniation and brainstem compression
• Histologic changes are strongly definitive
• Meningoencephalomyelitis with neuronal degeneration, gliosis, perivascular and neuroparenchymal infiltrates, and meningitis are highly suggestive for this disease group
• The gliosis is extremely widespread, especially in the cortex extending into the corona radiata with cells composed primarily of nondegenerate neutrophils
• Lesions can be observed in the heart and antigen has been found

TREATMENT

AIMS
• Treatment is supportive and should be aimed at metabolic maintenance and care and prophylaxis of self-induced trauma
• No specific treatment will reduce morbidity and mortality. Prognosis for EEE survival extremely poor
• Prognosis for any recumbent and comatose horse extremely poor with death imminent

NURSING CARE
Many horses, if they survive, have residual neurologic deficits—the ethics of nursing these cases should be discussed with owners.

CLIENT EDUCATION
Appropriate vaccination and vector control.

E

EASTERN (EEE), WESTERN (WEE), AND VENEZUELAN (VEE) EQUINE ENCEPHALITIDES (CONTINUED)

MEDICATIONS

DRUG(S) OF CHOICE
• Fluid and metabolic support can be useful
• No specific drug treatment is likely to alter morbidity or mortality
• Early treatment with corticosteroids—considered anecdotally to lead to improvement in less severe cases

FOLLOW-UP

PATIENT MONITORING
Regular detailed neurologic examinations in horses demonstrating fever, inappetence, and depression during peak seasons.

PREVENTION/AVOIDANCE
• Strict mosquito control and vaccination can prevent both human and equine cases
• All equine cases must be reported to state health officials

POSSIBLE COMPLICATIONS
Self-induced trauma may be severe.

EXPECTED COURSE AND PROGNOSIS
• Complete recoveries from the neurologic deficits associated with EEEV are reported, but they are rare with mortality ranging from 85% to 100%
• Animals that have recovered from EEEV often have residual neurologic deficits that commonly include clumsiness, depression, and abnormal behavior
• Neurologic sequelae are similar but less common in horses that recover from WEEV and the mortality rate is similar to WNV at 20–40%
• Depending on the VEEV strain mortality can be quite variable spanning from 40% to 80%
• Reinfection is possible and survivors should be vaccinated

MISCELLANEOUS

ZOONOTIC POTENTIAL
• Horses do become viremic with EEEV and WEEV, but not high enough to transmit to feeding mosquitoes. Hence, they are dead-end hosts
• Brain and cranial spinal tissues of horses with EEEV and VEEV are laden with virus. Extreme caution and rabies protocol for necropsy required
• Horses with epizootic VEE have sufficient circulating viral concentrations and are the principal reservoirs
• Blood and ocular and nasal secretions from infected horses contain high concentrations of VEEV and personal protection equipment should be incorporated while treating equines during epizootics

SEE ALSO
• Hepatic encephalopathy
• Leukoencephalomalacia
• Rabies
• West nile virus

ABBREVIATIONS
• EEE = Eastern equine encephalomyelitis
• EEEV = Eastern equine encephalomyelitis virus
• ELISA = enzyme-linked immunosorbent assay
• MDV = Maradiaga virus
• VEE = Venezuelan equine encephalomyelitis
• VEEV = Venezuelan equine encephalomyelitis virus
• WEE = Western equine encephalomyelitis
• WEEV = Western equine encephalomyelitis virus
• WNV = West Nile virus

Internet Resources
International Veterinary Information Service. http://www.ivis.org/advances/Carter/toc.asp

Suggested Reading
Del Piero F, Wilkins PA, Dubovi EJ, et al. Immunohistochemical, and virologic findings of Eastern equine encephalomyelitis in two horses. Vet Pathol 2001;38:451–456.

Author Maureen T. Long
Consulting Editor Caroline N. Hahn
Acknowledgment The author acknowledges the prior contribution Caroline N. Hahn.

BASICS

DEFINITION
• A rare metabolic condition resulting from hypocalcemia in heavily lactating mares.
• Clinical signs are progressive and include muscle fasciculations; stiff, stilted gait; tachycardia with dysrhythmias

PATHOPHYSIOLOGY
• Loss of calcium in the milk, mainly in heavily milking mares kept on lush pasture.
• Also in well-muscled mares that are working while lactating, in lactating mares that are transported over long distances, or in mares 1–2 days post weaning

SYSTEMS AFFECTED
• Mammary. • Musculoskeletal.
• Cardiovascular

GENETICS
Draft breeds—Belgian, Percheron, Clydesdale, but not exclusively.

INCIDENCE/PREVALENCE
Rare

SIGNALMENT
• See Pathophysiology. • Draft mares. • No age predisposition. • Unlikely occurrence in primiparous mares

SIGNS
• Related to the level of serum calcium. • May include: ○ Muscle fasciculations of the temporal, masseter, and triceps muscles. ○ Generalized increased muscle tone; stiff, stilted gait; rear limb ataxia. ○ Trismus; dysphagia; salivation. ○ Profuse sweating; elevated rectal temperature; anxiety; tachycardia with dysrhythmias. ○ Synchronous diaphragmatic flutter, convulsions, coma, and death. ○ If untreated, the condition is progressive over a 24–48 h period. ○ Increased excitability with calcium levels that are below normal (normal range 11–13 mg/dL) but >8 mg/dL. ○ Calcium levels of 5–8 mg/dL usually produce signs of tetanic spasms and incoordination. ○ Serum calcium levels <5 mg/dL—often become stuporous and are recumbent

CAUSES
Loss of calcium in milk.

RISK FACTORS
Lactation, postpartum, heavier milking mares, exercise, transport, weaning or other stressful events.

DIAGNOSIS
Total serum calcium values <8 mg/dL, coupled with associated clinical signs.

DIFFERENTIAL DIAGNOSIS
• Colic. • Laminitis. • Myositis. • Tetanus.
• Other neuromuscular disorders

CBC/BIOCHEMISTRY/URINALYSIS
• Hyper-/hypophosphatemia and hyper-/hypomagnesemia may also be present.
• Hypomagnesemia/hypocalcemia with transport of heavily lactating mares

DIAGNOSTIC PROCEDURES
• No clinical signs if ionized calcium is within normal range. Normal ionized calcium is possible despite hypocalcemia, if a mare is severely hypoproteinemic. • There may be excess protein in the mare's urine

PATHOLOGIC FINDINGS
None

TREATMENT

APPROPRIATE HEALTH CARE
Therapy is recommended in nearly all cases. A few mildly affected cases will recover without treatment.

NURSING CARE
Occasionally, a mare may require a second calcium treatment, if relapse occurs.

ACTIVITY
Restrict transit of heavily lactating mares during the susceptible period, the first 10–12 days postpartum.

DIET
• Restrict access of heavily lactating mares to lush pasture if they have a history of eclampsia. • Feed high-protein, high-calcium diets post foaling for mares with a history of eclampsia

CLIENT EDUCATION
Reduce nutritional intake (quality) in heavily lactating mares for 1–2 weeks prior to weaning to reduce milk production.

MEDICATIONS

DRUG(S) OF CHOICE
• IV calcium, in the form of 20% calcium borogluconate or 23% calcium gluconate.
• Rate—250–500 mL per 500 kg body weight. • Calcium solutions should be diluted 1:4 with saline or dextrose

PRECAUTIONS
• Use caution when administering calcium solutions due to potential cardiotoxic effects.
• Imperative to monitor the heart for any alterations in rate or rhythm. If alterations occur, the treatment should immediately be stopped. • Dilution of the calcium with saline or dextrose reduces the potential for cardiotoxic effects

FOLLOW-UP

PATIENT MONITORING
• A reduction in the clinical signs and a positive inotropic effect indicate treatment is effective. • If no response is evident after the initial treatment, a second treatment may be necessary in 30 min

PREVENTION/AVOIDANCE
• Decreasing high-protein feeds in the mare's diet late in gestation may decrease incidence in susceptible mares. • In previously affected mares, decrease intake of calcium 2–5 weeks before foaling. • High-protein, high-calcium diets after foaling for mares prone to eclampsia. • See Diet and Client Education for susceptible mares

POSSIBLE COMPLICATIONS
Cardiovascular effects.

EXPECTED COURSE AND PROGNOSIS
• Most mares respond to treatment with a full recovery; however, relapses can occur, necessitating additional therapy. • Recurrence possible if no changes in the management conditions

MISCELLANEOUS

PREGNANCY/FERTILITY/BREEDING
Occurs either late in gestation or during the peripartum period.

SYNONYMS
• Lactation tetany. • Puerperal tetany.
• Transit tetany

SEE ALSO
Dystocia

Suggested Reading
Baird JD. Lactation tetany (eclampsia) in a Shetland Pony mare. Aust Vet J 1971;47:402–404.
Fenger CK. Disorders of calcium metabolism. In: Reed SM, Bayly WM, eds. Equine Internal Medicine. Philadelphia, PA: WB Saunders Co., 1998:930–931.
Valberg SJ, Hodgson DR. Diseases of muscle. In: Smith BP, ed. Large Animal Internal Medicine, 2e. St. Louis, MO: Mosby, 1996:1498–1499.
Author Carla L. Carleton
Consulting Editor Carla L. Carleton

ECTOPARASITES

BASICS

DEFINITION
Chorioptes (equi) bovis, Psoroptes (equi) bovis, and lice (*Werneckiella equi* and *Haematopinus asini*) are ectoparasites that affect horses. They complete their life cycle on the horse and are transmitted to other horses by contact.

PATHOPHYSIOLOGY
The mites cause disease by direct irritation and inducing a cutaneous hypersensitivity reaction while the sucking lice (*H. asini*) can induce anemia.

SYSTEMS AFFECTED
Skin

GENETICS
N/A

INCIDENCE/PREVALENCE
• Incidence is sporadic and secondary to contact with another infested horse or the immediate environment containing scabs or hair shafts with eggs or larvae present
• More common in barns with horses that are hauled frequently and return with subclinical infestations

GEOGRAPHIC DISTRIBUTION
Worldwide

SIGNALMENT
Chorioptic acariosis is more common in breeds with feathered fetlocks, such as draft breeds.

Mean Age and Range
Young and geriatric animals may be more prone to severe lice infestations.

SIGNS

General Comments
Mite and lice infections are more severe in colder months. Weight loss can be seen due to the chronic irritation. Infestations may produce typical clinical signs in some animals whereas others may exhibit few clinical signs or may be asymptomatic carriers.

Historical Findings
Often involves travel to an equestrian event where exposure had occurred.

Physical Examination Findings
Lice Infestation
• Common in sick, old, or otherwise debilitated animals
• Secondary seborrhea can camouflage the lice from detection. As the louse hangs onto the hair shaft when feeding, do not expect to find lice in alopecic areas
• Hair coat is of poor quality, represented by multifocal areas of alopecia and scale
• Pruritus is variable and affects the neck, shoulders, mane, tail, and less often the legs
• Lice glue their nits to hair shafts.
• *W. equi*, the biting louse of equids, prefers sites on the body such as the forehead, neck,

and dorsolateral trunk rather than the neck and tail
Chorioptes (leg mange)
• *Chorioptes* is an important cause of pastern dermatitis, particularly in draft horses (Figure 1. Mites live on the surface of the skin. These infections are generally less severe and less pruritic than *Psoroptes*
• Chorioptic acariosis starts with pruritus, irritation, and restlessness. Pruritus may be mild or absent in some cases. A mildly erythematous papular to crusted dermatitis involving the distal legs is the first sign. Exudation of serum with matting of leg hair and thick adherent crusts may develop over limited or extensive areas. Self-trauma results in secondary bacterial dermatitis
bovis (ear and body mange)
• *P. equi* is rare but highly contagious. Psoroptic mites do not burrow, and feeding results in exudation and crusting
• Lesions are found on regions such as under the forelock, base of the mane and tail, and the axillary region. The mites prefer areas with thick hair such as the ears, mane, tail, and intermandibular areas
• Intense pruritus is the hallmark resulting in marked head shaking and tail rubbing. Papules, vesicles, crusts, scaling, alopecia, excoriations, and exudation on the skin and ear margins are common. Lichenification of the ears, mane, and tail-head is seen in chronic cases
• The species *Psoroptes hippotis* and *Psoroptes cuniculi* cause otoacariosis, which results in aural discharge, head rubbing, head shaking, and carrying the ears in a downward droopy flat position
Trombiculidiasis (harvest mite, chiggers)
Trombicula autumnalis infestation leads to papular dermatitis and seasonal pruritus of the sides of the face (peri ocular, perioral, and muzzle), feathers of the fetlocks, mane and tail, and sometimes the ventrum in pasture-grazed horses. Pruritus is typically intense, leading to significant self-trauma.

CAUSES
Opportunistic infestations secondary to contact with another infested horse.

RISK FACTORS
• Travel to equestrian events or trail rides
• Asymptomatic carriers of *C. bovis* serve to perpetuate the infection from season to season as *Chorioptes* may survive off the host for months
• Horses put out to pasture with tall grass in the late spring to late summer are a risk for development of trombiculidiasis

DIAGNOSIS

DIFFERENTIAL DIAGNOSIS
Differential diagnoses for crusting and pruritus on the legs besides *Chorioptes* include:
• *Culicoides* hypersensitivity
• *Staphylococcus* infection
• Contact dermatitis
• Dermatophytosis
• Vasculitis
• Food allergy
Differential diagnoses for crusting and pruritus on the body besides *Psoroptes* include:
• *Culicoides* hypersensitivity
• *Staphylococcus* infection
• Atopic dermatitis
• Food allergy
• Dermatophytosis
• Dermatophilosis
• Pemphigus
Differential diagnoses for tail and mane pruritus besides *Psoroptes* include:
• *Culicoides* hypersensitivity
• *Onchocerca*
• *Oxyuris equi* infestation (for tail pruritus)
• Tail pyoderma (for tail pruritus)
• Food allergy
Differential diagnoses for pruritic otitis besides *Psoroptes* include:
• *Culicoides* hypersensitivity

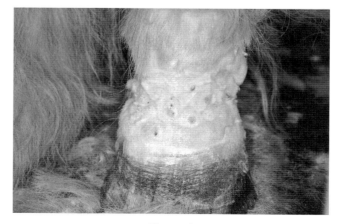

Figure 1.

Chorioptes.

- Atopic dermatitis
- Food allergy

CBC/BIOCHEMISTRY/URINALYSIS
- Anemia with heavy *H. asini* infestations
- Nonspecific eosinophilia with mange infestations

OTHER LABORATORY TESTS
N/A

IMAGING
- Microscopy for differentiating the causative arthropod
- *W. equi* are 1–2 mm in size, have a relatively broad body, and a square head, while *H. asini* are 3–3.5 mm in size, have a longer narrower body, with a sharp conical head and piercing mouth parts
- *Chorioptes* can be easily seen with a magnifying lens. This mite is 0.3–0.5 mm and has an oval body, a small head with blunt mouthparts, and long legs with suckers directly fixed to the extremity
- *Psoroptes* are 0.4–0.8 mm in size with an oval body and elongated mouthparts and long legs with triarticulate sucker-bearing peduncles
- Trombiculid larvae are orange to red and 0.25–1.0 mm, have 6 long legs and an oval body, and can sometimes be seen by the naked eye

OTHER DIAGNOSTIC PROCEDURES
- Clipping of the affected area before skin scraping is helpful. Use a no. 10 blade coated with mineral oil to help collect the mites when performing superficial skin scrapes
- Multiple superficial skin scrapings are needed to recover mites such as *Chorioptes* and *Psoroptes.* Skin scrapings can be negative in asymptomatic carriers or in chronic disease. *Trombicula* are found in crusts of dried serum. Soften crusts in 10% KOH before examination under the microscope. The orange-colored larval stages are seen under low power
- Other collection methods include acetate tape preparations or a firm toothbrush used to brush material downward onto a glass slide or Petri dish
- An otoscope provides both a magnifying lens and good light in 1 tool and is useful for ectoparasite identification among the hairs

PATHOLOGIC FINDINGS
Skin biopsies are nonspecific unless fragments or entire parasites are present. Findings include varying degrees of superficial perivascular dermatitis with numerous eosinophils and possible deep lymphoid nodules, a description compatible with both ectoparasites and hypersensitivities.

TREATMENT
- Prevent reinfestations with use of long-acting insecticides or acaricides. Treat all horses on the premises to prevent a single

reservoir supplying the mites or lice for reinfestation
- Outpatient medical management is appropriate for most cases
- As additional dispersal is by host mobility and transportation of infested hosts, limit the horse's contact with others in pastures, barns, and transportation vehicles
- Poor nutrition predisposes to many illnesses beyond lice and mites
- Prevention is achieved by the use of pyrethroid sprays or wipes during periods off premises and aids in avoiding infestations when the horse returns to the barn

SURGICAL CONSIDERATIONS
N/A

MEDICATIONS
DRUG(S) OF CHOICE
- Shampooing the mane and tail with pyrethrin, pyrethroids, lime sulfur, or selenium sulfide products is an initial step in removal of adult lice, or washing the fetlocks in the case of a chorioptic mange infestation. Clipping of the feathers is important in cases of *Chorioptes*. This in itself is insufficient as eggs will hatch after bathing. Removal of the nits from the mane and tail is beneficial. Long-acting pyrethroid, cypermethrin, or resmethrin sprays or wipes must then be applied to kill hatching larval stages of the arthropod. Fly wipes or sprays with pyrethroid compounds may require weekly application to achieve success
- Fipronil is not approved for use on horses. Fipronil is highly effective against related arthropods. Application of the spray at 3 week intervals for 3 treatments should be completely effective
- Ivermectin 200 μg/kg PO given twice with a 14 day interval is effective against *H. asini* but not *W. equi*
- For chorioptic mange, clipping is advised before applying the antiparasitic agents. Ivermectin reduces mite numbers but is less effective. Treat the entire body as the mites can migrate to the neck, trunk, and face
- For psoroptic acariosis, ivermectin at 200 μg/kg PO given twice with a 14 day interval is effective
- For control of mange, a combination of a systemic macrocyclic lactone with the application of a topical acaricide is the best treatment
- Trombiculidiasis is self-limiting if the horse is removed from the pasture; however, using topical acaricides effectively kills the larvae and corticosteroid treatment may be necessary to provide immediate relief from the pruritus

CONTRAINDICATIONS
Amitraz use is contraindicated in horses.

PRECAUTIONS
- Feline susceptibility to pyrethroid compounds is dose dependent and the formulations for use on horses (0.05–0.10%) are rarely of a level to achieve this toxicity, but some topical formulations for dogs and horses reach >50% permethrin, which is toxic to a cat. After applying a pyrethroid product directly to horses, a 2 h drying time generally limits any toxic transfer from the horse to a cat
- Injectable ivermectin can cause serious side effects in some horses

POSSIBLE INTERACTIONS
Not known.

FOLLOW-UP
PATIENT MONITORING
Observe for clinical signs of reinfestation.

PREVENTION/AVOIDANCE
Treat all horses on the premises to prevent reinfestations. Parasiticidal treatments must be combined with isolation of all contaminated horses, avoidance of infested areas, and disinfection of barns and material.

POSSIBLE COMPLICATIONS
Reinfection can occur when using short-acting insecticides or acaricides.

EXPECTED COURSE AND PROGNOSIS
Excellent prognosis if all horses on a farm are treated.

MISCELLANEOUS
AGE-RELATED FACTORS
Exposure is required, thus more common in juveniles or adults rather than foals or weanlings, but infestation is possible if present on the breeding farm.

ZOONOTIC POTENTIAL
Lice are species specific. Transient infestations of mites on humans are possible for a matter of hours, but no establishment is possible.

SEE ALSO
- Atopic dermatitis
- Insect hypersensitivity
- Pastern dermatitis

Suggested Reading
Paterson S, Coumbe K. An open study to evaluate topical treatment of equine chorioptic mange with shampooing and lime sulphur solution. Vet Dermatol 2009;20(5-6):623–629.

Author Rosanna Marsella
Consulting Editor Gwendolen Lorch

EMBRYO TRANSFER

BASICS

DEFINITION

ET traditionally refers to the removal of an embryo from the uterus or oviduct of 1 mare (the donor) and placement into the uterus or oviduct of another (the recipient). Oocyte transfer and IVF are other, related assisted reproductive technologies also being further developed and used in horses.

SYSTEMS AFFECTED

Reproductive

SIGNS

General Comments

Indications/Potential Donors
• Mares >15 years with a history of conception failure, EED, and/or abortion
• Mares with systemic disease or structural abnormalities which prevent them from carrying a foal to term
• Young mares with valuable genetics or those in competition
• Certain extraspecific matings, e.g. zebra transferred into a horse recipient

DIAGNOSIS

DIAGNOSTIC PROCEDURES

Prebreeding/Embryo Collection Evaluations

• Indicated in individuals with a history of conception failure, EED, or abortion
• Transrectal US, vaginal examination (both digital manual and speculum), endometrial cytology/culture, and endometrial biopsy to detect evidence of anatomic defects, endometritis, and fibrosis, which may predispose a mare to conception failure or EED
• Similar procedures should be performed on mares being screened as potential ET recipients. These mares should have minimal reproductive abnormalities and physically be capable of carrying a foal to term

Transrectal/Transvaginal US Examinations

• Transrectal US is used to evaluate follicular development and ovulation and to determine the appropriate timing for donor mare insemination/breeding. The ovulations of the donor and recipient mares should be synchronized with one another, with the recipient mare ovulating within 48 h of (and preferably after) the donor; there is some clinician preference based on the individual's experience
• Transrectal US examination is indicated for the donor and recipient mares at the time of flushing and transfer, respectively, to determine the absence of intrauterine fluid and the presence of a CL

• Transvaginal US procedures have been used in the aspiration of oocytes

Other Diagnostic Procedures

• Checking the recipient's progesterone concentration may be indicated prior to transfer and at the recipient's initial pregnancy examination to check for a functional CL
• ELISA or radioimmunoassay for acceptable progesterone levels vary from >1 to >4 ng/mL, depending on the reference laboratory

PATHOLOGIC FINDINGS

An endometrial biopsy can demonstrate the presence of moderate to severe, chronic endometritis, endometrial periglandular fibrosis with decreased normal glandular architecture, and/or lymphatic lacunae.

TREATMENT

APPROPRIATE HEALTH CARE

Most ETs are best handled in a hospital setting with adequate facilities and personnel. It is important that all of the reusable and disposable equipment, as well as supplies that will potentially come into contact with the embryo, be free of bacterial contamination and embryocidal residues.

Embryo Recovery Procedures

• For optimal success embryos are collected 6–8 days post ovulation, depending on the circumstances, logistical considerations, and clinician preference
• The flushing solution used for ET is commonly a modified phosphate-buffered saline solution with added fetal or newborn calf serum, ± antibiotics
• Nonsurgical uterine flushing 6–8 days after ovulation
• Surgical oviductal flushing 2–4 days after ovulation
• Laparoscopic and, especially, transvaginal US-guided recovery of oocytes

Identification of Embryos

• After the flushing medium is run into the donor mare's uterus, it is collected, usually in conjunction with some type of filtering device
• Equine embryos can vary in size and appearance depending on their age
• Embryos are evaluated and graded using a standard grading scheme. Grade 1 denotes a high-quality embryo, and grade 4 denotes a very poor quality embryo
• Multiple embryos can be collected, if there are multiple ovulations, and unfertilized oocytes are also occasionally recovered
• Embryos are washed and can be transferred immediately

ET Procedures

• Embryos can be transferred immediately, or they can be cooled and shipped to an ET center that maintains recipient mares. The mares are examined regularly throughout the

breeding season to identify the best match (synchrony) with embryos as they are received. Smaller facilities may work closely with the shipping entity to ensure there will be multiple synchronized recipients close in ovulation time to the donor mares' embryos
• Embryos are shipped in containers developed to transport cooled semen or in specifically designed containers for embryos. The type of medium in which the cooled embryos are shipped might differ from that medium used to flush the donor mare (consult with the ET center prior to breeding the donor)
• Nonsurgical intrauterine transfer—most commonly used technique; logistically simpler and less expensive than surgical transfer
• Surgical intrauterine transfer—initially more successful than nonsurgical transfer before improved nonsurgical equipment and methods became available
• Oocyte collection and IVF, using intracytoplasmic sperm injection to produce a zygote, followed by laparoscopic or surgical oviductal transfer of zygotes (ZIFT)
• Oocyte collection followed by laparoscopic or surgical oviductal transfer of gametes (GIFT) into inseminated/bred recipient whose own follicles have been aspirated
• Cryopreservation of embryos and unfertilized oocytes; manipulation, transport, and cryopreservation schemes have improved greatly over the last 10 years

NURSING CARE

Generally required after more invasive procedures in donor and recipient mares.

ACTIVITY

• Generally restricted after more invasive procedures in donor and recipient mares
• Preference may be to restrict activity of donor mares in competition because of the possible impact of stress on pregnancy maintenance

DIET

Normal diet, unless contraindicated by concurrent maternal disease or exercise restriction.

CLIENT EDUCATION

• ET procedures are not approved by all breed registries
• Success rates can be less than expected when donor mares are older, subfertile mares
• Emphasize to the client that communication between the individuals breeding the donor mare and those performing the embryo collection and transfer is essential
• Recipient mares generally need to be fairly closely synchronized with donor mare, depending on the procedure (within 0–2 days)
• If the number of normal, synchronized recipients is limited, embryos can be transported to commercial facilities with large numbers of recipient mares
• Embryo-freezing procedures are improving

E

SURGICAL CONSIDERATIONS
• Surgical intervention might be indicated to repair anatomic defects predisposing a mare to endometritis
• Surgical oviductal recovery and implantation

MEDICATIONS

DRUG(S) OF CHOICE
• Progestins, antibiotics, anti-inflammatory medications, and/or intrauterine therapy may be used in donors and, possibly, in recipient mares, depending on the circumstances, procedures involved, and clinician preference
• Equine follicle-stimulating hormone has also been used with some success to superovulate mares for embryo collection. However, superovulation remains a challenge with horses

FOLLOW-UP

PATIENT MONITORING
• Accurate teasing records
• Reexamination of donors diagnosed and treated for endometritis before ET
• Early transrectal US of recipient mare for pregnancy
• Transrectal US to monitor embryonic and fetal development in the recipient mare

POSSIBLE COMPLICATIONS
• Recipient EED or abortion
• Endometritis in donor mares after the uterine flushing procedures
• Pregnancy in donor mare following an *unsuccessful flush* (i.e. no embryo retrieved and follow-up prostaglandin injection not administered post flush to the donor)

EXPECTED COURSE AND PROGNOSIS
• Prognosis for successful pregnancy depends on the quality of the oocyte and/or embryo

and the reproductive health of the recipient mare
• Prognosis for successful recovery of intrauterine embryo at 6–8 days after ovulation is ≈70% in normal mares (less in subfertile mares)
• Prognosis for successful surgical intrauterine transfer of embryos resulting in a successful pregnancy is ≈70–75% for embryos from normal mares (depends on facility and clinician; less from subfertile mares)
• Nonsurgical intrauterine transfer of embryos originally was less successful (large individual and facility variation) than surgical transfer, but has become very widespread, with improved equipment and techniques
• Other embryo, early zygote, and gamete procedures might have lower success rates than traditional ET, but still are being improved
• Embryo cryopreservation techniques have been developed and continue to be improved
• Oocyte collection, manipulation, and cryopreservation techniques are improving

MISCELLANEOUS

SYNONYMS
• GIFT
• IVF
• ZIFT

SEE ALSO
• Abortion, spontaneous, infectious
• Abortion, spontaneous, noninfectious
• Conception failure in mares
• Endometrial biopsy
• Endometritis
• Postpartum metritis
• Spermatogenesis and factors affecting sperm production

ABBREVIATIONS
• CL = corpus luteum
• EED = early embryonic death
• ELISA = enzyme-linked immunosorbent assay
• ET = embryo transfer
• GIFT = gamete intrafallopian tube transfer
• IVF = in vitro fertilization
• US = ultrasonography, ultrasound
• ZIFT = zygote intrafallopian tube transfer

Suggested Reading
Carnevale EM. Advances in collection, transport and maturation of equine oocytes for assisted reproductive techniques. Vet Clin North Am Equine Pract 2016;32(3):379–399.
Hartman DL. Embryo transfer. In: McKinnon AO, Squires EL, Vaala WE, Varner DD, eds. Equine Reproduction, 2e. Ames, IA: Wiley Blackwell, 2011:2455–2478, 2871–2879.
McCue PM, LeBlanc MM, Squires EL. eFSH in clinical equine practice. Theriogenology 2007;68(3):429–433.
McCue PM, DeLuca CA, Wall JJ. Cooled transported embryo technology. In: McKinnon AO, Squires EL, Vaala WE, Varner DD, eds. Equine Reproduction, 2e. Ames, IA: Wiley Blackwell, 2011:2455–2478, 2880–2886.
Moussa M, Duchamp G, Daels PF, et al. Effect of embryo age on the viability of equine embryos after cooled storage using two transport systems. J Equine Vet Sci 2006;26(11):529–534.
Rader K, Choi YH, Hinrichs K. Intracytoplasmic sperm injection, embryo culture, and transfer of in vitro-produced blastocysts. Vet Clin North Am Equine Pract 2016;32(3):401–413.
Squires EL. Breakthroughs in equine embryo cryopreservation. Vet Clin North Am Equine Pract 2016;32(3):415–424.

Author Tim J. Evans
Consulting Editor Carla L. Carleton

ENDOCARDITIS, INFECTIVE

BASICS

DEFINITION
• Infective endocarditis is a bacterial, or rarely fungal, infection of the valvular or mural endocardium
• A platelet fibrin thrombus attaches to endocardium in response to collagen exposure on a denuded endothelial surface and is colonized during periods of bacteremia. Proliferation of a vegetative mass of fibrin and platelets containing bacteria (or fungi) occurs
• Microorganisms are most likely to localize on areas of endocardial damage related to valve disease or intra-cardiac shunts
• The most common site is the mitral valve, followed by the aortic valve
• The tricuspid valve can be affected with septic jugular vein thrombophlebitis

PATHOPHYSIOLOGY
• Clinical signs depend on the site and severity of the infection, embolization of vegetations, constant bacteremia, and immune complex disease
• The vegetative lesion, if large, may obstruct the outflow of blood, and/or lead to permanent valvular damage and valvular incompetence
• There may also be concurrent myocarditis

SYSTEMS AFFECTED
• Cardiovascular—primary
• Respiratory—secondary
• Nervous—secondary
• Renal—secondary
• Hepatobiliary—secondary
• GI—secondary
• Musculoskeletal—secondary

GENETICS
N/A

INCIDENCE/PREVALENCE
Uncommon

SIGNALMENT
• All ages, but horses <3 years constitute the majority
• No breed or sex predilection

SIGNS
General Comments
Usually associated with fever.

Historical Findings
• Fever
• Shifting leg lameness
• Joint or tendon sheath distention
• Jugular thrombosis

Physical Examination Findings
• Fever
• Tachycardia
• Cardiac murmur; may be absent with right-sided infective endocarditis
• Other, less common findings—arrhythmias, weight loss, coughing, and CHF

CAUSES
Most frequently involves streptococci, *Pasteurella/Actinobacillus,* and *Pseudomonas* sp. But a wide range of bacterial species have been implicated, and fungal endocarditis is reported rarely.

RISK FACTORS
• Preexisting endocardial damage
• Septic jugular vein thrombophlebitis
• Bacteremia can be associated with dental disease or manipulation but has not been specifically linked with infective endocarditis

DIAGNOSIS

DIFFERENTIAL DIAGNOSIS
• Pericarditis—differentiate echocardiographically
• Myocarditis—can be concurrent; differentiate echocardiographically
• Degenerative valve disease—fever and depression are not present
• Other diseases causing fever of unknown origin (e.g. peritonitis, pleuropneumonia, abscesses, neoplasia)—murmurs and shifting leg lameness usually are not present; differentiate echocardiographically and with clinicopathology and ultrasonography

CBC/BIOCHEMISTRY/URINALYSIS
• Often, neutrophilic leukocytosis with elevated SAA hyperfibrinogenemia, hyperglobulinemia, and anemia
• BUN and creatinine may be increased in horses with infective endocarditis. Azotemia with renal emboli or maybe prerenal in horses with low cardiac output

OTHER LABORATORY TESTS
• Obtain 3 serial blood cultures at 1 h intervals before treatment with antimicrobials
• Antimicrobial therapy reduces likelihood of a positive blood culture
• Increased cardiac troponin I concentrations identify myocardial involvement

IMAGING
Echocardiography
• Identify oscillating masses associated with the valve apparatus or mural endocardium but small vegetative lesions and lesions in the atria may be difficult to detect with transthoracic echocardiography
• Determine the number of valve leaflets affected and size of the lesions
• Doppler examination documents valvular regurgitation

Thoracic Radiography
• Pulmonary edema indicates CHF
• Pneumonia may be present with right-sided endocarditis

OTHER DIAGNOSTIC PROCEDURES
ECG identifies concurrent arrhythmias.

PATHOLOGIC FINDINGS
• Focal or diffuse thickening or distortion of valve leaflets with vegetative masses on the leaflet, chordae tendineae, or mural endocardium
• Ruptured chordae tendineae
• Jet lesions usually are detected in the preceding chamber
• Enlargement and thinning of the walls of the chambers receiving the regurgitation
• Myocardial inflammatory cell infiltrate, necrosis, and fibrosis detected histopathologically
• Infarcts and abscesses secondary to septic embolization particularly in the lung, kidneys, spleen, myocardium, and brain

TREATMENT

AIMS
The goals of treatment are sterilization of the vegetations and provision of cardiovascular support.

APPROPRIATE HEALTH CARE
• Hospitalize horses with infective endocarditis, and treat with systemic, bactericidal, broad-spectrum antimicrobials that are initially empirical and subsequently based on results of blood culture and sensitivity and clopidogrel for its antiplatelet activity
• Horses with moderate to severe mitral or aortic regurgitation may benefit from long-term vasodilator therapy
• Treat horses with severe mitral, aortic, or tricuspid regurgitation and CHF with positive inotropic drugs, vasodilators, and diuretics
• Closely monitor response to therapy with clinical, clinicopathologic, and echocardiographic reevaluations

NURSING CARE
N/A

ACTIVITY
• Stall rest and hand-walking only while being treated for infective endocarditis
• Once a bacteriologic cure is achieved, rest with small paddock turnout is appropriate
• Ability of the horse to return to work successfully depends on severity of the residual valvular damage
• Horses with significant ventricular arrhythmias or pulmonary artery dilatation are no longer safe to ride

CLIENT EDUCATION
• Monitor the horse's temperature daily, preferably during the late afternoon or evening, during treatment of infective endocarditis and after discontinuation of antimicrobials
• Regularly monitor cardiac rhythm; any irregularities other than second-degree atrioventricular block should prompt ECG

• Carefully monitor for exercise intolerance, respiratory distress, prolonged recovery after exercise, increased resting respiratory or heart rate, cough, or edema; if detected, see Patient Monitoring.

MEDICATIONS

DRUG(S) OF CHOICE

Infective Endocarditis
• To cure endocarditis requires sterilization of the vegetation
• Bactericidal antimicrobials can be administered for 4–6 weeks
• Empirically, until blood culture and sensitivity results are available, penicillin and gentamicin are a good combination. Enrofloxacin is likely to penetrate vegetations and rifampin (rifampicin) may be added to improve penetration of the antimicrobial into the lesion
• Administer aspirin or clopidogrel to decrease platelet adhesiveness
• With life-threatening ventricular arrhythmias, institute appropriate antiarrhythmic drugs

Valvular Insufficiency
Treat affected horses in CHF with furosemide, vasodilators such as benazepril, quinapril, or the inodilator pimobendan.

PRECAUTIONS
• Evaluate creatinine and BUN before starting aminoglycoside antimicrobials and use therapeutic drug monitoring to individualize dosage regimens
• ACE inhibitors can cause hypotension; thus, do not give as a large dose without time to accommodate to this treatment

FOLLOW-UP

PATIENT MONITORING
• Assess CBC and in particular serum creatinine and fibrinogen concentrations
• Frequently monitor lesions echocardiographically during treatment with antimicrobials to assess the efficacy of treatment
• Once antimicrobials have been discontinued, monitor lesions echocardiographically 2 and 4 weeks later and periodically thereafter, depending on the valve

affected and the severity of the valvular regurgitation that has developed
• With severe valvular insufficiency, echocardiographic reevaluations are recommended at 3 month intervals

PREVENTION/AVOIDANCE
Institute aggressive treatment of septic jugular vein thrombophlebitis to minimize seeding of the tricuspid valve from septic emboli associated with the infected jugular vein.

POSSIBLE COMPLICATIONS
• Immune-mediated synovitis or tenosynovitis
• Right-sided infective endocarditis—pulmonary thromboembolism, pulmonary abscess, and pneumonia
• Left-sided infective endocarditis—hepatic, splenic, and renal abscess; myocardial and cerebral infarction

EXPECTED COURSE AND PROGNOSIS
• Prognosis for horses is primarily determined by the valve(s) affected and the severity of valvular damage that develops, and is also likely to be influenced by the organism(s) involved and the response to antimicrobial treatment
• Prognosis for horses with right-sided infective endocarditis is guarded and for left-sided infective endocarditis is grave
• Achieving bacteriologic cure can be difficult
• Even when bacteriologic cure is achieved, continued damage to the affected valve occurs. This usually results in worsening of the valvular regurgitation. These horses may develop clinical signs associated with the worsening valvular insufficiency that shortens both useful performance life and life expectancy

MISCELLANEOUS

ASSOCIATED CONDITIONS
• Septic jugular vein thrombophlebitis
• Preexisting valve damage
• Congenital cardiac disease

AGE-RELATED FACTORS
Infective endocarditis is more frequent in horses <3 years of age.

ZOONOTIC POTENTIAL
N/A

PREGNANCY/FERTILITY/BREEDING
• Pregnant mares are at risk for development of placentitis, and the fetus may become septic

• Treating pregnant mares with IV broad-spectrum bactericidal antimicrobials is important. Base the antimicrobial therapy on blood culture and sensitivity, if available, and choose antimicrobials that are safe for the developing fetus
• The volume expansion of late pregnancy places an additional load on the already volume-loaded heart and may precipitate CHF in mares with severe valvular insufficiency
• In pregnant mares with CHF, treat for the underlying cardiac disease with positive inotropic drugs and diuretics. ACE inhibitors are contraindicated because of potential adverse effects on the fetus

SYNONYMS
• Vegetative endocarditis
• Infective endocarditis

SEE ALSO
• Aortic regurgitation
• Mitral regurgitation
• Tricuspid regurgitation

ABBREVIATIONS
• ACE = angiotensin-converting enzyme
• BUN = blood urea nitrogen
• CHF = congestive heart failure
• SAA = serum amyloid A

Suggested Reading
Buergelt CD, Cooley AJ, Hines SA, Pipers FS. Endocarditis in 6 horses. Vet Pathol 1985;22:333–337.
Kasari TR, Roussel AJ. Bacterial endocarditis. Part I. Pathophysiologic, diagnostic and therapeutic considerations. Compend Contin Educ Pract Vet 1989;11:655–671.
Marr CM. Cardiovascular Infections. In Sellon DC, Long MT, eds. Equine Infectious Disease, 2e. St. Louis, MO: Elsevier, 2014:21–41.
Maxson ADM, Reef VB. Bacterial endocarditis in horses: a review of 10 cases (1984–1995). Equine Vet J 1997;29:394–399.
Porter SR, Saegerman C, van Galen G, et al. Vegetative endocarditis in equids (1994-2006). J Vet Intern Med 2008;22:1411–1416.

Author Celia M. Marr
Consulting Editor Celia M. Marr and Virginia B. Reef
Acknowledgment The author acknowledges the prior contribution of Virginia B. Reef.

E

ENDOMETRIAL BIOPSY

BASICS

DEFINITION
Histopathologic evaluation of the endometrium to predict a mare's ability to carry a foal to term and to identify pathologies to direct medical management of reproductive disease.

PATHOPHYSIOLOGY
Normal Architecture and Seasonal Variation
• The endometrium is the mucosal layer of the luminal surface of the uterus and consists of epithelium, stroma, glands, and vascular and lymphatic vessels. The stratum compactum and the stratum spongiosum are the superficial and deep layers, respectively
• Normal changes are driven by ovarian estrogen and P_4, with cycle and season—winter anestrus: atrophy; vernal (spring) transition: increasing estrogen stimulates activity; breeding season: estrus and diestrus variations:
   ○ *Estrus*—tall columnar luminal epithelium, stromal edema, PMNs marginate on vasculature, but do not enter stroma, straight glands
   ○ *Diestrus*—mostly columnar/cuboidal luminal epithelium, less edema, tortuous glands

Assessment for Inflammatory or Degenerative Pathologic Changes
• Endometritis—inflammation and type of cell infiltration; bacterial or fungal/yeast organisms
• Periglandular fibrosis, *endometriosis*
• Cystic glandular distention with/without periglandular fibrosis
• Lymphangiectasia
• Vascular damage, *angiosis*
• Endometrial maldifferentiation, inappropriate for season and/or cycle
• Inflammation from coitus, pregnancy, infectious organisms, pneumovagina, urovagina, DUC, and other unknown causes
• Other degenerative changes usually are progressive, associated with aging, exacerbated by parity and chronic inflammation
• Cumulative pathologies decrease probability of term pregnancy

SYSTEMS AFFECTED
Reproductive

GENETICS
N/A

SIGNALMENT
Aged mares and increased parity.

SIGNS
Historical Findings
• Infertility or subfertility
• Barren from previous/current season, though bred ≤48 h preovulation with proven semen

• Anestrus mare during breeding season
• Reproductive tract abnormalities
• EED, abortion
• Cytology and culture inconclusive for endometritis diagnosis
• Reproductive prepurchase examination of broodmare prospect

Physical Examination Findings
Perineal examination—poor vulvar conformation, associated pneumo- or urovagina.

CAUSES
Inflammation
• Most common abnormality, described by distribution—focal, diffuse; frequency—mild, moderate, severe; cell type—acute, chronic, chronic/active
   ○ Acute—PMNs predominate
   ○ Chronic—lymphocytes, plasma cells, macrophages
   ○ Chronic/active—PMNs, with lymphocytes, plasma cells
• Inflammatory cells in stratum compactum and in chronic cases also in stratum spongiosum
• Macrophages linked to irritating or poorly absorbed foreign matter
• Siderophages (macrophage with hemoglobin pigment) indicate past foaling, abortion, hemorrhage, within last 2–3 years
• Eosinophils due to pneumo- or urovagina, less often fungal endometritis

Fibrosis/Endometriosis
• Considered irreversible degenerative change
• Widespread distribution correlates with low foaling rate
• Stromal cells deposit collagen in response to inflammation, aging, or other stimuli
• Most collagen deposition is periglandular, resulting in fibrotic glandular nests, cystic glandular distention, epithelial atrophy, and decreased uterine milk secretion
• Uterine milk provides early nutrition; when insufficient—EED or fetal loss by 45–90 days of gestation
• Poorer prognosis with increased layers of collagen and frequency of nests

Cystic Glandular Distention without Periglandular Fibrosis
• Normal seasonal variation during anestrus and transition
• In breeding season, identified in old, pluriparous mares with repeat breeding
• Glands have impaired flow of secretions, inspissation of content
• Cystic glandular distention may precede periglandular fibrosis
• Glands are uniformly dilated after abortion or pregnancy

Lymphangiectasia
• Characterized by dilated dysfunctional lymphatic vessels
• Common in mares with pendulous uterus and DUC

• TRP may reveal thickened soft uterus with poor diestrous tone
• Widespread severe lymphangiectasia reduces foaling rates
• Lymphatic lacunae enlarge into gross lymphatic cysts, visible with US or endoscopy

Angiosis
• Sclerotic changes of uterine vessels primarily related to parity, secondarily with aging
• Younger maiden mares have intact vessels. Pluriparous mares have disruption of the intima with medial and adventitial elastosis and fibrosis
• Severe angiosis decreases perfusion, results in edema
• Negatively affects pregnancy outcome

Nonseasonal Glandular Atrophy, Hypoplasia, or Maldifferentiation
• Decreased gland density during breeding season is abnormal and associated with ovarian dysgenesis or granulosa–theca cell tumor
• Focal glandular atrophy in old pluriparous mares
• Ovarian dysgenesis

Prognostic Categories
Category I
• ≥80% of mares conceive and carry to term; endometrium is essentially normal
• Changes, if present, are only slight, focal, scattered
Category IIA
• Foaling rate of 50–80% with proper management
• Changes—slight to moderate and scattered
   ○ Diffuse cellular infiltration of superficial layers or foci
   ○ Periglandular fibrosis of branches, 1–3 layers, or ≤2 fibrotic nests/LPF in 5 fields
   ○ Endometrial atrophy in late breeding season
• Bred, but barren for ≥2 years, with a biopsy of category IIA change is downgraded to IIB
• Category may improve with treatment
Category IIB
• Foaling rate of 10–50% with proper management
• Changes are more diffuse and severe than IIA and may include:
   ○ Moderately severe cellular infiltration of superficial layers
   ○ Periglandular fibrosis of branches, ≥4 layers, or 2–4 fibrotic nests/LPF in 5 fields
   ○ Widespread lymphangiectasia only (without other pathology)
• A category IIB biopsy is downgraded to III when widespread lymphangiectasia present
• Category may improve with proper treatment
Category III
• ≤10% foaling rate, even with optimal management
• Greatly decreased conception rate and pregnancy maintenance

(Continued)

E

- Histologic changes are prominent, diffuse, and severe:
  - Cellular infiltration
  - Fibrotic glandular nests with ≥5 nests/LPF
  - Lymphangiectasia with palpable "jelly-like" texture
  - Endometrial glandular atrophy during the breeding season

RISK FACTORS
- Age
- Parity
- Anatomic abnormalities causing inflammation, e.g. pneumovagina or urovagina
- Repeated inflammation from coitus, DUC, infectious endometritis

 DIAGNOSIS

IMAGING
US for presence of intraluminal uterine fluid, edema, lymphatic cysts, foreign body, or other.

OTHER DIAGNOSTIC PROCEDURES
Breeding Soundness Examination
- Endometrial biopsy is performed as part of a complete examination, not as a sole diagnostic
- Swab or brush culture and cytology precede biopsy to avoid contamination
- Sterile biopsy forceps are carried through the cervix into the uterus, sampling at the caudal portion of the horn or junction of horn/body, preferably when the mare is cycling and in estrus. TRP guides placement of forceps, tissue is pressed into the opened forceps, which are closed to obtain tissue
- One sample is representative of the entire endometrium. If gross abnormality is present additional samples are obtained (pathologists prefer 2 or 3 samples)
- Preferred to fix in Bouin's solution for 4–24 h, then transfer into 70% ethanol or 10% BNF until processed. If Bouin's is unavailable, use 10% BNF
- Routine stain—H&E; may request others
- Include history, stage of cycle, TRP, and US findings on day of examination
- If performing cytology, roll biopsy specimen onto sterile slide, air dry, stain
- If performing culture from biopsy specimen, guarding the biopsy forceps is required
- Culture and cytology from biopsy may be more accurate than swab method

Endoscopy
Evaluate for intraluminal adhesions, endometrial cysts, focal lesions, and foreign body.

PATHOLOGIC FINDINGS
See I, IIA, IIB, and III category descriptions.

 TREATMENT

CATEGORY I
- Exclude bacterial endometritis
- Focus on estrus detection, timing of breeding and insemination with respect to ovulation, semen quality and type, mare anatomic or behavioral abnormalities
- Evaluate health—manage lameness or systemic disease; reproduction is a *luxury*

CATEGORIES IIA AND IIB
- Direct therapy at problems identified on biopsy, to improve category and prognosis
- Minimize contamination and inflammation at and after breeding
- Caslick's vulvoplasty for pneumovagina
- Bacterial or fungal infections—local/systemic antibiotic/antifungal
- Treat DUC with uterine lavage and oxytocin
- Impaired lymphatics and edema managed with cloprostenol (PGF$_{2\alpha}$ analog) at 12–24 h before and after breeding
- P + E improves uterine tone and may enhance vascular perfusion and lymphatic drainage
- Urethral extension surgery, if vulvo- or perineoplasty does not adequately improve urovagina
- Fibrosis and angiosis are irreversible

CATEGORY III
- May conceive, but EED or fetal loss at ≤90 days of gestation
- Aggressive therapy directed at problems identified on biopsy
- Extensive fibrosis—irreversible, category will not improve
- If no improvement is achieved, reproductively retire mare
- If allowed by breed registry, consider mares for embryo transfer or as oocyte donor

 MEDICATIONS

DRUG(S) OF CHOICE
- Antibiotic based on culture and sensitivity
- Normal saline or lactated Ringer's solution for uterine lavage
- Cloprostenol 100–250 µg IM
- P + E:
  - Combined P$_4$ (150 mg) + E (5–10 mg) IM daily for 10 days or 10 mL bio-release P + E IM once
  - Day 10 administer PGF$_{2\alpha}$ 10 mg IM
  - Day 5 after ovulation, if no fluid is in the uterus (indicating inflammation or infection), may resume treatment
  - If pregnant at 14 days, may continue to day 45 of gestation

CONTRAINDICATIONS
- Do not administer P$_4$ or progestins if mare is infected, as endometritis will worsen
- Cloprostenol or PGF$_{2\alpha}$ is generally not recommended post ovulation as it may harm luteal growth and P$_4$ production
- PGF$_{2\alpha}$ or cloprostenol is contraindicated during pregnancy

 FOLLOW-UP

PATIENT MONITORING
Repeat biopsy ≅2 weeks after treatment, as a means to determine effectiveness.

POSSIBLE COMPLICATIONS
- Rarely uterine perforation or excessive hemorrhage
- Pregnancy is a contraindication to biopsy

 MISCELLANEOUS

SYNONYMS
Uterine biopsy

SEE ALSO
Endometritis

ABBREVIATIONS
- BNF = buffered neutral formalin
- DUC = delayed uterine clearance
- EED = early embryonic death
- LPF = low-power field (5.5 mm)
- P$_4$ = progesterone
- P + E = P$_4$ + estradiol-17β
- PGF$_{2\alpha}$ = prostaglandin F$_{2\alpha}$ (dinoprost tromethamine; Lutalyse®)
- PMN = polymorphonuclear leukocyte
- TRP = transrectal palpation
- US = ultrasonography, ultrasound

Suggested Reading

Love CC. Endometrial biopsy. In: McKinnon AO, Squires EL, Vaala WE, Varner DD, eds. Equine Reproduction, 2e. Ames, IA: Wiley Blackwell, 2011:1929–1939.

McCue PM. Endometrial biopsy. In: Dascanio J, McCue P, eds. Equine Reproductive Procedures. Hoboken, NJ: Wiley Blackwell, 2014:68–70.

Snider TA, Sepoy C, Holyoak GR. Equine endometrial biopsy reviewed: observation, interpretation, and application of histopathologic data. Theriogenology 2011;75:1567–1581.

Wolfsdorf KE. How to utilize endometrial culture, cytology, and biopsy to manage the sub-fertile mare. Proc Am Assoc Equine Pract 2016;62:164–168.

Authors Audrey A. Kelleman and Maria E. Cadario
Consulting Editor Carla L. Carleton

ENDOMETRITIS

BASICS

DEFINITION
- Infectious/noninfectious endometrial inflammation
- Major cause of mare infertility
- Multifactorial disease classified in 1 of 4 groups:
  - Infectious (acute, chronic, or subclinical) endometritis
  - PMIE
  - Endometritis due to a sexually transmitted disease
  - Degenerative endometritis due to aging (angiosis, periglandular fibrosis)
- May involve more than 1 group/origin

PATHOPHYSIOLOGY
Infectious Endometritis
- Uterus repeatedly exposed to contamination at breeding, parturition, and gynecologic examinations
- Uterine defense mechanisms to clear contamination, combination of:
  - Anatomic (physical) barriers
  - Cellular phagocytosis
  - Physical evacuation of uterine contents

Chronic and Subacute Infectious Endometritis
- When treatments are unsuccessful in eliminating infectious agents or byproducts of inflammation
- Reinfection caused by persisting anatomic/functional defects
- Failure to identify the microorganisms
- Excess of endometrial mucus production or accumulation:
  - Precludes antibiotics for reaching therapeutic concentrations
- Bacterial biofilm:
  - Acts as a reservoir for microorganisms and increases resistance to antibiotics

PMIE
- Increased parity in aged mares and incomplete cervical dilation in old maiden mares predisposes to intrauterine fluid accumulation
- Breeding induces a normal, transient, endometritis
- Byproducts of inflammation normally are removed by uterine contractions through an open estrual cervix. Following ovulation, the cervix closes; fluids within the uterine lumen are cleared by the lymphatics (<12 h post mating)
- Fluid accumulation and lymphatic stasis increases if the uterus is suspended below the pelvic brim, uterine contractions are incomplete, or negligible cervical dilation during estrus

Low Pregnancy Rate
- Direct—interference with embryo survival
- Indirect—by premature luteolysis

SEXUALLY TRANSMITTED (VENEREAL) ENDOMETRITIS
- Coitus or AI with infected semen
- Most common bacteria are *Pseudomonas aeruginosa, Klebsiella pneumonia,* and *Streptococcus zooepidemicus*
  - All opportunistic organisms on the penile surface

SYSTEMS AFFECTED
Reproductive

GENETICS
N/A

INCIDENCE/PREVALENCE
Frequent

SIGNALMENT
Infectious Endometritis
Predisposition to contamination is caused by an inherent or acquired anatomic defect of the vulva, vestibular sphincter, or cervix.

PMIE
- Pluriparous mares—usually >12–14 years with pendulous uterus
- Nulliparous mares—young or old, having incomplete cervical dilation during estrus

SIGNS
Historical Findings
- Infertility
- Accumulation of uterine fluid (luminal) before and/or after breeding
- Failure to conceive after repeated breeding to a stallion of known fertility
- Early embryonic loss
- Hyperemia of the cervix/vagina
- Vaginal discharge

Physical Examination Findings
- Can be inconclusive
- Guarded swab, uterine brush or LVL to obtain samples for endometrial cytology and uterine culture
- Endometrial biopsy is indicated only in specific cases

Infectious Endometritis
- Abnormal vulvar conformation
- TRP often not diagnostic
- US usually reveals accumulation of echogenic (*Streptococcus*) or nonechogenic (*Klebsiella*) fluid in the uterine lumen
- Hyperemia of vaginal and cervical mucosa; discharge may be observed at the cervix
- Endometrial cytology and uterine culture reveal neutrophils; positive cytology when ≥1 PMNs/HPF (LVL) to ≥5 PMNs/HPF (swab, cup, brush)
- Usually isolate a pure bacterial growth, single organism
- Fungal endometritis usually follows excessive antibiotic uterine therapy
- Fungal or bacterial endometritis may be overshadowing another bacteria not detected until first microorganism is eradicated

PMIE
- External genitalia often normal

- TRP, US, cytology/culture results may be inconclusive in the spring, prior to onset of the breeding season
- Signs of persistent inflammation usually appear post breeding
- May be hyperemia of vaginal and cervical mucosa due to irritation, rarely infection
- Pendulous, edematous uterus in older mares
- Presence of >2 cm (height determined by US) intrauterine fluid during estrus is diagnostic/predictive of PMIE
- Postbreeding US reveals luminal fluid that persists for >12–24 h without treatment
- Endometrial cytology reveals significant inflammation (≥1–5 PMNs/HPF)
- Bacterial culture—usually negative

CAUSES
See Pathophysiology.

RISK FACTORS
See Pathophysiology.

DIAGNOSIS

DIFFERENTIAL DIAGNOSIS
For Vaginal Discharge
- Pneumovagina
- Bacterial vaginitis secondary to pneumovagina
- Treatment-induced vaginitis and/or necrosis
- Necrotizing vaginitis secondary to excessive manipulation or inadequate lubrication, or contamination during the delivery of a necrotic fetus
- Urine pooling
- Varicosities in the region of the vaginovestibular sphincter
- Lochia
- Postpartum metritis
- Pyometra
- During pregnancy, may be a sign of placentitis
- Ascending, infectious placentitis
- Serosanguineous cervical discharge with a negative bacterial swab indicates premature placental separation

CBC/BIOCHEMISTRY/URINALYSIS
N/A

OTHER LABORATORY TESTS
Microbiology
Aerobes
- Most common isolates—*S. zooepidemicus* and *Escherichia coli*
- An endometrial sample of the surface (swab), contents (swab, LVL) or a biopsy is obtained
- Contact (pressure with swab) the endometrial surface with a guarded swab for culture and identification of microorganism
Anaerobes
- *Bacteroides fragilis*
- May be recovered in some cases of postpartum metritis
Yeasts
- *Candida* spp., *Aspergillus* spp.

E

Cytology
- Sample is of endometrial cells and intraluminal content
- Contact (pressure with swab) endometrial surface with the swab tip or cap (if using a Kalayjian swab); gently roll the sample onto a slide; stain with Diff-Quik
- Presence of endometrial cells is necessary to be considered a valid/reliable cytology
- Presence and number of PMNs is diagnostic and indicates the severity of uterine irritation
- Microorganisms can be seen around cells or inside PMNs—branching and/or round structures are pathognomonic of fungal infection. *Actinomyces* cytology is also characterized by branching

Interpretation
- Persistent, positive cytology without bacterial growth most often suggests a recurrent, noninfectious cause
- Subclinical, chronic endometritis usually results from the inability to identify the microorganism due to focal location or difficult access deeper in a pendulous uterus
- Positive culture with positive cytology—diagnostic for uterine infection
- Positive culture with negative cytology—indicates contamination during uterine sampling in most cases
- Negative cytology results in 30% of subsequently confirmed endometritis, due to inability to reach the PMNs in the pendulous areas of the uterus or *E. coli* or *P. aeruginosa* infections characterized by poor neutrophilic influx

IMAGING
US
- Mares with DUC often have luminal fluid present before breeding and always retain fluid for 12–24 h post breeding
- Persistent edema during and after ovulation—only occurs post breeding due to lymphatic stasis or endometritis

OTHER DIAGNOSTIC PROCEDURES
Low-Volume Uterine Lavage
- Recommended for identification of chronic or subclinical endometritis
- Twice as sensitive as endometrial swabbing and nearly as efficient (90%) as endometrial biopsy
- In estrus or diestrus infuse the uterus with 60–150 mL of sterile saline or LRS, recover the effluent into a sterile container
- The effluent is evaluated for cloudiness and amount of mucus. Both parameters are highly associated with the isolation of microorganism (70% of cases)
- The sample settles for 30–60 min or is centrifuged at 400 *g* for 10 min. The pellet is sampled for culture and cytology
- Can identify the presence of bacteria in cases with otherwise poor clinical presentation, e.g. weak influx of PMNs and decreased uterine fluid production
- The cytologic evaluation includes the presence of PMNs (1 PMN/×40 field is

indicative of inflammation), epithelial cells, bacteria, and debris to be considered an appropriate sample and to rule out false-positive cultures due to contamination

Endometrial Biopsy
- Best method to determine the presence of endometritis when clinical and bacteriologic findings are inconclusive
- Bacteriologic and cytologic results obtained by endometrial biopsy are considered the "gold standard" in the diagnosis of endometritis
- Inflammatory cells (neutrophils) indicate active endometritis
- Low numbers of lymphocytes and plasma cells (indicative of chronic endometritis) are not always associated with infertility
- Lymphatic stasis is common in mares with a pendulous uterus and DUC

Endoscopy
- When other modalities fail to define the cause of infertility
- Better method to visualize intrauterine adhesions affecting uterine drainage, luminal tumors, or uterine abscess (rare)

PATHOLOGIC FINDINGS
Endometritis
- Cannot predict a mare's endometrial biopsy category, ranges from IIA to III (rarely)
- Category relates to the length of sexual rest, conformational abnormalities, and age
- Histopathology associated with endometritis—mild, diffuse lymphocytic or neutrophilic infiltration; focally moderate fibrosis (1–4 nests); lymphangiectasia, presence of bacteria (if infectious), excess mucus if recurrent irritation

PMIE
- Biopsy score at the beginning of the breeding season is not diagnostic
- Category may be IIA or IIB, with mild inflammation and moderate fibrosis
- After breeding, interstitial edema; lymphatic stasis; diffuse/acute/or subacute inflammation (PMNs) usually develop
- Serial sampling may be useful

TREATMENT
APPROPRIATE HEALTH CARE
Minimize contamination during breeding:
- Wash mare's perineum and stallion's penis with clean water; dry the stallion's penis prior to mating or semen collection for AI
- Limit to 1 breeding (live cover or AI) per estrus
- Breed as close to ovulation as possible
- In mares predisposed to infectious endometritis, immediately prior to natural breeding (live cover) infuse semen extender (60–120 mL) with nonspermicidal antibiotic (antibiotic concentration compatible with sperm viability); minimum contamination technique

NURSING CARE
N/A
ACTIVITY
N/A
DIET
N/A
CLIENT EDUCATION
N/A
SURGICAL CONSIDERATIONS
- Consider feasibility of surgical correction of predisposing causes before treating a uterine infection—Caslick's vulvoplasty (pneumovagina); vaginoplasty; urethral extension (urine pooling); repair of cervical tears
- Rectovaginal fistula and extensive cervical tears (foaling trauma—prudent to wait for results of endometrial biopsy before surgery if the broodmare has been barren for >1 year). Chronic endometritis may have seriously worsened the mare's biopsy category

MEDICATIONS
DRUG(S) OF CHOICE
General Principles
- Administer treatments during estrus, although this is controversial
- For infectious endometritis, organism is eliminated chemically (local antibiotics, antiseptics), and mechanically (uterine lavage, ecbolic drugs)
- Systemic treatment when 2 organisms with different sensitivity are isolated—local antibiotic for one microorganism and systemic for the other. Also, when access to the mare is limited, e.g. unsafe or unsanitary conditions, or when avoiding further uterine contamination
- Subclinical and chronic endometritis—unsuccessful in eliminating microorganism due to reinfection; failure to isolate microorganism due to method used; excessive mucus production, bacterial biofilm
- New methods for treatment include mucolytic drugs, buffered chelating agents, solvents, CSA and immune modulators in addition to uterine lavage, oxytocin, and the antibiotic of choice
- Uterine lavage is recommended for DUC and to evacuate debris from the uterus before antibiotic instillation, if necessary:
  - Uterine lavage with LRS (without oxytocin) can be performed 1 h prior to insemination if there is intrauterine fluid, e.g. rebreeding or multiple inseminations in a 24 h period
  - If oxytocin is used during/after the lavage, it is advisable to wait 4 h before inseminating the mare

Infectious Endometritis
Acute Endometritis
- Uterine lavage without oxytocin (daily or when intrauterine fluid ≥2 cm) followed by

ENDOMETRITIS   (CONTINUED)

E

intrauterine infusion of chosen antibiotics for 3–7 days. Oxytocin is administered 8–12 h later to stimulate uterine evacuation without interfering with the antibiotic's action
• Antibiotics based on culture and sensitivity; should be diluted in 60–120 mL of sterile saline (maximum volume infused)

Chronic Inflammation
Do not breed mare until 45–60 days after treatment.

Chronic Infectious Endometritis
Surgical correction of defective anatomic barriers before intrauterine treatment.

Subclinical Endometritis
Positive or negative cytology, no bacteria identified but clinical signs and subfertility/infertility present:
• Uterine lavage if intrauterine fluid is present, the antibiotic(s) of choice should be infused by diluting in LRS alone or in combination with mucolytic drugs if excessive mucus; buffer chelators to increase bacterial permeability; and/or nonantibiotics, anti-infectious agents (CSA)
• If history warrants, consider postbreeding treatment

Yeast Infection
• Correct anatomic defects; culture and treat uterus and reservoirs of infection, e.g. vagina and clitoral fossa
• Uterine lavage since fluid is frequently present. The antifungal of choice (nystatin, clotrimazole, etc.) should be infused by diluting in LRS alone or in combination with buffer chelators (Tris-EDTA, Tricide®) to increase microorganism permeability to the drug
• Alternatively, uterine lavage with diluted 0.01–0.05% povidone–iodine solution (to the approximate color of light iced tea), acetic acid/vinegar (2%), or peroxide (3% v/v = 30 mL H_2O_2 in 1 L of 0.9% saline) for 7–10 days
• Repeat culture and cytology in the following estrus (uterus, vagina, and clitoral fossa)

PMIE
• Manual cervical dilation before breeding with systemic (cloprostenol) or local application (misoprostol) may help intrauterine semen deposition and uterine clearance
• Foaling, at least once, is highly recommended to improve cervical relaxation and drainage in old maiden mares
• Promote uterine clearance by lavage and ecbolic drugs (oxytocin, carbetocin, cloprostenol)
• Control intrauterine fluid production and excessive edema by modulating inflammation and immune response (glucocorticoids) of mares with history of acute and persistent inflammation post breeding
• Mare with no history or characteristics of DUC:

○ Begin evaluation and treatment, if necessary, 12 h post breeding to let the normal mechanisms of clearance occur
• If the mare has been diagnosed with PMIE:
○ 4–8 h post breeding promote uterine clearance by uterine lavage with LRS or saline, followed by the administration of an ecbolic drug
○ 4 h interval ensures spermatozoa are in the oviduct, 8 h interval that bacteria have not yet adhered or multiplied in the uterus
• Oxytocin during or immediately after lavage stimulates strong uterine contractions, clears the remaining uterine contents, and promotes lymphatic drainage
• Administer oxytocin every 3–4 h in refractory cases, e.g. older maiden mares
• $PGF_{2\alpha}$ (Lutalyse®) and analogs (cloprostenol):
○ Sustains smoother uterine contractions longer than oxytocin (4–5 h vs. 45–60 min)
○ Reduce persistent uterine edema by stimulating lymphatic drainage
• Administration of glucocorticoids at the time of breeding (before, during, and/or after) increases pregnancy rate

US
• 4–8 h post AI or breeding (not ovulation)—check for uterine fluid:
○ If >2 cm free fluid, lavage uterus with 1–3 L of sterile saline or LRS
○ Administer oxytocin during or after lavage
○ If only a small amount of free fluid, administer only oxytocin
• If possible, 12 h after breeding—use cloprostenol if history includes dilated uterine lymphatics and poor drainage. Use dexamethasone if excessive edema
• 24 h after breeding—if mare has free intraluminal fluid, lavage and oxytocin
○ If free fluid and persistent edema in the walls—lavage the uterus/oxytocin and add a regimen of IV/IM oxytocin alternating with IM cloprostenol every 4–6 h
○ If only edema is present, cloprostenol every 4–12 h, up to 36 h post ovulation. Dexamethasone 20 mg IV once daily is also a good option before and after 36 h
• 48 h post breeding—if the mare has not ovulated, rebreed; oxytocin/cloprostenol sequence begins anew. Prebreeding uterine lavage may be indicated
• Treatment should continue, if necessary, no more than 3–4 days post ovulation:
○ Embryo enters the uterus day 5 + 20 h; allows treatment-induced uterine inflammatory response to subside

Drugs and Fluids
Intrauterine Antibiotics Most Frequently Used
• Amikacin (0.5–2 g)—Gram negative; *Pseudomonas* and *Klebsiella* spp. An intrauterine infusion of Tris-EDTA increases the permeability of the *Pseudomonas* capsule to the antibiotic
• Ampicillin (1–3 g)—Gram positive; streptococci

• Carbenicillin (2–6 g)—broad spectrum; persistent *Pseudomonas* spp.
• Gentamicin (0.5–2 g)—primarily Gram negative; streptococci
• K-penicillin (5×10^6 U)—Gram positive; streptococci
• Ticarcillin/Timentin® (3–6 g)—broad spectrum
• Ceftiofur sodium/Naxcel® (1 g)—broad spectrum
• Aminoglycosides must be buffered before infusion. Mix the antibiotic with an equal volume of sodium bicarbonate, then dilute in sterile saline

Systemic Antibiotics
• Ceftiofur in crystalline form—Excede®; very effective at treating endometritis due to *S. zooepidemicus*. Full therapy—2 doses (6.6 mg/kg) IM 4 days apart
• Trimethoprim–sulfamethoxazole
• Trimethoprim-sulfadiazine Equisul® (24 mg/Kg BID) provides drug concentrations above the MIC90 for at least 98% of the dosing interval
• K-penicillin
• Procaine penicillin G
• Gentamicin
• Amikacin
• Ampicillin

Antimycotics
• Nystatin (0.5–2.5 × 10^6 U)—*Candida* spp.
• Clotrimazole (500–700 mg)—*Candida* spp.
• Amphotericin B (100–200 mg)—*Aspergillus, Candida,* and *Mucor* spp.; tablets must be crushed and well suspended in 60–120 mL of sterile saline for intrauterine infusion

Others
New Methods
• Mucolytic agents (NAC), buffered chelating agents (Tris-EDTA), and solvents (DMSO) have been added to the uterine lavage treatment to dissolve exudates, mucus, or bacterial biofilm
• NAC—infuse a 3.3% solution of NAC (30 mL of a 20% solution in 150 mL of saline or LRS) on day 1 of the treatment followed by uterine lavage 24 h later. *In vitro* studies showed that mixing NAC with antibiotics in the same syringe, reduces the antibiotic efficacy. The removal of debris, secretions, exudate, mucus and the potential disruption of the bacterial biofilm may:
○ Expose otherwise inaccessible microorganisms, so culture of lavage effluent is recommended
○ Increase the level of antibiotic locally available
• Buffered chelating solutions or agents—Tris-EDTA in cases of failure of antimicrobial therapy in infectious endometritis due to the presence of biofilm produced by Gram-negative bacteria or fungi that confer microbial resistance

○ Biofilm-producing pathogens are *P. aeruginosa, Staphylococcus epidermis, E. coli, Enterobacter cloacae*, and some fungi
○ The initial volume of infusion should be sufficient to fill the uterine lumen (250–1000 mL, based on horn size) so that microorganisms are reached within minutes. The treatment-induced accumulation of bacterial/cellular debris should be cleared from the uterus by uterine lavage within 24 h
○ The recommended protocol consists of uterine lavage (LRS) followed by uterine infusion with 250–1000 mL of the buffered chelating solution. Advisable to repeat lavage 12–24 h later to remove cellular debris and dead bacteria
○ Mix the appropriate antibiotic with 30–40 ml of buffered chelating solution to a final volume of 60–80 ml in the days following the first treatment *or* from the first day (if bacteria have already been identified). This treatment can be repeated on subsequent days of the same estrus
• DMSO 30% (33 mL of DMSO at 90% in 64 mL of saline solution)
• CSA (Ceragyn®)—nonantibiotic, broad-spectrum antibacterial, antifungal, and antiviral agent. Good option when antibiotic resistance is present
  ○ Used for uterine infusion (60 mL vial) or for uterine lavage (mix 60 mL vial with LRS and flush the uterus 4 h before or 6–48 h after breeding)
Uterotonic/Ecbolic Drugs
• Oxytocin (10 IU or 20 IU IV or IM)
• Carbetocin (175 µg IV or IM), synthetic analog of oxytocin; its half-life is 2.5 times longer than oxytocin. Unavailable in the USA
  ○ Recommended for mares that accumulate intrauterine fluid before and after breeding and respond poorly to conventional dose and frequency of oxytocin
  ○ Useful when access to the mare is limited
• Cloprostenol (250–500 µg IM/500 kg mare, Estrumate®), a synthetic analog of PGF$_{2\alpha}$ which has uterotonic properties
  ○ Used to expel intrauterine fluid through a poorly dilated or inefficient cervix, i.e. older maiden mares, and to reduce edema due to dilated lymphatics by sustained uterine contractions of smooth muscle
  ○ Its effect lasts longer than oxytocin (4 h vs. 45–60 min) with fewer adverse effects
Cervical Dilation
• Synthetic prostaglandin E$_1$ (misoprostol 200 µg/3 mL ointment) is used for cervical relaxation
  ○ Applied onto cervical mucosa 2–4 h before breeding; achieves cervical relaxation for 8 h, favors not only breeding but also drainage post breeding
  ○ Buscopan® solution, a smooth muscle relaxant (3 ml mixed with sterile lube) is empirically used for cervical relaxation

Immunomodulators
• Glucocorticoids and immunomodulators—administered around the time of breeding, in combination with traditional postbreeding treatments; increase pregnancy rates
  ○ Prednisolone acetate (0.1 mg/kg every 12 h) beginning 48 h before breeding and continuing until ovulation
  ○ Single dose of dexamethasone (50 mg IV) administered 1 h after breeding
  ○ Common practice—dexamethasone (20 mg every 24 h) beginning 24 h before breeding and continuing until ovulation or up to 24–48 h after. Clinically may be some benefit to continue its use up to 72 h if edema persists or a small amount of fluid remains (refractory to oxytocin administration)
• Cell-mediated immunomodulators—mycobacterial cell wall extract, e.g. Settle® and EqStim®, believed to induce and increase cell-mediated immunity
  ○ Settle is effective to clear *S. zooepidemicus*-induced endometritis
  ○ Mares with persistent endometritis treated with EqStim had higher pregnancy rates than mares treated with conventional treatment

CONTRAINDICATIONS
• Do not administer prostaglandin or its analogs >36 h post ovulation; affects progesterone production by the CL; may result in EED
• Intrauterine infusion of enrofloxacin (Baytril®) is contraindicated; not labeled for horses; highly irritating for endometrium
• Glucocorticoids are only recommended in mares with a negative bacterial culture
• Do not mix NAC and antibiotics in the same syringe since reduces antibiotic activity

PRECAUTIONS
Adverse reactions may occur with natural or synthetic prostaglandin—transient sweating, ataxia, increased gastrointestinal motility.

FOLLOW-UP
PATIENT MONITORING
• Complete the gynecologic evaluation with special attention to uterine culture/cytology on day 1 or 2 of the estrus after treatment
• If no conception after several attempts, repeat the complete evaluation

POSSIBLE COMPLICATIONS
• Pyometra
• Secondary bacterial/yeast overgrowth due to excessive use of antibiotics
• Uterine adhesions

MISCELLANEOUS
AGE-RELATED FACTORS
See Risk Factors.

SEE ALSO
• Cervical lesions
• Endometrial biopsy
• Postpartum metritis
• Pyometra
• Urine pooling/urovagina

ABBREVIATIONS
• AI = artificial insemination
• CL = corpus luteum
• CSA = cationic steroid antimicrobial
• DMSO = dimethylsulfoxide
• DUC = delayed uterine clearance
• EED = early embryonic death
• HPF = high-powered field (microscopy)
• LRS = lactated Ringer's solution
• LVL = low-volume uterine lavage
• NAC = *N*-acetylcysteine
• PGF$_{2\alpha}$ = prostaglandin F$_{2\alpha}$
• PMIE = persistent mating-induced endometritis
• PMN = polymorphonuclear cell
• TRP = transrectal palpation
• US = ultrasonography, ultrasound

Suggested Reading
Asbury AC, Lyle SK. Infectious causes of infertility. In: McKinnon AO, Voss JL, eds. Equine Reproduction. Philadelphia, PA: Lea & Febiger, 1993:381–391.
Blanchard TL, Varner DD, Schumacher J. Uterine defense mechanisms in the mare. In: Manual of Equine Reproduction. St. Louis, MO: Mosby, 1998:47–58.
Brinsko S, Rigby SL, Varner DD, Blanchard TL. A practical method for recognizing mares susceptible to post-breeding endometritis. Proc Am Assoc Equine Pract 2003;49:363–365.
Bucca S, Carli A, Buckley T, et al. The use of dexamethasone administered to mares at breeding time in the modulation of persistent mating induced endometritis. Theriogenology 2008;70:1093–1100.
Hess MB, Parker NA, Purswell BJ, Dascanio JD. Use of Lufenuron as a treatment for fungal endometritis in four mares. J Am Vet Med Assoc 2002;221:266–267.
LeBlanc MM. How to perform and interpret findings from a low volume uterine flush. Proc Am Assoc Equine Pract 2011;57:32–36.
Lyle SK. Incorporating non-antibiotic anti-infective agents into the treatment of equine endometritis. Clin Theriogenol 2012;4(3):386–390.
Nielsen JM, Troedsson MHT, Pedersen MR, et al. Diagnosis of endometritis in the mare based on bacteriological and cytological examinations of the endometrium: comparison of results obtained by swabs and biopsies. J Equine Vet Sci 2010;30:27–30.
Vanderwall DK, Woods GL. Effect on fertility of uterine lavage performed immediately prior to insemination in mares. J Am Vet Med Assoc 2003;222:1108–1110.

Author Maria E. Cadario
Consulting Editor Carla L. Carleton

ENDOTOXEMIA

 BASICS

DEFINITION
- Endotoxemia is a clinical syndrome characterized by the presence of endotoxin in the blood, generalized inflammatory response, and systemic effects. Endotoxin (LPS) is a heat-stable toxin associated with the lipid portion of the outer layer of cell membranes in Gram-negative bacteria. Endotoxemia occurs when either Gram-negative bacteria or the LPS gain access to the systemic circulation
- The term *systemic inflammatory response syndrome (SIRS)* is used to describe the clinical manifestation of endotoxemia
- Endotoxemia occurs through a cascade of events. First, LPS is absorbed from severe localized or disseminated Gram-negative bacterial infection or as free LPS through hypoperfused or inflamed damaged epithelial surfaces. Once in the systemic circulation, LPSs interact with blood constituents or can be removed by macrophages in liver, spleen, or pulmonary vasculature. This is initiated when the LPS-binding protein complexes are bound by the pattern recognition receptors of the inflammatory cells. This complex activates the MyD88 adaptor protein in the equine monocytes, resulting in proinflammatory effects. Therefore, LPS is a potent stimulus of the host inflammation, leading to activation of defense mechanisms that initiate overzealous inflammatory processes causing the manifestations seen in endotoxemia, which are determined by the effects of inflammatory mediators (TNF, IL-1, IL-6, IL-8, IL-10, TXA_2, PGE_2, PAF, LTB_4, kinins, oxygen-derived free radicals, etc.)
- The main effects are endothelial dysfunction, hemodynamic changes, neutrophil activation, coagulopathy, complement activation, acute phase response, shock, and organ failure

SYSTEMS AFFECTED
Cardiovascular
- Reduced myocardial contractility
- Vascular endothelial damage resulting in permeability changes, fluid leakage, and DIC
GI
Impaired mucosal perfusion may cause mucosal sloughing, allowing bacterial translocation and further LPS absorption.
Hepatobiliary
Hepatic ischemia may cause hepatocellular enzyme increases, and alter hepatic function.
Renal
Acute renal failure may result from reduced renal blood flow.
Respiratory
Pulmonary edema and pulmonary thromboembolism may occur.

SIGNS
Early
- Fever
- Depression
- Tachycardia
- Pale mucous membranes
- Rapid CRT
- Tachypnea and/or labored respiration
Late
- Tachycardia or bradycardia
- Poor peripheral pulses
- Hypotension
- Dark mucous membranes
- Prolonged CRT
- Cool extremities
- Hypothermia
- Peripheral edema
- Abdominal pain
- Diarrhea
- Ileus
- Laminitis
- Abortion
- Petechial and ecchymotic hemorrhages
- Death
Neonates
Decreased suckling and weakness.

CAUSES
GI Disorders
LPS normally gains access to the blood through compromised mucosa that may also allow translocation of Gram-negative bacteria.
Neonatal Sepsis
Localized or disseminated infectious focus causing Gram-negative bacteremia or release of LPS into the circulation.

RISK FACTORS
- The equine is particularly susceptible to sepsis secondary to GI disease, metritis, pneumonia and pleuropneumonia, and neonatal sepsis
- Failure of transfer of passive immunity and high-risk pregnancies in neonatal septicemia

 DIAGNOSIS

The diagnosis is usually made based on appreciation of the primary disease process with a high risk of endotoxemia and the presence of the above-mentioned clinical signs in combination with clinicopathologic laboratory findings. A chemiluminescent endotoxin assay has been used to measure endotoxin activity in horses with colic.

DIFFERENTIAL DIAGNOSIS
- Hypovolemic shock
- Cardiogenic shock

CBC/BIOCHEMISTRY/URINALYSIS
- Initially, there is a neutropenia due to vascular margination (may be < 1000/μL; 10^9 cells/L). This is followed by a neutrophilic leukocytosis with a left shift, due to induction of myeloid proliferation in the bone marrow. Toxic changes are usually present in the neutrophils
- Hemoconcentration (increased PCV and total plasma protein)
- Hyperproteinemia initially due to hemoconcentration, but may decrease significantly with GI losses
- High hepatocellular enzymes and bilirubin due to ischemic hepatic injury
- Azotemia may be due to renal or prerenal azotemia associated with blood volume depletion
- Initial hyperglycemia followed by hypoglycemia

OTHER LABORATORY TESTS
Coagulation Profile
- Prolongation of the activated partial thromboplastin time and partial thromboplastin time
- Increased fibrinogen degradation products
- Thrombocytopenia
- Decreased plasma fibrinogen
- Decreased antithrombin III
Blood Gas Analysis
- Hypoxemia
- Acid–base disturbances; metabolic acidosis due to decreased peripheral perfusion and hypoxemia

DIAGNOSTIC PROCEDURES
Aerobic and anaerobic blood cultures.

 TREATMENT

The ideal treatment for endotoxemia is prevention. Close monitoring to prevent the development of the cascade of events should be instituted. Treatment should be initiated quickly and should be aimed at stabilization with aggressive symptomatic therapy, inhibition of endotoxin release into circulation, controlling the inflammatory response, and providing supportive care while establishing tissue perfusion, scavenging of LPS, and management of coagulopathy. If the source of sepsis can be identified, it should be addressed.

 MEDICATIONS

DRUG(S) OF CHOICE
Fluid Therapy and Cardiovascular Support
- Fluid therapy—restoration of the circulating blood volume is the most important factor in restoring peripheral perfusion. Balanced electrolyte solutions such as lactated Ringer's solution or 0.9% sodium chloride; in foals, dextrose should be added to the fluid therapy. Rates of 10–20 mL/kg/h to severely

compromised horses. Use caution not to overhydrate and cause pulmonary edema. Foals and adults with low plasma protein levels are particularly susceptible
• Colloidal solutions (whole blood, plasma, hetastarch, dextrans) can be used to maintain the fluid in the vascular space. They should be initiated when plasma proteins are <4 g/dL, 40 g/L
• Colloids should be from a commercial source or from appropriate donors (Aa and Qa isoantibody negative)
• 7.5% hypertonic saline solution 4 mL/kg for rapid volume expansion
• Sodium bicarbonate to treat severe metabolic acidosis that does not correct with volume expansion. Adult—0.5 mEq × body weight (kg) × (base deficit); give half the dose slowly IV over 20 min. Give the rest of the dose in crystalloid fluids over 4 h if necessary. Foals—0.7 mEq × body weight (kg) × (base deficit); then follow the same regimen as above
• Inotropic agents can be given to increase systemic blood pressure when it drops to <60 mmHg. Dopamine hydrochloride—1–5 µg/kg/min by continuous IV administration but its use in horses is questioned. Dobutamine—titrated from 0.5–1 µg/kg/min by continuous IV administration in adult horses and 1–3 µg/kg/min in foals
• Oxygen therapy if hypoxia and respiratory distress are present

Inhibition of Endotoxin Release
• Antimicrobials should be initiated soon after samples for culture have been obtained when a primary bacterial infection is suspected. Initially, broad-spectrum antimicrobials should be selected pending the results of the culture and susceptibility. Commonly used drugs include aminoglycosides, third-generation cephalosporins, potentiated sulfonamides, and expanded-spectrum penicillins. However, the use of aminoglycosides and carbapenems is suggested given they cause minimal LPS release from bacteria
• The use of antimicrobials for endotoxemia resulting from gastroenteritis is debatable
• Removal of infected tissues or fluids may be helpful

Inhibition of Mediator Synthesis
Corticosteroids
The use of corticosteroids is controversial in horses. In humans, low-dose corticosteroids are now used in the treatment of septic shock with an increase in survival rate without increasing adverse events, while administration of high-dose corticosteroids is discouraged. Whether corticosteroids will provide similar benefit in horses remains to be determined.

NSAIDs
• NSAIDs are used for attenuation of the inflammatory cascade by inhibiting cyclooxygenase
• Flunixin meglumine (0.5 mg/kg every 8–12 h or 0.25 mg/kg every 6–8 h) appears to have the most potent antiendotoxic effects
• NSAIDs inhibit vasodilator PGs; therefore, care must be taken with regard to renal damage

Scavenger of LPS
Immunotherapy (Hyperimmune Antisera or Plasma)
• O-chain-specific antiserum is not clinically useful due to the antigenic diversity in this region
• Different Gram-negative bacteria share common core antigens; therefore, antibodies are aimed at the LPS core. The use of J5 hyperimmune plasma (4.4 mL/kg) is controversial due to inconsistent efficacy in different studies
Polymyxin B
• Cationic polypeptide antibiotic used to bind the lipid A portion of LPS
• It is nephrotoxic and neurotoxic; caution is advised
• Reduced toxicity is achieved if the drug is administered as a conjugate with Dextran-70
• Current recommendation of IV administration of 1000–6000 U/kg every 8–12 h up to 4 or 5 times is based on experimental studies. Its efficacy in clinical equine cases has not been critically evaluated

CONTRAINDICATIONS
• Glucocorticoids may be contraindicated in horse with severe bacterial infection or exhibiting signs of laminitis
• Caution is advised when polymyxin B is administered to dehydrated, hypovolemic, and azotemic patients given its neurotoxicity and nephrotoxicity

PRECAUTIONS
NSAID toxicity may result in GI ulceration and renal ischemia.

POSSIBLE INTERACTIONS
Sodium bicarbonate and dopamine cannot be administered in the same IV line.

ALTERNATIVE DRUGS
• Pentoxifylline
• DMSO
• Lidocaine in CRI
• Ketamine in CRI

 FOLLOW-UP

PATIENT MONITORING
• Vital parameters should be closely monitored

• Blood gas analysis and pulse oximetry to measure oxygenation and acid–base balance
• PCV, serum total protein, albumin, serum electrolytes, hepatocellular enzymes, BUN, and serum creatinine should be monitored

POSSIBLE COMPLICATIONS
• Laminitis
• Electrolyte and acid–base disturbances
• Pulmonary edema
• Pulmonary thromboembolism
• DIC
• Renal dysfunction
• Hepatic dysfunction
• GI ischemia and bacterial translocation
• Vasculitis and peripheral edema
• Cardiac arrest

 MISCELLANEOUS

SYNONYMS
• Endotoxic shock
• Gram-negative sepsis

SEE ALSO
• Bacteremia/sepsis
• Disseminated intravascular coagulation
• Hypoxemia
• Septicemia, neonate

ABBREVIATIONS
• BUN = blood urea nitrogen
• CRI = constant rate infusion
• CRT = capillary refill time
• DIC = disseminated intravascular coagulation
• GI = gastrointestinal
• IL = interleukin
• LTB$_4$ = leukotriene B$_4$
• LPS = lipopolysaccharide
• NSAID = nonsteroidal anti-inflammatory drug
• PAF = platelet-activating factor
• PCV = packed cell volume
• PG = prostaglandin
• TNF = tumor necrosis factor
• TXA$_2$ = thromboxane A$_2$

Suggested Reading
Kelmer G. Update on treatments for endotoxemia. Vet Clin North Am Equine Pract 2009;25:259–270.
Moore JN, Vandenplas ML. Is it the systemic inflammatory response syndrome or endotoxemia in horses with colic? Vet Clin North Am Equine Pract 2014;30:337–351.
Author Olimpo Oliver-Espinosa
Consulting Editors Henry Stämpfli and Olimpo Oliver-Espinosa

ENTEROLITHIASIS

BASICS

DEFINITION
Enteroliths are calculi composed of struvite (magnesium ammonium phosphate hexahydrate) that form in the ampulla of the right dorsal colon and subsequently cause colic due to partial or complete obstruction of the right dorsal, transverse, or descending colon.

PATHOPHYSIOLOGY
• Enteroliths form and enlarge over a period of 1 or more years by deposition of concentric rings of struvite around a central nidus, which consists of a flint-like pebble (a piece of metal, or fibrous material, such as feed particles, nylon baling twine, or hair)
• Enterolithiasis appears to be facilitated by a combination of breed predisposition, type of feed, and environmental and management factors. Horses at risk for enterolithiasis have a pH of colonic contents that is more alkaline than normal, with higher calcium, magnesium, and phosphorus content in their right dorsal colon, and they have a high dietary intake of magnesium and protein (typical of alfalfa-rich diets)
• The valve-like effect of the enterolith at the junction of the right dorsal and transverse colon may intermittently cause partial colonic obstruction and colic. Complete colonic obstruction and persistent colic occur when enteroliths migrate aborally and become lodged at the junction of the right dorsal and transverse colon, or within the smaller diameter transverse or descending colon. Pressure from the lodged enterolith may cause necrosis and rupture of the bowel wall, resulting in septic peritonitis, followed by acute death

SYSTEMS AFFECTED
The GI system.

GENETICS
There is no proven genetic basis for this disease, although breed predilections do exist.

INCIDENCE/PREVALENCE
Enterolithiasis has a worldwide distribution, but is much more common in certain geographic areas.

GEOGRAPHIC DISTRIBUTION
A strong geographic predisposition for enterolithiasis exists, although sporadic cases occur throughout all parts of the USA and in other regions of the world. California appears to be the most commonly affected region, but Florida and Texas also experience moderate numbers of cases. The geographic distribution is likely related to the feeding of alfalfa hay with potential influences from mineral content in the ground water and alfalfa hay; however, there are areas of the world where enteroliths in equines occur with no alfalfa

feeding, suggesting other mechanisms are also involved in its development.

SIGNALMENT
Enteroliths occur in all breeds, but the most overrepresented breeds are Arabian and Arabian crosses and Morgans. In endemic areas, Thoroughbreds and Warmbloods are underrepresented. There is no apparent sex predilection. The mean age for affected horses is 11.5 years (age range 1–36 years).

SIGNS
Historical Findings
• A diet consisting of >50% alfalfa is common
• Recurrent mild to moderate colic occurs in 33.3% of horses and is more typical of the larger enteroliths within the right dorsal colon
• Horses with descending colon obstructions from an enterolith may have more severe signs without any past history of colic
• 15% of horses with obstructive enterolithiasis have a history of passing enteroliths in the feces
• Less frequently, attitude changes, lethargy, weight loss, intermittent anorexia, resentment of tightening the girth, impaired athletic performance, or reluctance to travel down hills

Physical Examination Findings
Typical signs in horses with enterolithiasis without intestinal rupture reflect mild to moderate colic signs. Horses with enterolith obstruction of the descending colon tend to be more tachycardic than those with ascending colon obstruction. Examination findings may sometimes be within normal limits for horses with ascending colon obstructions, necessitating abdominal radiography for confirmation of a diagnosis.

CAUSES
Enteroliths are caused by the deposition of concentric rings of struvite around a central nidus.

RISK FACTORS
Proven risk factors include residing in an endemic area, feeding alfalfa as the predominant or sole forage, and stall confinement with a lack of pasture grazing access. Arabian and Morgan horse breeds are overrepresented.

DIAGNOSIS

DIFFERENTIAL DIAGNOSIS
• All other causes of large intestinal nonstrangulating obstructions such as colonic impaction, colon displacements, and foreign body obstruction
• For those horses with recurrent colic (33%), differential diagnoses include other causes of chronic or recurrent colic such as sand impaction, internal abdominal abscess, gastric or colonic ulcers

CBC/BIOCHEMISTRY/URINALYSIS
Changes are nonspecific for enterolithiasis. Increased hematocrit and hyperproteinemia are common.

OTHER LABORATORY TESTS
In uncomplicated cases, peritoneal fluid is usually normal. Secondary bowel wall compromise leads to amber discoloration, increased turbidity, increased protein concentration, and increased cell count.

IMAGING
• Abdominal radiography is useful diagnostically in many but not all horses. Enteroliths are recognized by their spherical or tetrahedral shape and homogeneously increased density
• Sensitivity and specificity of digital abdominal radiography for diagnosis of enterolithiasis is 84% and 96%, respectively, with sensitivity for descending colon enteroliths being lower at 61.5% versus 88.9% for ascending colon obstructions
• Abdominal ultrasonography is of limited utility

OTHER DIAGNOSTIC PROCEDURES
Rectal examination findings may be within normal limits in up to 25% of horses with enterolithiasis; however, rectal examination frequently reveals distention of the large colon and, less often, tight mesenteric bands. Enteroliths are palpable on rectal examination in about 5% of cases.

PATHOLOGIC FINDINGS
N/A

TREATMENT

Surgical intervention is the only treatment documented to be effective for elimination of formed enteroliths and is best performed via ventral midline celiotomy within a few hours of the onset of signs or, preferably, before signs of complete colonic obstruction are present. The preferred approach is to evacuate the colon via an enterotomy created at the pelvic flexure, after which the enterolith is gently manipulated to this site or to a second enterotomy site for removal. Enteroliths obstructing the descending colon must be removed through a secondary enterotomy at the site of obstruction.

APPROPRIATE HEALTH CARE
Initial evaluation and treatment of horses with enterolithiasis is handled appropriately on an outpatient basis. Horses that do not have a complete colonic obstruction frequently respond favorably to medical approaches commonly used to treat colic. Transportation to a referral center is usually necessary for radiographic confirmation of the diagnosis and surgical management.

E

NURSING CARE
Prevention of rolling and self-induced trauma, provision of analgesia, and passage of a nasogastric tube is indicated before referral. IV fluid therapy is often indicated before, during, and after surgery.

ACTIVITY
After ventral midline celiotomy, stall rest with hand-walking is recommended for the first 4 weeks postoperatively followed by 4 weeks of small paddock turnout and a gradual return to work during weeks 8–12 postoperatively.

DIET
Alfalfa should be eliminated from the diet of horses that have had enteroliths removed surgically.

CLIENT EDUCATION
Restriction of exercise is necessary only in the immediate postoperative period. There is a high likelihood of recurrence if diet and management are not changed.

SURGICAL CONSIDERATIONS
If the patient shows evidence of complete colonic obstruction or has a large, nonobstructing enterolith in the large colon, surgical removal of the enterolith is the only effective treatment.

 MEDICATIONS

DRUG(S) OF CHOICE
See Appropriate Health Care.

CONTRAINDICATIONS
Repeated administration of potent pain-relieving medications in horses with enterolith obstruction are likely to result in fatal GI rupture.

PRECAUTIONS
Repeated use of potent analgesics such as flunixin meglumine, xylazine, detomidine, and butorphanol to control colic pain should be avoided unless appropriate diagnostic and therapeutic intervention is also pursued.

POSSIBLE INTERACTIONS
N/A

ALTERNATIVE DRUGS
N/A

 FOLLOW-UP

PATIENT MONITORING
Observe for signs of colic or inappetence. Follow-up annual abdominal radiographs may be helpful in detecting recurrence.

PREVENTION/AVOIDANCE
• Replace alfalfa hay in the diet with good quality grass or oat hay. Alfalfa should make up <50%
• Supplementation of hay with 8 fl oz (250 mL/450 kg) of apple cider vinegar daily, and/or mixed grain may help acidify colonic contents
• Provide regular exercise and access to pasture turnout
• Eliminate hard drinking water if possible

POSSIBLE COMPLICATIONS
Postoperative complications are similar to those encountered after colic surgery. The main complication specific to this condition is recurrence of enteroliths if dietary modification is not instituted.

EXPECTED COURSE AND PROGNOSIS
• Horses with small enteroliths in their large colon likely remain asymptomatic for months or years and often pass the enteroliths in their manure. Prognosis for horses with small nonobstructing enteroliths is good
• Prognosis for horses with large nonobstructing enteroliths in the large colon is guarded without surgical removal
• Prognosis for recovery for horses with a complete colonic obstruction detected before bowel compromise has occurred is excellent following surgical removal of the stone. Complete recovery can be anticipated in >90% of cases that undergo surgery before the bowel ruptures

 MISCELLANEOUS

ASSOCIATED CONDITIONS
Colonic rupture, colonic displacement, septic peritonitis, endotoxemia, and the postoperative complications listed previously.

AGE-RELATED FACTORS
Enterolithiasis is rarely a clinical problem in horses younger than 2 years of age. Peak incidence is in horses between 5 and 15 years of age.

ZOONOTIC POTENTIAL
N/A

PREGNANCY/FERTILITY/BREEDING
Pregnant mares are likely at increased risk for abortion, as is the case for other causes of colic requiring surgery.

SYNONYMS
• Intestinal calculi
• Intestinal stones

SEE ALSO
Colic, chronic/recurrent

ABBREVIATIONS
GI = gastrointestinal

Suggested Reading
Hassel DM, Langer DL, Snyder JR, et al. Evaluation of enterolithiasis in horses: 900 cases (1973–1996). J Am Vet Med Assoc 1999;214:233–237.
Hassel DM, Rakestraw PC, Gardner IA, et al. Dietary risk factors and colonic pH and mineral concentrations in horses with enterolithiasis. J Vet Intern Med 2004;18:346–349.
Hintz HF, Lowe JE, Livesay-Wilkins P, et al. Studies on equine enterolithiasis. Proc Am Assoc Equine Pract 1988;24:53–59.
Kelleher ME, Puchalski SM, Drake C, le Jeune SS. Use of digital abdominal radiography for the diagnosis of enterolithiasis in equids: 238 cases (2008-2011). J Am Vet Med Assoc 2014;245:126–129.
Lloyd K, Hintz HF, Wheat JD, Schryver HF. Enteroliths in horses. Cornell Vet 1987;77:172–186.

Author Diana M. Hassel
Consulting Editors Henry Stämpfli and Olimpo Oliver-Espinosa

EOSINOPHILIA AND BASOPHILIA

BASICS

OVERVIEW

Eosinophilia
• Blood test >800 cells/µL (>0.8 × 10⁹/L).
• Eosinophilopoiesis is stimulated by T-cell-derived lymphokines (IL-3, IL-5, GM-CSF, and eosinophilopoietin). IL-5 also promotes eosinophil differentiation, maturation, survival, and function.
• Eosinophils are found in subepithelial locations of tissues at sites of foreign particle entry (skin, respiratory, genitourinary, and gastrointestinal tracts). • Eosinophils have diverse functions: parasiticidal activity, and regulation of allergic, inflammatory, coagulation, and fibrinolytic processes.
• During recruitment, eosinophils migrate to tissues under the influence of chemoattractants and are activated by cytokines, complement, and immunoglobulins. • Recruitment of eosinophils is often associated with specific immune responses to antigens through release of constituents of mast cells, basophils, and/or lymphokines. • Protracted eosinophilic inflammation can result in tissue damage and organ dysfunction. • Tissue eosinophilia can occur without concurrent blood eosinophilia.
• Blood eosinophilia results from increased production or release from the bone marrow reserve pool, intravascular redistribution, or prolonged survival

Basophilia
• Basophil count in peripheral blood >300 cells/µL (>0.3 × 10⁹/L). • Production is antigen specific and regulated by IL-3, IL-5, and GM-CSF. • Basophils have functional similarities to mast cells—both elicit type I hypersensitivity reactions upon cross-linking of surface-bound IgE by specific antigens.
• Other functions—regulation of hemostasis, lipolysis, and parasite rejection

SIGNALMENT
N/A

SIGNS
Dependent on the underlying disease.

CAUSES AND RISK FACTORS

Eosinophilia
• Eosinophilia is most common in diseases involving tissues with high concentrations of mast cells and interactions between specific antigen, IgE, and mast cells/basophils. • In these diseases tissue eosinophilia is common, but blood eosinophilia is inconsistent

Parasitism
Endoparasites (e.g. *Parascaris* spp., *Strongylus* spp., and *Dictylocaulus arnfieldi*).

Fungal infection
Conidiobolus spp., *Basidiobolus* spp., or *Pythium insidiosum*.

Idiopathic
MEED, EE.

Neoplasia
Eosinophilic leukemia, paraneoplastic condition with lymphoma.

Immune
Type I hypersensitivity reactions—eosinophilia is rare.

Basophilia
• Hypersensitivity reactions—rare.
• Parasitism—rare. • Basophilic leukemia—rare

DIAGNOSIS

DIFFERENTIAL DIAGNOSIS
N/A

CBC/BIOCHEMISTRY/URINALYSIS
• Eosinophil and/or basophil count > laboratory reference intervals.
• Biochemical analysis may reveal evidence of organ dysfunction

OTHER LABORATORY TESTS
N/A

IMAGING
Thoracic radiography, thoracic and abdominal ultrasonography—lesions of lymphoma, MEED, or EE.

OTHER DIAGNOSTIC PROCEDURES
• Fecal flotation techniques—nematode parasite ova or larvae. • Baermann technique—*D. arnfieldi* larvae in feces.
• Abdominocentesis—eosinophils suggest parasitism, MEED, or EE; abnormal lymphocytes suggest lymphoma.
• Thoracocentesis—eosinophils suggest MEED; atypical lymphocytes suggest lymphoma. • Oral glucose absorption test—malabsorption in lymphoma, MEED, or EE. • Rectal biopsy—lymphoma, MEED, or EE. • Endoscopy of the airways—masses in cases of MEED or exudate in lung disease.
• Tracheal aspirate and/or bronchoalveolar lavage—eosinophilic inflammation. • Skin biopsy in cases of fungal infection or MEED.
• Bone marrow aspirate/biopsy—myeloproliferative disease. • Intradermal antigen testing—atopy

TREATMENT
Treatment should be directed at underlying disease.

MEDICATIONS

DRUG(S) OF CHOICE
• Immunosuppressive treatment with corticosteroids—e.g. dexamethasone (0.2 mg/kg IV or IM once daily for 5 days) then prednisolone (1 mg/kg PO once daily for 14 days, then 1 mg/kg PO every second day).
• Appropriate anthelmintics for parasitism

CONTRAINDICATIONS/POSSIBLE INTERACTIONS
Avoid corticosteroids in horses with laminitis or infectious disease.

FOLLOW-UP

PATIENT MONITORING
Periodic CBC to monitor eosinophil/basophil counts.

PREVENTION/AVOIDANCE
N/A

POSSIBLE COMPLICATIONS
Eosinophil infiltration can cause organ dysfunction.

EXPECTED COURSE AND PROGNOSIS
• Depends on underlying condition. • MEED and lymphoma—poor to grave prognosis.
• Parasitism and EE—guarded prognosis.
• Allergy—depends on ongoing antigen exposure

MISCELLANEOUS

ASSOCIATED CONDITIONS
N/A

AGE-RELATED FACTORS
Eosinophils are absent at birth, then counts increase to a mean of 353 cells/µL (0.353 × 10⁹/L) at 4 months.

ZOONOTIC POTENTIAL
N/A

PREGNANCY/FERTILITY/BREEDING
Corticosteroids should be avoided in the last trimester.

SEE ALSO
Anaphylaxis

ABBREVIATIONS
• EE = eosinophilic enterocolitis.
• GM-CSF = granulocyte–macrophage colony-stimulating factor.
• IgE = immunoglobulin E.
• IL = interleukin. • MEED = multisystemic eosinophilic epitheliotropic disease

Suggested Reading
Carrick JB, Begg AP. Peripheral blood leukocytes. Vet Clin North Am Equine Pract 2008;24:239–259.

Author Kristopher Hughes
Consulting Editors David Hodgson, Harold C. McKenzie, and Jennifer L. Hodgson

BASICS

Eosinophilic enteritis presents in 2 main forms—either acute, focal or chronic diffuse. In some cases there may be some overlap of these forms.

ACUTE, FOCAL

Definition
• These lesions are most frequently termed idiopathic focal eosinophilic enteritis and are characterized by 1 or more hyperemic, palpably thickened, circumferential or antimesenteric plaque-like lesions
• Variably termed inflammatory bowel disease, idiopathic eosinophilic enteritis, multifocal eosinophilic enteritis, and circumferential mural bands
• Impaction of ingesta can develop oral to a lesion, resulting in simple obstruction of the SI and acute colic. This is due to a reduction in luminal diameter at the site and localized ileus due to inflammation
• It can be difficult to establish a diagnosis without confirmation at laparotomy enabling other causes of SI obstruction to be ruled out
• Surgical management is required to decompress the SI and prevent gastric overload and sometimes rupture. Ongoing SI distention can result in venous occlusion and ischemia of distended SI proximal to the impaction and secondary SI volvulus can develop
• Relatively rare cause of SI obstruction. More frequent in certain geographic regions including parts of the USA, Ireland, and the UK; subjective increase in prevalence in northwest UK in the last 10–15 years

Signalment
Younger horses at greatest risk but can occur in any age.

Signs
Acute abdominal pain consistent with nonstrangulating obstruction of the SI.

Causes
• Unknown, speculated to be an acute inflammatory response to an antigen. There is no evidence that high parasite burdens are a cause. Lesions do not recur, so the cause appears to be different than the chronic, diffuse form
• Age and fall months in specific geographic regions are key risk factors

Risk Factors
See Causes.

CHRONIC DIFFUSE

Definition
• Diffuse infiltration of the SI mucosa with eosinophils and lymphocytes
• This is a subgroup of IBD lesions that may occur in the horse
• Eosinophil infiltration may affect other regions of the intestinal tract, including the large colon and other organs such as the skin and liver (MEED)

Pathophysiology
Inflammation and cell infiltration in the gut wall result in protein-losing enteropathy and SI malabsorption.

Systems Affected
Eosinophil infiltration may be confined to the SI and other areas of the intestinal tract, and in horses with MEED may involve the skin, liver, pancreas, esophagus, oral cavity, lungs, and mesenteric lymph nodes.

Genetics
N/A

Incidence/Prevalence
The true prevalence is unknown.

Geographic Distribution
Reported in multiple countries.

Signalment
Young horses (up to 4 years of age) are reported to be more commonly affected, as are Standardbred and Thoroughbred horses.

Signs
• Recurrent colic
• Weight loss
• Diarrhea (if infiltration of the large colon)
• In horses with MEED other clinical signs may be evident dependent on the organ affected, e.g. severe dermatitis in horses with extensive eosinophil infiltration in the skin

Causes
Unknown. A type 1 hypersensitivity reaction to an unknown antigen is suspected. Dietary, inhaled, or parasitic antigens have been proposed.

DIAGNOSIS

ACUTE, FOCAL

Differential Diagnosis
Other forms of nonstrangulating SI obstructions, e.g. ileal impaction, anterior enteritis.

CBC/Biochemistry/Urinalysis, Other Laboratory Tests
There are no key diagnostic tests characteristic of idiopathic focal eosinophilic enteritis—these are largely dependent on duration of SI obstruction and degree of systemic compromise.

Imaging
• Distention of SI confirmed using transabdominal ultrasonography. The intestinal wall is of normal thickness, but if lesions are visualized there is localized mural thickening
• Excess peritoneal fluid may be evident

Other Diagnostic Procedures
• *Nasogastric intubation*—net reflux of >2 L may be obtained depending on duration of SI obstruction and location of the obstruction in the SI
• *Rectal examination*—distended SI may be palpated
• *Abdominocentesis*—total protein, lactate, and white blood cells are usually within normal range (consistent with a nonstrangulating SI obstruction). Eosinophils may or may not be seen on cytologic examination of the fluid
• *Exploratory laparotomy*—the only way in which the cause of SI obstruction can be confirmed and other causes of SI obstruction ruled out. Lesions may be single but up to over 40 separate lesions may be evident

Pathologic Findings
Visual appearance of gross lesions and confirmation on histopathology.

CHRONIC, DIFFUSE

Differential Diagnosis
• Other forms of IBD, e.g. granulomatous enteritis, lymphocytic/plasmacytic enteritis, intestinal lymphosarcoma, infectious causes (*Lawsonia intracellularis, Rhodococcus equi*) in foals/weanlings
• Other causes of recurrent colic

CBC/Biochemistry/Urinalysis
• CBC—peripheral eosinophilia uncommon, may be normal or neutrophilia evident; hyperfibrinogenemia, anemia
• Biochemistry—hypoproteinemia due to hypoalbuminemia, globulins variable. In horses with MEED other abnormalities may be seen, e.g. elevated γ-glutamyltransferase if eosinophilic infiltration of the liver
• Urinalysis—rule out proteinuria

Other Laboratory Tests
N/A

Imaging
Abdominal ultrasonography—transcutaneous and per rectum. Identification of thickened SI wall (>3–5 mm thickness). Imaging of both sides of the abdomen to evaluate other areas of the gastrointestinal tract and other organs.

Other Diagnostic Procedures
• *Abdominocentesis*—to rule out neoplastic causes of SI disease, peritonitis. Increased eosinophils may be seen on cytology
• *Duodenal biopsy (gastroscopy)*—may not be helpful if this portion of the SI is not affected and also because full-thickness biopsies are required
• *Rectal biopsy*—may assist diagnosis
• *Absorption tests*—oral glucose or D-xylose absorption tests, results may be normal in horses with eosinophilic enteritis unlike other forms of IBD
• *SI biopsy*—definitive diagnosis. Multiple, full-thickness biopsies including visibly normal and abnormal intestine required. Usually performed by conventional laparotomy to inspect other areas of the gastrointestinal tract and obtain biopsies from the large colon but a standing flank laparotomy can be performed in horses with

E

EOSINOPHILIC ENTERITIS (CONTINUED)

severe systemic compromise (general anesthesia considered too risky)
• *Parasite testing*—determine intestinal parasite burden

Pathologic Findings
Confirmation of diagnosis on histopathologic examination of tissues.

TREATMENT

ACUTE, FOCAL
• Exploratory laparotomy to confirm the diagnosis, rule out other causes of SI obstruction, and to decompress SI
• Surgical resection of lesions is not required, unless there is marked compromise of the SI lumen due to stricture formation

CHRONIC, DIFFUSE

Appropriate Health Care
Rule out other causes of weight loss/failure to gain weight/recurrent colic, e.g. diet, dental disease.

Nursing Care
N/A

Activity
N/A

Diet
Dietary allergens have been proposed as a potential cause so dietary modification may be trialed. There is no evidence as to a specific diet that may be recommended. Oil may added to the diet—additional fat and calories.

Surgical Considerations
N/A

MEDICATIONS

ACUTE, FOCAL
• IV fluid therapy with isotonic fluids—depending on the degree of preoperative systemic compromise and development of POI/POR
• Flunixin meglumine 1.1 mg/kg IV every 12 h
• Antimicrobials as per clinic protocol following laparotomy
• IV 0.1 mg/kg dexamethasone may be given IV during surgery to reduce the inflammatory reaction. No evidence about optimal dose and duration, ongoing steroid therapy not normally recommended to avoid impaired healing of the laparotomy incision
• Prokinetic therapy if POR develops

CHRONIC, DIFFUSE

Drug(s) of Choice
• Steroid therapy—little evidence regarding the optimal dose and duration of administration
• Parenteral administration recommended initially (3 days to 3 weeks) with 0.05–0.1 mg/kg dexamethasone IM/IV followed by a tapering course of oral prednisolone or dexamethasone
• Ongoing medication may be required—response to treatment and relapse of clinical signs following reduction/cessation of steroid therapy
• Anthelmintics administered as required

Contraindications
N/A

Precautions
Complications associated with prolonged corticosteroid use.

Possible Interactions
N/A

Alternative Drugs
N/A

FOLLOW-UP

ACUTE, FOCAL
• The chronic dilation of the SI may result in venous occlusion of SI proximal to the site of obstruction, which may result in ischemia–reperfusion injury and development of POR
• Frequent nasogastric decompression required if POR develops to prevent gastric rupture
• Reobstruction of ingesta at lesions may occur in the early postoperative period (colic signs and development of nasogastric reflux), and care should be taken to reintroduce feed gradually, particularly in the first 7 days
• Lesions appear to resolve within 3–7 days and recurrence has not been documented. Ongoing medical therapy is not required
• Long-term survival is good provided complications do not occur in the early postoperative stage with rates of up to 100% reported

CHRONIC, DIFFUSE

Patient Monitoring
Ongoing monitoring of clinical progress and assessment of weight gain/reduction in colic episodes.

Prevention/Avoidance
N/A

Possible Complications
N/A

Expected Course and Prognosis
The prognosis is generally considered to be poor, some reports of successful management of chronic, diffuse eosinophilic enteritis.

MISCELLANEOUS

SYNONYMS
Inflammatory bowel disease

SEE ALSO
• Granulomatous enteritis
• Lymphocytic plasmacytic enterocolitis
• Protein-losing enteropathy (PLE)

ABBREVIATIONS
• IBD = inflammatory bowel disease
• MEED = multisystemic eosinophilic epitheliotropic disease
• POI = postoperative ileus
• POR = postoperative reflux
• SI = small intestine

Suggested Reading
Archer DC, Edwards GB, Kelly DF, et al. Obstruction of equine small intestine associated with focal idiopathic eosinophilic enteritis: an emerging disease? Vet J 2006;171:503–512.
Archer DC, Costain DA, Sherlock C. Idiopathic focal eosinophilic enteritis (IFEE), an emerging cause of abdominal pain in horses: the effect of age, time and geographical location on risk. PLoS One 2014;9(12):e112072.
Kalck KA. Inflammatory bowel disease in horses. Vet Clin North Am Equine Pract 2009;25:303–315.
Perez Olmos JF, Schofield WF, Dillon H, et al. Circumferential mural bands in the small intestine causing simple obstructive colic: a case series. Equine Vet J 2006;38:354–349.
Schumacher J, Edwards JF, Cohen ND. Chronic idiopathic inflammatory bowel diseases of the horse. J Vet Intern Med 2000;14:258–265.
Southwood LL, Kawcak CE, Trotter GW, et al. Idiopathic focal eosinophilic enteritis associated with small intestinal obstruction in 6 horses. Vet Surg 2000;29:415–419.

Author Debra C. Archer
Consulting Editors Henry R. Stämpfli and Olimpo Oliver-Espinosa

EOSINOPHILIC KERATITIS

BASICS

OVERVIEW
• EK is a relatively common disease of horses with an unknown etiology
• An accumulation of mainly eosinophils and a few mast cells in the affected cornea is characteristic
• Systems affected—ophthalmic

SIGNALMENT
All ages and breeds affected.

SIGNS
• The clinical appearance of EK in horses can be highly variable
• Mild to severe blepharospasm, epiphora, chemosis, conjunctival hyperemia, mucoid discharge, corneal ulcers, and associated raised, white, necrotic plaques
• A subset of horses with minimal discomfort and more chronic, nonulcerated, proliferative lesions of the cornea has been observed

CAUSES AND RISK FACTORS
• The true etiology of this condition is yet to be determined
• Possibly allergic or parasitic
• May be immune mediated

DIAGNOSIS

DIFFERENTIAL DIAGNOSIS
Allergic or hypersensitivity keratitis/keratoconjunctivitis; eosinophilic granuloma; bacterial, mycotic, or viral keratitis; foreign body reaction; onchocerciasis; habronemiasis; corneal neoplasia such as squamous cell carcinoma or mastocytoma; traumatic keratitis with scarring; calcium or lipid degeneration.

CBC/BIOCHEMISTRY/URINALYSIS
N/A

OTHER LABORATORY TESTS
• Rule out infectious causes (bacterial or fungal) with corneal scrapings for cytology and culture
• Corneal scrapings of EK typically contain degenerate collagen, numerous eosinophils, and a few neutrophils, macrophages, lymphocytes, and mast cells
• Cytology is usually diagnostic; however, biopsy for histology will help to confirm the diagnosis if corneal scrapings are not conclusive

• In cases with an associated conjunctivitis, the distribution of inflammatory cells in a sample from the conjunctiva resembles that from the cornea

IMAGING
N/A

OTHER DIAGNOSTIC PROCEDURES
N/A

PATHOLOGIC FINDINGS
Histologic examination finds eosinophilic, acellular granular material and subepithelial, fragmented degenerate collagen infiltrated by eosinophils, lymphocytes, plasma cells, and macrophages.

TREATMENT
• Medical therapy is aimed at decreasing the inflammatory response within the cornea
• Often combination therapy is necessary
• Superficial lamellar keratectomy to remove plaques may speed healing

MEDICATIONS

DRUG(S) OF CHOICE
• Topical corticosteroids (1% prednisolone acetate or 0.1% dexamethasone) 3 or 4 times a day in early stages (despite corneal ulcerations)
• Topical cyclosporine 0.2–2.0% BID or TID
• Topical mast cell stabilizers such as 4% cromolyn sodium (cromoglicic acid) and 0.01% lodoxamide or olopatadine can be helpful in some cases 3–4 times a day
• Topical antibiotics (e.g. bacitracin–neomycin–polymyxin B, chloramphenicol), 1% atropine, and 0.03% phospholine iodide (ecothiopate iodide) BID in combination with systemic NSAIDs (e.g. flunixin meglumine 0.25–1 mg/kg BID PO, IM, IV) to protect the corneal wounds from secondary infection and treat any associated uveitis
• Once improvement is noted, medical therapy should be tapered slowly

CONTRAINDICATIONS/POSSIBLE INTERACTIONS
• Phospholine iodide is an acetylcholinesterase inhibitor which may be larvicidal for parasites. Its use is controversial

• The use of topical NSAIDs may increase the severity of clinical signs in the horse since they do not inhibit and may potentiate leukotrienes
• Horses receiving topically administered atropine should be monitored for signs of colic

FOLLOW-UP

EXPECTED COURSE AND PROGNOSIS
• Although therapy is often prolonged and these lesions are often slow to heal, the prognosis for resolution with diligent treatment is good
• Scarring of the cornea may occur
• May recur. May be seasonal

MISCELLANEOUS

ASSOCIATED CONDITIONS
Uveitis

SEE ALSO
• Burdock pappus bristle keratopathy
• Corneal/scleral lacerations
• Corneal stromal abscesses
• Corneal ulceration
• Glaucoma
• Equine recurrent uveitis
• Superficial nonhealing ulcers

ABBREVIATIONS
• EK = eosinophilic keratitis/keratoconjunctivitis
• NSAID = nonsteroidal anti-inflammatory drug

Suggested Reading
Brooks DE. Ophthalmology for the Equine Practitioner, 2e. Jackson, WY: Teton NewMedia, 2008.
Brooks DE, Matthews AG. Equine ophthalmology. In: Gelatt KN, ed. Veterinary Ophthalmology, 4e. Ames, IA: Blackwell, 2007:1165–1274.
Gilger BC, ed. Equine Ophthalmology, 3e. Ames, IA: Wiley Blackwell, 2017.

Authors Caryn E. Plummer
Consulting Editor Caryn E. Plummer

E

EPIGLOTTIC ENTRAPMENT

BASICS

OVERVIEW
• A result of the loose aryepiglottic mucosa, which normally is on the ventral surface of the epiglottis, enveloping part or all of its dorsal surface
• Usually, the epiglottis remains in its normal position, but the condition can occur concurrently with DDSP
• Leads to varying degrees of respiratory compromise and exercise intolerance
• Most often diagnosed during resting endoscopy because the entrapment is persistent
• Also can occur intermittently
• Severity can significantly impact the outcome after treatment

SIGNALMENT
• Affects primarily Thoroughbred and Standardbred racehorses
• Other breeds or horses engaged in other activities rarely are affected
• Rarely seen in older noncompetitive horses, associated with a cough
• Can occur at any age
• No sex predilection

SIGNS
• Exercise intolerance is the most frequent chief complaint
• Abnormal respiratory noise may be present
• Other signs—coughing, dysphagia, nasal discharge

CAUSES AND RISK FACTORS
• The cause is unknown
• Racing is the most significant risk factor
• Horses with a small epiglottis are predisposed
• An association exists between epiglottic entrapment and DDSP

DIAGNOSIS

DIFFERENTIAL DIAGNOSIS
• Epiglottiditis—swelling of the epiglottis smooths out the normal edges and distorts the vascular pattern, but there is no membrane over the epiglottis
• Epiglottic deformity/hypoplasia—there may be varying degrees of deformity, but there is no membrane over the epiglottis
• DDSP—the outline of the epiglottis is not visible

IMAGING
• Upper airway endoscopy at rest—the most common diagnostic technique. The

triangular-shaped epiglottis remains visible, but the entrapping membrane obscures the normal serrated edge and vascular pattern of the epiglottis. The normal vasculature consists of 2 vessels that extend toward the apex and that arborize into smaller vessels toward the edge of the epiglottis. Swallowing may induce an intermittent entrapment. With chronicity, the membrane becomes thickened and, sometimes, ulcerated. Infrequently, entrapment can lead to epiglottic deformity that may not be apparent until after the entrapment is resolved
• With concurrent DDSP, it is difficult to see the entrapment. Close inspection may reveal another edge of membrane before the dorsal surface of the epiglottis is apparent. A bulge into the palate is sometimes present
• Skull radiography—the convex shape of the epiglottis is obscured on lateral radiographs

OTHER DIAGNOSTIC PROCEDURES
• Exercising endoscopy may be required for the diagnosis of intermittent entrapment
• Visualization of the membrane below the epiglottis with the use of sedation, local anesthetic, and bronchoesophageal graspers can reveal the presence of ulceration that could indicate previous intermittent entrapment
• Arterial blood gases during exercise are typically normal when concurrent abnormalities are not present

TREATMENT
• Surgical correction of the simple, nonulcerated entrapment entails axial division of the entrapping membrane in the standing horse with sedation and topical anesthetic. The division is performed with direct visualization, employing a laser fiber through the instrument portal of a videoendoscope. Axial division also can be performed with a hooked bistoury, typically under endoscopic guidance
• Very thickened, ulcerated entrapping membranes often require surgical resection of the tissue. This can be approached through a laryngotomy under general anesthesia, or via transendoscopic laser surgery in the sedated horse

MEDICATIONS

DRUG(S) OF CHOICE
• Anti-inflammatory drugs (dexamethasone, phenylbutazone) and throat sprays (10 mL of

a Furacin (nitrofurazone)-based solution with 2 mg of prednisolone in a 1 mL solution BID) for several days postoperatively
• Antimicrobials are advised in cases of thickened membranes or ulceration, but may not be necessary in an uncomplicated entrapment

FOLLOW-UP
• Perform endoscopy postoperatively and before resuming training; further examinations depend on change in performance
• It may be valuable to evaluate the ventral surface of the epiglottis prior to determining a return to exercise when the membranes are particularly thickened or ulcerated or a resection was performed
• Epiglottic entrapment has a very low recurrence rate

MISCELLANEOUS

SEE ALSO
• Acute epiglottiditis
• Dynamic collapse of the upper airways

ABBREVIATIONS
DDSP = dorsal displacement of the soft palate

Suggested Reading
Aitken MR, Parente EJ. Epiglottic abnormalities in mature nonracehorses: 23 cases (1990-2009). J Am Vet Med Assoc 2011;238(12):1634–1638.
Epstein KL, Parente EJ. Epiglottic fold entrapment. In: McGorum BC, Dixon PM, Robinson NE, Schumacher J, eds. Equine Respiratory Medicine and Surgery. Philadelphia, PA: WB Saunders, 2006:459–466.
Lacourt M, Marcoux M. Treatment of epiglottic entrapment by transnasal axial division in standing sedated horses using a shielded hook bistoury. Vet Surg 2011;40(3):299–304.

Author Eric J. Parente
Consulting Editors Mathilde Leclère and Daniel Jean

BASICS

OVERVIEW
• A noninfectious condition affecting the lower airways of horses. This terminology has been introduced because of the numerous and confusing terminologies that have been used in the past, and because of the similarities that these conditions share with human asthma
• Mild and moderate equine asthma is now used to describe the condition previously known as inflammatory airway disease, while severe equine asthma is used instead of heaves or recurrent airway obstruction
• This new terminology does not imply a common pathophysiology
• Results from the inhalation of antigens present in the environment of horses, primarily those found in hay (classic form) or pasture (summer form)
• Systems affected—respiratory
• Worldwide distribution. The severe form is rare in warm climates

SIGNALMENT
• No breed or sex predisposition
• All ages for mild and moderate equine asthma; horses with severe asthma are usually 7 years or older

SIGNS
• Suggestive of lower airway disease
• Exercise intolerance, cough, nasal discharge, increased breathing frequency
• Episodes of labored breathing at rest only in severe equine asthma
• Thoracic auscultation may be normal in the mild form, but wheezes and crackles are frequent when using a rebreathing bag, especially in the more severe cases

CAUSES AND RISK FACTORS
• Immune-mediated reaction to inhaled antigens suspected
• Genetic predisposition well documented in some families
• Stabling and hay feeding, or pasture in the summer form

DIAGNOSIS

DIFFERENTIAL DIAGNOSIS
Other causes of lung diseases.

CBC/BIOCHEMISTRY/URINALYSIS
Within normal limits.

OTHER LABORATORY TESTS
Arterial blood gases may reveal hypoxemia in the severe form.

IMAGING
Thoracic radiography may reveal a bronchointerstitial pattern.

OTHER DIAGNOSTIC PROCEDURES
• The diagnosis should ideally be based on the presence of lower airway obstruction, but is rarely performed due to the lack of portable and sensitive equipment
• Bronchoscopy—tracheal mucus is common
• Bronchoalveolar lavage cytology—increased neutrophils, mast cells, or eosinophils
• Tracheal aspirates—reveal inflammation but not considered diagnostic

PATHOLOGIC FINDINGS
• Chronic active bronchiolitis
• Airway remodeling characterized by smooth muscle thickening and increased collagen, at least in the severe form

TREATMENT
• Outpatient care
• Avoid hay feeding, straw bedding, and stabling when possible
• Favor pasture/paddock, pelleted hay, haylage, or pasteurized hay in the classic form
• Favor stabling and pelleted hay in the summer form

MEDICATIONS

DRUG(S) OF CHOICE

Corticosteroids
• The most potent drugs to control clinical signs
• Inhaled drugs are preferred for prolonged administration
• Improvement in clinical signs and airway obstruction within days (systemic) or days to weeks (inhaled). Cough may take longer to respond
• Few residual effects unless combined with antigen avoidance strategies

Bronchodilators
• Should not be used as sole therapy. To be combined with antigen avoidance strategies or corticosteroids
• Short-acting bronchodilators may be administered by inhalation prior to exercise, or orally for more sustained effects

Other Drugs
• Inhaled sodium cromoglycate (cromoglicic acid) with inflammation associated with mast cells
• In the absence of antigen avoidance strategies, no drugs normalize airway neutrophilic inflammation

CONTRAINDICATIONS/POSSIBLE INTERACTIONS
• Corticosteroids should not be administered systemically to horses with a history of laminitis or concurrent bacterial infection

• Vaccination against botulism when feeding haylage is recommended in some areas

FOLLOW-UP

PATIENT MONITORING
Repeat BAL fluid cytology and lung function (when possible) 6–8 weeks after implementation of antigen avoidance strategies to assess effectiveness.

PREVENTION/AVOIDANCE
Avoid exposure of all horses to moldy hay, especially when they are genetically susceptible.

EXPECTED COURSE AND PROGNOSIS
• Mild and moderate equine asthma may be self-limiting
• Severe equine asthma is incurable
• Removing the offending antigens normalizes BAL fluid cytology within 6 weeks but complete control of the clinical signs may take up to 3 months without drug therapy
• Currently it is not possible to predict which horses with mild/moderate asthma will progress to the severe form

MISCELLANEOUS

AGE-RELATED FACTORS
Severe asthma is rare in horses <7 years of age.

PREGNANCY/FERTILITY/BREEDING
Avoid systemic administration of corticosteroids and β_2-agonist bronchodilators during pregnancy.

SEE ALSO
• Cough, acute/chronic
• Expiratory dyspnea
• Heaves (severe equine asthma, RAO)
• Inflammatory airway diseases—IAD in performance horses (mild and moderate equine asthma)
• Summer pasture-associated equine asthma (pasture asthma)

ABBREVIATIONS
BAL = bronchoalveolar lavage

Suggested Reading
Pirie RS, Couëtil LL, Robinson NE, Lavoie JP. Equine asthma: an appropriate, translational and comprehendible terminology? Equine Vet J 2016;48:403–405.

Author Jean-Pierre Lavoie
Consulting Editors Mathilde Leclère and Daniel Jean

EQUINE CORONAVIRUS

E

BASICS

OVERVIEW
- In Coronaviridae family—single-stranded, positive-sense, nonsegmented, enveloped RNA viruses responsible for enteric, respiratory, hepatic, or neurologic disease in a variety of mammalian and avian species
- ECoV is classified within the *Betacoronavirus* genus, along with human OC43 and HKU1 coronavirus, BCoV, porcine hemagglutinating encephalomyelitis virus, canine respiratory coronavirus, mouse hepatitis virus, and sialodacryoadenitis virus
- A feco-oral transmission route has been experimentally documented. Clinically or asymptomatically infected horses appear to be responsible for direct and indirect transmission
- Sporadic cases and outbreaks have been reported with increased frequency since 2010 from Japan, the USA, and more recently from Europe
- Morbidity in affected herds is variable and has been reported to range between 10% and 83%

SIGNALMENT
All age groups are susceptible. Clinical disease is mainly seen in adult horses.

SIGNS
- Clinical disease develops 48–72 h after natural exposure
- Anorexia, lethargy, and fever. Soft formed to watery fecal consistency and colic can be present in less than 20% of infected horses
- Can occasionally develop signs of encephalopathy, including circling, head pressing, ataxia, proprioceptive deficits, nystagmus, recumbency, and seizure
- Persist for a few days to 1 week and generally resolve with minimal supportive care

CAUSES AND RISK FACTORS
- Outbreaks have predominantly been reported in riding, racing, and show horses and less frequently in breeding animals
- The case number is higher during the colder months

DIAGNOSIS

DIFFERENTIAL DIAGNOSIS
- Wide range of systemic diseases causing fever, lethargy, and anorexia

- Acute infectious diseases affecting the small and/or large intestine such as *Salmonella* spp., *Clostridium difficile*, *Neorickettsia risticii*

CBC/BIOCHEMISTRY/URINALYSIS
- Leukopenia due to neutropenia and/or lymphopenia
- Biochemical parameters may be unremarkable. Elevation of total and indirect bilirubin due to partial or complete anorexia, electrolyte changes consistent with enterocolitis, transient elevation of liver enzymes, and renal parameters suggestive of prerenal azotemia have been observed in some cases
- Hyperammonemia is likely due to increased ammonia production within or absorption from the GI tract due to GI barrier breakdown in severe necrotizing enteritis and septicemia

OTHER LABORATORY TESTS
qPCR for ECoV on feces (high sensitivity and specificity; quick turnaround time).

IMAGING
Abdominal ultrasonography may show increased small intestinal motility with fluid-filled content.

OTHER DIAGNOSTIC PROCEDURES
- Antemortem diagnosis—presence of clinical signs compatible with infection, neutropenia, and/or lymphopenia, the exclusion of other infectious causes, and molecular detection of ECoV in feces
- Postmortem diagnosis—histologic changes, qPCR detection of ECoV in small intestinal tissue, and/or content or detection of coronavirus-like viral particles via immunochemistry or direct fluorescent antibody testing of small intestinal tissue

PATHOLOGIC FINDINGS
Mild to moderate enteritis characterized by villus attenuation, villi tip epithelial cell necrosis, and neutrophilic and fibrin extravasation into the small intestinal lumen.

TREATMENT

Most adult horses recover spontaneously in a few days without specific treatment.

MEDICATIONS

DRUG(S) OF CHOICE
- Horses with persistent elevated rectal temperature, anorexia, and lethargy are

routinely treated with NSAIDs such as flunixin meglumine (0.5–1.1 mg/kg every 12–24 h IV or PO) or phenylbutazone (2–4 mg/kg every 12–24 h IV or PO) for 24–48 h, as long as their hydration status is believed normal
- Horses with colic, persistent lethargy, and anorexia and/or diarrhea should receive fluids and electrolyte per nasogastric intubation or IV administration of polyionic fluids until clinical signs have resolved

FOLLOW-UP

PREVENTION/AVOIDANCE
- Use of BCoV vaccine in horses for the prevention of ECoV has yet not been investigated and cannot be recommended at this time
- Because of the highly contagious nature of ECoV, any horse presenting with significant fever, anorexia, and lethargy with or without enteric signs should be strictly isolated until a diagnosis is secured
- Once ECoV infection is confirmed, strict isolation procedures and secondary quarantine of the source stable of the particular horse should be employed
- Fecal shedding of ECoV under natural conditions commonly resolves within 7–10 days of acute onset of clinical signs

MISCELLANEOUS

ABBREVIATIONS
- BCoV = bovine coronavirus
- ECoV = equine coronavirus
- GI = gastrointestinal
- NSAID = nonsteroidal anti-inflammatory drug
- qPCR = quantitative polymerase chain reaction

Suggested Reading
Pusterla N, Vin R, Leutenegger C, et al. Equine coronavirus: an emerging enteric virus of adult horses. Equine Vet Educ 2016;28:216–222.

Author Nicola Pusterla
Consulting Editor Ashley G. Boyle

Client Education Handout available online

E

BASICS

DEFINITION
Seasonal, tick-borne disease caused by a granulocytotropic rickettsial organism, *Anaplasma phagocytophilum* (previously *Ehrlichia equi*).

PATHOPHYSIOLOGY
• Caused by a Gram-negative bacteria, present inside granulocytes
• *Ixodes scapularis* (the black-legged tick or deer tick) is the likely primary vector for the disease in the eastern and midwestern USA and *Ixodes pacificus* (the western black-legged tick) in the west
• Existence of a maintenance or sylvatic host likely represents a wild reservoir, such as rodents; horses are considered dead-end hosts and are not directly contagious
• Disease transmission occurs when infected ticks feed on the horse for 2–36 h
• Incubation period is 8–25 days after experimental infection using ticks as vectors
• The agent affects granulocytes (both neutrophils and eosinophils) and causes a vasculitis and interstitial inflammation, leading to edema, petechial hemorrhages, ataxia, and hemolytic anemia
• Infection can result in pancytopenia, especially thrombocytopenia
• Severe myopathies have occurred concurrent with the infection

SYSTEMS AFFECTED
• Behavioral—mentation alteration (i.e. lethargy) of varying degrees
• Hemic/lymphatic/immune—vasculitis, leading to edema and mucosal hemorrhages; hemolytic anemia
• Musculoskeletal—reluctance to move, limb edema
• Nervous—vasculitis in the CNS, leading to ataxia and recumbency
• Cardiac—arrhythmias have been associated with myocarditis secondary to vasculitis within the myocardium
• Myopathy—rare

INCIDENCE/PREVALENCE
• High prevalence in the Sierra Nevada foothills and northern coastal range of California and many areas of eastern and midwestern USA. Anywhere the tick vector is present is at risk for the disease
• Seroprevalence studies in northern California show a prevalence of 3.1–10.3%, depending on geographic location, and >50% seropositivity among horses on premises known to be enzootic for the disease
• The disease is seasonal, having its highest occurrence during the late fall, winter, and spring

GEOGRAPHIC DISTRIBUTION
• USA—west and east coasts are regions most affected

• The disease has been diagnosed in Germany, Switzerland, Sweden, Norway, the UK, Denmark, Canada, Austria, Czech Republic, the Netherlands, France, Poland, and Italy, among other countries. Reports also exist from Asia and Africa

SIGNALMENT
• Primarily affects horses, but donkeys have been experimentally infected
• No breed or sex predilections
• Horses ≥4 years are most severely affected
• Has been reported in a foal as young as 2.5 months

SIGNS
Historical Findings
• Lethargy
• High fever
• Anorexia
• Limb edema
• Tick exposure

Physical Examination Findings
• Pyrexia
• Anorexia
• Depressed mentation
• Limb edema (absent in young animals)
• Mild petechiae and ecchymoses on mucous membranes and sclerae
• Icterus
• Ataxia
• Reluctance to move, stiffness, myopathy
• Arrhythmias (rare)
• Recumbency (rare)

CAUSES
• *A. phagocytophilum*
• Close antigenic and genetic similarity to the agent of HGE and to European tick-borne fever affecting ruminants

RISK FACTORS
• Geography
• Exposure to *Ixodes ricinus* complex ticks
• Age—horses ≥4 years are most severely affected
• Immune status

DIAGNOSIS

DIFFERENTIAL DIAGNOSIS
• Viral encephalitis
• Liver disease with hepatic encephalopathy
• Purpura haemorrhagica
• Equine infectious anemia
• Equine viral arteritis

CBC/BIOCHEMISTRY/URINALYSIS
• Leukopenia with neutropenia
• Less commonly leukocytosis
• Thrombocytopenia
• Increased icteric index
• Anemia
• Hyperfibrinogenemia
• Hyperbilirubinemia (high unconjugated bilirubin)

OTHER LABORATORY TESTS
• Giemsa-, new methylene blue-, or Wright-stained peripheral blood smears show inclusion bodies (i.e. morula) within the cytoplasm of neutrophils and eosinophils. Inclusions are pleomorphic and blue-gray to dark blue in color, have a spoke-wheel appearance, and occur in 3–75% of circulating granulocytes within 2–6 days of the onset of fever
• Buffy coat smears concentrate granulocytes and, therefore, increase the sensitivity of identifying inclusion bodies
• Indirect fluorescent antibody tests are available for serology. A titer ≥1:10 suggests exposure which may not be acute. An increasing titer documents active infection but requires an acute and convalescent sample. A single sample with a cutoff value of 1:40 can be seen from prior subclinical infection and is not diagnostic for acute infection
• PCR amplification of DNA from buffy coats of infected horses is a very sensitive diagnostic tool. PCR is positive before inclusion bodies are first observed in neutrophils and persists while the animal is febrile
• Immunohistochemistry of tissues from postmortem examination can be used for diagnosis

DIAGNOSTIC PROCEDURES
See Other Laboratory Tests.

PATHOLOGIC FINDINGS
• Mortality is rare, except for reasons of secondary complications. One recent report of mortality from the primary infection itself is thought to be due to severe vasculitis and DIC
• Inflammation of small arteries and veins (vasculitis), hemorrhage, edema
• Petechiae on mucous and serous membranes
• Mild inflammatory, vascular, or interstitial lesions in the heart, CNS, kidneys, spleen, liver, and lung

TREATMENT

APPROPRIATE HEALTH CARE
Hospitalize horses with severe ataxia or secondary complications; otherwise, uncomplicated cases can be managed in the field. The infection is often self-limiting, with horses recovering fully within 1–2 weeks.

NURSING CARE
• Supportive limb bandages for edema
• NSAIDs for antipyretic purposes
• Debilitated cases may benefit from IV fluid or electrolyte therapy
• Corticosteroids may benefit horses with severe ataxia by reducing the severity of vasculitis

EQUINE GRANULOCYTIC ANAPLASMOSIS   (CONTINUED)

ACTIVITY

Stall confinement for ataxic animals; otherwise, hand-walking may help to reduce edema.

CLIENT EDUCATION

When entering known *Ixodes* tick-infested areas, use tick repellents, and check horses closely for ticks upon return from these areas.

MEDICATIONS

DRUG(S) OF CHOICE

• Oxytetracycline (7 mg/kg IV every 24 h for 3–7 days diluted and administered slowly in 0.9% saline (1 L for an average-sized horse)). With this treatment, a marked decrease in rectal temperature and improvement in appetite and attitude should be observed within 12–24 h of the first administered dose
• Doxycycline (10 mg/kg PO every 12 h for 7–10 days) and minocycline (4 mg/kg PO every 12 h for 7–10 days) are alternatives used with success in field cases. For cases in which oxytetracycline is administered IV for 1–3 days, they can be switched to oral doxycycline or minocycline for a further 7 days
• Short-term corticosteroids (dexamethasone) have been used to reduce inflammation and ataxia and have been safe to use in the experimental setting

PRECAUTIONS

• Tetracyclines can retard fetal skeletal development and discolor deciduous teeth; therefore, use with caution and only for a short duration during the first half of gestation, then only when the benefits outweigh the fetal risks
• Tetracyclines have been associated with enterocolitis, photosensitivity, and nephrotoxicity
• IV oxytetracycline can result in perivascular swelling and phlebitis if administered perivascularly

FOLLOW-UP

PATIENT MONITORING

• Monitor temperature, attitude, and appetite for significant improvement within 12–24 h of treatment. In horses diagnosed in the very early stages of the disease and treatment administered for 5 days, relapses of the original infection have occurred

• Evaluate serial buffy coat smear for inclusion bodies
• Monitor hydration status and renal function while on oxytetracycline

PREVENTION/AVOIDANCE

• Minimize exposure to *Ixodes* or other transmitting ticks through application of topical tick repellents when entering infested areas, and carefully examine horses for ticks on their return from such areas
• Many horses may experience subclinical infections and develop subsequent immunity

POSSIBLE COMPLICATIONS

• Rare, secondary bacterial infections, especially bronchopneumonia
• Horses with severe ataxia may suffer traumatic injury (e.g. fractures)
• Cardiac arrhythmias, including ventricular tachycardia, may be associated with myocarditis
• DIC—very rare
• Recumbency
• Immune-mediated myopathy (rare)

EXPECTED COURSE AND PROGNOSIS

• Excellent prognosis in uncomplicated cases
• Horses are immune to reinfection for at least 2 years; no carrier or latent state has been documented
• With therapy, horses show rapid improvement—a decrease in rectal temperature, increase in appetite, and improvement in overall demeanor should be noted in 12–24 h; the ataxia should resolve within 2–3 days and the edema within several days
• Left untreated, the disease is self-limiting in 2–3 weeks; however, affected horses exhibit more severe weight loss, edema, and ataxia and are at greater risk for secondary complications than horses treated with tetracycline. Laminitis is not associated with infection
• Mortality due solely to acute infection is rare

MISCELLANEOUS

AGE-RELATED FACTORS

Severity of clinical signs is associated with age—horses <1 year generally do not show signs of infection or only slight lethargy and fever; 1–3 years of age show mild to moderate signs; and ≥4 years are affected most severely, with ataxia, icterus, edema, and petechial hemorrhages.

ZOONOTIC POTENTIAL

• The agent of HGE may represent 1 or more strains of the equine pathogen; however, horses are considered dead-end hosts and do not act as a source of human infection directly
• Ticks are required as intermediate hosts

PREGNANCY/FERTILITY/BREEDING

• 2 pregnant mares are reported to have been naturally infected with *A. phagocytophilum* during gestation and to have subsequently delivered live foals at full term. Experimental infection in pregnant mares produces no abortion, and live foals have resulted
• No abortions or congenital abnormalities have been described
• Passive immunity is transferred to suckling foals but is short-lived in duration

SYNONYMS

Equine ehrlichiosis

SEE ALSO

• Infectious anemia (EIA)
• Thrombocytopenia

ABBREVIATIONS

• CNS = central nervous system
• DIC = disseminated intravascular coagulation
• HGE = human granulocytic ehrlichiosis
• NSAID = nonsteroidal anti-inflammatory drug
• PCR = polymerase chain reaction

Suggested Reading

Dziegiel B, Adaszek L, Kalinowski M, Winiarczyk S. Equine granulocytic anaplasmosis. Res Vet Sci 2013;95:316–320.

Madigan JE, Gribble D. Equine ehrlichiosis in northern California: 49 cases (1968–1981). J Am Vet Med Assoc 1987;190:445–448.

Nolen-Walston RD, D'Oench SM, Hanelt LM, et al. Acute recumbency associated with *Anaplasma phagocytophilum* infection in a horse. J Am Vet Med Assoc 2004;224:1964–1966.

Reubel GH, Kimsey RB, Barlough JE, Madigan JE. Experimental transmission of *Ehrlichia equi* to horses through naturally infected ticks (*Ixodes pacificus*) from northern California. J Clin Microbiol 1998;36:2131–2134.

Authors K. Gary Magdesian and John E. Madigan
Consulting Editor Ashley G. Boyle

BASICS

OVERVIEW
• EHV-5 is an equine gammaherpesvirus that establishes a lifelong latent infection in peripheral blood mononuclear cells, predominantly in equine B lymphocytes
• EHV-5 is frequently detected in respiratory samples, ocular samples, and blood cells, sites of both primary infection and latency
• Although EHV-5 has been detected in clinical samples from horses with no clinical disease, it has recently been associated with EMPF, a progressive nodular fibrotic lung disease. EHV-5 has been detected in bronchoalveolar lavage samples and postmortem tissue, and the highest loads of EHV-5 were detected in the most severe EMPF lesions
• Whether the EHV-5 causes EMPF or the local pulmonary microenvironment associated with EMPF increases the EHV-5 load in the vicinity of the EMPF lesions is not yet clear
• Systems affected—respiratory
• EHV-5 has been commonly detected in clinical samples from clinically normal and diseased adult horses
• EMPF should be considered in cases with presenting clinical signs of chronic weight loss, ill thrift, and/or tachypnea
• EHV-5 has been detected in horse populations around the world

DIAGNOSIS

DIFFERENTIAL DIAGNOSIS
Chronic, long-term, lower respiratory tract diseases such as interstitial or infectious pneumonia, pulmonary neoplastic disease, idiopathic pulmonary fibrosis.

CBC/BIOCHEMISTRY/URINALYSIS
EMPF cases present with nonspecific clinicopathologic abnormalities, including anemia, leukocytosis, hyperfibrinogenemia, and/or hypoalbuminemia.

OTHER LABORATORY TESTS
• Histopathology on lung biopsy or postmortem samples have demonstrated marked pulmonary interstitial expansion by well-organized mature collagen with infiltration of mixed inflammatory cells and the preservation of "alveolar-like" architecture
• There are a variety of molecular diagnostic tests available to detect EHV-5 in clinical samples

IMAGING
Thoracic ultrasonography to demonstrate generalized nodular consolidation and thoracic radiography to confirm the generalized distribution of the nodules and interstitial pattern.

MEDICATIONS

DRUG(S) OF CHOICE
While supportive therapy is indicated, there is no evidence to support the use of any specific therapeutic regimen to treat EMPF, including administration of antiherpetic drugs such as valacyclovir (valaciclovir) or acyclovir (aciclovir).

FOLLOW-UP

EXPECTED COURSE AND PROGNOSIS
Some cases will recover, but generally the prognosis for cases of EMPF is guarded to poor.

MISCELLANEOUS

SEE ALSO
• Fungal pneumonia
• Heaves (severe equine asthma, RAO)
• Lungworm—parasitic bronchitis and pneumonia
• Pleuropneumonia
• Tumors of the respiratory system

ABBREVIATIONS
• EHV-5 = equine herpesvirus 5
• EMPF = equine multinodular pulmonary fibrosis

Suggested Reading
Hartley CA, Dynon KJ, Mekuria ZH, et al. Equine gammaherpesviruses: perfect parasites? Vet Microbiol 2013;167:86–92.
Williams KJ, Maes R, Del Piero F, et al. Equine multinodular pulmonary fibrosis: a newly recognized herpesvirus-associated fibrotic lung disease. Vet Pathol 2007;44:849–862.

Author James R. Gilkerson
Consulting Editor Ashley G. Boyle

E

EQUINE HERPESVIRUS MYELOENCEPHALOPATHY

BASICS

OVERVIEW
- EHM is an uncommon CNS disease associated with EHV-1 infection
- The disease can occur sporadically or in outbreaks and is seen worldwide, mainly in northern Europe and North America
- There is no breed or sex predilection; however horses >3 years old seem to be more likely to be affected
- EHV-1 is a species-specific enveloped DNA that typically causes lifelong infection of the host
- EHM is a rare outcome of an infection that typically causes respiratory disease and abortions
- EHM is caused by multifocal hemorrhages due to disease of the CNS vasculature, particularly in the lumbosacral spinal cord
- Infection of the respiratory tract and subsequent local virus multiplication results in peripheral blood mononuclear cell-associated viremia and infection of endothelial cells in the CNS (as well as gonads and the fetal–maternal interface, the latter resulting in abortion). Infection of the endothelial cells results in cell lysis with secondary ischemic and hemorrhagic infarction of neutropils

SIGNS

Historical Findings
Index case is often a horse that recently attended a competition. Horses may or may not have a current vaccination record. Respiratory disease or abortion may, or may not, be evident in exposed horses and herd mates.

Physical Examination Findings
- The latent period before the onset of viremia with pyrexia is approximately 7 days, during which there may be nasal shedding. Neurologic signs occur subsequent to the viremia
- Pelvic limb ataxia and paresis is usually symmetric but thoracic limb ataxia can rarely be seen, as can brainstem signs more often due to vestibular dysfunction
- Neurologic signs develop rapidly between 24 and 48 h following the cessation of pyrexia, and will be most severe 24–48 h after onset of clinical signs. Relatively fast improvement of the ataxia and urinary signs might be seen within the next 5–7 days

DIAGNOSIS
- A presumptive diagnosis of EHM can be made in horses with peracute spinal cord deficits, dysuria, and bladder distention, particularly if the patient has recently returned from mixing with outside horses
- Antemortem diagnosis can be made quickly with high sensitivity using real-time quantitative PCR of nasal swabs and EDTA venous blood samples
- Serum samples should be banked during an outbreak for ELISA or virus neutralization testing on acute and 3–4 week convalescent samples
- Cerebrospinal fluid, especially from the lumbosacral space, may have xanthochromia and elevated protein content (0.01–0.04 g/L), reflecting the leakage of blood pigments from vasculitis

DIFFERENTIAL DIAGNOSIS
Trauma, equine protozoal myeloencephalitis, other viral encephalitis.

TREATMENT
- Once a diagnosis has been made, the entire farm and, separately, individual cases should be strictly quarantined
- Severely affected clinical cases require excellent nursing care, including bladder catheterization and preferably slinging of paraplegic cases
- Dexamethasone (0.05–0.1 mg/kg IM BID for 1–3 days) in the early stages of showing clinical signs may be efficacious

TRANSMISSION OUTBREAK PREVENTION
- Virus transmitted by contact, especially with affected herd mates
- Neurologically affected horses can be the source of new transmission of EHM up to a week or more from the onset of clinical neurologic signs and strict isolation protocols must remain in place for 21 days after evidence of active (i.e. new cases) of EHV-1 disease
- While vaccination decreases viral shedding and is encouraged, vaccination of herd mates is controversial due to the associated immunosuppression

- Antiviral agents such as valaciclovir (30 mg/kg TID for 48 h then 20 mg/kg PO BID) has been shown to decrease viral transmission in febrile horses before the onset of clinical signs. Gastrointestinal-sparing NSAIDs such as firocoxib (administered at the first detection of pyrexia and continuing for 3–5 days after the fever has ceased) have been shown to prevent viral entry into the endothelial cells

FOLLOW-UP

EXPECTED COURSE AND PROGNOSIS
Mildly affected horses, and rarely even paraplegic patients, can return to full function after several days to more than 1 year.

MISCELLANEOUS

SEE ALSO
- Eastern (EEE), western (WEE), and Venezuelan (VEE) equine encephalitides
- Equine herpesvirus myeloencephalopathy
- Equine protozoal myeloencephalitis (EPM)
- Head trauma
- Rabies
- West nile virus

ABBREVIATIONS
- CNS = central nervous system
- EHM = equine herpesvirus myeloencephalopathy
- EHV-1 = equine herpesvirus 1
- ELISA = enzyme-linked immunosorbent assay
- NSAID = nonsteroidal anti-inflammatory drug
- PCR = polymerase chain reaction

Suggested Reading
Goehring LS. Equid herpesvirus-associated myeloencephalopathy. In: Furr M, Reed S, eds. Equine Neurology, 2e. Ames, IA: Wiley Blackwell, 2016:225–232.
Mayhew IG. Large Animal Neurology, 2e. Chichester, UK: Wiley Blackwell, 2008.
Walter J, Seeh C, Fey K, et al. Clinical observations and management of a severe equine herpesvirus type 1 outbreak with abortion and encephalomyelitis. Acta Vet Scand 2013;55:19.

Author Caroline N. Hahn
Consulting Editor Caroline N. Hahn

EQUINE METABOLIC SYNDROME (EMS)/INSULIN DYSREGULATION (ID)

E

BASICS

DEFINITION
• EMS is a collection of risk factors for laminitis that includes ID, generalized obesity and/or regional adiposity, dyslipidemia, and altered adipokine concentrations
• Insulin abnormalities detected in equids with EMS include fasting hyperinsulinemia, excessive insulin responses to oral sugars, and insulin resistance. These problems are collectively referred to as ID

PATHOPHYSIOLOGY
• EMS results from an interaction between genetics and environment, and the risk of laminitis in the individual animal depends on both genetic and environmental influences. Consumption of high-sugar feeds, obesity, and PPID are exacerbating factors
• Hyperinsulinemia occurs in affected horses and increases the risk of laminitis developing. Laminitis has been experimentally induced in horses by infusing high doses of insulin IV. The risk of laminitis is likely to increase as blood insulin concentrations increase. Mechanisms involved in hyperinsulinemia-induced laminitis include binding of insulin to insulin-like growth factor-1 receptors and altered blood flow or endothelial cell function within the hoof vessels as a result of hyperinsulinemia
• Incretin hormones (glucagon-like peptide-1 and glucose-dependent insulinotropic peptide) likely play a role in EMS. Both hormones are secreted by intestinal cells in response to amino acids and sugars, and stimulate the release of insulin from pancreatic beta cells

SYSTEMS AFFECTED
• Musculoskeletal
• Endocrine/metabolic

GENETICS
Genetic component of EMS in Morgan horses, Arabians and Welsh ponies.

INCIDENCE/PREVALENCE
• Pasture-associated laminitis accounts for approximately 45% of laminitis cases occurring on United States farms
• Laminitis episodes occur more frequently in the spring as pastures turn green. Episodes also occur when the grass is challenged by dry conditions, growing quickly after summer rains, or adapting to the cooler temperatures of the fall season

GEOGRAPHIC DISTRIBUTION
EMS may be more common in regions with heavier rainfall and greener pastures. Geographic distribution of EMS is unknown.

SIGNALMENT
• Predisposed breeds include Morgan horses, Paso Fino, Andalusian, and pony breeds. Arabian, Quarter Horse, Saddlebred,

Tennessee Walking Horse, and Warmblood breeds of horse are also affected. Standardbreds and Thoroughbreds are less likely to be affected
• EMS may only be recognized when a horse becomes middle aged
• Hyperinsulinemia may be exacerbated by PPID
• No known sex predilection

SIGNS
• Many horses with EMS exhibit generalized obesity and/or regional adiposity, but others have a leaner phenotype and can only be identified by testing for ID
• Regional adiposity, including a "cresty neck" and/or fat deposits next to the tail-head, in the sheath, within the supraorbital fossae, or randomly distributed throughout the trunk region as subcutaneous masses
• Divergent growth rings that are wider at the heel than the toe (founder lines) may indicate historical laminitis and may be detected in horses that do not have a history of lameness
• "Easy keepers"

CAUSES
• Environmental factors include high NSC diet (e.g. concentrates or pasture with abundant grass) and insufficient exercise
• Laminitis episodes are likely be triggered by hyperinsulinemia

RISK FACTORS
• See Genetics
• Offspring of a mare or stallion with EMS
• "Easy keeper"

DIAGNOSIS

DIFFERENTIAL DIAGNOSIS
• Some horses can be obese without ID
• PPID (also called equine Cushing disease) is distinguished from EMS by the presence of muscle wasting, an increased caloric requirement to maintain body mass, and delayed haircoat shedding. PPID has a higher frequency in aged horses

CBC/BIOCHEMISTRY/URINALYSIS
• Blood glucose concentrations may be high normal
• Mildly increased triglyceride concentrations (hypertriglyceridemia)
• Mildly increased γ-glutamyltransferase concentrations
• Glucosuria is not detected unless diabetes mellitus has developed

OTHER LABORATORY TESTS
• Serum or plasma insulin concentrations—blood can be collected when hay is available or as horses graze on pasture, but do not feed grain within 4 h of sample collection. Fasting is no longer recommended. Interpretation—no evidence of ID if insulin concentration <20 μU/mL (also written as

mU/L); ID suspected if 20–50 μU/mL; and ID is present if the insulin is >50 μU/mL. Suspect horses with insulin values <20 μU/mL should undergo further testing to rule out ID. Concentrations may be reported in pmol/L and the conversion factor is approximately 7
• Serum leptin concentrations—increased in equids with EMS due to increased body fat
• High-molecular-weight adiponectin—decreased in equids with EMS, and this variable may be useful for assessing laminitis risk

IMAGING
Horses with EMS often show radiographic evidence of laminitis, including rotation and bony remodeling of the third phalanx. These abnormalities may be detected in the absence of any discernable lameness and provide evidence of prior subclinical laminitis events.

OTHER DIAGNOSTIC PROCEDURES
OST—often used to detect ID. Withhold feed for 3–8 h before testing. It is common practice to leave 1 flake of hay with the horse after 10:00 PM and then withhold feed until the test is completed the following morning. Administer 0.15 mL Karo Light syrup per kilogram body weight (75 mL for a 500 kg horse) orally via a dose syringe and collect blood at 60–90 min. Measure insulin and glucose concentrations. An insulin concentration >45 μU/mL provides evidence of ID. Glucose values are assessed to detect diabetes mellitus, which may occur in horses with EMS. Other glucose or insulin tolerance tests are available (see chapters Glucose tolerance tests and Insulin levels/insulin tolerance test).

PATHOLOGIC FINDINGS
• Regional adiposity, including enlarged adipose tissue deposits in the neck region or distributed throughout the subcutaneous tissues as masses
• Gross or histopathologic evidence of laminitis is often present

TREATMENT

AIMS
• Weight loss in horses with generalized obesity
• Improve insulin sensitivity through weight loss, diet, and exercise
• Avoid dietary triggers for laminitis

NURSING CARE
See chapter Laminitis.

DIET
• Obese horses that are easy keepers can be placed on a diet of hay and a vitamin/mineral supplement
• Obese horses can be fed 1.5% of ideal body weight in hay to induce weight loss

EQUINE METABOLIC SYNDROME (EMS)/INSULIN DYSREGULATION (ID) (CONTINUED)

• Hay fed to EMS horses should have a lower (<12%) NSC content. Samples can be tested by commercial laboratories. Hay with NSC content >12% should be soaked in cold water for 30 min to lower the sugar content
• Horses with EMS should be supplemented with 1000 IU vitamin E daily
• Avoid feeds that exacerbate hyperinsulinemia. Restrict or eliminate pasture access, or use a grazing muzzle if on pasture
• Thinner EMS horses may be supplemented with low-sugar/low-starch feeds

CLIENT EDUCATION
• Obesity is likely to be an important risk factor for EMS. In obese horses, limit dietary intake, increase exercise, and limit pasture access, particularly at high-risk times of the year
• Body condition scoring should be routinely performed
• Development of regional adiposity (e.g. cresty neck) should prompt diagnostic testing for ID
• PPID is thought to exacerbate ID and increase the risk of laminitis

SURGICAL CONSIDERATIONS
In some cases of severe, chronic laminitis, dorsal hoof wall resection and deep digital tenotomy.

MEDICATIONS
DRUG(S) OF CHOICE
• Levothyroxine sodium (Thyro-L; Vet-A-Mix, Lloyd, Inc., Shenandoah, IA) 12 mg/5 mL (1 teaspoon)
• Used when rapid weight loss is required in a horse that has suffered from laminitis and is threatened by subsequent episodes, and in horses that remain obese despite stringent diet and exercise interventions
• Administered at a dosage of 0.1 mg/kg body weight every 24 h, which is equivalent to a total dose of 48 mg or 20 mL (4 teaspoons) daily for a 500 kg horse, administered by mouth or in the feed for 3–6 months
• Serum thyroxine concentrations are usually between 60 and 100 ng/mL in treated horses. This range can be targeted when lower dosages are selected for smaller patients
• Taper carefully—halve the dose for 2 weeks and then halve again for 2 weeks in order to allow endogenous thyroid hormone production to resume
• Metformin hydrochloride 500 mg or 1000 mg tablets

• Used to blunt the increase in insulin concentrations that follows ingestion of sugars
• Indicated when hyperinsulinemia persists after obesity has been addressed, PPID managed (if present), and dietary changes have been made
• Administer 30–60 min before feeding. Starting dosage of 30 mg/kg body weight orally 2 or 3 times daily, depending on feeding schedule. Can be increased to 50 mg/kg every 8–12 h orally in refractory cases
• Treatment of PPID is indicated if this endocrine disorder has developed

CONTRAINDICATIONS
• The levothyroxine dosages recommended above are not appropriate for thin horses with ID because weight loss will be induced
• Neither treatment has been evaluated in pregnant mares

PRECAUTIONS
• Cardiac hypertrophy and bone resorption have been associated with levothyroxine sodium use in humans, but not horses
• Metformin can cause oral irritation, especially when administered at higher dosages

POSSIBLE INTERACTIONS
No known interactions.

ALTERNATIVE DRUGS
Supplements that are thought to improve insulin sensitivity are also available to horse owners.

FOLLOW-UP
PATIENT MONITORING
• An OST should be repeated after diet, exercise, or treatment interventions
• Patients should be reevaluated at different times of the year because seasonal and dietary influences vary

PREVENTION/AVOIDANCE
• Avoid overfeeding
• Regular exercise
• Currently, it is only possible to recognize that the offspring of affected horses may be predisposed to EMS, but genetic tests may be available in the future

POSSIBLE COMPLICATIONS
Chronic damage to the hoof laminae and structures of the foot.

EXPECTED COURSE AND PROGNOSIS
EMS is a manageable condition if recognized.

MISCELLANEOUS
ASSOCIATED CONDITIONS
N/A

AGE-RELATED FACTORS
N/A

ZOONOTIC POTENTIAL
N/A

PREGNANCY/FERTILITY/BREEDING
N/A

SYNONYMS
• Insulin resistance syndrome
• Peripheral Cushing syndrome

SEE ALSO
• Glucose tolerance tests
• Hyperlipidemia/hyperlipemia
• Insulin levels/insulin tolerance test
• Laminitis
• Pituitary pars intermedia dysfunction

ABBREVIATIONS
• EMS = equine metabolic syndrome
• ID = insulin dysregulation
• NSC = nonstructural carbohydrates
• OST = oral sugar test
• PPID = pituitary pars intermedia dysfunction

Internet Resources
Equine Endocrinology Group, Equine metabolic syndrome. http://sites.tufts.edu/equineendogroup/equine-metabolic-syndrome/

Suggested Reading
Menzies-Gow NJ, Harris PA, Elliott J. Prospective cohort study evaluating risk factors for the development of pasture-associated laminitis in the UK. Equine Vet J 2017;49(3):300–306.
Schuver A, Frank N, Chameroy KA, et al. Assessment of insulin and glucose dynamics by using an oral sugar test in horses. J Equine Vet Sci 2014;34:465–470.

Author Nicholas Frank
Consulting Editors Michel Lévy and Heidi Banse

BASICS

DEFINITION
An acquired neurodegenerative disease primarily affecting somatic motor neurons.

PATHOPHYSIOLOGY
The cause of EMND is unproven, although there is a strong association between the disease and vitamin E deficiency. Lower motor neuron cell bodies in the spinal cord and brainstem degenerate, presumably from oxidative damage. The oxidative damage is likely a result of an imbalance in pro-oxidants and antioxidants and the disease is associated with a low vitamin E status. Early dysfunctional changes in the motor neuron cells may be associated with mitochondrial damage, followed by disintegration of the nucleus and neurofibrillary accumulation. Dead motor neurons may eventually be removed by glial cells. Clinical signs only become apparent when approximately 30% of the motor neurons become dysfunctional. Ventral horn motor neurons that supply postural muscles (those muscles with predominantly type 1 fibers) are preferentially affected; this is believed to occur because of the higher oxidative activity of predominant type 1 muscle and its corresponding parent motor neuron. The oxidative disease causes lipopigment (ceroid) accumulation in the endothelium of spinal cord capillaries, neurons, and RPE. The RPE ceroid can generally be seen on fundoscopic examination as brown streaks. Excessive lipopigment may also, on occasion, be found in the liver of affected horses.

SYSTEMS AFFECTED
• Neuromuscular—motor neuron cell dysfunction causing neurogenic muscular atrophy and weakness
• Ophthalmic—lipopigment accumulation in the RPE causes electroretinographic abnormalities; vision is likely affected
• Gastrointestinal—a functional abnormality in carbohydrate absorption occurs in severely affected horses and may be related to a mitochondrial dysfunction in the enterocyte. There are rarely abnormal light microscopic changes

GENETICS
There is no known genetic basis to the disease. Although SOD activity is abnormally low in red blood cells and nervous tissue, this is believed to be a result of excessive oxidative stress. Abnormal polymorphisms in the *SOD* gene in affected horses versus controls have not been found.

INCIDENCE/PREVALENCE
Affects approximately 1 horse per 10 000 per year in the northeastern USA (between 1990 and 1996).

GEOGRAPHIC DISTRIBUTION
EMND is seen worldwide but is most common in those geographic areas less likely to have alfalfa hay, e.g. northeastern USA and Canada, and lack of pasture (urban areas). Clusters may occur on certain premises.

SIGNALMENT
Environment. Most horses have a history of being kept without pasture and leafy green hay for at least 1 year; however, increasingly horses in Europe are presented with EMND even though they have had access to grass (those tested, however, are still low in vitamin E).
• Breed predilection—all breeds of horses and ponies may be affected
• Age—mean age is 12 years; range 2–25 years. Rarely, and in younger horses, EMND is diagnosed along with equine degenerative myeloencephalopathy
• No gender predisposition

SIGNS

Historical Findings
In many but not all cases there is a history of lack of access to grass.

Physical Examination Findings
Findings vary depending upon the stage/duration of the disorder and are due to neuromuscular weakness. EMND cases do not have proprioceptive deficits, i.e. they are not ataxic. Signs are best summarized by dividing into subacute and chronic forms.
Subacute Form
Horses develop an acute onset of trembling, fasciculations, lying down more than normal, frequent shifting of weight in the pelvic limbs, and abnormal sweating. Head carriage may be abnormally low. Horses may appear less comfortable when standing than walking. Appetite and gait are usually not noticeably affected. The owners may mention that the horses had been losing weight (loss of muscle mass) for 1 month prior to the trembling, etc.
Chronic Form
The trembling and fasciculations subside and the horse stabilizes but with varying degrees of muscle atrophy. With fibrosis of postural muscles the pelvic limbs have a shortened cranial phase of the stride reminiscent of fibrotic myopathy. In some cases, the atrophy is so severe that the horse looks emaciated. In other cases, there is noticeable improvement in muscle mass and/or fat deposition. The tail-head is frequently in an abnormally high resting position.

RISK FACTORS
Low access to vitamin E or increased exposure to putative oxidant.

DIAGNOSIS
• Finding evidence of neurogenic atrophy in a muscle biopsy of the sacrocaudalis dorsalis

medialis muscle (tail-head muscle) is a sensitive and specific test for EMND. Rarely, very early cases many not show neurogenic atrophy but have a moth-eaten appearance on staining for mitochondria when frozen muscle biopsies are stained with NADH-Tr
• Degeneration of the myelinated fibers of the spinal accessory nerve also has high specificity and sensitivity for the diagnosis of EMND

DIFFERENTIAL DIAGNOSIS
• Colic is often considered because of the propensity of the horses to stand for only brief periods during the subacute form. The normal appetite and fecal production should serve to rule out an abdominal disorder
• Laminitis is another consideration because of the almost constant shifting of weight in the subacute form. The ease of motion and even desire to walk as seen in EMND is contradictory to the diagnosis of laminitis
• Other neuromuscular disorders such as botulism and myositis/myopathy may have similarities to EMND. The normal appetite, elevated tail-head, and lack of cranial nerve dysfunction should separate EMND from botulism. Chronic myopathies, e.g. polysaccharide storage myopathy, may appear very similar to EMND, and a muscle biopsy may be required to delineate between the two. EMND causes symmetric muscle weakness and atrophy without ataxia and elevation of muscle enzymes (in the subacute cases) as opposed to equine protozoal myeloencephalitis
• The severe muscle wasting with a normal appetite in the chronic form may look similar to intestinal malabsorption syndrome. Plasma albumin is low in most infiltrative bowel syndromes but is normal in EMND

CBC/BIOCHEMISTRY/URINALYSIS
The CBC is generally within normal range. The most common abnormal biochemical finding is a moderate elevation in muscle enzymes in the subacute case. A few horses may have elevated liver enzymes. The urinalysis is normal in most cases, although some may have myoglobinuria. CBC, biochemistry, and urinalysis are all normal in the chronic cases.

OTHER LABORATORY TESTS
• In the subacute cases, plasma or serum vitamin E (alpha tocopherol) is abnormally low (mean 0.56 µg/mL). Serum ferritin and lipid peroxidases are often abnormally high
• In chronic cases, alpha tocopherol values may have returned to normal
• Fundoscopic examination frequently reveals brown streaking of the retina. This is specific for vitamin E deficiency and only supportive for EMND
• Glucose malabsorption is generally present in subacute cases, but is only supportive for EMND

E

EQUINE MOTOR NEURON DISEASE

PATHOLOGIC FINDINGS
- An abnormal paleness of some muscles (e.g. vastus intermedius) containing most type 1 fibers may be observed. Body fat stores are variable
- Microscopically, central nervous system lesions are confined to the spinal cord ventral horn cells, and cranial nerves nuclei V, VII, VIII, IX, X, XI, and XII. Degeneration of corresponding motor nerves and neurogenic muscle atrophy is found
- There is lipofuscinosis of the retinal pigment epithelial layer and spinal cord endothelium in all cases and of the liver in a few cases
- There are no light microscopic lesions in the intestine in 90% of cases, but ultrastructural changes may be seen

TREATMENT
Horses with EMND can be treated either on the farm or in the hospital. Transporting can worsen the clinical signs.

ACTIVITY
The affected horse should not have free movement restricted but should not be exercised and/or ridden.

DIET
Leafy green hay or grass with additional vitamin E (2000–7000 units/day) should be provided.

CLIENT EDUCATION
Regular access to grass for all horses if this is deficient.

MEDICATIONS
Oral vitamin E supplements.

FOLLOW-UP

PATIENT MONITORING
With the subacute form, improvement in clinical signs often corresponds to return of serum muscle enzymes to normal values. Vitamin E concentrations should be monitored to determine that levels return to normal. It should be kept in mind, however, that neurons that have been lost will never be replaced, and an increase in weight is likely to be due to fat deposition rather than muscle hypertrophy.

PREVENTION/AVOIDANCE
All other horses kept under similar conditions should be supplemented with vitamin E.

EXPECTED COURSE AND PROGNOSIS
- Of horses subacutely affected with EMND approximately 40% will stabilize within 3–8 weeks and regain some loss of muscle mass. Other horses will have progressive deterioration in clinical signs or no improvement, in spite of vitamin E treatment
- Horses with the chronic and more stabilized form may have several years of quality life but not performance. Their life expectancy would be shorter than normal and another acute onset of clinical signs may occur years later (similar to the human postpolio paresis). Horses diagnosed with EMND should not be ridden as they can be unsafe and moderate to severe exercise will likely shorten their life expectancy

MISCELLANEOUS

SEE ALSO
Neuroaxonal dystrophy/equine degenerative myeloencephalopathy

ABBREVIATIONS
- EMND = equine motor neuron disease
- NADH-Tr = nicotinamide adenine dinucleotide tetrazolium reductase
- RPE = retinal pigment epithelium
- SOD = superoxide dismutase

Suggested Reading
Bedford HE, Valberg SJ, Firshman AM, et al. Histopathologic findings in the sacrocaudalis dorsalis medialis muscle of horses with vitamin E-responsive muscle atrophy and weakness. J Am Vet Med Assoc 2013;242:1127–1137.
Finno CJ, Miller AD, Sisó S, et al. Concurrent equine degenerative myeloencephalopathy and equine motor neuron disease in three young horses. J Vet Intern Med 2016;30:1344–1350.
Ledwith A, McGowan CM. Muscle biopsy: a routine diagnostic procedure. Equine Vet Educ 2004;16:62–67.
McGorum BC, Mayhew IG, Amory H, et al. Horses on pasture may be affected by equine motor neuron disease. Equine Vet J 2006;38:47–51.

Author Caroline N. Hahn
Consulting Editor Caroline N. Hahn

EQUINE ODONTOCLASTIC TOOTH RESORPTION AND HYPERCEMENTOSIS

BASICS

DEFINITION
EOTRH is a severe form of dental disease of older horses affecting the incisor and canine teeth most often. EOTRH shares many features with similar dental syndromes described in humans (multiple idiopathic root resorption) and cats (feline odontoclastic root resorption syndrome). EOTRH is characterized by internal and external resorption of the dental structures and adjacent alveolar bone and is often associated with excessive irregular cementum production of the tooth.

PATHOPHYSIOLOGY
• The exact etiology remains unknown. Excessive strain on the periodontal ligaments of aging incisors due to shorter reserve crowns is proposed to be an inciting cause
• Periodontal inflammation is thought to be the initial lesion. Inflammatory mediators stimulate osteoclasts, leading to tooth resorption. A reparative process ensues with fibroblasts, odontoblasts, and cementoblasts invading the resorbed dental surface. Irregular cementum is deposited to repair the defects; however, it may also proliferate excessively. Depending on the resorption and repair at the individual teeth, a mouth may have different stages of disease simultaneously
• A recent study detected red complex bacteria (*Treponema* and *Tannerella spp.*) in gingival crevicular fluid of EOTRH-affected horses, suggesting an etiological role of these pathogens

SYSTEMS AFFECTED
Gastrointestinal

GENETICS
N/A

INCIDENCE/PREVALENCE
The prevalence is unknown.

SIGNALMENT
Horses with EOTRH are generally >15 years. Male sex and breed predisposition towards Islandic horses have been proposed.

SIGNS
Clinical signs include reduced ability to grasp hard feed, decreased use of incisor teeth for grazing, ptyalism, head shyness, sensitivity to biting, headshaking, and weight loss. Some horses will also lay their tongue between their incisors.

RISK FACTORS
• Biomechanical factors, husbandry (confinement, grazing), and behavior (cribbing), which lead to excessive strain on the periodontal ligaments, are thought to play a role in the etiology
• Cushing syndrome and other systemic conditions may play a role in the etiology

DIAGNOSIS

DIFFERENTIAL DIAGNOSIS
Periodontal disease, endodontic infections, epulides, and neoplastic disorders.

CBC/BIOCHEMISTRY/URINALYSIS
Nonspecific

OTHER LABORATORY TESTS
N/A

IMAGING
• Standard views include occlusal intraoral radiographs of the mandibular/maxillary incisor and canine teeth obtained with the plate/sensor placed in the mouth as well a laterolateral extraoral view of the incisor and canine teeth. Radiographic changes include dental resorption, loss of the periodontal space, disruption of the alveolar and regional cancellous bone, evidence of osteomyelitis, bulbous enlargement of the tooth root by a radiopaque mass (hypercementosis), and fractures of the teeth and/or alveolar bone
• Radiographic evidence of disease possible even in clinically normal teeth

OTHER DIAGNOSTIC PROCEDURES
• A general physical examination, a close examination of the head, and a thorough oral examination should be performed. The oral examination can be challenging because patients are resistant to manipulations of the lips and resent pressure on their incisor teeth
• Oral examination may show severe regional inflammation, gingival recession, hyperplastic gingiva, gingival and mucogingival fistulation and purulent drainage, calculus formation, feed material accumulation, dental mobility, bulbous enlargement of dental structures, and decreased incisor angle (Figure 1)

PATHOLOGIC FINDINGS
Histopathology of resorptive lesions has shown osteoclasts and odontoclasts residing in large, atypical lacunae within bone, cementum, enamel, and dentin. Inflammatory cell infiltration caused by neutrophils and mononuclear cells leading to a granulomatous or suppurative inflammation in the periodontal area has been noted. Bacteria and plant material may also be found. An abnormal type of cementum with intrinsic collagen fiber bundles is seen invading not only the lacunae but also the normal cementum, dentin, enamel, and pulp.

TREATMENT

• In horses with mild subgingival resorption, no involvement of the alveolar bone, and little pain the disease can be monitored biannually to annually clinically and radiographically
• In mild and early diagnosed disease crown reduction and removing affected incisor teeth

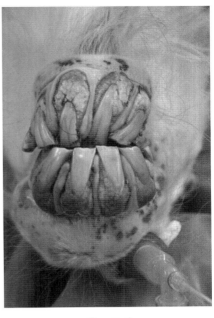

Figure 1.

Pony with severe EOTRH in dorsal recumbency under general anesthesia intubated with a nasotracheal tube. Note the severe bulbous enlargement of dental structures.

out of occlusion will eliminate forces acting upon them; subsequently inflammation and pain will decrease
• Medical management using Brazilian mushrooms (*Agaricus blazei* Murrill) in conjunction with vitamin D (EquiSANO D™) has been advocated to be successful in slowing down the disease process
• Once disease worsens (lesions appear supragingival, tooth resorption, alveolitis, osteomyelitis, and tooth fractures become apparent) affected incisor and canine teeth need to be extracted. This may be done in a staged process, or in severe cases all teeth may be extracted at once. Generally once the affected teeth are completely removed infection, inflammation, and pain subside

NURSING CARE
N/A

ACTIVITY
N/A

DIET
Following incisor removal horses may initially have problems grasping feed; however, they may learn to grasp it with their lips and to pass the feed into the back of their mouths with their tongues. Following complete teeth extraction horses should not solely be pasture fed, but supplemented with dietary roughage and/or processed feed because they will have problems grazing in the early postoperative period.

CLIENT EDUCATION
Routine dental prophylaxis is the best method for monitoring and detecting the disease at an

EQUINE ODONTOCLASTIC TOOTH RESORPTION AND HYPERCEMENTOSIS   (CONTINUED)

early stage. Following complete incisor and canine teeth extraction some horses will play with their tongue more often. The tongue commonly hangs loosely out of the mouth after incisor teeth extraction. Clients should be informed of this prior to removal of these teeth.

SURGICAL CONSIDERATIONS
In most cases incisors can be extracted standing under sedation and perineural (mental and/or infraorbital nerve blocks) and/or local anesthesia. Following extraction the gingiva and vacated alveoli should be debrided and potential tooth root fragments should be removed. Intraoperative radiography is helpful to confirm complete tooth removal. The vacated alveoli should be lavaged and packed. Packing materials such as swabs, dental wax, plaster of Paris in addition to local honey, antiseptic, or antimicrobial agents may be used. Following dental extraction grazing should be restricted until the alveoli have completely healed.

MEDICATIONS

DRUG(S) OF CHOICE
• *Sedatives* required to complete a thorough and safe oral examination. α_2-Agonists (xylazine, detomidine, romifidine) provide adequate sedation. Premedication with acepromazine and the addition of an opioid such as butorphanol can increase the reliability of the sedation
• NSAIDs (phenylbutazone, flunixin meglumine) after dental work is often recommended in cases of incisor and canine teeth extraction
• There are no published benefits of using systemic antibiotics to treat EOTRH. Following incisor and canine teeth extractions systemic antibiotics may be administered until alveolar bone is covered by granulation tissue

CONTRAINDICATIONS
N/A

PRECAUTIONS
N/A

POSSIBLE INTERACTIONS
N/A

ALTERNATIVE DRUGS
N/A

FOLLOW-UP

PATIENT MONITORING
Some horses may appear uncomfortable and have a decreased appetite for the first 2–3 weeks following extraction until the alveoli have healed. Weight gain in horses should be monitored. Otherwise, a good appetite, without evidence of quidding, should be noted following treatment.

PREVENTION/AVOIDANCE
To date there are no clear recommendations to avoid this disease; however, early diagnosis by regular dental prophylaxis ensures early management.

POSSIBLE COMPLICATIONS
When performing single incisor extractions care must be taken not to damage or loosen adjacent teeth. As fracture of the tooth roots is a common complication care should be taken to ensure complete removal of the teeth. Visual inspection of the vacated alveolus, probing, and intraoperative radiographs will help identify residual dental fragments. These fragments can be removed with instruments via the alveolus. In rare cases of EOTRH of the incisors, but more commonly when the canine teeth are affected, the labial alveolar wall may need to be opened using an osteotome to remove the remaining fragments. This may also be necessary in cases of large masses of cementum deposition at the root, where the extraction through the alveolus is not possible due to the bulbous-like shape of the tooth root. Injury of the major palatine artery and vein is a complication rarely encountered. When loosening canine teeth before extraction regional bone unavoidably gets damaged; bone sequestrum formation can be a complication as well as damage to the mental nerve. When extracting canine teeth of the maxilla, care should be taken not to damage the thin bony lamellae to the nasal cavity, creating an alveolar–nasal fistula.

EXPECTED COURSE AND PROGNOSIS
• When the stage of disease is mild, appropriate crown reduction and removing the affected incisor teeth out of occlusion is recommended. In these cases tooth extraction can be postponed, but it will become inevitable
• Complete incisor and canine extraction is often necessary; however, healing is generally uncomplicated and completed in 3–4 weeks. Extraction of affected teeth carries a good prognosis

MISCELLANEOUS

ASSOCIATED CONDITIONS
Weight loss and decreased social interaction.

AGE-RELATED FACTORS
At 13–15 years, incisor eruption stops, while incisor wear continues. This leads to a more acute angle between the upper and the lower incisors and in turn leads to greater stresses on the periodontal ligament attachment in older horses.

SEE ALSO
Oral neoplasia

ABBREVIATIONS
• EOTRH = equine odontoclastic tooth resorption and hypercementosis
• NSAID = nonsteroidal anti-inflammatory drug

Suggested Reading
Earley E, Rawlinson JT. A new understanding of oral and dental disorders of the equine incisor and canine teeth. Vet Clin North Am Equine Pract 2013;29:273–300.
Lorello O, Foster DL, Levine DG, et al. Clinical treatment and prognosis of equine odontoclastic tooth resorption and hypercementosis. Equine Vet J 2016;48(2):188–194.
Smedley RC, Earley ET, Galloway SS, et al. Equine odontoclastic tooth resorption and hypercementosis: histopathologic features. Vet Pathol 2015;52(5):903–909.
Staszyk C, Bienert A, Kreutzer R, et al. Equine odontoclastic tooth resorption and hypercementosis. Vet J 2008;178(3):372–379.
Sykora S, Pieber K, Simhofer H, et al. Isolation of *Treponema* and *Tannerella* spp. from equine odontoclastic tooth resorption and hypercementosis related periodontal disease. Equine Vet J 2014;46(3):358–363.

Authors Andrea S. Bischofberger and Felix Theiss
Consulting Editors Henry Stämpfli and Olimpo Oliver-Espinosa

EQUINE OOCYTES AND INTRACYTOPLASMIC SPERM INJECTION (ICSI)

BASICS

DEFINITION
ICSI is a method for in vitro fertilization in which a single sperm is injected into the cytoplasm of a mature oocyte to achieve fertilization. The resulting fertilized oocytes are cultured for 7–10 days to allow development into blastocysts, which can then be transferred transcervically into a recipient mare, as for standard embryo transfer.

Advantages of ICSI over OT
• OT is the surgical transfer of matured oocytes to the oviducts of inseminated recipient mares; ICSI avoids the need for surgery on the recipient mare
• Fresh, frozen, or cooled semen and semen of low quality can be used to perform ICSI; for OT a dose of good quality semen is needed to inseminate the recipient mare

PATHOPHYSIOLOGY
N/A

SYSTEMS AFFECTED
Reproductive

GENETICS
N/A

INCIDENCE/PREVALENCE
N/A

GEOGRAPHIC DISTRIBUTION
N/A

SIGNALMENT
• Oocytes can be recovered from mares of any age, although recovery is more commonly performed in older mares that are unable to carry foals to term or deliver foals themselves or when pregnancies are sought from stallions with limited supplies of spermatozoa
• Any breed. Owners should consult individual breed registries for guidelines regarding the possibility of registering any resulting foals

SIGNS
N/A

CAUSES
N/A

RISK FACTORS
N/A

DIAGNOSIS

DIFFERENTIAL DIAGNOSIS
N/A

CBC/BIOCHEMISTRY/URINALYSIS
N/A

OTHER LABORATORY TESTS
N/A

IMAGING
• Transrectal US to monitor follicular growth and determine timing of hCG administration if aspirating a dominant stimulated follicle
• Transvaginal US for aspiration of immature follicles via TVA

OTHER DIAGNOSTIC PROCEDURES
N/A

PATHOLOGIC FINDINGS
N/A

TREATMENT

APPROPRIATE HEALTH CARE
• Oocyte recovery from live mares is best performed in a hospital setting with adequate facilities for mare restraint and trained personnel experienced in follicular aspirations
• ICSI is performed at a laboratory equipped with the proper equipment (micromanipulator, incubator, hood, microscope, etc.) by trained personnel knowledgeable in embryo culture medium preparation and experienced in oocyte and embryo handling, sperm preparation, and micromanipulation
• Ovaries from euthanized mares can be shipped to the ICSI laboratory for oocyte recovery, maturation, and ICSI. Alternatively, the referring veterinarian can recover oocytes from the ovaries and ship the oocytes to the ICSI laboratory for maturation and ICSI

INDICATIONS
• Subfertile mares that cannot provide embryos for transfer due to chronic endometritis, pyometra, uterine adhesions, cervical tears, persistent anovulatory follicles, oviductal blockage, or idiopathic causes
• Subfertile stallions with very low sperm numbers or quality
• When only a few straws of frozen semen exist from deceased stallions
• When oocytes are recovered from mares' ovaries after euthanasia

OOCYTE RECOVERY PROCEDURES

Dominant Stimulated Follicle
• Must monitor follicular growth; predict the first day of responsiveness as indicated by size, shape, and wall thickness of dominant follicle, and administer hCG or deslorelin
• Aspirate follicle 24–35 h after hCG administration
• Can aspirate follicle via flank aspiration
Advantages
• High recovery rate (>80%)
• Essentially all recovered oocytes are mature
• High embryonic developmental competence
Disadvantages
• Only 1 or 2 follicles/oocytes available per cycle
• Must accurately time hCG stimulation and aspiration

• In vivo matured oocytes are sensitive to temperature and difficult to ship

Immature Follicles
• All follicles ≥5 mm in diameter on the ovary can be aspirated
• Must aspirate via US-guided TVA
Advantages
• Many follicles are available for aspiration (average 9 follicles per mare per TVA)
• Immature oocytes are easy to ship
Disadvantages
• Lower recovery rates (54% or 5 oocytes per TVA)
• Lower maturation rates (66% or 3 mature oocytes per TVA)

Postmortem
• Mare is anesthetized with xylazine/ketamine, ovaries are removed and the mare is euthanized immediately after
• Best results when oocytes are recovered from ovaries within 6 h of euthanasia
• If transporting ovaries <2 h, maintain at body temperature (37°C); if transporting >2 h, cool to room temperature (20°C). Do not refrigerate ovaries

NURSING CARE
May be required if complications (see Possible Complications) occur during the procedure.

ACTIVITY
Restricted while the mare is under sedation.

DIET
Normal diet.

CLIENT EDUCATION
• Oocyte recovery by flank aspiration or TVA is a relatively benign procedure; however, certain complications (see Possible Complications) can occur
• Performing ICSI is much more labor intensive and expensive than standard embryo transfer
• ICSI is a procedure that should only be used when the indications listed above are present, and it is not a recommended means of obtaining more foals in a given season from normally fertile mares using good quality semen

SURGICAL CONSIDERATIONS
If an ovarian abscess develops following oocyte recovery, surgery may be indicated to remove the affected ovary.

MEDICATIONS

DRUG(S) OF CHOICE

For Oocyte Recovery via Flank Aspiration or TVA
• Detomidine for sedation
• Butorphanol tartrate for analgesia
• N-butylscopolamine bromide as an antispasmodic

E

EQUINE OOCYTES AND INTRACYTOPLASMIC SPERM INJECTION (ICSI) (CONTINUED)

• Flunixin meglumine for analgesia; administered after oocyte recovery
• Antibiotics if complications occur during the procedure

For Oocyte Recovery from Ovaries Postmortem
• Xylazine/ketamine for anesthesia, and after ovary removal, followed by
• Pentobarbital or KCl for euthanasia

CONTRAINDICATIONS
N/A

PRECAUTIONS
N/A

POSSIBLE INTERACTIONS
N/A

ALTERNATIVE DRUGS
N/A

FOLLOW-UP

PATIENT MONITORING
Follicular aspirations of immature or dominant stimulated follicles can be performed once every 2 weeks. If aspirating a dominant stimulated follicle, follicular growth must be monitored by transrectal US.

PREVENTION/AVOIDANCE
N/A

POSSIBLE COMPLICATIONS
• Rectal bleeding
• Ovarian abscess
• Peritonitis
• Death from puncture of uterine artery

EXPECTED COURSE AND PROGNOSIS
Expected outcomes may vary by laboratory because different laboratories use different procedures and media for the different steps involved with in vitro embryo production. The expected outcomes at the Texas A&M Equine Embryo Laboratory are:
• 66% of immature oocytes mature in culture
• 75% of oocytes undergo cleavage after ICSI
• 23% of oocytes, recovered from immature follicles, subjected to ICSI will develop blastocysts
• 38% of oocytes, recovered from dominant stimulated follicles, subjected to ICSI will develop blastocysts
• 52% foaling rate per transferred blastocyst

MISCELLANEOUS

ASSOCIATED CONDITIONS
Subfertility

AGE-RELATED FACTORS
• For mares ≤24 years of age, age does not affect oocyte recovery rate, blastocyst rate, or pregnancy or foaling rates. However, older mares tend to have fewer follicles and therefore there are fewer oocytes to recover and fewer blastocysts are produced
• Stallions do have an effect on the cleavage and blastocyst rates after ICSI; embryo development rates may be altered by the method used to prepare sperm prior to ICSI

ZOONOTIC POTENTIAL
N/A

PREGNANCY/FERTILITY/BREEDING
See Expected Course and Prognosis.

SYNONYMS
N/A

SEE ALSO
• Embryo transfer
• Vitrification of equine embryos

ABBREVIATIONS
• hCG = human chorionic gonadotropin
• ICSI = intracytoplasmic sperm injection
• OT = oocyte transfer
• TVA = transvaginal aspiration
• US = ultrasonography, ultrasound

Suggested Reading
Brinsko SP, Blanchard TL, Varner DD, et al. Assisted reproductive technology. In: Manual of Equine Reproduction, 3e. St. Louis, MO: Mosby Elsevier, 2011:302–312.
Hinrichs K, Choi YH. Factors influencing the success of equine intracytoplasmic sperm injection in a clinical program. Reprod Fertil Dev 2015;28(2):258.
Hinrichs K, Choi YH, Love CC, et al. Use of intracytoplasmic sperm injection and *in vitro* culture to the blastocyst stage in a commercial equine assisted reproduction program. J Equine Vet Sci 2014;34:176.

Author Sicilia T. Grady
Consulting Editor Carla L. Carleton

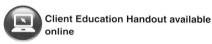
Client Education Handout available online

EQUINE PROTOZOAL MYELOENCEPHALITIS (EPM)

BASICS

DEFINITION
Multifocal neurologic disease of horses caused by *Sarcocystis neurona* and *Neospora hughesi*.

PATHOPHYSIOLOGY
• Infection results from ingestion of sporocysts of *S. neurona* in feed and water contaminated with feces of opossums, the definitive host
• Sporocysts can be transmitted by vectors such as birds, rodents, and insects
• Sporocysts excyst in the horse's small intestine, releasing sporozoites that penetrate the enterocytes and enter the bloodstream
• 2 rounds of replication (i.e. merogony) occur, and *S. neurona* invade the entire organism before forming sarcocysts in the muscles of intermediate hosts, including horses
• Parasites appear to gain access to the CNS either by direct penetration of the blood–brain barrier or through infected white blood cells. Merozoites multiply within neurons and leukocytes, resulting in cell death
• Clinical signs are caused by neuronal loss and inflammation and swelling, which disrupt normal CNS architecture, compromise blood flow, and reduce oxygen delivery
• Incubation time can be as short as 10 days but latent infections can persist for months
• Life cycle of *N. hughesi* is not well understood but infection can occur transplacentally (or vertical infection was described)

SYSTEMS AFFECTED
• Nervous—multifocal CNS infection results in variable sensory, motor, and cognitive dysfunction; cranial nerve deficits can occur
• Neuromuscular—discrete, neurogenic muscle atrophy and weakness are common
• Musculoskeletal—occasional secondary injuries and soreness from ataxia; asymmetric muscle weakness/atrophy
• Gastrointestinal—cranial nerve signs associated with prehension, mastication, and swallowing; loss of anal tone
• Skin—hyporeflexia, discrete areas of sensory loss and hyperhidrosis
• Respiratory—laryngeal hemiplegia and pneumonia secondary to dysphagia
• Ophthalmic—loss of ocular reflexes and blindness
• Renal/urologic—urinary incontinence

GENETICS
No apparent genetic predisposition.

INCIDENCE/PREVALENCE
• Seroprevalence of *S. neurona* reaches approximately 50% in many parts of the USA, 70% in Brazil, and 35% in Argentina
• Incidence of the disease is low, with 0.014% of the population of horses affected in the USA

• Seroprevalence of *Neospora* spp. in North and South America is very low—3.4% and 2.5%, respectively

GEOGRAPHIC DISTRIBUTION
• The geographic range of EPM cases is defined by the distribution of the opossum
• Native cases of EPM have only been reported in North and South America
• Cases of neosporosis have been described in the USA and in France

SIGNALMENT
Breed Predilections
Thoroughbreds, Standardbreds, and Quarter Horses are most frequently affected.

Mean Age and Range
Horses may be affected at any age (3 months to 30 years of age). The majority of the cases confirmed at postmortem were <4 years old.

Predominant Sex
Male Standardbreds might be at greater risks.

SIGNS
General Comments
• There is a great variation in clinical signs due to multifocal localization of the parasites in the CNS
• The onset of the disease may be acute or insidious and can progress rapidly or remain stable for a long period of time

Historical Findings
• Apparent lameness from asymmetrical ataxia and muscle weakness is the most common clinical complaint
• Muscle atrophy, sore back, and cranial nerve deficits also may be reported

Physical Examination Findings
• Affected horses are usually bright and alert
• Clinical signs suggestive of spinal cord lesions, with variable degrees of ataxia and paresis in 1 or more limbs, are the most frequent finding (see Web Video 1)
• Localized muscle atrophy, head tilt, facial paralysis, diminished ocular reflexes, poor prehension, mastication or dysphagia, laryngeal hemiplegia, urinary incontinence, localized sweating, seizure, and head shaking are also common

CAUSES
• *S. neurona*
• *N. hughesi*

RISK FACTORS
• Opossums or previous diagnosis of EPM on the premises
• Stress or adverse health event <90 days before presentation

DIAGNOSIS

DIFFERENTIAL DIAGNOSIS
• Ataxia and paresis often confused with lameness

• Cervical vertebral malformation—has similar breed predilection and usually produces symmetric ataxia
• Trauma—history, external evidence of injury, and anatomic localization to a single area of the CNS are common
• Equine degenerative myeloencephalopathy—progressive, symmetrical ataxia, and paresis in horses <2 years
• Equine herpesvirus 1 myeloencephalopathy—typically affects more than 1 horse in a group and often follows respiratory disease. It is commonly associated with symmetric, posterior ataxia and paresis, bladder dysfunction, and loss of tail and anal tone
• Equine viral encephalitis (West Nile virus, Eastern equine encephalitis, Western equine encephalitis, Venezuelan equine encephalitis)—depression and fever
• Any conditions causing central and peripheral nervous system dysfunctions

CBC/BIOCHEMISTRY/URINALYSIS
CBC and serum biochemistry are usually unremarkable.

OTHER LABORATORY TESTS
• Gold standard remains postmortem identification of characteristic lesions and parasites within the CNS. Immunohistology can help identify the parasites on fixed tissues
• WB—positive serology is only indicative of exposure to the parasite. Negative tests indicate a high probability that the horse is not infected with *S. neurona*
• In a study on 234 horses, sensitivity of WB on CSF was 87–88% regardless of whether the horses showed signs of neurologic diseases. Specificity reported on CSF varies from 44% to 60% depending on the presence or absence of neurologic signs, respectively
• False-positive results on CSF samples may occur due to blood contamination of the CSF, subclinical infection with other concurrent neurologic disease, crossreactivity with other *Sarcocystis* or *Neospora* spp., or natural passage of antibody from the blood to the CSF after vaccination or colostrum ingestion
• IFAT—sensitivity and specificity using serum samples of horses naturally infected with *S. neurona* are 83.3% and 96.9%, respectively. Using CSF, sensitivity is 100% and specificity is 99%
• ELISA to detect *S. neurona*-specific immunoglobulin G has been described. Sensitivity and specificity are 95.5% and 92.9%, respectively
• PCR detection of *S. neurona* DNA on the CSF has a high specificity but poor sensitivity
• IFAT is more accurate to diagnose *N. hughesi*-infected horses than ELISA and direct agglutination test. Sensitivity is 100% and specificity varies from 71.5% to 100% depending on the cutoff value

EQUINE PROTOZOAL MYELOENCEPHALITIS (EPM)   (CONTINUED)

IMAGING
Lesions localized in the brain, brainstem, and cervical spinal cord can be visualized using CT/MRI.

OTHER DIAGNOSTIC PROCEDURES
• CSF is usually within normal limits, although its analysis may help rule out other diseases
• Cytology on the CSF—more than 50 red blood cells per μL indicates blood contamination and prevents interpretation of a positive WB

PATHOLOGIC FINDINGS
• Gross lesions not always visible at necropsy
• CNS lesions due to *S. neurona* are commonly multifocal, characterized by hemorrhage and necrosis in the brain, brainstem, and spinal cord. Infective organisms are found primarily in neurons but also occasionally in leukocytes and vascular endothelium
• *N. hughesi* causes multifocal granulomas in the CNS

TREATMENT

AIMS
• Stopping progression of the disease
• Improving the neurologic status of the horse
• Preventing lesions from self-trauma
• Preventing relapse when possible

APPROPRIATE HEALTH CARE
General supportive care in horses with severe neurologic dysfunction primarily aimed at avoiding self-traumatic injuries (deep bedding, sling support, and protective gear).

NURSING CARE
• Severely ataxic horses should be confined in a heavily bedded box stall
• Turning of the recumbent horse must be attempted every 2–6 h
• Legs should be bandaged to avoid traumatic injuries
• Adequate nutritional support must be provided. Diets and routes of administration must be adapted to each patient

ACTIVITY
• Prolonged inactivity does not enhance recovery
• However, premature return to heavy work may prolong the time to recovery and promote relapse

DIET
• Use of folate inhibitors may result in bone marrow suppression and anemia. If life-threatening anemia develops, discontinue medication for 2–3 weeks to allow recovery or switch to an alternative medication. High-quality pasture and alfalfa hay are excellent sources of folinic acid and highly recommended during treatment. Folic acid is poorly absorbed by the horse and has been associated with toxicity
• Supplementation with vitamin E 6000–10 000 IU PO daily has been recommended during therapy and rehabilitation

MEDICATIONS

DRUG(S) OF CHOICE
• Ponazuril (Marquis, Bayer) is administered orally at 5 mg/kg daily for 28 days and is well tolerated in horses. Few adverse effects have been described at recommended dosages
• Oral administration of nitazoxanide (Navigator, Idexx Pharmaceuticals) starts at 25 mg/kg daily for 5 days and then 50 mg/kg daily for a total of 28 days
• Folate inhibitors are still widely used at 20 mg/kg sulfadiazine and 1.0 mg/kg pyrimethamine orally daily for 4–6 months or at least 1 month after the horse stops showing further improvement. Many veterinarians now recommend 1.5–2.0-fold the standard dose of pyrimethamine for the initial treatment or after 30 days without satisfactory progress. The combination should be given on an empty stomach to prevent interference with absorption from the gut
• Administration of flunixin meglumine (1.1 mg/kg BID) or phenylbutazone (2.2 mg/kg BID) during the first 1–2 weeks of treatment and any time the condition appears to worsen may help minimize further damage due to parasite death and the host response
• DMSO (1.0 g/kg in 10% saline IV daily for 3 days) may be beneficial
• Use of dexamethasone (0.05 mg/kg IV daily or BID) in severely affected horses may help reduce CNS inflammation but remains controversial
• Treatment of *N. hughesi* remains a challenge. In 1 report, the parasite was not affected by treatment with folate inhibitors and nitazoxanide, while in vitro studies indicate its susceptibility to those compounds

CONTRAINDICATIONS
Known sensitivity to 1 of the drugs.

PRECAUTIONS
• Corticosteroids should be used with caution because they can suppress the immune response to the parasite. Their use should not exceed 1–3 days to avoid exacerbating the disease
• Fatal enterocolitis, anorexia, weight loss, depression, colic, discoloration of the urine, fever, peripheral edema, and laminitis have been described in horses treated with nitazoxanide
• Stallions may be at increased risks of developing laminitis while treated with nitazoxanide
• Folic acid supplementation in horses treated with folate inhibitors may paradoxically exacerbate the deficiency
• Abortion and decreased stallion fertility may occur using folate inhibitors

POSSIBLE INTERACTIONS
Use of potentiated sulfas and pyrimethamine may increase the side effects of folic acid depletion.

ALTERNATIVE DRUGS
• Diclazuril and toltrazuril (5–10 mg/kg PO daily for 28 days) have been used in the treatment of EPM in the horse. Their efficacy appears to be comparable to folate inhibitors
• Immunostimulants such as levamisole, killed *Propionibacterium acnes,* and mycobacterial cell wall extract have been recommended, but their efficacy has not been documented

FOLLOW-UP

PATIENT MONITORING
• Neurologic examination of affected horses is recommended at regular intervals during treatment
• Relapse may occur in 10–25% of horses
• To reduce the relapse rate, medication should not be discontinued until CSF becomes negative, but some horses remain CSF positive for an extended period after full recovery or stabilization
• The relapse rate among horses with negative CSF at the time treatment is stopped has been extremely low
• When using folate inhibitors, monthly CBCs are recommended to monitor anemia

PREVENTION/AVOIDANCE
• Ataxic horses represent a risk for themselves and their handlers
• Management should aim at preventing physical stress from injury and bacterial infection. Long trailer rides are stressful and commonly mentioned in clinical histories of affected horses
• Prevention should aim at limiting the access of opossums and other wildlife to the horse's environment, feed, and water supply

POSSIBLE COMPLICATIONS
Secondary injuries may occur from ataxia. Keep performance animals out of training during therapy.

EXPECTED COURSE AND PROGNOSIS
• Regardless of treatment used, improvement usually varies between 60% and 75%
• Full recovery rate are <25%. Mildly affected horses treated early in the course of infection have a better prognosis. Improvement often is observed during the first week of therapy and frequently progresses steadily for several weeks. The rate of improvement typically slows as the horse gradually improves over many weeks, until a plateau is reached.

Chronic signs of CNS damage (e.g. muscle atrophy) rarely improve

MISCELLANEOUS

ASSOCIATED CONDITIONS
Secondary injuries.

ZOONOTIC POTENTIAL
N/A

PREGNANCY/FERTILITY/BREEDING
Transplacental transmission of *N. hughesi* is documented but not of *S. neurona*. Abortion and death of foals born from mares treated with folate inhibitors and supplemented with folic acid and vitamin E are reported.

SEE ALSO
- Cervical vertebral malformation
- Eastern (EEE), western (WEE), and Venezuelan (VEE) equine encephalitides
- Equine herpesvirus myeloencephalopathy
- Neuroaxonal dystrophy/equine degenerative myeloencephalopathy
- Verminous meningoencephalomyelitis
- West nile virus

ABBREVIATIONS
- CNS = central nervous system
- CSF = cerebrospinal fluid
- CT = computed tomography
- DMSO = dimethyl sulfoxide
- ELISA = enzyme-linked immunosorbent assay
- EPM = equine protozoal myeloencephalitis
- IFAT = immunofluorescence antibody test
- MRI = magnetic resonance imaging
- PCR = polymerase chain reaction
- WB = western blot test

Suggested Reading
Furr M, MacKay R, Granstorm D. Clinical diagnosis of equine protozoal myeloencephalitis (EPM). J Vet Intern Med 2002;16:618–621.

Packham AE, Conrad PA, Wilson WD, et al. Qualitative evaluation of selective tests for detection of *Neospora hughesi* antibodies in serum and cerebrospinal fluid of experimentally infected horses. J Parasitol 2002;88:1239–1246.

Sellon DC, Dubey JP. Equine protozoal myeloencephalitis. In: Sellon DC, Long MT, eds. Equine Infectious Diseases. St. Louis, MO: Saunders, 2006:453–464.

Author Laureline Lecoq
Consulting Editor Caroline N. Hahn

EQUINE RECURRENT UVEITIS

BASICS

DEFINITION
• ERU is a common cause of blindness and chronic discomfort in a wide variety of horses. ERU is used, confusingly, to refer to a group of recurrent or persistent immune-mediated diseases of multiple origins, as well as a specific diagnosis. Recurrent attacks of uveitis are the hallmark of ERU. Additionally, some horses will present with a chronic and persistent course of disease
• ERU is characterized by recurrent episodes of intraocular inflammation of variable degrees of intensity that are interrupted by periods of quiescence

PATHOPHYSIOLOGY
ERU appears to have characteristics of an infection-mediated autoimmune disease. The triggers for ERU are not completely understood. ERU can occur as a late sequela to systemic infection with ocular signs developing months after exposure. Hypersensitivity to infectious agents such as *Leptospira interrogans* is possible.

SYSTEMS AFFECTED
Ophthalmic

GENETICS
Unknown but some genetic predisposition has been shown in German Warmblood and Appaloosa horses. There is evidence of a genetic link between ERU and IL-17A and IL-17F in German Warmblood horses.

INCIDENCE/PREVALENCE
1–2% of American horses are affected.

SIGNALMENT

Breed Predilection
L. interrogans-seropositive Appaloosas were 8.3 times as likely to develop uveitis as other breeds, and 3.8 times more likely as other breeds to lose vision following development of uveitis.

Mean Age and Range
While all ages can be affected, a large proportion of horses present before the age of 12 years.

Predominant sex
None

CLASSIFICATION
ERU is currently classified as follows:
• *Classic ERU* is characterized by active bouts of intraocular inflammation followed by periods of quiescence or minimally detectable inflammation. The iris, ciliary body, and choroid are primarily affected
• *Insidious ERU* has the hallmark feature of low-grade intraocular inflammation that does not appear to be outwardly painful but that results in a gradual and steady level of destruction, which culminates in the degeneration of multiple intraocular

structures. Breed predisposition: Appaloosa, draft, and Knabstrupper breeds
• *Posterior ERU* is characterized by predominately posterior segment inflammation (e.g. vitreous, retina, and choroid), but mild anterior inflammation is commonly present

SIGNS
• *Classic ERU*—lacrimation, blepharospasm, photophobia, and miosis, as well as variable degrees of corneal edema, conjunctival hyperemia, ciliary injection, aqueous flare, hyphema, intraocular fibrin, and hypopyon. Miosis may result in secondary posterior synechiae and/or dyscoria. Acute cases generally have low IOP, while chronic and/or insidious ERU may be associated with intermittent elevations in IOP. Recurrent bouts of inflammation may cause cataracts, intraocular adhesions, phthisis bulbi, eventually resulting in vision loss
• *Insidious ERU*—conjunctival and episcleral vascular hyperemia, mild to moderate blepharitis, focal or diffuse corneal edema, corneal vascularization, aqueous flare, iris discoloration (hyperpigmentation and/or depigmentation), and corpora nigra degeneration, as well as iris atrophy and miosis, corneal fibrosis, posterior synechia, and pigment of the anterior lens capsule. Focal and/or diffuse cataracts and lens sub/luxations are possible. Secondary glaucoma is common
• *Posterior ERU*—vitritis (cloudy or hazy vitreous), chorioretinal scarring, retinal detachments (peripapillary linear traction band detachments are most common), and retinal degeneration
• In chronic cases, regardless of which type of ERU, corneal vascularization, endothelial degeneration resulting in persistent corneal edema, band keratopathy, synechiae, cataract formation, and alterations in iris color may occur. Secondary glaucoma and phthisis bulbi can occur and irreversible blindness is a common sequela in many cases of ERU

CAUSES
• While the pathogenesis is clearly immune mediated, the true underlying cause often remains unknown
• Hypersensitivity to infectious agents such as *L. interrogans* serovar *pomona* is commonly implicated as a possible cause
• Toxoplasmosis, salmonellosis, *Streptococcus*, *Escherichia coli*, *Rhodococcus equi*, borreliosis, strongyles, onchocerciasis, parasites, and viral infections have also been implicated

RISK FACTORS
• Appaloosa or Warmblood breed
• *Leptospira* infections increase the risk for ERU

DIAGNOSIS

DIFFERENTIAL DIAGNOSIS
• Ulcerative keratitis
• Corneal stromal abscess
• Glaucoma
• Endothelial immune-mediated keratitis
• Heterochromic iridocyclitis with keratitis

CBC/BIOCHEMISTRY/URINALYSIS
None

OTHER LABORATORY TESTS
• Antibody titer evaluation from both aqueous humor and serum can be useful to determine the degree of intraocular antibody production or if a horse has systemic leptospirosis
• The ratio of aqueous humor to serum antibody titers (i.e. Goldmann–Witmer coefficient) to determine if intraocular antibody production is taking place as opposed to leakage of serum antibodies into the eye. A *c*-value >1 suggests local antibody production and >4 provides greater confidence of active leptospiral uveitis. Detection of *Leptospira* organisms by culture or PCR in aqueous or vitreous humor samples may be considered.
• Leptospiral titers for *L. pomona, L. bratislava,* and *L. autumnalis* should be requested in the USA. Additionally, *L. grippotyphosa* titers should be evaluated in Europe. Positive titers for serovars of 1:400 or greater are of importance

IMAGING
Ocular ultrasonography to assess the condition of the posterior segment or to evaluate for cataract and luxation or subluxation of the lens and to look for retinal degeneration and detachments.

PATHOLOGIC FINDINGS
• In acute stages, lymphocytic infiltration with neutrophils can be found in the uveal tract, resulting in edema and plasmoid vitreous and aqueous
• The chronic stages manifest by corneal scarring, cataract formation, and chorioretinitis and retinal degeneration

TREATMENT

APPROPRIATE HEALTH CARE
• The major goals of treatment of ERU are to suppress inflammation, prevent or minimize the frequency and intensity of recurrent bouts of uveitis, decrease or eliminate pain and discomfort, and preserve vision
• Specific prevention and targeted therapy are often not possible as the etiology remains elusive in many cases
• Therapy will last for weeks, and often requires months of slow and deliberate tapering-off of medications

(CONTINUED)

E

• Initially, stall rest with minimal turn out and avoidance of bright sunlight is recommended

ACTIVITY

Activity should be reduced pending resolution of clinical signs.

CLIENT EDUCATION

• A complete cure is not possible in most affected horses
• Medical treatment of the disease can be both time-consuming and expensive. The owner should be educated about the potential for recurrence and the debilitating and blinding nature of this disease

SURGICAL CONSIDERATIONS

• Pars plana vitrectomy in horses with ERU has been used successfully to remove vitreal debris and infectious organisms
• A sustained release cyclosporine A (ciclosporin) drug-releasing device surgically inserted into the suprachoroidal space can effectively suppress the intensity of the uveitis in many eyes with ERU. The drug should theoretically be released for a period of 3–5 years
• Low-dose intravitreal gentamicin (4 mg) injections have been utilized over the past few years with increasing success

MEDICATIONS

DRUG(S) OF CHOICE

• Topical prednisolone acetate (1%) or dexamethasone (0.1%) should be applied a minimum of 4–6 times per day initially
• Systemic corticosteroids may be beneficial in severe, refractory cases of ERU but should be used with caution
• Topical NSAIDs (flurbiprofen, indomethacin (indometacin), diclofenac, suprofen, bromfenac every 24 h to every 8 h) are effective at reducing the intraocular inflammation when a corneal ulcer is present
• Flunixin meglumine (0.25–1.1 mg/kg PO every 12 h) and phenylbutazone (1 g IV or PO every 12 h) are frequently used systemically. Aspirin (15 mg/kg/day) is still commonly used to manage chronic uveitis; however, its efficacy is questionable
• Mydriatic and cycloplegic medications (atropine 1%) minimize synechiae formation by inducing mydriasis, and alleviate some of the pain of ERU by relieving spasm of ciliary body muscles (cycloplegia)
• Antibiotic treatment for horses with positive titers for *Leptospira* remains speculative but streptomycin (11 mg/kg IM BID) or

enrofloxacin (7.5 mg/kg SID) may be a good choice for horses at acute and chronic stages of the disease. Penicillin G sodium (10 000 U/kg IV or IM QID) and oxytetracycline (5–10 mg/kg IV BID) may be beneficial. Oral doxycycline (10 mg/kg BID) does not enter the aqueous or vitreous of normal horse eyes at therapeutic levels, but might reach higher levels in inflamed eyes
• Preservative-free, low-dose (4 mg) gentamicin has been demonstrated to suppress recurrent episodes of uveitic attacks.

PRECAUTIONS

Horses receiving topical atropine should be monitored for colic.

FOLLOW-UP

PATIENT MONITORING

• Regularly scheduled follow-up examinations should be carried out at least weekly during the first 2–3 weeks once a positive response to treatment has been established
• Once tapering off of topical and systemic medical therapy is initiated, the horse should be carefully monitored for signs of recurrent inflammation

PREVENTION/AVOIDANCE

• In horses where the disease tends to flare up after routine vaccination or deworming, prophylactic treatment of the eye may be beneficial
• While a *Leptospira* vaccine is presently available, no proof exists that it will prevent the development of *Leptospira*-induced ERU

POSSIBLE COMPLICATIONS

ERU can potentially result in blindness.

EXPECTED COURSE AND PROGNOSIS

The prognosis for ERU is usually poor, but the disease may be controlled with medical (conventional or suprachoroidal cyclosporine-releasing devices) or surgical (i.e., low-dose intravitreal gentamicin [4 mg] injection) intervention.

MISCELLANEOUS

ASSOCIATED CONDITIONS

Systemic infection by the ERU-causing organism.

AGE-RELATED FACTORS

N/A

ZOONOTIC POTENTIAL

Infectious agents such as *Leptospira* can be a health risk for people.

PREGNANCY/FERTILITY/BREEDING

Leptospira infection may lead to abortion.

SYNONYMS

• Periodic ophthalmia
• Moon blindness
• Iridocyclitis

SEE ALSO

• Calcific band keratopathy
• Chorioretinitis
• Corneal stromal abscesses
• Corneal ulceration
• Glaucoma
• Immune-mediated keratitis
• Stationary night blindness

ABBREVIATIONS

• ERU = equine recurrent uveitis
• IL = interleukin
• IOP = intraocular pressure
• NSAID = nonsteroidal anti-inflammatory drug
• PCR = polymerase chain reaction

Suggested Reading
Brooks DE. Ophthalmology for the Equine Practitioner, 2e. Jackson, WY: Teton NewMedia, 2008.
Dwyer AE, Crockett RS, Kalsow CM. Association of leptospiral seroreactivity and breed with uveitis and blindness in horses: 372 cases (1986–1993). J Am Vet Med Assoc 1995;207:1327–1331.
Fischer BM, McMullen Jr RJ, Reese S, Brehm W. Intravitreal injection of low-dose gentamicin for the treatment of recurrent or persistent uveitis in horses: Preliminary results. BMC Veterinary Research, 2019; doi.org/10.1186/s12917-018-1722-7
Gilger BC, Hollingsworth SR. Diseases of the uvea, uveitis, and recurrent uveitis. In: Gilger BC, ed. Equine Ophthalmology, 3e. Ames, IA: Wiley Blackwell, 2017:369–415.
McMullen Jr RJ, Fischer BM. Medical and surgical management of equine recurrent uveitis. Vet Clin Equine 2017;33:465–481.

Author Richard J. McMullen Jr.
Consulting Editor Caryn E. Plummer
Acknowledgment The author and editor acknowledge the prior contribution of Andras M. Komaromy and Dennis E. Brooks.

EQUINE SARCOIDOSIS

BASICS

OVERVIEW
• ES is an uncommon disease and is also called idiopathic systemic granulomatous disease. ES occurs locally, partially generalized, and generalized. The generalized form is often only in a later stage and has started with exfoliative dermatitis or with subcutaneous nodules. • Localized ES is limited to the skin without systemic signs. Horses with the PGF often progress to the GF. The GF of ES may start with an exfoliative dermatitis or with granulomatous inflammatory nodules in multiple organs. Horses with the exfoliative form almost invariably develop nodules and vice versa.

SIGNALMENT
No apparent age, breed, or sex predilections.

SIGNS
• Clinical signs vary depending on the form, the localized form is the most common.
• Onset is typically slowly progressive but may be explosive. • Nonpruritic exfoliative dermatitis is often the primary clinical sign; however, sometimes the disease starts with granulomatous nodules or by severe wasting.
• Skin lesions in the localised form consist of scaling, crusting, and alopecia representing the most common form (Figure 1). Lesions usually start on the lower limbs and only rarely progress to generalized disease. In PGF or GF the mane and tale are usually unaffected. • Horses with the PGF or GF may develop exercise intolerance, weight loss, and low-grade fever. Many have granulomatous

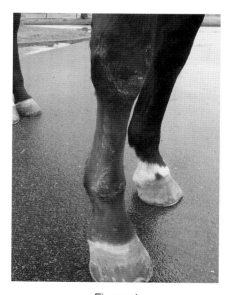

Figure 1.

Localized sarcoidosis.

inflammation of the internal organs confirmed at necropsy

CAUSES AND RISK FACTORS
The etiologic agent or the initiating pathophysiologic mechanism is unknown. Disease may occur from an abnormal immune response to an ingested or inhaled environmental antigen, or an underlying infectious or neoplastic process resulting in chronic antigenic stimulation.

DIAGNOSIS

DIFFERENTIAL DIAGNOSIS
• Nonpruritic scaling and crusting dermatoses. • Dermatophilosis.
• Dermatophytosis. • Idiopathic seborrhea.
• Pemphigus foliaceus. • Lower limb vasculitis. • Leucocytoclastic pastern vasculitis

CBC/BIOCHEMISTRY/URINALYSIS
Horses with generalized disease may have leukocytosis, mild nonregenerative anemia, hyperfibrinogenemia, hyperglobulinemia, and hypoalbuminemia depending on the organs involved and chronicity.

OTHER LABORATORY TESTS
• Multiple, full-thickness punch biopsies of the affected skin or of the subcutaneous nodules. • Confirmation of a diagnosis is obtained when typical granulomatous changes exist with multinucleated Langhans-type giant cells, and other granulomatous diseases secondary to bacterial or fungal organisms have been ruled out by appropriate cultures and/or special stains

TREATMENT
Topical therapies include antibacterial and antiseborrheic shampoos but are often unsuccessful.

MEDICATIONS

DRUG(S) OF CHOICE
• CS at immunosuppressive doses are the preferred treatment. Administration should be continued for several weeks to months with a slow taper when in remission. Consider benefits and risks of long-term CS therapy in cases with only cutaneous involvement as spontaneous resolution may occur.
• Prednisolone at 1–2 mg/kg PO every 24 h.
• Dexamethasone 0.04–0.08 mg/kg IM, IV, or PO every 24 h. • Always give CS before 9:00AM as it may decrease the risk of laminitis

CONTRAINDICATIONS/POSSIBLE INTERACTIONS
In cases with a history of laminitis, corticosteroids should be used with care. Anecdotal reports of an increased risk of laminitis exists.

FOLLOW-UP

PATIENT MONITORING
Evaluate response to therapy to allow for tapering of CS to lowest effective dose.

POSSIBLE COMPLICATIONS
Secondary to CS.

EXPECTED COURSE AND PROGNOSIS
Response to therapy in the localized form is reasonable and in the PGF and GF poor.

MISCELLANEOUS

ASSOCIATED CONDITIONS
None

AGE-RELATED FACTORS
None

ZOONOTIC POTENTIAL
None documented.

PREGNANCY/FERTILITY/BREEDING
Corticosteroid treatment is contraindicated.

SEE ALSO
• Dermatophilosis. • Leucocytoclastic pastern vasculitis. • Pemphigus foliaceus

ABBREVIATIONS
• CS = corticosteroids. • ES = equine sarcoidosis. • PGF = partially generalized form. • GF = generalized form

Suggested Reading
Reijerkerk EPR, Veldhuis Kroeze EJB and Sloet van Oldruitenborgh-Oosterbaan MM. Generalized sarcoidosis in two horses. Tijdschr Diergeneeskd 2008;133:654–661.
Sloet van Oldruitenborgh-Oosterbaan MM, Grinwis GCM. Equine sarcoidosis. Vet Clin North Am Equine Pract 2013;29:615–627.

Author Marianne M. Sloet van Oldruitenborgh-Oosterbaan
Consulting Editor Gwendolen Lorch
Acknowledgment The author and editor acknowledge the prior contribution of Sandra J. Sargent.

ESOPHAGEAL OBSTRUCTION (CHOKE)

 ## BASICS

DEFINITION
A partial or complete obstruction of the esophageal lumen by feed or foreign body that results in an inability to swallow. The disorder may occur as a single acute episode or as a chronic, intermittent problem.

PATHOPHYSIOLOGY
• Esophageal obstruction occurs with higher frequency at sites with naturally decreased esophageal distensibility—the mid-cervical region, the thoracic inlet, and the terminal esophagus
• The most common type of obstruction is impaction with feed material
• Wood shavings and various foreign bodies can also cause obstruction of the esophagus
• A frequent predisposing factor is improper mastication by older or younger horses caused by defective and erupting teeth, respectively. Improper mastication can also occur in gluttonous, sedated, or exhausted horses or in horses recovering from general anesthesia
• Horses with preexisting lesions such as external esophageal compression, megaesophagus, and esophageal diverticulum or stricture experience recurrent obstructions at the affected site
• Choke can also occur secondarily to neurologic disorders causing dysphagia

SYSTEMS AFFECTED
Gastrointestinal
Choke causes dysphagia. Sequelae to choke include esophageal perforation or stricture formation and megaesophagus.

Respiratory
Aspiration of feed material and saliva frequently occurs in horses with esophageal obstruction. This can lead to aspiration pneumonia and pleuropneumonia. Other less common sequelae to choke are pleuritis and mediastinitis secondary to esophageal perforation.

Cardiovascular
The inability to drink water may result in dehydration.

Skin/Exocrine
Esophageal perforation can result in cervical cellulitis and fistula formation.

GENETICS
N/A

SIGNALMENT
Mean Age and Range
Younger and older horses.

SIGNS
General Comments
Ptyalism and feed-containing nasal discharge are the most common clinical signs of choke. Other clinical signs vary with the duration and the degree of the obstruction. Partial obstruction might cause intermittent clinical signs depending on the diet.

Historical Findings
• Frequent, ineffectual attempts to swallow
• Retching
• Repeated extension of the head and neck
• Coughing during swallowing
• Nasal discharge of saliva mixed with feed
• Restlessness
• Sweating
• Anxiety

Physical Examination Findings
• Dysphagia, coughing, ptyalism, and regurgitation of saliva and feed material through the mouth and nostrils
• If the obstruction is located in the cervical esophagus, focal swelling may be palpated or visible
• The presence of subcutaneous emphysema and/or cellulitis over the cervical region may indicate esophageal rupture
• In cases of aspiration pneumonia, abnormal lung sounds such as crackles and wheezes can be present
• In pleuropneumonia, no respiratory sounds are heard ventrally and chest percussion is dull ventrally too

CAUSES
• Obstruction of the esophagus is most frequently caused by intraluminal impaction of feed material or, less commonly, by foreign bodies
• Improper mastication due to erupting or defective teeth, sedation, exhaustion, and fracture of the hyoid bone are potential predisposing factors to intraluminal feed obstruction
• Dry feeds (e.g. beet pulp, pelleted feeds, oats) are most often associated with the condition
• Defects in the esophageal wall (intramural lesions) such as strictures, intramural abscesses or cysts, esophageal diverticula, and neoplasia (especially squamous cell carcinoma) usually result in recurrent esophageal obstructions
• Acquired lesions causing external esophageal compression are relatively rare and include abscesses, tumors, cervical cellulitis, and diaphragmatic hernia
• Congenital disorders such as megaesophagus, achalasia, vascular ring anomalies, and right aortic arch are rare causes of esophageal obstruction
• Esophageal motility disorders can result in esophageal obstruction and megaesophagus

RISK FACTORS
• Poor dental care
• Rapid ingestion of feed
• Poor quality feed; pelleted or dry feeds such as beet pulp and oats
• Inadequate water intake
• Previous episode of choke

 ## DIAGNOSIS

DIFFERENTIAL DIAGNOSIS
• Other causes of bilateral nasal discharge, e.g. guttural pouch empyema, strangles, and lung edema
• Neurologic disorders causing dysphagia, e.g. rabies, botulism, and guttural pouch mycosis affecting cranial nerves IX, X, and XII
• Foreign bodies in the pharynx or oral cavity

CBC/BIOCHEMISTRY/URINALYSIS
• Neutrophilia or neutropenia as well as increased serum amyloid A protein and fibrinogen may be seen in cases that develop aspiration pneumonia
• Prolonged excessive salivary loss may cause hyponatremia, hypochloremia, and metabolic alkalosis

OTHER LABORATORY TESTS
N/A

IMAGING
Ultrasonography
Ultrasonography can be used to provide information about the location and extent of a cervical esophageal impaction.

Radiography
• Radiographic evaluation of the esophagus supplies information concerning the nature and degree of the obstruction but is more commonly used for evaluation of patients with recurrent episodes
• After relief of the impaction, contrast radiographic studies are useful to evaluate diverticulum formation, strictures, esophageal dilation, megaesophagus, and luminal narrowing secondary to extraluminal compression

OTHER DIAGNOSTIC PROCEDURES
• Passage of a nasogastric tube can confirm a tentative diagnosis of esophageal obstruction and determine the approximate location of the obstruction
• Endoscopic evaluation of the esophagus gives further information about the nature of the obstruction

PATHOLOGIC FINDINGS
N/A

 ## TREATMENT

APPROPRIATE HEALTH CARE
• Although some cases of esophageal obstruction resolve spontaneously, they should be treated as emergencies
• Most cases of esophageal obstruction can be successfully treated on the farm. Only a few cases require referral to an animal hospital

E

ESOPHAGEAL OBSTRUCTION (CHOKE)   (CONTINUED)

NURSING CARE
- The basic approaches to treatment of esophageal obstruction are gentle esophageal lavage in conjunction with administration of drugs that result in relaxation of the esophageal musculature and a reduced level of anxiety
- In cases of mild obstruction, administration of these drugs alone may result in muscular relaxation to allow the obstruction to pass
- A nasogastric tube is advanced to the level of the obstruction and small amounts of water are used for gentle lavage of the impaction site. The patient's head should be kept at a low level to facilitate the exit of fluid and prevent aspiration. The procedure requires patience and gentleness
- Continuous lavage can be performed by passing a cuffed endotracheal tube into the esophagus and passing a smaller tube through the larger cuffed tube. Alternatively, a specially designed cuffed tube for treatment of esophageal obstruction (esophageal flush tube) can be used
- If the impaction is not relieved, the lavages can be performed intermittently with the horse placed in a stall without access to feed, water, and bedding between the attempts
- Refractory cases may be lavaged during general anesthesia with endotracheal intubation. General anesthesia provides optimal relaxation of the esophageal musculature
- Most cases of esophageal obstruction do not require IV fluid therapy but should be given if the horse is dehydrated or water consumption is restricted

DIET
- The owner should be instructed to remove feed and water from the stall while waiting for the veterinarian to arrive
- Esophageal dilatation post obstruction increases the likelihood of reimpaction for at least 48 h
- In case with mild impactions without esophageal mucosal damage, horses can be fed small amounts of moistened pellets (soup) after 12–24 h. The amount can be increased as the condition improves
- Small amounts of hay presoaked in water can be gradually introduced after a few days
- In horses with more complicated impactions with mucosal damage and/or remaining dilated esophagus, feed should not be provided until these problems have resolved

CLIENT EDUCATION
- The feeding regime after treatment is important in order to decrease the risk for reobstruction

- There is a risk for aspiration pneumonia and the owner is advised to monitor the horse's body temperature for a couple of days after the treatment

MEDICATIONS
DRUG(S) OF CHOICE
- Administration of xylazine (0.25–0.5 mg/kg IV), detomidine (0.01–0.02 mg/kg IV), or acepromazine (0.05 mg/kg IV) provides sedation and muscle relaxation of the esophagus
- The use of α_2-adrenergic agonists has the advantage of causing lowering of the head, thereby facilitating the lavage and decreasing the likelihood of aspiration
- Butorphanol can be used in combination with α_2-adrenergic agonists
- Anti-inflammatory drugs (e.g. flunixine meglumine) are used to control pain and treat inflammation

CONTRAINDICATIONS
Administration of lubricating agents, such as mineral oil, or softening agents, such as dioctyl sodium succinate, in order to facilitate the removal of an esophageal obstruction are contraindicated because they might be aspirated.

PRECAUTIONS
NSAIDs should be administered cautiously to dehydrated animals due to their potentially nephrotoxic effects.

ALTERNATIVE DRUGS
Oxytocin (0.11–0.22 IU/kg IV) can be used to relax the esophagus but it may be associated with transient abdominal discomfort, sweating, and muscle tremors. Oxytocin should not be used in pregnant mares.

FOLLOW-UP
PATIENT MONITORING
- Endoscopy of the esophagus should be performed after the obstruction has been relieved in order to determine the presence and extent of esophageal lesions, establish the prognosis, and make recommendations for additional treatments and feeding regimen
- Repeated esophageal endoscopies are indicated if mucosal damage has occurred. Strictures most often occur 15–30 days after mucosal damage
- Thoracic auscultation and monitoring of body temperature may help identify aspiration

pneumonia. Thoracic radiographs are indicated if aspiration pneumonia is suspected

POSSIBLE COMPLICATIONS
- Recurrent esophageal obstructions
- Esophageal diverticulum
- Esophageal stricture
- Esophageal ulceration
- Esophageal perforation
- Cellulitis
- Esophageal dilation
- Mediastinitis
- Aspiration pneumonia
- Pleuritis

MISCELLANEOUS
ASSOCIATED CONDITIONS
Aspiration pneumonia.

AGE-RELATED FACTORS
Younger and older horses are most commonly affected.

ZOONOTIC POTENTIAL
N/A

PREGNANCY/FERTILITY/BREEDING
α_2-Adrenergic agonists may induce premature parturition if used during the last trimester of pregnancy.

SYNONYMS
Choke

SEE ALSO
- Aspiration pneumonia
- Cleft palate

ABBREVIATIONS
NSAID = nonsteroidal anti-inflammatory drug

Internet Resources
https://www.merckvetmanual.com/digestive-system/diseases-of-the-esophagus-in-large-animals/esophageal-obstruction-in-large-animals

Suggested Reading
Sanchez CL. Esophageal disease. In: Reed SM, Bayly WM, Sellon DC, eds. Equine Internal Medicine, 3e. St. Louis, MO: WB Saunders, 2010:830–838.
Whithair KJ, Cox JH, Coyne CP, DeBowes RM. Esophageal obstruction in the horse. Compend Contin Educ Vet Pract 1990;1:91–96.

Author Johan Bröjer
Consulting Editors Henry Stämpfli and Olimpo Oliver-Espinosa

EXCESSIVE MATERNAL BEHAVIOR/FOAL STEALING

BASICS

OVERVIEW
• Uncommon
• Mares may show maternal behavior for a foal that is not her own without preventing care by the foal's biological mother. Such mares may stay closer to the foal than other herd members (except for the mother) and may stand for the foal to suckle
• Mares that are not pregnant and currently have no foals of their own occasionally produce milk for a foal they have spontaneously adopted, but this phenomenon is rare
• Some mares may prevent the foal's biological mother from caring for it
• Endocrine changes that prepare prepartum mares to care for their own foals may prompt them to steal the foals of subordinate mares. Maternal behavior is under neural and hormonal control, with estrogen, progesterone, and oxytocin being most significant; however, the exact neuroendocrine mechanism for mis-mothering is unknown

SIGNALMENT
Mares that are dominant to most other mares in the herd are the most likely to be successful in stealing foals of subordinate mares.

SIGNS
• A mare other than the mother remaining near a foal and standing for the foal to suckle
• In cases of true foal stealing, a mare remains between the foal and its biological mother and shows aggressive behavior (e.g. biting and kicking, or threatening such) toward the mother and may chase the mother away from the vicinity of the foal

CAUSES AND RISK FACTORS
• Neuroendocrine mechanisms that prepare a prepartum mare to care for her own foal
• Parturition by a low-ranking mare within 48 h of parturition by a high-ranking mare provides the stimulus of a neonatal foal to the higher ranking mare
• Very timid, nonaggressive, low-ranking biological mothers are most likely to have their foals stolen
• Very aggressive nonmothers that are hormonally ready to care for a neonate are most likely to steal foals

DIAGNOSIS

DIFFERENTIAL DIAGNOSIS
N/A

CBC/BIOCHEMISTRY/URINALYSIS
N/A

OTHER LABORATORY TESTS
N/A

IMAGING
N/A

OTHER DIAGNOSTIC PROCEDURES
In herds that are surveyed only periodically and for which the actual birth was not observed, it may be superficially unclear which of 2 mares fighting over a foal is the biological mother. Examine both mares to determine which has recently given birth and which is still pregnant. DNA analyses can be done later to positively identify the mother.

TREATMENT
• Isolate the foal and its biological mother from the mare attempting to steal the foal. Isolating the mother and foal from herd members not attempting to steal the foal may not be necessary, unless the foal requires medical attention
• The foal that was stolen and/or the foal of the stealing mare, if the history suggests that, may be unable to get colostrum from its mother
• If the foal is dry when the problem is discovered, try to find the placenta and determine if there is any moisture left in it. If so, smear it on the foal to trigger licking by the biological mother, as licking placental fluids off the neonate is part of the process of the mare bonding to her foal
• Fluid therapy if dehydrated

MEDICATIONS

DRUG(S) OF CHOICE
N/A

CONTRAINDICATIONS/POSSIBLE INTERACTIONS
N/A

FOLLOW-UP

PATIENT MONITORING
Once the stealing mare has her own foal, she is unlikely to attempt to steal a foal again; nevertheless, both mares should be observed carefully once returned to the herd to ensure no resumption of conflict.

PREVENTION/AVOIDANCE
Daily monitoring of herds of pregnant and nursing mares. Watch for signs suggestive of possible foal stealing.

POSSIBLE COMPLICATIONS
If a foal has been suckling a prepartum mare, it may have consumed her colostrum. Alternatively, its mother may have lost her colostrum during several hours of conflict with the foal-stealing mare, during which time the foal may have been unable to suckle. Be prepared to assess foals for dehydration and exhaustion. Provide stored colostrum, if available.

E

MISCELLANEOUS

ASSOCIATED CONDITIONS
Mares that steal foals may be more likely to engage in excessive aggression toward other herd members, regardless of the presence or absence of foals.

AGE-RELATED FACTORS
N/A

ZOONOTIC POTENTIAL
N/A

PREGNANCY/FERTILITY/BREEDING
Mares in late pregnancy have the greatest risk of this behavior.

SYNONYMS
• Misdirected maternal behavior
• Mis-mothering

SEE ALSO
Aggression

Suggested Reading
Crowell-Davis SL. Normal behavior and behavior problems. In: Kobluk CN, Ames TR, Geor RJ, eds. The Horse: Diseases and Clinical Management. Philadelphia, PA: WB Saunders, 1995:1–21.
Crowell-Davis SL, Houpt KA. Maternal behavior. Vet Clin North Am Equine Pract 1986;2:557–571.
Author Sharon L. Crowell-Davis
Consulting Editor Victoria L. Voith

EXERCISE-ASSOCIATED ARRHYTHMIAS

E

BASICS

OVERVIEW
EAAs are common in athletic horses, often as the heart rate speeds up or slows down following intense exercise. Arrhythmias during strenuous exercise are of greatest significance.

SIGNALMENT
EAAs are detected most often in performance animals and are occasionally identified in horses engaged in lower level athletic performance.

SIGNS
• EAAs can be associated with signs of poor athletic performance or found incidentally
• Some individuals with the more severe arrhythmias such as ventricular tachycardia or paradoxical atrial fibrillation present with marked exercise intolerance, distress, or collapse at exercise
• Cardiac arrhythmias are often assumed to account for sudden death at exercise, but this is difficult to prove

CAUSES AND RISK FACTORS
• Some EAAs, particularly in the pre- and postexercise periods, represent physiologic variants as the heart rate speeds up and slows down
• Dynamic airway obstruction, arterial hypoxemia, electrolyte disturbances, particularly depletion of total body magnesium, calcium, and potassium, are potential risk factors
• Some horses with hyperkalemic periodic paralysis develop ventricular arrhythmias at exercise and these horses may also have dynamic airway obstruction
• Myocardial pathology can lead to arrhythmias at rest and exercise

DIAGNOSIS

DIFFERENTIAL DIAGNOSIS
Upper airway disorders, exercise-induced pulmonary hemorrhage, lameness, and myopathy.

CBC/BIOCHEMISTRY/URINALYSIS
• Cardiac troponin I is increased only with myocardial necrosis
• Arterial oxygen measurements, taken during treadmill exercise, may reveal hypoxemia
• Serum electrolyte concentrations and fractional excretion of electrolytes can identify electrolyte disturbances

IMAGING
• ECG during exercise is mandatory to identify the specific form of arrhythmia
• Once EAAs have been identified, 24 h continuous ECG is used to determine whether the arrhythmia is also present at rest
• Owing to their portability smartphone ECG devices can be useful. Recording after exercise may identify individuals that warrant more extensive ECG studies

OTHER DIAGNOSTIC PROCEDURES
Dynamic airway endoscopy can identify predisposing respiratory disorders.

PATHOLOGIC FINDINGS
Gross and histologic examination of the heart is often unremarkable but myocardial necrosis, fibrosis, or inflammation may be identified.

TREATMENT
• With arrhythmias confined to the warmup and postexercise periods, no treatment may be necessary
• In horses that have multiple premature depolarizations during maximal exercise, the possibility of collapse during exercise and consequent risk to a rider must be considered
• Treatment should be aimed at predisposing diseases
• In the absence of obvious causes, rest and corticosteroids are recommended with around a 40% chance that the arrhythmia will resolve

MEDICATIONS

DRUG(S) OF CHOICE
• For treatment of myocardial pathology, corticosteroids such as prednisolone (1 mg/kg PO every 48 h) or dexamethasone (0.05–0.1 mg/kg IV or 0.1 mg/kg PO every 24 h for 3–4 days and then continued every 3–4 days in decreasing dosages) are recommended
• Vitamin C (20 mg/kg PO every 24 h) and vitamin E (10 IU/kg PO every 24 h) may also be beneficial owing to their antioxidant effect

CONTRAINDICATIONS/POSSIBLE INTERACTIONS
High-dose corticosteroid therapy has been associated with laminitis, particularly in cases in which other laminitis risk factors such as systemic illness and excessive body condition are present.

FOLLOW-UP

PATIENT MONITORING
Exercising ECGs following treatment are used to assess efficacy.

POSSIBLE COMPLICATIONS
• Ventricular arrhythmias at exercise can lead to collapse or sudden death with consequent risk to a rider
• Frequent supraventricular arrhythmias may predispose the horse to the development of atrial fibrillation and more severe exercise intolerance

EXPECTED COURSE AND PROGNOSIS
• Many apparently healthy horses have EAAs consisting of atrioventricular block, usually immediately after strenuous exercise, sinus arrhythmia in the warmup and postexercise phases, or isolated supraventricular or ventricular premature depolarizations at any stage, providing there are no more than 2 at strenuous exercise
• Horses with frequent premature depolarizations during strenuous exercise or with paroxysmal atrial fibrillation will show more severe signs. Paroxysmal atrial fibrillation often occurs only once but frequent premature depolarizations tend to persist and will cause ongoing performance problems if they cannot be treated successfully

MISCELLANEOUS

SEE ALSO
• Atrial fibrillation
• Dynamic collapse of the upper airways
• Myocardial disease
• Supraventricular arrhythmias
• Ventricular arrhythmias

ABBREVIATIONS
EAA = exercise-associated arrhythmia

Suggested Reading
Slack J, Boston RC, Soma LR, Reef VB. Occurrence of cardiac arrhythmias in Standardbred racehorses. Equine Vet J 2015;47:398–404.

Author Celia M. Marr
Consulting Editor Celia M. Marr and Virginia B. Reef

EXERCISE-INDUCED PULMONARY HEMORRHAGE (EIPH)

BASICS

OVERVIEW
• EIPH is defined as the presence of blood in the airways after exercise
• Pathophysiology unknown. Current speculation—exercising horses have high cardiac outputs and vascular pressures. Repeated bouts of venous hypertension during strenuous exercise cause intrapulmonary vein wall remodeling and collagen accumulation, venous occlusion, and pulmonary capillary hypertension in the caudodorsal regions of the lung. Subjected to high pressures, there is capillary stress failure and bleeding into the interstitium and alveolar spaces. Blood in the interstitium or alveoli elicits an inflammatory reaction that contributes to bronchointerstitial fibrosis and arterial neovascularization, which may also be a source of hemorrhage during subsequent exercise
• Worldwide distribution

SIGNALMENT
• Most commonly described in horses that run at high speed
• Reported frequency based on postexercise endoscopy—>80% in racing Thoroughbreds, 87% in Standardbreds, 62% in racing Quarter Horses
• Other breeds could be affected—associated with exercise
• Occurs with onset of strenuous exercise and training, thus from 2 years of age
• Males, geldings, and females are equally affected

SIGNS
• Commonly, no external clinical signs
• Rarely, epistaxis can occur during or after exercise (0.1–9%)
• Performance could be impaired

CAUSES AND RISK FACTORS
• Strenuous exercise
• Less commonly, underlying parenchymal disease

DIAGNOSIS

DIFFERENTIAL DIAGNOSIS
• Epistaxis—ethmoid hematoma, guttural pouch mycosis, trauma, coagulopathy
• Airway blood—pulmonary abscess, pneumonia, foreign body, neoplasia

CBC/BIOCHEMISTRY/URINALYSIS
Usually, no significant abnormalities.

OTHER LABORATORY TESTS
Tracheal wash or bronchoalveolar lavage fluid cytology (high sensitivity and specificity)—presence of red blood cells and macrophages with intracytoplasmic hemosiderin (hemosiderophages). Provides information on severity and duration of EIPH.

IMAGING
• Thoracic ultrasonography—comet tail artifacts caudodorsally (high sensitivity, low specificity)
• Thoracic radiography—increased homogeneous parenchymal density in caudodorsal lung fields (low sensitivity)

OTHER DIAGNOSTIC PROCEDURES
Tracheal endoscopy 30–120 min after strenuous exercise. Severity is assessed with a 0–4 scoring system. Repeated endoscopies increase sensitivity.

PATHOLOGIC FINDINGS
Gross
• Characteristic patchy to multifocal, symmetric, blue-brown staining of the parenchyma in the caudodorsal regions of the caudal lung lobe
• Foci of subpleural scarring with enhanced subpleural vasculature

Histopathologic
• Remodeling of small pulmonary veins characterized by accumulation of adventitial collagen
• Bronchiolitis
• Hemosiderophages in the alveolar lumen and interstitial spaces
• Fibrosis of interlobular septa, pleura, and around vessels and bronchioles

TREATMENT
• No known treatment
• Rest (30 days to 1 year) may help parenchymal repair
• Reduce the intensity of athletic activity if exercise is continued

MEDICATIONS

DRUG(S) OF CHOICE
• Furosemide (0.5–1 mg/kg IV) 4 h before strenuous exercise. There is high-quality evidence that furosemide decreases the severity and incidence of EIPH
• Other treatments (aminocaproic acid, bronchodilators, corticosteroids, NSAIDs, pentoxifylline, nasal strip)—low-quality evidence that EIPH severity is affected
• Treat lower airway disease if present—see chapter Inflammatory airway diseases—IAD in performance horses (mild and moderate equine asthma)

CONTRAINDICATIONS/POSSIBLE INTERACTIONS
Chronic furosemide administration, especially if the horse is dehydrated, may predispose to electrolyte disorders. The use of furosemide is prohibited by many racing jurisdictions.

FOLLOW-UP

PATIENT MONITORING
• Repeat endoscopy after subsequent strenuous activities provides information on the frequency and severity of the condition
• If severe bleeding, repeat examination in 24–48 h to make sure bleeding has stopped; may indicate intercurrent disease

PREVENTION/AVOIDANCE
Administration of furosemide during training helps to reduce incidence and severity of EIPH episodes.

POSSIBLE COMPLICATIONS
The link between EIPH and sudden death has yet to be clarified.

EXPECTED COURSE AND PROGNOSIS
• There is evidence that EIPH is a progressive pathology and that affected horses have shorter racing careers
• Resolution of lung pathology especially with continued strenuous exercise is unlikely

MISCELLANEOUS

SEE ALSO
• Hemorrhagic nasal discharge
• Inflammatory airway diseases—IAD in performance horses (mild and moderate equine asthma)

ABBREVIATIONS
• EIPH = exercise-induced pulmonary hemorrhage
• NSAID = nonsteroidal anti-inflammatory drug

Suggested Reading
Hinchcliff KW, Couetil LL, Knight PK, et al. Exercise induced pulmonary hemorrhage in horses: American College of Veterinary Internal Medicine consensus statement. J Vet Intern Med 2015;29:743–758.

Author Francesco Ferrucci
Consulting Editors Mathilde Leclère and Daniel Jean
Acknowledgment The author and editors acknowledge the prior contribution of John R. Pascoe.

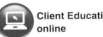
Client Education Handout available online

E

EXERCISE INTOLERANCE IN SPORT HORSES

BASICS

DEFINITION
• "Sport horses" are horses involved in equestrian sports such as dressage, show jumping, eventing, endurance, driving, and polo
• Exercise intolerance is the inability of the horse to accomplish work at its intended level, during either training or competition

PATHOPHYSIOLOGY
• Performance results from the capacity of all body systems to coordinate and function optimally
• Exercise intolerance can be caused by an insufficiency in any one or several of the body systems participating to exertion. It can also be related to poor genetic potential, incapacity of the rider or an inadequate level of training or competition, inadequate diet, or environment
• Limiting factors to performance vary according to the equestrian discipline in which the horse is involved (i.e. impaired oxygen transport chain or thermoregulation in eventers, dehydration, electrolyte, or substrate depletion in endurance horses)

SYSTEMS AFFECTED
• Behavioral
• Musculoskeletal
• Neuromuscular
• Respiratory
• Cardiovascular
• Dental
• Gastrointestinal
• Endocrine/metabolic
• Hemic/lymphatic/immune
• Nervous

SIGNALMENT
Young horses are more likely to suffer from inexperience or lack of fitness and infectious and congenital diseases (cardiac or upper airway). Older horses are more likely to have chronic or degenerative diseases (musculoskeletal, lower airway, or cardiac).

SIGNS

General Comments
• Can be subclinical or accompanied by overt signs such as lameness, respiratory noise, tying-up, etc.
• Lameness or irregular gait
• Defensive behavior, reluctance to work
• Inability to gain fitness or improve body condition, muscle wastage
• Labored breathing or breathlessness
• Respiratory noise
• Premature fatigue
• Excessive sweating
• Prolonged cardiorespiratory recovery

Historical Findings
• Competitive records should be examined to evaluate if the horse has had consistent previous performances
• Are symptoms evident only during regular training or during competition? Timing of the symptoms (onset, mid-, or end of exercise)
• Is there evidence of concomitant disease?

Physical Examination Findings
• Body condition score, general conformation, and attitude
• HR, pulse, mucosa, capillary refill time. Is there a jugular pulse, pathologic arrhythmias, or murmurs on auscultation?
• Breathing pattern, respiratory rate, lymph node size, laryngeal palpation, tracheobronchial and lung auscultation (rebreathing bag)
• Musculoskeletal—symmetry, conformation, and stance of limbs or articulations, digital pulse, areas of heat, swelling, stiffness, pain, amyotrophy, or decreased range of motion
• Lameness examination
• Ridden examination

CAUSES

Musculoskeletal
• Lameness (can be subclinical)
• Neurologic disorders (can be subclinical)
• Rhabdomyolysis
• Vitamin E, selenium deficiency

Respiratory
• Upper airway disorders
• Dynamic upper airway obstruction (can be noiseless)
• Lower airway diseases
   ○ Equine asthma (Inflammatory airway disease)
   ○ EIPH
   ○ Pulmonary edema—cardiogenic or noncardiogenic

Cardiovascular
• Acquired cardiovascular defects (valvular regurgitation, chamber dilation)
• Congenital cardiovascular defects (ventricular septal defect)
• Exercising arrhythmia (e.g. atrial fibrillation, ventricular premature contraction, supraventricular premature contraction)
• Anemia

Digestive System
• Inadequate diet
• Dental disorders
• Gastric ulcers
• Parasitic infection
• Inflammatory bowel disease

Other
• Endocrine disorders
• Poor equitation
• Inadequate training (under- or overtraining)
• Infectious diseases (can be subclinical)

RISK FACTORS

Environment
• Hygiene of the buildings (e.g. exposure, volume, ventilation, dust, drainage)
• Quality of transport vehicles
• Access to paddocks, walker, outdoor tracks
• Quality of footing

Rider and Equipment
• Rider proficiency and competitive records
• Ill-fitting and hygiene of tack or protections
• Farriery

Training and Management
• Diet and forage
• Training and competitive schedule

DIAGNOSIS

CBC/BIOCHEMISTRY/URINALYSIS
• Hematology, inflammatory proteins (serum proteins, fibrinogen, serum amyloid A)
• Electrolytes, urea, creatinine
• Muscle enzyme activity (aspartate aminotransferase, creatine kinase), vitamin E, glutathione peroxidase
• Cardiac troponin I

OTHER LABORATORY TESTS
• Functional variables—lactates (over a standardized exercise test), arterial blood gas analysis
• Respiratory viruses
• Serology for leptospirosis, piroplasmosis, borreliosis, or ehrlichiosis
• Adrenocorticotropic hormone for suspected subclinical pituitary pars intermedia dysfunction

IMAGING

Radiography
• According to lameness examination
• Skeletal, articular, or synovial abnormalities of foot, limbs, neck, back

Ultrasonography
• Tendon, ligament, muscular, or articular imaging
• Doppler echocardiography

Endoscopy
• Endoscopy is essential for diagnosing obstructive upper airway diseases
• Resting endoscopy is useful to identify anatomic defects, masses, mucus, or blood in the airways
• Exercising videoendoscopy is necessary to assess upper airway function and patency, especially when noise is absent. Overground endoscopy during a ridden exercise should be preferred as it allows assessment of the effect of rider and equitation. Sufficient exertion is necessary to elicit symptoms and reproduction of competitive exercise might be indicated
• Gastroscopy

OTHER DIAGNOSTIC PROCEDURES

Exercise Testing
• Standardized exercise test with measurement of HR, lactates, speed, incline either ridden or on a treadmill to evaluate physiologic response of the horse to exercise and help orientate diagnosis. Can be associated with upper airway endoscopy
• Abnormal increase in lactates can be caused by lack of training or disturbance in the oxygen transportation chain (respiratory system, cardiovascular system, anemia, muscular metabolism), exercise in hot or hot and humid conditions. Increased HR can also be caused by the latter as well as pain (of musculoskeletal, gastric or urogenital origin)
• Both lactates and HR are influenced by level of training and athleticism

ECG
Ideally during sufficient exertion to elicit and detect pathologic arrhythmias.

Respiratory Samples
• Cytology, bacterial and fungal culture of tracheal wash to diagnose airway infection
• Cytology of bronchoalveolar lavage to diagnose lower airway inflammation and EIPH

MEDICATIONS

• Depend on cause of exercise intolerance
• Use of medication during competition is strictly regulated and most drugs are prohibited in sport horses participating in competitions. There are some regional, national, or international variations according to the competent regulatory authority
• Thorough knowledge of antidoping rules is essential. Sufficient withdrawal times should be applied

FOLLOW-UP

Regular veterinary follow-up examinations in healthy and performing individuals are useful to prevent the occurrence of disease and monitor training and recovery from competition and to adapt competitive schedule.

EXPECTED COURSE AND PROGNOSIS
Dependent on cause of exercise intolerance.

MISCELLANEOUS

SEE ALSO
• Atrial fibrillation
• Dorsal displacement of the soft palate (DDSP)
• Dynamic collapse of the upper airways
• Exercise-associated arrhythmias
• Exercise-induced pulmonary hemorrhage (EIPH)
• Exertional rhabdomyolysis syndrome
• Inflammatory airway diseases—IAD in performance horses (mild and moderate equine asthma)
• Laryngeal hemiparesis/hemiplegia (recurrent laryngeal neuropathy)
• Osteoarthritis
• Tendonitis

ABBREVIATIONS
• EIPH = exercise-induced pulmonary hemorrhage
• HR = heart rate
• RR = respiratory rate

Internet Resources
Fédération Equestre Internationale (FEI). www.fei.org

Suggested Reading
Hinchcliff KW, Kaneps AJ, Geor RJ. Equine Sports Medicine and Surgery, 2e. Edinburgh, UK: Saunders Elsevier, 2013.
Hodgson DR, McKeever KH, McGowan CM. The Athletic Horse: Principles and Practice of Equine Sports Medicine, 2e. St. Louis, MO: Elsevier Saunders, 2013.
Marlin D, Nankervis KJ. Equine Exercise Physiology. Oxford, UK: Wiley Blackwell, 2013.
Parente EJ. Diagnostic techniques for upper airway obstruction. In: Robinson NE, ed. Current Therapy in Equine Medicine, 4e. Philadelphia, PA: WB Saunders, 1997:401–403.

Author Emmanuelle van Erck-Westergren
Consulting Editor Jean-Pierre Lavoie

E

EXERTIONAL RHABDOMYOLYSIS

 BASICS

DEFINITION
Exercise-induced muscle necrosis.

PATHOPHYSIOLOGY
• Exercise-induced skeletal muscle necrosis results in release of CK and myoglobin into circulation, often with stiffness, cramping, and pain; severe myoglobinuria can result in renal tubular damage and renal insufficiency. • ER can occur as an acquired disorder associated with overexertion, heat exhaustion, viral infections, and other factors; however, it is most commonly associated with heritable muscular disorders including RER and PSSM.

SYSTEMS AFFECTED
• Musculoskeletal • Renal

GENETICS
• In Thoroughbreds, RER is an autosomal dominant trait potentially associated with disturbed intracellular calcium regulation. Causative genetic defect is currently unknown. • In Quarter Horses and related breeds, and Belgian drafts, PSSM is an autosomal dominant trait related to a mutation in the glycogen synthase 1 gene (*GYS1*). Homozygotes and horses that concurrently carry the malignant hyperthermia-associated mutation of the ryanodine receptor gene (*RYR1*) tend to have more severe clinical signs.

INCIDENCE/PREVALENCE
• RER affects ~5–7% of racing Thoroughbreds. • PSSM affects ~6–10% of Quarter Horses, higher prevalence in halter Quarter Horses (~28%). In Belgian drafts, prevalence approaches 40%

GEOGRAPHIC DISTRIBUTION
Worldwide

SIGNALMENT
Breed Predilections
Thoroughbreds, Quarter Horses, Appaloosa, Paint, Belgian draft, Percheron, Arabian, Standardbred, Warmblood, many other light breeds.

Mean Age and Range
• For PSSM, mean age of onset of signs in Quarter Horses is ~5 years (range 1 day to late maturity). • In Thoroughbred racehorses, 2-year-olds most frequently affected. • In Arabian endurance horses, clinical disease >5 years of age and often in older horses

Predominant Sex
• In Thoroughbreds and Standardbred racehorses, 2–3-year-old females more likely to be affected. Sex bias resolves with increasing age. • Sex predilection not reported for the other disorders

SIGNS
General Comments
• Frequency and severity of rhabdomyolysis episodes can be very variable between and within individuals. • Clinical signs can occur any time from immediately before exercise until sometimes hours after exercise. • Subclinical disease (elevated CK/AST only) can occur with few clinically visible abnormalities, and may be a particular risk in endurance horses

Historical Findings
• Possible triggering factors—training regime changes, ration changes, prior rest period. • Variable signs from mild stilted gait to severe sweating, stiffness, and recumbency. • Repeated episodes may be observed

Physical Examination Findings
• Exercise intolerance. • Stiffness, stilted gait. • Sweating. • Reluctance to move. • Swollen and/or fasciculating muscles. • Tachycardia, tachypnea. • Distress. • Recumbency. • Pawing, stretching, discomfort. • Discolored (red/brown) urine. • Muscle atrophy. • Usually normal between episodes

CAUSES
Acquired Causes
• Exercise exceeding level of training. • Exhaustive exercise. • Dietary electrolyte and mineral imbalance. • Electrolyte depletion during exercise. • Vitamin E and/or selenium deficiency. • Influenza

Inherited Causes
• In Thoroughbred RER, defective calcium regulation resulting in a low threshold for muscle contraction; ±analogous disorder in Standardbreds. • In PSSM, heritable defect of glycogen metabolism recognized in Quarter Horses, Paints, some drafts, and related breeds

RISK FACTORS
• High starch (grain) diet. • >24 h of stall rest in horses with underlying muscle disease. • Sudden interruption of exercise routine. • Infectious respiratory disease. • Nervous temperament (Thoroughbreds, polo horses). • Lameness (Thoroughbreds). • Genetic predisposition. • High level of fitness (Thoroughbreds, Arabians)

 DIAGNOSIS

DIFFERENTIAL DIAGNOSIS
• Association between exercise and onset of signs in addition to physical examination and laboratory findings facilitates differentiation from other conditions. • Conditions causing reluctance to move, acute recumbency, and/or discolored urine, including:
◦ Lameness/laminitis. ◦ Colic.
◦ Pleuropneumonia. ◦ Tetanus. ◦ Lactation

tetany. ◦ Diseases causing intravascular hemolysis or bilirubinuria. ◦ Neurologic disease. ◦ Aortoiliac thrombosis. ◦ HYPP

CBC/BIOCHEMISTRY/URINALYSIS
• Elevated serum CK, AST, and lactate dehydrogenase. • Myoglobinuria. • ±Hypochloremia, hypocalcemia, hyponatremia, hyperkalemia (severe disease). • ±Metabolic alkalosis or acidosis. • ±Elevated serum creatinine and urea nitrogen

OTHER LABORATORY TESTS
• Urinary fractional excretion of electrolytes. • Blood selenium and serum/plasma vitamin E

IMAGING
N/A

OTHER DIAGNOSTIC PROCEDURES
• PCR testing of blood or hair for *GYS1* mutation in PSSM breeds. • Semimembranosus muscle biopsy in non-PSSM breeds (Warmbloods, Arabians). • Submaximal exercise test—serum CK activity before 15 min of walk and trot exercise, then 4–6 h later >2–3-fold CK increase is considered suspicious. This test has greatest utility in PSSM

PATHOLOGIC FINDINGS
• In RER, nonspecific muscle changes (increased centrally located nuclei, myocyte degeneration and regeneration). • In PSSM, abnormal polysaccharide inclusions if >2 years of age, subsarcolemmal vacuolations. • Arabian horses with ER—abnormal cytoplasmic desmin accumulation in myocytes

 TREATMENT

APPROPRIATE HEALTH CARE
• Aims of treatment—reduce discomfort and anxiety, prevent further damage, normalize hydration, acid–base and electrolyte status, and restore or protect renal function. • Severe rhabdomyolysis is an emergency. Inpatient management recommended to facilitate fluid therapy. Further muscle damage can occur with transport; less severe cases can be managed as outpatients

NURSING CARE
• IV or oral fluid therapy with balanced electrolyte solutions until myoglobinuria resolves. • Alkalinizing fluids in myoglobinuric horses with metabolic acidosis to protect against renal injury. • Deep bedding, particularly for recumbent patients. • ±Slinging to prevent prolonged recumbency and further muscle trauma

ACTIVITY
• After mild episode, commence gentle exercise (at reduced intensity and duration than prior to episode) in 24–48 h if clinical signs of stiffness have resolved. • With severe episode, remain stall confined until recovered. Low-intensity exercise (hand-walking) initiated when clinical signs and serial CK improves

DIET
• Low-starch diet (grass hay) according to caloric requirements. • In RER-susceptible horses, avoid >2.2 kg (5 lb) of grain per day. • In PSSM-susceptible horses, no grain. • ±Fat supplements (rice bran, vegetable oil) and soluble fibers (beat pulp) if higher caloric requirements exist. • Eliminate high-starch supplements (molasses)

CLIENT EDUCATION
• Susceptible horses should not be stall rested for >24 h at a time. Frequent exercise is preventative. • Daily turnout or forced daily exercise (riding or lunge work) is ideal. Interruption of routine exercise is a prominent risk factor. • Restrict dietary starch. High caloric requirements met with supplemental fat sources. • Discuss breeding management when underlying hereditary muscle disorder is suspected

SURGICAL CONSIDERATIONS
N/A

MEDICATIONS
DRUG(S) OF CHOICE
• For significant distress and pain, xylazine (0.2–0.4 mg/kg) or detomidine (0.01–0.02 mg/kg IM or IV); butorphanol (0.01–0.04 mg/kg IM or IV or as a CRI at 23.7 µg/kg/h after a loading dose of 17.8 µg/kg IV); or lidocaine (CRI at 30–50 µg/kg/min after a loading dose of 1.3 mg/kg IV slowly). Flunixin meglumine (1.1 mg/kg IV or PO) or phenylbutazone (2.2–4.4 mg/kg IV or PO). • Muscle relaxants—methocarbamol (5–22 mg/kg IV slowly every 6–12 h) or dantrolene sodium (4–6 mg/kg PO every 12–24 h). Give dantrolene within 4 h of feeding for adequate absorption. • Prevention—dantrolene 60–90 min prior to exercise

CONTRAINDICATIONS
• Avoid NSAIDs in azotemic or significantly myoglobinuric horses. • Avoid dantrolene in horses with hyperkalemia or HYPP

PRECAUTIONS
• Use caution with drugs that depress blood pressure in horses with myoglobinuria or azotemia, and correct dehydration prior to use

POSSIBLE INTERACTIONS
None

ALTERNATIVE DRUGS
Diazepam (0.05–0.5 mg/kg slow IV).

FOLLOW-UP
PATIENT MONITORING
• After mild to moderate ER, resume exercise after stiffness resolves. • Severe ER requires longer recuperation. Resume exercise after substantial CK and AST reduction. • In PSSM, mild elevations of CK and AST can persist; resume exercise when clinical signs resolve

PREVENTION/AVOIDANCE
• Daily exercise and avoiding stall rest are critically important for prevention in susceptible horses. • Eliminate/reduce high-starch feeds. Grass hay (1.5–2.0% body weight) with supplemental fat sources (rice bran, oil, commercial high-fat feeds) to meet higher caloric needs. Susceptible horses fed minimal grain. • Young anxious Thoroughbreds may benefit from stress-reducing management changes, such as feeding and exercising them before others and low-dose sedatives before training. • In sporadic ER, appropriate training regimes that prepare them for their intended athletic use

POSSIBLE COMPLICATIONS
• Acute or chronic renal insufficiency from myoglobinuria. • ± Atrophy of affected muscles weeks to months after severe episode

EXPECTED COURSE AND PROGNOSIS
• Horses with sporadic acquired ER have good prognosis with appropriate management. • Horses with mild to moderate signs of PSSM or RER usually respond to a disciplined routine of daily exercise and appropriate dietary changes. • PSSM horses with late onset of signs have good prognosis if the triggering management changes are identified and addressed. • PSSM horses developing signs early (<1 year of age) may have a less favorable prognosis for athletic function. • Horses with repeated and severe episodes of muscle necrosis have poor prognosis for athletic function if they display limited response to appropriate dietary and training changes. • Horses with acute or chronic renal insufficiency due to rhabdomyolysis have a good to guarded prognosis depending on severity and response to treatment

MISCELLANEOUS
ASSOCIATED CONDITIONS
Renal insufficiency.

AGE-RELATED FACTORS
Different disorders can vary in likely age of presentation.

ZOONOTIC POTENTIAL
None

PREGNANCY/FERTILITY/BREEDING
Avoid breeding horses with heritable disorders of muscle function.

SEE ALSO
Polysaccharide storage myopathy

ABBREVIATIONS
• AST = aspartate aminotransferase
• CK = creatine kinase
• CRI = constant rate infusion
• ER = exertional rhabdomyolysis
• HYPP = hyperkalemic periodic paralysis
• NSAID = nonsteroidal anti-inflammatory drug
• PCR = polymerase chain reaction
• PSSM = polysaccharide storage myopathy
• RER = recurrent exertional rhabdomyolysis

Suggested Reading
Piercy RJ, Rivero JL. Muscle disorders of equine athletes. In: Hinchcliff KW, Kaneps AJ, Geor RJ, eds. Equine Sports Medicine and Surgery, 2e. Edinburgh, UK: Saunders Elsevier, 2014:109–143.
Valberg SJ. Muscling in on the cause of tying-up. Proc Am Assoc Equine Pract 2012;58:85–123.
Valberg SJ. Diseases of muscle. In: Smith BP, ed. Large Animal Internal Medicine, 5e. St. Louis, MO: Elsevier Mosby, 2015:1276–1308.

Author Erica C. McKenzie
Consulting Editor Elizabeth J. Davidson

E

EXPIRATORY DYSPNEA

BASICS

DEFINITION
• In animals, dyspnea is used to describe clinical signs associated with difficult, labored breathing or respiratory distress, which can be present throughout the respiratory cycle or be primarily associated with either inhalation (i.e. inspiratory dyspnea) or exhalation (i.e. expiratory dyspnea)
• The lay term for expiratory dyspnea in horses (i.e. heaves) describes the prolonged abdominal push at the end of expiration

PATHOPHYSIOLOGY
• As a primary clinical sign, usually associated with obstruction of the lower (intrathoracic) airways by mucus, edema, or bronchospasm; the abdominal muscles are recruited to move air out of the lungs through partially obstructed airways and a forced abdominal exhalation is noticeable
• Can also accompany inspiratory dyspnea in any animal with severe impairment of gas exchange

SYSTEMS AFFECTED
• Respiratory
• Cardiovascular
• Hemic/lymphatic/immune

INCIDENCE/PREVALENCE
Unknown

GEOGRAPHIC DISTRIBUTION
Worldwide

SIGNALMENT
Depends on the underlying cause, but equine asthma usually occurs in mature to old animals.

SIGNS
• Expiratory dyspnea is a sign, but associated signs can indicate the source of dyspnea
• An accompanying cough indicates inflammation of the tracheobronchial tree
• Inflammation of the lower airway can result in bilateral mucopurulent nasal discharge
• Unilateral or bilateral nasal discharge, either purulent or hemorrhagic, can be a sign of a nasal or pharyngeal mass causing severe airway obstruction
• Accompanying inspiratory dyspnea and loud respiratory noises are indicative of a fixed airway obstruction (e.g. mass encroaching into the upper airways)

Historical Findings
Exposure to environmental risk factors (e.g. indoor housing, poor ventilation, dust, humidity, ammonia, use of hay or straw containing microorganisms such as microscopic molds and bacteria).

Physical Examination Findings
• Forced and prolonged abdominal component to expiration, particularly obvious at end exhalation. If severe, the horse may rock forward during the abdominal effort

• Bulging and mobilization of the anus, synchronous to breathing (abdominal effort raises intra-abdominal pressure)
• Hypertrophy of the external abdominal muscle can be seen ("heaves line")
• Flared nostrils and increased excursions of the thorax during breathing are common since dyspnea is often mixed (expiratory and inspiratory)
• Fixed airway obstruction—nasal discharge, sometimes foul breath, and both inspiratory and expiratory dyspnea
• Bronchitis/bronchiolitis—cough, wheezing audible on lung auscultation, increased breath sounds or crackles on both inhalation and exhalation,
• Anxiety and anorexia can occur
• Cyanotic mucosa in severe cases
• Fever is unusual without a viral or bacterial cause

CAUSES

Respiratory
• Extrathoracic causes are usually accompanied by inspiratory dyspnea—congestion of the nasal mucosa (e.g. Horner syndrome, inflammatory disease), deviation of the nasal septum, space-occupying lesion affecting the nasal cavity (e.g. foreign body, intraluminal mass, ethmoid hematoma, extraluminal mass or swelling), congenital pharyngeal cysts, space-occupying masses encroaching on the pharynx (e.g. enlarged lymph nodes), guttural pouch enlargement (usually by tympanites), deformity of the larynx (e.g. edema, epiglottiditis, chondritis), and tracheal obstruction caused by trauma, masses, or a foreign body (see chapter Inspiratory dyspnea)
• Lower respiratory tract—equine asthma (heaves, pasture asthma), pulmonary edema, infiltrative disease of the alveolar interstitium (interstitial pneumonia)

Nonrespiratory
Medical conditions causing heart failure.

RISK FACTORS
See the individual conditions causing expiratory dyspnea.

DIAGNOSIS

DIFFERENTIAL DIAGNOSIS

Differential Similar Signs
• Inspiratory dyspnea is characterized by an enhanced thoracic component to inhalation and is accompanied by a loud inspiratory noise (stridor)
• Tachypnea is not accompanied by prolonged exhalation
• Deep breathing after strenuous exertion has a marked inspiratory and expiratory component

Differential Causes
• Fixed upper airway obstructions produce severe respiratory distress on both inhalation and exhalation and are accompanied by a loud respiratory noise
• Fever, malaise, and inappetence can indicate infectious inflammatory disease
• Expiratory dyspnea of gradual onset, precipitated by an environmental cause and accompanied by cough in an afebrile mature horse, is indicative of equine asthma (heaves, recurrent airway obstruction, pasture asthma)
• Expiratory dyspnea of sudden onset in a febrile young horse is indicative of pulmonary edema or infectious bronchiolitis or pneumonia. The latter can include interstitial pneumonia (toxic ingestion or inhalation, smoke inhalation, EMPF, MEED)
• Once a fixed upper airway obstruction is ruled out, equine asthma is the most likely cause of expiratory dyspnea

CBC/BIOCHEMISTRY/URINALYSIS
Dependent on causes.

OTHER LABORATORY TESTS
• With fixed airway obstruction, arterial blood gas analysis identifies hypoventilation (i.e. increased $PaCO_2$) and hypoxemia (i.e. low PaO_2), with the increase in $PaCO_2$ being almost equal to the decrease in PaO_2
• Bronchitis/bronchiolitis usually is accompanied by obvious hypoxemia (i.e. PaO_2 <80 mmHg), with only a slightly elevated $PaCO_2$ (i.e. 45–50 mmHg)

IMAGING

Radiography
• May identify a mass causing a fixed obstruction in the nose, pharynx, larynx, or trachea
• Bronchitis/bronchiolitis may not produce diagnostic radiographic signs
• Edema and diffuse interstitial alveolar disease may be observed as a diffuse increase in density
• A miliary or nodular pattern can be seen in cases of MEED or EMNP

Endoscopy
• Essential for diagnosing a fixed airway obstruction
• Can be used to assess the presence of exudate in the trachea, which is a sign of inflammation of the lower airways and lung, or edema

OTHER DIAGNOSTIC PROCEDURES
• Cytology of the lower airways, preferably by BAL can be used to determine the presence of lower airway inflammation
• Bacterial and fungal culture of tracheal mucus or tracheal lavage revealing a relatively pure culture of a known pathogen is suggestive of infection
• PCR for EHV-5 on BAL

PATHOLOGIC FINDINGS
Dependent on the cause of the dyspnea.

TREATMENT

AIMS
Maintain ventilation and gas exchange.

APPROPRIATE HEALTH CARE
In- or outpatient medical management.

NURSING CARE
• Supplemental oxygenation via a nasotracheal or nasopharyngeal catheter relieves hypoxemia and accompanying distress when dyspnea results from lung disease
• With fixed airway obstruction, oxygen can be life-saving until the problem is surgically corrected
• Equine asthma—move horse to a low-dust environment

DIET
Equine asthma—use low-dust diet such as pasture (except for the pasture-associated form), complete pelleted feed, haylage, steamed hay, or treated hay.

CLIENT EDUCATION
If the cause of expiratory dyspnea is equine asthma, emphasize the importance of eliminating contact with dust and microorganisms, which can be coming from feed and bedding in a stable or from dusty paddocks.

SURGICAL CONSIDERATIONS
• Relieve a fixed upper airway obstruction sufficient to cause panic or life-threatening hypoxemia by tracheotomy. Tracheotomy is not useful for relief of dyspnea originating in the lower airways
• Nasotracheal intubation also can be used to bypass the obstruction, especially when it is to be corrected surgically within a short time

 MEDICATIONS

DRUG(S) OF CHOICE
• Dependent on cause of the dyspnea. Therapy should aim at insuring oxygen delivery to the tissues, reducing inflammation, and alleviating bronchoconstriction. Antimicrobial therapy should be undertaken in case of infection
• Bronchodilators—atropine, or the safer butylhyoscine (butylscopolamine) provides rapid relief from dyspnea but can have serious side effects; other bronchodilators, either oral (e.g. clenbuterol 0.8–3.2 mg/kg every 12 h) or inhaled (e.g. ipratropium bromide 2–3 µg/kg, albuterol (salbutamol) 1–2 µg/kg, fenoterol 2–3 µg/kg) should be used for maintenance
• Corticosteroids are the only anti-inflammatory drugs effective in equine asthma, systemic or inhaled treatments are advocated (see chapter Equine asthma)
• In cases of primary or secondary pulmonary edema, furosemide can be used for its diuretic, vasodilator, and bronchodilator effects (0.5–1 mg/kg every 12 h)
• EMPF—based on the association with EHV-5, antiviral agents such as valacyclovir (valaciclovir) have been used, with or without corticosteroids
• In case of severe dyspnea, oxygen therapy is indicated

 FOLLOW-UP

PATIENT MONITORING
Equine asthma is a chronic problem that recurs whenever horses are exposed to the dusts and antigens that initiate the hypersensitivity response.

POSSIBLE COMPLICATIONS
Atropine may cause ileus and colic signs.

 MISCELLANEOUS

PREGNANCY/FERTILITY/BREEDING
Fetal growth retardation and fetal death may be observed in mares with severely compromised respiratory function.

SEE ALSO
• Aspiration pneumonia
• Diaphragmatic hernia

• Equine asthma
• Equine herpesvirus 5
• Fungal pneumonia
• Heaves (severe equine asthma, RAO)
• Inspiratory dyspnea
• Multisystemic eosinophilic epitheliotropic disease
• Pleuropneumonia
• Pneumothorax
• Summer pasture-associated equine asthma (pasture asthma)

ABBREVIATIONS
• BAL = bronchoalveolar lavage
• EHV-5 = equine herpesvirus 5
• EMPF = equine multinodular pulmonary fibrosis
• MEED = multisystemic eosinophilic epitheliotropic disease
• $PaCO_2$ = partial pressure of carbon dioxide in arterial blood
• PaO_2 = partial pressure of oxygen in arterial blood
• PCR = polymerase chain reaction

Suggested Reading
Hannas CM, Derksen FJ. Principles of emergency respiratory therapy. In: Colahan PT, Mayhew IG, Merritt AM, Moore JM, eds. Equine Medicine and Surgery, 4e. Goleta, CA: American Veterinary Publications, 1991:372–374.
Lavoie J-P. Recurrent airway obstruction (heaves) and summer-pasture-associated obstructive pulmonary disease. In: McGorum BC, Dixon PM, Robinson NE, Schumacher J, eds. Equine Respiratory Medicine and Surgery. Philadelphia, PA: WB Saunders, 2006:565–589.
McGorum BC, Dixon PM. Clinical examination of the respiratory tract. In: McGorum BC, Dixon PM, Robinson NE, Schumacher J, eds. Equine Respiratory Medicine and Surgery. Philadelphia, PA: WB Saunders, 2006:103–117.

Author Emmanuelle van Erck-Westergren
Consulting Editors Mathilde Leclère and Daniel Jean
Acknowledgment The author and editors acknowledge the prior contribution of N. Edward Robinson.

EXUDATIVE OPTIC NEUROPATHY

BASICS

OVERVIEW
• Presents as white to gray, raised nodular masses spread across the surface of the optic disc, which is usually swollen/edematous. Large lesions may obscure the optic nerve head entirely
• Retinal and optic disc hemorrhages may also be present

SIGNALMENT
This rare condition is observed more frequently in older horses (>15 years).

SIGNS
• Sudden onset of total blindness in bilateral cases
• Dilated pupils

CAUSES AND RISK FACTORS
• Definitive cause is unknown
• Possible etiologies include trauma, acute massive systemic hemorrhage, and systemic infectious diseases, such as *Streptococcus equi* spp. *equi*, equine herpesvirus 1, and *Actinobacillus equuli*

DIAGNOSIS

DIFFERENTIAL DIAGNOSIS
Must be distinguished from:
• Benign proliferative optic neuropathy in aged horses with otherwise normal findings in a visual eye
• Other conditions presenting as masses on the optic nerve head, such as optic nerve neoplasia, traumatic optic neuropathy, and ischemic optic neuropathy

• Other causes of blindness, such as those due to cataracts, glaucoma, equine recurrent uveitis, retinal detachment, central nervous system disease

CBC/BIOCHEMISTRY/URINALYSIS
N/A

OTHER LABORATORY TESTS
N/A

IMAGING
N/A

OTHER DIAGNOSTIC PROCEDURES
Diagnosed by characteristic funduscopic appearance.

PATHOLOGIC FINDINGS
White nodules protruding from the optic nerve head anteriorly into the vitreous are observed macroscopically; gitter cells from the optic nerve are observed microscopically.

TREATMENT
N/A

MEDICATIONS
No known therapy has been effective.

CONTRAINDICATIONS/POSSIBLE INTERACTIONS
N/A

FOLLOW-UP

EXPECTED COURSE AND PROGNOSIS
Poor prognosis for vision.

MISCELLANEOUS

ASSOCIATED CONDITIONS
Dependent on cause.

AGE-RELATED FACTORS
Older horses.

SEE ALSO
• Equine recurrent uveitis
• Ischemic optic neuropathy
• Proliferative optic neuropathy

Suggested Reading
Brooks DE. Retinopathies and ocular manifestations of systemic diseases in the horse. In: Brooks DE, ed. Ophthalmology for the Equine Practitioner, 2e. Jackson, WY: Teton NewMedia, 2008:207–225.
Dubielzig RR, Ketring K, McLellan GJ, Albert DM. Veterinary Ocular Pathology. Philadelphia, PA: WB Saunders, 2010.
Gilger BC. Equine ophthalmology. In: Gelatt KN, Gilger BC, Kern TJ, eds. Veterinary Ophthalmology, 5e. Ames, IA: Wiley Blackwell, 2013:1560–1609.
Nell B, Walde I. Posterior segment diseases. Equine Vet J Suppl 2010;37:69–79.
Wilkie DA. Diseases of the ocular posterior segment. In: Gilger BC, ed. Equine Ophthalmology, 2e. Maryland Heights, MO: WB Saunders, 2011:367–396.

Author Bianca C. Martins
Consulting Editor Caryn E. Plummer
Acknowledgment The author and editor acknowledge the prior contribution of Maria Källberg.

BASICS

DEFINITION

• A variety of conditions lead to abnormal function of the upper and lower eyelids, predisposing the globe to secondary diseases such as conjunctivitis and keratitis
• Major categories of eyelid disease include congenital, inflammatory, neoplastic, and traumatic. Manifestation of each type of disease depends on age, environment, duration and progression of problem, and prior treatment
• Regardless of the etiology, all eyelid diseases disrupt normal eyelid function—to provide the lipid part of the tear film, to distribute the tear film across the cornea, to protect the globe
• SCC and sarcoids have separate topics devoted to each of them and are not discussed here

SYSTEMS AFFECTED

• Eye
• Skin

SIGNALMENT

• Eyelid melanomas are found in gray horses, with Arabians and Percherons at increased risk. Entropion is predominantly found in young foals
• Equine papillomas are common in immature horses
• Arabians may inherit juvenile Arabian leukoderma (unknown mechanism)

SIGNS

These are variable according to the disease process.
• Eyelid disease may be acute or chronic. The owner may not notice a change in the eyelids until the disease is advanced. Trauma, however, is usually acutely recognized
• Blepharospasm
• Epiphora
• Conjunctivitis
• Acute (ulcers, edema) or chronic (vascularization, fibrosis, pigmentation) keratitis
• Rubbing
• Blepharedema
• Periocular discharge ranging from frank blood to purulent or serosanguineous
• Asymmetry of eyelids can be due to raised firm or soft masses, erosive blepharitis, or overt trauma
• Lack of palpebral reflex may stem from a neurogenic disorder or trauma

CAUSES

• Entropion is an inward rolling of the eyelid margin. It can be a primary problem in foals or secondary to dehydration or emaciation. Prior eyelid damage that leaves scarring may lead to a cicatricial entropion. Acquired or blepharospastic entropion is a secondary

condition due to chronic irritation and pain, causing spasms of the orbicularis oculi muscle
• Some foals have eyelid abnormalities identified at birth. Microphthalmos causes a related macropalpebral fissure and secondary entropion requiring intervention. Dermoids (choristomas), aggregates of skin tissue aberrantly located within adnexal tissue, conjunctiva, and cornea, have been reported in the eyelids of foals. Eyelid colobomas are areas of eyelid agenesis leading to exposure keratitis. Faulty induction of the surface ectoderm by defective or absent neuroectoderm results in these congenital anomalies
• Blepharitis, or inflammation of the eyelids, has multiple causes, including viral, fungal, parasitic, allergic, and immune mediated. Traumatic blepharitis can develop into eyelid abscesses and may be associated with orbital fractures, penetrating and lacerating trauma, subpalpebral lavage system irritation, and bony sequestra
• *Trichophyton* or *Microsporum* spp. are known to cause blepharitis, as are *Histoplasma farciminosum* and *Cryptococcus mirandi*
• Equine viral papillomas cause focal eyelid inflammation in immature horses
• *Demodex* infestation may lead to lid alopecia, meibomianitis, and papulopustular blepharitis
• *Thelazia lacrimalis* is a spirurid nematode and a commensal parasite of the equine conjunctival fornices and nasolacrimal ducts. This parasite can cause diffuse blepharitis
• Habronemiasis, a common cause of granulomatous blepharitis, occurs mainly in the summer months when house and stable flies serve as vectors. Dying microfilariae in the eyelids, conjunctiva, lacrimal caruncle, medial canthus, and nictitans incite an immune-mediated hypersensitivity
• Fly-bite blepharitis, *Dermatophilus*, and staphylococcal folliculitis cause blepharitis, especially in young foals
• Juvenile Arabian leukoderma, or "pinky" syndrome, is a cutaneous depigmentation condition affecting 6–24-month-old Arabians. This disease may present with cycles of depigmentation and repigmentation
• Allergic blepharitis, eosinophilic granuloma with collagen degeneration, pemphigus foliaceous, bullous pemphigoid, solar blepharitis of nonpigmented skin, and St. John's wort photosensitization of the lids are also reported
• Topical chemical toxicities can cause a caustic blepharitis
• Eyelid lacerations are common in the horse. Upper eyelid damage is more significant because the upper lid provides the greater degree of coverage of the cornea. Medial canthal lid trauma can involve the nasolacrimal system

• Tumors of the eyelids other than SCC and sarcoids include but are not limited to melanoma, mast cell tumor, and lymphoma

RISK FACTORS
See Causes.

DIAGNOSIS

DIFFERENTIAL DIAGNOSIS

• Many conformational eyelid diseases are confirmed on clinical presentation and successful outcome of medical or surgical intervention. Careful examination of the eyelids and the eye is essential to proper management of diseases such as entropion and microphthalmos
• Inflammation and neoplasia can look similar on presentation; therefore, documenting an accurate history and performing diagnostics (see Other Diagnostic Procedures) will provide information and direct therapeutic efforts
• Quite often, blepharitis is nonspecific and may mask a specific infection, parasitism, or neoplasia.

CBC/BIOCHEMISTRY/URINALYSIS

These tests are usually normal for eyelid diseases unless there is systemic involvement.

OTHER LABORATORY TESTS

• Cytology
• Microbial culture and susceptibility if fungal or bacterial infection is suspected
• Biopsy if neoplasia is a primary differential

IMAGING
N/A

OTHER DIAGNOSTIC PROCEDURES

• Complete ophthalmic examination
• Instillation of topical anesthesia differentiates blepharospastic entropion from other causes
• Look under nictitans and in conjunctival fornices for signs of tumor, parasites, or foreign bodies
• Flush nasolacrimal duct if obstruction is suspected
• Fluorescein stain any painful eye

PATHOLOGIC FINDINGS

Findings may range from simple blepharitis with neutrophilic, lymphocytic/plasmacytic, or eosinophilic infiltrates, to specific descriptions of differentiated tumors.

TREATMENT

APPROPRIATE HEALTH CARE

• Lid trauma needs to be corrected as soon as possible to prevent undesirable scarring and secondary corneal desiccation and ulceration

E

EYELID DISEASES (CONTINUED)

• Papillomas may regress spontaneously, or require surgery, cryotherapy, or autogenous vaccination

NURSING CARE
• Most eyelid diseases are treated on an outpatient basis. Severe infections may require more intensive topical or systemic therapy
• If caught early, most eyelid diseases are amenable to treatment. During treatment, a protective eye covering may be worn to keep dirt out and prevent further self-trauma induced by rubbing, and to protect any sutures that may be present
• Foals with entropion can have temporary tacking sutures in a vertical mattress pattern (4–0 silk) or surgical staples placed 2–3 mm from the eyelid margin at the affected areas until the causative mechanism has resolved. Adult horses with entropion can receive permanent reconstructive surgeries
• Blepharoplastic measures may be necessary in horses with primary anatomic entropion, eyelid colobomas, or severe eyelid trauma
• Fly repellants or insecticide strips reduce the incidence of fly-strike blepharitis

ACTIVITY
If the pathology of the eyelids impairs vision or if a protective eye covering must be worn, activity should be restricted until the visual impairment resolves.

DIET
No specific change in diet is necessary. Dust and debris should be kept to a minimum by feeding the hay at ground level.

MEDICATIONS
DRUG(S) AND FLUIDS
• In cases of exposure keratitis or conjunctivitis, supplemental lubrication in the form of artificial tears or ophthalmic antibiotic ointment is recommended until the eyelid problem is corrected
• For eyelid swelling due to acute trauma, ophthalmic antibiotic/steroid combinations may be indicated. Therapy for severe, chronic, or aggressive bacterial blepharitis should be directed by results of culture and susceptibility

• Intralesional steroid injections (triamcinolone) may be effective against granulomatous diseases stemming from habronemiasis. Systemic avermectins are indicated for *Demodex* and habronemiasis
• Topical therapy for solitary, focal *Habronema* lesions consists of a topical mixture of 135 g of nitrofurazone ointment, 30 mL of 90% DMSO, 30 mL of 0.2% dexamethasone, and 30 mL of a 12.3% oral trichlorfon (metrifonate) solution (BID–TID)
• Topical 2% miconazole or thiabendazole (tiabendazole) is effective against eyelid ringworm, whereas systemic antifungals are effective against *Histoplasma* and *Cryptococcus*

CONTRAINDICATIONS
In cases involving ulcerative keratitis, all steroid preparations are contraindicated.

PRECAUTIONS
• Antifungal drugs, antiparasitic drugs, and chemotherapy may all be irritating to local tissues. If a drug hypersensitivity is suspected, it should be temporarily discontinued and restarted with caution if necessary
• Many topical skin antibiotic preparations used in eyelid trauma can be highly irritating to the cornea

POSSIBLE INTERACTIONS
N/A

FOLLOW-UP
• Careful monitoring of the response to therapy is critical, as the correct diagnosis may not be evident initially and ocular health is dependent on normal eyelid function. A clean, dust-free environment minimizes the likelihood of irritant or allergic blepharitis. However, allergies to wood shavings and certain types of hay are not uncommon
• Loss of eyelid tissue or extreme postsurgical scarring can be detrimental to corneal health and without correction may lead to severe keratitis and vision loss
• Eyelids have a tremendous blood supply and heal readily when treated appropriately. Because this tissue is highly mobile, sutures in the eyelids may be left for 2–4 weeks to ensure proper wound healing

• Most eyelid tumors are locally invasive but metastasize infrequently
• Certain types of tumors if left unchecked will be invasive and destroy adnexal tissue and the globe

MISCELLANEOUS
ASSOCIATED CONDITIONS
Conjunctivitis, nasolacrimal disease, nictitans disease.

AGE-RELATED FACTORS
Horses known to have a difficult temperament or who are untrained (i.e. foals and yearlings) may be more likely to present for eyelid trauma.

PREGNANCY/FERTILITY/BREEDING
• Systemic absorption of topical medication is possible
• General anesthesia versus sedation and local akinesia must always be contemplated in pregnant mares

SEE ALSO
• Burdock pappus bristle keratopathy
• Calcific band keratopathy
• Conjunctival diseases
• Dacryocystitis
• Ocular/adnexal squamous cell carcinoma
• Ocular problems in the neonate
• Periocular sarcoid

ABBREVIATIONS
• DMSO = dimethylsulfoxide
• SCC = squamous cell carcinoma

Suggested Reading
Brooks DE. Ophthalmology for the Equine Practitioner, 2e. Jackson, WY: Teton NewMedia, 2008.
Brooks DE, Matthews AG. Equine ophthalmology. In: Gelatt KN, ed. Veterinary Ophthalmology, 4e. Ames, IA: Blackwell, 2007:1165–1274.
Gilger BC, ed. Equine Ophthalmology, 3e. Ames, IA: Wiley Blackwell, 2017.

Author Caryn E. Plummer
Consulting Editor Caryn E. Plummer
Acknowledgment The author/editor acknowledges the prior contribution of Dennis E. Brooks.

FAILURE OF TRANSFER OF PASSIVE IMMUNITY (FTPI)

BASICS

DEFINITION
• Inadequate passive immunity in neonates evidenced by abnormally low concentrations of immunoglobulins in serum at >18 h of age. Normal, healthy foals that ingest an adequate volume of high-quality colostrum and absorb the immunoglobulins have serum IgG >1500 mg/dL (>15 g/L) and often >2000 mg/dL (>20 g/L)
• IgG concentrations in serum <800 mg/dL (<8 g/L) represent FTPI. IgG concentrations in serum <400 mg/dL (<4 g/L) represent complete FTPI. IgG concentrations in serum of 400–800 mg/dL (4–8 g/L) represent partial FTPI

PATHOPHYSIOLOGY
• Because of diffuse epitheliochorial placentation in mares, immunoglobulins do not cross the placenta during gestation
• Foals are born immunologically competent but without significant concentrations of immunoglobulins in the blood. Humoral immunity is therefore dependent on absorption of colostral immunoglobulin. Autogenously produced gamma-globulins do not reach adult levels until about 4 months of age
• Immunoglobulins are concentrated by selective secretion in the mare's udder during the last 2 weeks of gestation. Specialized epithelial cells in the foal's small intestine pass macromolecules via pinocytosis into local lacteals and, subsequently, into the blood. These cells are replaced by nonspecialized intestinal epithelial cells; maximal absorption occurs after birth, decreases in efficiency by 12 h, and is gone by 24 h
• Foals require approximately 2 g/kg of IgG to achieve a serum IgG concentration of 2000 mg/dL (2 g/L)
• Foals (45 kg) need to ingest >1.5 L of acceptable quality colostrum to have a reasonable expectation of serum IgG > 800 mg/dL (>8 g/L)

SYSTEMS AFFECTED
FTPI places the foal at risk of systemic illness associated with infectious, usually bacterial, disease, with localization in the lungs (pneumonia), gastrointestinal tract (diarrhea), or joints (septic arthritis).

GENETICS
N/A

INCIDENCE/PREVALENCE
• FTPI has been reported to occur in 3–24% of otherwise normal Thoroughbreds, Standardbreds, and Arabians in the USA, UK, and Australia
• Out of a large population of neonatal foals, 61% of hospitalized foals had FTPI in a recent study

SIGNALMENT
Breed Predilections
N/A

Mean Age and Range
Affected foals are neonates, although signs of disease secondary to FTPI might not develop for days to weeks.

Predominant Sex
N/A

SIGNS
General Comments
• There are no clinical signs pathognomonic of FTPI because it is a measure of the strength of the immune system, not a pathologic process
• Foals with FTPI are at increased risk of developing sepsis, pneumonia, septic arthritis, diarrhea, and omphalophlebitis, among other infectious diseases. The signs are typical of these diseases

Historical Findings
• Foals born to mares >15 years of age are at increased risk
• Premature lactation diminishes the quantity of colostrum
• Mares kept on endophyte-infected tall fescue pasture or hay often fail to produce colostrum and milk
• Foals must ingest an adequate amount of colostrum within 12–18 h of birth, preferably within 3 h, in order to absorb sufficient IgG. Foals that are slow to stand and nurse, or that are unable to stand and nurse, are unable to ingest colostrum

Physical Examination Findings
• Normal unless they develop infectious disease
• Many foals with partial FTPI kept in optimal conditions with environmental cleanliness and good farm management do not become sick

CAUSES
• Insufficient volume of colostrum, loss of colostrum through premature lactation, or colostrum that contains insufficient amounts of immunoglobulins
• Colostrum with a specific gravity <1.060 (as measured with a colostrometer) has IgG concentration <3000 mg/dL (<30 g/L) and is associated with an increased risk of FTPI
• Failure of the foal to nurse by 3–6 h after birth is associated with complete or partial FTPI; foals that fail to nurse by 12 h usually have complete FTPI

RISK FACTORS
• Illness or chronic debilitating disease in the mare during gestation, mares >15 years, mares that lactate prematurely, mares with poor mothering behavior
• Foals born in cold, overcast climates have an increased incidence compared with foals born in climates with more total solar radiation
• Premature foals and foals from prolonged gestation

• Any foal that is weak or otherwise poorly adapted to extrauterine life

DIAGNOSIS

CBC/BIOCHEMISTRY/URINALYSIS
Foals with serum total protein concentrations <4.0 g/dL are 2.5 times more likely to have FTPI. However, unlike the situation in calves, this is not a good screening test for FTPI in foals. A CBC should be evaluated in any foal with FTPI to evaluate for evidence of systemic disease.

OTHER LABORATORY TESTS
• Serum IgG is detectable at 6 h of age in foals that nursed by 2 h and is almost maximal at 12–16 h of age in these foals
• The gold standard for measurement of serum IgG concentrations is the SRID. However, this test requires up to 24 h to complete and is therefore of minimal clinical utility. The turbidometric immunoassay is more rapid and correlates highly with the SRID
• An ELISA kit (CITE Foal IgG Test Kit, IDEXX Laboratories, Westbrook, ME) uses serum, plasma, or whole blood and provides semiquantitative measurement of IgG. The test has approximate sensitivity and specificity of 53% and 100%, respectively
• The zinc sulfate turbidity test has sensitivity and specificity of 97% and 57%, respectively, making a good screening test
• The glutaraldehyde clot test has sensitivity and specificity of 100% and 59%, respectively, making it also a good screening test
• The latex agglutination test (Foalcheck, Centaur, Overland Park, KS) estimates the amount of IgG from the degree of agglutination of serum or blood with latex beads coated with anti-equine IgG antibody. The test has low sensitivity and specificity (72% and 79%, respectively), so it is not recommended

DIAGNOSTIC PROCEDURES
Based upon the presence of signs of disease.

TREATMENT

AIMS
• Raise the serum IgG concentration to *at least* 800 mg/dL (8 g/L) for a foal that has any risk factors for sepsis
• Foals with serum IgG 400–800 mg/dL (4–8 g/L) may not require plasma transfusion if they are on a well-managed farm and are at low risk of sepsis

APPROPRIATE HEALTH CARE
• Colostrum and plasma can be given in the field, but if signs of septicemia or other

FAILURE OF TRANSFER OF PASSIVE IMMUNITY (FTPI)   (CONTINUED)

systemic illness are apparent referral is recommended
• Any neonatal foal with FTPI should be maintained in sanitary environmental conditions

NURSING CARE
• Foals <12 h of age—oral administration of colostrum with a specific gravity >1.060 is the preferred treatment. 2–4 L of colostrum administered in 500 mL increments every 1–2 h during the first 6–8 h of life is desirable. Administration of bovine colostrum results in equine-specific passive immunity that is less than optimal and is not recommended
• In foals >12 h, adequate absorption for optimal IgG concentrations is unlikely and serum or plasma should be administered IV
• Concentrated equine serum and lyophilized equine immunoglobulins are not recommended
• Plasma—use of commercial frozen plasma is preferred. Fresh plasma can also be harvested from the mare or another horse with neither lysins nor agglutinins to equine RBC antigens
• Plasma should be transfused at a rate of 40 mL/kg to foals with serum IgG <400 mg/dL and at a rate of 20 mL/kg to foals with serum IgG of 400–800 mg/dL. Generally, a 45 kg foal with IgG <400 mg/dL will require 2 L of plasma, and a foal with serum IgG of >400 mg/dL but <800 mg/dL will require 1 L of plasma. Most commercially available hyperimmune plasma products contain an IgG concentration of 1500–2500 mg/dL (15–25 g/L). Measurement of serum IgG should be performed after transfusion (as soon as 30–90 min post transfusion) to confirm that adequate IgG concentrations have been achieved
• Administer IV plasma through an inline filter. Thaw frozen plasma slowly in a water bath at 39–45°C (102–113°F), and warm to at least 20°C before administration. The initial plasma or serum infusion should be slow and the foal observed for adverse reactions. Subsequently, the infusion may be given at 20–30 mL/kg/h

CLIENT EDUCATION
Treatment of FTPI should be pursued as there is evidence of higher rates of nonsurvival in foals with any degree of FTPI compared with those with adequate IgG concentrations.

MEDICATIONS

CONTRAINDICATIONS
• No contraindications to commercially available, fresh-frozen plasma
• Use of fresh plasma from horses with agglutinins or lysins to equine RBC carries a risk for neonatal isoerythrolysis

PRECAUTIONS
• Frozen plasma thawed at too high a temperature or in a microwave oven contains denatured proteins that can subsequently cause severe reactions during transfusion
• If adverse reactions occur during administration of plasma or serum products, discontinue the infusion until signs abate, and then continue the infusion at a slower rate. If adverse reactions continue, terminate the infusion

FOLLOW-UP

PATIENT MONITORING
Foals with sepsis appear to have a reduced half-life of exogenous IgG and may need multiple transfusions to maintain serum concentrations above 800 mg/dL (8 g/L).

PREVENTION/AVOIDANCE
• Ensure that newborn foals are able to stand and nurse within 2–3 h of birth. If unable to nurse on own, supplement with at least 1.5 L good quality colostrum via bottle or nasogastric tube (in 500 mL increments)
• If the mare has dripped milk prior to delivery or has been exposed to fescue, the foal should receive a good quality colostrum or plasma transfusion shortly after birth

POSSIBLE COMPLICATIONS
Foals with FTPI should be monitored for signs of sepsis.

EXPECTED COURSE AND PROGNOSIS
• Foals with uncomplicated FTPI have an excellent prognosis with appropriate treatment
• Complications with sepsis will lower the prognosis

MISCELLANEOUS

ASSOCIATED DISEASES
• Neonatal sepsis
• Perinatal asphyxia syndrome

PREGNANCY/FERTILITY/BREEDING
Ensure pregnant mares are on an appropriate vaccination schedule.

SEE ALSO
Septicemia, neonate

ABBREVIATIONS
• ELISA = enzyme-linked immunosorbent assay
• FTPI = Failure of transfer of passive immunity
• IgG = Immunoglobulin G
• RBC = red blood cell
• SRID = single radial immunodiffusion assay

Internet Resources
Case File: Failure of Passive Transfer in a Foal. http://csu-cvmbs.colostate.edu/Documents/equine-medicine-surgery-case-study-2013-01-ERL.pdf

Suggested Reading
Giguère S, Polkes AC. Immunologic disorders in neonatal foals. Vet Clin North Am Equine Pract 2005;21(2):241–272.
Liepman R, Dembek K, Slovis N, et al. Validation of IgG cut-off values and their association with survival in neonatal foals. Equine Vet J 2015;47(5):526–530.

Author Rachel S. Liepman
Consulting Editor Margaret C. Mudge
Acknowledgment The author and editor acknowledge the prior contribution of Kenneth W. Hinchcliff.

BASICS

DEFINITION
An emotion of alarm and agitation caused by real or perceived danger and manifested by physiologic and behavioral responses.

PATHOPHYSIOLOGY
• Medical explanations of fearful behavior must be considered, particularly in horses showing an acute change in their behavior or those that exhibit concomitant neurologic abnormalities. Pain, toxin exposure, infectious conditions (e.g. rabies, tetanus, equine protozoal myelitis), and some ophthalmic conditions can cause animals to exhibit hyperreactive responses that may mimic fear
• Chronic conditions, such as pain, may affect responses to stimuli as horses attempt to avoid conditions previously associated with pain

SYSTEMS AFFECTED
• Nervous—restlessness, pacing, attempts to escape restraint or confinement, inattentiveness during training, inadequate performance, or aggression to handlers
• Neuromuscular—trembling
• Gastrointestinal—inappetence or altered eating habits and increased defecation rate when fearful/reactive; gastric ulceration may be associated with chronic fearful states
• Cardiovascular—horses rated as reactive (fearful) in behavioral tests exhibited high mean heart rate and low heart rate variability
• Respiratory—tachypnea or frequent snorting when exposed to fearful stimulus
• Endocrine/metabolic—chronic fear may increase metabolic rate and elevate endogenous cortisol levels
• Hemic/lymphatic/immune—conditions of chronic fear may reduce immune competence
• Musculoskeletal—traumatic injuries may occur during escape attempts or restraint
• Ophthalmic—rule out visual abnormalities, especially in cases of adult-onset fear responses
• Skin/exocrine—sweating may occur due to autonomic arousal
• Reproductive—fear may affect breeding performance and tractability by stallions and mares

GENETICS
• There is a genetic component to fearful responses. Although selective breeding for attenuated fear responses is part of the domestication process, some ancestral characteristics remain, including heritable tendencies to monitor the environment and react to novel stimuli
• In adult horses, fearfulness, as measured on personality tests, tends to be stable over years

INCIDENCE/PREVALENCE
• Common
• Aversion to veterinary and handling procedures may be a manifestation of fear

GEOGRAPHIC DISTRIBUTION
Regional conventions for horse handling may affect the prevalence of fearful responses.

SIGNALMENT
Breed Predilections
May be breed-specific differences in fear response to novel stimuli and attempts to flee.

Mean Age and Range
Common in young animals lacking positive experiences with humans or novel situations.

SIGNS
Historical Findings
• Horses raised without exposure to humans may have a large flight distance compared with handled horses
• Lack of systematic, positive training is associated with more reactive responses, especially in novel environments
• Affected horses described as "spooky" or "flighty"

Physical Examination Findings
• Usually unremarkable, may sweat, defecate excessively
• Acute—orientation toward the stimulus, head-up alert/immobility stance, spin, retreat
• Chronic—poor body condition, postural effects, often the opposite of acute reactions, such as droopy head position
• Self-inflicted trauma, secondary to attempts to escape
• May be difficult to examine, attempting escape or engaging in reactive/defensive/aggressive behavior when approached or restrained

CAUSES
• Strongly influenced by individual temperament, experiences, and expertise of handler/trainer
• Neonatal handling has not been shown to reduce adult reactions to novel situations any more than systemic exposure to novel stimuli and positive training

RISK FACTORS
• Horses with minimal exposure to humans and their activities
• Excessive arousal or frustration
• Previous or current mismanagement, abuse, and/or harsh, inadequate, or incompetent training

DIAGNOSIS

DIFFERENTIAL DIAGNOSIS
Identify associated pathologic conditions before seeking a purely behavioral diagnosis.

CBC/BIOCHEMISTRY/URINALYSIS
• Usually normal; possible stress leukogram
• Abnormalities may suggest metabolic or endocrine explanations

OTHER LABORATORY TESTS
May be indicated to rule out medical explanations.

IMAGING
May be indicated to identify sources of pain, congenital abnormalities, or cerebral neoplasia.

OTHER DIAGNOSTIC PROCEDURES
• Risk analysis involves historical information, observation of the horse, and supporting medical and legal data. Goals are to prevent injury, reduce client's and veterinarian's liability risk, and establish a rational management/rehabilitation plan
• "Flighty" horses that unpredictably exhibit fearful behavior (e.g. bolting) and horses that exhibit fear-motivated aggression are dangerous and should be handled only by experienced personnel

TREATMENT

AIMS
Reduce fear responses in order to safely manage and improve the horse's usefulness and welfare.

Environmental Management
• Use adequate barriers and sufficient restraint to prevent injuries and horse's escape
• Use well-fitting, sturdy halters with leads and other necessary restraint devices; competent, patient handler
• In some situations, a calm companion horse may attenuate physiological and fear responses of a frightened horse
• Establish safe, quiet environment to practice behavior modification techniques. Start in a familiar environment; then with success, progress to unfamiliar environments

Behavior Modification
• Training methods. "Sympathetic (positive) horsemanship"
• Desensitization/counterconditioning—list all situations in which the horse is fearful and align them along a continuum from least to most fearful. Initially, *avoid* all these situations. Teach the horse basic exercises in nonfearful, familiar conditions. Reward the horse for being calm and obedient. Then, practice these exercises in a range of environmental conditions and situations. Escape behavior must be avoided since it is strongly reinforced by the diminished fear that results from greater distance from the stimulus
• Next, when practicing control exercises, expose the horse, while in a calm state, to the least fearful stimulus on the fear continuum. Reward the horse for calm, tractable behavior. If necessary reduce the intensity of the fearful stimulus and more gradually move it closer as the horse acclimates to it

F

• A "target," such as a tennis ball affixed to a wooden dowel, can be used in a counterconditioning process. Initially, the target is associated with something of value to the horse. Position the target so that the horse voluntarily touches it. Immediately, this response is paired with a sound such as praise or a handheld clicker followed by a coveted reward, such as a small food treat. Repeat this sequence until the horse learns that when it touches the target, a reward is delivered. With time, the target can be used to teach the horse to move forward under potentially fearful conditions, such as walking into a transport trailer

APPROPRIATE HEALTH CARE
Positive-based, species-appropriate handling should be part of routine health care of all horses.

ACTIVITY
Regular exercise.

DIET
Vitamin B complex supplementation is allegedly helpful.

CLIENT EDUCATION
• Recommend handling of the affected horse by experienced persons
• Recommend safe, quiet housing. Extreme fear reactions can result in self-trauma during escape attempts
• Chronic fear responses constitute a welfare issue. Horses in a chronic, high-fear state may eat or drink poorly, exhibit stereotypic behaviors, or develop gastric ulcers. Wild mustangs transported for long distances have died from acidosis and dehydration associated with such a state

SURGICAL CONSIDERATIONS
Possibly castration to prevent reproduction.

MEDICATIONS

DRUG(S) OF CHOICE
Generally, drugs are not used for treatment. However, when used with a behavioral management program, may decrease arousal or anxiety and facilitate learning and safe handling.

CONTRAINDICATIONS
For ethical, legal, and safety reasons, the drugs listed below are not recommended for use in performance animals, e.g. while racing, showing, or sporting activities.

PRECAUTIONS
No drugs are approved by the FDA for treatment of fearful behaviors in horses. No clinical trials have been performed on these extralabel drugs; our knowledge is based on evidence from other species and anecdotal information from a few, individual cases. Inform the client regarding the experimental

nature of these treatments and the risk involved; document the discussion in the medical record.

POSSIBLE INTERACTIONS
To avoid risk of serotonin syndrome, SSRIs generally should not be used concurrently with tricyclic antidepressants or monoamine oxidase inhibitors.

ALTERNATIVE DRUGS
• Acepromazine, a phenothiazine tranquilizer, is used widely, and is valuable to reduce the effect of environmental stimuli, if acute fear-inducing situations are anticipated. Side effects include priapism and paraphimosis in stallions
• Fluoxetine, an SSRI with anxiolytic effects, may require 1–4 weeks of daily administration. Fluoxetine may decrease libido; high doses of fluoxetine may result in serotonin effects in the gastrointestinal tract
• Fluphenazine decanoate, a phenothiazine dopamine antagonist, has been used to reduce reactivity. Serious extrapyramidal side effects (motor restlessness, altered mentation) have been reported. Diphenhydramine has been used successfully as an antidote
• Tricyclic antidepressants, such as amitriptyline or imipramine, have serotonin and norepinephrine reuptake inhibitor effects; may enhance behavioral calming; side effects can include mild sedation and anticholinergic effects. Imipramine is associated with masturbation and erection in males. At high doses, imipramine (2–4 mg/kg PO every 24 h) can cause muscle fasciculations, tachycardia, and hyperresponsiveness to sound, likely due to norepinephrine effects
• A synthetic equine appeasing pheromone (Modipher EQ, VPL), commercially available and administered via intranasal spray, prior to exposure to an anxiety-producing situation has been reported to reduce fear responses and tachypnea in a test situation
• Sublingual detomidine hydrochloride (Dormosedan Gel, Zoetis) has anxiolytic and sedative effects; may be helpful prior to examination or handling fearful animals. Consult package insert for contraindications
• NSAIDs may be used for 2 weeks to help assess pain as an etiologic factor

FOLLOW-UP

PATIENT MONITORING
• Weekly to biweekly contact during the initial phases
• Clients frequently need feedback and assistance with behavior modification plans and medication management

PREVENTION/AVOIDANCE
Helpful examination strategies:
• Rapid recognition of fearful/phobic behavior by the examiner

• Suitable restraint equipment and environment
• A familiar, tractable horse within visual range
• Familiar, experienced handler using rewards for acceptable responses
• Familiar location, with nonslippery floor, that prevents escape or injury
• Avoid erratic movements and speech
• Allow the horse visual and olfactory inspection
• Chemical restraint, if necessary, to prevent injury and negative associations with the veterinarian

POSSIBLE COMPLICATIONS
• Injuries caused by a horse exhibiting fearful behavior
• Consider euthanasia for high-risk cases in which all other treatment options have failed or are not an option

EXPECTED COURSE AND PROGNOSIS
• The knowledge and patience of the handler greatly influence treatment success
• Individual temperament of horses may limit treatment success

MISCELLANEOUS

ASSOCIATED CONDITIONS
Pain may exacerbate fear responses.

AGE-RELATED FACTORS
• Fear-motivated behavior problems are common in young horses with little training
• Adult- or acute-onset fear-motivated behavior, particularly in previously well-handled animals, suggests a medical etiology or a severe emotional experience

ZOONOTIC POTENTIAL
Rabies is a potential cause of fearful behavior or aggression.

PREGNANCY/FERTILITY/BREEDING
Chronic use of behavioral medications is not recommended in pregnant animals.

SEE ALSO
Learning, training, and behavior problems

ABBREVIATIONS
• USFDA = United States Food and Drug Administration
• NSAID = nonsteroidal anti-inflammatory drug
• SSRI = selective serotonin reuptake inhibitor

Suggested Reading
Beaver BV. Equine Behavioral Medicine. Cambridge, MA: Academic Press, 2019.
Christensen JW, Keeling LJ, Nielsen BL. Responses of horses to novel visual, olfactory and auditory stimuli. Applied Animal Behaviour Science 2005;93(1–2):53–65.
Christensen JW, Malmkvist J, Nielsen BL, Keeling LJ. Effects of a calm companion on

fear reactions in naive test horses. Equine Veterinary Journal 2010;40(1):46–50.

DeAraugo J, McLean A, McLaren S, et al. Training methodologies differ with the attachment of humans to horses. J Vet Behav 2014;9(5):235–241.

Falewee C, Gaultier E, Lafont C, et al. Effect of a synthetic equine maternal pheromone during a controlled fear-eliciting situation. Appl Anim Behav Sci 2006;101:144–153.

Gorecka-Bruzda A, Jastrzebska E, Sosnowska Z, et al. Reactivity to humans and fearfulness tests: field validation in Polish cold blood horses. Appl Anim Behav Sci 2011;133(3-4):207–215.

Heleski C, Wickens C, Minero M, et al. Do soothing vocal cues enhance horses' ability to learn a frightening task? J Vet Behav 2015;10:41–47.

Hintze S, Smith S, Patt A, et al. Are eyes a mirror of the soul? What eye wrinkles reveal about a horse's emotional state. PLoS One 2016;11(10):e0164017.

Karrasch S, Karrasch V, Newman A. You Can Train Your Horse to Do Anything: Target Training, Clicker Training, and Beyond. North Pomfret, VT: Trafalgar Square Publishing, 2000.

Lansade L, Bouissou M-F, Erhard HW. Fearfulness in horses: a temperament trait stable across time and situations. Applied Animal Behaviour Science 2008;115(3–4):182–200.

Lansade L, Pilippon P, Herve L, Vidament M. Development of personality tests to use in the field, stable over time and across situations, and linked to horses' show jumping performance. Appl Anim Behav Sci 2016;176:43–51.

Leiner L, Fendt M. Behavioural fear and heart rate responses of horses after exposure to novel objects: Effects of habituation. Science Direct 2011;131(3–4):104–109.

Mansmann RA, Currie MC, Correa MT, et al. Equine behavior problem around farriery: foot pain in 11 horses. J Equine Vet Sci 2011;31:44–48.

McDonnell SM. Oral imipramine and intravenous xylazine for pharmacologically-induced ex copula ejaculation in stallions. Anim Reprod Sci 2001;68(3–4):153–159.

Momozawa Y, Ono T, Sata F, et al. Assessment of equine temperament by a questionnaire survey to caretakers and evaluation of its reliability by simultaneous behavior test. Appl Anim Behav Sci 2003;84:127–138.

Voith VL. Fears and phobias. In: Voith V, Borchelt P, eds. Readings in Companion Animal Behavior. Trenton, NJ: Veterinary Learning Systems, 1996:140–152.

Wathan J, Burrows AM, Waller BM, McComb K. EquiFACS: The Equine Facial Action Coding System. PLoS One 2015:10(8);e0131738.

Authors Victoria I. Voith and Barbara L. Sherman
Consulting Editor Victoria L Voith
Acknowledgment The authors acknowledge the prior contribution of Richard A. Mansmann.

FESCUE TOXICOSIS

BASICS

DEFINITION
• Toxicosis in pregnant mares associated with ingestion of endophyte-infected tall fescue (*Festuca arundinacea* Schreb.) during late gestation (i.e. post gestation day 300)
• The endophyte is a fungus (*Neotyphodium coenophialum*) that lives in a mutualistic relationship within the intercellular spaces of the plant. Previous names for the fungus include *Acremonium coenophialum* and *Epichloë typhina*
• The endophyte produces ergot peptide alkaloids, the most prominent being ergovaline
• The ergot peptide alkaloids produced by the endophyte are mycotoxins—secondary metabolites of a fungus

PATHOPHYSIOLOGY
• Ergot peptides act as dopamine agonists, binding D_2-dopamine receptors and suppressing prolactin secretion
• Prolactin affects not only mammary development and milk production but also lipogenesis, immunity, and reproductive hormones

SYSTEMS AFFECTED
Reproductive system and mammary gland.

GENETICS
N/A

INCIDENCE/PREVALENCE
• Tall fescue occupies >35 million acres in the USA and is especially prominent in the southeast
• Most tall fescue pastures derive from a Kentucky 31 variety released in 1943 that was contaminated by an endophyte; >95% of tall fescue pastures are estimated to contain this endophyte
• An estimated 688 000 horses are maintained on tall fescue pastures
• 1 survey indicated that 53% of pregnant mares maintained on fescue pastures were agalactic, 38% had prolonged gestation, and 18% had stillborn or weak foals that died

GEOGRAPHIC DISTRIBUTION
Tall fescue is most prominent in the southeastern USA, but it can be found over much of the eastern USA and is grown for grass seed in the Pacific Northwest.

SIGNALMENT
Pregnant mares during late gestation, with the last 30 days of pregnancy (i.e. post gestation day 300) being the most critical.

SIGNS
Historical Findings
• Lack of udder development in mare
• Mare is past her due date
• "Red bag presentation" with premature placental separation of chorioallantois preceding foal through birth canal
• Mare is having foaling problem
• Weak foal with "dummy-like" behavior
• Lower average daily gain is possible in yearlings not supplemented with concentrates

Physical Examination Findings
• Typically, mares are 3–4 weeks past their due date
• Agalactia in mares; milk appears brown or straw-colored rather than white
• Larger-than-normal foal or inadequate preparation of the reproductive tract may cause dystocia; foal may be turned 90° in the pelvis
• Placenta may be thickened enough that the foal has trouble breaking through, and the mare may retain the placenta
• Foals are weak or stillborn
• Foals are large and gangly, with long and fine hair coats, poor muscle mass, overgrown hooves, and nonerupted incisor teeth (i.e. dysmature)
• Foals may be hypothyroid, with signs of incoordination and poor suckling reflex
• Foals may suffer from failure of passive transfer of colostral antibodies due to mare agalactia; septicemia in foals is common

CAUSES
• Any tall fescue should be considered infected by the endophyte unless the owner has purposely planted an endophyte-free variety
• Lower percentages of fescue in mixed pastures decrease the severity or likelihood of problems; however, minimal toxic concentrations of ergovaline in endophyte-infected tall fescue have not been determined for horses; any tall fescue exposure should be considered potentially toxic for mares

RISK FACTORS
• Ergovaline concentrations are highest in seed heads during summer months; concentrations are increased by drought, excessive rain, and fertilization
• Fescue hay retains its toxicity
• Non-endophyte-infected fescue cannot become infected; however, endophyte-infected fescue will outcompete non-endophyte-infected fescue and will eventually take over a pasture

DIAGNOSIS

DIFFERENTIAL DIAGNOSIS
• Other causes of dystocia, placentitis, and dysmature foals
• Ergot alkaloids associated with ergot sclerotia from *Claviceps purpurea* in small grains or hay can mimic fescue toxicosis

CBC/BIOCHEMISTRY/URINALYSIS
No major changes are likely, unless a stress leukogram caused by prolonged parturition is present.

OTHER LABORATORY TESTS
• Mares—decreased serum prolactin and progesterone concentrations; increased serum estradiol-17β
• Foals—decreased serum triiodothyronine and plasma adrenocorticotropin hormone and cortisol concentrations

IMAGING
Ultrasonography may show a thickened placenta and large foal.

OTHER DIAGNOSTIC PROCEDURES
• Pasture or hay concentrations of ergovaline likely are >200 ppb dry weight
• Endophyte contamination can be checked qualitatively by staining plant tillers at plant pathology laboratories or by ELISA testing

PATHOLOGIC FINDINGS
• Thickened, congested, and edematous placenta, with no significant bacterial cultures
• Edema is most severe in allantochorion at the area of the cervical star
• The amnion is edematous throughout and the umbilical cord also may be edematous
• Placenta may be ruptured in the uterine body rather than the typical location at the cervical star
• Foals may have overgrown hooves and nonerupted incisor teeth
• An enlarged thyroid in a foal is not apparent grossly, but large, distended thyroid follicles lined by flat, cuboidal epithelial cells can be seen histopathologically
• If a mare dies from dystocia, uterine rupture may be present and the mammary gland undeveloped

TREATMENT

APPROPRIATE HEALTH CARE
N/A

NURSING CARE
N/A

ACTIVITY
N/A

DIET
N/A

CLIENT EDUCATION
N/A

SURGICAL CONSIDERATIONS
N/A

MEDICATIONS

DRUG(S) OF CHOICE
• Oxytocin, uterine infusion of fluids, and possibly antibiotics/anti-inflammatory drugs for retained placentas
• Stored colostrum or plasma as immunoglobulin sources for foals not receiving enough colostrum; antibiotics for septicemia in foals
• Domperidone, a D_2-dopamine antagonist, is marketed as an oral gel for mares; it is given at 1.1 mg/kg once a day for 7–10 days before anticipated parturition if the mare exhibits no signs of milk production; domperidone may be continued 5–10 days after foaling at the same dosage; agalactia in a mare that has already foaled can be treated twice a day at 1.1 mg/kg for 2 days and then once a day at 1.1 mg/kg for at least 3 more days

CONTRAINDICATIONS
Domperidone stimulates GI motility; avoid use in mares with GI blockage or perforation.

PRECAUTIONS
• Domperidone may cause leaking of milk and loss of colostrum prior to foaling; if this occurs, administer one-half the regular dose twice a day; if milk loss continues with the split dose, administer one-third or less of the regular dose twice a day; collect and save colostrum; if significant colostrum is lost, monitor serum IgG levels in the foal
• Domperidone may cause a false-positive result for the milk calcium test that is used to predict foaling date

POSSIBLE INTERACTIONS
N/A

ALTERNATIVE DRUGS
N/A

FOLLOW-UP

PATIENT MONITORING
• Monitor serum IgG concentration in foals to assess adequate passive transfer
• Keep mares away from fescue for $\cong$ 1 week until lactating well
• Bucket- or bottle-feeding of milk replacers or a nurse mare may be needed for foals
• Mares may have rebreeding problems

PREVENTION/AVOIDANCE
• Prevention is much more feasible than treatment
• Remove mares from fescue pastures and fescue hay a minimum of 3–4 weeks before their foaling date; some practitioners recommend 6–8 weeks before foaling; mares should not be exposed to tall fescue beyond day 300 of gestation
• If removal from fescue pasture is not possible, domperidone can be administered orally at 1.1 mg/kg/day during the last 10–14 days of gestation
• Endophyte-infected tall fescue pastures can be replanted with other grasses or new novel varieties of endophyte-infected fescue, which do not produce ergovaline; new novel varieties of endophyte-infected fescue retain their resistance to overgrazing, insect damage, and drought stress without causing adverse effects in animals; non-endophyte-infected tall fescue is not very hardy or persistent
• A glucomannan product produced from yeast cell walls is marketed as a binder of ergovaline in the GI tract

POSSIBLE COMPLICATIONS
Dystocia or uterine rupture in mares.

EXPECTED COURSE AND PROGNOSIS
Guarded prognosis for dysmature foals.

MISCELLANEOUS

ASSOCIATED CONDITIONS
N/A

AGE-RELATED FACTORS
N/A

ZOONOTIC POTENTIAL
N/A

PREGNANCY/FERTILITY/BREEDING
See Patient Monitoring section and Possible Complications section.

SEE ALSO
• Agalactia/hypogalactia
• Failure of transfer of passive immunity (FTPI)
• Prematurity/dysmaturity in foals
• Retained fetal membranes

ABBREVIATIONS
• ELISA = enzyme-linked immunosorbent assay
• GI = gastrointestinal
• IgG = immunoglobulin G

Suggested Reading
Blodgett DJ. Fescue toxicosis. Vet Clin North Am Equine Pract 2001;17(3):567–577.
Boosinger TR, Brendemuehl JP, Bransby DL, et al. Prolonged gestation, decreased triiodothyronine concentration, and thyroid gland histomorphologic features in newborn foals of mares grazing *Acremonium coenophialum*-infected fescue. Am J Vet Res 1995;56:66–69.
Cross DL. Fescue toxicosis in horses. In: Bacon CW, Hill NS, eds. Neotyphodium/Grass Interactions. New York: Plenum Press, 1997:289–309.

Author Tim J. Evans
Consulting Editors Wilson K. Rumbeiha and Steve Ensley
Acknowledgment The author and editors acknowledge the prior contribution of Dennis J. Blodgett.

F

FETAL STRESS/DISTRESS/VIABILITY

BASICS

DEFINITION
Often found in conjunction with *high-risk pregnancies* and impaired placental function; compromise fetal survival. Fetal stress is a normal physiologic response to potentially life-threatening situations. If not addressed, quickly progressed to distress, a pathophysiologic condition leading to fetal demise or delivery of a severely compromised foal.

PATHOPHYSIOLOGY
Maternal disease and/or compromised placental function including the following.

Preexisting Maternal Disease
- PPID (formerly equine Cushing-like disease)
- EMS/IR
- Laminitis
- Chronic, moderate to severe endometrial inflammation, endometrial periglandular fibrosis, and/or lymphatic cysts leading to impaired placental function

Gestational Maternal Conditions
- Malnutrition
- Colic
- Enterocolitis
- Hyperlipemia
- Prepubic tendon rupture
- Uterine torsion
- Dystocia
- Granulosa cell tumor
- Laminitis
- Musculoskeletal disease
- Exposure to ergopeptine alkaloids in endophyte-infected fescue or ergotized grasses and/or grains
- Exposure to other xenobiotics
- Exposure to abortigenic infections, especially equine herpesvirus; bacterial contaminants on Eastern tent caterpillar setae

Placental Conditions
- Placentitis; insufficiency; early separation; placental abnormalities reported with foals resulting from SCNT cloning procedures
- Umbilical cord torsion or torsion of the amnion
- Hydrops of fetal membranes
- Mare reproductive loss syndrome

Fetal Conditions
- Twins
- Fetal abnormalities
- Delayed fetal development, intrauterine growth retardation
- Fetal trauma
- Foals resulting from SCNT cloning procedures
- Depending on the specific cause, the mechanisms can involve 1 or more of the following:
  - Maternal systemic disease; placental infection, insufficiency, torsion, separation; fetal abnormalities, all of which impede efficient fetal gas exchange and nutrient transfer
  - If impairment/stress is not resolved quickly the fetus responds pathophysiologically (i.e. distress) to alterations in oxygenation/nutrient supply (e.g. passing/aspirating meconium pre- or perinatally, decreased respiratory movements, irregular heartbeat), potentially leading to fetal compromise and death
  - Acute fetal stress may be premature birth of a nonviable foal
  - Fetal stress to distress results in fetal death and/or delivery of a severely compromised foal

SYSTEMS AFFECTED
- Maternal—reproductive
- Fetal—all organ systems

RISK FACTORS
- May be nonspecific
- Thoroughbreds, Standardbreds, draft and American Miniature Horse mares, and related breeds predisposed to twinning
- >15 years of age

Historical Findings
- Previous examination with placentitis or fetal compromise
- Previous abortion, high-risk pregnancy, or dystocia
- History of delivering a small, dysmature, septicemic, and/or congenitally malformed foal
- Preexisting maternal disease at conception (see Pathophysiology)
- Previous exposure to endophyte-infected fescue or ergotized grasses and/or grains; abortigenic xenobiotics or infections

Physical Examination Findings
Maternal and Placental Signs
- Anorexia, fever, other signs of concurrent, systemic disease
- Abdominal discomfort
- Mucoid, mucopurulent, hemorrhagic, serosanguineous, or purulent vulvar discharge
- Premature udder development, dripping milk (except in cases of fescue toxicosis)
- Premature placental separation (*red bag*)
- Placentitis, placental separation, or hydrops of fetal membranes by TRP or transabdominal US
- Excessive swelling along the ventral midline and evidence of ventral body wall weakening by TRP or transabdominal US
- Excessive abdominal distention
- Alterations in maternal circulating levels of progestins, estrogens, and/or relaxin reflect changes in fetal wellbeing and/or placental function
Fetal Signs
- Clinical sign of fetal stress and/or distress might be premature delivery of a live or dead foal or late delivery of a severely compromised foal, unable to stand and suckle. Fetal hyperactivity or inactivity (concurrent with maternal or placental abnormalities) may suggest a less than ideal fetal environment and/or fetal compromise
- Can be assessed by visual inspection or by TRP of the mare
- Alterations in parameters assessed using TRP or transabdominal US

DIAGNOSIS

DIFFERENTIAL DIAGNOSIS
Normal, uncomplicated, pregnancy with an active, normal fetus as assessed by TRP, transrectal or transabdominal US, and/or various laboratory tests.

CBC/BIOCHEMISTRY/URINALYSIS
Maternal Assessment
- Complete physical examination
- CBC, serum biochemistry, determine inflammatory or stress leukocyte response, as well as other organ system involvement
- Test for PPID or EMS/IR
- ELISA or RIA analyses for maternal P_4 may be useful at <80 days of gestation (normal levels vary from >1 to >4 ng/mL, depending on reference laboratory). At >100 days, RIA detects both P_4 (very low > day 150) and cross-reacting 5α-pregnanes of uterofetoplacental origin. Acceptable levels of 5α-pregnanes vary with stage of gestation and the laboratory used. Decreased maternal 5α-pregnane concentrations during late gestation are associated with fescue toxicosis and ergotism and are reflected in RIA analyses for progestagens
- Maternal estrogen concentrations can reflect fetal estrogen production and viability, especially conjugated estrogens, e.g. estrone sulfate
- Decreased maternal relaxin concentration: with abnormal placental function
- Decreased maternal prolactin secretion during late gestation—associated with fescue toxicosis and ergotism
- Anecdotal reports of lower T_3/T_4 levels in mares with history of conception failure, EED, high-risk pregnancies, or abortion. The significance of low T_4 levels is unknown
- Feed or environmental analyses might be indicated for specific xenobiotics, ergopeptine alkaloids, phytoestrogens, heavy metals, or fescue endophyte (*Epichloë coenophiala*, formerly *Neotyphodium coenophialum*)

Fetal Assessment
- Transrectal and transabdominal US can be useful in diagnosing twins, assessing fetal stress, distress, and/or viability, monitoring fetal development, evaluating placental health and diagnosing other gestational abnormalities, e.g. hydrops of fetal membranes
- Predisposed individuals, i.e. barren, older mares, mares with prior high-risk pregnancy, placentitis, abortion, EED, conception

failure, or endometritis, transrectal or transabdominal US should be performed on a routine basis during the entire pregnancy to assess fetal stress and viability
• Confirmation of pregnancy and diagnosis of twins should be performed any time serious maternal disease occurs or surgical intervention is considered for a mare bred within the last 11 months
• Twins confirmed by identifying 2 fetuses (easier by transrectal US when gestational age is <90 days) or by presence of a nonpregnant uterine horn (transabdominal US during late gestation)
• By transabdominal US during late gestation—view fetus in both active and resting states for at least 30 min. Note abnormal fetal presentation and position
• Abnormally high FHR after activity >100 bpm or >40 bpm difference between resting and active rates reflects fetal stress, rather than distress
• Abnormal fetal heart rhythm by echocardiography may occur immediately before, during, or after foaling and might indicate distress from acute hypoxia
• Abnormally low resting FHR is <60 bpm or <50 bpm after day 330 of gestation
• Bradycardia and absence of heart rate variation with activity indicate central nervous system depression, probably from acute hypoxia. If persistent, correlates well with poor prognosis
• Absence of fetal heartbeat is a reliable sign of fetal death
• Absence of fetal breathing movements correlates well with fetal distress
• Alterations in fetal fluid amounts
  ○ Normal range for maximal allantoic fluid depth, 4.7–22.1 cm
  ○ Normal range for maximal amniotic fluid depth, 0.8–14.9 cm; increased amounts reflect hydrops; low amounts indicate fetal distress and longstanding, chronic hypoxia
• Increased echogenicity of fetal fluids may reflect distress earlier in pregnancy; can be normal during later gestation
• Fetal ECG has been used to detect twins and to assess fetal viability and distress but largely has been replaced by transabdominal US with ECG capabilities
• While a higher risk technique in horses than in humans, US-guided amniocentesis and/or allantocentesis and analysis of the collected fluids might become a future means to assess fetal karyotype, pulmonary maturity, and to measure fetal proteins
• Samples might reveal bacteria, meconium, or inflammatory cells

PATHOLOGIC FINDINGS
• Evidence of villous atrophy or hypoplasia on the chorionic surface of the fetal membranes
• Thickening/edema of the chorioallantois or allantochorion

• Endometrial biopsy (of nonpregnant mare)—presence of moderate to severe, chronic endometritis, endometrial periglandular fibrosis, decreased normal glandular architecture, lymphatic lacunae

TREATMENT
APPROPRIATE HEALTH CARE
• Monitoring/managing fetal stress/distress, including prolonged examination times required for complete serial transabdominal fetal assessments, is best performed at a facility prepared to manage high-risk pregnancies, especially if distress is severe and parturition (induction or cesarean section) is imminent
• Early diagnosis is essential
• Balance fetal distress and maintenance of pregnancy with the need to induce parturition (with or without cesarean section) if necessary to stabilize mare's health
• Parturition requires close supervision in cases of fetal stress and distress. The neonatal foal will very likely require intensive care
• Foal resuscitation during delivery or immediately postpartum, attention to airways, breathing, and circulation
  ○ Complications with dystocia or RFM

ACTIVITY
• For most cases, exercise will be limited and supervised
• Prepubic tendon rupture, laminitis, fetal hydrops may necessitate severe restrictions/complete elimination of exercise

CLIENT EDUCATION
• Discuss risk factors
• Early diagnosis is essential for fetal survival
• Predisposing conditions compromise fetal wellbeing, correct/manage for positive outcome
• Induction of parturition and cesarean section are not without risk to dam and foal

SURGICAL CONSIDERATIONS
• Cesarean section may be indicated when vaginal delivery is not possible, or dystocia not amenable to resolution by manipulation alone
• Surgical intervention indicated for repair of anatomic defects predisposing mares to endometritis
• Certain diagnostic and therapeutic procedures might also involve some surgical intervention

MEDICATIONS
DRUG(S) OF CHOICE
See specific conditions.

FOLLOW-UP
PATIENT MONITORING
Mare and fetus need frequent monitoring until termination of pregnancy.

PREVENTION/AVOIDANCE
• Recognition of at-risk mares
• Correction of perineal conformation to prevent placentitis
• Manage preexisting endometritis before breeding
• Early monitoring of mares with a history of fetal stress, distress, and/or viability concerns
• Complete breeding records, especially for recognition of double ovulations, early diagnosis of twins, embryonic or fetal reduction
• Careful monitoring of pregnant mares for vaginal discharge/premature mammary secretions
• Removal of pregnant mares from fescue pasture or ergotized grasses or grains during last trimester (60 days optimal, especially if bred on multiple cycles, with no US confirmation of pregnancy; minimum of 30 days prepartum, with adequate breeding dates and confirmation of pregnancy using US)
• Use ET procedures with mares predisposed to EED or high-risk pregnancies
• Avoid breeding or using ET procedures in mares which have produced multiple stressed, distressed, or dead foals due to congenital and potentially inheritable conditions
• Prudent use of medications in pregnant mares
• Avoid exposure to known toxicants

POSSIBLE COMPLICATIONS
• Abortion, dystocia, RFM, endometritis, metritis, laminitis, septicemia, reproductive tract trauma, and/or impaired fertility—all affect the mare's wellbeing and reproductive value
• Neonatal foals compromised during pregnancy are more likely to be dysmature, septicemic, subject to angular limb deformities than foals from normal pregnancies

EXPECTED COURSE AND PROGNOSIS
• The ability to prevent and treat conditions leading to stress/distress have improved. Successful management of at-risk pregnancies requires rigorous monitoring of mare, fetus, neonate
• If predisposing conditions can be treated/managed, pregnancies diagnosed as stressed have a guarded prognosis for normal term gestation
• If evidence of stress progresses to distress and distress continues during treatment the prognosis for successful term gestation is guarded to poor

F

FETAL STRESS/DISTRESS/VIABILITY

MISCELLANEOUS

SYNONYMS
- Abortions, spontaneous infectious and noninfectious
- High-risk pregnancy
- Placental insufficiency
- Twins

SEE ALSO
- Abortion, spontaneous, infectious
- Abortion, spontaneous, noninfectious
- Dystocia
- Early embryonic death
- Endometrial biopsy
- Endometritis
- High-risk pregnancy
- Hydrops allantois/amnion
- Placental insufficiency
- Placentitis
- Twin pregnancy

ABBREVIATIONS
- EED = early embryonic death
- ELISA = enzyme-linked immunosorbent assay
- EMS = equine metabolic syndrome
- ET = embryo transfer
- FHR = fetal heart rate
- IR = insulin resistance
- P_4 = progesterone
- PPID = pituitary pars intermedia dysfunction
- RFM = retained fetal membranes
- RIA = radioimmunoassay
- SCNT = somatic cell nuclear transfer
- T_3 = triiodothyronine
- T_4 = thyroxine
- TRP = transrectal palpation
- US = ultrasonography, ultrasound

Suggested Reading

Bucca S. Ultrasonographic monitoring of the fetus. In: McKinnon AO, Squires EL, Vaala WE, Varner DD, eds. Equine Reproduction, 2e. Ames, IA: Wiley Blackwell, 2011:39–54.

Burns TA. Effects of common equine endocrine diseases on reproduction. Vet Clin North Am Equine Pract 2016;32(3):435–449.

Evans TJ, Blodgett DJ, Rottinghaus GE. Fescue toxicosis. In: Gupta RC, ed. Veterinary Toxicology: Basic and Clinical Principles, 2e. San Diego, CA: Elsevier, 2012:1166–1177.

McKinnon AO, Pycock JF. Maintenance of pregnancy. In: McKinnon AO, Squires EL, Vaala WE, Varner DD, eds. Equine Reproduction, 2e. Ames, IA: Wiley Blackwell, 2011:2455–2478.

Powell DG. Mare reproductive loss syndrome. In: McKinnon AO, Squires EL, Vaala WE, Varner DD, eds. Equine Reproduction, 2e. Ames, IA: Wiley Blackwell, 2011:2410–2417.

Pozor MA, Sheppard B, Hinrichs K, et al. Placental abnormalities in equine pregnancies generated by SCNT from one donor horse. Theriogenology 2016;86(6):1573–1572.

Vaala WE. Monitoring the high risk pregnancy. In: McKinnon AO, Squires EL, Vaala WE, Varner DD, eds. Equine Reproduction, 2e. Ames, IA: Wiley Blackwell, 2011:16–38.

Author Tim J. Evans
Consulting Editor Carla L. Carleton

BASICS

DEFINITION
- A regulated elevation in the thermal set point. Body temperature is actively maintained at this new set point by the body's thermoregulatory mechanisms. Hyperthermia is differentiated from fever as it involves a loss of thermoregulation, resulting in an unregulated rise in body temperature
- Normal rectal temperature—adult 99.1–100.5°F (37.3–38°C); foal 100–102°F (37.8–39°C)

PATHOPHYSIOLOGY
- A physiologic reaction involving communication between the periphery and the central nervous system
- Involves complex interactions between cytokines, acute-phase reactants, and the neuroendocrine system
- Induced by endogenous (including cytokines that are released from cells of the immune system in response to infectious, inflammatory, neoplastic, traumatic, or immunologic stimuli) or exogenous (bacterial products, foreign antigens) pyrogens
- Endogenous pyrogens act on the organum vasculosum laminae terminalis (cluster of neurons surrounded by the anterior hypothalamus and preoptic nucleus) to stimulate the production of prostaglandins within the central nervous system. Prostaglandin E_2 initiates a cascade that results in an increase in the set point for thermoregulation. Toll-like receptors bind exogenous pyrogens resulting in a similar intracellular cascade

SYSTEMS AFFECTED
All body systems can be affected.

GENETICS
Certain breeds are predisposed to associated disorders—Fell Ponies (Fell Pony syndrome), Arabians (severe combined immunodeficiency).

SIGNALMENT
Nonspecific

SIGNS

Historical Findings
Investigate recent exposure to new animals, recent travel, vaccination history, health of in-contact animals, diet, housing, previous medical history, medication administration, and course.

Physical Examination Findings
- Thorough physical examination is essential, including oral, rebreathing, rectal, and neurologic examinations as well as lymph node palpation and gait analysis
- Nonspecific signs such as lethargy, anorexia, and weight loss, or physical examination may identify a suspected source

CAUSES

Infectious
Respiratory
- Upper respiratory tract—EHV-1, EHV-4, equine influenza virus, *Streptococcus equi*
- Guttural pouch empyema—secondary to upper respiratory tract infection or retropharyngeal lymph node abscessation, *S. equi, Streptococcus zooepidemicus*
- Retropharyngeal lymph node abscessation—*S. equi, S. zooepidemicus, Corynebacterium pseudotuberculosis, Actinobacillus, Mycobacterium avium*
- Sinusitis—primary (bacterial, fungal, mixed); secondary to dental disease, trauma, neoplasia
- Lower respiratory tract—*S. zooepidemicus, S. equi, Streptococcus pneumoniae, Pasteurella, Escherichia coli, Klebsiella, Pseudomonas, Bacteroides* spp., *Mycoplasma, Aspergillus,* phycomycetes, *Pneumocystis carinii, Coccidioides immitis, Histoplasma capsulatum, Cryptococcus neoformans,* EHV-5 (equine multinodular pulmonary fibrosis), African horse sickness, *M. avium, Mycobacterium bovis, Mycobacterium tuberculosis, Nocardia asteroides,* adenovirus, Hendra virus
- Pleuropneumonia—*S. zooepidemicus, Pasteurella, Actinobacillus, E. coli, Klebsiella, Bacteroides*
- Foals—*Rhodococcus equi, S. zooepidemicus, S. equi, Staphylococcus epidermidis, Pasteurella, P. carinii*

Gastrointestinal
- Peritonitis—primary: *Actinobacillus equuli;* secondary: gastrointestinal trauma, perforation, ischemia or vascular compromise; abdominal abscess rupture, common variable immunodeficiency
- Colitis—*Salmonella* spp., *Clostridium difficile, Clostridium perfringens, Neorickettsia risticii,* equine coronavirus, cyathostomiasis. Foals—*Salmonella* spp., *C. perfringens, C. difficile,* rotavirus, *Cryptosporidium, R. equi*
- Duodenitis—proximal jejunitis
- Abdominal abscessation—*S. equi, R. equi, C. pseudotuberculosis*
- Vesicular stomatitis

Neurologic
- Cerebrum/brainstem—EEE, WEE, VEE, WNV, rabies, bacterial meningitis, brain abscess, mycotic encephalitis, listeriosis, hyperammonemia (enteric disease)
- Spinal cord disease—EHV-1, vertebral osteomyelitis (*R. equi, Streptococcus* spp., *Staphylococcus* spp., *Actinobacillus, Aspergillus, Brucella abortus*)
- Otitis media/interna—*Actinobacillus, Salmonella* spp., *Enterobacter, Pseudomonas, Streptococcus* spp., *Staphylococcus* spp., *Aspergillus*

Hepatic
- Cholelithiasis—associated with *Salmonella* spp., *E. coli, Aeromonas, Citrobacter,* group D *Streptococcus*
- Cholangiohepatitis—Gram-negative enteric bacteria (*Salmonella* spp., *E. coli, Citrobacter*), *Aeromonas, Acinetobacter*
- Infectious necrotic hepatitis
- Tyzzer disease
- Chronic active hepatitis
- Liver abscess

Musculoskeletal
- Clostridial myonecrosis—*Clostridia* spp.
- *Streptococcus*-associated rhabdomyolysis
- Osteomyelitis/septic arthritis (bacterial, fungal)
- Fistulous withers

Integument
- Cellulitis—*Staphylococcus* spp., *Streptococcus* spp., *Clostridia* spp.
- Dermatophilosis—*Dermatophilus congolensis*
- Subcutaneous abscess—*C. pseudotuberculosis,* foreign body, *S. equi*
- Urticaria—equine Getah virus

Hematologic
Anemia—equine infectious anemia, piroplasmosis.

Cardiovascular
- Vasculitis—equine viral arteritis, equine infectious anemia, *Anaplasma phagocytophilum*
- Phlebitis—thrombophlebitis (*Streptococcus* spp., *Staphylococcus* spp., *Pasteurella, Actinobacillus, E. coli, Klebsiella pneumoniae*)
- Omphalophlebitis—many organisms can be involved, i.e. *E. coli, Proteus, Streptococcus* spp.
- Endocarditis—*Streptococcus* spp., *A. equuli, R. equi, Pasteurella* spp., *Candida parapsilosis, Erysipelothrix rhusiopathiae, Staphylococcus aureus*
- Pericarditis—idiopathic
- Septic—*A. equuli, Enterococcus faecalis, Streptococcus faecalis, C. pseudotuberculosis*
- African horse sickness

Renal
Pyelonephritis—Gram-negative infections common.

Reproductive
Abortion—bacterial and viral causes.

Systemic
Septicemia

Inflammatory
Respiratory
- Smoke inhalation
- Acute respiratory distress syndrome

Gastrointestinal
- Ulcerative duodenitis (foals)
- Right dorsal colitis (NSAID toxicity)
- Sterile peritonitis (uroperitoneum)

Hepatic
- Chronic active hepatitis—etiology unknown
- Idiopathic acute hepatitis disease (Theiler disease)

Integument
- Purpura haemorrhagica—secondary to viral disease, bacterial disease, drug administration, or toxin exposure. Most commonly associated with *S. equi*
- Thermal burns
- Generalized granulomatous disease

F

• Pemphigus foliaceus—autoantibody formation against a desmosomal glycoprotein
• Bullous pemphigoid—autoantibody formation against epithelial basement membrane
• Systemic lupus erythematous—type III hypersensitivity reaction
• Panniculitis—trauma, infection, autoimmune disease, vasculitis
Hematologic
• Immune-mediated hemolytic anemia—primary; secondary (associated with drugs, infection, neoplasia)
• Neonatal isoerythrolysis
• Transfusion reaction—immunologic; nonimmunologic—due to contamination of donor product during collection, storage, or administration
Cardiovascular
Myocarditis—inflammation secondary to viral, bacterial, or parasitic disease.
Systemic
Systemic inflammatory response syndrome—can occur secondary to many diseases and injuries.

Nutritional
• Nutritional myodegeneration—vitamin E and selenium deficiency (cardiac and skeletal forms)
• Hyperlipemia

Neoplasia
With any form of neoplasia.

Iatrogenic
• Myelogram (e.g. pneumonia, septic or aseptic meningitis)
• Transport (respiratory infections)
• Transfusion reactions
• Adverse drug reaction
• Antibiotic-associated colitis
• Thrombophlebitis

Trauma
Traumatic inflammation.

Immunodeficiency
• Result of increased susceptibility to infection
• Severe combined immunodeficiency
• Selective immunoglobulin M deficiency
• Transient hypogammaglobulinemia
• Agammaglobulinemia
• Fell Pony syndrome
• Common variable immunodeficiency

Toxins
• Fescue toxicosis
• Blister beetle toxicosis (cantharidin)
• Snake bite
• Castor bean toxicity *(Ricinus communis)*
• Arsenic
• Mercury
• Chlorinated hydrocarbons
• Dinitrophenol
• Trichloroethylene extracted feed
• Propylene glycol
• Algae
• Pyrrolizidine alkaloid
• Water hemlock *(Cicuta* spp.)

• Jimson weed
• Mycotoxicosis

RISK FACTORS
• Exposure to infected animals
• Poor biosecurity/husbandry/management
• Transportation
• Immunodeficiency
• Intense exercise

DIAGNOSIS

DIFFERENTIAL DIAGNOSIS
In 1 retrospective study of fever, cause was—43% infectious, 22% neoplastic, 6.5% immune mediated, 19% miscellaneous; 9.5% cause was not identified.

FURTHER DIAGNOSTICS
Depending on the abnormalities identified on initial clinical evaluation, ancillary testing will likely be required.

CBC/CHEMISTRY/URINALYSIS
• Hematology—fibrinogen and serum amyloid A: markers of infection/inflammation (fibrinogen >1000 mg/dL often indicates abscess, osteomyelitis, pyelonephritis)
• White blood cell count/differential—increases often with bacterial infections or decreases with severe acute infections
• Blood smear—*A. phagocytophilum* in neutrophil cytoplasmic vacuoles, red blood cell parasites, and assess cell morphology
• Packed cell volume and total protein—assess for evidence of hemoconcentration, anemia, hypoproteinemia, or hyperproteinemia
• Serum chemistry—specific organ compromise
• Urinalysis—identifying renal protein loss, urinary tract infection, and hematuria/hemoglobinuria; cantharidin toxin and leptospirosis

OTHER LABORATORY TESTS
• Blood culture (bacteremia, fungemia)
• Immunoglobulin levels (neonates)
• Coggins test (equine infectious anemia)
• Direct Coombs test (hemolytic anemia)
• Antinuclear antibody test
• Virus isolation (from blood, nasopharynx)
• Serology—paired titers most useful
• Fungal serology
• PCR—*S. equi, Neorickettsia, A. phagocytophilum,* piroplasmosis
• Vitamin E level—whole blood levels in suspected nutritional myodegeneration

IMAGING
Ultrasonography
• Thorax—assess effusion, consolidation, pleural masses
• Abdomen—assess internal organs, intestinal wall thickness, peritoneal fluid, lymph nodes
• Jugular veins (thrombosis)

• Heart—assess valves (endocarditis), pericardium (effusion)
• Abscess/mass—useful to assess nature and extent of unidentified masses

Radiography
• Thorax—useful in cases of pneumonia, neoplasia, pleural effusion, masses
• Abdomen—limited usefulness, especially in adults; can do contrast studies to assess swallowing and gastric emptying
• Skull—sinusitis, masses
• Musculoskeletal—assess physitis, osteomyelitis, osteosarcoma, vertebral body abscessation

Endoscopy
• Upper respiratory tract—assess guttural pouches, pharyngeal region, nasomaxillary opening
• Lower respiratory tract—identify tracheitis, abnormalities in distal airways
• Gastroscopy—assess esophageal and gastric mucosa for ulceration, masses, biopsy (gastric, duodenal)
• Other—cystoscopy, sinoscopy, rectum

Nuclear Scintigraphy
• Identify regions of active inflammation
• Can perform with radiolabeled white cells or radiolabeled albumin

MRI/CT
Perform studies of head in cases of suspected intracranial or brainstem disease or in cases of otitis interna/media or sinusitis.

OTHER DIAGNOSTIC PROCEDURES
• Transtracheal wash—culture, cytology, Gram stain: lower respiratory tract disease suspected
• Bronchoalveolar lavage—cytology, Gram stain: diffuse lower airway disease suspected
• Guttural pouch lavage—culture, cytology, PCR
• Abdominocentesis—culture, cytology, Gram stain: peritonitis, bowel compromise, or neoplasia
• Thoracocentesis—culture, cytology, Gram stain
• Sinocentesis—culture, Gram stain, cytology
• Cerebrospinal fluid analysis—assess nucleated cell count, protein, culture, cytology, and specific disease testing
• Lymph node aspiration—culture, Gram stain, cytology
• Abscess aspiration—culture, Gram stain, cytology
• Fecal assessment—*Salmonella* PCR/culture, *C. perfringens* toxin assay, *C. difficile* toxin assay, rotavirus ELISA/latex agglutination, fecal egg count. Perform similar cultures and toxin assays on gastric reflux
• Biopsy—lung (parenchymal disease), liver, skin, muscle (immunofluorescent stain for *S. equi*), lymph nodes, bone
• Synoviocentesis—cytology, cell count, total protein level, culture
• Pericardiocentesis—cytology and culture

- Bone marrow aspirate/biopsy—assess progenitor cells in selected cases of anemia, thrombocytopenia, or leukogram abnormalities

PATHOLOGIC FINDINGS
Dependent on cause.

TREATMENT
- Target at known source. Supportive nursing care, rest, temperature-controlled environment, food and water
- IV fluid therapy
- Enteral or parenteral nutritional support. Pyrexia is a catabolic state and weight loss should be closely monitored

CLIENT EDUCATION
- Identify clinical signs in contact horses
- Monitor horses' temperature daily
- Biosecurity

SURGICAL CONSIDERATIONS
Exploratory laparotomy may be indicated. Surgery may be necessary as an adjunct to medical therapy in some disease processes, i.e. sinusitis secondary to tooth root abscessation, septic arthritis.

MEDICATIONS
There is some debate as to whether treatment of fever is beneficial.
- Beneficial effects of fever include enhancement of host defenses and inhibition of certain neoplastic cells. Several animal studies looking at serious infection have shown an inverse correlation between mortality and temperature
- Detrimental effects of fever include muscle atrophy and weakness due to increased catabolism, increased metabolic rate, anorexia, seizures (>108°F, 42°C) and prolonged fever can result in cardiovascular collapse
- Reducing fever is often thought to improve patient comfort, but it is difficult to discern if this effect is due to reducing fever or secondary to the analgesic effects of most antipyretic medications
- External cooling has been shown in humans to increase discomfort. This should be considered prior to administering alcohol baths

DRUG(S) OF CHOICE

NSAIDs
Weigh benefits, disadvantages, and potential side effects.

Corticosteroids
- Anti-inflammatory agents, and at higher doses immunosuppressive agents (dexamethasone, prednisolone, and prednisolone sodium succinate). These drugs can be useful in the treatment of selected

nonseptic inflammatory and immune-mediated diseases. Occasionally used as a powerful anti-inflammatory in the presence of infections (*R. equi* pneumonia and acute respiratory distress syndrome)
- Other anti-inflammatory drugs that are in use include azathioprine, cyclophosphamide, aurothioglucose, and pentoxifylline

Antimicrobials
- Ideally, the source of fever and etiologic agent should be identified before antimicrobial therapy is initiated. Bacterial sources of fever should be treated with antibiotics based on culture and sensitivity results. The location of infection must be taken into consideration with appropriate antimicrobials chosen to target this location. In circumstances where empirical treatment must be initiated without the benefit of culture and sensitivity results, broad-spectrum antimicrobial cover should be initiated
- Local therapy may be more appropriate than systemic therapy (i.e. intra-articular and regional administration in septic joints/osteomyelitis)
- Fungal disease can be difficult to treat in the horse due to the lack of availability of antifungal agents and the expense of treatment. Therapy should ideally be initiated based on culture and sensitivity results
- Parasitism should be treated with institution of a comprehensive deworming program based on the needs and facilities of the individual horse and property. It is important to monitor for development of resistance and to treat for encysted cyathostomes and tapeworms
- Viral disease rarely has directed therapeutic options and care normally involves supportive therapy. Acyclovir (aciclovir) has been used in treatment of the neurologic form of EHV-1, and interferon therapy has been tried in the treatment of WNV

PRECAUTIONS

NSAIDs
Can result in nephrotoxicity, right dorsal colitis, gastric ulceration. Side effects are more common in dehydrated or hypovolemic animals, and when administered concurrently with other nephrotoxic agents such as aminoglycosides, tetracyclines, and amphotericin B.

Corticosteroids
- Can induce hypothalamic–pituitary–adrenal system suppression or immunosuppression
- Have been associated with development, or worsening, of laminitis

Antimicrobials
- Can result in antibiotic-induced colitis. Aminoglycosides, oxytetracycline, and amphotericin B are potentially nephrotoxic. Aminoglycoside therapeutic drug monitoring is recommended
- Itraconazole—use with care in cases with hepatic impairment

POSSIBLE INTERACTIONS
- Care should be taken in using multiple drugs that are potentially nephrotoxic in patients that are dehydrated or hypovolemic
- α_2-Agonist drugs (e.g. xylazine, detomidine) may induce tachypnea and nostril flaring in horses with pyrexia

FOLLOW-UP
PATIENT MONITORING
Therapeutic efficacy should be monitored by assessing clinical abnormalities on a regular basis (i.e. fibrinogen, ultrasonographic or radiographic findings). While receiving medications, monitoring should be used to assess for side effects; i.e. monitor total protein, albumin, and creatinine while undergoing NSAID treatment.

PREVENTION/AVOIDANCE
- Follow simple biosecurity rules when working with horses
- Maintain current vaccination status on all horses

POSSIBLE COMPLICATIONS
- Many disease processes that cause fever have been associated with a risk for the development of laminitis
- Many horses with severe infectious disease such as colitis or pleuropneumonia have subclinical coagulopathies and are at risk for jugular thrombophlebitis and disseminated intravascular coagulopathy
- Anorexia can predispose horses, ponies, and donkeys to hyperlipemia

MISCELLANEOUS
AGE-RELATED FACTORS
- Neonates are immunodeficient prior to receiving colostrum
- Foals
  ○ Increased susceptibility to disease when maternal immunity wanes
  ○ *R. equi*—signs of disease are seen between 1 and 6 months of age
- Racehorses
  ○ Transportation and exercise can both contribute to compromised immune function. Populations are often transient, with constant exposure to new horses occurring
  ○ Pleuropneumonia
  ○ Viral respiratory disease
- Older horses—neoplasia

ZOONOTIC POTENTIAL
- Rabies
- *Salmonella* spp.
- Brucellosis
- Leptospirosis
- EEE, WEE, VEE

F

- Anthrax
- *Cryptosporidium*
- *C. difficile*
- *R. equi* (immunocompromised individuals)
- Hendra virus

PREGNANCY/FERTILITY/BREEDING
Fever and the associated inflammatory response can be detrimental to pregnancy; fetal evaluations should be performed in febrile pregnant mares. Foaling should be attended and the foal carefully assessed for signs of in utero compromise. Drug therapy should be carefully considered in the late term mare to ensure there are no contraindications.

SYNONYMS
Pyrexia

ABBREVIATIONS
- CT = computed tomography
- EEE –Eastern equine encephalitis
- EHV = equine herpesvirus
- ELISA = enzyme-linked immunosorbent assay
- MRI = magnetic resonance imaging
- NSAID = nonsteroidal anti-inflammatory drug
- PCR = polymerase chain reaction
- VEE = Venezuelan equine encephalitis
- WEE = Western equine encephalitis
- WNV = West Nile virus

Suggested Reading

Dinarello CA. Infection, fever, and exogenous and endogenous pyrogens: some concepts have changed. J Endotoxin Res 2004;10:201–222.
Greisman LA, Mackowiak PA. Fever: beneficial and detrimental effects of antipyretics. Curr Opin Infect Dis 2002;15:241–245.

Author Michelle Abraham Linton
Consulting Editor Ashley G. Boyle
Acknowledgment The author and editor acknowledge the prior contribution of Julie Ross.

FLEXURAL LIMB DEFORMITY

 BASICS

DEFINITION
• FLD is a conformational limb abnormality that can be defined as a deviation of the limb in the sagittal plane, described as either persistent hyperflexion or persistent hyperextension of the joint region. • The flexural deformity is named according to the joint involved. Joints commonly involved include distal interphalangeal, metacarpophalangeal/metatarsophalangeal, and carpus. • Flexural limb deformities may be congenital or acquired

PATHOPHYSIOLOGY
Congenital
Present at birth. Thought to involve genetic predisposition, intrauterine malpositioning, and teratogens (i.e. ingestion of locoweed and hybrid sudangrass by the mare, maternal influenza infection, collagen cross-linking abnormality, and equine goiter).

Acquired
• Nutrition—excessive intake and abrupt changes in quality and quantity of feed can lead to accelerated growth in foals. It is believed that, during the rapid growth phase, the longitudinal growth rate of the bone exceeds the ability of the tendons to lengthen passively, pulling the respective joint into flexion. • Polyarthritis and trauma—both are painful conditions that result in the "flexion result reflex," leading to an acquired hyperflexural deformity

SYSTEMS AFFECTED
Musculoskeletal—FLD is commonly found in the distal interphalangeal joint, metacarpophalangeal joint, metatarsophalangeal joint, and carpus.

GENETICS
Congenital FLD is thought to have a genetic predisposition.

INCIDENCE/PREVALENCE
N/A

GEOGRAPHIC DISTRIBUTION
Worldwide

SIGNALMENT
Breed Predilections
Any. Glycogen branching enzyme deficiency may cause transient flexural deformities in Quarter Horses.

Mean Age and Range
• Congenital deformity—present at birth. • Acquired deformity—flexural deformities at the distal interphalangeal joint usually occur at 1–4 months of age; deformities at the metacarpophalangeal joint usually occur at 12–14 months of age

Predominant Sex
N/A

SIGNS
General Comments
FLD is a common orthopedic problem in foals.

Historical Findings
• Dystocia in the mare may occur secondary to flexural deformity in the foal. • The foal may have difficulty rising or ambulating. There is sometimes a history of failure to stand and nurse

Physical Examination Findings
• Congenital
  ◦ Digital hyperextension—toes lift off the ground due to flaccidity of the flexor tendons and the foot may rock back on the heel. More severe cases result with the foal walking on the palmar/plantar surface of the phalanges, especially in the hind limbs, which can result in severe skin abrasions.
  ◦ Hyperflexural deformities—foals with hyperflexion usually have no voluntary extension of the affected limb. Often occurs bilaterally. If the deformity is located at the distal interphalangeal joint, the foals walk on their toes. If the metacarpophalangeal joint is involved, the foal will often have difficulty standing and will knuckle over at the fetlock. If the carpus is affected, the foals can be observed to buckle forward.
• Acquired
  ◦ Hyperflexural deformity of the distal interphalangeal joint—short toe and steep dorsal hoof wall angle. Over time, a "boxy" appearance is observed as the heel increases in length relative to the toe. Stage I—angle of the dorsal hoof wall is less than 90°. Stage II—angle of the dorsal hoof wall is >90°. ◦ Hyperflexural deformity of the metacarpophalangeal/metatarsophalangeal joint—characterized from a straight angle to "knuckled-over" appearance at the fetlock. More common in the front limbs but can occur in the hindlimbs. ◦ Hyperflexural deformity of the proximal interphalangeal joint. Dorsal subluxation with audible click heard as the foal walks

CAUSES
Congenital
• Genetic predisposition. • Uterine malpositioning. • Teratogens. • Multifactorial. • Prematurity/dysmaturity (hyperextension/laxity)

Acquired
• Pain. • High plane of nutrition. • Rapidly growing foals. • Infectious polyarthritis. • Genetics. • Inability to bear weight of affected limb. • Overload of unaffected limb. • Trauma

RISK FACTORS
• Multifactorial. • Nutrition offering high energy and protein

 DIAGNOSIS

DIFFERENTIAL DIAGNOSIS
• Rupture of the common digital extensor or lateral digital extensor—swelling over the dorsolateral carpus: ends of the extensor tendon can be palpated within the tendon sheath. • Rupture of the SDFT or DDFT could mimic digital hyperextension—palpation and ultrasonography of the flexor tendons should differentiate

CBC/BIOCHEMISTRY/URINALYSIS
Complete biochemistry/CBC workup prior to administration of oxytetracycline.

OTHER LABORATORY TESTS
N/A

IMAGING
Radiography and ultrasonography commonly show no abnormal findings. Radiographs may be helpful in detection of bony abnormalities such as osteochondrosis and degenerative joint disease. Premature foals with significant tendon/ligament laxity should have radiographs of the carpus and tarsus to assess for ossification of the cuboidal bones.

OTHER DIAGNOSTIC PROCEDURES
• Observation of the foal standing and walking. • Manipulation/palpation of the limb, in both weight-bearing and non-weight-bearing positions. Palpation of the flexor tendons while attempting to straighten a limb with hyperflexion can help to determine which tendon is involved

PATHOLOGIC FINDINGS
N/A

 TREATMENT

AIMS
• Pain management to encourage weight-bearing for hyperflexural deformities. • Bandages/splints/casts/oxytetracycline to induce laxity and straighten the limb for hyperflexural deformities. • Strengthening of the musculotendinous unit for hyperextension deformities

APPROPRIATE HEALTH CARE
N/A

NURSING CARE: CONSERVATIVE TREATMENT
Congenital Deformities
Digital Hyperextension Deformity
• Moderate exercise. • Light bandages (protection of the palmar/plantar aspect of the phalanges). • Corrective shoeing, application of glue-on shoes with heel extensions
Hyperflexural Deformity
• Encourage restricted weight-bearing exercise; physical therapy manipulation of the

F

FLEXURAL LIMB DEFORMITY   (CONTINUED)

limbs in recumbent foals. • Correct nutrition.
• Corrective shoeing, toe extensions. • Splints and casts, used to relax the muscle–tendon unit

Acquired Deformities
Distal Interphalangeal Joint
• Balanced nutrition. • Exercise. • Analgesia.
• Toe extensions increase tension in the DDFT, resulting in stretching of the tendon unit. • Casts also have been used to aid correction of the deformity
Metacarpophalangeal Joint
• Balanced nutrition. • Physical therapy.
• Analgesia. • Corrective shoeing—wedge pads used to raise the heel, alleviating the DDFT while bringing the fetlock into a more normal position
Carpal Joint
Physical therapy and splints have been used to manage carpal region deformities.
Proximal Interphalangeal Joint
Trimming of the hoof.

ACTIVITY
See Nursing Care.

DIET
• Balanced nutrition is very important. Early weaning may be necessary for foals with acquired flexural deformities (lower plane of nutrition). • Creep feeding of young foals and high-energy diets in weanlings may contribute to the development of angular limb deformity/FLD

SURGICAL CONSIDERATIONS
Congenital
• Digital hyperextension deformity—historically, tenoplasty as surgical management for small or miniature foal patients has been described. • Contractural deformity—see Acquired Contractural Deformities

Acquired Contractural Deformities
• Distal interphalangeal joint
  ◦ Desmotomy of the accessory check ligament of the DDFT indicated for stage I hyperflexural deformities. Correction observed immediately up to a few days following surgery. ◦ Tenotomy of the DDFT recommended for stage II hyperflexural deformities, may limit athletic prognosis significantly.
• Metacarpophalangeal joint
  ◦ Desmotomy of the accessory ligament of the DDFT or the SDFT, depending on which tendon palpates tighter, in order to allow for release. Transection of both accessory ligaments as well as the suspensory ligament may be required in severe cases; however, the prognosis for athletic soundness is poor

• Carpal joint
  ◦ Tenotomy of the ulnaris lateralis and flexor carpi ulnaris tendons. Transection of the palmar carpal ligament and palmar joint capsules has also been described, but with limited success. These procedures can also be used for refractory congenital carpal hyperflexion.
• Proximal interphalangeal joint
  ◦ Transection of the accessory ligament of the DDFT and the medial head of the deep digital flexor muscle has been described. Dorsal subluxation of the pastern that is not reducible may require realignment and surgical arthrodesis to achieve soundness

MEDICATIONS

DRUG(S) OF CHOICE
• Oxytetracycline (for a 50 kg foal 3 g in 250 or 500 mL saline IV, may be repeated 2 or 3 times given 24 h apart); may be beneficial for congenital hyperflexural cases in the first few days of life. • For surgical cases, NSAIDs and antibiotics can be given as needed perioperatively. • Aggressive pain relief including NSAIDs, opioids, sedation, and short-term anesthesia during splint application is imperative as ongoing pain may potentiate hyperflexural deformity

CONTRAINDICATIONS
N/A

PRECAUTIONS
• NSAIDs can have an ulcerogenic effect on foals—can administer omeprazole or ranitidine during NSAID administration.
• Monitor renal values in foals prior to use of oxytetracycline

POSSIBLE INTERACTIONS
N/A

ALTERNATIVE DRUGS
N/A

FOLLOW-UP

PATIENT MONITORING
• Monitor foals in splints and casts closely in order to avoid pressure sores. • Monitor renal values in foals receiving oxytetracycline

PREVENTION/AVOIDANCE
Balanced nutrition (avoid high-energy and excessive protein diets).

POSSIBLE COMPLICATIONS
• Renal failure from oxytetracycline given to a neonate. • Rupture of the common digital

extensor tendon secondary to flexor tendon hyperflexion splinting (usually just a cosmetic defect). • Nonsurgical management—pressure sores. • Surgical management—hematoma/seroma formation at surgery site, incisional infection, wound dehiscence

EXPECTED COURSE AND PROGNOSIS
• If the deformity is corrected easily with manual reduction, the prognosis with medical treatment is generally good. Laxity of tendinous and ligamentous structures usually resolves even if severe, but can take many months. • If medical management does not result in improvement of FLD, surgical intervention should be considered.
• Reasonable prognosis for desmotomy of the inferior check ligament with hyperflexion at the distal interphalangeal joint. • Poor athletic prognosis for moderate to severe FLD

MISCELLANEOUS

ASSOCIATED CONDITIONS
N/A

AGE-RELATED FACTORS
N/A

ZOONOTIC POTENTIAL
N/A

PREGNANCY/FERTILITY/BREEDING
N/A

SYNONYMS
Contracted tendons

SEE ALSO
Angular limb deformity

ABBREVIATIONS
• DDFT = deep digital flexor tendon
• FLD = flexural limb deformity
• NSAID = nonsteroidal anti-inflammatory drug
• SDFT = superficial digital flexor tendon

Suggested Reading
Adams SB, Santschi ES. Management of congenital and acquired flexural limb deformities. Proc Am Assoc Equine Pract 2000;46:117.
Kidd JA. Flexural limb deformities. In: Auer JA, Stick JA, eds. Equine Surgery, 4e. St. Louis, MO: WB Saunders, 2012:1221–1239.
Trumble T. Orthopedic disorders in neonatal foals. Vet Clin North Am Equine Pract 2005;21:357–385.

Authors Alison K. Gardner and Shannon J. Murray
Consulting Editor Margaret C. Mudge

BASICS

DEFINITION
- Fluid therapy consists of oral or IV fluids administered for treatment of shock, fluid replacement, or fluid maintenance
- This chapter will focus on IV fluid therapy in the foal, although in less debilitated foals fluid requirements should be supplied by nursing or enteral feeding of mare's milk

PATHOPHYSIOLOGY
- Neonates distribute fluids to the interstitial space rapidly owing to a high capillary filtration coefficient. Because of this filtration as well as immature renal function, neonates do not handle large fluid volumes as well as adults. Sepsis and hypoxia may exacerbate leakage of fluids into the interstitial space
- Neonatal foals have low urinary fractional excretion of sodium, and this normal physiologic sodium conservation is well suited to the low-sodium milk diet. However, the sodium in isotonic IV fluids will lead to sodium overload and retention of free water
- Hypovolemia—a decrease in circulating blood volume will lead to decreased perfusion of tissues. If perfusion impairment is severe or prolonged, organ failure may result

SYSTEMS AFFECTED
- Cardiovascular—hypovolemia can reduce cardiac output, ejection fraction, and end-organ tissue perfusion
- Renal/urologic—hypovolemia and poor systemic perfusion will decrease renal blood flow and renal perfusion, leading to azotemia, and, if the insult is severe enough, acute kidney injury
- GI—poor perfusion can result in loss of mucosal barrier function and secondary bacterial translocation

GENETICS
N/A

INCIDENCE/PREVALENCE
N/A

GEOGRAPHIC DISTRIBUTION
N/A

SIGNALMENT
N/A

SIGNS
Historical Findings
- Decreased nursing or lack of nursing for 4 h or longer. Mare will have a full udder and may be streaming milk
- Fluid losses though diarrhea or third-spacing in the intestinal tract or abdomen

Physical Examination Findings
- Signs of dehydration include prolonged skin tent, sunken eyes, tacky mucous membranes, increased urine specific gravity,

hypercreatinemia, and prolonged capillary refill time
- Signs of hypovolemia include tachycardia, cold extremities, decreased urine production, depressed mentation, and poor pulse pressure

CAUSES
Indications for Fluid Therapy
- Correct dehydration
- Increase perfusion, treat hypovolemia
- Sepsis/septic shock
- Diarrhea or other GI fluid losses
- GI disease preventing enteral intake
- Volume replacement after acute blood loss (e.g. umbilical bleeding)

RISK FACTORS
N/A

DIAGNOSIS

DIFFERENTIAL DIAGNOSIS
N/A

CBC/BIOCHEMISTRY/URINALYSIS
- Hemoconcentration (elevated packed cell volume and TP) is common with dehydration
- Elevated blood lactate concentration may indicate poor perfusion or tissue hypoxia
- Urine specific gravity in normal foals is usually <1.008. Urine concentration will increase with dehydration and hypovolemia, provided renal function is normal

OTHER LABORATORY TESTS
Immunoglobulin G should be checked in the neonatal foal—if plasma transfusion is required, this will need to be accounted for in the fluid therapy plan.

IMAGING
Vessel appearance on thoracic radiographs, ultrasonographic imaging of the size of the right atrium and ventricle.

OTHER DIAGNOSTIC PROCEDURES
- Central venous pressure
- Blood pressure
- Urine output measurements
- Cardiac output

PATHOLOGIC FINDINGS
N/A

TREATMENT

AIMS
Replacement Fluids
- Boluses up to 80 mL/kg crystalloid fluid may be needed for treatment of shock. Fluids can be administered as boluses of 10–20 mL/kg (0.5–1 L in a 50 kg foal), with reassessment after each bolus. A foal that has received 60–80 mL/kg fluid boluses and is

persistently hypotensive should receive vasopressor/catecholamine therapy
- Rehydration—volume needed can be estimated by the formula (% dehydration × weight (kg))

Maintenance Fluids
- Fluids with lower sodium and higher potassium than that of plasma (e.g. Plasma-Lyte 56) are more appropriate for maintenance requirements. Half-strength saline (0.45% NaCl) with dextrose (2.5%) can be used as well
- Daily requirements for maintenance fluid administration can be calculated using the Holliday–Segar formula:
  - 100 mg/kg/day for the first 10 kg body weight
  - 50 mL/kg for the second 10 kg body weight, and
  - 25 mL/kg for body weight above 20 kg
  - A 50 kg foal would therefore require 2250 mL/day. The use of this formula results in substantially lower volume delivered than with a more traditional estimate of 60–80 mL/kg/day
- Fluids can be administered as a constant rate infusion or as boluses given every 1–4 h
- Additional fluid losses (diarrhea, reflux) should also be considered when determining fluid rates
- Enteral and parenteral nutrition should be considered—increasing volumes of nutrition will lower the IV fluid requirements

APPROPRIATE HEALTH CARE
IV fluids are generally administered as inpatient medical management. Foals with severe systemic disease or hypovolemic shock will require emergency inpatient intensive care management.

NURSING CARE
IV catheter care—over-the-wire flexible polyurethane 14- or 16-gauge catheters placed in sterile fashion are preferred for long-term fluid and medication administration. Over-the-needle catheters can be placed for emergency administration of fluids.

ACTIVITY
Foals requiring IV fluids must be restricted to a stall or small pen in order to maintain the IV catheter and deliver fluids. Foals may need to be separated from the mare (by a divider or in a pen) if they are receiving continuous IV fluids.

DIET
See chapter Nutrition in foals.

CLIENT EDUCATION
N/A

SURGICAL CONSIDERATIONS
N/A

F

FLUID THERAPY, NEONATE

MEDICATIONS

DRUG(S) OF CHOICE

IV Fluids
- Crystalloids
  ∘ Lactated Ringer's, 0.9% saline, Plasma-Lyte 148, and Normosol-R are isotonic crystalloid solutions that can be used for fluid replacement. Normal saline is acidifying due to the high chloride concentration (154 mEq/L), and is generally preferred only if a potassium-free crystalloid is needed for resuscitation (as with uroperitoneum)
  ∘ Plasma-Lyte 56 and Normosol-M are crystalloid maintenance solutions that are more appropriate for long-term fluid therapy. These solutions may not be readily available, but maintenance solutions low in sodium (40–80 mEq/L) and high in potassium (13 mEq/L) can be made using 0.45% saline or a combination with 2.5% dextrose in water with potassium supplementation
- Colloids
  ∘ Hetastarch 6% (3–10 mL/kg) is an example of a synthetic colloid that will remain in the vasculature for a longer period of time due to the large molecule size. There is no evidence of superiority of colloid fluids for resuscitation, but colloids are indicated when colloid oncotic pressure is low and volume resuscitation is needed
- Plasma
  ∘ Plasma is a natural colloid and is the most commonly used colloid in neonatal foals due to the frequent need for immunoglobulin supplementation
- Whole blood
  ∘ It should not be a first-line fluid for resuscitation unless hemorrhagic shock is present

Fluid Supplementation
- Glucose—start with a rate of 4–8 mg/kg/min (in a 50 kg foal, ≈250 mL/h of a 5% dextrose solution) if enteral or parenteral feedings have been initiated. Dextrose solution should not exceed 10%. Blood glucose should ideally be <150 mg/dL and >80 mg/dL. If hyperglycemia persists, treatment with insulin may be needed
- Potassium—supplementation of a maintenance fluid may range from 10 to 40 mEq/L. The rate of potassium administration should not exceed 0.5 mEq/kg/h
- Bicarbonate—should not be used routinely to correct metabolic acidosis since lactic acidosis may resolve readily with fluid

resuscitation. If pH < 7.2 or there is significant loss of bicarbonate, a combination of IV and oral supplementation may be needed. Formula for bicarbonate supplementation: base deficit × 0.3 × body weight (kg), with half the calculated amount given initially, then blood gas reassessed
- Calcium and magnesium supplementation should be guided by ionized values. Systemic inflammatory response syndrome appears to produce hypocalcemia and hypomagnesemia; therefore, septic neonates may require supplementation

CONTRAINDICATIONS
- Hypertonic saline is generally not recommended for use in neonatal foals, since it causes rapid changes in osmolarity and foals have less ability to handle large sodium loads resulting in fluid retention and a hyperchloremic metabolic acidosis
- Bicarbonate is contraindicated with hypoventilation/abnormal respiratory function because the CO_2 produced cannot be eliminated

PRECAUTIONS
Hetastarch can prolong clotting times at doses ≥20 mL/kg. Once Hetastarch has been administered, TP is no longer a good estimate of oncotic pressure, so colloid oncotic pressure should be directly measured with a colloid osmometer.

POSSIBLE INTERACTIONS
Bicarbonate- and calcium-containing solutions are incompatible.

ALTERNATIVE DRUGS
N/A

FOLLOW-UP

PATIENT MONITORING
- Volume and perfusion status—monitor for improvement in mentation, return of peripheral pulse and warmer extremities, urine production, and improvement in mucous membrane color and capillary refill time. Monitor blood work every 4–24 h, and adjust fluid composition and rate accordingly
- Catheter complications—examine IV catheter site at least daily for any heat, swelling, pain, discharge, phlebitis, or kinking/pulling out of the catheter
- Body weight every 24 h to estimate fluid balance and adequate nutrition

PREVENTION/AVOIDANCE
Frequent nursing is imperative for maintenance of normal hydration in neonatal foals. Any foal that has not been seen to nurse

during a period of 4 h is at high risk of dehydration. Careful monitoring of nursing behavior and fluid losses (e.g. diarrhea) may help to prevent life-threatening hypovolemia.

POSSIBLE COMPLICATIONS
- Fluid overload
- Hypernatremia
- Thrombophlebitis

EXPECTED COURSE AND PROGNOSIS
- Foals with uncomplicated dehydration should respond rapidly to fluid therapy, although they may require continued fluid replacement if there are ongoing fluid losses or reduced intake
- Prognosis depends on the underlying disease

MISCELLANEOUS

AGE-RELATED FACTORS
Neonatal foals (<2 weeks old) have a large interstitial fluid reserve and altered handling of sodium loads compared with adults.

ZOONOTIC POTENTIAL
N/A

PREGNANCY/FERTILITY/BREEDING
N/A

SYNONYMS
- Rehydration
- Fluid resuscitation

SEE ALSO
- Hemorrhage, acute
- Nutrition in foals
- Septicemia, neonate

ABBREVIATIONS
TP = total protein

Suggested Reading
Buchanan BR, Sommardahl CS, Rohrback BW, Andrews FM. Effect of a 24-hour infusion of an isotonic replacement fluid on the renal clearance of electrolytes in healthy neonatal foals. J Am Vet Med Assoc 2005;227:1123–1129.
Magdesian GE. Fluid therapy for neonatal foals. In: Fielding CL, Magdesian GE, eds. Equine Fluid Therapy. Ames, IA: Wiley Blackwell, 2014:279–298.
Palmer JE. Fluid therapy in the neonate: not your mother's fluid space. Vet Clin North Am Equine Pract 2004;20:63–75.

Author Eric L. Schroeder
Consulting Editor Margaret C. Mudge
Acknowledgment The author acknowledges the prior contribution of Margaret C. Mudge.

FOAL IMMUNODEFICIENCY SYNDROME

BASICS

OVERVIEW
• Familial disease of Fell and Dale Ponies that is characterized by B-lymphocyte immunodeficiency, progressive anemia, peripheral ganglionopathy, secondary opportunistic infection, and death (100%) usually by 3 months of age
• Formerly termed Fell Pony syndrome

SIGNALMENT
• Fell and Dale Pony breeds and their interbred crosses
• Colts and fillies equally affected

SIGNS
• Nonspecific signs usually begin at approximately 2–3 weeks of age, including weight loss, depression, ill thrift, and lethargy
• Pale membranes
• Fever secondary to opportunistic infection
• Tachycardia and tachypnea due to severe anemia and/or concurrent illness
• Opportunistic infections, e.g. cryptosporidial enteritis, adenoviral bronchopneumonia, and/or pancreatitis

CAUSES AND RISK FACTORS
• A single recessive genetic mutation in the sodium/myoinositol cotransporter gene
• 39–48% of Fell Ponies and 11–18% of Dale Ponies carry the defective gene. Affected foals are homozygous for the defective gene. Heterozygotes (carriers) are unaffected clinically

DIAGNOSIS

• Genetic testing on hair to identify affected foals and/or carrier parents
• Immunologic testing:
  ○ B-lymphocyte depletion
  ○ T-lymphocyte function tests are typically normal
  ○ Normal distribution of CD4 + and CD8 + lymphocyte populations
  ○ Low serum IgM and IgA concentrations when measured at >3–4 weeks of age
  ○ IgG concentration may be normal due to maternally derived acquisition

DIFFERENTIAL DIAGNOSIS
• Sepsis
• Infectious enteritis
• Other immune deficiency syndromes (see Associated Conditions)

CBC/BIOCHEMISTRY/URINALYSIS
• Severe nonregenerative anemia with packed cell volume often <15% and lymphopenia
• Thrombocytopenia
• Plasma protein concentrations and blood lymphocyte counts may be normal or low

OTHER LABORATORY TESTS
• Bone marrow biopsy—marked erythroid hypoplasia with myeloid to erythroid ratios 21–62:1
• Flow cytometry on peripheral blood leukocytes—severe B-cell lymphopenia with normal to increased functional T-lymphocyte concentrations
• T lymphocytes may have decreased expression of major histocompatibility complex class II
• Decreased IgM concentration

IMAGING
N/A

OTHER DIAGNOSTIC PROCEDURES
N/A

PATHOLOGIC FINDINGS
• Hypoplasia of lymphoid tissue including the thymus and an absence of secondary lymph node follicles and plasma cells
• Low numbers of plasma cells in the spleen
• Peripheral ganglionopathy characterized by neuronal chromatolysis in the cranial mesenteric, dorsal root, and trigeminal ganglia

TREATMENT

• This condition is uniformly fatal; most foals die by 3 months of age
• Supportive care with IV fluids and parenteral nutrition
• Treat secondary infections with appropriate antimicrobials
• Blood transfusion with packed red blood cells may prolong survival temporarily
• Affected foals often respond initially to targeted supportive therapy but soon succumb to severe anemia and immunodeficiency
• Humane euthanasia should be considered in affected foals

MEDICATIONS

DRUG(S) OF CHOICE
Broad-spectrum antimicrobials—penicillin (22 000 IU/kg every 6 h) and amikacin (25 mg/kg IV every 24 h) or ceftiofur (10 mg/kg IV every 6 h).

CONTRAINDICATIONS/POSSIBLE INTERACTIONS
N/A

FOLLOW-UP

PATIENT MONITORING
• Repeat bloodwork to assess for worsening of anemia or efficacy of transfusions
• Monitor for development of opportunistic infections
• Diagnosis of foal immunodeficiency syndrome should be pursued, as further treatment is likely futile, and humane euthanasia is recommended

PREVENTION/AVOIDANCE
Avoid carrier–carrier matings of Fell and Dale Ponies and their inbred crosses. Genetic screening of dam and sire to determine carrier status.

POSSIBLE COMPLICATIONS
N/A

EXPECTED COURSE AND PROGNOSIS
• Severe nonregenerative anemia, immunodeficiency, and overwhelming secondary infection occur rapidly in early life, ultimately causing death
• Many foals will die from disseminated intravascular coagulation related to severe septic shock

MISCELLANEOUS

ASSOCIATED CONDITIONS
Other humoral immunity deficiencies exist in horses, including failure of transfer of passive immunity, transient hypogammaglobulinemia of young horses, severe combined immunodeficiency syndrome of Arabian foals, primary agammaglobulinemia, selective IgM deficiency, and common variable immunodeficiency.

AGE-RELATED FACTORS
Foals begin showing signs as maternally derived immunity begins to wane. The clinical course is typically rapid thereafter.

PREGNANCY/FERTILITY/BREEDING
N/A

SEE ALSO
• Immunoglobulin deficiencies
• Septicemia, neonate

ABBREVIATIONS
Ig = immunoglobulin

Suggested Reading
Fox-Clipsham LY, Brown EE, Carter SD, Swinburne JE. Population screening of endangered breeds for the foal immunodeficiency syndrome mutation. Vet Rec 2011;169:655–658.
Gardner RB, Hart KA, Stokol T, et al. Fell Pony syndrome in a pony in North America. J Vet Intern Med 2006;20:198–203.
Scholes SF, Holliman A, May PD, Holmes MA. A syndrome of anaemia, immunodeficiency and peripheral ganglionopathy in Fell Pony foals. Vet Rec 1998;142:128–134.

Author Samuel D.A. Hurcombe
Consulting Editor Margaret C. Mudge

F

FRACTURES IN ENDURANCE HORSES

F

BASICS

DEFINITION
• Endurance is the fastest growing FEI discipline. As the sport has become more competitive, training has become more rigorous and speeds have increased
• Fractures similar to those seen in flat-racing horses have become more common

PATHOPHYSIOLOGY
Stress-related maladaptive response of bone to training and competition.

SYSTEMS AFFECTED
Musculoskeletal

GEOGRAPHIC DISTRIBUTION
• Injuries of this nature may occur anywhere in the world, but are most common in areas where courses are flat and fast: the Middle East and South America, especially
• Fractures in endurance horses are becoming increasingly common in Europe

SIGNALMENT
• Arabian horses and Arab crosses are most commonly used for endurance competitions
• They are not permitted to compete until they are 6 years of age and may race until they are in their late teens, but most affected horses are 10–18 years old
• No sex predilection or genetic basis has been noted

SIGNS
• The horse may exhibit sudden non-weight-bearing lameness during competition, sometimes accompanied by collapse
• Open fractures are obvious (presence of blood and disruption of the integument)
• Less obvious fractures occur in horses that complete a phase of the course, but lameness becomes apparent in the cooling, inspection, or crewing area
• Joint effusion is often present if the fracture extends into the joint, but may not occur immediately

CAUSES
• Unrecognized or subclinical bone injury
• Maladaptation of bone to rigors of training
• Inadequate time given for bone to remodel to accommodate stress
• Continued training of unsound horses
• Use of systemic or regional analgesics to allow unsound horses to train and compete
• Muscular fatigue
• Pushing horses beyond their physiologic limits

RISK FACTORS
See Causes.

DIAGNOSIS

DIFFERENTIAL DIAGNOSIS
• Myopathy (exertional rhabdomyolysis)
• Muscle rupture

CBC/BIOCHEMISTRY/URINALYSIS
Depending on the phase of competition in which the fracture occurs, hemoconcentration and azotemia may be present.

IMAGING
• Fractures of the distal limb are often easily discernible on radiographs
• The most common types of fractures are of the metacarpal/tarsal condyles and sagittal fractures of the first phalanx
• Proximal third metacarpal fractures and compression fractures at the level of the distal metacarpal physeal scar are also not uncommon
• Incomplete fractures of the upper limb are difficult to image radiographically, and ultrasonography may help in the diagnosis, especially with pelvic, tibial, humeral, and scapular fractures
• If the problem is not identifiable with conventional imaging techniques, scintigraphy and MRI can be useful adjuncts to diagnosis
• Advanced imaging modalities may help to identify occult fractures or bone damage that could propagate to become catastrophic if undiscovered

OTHER DIAGNOSTIC PROCEDURES
Displaced fractures of the humerus, radius, femur, and tibia, can usually be diagnosed clinically by abnormal limb movement, auscultation of crepitus, and hematoma.

PATHOLOGIC FINDINGS
Histopathology has not been performed, but gross examination of some specimens, review of previous radiographs, and clinical history, when available, point to preexisting stress pathology.

TREATMENT

AIMS
• The primary aims are to stabilize those fractures that are amenable to repair or healing and to prevent suffering, by means of euthanasia, when the horses have fractures with a hopeless prognosis
• Appropriate stabilization of the distal limb using accepted splinting techniques is an essential part of emergency care
• Veterinarians should be familiar with the principles of field splinting and fracture stabilization, and should ensure that appropriate materials are available
• Kimzey splints, "monkey splints," and PVC pipe cut to various lengths should be available *before* they are needed
• Good preparation and stabilization of repairable fractures ensures that a potentially repairable fracture does not become irreparable
• Most distal limb fractures are amenable to surgical repair, and conservative treatment (casting) may be an option for certain nondisplaced fractures
• Surgical repair requires referral to a tertiary care facility
• Nondisplaced fractures treated by cast fixation must be carefully monitored to avoid damage to underlying soft tissue structures
• Most open fractures of the distal limb and displaced long bone fractures of the upper limb (radius, humerus, tibia, and femur) have a poor prognosis, and horses should be euthanized
• Horses with irreparable injuries should not be transported long distances for euthanasia
• A second opinion confirming the need for euthanasia should be sought, when practical, but the procedure must not be delayed, especially in the case of open fractures
• Support of the President of the Veterinary Commission, Foreign Veterinary Delegate, and President of the Ground Jury should be obtained at FEI rides, and all reporting requirements met
• Most endurance horses are subject to some degree of hypovolemia and dehydration during competition
• Close attention must be paid to restoring fluid deficits prior to shipping or subjecting patients to general anesthesia for surgical repair
• Hematocrit levels are easily monitored in the field, and are helpful in determining the number of liters of IV fluids needed for restoration of circulating blood volume
• Normal saline (0.9%) is used routinely, but if it is not available any isotonic fluid can be used
• At least 10 L is administered IV prior to transport
• Restoration of fluid deficits via nasogastric intubation is not recommended, because many endurance horses have ileus, and there is a danger of gastric rupture using this method

MEDICATIONS
• Horses with fractures should be provided with analgesia
• Volume depletion and prerenal azotemia are common in endurance horses, necessitating

that NSAIDs be used judiciously, following restoration of fluid volume
• Flunixin meglumine (1 mg/kg IV) or phenlybutazone (4 mg/kg IV) should be readily available and are appropriate to use after administration of IV fluids
• If serum creatinine levels are high, butorphanol (0.01–0.02 mg/kg) combined with xylazine (0.3–0.5 mg/kg) or detomidine (0.01 mg/kg) can be used to provide analgesia until creatinine levels return to normal
• If xylazine and butorphanol are used, start with a lower dose to avoid ataxia

CONTRAINDICATIONS

• Serious complications (renal failure) may occur if NSAIDs are used in endurance horses prior to volume expansion
• It is contraindicated to give NSAIDs to an endurance horse that has sustained a fracture without first checking hydration status and creatinine levels, unless the decision for euthanasia has been made
• If this is not possible, at least 10 L of IV fluids should be administered prior to any NSAID administration
• Many horses recover after sustaining fractures of the lower limb, but if the treating veterinarian does not follow guidelines for volume expansion prior to administering nephrotoxic drugs, or if dosages are excessive, irreparable renal damage may occur
• If elevated creatinine levels do not return to normal following fluid therapy, acute renal failure is suspected and the prognosis is guarded

POSSIBLE INTERACTIONS

See Contraindications.

 FOLLOW-UP

PATIENT MONITORING

• Patient's progress should be reviewed and fracture healing assessed radiographically after fracture repair and again prior to release from the hospital
• Horses are expected to walk comfortably immediately following successful fracture repair

• After release, box rest and follow-up radiographs every 4 weeks are recommended to monitor healing
• Most horses that have undergone lag screw fixation of uncomplicated phalangeal or condylar fractures can begin hand-walking at 6–8 weeks postoperatively
• Nondisplaced, unilateral fractures of the ilium usually heal with 12–16 weeks of box rest
• Ultrasonography of fractures of the ilium is also performed approximately every 4 weeks
• Whether treatment is surgical or nonsurgical, exercise must be carefully monitored and gradually introduced after fracture healing

PREVENTION/AVOIDANCE

• Lameness should be investigated prior to return to training or competition to decrease the likelihood of fracture occurrence
• Horses that are not sound enough to train or compete without the use of medication are at high risk for fracture formation

POSSIBLE COMPLICATIONS

• Some fractures, especially condylar fractures of the third metacarpus and metatarsus, may be bilateral, but present as a unilateral lameness
• Radiographing the contralateral limb prior to surgical repair is mandatory to prevent complete fracture of an undiagnosed fracture of the opposite limb during recovery from anesthesia
• Laminitis in the contralateral limb, enterocolitis, and cecal impaction are also possible complications

EXPECTED COURSE AND PROGNOSIS

• Return to athletic function is dependent on fracture type, location, and presence or absence of joint involvement, but, in general, fewer endurance horses return to their former level of competition than their flat-racing counterparts
• Whether the less successful return to the former level of athletic function is a result of the more advanced age of endurance horses as compared with flat-racing horses or the rigors of training required to achieve sufficient levels of fitness for endurance competition is undetermined

 MISCELLANEOUS

ASSOCIATED CONDITIONS

A number of endurance horses may have subclinical renal disease. It is prudent to monitor serum creatinine levels prior to shipping and during treatment and hospitalization. The use of NSAIDs should be minimized, and fluid therapy provided as needed.

AGE-RELATED FACTORS

• Endurance horses are skeletally mature before they are eligible for competition
• It is unlikely that age differences in the population are likely to affect prognosis in fracture healing, although older horses may be expected to have a greater number of other musculoskeletal issues that may affect overall return to function

ZOONOTIC POTENTIAL

None

PREGNANCY/FERTILITY/BREEDING

N/A

SEE ALSO

• Azotemia and uremia
• Exertional rhabdomyolysis syndrome
• Polycythemia

ABBREVIATIONS

• FEI = Fédération Equestre Internationale
• MRI = magnetic resonance imaging
• NSAID = nonsteroidal anti-inflammatory drug
• PVC = polyvinylchloride

Suggested Reading
Misheff MM, Alexander GR, Hirst GR. Management of fractures in endurance horses. Equine Vet Educ 2010;22:623–630.
Mudge M, Bramlage LR. Field fracture management. Vet Clin North Am Equine Pract 2007;23:117–133.

Author Martha M. Misheff
Consulting Editor Jean-Pierre Lavoie

F

FUMONISINS

BASICS

DEFINITION
Fumonisins are a group of mycotoxins produced by the fungus *Fusarium verticillioides* (formerly *Fusarium moniliforme*), which are responsible for the disease ELEM, also referred to as moldy corn disease. The most important of these is fumonisin B_1. ELEM is a fatal disease characterized by rapidly progressing neurologic impairment in horses and other equids. Distinctive lesions include softening and necrosis of cerebral white matter, as well as swollen and discolored livers.

PATHOPHYSIOLOGY
• Fumonisins are structurally similar to the sphingolipids sphingosine and sphinganine, which are necessary for cellular membrane function and cellular regulation. Fumonisins inhibit ceramide synthase, a sphingolipid metabolizing enzyme, resulting in accumulations of sphingosine and sphinganine and disruption of sphingolipid-dependent processes. Clinical and pathologic effects are thought to be due to sphingolipid alterations on the vasculature of the brain, cardiovascular dysfunction, and, in some individuals, hepatocellular necrosis. In vitro work suggests that fumonisins may have the ability to affect hoof lamellar integrity
• There are few data on the toxicokinetics of fumonisins in horses. For most species, fumonisins are poorly absorbed following oral administration and are rapidly eliminated. Fumonisin tissue concentrations are usually undetectable

SYSTEMS AFFECTED
In horses, the nervous system is the target organ, followed by the hepatobiliary system.

GENETICS
N/A

INCIDENCE/PREVALENCE
• Fumonisin outbreaks occur sporadically throughout all regions of the world
• Insect damage and adverse weather conditions are associated with increased fumonisin production. Conditions favoring fumonisiin generation include a period of drought during the growing season, followed by cool and moist conditions during pollination and kernel formation. Clinical outbreaks occur seasonally, generally from late fall to early spring. As many as 15–25% of animals within a group may be affected
• ELEM outbreaks occur under environmental conditions favoring mold production in corn crops, as well as from contaminated corn shipped to other locations

SIGNALMENT
• Horses, ponies, donkeys, and mules can be affected
• Any ages, but mature horses may be more susceptible

SIGNS
• Both neurotoxic and hepatotoxic syndromes have been described, but generally only some aspects of both syndromes are noted. The predominance of each syndrome is related to the concentration of fumonisin in the feed, the duration of toxin consumption, and individual susceptibility
• The neurologic syndrome is considered the most common. Signs of a fumonisin toxicosis are usually first noticeable following several weeks of daily ingestion of contaminated feed. Clinical signs often have a sudden onset and are rapidly progressive
• Depression, anorexia, blindness, ataxia, aimless wandering, lowered head and/or head pressing, circling, hyperexcitability, facial paralysis, paresis, recumbency, coma, and death
• Severely affected animals may die within 2–3 days; others may survive a week or more after onset of signs
• Horses may be found dead without the owner noticing any unusual clinical signs
• Body temperature usually remains normal
• Depressed horses are usually unresponsive. However, some may become hyperexcitable and unpredictable when disturbed
• Icterus, hemorrhages, and edema are possible with liver failure

CAUSES
• Ingestion of corn and corn products contaminated with fumonisins, or foraging on damaged or moldy corn
• Rarely, fumonisins have been reported in "black oats" feed from Brazil, hay from Brazil, and in New Zealand forage grasses
• Horses are the most sensitive species to fumonisins
• The highest concentrations of fumonisins can be found in broken kernels and screenings
• The minimum dietary concentration associated with induction of ELEM is about 8–10 ppm ingested for a period of approximately 30 days. Higher dosages result in signs as early as 7–10 days. High dosages seem to cause predominantly ELEM and lower exposures for longer periods favor the development of hepatotoxicosis
• Fumonisins are water soluble, heat stable, and resistant to alkali treatments that render many other mycotoxins inactive during feed processing

RISK FACTORS
See Causes.

DIAGNOSIS

DIFFERENTIAL DIAGNOSIS
• Rabies—brain positive for rabies virus antigen using fluorescent antibody techniques, histopathology
• Encephalitis—rapid progression of febrile syndrome with CNS inflammation, high serum antibody titers (especially if acute and convalescent serum samples are available), no history of appropriate vaccination, CSF analysis, pathologic changes in CNS
• Botulism—paralytic syndrome, detection of botulinum toxin via mouse bioassay or ELISA in feed, gastrointestinal contents, or liver
• Head trauma—history of trauma, physical examination, imaging
• Hepatic encephalopathy—underlying liver dysfunction, clinical pathology
• Aflatoxicosis—clinical pathology compatible with liver disease, liver pathology, detection of aflatoxins in feed or liver
• PA hepatotoxicosis—history of exposure to PA-containing plants, signs related to chronic wasting, clinical pathology compatible with liver disease, liver pathology, detection of PAs in feed

CBC/BIOCHEMISTRY/URINALYSIS
• Serum biochemistry results are reflective of hepatic disease. Increases in serum lactate dehydrogenase, alkaline phosphatase, aspartate aminotransferase, γ-glutamyltransferase, and bilirubin may be seen
• Urinalysis is often normal

OTHER LABORATORY TESTS
• Elevations in serum sphinganine to sphingosine ratios are often pronounced. This assay is performed only by select diagnostic laboratories
• Detection of fumonisins in feed specimens can be performed at many veterinary diagnostic laboratories. Representative feed samples can be difficult to obtain because of the long duration from consumption until clinical manifestations occur
• To date reliable assays for detection of fumonisins in blood or tissues are not available
• Culturing of the feed samples for the *Fusarium* fungus does not correlate to fumonisin concentrations, because high fumonisin concentrations have been found without the presence of the fungus while other samples have demonstrated large amounts of fungus without concomitant toxin production. Therefore, testing for the toxin is required to diagnose intoxication
• When testing feed, it is important to obtain representative samples of the entire batch, at various locations and depths within the batch, in order to catch potential "hot spots"

IMAGING
N/A

OTHER DIAGNOSTIC PROCEDURES
CSF findings may include elevated protein concentrations, albumin, and immunoglobulin G concentrations.

PATHOLOGIC FINDINGS
• Evaluation of the brain can reveal massive softening and liquefaction of subcortical cerebral white matter. Lesion size may range from a few millimeters to involving large portions of the white matter of either or both sides of the cerebral hemispheres. Areas surrounding the necrosis are usually edematous and hemorrhagic. These lesions have only been found in horses
• The liver can appear swollen and brownish on gross examination
• Histologic examination may reveal fatty change of hepatocytes, loss of hepatic architecture, scattered liver cell necrosis, portal fibrosis, bile stasis, and bile duct proliferation

TREATMENT
• There is currently no successful treatment for horses with ELEM. Most horses die or are euthanized
• Treatment is aimed at providing supportive care for animals with neurologic and/or hepatic disease and reducing further exposure to the source of contamination
• Outpatient medical management
• Because of the long latent period involved, gastrointestinal decontamination is of limited value
• Horses with hepatic dysfunction should be treated with fluids and hepatoprotectants
• Activity should be decreased to prevent injury in those horses exhibiting neurologic signs. Excitable horses should be sedated to prevent injury to the horse or handler
• Contaminated feed should be replaced with laboratory-confirmed mycotoxin-free feed

MEDICATIONS
DRUG(S) OF CHOICE
There is no antidote for fumonisin intoxication.

CONTRAINDICATIONS
N/A

PRECAUTIONS
N/A

POSSIBLE INTERACTIONS
N/A

ALTERNATIVE DRUGS
N/A

FOLLOW-UP
PATIENT MONITORING
• Neurologic function and hepatic enzymes should be monitored following removal from contaminated feed
• Animal handlers should take caution around affected horses because their behavior may be unpredictable and serious injury may result

PREVENTION/AVOIDANCE
• Animal owners should be informed about the conditions favoring toxin production, and the risks involved in feeding corn or corn-based products
• Corn intended to be fed to horses should be periodically tested so that fumonisin concentrations are below FDA recommended guidelines. Currently, equine feeds should contain no more than 5 ppm dietary fumonisins, which, in turn, should constitute no more than 20% of the total diet
• No binding agents are currently available to decrease fumonisin absorption following ingestion
• Contaminated feeds should be either diluted with clean feed and retested prior to feeding or fed to a less sensitive species, such as ruminants

POSSIBLE COMPLICATIONS
N/A

EXPECTED COURSE AND PROGNOSIS
Horses with ELEM have a poor prognosis and are not likely to recover despite treatment.

MISCELLANEOUS
ASSOCIATED CONDITIONS
N/A

AGE-RELATED FACTORS
N/A

ZOONOTIC POTENTIAL
N/A

PREGNANCY/FERTILITY/BREEDING
Ingestion of fumonisin-contaminated corn has been associated with neural tube defects in humans. The significance of these findings to the pregnant mare and fetus has yet to be determined.

SYNONYMS
• ELEM
• Cornstalk disease
• Moldy corn disease

SEE ALSO
N/A

ABBREVIATIONS
• CFS = cerebral spinal fluid
• CNS = central nervous system
• ELEM = equine leukoencephalomalacia
• ELISA = enzyme-linked immunosorbent assay
• FDA = United States Food and Drug Administration
• PA = pyrrolizidine alkaloid

Suggested Reading
Marasas WFO, Riley RT, Hendricks KA, et al. Fumonisins disrupt sphingolipid metabolism, folate transport, and neural tube development in embryo culture and in vivo: a potential risk factor for human neural tube defects among populations consuming fumonisin-contaminated maize. J Nutr 2004;134:711–716.
Reisinger N, Dohnal I, Nagl V, et al. Fumonisin B1 (FB1) induces lamellar separation and alters sphingolipid metabolism of *in vitro* cultured hoof explants. Toxins (Basel) 2016;8:89.
Smith GW. Fumonisins. In: Gupta RC, ed. Veterinary Toxicology: Basic and Clinical Principles, 2e. San Diego, CA: Elsevier, 2012:1205–1219.
Vendruscolo CP, Frias NC, de Carvalho CB, et al. Leukoencephalomalacia outbreak in horses due to consumption of contaminated hay. J Vet Intern Med 2016;30(6):1879–1881.
Voss KA, Smith GW, Hashek WM. Fumonisins: toxicokinetics, mechanism of action and toxicity. Anim Feed Sci Technol 2007;137:299–325.

Author Petra A. Volmer
Consulting Editors Wilson K. Rumbeiha and Steve Ensley

 Client Education Handout available online

FUNGAL PNEUMONIA

BASICS

OVERVIEW
• Primary fungal pneumonia is caused by pathogens with discrete geographic restrictions
• Secondary fungal pneumonia is caused by ubiquitous environmental fungal agents such as *Aspergillus* and affects horses with immune compromise or with significant gastrointestinal comorbidities such as colitis

SIGNALMENT
• Horses with fungal pneumonia may be any age
• *Pneumocystis jiroveci* (previously *Pneumocystis carinii*) has only been reported in foals 1.5–4 months of age

SIGNS
• Fungal pneumonia—weight loss, exercise intolerance, and cough are common and fever, tachypnea, hemoptysis, and nasal discharge have also been noted
• Foals with *P. jiroveci* pneumonia typically present with severe respiratory distress and pneumonia

CAUSES AND RISK FACTORS
• Primary fungal pneumonia is caused by inhalation of the infectious form of pathogen fungi such as *Blastomyces dermatitidis, Coccidioides immitis, Cryptococcus neoformans*, and *Histoplasma capsulatum*
• Secondary fungal pneumonia is caused by environmental (ubiquitous) fungi, and occurs only in horses profoundly immunocompromised by other diseases or the use of immunosuppressive drugs. Agents identified in horses with secondary pneumonia include *Aspergillus, Phycomycetes, Rhizopus, Mucor, Acremonium, Paecilomyces*, and *P. jiroveci* in foals

DIAGNOSIS

DIFFERENTIAL DIAGNOSIS
• Bacterial pneumonia/pleuritis
• Equine multinodular fibrosis
• Severe equine asthma
• Intrathoracic neoplasia

CBC/BIOCHEMISTRY/URINALYSIS
Nonspecific inflammatory leukogram.

OTHER LABORATORY TESTS
• Serology for *C. neoformans, C. immitis*, and *H. capsulatum* can be supportive of the diagnosis, but previous exposure can cause titers in unaffected animals

• Panfungal PCR assays are available to identify fungal DNA in fluid or tissue samples

IMAGING
Thoracic radiographs typically show significant abnormalities. Interstitial, miliary, nodular, and patchy bronchoalveolar patterns have all been described.

OTHER DIAGNOSTIC PROCEDURES
• Special care should be taken not to overdiagnose this disease in the field; up to 70% of transtracheal washes have evidence of fungal elements which are considered normal
• Lung biopsy is frequently diagnostic. Special stains are often needed to visualize fungal organisms
• Fungal culture may identify specific pathogens but 16% of healthy horses will have fungal growth on transtracheal wash culture

TREATMENT
• Antifungal medications form the mainstay of treatment
• Supportive care for pneumonia is indicated

MEDICATIONS

DRUG(S) OF CHOICE
• Itraconazole, fluconazole, ketoconazole, and voriconazole have all been investigated in horses. Voriconazole is the newest (4 mg/kg PO SID) and is considered broad spectrum; itraconazole (5 mg/kg PO SID) is effective against *Aspergillus* spp. Fluconazole (loading dose of 14 mg/kg followed by 5 mg/kg PO SID) is ineffective against the filamentous fungi such as *Aspergillus* and *Fusarium*
• Amphotericin B (0.1–0.5 mg/kg IV every 48 h) has been used when other drugs are ineffective
• Iodides and 5-fluorocytosine (flucytosine) have also been used
• For *Pneumocystis* infection in foals, trimethoprim–sulfamethoxazole (25 mg/kg PO BID) can be used. Oral dapsone can be an alternative treatment

CONTRAINDICATIONS/POSSIBLE INTERACTIONS
• Fluconazole (and other azole drugs) have been associated with hepatoxicity, but are generally well tolerated
• Amphotericin B is potentially nephrotoxic; kidney function should be monitored closely

FOLLOW-UP

PATIENT MONITORING
• Repeated radiographs are useful for monitoring course of disease
• Decreasing serum titers (where applicable) may also be helpful

PREVENTION/AVOIDANCE
Horses should be housed in areas with low dust levels, as the majority of dust particles are of fungal origin.

POSSIBLE COMPLICATIONS
Most complications are associated with the chronic, severe pneumonia, or the primary cause of immunodeficiency.

EXPECTED COURSE AND PROGNOSIS
• The prognosis for fungal pneumonia is generally poor, although mild infection with some of the primary pathogens may be self-limiting
• Treatment is often unrewarding and expensive, and involves long-term (2–4 months) administration of antifungal agents and supportive care

MISCELLANEOUS

ASSOCIATED CONDITIONS
Many of the primary fungal pathogens also cause disease of other organs such as the skin, liver, meninges, or bone.

AGE-RELATED FACTORS
P. jiroveci has been diagnosed in foals only.

ZOONOTIC POTENTIAL
Organisms are of low virulence to humans. Nonetheless, immunocompromised humans should be advised to avoid contact with these patients.

PREGNANCY/FERTILITY/BREEDING
H. capsulatum and *C. neoformans* are associated with abortion in mares. Many antifungals are teratogens, and should be avoided during pregnancy.

ABBREVIATIONS
PCR = polymerase chain reaction

Suggested Reading
Stewart AJ, Cuming RS. Update on fungal respiratory disease in horses. Vet Clin North Am Equine Pract 2015;31(1):43–62.

Author Rose D. Nolen-Walston
Consulting Editors Daniel Jean and Mathilde Leclère

BASICS

OVERVIEW
• The *Fusarium* spp. produce a number of mycotoxins, including the trichothecenes, zearalenone, and fumonisins (see chapter Fumonisins)
• The trichothecene class is produced predominantly by *Fusarium sporotrichioides,* and consists of approximately 150 mycotoxins including DON (vomitoxin), T-2 toxin, DAS, and nivalenol
• The trichothecenes are potent inhibitors of protein synthesis most commonly found in Canada and north-central USA and primarily in corn and wheat
• Zearalenone, a weak estrogen, is produced primarily *Fusarium roseum* (*Fusarium graminearum*) in corn, but has also been reported in wheat, barley, rice, and *Sorghum.* Zearalenone toxicosis is uncommon in horses
• Feeds may be co-contaminated with multiple mycotoxins. Fungal infection of grain, with or without toxin production, reduces nutrient quality, leading to poor production and nutritional impairment of animals

SIGNS
• Horses appear to be resistant to the effects of DON; feed refusal is reported in sensitive animals
• Experimentally, T-2 and DAS can cause dermal irritation and necrosis, lymphoid depletion, gastroenteritis, cardiovascular failure, and death at concentrations which are unlikely to occur in the field
• In 1 case report, zearalenone was associated with edema and flaccidity of the equine genitals

CAUSES AND RISK FACTORS
• Ingestion of contaminated grain or processed feed, or inhalation of contaminated bedding. Trichothecene mycotoxins and zearalenone are resistant to heat and pressure of food processing, and are stable in the environment
• Unusually cool weather conditions in late summer and early fall coupled with heavy rainfall can result in trichothecene production
• High concentrations of zearalenone usually result from improper storage at high moisture concentrations (greater than 30–40%)

DIAGNOSIS

DIFFERENTIAL DIAGNOSIS
• For the GI effects of the trichothecenes
  ○ Cantharidin toxicosis—detection of cantharidin in gastric contents or urine, evidence of insects in hay or GI contents, characteristic lesions
  ○ *Ranunculus* spp.—blistering of skin and mouth, erythema and swelling of muzzle and lips, evidence of ingestion
  ○ NSAIDs
  ○ Arsenic—arsenic concentration in liver, kidney, urine, hair, feed, hemorrhagic gastroenteritis
  ○ Castor bean (*Ricinus communis*) and other toxic lectins—clinical signs, detection of ricin in tissues, evidence of beans in GI contents, histopathology
  ○ Gastroenteritis
• For the reproductive effects of zearalenone
  ○ Fescue toxicosis
  ○ Endometritis and pyometra

CBC/BIOCHEMISTRY/URINALYSIS
No clinically significant changes.

OTHER LABORATORY TESTS
Feed can be tested for mycotoxins.

PATHOLOGIC FINDINGS
• No pathognomonic lesions for DON
• T-2 and DAS—dermal and mucosal irritation, necrosis, intestinal inflammation
• Zearalenone—swelling of vulva and uterus, ovarian atrophy

TREATMENT
• Removal of contaminated feed and/or bedding. Animals should return to normal performance in weeks to months following removal from toxin
• There is no specific treatment for the trichothecenes or zearalenone. Symptomatic and supportive treatment is recommended

MEDICATIONS

DRUG(S) OF CHOICE
N/A

FOLLOW-UP

PREVENTION/AVOIDANCE
• Feed should be visually inspected and tested for the presence of mycotoxins
• Avoiding late harvests, removing overwintered stubble from fields, and avoiding a corn/wheat rotation that favors *Fusarium* growth in crop residue can reduce contamination of grains
• Store grains at less than 13–14% moisture to prevent mycotoxin production

• Once produced, the trichothecenes and zearalenone are environmentally stable compounds

POSSIBLE COMPLICATIONS
Poor performance in exposed animals.

EXPECTED COURSE AND PROGNOSIS
The clinical effects are expected to resolve following removal of the toxin.

MISCELLANEOUS

AGE-RELATED FACTORS
Neonatal animals are more susceptible to effects of the trichothecenes.

ZOONOTIC POTENTIAL
N/A

PREGNANCY/FERTILITY/BREEDING
Failure of implantation and early embryonic death were reported in swine administered zearalenone.

SEE ALSO
Fumonisins

ABBREVIATIONS
• DAS = diacetoxyscirpenol
• DON = deoxynivalenol
• GI = gastrointestinal
• NSAID = nonsteroidal anti-inflammatory drug

Suggested Reading
Caloni F, Cortinovis C. Effects of fusariotoxins in the equine species. Vet J 2010;186:157–161.
Mostrom MS. Zearalenone. In: Gupta RC, ed. Veterinary Toxicology: Basic and Clinical Principles, 2e. San Diego, CA: Elsevier, 2012:1266.
Mostrom MS, Raisbeck MF. Trichothecenes. In: Gupta RC, ed. Veterinary Toxicology: Basic and Clinical Principles, 2e. San Diego, CA: Elsevier, 2012:1239.
Osweiler GD. Mycotoxins. Vet Clin North Am Equine Pract 2001;17:547–566.
Songsermsakul P, Bohm J, Aurich C, et al. The levels of zearalenone and its metabolites in plasma, urine and faeces of horses fed with naturally, Fusarium toxin-contaminated oats. J Anim Physiol Anim Nutr (Berl) 2013;97:155–161.
Villar D, Carson TL. Trichothecene mycotoxins. In: Plumlee KH, ed. Clinical Veterinary Toxicology. St. Louis, MO: Mosby, 2004:270.

Author Petra A. Volmer
Consulting Editors Wilson K. Rumbeiha and Steve Ensley

Client Education Handout available online

F

GAMMA-GLUTAMYLTRANSFERASE (GGT)

BASICS

DEFINITION
• Serum GGT concentration is one of the most sensitive markers of hepatobiliary disease, but normal values do *not* rule out significant disease
• Serum increases may be associated with overtraining or poor racing performance
• Urine GGT can be used as a marker for renal tubular degeneration or necrosis

PATHOPHYSIOLOGY
• GGT is a membrane-bound carboxypeptidase that plays a major role in glutathione metabolism
• High tissue concentrations in kidney, liver, and pancreas
• Liver GGT activity is greatest along the brush border of biliary epithelial cells
• Increased membrane release or increased synthesis (i.e. induction) contributes to increased serum activity
• Mechanism of release into the blood is proposed to involve membrane solubilization by bile salts, release of membrane fragments/vesicles, or biliary regurgitation
• Serum half-life is $\cong$3 days
• Greatest serum GGT elevations are associated with cholestasis or chronic liver disease, but acute hepatocellular injury also increases serum activity. Experimentally, bile duct ligation causes 8–10-fold increases by 10 days; cellular injury is associated with peak increases (4–5-fold) within 2 days. In acute cholestasis, bile acids and conjugated bilirubin may precede serum GGT elevations, since GGT increases depend in part on enzyme induction. Serum GGT activity also increases with biliary epithelial hyperplasia. In chronic diseases, serum GGT concentration can be markedly elevated
• With renal injury, GGT is released into urine
• Equine pancreatitis is uncommon, and its contribution to increased serum GGT concentration is equivocal. Thus, increases in serum GGT concentration are considered relatively specific for hepatobiliary disease
• Mechanism for increased serum GGT concentration associated with overtraining is unclear, but GGT values >100 U/L tend to be associated with compromised performance

SYSTEMS AFFECTED
• Hepatobiliary—increases are associated with cholestasis (with or without biliary hyperplasia) and cell injury
• Renal—tubular epithelial injury increases urinary, but not serum, GGT concentration
• Musculoskeletal—increases are associated with overtraining; GGT source is equivocal
• GI/Endocrine—pancreatitis (uncommon) is a potential source of increased serum GGT concentration

GENETICS
N/A

INCIDENCE/PREVALENCE
N/A

GEOGRAPHIC DISTRIBUTION
N/A

SIGNALMENT
• Neonates—healthy neonatal values during the first 2–3 weeks of life may exceed adult values by 2–3-fold. The increase may reflect biliary proliferation. Foals do not absorb GGT from colostrum, as occurs in ruminants
• Healthy donkeys, burros, and asses may have 2–3-fold higher GGT activity than horses

SIGNS

Historical Findings
• Icterus, dark-yellow/orange urine, anorexia, weight loss, and/or listlessness with hepatobiliary disease
• Behavioral changes may reflect hepatic failure
• Colic may occur with acute hepatopathies (i.e. capsular swelling) or biliary obstructions

Physical Examination Findings
• Icterus is common
• Increased pulse and respiratory rates, fever, photosensitization, weight loss, and obesity vary and depend on the underlying disease process

CAUSES

Hepatobiliary System
• Metabolic—secondary to severe anemia, hyperlipemia, fasting (<50% increase in 2–3 days, nonpathologic), or diabetes mellitus
• Immune mediated, infectious—chronic active hepatitis, Theiler's disease, amyloidosis, endotoxemia, viral (e.g. EIA, equine viral arteritis, equine herpesvirus 1 in perinatal foals), bacterial (e.g. Tyzzer's disease, salmonellosis), fungal, protozoal (*Theileria equi, Babesia caballi*), and parasitic (e.g. liver flukes, strongyle larval migrans)
• Nutritional—hepatic lipidosis, ferrous fumarate toxicity in neonates
• Degenerative—cirrhosis, cholelithiasis
• Toxic—pyrrolizidine alkaloid-containing plants (e.g. *Senecio, Crotalaria*), alsike clover, kleingrass, aflatoxin, rubratoxin, *Fusarium* mycotoxins, chemical toxins (e.g. arsenic, chlorinated hydrocarbons, monensin, phenol, paraquat); mild increases are inconsistently reported with halothane anesthesia
• Anomaly—biliary atresia, portovascular shunts
• Neoplastic—primary liver tumors, metastatic neoplasia

Musculoskeletal System
Mild increases with overtraining.

GI System
• Potentially associated with pancreatitis
• Proximal enteritis—GGT concentration elevated 12-fold more likely (vs. small intestine strangulating obstruction)

• Right displacement of descending large colon—compresses bile duct, causing increased GGT activity in ~50% of cases, versus 2% for left colon displacement

Hematopoietic System
• Severe anemia (e.g. acute EIA, red maple leaf toxicity, onion toxicity, postparturient hemorrhage) leads to hypoxic injury and hepatocellular swelling with subsequent cholestasis
• Hepatic lymphoma, leukemias, etc.

RISK FACTORS
• Theiler's disease—equine biologic administration (e.g. tetanus antitoxin, plasma) within previous 40–90 days
• Ponies and donkeys—particularly susceptible to hyperlipemia and hepatic lipidosis
• Horses used long term as hyperimmunized serum donors might develop amyloidosis
• Fasting—see Causes

DIAGNOSIS

DIFFERENTIAL DIAGNOSIS
• Consider pancreatitis and overtraining. Otherwise, increased serum GGT activity is considered specific for hepatobiliary disease. However, it is not specific for the type of hepatobiliary condition
• Highest elevations are associated with longstanding conditions with severe cholestasis or biliary hyperplasia (e.g. chronic active hepatitis, cirrhosis, cholelithiasis, lipidosis)
• Concurrent obesity and high enzyme activities suggest hyperlipemia/lipidosis; anorexia and weight loss are typical of most other differentials

CBC/BIOCHEMISTRY/URINALYSIS
• Serum is the preferred sample type, but heparin, EDTA, or citrated plasma potentially can be used if validated by laboratory
• Serum samples are stable for 3 days at 4°C or for at least 1 month at −20°C
• Extreme icterus, severe lipemia, and marked hemolysis may affect values

Erythrocytes
• Nonregenerative anemia may be seen with liver disease
• Microcytosis is associated with portosystemic shunts
• Acanthocytes, schistocytes (from liver microvascular disease) are associated with decreased RBC survival and may contribute to mild hemolytic anemia
• Severe hemolytic anemia can cause hypoxic injury
• A severe hemolytic crisis can occur terminally with liver failure

Leukocytes
• Neutrophilia, neutropenia, or monocytosis may occur with inflammatory hepatobiliary disease
• Evidence of antigenic stimulation may be seen (e.g. lymphocytosis, reactive lymphoid cells)

Glucose
Postprandial hyperglycemia or fasting hypoglycemia may occur with hepatic insufficiency/shunts.

Albumin
• Decreased production with hepatic insufficiency may decrease serum concentrations
• Albumin is a negative acute-phase reactant; mild decreases may occur with chronic inflammation

Blood Urea Nitrogen
Decreases with hepatic insufficiency/shunts because of decreased conversion of ammonia to urea.

Sorbitol Dehydrogenase
Increases specifically with hepatocellular injury.

Aspartate Aminotransferase
Increases with hepatocellular or muscle injury.

Alkaline Phosphatase
Increases primarily with cholestasis.

Bilirubin
• Conjugated—increases with cholestasis
• Unconjugated—increases with increased RBC destruction (i.e. hemolysis) and defective hepatocellular uptake (e.g. injured hepatocytes, hepatic insufficiency, vascular shunting); increases with fasting because of a physiologic decrease in hepatocellular uptake

Triglycerides
Increases with hyperlipemia.

Urinalysis
• Bilirubinuria indicates cholestasis
• Ammonia urates may be observed with hepatic insufficiency/shunt

OTHER LABORATORY TESTS
Bile Acids
• Sensitive indicator of decreased hepatobiliary function, but not specific
• Concentrations depend on adequate enterohepatic circulation, hepatobiliary function, and hepatocellular perfusion
• More sensitive than serum GGT concentration for acute cholestasis

Ammonia
Serum concentrations are affected by hepatic uptake and conversion to urea; ammonia correlates inversely with hepatic functional mass.

Clearance Tests (Sulfobromophthalein, Indocyanine Green)
• Prolonged clearance intervals occur with decreased functional mass or cholestasis
• Accelerated clearance (possibly masking insufficiency) occurs with hypoalbuminemia

Coagulation Tests
May be prolonged with hepatic insufficiency/shunting.

IMAGING
Ultrasonography is useful for assessing liver size, shape, position, and parenchymal texture.

OTHER DIAGNOSTIC PROCEDURES
Aspiration cytology or biopsy for microbiologic testing, cytologic imprints, and histopathologic evaluation.

TREATMENT
Treatment is directed at the underlying disease process.

MEDICATIONS
DRUG(S) OF CHOICE
N/A

CONTRAINDICATIONS
N/A

PRECAUTIONS
With suspected hepatic insufficiency, assess coagulation profiles before invasive procedures.

POSSIBLE INTERACTIONS
N/A

ALTERNATIVE DRUGS
N/A

FOLLOW-UP
PATIENT MONITORING
• Serial biochemistries to characterize disease progression and identify evidence of improvement

• Cholangiohepatitis/cholelithiasis—consider use of antibiotics until serum GGT concentration is normal. Clinical improvement may precede this by days to weeks

PREVENTION/AVOIDANCE
N/A

POSSIBLE COMPLICATIONS
NA

EXPECTED COURSE AND PROGNOSIS
• Dependent on the underlying cause
• Risk of nonsurvival is variably reported to increase with GGT > 399 IU/L (hazard ratio = 4.54) or with GGT > 224 IU/L, predicting nonsurvival with sensitivity of 54% and specificity of 95%
• Hypoglycemia with liver disease carries a guarded prognosis

MISCELLANEOUS
ASSOCIATED CONDITIONS
Dependent on the underlying cause.

AGE-RELATED FACTORS
See Signalment.

ZOONOTIC POTENTIAL
N/A

PREGNANCY/FERTILITY/BREEDING
N/A

SYNONYMS
γ-Glutamyltranspeptidase

SEE ALSO
See Causes.

ABBREVIATIONS
• EIA = equine infectious anemia
• GGT = γ-glutamyltransferase
• RBC = red blood cell

Suggested Reading
Barton MH. Disorders of the liver. In: Reed S, Bayly W, Sellon D, eds. Equine Internal Medicine, 3e. St. Louis, MO: WB Saunders, 2010:939–975.
Smith GW, Davis JL. Diseases of the hepatobiliary system. In: Smith B, ed. Large Animal Internal Medicine, 5e. St. Louis, MO: Elsevier Mosby, 2015:843–872.

Author John A. Christian
Consulting Editor Sandra D. Taylor

G

GASTRIC DILATION/DISTENTION

 BASICS

DEFINITION
Accumulation of excessive amounts of gas, fluid, or solid material in the stomach, resulting in dilation.

PATHOPHYSIOLOGY
• The position of the stomach as well as the high resting tone of the esophageal sphincter result in the inability of the horse to regurgitate or vomit. Furthermore, if this occurs, the horse will be at risk of aspiration pneumonia owing to its upper airway anatomy. For this reason, horses are predisposed to excessive distention of the stomach followed by possible rupture
• Causes of gastric dilation can be primary, secondary, or idiopathic
• Primary causes of gastric dilation include diseases of the stomach, aerophagia, feed engorgement, and rapid intake of water. The dilation results in decreased motility and a failure to discharge the stomach contents into the proximal duodenum. Overeating of easily fermentable food such as grain, fresh grass, beets, or beet pulp can lead to production of lactic acid and volatile fatty acids by the gastric flora. Gastric emptying is inhibited by increased concentrations of volatile fatty acids, resulting in further fermentation and production of gas. Primary gastric dilation may also result from local infestation of *Gasterophilus* larvae or habronemiasis, especially in the area of the pylorus. Primary gastric distention can also be caused iatrogenically following passage of a nasogastric tube and overloading the stomach with liquids
• Gastric dilation can be secondary to an obstructive lesion of the small intestine, resulting in retrograde movement of intestinal fluid and bile, or nonobstructive small intestinal ileus (e.g. proximal duodenojejunitis). The time of development of gastric reflux is proportional to the distance to the obstructed small intestine segment. It may also be secondary to colonic displacement (left and right dorsal displacement), which most likely obstructs duodenal outflow. Improper mastication, poorly digestible ingested material, and eating behaviors may result in gastric impaction
• Gastric dilation may lead to gastric rupture, usually along its greater curvature. Gastric rupture may be secondary to mechanical obstruction, gastric ulceration, ileus, as well as overload and idiopathic causes

SYSTEMS AFFECTED
• Gastrointestinal
• Cardiovascular—affected if horse is dehydrated. Gastric rupture results in endotoxemia, shock, and death

• Respiratory—abdominal distention and pressure on the diaphragm may affect breathing

INCIDENCE/PREVALENCE
Not common.

SIGNALMENT
No sex or breed disposition, but the age might assist in the identification of a primary cause. For example, foals are more predisposed to gastric ulceration.

SIGNS
General Comments
A gastric dilation/distention can lead to gastric rupture.

Historical Findings
Depend on the severity of the dilation/distention. Signs of abdominal pain may occur abruptly following excessive or rapid consumption of a large amount of liquid or food. There may be a history of ingestion of highly fermentable food. If secondary to a distal obstruction, the clinical signs are initially related to the primary problem. Mild to severe signs of abdominal pain may be observed. The animal may assume a dog sitting position and present with retching or gurgling sounds. Gastric rupture results in relief, depression, and eventually a reluctance to move.

Physical Examination Findings
Increase in heart and respiratory rates, may have sour smell to the breath, and possibly some ingesta at the nares. Cyanosis and pale mucous membranes may be present, likely due to the local increase in gastric space occupation, thus reducing venous return. There may be dehydration or toxic shock as the disease progresses. Rectal examination may reveal the spleen to be displaced caudally. If the condition is secondary to an aboral obstruction, other abnormalities such as distention of the small intestines may be palpated. On nasogastric intubation, large amounts of gas, fluid, or ingesta may escape. Net gastric reflux of more than 2 L is significant. Spontaneous reflux may also be present in severe cases. Passage of the nasogastric tube may be difficult due to distortion of the cardia. If gastric rupture occurs, the signs of colic will initially subside. Depression, tachycardia, tachypnea, sweating, muscle fasciculations, blue or purple mucous membranes, and severe signs of shock will quickly develop; colic may return.

CAUSES
See Pathophysiology.

RISK FACTORS
• Overeating
• Poor mastication
• Intestinal obstructions
• Ingestion of fermentable food

 DIAGNOSIS

DIFFERENTIAL DIAGNOSIS
Any other cause of colic.

CBC/BIOCHEMISTRY/URINALYSIS
• May have an elevated packed cell volume and total protein due to dehydration or endotoxic shock. Horses with severe dehydration may have prerenal azotemia
• Hypoproteinemia if protein loss
• Hypochloremia if gastric reflux is present, resulting in metabolic alkalosis
• Metabolic acidosis secondary to severe endotoxemic shock and progressive dehydration possible
• If gastric rupture occurs, a moderate to severe leukopenia will be noticed secondary to the acute peritonitis

OTHER LABORATORY TESTS
pH
pH of reflux might assist to determine the origin of the problem. Normal gastric pH varies between 3 and 6. pH of fluid originating from the small intestine is between 5 and 7 and has a bilious color.

Abdominocentesis
• Abdominocentesis is usually normal if there is a primary gastric dilation without rupture
• There may be an increase in protein concentrations and leukocytes with devitalized bowel (stomach or small intestine)
• Sanguineous fluid may be indicative of a strangulated obstructive lesion of the small intestine or devitalization of the stomach
• Plant material in the sample in the absence of an enterocentesis suggests intestinal rupture
• No leukocytes or cells should be present if an enterocentesis was performed

IMAGING
Radiology
Radiography may identify an impacted stomach pushing on the diaphragm. In foals, a contrast study can help in outlining the gastric wall for detection of gastric ulcers and possibly strictures and determining the gastric emptying time.

Gastroscopy
Gastroscopy is useful for identification of impacted stomach, parasites, gastric ulcer, and neoplasm. In small horses, the duodenum also may be inspected for presence of ulceration and strictures.

Abdominal Laparoscopy
Abdominal laparoscopy is useful for visual inspection of the visceral part of the stomach and small intestine for lesions.

Ultrasonography
Stomach outline is usually seen between the 10th and 15th intercostal spaces. The wall

thickness is less than 0.75 cm. May be able to evaluate distention if expand to other intercostal spaces. There is a correlation between the volume in the stomach and its height at the level of the 12th intercostal space. May be useful to identify a primary lesion in the small intestine by evaluation of its wall thickness and diameter. Abnormal findings such as intussusception, mass, abscess, and adhesions may sometimes be identified. The evaluation of the amount, quality, and characteristics of abdominal fluid is also possible.

OTHER DIAGNOSTIC PROCEDURES
Exploratory laparotomy is useful to treat small intestinal lesions and possibly some gastric problems.

 TREATMENT

Supportive therapy for treatment of shock.

Primary Gastric Dilation/Impaction
Primary gastric dilation consists of deflating the stomach regularly by passage of the nasogastric tube. If impaction is present, lavage of the stomach followed by administration of DSS (10–30 mg/kg of a 10% solution), which acts as a surfactant and allows water to penetrate the impaction to soften it. It may be necessary to repeat this procedure. Care should be taken not to give too much DSS. Following resolution of an impaction the horse should be kept off feed for 48–72 h. Alternatively, repeated intragastric administration of saline carbonated drinks ("soft drinks") may be useful.

Secondary Gastric Dilation
Treatment consists of leaving the nasogastric tube in place and performing periodic decompression until resolution of the primary problem by medical or surgical treatment. Gastric rupture may occur despite periodic emptying of the stomach. Ultrasonographic monitoring may be useful to monitor the decompression.

Fluidotherapy
May be necessary in the presence of dehydration.

 MEDICATIONS

DRUG(S) OF CHOICE
Analgesics may be necessary to control the abdominal pain. They include:
• NSAIDs—flunixin meglumine (0.5–1.1 mg/kg IV, IM every 8 or 12 h); and α_2-blockers, such as xylazine (0.25–0.5 mg/kg IV or IM), detomidine (5–10 μg/kg IV or IM), or romifidine (0.02–0.05 mg/kg IV or IM)
• Narcotic or narcotic-derivative analgesics such as butorphanol (0.02–0.04 mg/kg IV), which can be given alone or in combination with xylazine. There is potentiation of these 2 drugs. Analgesics should be used judiciously as they may mask clinical signs and may lead to postponement of surgery
• Parenteral fluid treatments (100–200 mL/kg/day)
• When cardiovascular shock is present, hypertonic saline IV (in the adult horse 2 L of 7% NaCl; 4 mL/kg) prior to balanced electrolyte solutions (e.g. lactated Ringer's solution)
• In case of grain overload, secondary endotoxemia may result in laminitis; see chapter Laminitis

PRECAUTIONS
The nasogastric tube should be manipulated gently; avoid overloading the stomach.

 FOLLOW-UP

PATIENT MONITORING
The patient should be monitored for any increase in heart rate or discomfort indicating that the stomach may need to be further decompressed. If the condition is secondary to gastric ulcer, the use of NSAIDs may aggravate the problem.

POSSIBLE COMPLICATIONS
• Gastric rupture
• Endotoxemic shock

 MISCELLANEOUS

ASSOCIATED CONDITIONS
Primary Condition
• Gastric ulceration
• Parasitism
• Neoplasia

Secondary Condition
• Small intestinal obstruction (strangulated or nonstrangulated)
• Proximal duodenojejunitis

AGE-RELATED FACTORS
Gastric ulceration is often the primary cause of gastric dilation/distention in young foals.

ZOONOTIC POTENTIAL
N/A

PREGNANCY/FERTILITY/BREEDING
N/A

SEE ALSO
• Acute adult abdominal pain—acute colic
• Gastric impaction
• Small intestinal obstruction

ABBREVIATIONS
• DSS = dioctyl sodium succinate (docusate sodium)
• NSAID = nonsteroidal anti-inflammatory drug

Suggested Reading
Carter GK. Gastric diseases. In: Robinson NE, ed. Current Therapy in Equine Medicine, 2e. Philadelphia, PA: WB Saunders, 1987:41–44.

Hackett ES. Specific causes of colic. In: Southwood LL, ed. Practical Guide to Equine Colic. Ames, IA: Wiley Blackwell, 2013:204–207.

Kiper ML, Traub-Dargatz J, Curtis CR. Gastric rupture in horses: 50 cases (1979–1987). J Am Vet Med Assoc 1990;196:333–336.

Murray MJ. Diseases of the stomach. In: Mair T, Divers T, Ducharme N, eds. Manual of Equine Gastroenterology. Philadelphia, PA: WB Saunders, 2002:241–248.

Todhunter RJ, Erb HN, Roth L. Gastric rupture in horses: a review of 54 cases. Equine Vet J 1986;18:288–293.

Author Nathalie Coté
Consulting Editor Henry Stämpfli and Olimpo Oliver-Espinosa

G

GASTRIC IMPACTION

 BASICS

DEFINITION
Distention of the stomach due to accumulation of dehydrated ingesta that does not clear after an appropriate fasting period.

PATHOPHYSIOLOGY
• Can be primary or secondary; however, this definition is not used consistently.
• Primary gastric impactions can result from disturbance of the motility of the GI tract. These can include abnormal motility patterns, abnormal gastric secretion, or functional outflow obstructions. Thickening of the muscular layers without obvious cause has been reported.
• Secondary gastric impactions can be due to ingestion of expandable feeds, persimmon seeds, dental disease, mechanical outflow obstruction, inadequate water intake, or reduced GI motility due to systemic disease. Persimmon seed has a water-soluble tannin that polymerizes in the presence of gastric acid to form an adhesive coagulum. The coagulum reacts with cellulose and hemicellulose to form a hard solid mass. Hepatic disease, particularly caused by ragwort poisoning, has also been described as a cause of gastric impaction.
• Dehydrated gastric impaction can be an incidental finding during surgery for intestinal obstruction.
• Chronic impaction can result in thickening and severe dilation of the stomach wall. Up to 60 kg of ingesta has been removed from gastric impactions during surgery or at necropsy

SYSTEMS AFFECTED
• GI—the main signs are acute or chronic colic, anorexia, weight loss, and abnormal fecal output
• Cardiovascular—dehydration can be present

GENETICS
No genetic predisposition.

INCIDENCE/PREVALENCE
There is no prevalence data but the condition is rare. Engorgement with ripe persimmon fruit is more likely in the fall.

GEOGRAPHIC DISTRIBUTION
Worldwide

SIGNALMENT
There is no reported breed, age, or sex predilection. Foals may also be affected.

SIGNS
Historical Findings
Anorexia is the predominant reported clinical sign, often accompanied by weight loss and signs of colic. The duration of clinical signs at presentation can range from days to months. Colic signs can be acute or chronic, constant or intermittent, and can range from mild to severe. Fecal output is sometimes reduced and can be abnormal in consistency.

Physical Examination Findings
• Horses can be lethargic and show varying degrees of anorexia and colic.
• In acute cases tachycardia and tachypnea can be present; however, in chronic cases this is usually not seen.
• Abdominal wall tension may be increased and GI sounds decreased. Affected horses often have a decreased body condition score.
• Cardiovascular parameters are usually normal. Signs of dehydration can be present. Rarely, in acute cases horses have GI reflux, which can be visible at the nares or is diagnosed upon nasogastric intubation

CAUSES
• Primary impaction of unknown origin
• Secondary to
  ○ Gastric masses (neoplasia, polyp)
  ○ Pyloric masses (neoplasia, polyp)
  ○ Pyloric thickening (chronic ulcer disease)
  ○ Obstruction due to expandable feeds (wheat, barley, and sugar beet pulp)
  ○ Phytobezoar (persimmon seeds, mesquite beans)
  ○ Any systemic disease affecting GI motility
  ○ Hepatic disease
• In some cases an obvious cause cannot be found

RISK FACTORS
• Ingestion of certain feeds that swell or form a mass after ingestion
• Dental disease resulting in improper chewing of the food
• Inadequate water supply
• Rapid eating

 DIAGNOSIS

DIFFERENTIAL DIAGNOSIS
Delayed gastric emptying due to systemic disease.

CBC/BIOCHEMISTRY/URINALYSIS
Abnormalities are inconsistent and depend on the duration of the disease as well as the underlying cause.

OTHER LABORATORY TESTS
None

IMAGING
Abdominal US
Should be performed to evaluate the stomach. The normal equine stomach usually extends over 5 ICSs (10th–15th ICS) and is visible dorsal to the spleen and ventral to the lung on the left side. In horses with gastric distention the stomach is displaced dorsocaudally, extends >5 ICSs and can be visible from both sides, sometimes up to the paralumbar fossa. Care has to be taken not to overinterpret findings from US. Repeated US should be performed to assess whether findings are consistent. Gastric wall thickness of >10–35 mm has been reported (normal 1–5 mm).

Abdominal Radiographs
Often inconclusive and are mainly used to rule out differential diagnosis for recurrent colic.

OTHER DIAGNOSTIC PROCEDURES
Rectal Examination
The spleen is often displaced medially and caudally in the abdomen. In chronic cases with severe gastric dilation the enlarged stomach can be felt on rectal examination.

Nasogastric Intubation
Should be performed to rule out or relieve gastric distention. While reflux is not a feature in chronic cases, it can occur in acute cases. Difficulties passing the nasogastric tube beyond the cardia have been reported.

Gastroscopy
Visualization of the stomach, in particular of the margo plicatus, is precluded owing to dehydrated feed material. The horse should have been fasted for a minimum of 16 h to diagnose this condition. In the case of persimmon fruit phytobezoars the seeds can often be seen on the surface of the gastric impaction

Laparoscopy or Exploratory Laparotomy
The only definitive method to diagnose a gastric impaction is exploratory celiotomy.

Liver Biopsy
Should be performed when clinical or laboratory findings suggest an underlying hepatic cause.

 TREATMENT

APPROPRIATE HEALTH CARE
Horses can be managed on the farm. As diagnosis often requires specialized equipment referral to a hospital may be indicated. Medical and surgical treatment has been described.

NURSING CARE
• IV fluid therapy using an electrolyte solution (e.g. lactated Ringer's solution) should be instituted if dehydration is present and to attempt to soften the gastric contents. The rate of fluid administration depends on the degree of dehydration and should exceed maintenance requirements (2–4 mL/kg/h). Once the gastric impaction resolves, IV fluid therapy should be discontinued. If no improvement or resolution within 3–5 days, IV fluid therapy should be discontinued; it likely will not have further benefits.
• Enteral fluid therapy should be instituted to attempt to resolve the gastric impaction. Care should be taken to avoid rupture of the stomach. Note that rupture can occur even if fluid therapy is done correctly. The amount of

fluid administered depends on the fill and size of the stomach (2–6 L every 2–4 h over 1.5 days).
• Gastric lavage can be attempted using water alone or with mineral oil or magnesium sulfate. The use of carbonated cola has also been reported to be successful to resolve gastric impactions. In most cases gastric lavage has to be performed repeatedly. Gastric rupture can occur during gastric lavage. Gastric lavage should therefore be started conservatively using small amounts (1–2 L of fluid at a time). If this is tolerated well, the amount of fluid used can be increased gradually

DIET
• Fasting is indicated until a diagnosis is reached and during resolution of the gastric impaction. Once the impaction is resolved, feeding should be reinstituted gradually.
• Animals that are held off feed for prolonged periods of time and present in poor body condition may benefit from parenteral nutrition

CLIENT EDUCATION
Clients should be made aware of:
• The guarded prognosis in cases where the impaction cannot be resolved or the stomach shows signs of thickening and enlargement
• The risk of gastric rupture, which could occur spontaneously or during treatment with gastric lavage or enteral fluid therapy

MEDICATIONS

DRUG(S) OF CHOICE
• The use of laxatives is suggested in the literature; however, there is no conclusive evidence for the effectiveness. Mineral oil (1–5 L every 4–6 h per nasogastric tube for 1–5 days) or magnesium sulfate (1 g/kg every 12–24 h per nasogastric tube for 1–5 days) can be used. Carbonated cola has been reported to resolve gastric impactions in humans and horses, although its effect is questionable.
• Flunixin meglumine (1.1 mg/kg every 12 h IV) if needed to control signs of colic.
• Prokinetic drugs such as bethanechol (0.2–0.4 mg/kg PO every 6–8 h or 0.03–0.04 mg/kg SC or IV every 6–8 h) or metoclopramide (0.6 mg/kg PO every 4–6 h or 0.04 mg/kg/h CRI) can be used in an

attempt to facilitate gastric emptying. They are unlikely to show effect without lavaging the stomach and breaking up the impaction

CONTRAINDICATIONS
None

PRECAUTIONS
Caution should be used when treating horses with preexisting renal disease with NSAIDs.

POSSIBLE INTERACTIONS
None

ALTERNATIVE DRUGS
• Other NSAIDs can be used as analgesics. An alternative to NSAIDs for analgesia is butorphanol (0.01–0.1 mg/kg every 4–6 h IM or IV or as CRI)
• Sodium sulfate (1 g/kg) or dioctyl sodium succinate (20 mg/kg, 2 doses over 48 h) can be used instead of magnesium sulfate as a laxative

FOLLOW-UP

PATIENT MONITORING
The horse should be monitored closely during enteral fluid therapy or lavage as gastric rupture can occur. If signs of colic worsen or persist nasogastric intubation should be performed to check for reflux.

PREVENTION/AVOIDANCE
Depends on underlying cause. Instruction should be given to owners on how to correctly feed expandable feedstuffs to horses.

POSSIBLE COMPLICATIONS
• Gastric rupture
• Peritonitis

EXPECTED COURSE AND PROGNOSIS
• If gastric impaction does not resolve within 5 days after instituting medical treatment, it is unlikely to be successful. Surgical therapy should then be considered. If surgery is not feasible or declined by the owner the horse can potentially be managed with dietary recommendations. The surgery is difficult to perform and has a guarded prognosis.
• Once dilation of the stomach has occurred, success of treatment (medical or surgical) is unlikely. Even if the impaction can be resolved, recurrence is likely.
• Depending on the underlying cause prognosis varies. Recurrence has been reported and likely depends on the underlying cause

MISCELLANEOUS

ASSOCIATED CONDITIONS
Chronic gastric ulceration (pyloric outflow stenosis).

AGE-RELATED FACTORS
• Pyloric outflow stenosis due to gastric and pyloric ulcers is more common in foals <6 months of age.
• Neoplasia of the stomach and resulting outflow obstruction is more common in older horses

PREGNANCY/FERTILITY/BREEDING
N/A

SEE ALSO
• Acute adult abdominal pain—acute colic
• Anorexia and decreased food intake
• Chronic weight loss
• Colic, chronic/recurrent
• Gastric dilation/distention
• Gastric neoplasia
• Gastric ulcers and erosions (equine gastric ulcer syndrome, EGUS)

ABBREVIATIONS
• CRI = constant rate infusion
• GI = gastrointestinal
• ICS = intercostal space
• NSAID = nonsteroidal anti-inflammatory drug
• US = ultrasonography, ultrasound

Suggested Reading
Bird AR, Knowles EJ, Scherlock CE, et al. The clinical and pathological features of gastric impaction in twelve horses. Equine Vet Educ 2012;44(Suppl.):105–110.
Hurtado IR, Stewart A, Pellegrini-Masini A. Successful treatment for a gastric persimmon bezoar in a pony using nasogastric lavage with carbonated cola soft drink. Equine Vet Educ 2007;19:571–574.
LeJeune S, Whitcomb MB. Ultrasound of the equine abdomen. Vet Clin North Am Equine Pract 2014;30(2):353–381.
Vainio K, Skyes BW, Bilkslager AT. Primary gastric impaction in horses: a retrospective study of 20 cases (2005-2008). Equine Vet Educ 2011;23:186–190.

Author Angelika Schoster
Consulting Editors Henry Stämpfli and Olimpo Oliver-Espinosa

G

GASTRIC NEOPLASIA

BASICS

OVERVIEW
- Gastric neoplasia of horses is rare; SCC, adenocarcinoma, lymphoma, leiomyosarcoma, and leiomyoma account for 1.5% of all equine neoplasms
- SCC usually originates in the squamous portion of the stomach, infiltrates the wall, and projects into the lumen. There are 2 types of SCC: erosive and productive/proliferative. Both types may be present simultaneously
- Although SCC is the most common gastric neoplasm, only 3% of carcinomas in horses are of gastric origin
- SCC lesions of the stomach may reach a considerable size owing to local invasiveness and have a proliferative appearance. They are often ulcerated and secondarily infected. The surface may then have a grayish-white and hemorrhagic appearance. There may be adhesions of the stomach to adjacent liver, spleen, or diaphragm, and there are frequently metastatic nodules in the abdominal and thoracic cavities; however, this metastatic form progresses slowly. The tumors may cause physical obstruction in the stomach and may occasionally be associated with severe intraluminal hemorrhage
- Adenocarcinoma of the glandular part is very rare in horses and it may affect the pylorus and the fundic region. Although adenocarcinomas may project into the gut lumen, the predominant feature is growth from the mucosa into the submucosa and the muscularis to the serosa
- Leiomyosarcoma affects the cranial aspects of the stomach
- Other signs may be related to the effects of metastases (e.g. pleural effusion)

SIGNALMENT
- Horses of middle age and older (range 8.6–14.6 years with an increased risk between 11 and 12 years) are susceptible to SCC, and a 4:1 male to female ratio has been reported
- Breeds with an increased risk of developing SCC are draft horses, Appaloosas, American Paints, Pintos, and mixed breeds
- Adenocarcinoma and lymphoma have a similar age distribution

SIGNS
- Clinical signs are usually vague and rarely lead to the stomach as the affected organ
- Affected horses have a history of gradual weight loss, anorexia, halitosis, dysphagia, ptyalism, and lethargy extending over 2–6 weeks
- Abdominal pain and difficulty in eating or swallowing are not usually features of gastric neoplasia
- Pallor of mucous membranes and an increase in heart rate may be seen due to anemia resulting from gastric hemorrhage or depressed erythrogenesis
- Recurrent episodic pyrexia up to 40°C may occur as the result of necrosis in the neoplasm, and the respiratory rate may be raised in response to metastatic masses or pleural effusion in the thorax
- Ascites and ventral edema may be primary signs in a few horses, so that despite the weight loss the abdomen appears distended
- Fecal consistency is variable

CAUSES AND RISK FACTORS
None determined, but dietary excesses, mineral and vitamin deficiencies, and chronic irritation have been suggested such risk factors.

DIAGNOSIS

A definitive diagnosis is made on histologic examination of tissue obtained by endoscopic biopsy or at autopsy.

DIFFERENTIAL DIAGNOSIS
See chapter Chronic weight loss.

CBC/BIOCHEMISTRY/URINALYSIS
The packed cell volume may be low at 12–28% with gastric carcinoma.

OTHER LABORATORY TESTS
- Feces may test positive for occult blood
- Neoplastic cells may be found in fluid recovered by gastric lavage, in peritoneal fluid, or in pleural fluid

IMAGING
- Endoscopy using a video or fiber endoscope of 2 m in length or more enables direct visualization and biopsy of the gastric growth in adult horses
- Exploratory laparotomy or standing laparoscopy allows an examination of the serosal surface of the stomach, determines the extent of the spread of the tumor if any, and allows biopsy of the primary mass or metastatic nodules
- Radiographs of the thorax may reveal pleural effusion. A pneumogastrogram may be of value in delineating the intraluminal portion of the tumor
- Ultrasonography from the left cranial abdomen may show thickening and abnormal echogenicity of the stomach wall

OTHER DIAGNOSTIC PROCEDURES
Rectal examination may indicate metastatic masses or increased abdominal fluid. Abdominocentesis is normal when the tumor is confined in the stomach but may be an exudate if it has spread.

TREATMENT

By the time a diagnosis is made the tumors have usually progressed beyond the point where any treatment is feasible, and euthanasia is the only option. No report of successful therapy was found.

MEDICATIONS

DRUG(S) OF CHOICE
N/A

CONTRAINDICATIONS/POSSIBLE INTERACTIONS
N/A

FOLLOW-UP
N/A

MISCELLANEOUS

SEE ALSO
- Chronic weight loss
- Gastric dilation/distention
- Gastric impaction
- Gastric ulcers and erosions (equine gastric ulcer syndrome, EGUS)

ABBREVIATIONS
SCC = squamous cell carcinoma

Suggested Reading
East LM, Savage CJ. Abdominal neoplasia (excluding urogenital tract). Vet Clin North Am Equine Pract 1998;14:475–493.
Head KW, Else RW, Dubielzig RR. Tumors of the alimentary tract. In: Meuten DJ, ed. Tumors in Domestic Animals, 4e. Ames, IA: Iowa State Press, 2002:401–481.
Knottembelt DC, Patterson-Kane JC, Snalune JC. Clinical Equine Oncology. Edinburgh, UK: Elsevier, 2015:429–479.

Author Olimpo Oliver-Espinosa
Consulting Editors Henry Stämpfli and Olimpo Oliver-Espinosa

GASTRIC ULCERS AND EROSIONS (EQUINE GASTRIC ULCER SYNDROME, EGUS)

 BASICS

DEFINITION
Gastric ulcers are defects in the gastric mucosa that extend into the muscularis mucosa. Erosions are less severe and do not extend into the muscularis mucosa. Ulcers and/or erosions in the glandular mucosa of the stomach are referred to as EGGD. Lesions affecting the squamous portion of the equine stomach are referred to as ESGD.

PATHOPHYSIOLOGY
• The proximal third of the equine stomach or nonglandular region is covered by stratified squamous epithelium and has no mucous or bicarbonate layer to protect it against acid-induced injury
• Primary ESGD is common in horses in training and racing, probably because of an increased exposure of the nonglandular region to acidic gastric contents during exercise. It is also possible that diets high in fermentable carbohydrates cause production of short-chain fatty acids by resident bacteria acting synergistically with HCl in destruction of the squamous epithelium
• Secondary ESGD develops in animals with delayed gastric emptying due to gastric ulceration, pyloric stenosis, equine dysautonomia, ileus, gastric impaction, and/or idiopathic recurrent colic
• EGGD is thought to occur when the imbalance between aggressive and protective factors causes back-diffusion of HCl. The aggressive factors are primarily HCl and pepsin with their acidic and proteolytic properties. Protective factors include the gastric mucosal barrier (mucus, sodium bicarbonate), prostaglandins, mucosal blood flow, and mucosal restitution
• NSAIDs cause EGGD by topical irritation given PO or parenterally, by inhibiting the biosynthesis of gastric prostaglandins. GI damage is dose dependent. NSAIDs more selective for COX-2 than COX-1 are less likely to cause GI mucosa damage
• Stress-induced gastric ulcerations in patients that are critically ill or under extreme physiologic stress probably develop as a result of reduced splanchnic blood flow

SYSTEMS AFFECTED
GI
EGUS has been adopted in reference to a number of specifically unique problems that describe erosive and ulcerative diseases of the stomach.

Respiratory
Foals with gastroesophageal reflux may develop aspiration pneumonia.

Hepatobiliary
Ascending cholangitis is possible with duodenal ulceration.

INCIDENCE/PREVALENCE
• The reported prevalence in foals is 25–50%
• Depending on breed and/or the level of work, the prevalence of ESGD is 11–100%, and the prevalence of EGGD is 16–64%

SIGNALMENT
Breed Predilections
No sex, age, or breed predilections.

SIGNS
General Comments
Asymptomatic in many animals. Signs may vary with the age group and are not specific for the condition.

Historical Findings
• Poor appetite
• Decrease in performance
• Weight loss
• Low-grade colic or abdominal discomfort (rare—depends on the severity of the ulceration)
• Poor performance

Physical Examination Findings
• Foals—often asymptomatic. Clinical signs include poor appetite, inappetence, intermittent nursing (may nurse for short period and then act mildly uncomfortable), episodes of mild colic, diarrhea, pot-bellied appearance, bruxism, salivation, and dorsal recumbency. Salivation and bruxism are usually indicative of severe glandular or duodenal ulcers with concurrent gastroesophageal reflux and delayed gastric emptying
• Adults—often asymptomatic. Clinical signs include poor appetite, inappetence, poor body condition, rough haircoat, low-grade colic, behavior change, weight loss, and poor performance

CAUSES
Multifactorial. *Helicobacter* species or any other bacteria are currently not considered as an etiological factor.

RISK FACTORS
• Significant illness
• Intense training
• Halter breaking, confining and handling of young horses
• Administration of NSAIDs
• Hospitalization
• High-grain, low-roughage diet
• Fasting
• Water deprivation

 DIAGNOSIS

A definitive diagnosis can only be reached with gastroscopy. Although a tentative diagnosis can be made based on clinical signs and response to therapy, the initiation of treatment without prior gastroscopy is not recommended.

DIFFERENTIAL DIAGNOSIS
The clinical signs and physical examination findings with gastric ulcers are not pathognomonic and can be associated with many other conditions. EGUS often occurs secondary to other diseases.

CBC/BIOCHEMISTRY/URINALYSIS
There are no changes associated with EGUS. Anemia and hypoproteinemia are uncommon and, when present, other causes should be pursued.

OTHER LABORATORY TESTS
Fecal occult blood tests are often negative because colonic microflora digest hemoglobin.

IMAGING
Although, in foals, positive contrast studies might outline gastric ulcers, abdominal radiography is not a reliable diagnostic tool.

OTHER DIAGNOSTIC PROCEDURES
Gastroscopic examination is the most effective diagnostic procedure. For foals, a ≤10 mm diameter, 1 m endoscope is adequate. In adult horses, a 2–3 m gastroscope is necessary. Fasting is necessary to ensure gastric emptying for adequate visualization. Young foals require minimum fasting. However, older foals and adults eating roughage require a fasting period of 8–18 h.

 TREATMENT

APPROPRIATE HEALTH CARE
Treat as outpatient if stable and underlying conditions causing EGUS have been corrected.

NURSING CARE
N/A

ACTIVITY
Decrease level of intense training if possible.

DIET
Turn out to pasture if practical.

CLIENT EDUCATION
• Decrease intensity of training
• Allow as much pasture time as possible
• Minimize NSAID administration
• Minimize periods of fasting
• Ulcers will likely recur when intense training is resumed

SURGICAL CONSIDERATIONS
Foals with chronic gastric outflow disease caused by stricture of the pylorus or duodenum after ulcer healing may require gastrojejunostomy.

 MEDICATIONS

DRUG(S) OF CHOICE
• PPIs (omeprazole) significantly decrease gastric acid secretion by specifically inhibiting

G

GASTRIC ULCERS AND EROSIONS (EQUINE GASTRIC ULCER SYNDROME, EGUS) (CONTINUED)

the activity of proton pumps in the canalicular membrane of gastric parietal cells. Omeprazole is administered 1–4 mg/kg PO once daily for at least 28 days. Omeprazole has a time- and dose-related effect on healing of gastric ulcers. Higher doses result in more rapid and complete healing, whereas lower doses are appropriate for prevention of EGUS. Omeprazole requires 3–5 days of treatment for maximum antisecretory effect to occur. Control gastroscopy should be performed before the discontinuation of treatment
• Histamine H_2 receptor antagonists (cimetidine, ranitidine, and famotidine) inhibit gastric acid secretion by blocking the effect of histamine on the parietal cells. These compounds rapidly inhibit secretion after oral or IV administration. However, the effect is short-lived and they must be administered at least every 6–8 h. Cimetidine is administered at 20–25 mg/kg PO or at 4–6 mg/kg IV body weight every 6–8 h. Ranitidine is administered at 6–8 mg/kg PO or 1.5–2.0 mg/kg IV every 6–8 h
• The use of mucosal protectants, especially in foals, is warranted. Sucralfate is administered at 10–20 mg/kg PO every 6–8 h and 20–40 mg/kg PO every 8 h in foals and adults, respectively. Sucralfate is less likely to be effective in the treatment of ESGD but could possibly be effective in EGGD
• Antimicrobial therapy is presently not recommended as a routine therapy for EGUS

CONTRAINDICATIONS
Use NSAIDs with caution. These compounds may increase the severity of EGUS and prevent mucosal healing.

PRECAUTIONS
Clinical signs of gastric ulcers usually diminish quickly with appropriate therapy. If signs or condition worsen while on appropriate treatment, pursue a concurrent disease.

POSSIBLE INTERACTIONS
Cimetidine and, to a lesser extent, omeprazole are hepatic cytochrome P450 inhibitors and might slow the metabolism of concurrently administered compounds that require this enzyme for metabolism and elimination. Treatment with PPIs and/or sucralfate may also have a negative impact on other medications.

ALTERNATIVE DRUGS
Antacid Compounds
Antacid compounds buffer gastric acid. Their effect is short lived (≤2 h). Bismuth subsalicylate paste is given at 1000 mg/45 kg (100 lb); application via the nasogastric tube is recommended.

Nutraceuticals
Nutraceuticals alone or together with antacids are currently being investigated for prevention of EGUS.

FOLLOW-UP

PATIENT MONITORING
Clinical Signs
• Diminished appetite
• Interrupted nursing
• Teeth grinding
• Mild to moderate colic—if colic is more than low grade or persists for >24–48 h, an alternate diagnosis should be pursued

PREVENTION/AVOIDANCE
Susceptible horses may require prophylactic treatment with omeprazole or H_2 receptor antagonists during periods of intense training/racing. Horses with access to pasture have fewer gastric ulcers than horses in confinement. Avoid chronic administration of NSAIDs and minimize periods of fasting.

POSSIBLE COMPLICATIONS
Pyloric or duodenal stricture in foals. Gastric or duodenal perforation, with severe hemorrhage, is rare.

EXPECTED COURSE AND PROGNOSIS
The prognosis is generally good for uncomplicated cases. However, recurrence is frequent when intense training is resumed. Foals that develop pyloric or duodenal strictures and require surgical intervention have a guarded prognosis.

MISCELLANEOUS

ASSOCIATED CONDITIONS
Any disease process has the potential to cause secondary gastric ulceration.

AGE-RELATED FACTORS
Foals have a higher incidence of glandular mucosal and duodenal ulcers.

ZOONOTIC POTENTIAL
N/A

PREGNANCY/FERTILITY/BREEDING
There are inadequate data on the use of histamine H_2 receptor antagonists or omeprazole in pregnant mares. However, clinical cases of gastric ulcers in pregnant mares have been treated successfully with these compounds with no apparent adverse effects on the mare or the fetus.

SYNONYMS
N/A

ABBREVIATIONS
• COX = cyclooxygenase
• EGGD = equine glandular gastric disease
• EGUS = equine gastric ulcer syndrome
• ESGD = equine squamous gastric disease
• NSAID = nonsteroidal anti-inflammatory drug
• PPI = proton pump inhibitor

Suggested Reading
Hunt RH, Camilleri M, Crowe SE, et al. The stomach in health and disease. Gut 2015;64:1650–1668.
Martineau H, Thompson H, Taylor D. Pathology of gastritis and gastric ulceration in the horse. Part 1: range of lesions present in 21 mature individuals. Equine Vet J 2009;41:638–644.
Martineau H, Thompson H, Taylor D. Pathology of gastritis and gastric ulceration in the horse. Part 2: a scoring system. Equine Vet J 2009;41:646–651.
Sykes BW, Hewetson M, Hepburn RJ, et al. European College of Equine Internal Medicine consensus statement—equine gastric ulcer syndrome in adult horses. J Vet Intern Med 2015;29:1288–1299.
Sykes BW, Underwood C, Greer R, et al. The effects of dose and diet on the pharmacodynamics of omeprazole in the horse. Equine Vet J 2016;49(4):525-531.

Author Modest Vengust
Consulting Editors Henry Stämpfli and Olimpo Oliver-Espinosa

BASICS

DEFINITION
Areas of mucosal disruption in the nonglandular stratified squamous mucosa, margo plicatus, and glandular mucosa (fundus and pylorus) of the stomach.

PATHOPHYSIOLOGY
• Gastric ulcers are caused by an imbalance between mucosal aggressive factors (HCl, pepsin, bile acids) and mucosal protective factors (mucosal blood flow, mucus–bicarbonate layer, mucosal PGE_1 and motility)
• Ulcers in the squamous mucosa are related to prolonged exposure to gastric acids. Delayed gastric emptying and recumbency can increase this exposure. Milk buffers gastric acid, so infrequent nursing may lead to increased acid exposure
• Gastric ulcers may be related to desquamation of the squamous epithelium that occurs in 80% of normal foals up to 40 days of age
• Endogenous corticosteroids and NSAID treatment can decrease mucosal blood flow, inhibit bicarbonate secretion, and stimulate gastric acid secretion by blocking prostaglandin synthesis
• Glandular ulceration is considered the most clinically significant. The mucus–bicarbonate layer covers the surface of the glandular mucosa. Ulcers in this region are primarily due to disruption of blood flow and decreased secretion of mucus and bicarbonate. Septic shock and hypovolemia leading to hypoperfusion and reduced oxygen delivery may be involved in the pathogenesis of glandular mucosal injury
• Foals may also have ulcers in the pylorus or proximal duodenum that can lead to squamous gastric and esophageal ulcers from delayed gastric emptying

SYSTEMS AFFECTED
Gastrointestinal

INCIDENCE/PREVALENCE
• The reported prevalence in foals varies from 25% to 57%
• Endoscopic surveys of normal foals 2–85 days of age revealed that 50% had squamous ulcers and 4–9% had glandular ulcers

SIGNALMENT
No breed or sex predilection.

SIGNS
General Comments
In foals, there appear to be 4 separate clinical syndromes:
1. Silent (subclinical) ulcers are most common
   ◦ Most commonly found in foals <4 months of age
   ◦ Usually seen in foals with concurrent illness
   ◦ Ulcers may heal spontaneously or may be found incidentally at necropsy
2. Active (clinical) ulcers
   ◦ Primarily in the squamous mucosa
   ◦ Clinical signs include depression, anorexia, bruxism, ptyalism, dorsal recumbency, and colic
3. Perforating ulcers with diffuse peritonitis are uncommon
   ◦ Most frequent in the squamous mucosa
   ◦ Clinical signs usually absent until just before rupture
   ◦ Severity poorly predicted by endoscopic appearance
   ◦ Once ruptured, foals show progressive evidence of endotoxemia and may have abdominal distention and colic
4. Pyloric strictures associated with gastric outflow obstruction are uncommon
   ◦ Bruxism, ptyalism, postprandial colic, aspiration pneumonia, dehydration, systemic hypochloremic alkalosis
   ◦ Most common in foals 3–5 months of age

Historical Findings
Poor growth, rough haircoat, pot-bellied appearance, and history of prior illness, including diarrhea, colic, lethargy, or anorexia.

Physical Examination Findings
• Depression and intermittent nursing are the most commonly observed clinical signs
• Colic
• Diarrhea
• Bruxism and ptyalism

CAUSES
• Increased mucosal exposure to gastric acid
• Mucosal blood flow disruption

RISK FACTORS
• Fasting, decreased gastric motility, and delayed gastric emptying may lead to squamous ulcers
• Disruption of mucosal blood flow due to hypovolemia, shock, stress, and/or NSAID use may cause glandular ulcers

DIAGNOSIS

DIFFERENTIAL DIAGNOSIS
Any disorder resulting in signs of colic, e.g. small intestinal intussusception, small intestinal volvulus, pyloric stenosis, enterocolitis.

CBC/BIOCHEMISTRY/URINALYSIS
• Hematology values are usually normal but may reveal a stress leukogram
• Anemia may be present with blood loss

OTHER LABORATORY TESTS
Fecal or gastric occult blood may suggest bleeding ulcers; these tests are neither sensitive nor specific.

IMAGING
• Abdominal radiographs may help rule out other causes of colic
• Barium contrast radiographs should be taken in foals with suspected gastric outflow obstruction
• Abdominal ultrasonography should be performed to evaluate intestinal wall thickness and to evaluate for ileus and peritoneal effusion

OTHER DIAGNOSTIC PROCEDURES
• Gastroscopy or gastroduodenoscopy will definitively confirm the diagnosis. Use a 1 m long endoscope with a maximal outer diameter of 9 mm
• Nuclear scintigraphy, acetaminophen (paracetamol) absorption, and postconsumption [^{13}C]-octanoic acid blood or breath testing can be used to diagnose delayed gastric emptying

PATHOLOGIC FINDINGS
NSAID toxicity produces ulcers in the glandular and nonglandular stomach. Ulcer size is highly variable, ranging from 2 mm to >2 cm in diameter. Larger ulcers may be 1–2 mm in depth and surrounded by hyperemia.

TREATMENT

AIMS
• Suppression or neutralization of gastric acid
• Supportive therapy
• Foals with mild to moderate gastric ulcers should respond to treatment within 24–48 h

APPROPRIATE HEALTH CARE
• Patients with gastric ulcers can be treated in the field
• Hospitalization is recommended for foals with dehydration or electrolyte imbalance, peritonitis, signs of sepsis, esophageal reflux, or uncontrolled pain

NURSING CARE
In severely compromised critically ill foals, supportive care (including fluid therapy and inotropic support) is needed to maintain perfusion.

ACTIVITY
Normal

DIET
• Normal diet in cases without reflux
• In case of reflux, parenteral nutrition is sometimes necessary

CLIENT EDUCATION
Avoid use of NSAIDs without veterinary supervision.

SURGICAL CONSIDERATIONS
• Foals with severe gastroduodenal ulcer disease can develop duodenal strictures. If medical therapy is unsuccessful, then surgical correction is necessary

GASTRIC ULCERS, NEONATE (CONTINUED)

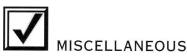

• Surgical techniques include pyloroplasty or bypass techniques

MEDICATIONS

DRUG(S) OF CHOICE

Histamine H₂ Receptor Antagonists
Suppress HCl secretion by binding and competitively inhibiting the histamine H_2 receptor on parietal cells:
• Cimetidine—6–20 mg/kg PO every 6–8 h or 6.6 mg/kg IV every 6 h
• Ranitidine—6.6 mg/kg PO every 8 h or 1.5–2 mg/kg IV every 6–8 h
• Famotidine—2–3 mg/kg PO every 12 h

Proton Pump Inhibitors
• Block secretion of H^+ by parietal cell membrane H^+/K^+-ATPase pump (proton pump)
• Acid secretion is effectively suppressed for up to 27 h
• Omeprazole—4.0 mg/kg PO every 24 h for treatment of gastric ulcers; 1.0–2.0 mg/kg PO every 24 h for prophylaxis

Antacids
• Aluminum hydroxide, magnesium hydroxide, and calcium carbonate (200–250 mL PO every 6 h)
• Can be used to ameliorate clinical signs or to prevent recurrence; efficacy not determined

Sucralfate
• Adheres to ulcerated mucosa, forms a proteinaceous barrier, and stimulates PGE_1 synthesis and mucus secretion
• Efficacy in treatment of squamous mucosal lesions has not been determined
• Best used as an adjunct in addition to H_2 antagonists or proton pump inhibitors
• Dose is 10–20 mg/kg PO TID or QID
• Do not administer at the same time as other oral medications (may inhibit absorption of other drugs)

Prostaglandin Analogs
• Misoprostol (Cytotec™)—1–4 µg/kg PO every 12–24 h
• Synthetic PGE_1 analog
• PGE_1 inhibits HCl and gastrin secretion; increases gastric mucus formation and mucosal blood flow
• May aid in the treatment/prevention of gastric ulcers induced by NSAIDs

Prokinetics
• May be administered to foals with duodenal ulcers, with gastroesophageal reflux, and when delayed gastric emptying without a physical obstruction is suspected
• Bethanechol—0.02 mg/kg SC every 6–8 h; cholinergic agonist that increases the rate of gastric emptying in horses

CONTRAINDICATIONS
Prokinetics should not be used if mechanical obstruction is suspected.

PRECAUTIONS
• Side effects of prostaglandin analog use may include abdominal pain, diarrhea, bloating, and cramping
• Bethanechol—adverse effects include diarrhea, inappetence, salivation, and colic

POSSIBLE INTERACTIONS
• Cimetidine may inhibit hepatic microsomal enzyme systems and thereby reduce metabolism, prolong half-lives, and increase serum levels of some drugs, e.g. metronidazole
• Do not use bethanechol concomitantly with other cholinergic or anticholinesterase agents

FOLLOW-UP

PATIENT MONITORING
• Recheck gastroscopy 14–28 days after initiating treatment
• If gastroscopy is unavailable, the efficacy of treatment can be based on clinical signs
• Signs of colic or diarrhea that result from gastric ulcers usually resolve within 48 h. Appetite, body condition, and attitude improve within 1–3 weeks

PREVENTION/AVOIDANCE
• Prophylactic antiulcer therapy is routinely administered in critically ill foals. Some critically ill foals have a predominantly alkaline gastric pH profile, and because gastric acidity may be protective against bacterial translocation in neonates the need for prophylactic ulcer therapy is controversial (this practice has been associated with diarrhea in neonatal foals)
• Avoid unnecessary NSAID use in foals

POSSIBLE COMPLICATIONS
• Pyloric stricture
• Acute hemorrhage
• Gastric, duodenal rupture, and peritonitis

EXPECTED COURSE AND PROGNOSIS
• Outcome is variable
• Foals with gastric ulcers that respond favorably to therapy for a primary problem have a good prognosis. Ulcers may heal in 2–3 weeks
• Foals with duodenal ulcers have a guarded prognosis due to potential for duodenal stricture, fibrosis, and gastric outflow obstruction
• Foals with perforating ulcers have a grave prognosis
• Mortality from gastric ulceration has been reported to range from 7.1% to 16.2% in foals

MISCELLANEOUS

ASSOCIATED CONDITIONS
• Septicemia
• Neonatal maladjustment syndrome

AGE-RELATED FACTORS
Frequently seen in neonatal foals with other comorbidities

SYNONYMS
• Gastroduodenal ulcer syndrome
• Peptic ulcers

SEE ALSO
Gastric ulcers and erosions (equine gastric ulcer syndrome, EGUS)

ABBREVIATIONS
• NSAID = nonsteroidal anti-inflammatory drug
• PGE_1 = prostaglandin E_1

Suggested Reading
Elfenbein JR, Sanchez LC. Prevalence of gastric and duodenal ulceration in 691 nonsurviving foals (1995–2006). Equine Vet J Suppl 2012;41:76–79.
Furr M, Cohen ND, Axon JE, et al. Treatment with histamine-type 2 receptor antagonists and omeprazole increase the risk of diarrhea in neonatal foals treated in intensive care units. Equine Vet J Suppl 2012;41:80–86.
Magdesian G. Gastrointestinal problems in the neonatal foal. In: Paradis MR, ed. Equine Neonatal Medicine: A Case-Based Approach. Philadelphia, PA: Saunders, 2006:208.
Ryan CA, Sanchez LC. Nondiarrheal disorders of the gastrointestinal tract in neonatal foals. Vet Clin North Am Equine Pract 2005;21:313–332.

Author Teresa A. Burns
Consulting Editor Margaret C. Mudge
Acknowledgment The author and editor acknowledge the prior contribution of Sandra C. Valdez-Almada.

GETAH VIRUS INFECTION

BASICS

OVERVIEW
• Getah virus is a mosquito-borne arbovirus classified in the Semliki Forest complex genus *Alphavirus*, family Togaviridae. The virus or one related to it (Sagiyama, Ross River, or Bebaru, which are also included in the Getah virus subgroup) can be found over a wide geographic range, extending from Eurasia to Australia
• Although serologic studies suggest widespread exposure to the virus among vertebrates (mammals, birds, and reptiles) including humans, naturally occurring disease due to Getah virus has only been reported infrequently in horses and very uncommonly in swine
• Racetrack outbreaks have been reported in Japan (1978, 1979, 1983, 2014, 2015, 2016) and on a breeding farm in India (1990)
• In areas of the world considered endemic for Getah virus, it is thought to be maintained in a mosquito-swine-mosquito cycle. Pigs and perhaps other vertebrates are regarded as amplifying hosts of the virus

SIGNALMENT
Whereas experimental infection with Getah virus can be established in various horse breeds, the majority of reported outbreaks have been in Thoroughbreds at racetracks, frequently in 2-year-old horses in training, with spread of infection recorded over a 4–6 week period.

SIGNS
• Most cases of primary Getah virus infection are asymptomatic
• The virus can cause extensive outbreaks of mild illness that is self-limiting, nonfatal, and apparently without sequelae
• Clinical signs appear 2–6 days after exposure. They can include some or all of the following—fever (3–4 days' duration), anorexia, depression, limb and preputial edema, skin rash, serous nasal discharge, submandibular lymphadenopathy, stiff gait, and mild icterus. Limb edema and rash supervene several days after onset of fever
• Complete clinical recovery occurs within 7–14 days
• Getah virus can frequently cause a peracute fatal illness in neonatal piglets

CAUSES AND RISK FACTORS
• Getah virus infection is primarily transmitted by certain species of *Culex* and *Aedes* mosquitos in regions of the world where the virus is endemic
• Since the virus can be shed into the respiratory tract of some acutely infected horses, there is the potential for horse-to-horse transmission via the respiratory route, either by direct animal contact or indirectly, through virus-contaminated fomites

DIAGNOSIS

DIFFERENTIAL DIAGNOSIS
• The clinical signs can readily be confused with those of equine viral arteritis. Unlike the latter, Getah virus has never been associated with abortion or illness/death in neonatal foals
• There is also some clinical resemblance to African horse sickness fever, equine encephalosis, and toxicosis due to ingestion
• Toxicosis due to ingestion of hoary alyssum (*Berteroa incana*)

CBC/BIOCHEMISTRY/URINALYSIS
Lymphopenia is invariably present early in the acute phase of the disease.

OTHER LABORATORY TESTS
• Confirmation is based on virus detection by RT-PCR or virus isolation in cell culture or by serologic testing of acute and convalescent (paired) sera
• Blood, nasal secretions, and even saliva are appropriate specimens for attempting virus detection. Viremia can last for 3–5 days
• Samples should be taken early after the onset of fever

IMAGING
N/A

OTHER DIAGNOSTIC PROCEDURES
N/A

PATHOLOGIC FINDINGS
Grossly, moderate lymphadenomegaly, scattered maculae, and subcutaneous edema. Histologically, lymphoid hyperplasia in lymph nodes and spleen. Perivascular lymphoid infiltration, edema of blood vessel walls, and hemorrhagic foci in dermal maculae.

TREATMENT
Not usually indicated because of the mild nature of the disease.

MEDICATIONS

DRUG(S) OF CHOICE
Administration of NSAIDs may be called for in more severely affected horses.

CONTRAINDICATIONS/POSSIBLE INTERACTIONS
N/A

FOLLOW-UP

PREVENTION/AVOIDANCE
• Recommended use of an inactivated vaccine prior to onset of mosquito season. It is very important to ensure that horses at risk are fully vaccinated annually against the disease
• Accommodate horses indoors from dusk to dawn to minimize risk of mosquito exposure

EXPECTED COURSE AND PROGRESS
Clinical course 7–14 days; excellent prognosis.

MISCELLANEOUS

ABBREVIATIONS
• NSAID = nonsteroidal anti-inflammatory drug
• RT-PCR = reverse transcription polymerase chain reaction

Suggested Reading
Bannai H, Ochi A, Nemoto M, et al. A 2015 outbreak of Getah virus infection occurring among Japanese racehorses sequentially to an outbreak in 2014 at the same site. BMC Vet Res 2016;12:98.

Author Peter J. Timoney
Consulting Editor Ashley G. Boyle

Client Education Handout available online

G

GLANDERS

 ## BASICS

OVERVIEW
• Contagious zoonotic disease of equids caused by bacterium *Burkholderia mallei*
• Characterized by ulcerative nodules of the skin and respiratory tract with signs of pneumonia
• Mortality rate is high; some animals remain asymptomatic and serve as a source and risk for (re-)introduction into susceptible horse populations
• Disease has been eradicated from most countries in the world; still endemic in parts of the Middle East (i.e. Iraq), Asia (i.e. Iran, India, Pakistan, Mongolia), North Africa, and South America (i.e. Brazil)
• Has been classified as a re-emerging disease, as evidenced by a recent outbreak in Germany

SIGNALMENT
Horses, donkeys, mules of all ages and camels.

SIGNS
• Acute cases—fever, depression, septicemia, rapid weight loss, cough, mucopurulent or sanguineous nasal discharge, and death occurs within a few days
• Chronic glanders is more common; typically seen in horses and is characterized by periods of fever, cough, weight loss, purulent nasal discharge with crusting in the nasal passages and epistaxis. Horses appear to recover but disease gradually progresses over months to years
• Cutaneous—known as *farcy*; characterized by nodules and thickened cord-like lymphatic vessels (Web Figure 1). The nodules frequently ulcerate and drain a honey-like fluid. Limb edema is a common sequela
• Many cases may have both respiratory and cutaneous involvement
• Recently, asymptomatic cases are reported as "carriers," "latent," or "occult" disease

CAUSES AND RISK FACTORS
• Source of infection—nasal and cutaneous discharges from infected equids. Ingestion of feed or water contaminated by *B. mallei* is believed to be the primary route of infection. Transmission is facilitated if animals share feeding or watering facilities
• *B. mallei* does not survive in a dry environment for more than a few weeks, but can remain viable for several months in a warm moist environment
• Chronic cases may not be detected by diagnostic tests and, coupled with international travelling, indicate a risk for re-emerging of this disease

 ## DIAGNOSIS

DIFFERENTIAL DIAGNOSIS
Lymphangitis caused by *Histoplasma farciminosum, Corynebacterium pseudotuberculosis, Sporothrix schenckii*; melioidosis caused by *Burkholderia pseudomallei*; or strangles caused by *Streptococcus equi* ssp. *equi*.

CBC/BIOCHEMISTRY/URINALYSIS
Hematology is consistent with a chronic inflammatory process (i.e. neutrophilia, hyperfibrinogenemia, hyperglobinemia, and anemia).

OTHER LABORATORY TESTS
• *B. mallei* is a Gram-negative, nonencapsulated, nonmotile rod. Diagnosis relies on identification of the bacteria from exudate or nodules by staining, bacterial culture, and PCR
• A variety of serologic tests are available but antibody titers may only be detected 4–12 weeks post infection. Complement fixation is the OIE recommended test and is considered the most reliable serologic test, although its low specificity may result in false-positive test results. ELISA and western blot have a higher specificity and can be used in case a false-positive result is suspected

IMAGING
N/A

OTHER DIAGNOSTIC PROCEDURES
A positive intradermal mallein test will result in fever, pain, or swelling of the injection site within 48–72 h post application.

PATHOLOGIC FINDINGS
B. mallei infection causes nodules in lymph nodes and lungs. The upper airway, skin, liver, and other organs may also be involved. Miliary nodules and characteristic stellate scars in the nasal mucosa mark the chronic form.

 ## TREATMENT

Glanders is a class B bioterrorism agent and a reportable disease (WHO/OIE). Regulatory officials should be notified if glanders is suspected. Affected animals should be destroyed and all exposed animals quarantined for further testing. Treatment of animals should not be attempted.

 ## MEDICATIONS

DRUG(S) OF CHOICE
Treatment is not usually permitted.

 ## FOLLOW-UP

• Management of an outbreak includes destruction of clinical cases, bedding, and equipment associated with infected horses and diagnostic testing of all exposed horses
• No vaccine is available for glanders
• All equids from endemic areas should be tested prior to entering a glanders-free area during (inter)national movement

 ## MISCELLANEOUS

ZOONOTIC POTENTIAL
Glanders is a zoonotic disease that can rarely cause disease in humans with a high case fatality rate. People who handle infected horses and laboratory personnel working with *B. mallei* should take special biosecurity measures.

SYNONYMS
Farcy or malleus.

ABBREVIATIONS
• ELISA = enzyme-linked immunosorbent assay
• OIE = Office International Epizooties/World Organisation for Animal Health
• PCR = polymerase chain reaction
• WHO = World Health Organization

Internet Resources
World Organisation for Animal Health (Office International des Epizooties (OIE)), World Animal Health Information Database (WAHID). http://www.oie.int

Author Elisabeth-Lidwien J.M.M. Verdegaal
Consulting Editor Ashley G. Boyle
Acknowledgment The author and editor acknowledge the prior contribution of Laura K. Reilly.

 Client Education Handout available online

BASICS

OVERVIEW
• The glaucomas are a group of diseases resulting from alterations of aqueous humor dynamics that cause an IOP increase above that which is compatible with normal function of the retinal ganglion cells and optic nerve
• Glaucoma in horses is being recognized with increased frequency, although the prevalence of glaucoma in the horse is surprisingly low given the horse's propensity for ocular injury and marked intraocular inflammatory responses
• All glaucomas consist of 5 stages: (1) an initial event or series of events that influence the aqueous humor outflow system; (2) morphologic alterations of the aqueous outflow system that eventually lead to aqueous outflow obstruction and IOP elevation; (3) elevated IOP or ocular hypertension that severely reduces retinal ganglion cell sensitivity and function; (4) subsequent retinal ganglion cell and optic nerve axon degeneration; and (5) progressive visual deterioration that eventually leads to blindness
• The glaucomas are frequently categorized into primary, secondary, and congenital types. While all types of glaucoma have a causative mechanism, primary glaucomas possess no overt ocular abnormality to account for the increase in IOP, whereas secondary glaucomas have an identifiable cause, such as intraocular inflammation, neoplasia, or lens luxation
• Primary bilateral glaucoma has been rarely reported in the horse
• Secondary glaucomas due to anterior uveitis and intraocular neoplasia are most commonly recognized in the horse
• Congenital glaucoma is reported in foals and associated with developmental anomalies of the iridocorneal angle

SIGNALMENT
• Glaucoma is reported in the Appaloosa, Paso Fino, Thoroughbred, and Warmblood, although all ages and breeds of horses are at risk
• There appears to be an increased incidence of glaucoma in horses with chronic uveitis, such as those with ERU, horses >15 years old, and Appaloosas

SIGNS
• Equine glaucoma may not be easily recognized in the early stages of the disease due to the subtle nature of the clinical signs
• Initially, the pupils of affected eyes are often only slightly mydriatic, and overt discomfort is uncommon
• Afferent pupillary light reflex deficits, corneal striae, fibrosis of the drainage angle, decreased vision, lens subluxations and luxations, mild iridocyclitis, and optic nerve

atrophy/cupping may also be found in eyes of horses with glaucoma
• The presence of corneal striae, or corneal endothelial "band opacities," in non-buphthalmic horse eyes warrants a high degree of suspicion for the finding of elevated IOP, which may also be found in eyes that are normotensive at the time of examination. Corneal striae are linear, often interconnecting or branching, white opacities found deep in the cornea, caused by stretching or rupture of Descemet's membrane, and may be associated with increased IOP

CAUSES AND RISK FACTORS
• Aqueous humor is produced in the ciliary body by energy-dependent and -independent mechanisms. The ciliary enzyme carbonic anhydrase plays an important role in aqueous production. Aqueous humor passes into the posterior chamber, through the pupil into the anterior chamber, and then exits through the iridocorneal angle (conventional) outflow pathway or through the uveovortex and uveoscleral (unconventional) outflow pathways
• Perfusion and morphologic studies indicate potentially extensive unconventional aqueous humor outflow pathway involvement in the horse. The extensive low-resistance equine conventional aqueous humor outflow pathway and the prominent unconventional outflow pathways in the horse may minimize development of glaucoma in many cases of anterior uveitis
• However, anterior uveitis can lead to formation of preiridal fibrovascular membranes that limit aqueous absorption by the iris and to physical and functional obstruction of the iridocorneal angles with inflammatory cells and debris
• Iridal and ciliary body neoplasms and endophthalmitis can cause secondary glaucoma by infiltration of the outflow pathways

DIAGNOSIS

DIFFERENTIAL DIAGNOSIS
ERU, corneal ulceration, and endotheliitis may be associated with corneal edema, ocular pain, and vision loss in horses.

CBC/BIOCHEMISTRY/URINALYSIS
N/A

OTHER LABORATORY TESTS
Serologic tests for infectious diseases causing the anterior uveitis in horses with glaucoma may or may not identify the causative organism.

IMAGING
B-scan ultrasonography can demonstrate intraocular tumors associated with glaucoma in horses.

OTHER DIAGNOSTIC PROCEDURES
• The diagnosis of equine glaucoma is made with the tonometric documentation of elevated IOP, and the presence of clinical signs specific to glaucoma, such as a mydriatic pupil and buphthalmia. ERU alone, in contrast, generally has a low IOP and a miotic pupil
• The accurate measurement of IOP in the horse requires applanation or rebound tonometry. The mean IOP in the horse ranges from 17 to 28 mmHg. The IOP can vary at different times of day in horses with glaucoma and horses with ERU. It is important to measure IOP with the horse's head held above its heart to prevent falsely elevated readings

PATHOLOGIC FINDINGS
Preiridal fibrovascular membrane formation with secondary iridocorneal angle closure and trabecular meshwork sclerosis and collapse are noted. Since most cases of glaucoma in horses are secondary to uveitis, there is often infiltration of the uveal tissues with inflammatory cells and exudates.

TREATMENT

Various combinations of drugs and surgery may be necessary to reduce the IOP to levels that are compatible with preservation of vision in horses with glaucoma. Glaucoma is particularly aggressive and difficult to control in the Appaloosa.

MEDICATIONS

DRUG(S) OF CHOICE
• Aqueous production may be reduced with the systemically administered carbonic anhydrase inhibitor acetazolamide (1–3 mg/kg QD PO), a β-adrenergic blocker such as 0.5% BID or TID timolol maleate, and a topical carbonic anhydrase inhibitor such as 2% dorzolamide BID or TID. Topical cholinergics and prostaglandin drugs may exacerbate iridocyclitis and should only be used with caution
• Anti-inflammatory therapy, consisting of topically and systemically administered corticosteroids and/or topically and systemically administered NSAIDs (phenylbutazone 1 mg/kg BID PO; flunixin meglumine 250 mg BID PO) also appears to be beneficial in the control of IOP
• When medical therapy is inadequate, Nd:YAG or diode laser cyclophotoablation may be a viable alternative for long-term IOP control. Nd:YAG laser cyclophotoablation is very effective at controlling IOP and maintaining vision in the horse. The author recommends 55 laser sites per eye for contact Nd:YAG laser cyclophotoablation in the horse, 5–6 mm posterior to the limbus, at a

GLAUCOMA (CONTINUED)

power setting of 12 W for 0.3 s duration per site. Diode lasers may be used in 55–70 sites at 1500 mW for 1500 ms per site. Laser cyclophotoablation may be performed in the standing horse. Endoscopic cyclophotoablation, wherein the ciliary processes are directly visualized and ablated with a diode laser, requires general anesthesia and an intraocular approach

CONTRAINDICATIONS/POSSIBLE INTERACTIONS

Conventional glaucoma treatment with miotics may provide varying amounts of IOP reduction in horses. A number of horses have *increased* IOP when administered topical miotics. As miotics can potentiate the clinical signs of uveitis, miotic therapy is generally considered to be contraindicated in glaucoma secondary to uveitis, and should be used cautiously, with careful IOP monitoring, in horses with mild or quiescent anterior uveitis.

 FOLLOW-UP

PATIENT MONITORING

• Serial tonometry is required to document IOP spikes in horses with anterior uveitis and secondary glaucoma
• Continued pupillary dilation is a sign of continued IOP elevation and optic nerve damage

• Horses with glaucoma should be stall-rested until the condition is under control. Intraocular hemorrhage and increased severity of uveitis are sequelae to overexertion
• Diet should be consistent with the activity and training level of the horse
• Self-trauma should be avoided by use of hard- or soft-cup hoods

PREVENTION/AVOIDANCE

Breeding of horses with glaucoma is not recommended.

POSSIBLE COMPLICATIONS

Chronic pain and blindness are complications.

EXPECTED COURSE AND PROGNOSIS

The horse eye seems to tolerate elevations in IOP for many months to years that would blind a dog; however, blindness is ultimately the end result. Buphthalmia can be associated with exposure keratitis.

 MISCELLANEOUS

ASSOCIATED CONDITIONS

• ERU
• Exposure keratitis and persistent corneal ulcerations

AGE-RELATED FACTORS

Older horses are at risk of developing glaucoma.

ZOONOTIC POTENTIAL
N/A

PREGNANCY/FERTILITY/BREEDING
N/A

SYNONYMS
N/A

SEE ALSO
Equine recurrent uveitis

ABBREVIATIONS

• ERU = equine recurrent uveitis
• IOP = intraocular pressure
• Nd:YAG = neodymium:yttrium–aluminum–garnet
• NSAID = nonsteroidal anti-inflammatory drug

Suggested Reading
Brooks DE. Ophthalmology for the Equine Practitioner, 2e. Jackson, WY: Teton NewMedia, 2008.
Brooks DE, Matthews AG. Equine ophthalmology. In: Gelatt KN, ed. Veterinary Ophthalmology, 4e. Ames, IA: Blackwell, 2007:1165–1274.
Gilger BC, ed. Equine Ophthalmology, 3e. Ames, IA: Wiley Blackwell, 2017.

Author Caryn E. Plummer
Consulting Editor Caryn E. Plummer
Acknowledgment The author/editor acknowledges the prior contribution of Dennis E. Brooks.

GLUCOSE, HYPERGLYCEMIA

BASICS

DEFINITION
The glucose concentration is greater than the laboratory reference interval.

PATHOPHYSIOLOGY
• Serum glucose concentration depends on a variety of factors, including intestinal absorption, hepatic production, hormonal regulation, and tissue utilization
• Hyperglycemia may result from insulin-dependent diabetes mellitus (type 1) due to lack of insulin production
• Hyperglycemia may result from insulin resistance due to EMS or PPID (formerly referred to as equine Cushing's disease). Sometimes the 2 syndromes may coexist
• EMS is characterized by insulin resistance/dysregulation, which can lead to hyperglycemia
• PPID is due to functional adenomas or adenomatous hypertrophy and hyperplasia of the pars intermedia of the pituitary gland. Decreased release of dopamine from the hypothalamus is thought to result from oxidative damage; decreased dopaminergic inhibition of the pars intermedia leads to increased secretion of POMC by melanotropes. POMC is cleaved into ACTH, α-melanocyte-stimulating hormone, β-endorphin, and corticotropin-like intermediate lobe peptide. ACTH causes increased cortisol release from the adrenal glands, which can lead to hyperglycemia through increased hepatic gluconeogenesis
• Epinephrine causes hyperglycemia by inhibiting insulin secretion and stimulating glucagon secretion in the pancreas. Epinephrine also stimulates glycogenolysis and gluconeogenesis in the liver. Therefore, the "fight or flight" response and, rarely, pheochromocytomas, can cause hyperglycemia
• Physiologic, transient, postprandial hyperglycemia may occur
• Hyperglycemia may be associated with SIRS (e.g. sepsis [colitis, pleuropneumonia, metritis] trauma, acidosis, burns) owing to dysregulation of glucose homeostasis
• Early in septic or hypovolemic shock, increased catecholamines, glucagon, and glucocorticoids can increase hepatic gluconeogenesis, leading to hyperglycemia

SYSTEMS AFFECTED
• Endocrine/metabolic—hormonal regulation of gluconeogenesis and glycogenolysis
• Renal/urologic—PU/PD caused by glucosuria, resulting in osmotic diuresis
• Nervous—may result in CNS dysfunction due to increased osmolality

GENETICS
Ponies, Miniature horses, and some horse breeds (e.g. Warmbloods, Morgans, and Saddlebreds) may be predisposed to EMS.

INCIDENCE/PREVALENCE
N/A

GEOGRAPHIC DISTRIBUTION
N/A

SIGNALMENT
• Any breed, age, or sex
• PPID is seen in older horses (>15 years)
• See Genetics

SIGNS

Historical Findings
Dependent on the underlying cause. See Physical Examination Findings.

Physical Examination Findings
• EMS—obesity, regional adiposity (e.g. cresty neck, tail-head fat), infertility, and laminitis
• PPID—generalized hypertrichosis (hirsutism), abnormal fat distribution, weight loss, muscle wasting, pendulous abdomen, PU/PD, recurrent infections (e.g. sinusitis, hoof abscess, dental disease, dermatitis), or laminitis. Horses with early PPID may be subclinical
• Anxiety—tachycardia, tachypnea, sweating

CAUSES
• Absolute insulin deficiency (i.e. hypoinsulinemia)/type 1 diabetes mellitus—uncommon in horses; may be secondary to destruction of pancreatic islets from chronic pancreatitis or immune-mediated polyendocrinopathy (rare)
• EMS—genetic predisposition to insulin dysregulation/insulin resistance with resulting hyperglycemia; there is possible overproduction of cortisol from adipose tissue
• PPID—excessive ACTH leads to overproduction of cortisol, which stimulates hepatic gluconeogenesis, decreases peripheral glucose utilization, and causes insulin resistance, all of which lead to hyperglycemia
• Pheochromocytoma—excessive catecholamine release
• Physiologic hyperglycemia can occur postprandially due to epinephrine-mediated excitement or cortisol-mediated stress responses
• SIRS—insulin resistance with reduced glucose utilization and increased gluconeogenesis from release of epinephrine and cortisol
• Iatrogenic hyperglycemia can result from administration of dextrose-containing fluids, parenteral nutrition, corticosteroids, α_2-agonists (xylazine or detomidine)

RISK FACTORS
See Genetics and Signalment.

DIAGNOSIS

DIFFERENTIAL DIAGNOSIS
• See Causes
• Colic—hyperglycemia has been reported in cases of colic (epinephrine from pain/anxiety, cortisol from stress)

CBC/BIOCHEMISTRY/URINALYSIS

CBC
• Inflammatory leukogram if underlying inflammatory disease
• Stress leukogram with neutrophilia, lymphopenia, and monocytosis if cortisol mediated
• Mature neutrophilia if epinephrine induced

Biochemistry
• Hyperglycemia
• Diabetes mellitus—hyperglycemia; glucosuria
• EMS—hypertriglyceridemia is possible
• PPID—elevated creatine kinase and aspartate aminotransferase concentrations because of muscle catabolism; electrolyte abnormalities due to PU/PD or anorexia

Urinalysis
Glucosuria if renal threshold (180–200 mg/dL) is exceeded.

OTHER LABORATORY TESTS
Type 1 diabetes mellitus—serum insulin concentrations are typically low.

EMS
• Insulin—glucose sensitivity testing (dynamic testing) is used to evaluate insulin resistance. Options include oral sugar test, 2-step insulin test, IV glucose tolerance test, and combined glucose–insulin test. With insulin resistance, blood glucose fails to decrease adequately as expected
• Serum leptin may be increased in horses with EMS since leptin is produced by adipocytes

PPID
• Serum insulin concentrations are typically high–normal or elevated
• Plasma ACTH concentration may be elevated in PPID
• Thyrotropin-releasing hormone stimulation of ACTH—exaggerated increase in ACTH
• Dexamethasone suppression test (overnight)—cortisol concentration will be suppressed below 1 μg/dL in normal horses; horses with PPID fail to suppress due to endogenous ACTH production. Poor sensitivity in early stages of PPID (note that steroid administration may worsen laminitis)

IMAGING
Radiography to diagnose laminitis.

OTHER DIAGNOSTIC PROCEDURES
N/A

G

GLUCOSE, HYPERGLYCEMIA (CONTINUED)

PATHOLOGIC FINDINGS
Pancreatitis or pancreatic fibrosis in type 1 diabetes mellitus; laminitis; pituitary adenomas; pheochromocytoma.

TREATMENT
Dependent on the underlying cause.

MEDICATIONS

DRUG(S) OF CHOICE
• Type 1 diabetes mellitus—insulin; long-term therapeutic success has been limited
• PPID—dopamine agonist (pergolide)

CONTRAINDICATIONS
• Corticosteroids
• Dextrose-containing fluids

PRECAUTIONS
• Hyperinsulinemia may contribute to laminitis
• Sustained high glucose concentrations above the renal threshold can lead to cell deprivation of glucose for energy and may indicate a poorer prognosis for recovery
• Ketoacidosis may develop with diabetes mellitus

POSSIBLE INTERACTIONS
N/A

ALTERNATIVE DRUGS
N/A

FOLLOW-UP

PATIENT MONITORING
Monitor blood glucose concentrations.

PREVENTION/AVOIDANCE
Prevent overconditioning in horses predisposed to EMS.

POSSIBLE COMPLICATIONS
• Immunosuppression associated with PPID can lead to recurrent infections
• Severe hyperglycemia can result in hyperosmolality and possible CNS depression
• Laminitis
• Infertility

EXPECTED COURSE AND PROGNOSIS
• Dependent on the underlying cause
• Guarded if prolonged hyperglycemia, since cells are deprived of glucose for energy
• In cases of colic (pain, stress), glucose concentrations >250–300 mg/dL indicate a poor prognosis

MISCELLANEOUS

ASSOCIATED CONDITIONS
N/A

AGE-RELATED FACTORS
Middle-aged to older horses have increased incidence of PPID.

ZOONOTIC POTENTIAL
N/A

PREGNANCY/FERTILITY/BREEDING
Infertility or lack of estrus cycles.

SYNONYMS
• EMS—insulin dysregulation
• PPID—equine Cushing's disease

SEE ALSO
• Equine metabolic syndrome (EMS)/insulin resistance (IR)
• Laminitis
• Pituitary pars intermedia dysfunction

ABBREVIATIONS
• ACTH = adrenocorticotropic hormone
• CNS = central nervous system
• EMS = equine metabolic syndrome
• POMC = pro-opiomelanocortin
• PPID = pituitary pars intermedia dysfunction
• PU/PD = polyuria/polydipsia
• SIRS = systemic inflammatory response syndrome

Internet Resources
Cornell University College of Veterinary Medicine, Eclinpath, glucose. http://www.eclinpath.com/chemistry/energy-metabolism/glucose
American College of Veterinary Internal Medicine, Pituitary Pars Intermedia Disease in Horses. http://www.acvim.org/Animal-Owners/Animal-Education/Health-Fact-Sheets/Large-Animal-Internal-Medicine/Pituitary-Pars-Intermedia-Disease-in-Horses
American Association of Equine Practitioners. http://www.aaep.org/info/horse-health?publication=747

Suggested Reading
Frank N. Disorders of the endocrine system: insulin resistance and equine metabolic syndrome. In: Reed SM, Bayly WM, Sellon DC, eds. Equine Internal Medicine, 3e. St. Louis, MO: WB Saunders, 2010:1270–1277.
Hassel DM, Hill AE, Rorabeck RA. Association between hyperglycemia and survival in 228 horses with acute gastrointestinal disease. J Vet Intern Med 2009;23:1261–1265.
McFarlane D. Equine endocrine and metabolic disorders: pituitary and hypothalamus. In: Smith BP, ed. Large Animal Internal Medicine, 5e. St. Louis, MO: Elsevier Mosby, 2015:1223–1228.
Toribio RE. Disorders of the endocrine system: endocrine pancreas. In: Reed SM, Bayly WM, Sellon DC, eds. Equine Internal Medicine, 3e. St. Louis, MO: WB Saunders, 2010:1260–1262.

Author Claire B. Andreasen
Consulting Editor Sandra D. Taylor

BASICS

OVERVIEW
- Hypoglycemia is a decreased concentration of glucose in blood, plasma, or serum
- Glucose is a major source of energy, especially for the central nervous system
- Glucose is acquired from the diet and stored as glycogen in liver and muscle
- Insulin moves glucose from plasma into cells
- Hypoglycemia results from decreased glycogen availability, excessive cellular use of glucose, decreased feed intake, or excessive insulin or IGFs
- Bacterial utilization of glucose can cause hypoglycemia, especially in neonates
- Systems affected—nervous, neuromuscular, cardiovascular, behavioral

SIGNALMENT
Neonates are very susceptible to hypoglycemia from decreased intake because of limited energy reserves.

SIGNS
- Depression, weakness, tachycardia, muscle fasciculations, tremors, ataxia, collapse, and seizures
- Additional signs depending on the underlying cause

CAUSES AND RISK FACTORS
- Neonates—anorexia, sepsis/septicemia, ischemic hepatopathy (e.g. perinatal asphyxia)
- Sepsis/endotoxemia
- Exhaustion after prolonged exercise
- Hepatic failure—toxins (pyrrolizidine alkaloid-containing plants, Alsike clover, *Panicum* grasses, aflatoxins, *Indigofera*, iron, copper), infections (*Clostridium*, *Fasciola*, *Parascaris*), hepatic lipidosis, chronic active hepatitis, cholangiohepatitis, Theiler's disease, neoplasia, Tyzzer's disease in neonates
- Iatrogenic—e.g. treatment of hyperlipidemia/hyperlipemia
- Pancreatic islet B-cell neoplasia (rare)
- Renal or hepatic carcinomas that secrete IGF (rare)

DIAGNOSIS

DIFFERENTIAL DIAGNOSIS
- Obtundation in neonates—perinatal asphyxia, meningitis, septicemia, Tyzzer's disease, neonatal isoerythrolysis

- Weakness—equine motor neuron disease, botulism, hypocalcemia, hypomagnesemia
- Seizures—perinatal asphyxia (neonates), space-occupying brain mass (e.g. tumor, abscess, pituitary adenoma), equine protozoal myeloencephalitis, epilepsy

CBC/BIOCHEMISTRY/URINALYSIS
Note that in vitro glucose consumption by RBCs occurs with delayed sample processing.

CBC
In cases of acute sepsis, leukopenia characterized by neutropenia and a degenerative left shift might be observed.

Biochemistry
- Infection or neoplasia—increased serum globulin concentrations
- Hepatopathy—increased liver enzyme concentrations (sorbitol dehydrogenase, aspartate aminotransferase, γ-glutamyltransferase, alkaline phosphatase) and bilirubin concentration; decreased blood urea nitrogen and albumin concentrations
- Exhaustion—hyponatremia, hypochloremia, hypokalemia, increased TCO_2

OTHER LABORATORY TESTS
- Arterial blood gas analysis if suspect perinatal asphyxia (respiratory acidosis) or exhausted horse syndrome (metabolic alkalosis)
- Serum or plasma insulin concentration

IMAGING
- Ultrasonography to evaluate liver in cases of hepatopathy
- Ultrasonography to evaluate umbilicus in cases of neonatal septicemia

OTHER DIAGNOSTIC PROCEDURES
- Dependent on the underlying cause
- Blood culture if suspect septicemia
- Liver biopsy if suspect hepatopathy

TREATMENT
Dependent on the underlying cause.

MEDICATIONS

DRUG(S) OF CHOICE
- Dextrose-containing fluids IV (4–8 mg/kg/min)
- Administer enteral and/or parenteral nutrition when appropriate

CONTRAINDICATIONS/POSSIBLE INTERACTIONS
- Insulin is contraindicated
- Administration of 5% dextrose in water acts as a hypotonic solution once administered because glucose is metabolized immediately

FOLLOW-UP

PATIENT MONITORING
Serial blood glucose measurements.

POSSIBLE COMPLICATIONS
- Perivascular leakage of IV dextrose can cause tissue necrosis
- Parenteral nutrition may cause hyperosmolar syndrome or hyperlipidemia

EXPECTED COURSE AND PROGNOSIS
- Dependent on the underlying cause
- Survival rates for septic foals treated with intensive care vary from 60% to 75%

MISCELLANEOUS

PREGNANCY/FERTILITY/BREEDING
Placentitis can lead to in utero sepsis of the foal.

SEE ALSO
- Acute hepatitis in adult horses (Theiler disease)
- Bacteremia/sepsis
- Endotoxemia
- Nutrition in foals
- Seizure disorders
- Seizures in foals
- Septicemia, neonate
- Septic meningoencephalomyelitis
- Toxic hepatopathy
- Tyzzer disease (*Clostridium piliformis*)

ABBREVIATIONS
- IGF = insulin-like growth factor
- RBC = red blood cell
- TCO_2 = total carbon dioxide

Suggested Reading
McKenzie III HC, Geor RJ. Feeding management of sick neonatal foals. Vet Clin North Am Equine Pract 2009;25:109–119.
Smith GF, Davis JL. Diseases of the hepatobiliary system. In: Smith BP, ed. Large Animal Internal Medicine, 5e. St. Louis, MO: Elsevier Mosby, 2015:843–872.

Author Katie M. Boes
Consulting Editor Sandra D. Taylor

G

GLUCOSE TOLERANCE TESTS

BASICS

DEFINITION
• Performed to evaluate a horse's ability to metabolize glucose appropriately. Glucose tolerance tests evaluate response to a glucose load, and are 1 method of testing for insulin dysregulation. Insulin tolerance tests may also be used (see chapter Insulin levels/insulin tolerance test)
• In normal horses, insulin secretion is closely tied to blood glucose concentrations. Fasted insulin concentrations are quite low (<20 μU/mL) but increase rapidly when the horse receives glucose. In turn, this rapidly causes blood glucose to return to the normal range
• Several glucose tolerance tests have been developed:
  ◦ Oral sugar test—administer 0.15–0.45 mL/kg Karo Light Syrup and assess insulin and glucose at 60–90 min. Insulin <45 μU/mL is considered normal. Insulin 45–60 μU/mL is considered equivocal, and insulin >60 μU/mL is abnormal
  ◦ The in-feed glucose test—administer 1 g/kg oral glucose in 0.5 g/kg chaff. Insulin >85 μU/mL at 2 h is considered abnormal
  ◦ IV glucose tolerance test—administer dextrose (0.5 g/kg as a 50% solution IV). Either blood glucose alone or glucose and insulin are determined before and every 30 min after administration for 3 h. Glucose is not given orally to remove the confounding effects of poor intestinal absorption or delayed gastric emptying. Serum glucose should be normal within 2 h of administration and an elevated glucose 3 h after beginning the test is clear evidence of insulin dysregulation
  ◦ The combined glucose-insulin test—administer dextrose (150 mg/kg 50% solution IV), immediately followed by 0.10 U/kg regular insulin. Collect blood at 45 min. Insulin resistance if blood glucose is above baseline and/or insulin above 100 μU/mL
• Common diseases causing abnormal results include insulin dysregulation in horses with EMS or PPID (equine Cushing disease). Results will also be abnormal in cases of diabetes mellitus caused by insulin deficiency

PATHOPHYSIOLOGY
• In oral glucose tolerance tests, increased serum insulin levels in euglycemic or hyperglycemic horses may result from insulin dysregulation, which may be due to peripheral (tissue) insulin resistance, increased pancreatic secretion (primary or secondary to increased stimulation by incretins), or alterations in insulin clearance

• In IV glucose tolerance, increased serum insulin levels in euglycemic or hyperinsulinemic horses may be due to peripheral (tissue) insulin resistance, or alterations in pancreatic function or insulin clearance. IV glucose tolerance tests will not evaluate the role of incretin stimulation
• Diabetes mellitus is associated with decreased circulating insulin and increased glucose tolerance test times. Type 2 is due to pancreatic exhaustion and type 1 is due to autoimmune pancreatic destruction. Diabetes mellitus is very rare in equids

SYSTEMS AFFECTED
Endocrine system—slow return of blood glucose to the normal range indicates abnormal insulin regulation.

GENETICS
EMS is thought to be in part heritable.

INCIDENCE/PREVALENCE
Prevalence of abnormal glucose tolerance is not known.

GEOGRAPHIC DISTRIBUTION
N/A

SIGNALMENT
• There are breed differences in response to an oral glucose load. Ponies and thrifty breeds (e.g. Andalusians) tend to have a physiologic degree of insulin resistance; thus, blood glucose returns to normal levels more slowly than in other horses
• No sex differences
• Frequently obese
• PPID can be associated with alterations in glucose metabolism and tends to occur in old horses (>18 years)

SIGNS
• In horses with PPID—lethargy, exercise intolerance, hypertrichosis and failure to shed (or delayed shedding of) winter coat, tendency for chronic infections, pendulous abdomen, polyuria and polydipsia, laminitis
• In horses with EMS—exercise intolerance, obesity, abnormal fat distribution (neck, tail-head, supraorbital), laminitis
• In horses with diabetes mellitus—weight loss, polyuria and polydipsia, and lethargy or depression

CAUSES
• The primary cause for abnormal results is insulin dysregulation
• Hyperglycemia and hypoinsulinemia indicate diabetes mellitus
• Diet and fed status can influence oral glucose tolerance test results. Thus, the tests should be performed on horses consuming grass hay or other low-carbohydrate feeds (not grain). Fasting duration may influence results

RISK FACTORS
• PPID
• Obesity

DIAGNOSIS

DIFFERENTIAL DIAGNOSIS
Polyuria, polydipsia, and glucosuria in horses with suspected endocrine disorders indicate a disorder in glucose homeostasis, and are generally consistent with diabetes mellitus.

LABORATORY FINDINGS
Drugs That May Alter Laboratory Results
• Corticosteroids
• α₂-Agonists (xylazine, detomidine)

Disorders That May Alter Laboratory Results
Delayed separation of serum from cells falsely lowers blood glucose values.

Valid if Run in a Human Laboratory?
Yes; however, note that there may be marked differences in insulin concentration depending upon which assay is used.

CBC/BIOCHEMISTRY/URINALYSIS
• Horses with abnormal glucose response associated with PPID may exhibit a stress response with mature neutrophilia, lymphopenia, and eosinopenia. They also may have glucosuria
• Horses with type 1 or 2 diabetes mellitus have hyperglycemia. Horses with EMS have normal blood glucose levels in the face of increased insulin concentrations

OTHER LABORATORY TESTS
Pituitary function—TRH stimulation (non-fall) or endogenous ACTH (fall) tests. If these results are consistent with PPID, that diagnosis is supported; if these results do not indicate PPID, suspect either a stress response or EMS.

IMAGING
• Not diagnostic for abnormalities of glucose metabolism
• Increased pituitary gland size may be visualized with specialized modalities—CT or venous contrast

OTHER DIAGNOSTIC PROCEDURES
N/A

TREATMENT

APPROPRIATE HEALTH CARE
• Horses with hyperlipemia require inpatient treatment with IV dextrose, balanced electrolyte solutions, caloric replacement, heparin, and exogenous insulin
• All other horses with abnormal test results can be treated as outpatients

NURSING CARE
Horses with laminitis need corrective hoof trimming and shoeing and dietary management.

ACTIVITY
• Limit the activity of horses with laminitis
• Increase the activity of sound, obese horses in an effort to lose weight

DIET
• Horses with laminitis generally benefit from a low-carbohydrate, high-fiber diet
• Keep horses with insulin dysregulation on a low-carbohydrate diet
• Restrict or increase caloric intake in all horses until a condition score of 4–6 out of 9 is achieved

CLIENT EDUCATION
• Horses with PPID may be managed with medication and nursing care, but their prognosis is quite variable. Some do well for several years; others are refractory to treatment. Inform owners that treatment of such horses is palliative and required for life
• Encourage clients to maintain horses at condition scores of 4–6 out of 9 and to prevent obesity

SURGICAL CONSIDERATIONS
N/A

MEDICATIONS
DRUG(S) OF CHOICE
• Metformin may help improve insulin and glucose responses to an oral glucose test (15–30 mg/kg PO before feeding every 12–24 h)
• The agent most commonly used to alter symptoms of PPID is pergolide (0.50–2 mg/horse/day PO)
• Horses with insulin deficiency (i.e. diabetes mellitus) require insulin supplementation. Protamine zinc insulin (0.5 IU IM every 12 h) was reported to normalize blood glucose in a case report of a pony
• Hyperlipemia—protamine zinc insulin (0.075–0.4 IU/kg SC or IM every 12–24 h). Regular insulin (0.4 IU/kg) has also been recommended

• Regard these doses as starting points that should be changed in response to blood glucose levels

CONTRAINDICATIONS
N/A

PRECAUTIONS
Horses that receive overdoses of pergolide may exhibit anorexia, lethargy, and ataxia.

POSSIBLE INTERACTIONS
N/A

ALTERNATIVE DRUGS
N/A

FOLLOW-UP
PATIENT MONITORING
• Upon initial diagnosis, test horses with PPID in 4–6 weeks to determine treatment efficacy by endogenous ACTH determination or TRH stimulation test. Abnormal results indicate the need for an increased dose of the compound the horse is receiving or change in medication
• Once stable, test horses with PPID less frequently (every few months)
• For horses with abnormal glucose tolerance test results associated with EMS or PPID, monitor glucose tolerance in 3–4 months following implementation of therapy
• Check the blood glucose level of horses with diabetes mellitus on insulin therapy twice a day. Increase or decrease insulin doses in response to blood glucose values outside the normal range

POSSIBLE COMPLICATIONS
N/A

MISCELLANEOUS
ASSOCIATED CONDITIONS
• Hypertrichosis, chronic infections, and laminitis are commonly associated with PPID

• Obesity, laminitis, and dyslipidemia are commonly associated with EMS

AGE-RELATED FACTORS
N/A

ZOONOTIC POTENTIAL
N/A

PREGNANCY/FERTILITY/BREEDING
N/A

SYNONYMS
N/A

SEE ALSO
• Equine metabolic syndrome (EMS)/insulin resistance (IR)
• Insulin levels/insulin tolerance test
• Pituitary pars intermedia dysfunction

ABBREVIATIONS
• ACTH = adrenocorticotrophic hormone
• CT = computed tomography
• EMS = equine metabolic syndrome
• PPID = pituitary pars intermedia dysfunction
• TRH = thyrotropin-releasing hormone

Suggested Reading
Bertin FR, Taylor SD, Bianco AW, Sojka-Kritchevsky JE. The effect of fasting duration on baseline blood glucose concentration, blood insulin concentration, glucose/insulin ratio, oral sugar test, and insulin response test results in horses. J Vet Intern Med 2016;30(5):1726–1731.
Frank N. Equine metabolic syndrome. Vet Clin North Am Equine Pract 2011;27:73–92.
Frank N, Tadros EM. Insulin dysregulation. Equine Vet J 2014;46:103–112.
Freestone JF, Shoemaker K, Bessin R, Wolfsheimer JK. Insulin and glucose response following oral glucose administration in well conditioned ponies. Equine Vet J Suppl 1992;11:13–17.

Authors Janice Kritchevsky and Heidi Banse
Consulting Editors Michel Lévy and Heidi Banse

G

GLYCOGEN BRANCHING ENZYME DEFICIENCY

BASICS

OVERVIEW
• This is an inherited autosomal recessive genetic disease of Quarter Horses and related crosses that results in a nonsense mutation in the gene coding for GBE, rendering the enzyme ineffective
• Also known as glycogen storage disease IV, which is also reported in humans and Norwegian forest cats
• GBE is needed for the formation of the 1,6 branch points in glycogen. This defect in glycogen can lead to abnormal glucose homeostasis in cardiac and skeletal muscle and liver
• Foals typically exhibit weakness and hypotonia and die shortly after birth

SIGNALMENT
• Quarter Horse and Paint neonatal foals
• Clinical signs are generally seen from the time of birth
• Late term abortion in mares carrying an affected fetus

SIGNS
• Many affected foals present for other illness such as septicemia. Concurrent disease such as pneumonia is common in this age group of foals
• Late-term abortion (up to 3% of all abortions in Quarter Horses)
• Stillbirths or persistent recumbency
• Transient flexural limb deformities
• Seizures—due to inadequate glucose metabolism in neurons
• Cardiorespiratory failure—due to muscular weakness and cardiomyopathy

CAUSES AND RISK FACTORS
• Heritable trait among certain Quarter Horse and Paint lines
• Defective gene is on chromosome 26, which encodes the GBE
• In 2004, the genetic basis of the defective GBE gene was identified by cDNA sequences—a single C-to-A substitution at base 102 of codon 34 of exon 1
• When evaluated in 11 affected foals, all were homozygous for the defective *X34* allele. When the gene is expressed, the mRNA product encodes for a 699 amino acid protein with a nonsense mutation, rendering the GBE ineffective. The affected foal pedigrees had a common ancestry and contained prolific stallions who are likely to be heterozygous for the recessive *X34* allele
• Up to 10% of all Quarter Horses may have at least 1 defective gene

DIAGNOSIS
• Genetic testing using DNA from tail/mane hair (PCR technique)

• Muscle biopsy—PAS stain is decreased; polysaccharide accumulates in skeletal muscle with amorphous PAS-positive inclusions
• Pedigree analysis—inherited as a simple autosomal recessive condition

DIFFERENTIAL DIAGNOSIS
• Neonatal septicemia—may also exhibit weakness and hypoglycemia, but should have changes in leukogram (neutropenia or neutrophilia), fever, and signs of infection
• Congenital myotonia—progressive myotonia may have similar weakness, but progresses to muscle stiffness and atrophy with prolonged contraction of the affected muscles after stimulation. Apparent as early as 1 month of age, but usually not apparent from birth. Specific histologic changes in muscle
• Hyperkalemic periodic paralysis—muscular weakness is episodic rather than progressive; clinical signs rarely seen in neonatal foals. Serum potassium may be increased during episodes of muscle fasciculation. Autosomal dominant condition of Quarter Horses—genetic testing (DNA) indicated if hyperkalemic periodic paralysis is suspected

CBC/BIOCHEMISTRY/URINALYSIS
• CBC may be normal but often has leukopenia with neutropenia
• Biochemistry—affected foals tend to have intermittent or persistent hypoglycemia, elevated serum liver enzyme activities, and increases in creatine kinase, aspartate aminotransferase, and γ-glutamyltransferase

OTHER LABORATORY TESTS
N/A

IMAGING
N/A

OTHER DIAGNOSTIC PROCEDURES
N/A

PATHOLOGIC FINDINGS
• Skeletal and cardiac muscle specimens show an absence of normal glycogen staining with PAS stain and myonecrosis
• Accumulation of unbranched glycogen inclusion bodies in many tissues, including skeletal muscle, liver, myocardium, and Purkinje fibers
• Paucity of any normal glycogen content in skeletal muscle. Often normal glycogen content in liver

TREATMENT
This is a fatal condition of neonatal foals, with no known treatment.

MEDICATIONS
DRUG(S) OF CHOICE
N/A

CONTRAINDICATIONS/POSSIBLE INTERACTIONS
N/A

FOLLOW-UP
PATIENT MONITORING
N/A

PREVENTION/AVOIDANCE
N/A

POSSIBLE COMPLICATIONS
N/A

EXPECTED COURSE AND PROGNOSIS
• Grave prognosis
• Most foals die during hospitalization or shortly after discharge. This is a fatal disease of neonates

MISCELLANEOUS
ASSOCIATED CONDITIONS
N/A

AGE-RELATED FACTORS
Clinical signs are seen from the time of birth.

ZOONOTIC POTENTIAL
N/A

PREGNANCY/FERTILITY/BREEDING
N/A

SEE ALSO
• Hyperkalemic periodic paralysis
• Seizures in foals

ABBREVIATIONS
• GBE = glycogen branching enzyme
• PAS = periodic acid–Schiff
• PCR = polymerase chain reaction

Suggested Reading
Valberg SJ, Ward TL, Rush B, et al. Glycogen branching enzyme deficiency in Quarterhorse foals. J Vet Intern Med 2001;15:572–580.
Wagner ML, Valberg SJ, Ames EG, et al. Allele frequency and likely impact of the glycogen branching enzyme deficiency gene in quarter horse and paint horse populations. J Vet Intern Med 2006;20:1207–1211.

Author Samuel D.A. Hurcombe
Consulting Editor Margaret C. Mudge

BASICS

OVERVIEW
- Goiter is enlargement of the thyroid gland
- Goiter can be either diffuse or nodular. Nodular may be either uninodular or multinodular and either functional or nonfunctional. Nodular goiter is the result of thyroid tumors within the parenchyma of the gland. Diffuse goiter is caused by either excess or deficient iodine in the diet or by ingestion of goitrogens, which make ingested iodine unavailable
- Goiter can occur in foals as part of the CHD syndrome or when born to mares ingesting excess amounts of iodine throughout pregnancy
- Horses with diffuse goiter are generally hypothyroid. Nodular goiter is usually caused by thyroid adenomas that are nonfunctioning and are not associated with clinical signs

SIGNALMENT
- There are no breed or sex predilections. Most horses with goiter are foals born with congenital goiter
- Goiter is not a genetic condition

SIGNS
The defining characteristic of a goiter is a thyroid gland enlarged to 2 times its normal size.

CAUSES AND RISK FACTORS
- The cause of diffuse goiter in foals is ingestion of too much or too little iodine by the dam. If pregnant mares receive high-iodine diets, they will be clinically normal while their offspring will have goiter
- Thyroid adenoma or adenocarcinoma most often causes nodular goiter
- Goiter is uncommon in horses
- Endemic goiter may occur in broodmare farms if dietary iodine is unbalanced
- Goiter can occur in foals with CHD syndrome. A case–control study found that mares being fed green feed, irrigated pastures, receiving no supplemental minerals, and leaving their "home" pastures were more likely to produce affected foals than mares not exposed to those conditions. Ingesting high-nitrate and low-iodine levels may affect fetal thyroid function and has been implicated as an important predisposing factor

DIAGNOSIS

- Diagnosis can be made on physical examination by observing and palpating a grossly enlarged thyroid gland
- Differential diagnosis includes other structures that might cause swelling in the proximal neck, including abscess, enlarged lymph node, guttural pouch enlargement, generalized edema, or cellulitis

CBC/BIOCHEMISTRY/URINALYSIS
These tests are generally normal.

OTHER LABORATORY TESTS
Blood total and free triiodothyronine and thyroxine levels may be low if the animal is hypothyroid.

IMAGING
An enlarged thyroid gland may be seen as a soft tissue mass on radiographs of the proximal neck. The enlarged thyroid can also be imaged via ultrasonography.

OTHER DIAGNOSTIC PROCEDURES
Fine needle biopsy or aspirate of the goiter may be performed to confirm that the structure in question is the thyroid gland.

PATHOLOGIC FINDINGS
- Nodular goiter—a tumor in the thyroid gland is often found on pathologic examination
- Diffuse goiter—enlarged follicles filled with colloid and few or no resorption vesicles are seen on histopathologic examination

TREATMENT

- The dietary iodine concentration of affected foals and their dams should be determined
- From 35 to 40 mg/day iodine in a pregnant mare's diet may cause congenital goiter in her foal. NRC recommendations for daily iodine intake are 1–2 mg/day
- Once the diet is corrected to a proper iodine level, the goiter general resolves
- If a pregnant mare is pastured in the geographic area associated with CHD syndrome (northwestern USA, particularly the states of Washington and Oregon, and northwestern Canada), removal from irrigated or green feed pasture or supplementation with hay and minerals may be preventative
- Removal of a thyroid tumor in instances of nodular goiter is curative

MEDICATIONS

If the horse is hypothyroid, supplementation with thyroxine is curative. Synthetic thyroxine at a dose of 20 μg/kg will maintain normal thyroid hormone levels for 24 h.

CONTRAINDICATIONS/POSSIBLE INTERACTIONS
N/A

FOLLOW-UP

- If goiter is due to a benign tumor, removal of the tumor will be curative
- If goiter is due to excess or deficient iodine, correcting the diet to an acceptable level should result in resolution of the symptoms
- Foals with goiter should be carefully monitored to make sure that any skeletal abnormalities associated with hypothyroidism do not cause angular limb deformities
- Most foals with CHD syndrome are euthanized due to severe musculoskeletal deformities
- The expected course is for the goiter to resolve and for the thyroid gland to regain its normal size once the cause has been removed

MISCELLANEOUS

SEE ALSO
- Disorders of the thyroid, hypo- and hyperthyroidism
- Thyroid tumors

ABBREVIATIONS
- CHD = congenital hypothyroidism and dysmaturity
- NRC = National Research Council

Suggested Reading
Allen AL. Congenital hypothyroidism in horses: looking back and looking ahead. Equine Vet Educ 2014;26:190–193.
Allen AL, Townsend HG, Doige CE, Fretz PB. A case-control study of the congenital hypothyroidism and dysmaturity syndrome of foals. Can Vet J 1996;37:349–358.
Driscoll J, Hintz HF, Schryer HF. Goiter in foals caused by excessive iodine. J Am Vet Med Assoc 1968;153:1618–1630.

Author Janice Kritchevsky
Consulting Editors Michel Lévy and Heidi Banse

G

GRANULOMATOUS ENTERITIS

BASICS

OVERVIEW
GE represents 1 of several types of chronic inflammatory bowel diseases affecting the mature horse. The disease is characterized by a diffuse and circumscribed infiltration of the lamina propria and submucosa of the gastrointestinal tract with lymphocytes, macrophages, and epithelioid cells with occasional plasma cells and multinucleated giant cells. The ileum is the most consistently affected site. The presence of marked villous atrophy and clubbing contributes to malabsorption of carbohydrates due to the loss of absorptive surface area and the loss of absorptive epithelial cells at the tips of the villi. Other features of the small bowel mucosa include ulceration, lymphoid hyperplasia, crypt abscesses, and lymphangiectasia.

SIGNALMENT
Granulomatous enteritis can occur at any age or in any breed, or either sex. It is most common in young adult horses, and Standardbreds are predisposed.

SIGNS
• Chronic, insidious weight loss of several months' duration is the most common presenting sign. Horses present in thin or emaciated body condition
• Bright and alert initially, but become depressed with debilitation
• Decreased exercise tolerance may be the first clinical sign observed
• Appetite variable; is usually increased initially
• Roughened haircoat; alopecia; skin dry and flaky
• Dependent edema may develop as animal becomes hypoproteinemic
• Diarrhea is not usually present unless there is involvement of the large intestine and rectum
• Multiple, firm nodules or masses within the mesentery or small intestine may be palpated consistently on per rectal examination

CAUSES AND RISK FACTORS
Unknown. It has been hypothesized that it may result from an aberrant host immune-mediated response to dietary, parasitic, or bacterial antigens.

DIAGNOSIS

DIFFERENTIAL DIAGNOSIS
Rule out other diseases that cause significant protein loss into body cavities or urinary system, and other causes of chronic weight loss including:
• Chronic eosinophilic gastroenteritis
• Intestinal lymphosarcoma
• Abdominal abscessation
• Lymphocytic–plasmacytic enterocolitis

CBC/BIOCHEMISTRY/URINALYSIS
• Hypoalbuminemia (moderate to severe) is the most consistent laboratory finding, being reported in 90% of cases
• Hypoproteinemia reported in approximately 65% of GE cases
• Mild to moderate hypoglobulinemia. Varying serum gamma-globulin levels
• Anemia reported in 87% of GE cases or normal CBC
• Moderate neutrophilia with mild left shift
• Urinalysis normal

DIAGNOSTIC PROCEDURES
• Decreased D-xylose or glucose absorption tests if there is significant small intestine involvement
• Ultrasonography of abdomen to confirm small intestinal thickening
• Abdominocentesis is usually normal, except occasionally peritoneal macrophages may exhibit evidence of decreased phagocytic activity
• Rectal mucosal biopsy provides a diagnosis in approximately 50% of GE cases and depends on whether rectum is involved
• Ileal biopsy through a standing left-flank laparotomy is necessary for a definitive diagnosis; however, surgery on a debilitated, hypoproteinemic animal is not without risk

TREATMENT
Poor prognosis.

MEDICATIONS

DRUG(S) OF CHOICE
• Medical therapies have been generally unsuccessful
• Long-term parenteral dexamethasone sodium phosphate administration has been used successfully in 1 case reported in the literature. Parenteral administration of corticosteroids believed to be more effective than oral administration
• Total parenteral nutrition may be indicated in very valuable patients

CONTRAINDICATIONS/POSSIBLE INTERACTIONS
Alleged risk of laminitis following parenteral dexamethasone administration.

FOLLOW-UP
• Monitor body weight, total serum protein, and serum albumin levels following corticosteroid therapy
• Repeat per rectum examinations and D-xylose absorption test
• Feed free-choice, highly digestible, and well-balanced ration
• Prognosis—poor in the long term

MISCELLANEOUS

SEE ALSO
• Eosinophilic enteritis
• Internal abdominal abscesses
• Lymphocytic–plasmacytic enterocolitis
• Lymphosarcoma
• Protein-Losing Enteropathy (PLE)

ABBREVIATIONS
GE = granulomatous enteritis

Suggested Reading
Barr BS. Infiltrative intestinal disease. Vet Clin North Am Equine Pract 2006;22:e1–7.
Cimprich RE. Equine granulomatous enteritis. Vet Pathol 1974;11:535–547.
Duryea JH, Ainsworth DM, Mauldin EA, et al. Clinical remission of granulomatous enteritis in a Standardbred gelding following long term dexamethasone administration. Equine Vet J 1997;29:164–167.
Kalck KA. Inflammatory bowel disease in horses. Vet Clin North Am Equine Pract 2009;25:303–315.
Lindberg R. Pathology of equine granulomatous enteritis. J Comp Pathol 1984;94:233–247.
Merritt AM, Cimprich RE, Beech J. Granulomatous enteritis in nine horses. J Am Vet Med Assoc 1976;169:603–609.
Platt H. Chronic inflammatory and lymphoproliferative lesions of the equine small intestine. J Comp Pathol 1986;96:671–684.
Schumacher J, Edwards JF, Chen ND. Chronic idiopathic inflammatory bowel disease of the horse. J Vet Intern Med 2000;14:258–265.

Author John D. Baird
Consulting Editors Henry Stämpfli and Olimpo Oliver-Espinosa

BASICS

DEFINITION
GS (equine dysautonomia) is a frequently fatal multisystem neuropathy of equids characterized by chromatolysis of autonomic, enteric, and somatic neurons.

PATHOPHYSIOLOGY
• Clinical signs reflect dysfunction of autonomic, enteric, and somatic neurons
• The dominant clinical signs reflect functional paralysis of the entire GI tract. This is attributable to degeneration of enteric neurons, which is typically most severe in the ileal myenteric and submucosal plexi

SYSTEMS AFFECTED
• GI
• Nervous

INCIDENCE/PREVALENCE
It is estimated that GS kills 1–2% of horses in the UK annually.

GEOGRAPHIC DISTRIBUTION
GS occurs in most Northern European countries, with the highest incidence in the UK. An identical disease termed "mal seco" occurs in Argentina, Chile, and the Falkland Islands. A clinically similar disease termed "tambora" occurs in Colombia; further investigation is required to determine whether this is identical to GS.

SIGNALMENT
• While GS has been reported in horses between 12 days and 47 years old, it predominantly affects 2–9-year-old horses
• There is an increased risk of GS in native Scottish pure breeds
• There is no apparent gender predisposition

SIGNS
GS is categorized into acute, subacute, and chronic forms based on disease severity. This classification is somewhat artificial, since disease severity is a continuum, but it can aid prediction of case outcome. Acute and subacute GS is invariably fatal, with affected horses typically being euthanized within, respectively, 48 h and 7 days after the onset of clinical signs. Approximately 55% of horses with chronic GS survive with supportive care.

Acute GS
Horses commonly present with inappetence and profound depression, but soon develop generalized GI stasis with resultant dysphagia, salivation, dehydration, colic, and distention of the stomach and small intestine with malodorous green-brown fluid and firm, corrugated secondary large intestinal impactions. Despite the severity of these GI abnormalities, signs of abdominal pain are typically mild to moderate. This apparent discrepancy may reflect dysfunction of visceral afferent sympathetic neurons that mediate GI

pain. Dysphagia reflects oral, pharyngeal, and esophageal dysfunction and may be evident as prolonged mastication, quidding, pouching of food in the cheeks, salivation, and reflux of water from the mouth during drinking. Food and water do not reflux via the nares, but spontaneous nasal reflux of gastric fluid occasionally occurs. Per rectum examination may reveal small intestinal distention, large bowel impaction, a dry and tacky rectal mucosa, and small, firm, dry fecal pellets coated with inspissated mucus. Other manifestations of dysautonomia in acute GS include tachycardia (typically 70–120 bpm), sweating, piloerection, and bilateral ptosis. Fasciculations of the triceps, shoulder, and flank muscles are common. Fasciculations are exaggerated by stressful stimuli, and, in contrast to those of botulism and equine motor neuron disease, do not cease when muscles are rested.

Subacute GS
Horses have less severe GI stasis and tachycardia (typically 60–80 bpm), but have an obvious generalized loss of body condition and a tucked up abdomen. Gastric and small intestinal distention is absent, but secondary large intestinal impactions are common. Mild diffuse weakness of the skeletal muscles of the neck, trunk, and limbs causes horses to adopt a base narrow stance, low head and neck carriage, and with the hindquarters supported against the stable wall. Horses attempt to relieve weak postural muscles by spending increased time recumbent and by frequently shifting weight among all 4 limbs while standing. Rhinitis sicca, which appears to be pathognomonic for GS, is common in subacute and chronic GS, but may be absent in the early stages of GS.

Chronic GS
Chronic GS is characterized by profound cachexia, generalized myasthenia, tachycardia (typically 50–60 bpm), and mild signs of GI dysfunction. Rhinitis sicca may cause overt nasal obstruction, and "snuffling" inspiratory and expiratory noise.

CAUSES
While the etiology is unknown, proposed causes include pasture-derived mycotoxins and toxico-infection with *Clostridium botulinum* types C or D.

RISK FACTORS
• Horse factors—peak incidence in 2–9-year-old horses. Increased risk with low serum concentrations of antibodies to surface antigens of *C. botulinum* type C and *Clostridium novyi* type A, and to *C. botulinum* type C neurotoxin complex toxoid
• Premise factors—increased risk in certain geographic locations and on "high-risk" fields. GS occurs more commonly on sand and loam soils than on chalk soils. Increased risk with high soil nitrogen content, large number of

horses on premise, and recent occurrence of GS on the premise
• Management factors—increased risk with grazing, recent stressful procedures, dietary change, moving pasture, recent administration of ivermectin, frequent chain harrowing, soil disturbance, and lack of supplementary feeding with forage while at pasture. Mechanical removal of feces from pastures increases the risk of GS while manual removal of feces reduces the risk
• Other factors—peak incidence in spring and fall and following cool (7–11°C) dry weather

G

DIAGNOSIS

DIFFERENTIAL DIAGNOSIS
Acute GS should be differentiated from other forms of colic, in particular those associated with small intestinal distention. Subacute and chronic GS should be differentiated from botulism and equine motor neuron disease.

CBC/BIOCHEMISTRY/URINALYSIS
• As GS is not associated with specific laboratory abnormalities, these analyses are mainly useful to rule out other diseases
• Acute-phase proteins are often elevated in GS

OTHER LABORATORY TESTS
Definitive antemortem diagnosis is generally considered to require histologic demonstration of the characteristic enteric neurodegeneration in ileal biopsies obtained via midline or, less commonly, flank laparotomy. While laparotomy may be indicated to facilitate prompt differentiation of acute GS and surgical colic cases, this invasive procedure is not advocated for the diagnosis of subacute and chronic GS.

IMAGING
Abdominal ultrasonography is useful to identify gastric and small intestinal distention in acute GS.

OTHER DIAGNOSTIC PROCEDURES
• Clinicians with previous experience of GS can accurately diagnose most cases of GS solely using clinical examination and historical data. However, some acute GS cases present a diagnostic challenge because clinical signs are variable and common to many other diseases
• The discrepancy between the severity of abdominal pain (mild), the severity of the GI dysfunction (severe), and the elevation in heart rate (marked) may aid differentiation of acute GS and surgical colic cases
• Detection of a large intestinal impaction in a grazing horse should alert the clinician to the possibility of GS
• Rhinitis sicca is considered pathognomonic of GS

GRASS SICKNESS

• Detection of subtle bilateral ptosis is facilitated by topical application of 0.5 mL 0.5% phenylephrine eye drops into 1 conjunctival sac. A positive test is evidenced by restoration of normal eyelash angulation within 20–30 min, but is not pathognomonic for GS. False-negative and -positive responses occur, with the latter occurring in some sedated horses and horses with botulism

PATHOLOGIC FINDINGS
• Gross postmortem findings in acute GS include gastric and small intestinal distention with malodorous green-brown fluid, linear ulceration of the distal esophagus, gastric ulceration, and dry firm mucus-coated fecal balls within the small colon and rectum. Gastric rupture may occur. Secondary large intestinal impactions occur in acute and subacute GS. Chronic GS is characterized by a relatively empty GI tract, rhinitis sicca, cachexia, and possibly aspiration pneumonia
• Neuronal pathology in GS has an exquisitely specific neuroanatomic distribution. There is degeneration and loss of enteric neurons in myenteric and submucosal plexi, especially those in the ileum. Neuronal pathology also occurs in the celiacomesenteric, cranial mesenteric, caudal mesenteric, cranial cervical, caudal cervical, thoracic sympathetic chain, and parasympathetic terminal cardiac ganglia. Affected neurons have loss of Nissl substance and cytoplasmic eosinophilia (chromatolysis), nuclear eccentricity and pyknosis, cytoplasmic vacuolation, and intracytoplasmic eosinophilic bodies. Central lesions include chromatolysis of autonomic neurons in the intermediolateral horn of spinal cord and in the nuclei of CN III and CN X, and the somatic lower motor neurons in the ventral horn of the spinal cord and in the nuclei of CN III, CN V, CN VI, CN VII, and CN XII. Early ultrastructural features of GS include disruption of the cytoskeleton and loss of the Golgi apparatus.

TREATMENT
Acute and subacute GS is invariably fatal and affected horses should be euthanized as soon as a confident diagnosis is made. Approximately 55% of chronic GS cases survive. Intensive nursing is the mainstay of treatment. Administration of analgesics, omeprazole, fluids, and electrolytes may be beneficial. The rapidity and magnitude of body weight loss may aid prediction of survival. Complications occurring during the recovery phase of GS include continued weight loss, debility and muscular weakness, colic, esophageal choke, intestinal bacterial overgrowth, diarrhea, penile prolapse, inappropriate sweating, and aspiration pneumonia.

DIET
• The greatest obstacle to survival is generally profound inappetence. Consequently a selection of highly palatable feeds (ideally high in energy and protein) should be offered
• Supplementing the diet with vegetable oil will increase the energy density
• Prolonged feeding via nasogastric tube does not appear to improve survival

MEDICATIONS
Analgesics, omeprazole, fluids, and electrolytes may be beneficial.

FOLLOW-UP
PREVENTION/AVOIDANCE
There are no known guaranteed methods to prevent GS in high-risk areas. After an occurrence of GS, co-grazing horses may be housed for 2–4 weeks to prevent them developing GS. If this is not practical, co-grazers may be moved to a separate field. Factors which increase the risk of GS (see Risk Factors) should be avoided, particularly during spring and fall.

MISCELLANEOUS
SEE ALSO
• Acute adult abdominal pain—acute colic
• Chronic weight loss
• Colic, chronic/recurrent
• Inspiratory dyspnea
• Regurgitation/vomiting/dysphagia

ABBREVIATIONS
• CN = cranial nerve
• GI = gastrointestinal
• GS = grass sickness

Suggested Reading
Jago RC, Handel I, Hahn CN, et al. Bodyweight change aids prediction of survival in chronic equine grass sickness. Equine Vet J 2015;48(6):792–797.
Pirie RS, Jago RC, Hudson NPH. Equine grass sickness. Equine Vet J 2014;46:545–553.

Authors Olimpo Oliver-Espinosa and Bruce McGorum
Consulting Editors Henry Stämpfli and Olimpo Oliver-Espinosa

Client Education Handout available online

BASICS

OVERVIEW
• GPs are diverticula of the auditory tubes that communicate with the pharynx. Infection within the GP causes accumulation of mucopurulent material (GPE)
• Uni- or bilateral GPE often occurs secondarily to upper respiratory tract infection, abscessation, and rupture of the retropharyngeal lymph nodes into the GP

SIGNALMENT
Affects horses of any breed, sex, or age.

SIGNS
Historical Findings
• Previous history of strangles
• Chronic, mucopurulent nasal discharge of unknown cause

Physical Examination Findings
• Unilateral or bilateral nasal discharge; may be abundant
• Occasional swelling of adjacent lymph nodes
• May present with cough, fever, difficulty swallowing, and/or breathing
• Abnormal carriage of the head and neck
• Empyema may occur without other clinical abnormalities

CAUSES AND RISK FACTORS
• Frequently associated with *Streptococcus equi* var. *equi* and var. *zooepidemicus*
• Infusion of irritants (therapeutics)
• Congenital stenosis of the pharyngeal orifice of the auditory tube
• Fracture of the stylohyoid bone
• Pharyngeal perforation during nasogastric intubation

DIAGNOSIS

DIFFERENTIAL DIAGNOSIS
• GP mycosis
• Trauma to GPs
• Diseases causing mucopurulent nasal discharge (pneumonia, sinusitis)

CBC/BIOCHEMISTRY/URINALYSIS
May be within normal limits; occasionally leukocytosis and fibrinogenemia.

OTHER LABORATORY TESTS
Bacterial culture and sensitivity and cytology from GP aspirations or lavages.

IMAGING
• Radiography of the pharynx—standing, lateral projection to identify a distinct fluid line

• Ultrasonography—potential diagnostic value

OTHER DIAGNOSTIC PROCEDURES
• Pharyngeal endoscopy to identify affected GP and intra-GP endoscopy to confirm the diagnosis
• Passing of a sterile polyethylene catheter through the biopsy channel of the endoscope to collect samples for cytology and bacterial culture

PATHOLOGIC FINDINGS
Mucosal ulcerations with exudate accumulation, chondroids, and occasionally rupture and drainage of adjacent lymph nodes into the GP.

TREATMENT

• Placement of an indwelling catheter to allow gentle irrigation of the GP with isotonic saline (500 mL) daily until debris no longer present
• Avoid high-pressure/large-volume lavage to minimize risk of pouch rupture and the use of irritating solutions until debris is no longer present
• Use of antibiotics based on bacterial culture and sensitivity results
• Noninvasive methods for chrondroid removal include maceration, endoscopically guided grasping forceps, basket snare, or wire loop (best performed at a referral facility)

MEDICATIONS

DRUG(S) OF CHOICE
• Antibiotics based upon bacterial culture and sensitivity results for a period of 10 days may be necessary
• NSAIDs

CONTRAINDICATIONS/POSSIBLE INTERACTIONS
Avoid irrigation with irritating solutions such as a strong iodine solution and traumatic placement of the lavage catheter, which may cause damage to cranial nerves.

FOLLOW-UP

PATIENT MONITORING
• Repeat endoscopy 1–2 weeks after the last irrigation therapy
• Ground feeding to facilitate natural drainage
• Provide appropriate care for dysphagic or dyspneic horses

PREVENTION/AVOIDANCE
• Avoid exercise during treatment period
• Biosecurity practices to prevent the introduction of strangles on a farm or to contain strangles once suspected/diagnosed
• Vaccination protocols

POSSIBLE COMPLICATIONS
• Chondroid formation
• Neurologic injury to the glossopharyngeal, vagus, accessory, and hypoglossal nerves

EXPECTED COURSE AND PROGNOSIS
• Duration depends on the cause of the empyema
• Prognosis is favorable with early diagnosis and treatment
• Chondroids requiring surgical removal carry a poorer prognosis than medical treatment alone
• Neurologic dysfunction carries a poor prognosis

G

MISCELLANEOUS

ASSOCIATED CONDITIONS
• Strangles
• *S. equi* var. *zooepidemicus* sinusitis or laryngitis

AGE-RELATED FACTORS
Retropharyngeal lymph node abscessation due to strangles in foals and yearlings.

SEE ALSO
Guttural pouch mycosis

ABBREVIATIONS
• GP = guttural pouch
• GPE = guttural pouch empyema
• NSAID = nonsteroidal anti-inflammatory drug

Suggested Reading
Freeman DE. Complications of surgery for diseases of the guttural pouch. Vet Clin North Am Equine Pract 2009;24:485–497.
Freeman DE. Update on disorders and treatment of the guttural pouch. Vet Clin North Am Equine Pract 2015;31:63–89.
Pascoe JR. Guttural pouch diseases. In: Smith BP, ed. Large Animal Internal Medicine, 5e. St. Louis, MO: Elsevier Mosby, 2015:555–558.

Authors Mary Catherine Furness and Laurent Viel
Consulting Editors Daniel Jean and Mathilde Leclère

GUTTURAL POUCH MYCOSIS

BASICS

OVERVIEW
• Fungal infection which usually affects 1 GP, but bilateral lesions are possible (20%)
• Clinical signs relate to damage to the arteries and nerves underlying the GP mucosa
• Spontaneous epistaxis in a resting horse usually is the first sign

SIGNALMENT
• More common in mature horses but also reported in foals
• No breed, sex, genetic, or geographic predisposition
• Not contagious

SIGNS
• Epistaxis—reason for consultation in 74% of horses affected by mycosis; not related to exercise; severity varies from a mild, unilateral, blood-tinged nasal secretion to fatal hemorrhage. Bleeding may be bilateral with severe hemorrhage. Premonitory bleeding often, but not always, precedes fatal hemorrhage
• Dysphagia—results from lesions involving the vagus, glossopharyngeal, or hypoglossal nerve
• Other neurologic deficits—abnormal respiratory noise (laryngeal hemiplegia, dorsal displacement of the soft palate, pharyngeal collapse), facial paralysis, and Horner syndrome
• Less commonly observed—headshaking, abnormal head posture, visual disturbances, neck stiffness (parotid pain, septic arthritis of the atlanto-occipital joint)
• May be asymptomatic

CAUSES AND RISK FACTORS
• No evidence of initiating factor predisposing to growth of opportunistic fungi in the affected GP. *Aspergillus fumigatus* is the most frequently isolated fungus
• Erosion of the arterial wall by fungus will cause epistaxis; internal carotid will be affected in 2/3 cases. The external carotid or 1 of its branches will be affected in 1/3 cases
• Fungus can also cause nerve damage either by inflammation and infiltration of nerves by mycelium or by diffusion of fungal toxins. Nerve damage can also result from sequestration of nerves in scar tissue. Cranial nerves (VII, IX, X, XI, XII) and their branches, cranial cervical ganglion, and sympathetic trunk may be affected

DIAGNOSIS

DIFFERENTIAL DIAGNOSIS
• Epistaxis—exercise-induced pulmonary hemorrhage, ethmoid hematoma, head trauma, foreign bodies, upper airway neoplasia, longus capitis muscle rupture, and coagulopathy
• Dysphagia—esophageal obstruction, megaesophagus, fracture of the hyoid apparatus, inflammatory reaction, pharyngeal mass, empyema or tympanism of the guttural pouch, central nervous system affections

CBC/BIOCHEMISTRY/URINALYSIS
• Hypoproteinemia and anemia in cases of significant blood loss
• Leukocytosis and hyperfibrinogenemia in cases of aspiration pneumonia

IMAGING
Endoscopy
• Critical for diagnosis, but risky in case of epistaxis
• In case of bleeding from pharyngeal orifices or nostril, prepare surgical facilities and scope the horse in the induction stall. The endoscope should not be introduced into the GP in case of active bleeding as this could dislodge the thrombus. Large amount of blood in the GP may preclude visualization of affected nerves and arteries
• If no bleeding seen from pharyngeal orifices, perform a thorough examination of both GPs to determine which vessels are affected. Mycotic lesions appear as a diphtheritic membrane on the surface of the mucosa. No relationship exists between lesion size and severity of the clinical signs
• In cases of dysphagia or abnormal respiratory noise, examine for food material, pharyngeal collapse, laryngeal hemiplegia, soft palate displacement

TREATMENT

• The first goal is to prevent spontaneous fatal hemorrhage and the treatment is surgical. Perform arterial occlusion as soon as possible. In life-threatening emergency, ligature of the common carotid artery may in some cases prevent fatal bleeding. However, this does not eliminate completely the risk of fatal hemorrhage due to retrograde blood flow

• The aim is to stop blood flow distally and proximally to the lesion. Different techniques of internal occlusion have been described—balloon catheter occlusion (first described technique, high complication rate), transarterial coil or nitinol plug embolization under fluoroscopic guidance (less invasive, low complication rate, specialized equipment)

MEDICATIONS

DRUG(S) OF CHOICE
Medical treatment provides doubtful results.

CONTRAINDICATIONS/POSSIBLE INTERACTIONS
• Use α_2-agonists with caution if epistaxis; they may worsen hemorrhage by increasing the arterial pressure
• Possible irritating or neurotoxic effect of topical drugs

FOLLOW-UP

• Surgical treatment in cases of epistaxis provides an excellent prognosis for survival (84%)
• Guarded prognosis for recovery of neurologic dysfunction (50%)
• Rare spontaneous regression
• 50% have fatal hemorrhage if left untreated

MISCELLANEOUS

ABBREVIATIONS
GP = guttural pouch

Suggested Reading
Lepage OM, Picot-Crézollet C. Trans-arterial coil embolization in 31 horses (1999–2002) with guttural pouch mycosis: a 2-year follow-up. Equine Vet J 2005;37:430–434.
Author Perrine Piat
Consulting Editors Daniel Jean and Mathilde Leclère
Acknowledgment The author and editors acknowledge the prior contribution of Vincent J. Ammann.

BASICS

OVERVIEW
Nonpainful and tympanic swelling in the parotid and laryngeal region due to distention of 1 or both GPs with air. The enlarged GP may displace the pharynx, larynx, and trachea ventrally and to the contralateral side.

SIGNALMENT
• Observed only in foals and weanlings; most common between 2 and 4 months of age
• Fillies are predominantly affected with a female-to-male ratio of 2:1 to 4:1
• Most frequently reported in Standardbreds, Thoroughbreds, Arabians, Quarter Horses, Appaloosas, Paints, American Saddle Horses, and Warmbloods
• A genetic predisposition has been reported in Arabian horses

SIGNS
• Nonpainful and tympanic swelling over the parotid region
• In severe cases, stertorous breathing and dysphagia may develop
• Secondary GP empyema and aspiration pneumonia are common findings
• Unilateral involvement of the GPs is most frequently observed, although the parotid region is usually bilaterally distended

CAUSES AND RISK FACTORS
• Exact etiology of the condition is unknown
• It is considered to be a congenital dysfunction of the pharyngeal orifice of the affected GP

DIAGNOSIS

DIFFERENTIAL DIAGNOSIS
• *Streptococcus equi* infection (strangles) causing extreme swelling of the submandibular or retropharyngeal lymph nodes, retropharyngeal abscesses, and cellulitis is easily distinguished from GP tympany because these former conditions are associated with pain, fever, leukocytosis, and hyperfibrinogenemia
• Primary GP empyema with *Streptococcus zooepidemicus*

CBC/BIOCHEMISTRY/URINALYSIS
• Stress leukocytosis may be present
• Leukocytosis and hyperfibrinogenemia are found in the presence of aspiration pneumonia

OTHER LABORATORY TESTS
N/A

IMAGING
Endoscopic Examination
• Decreased airway size is observed when the nasopharynx and oropharynx are examined
• Protrusion of either the roof alone or the roof and the wall of the pharynx on the affected side into the pharyngeal lumen is present
• Introduction of the endoscope in the affected GP will deflate it and help to distinguish between unilateral and bilateral tympany

Radiography
• Enlargement of air-filled GPs is noticed on lateral radiographic examination of the head and neck (rostral portion). With GP tympany, the affected pouch extends caudally
• Collapse of the pharynx can also be noted

Thoracic Radiography
Rule out aspiration pneumonia.

OTHER DIAGNOSTIC PROCEDURES
Bacterial culture and antimicrobial sensitivity of fluid accumulated in the GP may be performed.

TREATMENT
• External deflation of the GP by needle aspiration is not recommended because of the possibility of causing hemorrhage or damaging the nerves
• Temporary alleviation can be achieved by applying a gentle but firm pressure bilaterally on the parotid area or through an indwelling catheter placed in the pharyngeal orifice of the affected pouch. Definitive treatment is surgical
• 2 surgical treatments performed under general anesthesia are described. 1 consists of the fenestration of the median septum that separates the 2 GPs. The other consists of the resection of a small segment of the medial lamina of the eustachian tube and its associated mucosal fold to create a larger opening of the affected GP into the pharynx. Fenestration of the median septum is used in unilateral GP tympany; both procedures are performed when bilateral involvement
• Fenestration of the median septum and creation of a fistula between the pharynx and the Eustachian tube with the use of laser equipment or electrosurgery can also be performed

MEDICATIONS

DRUG(S) OF CHOICE
• Preoperative and postoperative medication consists of the administration of systemic antibiotics (procaine penicillin G 20 000 U/kg IV BID or trimethoprim–sulfamethoxazole 30 mg/kg IV BID) and NSAIDs (flunixin meglumine 1 mg/kg IV BID)
• In cases complicated by aspiration pneumonia or GP empyema, administration of broad-spectrum antibiotics

CONTRAINDICATIONS/POSSIBLE INTERACTIONS
α_2-Agonist agents should be used with caution in horses with GP tympany as they may worsen upper airway obstruction.

FOLLOW-UP
• In the absence of aspiration pneumonia or GP empyema, the prognosis for a unilateral GP tympany is favorable
• Recurrence rate following a surgical correction is 30%. The prognosis for a bilateral GP tympany is guarded

MISCELLANEOUS

ABBREVIATIONS
• GP = guttural pouch
• NSAID = nonsteroidal anti-inflammatory drug

Suggested Reading
Blazyczek I, Hamann H, Deegen E, et al. Retrospective analysis of 50 cases of guttural pouch tympany in foals. Vet Rec 2004;154:261–264.
Blazyczek I, Hamann H, Ohnesorge B, et al. Inheritance of guttural pouch tympany in the Arabian horse. J Hered 2004;95:195–199.
Ragle CA. Guttural pouch disease. In: Robinson NE, ed. Current Therapy in Equine Medicine, 5e. Philadelphia, PA: WB Saunders, 2003:386–390.

Author Ludovic P. Bouré
Consulting Editors Daniel Jean and Mathilde Leclère

G

HEADSHAKING

BASICS

DEFINITION
Headshaking as a result of sensitization (abnormally low threshold for activation) of the trigeminal nerve, thought to cause neuropathic facial pain. A subset of horses appear to have headshaking in response to light stimulus; see chapter Photic headshaking.

PATHOPHYSIOLOGY
Sensitization of the trigeminal nerve appears to be acquired and to be the result of a functional, rather than structural, change. Cause and mechanism are unknown.

SYSTEMS AFFECTED
Neurologic—trigeminal nerve and/or central.

GENETICS
Unknown

INCIDENCE/PREVALENCE
1–4% of the UK equine population

SIGNALMENT
• Onset is usually in young adulthood (5–10 years)
• Geldings may be overrepresented

SIGNS
• Predominantly vertical headshaking, often with smaller, sharp vertical head movements, and accompanied by nasal irritation (rubbing the nose, snorting)
• At rest, but usually worse at exercise
• Severity may be graded—0/3, no headshaking; 1/3, headshaking but not so severely as to interfere with ridden exercise; 2/3, headshaking of sufficient severity as to make ridden exercise impossible or unsafe; 3/3, headshaking even at rest
• Some horses are only affected seasonally; if so, usually in the spring and summer

CAUSES
Unknown

RISK FACTORS
Unknown

DIAGNOSIS

DIFFERENTIAL DIAGNOSIS
Headshaking from any other causes of facial pain, such as dental disease, temporohyoid osteopathy, iris cyst, bit and tack problems.

CBC/BIOCHEMISTRY/URINALYSIS
N/A

OTHER LABORATORY TESTS
N/A

IMAGING
CT of the head and endoscopy of the upper respiratory tract and guttural pouches to rule out other causes for headshaking.

OTHER DIAGNOSTIC PROCEDURES
• History and observation are key. Ophthalmic and oral examinations to rule out other cause for headshaking
• Infiltration of local anesthetic around the caudal portion of the infraorbital nerve may alleviate signs, confirming headshaking due to facial pain, although not the cause for facial pain. A negative response does not refute facial pain
• Somatosensory-evoked potential testing under general anesthesia could confirm sensitization of the trigeminal nerves but this would not be a mainstream diagnostic test

PATHOLOGIC FINDINGS
Unremarkable

TREATMENT

APPROPRIATE HEALTH CARE
• A nose net provides 70% relief in 25% of cases and is the first treatment to try. Cheap, noninvasive, and suitable for most competitions
• Other products and supplements claim to alleviate headshaking but without scientific evidence or with scientific evidence to show they are ineffective for trigeminal-mediated headshaking

NURSING CARE
N/A

ACTIVITY
Signs usually worse at exercise and some horses may not be safe to ride or even handle.

DIET
No evidence for effect.

CLIENT EDUCATION
Headshaking may occur as a result of neuropathic pain and requires veterinary investigation.

SURGICAL CONSIDERATIONS
• There is no one good treatment for trigeminal-mediated headshaking as yet
• EquiPENS™ neuromodulation currently has the best results with no significant side effects. Under standing sedation, the trigeminal nerve is stimulated using an electrically conductive probe. At least three procedures are required initially. If remission is attained it may only be short term with about 25% of cases showing long-term remission, although the procedure and data are still in their infancy
• Placement of platinum coils in the nerve can alleviate signs long term in 25% of cases but with a significant risk of potentially fatal complications

MEDICATIONS

DRUG(S) OF CHOICE
• Carbamazepine and/or cyproheptadine, which have central effects, may be used although results are inconsistent and may only be short term
• Gabapentin, used for neuropathic pain, may also be used although there are no published results
• Pulsed high-dose corticosteroids have been shown to be ineffective

CONTRAINDICATIONS
Not for use in competition animals.

PRECAUTIONS
May cause side effects of drowsiness, which could have safety implications.

POSSIBLE INTERACTIONS
Unknown

ALTERNATIVE DRUGS
None with evidence of efficacy.

MISCELLANEOUS

ASSOCIATED CONDITIONS
None suspected.

AGE-RELATED FACTORS
Acquired usually in early adulthood (5–10 years). There are few longitudinal data. Some individuals may experience remission, but it is likely most remain affected and may progress.

ZOONOTIC POTENTIAL
None

PREGNANCY/FERTILITY/BREEDING
There is no evidence that these horses are at directly increased risk of having affected offspring.

SYNONYMS
• Headshaking
• Idiopathic headshaking

SEE ALSO
Photic headshaking

ABBREVIATIONS
CT = computed tomography

Suggested Reading
Pickles K, Madigan J, Aleman M. Idiopathic headshaking: is it still idiopathic? Vet J 2014;201:21–30.
Roberts VL, Patel NK, Tremaine WH. Neuromodulation using percutaneous electrical nerve stimulation for the management of trigeminal-mediated headshaking: a safe procedure resulting in medium-term remission in five of seven horses. Equine Vet J 2016;48(2):201–204.
Author Veronica L.H. Roberts
Consulting Editor Caroline N. Hahn

BASICS

DEFINITION
Trauma to the skull and/or associated soft tissues results in primary damage to the brain. Secondary brain injury results from the primary injury and causes physiologic changes in brain tissue. Secondary brain injury can be prevented or lessened, whereas primary injury cannot.

PATHOPHYSIOLOGY
• Following a traumatic insult to the brain, a cycle of cellular events occurs, including membrane disruption, ischemia, hypoxia, edema, and hemorrhage. The severity of these abnormalities is dependent on the type and extent of the initial primary injury. The traumatic insult is also responsible for increased permeability of brain capillary endothelial cells, resulting in vasogenic edema. This is the most common type of edema found following head trauma, and white matter is especially prone to vasogenic edema. Vasogenic edema results in displacement of cerebral tissue and increased ICP. Ultimately, these changes may produce brain herniation
• Cytotoxic edema results from swelling of the cellular elements of the brain. This type of edema occurs in gray and white matter and often results in decreased cerebral function, with stupor and coma as signs. A cycle occurs when increased ICP leads to decreased cerebral blood flow, resulting in further ischemia and brain swelling
• The types of cranial trauma from least to most severe are concussion, contusion, laceration, and hemorrhage. Concussion is short-term loss of consciousness and is often reversible and occurs without anatomic lesions. Contusion is associated with vascular and neural tissue damage without major structural disruption. Laceration and hemorrhage result from penetrating wounds, fractures, or direct blunt trauma. Cerebral hemorrhage in horses may be subdural (rare), intracerebral, or subarachnoid (common)
• Fracture of the basisphenoid/basioccipital bones is not uncommon after poll trauma (falling over backward)
• Hematoma formation is potentially devastating as hemorrhage results in expansion within the rigid skull with herniation, pressure necrosis, and brainstem compression possible

SYSTEMS AFFECTED
• Behavioral—altered mentation
• Cardiovascular—arrhythmias/bradycardia due to dysfunction of central cardiovascular centers
• Musculoskeletal—skull fracture(s); postural/gait abnormalities due to disruption of central motor pathways; other lacerations/fractures from traumatic episode

• Nervous—disruption of neural pathways resulting in changes in behavior, heart rate and rhythm, respiratory rate and rhythm, and neurologic testing
• Ophthalmic—abnormal eye position, movements, and reflexes, and changes in vision
• Respiratory—apneustic and/or erratic breathing due to dysfunction of respiratory regulatory center in the caudal medulla oblongata

SIGNALMENT
No age, breed, or sex predilections.

SIGNS

Historical Findings
• Ascertain if any known episode of trauma or physical evidence of trauma to the horse or its environment
• Potentially abnormal behavior, gait changes, sudden blindness, or recumbency

Physical Examination Findings
• The initial evaluation should be directed toward identification and stabilization of life-threatening problems such as open skull fractures, airway obstruction, hemorrhage, cardiovascular collapse, pneumothorax, and other fractures
• Look for evidence of head trauma. Palpation of the skull may reveal fractures
• Blood from the ears, mouth, or nostrils suggests potential basisphenoid or basioccipital fractures
• Occasionally, CSF may be seen draining from the ears with basilar fractures
• Bradycardia and/or arrhythmias may be present with apneustic or erratic breathing

Neurologic Examination
Neurologic deficits may range from inapparent to recumbency with profound depression, dementia, and tetraparesis. Injury to the:
• *Cerebrum* may manifest as behavior changes, obtundation, coma, circling or wandering, seizures, and blindness with normal pupillary reflexes
• *Cerebellum* may manifest as altered behavior, ataxia, hypermetria, intention tremor, hypertonicity, and lack of menace without blindness
• *Diencephalons (thalamus)* may manifest as depression to stupor, normal to mild tetraparesis, deviation of the head and eyes with circling toward the side of a unilateral lesion, and bilateral nonreactive pupils with blindness
• *Midbrain* may demonstrate stupor to coma with hemiparesis, tetraparesis or tetraplegia, and changes in pupils such as miosis, mydriasis (if mydriatic and unresponsive, sign of poor prognosis) or anisocoria
• *Pons and rostral medulla oblongata* (including the inner ear) often shows obtundation, ataxia with tetraparesis or tetraplegia, and head tilt, nystagmus, facial paralysis, and medial strabismus

• *Caudal medulla oblongata* may manifest as obtundation, ataxia with hemiparesis to tetraparesis, abnormal respiratory patterns, and dysphagia with a flaccid tongue

CAUSES
Head trauma.

RISK FACTORS
• Young age
• Fractious behavior
• Unsafe environment

DIAGNOSIS

DIFFERENTIAL DIAGNOSIS
• Consider other primary brain disorders such as seizures, infection, inflammation, neoplasia, degenerative disease, and congenital problems
• Syncope from cardiovascular disease, metabolic diseases, toxin exposure, adverse drug reactions, and nutritional deficiencies may also affect brain function

CBC/BIOCHEMISTRY/URINALYSIS
Changes in any of these tests may reflect changes in other organ systems secondary to the effects of trauma or due to other underlying disease processes. There are no specific changes in any of these tests for head trauma.

IMAGING
• Skull radiographs may reveal fractures, luxations, and subluxations. Radiography of other areas of the body (long bones, chest) that have evidence of trauma is warranted
• Ultrasonography can be extremely useful for diagnosing skull fractures
• CT or MRI of the head may reveal fractures, hemorrhage, or foreign bodies lodged in the skull or brain
• Scintigraphy is useful for diagnosis of nondisplaced and occult fractures and soft tissue lesions

OTHER DIAGNOSTIC PROCEDURES
• CSF analysis may show xanthochromia with mild to moderate increases in protein. In acute or chronic cases, CSF may be normal. A cisternal (atlanto-occipital) CSF tap is contraindicated if increased ICP is suspected due to the possibility of brain herniation
• Lumbosacral tap safer but may not reflect changes in intracranial CSF
• Brainstem auditory-evoked potentials are evaluated to determine brainstem function
• ECG evaluation aids in determining cardiac rhythm dysfunction

PATHOLOGIC FINDINGS
• Gross and histopathologic findings may include skull fractures, brain laceration/foreign body, hemorrhage, edema, and evidence of hypoxia
• Contusion and concussion may be seen

H

HEAD TRAUMA (CONTINUED)

TREATMENT

APPROPRIATE HEALTH CARE
Usually requires intensive inpatient care—often on an emergency basis.

NURSING CARE
• Treat shock first as neurologic status may improve once the shock is corrected
• Adhere to the ABCs of trauma management
• Monitor oxygenation with pulse oximetry and supplement oxygen as necessary
• Consider controlled ventilation of horse if stuporous, comatose, or if rapid neurologic deterioration occurs
• Maintain normal PCO_2 and PO_2
• Elevate the head up to an angle of 20° to help prevent increased ICP. Do not put the head at an angle greater than this to avoid pressure on the jugular vein as this increases ICP
• Institute fluid therapy to avoid hypotension. Overzealous administration of crystalloids (shock doses of 40–90 mL/kg/h) may exacerbate increased ICP. The use of colloids is contraindicated if intracranial hemorrhage is ongoing. Hypertonic saline (4–6 mL/kg IV over 15 min) is the preferred fluid choice for head trauma horses in shock; shown in people to be superior to mannitol for treating raised intracranial pressure. Isotonic fluids may then be used for maintenance requirements (60 mL/kg/day). In recumbent horses, physical therapy is critical to prevent myositis, decubital sores, and hypostatic pulmonary congestion
• Lubricate the eyes and turn the horse every 2–4 h
• Use deep bedding
• Hydro/massage therapy and therapeutic ultrasonography are useful to maintain circulation to the large muscle groups
• Ensure normothermia and especially avoid hyperthermia

ACTIVITY
• Restricted with strict stall confinement
• Once stable, controlled exercise is useful for physical therapy/rehabilitation

DIET
• Allow access to food and water if the mental status allows
• Provide supplemental tube feeding or parenteral nutrition if the horse is unable/unwilling to eat and drink

CLIENT EDUCATION
• True neurologic status may not be evident for several days, and intensive and potentially costly care may be required
• Full recovery may take months and residual deficits may persist
• An ataxic and demented horse is a potential hazard to humans

SURGICAL CONSIDERATIONS
• Consider surgical intervention of open or depressed skull fractures, and for retrieval of foreign bodies
• The horse needs to be fully stabilized before general anesthesia is contemplated. Perform standing procedure if possible
• Consider craniectomy if increased ICP persists despite medical treatment, and for midbrain signs with a history of cerebral trauma or bleeding

MEDICATIONS

DRUG(S) OF CHOICE
• Sedation with α_2-agonist if patient delirious and thrashing
• Diuretics if horse remains in a coma or semicoma and recumbent for more than a few minutes—mannitol 0.25–2 mg/kg IV over 20 min is favored over furosemide
• If fracture of cranium obvious, tetanus prophylaxis and systemic antibiotics such as penicillin should be considered

CONTRAINDICATIONS
• Glucocorticoid use in human head trauma is no longer recommended and should therefore be avoided
• Avoid drugs that may increase ICP such as ketamine or cause hypertension

FOLLOW-UP

PATIENT MONITORING
Evaluate progress with serial neurologic examinations several times a day initially and taper the frequency based on the stability of the horse.

PREVENTION/AVOIDANCE
Keep area where horses are housed free of clutter.

POSSIBLE COMPLICATIONS
• Increases in ICP may lead to further hemorrhage and ultimately herniation
• Problems associated with recumbent horses (myositis, decubital sores, corneal lacerations, hypostatic pulmonary congestion leading to pneumonia, fecal and urine scalding)

EXPECTED COURSE AND PROGNOSIS
The best prognosis is with minimal injury that is identified early post injury in which prompt treatment is sought. Horses that show rapid improvement with stabilization of signs have a better prognosis.

MISCELLANEOUS

SYNONYMS
• Brain injury
• Brain trauma
• Traumatic brain injury

SEE ALSO
• Aortic rupture
• Botulism
• Eastern (EEE), western (WEE), and Venezuelan (VEE) equine encephalitides
• Equine herpesvirus myeloencephalopathy
• Hepatic encephalopathy
• Hydrocephalus
• Ionophore toxicosis
• Meningitis, neonate
• Neonatal isoerythrolysis
• Neonatal maladjustment syndrome
• Nutritional myodegeneration
• Seizure disorders
• Septicemia, neonate
• Tyzzer disease (*Clostridium piliforme*)

ABBREVIATIONS
• CSF = cerebrospinal fluid
• CT = computed tomography
• ICP = intracranial pressure
• MRI = magnetic resonance imaging
• PCO_2 = partial pressure of carbon dioxide
• PO_2 = partial pressure of oxygen

Suggested Reading
Alderson P, Roberts I. Corticosteroids for acute traumatic brain injury. Cochrane Database Syst Rev 2005;(1):CD000196.

Author Dylan Gorvy
Consulting Editor Caroline N. Hahn
Acknowledgment The author acknowledges the prior contribution of Caroline N. Hahn.

HEAVES (SEVERE EQUINE ASTHMA, RAO)

BASICS

DEFINITION
An inflammatory condition of the lower airways characterized by bronchospasm, excess mucus production, and airway remodeling leading to reversible airway obstruction.

PATHOPHYSIOLOGY
• Stabling and feeding dusty hay leads to inflammation and obstruction of the lower airways in susceptible horses
• Hypoxemia is common
• A hypersensitivity reaction to thermophilic molds and *Actinomyces* antigens is suspected
• The role of endotoxins and nonspecific environmental dust particles on the induction and maintenance of heaves is currently ill defined

SYSTEMS AFFECTED
Respiratory

GENETICS
• A genetic susceptibility has been demonstrated in selected breeds
• Multiple genes may be involved but differ between affected families
• Genes and environment interactions contribute to the expression of the disease

INCIDENCE/PREVALENCE, GEOGRAPHIC DISTRIBUTION
10–20% of horses in countries with temperate and cold climates, where horses are stabled for prolonged periods

SIGNALMENT
• No clear sex or breed predilections
• Incidence increases with age; uncommon in horses <7 years

SIGNS
• During clinical exacerbation, respiratory distress at rest and biphasic expiratory efforts define the syndrome. Increased respiratory rate and flared nostrils are also present. Emaciation and hypertrophy of the external abdominal oblique muscles ("heaves line") may develop
• Signs may be limited to exercise intolerance and occasional cough when horses are in remission. Coughing generally increases as the disease progresses, becoming paroxysmal
• Clinical signs often wax and wane. Clinical signs can worsen in hot and humid summer days

CAUSES
Inhalation of dust particles from moldy hay and straw induces clinical exacerbation in susceptible horses.

RISK FACTORS
• Moldy hay and straw
• Prolonged stabling

DIAGNOSIS

DIFFERENTIAL DIAGNOSIS
• Pharyngitis and mild dysphagia can cause chronic cough—lung auscultation and endoscopy should identify the upper airways as the site of the problem
• Inflammatory airway disease—no history of episodes of labored breathing
• Viral and bacterial airway infections—can be differentiated from heaves on the basis of febrile episodes, other signs of infection, and duration of clinical signs
• Summer pasture-associated equine asthma—occurs when horses are pastured rather than stabled and fed hay
• Lungworm infection—larvae in feces or tracheal secretions

CBC/BIOCHEMISTRY/URINALYSIS
Usually within normal ranges. Blood neutrophils and total proteins can increase during disease exacerbation.

OTHER LABORATORY TESTS
• Generally >25% neutrophils in BALF cytology. Can be normal when horses are asymptomatic. Presence of bacterial and fungal elements in BALF cytology are common but indicate impaired mucociliary clearance rather than an ongoing intrapulmonary septic process
• Cytology of tracheal aspirates also reveals neutrophilia, but this is less specific than BALF. Bacterial culture of tracheal secretions may yield bacterial growth, but without other signs of infection. This may represent colonization of the lower airways because of impaired mucociliary clearance
• Arterial blood gases—PaO_2 values are <80 mmHg and can be as low as 40 mmHg during exacerbation; $PaCO_2$ values may be elevated
• Histologic scores performed on endobronchial biopsies correlate with the degree of airway obstruction
• Transcutaneous lung biopsies for diagnosis of heaves is not recommended

IMAGING
• During exacerbation, endoscopy reveals copious mucopurulent exudate
• Thoracic radiography can reveal an increased bronchointerstitial pattern. Bronchiectasis may also be present
• Thoracic ultrasonography is usually unremarkable
• Endobronchial ultrasonography reveals thickening of the bronchial wall

OTHER DIAGNOSTIC PROCEDURES
• The diagnosis is established on the basis of signalment, history, and clinical findings combined with the exclusion of other common diseases affecting the respiratory tract, and response to therapy
• Thoracic auscultation—wheezes and expiratory crackles are common findings. Bronchovesicular lung sounds can be decreased during severe episodes. Auscultation can be normal during remission
• Thoracic percussion may reveal hyperresonance of the ventral and caudal borders of the lung fields because of air trapping
• Lung function measurements reveal increased resistance and elastance—to date, few techniques are adapted to clinical settings

PATHOLOGIC FINDINGS
• Chronic active bronchiolitis, with intraluminal accumulation of mucus and neutrophils, and epithelial hyperplasia with goblet cell metaplasia. Histomorphometry reveals deposition of extracellular matrix and increased airway smooth muscle mass in the airway wall
• Interstitial emphysema, mostly in the cranial regions, and patchy areas of alveolar hyperinflation may be seen

TREATMENT

AIMS
Control airway inflammation and decrease airway obstruction.

APPROPRIATE HEALTH CARE
In- or outpatient medical management.

NURSING CARE
• Incurable, but the clinical signs and airway inflammation are reversible with proper control of environmental dust, which is best achieved by keeping horses outdoors, preferably on pasture or replacing hay with cubed or pelleted food, or haylage, and use of shredded paper or good quality wood shavings instead of straw. Pasteurized (steam) hay improves the clinical signs in some horses, but inflammation may be incompletely controlled
• Airway remodeling is only partially reversible
• Respiratory signs recur within days to weeks of re-exposure to dusty hay and bedding
• Without drug therapy, a few weeks to months of environmental dust control may be required before affected horses become free of respiratory signs
• In horses with profound hypoxemia (PaO_2 <60 mmHg), inhaled oxygen supplementation via a nasopharyngeal tube improve breathing, but is rarely required

ACTIVITY
Adjust exercise level according to the degree of respiratory dysfunction.

H

HEAVES (SEVERE EQUINE ASTHMA, RAO)   (CONTINUED)

H

DIET
- Cubed or pelleted food, haylage/silage, or pasteurized hay is preferred if pasture not available
- Soaked hay may be an adequate alternative for some horses, but is usually less effective

CLIENT EDUCATION
- A dust-free environment is paramount for the long-term management
- Never feed moldy hay to horses

MEDICATIONS
DRUG(S) OF CHOICE
Corticosteroids
- Allow effective control of the clinical signs and airway obstruction, but the airway neutrophilia persists if horses are stabled and fed hay. The effects are also short lived after treatment cessation in absence of proper dust control
- When systemically administered, expect a delay of 3–7 days between initiation of therapy and maximal clinical response
- For severe attacks, dexamethasone (initial dose of 0.05 mg/kg PO, IV, IM, until control of clinical signs and then decrease and administer on alternate days for 10–20 days) is most effective
- A single dose of triamcinolone acetonide (20–40 mg IM/500 kg) also improves clinical signs and airway obstruction for 3–5 weeks, but is less desirable because of increased risk of side effects
- Oral prednisolone (1–4 mg/kg) may also be used, but its efficacy is less than with dexamethasone, without demonstrated better toxicity profile. Prednisone is poorly absorbed orally in horses and should not be used
- Inhaled corticosteroids allow maximal concentration of drugs at the effector sites and minimize side effects. Nebulization chambers or masks have been designed for use of MDIs in horses
- Inhaled beclomethasone diproprionate (beclometasone diproprionate) (2000–3500 µg/500 kg every 12–24 h) and fluticasone propionate (2000–3000 µg/500 kg every 12–24 h) are efficacious and well tolerated but have few residual effects. A delay in response of 7 days or longer should be expected

Bronchodilators
- Bronchodilators are symptomatic treatments used to relieve lower airway obstruction

caused by the airway smooth muscle contraction. They may also improve delivery of inhaled corticosteroids to the distal airways
- Long-term administration should be combined with environmental dust control or corticosteroids, because inflammation could progress despite the improvement of clinical signs
- Clenbuterol (0.8–3.2 µg/kg every 12 h) has bronchodilator effects and increases mucociliary transport. Clinical efficacy is inconsistent if exposure to dust is maintained. Decreased efficacy is expected after 2 weeks of treatments due to tachyphylaxis
- Ipratropium bromide (0.4–1 µg/kg every 6 h), albuterol (salbutamol) (1–2 µg/kg), salmeterol (0.5 µg/kg every 8 h), and pirbuterol (1.3 µg/kg every 6 h) are bronchodilators that can be used by inhalation with MDIs
- Atropine and Buscopan (hyoscine butylbromide) administered systemically have been used to assess the reversibility of clinical signs. However, they have limited therapeutic use because their effects are transient. Atropine may also be associated with severe side effects
- Aminophylline has limited efficacy in heaves

Expectorant, Mucolytic, and Mucokinetic Agents
Evidence of efficacy for these agents in improving clinical signs is sparse.

CONTRAINDICATIONS
Corticosteroid administration in the face of sepsis or laminitis, or in horses prone to laminitis.

ALTERNATIVE DRUGS
- Inhaled sodium cromoglycate (cromoglicic acid) (200 mg every 12–24 h) in some horses in clinical remission prevents the appearance of clinical signs
- Nedocromil sodium (24–60 mg every 12 h), another cromone, may be used by inhalation

FOLLOW-UP
PATIENT MONITORING
Sequential PaO_2 determination to monitor response to therapy in horses with severely compromised respiratory function.

PREVENTION/AVOIDANCE
Hay substitutes and dust-free environment.

POSSIBLE COMPLICATIONS
- Heaves is a wasting disease that may rarely lead to death in severe cases if not treated

- Bronchiectasis and right heart failure rare complications in severe cases
- Risk of botulism with haylage and silage in unvaccinated horses

EXPECTED COURSE AND PROGNOSIS
The clinical signs at rest are reversible with prolonged environmental control and therapy. Some degrees of exercise intolerance may persist.

MISCELLANEOUS
AGE-RELATED FACTORS
- Rarely seen in horses <7 years
- Severity may increase with age

PREGNANCY/FERTILITY/BREEDING
- Anecdotal reports suggest clinical signs may improve in some mares during pregnancy
- Fetal growth retardation may occur in mares with severely compromised respiratory function

SYNONYMS
- Severe equine asthma
- RAO
- Improper terminologies—equine chronic obstructive pulmonary disease, chronic bronchitis, chronic bronchiolitis, broken wind, pulmonary emphysema

SEE ALSO
- Equine asthma
- Expiratory dyspnea
- Inflammatory airway diseases—IAD in performance horses (mild and moderate equine asthma)
- Summer pasture-associated equine asthma (pasture asthma)

ABBREVIATIONS
- BALF = bronchoalveolar lavage fluid
- MDI = metered dose inhaler
- $PaCO_2$ = partial pressure of carbon dioxide in arteral blood
- PaO_2 = partial pressure of oxygen in arteral blood
- RAO = recurrent airway obstruction

Suggested Reading
Leclère M, Lavoie-Lamoureux A, Lavoie JP. Heaves, an asthma-like disease of horses. Respirology 2011;16:1027–1046.
Ramseyer A, Gaillard C, Burger D, et al. Effects of genetic and environmental factors on chronic lower airway disease in horses. J Vet Intern Med 2007;21:149–156.

Author Jean-Pierre Lavoie
Consulting Editors Mathilde Leclère and Daniel Jean

BASICS

DEFINITION
• A malignant neoplasm originating from vascular endothelial cells. • May occur as a single mass, with or without local invasion, or disseminated through multiple organs

PATHOPHYSIOLOGY
Malignant transformation of endothelial cells.

SYSTEMS AFFECTED
All

GENETICS
No breed predilection identified.

INCIDENCE/PREVALENCE
Rare

GEOGRAPHIC DISTRIBUTION
Worldwide

SIGNALMENT
• Disseminated—more common in middle-aged horses (age range 3–26 years; mean 12 years). • Juvenile hemangiosarcoma seen in horses ≤3 years of age. • Congenital hemangiosarcoma has been reported

SIGNS
• Vary depending on location and often attributable to hemorrhage or mass effect/swelling. • Predominantly referable to respiratory and musculoskeletal systems including dyspnea, tachypnea (hemothorax), epistaxis, cough, subcutaneous edema/swelling, lameness, tachycardia, and pale/icteric mucous membranes. • Cutaneous form includes generally solitary dermal or subcutaneous lesions that are poorly circumscribed with necrosis, ulceration, or bleeding

CAUSES
Unknown

RISK FACTORS
Unknown

DIAGNOSIS

DIFFERENTIAL DIAGNOSIS
• Hemangiomas—benign endothelial cell tumors, generally in horses <1 year old. • With dyspnea—consider infectious or obstructive respiratory. • With epistaxis—consider trauma, infection including guttural pouch mycosis, neoplasia, coagulopathy, and exercise-induced pulmonary hemorrhage. • With lameness and/or muscular swelling—consider multiple causes including trauma (hematoma) and degenerative conditions, abscessation, or other forms of neoplasia

CBC/BIOCHEMISTRY/URINALYSIS
• Most common finding is anemia. • Neutrophilic leukocytosis and thrombocytopenia are common. • Variable total protein—hypoproteinemia accompanied by hypoalbuminemia is common. • Elevated globulin fractions (>4.0 g/dL) with normal to slightly elevated fibrinogen. • Biochemical abnormalities are nonspecific and may include mild to moderate azotemia and hyperbilirubinemia, increases in muscle enzyme activities, and mild electrolyte abnormalities

OTHER LABORATORY TESTS
Immunohistochemistry using factor VIII-related antigen (von Willebrand factor) has been successfully used to identify endothelial cell origin cutaneous tumors.

IMAGING
May be useful (endoscopy, radiography, ultrasonography, and pleuroscopy) but typically lack specificity.

OTHER DIAGNOSTIC PROCEDURES
• Antemortem diagnosis is difficult without direct visualization and biopsy. • Cytologic evaluation of various biologic fluids is often consistent with hemorrhage or inflammation and not specifically diagnostic. • Localization of signs to a specific system may allow for endoscopically guided biopsy. • Biopsy or fine needle aspiration may be diagnostic. Both histopathology (endothelial cells with numerous mitotic figures) and immunohistochemistry are helpful in differentiating hemangiosarcoma from hemorrhage and inflammation. • Diagnosis often established during postmortem examination

PATHOLOGIC FINDINGS
• Common primary sites for disseminated hemangiosarcoma include lung, pleura, skeletal muscle, heart, and spleen.
• Postmortem findings commonly include severe hemothorax and hemoabdomen, and hemorrhage within affected muscle groups. Tumors are friable, dark red to black masses within the affected organ or tissue.
• Histologically, tumors consist of multiple, poorly organized vascular channels lined by plump, spindle-shaped cells. Neoplastic endothelial cells have large, ovoid, vesicular hyperchromic nuclei and prominent nucleoli with multiple, bizarre mitotic figures

TREATMENT

APPROPRIATE HEALTH CARE
N/A

NURSING CARE
General supportive care.

ACTIVITY
N/A

DIET
Horses with disseminated disease likely have poor appetite, so encouraging the horse to eat is important.

CLIENT EDUCATION
Warn owners of rapid deterioration in the disseminated form, and possibility of metastases if the localized mass is excised.

SURGICAL CONSIDERATIONS
Surgical excision may be beneficial for cutaneous or well-localized lesions.

MEDICATIONS

DRUG(S) OF CHOICE
No established protocols.

FOLLOW-UP

PATIENT MONITORING
Horses should be carefully monitored for recurrence/metastases following surgical excision.

PREVENTION/AVOIDANCE
N/A

POSSIBLE COMPLICATIONS
Severe hemorrhage following biopsy.

EXPECTED COURSE AND PROGNOSIS
Clinical deterioration typically rapid with the disseminated form and the long-term prognosis is poor. Surgical excision has resulted in resolution in a small number of reported cases.

MISCELLANEOUS

ASSOCIATED CONDITIONS
N/A

AGE-RELATED FACTORS
N/A

ZOONOTIC POTENTIAL
N/A

PREGNANCY/FERTILITY/BREEDING
N/A

SYNONYMS
• Angiosarcoma. • Malignant hemangioendothelioma

SEE ALSO
N/A

Suggested Reading
Johns I, Stephen JO, Del Piero F, et al. Hemangiosarcoma in 11 young horses. J Vet Intern Med 2005;19:564–570.
Taintor J. Haemangiosarcoma in the horse. Equine Vet Educ 2014;26:499–503.

Author Imogen Johns
Consulting Editors David Hodgson, Harold C. McKenzie, and Jennifer L. Hodgson
Acknowledgment The author and editors acknowledge the prior contribution of Mark V. Crisman.

H

HEMORRHAGE, ACUTE

 BASICS

DEFINITION
Rapid loss of blood, usually over <24 h.

PATHOPHYSIOLOGY
• Acute loss of >30% of circulating blood volume (≈12 L/500 kg) results in hypovolemic shock; immediate triggering of compensatory mechanisms
• Rapid loss of >40–50% of circulating blood volume is a severe, irreversible physiologic insult; death is common
• Compensatory mechanisms include vasoconstriction, increased cardiac contractility and rate, expansion of blood volume via increased water and sodium resorption, and fluid movements from the intracellular/interstitial spaces to the vascular pool
• RBCs are released into the circulation via splenic contraction
• PCV may not reflect total blood loss for up to 24 h. TP decreases in ≈6 h. With internal hemorrhage ≈$\frac{2}{3}$ of RBCs are autotransfused to the circulation within 24–72 h
• A regenerative bone marrow response is demonstrable from 3 to 42 days. Complete restoration of RBC mass requires 1–3 months
• Replacement of plasma proteins is more rapid, with albumin taking ≈5–10 days and globulins ≈3–4 weeks

SYSTEMS AFFECTED
• Cardiovascular and respiratory
• Hemic/lymphatic/immune
• Hepatobiliary, renal, GI, musculoskeletal, and central nervous

GENETICS
N/A

INCIDENCE/PREVALENCE
N/A

GEOGRAPHIC DISTRIBUTION
N/A

SIGNALMENT
All ages/breeds.

SIGNS
General Comments
Signs vary with the duration and severity of blood loss, site of hemorrhage, and underlying disease.

Historical Findings
• Evidence of trauma
• Recent dystocia in neonatal foals with hemothorax
• Recent foaling; uterine artery rupture
• Sudden collapse or distress in stallions; aortic root rupture
• Recent intense exercise in racehorses (EIPH)

Physical Examination Findings
• Signs of shock (loss of >30% of circulating blood volume) include tachycardia, tachypnea, mucous membrane pallor, systolic

heart murmur, slowed jugular filling, reduced pulse pressure, and oliguria. Agitation, generalized weakness, and sweating may occur
• Ataxia and collapse with >40% blood volume loss
• Epistaxis, respiratory distress, decreased or absent ventral lung sounds, and pleurodynia if lung/thorax are involved
• Signs of low-grade colic and decreased GI tract motility may occur with diminution of organ perfusion or intra-abdominal hemorrhage
• Sudden death may be the only sign with aortic root rupture

CAUSES
Internal Abdominal Hemorrhage and Hemoperitoneum
• Splenic and hepatic rupture following trauma
• Rupture of caudal vena cava (after incarceration of the small intestine in the epiploic foramen)
• Rupture of the middle uterine artery following dystocia or uterine eversion/prolapse
• Hemorrhage from ovarian arteries.
• Iliac arterial rupture secondary to a displaced pelvic fracture. Neoplasia, e.g. hemangiosarcoma
• Recent surgery or biopsy

Internal Thoracic Hemorrhage
• Thoracic trauma, e.g. rib fractures, lacerated heart or vessels during lung biopsy
• Aortic root/other large vessel rupture
• Diaphragmatic hernia with vascular tearing
• Pulmonary hemorrhage
• Neoplasia
• Coagulopathy

External Hemorrhage
• Epistaxis due to guttural pouch mycosis with erosion of the carotid artery, EIPH, severe trauma
• Trauma, e.g. wounds
• Surgical complications, e.g. post castration
• Umbilical hemorrhage
• Coagulopathy

RISK FACTORS
• High-intensity exercise; risk of EIPH
• Previous periparturient hemorrhage in mares; a risk in future pregnancies
• Older breeding stallions and Friesians at higher risk for acute aortic root rupture
• Neonatal foals at risk of rib fractures and umbilical hemorrhage

 DIAGNOSIS

DIFFERENTIAL DIAGNOSIS
• Low-grade colic differentiated by rectal examination, abdominal US, and abdominocentesis
• Acute severe hemolytic anemia differentiated on basis of history, biochemistry, serology

(Coggins), examination of blood smears, or Coombs test
• Sudden death differentiated by history, physical, and postmortem examinations

CBC/BIOCHEMISTRY/URINALYSIS
• Decreases in TP usually precede decreases in PCV due to splenic contraction
• Few changes in mean cell volume, mean cell hemoglobin, and mean cell hemoglobin concentration. Transient leukocytosis with neutrophilia
• Increased serum creatinine and urea nitrogen concentrations reflect prerenal or renal azotemia. Increased aspartate aminotransferase and creatine kinase activities if significant musculoskeletal trauma has occurred
• Oliguria and increased urine specific gravity (>1.040) with hypovolemic shock

OTHER LABORATORY TESTS
• Coagulation tests (e.g. platelet count, prothrombin time, activated partial thromboplastin time) should be performed if a coagulopathy is suspected
• Blood lactate ≥4 mmol/L and oxygen extraction ratio ≤40%, with clinical signs of acute or ongoing blood loss, support a decision to transfuse

IMAGING
Radiography
Thoracic radiography if hemothorax, rib fractures, or pneumothorax are suspected.

US
US to demonstrate hemoabdomen/hemothorax or identify thoracic or abdominal masses and suspected aortic root rupture.

OTHER DIAGNOSTIC PROCEDURES
• Abdominocentesis and thoracocentesis. Erythrophagocytosis rules out inadvertent splenic or subcutaneous vessel puncture during sampling
• Rectal palpation if intra-abdominal hemorrhage suspected
• Airway endoscopy to localize the source of epistaxis
• Laparoscopy to differentiate causes of intra-abdominal hemorrhage
• Systolic blood pressure <80 mmHg or mean pressure <60 mmHg indicates hypotension

PATHOLOGIC FINDINGS
Depends on underlying cause. Wounds, hemothorax, hemoperitoneum, ruptured vessels, broad ligament rupture, broken ribs, epistaxis, melena, cardiac tamponade.

 TREATMENT

APPROPRIATE HEALTH CARE
• Aims—preserve life; stop hemorrhage; restore vascular fluid and blood volumes; treat associated injuries/problems

(CONTINUED)

• Severe acute hemorrhage often constitutes an emergency
• Controlling hemorrhage and replacing blood volume are priorities
• External hemorrhage may be controlled by pressure bandages or ligating ruptured vessels
• Control of internal hemorrhage is more difficult; use a "wait and see" approach

Fluid Therapy
• Balanced isotonic IV fluid therapy (initially 20 mL/kg; 10 L/500 kg) indicated if tachycardia, poor pulse quality, and cool extremities and low blood pressure present. Total volume administered should be ≥2–3 times the estimated loss
• If high-volume isotonic fluid replacement is not practical, give small volumes of hypertonic saline (7% NaCl at 2–4 mL/kg IV) over 15 min *if hemorrhage has been controlled*. Isotonic fluids in sufficient volume to replace estimated deficits should follow within a few hours
• Hydroxyethyl starch (6%) (8–10 mL/kg IV) may be used *when hemorrhage has been controlled*

Blood Transfusion
• Indications for blood transfusion include poor response to fluids, persistent severe tachycardia, profound hypotension, ongoing hemorrhage, PCV decreasing to <20% within 12 h or if it falls to <12% over 24–48 h
• Donors should be selected based on compatibility testing. If an immediate transfusion is needed blood may be collected from a gelding of similar breed with no history of blood/plasma therapy. Initial transfusions rarely cause adverse reactions, but subsequent transfusions (after ≈3 days) may cause severe reactions. An adult horse can donate 8–10 L of blood (or 20–25% of total blood volume) every 4–5 weeks without adverse clinical or physiologic consequences. Blood should be collected into bags containing citrate anticoagulant, with acid–citrate–dextrose (ACD), citrate–phosphate–dextrose (CPD), or CPD with supplemental adenine
• Transfusion volume should be based on degree of hypovolemia and estimates of blood loss. For adult horses weighing ≈500 kg, 6–8 L (or 15 mL/kg) usually is required. The initial transfusion volume should be ≈50% of the estimated blood loss. Transfusion should be slow for the first 15 min (0.1 mL/kg/min); if no adverse reactions occur increase to 20 mL/kg/h

NURSING CARE, ACTIVITY
• Box stall rest with severe blood loss
• Horses with severe, acute hemorrhage require inpatient care

• With hemothorax and respiratory distress blood can be removed by thoracocentesis; rapid refilling may occur
• Administration of oxygen is indicated in hypoxemic patients; this is not a replacement for blood transfusion

DIET
Good quality.

CLIENT EDUCATION
Monitoring and adhere to treatment plan.

SURGICAL CONSIDERATIONS
Horses with acute severe hemorrhage are poor anesthetic risks and should be stabilized prior to surgery.

MEDICATIONS
DRUG(S) OF CHOICE
Aminocaproic acid (10–40 mg/kg IV diluted in 0.9% saline and administered over 30–60 min, every 6 h) and tranexamic acid (5 g IV every 12 h). Smaller doses may be effective. *Yunnan baiyao* (Chinese herbal mixture) has been used. Flunixin meglumine (0.5–1.0 mg/kg every 8–12 h) for anti-inflammatory/analgesic activity.

CONTRAINDICATIONS
• Oxytocin is contraindicated with hematoma of the broad ligament
• Parenteral iron dextran preparations can cause death

PRECAUTIONS
• Synthetic colloidal products (dextrans, hetastarch) may reduce platelet aggregation and coagulation protein efficacy
• Acepromazine should be used with extreme caution in hypotensive animals.
• Hypertonic saline in horses with uncontrolled hemorrhage may increase blood loss

ALTERNATIVE DRUGS
Stroma-free bovine hemoglobin (30 mL/kg) has been used as an alternative to whole-blood transfusion.

FOLLOW-UP
PATIENT MONITORING
• Heart rate, pulse quality, and blood pressure should be monitored frequently during the initial 12–24 h
• Ongoing hemorrhage and bone marrow response can be assessed by determining PCV for 1–3 days after hemorrhage
• A regenerative response is indicated by increases in PCV; PCV remaining low suggests continuing bleeding

PREVENTION/AVOIDANCE
Problematic due to myriad causes of hemorrhage.

POSSIBLE COMPLICATIONS
Blood transfusion should be stopped if an immediate transfusion reaction occurs and appropriate therapy administered.

EXPECTED COURSE AND PROGNOSIS
• Prognosis for acute hemorrhage depends on severity, rate, and cause of blood loss
• Anemia can resolve within 4–12 weeks when hemorrhage is controlled
• Rupture of major vessels (e.g. aorta, middle uterine artery) has a higher fatality rate

MISCELLANEOUS
ASSOCIATED CONDITIONS
N/A

AGE-RELATED FACTORS
Severe hypovolemic shock may compromise the fetus, particularly during the last trimester. Follow-up monitoring should include evaluation of fetal viability.

ZOONOTIC POTENTIAL
N/A

PREGNANCY/FERTILITY/BREEDING
Mares with previous rupture of the broad ligament are at risk of hemorrhage during subsequent pregnancies.

SYNONYMS
Severe bleeding; major blood loss.

SEE ALSO
• Anemia
• Blood and plasma transfusion reactions
• Hemorrhage, chronic

ABBREVIATIONS
• EIPH = exercise-induced pulmonary hemorrhage
• GI = gastrointestinal
• PCV = packed cell volume
• RBC = red blood cell
• TP = total protein
• US = ultrasonography, ultrasound

Suggested Reading
Mudge MC. Acute hemorrhage and blood transfusions in horses. Vet Clin North Am Equine Pract 2014;30:427–436.

Author Margaret C. Mudge
Consulting Editors David Hodgson, Harold C. McKenzie, and Jennifer L. Hodgson
Acknowledgment The author and editors acknowledge the prior contribution of Nicholas Malikides.

HEMORRHAGE, CHRONIC

BASICS

OVERVIEW
- Chronic hemorrhage is rare in horses
- May arise from the GI, urinary, or respiratory tract
- Physiologic adaptations often obscure clinical signs until the PCV is <0.12 L/L
- Regenerative responses usually compensate for losses until the rate of erythropoiesis is exceeded by the rate of blood loss, or if chronic blood loss occurs externally, when iron deficiency causes maturation arrest of marrow erythroid precursors
- Chronic internal hemorrhage allows reutilization of some red blood cells, iron, and plasma protein
- Chronic external hemorrhage often causes deficiencies of these blood constituents

SIGNALMENT
No breed, sex, or age predilection.

SIGNS
- Overt signs (e.g. tachycardia, tachypnea, or weakness) may not occur until PCV <0.12 L/L
- Pale mucous membranes, exercise intolerance, and marked increases in heart and respiratory rates may occur with stress
- Other signs of an underlying disease process may be present

CAUSES AND RISK FACTORS
Depends on the primary disease process:
- GI tract—severe parasitism, GI tract ulceration, neoplasia
- Renal/urologic—hemorrhagic cystitis, urolithiasis, trauma, neoplasia, pyelonephritis
- Respiratory—exercise-induced pulmonary hemorrhage, ethmoid hematoma, guttural pouch mycosis, fungal rhinitis, neoplasia
- Miscellaneous—immune-mediated thrombocytopenia, coagulopathies

DIAGNOSIS

DIFFERENTIAL DIAGNOSIS
- Anemia of chronic disease
- Low-grade chronic hemolytic anemia

CBC/BIOCHEMISTRY/URINALYSIS
- Macrocytosis or increased mean cell volume may occur with regenerative anemia. Microcytic, hypochromic anemia with low serum iron, low marrow iron stores, and increased total iron-binding capacity may occur with chronic blood loss
- Hypoproteinemia may reflect external blood loss although plasma total protein

concentration may be normal due to compensation
- Increased total and indirect bilirubinemia indicates internal blood loss
- Chronic tissue hypoxia may cause increased serum hepatic enzyme activities and serum creatinine concentrations
- Microscopic or gross hematuria may indicate a primary renal/urologic problem

OTHER LABORATORY TESTS
See CBC/Biochemistry/Urinalysis.

IMAGING
- Ultrasonography may identify NSAID-induced right dorsal colitis; intra-abdominal or intrathoracic masses
- Upper respiratory tract radiography for sinus or ethmoidal masses

OTHER DIAGNOSTIC PROCEDURES
- Bone marrow aspirate. If the myeloid to erythroid ratio is <0.5, the anemia is regenerative
- Positive fecal occult blood indicates GI hemorrhage or blood swallowed
- Positive fecal examination for parasitic ova supports a diagnosis of parasitism when accompanied by weight loss, diarrhea, or poor deworming history
- Gastroscopy may reveal gastroduodenal ulceration or gastric squamous cell carcinoma
- Cystoscopy may identify urethral, bladder, or ureteral hemorrhage
- Upper airway endoscopy may demonstrate rhinitis, neoplasia, guttural pouch mycosis, ethmoid hematoma, or blood in the trachea
- Erythrocytophagia and hemosiderophages may be identified in abdominal fluid, tracheal aspirate, or bronchoalveolar lavage fluid
- Ultrasonography-guided biopsies of masses may help characterize the primary disease process

TREATMENT
- Should be based on identification and elimination of the source of the underlying disease, which may necessitate inpatient care
- Blood transfusion usually is unnecessary unless PCV is <0.10 L/L or there are signs of tissue hypoxia

MEDICATIONS

DRUG(S) OF CHOICE
If there is evidence of true iron deficiency, ferrous sulfate can be administered (2 mg/kg PO daily).

CONTRAINDICATIONS/POSSIBLE INTERACTIONS
Avoid parenteral iron dextran solutions; they can cause fatal reactions.

FOLLOW-UP

PATIENT MONITORING
- Response to treatment of the underlying disease should be assessed
- Monitor response by weekly evaluation of PCV. Increase of PCV to the reference range should occur over 6–12 weeks
- Serial bone marrow aspiration is rarely necessary
- Client education should include recommendations regarding the underlying disease (e.g. parasite control)
- Prognosis depends on identifying the underlying disease

PREVENTION/AVOIDANCE
- Ensure correct dosing of NSAIDs
- Parasite control program

EXPECTED COURSE AND PROGNOSIS
Dependent on the cause of chronic anemia.

MISCELLANEOUS

ASSOCIATED CONDITIONS
- Anemia
- Hemorrhage, acute

AGE-RELATED FACTORS
N/A

ZOONOTIC POTENTIAL
N/A

PREGNANCY/FERTILITY/BREEDING
Depends on the cause of chronic anemia.

ABBREVIATIONS
- GI = gastrointestinal
- NSAID = nonsteroidal anti-inflammatory drug
- PCV = packed cell volume

Suggested Reading
Meindel MJ, Wilkerson MJ. Anemia. In: Sprayberry KA, Robinson NE, eds. Robinson's Current Therapy in Equine Medicine, 7e. St. Louis, MO: WB Saunders, 2015:471–475.

Author Margaret C. Mudge
Consulting Editors David Hodgson, Harold C. McKenzie, and Jennifer L. Hodgson
Acknowledgment The author and editors acknowledge the prior contribution of Nicholas Malikides.

BASICS

OVERVIEW
• Caused by lesions within the respiratory tract but can be secondary to hemostatic dysfunctions (rare)
• Unilateral discharge—often lesions rostral to the nasopharynx
• Bilateral discharge—often lesions caudal to the nasopharynx or from hemostatic dysfunctions
• Systems affected—respiratory and hemic

SIGNS
• Blood trickle at the nostril(s) to severe hemorrhage
• Unilateral trickle; upper respiratory origin; nasal passage, turbinates, or paranasal sinuses. Sometimes ipsilateral guttural pouch hemorrhage
• Bilateral trickle or severe hemorrhage; origin caudal to the nasopharynx (guttural pouch, lower respiratory tract) or hemostatic disorders
• Mucopurulent or foul-smelling discharges suggest an infectious or necrotic origin
• Bilateral frothy discharge is consistent with pulmonary edema
• Thrombocytopenia and DIC often are associated with mucosal petechiation, prolonged bleeding from venipuncture sites, and occult blood from the GI or urinary tracts

CAUSES AND RISK FACTORS
• Hemostatic dysfunction—thrombocytopenia, DIC, coagulation factor deficiency, or envenomation
• Respiratory tract disease—upper respiratory disease may result from primary bacterial or fungal infections (guttural pouch mycosis, sinusitis), neoplasia or idiopathic diseases (nasal polyp, nasal amyloidosis, ethmoid hematoma). Lower respiratory diseases include EIPH, pleuropneumonia, pulmonary edema, lung neoplasia
• Trauma—nasal intubation, fractures, longus capitis muscle rupture secondary to falling backward, and lung biopsy
• Other—vasculitis (purpura haemorrhagica), fibrous dysplasia, periocular bleeding

DIAGNOSIS

CBC/BIOCHEMISTRY/URINALYSIS
• Usually within normal range, however anemia may result from blood loss

• Neutrophilia or neutropenia may accompany inflammatory diseases
• Leukemia may be evident with myeloid neoplasia

OTHER LABORATORY TESTS
Assessment of hemostasis requires platelet count, plasma fibrinogen, prothrombin and activated partial thromboplastin time, and D-dimer concentration.

IMAGING
• Skull radiography may reveal bone fracture, mass, or fluid accumulation in the sinuses or guttural pouches
• Thoracic radiography may help to identify pleuropneumonia, EIPH, pulmonary edema, and lung tumors
• Thoracic ultrasonography is sensitive to detect pleural blood or effusion

OTHER DIAGNOSTIC PROCEDURES
• Endoscopy of the respiratory tract is helpful to identify the site of bleeding; nasal passages, pharynx, guttural pouches (needs a stylet), and lower airways examination
• Trephination to access paranasal sinuses using a flexible or rigid endoscope
• Fluid cytology from bronchoalveolar lavage (for EIPH) or thoracocentesis may reveal the source of bleeding
• Biopsy to identify the nature of a mass

PATHOLOGIC FINDINGS
• Depend on the primary disease process
• Nasal and paranasal neoplasms are malignant in 68% of cases

TREATMENT
• Emergency if severe bleeding or guttural pouch hemorrhage is suspected
• Treat the primary disease
• Stall rest is recommended and sedation if horse is agitated
• Treat severe blood loss with IV administration of sodium-containing crystalloid solutions. However, if the hemorrhage is not controlled, volume expansion may worsen blood loss. Perform blood transfusion when the red blood cell mass is insufficient to maintain tissue oxygenation (e.g. >30% blood volume lost acutely)
• Patients with hemostatic disorders may benefit from fresh plasma transfusion
• Consider surgical or laser resection of a nasal or paranasal mass
• Guttural pouch mycosis may be treated surgically by occlusion of the affected artery

MEDICATIONS

DRUG(S) OF CHOICE
• Immunosuppressive therapy with corticoids (dexamethasone 0.05–0.2 mg/kg IM or IV every 24 h) in cases of immune-mediated coagulopathy or vasculitis
• Heparin (20–80 IU/kg SC or IV every 6–12 h) and low-dose aspirin (15 mg/kg PO every 24–48 h) may reduce complications of DIC
• Warfarin and sweet clover toxicosis—treat with vitamin K1 (0.5–1 mg/kg SC every 6 h)
• Antifibrinolytics may help decrease blood loss (aminocaproic acid 10–20 mg/kg IV)
• Pulmonary edema—treat with furosemide (1 mg/kg IV) and respiratory support

FOLLOW-UP

PATIENT MONITORING
Monitor hematocrit and hydration status.

POSSIBLE COMPLICATIONS
Severe, fatal bleeding may occur if a major artery is involved.

EXPECTED COURSE AND PROGNOSIS
Depend on the underlying cause.

MISCELLANEOUS

SEE ALSO
• Exercise-induced pulmonary hemorrhage (EIPH)
• Guttural pouch mycosis
• Pleuropneumonia
• Sinusitis (paranasal)

ABBREVIATIONS
• DIC = disseminated intravascular coagulation
• EIPH = exercise-induced pulmonary hemorrhage
• GI = gastrointestinal

Suggested Reading
Collatos C. Blood loss anemia. In: Robinson NE, ed. Current Therapy in Equine Medicine, 5e. Philadelphia, PA: WB Saunders, 2003:340–342.

Author Renaud Leguillette
Consulting Editors Daniel Jean and Mathilde Leclère
Acknowledgment The author and editors acknowledge the prior contribution of Laurent Couëtil.

HEMOSPERMIA

BASICS

OVERVIEW
- Contamination of an ejaculate with blood
- Blood may originate from an external lesion, i.e. injury to the urethral process or penis, or an internal lesion
- May lower conception rate

SIGNALMENT
- All stallions
- Quarter Horses are overrepresented for tear of the urethral mucosa

SIGNS
- Physical examination at rest is usually unremarkable
- Discoloration of semen ranging from pink-tinged to frank hemorrhage is the most common sign
- In natural breeding situations, blood may be seen dripping from the penis on dismount, at the vulvar lips of the mare following breeding, or mares may not become pregnant following breeding
- Some stallions will concurrently have hematuria

CAUSES AND RISK FACTORS
- Top 2 causes:
  - *Trauma*—laceration of the urethral process, glans penis, or body of the penis (usually from tail hair); stricture of the urethra from chronic placement without monitoring/cleaning of a stallion ring
  - *Urethral defects*
- Urethritis
- Infection/inflammation of the accessory sex glands
- Neoplasia
  - Squamous cell carcinoma
  - Papilloma
- Risk factors—breeding activity (infection, lacerations to external penis)
- Hot, humid environmental conditions (cutaneous habronemiasis)

DIAGNOSIS

DIFFERENTIAL DIAGNOSIS
- Diagnosis is based on ejaculate color collected by AV; presence of RBCs on cytologic examination
- Fractionation of the ejaculate, using an open-ended AV, may help determine the source of blood
- Exact determination of the source of bleeding requires careful examination of the penis and urethra

CBC/BIOCHEMISTRY/URINALYSIS
- CBC and chemistry panel are generally unaffected
- Urinalysis might reveal RBCs

IMAGING
US
Transrectally to assess the vesicular glands:
- Normal glands can vary significantly in appearance. Range from flat in the nonaroused state to enlarged and filled with hypoechoic fluid after sexual stimulation
- Inflamed vesicular glands may be thickened and filled with echogenic fluid
- Note that some stallions produce normal gel that is echogenic on US examination

OTHER DIAGNOSTIC PROCEDURES
- Endoscopy—useful tool to diagnose urethral abnormalities (urethritis, rents) and vesicular gland inflammation
- Bacterial culture and cytology of semen are beneficial for determination of accessory sex gland infection
- Biopsy and histopathology for diagnosis of neoplasia or cutaneous habronemiasis

TREATMENT

All conditions warrant sexual rest.
- *Trauma*—usually outpatient care, palliative therapy aimed at hygiene and parasite control
- *Urethral defects*
  - Conservative approach—sexual rest (limited success)
  - Surgical approach—ischial urethrotomy, laser or reconstructive surgery, and a minimum of 2 months of sexual rest
- *Urethritis*—antibiotic therapy
- *Infection/inflammation of the accessory sex glands*
  - Antibiotic therapy (local, systemic)
  - Lavage of the glands (endoscopically)
  - Intrauterine infusion of semen extender containing appropriate antibiotics
- *Neoplasia*
  - Cryotherapy
  - Hyperthermia
  - Local excision
  - Reefing operation
  - Phallectomy
- *Cutaneous habronemiasis*
  - Parasite control
  - Cryotherapy
  - Surgical removal of affected sites

SURGICAL CONSIDERATIONS
Refer to individual etiologies in Treatment.

MEDICATIONS

DRUG(S) AND FLUIDS
- NSAID (phenylbutazone, flunixin meglumine) indicated in most cases
- Antibiotic therapy is directed at the organism identified to cause bacterial urethritis, culture and sensitivity

- Systemic antibiotic therapy for vesicular gland infection is often ineffective due to poor diffusion of the drug into the affected area
- Antibiotic of choice for systemic treatment is trimethoprim–sulfamethoxazole (15–30 mg/kg PO BID) if the identified organism is susceptible to it
- Lavage of the glands and infusion of an antibiotic directly into the vesicular glands may be a more effective treatment
- Antiparasitic therapy for cutaneous habronemiasis (ivermectin 0.2 mg/kg PO every 30 days until resolution of lesions)

FOLLOW-UP

PATIENT MONITORING
Sexual rest followed by semen collection and evaluation.

PREVENTION/AVOIDANCE
Parasite control, good management of stallions for semen collection, regular examination.

POSSIBLE COMPLICATIONS
- Infertility
- Urethral stricture or adhesions
- Adhesions of the vesicular glands
- Ruptured urinary bladder

EXPECTED COURSE AND PROGNOSIS
Dependent on etiology and severity of lesions.

MISCELLANEOUS

ASSOCIATED CONDITIONS
Hematuria

PREGNANCY/FERTILITY/BREEDING
Blood in the ejaculate can be harmful to spermatozoa and thus conception rates may decrease.

ABBREVIATIONS
- AV = artificial vagina
- NSAID = nonsteroidal anti-inflammatory drug
- RBC = red blood cell
- US = ultrasonography, ultrasound

Suggested Reading
Pearson LK, Campbell AJ, Tibary A. How to diagnosis and treat hemospermia: a review and case series. Proc Am Assoc Equine Pract 2013;59:40–50.

Author Ahmed Tibary
Consulting Editor Carla L. Carleton
Acknowledgment The author and editor acknowledge the prior contribution of Margo L. Macpherson.

HENDRA VIRUS

BASICS

OVERVIEW
• HeV (formerly known as equine morbillivirus) is an acute and frequently fatal viral disease of horses that causes respiratory and/or neurologic signs and is zoonotic
• An outbreak of HeV in 1994 (Hendra, Queensland, Australia) was characterized by rapidly progressive primarily respiratory signs and death/euthanasia in 14 of 21 Thoroughbred horses. Most cases since have displayed primarily neurologic signs. There have now been 72 confirmed equine cases, confined to Queensland and New South Wales, all of which have died/been euthanized
• There have been 7 confirmed human cases of HeV, 4 of these fatal
• Natural asymptomatic seroconversion was confirmed in 1 dog
• Apart from the 1994 Hendra outbreak and an outbreak in 2008, most other incidences have involved single horses, occasionally 2–4 horses. Individual cases have been easily isolated and the virus does not appear to be highly contagious
• HeV is a member of the genus *Henipavirus* in the Paramyxoviridae family
• Flying foxes (fruit bats or Pteropodidae) are the natural reservoir of HeV

SIGNALMENT
Nonspecific

SIGNS
• The incubation period in experimentally infected horses is 5–16 days (possibly up to 31 days)
• The clinical course is very acute, with death occurring within 48–72 h of onset in approximately 75% of cases
• Initial signs are nonspecific—anorexia, depression, fever (up to 41°C), and restlessness, with progression to acute respiratory and/or neurologic signs that are rapidly progressive
• Commonly reported signs in natural cases include tachycardia and tachypnea, nasal discharge, congested/hyperemic mucous membranes, muscle fasciculations, ataxia, circling, blindness, seizures, and recumbency
• Sudden death of 1 or more horses in an affected region should be treated with high suspicion

CAUSES AND RISK FACTORS
• HeV is not endemic in the Queensland horse population—flying foxes (fruit bats or Pteropodidae) are the natural reservoir for HeV, with sporadic "spillover" of HeV to horses causing natural cases of infection

• No outbreaks of HeV have been identified outside Australia
• HeV has been isolated from flying fox urine, uterine fluid, and fetal tissue. The source of infection for the horse is likely food or water contaminated with these materials
• Unvaccinated horses kept outside in areas attractive to flying foxes are at higher risk
• Close contact appears necessary for disease transmission between horses or from horses to humans, via infected body fluids or on fomites

DIAGNOSIS

DIFFERENTIAL DIAGNOSIS
• Other causes of acute death, including toxicoses (paraquat, monensin, heavy metals, mycotoxins, avocado, crofton weed), botulism
• Bacterial pneumonia
• Intestinal lesions (colitis, peritonitis, strangulating lesions)
• Viral encephalitis/meningoencephalitis (including equine herpesvirus 1, flavivirus infection, exotic encephalitides—Eastern, Western, and Venezuelan)
• Purpura haemorrhagica
• Snake bite
• Paralysis tick (*Ixodes holocyclus*)
• African horse sickness, equine influenza (exotic/eradicated from Australia)

CBC/BIOCHEMISTRY/URINALYSIS
Nonspecific

OTHER LABORATORY TESTS
• PCR of blood, swabs (nasal, oral, rectal), urine, and tissue samples
• ELISA and virus neutralization tests

IMAGING
N/A

OTHER DIAGNOSTIC PROCEDURES
N/A

PATHOLOGIC FINDINGS
• Gross postmortem lesions include dilated pulmonary lymphatics, severe pulmonary edema, congestion and consolidation, airways filled with blood-tinged foam and congestion and edema of lymph nodes
• Histologically, vasculitis affects a wide range of tissues, including lung, brain, lymphoid tissues, and kidney, with syncytial cells

TREATMENT

Suspected cases should be quarantined during testing, personnel in contact should wear protective equipment as per relevant local

guidelines. Confirmed cases will be euthanized.

MEDICATIONS

Horses in affected areas should be vaccinated—there is an effective subunit vaccine registered in Australia; an initial course is followed by annual boosters.

CONTRAINDICATIONS/POSSIBLE INTERACTIONS
N/A

FOLLOW-UP

• Notify and work with relevant local authorities
• Control of outbreak by quarantine, containment, early identification of the causal agent, and disinfection of the area

MISCELLANEOUS

ZOONOTIC POTENTIAL
• Infections and deaths have occurred from close contact with HeV-infected body fluids in live and dead horses
• Personnel should wear protective equipment and avoid contact with body fluids—refer to relevant local guidelines

ABBREVIATIONS
• ELISA = enzyme-linked immunosorbent assay
• HeV = Hendra virus
• PCR = polymerase chain reaction

Internet Resources
Queensland Government, Department of Agriculture and Fisheries. Hendra virus. https://www.daf.qld.gov.au/animal-industries/animal-health-and-diseases/a-z-list/hendra-virus

Suggested Reading
Middleton D. Hendra virus. Vet Clin North Am Equine Pract 2014;30:579–589.

Author Andrew W. van Eps
Consulting Editor Ashley G. Boyle

H

HEPATIC ABSCESS AND SEPTIC CHOLANGIOHEPATITIS

 OVERVIEW

Discrete hepatic abscesses are uncommon but ascending septic cholangiohepatitis is common in the horse.

SIGNALMENT
• Cholangiohepatitis is most commonly diagnosed in adult horses without additional age or sex predilection
• Focal abscesses are sporadic and may rarely affect foals, e.g. *Rhodococcus*, umbilical vein infection, or an adult horse, e.g. tumor necrosis

SIGNS
• The signs of cholangiohepatitis may include weight loss, icterus, abdominal pain, fever, and dermatitis
• In severe cases, there may be fulminant hepatic failure evidenced by encephalopathy and photosensitization
• Focal hepatic abscesses may cause ill thrift and sometimes colic

CAUSES
• Cholangiohepatitis—thought to be the result of ascending infection from enteric Gram-negative bacteria. There is generally no historical intestinal disease to explain the ascending infection. The inflammation of the bile epithelium and enzymes released from the bacteria may cause calcium bilirubinate calculi to form
• Discrete abscesses—may occur, although rarely, from intestinal–hepatic adhesions with necrosis, parasite migration, *Corynebacterium pseudotuberculosis*-, *Rhodococcus*-, or *Streptococcus*-disseminated infections in younger horses, neoplastic abscessation, septic portal vein thrombosis, extension of an umbilical vein abscess into the liver, or as a result of local vascular compromise (from hepatic lobe torsion or hepatic vessel thrombosis) leading to a focal region of tissue hypoxia and liver lobe necrosis. Infectious necrotic hepatitis (*Clostridium novyi* or Black disease) will also result in hepatic abscessation or necrosis

 DIAGNOSIS

DIFFERENTIAL DIAGNOSIS
• The differential diagnosis for chronic colic is extensive. However, the differential diagnosis for colic with marked jaundice and moderately to markedly elevated liver enzymes includes cholangiohepatitis, right dorsal displacement of the large colon, and neoplasia
• Fever, leukocytosis, and elevated serum globulin, in addition to the above, would be nearly pathognomonic for cholangiohepatitis

CBC/BIOCHEMISTRY/URINALYSIS
• Serum laboratory abnormalities in horses with cholangiohepatitis include marked elevations in GGT (generally >300 U/L), less marked elevation in hepatocellular enzymes, elevations in conjugated bilirubin (which may, on a few occasions, approach ≥50% of the total bilirubin), increased serum bile acids, and elevated serum globulins
• CBC generally reveals a mature neutrophilia with mild elevation in plasma fibrinogen
• Foals and horses with discrete hepatic abscess(es) may have mild elevations only in GGT without increases in hepatocellular enzymes or bilirubin
• Neutrophil counts in peripheral blood are generally increased and may be dramatic with *Rhodococcus equi* abscess(es)
• Blood fibrinogen and globulins are generally increased with any abscess, although they may not be abnormal with neoplasia-related abscess and *R. equi*

IMAGING
• US examination of the liver (both right and left side) is the imaging procedure of choice. Only a small percentage of the liver can be visualized on abdominal US in the adult; a greater percentage can be visualized in the foal
• Cholangitis may cause distended bile ducts (in ≈60% of cases), calculi with acoustic shadowing, sludge with acoustic enhancement, and a subjective hepatomegaly
• In acute cases, hepatomegaly may be present, whereas in more longstanding cases increased echogenicity (fibrosis) may be apparent
• In horses or foals with focal abscesses, the echogenicity of the abscess is variable
• CT can be used to image the liver in foals if discrete lesions are suspected

OTHER DIAGNOSTIC PROCEDURES
• The most important invasive diagnostic procedure is needle aspirate and/or biopsy for aerobic/anaerobic culture and sensitivity and microscopic examination of the liver
• This can be safely performed using a biopsy needle after outlining the location of the liver via US
• If obstruction of the common bile duct is suspected, duodenal endoscopy may allow visualization of the stone or a large bulge at the opening of the duct

 TREATMENT

• Hospitalization may not be required unless IV fluids are needed
• Antimicrobials are the mainstay of treatment, with surgery as a secondary option to remove obstructing calculi if not responsive to medical therapy
• If a focal hepatic abscess is in a surgically accessible area and medical management is not yielding results, then rib resection can be

performed to facilitate surgical intervention and draining
• Icteric horses should not be exposed to sunlight until bilirubin has returned to a normal range
• Since hepatoencephalopathy rarely occurs, a normal diet can be fed

 MEDICATIONS

DRUGS AND FLUIDS
• The primary treatment for septic cholangiohepatitis is long-term, appropriate treatment with antibiotics (based upon culture and sensitivity). Several drugs have been used successfully in treating the condition. These include appropriate combinations of trimethoprim–sulfa (30 mg/kg every 12 h) (>50% of the organisms may be resistant), enrofloxacin (7.5 mg/kg every 24 h), metronidazole (15 mg/kg every 8-12 h), ceftiofur sodium (3 mg/kg every 12 h), gentamicin (6.6 mg/kg every 24 h), and sodium penicillin IV (20,000 U/kg every 6 h) or procaine penicillin IM (25,000 U/kg every 12 h). Antimicrobials that can be given PO are preferred since long-term treatment (3 weeks to 6 months) is generally required. If culture and sensitivity cannot be performed or is inconclusive then empirical antibiotic therapy may have to be instituted and changed based on clinical response
• Parenterally administered antibiotics, fluids, pentoxifylline, and DMSO may be required for some cases with severe anorexia, biliary sludge, and persistent fevers
• NSAID treatment (e.g. flunixin meglumine) should be used at routine dosages for abdominal pain and during the first 3–5 days of antimicrobial therapy
• Horses with marked hepatic fibrosis have a poor prognosis and are not surgical candidates
• Discrete or focal abscess(es) should be treated with appropriate antibiotics based upon culture and sensitivity of aspirated fluid or knowledge of suspected pathogen
• Large abscess(es) or infected umbilical veins should be drained or removed

 FOLLOW-UP

• Clinical improvement is seen before normalization of GGT; it is recommended to continue antimicrobial therapy until the GGT has returned to normal range or at least <100 U/L
• After discontinuing antimicrobials, a follow-up measurement of GGT should be performed
• In cases of hepatic abscesses, follow-up with US is recommended for monitoring

EXPECTED COURSE AND PROGNOSIS

The prognosis of septic suppurative cholangitis is good with medical therapy if no obstructing calculi are found and echogenicity of the liver is normal. Horses with GGT >2500 U/L have recovered.

MISCELLANEOUS

SEE ALSO

- Acute adult abdominal pain—acute colic
- Cholelithiasis
- Colic, chronic/recurrent

ABBREVIATIONS

- CT = computed tomography
- DMSO = dimethylsulfoxide
- GGT = γ-glutamyltransferase
- NSAID = nonsteroidal anti-inflammatory drug
- US = ultrasonography, ultrasound

Suggested Reading

Cypher EE, Kendall AT, Panizzi L, et al. Medical and surgical management of an intra-abdominal abscess of hepatic origin in a horse. J Am Vet Med Assoc 2015;247(1):98–105.

Divers TJ. The equine liver in health and disease. Proc Am Assoc Equine Pract 2015;61:66–103.

Johnston JK, Divers TJ, Reef VB, Acland H. Cholelithiasis in horses: ten cases (1982-1986). J Am Vet Med Assoc 1989;194:405–409.

Peek SF. Cholangiohepatitis in the mature horse. Equine Vet Educ 2004;16(2):72–75.

Peek SF, Divers TJ. Medical treatment of cholangiohepatitis and cholelithiasis in mature horses: 9 cases (1991-1998). Equine Vet J 2000;32(4):301–306.

Authors Thomas J. Divers and Nikhita P. De Bernardis

Consulting Editors Henry Stämpfli and Olimpo Oliver-Espinosa

H

HEPATIC ENCEPHALOPATHY

BASICS

OVERVIEW
• Hepatic insufficiency causes altered behavior and conscious proprioception. • >80% of liver function must be impaired; can be acute, subacute, or chronic. • Possible mechanisms: ◦ Toxic metabolites act as false neurotransmitters (i.e. ammonia, mercaptans, phenols, fatty acids). ◦ Imbalance between excitatory and inhibitory neurotransmitters. ◦ Increase in aromatic amino acids increases false neurotransmitters, some of which cause sedation with decrease in branched chain amino acids, which decreases neurotransmitters. ◦ Increased expression benzodiazepine receptors, increased neurosteroid synthesis. ◦ Potential increased permeability of blood–brain barrier. ◦ Role for inflammation in disease

SIGNALMENT
No breed or sex predilection.

SIGNS
• Behavior changes (depression, somnolence, aggressive or violent behavior mixed with stupor). • Head pressing. • Circling. • Ataxia. • Wandering/aimless movement. • Anorexia. • Recumbency. • Icterus. • Photosensitization. • Pyrexia. • Weight loss. • Colic—chronic. • Coagulopathy. • Blindness. • Yawning. • Inspiratory stridor (laryngeal paralysis)

CAUSES AND RISK FACTORS
• Toxic hepatopathy, including pyrrolizidine alkaloids, mycotoxins, iron. • Acute necrotizing hepatitis—Theiler disease. • Cholelithiasis. • Chronic active hepatitis. • Tyzzer disease. • Hyperlipemia—ponies; miniature horses more at risk. • Neoplasia. • Hyperammonemia (adult horses, portosystemic shunts, Morgans)

DIAGNOSIS

DIFFERENTIAL DIAGNOSIS
• Viral encephalitis (e.g. Eastern equine encephalopathy, Western equine encephalopathy, West Nile virus, rabies). • Trauma. • Verminous encephalitis. • Electrolyte abnormalities—hyponatremia, hypernatremia, hypocalcemia, hypomagnesemia. • Brain abscess. • Meningitis. • Neonatal Maladjustment Syndrome, history. • Metabolic (foals—hypoglycemia, acidosis)
Progression of these diseases can lead to HE: • Theiler disease—history of antitoxin 4–10 weeks prior. • Cholangiohepatitis—adults, most >9 years old

CBC/BIOCHEMISTRY/URINALYSIS
• Azotemia. • Blood urea nitrogen and glucose—may be decreased in liver failure. • Liver-specific changes—elevated bilirubin, increased γ-glutamyltransferase, sorbitol dehydrogenase, glutamate dehydrogenase, hypoalbuminemia, hypoproteinemia, elevated resting ammonia levels, and elevated bile acids. • Hyperlipemia—may have increased cholesterol and triglycerides. • Secondary hypocalcemia, hypokalemia, and metabolic acidosis. • Delayed bromsulphthalein (bromosulfophthalein) clearance

OTHER LABORATORY TESTS
Coagulation profiles may be prolonged.

IMAGING
• Ultrasonography of the liver. Biopsy results help predict prognosis. • Radiographs—rule out fractures. • CT/MRI—assess for trauma, abscesses, tumors, hydrocephalus

OTHER DIAGNOSTIC PROCEDURES
• Cerebrospinal fluid tap—to rule out other infectious causes. • Feed analysis to assess for toxins

TREATMENT

• Prognosis is poor, but potentially reversible depending on cause. • Decrease inflammation (i.e. flunixin meglumine, DMSO, colchicine, cyclosporine (ciclosporin)). • Sedation may be necessary. Xylazine and detomidine can occasionally exacerbate signs. Valium and/or phenobarbital for seizures but can potentiate GABA effect and exacerbate HE signs. • Correct fluid, electrolyte, and acid–base deficits. • For anorectic or hypoglycemic animals, give 5% dextrose (2 mL/kg/h) to start, then 2.5% in half-strength saline. • High-carbohydrate, low-protein (i.e. 10%) diet with branched chain amino acids; need some fiber (i.e. oat, grass hay, beet pulp) to decrease gastrointestinal dysfunction. • Feed small amounts frequently (every 2–4 h). • Vitamin B1, K, folic acid, and C supplementation. • Protect from sunlight to prevent photosensitization

MEDICATIONS

DRUG(S) OF CHOICE
• Lactulose (0.3 mL/kg every 6 h). • Hyperlipemic horses can be given insulin, glucose/galactose, and heparin. • Mannitol for cerebral edema. • Mineral oil or magnesium sulfate if suspect toxins ingested. • Septic cholangiohepatitis—antibiotics are warranted. • *S*-adenosylmethionine if expect oxidative injury

CONTRAINDICATIONS/POSSIBLE INTERACTIONS
Avoid drugs that require hepatic metabolism.

FOLLOW-UP

• Prognosis depends on the primary cause. • Severe fibrosis associated with poor prognosis. • Animals with hyperlipidemia/hyperlipemia may respond well to aggressive treatment. • Animals with HE from toxins probably experienced the initial insult several weeks/months prior; determine if signs are still progressing. These animals may be stabilized, but if signs continue to progress or recur, a poor prognosis is indicated. • Poor prognosis for recumbent animals

MISCELLANEOUS

PREGNANCY/FERTILITY/BREEDING
Small percentage of pregnant animals will be hyperlipemic.

SEE ALSO
• Acute hepatitis in adult horses (Theiler disease)
• Calcium, hypocalcemia
• Eastern (EEE), western (WEE), and Venezuelan (VEE) equine encephalitides
• Equine herpesvirus myeloencephalopathy
• Head trauma
• Meningitis, neonate
• Neonatal maladjustment syndrome
• Sodium, hypernatremia
• Sodium, hyponatremia
• West nile virus

ABBREVIATIONS
• CT = computed tomography
• DMSO = dimethylsulfoxide
• GABA = γ-aminobutyric acid
• HE = hepatic encephalopathy
• MRI = magnetic resonance imaging

Suggested Reading
Reed SM, Bayly WM, Sellon DC, eds. Equine Internal Medicine, 3e. St. Louis, MO: WB Saunders, 2010.

Author Sharon G. Witonsky
Consulting Editor Caroline N. Hahn

HEREDITARY EQUINE REGIONAL DERMAL ASTHENIA

 BASICS

OVERVIEW
• HERDA results from a genetic mutation that affects the skin and other tissues
• Affected horses appear normal at birth but usually develop loose skin and wounds and disfiguring scars spontaneously or from minor trauma by the time they are two years old (see Web figures 1–3)
• Organ systems affected by this disease include cardiovascular, immune, musculoskeletal, ophthalmic, renal, and skin
• Palliative therapy is the only treatment
• Selective breeding strategies based on DNA testing should be used to minimize the number of affected horses produced

SIGNALMENT
HERDA is a specific form of EDS. EDS can be caused by a number of different mutations in genes important for collagen formation. EDS occurs in a large number of species including cats, dogs, and humans. The name HERDA is used when a specific mutation occurs in the *PPIB* gene, which encodes cyclophilin B and is important in collagen formation. This specific mutation only affects Quarter Horses and related horses (American Paint Horses, Appaloosas, etc.) to date but EDS can occur in any breed of horse. Of importance, not all Quarter Horses with EDS share the HERDA mutation (*PPIB*).

SIGNS
The hallmark of the disease is the presence of loose, hyperextensible skin that is not well attached to the horse in multiple areas ranging from 2–3 cm in diameter to more than 80% of the horse's body. Lesions are most common on the dorsal aspect of the horse's body but can occur anywhere. Fragile skin that sloughs and results in disfiguring scars is common. An unusual amount of joint flexibility may be present.

CAUSES AND RISK FACTORS
HERDA has an autosomal recessive mode of inheritance, for the foal to be affected *both* the sire and the dam *must* carry at least 1 copy of the gene. When 2 carriers (N/HRD) are mated an affected foal (HRD/HRD) will be produced 25% of the time. HERDA has become a significant concern in the Quarter Horse industry owing to the high frequency of heterozygote carriers. Although HERDA occurs most frequently in cutting horse bloodlines (28.3% carrier frequency), horses in other disciplines have also produced a significant number of affected individuals—30% of the top 10 leading lifetime sires are confirmed carriers. The performance traits of these select carrier bloodlines are highly desired, likely increasing the prevalence of HERDA.

 DIAGNOSIS

DIFFERENTIAL DIAGNOSIS
Trauma; hereditary junctional epidermolysis bullosa in the American Saddlebred, Belgian, and other draft horses; and other bullous immune-mediated diseases.

CBC/BIOCHEMISTRY/URINALYSIS
N/A

OTHER LABORATORY TESTS
DNA testing for the HERDA mutation, hair from the mane or tail with roots attached should be submitted (www.vgl.ucdavis.edu/service/horse/index.html). Deoxypyridinoline levels and deoxypyridinoline to pyridinoline ratios are significantly higher in the urine, skin, and other tissues of horses with HERDA than in control horses due to collagen cross-linking abnormalities.

IMAGING
N/A

OTHER DIAGNOSTIC PROCEDURES
Skin biopsies submitted for histopathology may be suggestive of HERDA but the diagnosis should be confirmed by DNA testing.

PATHOLOGIC FINDINGS
In addition to skin and joint abnormalities, affected horses have an increased incidence of corneal ulcers and other ocular abnormalities, with altered biochemical and molecular characteristics of many tissues including tendons, ligaments, heart valves, and bones.

 TREATMENT

Treatment is palliative and includes minimizing trauma, careful wound management, and restriction from sunlight. Meeting NRC requirements and adding supplemental vitamin C, lysine, and nutraceuticals containing glucosamine and chondroitin sulfate may improve the quality of the affected horse's life. Mildly affected horses may still be ridden, with an unknown percentage of these horses being competition sound. With excellent care affected horses can live a normal lifespan; however, most HERDA horses are humanely destroyed by age 3 years because they are unable to be ridden.

 MEDICATIONS

DRUG(S) OF CHOICE
N/A

CONTRAINDICATIONS/POSSIBLE INTERACTIONS
N/A

 FOLLOW-UP

PATIENT MONITORING
N/A

PREVENTION/AVOIDANCE
Selective breeding strategies based on DNA testing.

POSSIBLE COMPLICATIONS
N/A

EXPECTED COURSE AND PROGNOSIS
• For affected horses—poor; although some horses are successful competitors, most horses with HERDA are unable to be ridden
• For carriers—excellent

H

 MISCELLANEOUS

ASSOCIATED CONDITIONS
N/A

AGE-RELATED FACTORS
N/A

ZOONOTIC POTENTIAL
N/A

PREGNANCY/FERTILITY/BREEDING
Mares with HERDA have had successful full-term pregnancies.

ABBREVIATIONS
• EDS = Ehlers–Danlos syndrome
• HERDA = hereditary equine regional dermal asthenia
• NRC = National Research Council

Suggested Reading
Rashmir-Raven AM, Spier SJ. Hereditary equine regional dermal asthenia (HERDA) in Quarter Horses: a review of clinical signs, genetics and research. Equine Vet Educ 2015;27(11):604–611.

Author Ann Rashmir
Consulting Editor Gwendolen Lorch
Acknowledgment The author and editor acknowledge the prior contribution of Stephen D. White.

HERNIAS (UMBILICAL AND INGUINAL)

 BASICS

DEFINITION
- *Hernias* are abdominal wall defects through which fluid or GI contents can pass depending on the size
- *Umbilical hernias* are defects at the site of the umbilicus after umbilical structures regress
- *Inguinal hernias* are defects where intestines traverse through the inguinal rings or rupture through the adjacent peritoneum
- *Simple/reducible hernias* indicate contents can be pushed back into abdomen
- *Complicated/nonreducible hernias* indicate herniated tissue is incarcerated with potential strangulation of associated blood supply and emergency surgery is necessary

PATHOPHYSIOLOGY
Umbilical
- Umbilical hernias are the most common type of abdominal hernia in the horse
- The linea alba is discontinuous at birth, but the umbilical ring normally closes within the first few days of life by a fibrous plate
- Failure of this closure leads to herniation
- Small (<5 cm) hernias usually close within a few weeks
- Large defects (>10 cm) or those persisting at the age of 4 months warrant surgical correction

Inguinal
- Usually unilateral
- *Direct* inguinal hernias result from weakness of the transverse fascia adjacent to the inguinal rings, resulting in diverticulum of the peritoneum and associated bowel, and are reported in humans but not equids
- *Indirect* inguinal hernias result from GI contents penetrating the vaginal tunic; if contents pass through the internal and external rings into the scrotum the term *scrotal hernia* may be used
- *Ruptured* inguinal hernias occur when the vaginal tunic or peritoneum tears, resulting in bowel traveling subcutaneously

SYSTEMS AFFECTED
GI
- Small intestine most often herniates through an umbilical or inguinal hernia. Omentum, bladder, small colon, and large colon herniations are also reported
- The entire loop of small intestines may become incarcerated and strangulated, necessitating resection
- If only 1 wall of a viscus becomes incarcerated, it may become necrotic and develop into a Richter's hernia

Reproductive
In the case of inguinal hernias, the testicle on the affected side, and sometimes the adjacent testicle, usually becomes compromised enough to necessitate castration (unilateral or bilateral) due to pressure on the testicular

blood supply caused by pressure of incarcerated viscera on the spermatic cord.

Skin
Integument is usually healthy and resection of loose skin associated with herniorrhaphy is for cosmetic benefit only. In rare cases the skin may become irritated to the point of sloughing with pathologic hernias, particularly direct or ruptured scrotal hernias.

Urologic
Herniation of the urinary bladder has been reported.

GENETICS
Umbilical
May have a genetic predisposition (see Breed Predilections).

Inguinal
Some breeds overrepresented (see Breed Predilections).

INCIDENCE/PREVALENCE
Umbilical
0.5–2% incidence with only 4% progression to incarcerated bowel.

GEOGRAPHIC DISTRIBUTION
N/A

SIGNALMENT
Breed Predilections
Umbilical
Any, but some suggestion that Warmbloods and Friesians are overrepresented.
Inguinal
Any, but Standardbreds, American Saddlebreds, Tennessee Walking Horses, and draft breeds are overrepresented.

Mean Age and Range
Simple, congenital hernias <10 cm (umbilical) or indirect (scrotal) may resolve with age. Surgical fixation is recommended for simple hernias that persist past the age of 4 months.

Predominant Sex
Umbilical
Any gender.
Inguinal
Almost exclusively in colts, although cases of geldings and mares exist.

SIGNS
General Comments
Signs differ significantly when a simple hernia becomes irreducible.

Historical Findings, Physical Examination Findings
- Soft, fluctuant swelling that is completely reducible in a nonpainful animal is indicative of a simple hernia
- Complicated hernias involve incarceration of bowel, resulting in abdominal discomfort
- Swollen, firm, warm, and painful hernia sac—typical signs when incarceration is present
- Inguinal hernias often have swelling and peristaltic activity visible in the bowel under

the skin if peritoneum and/or vaginal tunic is ruptured

CAUSES, RISK FACTORS
Umbilical
Increased abdominal pressure at birth, umbilical infection, umbilical trauma especially during parturition, excessive straining due to abdominal discomfort.

Inguinal
- Excessive pressure during parturition may predispose to inguinal hernia
- Enlarged inguinal rings in some breeds have been proposed as a risk factor

 DIAGNOSIS

DIFFERENTIAL DIAGNOSIS
Umbilical
Omphalophlebitis—often accompanied by signs of systemic illness (fever, lethargy, leukocytosis), thickened and warm umbilicus on palpation, and abnormally large umbilical remnants on US.

Inguinal
Swelling due to trauma or other testicular pathology.

CBC/BIOCHEMISTRY/URINALYSIS
N/A

OTHER LABORATORY TESTS
N/A

IMAGING
US
Umbilical
- US allows evaluation of the hernia size and contents
- Abdominal US can identify secondarily distended intestines or enlarged umbilical structures consistent with omphalophlebitis
Inguinal
US may be beneficial in confirming abdominal structures involved.

OTHER DIAGNOSTIC PROCEDURES
Abdominocentesis
Serohemorrhagic peritoneal fluid with a lactate consistently higher than peripheral L -lactate is consistent with ischemic bowel, potentially secondary to an incarcerated hernia.

PATHOLOGIC FINDINGS
N/A

 TREATMENT

APPROPRIATE HEALTH CARE, NURSING CARE
- *Daily* monitoring of the hernia for reduction and comfort of the patient must be mandated
- Hernia clamps are successfully used by some practitioners in cases of small, simple

HERNIAS (UMBILICAL AND INGUINAL)

umbilical hernias, but intestines may become entrapped by the band
• A figure-of-eight bandage is recommended for colts with reducible nonruptured inguinal hernias until resolution

ACTIVITY

Umbilical
Activity does not need to be restricted as long as daily monitoring can be achieved.

Inguinal
Stall rest or controlled exercise is recommended if a figure-of-eight bandage is applied.

DIET
N/A

CLIENT EDUCATION
Ensure clients monitor daily for reducibility of the hernia.

SURGICAL CONSIDERATIONS

Umbilical
Surgery should be considered if the hernia is >10 cm in size or does not resolve by 4 months of age. A closed or open (resection of the umbilical sac) approach may be utilized.

Inguinal
• In cases of reducible nonruptured inguinal hernias, resolution may be obtained with castration of the affected side and transfixation ligature of the vaginal tunic and/or closure of the external inguinal ring. Bilateral castration should be performed if the owner does not want to use the animal for breeding, as herniation may occur bilaterally
• Laparoscopic herniorrhaphy of the internal inguinal ring with preservation of the spermatic cord may be performed when owners want to retain the animal for breeding. Good results have been obtained using either staples, suture, or peritoneal flap with careful closure of the caudomedial aspect of the ring
• Nonreducible hernias, either umbilical or inguinal, require emergency surgery for correction and potentially resection of affected bowel if strangulated

 MEDICATIONS

DRUG(S) OF CHOICE
• No drug therapy needed for nonsurgical hernias

• Perioperative antibiotics may be used as a prophylactic measure, especially if strangulated bowel is suspected

CONTRAINDICATIONS
None

PRECAUTIONS
None

POSSIBLE INTERACTIONS
None

ALTERNATIVE DRUGS
None

 FOLLOW-UP

PATIENT MONITORING

Umbilical
• Simple, small umbilical hernias should be evaluated on a daily basis until the ring is closed in order to allow early recognition of changes in size or consistency of the umbilical sac
• If colic occurs, consider the hernia as a possible cause

Inguinal
• Also monitor and reduce daily
• If colic occurs, consider hernia as a possible cause

PREVENTION/AVOIDANCE
A figure-of-eight bandage may help resolve nonruptured indirect inguinal hernia.

POSSIBLE COMPLICATIONS
The most common complication in both hernias is colic and entrapment of bowel.

EXPECTED COURSE AND PROGNOSIS
Most foals with small umbilical or inguinal hernias have a good prognosis for resolution within the first few weeks to months of life. Larger hernias may not resolve without surgery

 MISCELLANEOUS

ASSOCIATED CONDITIONS

Umbilical
Omphalophlebitis

AGE-RELATED FACTORS
Hernias that persist past the age of 4 months are unlikely to resolve without surgical treatment.

ZOONOTIC POTENTIAL
None

PREGNANCY/FERTILITY/BREEDING

Inguinal
Laparoscopic closure of the internal inguinal rings is required for closure of the inguinal canal if the animal is to retain the testicle on the affected side. Bilateral closure is recommended, as hernias can occur on the right and left.

SYNONYMS
None

SEE ALSO
Omphalophlebitis

ABBREVIATIONS
• GI = gastrointestinal
• US = ultrasonography, ultrasound

Suggested Reading
Gracia-Calvo LA, Ortega C, Ezquerra J. Laparoscopic closure of the inguinal rings in horses: literature review. J Equine Vet Sci 2014;34(10):1149–1155.
Kummer M, Stick JA. Abdominal hernias. In: Auer JA, Stick JA, eds. Equine Surgery, 4e. St. Louis, MO: WB Saunders, 2012:506–514.

Author Alison K. Gardner
Consulting Editor Margaret C. Mudge
Acknowledgment The author and editor acknowledge the prior contribution of Laura Hirvinen.

H

HERPESVIRUS 3

BASICS

OVERVIEW
EHV-3 is the causative agent in equine coital exanthema, a highly contagious venereal disease that results in vesicular lesions on the penis and prepuce of stallions and the vestibule and vulva of mares. The disease is generally limited to the reproductive tract, and infection does not appear to affect fertility. Horse-to-horse transmission in the absence of coitus is rare. Although coital exanthema is uncommon and the lesions resolve spontaneously, affected stallions may be unwilling to breed mares, leading to economic losses. Like other herpesviruses, a short-lived immunity develops after infection. Infected animals maintain a lifelong carrier state and virus may be shed by asymptomatic mares. The disease occurs sporadically worldwide.

SIGNALMENT
Horses most frequently affected are of breeding age and viral transmission occurs through genital contact.

SIGNS
• In stallions, vesicles appear on the penis within 5–9 days of exposure and later on the prepuce. Vesicles progress to pustules, which then slough, leaving ulcerated areas up to 1.5 cm in diameter. Ulcers heal within a few weeks and result in depigmented areas. Stallions may be more severely affected than mares and can become dull, anorectic, and febrile
• Mares develop multifocal areas of sharply demarcated erosions on the vestibular mucosa and vulval lips that subsequently ulcerate and then heal in a similar manner. Other clinical signs in mares may include tail swishing, frequent urination, and vulval discharge. Aged broodmares may develop recurrent coital exanthema during late gestation or in the early postparturient period, but a relationship with viral recrudescence has not been established. Lesions occur rarely on the oral and nasal mucosa. Following acute infection, mares may undergo a reactivation and re-excretion phase when, though asymptomatic, virus may still be shed

CAUSES AND RISK FACTORS
• Coital exanthema is caused by EHV-3, an alphaherpesvirus

• Horses of breeding age are at risk due to viral transmission by genital contact. Iatrogenic transmission by contaminated instruments may also be possible
• Shedding of EHV-3 by asymptomatic or subclinically infected mares is also possible

DIAGNOSIS

DIFFERENTIAL DIAGNOSIS
Vesicular or pustular lesions on the penis or vulva are characteristic for coital exanthema. However, inflammation of the penis or vulva may also occur due to trauma, bacterial infection, or contact hypersensitivities. Vesicular stomatitis may also uncommonly affect genitalia.

CBC/BIOCHEMISTRY/URINALYSIS
N/A

OTHER LABORATORY TESTS
• Diagnosis can commonly be made based only on clinical signs. Serum neutralizing antibodies peak 2–3 weeks after infection and may remain detectable for up to 1 year later; however, complement fixing antibodies are not present beyond 60 days after infection
• Virus detection can be performed using PCR

IMAGING
N/A

OTHER DIAGNOSTIC PROCEDURES
• Evaluation of the affected area is usually diagnostic
• Further testing may include virus isolation from erosions
• Characteristic herpesvirus inclusions can also be seen during histologic evaluation of biopsy samples
• Antibodies can be detected using seroneutralizing antibodies

TREATMENT
• Lesions are generally self-limiting, though daily cleaning with noncaustic antiseptics may reduce inflammation
• Application of topical antimicrobial ointments to affected areas may reduce the chances of secondary bacterial infections. Secondary infection with *Streptococcus zooepidemicus* is also possible and may increase time to healing

MEDICATIONS
No specific antiviral therapy has been evaluated for the treatment of EHV-3 infections. The use of topical antimicrobial ointments may decrease secondary bacterial infections.

FOLLOW-UP
• Clinically infected stallions should have sexual rest for at least 3 weeks after infection decreases to decrease spread of EHV-3
• If the breed registry permits, semen may be collected using an open-ended artificial vagina and artificially inseminated, so as to reduce the chance of viral transmission to the mare
• Silent recrudescence of the virus in stallions is likely, and may contribute to propagation of the disease. Using best practices for breeding, which should include washing the mare's perineum with plain water and povidone–iodine solution and cleaning the stallion's penis with plain water both before and after mating, will aid in decreasing the spread of EHV-3 from asymptomatic carriers
• Iatrogenic transmission is possible; therefore, instruments that are disposable or easily cleaned should be used when working with affected horses
• The number of subclinically affected horses may be underestimated

MISCELLANEOUS

ABBREVIATIONS
• EHV = equine herpesvirus
• PCR = polymerase chain reaction

Suggested Reading
Blanchard TL, Kenney RM, Timoney PJ. Venereal disease. Vet Clin North Am Equine Pract 1992;8:191–203.

Author Jennifer K. Linton
Consulting Editor Ashley G. Boyle
Acknowledgment The author and editor acknowledge the prior contribution of Pamela A Wilkins.

BASICS

DEFINITION
Ubiquitous, contagious viral equine pathogen that most frequently causes respiratory tract disease; may also cause abortion, fatal neonatal illness, or neurologic disease.

PATHOPHYSIOLOGY
EHV-1 and EHV-4 infect the respiratory tract; EHV-1 infects white blood cells, causing a viremia and dissemination of the virus to the reproductive tract or CNS. EHV-4 infections are usually limited to the upper respiratory tract and are a common cause of respiratory disease in young horses. Following resolution of clinical signs, either virus may become dormant (latent infection), only to recrudesce during periods of stress, such as shipping, weaning, training, or competition. The ability of the virus to evade the immune system and establish latent infection is important in the propagation of the disease and has made control by immunization difficult. It is unknown why EHV-1 periodically induces reproductive tract or CNS disease; infectious dose, immune status of the horse, and viral strain are likely factors. Neurotropic strains share a common mutation in their genetic code and result in more prolonged viremia, perhaps contributing to the development of neurologic disease.

SYSTEMS AFFECTED
Respiratory
The upper respiratory tract is primarily affected.

Reproductive
Following infection of the upper respiratory tract and subsequent viremia, EHV-1 may infect endometrium and fetal tissues, resulting in fetal death and abortion.

Nervous
Isolated cases and outbreaks of CNS disease occur. Viremic spread of EHV-1 to the CNS endothelium leads to thrombosis, ischemic neural damage, and characteristic clinical signs.

INCIDENCE/PREVALENCE
Worldwide wherever large groups of horses are present.

SIGNALMENT
The median age of horses hospitalized for the neurologic form of EHV-1 infection is 3 years. Any age or breed are susceptible to EHV-related diseases. Respiratory tract disease due to EHV-4 is extremely common in young horses.

SIGNS
• With partial immunity, silent infections occur (only signs are fever and depression)
• Distal limb edema due to associated vasculitis and decreased ambulation

Respiratory Disease
• Most common form: cough, mucopurulent nasal discharge, fever (102–106°F, 38.9–41°C), depression, and abnormal lung sounds
• Rare "pulmonary vasculotropic form"—infection of the respiratory vascular endothelium, resulting in severe disease that is potentially fatal

Reproductive Tract Disease
• Sporadic or multiple late term abortions (7–11 months) with or without other signs
• Aborted infected fetus lesions—pulmonary edema, pleural and peritoneal effusions, multifocal hepatic necrosis, icterus, and petechiation
• Uninfected fetus—no lesions
• Fetus, placenta, and fetal fluids may contain very large viral loads and be sources of additional infections

Neurologic Disease
• Deficits—symmetric or asymmetric
• Fever usually precedes an acute onset of hindlimb ataxia, proprioceptive deficits, and weakness
• Severe form—hindlimb paralysis leads to a dog-sitting posture or recumbency
• Cranial nerve abnormalities (head tilt, tongue weakness, nystagmus, blindness) also occur
• Common—bladder atony, fecal retention, perineal sensory deficits, and decreased tail tone
• Ophthalmologic examination—retinal hemorrhages due to optic neuritis

CAUSES
EHV-1 and EHV-4.

RISK FACTORS
• Stress—transportation, weaning, overcrowding, surgery, other illnesses, or competition
• Poor ventilation and crowding

DIAGNOSIS

DIFFERENTIAL DIAGNOSIS
Respiratory Disease
• Influenza
• Equine viral arteritis
• Adenovirus
• Bacterial pneumonia
• Severe equine asthma (heaves)

Reproductive Tract Disease
Abortion—equine viral arteritis, bacterial or fungal placentitis.

Neurologic Disease
• Equine protozoal myeloencephalitis, other viral encephalitides, aberrant parasite migration, trauma, cauda equina syndrome
• Fever is an aspect of herpesvirus myeloencephalopathy that is uncommon in the equine neurologic diseases above, except West Nile virus

CBC/BIOCHEMISTRY/URINALYSIS
CBC and serum biochemistry—normal at the onset of clinical signs.

OTHER LABORATORY TESTS
• PCR testing—nasopharyngeal swabs and whole blood at first examination may be diagnostic, frequently within 24–48 h of submission
• Test for both neurologic and wild-type strains (both can cause neurologic disease)
• Virus isolation
• 4-fold increase in antibody titer collected over a 2 week period
• Single positive titer can be exposure or vaccination
• Natural infection—rapid and dramatic increase in titer (serum must be collected early in the course of the disease to demonstrate an increasing titer)

IMAGING
Thoracic ultrasonography or radiology (secondary bacterial pneumonia).

OTHER DIAGNOSTIC PROCEDURES
PCR Testing
As described in Other Laboratory Tests.

Virus Isolation
• Contact diagnostic laboratory for transport media and specific collection and transportation procedures
• Place nasopharyngeal swabs immediately in media and refrigerate or freeze until transported to the laboratory
• Buffy coat of whole blood preserved with EDTA
• Viremia occurs during clinical signs

Cerebrospinal Fluid Aspirate
• Increase in protein concentration
• Normal or only mildly increased nucleated cell concentration
• Xanthochromia (yellow discoloration of CSF due to breakdown of red blood cells)
• Rarely isolated from CSF

PATHOLOGIC FINDINGS
• Respiratory epithelium—inapparent or cause epithelial necrosis, thrombus formation, and petechiation
• Reproductive tract—lesions in endometrium and fetus, resulting in abortion, typically showing evidence of vasculitis
• CNS endothelium—vasculitis of the small arteries and veins of the white matter of the spinal cord resulting in hemorrhage, thrombosis, and secondary ischemic degeneration

TREATMENT

APPROPRIATE HEALTH CARE
Rhinopneumonitis
• Fever lasting more than 3 days, persistent cough, abnormal lung sounds, depression, or

HERPESVIRUS TYPES 1 AND 4

anorexia may indicate secondary bacterial bronchopneumonia
• Recovering horses—no training, house in well-ventilated areas, caution in transporting long distances (severe pleuropneumonia risk)

Abortion
Reproductive tract examination to rule out retained fetal membranes or trauma.

Neurologic Disease
• Recumbent horses—isolate to well-bedded stall, keep sternal, and reposition frequently
• Many horses remain standing or stand with the assistance of a sling
• Monitor for urinary incontinence—palpation per rectum may reveal a distended bladder. Perform urinary catheterization at least twice daily by aseptic technique or place an indwelling urinary catheter
• Evacuate feces manually
• Dysphagia—give fluids IV or by nasogastric tube

ACTIVITY
Severe respiratory infections:
• 1 month to regain normal epithelial function
• Mucociliary clearance is impaired, leading to accumulation of respiratory secretions and inhaled antigens in the lower airways
• Persistent airway inflammation may occur when training is resumed prematurely
• Lung sounds should be normal and spontaneous cough resolved prior to training
• Uncomplicated rhinopneumonitis—2–4 weeks of rest

CLIENT EDUCATION
• Neurologic EHV-1/4 is reportable in many states in the USA
• Requires prolonged quarantine of affected facilities
• Affected horses—place in strict isolation as these horses are frequently actively shedding virus at the time of diagnosis
• Vaccination—effective in reducing severity and frequency of EHV-1/4-associated respiratory and reproductive tract disease

MEDICATIONS

DRUG(S) OF CHOICE

Respiratory Disease
• No specific antiviral therapy has been proven effective
• NSAIDs for inflammation and fever
• Antimicrobials (trimethoprim–sulfamethoxazole 30 mg/kg, PO, every 12 h) should be administered if secondary bacterial infections are suspected

Abortion
No specific drug therapy.

Neurologic Disease
• Severely affected—corticosteroids (dexamethasone 0.05–0.25 mg/kg IV or IM every 12 h in decreasing doses for 7–14 days)
• Recumbent—NSAIDs (flunixin meglumine 1 mg/kg PO or IV every 12 h) and broad-spectrum antimicrobials (ceftiofur 5 mg/kg IV or IM every 12 h) due to potential for pneumonia, cystitis, and decubital ulceration
• Acyclovir (aciclovir) (10 mg/kg twice daily IV given in 1 L of crystalloid fluid (*not* 5% dextrose) over 1 h) and valacyclovir (valaciclovir) (orally at 30–40 mg/kg PO BID–TID); effective against some equine herpesvirus isolates

PRECAUTIONS
Laminitis is a rare complication of corticosteroid administration in horses. Acyclovir may result in anaphylactic-like reaction if administered IV in large concentrations rapidly.

ALTERNATIVE DRUGS
Administration of acyclovir at 20 mg/kg PO 3 times daily appears to be safe although of unknown efficacy owing to poor oral bioavailability.

FOLLOW-UP

PATIENT MONITORING
• Most horses recover from rhinopneumonitis uneventfully
• Aborting mares—isolate for at least 2 weeks but may be bred in 1 month
• Neurologic recumbent horses—monitor for dehydration, decubital ulcers, pneumonia, bladder atony, cystitis, fecal incontinence, and self-trauma

PREVENTION/AVOIDANCE
• Adequate ventilation, decreasing stress, and quarantine of new horses
• Vaccination of animals at risk every 3 months is effective at reducing the severity and frequency of respiratory disease and decreases the likelihood of abortion. United States Equestrian Federation requires every 6 months
• Broodmares—vaccinate at months 5, 7, 9, of pregnancy
• Vaccination of unexposed horses in the face of the outbreak may decrease the spread of disease
• Currently available vaccines do not claim protection against neurologic disease

• Vaccination of animals with the neurologic syndrome is contraindicated
• Horses recovering from herpesvirus infections may shed the virus from nasal secretions for 2 weeks after infection and therefore should remain quarantined
• Aborted fetus and fetal membranes are major sources of virus and therefore should be placed in a sealed container and removed to decrease contamination of the environment

EXPECTED COURSE AND PROGNOSIS

Respiratory Disease
Most horses recover from an uncomplicated infection in 2–4 weeks.

Reproductive Tract Disease
Mares recover readily and subsequent fertility is not impaired.

Neurologic Disease
Many horses stabilize in 24–48 h and, if they remain standing, slow improvement usually occurs over a period of weeks to months. Some horses may have long-term residual neurologic deficits. Horses that become recumbent and cannot rise with assistance have a poorer prognosis. There is no apparent correlation between outcome and CSF characteristics.

MISCELLANEOUS

PREGNANCY/FERTILITY/BREEDING
Caution should be used when administering corticosteroids to pregnant mares.

SYNONYMS
Rhinopneumonitis

ABBREVIATIONS
• CNS = central nervous system
• CSF = cerebrospinal fluid
• EHV = equine herpesvirus
• NSAID = nonsteroidal anti-inflammatory drug
• PCR = polymerase chain reaction

Suggested Reading
Pusterla N, Hussey GS. Equine herpesvirus 1 myeloencephalopathy. Vet Clin North Am Equine Pract 2014;30:489–506.
Wilkins PA, Papich M, Sweeney RW. Acyclovir pharmacokinetics in adult horses. J Vet Emerg Crit Care 2005;15:174–178.

Author Pamela A. Wilkins
Consulting Editor Ashley G. Boyle

BASICS

DEFINITION
Pregnancy prone to early termination, delivery of a compromised foal, and/or prolongation due to maternal, fetal, and/or placental abnormalities.

PATHOPHYSIOLOGY
• Premature initiation of labor and/or prolonged gestation
• Specific conditions are similar to those resulting in fetal stress, distress, and/or viability

Preexisting Maternal Disease
• PPID
• EMS/IR
• Laminitis
• Chronic, moderate to severe endometritis, endometrial periglandular fibrosis, and/or lymphatic cysts (impaired placental function)

Gestational Maternal Conditions
• Malnutrition
• Colic
• Endotoxemia
• Hyperlipemia
• Prepubic tendon rupture
• Uterine torsion
• Dystocia
• Ovarian granulosa cell tumor
• Laminitis
• Musculoskeletal disease
• Ergopeptine alkaloid exposure (endophyte-infected fescue, ergotized grasses and/or grains)
• Xenobiotic exposure
• Abortigenic infection exposure, especially equine herpesvirus and bacterial contaminants on ETC setae

Placental Conditions
• Placentitis; placental insufficiency, early separation
• Umbilical cord torsion or torsion of the amnion
• Hydropic conditions
• MRLS
• Placental abnormalities reported with foals resulting from SCNT cloning procedures

Fetal Conditions
• Twins
• Fetal abnormalities, e.g. hydrocephalus
• IUGR
• Fetal trauma
• Foals resulting from SCNT cloning procedures
• Fetal stress and distress can involve 1 or more of the following:
  ◦ Maternal systemic disease; placental infection, insufficiency, torsion, and/or separation; fetal abnormalities, all of which impede efficient fetal gas exchange and nutrient transfer

◦ With placental insufficiency, fetal growth and development are slowed, resulting in IUGR
◦ Equine fescue toxicosis causes decreased maternal prolactin concentrations and impaired late-gestational 5α-pregnane secretion by the uterofetoplacental unit, resulting in prolonged gestation and fetal dysmaturity at the time of parturition

SYSTEMS AFFECTED
• Maternal—reproductive and other organ systems, depending on the nature of maternal systemic disease and complications, e.g. dystocia, RFM
• Fetal—all organ systems

SIGNS

Historical Findings
1 or more of the following:
• Maternal disease during gestation, e.g. colic, hyperlipemia, body wall or prepubic tendon rupture, uterine torsion, etc
• Mucoid, hemorrhagic, serosanguineous, or purulent vulvar discharge
• Premature udder development, dripping of milk
• Complete lack of late gestational udder development
• Previous examination indicating placentitis or fetal compromise
• Previous abortion, high-risk pregnancy, or dystocia
• History of delivering a small, dysmature, septicemic, and/or congenitally malformed foal
• Preexisting maternal disease at conception, such as laminitis, PPID, EMS/IR, endometritis, fibrosis and/or cysts
• Previous exposure to endophyte-infected fescue or ergotized grasses and/or grains
• Previous exposure to abortigenic xenobiotics or infections

Physical Examination Findings
Maternal and Placental Signs
• Laminitis
• Anorexia, fever, or other signs of concurrent, systemic disease
• Abdominal discomfort
• Mucoid, mucopurulent, hemorrhagic, serosanguineous, or purulent vulvar discharge
• Premature udder development and dripping of milk (except in cases of fescue toxicosis presenting with agalactia and little or no udder development)
• Premature placental separation (*red bag*)
• Placentitis, placental separation, or hydrops of fetal membranes
• Excessive abdominal distention
• Excessive swelling along the ventral midline, evidence of body wall weakening or rupture
• Alterations in maternal circulating levels of progestins, estrogens, and/or relaxin, reflecting changes in fetal wellbeing and/or placental function

Fetal Signs
• Fetal stress and/or distress might first be recognized upon premature delivery of a live or dead foal; the late delivery of a severely compromised foal, unable to stand and suckle
• Fetal hyperactivity or inactivity (concurrent with maternal or placental abnormalities) may suggest a less-than-ideal fetal environment and/or fetal compromise
• Can be assessed by visual inspection or by TRP of the mare
• Parameters are assessed using transrectal or transabdominal US:
  ◦ Fetal activity and normal muscle tone:
    ▪ <330 days of gestation, the normal FHR is ≤100 bpm after activity and ≥60 bpm at rest
    ▪ >330 days of gestation, the normal FHR is ≥50 bpm at rest and difference between resting and active rates is ≤40 bpm
    ▪ Normal fetal heart rhythm, as assessed by US and/or ECG
    ▪ Normal fetal breathing movements
  ◦ Increased volumes of amniotic fluid reflect hydrops amnion (*hydramnios*); low volumes indicate fetal distress, longstanding chronic hypoxia
  ◦ Sudden changes in the echogenicity of the amniotic fluid in late gestation can indicate meconium expulsion and fetal distress
  ◦ Appropriately sized fetus for gestational stage
    ▪ Fetal aortic diameter ≈ 2.1 cm at 300 days of gestation and 2.7 cm at 330 days of gestation
    ▪ Record length and width of fetal orbit
Placental Health
• Normal CTUP, by transabdominal US—12.6 ± 3.3 mm
  ◦ Uteroplacental thickness >19.2 mm indicative of placentitis
• Normal CTUP by transrectal US:
  ◦ 271–300 days of gestation ≤8 mm
  ◦ 300–330 days of gestation ≤10 mm
  ◦ >330 days of gestation ≤12 mm
• Look for evidence of absence or very small areas of uteroplacental detachment
• Increased echogenicity of allantoic fluid >44 days prior to anticipated foaling date may reflect fetal distress; floating particulate matter becomes gradually larger 10–36 days prior to foaling; sudden increases in the echogenicity of the allantoic fluid may indicate fetal and/or placental abnormalities
• The mean vertical distance of allantoic fluid in uncomplicated pregnancies from <300 days to term is generally 19 ± 9 mm

RISK FACTORS
• May be nonspecific
• Thoroughbreds, Standardbreds, draft, and American Miniature Horse mares, and related breeds predisposed to twinning
• >15 years of age

H

HIGH-RISK PREGNANCY   (CONTINUED)

- Other organ system involvement depends on the presence of placentitis, stage of gestation, presence of maternal disease, infection, and/or toxemia
- Hyperlipidemia is of special concern for overconditioned American Miniature Horses, ponies, and donkeys

Preexisting Maternal Disease
- PPID
- EMS/IR
- Laminitis
- Chronic, moderate to severe endometritis, endometrial periglandular fibrosis, and/or lymphatic cysts, leading to impaired placental function

DIAGNOSIS

DIFFERENTIAL DIAGNOSIS
Normal, uncomplicated pregnancy with an active, normal fetus as assessed by TRP, transrectal or transabdominal US, and/or various laboratory tests.

DIAGNOSTIC PROCEDURES

Maternal Assessment
- Complete physical examination
- CBC/differential serum biochemistry for inflammatory or stress leukocyte response, evidence of other organ system involvement
- Specific tests to confirm suspected predisposing cause (see Preexisting Maternal Disease)
- Test for EMS/IR, including basal glucose and insulin analyses, oral sugar test, and combined glucose and insulin test
- ELISA or RIA analyses for maternal P_4 useful at <80 days of gestation (normal levels vary from >1 to >4 ng/mL, depending on reference laboratory). At >100 days, RIA detects both P_4 (very low >day 150) and cross-reacting 5α-pregnanes of uterofetoplacental origin. Acceptable levels of progestins, including 5α-pregnanes, vary with stage of gestation and laboratory used. Decreased maternal 5α-pregnane concentrations during late gestation are associated with fescue toxicosis and ergotism and are reflected in RIA analyses for progestagens
- Maternal estrogen concentrations can reflect fetal estrogen production and viability, especially conjugated estrogens, e.g. estrone sulfate
- Decreased maternal relaxin concentration may be associated with abnormal placental function
- Decreased maternal prolactin secretion during late gestation is associated with fescue toxicosis and ergotism

Fetal Assessment
- Transrectal and transabdominal US useful in diagnosing twins, assessing fetal stress, distress, and/or viability, monitoring fetal development, evaluating placental health and diagnosing other gestational abnormalities
- In barren, older mares, mares with history of high-risk pregnancy (placentitis, abortion, EED, conception failure, or endometritis), transrectal or transabdominal US should be performed on a routine basis during the entire pregnancy to assess fetal stress and viability
- Confirmation of pregnancy and diagnosis of twins should be performed any time serious maternal disease occurs
- Twin pregnancy is confirmed by 2 fetuses (transrectal US when gestational age is <90 days) or ruled out by presence of a nonpregnant uterine horn (transabdominal US during late gestation)
- Fetal stress, distress, and/or viability can best be determined by transabdominal US during late gestation. View fetus in both active and resting states for at least 30 min. Note abnormal fetal presentation and position
- Fetal ECG can detect twins and assess fetal viability and distress, but largely has been replaced by transabdominal US with ECG capabilities
- While a higher risk technique in horses than in humans, US-guided amniocentesis and/or allantocentesis and analysis of the collected fluids might become a future means to assess fetal karyotype, pulmonary maturity, and to measure fetal proteins
  - Samples might reveal bacteria, meconium, or inflammatory cells

PATHOLOGIC FINDINGS
- Evidence of villous atrophy or hypoplasia on the chorionic surface of the fetal membranes
- Thickening and edema of the chorioallantois
- Various placental abnormalities reported with foals resulting from SCNT/cloning procedures
- An endometrial biopsy can demonstrate the presence of moderate to severe, chronic endometritis, endometrial periglandular fibrosis with decreased normal glandular architecture, and/or lymphatic lacunae

TREATMENT

APPROPRIATE HEALTH CARE
Depending on the circumstances, monitoring/managing high-risk pregnancies (especially close to anticipated foaling date), including prolonged examination times required for complete serial transabdominal fetal assessments, is best performed at a facility prepared to manage these types of pregnancies, especially if distress is severe and parturition (induction or cesarean section) is imminent.
- Early diagnosis of at-risk pregnancies is essential for successful treatment. Do not underestimate the impact of maternal disease on fetal and placental health

- Foal survival is improved with maternal body wall tears, when circumstances allow conservative management, without induction of parturition or elective cesarean section
- With prolonged fetal stress and/or distress, maintenance of pregnancy must be balanced with the need to induce parturition (with or without cesarean section), if necessary to stabilize the mare's health
- Parturition requires close supervision in cases of fetal stress and distress. The neonatal foal will likely require intensive care
- Foal resuscitation during delivery or immediately postpartum; pay close attention to airways, breathing, circulation
- Consider individual circumstances/their sequelae to determine nature and timing of treatment:
  - PE
  - CBC/biochemistry profile
  - Stage of gestation
  - Nature of maternal disease
  - Hydrops
  - Evidence of fetal stress, distress, or impending demise
  - Maternal mammary development
  - Maternal health risks and/or impending maternal demise
  - Occurrence of complications such as dystocia, RFM, FTPI (necessitating a plasma transfusion), and/or fetal dysmaturity, with or without septicemia
  - Financial—relative value of mare and foal

NURSING CARE
Depending on maternal disease, fetal stress/distress, the necessity for surgical intervention, intensive nursing care might very well be required for the neonatal foal and mare.

ACTIVITY
- For most cases, exercise will be somewhat limited and supervised. However, for EMS/IR exercise may an important part of the therapeutic regimen
- Body wall tears, prepubic tendon rupture, laminitis, and/or fetal hydrops may necessitate severe restrictions or complete elimination of exercise

DIET
Feed the mare an adequate, late gestational diet with proper levels of energy, protein, vitamins, and minerals, unless contraindicated by concurrent maternal disease, e.g. EMS/IR.

CLIENT EDUCATION
- Early diagnosis is essential for fetal survival
- Correct/manage predisposing conditions to improve outcomes
- Induction of parturition and cesarean section also have inherent risks

SURGICAL CONSIDERATIONS
- Cesarean section may be indicated when vaginal delivery is not possible or if dystocia is not amenable to resolution by manipulation alone

• Surgical intervention might be indicated for future repair of anatomic defects predisposing mares to endometritis and placentitis

MEDICATIONS

DRUG(S) OF CHOICE

See recommendations for specific conditions associated with high-risk pregnancies. Oxygen, epinephrine, vasopressin (argipressin), and atropine may be necessary for foal resuscitation

Altrenogest

• Depending on clinical circumstances, risk factors, and clinician preferences, administration can start at various stages of pregnancy, continue until near term or at parturition, be used for only short periods (based on maternal progestin concentrations), and/or be decreased over time or discontinued abruptly
• History of endometritis/previously aborted mare (without active infectious component) and/or mare with fibrosis—0.044–0.088 mg/kg PO daily; commence 2–3 days after ovulation or upon diagnosis of pregnancy; continue to ≥100 days of gestation; can decrease dose over 14 days at end of treatment period
• Endotoxic/Gram-negative septicemic mares <80 days of gestation—0.088 mg/kg PO daily, initially, then 0.044 mg/kg daily to ≥100 days of gestation; can decrease dose over 14 days at end of treatment period
• To prevent premature parturition and promote uterine quiescence, following diagnosis of maternal disease, placentitis, or late gestational twins—0.088 mg/kg PO daily, initially, then 0.044 mg/kg daily
• Near term, discontinue 7–14 days before expected foaling date, unless otherwise indicated by assessment of fetal maturity/viability, questions regarding accuracy of gestational age, and/or clinician preference

Antibiotic or Antibacterial Therapy

• Indicated with a diagnosis of or potential for diagnosis of maternal, placental, and/or fetal infection
• The specific antibiotics used depend on clinical circumstances, suspect organisms, therapeutic goals, clinician preferences, and, potentially, financial considerations

Domperidone

• Indicated for agalactia and late gestational fetal maturation
• When fescue toxicosis is diagnosed or when there is confirmation of prolonged gestation, based on breeding records—1.1 mg/kg PO daily
• Continue domperidone to parturition, with anticipated normal mammary development and lactation

Flunixin Meglumine

• Prophylaxis if endotoxin release is anticipated—0.25 mg/kg IM (potential for injection reactions) or, preferably, IV or PO (daily to QID)
• Dose can be doubled for analgesia and anti-inflammatory effect
• May help decrease premature uterine contractions

Pentoxifylline

• Anti-inflammatory and anticytokine effects, especially during endotoxemia
• Dosing regimens used vary from 4.4 mg/kg PO every 8 h for laminitis to 8.5 mg/kg PO twice daily to reduce cytokine effects in endotoxemia

PRECAUTIONS, POSSIBLE INTERACTIONS

Altrenogest

• Only to prevent abortion or premature delivery in confirmed pregnancies, where a live fetus is present in utero
• Not recommended to prevent spontaneous, infectious abortion other than those caused by placentitis and endotoxemia
• Initially, weekly monitoring of fetal viability—retention of dead fetuses has been reported to result from continued treatment with supplemental progestins
• Altrenogest is absorbed across skin; wear nitrile or rubber gloves and wash hands
• Dependent on the etiology of the high-risk pregnancy, progestin supplementation might be unsuccessful

Antibiotic or Antibacterial Therapy

• Depends on the specific drug
• Some are potentially *teratogenic*

Domperidone

Premature lactation; loss of colostrum—can generally be addressed by adjusting the treatment regimen.

Flunixin Meglumine

Can cause gastric ulcers and kidney problems.

Pentoxifylline

Potentially, adverse GI, CNS, and cardiovascular effects.

ALTERNATIVE DRUGS

• Injectable P_4 (150–500 mg/day, oil base) can be administered IM daily, instead of the oral formulation. Variations, contraindications, and precautions are similar to those associated with altrenogest
• Other injectable and implantable progestin preparations are available commercially for use in other species. Any use in horses of these products is off-label, and few scientific data are available regarding their efficacy
• Newer, repository forms of P_4 are occasionally introduced; however, some evidence of efficacy should be provided prior to use
• See recommendations for specific conditions, e.g. dystocia, fescue toxicosis,

high-risk pregnancy, induction of parturition, prepubic tendon rupture, RFM, hydrops
• Phenylbutazone can be used as an alternative to flunixin meglumine. Variations, contraindications, and precautions are similar to those associated with flunixin meglumine
• Thyroxine supplementation has been successful (anecdotally) for treating mares with histories of subfertility and high-risk pregnancy, especially obese mares with EMS; its use remains controversial; considered deleterious by some clinicians. Few clinical data available, metformin has been suggested for mares with IR, where exercise and diet are insufficient for successful management
• Medications for other maternal diseases—potential risks are dependent on the specific drug. Pergolide is currently the drug of choice for treating PPID. However, its effects will mimic those of fescue toxicosis, with agalactia/dysgalactia and possibly prolonged gestation. It may be appropriate to consider treating these mares as for fescue toxicosis

FOLLOW-UP

PATIENT MONITORING

• Monitor mare and fetus until termination of pregnancy
• Monitor for premature or inadequate udder development
• Within no more than 24 h after delivery, the foal should be assessed; if necessary, treat for FTPI
• Vaginal speculum examination, uterine cytology, and culture (as indicated) can be performed 7–10 days postpartum
• Endometrial biopsy may be indicated as part of the postpartum examination; a prognostic tool for future reproduction

PREVENTION/AVOIDANCE

• Early recognition of at-risk mares and potential high-risk pregnancies
• Correction of perineal conformation; prevent placentitis
• Management of preexisting endometritis before breeding
• Early monitoring of mares with a history of fetal stress, distress, and/or viability concerns
• Complete breeding records, especially for double ovulations, early diagnosis of twins (<25 days; ideally, days 14–15); selective embryonic or fetal reduction
• Careful monitoring of pregnant mares for vaginal discharge and premature mammary secretion
• Removal of pregnant mares from fescue pasture or ergotized grasses or grains during last trimester (60 days optimal, especially if bred on multiple cycles, with no US confirmation of pregnancy; minimum of 30 days prepartum, with adequate breeding

dates and confirmation of pregnancy using US)
• Use ET procedures with mares predisposed to EED or high-risk pregnancies
• Avoid breeding or using ET procedures in mares that have produced multiple stressed, distressed, or dead foals due to congenital and potentially inheritable conditions
• Prudent use of medications in pregnant mares
• Avoid exposure to known toxicants
• Management of ETCs for prevention of MRLS
• If history of abortion, evidence of moderate to severe endometritis and/or fibrosis, evaluate and treat before breeding

POSSIBLE COMPLICATIONS
• Abortion, dystocia, RFM, endometritis, metritis, laminitis, septicemia, reproductive tract trauma, and/or impaired fertility, which will all affect the mare's wellbeing and reproductive value
• Fetal stress and/or distress; fetal death; stillbirth; neonatal death
• Neonatal foals from high-risk pregnancies have potentially been compromised during gestation and are more likely to be dysmature, septicemic, and subject to FTPI, and/or angular limb deformities than foals from normal pregnancies

EXPECTED COURSE AND PROGNOSIS
• The ability to prevent and treat the conditions associated with high-risk pregnancies has improved dramatically. Successful management requires rigorous monitoring of mare, fetus, and neonatal foal. Address treatable health concerns as soon as possible during the pregnancy and to avoid

and/or minimize challenges to maternal, fetal, and placental health
• If the predisposing conditions can be treated and/or managed, pregnancies in which fetal stress has been diagnosed have a guarded prognosis for successful completion
• If there is evidence of fetal stress progressing to distress and the distress continues in the face of treatment, fetal viability and maternal health become major concerns and the prognosis for a healthy, term gestation under these circumstances is guarded to poor

☑ MISCELLANEOUS

SYNONYMS
• Abortions, spontaneous infectious and noninfectious
• Fetal stress, distress, and viability
• Placental insufficiency
• Twins

SEE ALSO
• Abortion, spontaneous, infectious
• Abortion, spontaneous, noninfectious
• Dystocia
• Early embryonic death
• Embryo transfer
• Endometrial biopsy
• Endometritis
• Fetal stress/distress/viability
• Hydrops allantois/amnion
• Placental insufficiency
• Placentitis
• Twin pregnancy

ABBREVIATIONS
• CNS = central nervous system
• CTUP = combined thickness of uterus and placenta
• EED = early embryonic death
• ELISA = enzyme-linked immunosorbent assay
• EMS = equine metabolic syndrome
• ET = embryo transfer
• ETC = eastern tent caterpillar
• FHR = fetal heart rate
• FTPI = failure of transfer of passive immunity
• GI = gastrointestinal
• IR = insulin resistance
• IUGR = intrauterine growth retardation
• MRLS = mare reproductive loss syndrome
• P_4 = progesterone
• PPID = pituitary pars intermedia dysfunction
• RIA = radioimmunoassay
• RFM = retained fetal membranes
• SCNT = somatic cell nuclear transfer
• TRP = transrectal palpation
• US = ultrasonography, ultrasound

Suggested Reading
Vaala WE. Monitoring the high risk pregnancy. In: McKinnon AO, Squires EL, Vaala WE, Varner DD, eds. Equine Reproduction, 2e. Ames, IA: Wiley Blackwell, 2011:16–38.

Author Tim J. Evans
Consulting Editor Carla L. Carleton

BASICS

OVERVIEW
• Hydrocephalus is an increase in the volume of CSF, either compensatory after tissue loss or obstructive due to blockage within the ventricular system. In horses, hydrocephalus is generally obstructive
• Since CSF production is independent of CSF pressure, any obstruction of the ventricular system results in enlargement of the ventricular system within the brain
• Obstructive hydrocephalus can be observed following congenital aqueductal stenosis or may be secondary to suppurative meningitis or space-occupying lesions such as cholesterol granuloma or abscesses in older animals
• Hydrocephalus is unusual in horses compared with dogs, but it can be an inherited trait in Friesian horses, rarely in Standardbred horses, or an isolated occurrence in all breeds
• Hydrocephalus in Friesian horses has been shown to be due to an autosomal recessive nonsense mutation in a gene which in humans is associated with muscular dystrophy–dystroglycanopathy
• Systems affected—central nervous system

SIGNALMENT
Acquired disease is evident at any age, but congenital disease can vary from foals born dead to developing clinical signs hours to days later.

SIGNS
Historical Findings
• A history of CNS disease and/or trauma can be seen with acquired disease. However, there may be no historical association

• In foals, severe hydrocephalus can on occasion be noted as an incidental finding after sudden death due to vascular instability in the hydrocephalic brain

Physical Examination
• Clinical signs can be very subtle even with minimal cerebral mantle remaining, but usually include failure to thrive, somnolence and aimless activity, poor suck reflex, poor swallowing, and central blindness
• Additional signs can accompany additional lesions present in individual disease types
• Just like in dogs, a ventrolateral deviation of the eyeballs can also occur. Presumably, this is the result of a change in shape and position of the bony orbits. Normal eyeball movements may be seen
• Note that Arabian foals may be born with a very "domed" head at birth but may not have hydrocephalus

CAUSES AND RISK FACTORS
Similar for the primary CNS disease processes that may be associated with acquired disease. There may be a genetic relationship in congenital disease.

DIAGNOSIS

Plain lateral radiographs classically have a homogeneous ground-glass appearance of the calvaria. CT or MRI imaging is definitive.

TREATMENT

There is no viable treatment in horses. Euthanasia should be considered.

MISCELLANEOUS

SEE ALSO
• Congenital cardiac abnormalities
• Meningitis, neonate
• Neonatal maladjustment syndrome

ABBREVIATIONS
• CNS = central nervous system
• CSF = cerebrospinal fluid
• CT = computed tomography
• MRI = magnetic resonance imaging

Suggested Reading
Furr M. Congenital malformation of the nervous system. In: Furr M, Reed S, eds. Equine Neurology, 2e. Ames, IA: Wiley Blackwell, 2016:401–405.
Ojala M, Huikku I. Inheritance of hydrocephalus in horses. Equine Vet J 1992;24:140–143.
Sipma KD, Cornillie P, Saulez MN, et al. Phenotypic characteristics of hydrocephalus in stillborn Friesian foals. Vet Pathol 2013;50:1037–1042.

Author Caroline N. Hahn
Consulting Editor Caroline N. Hahn

H

HYDROPS ALLANTOIS/AMNION

BASICS

DEFINITION
- Excessive fluid accumulation in either the allantoic or amniotic cavity of the pregnant uterus
- Hydrops allantois is related primarily to placental dysfunction/insufficiency, contributing to fluid accumulation within the allantoic space of the fetal membranes
- Hydrops amnion is attributable to abnormalities of the fetus, contributing directly to fluid accumulation by virtue of congenital anomalies. Segmental aplasias (primarily GI in origin) preclude swallowing and processing and/or recycling of amniotic fluid. The fetus may be delivered alive but rarely is viable

PATHOPHYSIOLOGY
- Dysfunction of either the placenta or the fetus results in accumulation of excessive amounts of allantoic or amniotic fluid, undermining the dam's health by excessive weight of modest to rapid accumulation, contributing to her dehydration, compromised GI function, and labored respiration
- There is a possibility that a hydropic condition may in some cases be related or secondary to the development of placentitis. A link has been proposed in human medicine and as a potential etiology in areas where leptospirosis is endemic (equids)
- Clinical management for both conditions is the same—induction of parturition, to save the dam's life, and to prevent rupture of the ventral abdominal wall and/or the uterus

SYSTEMS AFFECTED
Reproductive—dam and fetus.

GENETICS
There may be a hereditary role in development of hydropic conditions.

INCIDENCE/PREVALENCE
Rare

SIGNALMENT
- No breed or age predisposition, although more cases have been reported in draft mares
- Abnormal accumulation of fluid (up to 100 L) in the allantoic cavity; abdominal size is abnormally large for stage of gestation
- Commonly occurs from 6 to 10 months of gestation
- Frequently has a rapid onset occurring over a few days to a few weeks
- Most mares develop a tremendous amount of ventral abdominal edema
- Abdominal and/or uterine rupture can result due to the excessive weight of allantoic or amniotic fluid

SIGNS
- Modest to rapid accumulation of fluid within the uterus (allantoic or amniotic)

- Rapid increase in abdominal size/shape
- Abdominal pain (moderate to severe), severe ventral edema, elevated pulse, labored respiration due to pressure on the diaphragm, difficulty walking, recumbency as the condition progresses
- TRP reveals an abnormal accumulation of fluid
- The fetus is difficult or impossible to detect (transrectal palpation or ballottement)

CAUSES
N/A

RISK FACTORS
Draft mares.

DIAGNOSIS

DIFFERENTIAL DIAGNOSIS
- Twin pregnancy—mid-to-late gestation
- Prepubic tendon rupture
- Herniation or rupture of ventral abdominal wall
- Possibly, uterine torsion

CBC/BIOCHEMISTRY/URINALYSIS
- Possible increased or decreased PCV (secondary to hypovolemia or dehydration, respectively)
- Possible increase in blood urea nitrogen and creatinine secondary to dehydration
- Serum titer for leptospirosis. Interpretation of a titer's significance is made with caution, i.e. a 4-fold increase in the antibody titer would provide strong support for a leptospirosis diagnosis

OTHER LABORATORY TESTS
N/A

IMAGING
US
- Fluid compartments are grossly enlarged, either allantoic or amniotic
- Torso/abdomen of the hydramnios fetus may have a grossly widened diameter as a result of ascites
- Fetal activity and its heart beat/rate may be difficult to monitor or detect because of the enlarged fluid volume within which it is located

OTHER DIAGNOSTIC PROCEDURES
- US and TRP
- Abdominocentesis, US guided, may be of use to detect abnormal free fluid in abdomen and in cases of uterine rupture

PATHOLOGIC FINDINGS
- Placental insufficiency secondary to placentitis
- Hydrops amnion—fetal swallowing defects (segmental aplasia(s) preventing swallowing and processing of amniotic fluid, which leads to its accumulation in excessive amounts)
- Fetal defects such as growth retardation and hydrocephalus have been reported, as well as brachygnathia

- Torsion of the umbilical cord and amnion has been reported

TREATMENT

APPROPRIATE HEALTH CARE
- Manual dilation of the cervix, completed gradually over a 10–20 min period
- Measured, controlled drainage of allantoic/amniotic fluid via aseptic insertion of a sterile drain tube through the cervix and fetal membranes.
- Slow removal of fluid is important to prevent hypovolemic shock in the mare
  - A sudden loss of pressure on the abdominal vessels may result as the uterus is drained, and lead to vascular pooling. Monitor PCV and plasma proteins throughout
  - If removal can be well-managed, achieving a gradual decrease in volume over a 12–24 h period is best
  - 1 method—manually dilate cervix, serial cloprostenol administration (250 μg at 12 h interval; 2–4 doses). Place nasogastric tube through membranes, tying off around tubing to facilitate controlled fluid removal, 5–10 L at a time, clamping off in between increments to keep mare stabilized
  - Continue with IV fluid delivery and care, as follows
- For the dam:
  - IV fluids—balanced electrolyte solutions, lactated Ringer's solution, or hypertonic saline solution
  - Corticosteroids—prednisolone sodium succinate. Initial dose is 50–100 mg IV or IM. Initial IV should be given slowly (30 s to 1 min)
  - Flunixin meglumine (0.7 mg/kg IV every 24 h) to decrease the likelihood of hypovolemic shock
  - Oxytocin is often ineffective due to chronic stretching (uterine atony/inertia)
- Once sufficient fluid has been removed by a slow, controlled rate removal, the CA membrane should be ruptured and the fetus removed by forced extraction
  - Note—in some cases the CA membrane may be thickened and difficult to rupture, in which case, the membrane should be pulled caudally, into the anterior vagina, to facilitate easier opening of the membrane and extraction of the fetus
  - Continue monitoring the mare, fluids, and antibiotic administration, as indicated

NURSING CARE
Close monitoring of the mare for signs of shock and/or infection after removal of fluids and fetus.

ACTIVITY
Limited by inability of dam to move.

DIET
N/A

CLIENT EDUCATION
Mares that appear excessively large for stage of gestation should be evaluated, particularly if signs of systemic disease or disability develop.

SURGICAL CONSIDERATIONS
• Induction of parturition
• Caesarean section, but keep in mind that fetal survival is uncommon/unlikely

MEDICATIONS

DRUG(S) OF CHOICE
• Since most hydrops mares spontaneously abort, treatment should be directed at terminating the pregnancy
• The use of oxytocin is usually not effective since most of these mares will have uterine inertia (atony) due to the stretching of the uterine musculature
• During or soon after attempted slow, controlled drainage of allantoic fluid, treatment for hypotensive shock may be necessary:
  ○ Hypertonic saline solution 2–4 mL/kg (7.2%) IV (Bimeda Inc., Le Sueur, MN)
  ○ Hetastarch (colloids) 10 mL/kg IV (Hespan; Braun Medical Inc., Irvine, CA)
  ○ Plasma-Lyte A 30 mL/kg/h IV (Baxter Healthcare Corp., Deerfield, IL)

CONTRAINDICATIONS
N/A

PRECAUTIONS
N/A

POSSIBLE INTERACTIONS
N/A

ALTERNATIVE DRUGS
N/A

FOLLOW-UP

PATIENT MONITORING
• Once a diagnosis is made, termination of pregnancy is appropriate
• In a few rare cases that do not become dramatically enlarged until nearer term, the vertical depth of allantoic fluid can be monitored at weekly intervals, with delivery of a smaller than normal, but viable, foal
• It is imperative to monitor the dam for signs of respiratory distress, as well as for her general health and stability of her vital signs
• Fetal biophysical parameters, including serial recording of fetal heart rate (resting and notation of accelerations during periods of fetal activity)
• Serial measures of the combined thickness of the uterus and placenta at/near the cervical star and for areas of possible placental separation

PREVENTION/AVOIDANCE
• Hydrops amnion—breed to different sire once mare recovers from either controlled vaginal delivery or C-section
• Hydrops allantois—as the abnormal placentation may reflect ineffective placental attachment because of an abnormal endometrium, placentitis, or primary placental failure, rebreeding may result in a similar outcome
• Adventitious placentation has been reported in cattle and is an effort by the placenta to generate additional, however ineffective, sites for placental transfer (oxygen in, removal of fetal waste)

POSSIBLE COMPLICATIONS
• Loss of pregnancy
• Prepubic tendon rupture
• Rupture of ventral belly wall
• Maternal death

EXPECTED COURSE AND PROGNOSIS
• Prognosis for fetal survival is poor
• Prognosis for survival of the dam is guarded, if parturition is induced before more serious damage occurs
• Prognosis for future reproduction:
  ○ Guarded for a mare with a hydrops allantois as it is a reflection of insufficient placental attachment sites and more likely to be repeated with a subsequent pregnancy. If the breed permits embryo transfer, the mare could be flushed for embryos following breeding
  ○ Guarded for the pregnancy of a hydrops amnion mare. The recommendation would be for her to be bred to a different stallion once she has recovered from the delivery/abortion

MISCELLANEOUS

ASSOCIATED CONDITIONS
• Placentitis
• Adventitious placentation has been reported in cattle

AGE-RELATED FACTORS
Older, multiparous mares, but has been reported in all ages.

ZOONOTIC POTENTIAL
N/A

PREGNANCY/FERTILITY/BREEDING
A pregnancy-related condition.

SYNONYMS
N/A

SEE ALSO
• Dystocia
• Placental basics
• Placental insufficiency
• Placentitis
• Premature placental separation

ABBREVIATIONS
• CA = chorioallantoic
• GI = gastrointestinal
• PCV = packed cell volume
• TRP = transrectal palpation
• US = ultrasonography, ultrasound

Suggested Reading
Baker LP, Bridges ER, Lovelady A. Hydrops allantois in a mare with twin pregnancy. Clin Theriogenol 2016;8(3):368.
Canisso IF, Schnobrich MR. Disorders of the reproductive tract: hydrops of the fetal membranes. In: Reed SM, Bayly WM, Sellon DC, eds, Equine Internal Medicine. St. Louis, MO: Elsevier, 2018: 1289–1290.
Christensen BW, Troedsson MH, Murchie TA, et al. Management of hydrops amnion in a mare resulting in birth of a live foal. J Am Vet Med Assoc 2006;228(8):1228–1233.
Honnas CH, Spensley MS, Laverty S, Blanchard PC. Hydramnios causing uterine rupture in a mare. J Am Vet Med Assoc 1988;193:332–336.
Löfstedt RM. Abnormalities of Pregnancy. In: McKinnon AO, Squires EL, Vaala WE, Varner DD, eds. Equine Reproduction, 2e. Philadelphia, PA: Wiley-Blackwell, 2011:2441–2445.
Morrison MJW, Back B, McClure JT, et al. Hydroallantois and prepubic tendon rupture in a Standardbred mare. Clin Theriogenol 2016;8(3):359.
Shanahan LM, Slovis NM. Leptospira interrogans associated with hydrallantois in 2 pluriparous Thoroughbred mares. J Vet Intern Med 2011;25(1):158–161.
Vandeplassche M, Bouters R, Spincemaille J, Bonte P. Dropsy of the fetal sacs in the mare: induced and spontaneous abortion. Vet Rec 1976;99:67–69.
Waelchli RO. Hydrops. In: McKinnon AO, Squires EL, Vaala WE, Varner DD, eds. Equine Reproduction. Wiley-Blackwell, 2011:2368–2372.

Author Carla L. Carleton
Consulting Editor Carla L. Carleton

H

HYPERKALEMIC PERIODIC PARALYSIS

BASICS

DEFINITION
An inherited muscle disease, affecting Quarter Horses and related breeds, resulting in sporadic episodes of muscle tremors or paralysis.

PATHOPHYSIOLOGY
Caused by a point mutation in skeletal muscle sodium channel.

SYSTEMS AFFECTED
• Neuromuscular
• Respiratory
• Cardiovascular
• Ophthalmic

GENETICS
• Autosomal dominant trait
• Linked to Quarter Horse stallion named "Impressive"

INCIDENCE/PREVALENCE
Approximately 4% of Quarter Horses.

GEOGRAPHIC DISTRIBUTION
Worldwide

SIGNALMENT
• Quarter Horses or Quarter Horse-related breeds that are descendants of a sire or dam with the genetic mutation
• Horses with hypertrophied muscles. Clinical signs usually noted by 2–3 years of age

SIGNS
• Asymptomatic to daily muscle fasciculations and weakness
• In mild disease—muscle fasciculations in flanks, neck, shoulders, and/or facial muscle spasm and generalized muscle tension
• In severe disease—severe muscle cramping, weakness with swaying, staggering, dog sitting, or recumbency, ± tachycardia
• Third eyelid prolapse
• Tachypnea, respiratory stridor, or distress
• Death

CAUSES
Genetic mutation—phenylalanine/leucine substitution in skeletal muscle sodium channel causing excessive inward flux of sodium and outward flux of potassium, resulting in persistent depolarization and muscle weakness.

RISK FACTORS
• Sudden dietary change or ingestion of feeds high in potassium (>1.1%) (e.g. alfalfa hay, molasses, electrolyte supplements, kelp-based supplements), fasting, anesthesia or heavy sedation, trailer rides, and stress
• Exercise does not stimulate clinical signs, may relieve them

DIAGNOSIS

DIFFERENTIAL DIAGNOSIS
• Differentials for clinical signs—colic, exertional rhabdomyolysis, tetanus, botulism, laminitis, seizures, upper airway obstruction
• Differentials for hyperkalemia—delay before serum centrifugation, hemolysis, ruptured bladder, chronic renal failure, severe rhabdomyolysis

CBC/BIOCHEMISTRY/URINALYSIS
• Hyperkalemia (6–9 mEq/L) during an episode
• Hemoconcentration
• Hyponatremia
• ± Serum creatine kinase mildly increased

OTHER LABORATORY TESTS
DNA testing of mane or tail hair samples (including hair bulb) or whole blood (EDTA).

IMAGING
N/A

OTHER DIAGNOSTIC PROCEDURES
Electromyography between episodes reveals abnormalities.

PATHOLOGIC FINDINGS
N/A

TREATMENT

APPROPRIATE HEALTH CARE
• ± Spontaneous recovery in 20 min
• Early mild episodes may be halted using low-grade exercise or feeding grain or corn syrup to stimulate insulin-mediated movement of potassium across cell membranes
• With severe signs, aggressive medical therapy may be needed

NURSING CARE
N/A

ACTIVITY
Regular exercise and/or frequent access to a large paddock.

DIET
• Low dietary potassium (0.6–1.1% of total ration)
• Small meals of low-potassium diets (grass hay—later cuts of Timothy or Bermuda; grains—oats, corn, wheat, barley, beet pulp)
• Commercial complete feeds for hyperkalemic periodic paralysis

CLIENT EDUCATION
Dietary management as above.

SURGICAL CONSIDERATIONS
With severe respiratory obstruction, ± tracheostomy.

MEDICATIONS

DRUG(S) OF CHOICE
• During an episode, epinephrine (3 mL/500 kg 1:1000 formulation IM)
• In severe cases, IV calcium gluconate (0.2–0.4 mL/kg 23% solution diluted in 1 L of 5% dextrose) or IV dextrose (6 mL/kg of a 5% solution) alone or combined with sodium bicarbonate (1–2 mEq/kg)
• If clinical signs cannot be controlled with dietary changes, acetazolamide (2–4 mg/kg PO every 8–12 h) or hydrochlorothiazide (0.5–1 mg/kg PO every 12 h)

CONTRAINDICATIONS
N/A

PRECAUTIONS
Anesthesia or heavy sedation may precipitate signs.

POSSIBLE INTERACTIONS
Glucocorticoids may be contraindicated in susceptible horses as they induce episodes in humans with similar disorders.

ALTERNATIVE DRUGS
N/A

FOLLOW-UP

PATIENT MONITORING
• Serum potassium concentrations are usually normal between episodes
• Success of therapy is based on the absence of clinical signs
• Affected horses require frequent monitoring for clinical signs

PREVENTION/AVOIDANCE
See Treatment and Medications.
• Avoid high-potassium feeds (alfalfa hay, brome hay, canola oil, soybean meal or oil, sugar and beet molasses)
• General anesthesia appears to be a risk
• Owners should be discouraged from breeding these animals

POSSIBLE COMPLICATIONS
• Death during acute severe episodes
• Respiratory distress due to paralysis of upper respiratory muscles
• ± Aspiration pneumonia due to laryngeal dysfunction, particularly in foals
• ± Cardiac arrhythmias (ventricular fibrillation)

EXPECTED COURSE AND PROGNOSIS
• Prognosis for most is good with low-potassium diet ± diuretic therapy
• ± Recurrence of clinical signs
• Severe episodes may be fatal

MISCELLANEOUS

AGE-RELATED FACTORS
N/A

ZOONOTIC POTENTIAL
N/A

PREGNANCY/FERTILITY/BREEDING
Owners should be discouraged from breeding affected horses.

SYNONYMS
N/A

SEE ALSO
Polysaccharide storage myopathy

Suggested Reading
MacLeay JM. Diseases of the musculoskeletal system. In: Reed SM, Bayly WM, Sellon DC, eds. Equine Internal Medicine, 3e. St. Louis, MO: WB Saunders, 2010:506–508.

Author Anna M. Firshman
Consulting Editor Elizabeth J. Davidson

HYPERLIPIDEMIA/HYPERLIPEMIA

 BASICS

DEFINITION
• *Hyperlipidemia* refers to elevated blood concentrations of lipids including TG or cholesterol
• *Hypertriglyceridemia* refers to abnormally high serum or plasma TG concentrations
• *Equine hyperlipemia* is a clinical condition characterized by markedly increased serum TG concentrations (>500 mg/dL), depression, anorexia, and organ dysfunction
• Mild hyperlipidemia is an incidental finding in healthy nursing foals and results from normal chylomicron production after feeding
• Congenital hyperlipidemia characterized by marked hyperlipidemia can occur in newborn foals born to mares affected by EH prior to parturition
• DM is a cause of EH. Aged horses should be tested for PPID if DM is detected. Hypertriglyceridemia often improves with pergolide treatment
• Rarely, hypertriglyceridemia is detected in healthy animals; these may be hereditary hyperlipidemia cases

PATHOPHYSIOLOGY
• Negative energy balance stimulates lipolysis within adipose tissues, causing mobilization of FFAs (also called nonesterified fatty acids) and glycerol
• Lipolysis is catalyzed by HSL. Glucagon, glucocorticoids, catecholamines, and growth hormone increase HSL activity, whereas insulin inhibits it
• Mobilization of FFAs from adipose tissues is a normal physiologic response to negative energy balance
• EH is driven by excessive mobilization of FFAs from adipose tissue TG stores and is caused by an overabundance of substrate (i.e. TG) in the obese animal and ID
• Insulin normally inhibits the activity of HSL after feeding
• Most circulating FFAs are removed from the blood by the liver and serve as substrates for energy production or are esterified to TG. In turn, TG is stored within hepatocytes or packaged into VLDLs and exported to other tissues via the blood. The transported TG is hydrolyzed by LPL into FFAs, which are used as a source of energy
• If a high rate of lipolysis within adipose tissue persists, blood FFA concentrations rise and uptake of FFAs into the liver accelerates. Rates of TG-rich VLDL synthesis and export substantially increase, accumulation of TG-rich VLDL within the blood (i.e. hyperlipidemia) develops as hepatic production exceeds the clearance by LPL
• In severe cases, accumulation of TG within the liver results in hepatic lipidosis and TG

deposits in other tissues, causing fatty infiltration followed by organ dysfunction. A vicious cycle then develops as elevated serum TG concentrations further suppress appetite

SYSTEMS AFFECTED
• Endocrine/metabolic
• Hemic
• Hepatobiliary
• Renal
• GI

GENETICS
There is a genetic component of EMS in Arabians, Morgans, and Welsh ponies and this may also contribute to a predisposition towards hyperlipidemia

INCIDENCE/PREVALENCE
Low—dependent upon the breed of horse and feeding practices.

GEOGRAPHIC DISTRIBUTION
N/A

SIGNALMENT
• Breeds—ponies, miniature horses, and donkeys
• Occurs at all ages
• Foals may be born with congenital hyperlipidemia
• Mares are more susceptible during pregnancy and lactation
• Aged horses with PPID can develop hyperlipidemia more readily if DM is present

SIGNS
• Early signs are nonspecific—lethargy, inappetence, and depression
• As the disease progresses, patients cease eating and drinking. Fetid, fat-covered feces (steatorrhea) are produced (eventually in the form of diarrhea). Clinical signs associated with organ dysfunction may develop, including neurologic signs consistent with hepatic encephalopathy (depression, head pressing, ataxia, and sham drinking)
• Mild colic caused by stretching of the liver capsule may be observed
• Pregnant mares may abort
• Polyuria/polydipsia is reported when DM and/or PPID are present
• Newborn foals with congenital hyperlipemia are normal in appearance

CAUSES
• Negative energy balance, particularly in obese animals
• Recent stress

RISK FACTORS
• Breeds—ponies, donkeys, and miniature horses
• EMS
• PPID
• Pregnancy
• Stress
• Concurrent disease

• Endotoxemia
• Parasitism
• Lactation

 DIAGNOSIS

DIFFERENTIAL DIAGNOSIS
• Acute infectious diseases with nonspecific signs of depression and inappetence
• Hepatic, neurologic, or GI disease

CBC/BIOCHEMISTRY/URINALYSIS
Note that markedly elevated blood lipid concentrations may interfere with analyzer functions, particularly biochemical analysis.
• When the TG concentration is >500 mg/dL, it is not possible to read newsprint through the tube of a gravity-sedimented or centrifuged plasma sample
• TG concentrations may be reported in mmol/L and the conversion factor is approximately 89 (500 mg/dL = 5.6 mmol/L)
• Reference range for adult horses is 11–65 mg/dL. Higher concentrations are detected in healthy donkeys and pregnant ponies
• Hypoglycemia or hyperglycemia
• Increased total bilirubin, γ-glutamyltransferase, alkaline phosphatase, aspartate aminotransferase, and sorbitol dehydrogenase
• Azotemia with normal urinalysis. Blood urea nitrogen may be lower than expected because of hepatic failure
• Metabolic acidosis may be detected

OTHER LABORATORY TESTS
• Elevated serum insulin concentration or a low insulin to glucose ratio
• ID detected using the oral sugar test or other glucose or insulin tolerance tests
• Elevated blood ammonia concentration if hepatic lipidosis
• Elevated serum bile acid concentration if hepatic lipidosis
• Prolonged coagulation profile—advanced liver failure
• Diagnostic evaluation for PPID

IMAGING
Ultrasonography—liver enlargement and alterations in echogenicity are associated with hepatic lipidosis.

OTHER DIAGNOSTIC PROCEDURES
Liver biopsy to confirm hepatic lipidosis in advanced cases.

PATHOLOGIC FINDINGS
• Findings are consistent with fatty infiltration of tissues
• Pituitary hyperplasia or adenoma(s) may be present in older horses

(CONTINUED)   **HYPERLIPIDEMIA/HYPERLIPEMIA**

TREATMENT

APPROPRIATE HEALTH CARE
• In mild cases detected early, appropriate care can be provided on the farm
• Patient assessment is based on plasma/serum TG concentrations, duration of inappetence, and seriousness of concurrent disease conditions
• Provide treatment early in the course of disease
• Hospitalize severely affected patients immediately

NURSING CARE
Increase Feed Intake
• Mildly affected patients improve as their feed intake increases
• Provide a large variety of feedstuffs or treats until a preferred diet is identified
• Provide access to pasture.

Enteral and Parenteral Feeding
• A commercial enteral diet can be used for smaller patients
• Liquid preparations of alfalfa meal or soaked, pelleted feedstuffs with added dextrose can be administered via nasogastric tube. Administer small quantities frequently (as often as every 4 h)

IV Fluid/Nutritional Support
• Administer 5–10% dextrose within polyionic fluids as a continuous infusion. An initial rate of 60 mL/kg body weight per day is recommended
• Ideally, blood glucose measurements and urine dipstick testing should be used to establish a rate that minimizes renal overflow of glucose. Administer insulin if blood glucose concentrations exceed 200 mg/dL
• Partial parenteral nutrition can be provided using a solution composed of 50% dextrose and amino acids

ACTIVITY
No specific restrictions but minimize stress.

DIET
See Nursing Care.

CLIENT EDUCATION
• Clients should seek veterinary advice if inappetence develops in at-risk equids
• Obesity as a serious predisposing factor, particularly in pregnant animals

SURGICAL CONSIDERATIONS
N/A

MEDICATIONS

DRUG(S) OF CHOICE
Insulin
• Administer if blood glucose concentrations are above 200 mg/dL

• If dextrose is being administered IV, a constant rate infusion of regular (short-acting) insulin is prepared by adding 10 mL (100 IU/mL) Humulin R® to a 1 L bag of fluids and administering IV to effect (maintain blood glucose <200 mg/dL)
• Intermediate-acting insulin can be administered SC at a starting dosage of 0.10 IU/kg every 8–12 h

Heparin Sulfate
• Potentiates LPL activity. However, if LPL activity is already maximized, administration of heparin is ineffective
• Can be administered at a dose of 10–20 IU/kg body weight IV or SC TID
• Note that heparin lowers hematocrit levels and can inhibit hemostasis

Other Drugs
Pergolide should be administered to equids with PPID. It may be necessary to increase the dose in patients that are already receiving treatment. Starting dosage for pergolide is 0.002 mg/kg PO every 24 h. Treatment should be initiated if DM and hyperlipidemia are detected, even in anorexic patients.

CONTRAINDICATIONS
• Insulin administration in hypoglycemic patients
• Use of heparin sulfate in patients that may require surgery (e.g. cesarean section)
• Corticosteroids are contraindicated as they can exacerbate ID and lipolysis

PRECAUTIONS
Monitor blood glucose concentrations.

POSSIBLE INTERACTIONS
N/A

ALTERNATIVE DRUGS
N/A

FOLLOW-UP

PATIENT MONITORING
Repeated measurement of serum TG concentration.

PREVENTION/AVOIDANCE
• Maintain appropriate body condition (avoid obesity)
• Minimize stressful conditions for high-risk breeds, particularly when metabolic demands are high—pregnancy or lactation
• Early intervention when feed intake is reduced

POSSIBLE COMPLICATIONS
Liver and renal failure.

EXPECTED COURSE AND PROGNOSIS
• The course of this disease is rapid
• Mildly affected patients can recover quickly if the negative energy balance is reversed
• Prognosis is fair. Severely affected patients with signs of organ failure or neurologic deficits have a poorer prognosis

• Mortality rates of 57–85% have been reported, but these figures do not reflect recent advances in the treatment of this disorder. Patients may be successfully managed with IV dextrose and insulin treatment

MISCELLANEOUS

ASSOCIATED CONDITIONS
• Hepatic lipidosis and subsequent liver failure
• Hepatic encephalopathy
• Renal failure

AGE-RELATED FACTORS
N/A

ZOONOTIC POTENTIAL
N/A

PREGNANCY/FERTILITY/BREEDING
In pregnant animals, organ failure, metabolic acidosis, and stress may compromise the fetus, resulting in abortion.

SYNONYMS
• Hyperlipoproteinemia
• Hypertriglyceridemia

SEE ALSO
• Equine metabolic syndrome (EMS)/insulin resistance (IR)
• Hepatic encephalopathy
• Pituitary pars intermedia dysfunction

ABBREVIATIONS
• DM = diabetes mellitus
• EH = equine hyperlipemia
• EMS = equine metabolic syndrome
• FFA = free fatty acid
• GI = gastrointestinal
• HSL = hormone-sensitive lipase
• ID = insulin dysregulation
• LPL = lipoprotein lipase
• PPID = pituitary pars intermedia dysfunction
• TG = triglyceride
• VLDL = very-low-density lipoprotein

Suggested Reading
Dunkel B, Wilford SA, Parkinson NJ, et al. Severe hypertriglyceridaemia in horses and ponies with endocrine disorders. Equine Vet J 2014;46:118–122.
McKenzie 3rd HC. Equine hyperlipidemias. Vet Clin North Am Equine Pract 2011;27:59–72.
Waitt LH, Cebra CK. Characterization of hypertriglyceridemia and response to treatment with insulin in horses, ponies, and donkeys: 44 cases (1995-2005). J Am Vet Med Assoc 2009;234:915–919.

Author Nicholas Frank
Consulting Editors Michel Levy and Heidi Banse

H

HYPERTHERMIA

 BASICS

DEFINITION
• An abnormally high body temperature in which the hypothalamic temperature setpoint is not altered but the heat-dissipating mechanisms are overwhelmed or fail.
• Different from a fever, in which the body temperature is elevated because of upward resetting of the setpoint with the heat-dissipating mechanisms usually remaining intact. • Heat stroke occurs when hyperthermia is combined with CNS dysfunction. • Exertional heat illness, or post-race distress syndrome, is a severe hyperthermic state in performance horses that occurs following exercise in adverse environmental conditions and results in CNS and GI system dysfunction

PATHOPHYSIOLOGY
• The normal physiologic body temperature is set by the hypothalamic thermoregulatory center at 37.5–38.5°C (99.5–101.5°F). • With hyperthermia, mechanisms of heat dissipation are overwhelmed or inadequate. • Body heat is generated by metabolic processes, working muscles, and absorption of solar radiation. • During exercise, massive heat loads are produced by muscles. In the horse, approximately 80% of energy expended is in the form of heat. • Heat can be dissipated by conduction, convection, radiation, and evaporation. • Horses have a low surface area to body mass ratio and an insulating haircoat. Loss of heat is primarily evaporative through sweating and breathing. • Heat can also be dissipated in part by transfer of heat from the body surface through convection and radiation. • Heat from the body core is conducted to the cooler surface tissues by circulation of blood. • A body temperature >39.5°C (103°F) can be considered hyperthermia. • A body temperature >41–42°C (106–108°F) leads to heat denaturation of cellular proteins. • The CNS is most sensitive to hyperthermic damage. As the temperature continues to increase and/or persist, other organs and systems also become affected, leading to MODS-L. • Decreased perfusion of the GI tract as blood is shunted to muscles and the periphery can lead to translocation of bacteria and endotoxins, resulting in systemic signs of endotoxemia and systemic inflammatory response syndrome. • Profuse sweating during hyperthermia results in loss of water and electrolytes, leading to dehydration and metabolic derangements

SYSTEMS AFFECTED
All systems are susceptible to damage by hyperthermia.

GENETICS
Genetic predisposition to hyperthermia and rhabdomyolysis during anesthesia (i.e. MH).

INCIDENCE/PREVALENCE
Greater in hot, humid weather.

GEOGRAPHIC DISTRIBUTION
Any area, especially those that have hot, humid weather.

SIGNALMENT
• Breeds with a higher body size to skin ratio have increased heat production and a smaller surface area for heat dissipation.
• Dark-colored haircoats (increased absorption of radiant heat). • Long, thick haircoat (reduces evaporative and conductive heat loss)

SIGNS
Historical Findings
• Excessive sweating or lack of sweating. • Prolonged muscular exertion (endurance rides). • Maximal exercise in warm/humid environmental conditions. • Weakness. • Stilted gait. • Fatigue. • Depression. • Impaired performance. • Respiratory distress. • Seizures. • Anesthesia. • Transport. • Foal on macrolide antibiotic

Physical Examination Findings
• Elevated temperature associated with dyspnea, tachypnea, tachyarrhythmia, and tachycardia. • Parameters remain elevated in spite of exercise cessation. • Excessive, patchy, or lack of sweating. • Dull mentation. • Weakness. • Congested mucous membranes. • Prolonged capillary refill time. • Dehydration. • Dilated cutaneous vasculature. • Muscle rigidity. • Ataxia. • SDF. • Colic. • Ileus. • Signs of endotoxemia. • Seizures. • Collapse

CAUSES
• Excessive muscular activity, prolonged work. • Maximal exercise in warm/humid environmental conditions. • Generalized seizures. • Hypocalcemic tetany associated with transit or lactation. • Drugs—macrolides, halothane anesthesia (i.e. MH), phenothiazine tranquilizers, furosemide. • Endophyte-infested tall fescue. • Anhidrosis. • Confinement in closed trailers or buildings during hot weather

RISK FACTORS
• Poor physical fitness, insufficient conditioning, and lack of acclimatization. • High ambient temperature, especially >30°C (86°F), and high relative humidity. • No air movement and high solar radiation. • Dehydration—no access to drinking water during work. • Anhidrosis. • Foal on macrolide antibiotic, especially in hot ambient temperatures and exposed to direct solar heat. • Large body mass relative to body surface area. • Long haircoat (i.e. PPID). • Obesity. • Airway disease (cannot dissipate heat). • Possible risk of hyperthermia during anesthesia of horses with HYPP. • MH genetic predilection. • Halothane anesthesia

 DIAGNOSIS

DIFFERENTIAL DIAGNOSIS
• Fever from infectious, inflammatory, and neoplastic diseases (usually does not exceed 41°C or 106°F). • Rule out heaves (severe equine asthma), anhidrosis, exertional rhabdomyolysis, and PPID

CBC/BIOCHEMISTRY/URINALYSIS
• CBC—stress, hemoconcentration. • Biochemistry—elevated creatine kinase and aspartate aminotransferase with exertional rhabdomyolysis. • Decreased Ca^{2+}, Mg^{2+}. • Sodium can be increased or decreased. • Increased or decreased K^+. • Metabolic alkalosis or acidosis. • Respiratory alkalosis with hyperventilation. • Azotemia with dehydration, elevated renal and hepatic enzymes with organ damage. • Urinalysis (may be oliguric)—concentrated urine; possibly myoglobinuria

OTHER LABORATORY TESTS
• Intradermal epinephrine/terbutaline test for decreased sweating—anhidrosis. • Genetic marker blood test for HYPP or MH. • Blood gas disorders—possible alkalosis or acidosis. • Clotting profile—development of DIC, liver failure, thrombocytopenia, prolonged clotting time, and elevated fibrinogen degradation products. • Halothane—caffeine contracture test to identify individuals with MH

IMAGING
N/A

OTHER DIAGNOSTIC PROCEDURES
N/A

PATHOLOGIC FINDINGS
N/A

 TREATMENT

APPROPRIATE HEALTH CARE
Immediate emergency management on farm then, depending on severity, may require inpatient medical management.

NURSING CARE
• Provide shade or remove from direct sunlight. • Enhance cooling through fans or misting fans. • Repeatedly applying copious cold water can promote rapid cooling. Between applications of water, use sweat scraper to remove warmed water from haircoat. • Monitor rectal temperature and continue cooling until <40°C (104°F) for at least 30 min. • Correct dehydration by

providing drinking water if patient is not critical. • IV saline, lactated Ringer's solution to restore blood volume and perfusion. • Identify and correct electrolyte and acid–base derangements. Oral and IV sources of K^+, Na^+, Cl^-, Ca^{2+}, Mg^{2+} as indicated. • Clip long haircoat. • Identify and treat accordingly other conditions— rhabdomyolysis, renal failure. • SDF— administer 50–100 mL/L of 23% calcium borogluconate to isotonic fluids

ACTIVITY
Stop exercising/activity immediately.

DIET
Withhold feed until hyperthermia and relevant secondary complications (i.e. colic, ileus) are resolved.

CLIENT EDUCATION
• Ensure horses are acclimatized to high ambient temperature and humidity prior to prolonged or high exertional activity. • Ensure horses are hydrated and have ready access to water, especially during prolonged exercise. • If exercising in heat and humidity, ensure that cold water stations are readily available for rapid cooling of horses. If possible, avoid the hottest times of the day

SURGICAL CONSIDERATIONS
N/A

MEDICATIONS

DRUG(S) OF CHOICE
• NSAIDs, such as flunixin meglumine (1.1 mg/kg IV), may be used for their anti-inflammatory, antiendotoxic, and analgesic properties. Antipyretic properties of these drugs are not useful for nonpyrogenic hyperthermia. • Glucocorticoids have been used in other species and horses to decrease inflammation associated with heat damage and to aid in cell membrane stabilization; however, supportive research is sparse (dexamethasone 0.05–0.2 mg/kg IV). • Sedation may be necessary in many cases of hyperthermia, as horses become anxious, uncooperative, and/or dangerous to work around, thus making cooling efforts impossible. • Appropriate adjunctive therapy with rhabdomyolysis, muscle relaxants, anti-inflammatories. • MH, dantrolene sodium 10 mg/kg loading dose PO, then 2.5 mg/kg PO every 2 h

CONTRAINDICATIONS
Supplemental K^+ in cases of HYPP.

PRECAUTIONS
• Use NSAIDs cautiously in cases of renal compromise or dehydration. • Do not administer bicarbonate without knowing blood gas status. Note that these horses are most often alkalotic

POSSIBLE INTERACTIONS
N/A

ALTERNATIVE DRUGS
N/A

FOLLOW-UP

PATIENT MONITORING
• Monitor body temperature frequently. • Monitor renal function. • Assess hydration, packed cell volume, and total solids. • Assess response of electrolyte and blood gas adjustments

PREVENTION/AVOIDANCE
• A period of acclimation (recommend 15 days) to hot and humid conditions will help reduce the risk of heat-related disorders. • Condition animals appropriately for the level of work they are expected to do. • Avoid riding in hot and humid weather. • Identify MH and HYPP individuals prior to anesthesia. • Keep foals on macrolide antibiotics in a shaded, cool environment. • Clip long haircoats to improve evaporative heat loss

POSSIBLE COMPLICATIONS
• CNS disorders—seizures, coma, death. • MODS-L. • Renal and hepatic failure. • DIC. • Laminitis. • Pulmonary edema. • May be more prone to subsequent hyperthermia

EXPECTED COURSE AND PROGNOSIS
Favorable to grave—depending on early detection and reversal of hyperthermia, correction of dehydration and electrolyte derangements, and prevention of organ failure.

MISCELLANEOUS

ASSOCIATED CONDITIONS
N/A

AGE-RELATED FACTORS
N/A

ZOONOTIC POTENTIAL
N/A

PREGNANCY/FERTILITY/BREEDING
Abortions may occur with prolonged hyperthermia.

SYNONYMS
• Exertional heat illness. • Post-race distress syndrome. • Exhausted horse syndrome. • Heat exhaustion. • Heat stress. • Heat stroke

SEE ALSO
• Anhidrosis
• Exertional rhabdomyolysis syndrome
• Fever
• Hyperkalemic periodic paralysis
• Seizure disorders
• Synchronous diaphragmatic flutter

ABBREVIATIONS
• CNS = central nervous system
• DIC = disseminated intravascular coagulation
• GI = gastrointestinal
• HYPP = hyperkalemic periodic paralysis
• MH = malignant hyperthermia
• MODS-L = multiorgan dysfunction syndrome—laminitis
• NSAID = nonsteroidal anti-inflammatory drug
• PPID = pituitary pars intermediate dysfunction
• SDF = synchronous diaphragmatic flutter

Suggested Reading
Brownlow MA, Dart AJ, Jeffcott LB. Exertional heat illness: a review of the syndrome affecting racing Thoroughbreds in hot and humid climates. Aust Vet J 2016;94:240–247.
Cohn CW, Hinchcliff KW, McKeever KH. Evaluation of washing with cold water to facilitate heat dissipation in horses exercised in hot, humid conditions. Am J Vet Res 1999;60:299–305.
Hodgson DR, Davis RE, McConaghy FF. Thermoregulation in the horse in response to exercise. Br Vet J 1994;150:219–235.
McCutcheon LJ, Geor RJ. Thermoregulation and exercise-associated heat illnesses. In: Hinchcliff KW, Kaneps AJ, Goer RJ, eds. Equine Sports Medicine and Surgery, 2e. Philadelphia, PA: Saunders, 2013:901–918.

Author Ashley Whitehead
Consulting Editors Michel Levy and Heidi Banse
Acknowledgment The author and editors acknowledge the prior contribution of Wendy Duckett.

 Client Education Handout available online

H

HYPOXEMIA

 BASICS

DEFINITION
- Hypoxemia is a decreased amount of dissolved O_2 carried in blood
- PaO_2 <80 mmHg, PvO_2 <40 mmHg, or SO_2/SpO_2 <95% indicate hypoxemia

PATHOPHYSIOLOGY
- Hypoxemia may cause hypoxia, which is decreased O_2 delivery or utilization by tissues. Cellular function is adversely affected at a PaO_2 of <60 mmHg
- Hypoxia results from low levels of inspired O_2 (atmospheric hypoxia); impaired delivery of air to alveoli due to respiratory obstruction or failure of the lungs to inflate or deflate (tidal hypoxia); decreased alveolar function due to abnormal alveoli, pulmonary interstitium, or pulmonary blood flow (alveolar hypoxia); or abnormal hemoglobin function (hemoglobic hypoxia)
- More than one mechanism often is present
- Anemia may cause hypoxia, but does not cause hypoxemia

SYSTEMS AFFECTED
All (hypoxia).

GENETICS
N/A

INCIDENCE/PREVALENCE
N/A

GEOGRAPHIC DISTRIBUTION
At high altitudes, FIO_2, PaO_2, and SO_2 decrease.

SIGNALMENT
Any breed, age, or sex.

SIGNS

Historical Findings
History may include exercise intolerance, respiratory distress, coughing, lethargy, and other signs referable to the primary problem.

Physical Examination Findings
- Tachypnea, tachycardia, coughing, reluctance to move, abducted elbows, outstretched neck, nostril flare, fever
- Cyanosis develops when PaO_2 is <40 mmHg

CAUSES
- Diffusion impairment
  - Pneumonia (e.g. *Rhodococcus equi* in foals, aspiration, pleuropneumonia, esophageal rupture)
  - Pulmonary edema (e.g. smoke inhalation, anaphylaxis, cardiac failure, volume overload)
  - Interstitial disease (acute respiratory distress syndrome, mineral oil pneumonitis, silicosis, EMPF)
  - Severe equine asthma (i.e. heaves, recurrent airway obstruction)
  - Prematurity

- Hypoventilation (e.g. perinatal asphyxia, botulism, anesthesia, thoracic trauma, brainstem lesion). A PaO_2 <60 mmHg stimulates respiration and increases minute ventilation. This may correct hypercapnia but often does not improve O_2 levels because O_2 does not diffuse as quickly as CO_2 and is more dependent on the matching of blood flow to ventilation to maintain normal levels
- V/Q mismatch (e.g. pulmonary hypertension, systemic hypotension, atelectasis)
- Cardiac failure or right-to-left cardiac shunts (e.g. tetralogy of Fallot, truncus arteriosus, tricuspid atresia)
- High altitude reduces the inspired O_2 tension
- Methemoglobinemia (e.g. red maple leaf toxicity) may decrease SO_2, but does not directly affect PaO_2 and SpO_2

RISK FACTORS
- General anesthesia
- Foals born from dams with dystocia might develop perinatal asphyxia (hypoventilation)
- Foals on farms with endemic *R. equi*
- Young performance horses (e.g. racehorses) and horses that are trailered long distances are at higher risk of developing pleuropneumonia
- Infection with equine herpesvirus 5 is associated with development of EMPF
- Environmental dust and mold can trigger exacerbation of severe equine asthma

 DIAGNOSIS

DIFFERENTIAL DIAGNOSIS
See Causes.

LABORATORY FINDINGS

Disorders That May Alter Laboratory Results
- With poor peripheral perfusion or cardiovascular shunt, results of blood gas analysis on samples taken from peripheral arteries may not reflect the patient's overall systemic condition
- Falsely increased PO_2 results may occur with sample exposure to room air, excessive heparin dilution, and standard plastic syringes
- Falsely decreased PO_2 results may occur with delayed sample analysis, failure to adequately chill the sample, and severe neutrophilia

Valid if Run in a Human Laboratory?
Yes

CBC/BIOCHEMISTRY/URINALYSIS
N/A

OTHER LABORATORY TESTS
- Arterial blood gas analysis is the definitive method for documenting hypoxemia
  - Take a heparinized blood sample anaerobically, cap with a rubber stopper, and analyze within 15–20 min

- If the sample is stored on ice and collected in syringes dedicated for this use and containing powder heparin, results are valid for up to 3–4 h
- Blood lactate concentrations can be measured with a handheld analyzer; hyperlactatemia is consistent with hypoxia

IMAGING
Radiography or ultrasonography to evaluate cardiac and pulmonary disease.

OTHER DIAGNOSTIC PROCEDURES
- Pulse oximetry measures SpO_2
- The oximeter calculates the amount of oxygenated versus deoxygenated hemoglobin in blood based on light absorption
- Decreased blood flow to the area of oximeter probe attachment invalidates the results (e.g. hypotension, vasoconstriction, hypothermia)
- Oximeter probes can be used on the tongue of anesthetized horses
- Conscious horses require a nasal oximeter probe

 TREATMENT

Resolution of the primary cause of hypoxemia is paramount.

O_2 THERAPY
- O_2 therapy via nasal insufflation can be effective in elevating the PaO_2. Inspired concentrations are limited to 30–45% with nasal insufflation. Higher levels may be obtained via insufflation directly into the trachea
- Inspired gases must be humidified to avoid damage to mucous membranes from desiccation. This is accomplished by use of a humidifier or passing the O_2 through a bottle of sterile water before exposure to the airway. The bottle must be secured in an upright position to prevent inspiration of fluid
- To avoid O_2 toxicity, maintain the FIO_2 at the lowest level that produces a PO_2 of >80 mmHg. If insufflation eliminates hypoxemia, $PaCO_2$ levels may increase if the low PO_2 was the primary stimulus of respiratory drive
- Begin insufflation at 3–5 L/min in foals and 5–10 L/min in adults
- Not useful if right-to-left cardiac shunt, persistent fetal circulation, or severe V/Q mismatch is present

Postural Therapy and Thoracic Percussion
- Helpful to improve ventilation and drainage of secretions, especially in foals
- Maintenance in sternal recumbency helps prevent atelectasis; turning every few hours is necessary for those in lateral recumbency

Mechanical Ventilation
- Necessary in patients with severe hypoventilation ($PaCO_2$ persistently

>65 mmHg) and hypoxemia, and feasible in foals and anesthetized adults
• Conscious foals can be intubated nasotracheally and connected to the rebreathing circuit of a small-animal anesthesia machine or a human ventilator
• 2 flowmeters (or one that allows mixing of O_2 and room air) are necessary, as is a monitor that can measure the FIO_2 level
• Assisted rather than controlled ventilation is better, because most foals are more comfortable when respiratory drive is not eliminated
• Sedation may be necessary in some patients but many relax once ventilation improves
• Periodic suctioning of the nasotracheal tube is necessary to prevent obstruction from accumulated secretions
• After weaning from mechanical ventilation, temporary nasal insufflation of O_2 is recommended in foals because their functional residual capacity will decrease and hypoxemia may recur

MEDICATIONS

DRUG(S) OF CHOICE
Dependent on the underlying cause.

CONTRAINDICATIONS
• Do not use doxapram to improve respiratory function in healthy anesthetized patients, especially during weaning. Its effects are temporary, and if the patient's PaO_2 levels are low or the patient remains depressed once it wears off, apnea may occur
• Mechanical ventilation for meconium aspiration might cause alveolar damage because of air-trapping behind obstructed bronchioles

PRECAUTIONS
• Do not allow combustible materials or smoking near the patient or the O_2 tanks
• Securely attach tanks to an immovable structure because they can rupture or explode violently if knocked over. Wear safety glasses and keep face out of range of the valves during setup and disconnection
• Use aseptic techniques in handling endotracheal tubes
• Use fluid therapy carefully in neonates, cardiac patients, and patients with renal failure to avoid volume overload
• O_2 toxicity can occur with administration of >50% FIO_2 or maintenance of a PaO_2 >100 mmHg for long periods

• O_2 therapy may decrease the ventilator response and worsen hypoventilation

POSSIBLE INTERACTIONS
N/A

ALTERNATIVE DRUGS
N/A

FOLLOW-UP

PATIENT MONITORING
• Serial arterial blood gas evaluations
• Pulse oximetry can be used to monitor hemoglobin saturation
• As PaO_2 improves, provide decreasing levels of FIO_2. Eventually, periodic trials on room air can be attempted
• Evaluate patient demeanor and degree or quality of respiratory effort as blood gas levels change. When the patient can maintain a PO_2 of >70 mmHg (>60 mmHg in premature neonates) on room air, O_2 therapy can be discontinued

PREVENTION/AVOIDANCE
N/A

POSSIBLE COMPLICATIONS
• Damage to nervous tissue from prolonged periods of hypoxemia may result in brain damage (e.g. altered consciousness, blindness, seizures)
• Cardiac arrhythmias may be caused by hypoxemic damage to the myocardium

EXPECTED COURSE AND PROGNOSIS
Dependent on the underlying cause.

MISCELLANEOUS

ASSOCIATED CONDITIONS
Metabolic acidosis caused by accumulation of lactic acid from anaerobic glycolysis may develop with prolonged hypoxemia, especially if hypotension exists.

AGE-RELATED FACTORS
• Neonatal foals normally have lower PaO_2 (<60 mmHg) and higher $PaCO_2$ (>50 mmHg) values during the first hour of life. PaO_2 values increase to >80 mmHg by 2–4 days. $PaCO_2$ values decrease to adult reference intervals by 4–7 days

• Premature neonates are highly predisposed to hypoxemia

PREGNANCY/BREEDING/FERTILITY
• Heavily pregnant mares are at greater risk of hypoxemia under general anesthesia
• Prolonged hypoxemia during gestation may result in fetal growth retardation and perinatal asphyxia

SEE ALSO
• Acidosis, respiratory
• Equine herpesvirus 5
• Heaves (severe equine asthma, RAO)
• Neonatal maladjustment syndrome
• Pleuropneumonia
• Pneumonia, neonate

ABBREVIATIONS
• EMPF = equine multinodular pulmonary fibrosis
• FIO_2 = percent fractional inspired oxygen concentration
• $PaCO_2$ = partial pressure of arterial carbon dioxide tension, mmHg
• PaO_2 = partial pressure of arterial oxygen tension, mmHg
• PvO_2 = partial pressure of venous oxygen tension, mmHg
• SO_2 = percent hemoglobin saturation with oxygen
• SpO_2 = percent hemoglobin saturation with oxygen in peripheral tissues (pulse oximetry)
• V/Q = ventilation–perfusion ratio

Suggested Reading
Bettschart-Wolfensberger R. Anesthesia and analgesia for domestic species: horses. In: Grimm KA, Lamont LA, Tranquilli WJ, et al., eds. Veterinary Anesthesia and Analgesia, 5e. Ames, IA: Wiley Blackwell, 2015:857–866.
McDonnell WN, Kerr CL. Respiratory system: physiology, pathophysiology, and anesthetic management of patients with respiratory disease. In: Grimm KA, Lamont LA, Tranquilli WJ, et al., eds. Veterinary Anesthesia and Analgesia, 5e. Ames, IA: Wiley Blackwell, 2015:513–558.
Palmer J. Ventilatory support of the critically ill foal. Vet Clin North Am Equine Pract 2005;21:457–486.

Author Katie M. Boes
Consulting Editor Sandra D. Taylor
Acknowledgment The author and editor acknowledge the prior contribution of Jennifer G. Adams.

H

ICTERUS (PREHEPATIC, HEPATIC, POSTHEPATIC)

 ## BASICS

DEFINITION
Icterus is caused by hyperbilirubinemia with bilirubin deposition in tissues and is characterized by yellow discoloration of the sclerae, nonpigmented skin, and mucous membranes.

PATHOPHYSIOLOGY
• Bilirubin, from heme breakdown, is converted to biliverdin and then to unconjugated bilirubin, bound to plasma albumin for transfer to the liver, then conjugated by hepatocytes. • Conjugated bilirubin is secreted into bile and enters the intestine, where most is converted to urobilinogen. • Hyperbilirubinemia can result from increased bilirubin production, impaired hepatic uptake or conjugation, or impaired excretion

SYSTEMS AFFECTED
• Skin—bilirubin has an affinity for elastic tissues; thus icterus is most evident in the sclerae and vulva. • Hepatobiliary—accumulated bilirubin may contribute to hepatocellular injury, cholestasis. • Renal—bile casts may cause tubular injury. • Nervous—bilirubin accumulation may cause degenerative lesions (e.g. kernicterus)

SIGNS
• Depression. • Anorexia. • Severely altered mentation—HE due to hypoglycemia, hyperammonemia, decreased BCAA:AAA ratio. • Weight loss—anorexia, failure of hepatic metabolic functions in chronic hepatic insufficiency. • Acute or recurrent subacute abdominal pain—hepatic swelling or biliary obstruction (e.g. cholelithiasis)

Less Frequent
• Photodermatitis—phylloerythrin accumulation in skin. • Diarrhea—altered intestinal microflora, portal hypertension with chronic hepatic insufficiency. • Bleeding diathesis—inadequate hepatic synthesis of clotting factors. • Dependent edema—hypoalbuminemia or portal hypertension

CAUSES

Prehepatic/Hemolytic Icterus
• Intra- and/or extravascular hemolysis or massive intracorporeal hemorrhage; rate of bilirubin production exceeds hepatic conjugation and excretion. • Oxidative injury—red maple (*Acer rubrum*), wild onion (*Allium* spp.), phenothiazine toxicosis, nitrate poisoning. • Immune mediated—neonatal isoerythrolysis, IMHA (secondary to *Clostridium perfringens* septicemia, purpura haemorrhagica, lymphosarcoma, penicillin administration, etc.), disseminated intravascular coagulation. • Infectious—EIA, EVA, piroplasmosis, anaplasmosis, leptospirosis. • Iatrogenic—DMSO (>10%)

IV, hypotonic/hypertonic fluids, blood transfusion. • Miscellaneous—snake venom, bee/wasp venom, erythrocytosis

Hepatic/Retention Icterus
Impaired hepatic uptake and/or conjugation of bilirubin.

Hepatic Causes—Hepatic Icterus
Acute Hepatic Diseases—Adults
• Bacterial—cholangiohepatitis, endotoxemia, infectious necrotic hepatitis (*Clostridium novyi* type B). • Viral—EIA, EVA, serum hepatitis (Theiler's disease-associated virus). • Parasitic—migration of *Strongylus equinus* and *Strongylus edentatus, S. equinus* thromboembolic disease. • Toxic—arsenic, carbon tetrachloride, chlorinated hydrocarbons, monensin, pentachlorophenols, phenol, phosphorus, paraquat, aflatoxin, rubratoxin. • Drugs—anabolic steroids, erythromycin
Acute Hepatic Diseases—Foals
• Bacterial—Tyzzer's disease (*Clostridium piliforme*), septicemia, endotoxemia. • Viral—equine herpesvirus 1. • Parasitic—*Parascaris equorum*, strongyles. • Toxic—ferrous fumarate, toxins listed for adults
Chronic Hepatic Diseases—Adults
• Idiopathic—chronic active hepatitis. • Bacterial—hepatic abscessation. • Metabolic—hyperlipemia. • Neoplastic—primary (e.g. cholangiocarcinoma, hepatocellular carcinoma) or secondary (e.g. lymphosarcoma). • Immunologic—amyloidosis. • Toxic—chronic megalocytic hepatopathy due to pyrrolizidine alkaloids
Chronic Hepatic Diseases—Foals
• Bacterial—hepatic abscessation secondary to septicemia or omphalophlebitis. • Neoplastic—mixed hamartoma

Extrahepatic Causes—Hepatic Icterus
• Anorexia. • Heparin administration. • Prematurity

Posthepatic/Obstructive Icterus
Partial or complete obstruction of biliary tree that decreases excretion of conjugated bilirubin; usually accompanied by bilirubinuria. • Adults—cholelithiasis, large colon displacement, cholangitis, neoplastic infiltration, fibrosis or hyperplasia of biliary tract, hepatitis. • Foals—acquired biliary obstruction (e.g. healing duodenal ulcer adjacent to hepatopancreatic ampulla), congenital biliary atresia

RISK FACTORS
• Previous administration of equine-origin biologic. • Septicemia, omphalophlebitis (foals). • Duodenal ulceration. • Inadequate parasite control/vaccination. • Exposure to plant/environmental toxins. • Use of certain drugs. • Anorexic, obese pony/miniature horse/donkey

 ## DIAGNOSIS

DIFFERENTIAL DIAGNOSIS
Prehepatic Icterus
• Abrupt onset of exercise intolerance, weakness, fever, tachypnea, dyspnea, tachycardia, mucous membrane pallor, pigmenturia (some cases). • Hemolytic crisis that can occur with terminal liver failure resembles prehepatic icterus

Hepatic/Posthepatic Icterus
• Chronic weight loss, diarrhea, abdominal pain, altered mentation, photodermatitis, pruritus; usually not observed in prehepatic icterus. • Icterus more marked in posthepatic than hepatic icterus—conjugated bilirubin causes more pronounced icterus. • Recurrent abdominal pain and pyrexia secondary to bacterial cholangitis are frequently found in posthepatic icterus

CBC/BIOCHEMISTRY/URINALYSIS
Prehepatic Icterus
• Severe anemia (usually regenerative), Heinz bodies, spherocytes. • Marked increase in unconjugated, some increase in conjugated bilirubin. • Mildly increased ALP, SDH. • Normal to low glucose. • Normal to high BUN. • Bilirubinuria

Hepatic Icterus
• Mild nonregenerative anemia. • Moderate increase in unconjugated (rarely >25 mg/dL), mild to moderate increase in conjugated bilirubin ($\leq$25% of total). • Mild to moderate increases in GGT, AST, SDH; mild increase in ALP. • Normal to low glucose, BUN, albumin. • Normal to slight bilirubinuria. • Normal to low urinary urobilinogen

Posthepatic Icterus
• Mild nonregenerative anemia. • Normal to mild increase in unconjugated, marked increase in conjugated bilirubin (>25–50% of total). • Normal to mild increase in AST, SDH, moderate to marked increase in GGT and marked increase in ALP. • Marked bilirubinuria. • Urinary urobilinogen absent with complete bile duct obstruction

OTHER LABORATORY TESTS
Prehepatic Icterus
• Giemsa, new methylene blue stain for intraerythrocytic parasites. • Saline agglutination test. • Direct antiglobulin test. • Osmotic fragility test

Hepatic/Posthepatic Icterus
• Serum bile acids—highest in obstructive liver disease, not discriminating. • Blood ammonia—not correlated with severity of HE, not discriminating. • Serum prothrombin time may be prolonged, not discriminating. • Serology for infectious diseases (hepatic icterus). • Serum triglycerides—marked increased in hyperlipemia

IMAGING

US
• To determine liver size, presence of abscesses, cysts, choleliths, dilated bile ducts, neoplasms. • To demonstrate abnormal intra/extrahepatic blood flow. • To guide liver biopsy

OTHER DIAGNOSTIC PROCEDURES

Liver Biopsy
• Yields diagnostic, prognostic, and therapeutic information. • Samples obtained using US-guided or blind techniques; placed in formalin for histopathology, transport media for microbiology.
• Complications—hemorrhage, pneumothorax, spread of infectious hepatitis, peritonitis (due to bile or ingesta); minimized by performing hemostasis profile, using US guidance

PATHOLOGIC FINDINGS
• Yellow discoloration of mucous membranes, body fat stores. • Other findings depend on the primary condition

TREATMENT

APPROPRIATE HEALTH CARE
Depends on primary disease.

NURSING CARE
• In the first 24 h, use IV fluids (5% dextrose at 2 mL/kg/h) for hypoglycemic patients with signs of HE. • After 24 h, substitute 2.5–5% dextrose in LRS (60 mL/kg/day). • In anorexic patients, add potassium chloride (20–40 mEq/L) to fluids

ACTIVITY
Restrict activity and avoid sunlight.

DIET
For hepatic and posthepatic icterus, a diet with 40–50 kcal/kg in the form of low-protein, high-energy feeds rich in BCAAs (e.g. milo, *Sorghum*, beet pulp) is recommended.

CLIENT EDUCATION
Depends on primary disease.

SURGICAL CONSIDERATIONS
• Foals with acquired bile duct obstruction. • Horses with colonic displacement causing acute bile duct obstruction

MEDICATIONS

DRUG(S) OF CHOICE

Prehepatic Icterus
• Treatment of IMHA (corticosteroids).
• Whole-blood transfusion if indicated.
• Fluid therapy (LRS 60 mL/kg/day) to promote diuresis

Hepatic/Posthepatic Icterus
• Manage clinical signs of HE with sedation (e.g. xylazine, detomidine) if necessary, decrease production and absorption of toxic metabolites (mineral oil via nasogastric tube; lactulose 0.3 mL/kg PO every 6 h, neomycin 10–100 mg/kg PO every 6 h). Oral BCAA concentrates can be formulated, IV preparations are available. • Weekly supplementation with vitamin K1 (40–50 mg/450 kg), vitamin B1, and folic acid when cholestasis present. • Antimicrobial therapy based on results of culture and sensitivity. Empiric therapy for bacterial cholangitis includes potentiated sulfonamide or beta-lactam and aminoglycoside. Use metronidazole if anaerobic infection is suspected. • Chronic active hepatitis treated with corticosteroids—dexamethasone (0.05–0.1 mg/kg/day for 4–7 days, then gradually taper dose over 2–3 weeks) followed by prednisolone (1 mg/kg/day for several weeks)

CONTRAINDICATIONS
• Hepatotoxic drugs—anticonvulsants, anabolic steroids, phenothiazines, macrolides.
• Tetracyclines (suppress hepatic protein synthesis). • Drugs eliminated primarily by the liver—analgesics, anesthetics, barbiturates, chloramphenicol

PRECAUTIONS
• Use reduced doses of sedatives metabolized by the liver. • Use corticosteroids cautiously—may exacerbate intercurrent infections

POSSIBLE INTERACTIONS
Duration and intensity of action of many drugs may be increased in patients with hepatobiliary disease.

FOLLOW-UP

PATIENT MONITORING
• Recheck packed cell volume as needed.
• Repeat transfusions as needed

Hepatic/Posthepatic Icterus
• Monitor liver enzyme levels, serum bile acids, bilirubin concentration. • Repeat biopsies to monitor progression

PREVENTION/AVOIDANCE
Depends on primary disease.

POSSIBLE COMPLICATIONS
Horses icteric due to anorexia or cholestatic drugs do not suffer long-term complications.

EXPECTED COURSE AND PROGNOSIS
Depends on primary disease.

MISCELLANEOUS

ASSOCIATED CONDITIONS

Prehepatic Icterus
• Hemoglobinemic nephrosis. • Hemic murmur

Hepatic/Posthepatic Icterus
See Causes.

AGE-RELATED FACTORS
See Differential Diagnosis.

ZOONOTIC POTENTIAL
Leptospirosis may be transmitted to people.

PREGNANCY/FERTILITY/BREEDING
Pregnant or lactating obese ponies/miniature horses/donkeys are predisposed to hyperlipemia.

SYNONYMS
• Hyperbilirubinemia. • Jaundice

SEE ALSO
• Acute hepatitis in adult horses (Theiler disease)
• Anemia
• Anemia, Heinz body
• Anemia, immune mediated
• Bilirubin (hyperbilirubinemia)
• Cholelithiasis
• Hepatic abscess and septic cholangiohepatitis
• Pyrrolizidine alkaloid toxicosis
• Toxic hepatopathy

ABBREVIATIONS
• AAA = aromatic amino acids
• ALP = alkaline phosphatase
• AST = aspartate aminotransferase
• BCAA = branched-chain amino acid
• BUN = blood urea nitrogen
• DMSO = dimethyl sulfoxide
• EIA = equine infectious anemia
• EVA = equine viral arteritis
• GGT = γ-glutamyltransferase
• HE = hepatoencephalopathy
• IMHA = immune-mediated hemolytic anemia
• LRS = lactated Ringer's solution
• SDH = sorbitol dehydrogenase
• US = ultrasonography, ultrasound

Suggested Reading
Barton MH. Disorders of the liver. In: Reed SM, Bayly WM, Sellon DC, eds. Equine Internal Medicine, 3e. St. Louis, MO: WB Saunders, 2010:939–975.
Divers TJ. The equine liver in health and disease. Proc Am Assoc Equine Pract 2015;61:66–103.

Authors Emily E. John and Jeanne Lofstedt
Consulting Editors Michel Levy and Heidi Banse

I

IDIOPATHIC COLITIS/TYPHLITIS

 BASICS

DEFINITION
Idiopathic colitis/typhlitis is a severe inflammatory condition of the large intestine with unknown etiology.

PATHOPHYSIOLOGY
It is likely a consequence of disturbed microbiota, upsetting homeostasis of absorption, secretion, permeability, and motility. This results in net colonic fluid accumulation, intestinal wall inflammation, systemic electrolyte imbalances, protein loss, and disturbance of the coagulation cascade, resulting in diarrhea and systemic clinical signs.

SYSTEMS AFFECTED
GI
The main clinical sign is diarrhea. Varying signs of colic and ileus may be present.

Cardiovascular
Varying severity of dehydration, endotoxemia, and cardiovascular shock. Systemic and local thromboembolic events, including venous thrombosis of catheter sites, can occur.

Musculoskeletal
Laminitis may develop. Peripheral edema occurs with severe hypoproteinemia.

Respiratory
Septic emboli leading to pulmonary abscess formation may occur.

Renal
Acute renal insufficiency due to dehydration can occur.

GENETICS
N/A

INCIDENCE/PREVALENCE
Sporadic condition. If outbreaks occur, an infectious agent should be suspected.

GEOGRAPHIC DISTRIBUTION
Worldwide

SIGNALMENT
There is no reported breed, age, or sex predilection. Foals as young as 24 h of age may be affected.

SIGNS
Historical Findings
Animals may be presented before the development of diarrhea with colic, abdominal distention, depression, anorexia, and pyrexia. Recent antibiotic use, change of feeding management, recent deworming, transport, surgery, or other management changes (stressors) may be reported.

Physical Examination Findings
• Diarrhea is present in most cases and may vary from cowpat consistency to profuse and watery to hemorrhagic
• Dehydration, fever, and tachycardia are common

• GI sounds may be hypermotile or hypomotile
• Signs of endotoxemia may be present
• Marked intestinal distention, especially in peracute cases, may be seen and cause colic. Gastric reflux or cessation of fecal passage can occur due to ileus
• Ventral edema may be present secondary to hypoproteinemia

CAUSES
Disturbance of the colonic microbiota; inciting agents that have yet to be identified or are missed owing to low diagnostic test sensitivity.

RISK FACTORS
Antimicrobial use, transportation, dietary changes, surgery, and other GI disorders.

 DIAGNOSIS

DIFFERENTIAL DIAGNOSIS
• Salmonellosis
• *Clostridium difficile* colitis
• *Clostridium perfringens* colitis
• Potomac horse fever
• Cyathostomiasis
• NSAID-induced colitis
• Cantharidin toxicosis
• Coronavirus-associated diarrhea
• Chronic sand impaction
• Foals—rotavirus diarrhea
• Gastric ulcers
• Cryptosporidia
• *Strongyloides westeri*
• Sepsis

CBC/BIOCHEMISTRY/URINALYSIS
CBC
• Elevated PCV from dehydration and splenic contraction is common
• Serum protein levels may be increased due to hemoconcentration but hypoproteinemia due to protein loss into the GI wall and lumen is more frequent
• Leukopenia with neutropenia and a left shift is often present early. Toxic changes may be present in neutrophils. At later stages of disease or in milder cases, a leukocytosis and neutrophilia may be present

Biochemistry
• Serum sodium, chloride, and calcium concentrations are typically decreased, potassium concentrations are variable, likely due to electrolyte loss into the intestinal lumen
• Prerenal azotemia is common and can result in renal insufficiency
• Blood lactate is often elevated and severity can be a prognostic indicator
• Acute-phase proteins serum amyloid A and fibrinogen are often elevated

Urinalysis
Increased urine specific gravity due to dehydration.

OTHER LABORATORY TESTS
Acid–base assessment—marked metabolic acidosis due to electrolyte derangements and hyperlactatemia can develop.

IMAGING
Abdominal Ultrasonography
The large colon is fluid filled, walls are edematous, and excess motility occurs.

OTHER DIAGNOSTIC PROCEDURES
Diagnosis is based on exclusion of other causes; appropriate samples should be submitted to rule out the common causes of colitis.

PATHOLOGIC FINDINGS
Marked exfoliation of colonic and cecal mucosal epithelial cells and hemorrhagic colitis–typhlitis, with thrombosis of the intestinal mucosal capillaries, are common.

 TREATMENT

APPROPRIATE HEALTH CARE
This condition is best managed with intensive inpatient care. Cases with mild diarrhea and adequate hydration may be treated at the farm but require close monitoring as a rapid deterioration may occur.

NURSING CARE
• IV fluid therapy using a balanced electrolyte solution (e.g. LRS) is often mandatory. The rate of fluid administration depends on the degree of dehydration and the estimated fluid loss through diarrhea. The use of 2 large-bore catheters in separate veins may help deliver a large volume of fluid for the rapid correction of fluid deficits in severely dehydrated horses. After correction of dehydration, IV administration of maintenance fluids (50–100 mL/kg/day) plus the estimated fluid loss through diarrhea should be continued. Hydration status should be assessed frequently because affected animals may become dehydrated even in the presence of fluid therapy
• Mild to moderate cases of metabolic acidosis typically resolve with fluid therapy. In severely hypokalemic horses, 20–40 mEq/L of KCl can be added to LRS or saline. IV administration of KCl should not exceed 0.5 mEq/kg/h
• An oral electrolyte solution containing 35 g KCl and 70 g NaCl in 10 L of water should be provided, along with clean, fresh drinking water and a salt block
• IV administration of hypertonic saline (4–6 mL/kg of 5–7.5% NaCl) may be indicated in severely dehydrated animals. It is essential that isotonic fluid therapy follows the use of hypertonic saline
• Fecal microbial transplantation can be performed to re-establish a normal GI microbiota. Probiotics are likely not effective

• Owing to the high incidence of venous thrombosis in colitis, the catheter site should be monitored frequently
• If distal limb edema develops due to hypoproteinemia, leg wraps should be applied and changed daily
• Deep bedding should be provided if there are any signs of laminitis. Hooves should be iced for 72 h

ACTIVITY
Owing to the need for continuous IV fluid therapy in most cases, stall confinement is required. Diarrheic horses should be considered infectious.

DIET
• Affected horses should be provided with free-choice hay. It is recommended to feed hay in a hay net to prevent severe facial and head edema
• Higher energy feeds can also be provided, but should be introduced slowly and fed in small amounts
• Anorexic animals may benefit from forced enteral feeding. Partial or total parenteral nutrition may be indicated

CLIENT EDUCATION
Inform clients that colitis is a potentially life-threatening condition, often associated with development of secondary problems, such as laminitis and jugular vein thrombosis. In multi-horse environments, it is important to explain the risk of infection to other animals and humans (salmonellosis).

SURGICAL CONSIDERATIONS
N/A

MEDICATIONS
DRUG(S) OF CHOICE
Antimicrobial Agents
• The use of antimicrobial drugs is controversial
• Metronidazole 15–25 mg/kg every 6–8 h should be given if clostridial involvement cannot be ruled out
• Administration of broad-spectrum antibiotics to severely neutropenic patients has been suggested to prevent sepsis. Additional disturbance of the microbiota occurs with antimicrobial therapy and can worsen diarrhea. Options include ceftiofur sodium 2–5 mg/kg IV or IM every 12 h, trimethoprim–sulfamethoxazole 24 mg/kg IV every 12 h or gentamicin 6.6 mg/kg daily in combination with sodium penicillin (22 000–30 000 IU/kg every 6 h); the last combination should only be used if renal function is normal and fluid deficits are addressed
• Antimicrobial therapy should be discontinued when clinical and laboratory values improve

Flunixin Meglumine
A dose of 0.25–0.5 mg/kg every 8 h can be used for antiendotoxic effects. A higher dosage (1.1 mg/kg) is necessary for analgesia.

Endotoxin Binding Drugs
Administration of hyperimmune serum (hyperimmunized to *Escherichia coli* J5 strain and/or polymyxin B (6000 IU/kg every 6–8 h IV) to moderate the effects of endotoxemia.

Colloidal Therapy
Colloidal solutions (e.g. whole blood, plasma, hetastarch) can be used to maintain the fluid in the vascular space. Colloids should be considered when plasma proteins are less than 4 g/dL (40 g/L). Plasma provides the additional benefit of anticoagulants, and procoagulant substances.

Antidiarrhea Drugs
Di-tri-octahedral smectite (loading dose 3 g/kg PO then 0.5–3 g/kg every 6–8 h PO)—can cause impaction if administered beyond resolution of diarrhea.

Laminitis Treatment
See chapter Laminitis.

CONTRAINDICATIONS
See Pregnancy/Fertility/Breeding.

PRECAUTIONS
At a dose of 1.1 mg/kg, flunixin meglumine may be nephrotoxic in dehydrated animals.

POSSIBLE INTERACTIONS
None

ALTERNATIVE DRUGS
N/A

FOLLOW-UP
PATIENT MONITORING
• Patients should be monitored frequently. Initially, PCV and total plasma protein levels should be evaluated at least daily
• If azotemia was present, this should be reevaluated after rehydration to ensure it was prerenal
• Plasma electrolytes should be monitored to determine whether supplementation with potassium and calcium is required
• The IV catheter site should be monitored frequently for signs of thrombophlebitis
• The feet should be checked frequently for evidence of laminitis

PREVENTION/AVOIDANCE
None

POSSIBLE COMPLICATIONS
• Endotoxemia
• Laminitis
• Jugular vein thrombosis
• Renal failure
• Pulmonary abscessation

EXPECTED COURSE AND PROGNOSIS
This disease often has a very fulminant character and horses may succumb to it within 8–24 h. There is a wide variety in the severity. Mortality rates have been reported in the range 10–40%.

MISCELLANEOUS
ASSOCIATED CONDITIONS
• Laminitis
• Venous thrombosis

AGE-RELATED FACTORS
None

ZOONOTIC POTENTIAL
All affected horses should be treated as zoonotic until shown to be negative for *Salmonella* spp. and *C. difficile*.

PREGNANCY/FERTILITY/BREEDING
Metronidazole should not be administered to pregnant mares as it is teratogenic. An increased risk of abortion may be present due to endotoxemia and hypovolemic shock.

SYNONYMS
Undifferentiated colitis, acute diarrhea. Old—colitis X.

SEE ALSO
• Cantharidin toxicosis
• *Clostridium difficile* infection
• Endotoxemia
• Laminitis
• Potomac horse fever (PHF)
• Probiotics in foals and horses
• Salmonellosis
• Sand impaction and enteropathy

ABBREVIATIONS
• GI = gastrointestinal
• LRS = lactated Ringer's solution
• NSAID = nonsteroidal anti-inflammatory drug
• PCV = packed cell volume

Internet Resources
ACVIM Fact Sheet: Colitis in Adult Horses. http://www.acvim.org/Portals/0/PDF/ Animal%20Owner%20Fact%20Sheets/ LAIM/Colitis%20in%20Adult%20Horses. pdf

Suggested Reading
Shaw SD, Stäempfli HR. Diagnosis and treatment of undifferentiated and infectious diarrhea in the adult horse. Vet Clin North Am Equine Pract 2018;34:39–53.

Author Angelika Schoster
Consulting Editors Henry Stämpfli and Olimpo Oliver-Espinosa
Acknowledgment The author acknowledges the prior contribution of Olimpo Oliver-Espinosa and Henry Stämpfli.

Client Education Handout available online

I

ILEAL HYPERTROPHY

 BASICS

OVERVIEW

Hypertrophy of the muscular layers of the ileum results in luminal diameter reduction and partial or complete nonvascular intestinal obstruction. It can present as a primary idiopathic condition or secondary to an aboral stenosis forcing the muscular layer to enlarge. Suggested etiologies for the primary idiopathic hypertrophy include ileal mucosa inflammation and edema; an imbalance in the autonomic nervous system; and dysfunction of the ileocecal valve. Ileocecal intussusception can result in ileal muscular hypertrophy. There is an increased risk of ileal impaction and hypertrophy in horses with tapeworm burdens. Hemomelasma ilei is a common finding in horses with ileal hypertrophy. Abnormal cecal motility has also been proposed as an etiologic factor.

SIGNALMENT

Occurs in adult horses of all ages, but tends to be more frequent in horses 5 years and older. There is no sex or breed predilection.

SIGNS

Depend on the degree of luminal obstruction. Horses may have a history of recurrent, low-grade colic with decreased appetite and weight loss. If complete obstruction occurs, horses develop a more severe, continuous colic with ileus and nasogastric reflux.

CAUSES AND RISK FACTORS

Risk factors are unknown, although high parasite load and poor quality roughage may be contributory factors. With compensatory ileal hypertrophy, risk factors also include parasitism and poor quality roughage, as well as intestinal neoplasia, lipoma formation, previous abdominal surgeries (adhesions), and any aboral luminal obstruction.

 DIAGNOSIS

DIFFERENTIAL DIAGNOSIS

• Ileal impactions and ileocecal intussusception often present with a similar history and similar clinical signs. Ileocecal intussusception has a characteristic ultrasonographic "target" image
• Small intestinal displacement (epiploic foramen) and strangulating lipomas can be difficult to diagnose, but the acute onset and severe colic signs differentiate them from ileal hypertrophy
• Small intestinal inguinal herniation is diagnosed via scrotal palpation

CBC/BIOCHEMISTRY/URINALYSIS
N/A

OTHER LABORATORY TESTS

Biopsy of the ileum at the time of exploratory celiotomy may be used to confirm the diagnosis.

IMAGING

Transabdominal and transrectal ultrasonography of the ileum may detect ileal hypertrophy, the presence of an abnormal layering pattern of the intestinal wall, and small intestinal distention orally and small intestinal hypermotility. The hypertrophied wall of the ileum is usually between 15 and 25 mm thick, becoming less thick orally. Narrowing of the ileal lumen may also be discernible.

OTHER DIAGNOSTIC PROCEDURES

Rectal examination findings may include a thickened ileum palpable in the right dorsal quadrant and loops of distended small intestine. Not all cases have these findings, and the diagnosis may only be revealed after evaluation of a biopsy of the ileum taken during exploratory celiotomy.

PATHOLOGIC FINDINGS

There is muscular hypertrophy of both circular and longitudinal smooth muscle layers for variable lengths along the ileum, and possibly also the jejunum. Individual muscle cells are enlarged, with elongated vesicular nuclei. Mucosal diverticula through the muscularis layer were found in approximately half of the specimens from 1 study. Fibrosis of the mucosa is often present.

 TREATMENT

Conservative therapy is attempted, but progression of clinical signs and increasing small intestinal distention are indicators for surgical intervention. Surgical treatments include ileal myotomy, ileocecal bypass, and jejunocecostomy. Ileocecal bypass has been used, but ingesta may pass through the ileum, causing pain. In addition, complications associated with this anastomosis are more likely. A jejunocecostomy with blind stumping of the ileum distally and removal of the proximal ileum may be the treatment of choice. A laxative diet may be palliative in horses in which surgery is not an option.

 MEDICATIONS

DRUG(S) OF CHOICE

There is no specific medication for ileal hypertrophy.

CONTRAINDICATIONS/POSSIBLE INTERACTIONS

Prokinetics and gastrointestinal osmotic cathartics may exacerbate colic pain severity in partial or complete intestinal obstruction.

 FOLLOW-UP

Routine postsurgical monitoring for colic cases is required. Prognosis after surgical correction is considered good, provided that the hypertrophy is focal.

 MISCELLANEOUS

ASSOCIATED CONDITIONS

See Differential Diagnosis.

AGE-RELATED FACTORS

Possibly more common in mature horses. In 1 study of 11 cases of idiopathic ileal muscular hypertrophy, the age range was 5–18 years with a median age of 10 years.

SEE ALSO

• Acute adult abdominal pain—acute colic
• Colic, chronic/recurrent

Suggested Reading
Chaffin MK, Fuenteabla IC, Schumacher J, et al. Idiopathic muscular hypertrophy of the equine small intestine: 11 cases (1980–1991). Equine Vet J 1992;24: 372–378.

Author Antonio M. Cruz
Consulting Editors Henry Stämpfli and Olimpo Oliver-Espinosa

Acknowledgment The author and editors acknowledge the prior contribution of Judith Koenig and Simon G. Pearce.

BASICS

DEFINITION
Ileus is defined as intestinal obstruction that impairs aboral transit of ingesta, and includes both physical and mechanical obstructions. However, in the equine, it mostly refers to the functional inhibition of propulsive intestine activity, irrespective of its pathophysiology.

PATHOPHYSIOLOGY
• Regulation of motility occurs as a complex interaction of central innervation, autonomic innervation, and the enteric nervous system. The enteric nervous system acts on the GI tract either directly through neurotransmitters or indirectly through intermediate cells, such as the interstitial cells of Cajal, cells of the immune system, or endocrine cells
• Acetylcholine is the main excitatory neurotransmitter in the gut. Sympathetic stimulation (norepinephrine) inhibits acetylcholine release from the cholinergic fibers, resulting in inhibition of motility. Nonadrenergic–noncholinergic neurotransmitters like adenosine triphosphate, vasoactive intestinal peptide, substance P, nitric oxide, and others also play a role in regulating GI activity
• Many reflexes are present that are essential to the proper functioning of intestinal motility, some of which occur locally within the enteric nervous system and are responsible for peristalsis and mixing contractions. Other reflexes travel to sympathetic ganglia, the spinal cord, or the brainstem to coordinate more complex activities, such as the gastrocolic reflex
• Pain can cause a systemic release of norepinephrine, inhibiting acetylcholine release and decreasing intestinal motility. Ileus can develop from diseases directly involving the digestive system. Shock, electrolyte imbalances, hypoalbuminemia, peritonitis, endotoxemia, and distention, ischemia, or inflammation of the intestinal tract have all been implicated as contributing to the pathophysiology of ileus in the horse
• POI occurs in around 20–25% of horses after laparotomy, affects small intestine most commonly, and is more frequent after small intestinal resection and anastomosis (42% of horses)

SYSTEMS AFFECTED
• GI
• Cardiovascular—hypovolemia and endotoxemia can result in depressed cardiovascular function

SIGNALMENT
More common in Arabians and horses >10 years of age.

SIGNS

Historical Findings
Depression, mild to moderate signs of colic, anorexia, and constipation. Ileus can occur secondary to many diseases (see Causes) that can be associated with specific historical findings.

Physical Examination Findings
• Heart rate and respiratory rate are often elevated and mild to severe signs of colic are common. Clinical signs associated with dehydration are often present due to intestinal sequestration of fluids
• Abdominal auscultation reveals an absence or reduction of borborygmi
• On rectal palpation, distention of either the small or large intestine may be present
• Build-up of fluid in the stomach occurs because of a lack of progressive motility. Decompression with a nasogastric tube not only prevents gastric rupture and provides pain relief, but it also allows for the volume of fluid to be quantified for IV replacement fluid therapy

CAUSES
Ileus can be induced by virtually any intestinal insult, including intestinal distention or impaction, enteritis/colitis, abdominal surgery or peritonitis, vascular or obstructive intestinal injuries, endotoxemia, pain, shock, hypoproteinemia, or electrolyte imbalances.

RISK FACTORS
Any factors predisposing the development of a previously mentioned cause of ileus. Colic cases with PCV >45%; elevated serum protein, albumin or glucose; electrolyte imbalances (hypokalemia or hypocalcemia); >8 L reflux at admission; prolonged anesthesia; prolonged surgery; high pulse rate; strangulating or ischemic lesion; resection and anastomosis. Certain drugs (α_2-agonists or opioid analgesics) also inhibit intestinal motility.

DIAGNOSIS

DIFFERENTIAL DIAGNOSIS
Functional ileus should be differentiated from obstructive diseases that require immediate surgical intervention. Persistent discomfort despite gastric decompression should alert for serious tissue injury or obstructive conditions.

CBC/BIOCHEMISTRY/URINALYSIS
• Increased PCV due to dehydration and/or splenic contraction. Azotemia may also be present
• Hypoproteinemia in cases of colitis or enteritis. Hyperproteinemia if an inflammatory response is present
• Leukopenia if associated with an acute inflammatory response. A longstanding inflammatory response can cause leukocytosis
• Hypokalemia, hypocalcemia, hypomagnesemia, hypochloremia, and hyponatremia may be present due to sequestration of fluid in the intestines

OTHER LABORATORY TESTS

Abdominocentesis
No detectable abnormalities except in cases of duodenitis/proximal jejunitis, peritonitis, or obstructive ileus, where the peritoneal fluid can be serosanguineous due to intestinal compromise and the cellular and protein levels are often high.

IMAGING

Ultrasonography
The intestine can be assessed for presence of movement, mural thickness, and dilation.

I

TREATMENT

AIMS
To decompress the GI tract, reduce inflammation and pain, stimulate motility, maintain hydration, and keep electrolytes balanced to both promote motility and maintain the GI barrier, as well as to prevent cardiovascular impairment.

APPROPRIATE HEALTH CARE
Inpatient intensive care management with 24 h monitoring.

NURSING CARE
• Parenteral fluid therapy is vital due to the inability to absorb oral fluids. Fluid rates should equal fluid deficit + maintenance + ongoing loss
• Maintenance fluid requirements are 50–60 mL/kg/day for adult horses, and 70–80 mL/kg/day for foals. Ongoing losses can be determined by quantifying volume of gastric reflux
• Horses suffering from hypovolemic or endotoxemic shock may benefit from hypertonic saline administration to rapidly expand the vascular fluid volume. Hypertonic saline (5–7%) can be administered at a dose of 4 mL/kg as a rapid bolus, followed by isotonic fluids because the volume expansion by hypertonic fluids is short-lived (<30 min)
• Horses with severe hyponatremia (<120 mmol/L) should not be given hypertonic saline due to the potential for demyelination reported to occur in humans. Serum sodium replacement should be closely monitored

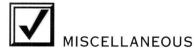

• Electrolyte imbalances should be addressed due to the negative effect of hypokalemia, hypomagnesemia, and hypocalcemia on motility. KCl may be added to parenteral fluids at a maximal rate of 0.5 mEq/kg/h due to the potential for cardiac effects
• To correct hypocalcemia, 200–500 mL of 23% calcium borogluconate can be administered slowly (diluted in LRS)
• To correct hypomagnesemia, 150 mg/kg per day of $MgSO_4$ (0.3 mL/kg of a 50% solution) is administered diluted in LRS
• Horses with hypoproteinemia (<35–40 g/L) require administration of plasma or colloids to increase oncotic pressure
• Gastric decompression via a nasogastric tube should be performed to relieve discomfort and to prevent gastric rupture

ACTIVITY
Frequent hand-walking (4–6 times daily) may help stimulate the GI tract.

DIET
Feed and water should be withheld.

CLIENT EDUCATION
If ileus persists or the horse deteriorates clinically, surgery is indicated owing to the potential for an obstructive/ischemic lesion.

SURGICAL CONSIDERATIONS
See Client Education.

MEDICATIONS
DRUG(S) OF CHOICE
Analgesics
• Pain relief is important when correcting ileus. NSAIDs are a good choice as they do not inhibit motility. If additional analgesia is needed, then α_2-agonists can be given alone or in conjunction with butorphanol (opioid). These drugs should be used judiciously as they can inhibit motility temporarily and mask signs of serious intestinal injury
• NSAIDs—flunixin meglumine 0.5–1.1 mg/kg IV every 8–12 h

Prokinetic Agents
• Bethanechol chloride—0.025 mg/kg IV or SC every 6 h. Side effects—salivation, abdominal cramps, diarrhea
• Cisapride—recommended dose 0.1 mg/kg IM every 8 h. Side effects in people are

cardiotoxicity. Related drugs like tegaserod or mosapride appear to be effective in horses as well
• Erythromycin lactobionate—its efficacy is questionable in the presence of inflammation of the intestine. Recommended dose 0.5 mg/kg IV every 6 h. Side effect—diarrhea
• Metoclopramide—recommended dose 0.04 mg/kg/h IV in saline as a CRI. Side effects—excitement, restlessness, sweating, abdominal cramps
• Lidocaine—suppresses sympathetic neurotransmission, has anti-inflammatory and analgesic properties, and ameliorates the negative effects of flunixin meglumine on injured intestinal mucosa. It is widely used as a prokinetic drug although its efficacy in horses has been under question. Recommended dose 1.3 mg/kg IV as a slow bolus, followed by 0.05 mg/kg/min IV in saline or LRS as a CRI over ≥24 h. Side effects—muscle fasciculations, trembling ataxia

CONTRAINDICATIONS
Oral drug administration is contraindicated in horses with ileus of the small intestine.

PRECAUTIONS
N/A

POSSIBLE INTERACTIONS
N/A

ALTERNATIVE DRUGS
Acupuncture may be successful in promoting motility in horses.

FOLLOW-UP
PATIENT MONITORING
The patient should be monitored closely to ensure that IV fluid therapy is appropriate and that decompression of gastric and small intestinal distention is adequate.

PREVENTION/AVOIDANCE
N/A

POSSIBLE COMPLICATIONS
• Circulatory shock
• GI rupture

EXPECTED COURSE AND PROGNOSIS
Survival of horses with POI has been reported to be around 60%.

✓ MISCELLANEOUS
AGE-RELATED FACTORS
N/A

ZOONOTIC POTENTIAL
N/A

SEE ALSO
• Acute adult abdominal pain—acute colic

ABBREVIATIONS
• CRI = constant rate infusion
• GI = gastrointestinal
• LRS = lactated Ringer's solution
• NSAID = nonsteroidal anti-inflammatory drug
• PCV = packed cell volume
• POI = postoperative ileus

Suggested Reading
Hardy J, Rakestraw PC. Postoperative care, complications and reoperation. In: Auer JA, Stick, JA, eds. Equine Surgery, 4e. St. Louis, MO: WB Saunders, 2012:499–506.
Lefebvre D, Hudson NPH, Elce YA, et al. Clinical features and management of equine post operative ileus (POI): survey of diplomates of the American Colleges of Veterinary Internal Medicine (ACVIM), Veterinary Surgeons (ACVS) and Veterinary Emergency and Critical Care (ACVECC). Equine Vet J 2016;48:714–719.
Lefebvre D, Pirie RS, Handel IG, et al. Clinical features and management of equine post operative ileus: survey of diplomates of the European Colleges of Equine Internal Medicine (ECEIM) and Veterinary Surgeons (ECVS). Equine Vet J 2016;48:182–187.
Salem SE, Proudman CJ, Archer DC. Has intravenous lidocaine improved the outcome in horses following surgical management of small intestinal lesions in a UK hospital population? BMC Vet Res 2016;12:157.
Sanchez LC, Lester GD. Gastrointestinal ileus. In: Smith B, ed. Large Animal Internal Medicine, 5e. St. Louis, MO: Elsevier Mosby, 2015:728–731.

Author Luis M. Rubio-Martinez
Consulting Editors Henry Stämpfli and Olimpo Oliver-Espinosa

I

BASICS

OVERVIEW
• IMMK is a diagnosis utilized to identify a group of corneoconjunctival diseases characterized by chronic (>3 months) corneal opacities associated with variable degrees of cellular infiltrate (mild, moderate, or severe) and corneal vascularization. In general, secondary uveitis and ocular discomfort are mild to moderate, if present. Associated infectious agents are rarely identified, generally only as a result of secondary corneal ulceration and subsequent infection
• Systems affected—ophthalmic

SIGNALMENT
All ages and breeds of horses can be affected.

SIGNS
• Corneal opacification with mild to moderate cellular infiltrate and variable degrees of vascularization
• Cellular infiltrate may appear yellow to white and may be associated with diffuse corneal discoloration and bullous corneal edema during phases of active, uncontrolled inflammation
• There are five currently recognized forms of IMMK, four of which are categorized based on their location within the cornea—epithelial, superficial stroma, midstromal, and endothelial
• Eosinophilic keratoconjunctivitis represents the fifth type. It demonstrates similarities to epithelial or anterior stromal forms of IMMK, but eosinophils are the predominant cells present
• Epithelial and subepithelial, anterior stromal keratopathies have also been suggested as being early manifestations of IMMK
• Endothelial IMMK is characterized by endothelial cellular infiltrates and focal or diffuse corneal edema without signs of anterior uveitis
• Equine IMMK is commonly a unilateral disease, but both eyes can be affected

CAUSES AND RISK FACTORS
Immune mediated.

DIAGNOSIS

DIFFERENTIAL DIAGNOSIS
• Other nonulcerative keratopathies such as onchocerciasis, bacterial or fungal stromal infections (stromal abscesses), viral keratitis, infiltrative neoplasia, corneal degeneration or dystrophy, calcific band keratopathy, and bullous keratopathy
• Chronic recurrent or persistent ulcerative keratitis or indolent ulcers
• Specific manifestations of anterior uveitis (e.g. equine recurrent uveitis)

• Acute or chronic glaucoma, and Descemet's membrane detachment (all of which present with variable degrees of corneal edema and ocular discomfort)
• Infectious keratitis, especially keratomycosis, is usually more acute in onset and associated with secondary anterior uveitis and more severe ocular discomfort. However, subtle and chronic forms of epithelial, subepithelial keratomycosis associated with minimal discomfort may be a challenge to differentiate based on clinical appearances only. Cytology is necessary to rule out an infectious process

CBC/BIOCHEMISTRY/URINALYSIS
N/A

OTHER LABORATORY TESTS
• Rule out infectious causes (bacterial or fungal) by corneal scrapings of superficial lesions for cytology, culture, and possibly histopathology
• Deeper lesions can only be sampled during surgical intervention (e.g. lamellar or penetrating keratoplasty)

IMAGING
Digital infrared photography can help to differentiate corneal fibrosis from cellular infiltration and may help to identify the presence of subtle corneal (ghost) vessels.

OTHER DIAGNOSTIC PROCEDURES
N/A

PATHOLOGIC FINDINGS
• Histopathology, in cases of non-eosinophilic keratoconjunctivitis, reveals stromal fibrosis, vascularization, and cellular infiltrates consisting mainly of lymphocytes and plasma cells
• In corneal biopsies obtained during keratectomy of anterior or midstromal IMMK, lymphoplasmacytic inflammation predominates. Concomitant histiocytic and polymorphonuclear cell inflammation may be present in variable degrees. Additionally, stromal necrosis, hyperplastic corneal epithelium, stromal edema, and hyalinization, as well as neovascularization, may be identified during histologic evaluation
• Recent immunohistochemical and immunopathologic evaluation of superficial stromal biopsy samples from horses with IMMK suggest that the pathogenesis is driven predominantly by T cells, with both helper and cytotoxic T cells being involved

TREATMENT
• While many cases of IMMK respond well to topical medication, they often require chronic, low-grade continuous treatment to prevent relapses. Horses that have frequent relapses or that do not respond favorably to topical medical therapy may require surgical intervention to remove cellular infiltrates with

or without a concomitant grafting procedure (e.g. amniotic membrane or conjunctival graft). Although once thought to be curative, relapses after surgical intervention in the form of a lamellar keratectomy ± conjunctival graft are being, anecdotally, more frequently identified. Thus, the search for an alternative intervention with long-term control of IMMK is a timely and important research topic
• Two promising interventions demonstrating the potential for long-term disease control with minimal risk of complication and without the need for chronic immune-suppressive medical therapy have recently been described:
  ◦ Bulbar subconjunctival injections of autologous bone marrow-derived mesenchymal stem cells showed promising results as it resulted in a notable reduction of corneal opacification and degeneration
  ◦ Photodynamic therapy utilizing intrastromal indocyanine green as the photosensitive agent activated by diffuse 810 nm infrared diode laser energy has been shown to suppress active inflammation and eliminate the need for long-term topical medical therapy for up to 1.5 years in the preliminary report
  ◦ Both treatments resulted in long-term corneal clearing and vascular regression over periods of up to 1.5 years without continual topical immune-suppressive therapy. While much research remains to be carried out before definitive answers become available, both treatment modalities have the potential to change the way that IMMK is managed in the future
• Additionally, the use of episcleral silicone matrix cyclosporine (ciclosporin) drug delivery devices have recently been shown to effectively control anterior and midstromal IMMK
• Of all types of IMMK, endothelial IMMK is the least amenable to medical treatment

MEDICATIONS

DRUG(S) OF CHOICE
• Topical corticosteroids (1% prednisolone acetate or 0.1% dexamethasone every 24 h to effect) is generally utilized initially, in combination with topical cyclosporine A every 12 h to achieve a state of quiescence. Once the clinical signs have been controlled, topical medications can be slowly tapered off (corticosteroids) or tapered down (cyclosporine A) to the lowest possible maintenance dosage (generally, this will be achieved with every 48–72 h dosage frequencies)
• Complete or incomplete clinical improvement with topical anti-inflammatory medication helps to confirm the diagnosis and

IMMUNE-MEDIATED KERATITIS (CONTINUED)

to decide when surgical or alternative intervention is indicated and/or warranted

CONTRAINDICATIONS/POSSIBLE INTERACTIONS
N/A

 FOLLOW-UP

EXPECTED COURSE AND PROGNOSIS
• Unless implemented surgical or alternative options achieve the desired results, long-term topical treatment every 12–72 h may be required to control the disease and prevent recurrences
• Routine follow-up examinations are essential in recognizing recurrence of inflammation or secondary ulcerative complications

 MISCELLANEOUS

ASSOCIATED CONDITIONS
• Superficial corneal ulcers may develop concurrently with any type of IMMK that is poorly controlled. These ulcers may become secondarily infected, especially if corticosteroids are concomitantly being utilized

• Superficial corneal ulcers may also develop secondary to chronic corneal edema associated with endothelial IMMK

SEE ALSO
• Calcific band keratopathy
• Corneal stromal abscesses
• Eosinophilic keratitis
• Equine recurrent uveitis
• Ocular/adnexal squamous cell carcinoma
• Viral (herpes) keratitis (putative)

ABBREVIATIONS
• IMMK = immune-mediated keratitis
• NSAID = nonsteroidal anti-inflammatory drug

Suggested Reading
Braus BK, Miller I, Kummer S, et al. Investigation of corneal autoantibodies in horses with immune mediated keratitis (IMMK). Vet Immunol Immunopathol 2017;187:48–54.
Brooks DE. Ophthalmology for the Equine Practitioner, 2e. Jackson, WY: Teton NewMedia, 2008.
Clode AB, Matthews AG. Diseases and surgery of the cornea. In: Gilger BC, ed. Equine Ophthalmology. Maryland Heights, MO: WB Saunders, 2011:183–266.

Gilger BC, Michau TM, Salmon JH. Immune-mediated keratitis in horses: 19 cases (1998–2004). Vet Ophthalmol 2005;8:233–239.
Gilger BC, Stoppini R, Wilkie DA, et al. Treatment of immune-mediated keratitis in horses with episcleral silicone matrix cyclosporine delivery devices. Vet Ophthalmol 2014;17(Suppl. 1):23–30.
Matthews AG, Gilger BC. Equine immune-mediated keratopathies. Vet Ophthalmol 2009;12(Suppl. 1):10–16.
McMullen Jr RJ, Clode AB, Gilger BC. Infrared digital imaging of the equine anterior segment. Vet Ophthalmol 2009;12:125–131.
Pate DO, Clode AB, Olivry T, et al. Immunohistochemical and immunopathological characterization of superficial stromal immune-mediated keratitis in horses. Am J Vet Res 2012;73:1067–1073.

Author Richard J. McMullen Jr.
Consulting Editor Caryn E. Plummer
Acknowledgment The author and editor acknowledge the prior contribution of Andras M. Komaromy.

BASICS

DEFINITION
Rare, primary disorders of the humoral immune system resulting in impaired antibody production and susceptibility to infections.

PATHOPHYSIOLOGY
• THY is associated with a transitory delay in immunoglobulin production in foals
• sIgMD is associated with decreased or absent serum IgM, with no abnormalities of other immunoglobulins
• AG is caused by a lack of mature B lymphocytes and plasma cells, with failure to synthesize immunoglobulins after immunization or infection
• FIS is associated with low concentration of IgM in serum, low numbers of B lymphocytes, and severe anemia
• CVID is a late-onset impairment of immunoglobulin production usually due to B-cell lymphopenia, but also with low normal B-cell distribution

SYSTEMS AFFECTED
The immune system and systems damaged by resulting infections.

GENETICS
• FIS involves a mutation in the gene *SLC5A3*
• CVID is an epigenetic aberrance involved in gene silencing

INCIDENCE/PREVALENCE
• Unknown for THY, sIgMD, AG (rare), and CVID
• For FIS, 43–54% of Fell Ponies, and 0–4% of Dales Ponies are carriers

GEOGRAPHIC DISTRIBUTION
• THY, sIgMD, AG, and CVID have been reported in the USA
• FIS has been reported in the UK, the Netherlands, and the USA

SIGNALMENT
• THY occurs in male and female foals of different breeds around 3 months and may persist for 18 months to 2 years of age
• Primary sIgMD has been described in many horse breeds and both sexes, usually before 2 years of age, but a secondary form can occur in adult horses
• AG has been described in Thoroughbred, Quarter Horse, and Standardbred male foals, usually before 1 year of age
• FIS has been described in male or female Fell and Dales Ponies that are usually <1 month of age
• CVID usually affects adult, male or female horses of many breeds, but also can occur in younger animals (range 2–23 years)

SIGNS

General Comments
• Infections are the most common clinical manifestation of these syndromes and include pneumonia, hepatitis, arthritis, enteritis, meningitis, and septicemia
• Foals or weanlings often present with ill thrift, nasal discharge, cough, and/or diarrhea
• Infections often involve encapsulated bacteria and other opportunistic organisms, e.g. adenovirus and *Cryptosporidium* spp.

Historical Findings
• A history of recurrent bacterial infections is common to all syndromes
• Infections may respond to aggressive antimicrobial therapy, but frequently relapse a few weeks after cessation of treatment

Physical Examination Findings
• Findings on a physical examination will vary depending on the site of infection
• THY presents as recurrent infections when colostrum-derived antibodies drop below protective levels around 2–3 months of age; delayed immunoglobulin production may persist for 18–24 months of age
• Primary sIgMD is observed in foals <10 months of age (usually 2–8); most foals die by 8 months, but if they survive >1 year they have poor growth rates and stunting; adult horses with secondary sIgMD present with ill thrift, weight loss, or chronic recurrent infections
• Foals with AG have intact T-lymphocyte function, which allows them to survive for months with appropriate therapy, but invariably they develop complications to recurrent infections and die
• Foals with FIS are normal at birth, but by 2–4 weeks develop depression, weight loss, bone marrow dysplasia/hypoplasia, severe anemia, and sepsis, and die or are submitted for euthanasia within a few weeks
• Horses with CVID show signs of recurrent bacterial infections and fevers in adult life; clinical signs consistent with pneumonia, hepatitis, and meningitis are the most common presentations

CAUSES
• The cause of THY is unknown; its transient feature suggests a delay in immune system development in young age
• The cause and effect of sIgMD are poorly defined since serum IgG and IgA concentrations are normal and surviving foals have been reported to resume IgM production; in adult horses (>2 years) sIgMD can be transitory or be secondary to poorly defined conditions including lymphoid neoplasia
• In humans, AG is due to a mutation in the gene encoding Bruton tyrosine kinase and is inherited as an X-linked trait; the occurrence of this disorder only in male horses suggests a similar X-linked mechanism in this species but is not yet confirmed

• FIS is associated with an autosomal recessive mutation in the gene *SLC5A3* on chromosome ECA26, but the pathologic implications of this mutation have not been completely resolved
• One mechanism of disease for CVID involves epigenetic hypermethylation of the *PAX5* gene, which encodes a B-cell essential transcription factor; silencing this gene results in impaired B-cell differentiation

RISK FACTORS
A risk factor for FIS is breeding Fell or Dales horses that tested positive as carriers (heterozygous) for the genetic mutation.

DIAGNOSIS

DIFFERENTIAL DIAGNOSIS
• Diagnosis of an immunodeficiency can be difficult in young horses before 6 months of age due to circulating maternal antibodies and age-dependent developmental changes in the immune system
• Differential diagnoses include SCID and FTPI
• SCID is diagnosed in young Arabian foals with low IgM and marked absolute lymphopenia (both B and T lymphocytes)
• FTPI often is observed in neonates with infections, and partial failure may cause increased susceptibility to infections in foals less than 2 months of age

CBC/BIOCHEMISTRY/URINALYSIS
• In general, CBC and biochemistry are normal or reflect an infectious or inflammatory process (i.e. leukocytosis with neutrophilia, mild anemia, hyperfibrinogenemia)
• In AG, FIS, and CVID, blood lymphocyte counts may be normal (due to presence of T lymphocytes) or decreased. Marked anemia occurs in foals with FIS; mild to moderate lymphopenia and thrombocytopenia occur in some cases

OTHER LABORATORY TESTS
• Serum IgM and IgG concentrations (and IgA when available) should be measured
• Serum IgM better reflects endogenous humoral function in the foal <3 months of age; serum IgG can be confounded by maternal antibodies up to 3–4 months of age; values should be compared with age-matched control foals and laboratory reference intervals
• Peripheral blood lymphocyte phenotyping informs the distribution of B and T cells; values are age dependent within the first 8–12 months of age
• In THY, sIgMD, AG, and FIS, serum IgM should be measured once the foal is >3 weeks of age; a result of <25 mg/dL is considered a deficiency

I

IMMUNOGLOBULIN DEFICIENCIES (CONTINUED)

• In THY, IgM, IgG, and IgA are transiently decreased; B and T cells are present; transient low CD4 T-cell distribution is also possible
• In sIgMD, only IgM is decreased; other immunoglobulins (i.e. IgG, IgA) are normal to increased; B-cell distribution is usually normal
• In AG, diagnosis is supported by IgG, IgM and IgA hypogammaglobulinemia, and marked B-cell (but not T) lymphopenia
• FIS is associated with decreased serum IgM and decreased circulating B (but not T) lymphocytes; serum IgG may be normal or low but reflects maternal origin
• In CVID, IgM and IgG are markedly low, IgA may be normal or low, and B cells undetectable or in low numbers

IMAGING
Radiographs and ultrasonography may reveal sites of infection.

OTHER DIAGNOSTIC PROCEDURES
• In adult horses with suspected secondary sIgMD the positive predictive value of serum IgM concentration is low for diagnosis of lymphoid neoplasia; therefore, alternate diagnostic tests are recommended to further investigate lymphosarcoma
• In vivo antigen-specific antibody production can be further tested using a serum sample before and 15–21 days after vaccination
• A genetic test is available for FIS (Animal Health Trust, UK)

PATHOLOGIC FINDINGS
• In THY and sIgMD lymphoid tissues are grossly and histologically normal
• In AG, FIS, and CVID lymphoid hypoplasia and lack of germinal centers are observed
• Gross and histologic findings of infection and inflammation in multiple organs are common
• Glossal hyperkeratosis, erythroid hypoplasia, and peripheral ganglionopathy are seen in foals with FIS

TREATMENT

AIMS
Therapy is supportive and aimed at controlling infections.

APPROPRIATE HEALTH CARE
• Plasma transfusions may provide an exogenous source of antibodies with short-term benefit
• In THY and sIgMD, appropriate antimicrobial therapy for treatment of bacterial infections is recommended until serum IgG concentrations reach protective levels (>800 mg/dL) and IgM production resumes
• No definitive treatment is available for AG, FIS, and CVID

NURSING CARE
N/A

ACTIVITY
N/A

DIET
N/A

CLIENT EDUCATION
• Clients should be advised to avoid breeding Fell or Dales horses that are carriers (heterozygous) for the genetic mutation for FIS
• If heterozygous animals are detected they should be used for nonreproductive pursuits

SURGICAL CONSIDERATIONS
N/A

MEDICATIONS

DRUG(S) OF CHOICE
Treat infections with appropriate antibiotics after culture and sensitivity testing.

CONTRAINDICATIONS
None

PRECAUTIONS
None

POSSIBLE INTERACTIONS
N/A

ALTERNATIVE DRUGS
None

FOLLOW-UP

PATIENT MONITORING
• Confirmation of clinical diagnosis should be made by repeating IgM and IgG assays
• In THY, low antibody values indicate the need for ongoing antibiotic coverage

PREVENTION/AVOIDANCE
• For FIS avoid production of affected foals by genetic testing both stallion and mare before breeding
• Breeding 2 carriers (heterozygous) will result in 25% of offspring with FIS, 50% carriers, and 25% normal
• Breeding a carrier with a normal horse will produce nonaffected foals but with 50% chance of being carrier

POSSIBLE COMPLICATIONS
Infections and organ dysfunction.

EXPECTED COURSE AND PROGNOSIS
• In general, prognosis is poor
• Cases of sIgMD have spontaneously recovered
• In THY, normal antibody production may resume by 12–24 months of age
• No cases of AG, FIS, or CVID have been reported to recover

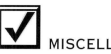

MISCELLANEOUS

ASSOCIATED CONDITIONS
Bacterial infections.

AGE-RELATED FACTORS
Predominantly observed in foals and weanlings, but late onset (adult age) is more common for CVID.

ZOONOTIC POTENTIAL
None

PREGNANCY/FERTILITY/BREEDING
For FIS avoid production of affected foals by genetic testing stallion and mare before breeding.

SYNONYMS
FIS was formerly known as Fell Pony syndrome.

SEE ALSO
• Failure of transfer of passive immunity (FTPI)
• Lymphopenia
• Lymphosarcoma
• Severe combined immunodeficiency

ABBREVIATIONS
• AG = agammaglobulinemia
• CVID = common variable immunodeficiency
• FIS = foal immunodeficiency syndrome
• FTPI = failure of transfer of passive immunity
• Ig = immunoglobulin
• SCID = severe combined immunodeficiency
• sIgMD = selective immunoglobulin M deficiency
• THY = transient hypogammaglobulinemia of the young

Suggested Reading
Bailey E. Screening for foal immunodeficiency syndrome. Vet Rec 2011;169:653.
Felippe MJB. Immunodeficiencies. In: Felippe MJB, ed. Equine Clinical Immunology. Ames, IA: Wiley Blackwell, 2016:193–204.

Author M. Julia B. Felippe
Consulting Editors David Hodgson, Harold C. McKenzie, and Jennifer L. Hodgson
Acknowledgment The author acknowledges the prior contribution of Jennifer L. Hodgson.

IMMUNOSUPPRESSION

BASICS

DEFINITION
The host's ability to mount an immune response to effect protection from pathogen challenge, which was initially normal, is diminished, rendering the animal at increased susceptibility to infection. Can involve any 1 or multiple of the components of the immune system—innate or adaptive arm, humoral, or CMI.

PATHOPHYSIOLOGY
• Protective immunity involves normal functioning and an orchestrated response of numerous cell types, including antigen-presenting cells, neutrophils, lymphocytes (B, CD4 + TH, CD8Tc), natural killer cells, monocytes/macrophages, mast cells, eosinophils, plus numerous soluble factors (cytokines, interleukins, interferons, chemokines, complement, immunoglobulins). • Immunologic defense mechanisms are described as innate and acquired. The innate immune system is a rapidly responding chemical and cellular defense mechanism that relies on pattern recognition of foreign antigens. Destruction involves cellular (neutrophils and macrophages) and soluble (complement system) factors. Innate immunity has no immunologic memory. • Acquired immunity is a defense mechanism characterized by immunologic memory and improved efficacy on reexposure. This system has 2 arms—humoral immunity ("Th2", B-lymphocyte produced, antibody mediated) directed against extracellular pathogens, and CMI ("Th1", T-lymphocyte mediated)

SYSTEMS AFFECTED
Hemic/lymphatic/immune.

GENETICS
N/A

INCIDENCE/PREVALENCE
Low

GEOGRAPHIC DISTRIBUTION
N/A

SIGNALMENT
Any age, breed, or gender.

SIGNS
• Onset of infectious disease during the first 6 postnatal weeks. • Recurrent infections that do not respond as expected to treatment. • Infections with organism with low pathogenicity, commensal organisms, or organisms rarely affecting immunocompetent animals (e.g. *Candida albicans, Cryptosporidium* spp., adenovirus). • Systemic illness following administration of attenuated live vaccine. • Failure to respond immunologically to vaccination. • Persistent, marked abnormalities in leukocyte numbers

CAUSES

Degenerative
Immunosenescence
• Innate, cell-mediated, and humoral immune responses all decline with age (>20 years). • Neutrophils and macrophages have reduced respiratory burst function and ability to produce nitrogen oxidants, decreasing their ability to kill phagocytized bacteria. Neutrophils have increased apoptosis. Dendritic cells have reduced numbers and B-lymphocyte stimulatory function
Pituitary Pars Intermedia Dysfunction
• Reduced neutrophil function, characterized by decreased oxidative burst activity and adhesion. • Likely effect of elevated α-melanocyte-stimulating hormone concentration

Anatomic
Neonate
Reduced ability to mount a Th1 CMI immune response, increasing susceptibility to pathogens.
Pregnancy
• Shift from a Th1 (CMI) to a Th2 (humoral) response. • Decreased neutrophil function

Metabolic
Strenuous High-Intensity Exercise, Prolonged Exhaustive Exercise, and Overtraining
• Decline in the ratio of CD4 + to CD8 + T lymphocytes. • Decreased proliferative response of blood lymphocytes after high-intensity exercise. • Suppression of innate immunity
Environmental Stressors
Rapid weaning, sleep deprivation, general anesthesia, prolonged transport, and overcrowding are all immunosuppressive.

Nutritional
Protein-Calorie Malnutrition
• Induces lymphopenia and reduces T-lymphocyte function. • B-lymphocyte function and humoral immunity unaffected. • Likely mediated through leptin deficiency associated with reduced adipose tissue stores. • Affected horses more commonly affected by bacterial diseases rather than viruses because bacteria can readily survive in malnourished tissue while viruses require healthy host cells in which to grow
Severe Obesity
Unknown mechanism.
Micronutrient Deficiencies Associated with Immunosuppression
• Copper—reduces neutrophil number and function by depression of superoxide production. Lymphopenia (T, B, and natural killer) and reduced lymphocyte function. Enhances mast cell histamine release. • Iron. • Magnesium—suppresses immunoglobulins. • Selenium—reduces neutrophil activity, T-, and natural killer lymphocyte responses and IgM production. • Vitamin A—loss of antioxidant action reduces lymphocyte proliferation, natural killer cell activity, and

cytokine and immunoglobulin production. • Vitamin B12 and folic acid—required for CMI. • Vitamin D—required for macrophage development. • Vitamin E—antioxidant in cell membranes and is important in regulating the oxidants produced by phagocytic cells. Depresses immunoglobulins through its effects on regulatory T cells. Decreased lymphocyte function. • Zinc—lymphoid atrophy, delayed CMI, reduced chemotaxis and microbial ingestion of phagocytic cells. Foals born to zinc-deficient mares are immunosuppressed

Neoplastic
Lymphosarcoma
Acquired selective IgM deficiency. Decreased lymphocyte blastogenesis response.
Plasma Cell Myeloma
Uncontrolled replication of single clones of plasma cells (differentiated B lymphocytes). Production of large quantities of a homogenous immunoglobulin or immunoglobulin fragment (monoclonal gammopathy). Normal immunoglobulins decreased.

Infectious
Perinatal EHV-1 Infection
In utero infection with EHV-1 associated with marked lymphoid damage resulting in perinatal development of interstitial pneumonia, lymphopenia, and immunosuppression.
Endotoxemia
Impairs CMI responses. Neutropenia and reduced neutrophil bactericidal function.
Chronic Diarrhea
Reduced IgA concentration and reduced lymphocyte response to mitogens.

Iatrogenic
Immunosuppressive Drugs
• Azathioprine and cyclophosphamide—act primarily to suppress activated lymphocytes. • Cyclosporine (ciclosporin) and tacrolimus—selective inhibition of T lymphocytes. Blocks CMI while preserving humoral responses
Corticosteroid-Induced Immunosuppression
• Endogenous (stress) or exogenous. • Suppression of CMI responses. • Eosinopenia, basopenia, and lymphopenia due to bone marrow sequestration. Circulating pool neutrophilia due to inhibition of adherence to vascular endothelium and emigration into tissues. Suppress neutrophil, monocyte, and eosinophil chemotaxis. • Induces T-cell lymphopenia. Suppress antigen-specific IgGa and IgGb responses while sparing IgG(T). • Inhibits proinflammatory cytokine synthesis and T-lymphocyte response by increasing the production of IκBα, the inhibitor of NF-κB. Inhibit the effects of phospholipases and prevent the production of prostaglandins and leukotrienes. • Enhanced catabolism of immunoglobulins. • Can induce

recrudescence of certain viral diseases (e.g. equine infectious anemia or EHV-1)

Traumatic and Toxic
Radiation
Kills dividing cells.
Environmental Toxins Inducing Immunosuppression
• Cadmium (cadmium chloride)—inhibits phagocytosis, inhibits T-cell and natural killer cell function and cell proliferation. • DDT. • Dieldrin. • Iodine. • Lead. • Methyl mercury. • Polybrominated and polychlorinated biphenyls. • Selenium
Plant Toxins Inducing Immunosuppression
Hairy vetch (*Vicia villosa*).
Mycotoxins Inducing Immunosuppression
• Aflatoxin mycotoxins—produced by fungal species including *Aspergillus, Penicillium, Rhizopus, Mucor*, and *Streptomyces*. Depress phagocytic activity. • Trichothecene mycotoxins—produced by the fungi *Fusarium, Myrothecium, Stachybotrys atra*, and *Trichothecium roseum* in grain. Depresses the response of lymphocytes and the chemotactic migration of neutrophils. Reduces IgM, IgA, and complement 3 concentrations.
• Fumonisin B1 inhibits division of both T and B lymphocytes
Severe Burn Injury
• Increased production of interleukin-10 and other immunosuppressive cytokines.
• Corticosteroid, prostaglandin, and suppressive active peptide release are all immunosuppressive. • Neutrophil and macrophage phagocytosis and respiratory burst activates impaired. • Reduced immunoglobulin synthesis

RISK FACTORS
See Causes.

DIAGNOSIS

DIFFERENTIAL DIAGNOSIS
• Neonatal sepsis. • Primary immunodeficiency

CBC/BIOCHEMISTRY/URINALYSIS
Leukopenia, neutropenia, lymphopenia, eosinopenia, and/or basopenia.

OTHER LABORATORY TESTS
• Lymphocyte subtyping via flow cytometry—normally 18% B lymphocytes, 62% CD4 + T cells, and 18% CD8 + T cells.
• Immunoglobulin subtype quantitation via radial immunodiffusion or serum electrophoresis tests B-lymphocyte function.
• Intradermal skin testing with the plant lectin phytohemagglutinin tests T-lymphocyte function. • Antibody response to novel vaccination and in vitro lymphocyte blastogenesis with pokeweed mitogen tests combined T- and B-lymphocyte function.
• Flow cytometric evaluation of phagocytosis by neutrophils and macrophages.

• Quantitation of complement, interferon, and various lymphokines

IMAGING
N/A

OTHER DIAGNOSTIC PROCEDURES
N/A

PATHOLOGIC FINDINGS
Perinatal EHV-1 infection—grossly small thymus and spleen, marked necrosis, and atrophy of the thymus and splenic lymphoid follicles, bilateral adrenocortical hyperplasia.

TREATMENT

APPROPRIATE HEALTH CARE
Culture and sensitivity of appropriate diagnostic specimen to identify secondary pathogen and instigation of treatment with appropriate antimicrobial/antifungal/anthelmintic/antiprotozoal agent as indicated.

NURSING CARE
Treatment of complications of secondary infection due to immunodeficiency.

ACTIVITY
Regular moderate exercise boosts immune function.

DIET
Appropriate dietary treatment of starved horse to avoid refeeding syndrome.

CLIENT EDUCATION
Depends on cause of immunosuppression.

SURGICAL CONSIDERATIONS
N/A

MEDICATIONS

DRUG(S) OF CHOICE
• Vitamin E (10–20 IU/kg RRR-α-tocopherol PO every 24 h, natural source higher biological activity) promotes B-cell proliferation. Mitigates pregnancy-induced immunosuppression. • Levamisole (2–3 mg/kg PO every 24 h for 3–5 days) stimulates T-cell differentiation and responses to antigens

CONTRAINDICATIONS
None

PRECAUTIONS
None

POSSIBLE INTERACTIONS
None

ALTERNATIVE DRUGS
N/A

FOLLOW-UP

PATIENT MONITORING
• Serial monitoring of CBC.
• Corticosteroid-induced lymphopenia usually resolves in 24 h

PREVENTION/AVOIDANCE
Conscientious use of drugs that may be immunosuppressive.

POSSIBLE COMPLICATIONS
Bacterial, viral, fungal, or parasitic infections.

EXPECTED COURSE AND PROGNOSIS
Prognosis is dependent upon the ability to address inciting cause and severity of the secondary infection at the time of diagnosis.

MISCELLANEOUS

ASSOCIATED CONDITIONS
Bacterial, fungal, and viral infections.

AGE-RELATED FACTORS
Any age.

ZOONOTIC POTENTIAL
Immunosuppressive drugs have identical biological effects in humans if absorbed.

PREGNANCY/FERTILITY/BREEDING
See Causes.

SYNONYMS
Immunologic disorder

SEE ALSO
• Failure of transfer of passive immunity (FTPI)
• Immunoglobulin deficiencies
• Lymphopenia
• Lymphosarcoma
• Pituitary pars intermedia dysfunction
• Severe combined immunodeficiency

ABBREVIATIONS
• CMI = cell mediated immunity
• EHV-1 = Equine herpesvirus-1 infection
• IgM/A/G = immunoglobulin M/A/G
• Th = T-helper cell

Suggested Reading
Tizzard IR. Secondary immunological deficits. In: Tizzard IR, ed. Veterinary Immunology, 8e. St. Louis, MO: WB Saunders, 2009:464–479.

Author Jamie G. Wearn
Consulting Editors David Hodgson, Harold C. McKenzie, and Jennifer L. Hodgson

BASICS

DEFINITION
An impaction is the obstruction of the GI tract, and depending on the portion affected may result in a variety of clinical signs. The obstruction may consist of feed material, fecal material, or foreign matter that slows or stops the movement of ingesta. This may result in distention of a viscus, causing abdominal pain. Impactions may be primary or secondary, and may cause partial to complete obstructions.

PATHOPHYSIOLOGY
Any disease that causes decreased gastric or intestinal motility may cause an impaction. There are feed-associated factors (coarse, high-fiber, low-digestible feedstuffs), and insufficient water intake, poor dentition, or a change in diet that may affect the breakdown of feed material resulting in delayed passage. Factors such as dehydration, change in exercise, and transport are thought to be important in initiating an obstruction. In addition, general anesthesia and surgical manipulations may affect the GI motility; therefore, postanesthetic impactions are not uncommon. Portions of the bowel where the intestinal lumen size narrows are common areas for impactions. These include the stomach, distal small intestine, cecum, pelvic flexure, right dorsal colon, transverse colon, and small colon. Impactions may also occur in areas where pacemakers controlling motility are located (cecum, pelvic flexure). In some cases, the cause of impactions may not be delineated.

SYSTEMS AFFECTED
GI
• Decreased appetite
• Decreased fecal output
• Increased or decreased borborygmi
• Abdominal distention
• Colic
• Diarrhea
• Other signs caused by primary disease

Behavioral
Vague changes in demeanor to severe signs of colic and toxemia.

Cardiovascular
• Normal to increased heart rate and capillary refill time
• Tacky mucous membranes
• Cardiovascular compromise as severity increases

Renal/Urologic
Changes associated with hypovolemia.

Respiratory
• Mild tachypnea
• Shallow respiration due to pain and abdominal distention

Skin/Exocrine
Sweating

SIGNALMENT
• Any age, breed, or sex
• Ascarid impactions—occurs in foals, weanlings, and yearlings
• Small colon impactions—may be more common in ponies and American Miniature Horses
• Cecal impaction—more common in postparturient mares and in horses following general anesthesia for nonabdominal surgeries

SIGNS
• Abdominal distention
• Anorexia (partial to complete)
• Decreased fecal output
• Diarrhea—sand impaction, small colon impaction, although may occur in course of treatment of other impactions
• Feces—firm/hard, dry, mucus covered
• Flank watching
• Frequent attempts to defecate
• Increased or decreased borborygmi
• Lethargy
• Nasogastric reflux
• Pawing
• Rectal prolapse
• Recumbency
• Rolling
• Straining to defecate
• Tail swishing

CAUSES
Gastric Impaction
Abrupt increase in amount of food, especially those that swell; outflow obstructions due to pyloric dysfunction or gastric mass, or small intestinal ileus or other disease that decreases small intestinal motility.

Small Intestine Impaction
Associated with coastal Bermuda grass, with mesenteric vascular disease, or with ileal wall thickening; ascarid impactions in young horses with heavy worm burdens are usually associated with anthelmintic treatments that cause sudden death or sudden paralysis of the parasites (organophosphates, piperazine, pyrantel pamoate), or cause hyperexcitability of the parasite prior to death (ivermectin, moxidectin).

Cecal Impaction
Multifactorial problem that occurs in the adult horse and is rare in foals. May occur as a primary problem due to an abrupt change in feed or may be secondary to altered motility due to general anesthesia, surgery, parturition, or sand ingestion. Parasitic or vascular damage affecting the cecal pacemaker may alter cecal motility.

Large Colon Impaction
• Decreased water intake
• Diet alteration
• Poor dentition
• Decreased exercise
• Sand ingestion

• Enteric parasitism

Small Colon Impaction
Similar to causes of large colon impaction.

DIAGNOSIS

DIFFERENTIAL DIAGNOSIS
Determination of the cause of colic should include a thorough collection of historical information, physical examination, abdominal palpation per rectum, and passage of a nasogastric tube.

Gastric Impaction
Rule out many other causes of colic, including causes of small intestinal/gastric reflux.

Small Intestine Impaction
Ileal hypertrophy, ileum-associated mass, small intestinal or ileal–cecal intussusception. Other causes of small intestinal distention include proximal duodenitis/jejunitis, small intestinal volvulus, entrapment, and strangulating lipoma.

Cecal Impaction
Differentials for cecal distention include cecocecal intussusception and cecocolic intussusception. For a "simple" cecal impaction, a cecum that is distended with ingesta should be palpable in the upper right abdominal quadrant. A medial and ventral band may be palpated. An apical impaction, early in the disease process, may not be palpable.

Large Colon Impaction
Colon displacements, early large colon/cecal torsions. Impaction of the left large colon should be palpable per rectum. The impacted pelvic flexure is usually located within the pelvic inlet and is positioned with the dorsal and ventral colon in a horizontal plane. A nephrosplenic entrapment may closely resemble a simple impaction of the left colon, but the position of the left colon is often reversed, and the colon and associated bands may be palpated from the pelvic brim to the nephrosplenic space. Ultrasonography is very helpful in making the diagnosis. Palpation of impactions of the right dorsal or transverse colon is not possible, and diagnosis would require a celiotomy or necropsy.

Small Colon Impaction
Major differential is impaction of the small intestine. Differentiation requires the detection of the large anti-mesenteric band on the small colon. Multiple loops of impacted small colon are usually palpable.

CBC/BIOCHEMISTRY/URINALYSIS
Usually normal; abnormalities may occur with progressive disease due to hypovolemia and debilitation of the bowel.

Abdominal Fluid Analysis
The fluid should be normal in appearance and have normal cytologic parameters.

I

IMPACTION

Abnormal cell count, cell differential, protein level, presence of bacteria or foreign material consistent with compromised bowel or another problem.

IMAGING

Radiographs
Helpful in assessing foal abdomens or searching for foreign bodies, enteroliths, or sand in adult horses.

Ultrasonography
A useful tool in evaluating foal and adult abdomens. Can be used transcutaneously or per rectum to assess intestinal distention (may include loss of sacculations with large colon impaction), intestinal wall thickness, and intestinal motility. Possible to detect intussusceptions and masses, but it has limitations in diagnosis of impaction.

TREATMENT

GI Impactions
• Resolve primary risk factors
• Medical therapy should include withholding feed; however, small amounts of feed may help maintain GI motility and may be considered in impactions of the large or small colon
• Further medical therapy may include IV crystalloid fluids given at a high rate to increase the fluid content in the bowel to break down impaction. If tolerated, fluids may be given via an indwelling nasogastric tube at rates up to 6 L/h in a 450 kg horse
• Medications may be given orally to soften the feces and analgesics may be administered as needed
• Exploratory surgery may be required depending on the type of disease and its severity, duration, and progression

Gastric Impactions
Medical therapy should include withholding feed and maintenance of the hydration status. The stomach may be lavaged through a nasogastric tube; however, caution must be used to prevent further gastric distention and rupture.

SURGICAL CONSIDERATIONS
Consider abdominal surgery for unmanageable pain, displacement of intestine, abnormal peritoneal fluid, or deterioration in condition.

MEDICATIONS

DRUG(S) OF CHOICE

Laxatives
• Mineral oil—2–4 L/450 kg horse, every 12 h via nasogastric tube
• DSS—120–240 mL/450 kg horse of 4% DSS with water

• Psyllium hydrophilic mucilloid— 0.25–0.5 kg/450 kg horse

Cathartics
• Magnesium sulfate (Epsom salts)— 0.5–1.0 kg every 24 h
• Sodium sulfate (Glauber's salts)— 0.25–0.5 kg every 24 h

Analgesia and Anti-inflammatory Drugs (NSAIDs)
• Flunixin meglumine—0.5–1.1 mg/kg IV every 24 h/12 h/8 h
• Ketoprofen—2.2 mg/kg IV every 24 h/12 h/8 h
• Phenylbutazone—2.2–4.4 mg/kg IV every 24 h/12 h

Analgesia and Sedation
• Xylazine—use α_2-adrenergic agonists sparingly due to decreased motility
• Romifidine—40–80 µg/kg IM, IV
• Detomidine—10–30 µg/kg IM, IV
• Butorphanol—0.01–0.05 mg/kg (some horses may need prior or concurrent α_2-adrenergic agonist)
• N-butylscopolammonium (spasmolytic)— 0.3 mg/kg IV

CONTRAINDICATIONS

NSAIDs
NSAIDs may cause renal papillary and tubular necrosis or GI ulceration; side effects may be worse in a dehydrated animal.

α_2-Adrenergic Agonists
Side effects include transient hypertension followed by longer lasting hypotension, bradycardia, secondary atrioventricular blockade, decreased GI motility, sweating, and diuresis.

Salt Cathartics
Animal must be well hydrated; may cause distention and more severe colic. Toxic to enterocytes with repeated administration.

FOLLOW-UP

POSSIBLE COMPLICATIONS
Magnesium sulfate therapy can lead to hypermagnesemia, especially if there is deficiency in renal function, hypocalcemia, or compromised vascular integrity.

EXPECTED COURSE AND PROGNOSIS
• Good for cecal impaction if primary and detected and treated early in disease
• Guarded for cecal impaction if it persists for >24–48 h
• Excellent for pelvic flexure impaction
• Guarded for ileal and small colon impactions

MISCELLANEOUS

SEE ALSO
Colic, chronic/recurrent

ABBREVIATIONS
• DSS = dioctyl sodium sulfosuccinate
• GI = gastrointestinal
• NSAID = nonsteroidal anti-inflammatory drug

Suggested Reading
Aitken MR, Southwood LL, Ross BM, Ross MW. Outcome of surgical and medical management of cecal impaction in 150 horses (1991-2011). Vet Surg 2015; 44(5):540–546.

Blikslager AT. Surgical disorders of the small intestine. In: Smith BP, ed. Large Animal Internal Medicine, 4e. St. Louis, MO: Mosby, 2009:732–733.

Blikslager AT. Surgical disorders of the large intestine. In: Smith BP, ed. Large Animal Internal Medicine, 4e. St. Louis, MO: Mosby, 2009:750–752.

Dart AJ, Snyder JR, Pascoe JR, et al. Abnormal conditions of the equine descending (small) colon: 102 cases (1979–1989). J Am Vet Med Assoc 1992;200:971–978.

Fleming K, Mueller PO. Ileal impaction in 245 horses: 1995-2007. Can Vet J 2011;52(7):759–763.

Frederico LM, Jones SL, Blikslager AT. Predisposing factors for small colon impaction in horses and outcome of medical and surgical treatment: 44 cases (1999-2004). J Am Vet Med Assoc 2006;229(10):1612–1616.

Furness MC, Snyman HN, Abrahams M, et al. Severe gastric impaction secondary to a gastric polyp in a horse. Can Vet J 2013;54(10):979–982.

Plummer AE, Rakestraw PC, Hardy J, Lee RM. Outcome of medical and surgical treatment of cecal impaction in horses: 114 cases (1994-2004). J Am Vet Med Assoc 2007;231(9):1378–1385.

White NA, Dabareiner RM. Treatment of impaction colics. Vet Clin North Am Equine Pract 1997;13:243–259.

Author Daniel G. Kenney
Consulting Editors Olimpo Oliver-Espinosa and Henry Stämpfli

I

BASICS

DEFINITION
• An infectious disease caused by the EIAV, a lentivirus of the family Retroviridae
• EIAV is closely related to HIV-1, the cause of AIDS in humans

PATHOPHYSIOLOGY
• EIAV is transmitted primarily by blood-feeding insects, especially tabanids (i.e. horseflies and deerflies); iatrogenic transmission can occur via contaminated needles, syringes, and surgical instruments as well as through contaminated semen and transfusion of contaminated blood or plasma
• Once infected, a horse remains so for life
• EIAV infects cells of the monocyte/macrophage lineage and can be detected in the cytoplasm of this cell type in the liver, spleen, lymph nodes, lung, bone marrow, and circulation
• EIAV also replicates in endothelial cells, which may serve as a viral reservoir; viral replication in endothelial cells may cause vasculitis
• EIAV can be characterized by 3 clinical syndromes—acute, chronic, and inapparent carrier; not all horses progress through all 3 syndromes
• Acute disease—usually occurs 1–4 weeks after infection; is associated with high levels of viremia; can be characterized by fever, anorexia, lethargy, ventral edema, thrombocytopenia, anemia, and, occasionally, epistaxis and death; and is usually <1 week in duration and sometimes mild enough to go completely unnoticed
• Chronic disease—associated with recurrent episodes of viral replication, causing repeated bouts of clinical signs; classic signs of anemia, ventral edema, and weight loss occur during this phase
• With time, episodes of clinical disease decrease in duration and severity, and most horses control the infection within 1 year, becoming inapparent carriers
• Inapparent carriers show no clinical signs, are seropositive, and are reservoirs of infection, capable of transmitting the virus to uninfected horses

SYSTEMS AFFECTED
• Hemic/lymphatic/immune—anemia caused by immune-mediated intravascular and extravascular hemolysis as well as bone marrow suppression. Likewise, thrombocytopenia is caused by both bone marrow suppression and enhanced platelet destruction; severe thrombocytopenia can lead to mucous membrane petechiae and epistaxis
• Cardiovascular—immune-mediated vasculitis leads to hemorrhage, thrombosis, and edema
• Hepatobiliary—accumulations of lymphocytes and macrophages in the liver can result in hepatomegaly, fatty degeneration, and hepatic cell necrosis
• Renal/urologic—immune complex deposition can result in glomerulonephritis
• Neurologic—vasculitis and lymphocyte accumulation in meninges occasionally result in ataxia

GENETICS
N/A

GEOGRAPHIC DISTRIBUTION
In the USA, since less than 25% of the total United States horse population is tested, the true prevalence is unknown and a reservoir of infected horses remains undetected. Prevalence varies by state, and ranges from 0% to 0.14% of horses tested. The prevalence is usually higher in the Gulf Coast states, because the climate is favorable for vectors and virus transmission.

SIGNALMENT
• Horses, ponies, mules, and donkeys are susceptible; however, donkeys and mules appear to be less severely affected
• No breed, age, or sex predilections

SIGNS
General Comments
• Clinical signs—vary, depending on the stage of disease
• Inapparent carriers—clinically normal
• Chronic stage—affected animals may show no signs between clinical episodes

Historical Findings
• Signs can go unnoticed
• May be a history of inappetence, lethargy, and fever
• Severely affected horses may have a history of high fever (40.5–41.5°C; 105–106°F), depression, ventral edema, weight loss, ataxia, and epistaxis

Physical Examination Findings
Normal, or could include poor body condition, lethargy, fever, mucosal petechiation, ventral edema, pale mucous membranes, epistaxis, and ataxia.

CAUSES
Infection with EIAV.

RISK FACTORS
Contact with other equids during warm weather, when tabanids are abundant. Transfusion of contaminated blood or plasma.

 DIAGNOSIS

DIFFERENTIAL DIAGNOSIS
• List of differential diagnoses depends on the predominant clinical signs
• Horses affected with these other diseases are seronegative for EIAV and easily differentiated from those infected with EIAV
• Anemia/thrombocytopenia—blood loss, anemia of chronic disease, red maple intoxication, immune-mediated thrombocytopenia/hemolytic anemia, and neoplasia
• Fever—other viral/bacterial/inflammatory diseases and neoplasia
• Fever/thrombocytopenia—*Anaplasma phagocytophilum* infection, trichothecene ingestion/toxicity
• Weight loss—inadequate feed intake, dental abnormalities, parasitism, other chronic diseases, and neoplasia
• Ventral edema—hypoalbuminemia, pleuropneumonia, vasculitis, neoplasia, protein-losing enteropathy, and peritonitis
• Ataxia—cervical stenotic myelopathy, equine herpesvirus 1 myeloencephalitis, and equine protozoal myeloencephalitis

CBC/BIOCHEMISTRY/URINALYSIS
• Thrombocytopenia—the first laboratory abnormality detected in acutely infected horses, occurs coincidentally with fever, resolves along with resolution of the clinical disease, but recurs with subsequent disease cycles
• Decreases in packed cell volume and red blood cells can occur shortly after infection but generally are more severe during the chronic stage; leukopenia, lymphocytosis, and monocytosis are observed in many infected horses
• Hypergammaglobulinemia may be present
• Increases in liver enzyme activities may occur

OTHER LABORATORY TESTS
• Diagnosis confirmed by serologic testing—AGID (Coggins test) and several ELISA tests are approved by the USDA and detect serum antibody to the EIAV core protein, Gag p26
• Acute infection produces detectable antibody within 45 days
• Coggins test—the most widely used and 95% accurate in diagnosing EIAV infection; occasional false-negative results may occur
• ELISA is more sensitive than AGID, but less specific, leading to possible false-positive results
• All horses testing positive with either test should be retested for confirmation

IMAGING
N/A

OTHER DIAGNOSTIC PROCEDURES
N/A

PATHOLOGIC FINDINGS
• In horses that die or are euthanized during a febrile episode, lesions include splenomegaly, hepatomegaly, accentuated hepatic lobular structure, lymphadenopathy, mucosal and visceral hemorrhages, ventral subcutaneous edema, and vessel thrombosis
• Accumulations of lymphocytes and macrophages in the periportal regions of the liver and in the spleen, lymph nodes, adrenal gland, lung, and meninges

I

INFECTIOUS ANEMIA (EIA)

- Lymphoproliferative lesions are thought to result from the spread of virus-reactive T lymphocytes to control infection
- Fatty degeneration of the liver and hepatic cell necrosis
- Glomerulitis can be present
- Necropsy of inapparent carriers—unremarkable

 TREATMENT

APPROPRIATE HEALTH CARE
- No effective treatment
- Immediately isolate seropositive horses from other equids and control vector populations

NURSING CARE
- Provide general supportive care during clinical episodes; the nature of this care varies, depending on the types and severity of signs
- Whole-blood transfusions may benefit horses with severe anemia or thrombocytopenia
- Standing leg wraps may benefit horses with ventral pitting edema
- Cold-water hosing may decrease the temperature in horses with high fever that is nonresponsive to NSAIDs

ACTIVITY
N/A

DIET
N/A

CLIENT EDUCATION
- A reportable disease in many countries, including the USA
- Federal law prohibits interstate travel of infected animals, except for slaughter, return to place of origin, or transport to a recognized research facility or diagnostic laboratory
- Individual states regulate intrastate travel, and most control measures include the following options for seropositive horses—euthanasia, permanent identification and lifelong quarantine, or transport to a recognized research facility

SURGICAL CONSIDERATIONS
N/A

 MEDICATIONS

DRUG(S) OF CHOICE
- Because no treatment for EIAV is effective and infected horses remain so for life, only rarely is treatment attempted

- NSAIDs may be administered for control of fever and inflammation during viremic, febrile episodes—flunixin meglumine (1.1 mg/kg IV every 12 h)

CONTRAINDICATIONS
Corticosteroids will exacerbate viremia and clinical disease, and are therefore contraindicated.

PRECAUTIONS
N/A

POSSIBLE INTERACTIONS
N/A

ALTERNATIVE DRUGS
N/A

 FOLLOW-UP

PATIENT MONITORING
N/A

PREVENTION/AVOIDANCE
- Federal and state control measures have lowered the prevalence of EIAV in the USA, but outbreaks still occur
- Veterinarians, horse owners, and others in the equine industry can reduce the chance of exposure by requiring an EIAV test as part of every prepurchase examination; a recent, negative EIAV test before admitting any new horse to a farm; recent, negative EIAV tests for horses entering shows, sales, race tracks, and other events; annual testing of all horses for EIAV exposure; never injecting different horses with a common needle or syringe; ensuring that blood and blood products used for transfusions are from EIAV-negative donors; thoroughly disinfecting instruments that come into contact with blood; and practicing rigorous fly control

POSSIBLE COMPLICATIONS
N/A

EXPECTED COURSE AND PROGNOSIS
- Occasionally, horses may die of EIAV, but most eventually control the infection and become lifelong, inapparent carriers
- Inapparent carriers are clinically normal but remain reservoirs of infection

 MISCELLANEOUS

ASSOCIATED CONDITIONS
N/A

AGE-RELATED FACTORS
N/A

ZOONOTIC POTENTIAL
N/A

PREGNANCY/FERTILITY/BREEDING
- EIAV can be transmitted transplacentally in pregnant mares and may cause abortion
- EIAV may be transmitted via colostrum or milk. Not all foals born to infected mares are infected; testing the foal after maternal antibody wanes should be considered

SYNONYMS
Swamp fever

ABBREVIATIONS
- AGID = agar gel immunodiffusion
- AIDS = acquired immunodeficiency syndrome
- EIAV = equine infectious anemia virus
- ELISA = enzyme-linked immunosorbent assay
- HIV = human immunodeficiency virus
- NSAID = nonsteroidal anti-inflammatory drug
- USDA = United States Department of Agriculture

Suggested Reading
Mealey RH. Equine infectious anemia virus. In: Sellon DC, Long MT, eds. Equine Infectious Diseases. St. Louis, MO: Saunders, 2006:213–219.
Montelaro RC, Ball JM, Rushlow KE. Equine retroviruses. In: Levy JA, ed. The Retroviridae. New York, NY: Plenum Press, 1993:257–360.
Sellon DC, Fuller FJ, McGuire TC. The immunopathogenesis of equine infectious anemia virus. Virus Res 1994;32:111–138.
Sponseller BA. Equine infectious anemia. In: Smith BP, ed. Large Animal Internal Medicine, 5e. St. Louis, MO: Elsevier Mosby, 2015:1060–1061.

Author Brett Sponseller
Consulting Editor Ashley G. Boyle
Acknowledgment The author and editor acknowledge the prior contribution of Robert H. Mealey.

INFECTIOUS ARTHRITIS (NONHEMATOGENOUS)

 BASICS

DEFINITION
Inflammatory intra-articular process caused by direct invasion of microorganisms such as bacteria or rarely viruses or fungi.

PATHOPHYSIOLOGY
Microorganisms invade joint by direct inoculation via intra-articular injections, traumatic wounds, joint surgery, or dissemination from periarticular infected tissue.

SYSTEMS AFFECTED
Musculoskeletal—joint.

INCIDENCE/PREVALENCE
Any breed.

SIGNALMENT
Breed Predilections
Standardbreds overrepresented due to frequent intra-articular injections.

Mean Age and Range
None

Predominant Sex
None

SIGNS
Historical Findings
• Lameness ± joint effusion. • Traumatic intra-articular wound. • Draining wound near joint. • Recent intra-articular injection

Physical Examination Findings
• Lameness, often severe. • Joint effusion. • Periarticular edema and/or cellulitis and heat. • Extreme pain on palpation and manipulation of affected joint. • With open joint lacerations, lameness and effusion are minimal

CAUSES
• Traumatic articular wounds. • Inoculation during intra-articular injection. • Postsurgical infection. • Idiopathic. • Common Gram-negative organisms— Enterobacteriaceae including *Escherichia coli, Pseudomonas, Acinetobacter, Proteus, Klebsiella, Citrobacter, Salmonella, Enterococcus.*
• Common Gram-positive organisms— coagulase-positive *Staphylococcus,* coagulase-negative *Staphylococcus,* β-hemolytic *Streptococcus,* non-β-hemolytic *Streptococcus, Rhodococcus equi, Corynebacterium.*
• *Staphylococcus aureus* is most common after surgery or injection. • Anaerobic organisms—*Clostridium, Bacteroides, Fusobacterium,* and *Peptostreptococcus* are common in wounds near the foot

RISK FACTORS
• Performance horse. • Intra-articular injection

 DIAGNOSIS

DIFFERENTIAL DIAGNOSIS
• Aseptic synovitis ("flare")—rule out with synovial fluid analysis. • Traumatic osteochondral fragmentation—rule out with radiography, synovial fluid analysis

CBC/BIOCHEMISTRY/URINALYSIS
• Increased SAA. • ± Hyperfibrinogenemia

OTHER LABORATORY TESTS
Synovial Fluid Analysis
• Gross abnormalities—watery, turbid, and cloudy fluid, ± flocculent material.
• Nucleated cells—>30 000 cells/μL, >80% neutrophils, ± toxic and degenerative changes. • Total protein—≥4.0 g/dL; in acute cases >3.5 g/dL. • Increased synovial SAA

Synovial Fluid Culture
• Only 60–75% of infected joints yield a positive culture. For this reason, synovial fluid cytology is imperative. • To increase likelihood of positive culture, obtain synovial sample prior to antibiotic administration and submit in broth culture medium with large synovial fluid volume (5–10 mL)

IMAGING
Radiography
• Often normal in early infection.
• ± Concomitant fracture. • ± Osteolysis or osteomyelitis. • Serial radiography to identify preexisting or developing osteoarthritis and to monitor progression, particularly in chronic infection

Ultrasonography
• Synovial effusion, intra-articular fibrinous material, synovial proliferation, ± cartilage defects. • Very helpful to confirm diagnosis when extensive edema, periarticular swelling, or joint location (hip or shoulder) make visual assessment of joint difficult

Nuclear Scintigraphy
• Increased radiopharmaceutical uptake in subchondral and/or periphyseal bone.
• Reduced radioactivity (photopenia) with sequestra

CT/MRI
Synovial proliferation, cartilage defects, subchondral bone changes.

OTHER DIAGNOSTIC PROCEDURES
Digital Exploration of the Wound
• Aseptically prepare wound and surrounding skin, explore with sterile gloves. • Confirms commination when articular cartilage is palpated. • Avoid creating a previously nonexistent communication between wound and joint

Joint Distention with Sterile Saline
• Easiest, most effective way to confirm wound communication. • Procedure—aseptic joint preparation, arthrocentesis at a location distant from wound, distend joint with sterile saline. • Leakage of fluid from the wound confirms joint communication

Contrast Radiography
Similar to saline joint distention, except iodinated contrast agent is injected into the joint. Radiopaque agent outside the joint confirms wound communication.

PATHOLOGIC FINDINGS
• Synovial thickening. • Hyperemic synovium. • Cartilage degradation. • Bone necrosis. • Intra-articular fibrin

 TREATMENT

AIMS
• Eliminate joint infection. • Avoid or minimize articular damage. • Reduce joint pain and inflammation. • Return horse to previous level of soundness

APPROPRIATE HEALTH CARE
• Should be regarded as a medical emergency.
• Inpatient medical management is desirable.
• Typical case management consists of antimicrobial therapy, joint lavage ± debridement, and pain management. Periodic synovial fluid analysis, lameness evaluation, and radiographic assessment are also performed. • Antimicrobial therapies:
◦ Systemic antimicrobials—broad spectrum until infection has completely resolved. Initial choices adjusted after bacterial culture and sensitivity results. Treatment continues for a minimum of 2–4 weeks beyond clinical resolution. ◦ Local therapy—intra-articular antimicrobials via single injection, constant rate infusion, and/or antimicrobial-impregnated polymethylmethacrylate beads; daily treatment initially, then as needed.
◦ Regional limb perfusion—delivery of high antimicrobial concentration via IV or interosseous delivery; procedure—place tourniquet proximal to affected joint, antimicrobials diluted into 60–100 mL of saline are administered slowly via venous or interosseous injection; remove tourniquet after 30–35 min; perform daily or every other day until infection resolves. • Pain management—systemic NSAIDs, intra-articular NSAIDs, topical NSAIDs, epidural narcotics, fentanyl transdermal patches

I

INFECTIOUS ARTHRITIS (NONHEMATOGENOUS) (CONTINUED)

NURSING CARE
• Bandaging—to reduce soft tissue swelling, edema, and joint effusion. Provides increased comfort, better visualization of infected structure(s). • Physical therapy—passive joint flexion once acute inflammation has resolved. • Cold therapy—<25 min per treatment; methods include cold hosing, ice wraps, cold/pressure delivery systems (Game Ready™)

ACTIVITY
• Rest and controlled exercise—minimum of 4 weeks of stall rest with hand-walking exercise. • Chronic cases, particularly those with associated degenerative changes, require extended convalescence

DIET
• Reduce high-energy feeds during convalescence. • Monitor hay intake to prevent large colon or cecal impactions

CLIENT EDUCATION
• It is a medical emergency and should be treated as such. • Any wound near a joint should be fully investigated. • Unexpected lameness and/or effusion after joint injections should be fully investigated. • Multiple therapies are common and treatment is frequently prolonged. • Without proper treatment, chronic lameness, refractory infection, and contralateral limb laminitis

SURGICAL CONSIDERATIONS
• Joint lavage—most important intervention along with antimicrobials; performed immediately and then as needed depending on infection severity; procedure—copious balanced electrolyte solution infused under pressure, ± antimicrobials or anti-inflammatories, multiple large (14–18)-gauge needles placed on opposite sides of joint; performed in the sedated standing horse with local anesthesia or anesthetized horse. • Arthroscopic lavage and debridement—allows joint visualization and removal of foreign debris, fibrin, infected synovium; also an effective method of lavage. • Joint drainage—considered in chronic cases and when lavage alone has not resulted in desired results; drainage via arthroscopic incisions, preexisting wound tract, open arthrotomy, or closed suction drainage systems

MEDICATIONS

DRUG(S) OF CHOICE
• Systemic antimicrobials—broad-spectrum combination (penicillin or cephalosporin and aminoglycoside) ○ Potassium penicillin

(22 000–44 000 IU/kg IV QID). ○ Ceftiofur sodium (2.2–4.4 mg/kg IV daily to BID). ○ Gentamicin sulfate (6.6–8.0 mg/kg IV SID). ○ Enrofloxacin (5 mg/kg PO SID). • Intra-articular antimicrobials ○ Amikacin sulfate (250–500 mg). ○ Gentamicin sulfate (500 mg). ○ Sodium penicillin (1×10^6 units). ○ Cefazolin (500 mg). ○ Ceftiofur sodium (500 mg). • Antimicrobials for regional limb perfusion ○ Amikacin sulfate, ceftiofur sodium, cefazolin, ceftazidime. ○ All at 1 g concentrations diluted into 60 mL of saline. • ± Dimethylsulfoxide as a 10% lavage solution as a free radical scavenger and anti-inflammatory agent. • Systemic NSAIDs—phenylbutazone (2.2–4.4 mg/kg IV or PO every 12–24 h). • Topical NSAIDs—1% diclofenac sodium cream (12.5 cm (5 inches) ribbon of cream over affected joint every 12 h for up to 10 days). • Epidural narcotics—morphine (0.1 mg/kg every 24 h) or detomidine (0.05 mg/kg every 6–24 h)

CONTRAINDICATIONS
• Systemic fluoroquinolones in neonates due to potential osteochondrosis. • Intra-articular fluoroquinolones due to their toxic effects on chondrocytes

PRECAUTIONS
• Systemic NSAIDs can be ulcerogenic. Monitor for inappetence, diarrhea, colic. • NSAIDs and aminoglycosides can be nephrotoxic; therefore, renal function (via serum creatinine levels) should be evaluated and rechecked periodically

POSSIBLE INTERACTIONS
None

ALTERNATIVE DRUGS
None

FOLLOW-UP

PATIENT MONITORING
• Joint evaluation during daily bandage change. Joint effusion, drainage, heat, and swelling are assessed. • General comfort and lameness are initially monitored daily and then as needed. • To assess disease progression and response to therapy, periodic synovial fluid analysis and synovial fluid culture and sensitivity are performed. • Periodic radiographic and ultrasonographic evaluations are also performed. CT scans allow early recognition of bone lesions, especially in foals

PREVENTION/AVOIDANCE
• Avoid unnecessary joint injections. • Good husbandry to reduce the likelihood of accidents and lacerations

POSSIBLE COMPLICATIONS
• Osteoarthritis. • Osteomyelitis. • Lameness, inability to return to previous level of performance. • Contralateral limb laminitis. • If severe, complications could necessitate euthanasia

EXPECTED COURSE AND PROGNOSIS
• Prognosis is good for survival and return to athletic soundness with early recognition and aggressive treatment. • Preexisting osteoarthritis or cartilage damage secondary to infection will decrease athletic performance. • Delayed recognition, minimal therapy, and drug-resistant organisms result in worse prognosis

MISCELLANEOUS

ASSOCIATED CONDITIONS
• Osteoarthritis. • Lameness. • Traumatic articular fracture

AGE-RELATED FACTORS
Infectious arthritis and osteomyelitis secondary to septicemia is common in newborn foals.

PREGNANCY/FERTILITY/BREEDING
None

SYNONYMS
Septic arthritis, joint infection.

SEE ALSO
• Laminitis
• Osteoarthritis
• Osteochondrosis

ABBREVIATIONS
• CT = computed tomography
• MRI = magnetic resonance imaging
• NSAID = nonsteroidal anti-inflammatory drug
• SAA = serum amyloid A

Suggested Reading
Bertone AL. Infectious arthritis. In: Ross MW, Dyson SJ, eds. Diagnosis and Management of Lameness in the Horse, 2e. St. Louis, MO: Elsevier Saunders, 2011:677–684.
Richardson DW, Ahern BJ. Synovial and osseous infections. In: Auer JA, Stick JA, eds. Equine Surgery, 4e. St. Louis, MO: WB Saunders, 2012:1189–1201.
van Weeren PR. Septic arthritis. In: McIlwraith CW, Frisbie DD, Kawcak CE, van Weeren PR, eds. Joint Disease in the Horse, 2e. St. Louis, MO: Elsevier, 2016:91–104.

Author José M. García-López
Consulting Editor Elizabeth J. Davidson

BASICS

DEFINITION
• A nonseptic inflammation of the lower airways caused by an accumulation of a variety of inflammatory cells leading to excess mucus production, coughing, and a reduction in exercise performance
• Some clinical features are similar to heaves/RAO
• The term "equine asthma" has recently been used when describing nonseptic inflammation of the lower airways with "severe equine asthma" for what was known as heaves/RAO, and mild to moderate equine asthma for IAD. This new terminology does not imply a common pathophysiology

PATHOPHYSIOLOGY
Horses develop an increased sensitivity to dust, molds, pollens, and other irritants, resulting in inflammatory cells such as mast cells, neutrophils, eosinophils, lymphocytes, and alveolar macrophages to release potent mediators. The relationship between the presence of increased populations of mast cells/eosinophils and airway hyperreactivity has been reported. Peribronchiolar inflammatory cell infiltration, goblet cell hyperplasia, and accumulation of mucus and neutrophils in the airway lumen has been demonstrated in lung biopsies.

SYSTEMS AFFECTED
• Respiratory
• Pathologic changes more severe in the peripheral airways (i.e. bronchioles); alveoli are not affected

GENETICS
Breed and sex-specific genetic linkages have not been consistently identified.

INCIDENCE/PREVALENCE
Widespread where horses are stabled or trained indoors.

GEOGRAPHIC DISTRIBUTION
Identified in North America, the UK, Australia, Iceland and Europe.

SIGNALMENT
• Any breed
• Typically first recognized in horses <12 years of age but older than 1 year

SIGNS
Historical Findings
• Reduced exercise tolerance or poor performance, with a prolonged recovery period after exercise is the most common reported clinical sign in performance horses
• Other observations include intermittent to frequent coughing while the horse is eating or early in exercise and nasal discharge

Physical Examination Findings
• Vital signs are within the normal range, except on occasion, when the resting

respiratory rate may exceed 18 breaths/min or when a prolonged return to normal respiratory rate after exercise is observed
• Nasal discharge is uncommon
• A significant increase in bronchial sounds over both lung fields easily heard on auscultation
• With a rebreathing bag, wheezes are frequently detected over the dorsal area of the lung field and coughing may be elicited in performance horses
• Lung-field percussion may identify dorsal and caudal areas of hyperresonance, detectable beyond the 16th rib

CAUSES
• A combination of airborne environmental allergens and endotoxins is considered to be the primary causative agents—mold and dust from hay and bedding and noxious gases such as ammonia from stagnant bedding
• The role of respiratory viral infections in the development of IAD remains under investigation
• Exacerbation of airway inflammation following a bacterial bronchitis in weanlings and occasionally yearlings
• Development and progressive airway inflammation following onset of exercise-induced pulmonary hemorrhage is a suspected cause

RISK FACTORS
• Predisposing and exacerbation of specific risk factors include respiratory viral infections (e.g. EIV and equine rhinitis viruses) and bacterial bronchitis (*Streptococcus zooepidemicus*) in young horses
• Higher incidence during hot summer days with high humidity
• High-intensity training and racing

 DIAGNOSIS

DIFFERENTIAL DIAGNOSIS
• Respiratory viral infections (e.g. EIV and equine herpesvirus) generally affect several horses in the same stable within a defined period of time, whereas IAD affects and persists in individuals and worsens over time
• Bacterial tracheitis and bronchitis, usually secondary to respiratory viral infection
• Localized pulmonary abscess may present with a similar history. However, pulmonary abscesses may be diagnosed based upon characteristic clinical signs including fever, inappetence, and pain on chest percussion over the anteroventral area of the lung fields

CBC/BIOCHEMISTRY/BLOOD GAS ANALYSIS/URINALYSIS
CBC and serum biochemistry profile are within normal limits.

OTHER LABORATORY TESTS
• Bronchoscopy and bronchoalveolar lavage to retrieve cells of the lower airways and alveoli

• Total count and differential of cell counts harvested from bronchoalveolar lavage fluid. These cells are analyzed quantitatively and qualitatively to determine major changes in the inflammatory cell population—neutrophils, mast cells, eosinophils, lymphocytes, and exfoliated epithelial cells
• Bronchoprovocation with histamine is a specific test that determines the degree of airway hyperresponsiveness (increased sensitivity to a variety of agents)
• Lung biopsies to evaluate histologic changes of the small airways and provide information on severity and prognosis. Lung biopsies are not routinely performed

IMAGING
Thoracic radiography has little value except to demonstrate noncharacteristic, small, 2–4-mm diameter, donut-shaped lesions in the periphery of bronchioles in some horses.

OTHER DIAGNOSTIC PROCEDURES
Pulmonary scintigraphy may have some potential as an adjunct diagnostic tool but is limited to most academic institutions or specialized equine clinics.

PATHOLOGIC FINDINGS
Persistent small airway inflammation has led to the term "airway remodeling," referring to dynamic pathologic changes during the course of persistent ongoing inflammation. Such changes have been recognized in heaves but have not been well characterized in IAD, where:
• Limited evidence suggests that lesions are generally restricted to the peripheral airways (<5 mm)
• Accumulation of inflammatory cells in the airways and mucus plugging of the airways caused by goblet cell hyperplasia may be early changes
• Increased smooth muscle mass suspected

 TREATMENT

AIMS
To control the airway inflammation, leading to improvement in pulmonary function and reduction in airway hyperreactivity and mucus production.

APPROPRIATE HEALTH CARE
• Environmental management is imperative to successfully treat and manage cases of IAD. Make all possible attempts to avoid environmental dust from low-quality hay and bedding. In susceptible horses, hay alternatives (e.g. pelleted/cube hay, haylage, and pasteurized hay ("hay steamer" such as Haygain)) are effective in reducing dust level
• Encourage outdoor living with opened shelter access

NURSING CARE
N/A

I

INFLAMMATORY AIRWAY DISEASE—IAD IN PERFORMANCE HORSES (MILD AND MODERATE EQUINE ASTHMA) (CONTINUED)

ACTIVITY
No limitations with proper therapeutic plans and environmental management control.

DIET
See Appropriate Health Care.

CLIENT EDUCATION
• IAD can be managed, allowing the horse to maintain an active and maximal performance athletic career
• Environmental management is imperative and includes a well-ventilated stall environment, rubber flooring with high-efficiency urine-absorbing materials and complete pelleted ration with small amount of steamed or soaked hay
• Turn out horses as much as possible
• Long-term therapy with an MDI is preferable as the medication is directly delivered to the lungs with minimal systemic effect. Alternatively, systemic therapy with corticosteroids (prednisolone/dexamethasone) at the minimum effective dose
• Maintain an up-to-date vaccination schedule for respiratory viral pathogens

SURGICAL CONSIDERATIONS
N/A

MEDICATIONS

DRUG(S) OF CHOICE
Corticosteroids (Mature Horses)
• Oral—prednisolone (400 mg BID for 15 days, then 300 mg once a day for 15 days, and a maintenance dose of 300 mg once a day on alternate days for as long as needed) or oral dexamethasone at a starting dose of 0.05 mg/kg daily or on alternate days
• MDIs with special delivery devices—fluticasone propionate (250 μg/puff; 8–12 puffs BID for 2 weeks, then on alternate days for as long as needed) or beclomethasone dipropionate (beclometasone dipropionate) (250 μg/puff; 12 puffs BID for 2 weeks, then on alternate days for as long as needed)

Mast Cell Stabilizer
Nedocromil sodium (2 mg/puff; 12 puffs BID for 2 weeks, then on alternate days for as long as needed).

Bronchodilators
• Clenbuterol (see the label recommendation; dosage varies from country to country)
• Ipratropium bromide (20 μg/puff; 5 or 6 puffs given 10–15 min before exercise)
• Albuterol (salbutamol) (100 μg/puff; 5–10 puffs given 10–15 min before exercise)

Corticosteroid and Bronchodilator Combination
Fluticasone propionate/salmeterol combination (2500/250 μg BID) has proven superior to fluticasone alone at improving lung function in heaves.

CONTRAINDICATIONS
Do not use high doses of corticosteroids in cases with suspected concomitant viral or bacterial infection, or when the administration of corticosteroids is contraindicated.

PRECAUTIONS
• Haylage has not been widely utilized in North America due to the fear of botulism
• Oral corticosteroids are not recommended in mares while in late gestation; however, inhaled corticosteroids appear safe because of their very low systemic effect
• *Verify medication regulations for withdrawal times before racing and/or competition*

POSSIBLE INTERACTIONS
N/A

FOLLOW-UP

PATIENT MONITORING
N/A

PREVENTION/AVOIDANCE
• Avoid moldy hay and bedding
• Maximize turnout periods and reduce stabling time. Outdoor living with shelter is an ideal environment
• Change diet—haylage, complete feed, or hay cubes with low-dust content and steamed/soaked flakes of hay

POSSIBLE COMPLICATIONS
Acute exacerbation similar to heaves.

EXPECTED COURSE AND PROGNOSIS
Prognosis largely depends on early diagnosis and owner compliance with maintaining a low-allergen environment and an appropriate therapeutic maintenance regimen.

MISCELLANEOUS

ASSOCIATED CONDITIONS
N/A

AGE-RELATED FACTORS
Presently there is little evidence in the scientific literature that the condition progresses with age.

ZOONOTIC POTENTIAL
N/A

PREGNANCY/FERTILITY/BREEDING
See Medications and Precautions.

SYNONYMS
• Nonseptic inflammatory airway disease (NSIAD)
• Allergic lower airway disease
• Allergic small airway disease

SEE ALSO
• Equine asthma
• Heaves (severe equine asthma, RAO)

ABBREVIATIONS
• EIV = equine influenza virus
• IAD = inflammatory airway disease
• MDI = metered dose inhaler
• RAO = recurrent airway obstruction

Suggested Reading
Couëtil LL, Cardwell JM, Gerber V, et al. Inflammatory airway disease of horses—revised consensus statement. J Vet Intern Med 2016;30:503–515.
Leguillette R, Tohver T, Bond SL, et al. Effect of dexamethasone and fluticasone on airway hyperresponsiveness in horses with inflammatory airway disease. J Vet Intern Med 2017;31:1193–1201.
Robinson NE. Inflammatory airway disease: defining the syndrome. Conclusions of the Havemeyer workshop. Equine Vet Educ 2003;15(2):61–63.

Authors Mary C. Furness and Laurent Viel
Consulting Editors Daniel Jean and Mathilde Leclère

BASICS

DEFINITION
- Infection of the respiratory tract by the EIV
- Highly contagious
- Most economically important contagious respiratory disease of the horse

PATHOPHYSIOLOGY
- Inhalation of aerosolized virus allows deposition of viral particles throughout respiratory tract
- Virus enters epithelial cells lining respiratory tract, replicates, and is released into the airways
- Infected cells undergo apoptosis
- Rapid spread of virus causes desquamation and denudation of respiratory epithelial cells and clumping of cilia
- Impaired mucociliary clearance results and may persist for 4 weeks post infection
- Secondary bacterial infections may occur

SYSTEMS AFFECTED
- Respiratory
- Musculoskeletal (rare)
- Cardiac (rare)

INCIDENCE/PREVALENCE
- Outbreaks occur among large groups of susceptible horses, often young racehorses
- Age and previous exposure (natural or vaccination) determine prevalence
- Morbidity can approach 100% in young naive horses

GEOGRAPHIC DISTRIBUTION
- Endemic in North and South America, Europe, the Middle East, and Asia
- First outbreak in Australia in 2007 (currently EIV free)
- Not present in New Zealand or Iceland

SIGNALMENT
- Equidae of all ages are susceptible
- Young horses (1–3 years) are more commonly affected

SIGNS
- 1–2 day incubation period
- Fever, anorexia, depression
- Frequent dry cough
- Mucoid nasal discharge. May become mucopurulent to purulent if secondary bacterial infection occurs
- Limb edema
- Conjunctivitis, epiphora
- Submandibular lymphadenopathy
- Muscle stiffness, soreness
- Clinical signs typically less severe in vaccinated horses

CAUSES
- Caused by an influenza A virus, family Orthomyxoviridae, genus *Influenza A virus* and *Influenza B virus*
- Subtypes identified by surface antigens HA and NA
- 2 subtypes of the virus exist:

  ○ A/equine/1 (H7N7)—has not been identified since 1979
  ○ A/equine/2 (H3N8)—currently identified virus
- Virus undergoes antigenic drift (minor changes of HA and NA surface proteins) and antigenic shift (major change)
- 2 antigenically distinct but related influenza A viruses currently co-circulate in America and Europe: Florida clade 1 and Florida clade 2

RISK FACTORS
- Where virus has been reported
- Age and immunity. Epidemics often occur when young, susceptible horses congregate
- Spread throughout the world, possibly facilitated by international transport of horses
- Donkeys are more severely affected

DIAGNOSIS

DIFFERENTIAL DIAGNOSIS
- Infections with EHV-1, EHV-4, EVA, and *Streptococcus equi* ssp. *equi* can look similar
- Influenza typically spreads more rapidly
- Cough is less commonly observed in animals infected with EHV, EVA, or *S. equi*
- The lymphadenopathy seen in cases of *S. equi* infection is typically more marked

CBC/BIOCHEMISTRY/URINALYSIS
- Early lymphopenia and eosinopenia followed by a monocytosis may be seen, although transient
- Leukocytosis and hyperfibrinogenemia may occur if a secondary bacterial pneumonia develops
- Increased creatine phosphokinase and aspartate aminotransferase have been rarely reported in horses which develop severe myopathies

OTHER LABORATORY TESTS
- Diagnosis based on classic clinical signs but can be confirmed by many methods—often needed in vaccinated horses with mild signs
- Virus isolation of nasopharyngeal swabs—infected, nonvaccinated horses may shed virus for up to 7–10 days. Take within 24–48 h of the development of clinical signs to maximize chances of isolating virus. Place in cool transport medium
- Antigen capture ELISAs (nasopharyngeal swab) used in diagnosis of human influenza are validated in horses. Rapid turnaround time. Useful in an outbreak situation
- RT-PCR of nasopharyngeal swabs—rapid, highly sensitive, specific, and widely available; first choice in outbreak control and screening programs for EI
- Seroconversion—4-fold increase in antibody titer between acute and convalescent samples obtained 10–14 days apart is considered diagnostic. hemagglutinin inhibition, virus neutralization, and single radial hemolysis tests can be used

IMAGING
Ultrasonographic or radiographic evaluation of the thorax can be used to diagnose pneumonia as a sequel.

PATHOLOGIC FINDINGS
- Foals more likely to die in an outbreak of naive horses than older animals
- Pregnant mares may abort or deliver stillborn fetus
- Tracheitis
- Bronchointerstitial bacterial pneumonia

TREATMENT

APPROPRIATE HEALTH CARE
- Affected animals should be isolated to prevent spread
- Most horses will recover from EI infection within 1–3 weeks

NURSING CARE
House in well-ventilated stalls.

ACTIVITY
- Stall rest or limited exercise until the respiratory epithelium has healed
- Early return to exercise can delay recovery. May lead to serious long-term and life-threatening complications (myocarditis)

DIET
Feed palatable feeds with low-dust content.

CLIENT EDUCATION
- Animals new to a population or potentially exposed horses returning to a group should be isolated for at least several days (ideally 2 weeks). Monitor closely for development of a fever or nasal discharge
- If an outbreak of influenza or other respiratory disease is suspected, a quarantine should be established. Arrivals and departures from the premise should be prevented
- Owners should be aware that vaccination of horses does not prevent infection

MEDICATIONS

DRUGS(S) OF CHOICE
- No antiviral drugs are marketed for the treatment of EI
- Antiviral drugs such as amantadine and rimantadine have been investigated but antivirals are typically not used
- Treatment is supportive—NSAIDs such as flunixin meglumine (1.1 mg/kg PO, IV every 12 h) or phenylbutazone (2.2–4.4 mg/kg IV, PO every 12 h) can be used to alleviate fever, depression, and muscle soreness
- Secondary bacterial pneumonia should be treated with antimicrobials based on sensitivity pattern of organisms identified

I

INFLUENZA   (CONTINUED)

from transtracheal wash. Pending culture results, broad-spectrum antimicrobial combinations targeted at commonly isolated organisms (*Streptococcus* spp. and *Actinobacillus* spp.) can be used (such as penicillin, tetracycline, ceftiofur, and gentamicin; trimethoprim–sulfamethoxazole)

CONTRAINDICATIONS

Corticosteroids are immunosuppressive. Recovery from influenza depends largely on an effective immune response. These drugs should not be used.

PRECAUTIONS

NSAIDs should be used judiciously in horses that are inappetent and dehydrated owing to the potential development of gastrointestinal and renal toxicity.

FOLLOW-UP

PATIENT MONITORING

Monitoring of vital signs, appetite, and attitude will allow horses that develop secondary sequelae such as bacterial pneumonia to be identified.

PREVENTION/AVOIDANCE

• Biosecurity measures and vaccination are the basis for prevention and control
• Hand-washing, minimizing horse-to-horse contact, and controlling fomites significantly reduce the risk of disease transmission
• Several vaccine types are available—all provide short-lived immunity compared with up to 12 months following natural infection
• Based on current OIE EI vaccine recommendations vaccines should include viral antigens of the currently circulating virus strains, including representatives of the Florida clade 1 and clade 2 lineages (both H3N8)
• Vaccines available (country dependent) include:
  ○ Whole inactivated virus vaccines, immuno-stimulating complex adjuvanted vaccines (ISCOM and ISCOM-Matrix), a live attenuated EIV vaccine, and a recombinant poxvirus-vectored vaccine
• Vaccination can be used in the face of an outbreak—most useful in previously vaccinated animals
• Foals
  ○ Schedule will depend on type of vaccine. AAEP guidelines:
    ▪ Inactivated—first dose at 6 months, second dose 3–4 weeks later, third dose at 10–12 months of age
    ▪ Modified live vaccine (intranasal)—first dose at 6–7 months; second dose at 11–12 months of age
    ▪ Canary pox vector vaccine—first dose at 6 months; second dose 5 weeks later

    ▪ ISCOM vaccine—first dose at 6 months; second dose 4 weeks later; third dose 5 months after dose 2
  ○ Broodmares—booster vaccination 4–6 weeks before foaling (do not use intranasal vaccine due to limited antibody production, limited transfer of passive immunity)
  ○ Adult horses at low risk—yearly booster
• Vaccination rules for competition horses vary depending on regulatory body governing the competition.
  ○ FEI/AAEP:
    ▪ Primary course—2 vaccinations not less than 21 days and not more than 92 days apart
    ▪ Booster vaccination within 7 months of second vaccination
    ▪ Boosters within 6 months + 21 days of previous vaccination
  ○ UK Thoroughbred racing:
    ▪ Primary course—2 vaccinations not less than 21 days and not more than 92 days apart
    ▪ Booster not less than 150 days and not more than 215 days after second vaccination
    ▪ Yearly booster

POSSIBLE COMPLICATIONS

• Secondary bacterial infections, causing pneumonia and pleuropneumonia, are potential sequelae. The destruction of the mucociliary apparatus by the virus removes 1 of the major defenses of the respiratory tract
• Auscultation of the thorax may reveal abnormal lung sounds such as wheezes and crackles in the case of pneumonia, or dull ventral sounds if pleural effusion develops
• Myocarditis and immune-mediated myositis—rarely reported as a sequela to influenza infection
• Persistent coughing has been anecdotally reported

EXPECTED COURSE AND PROGNOSIS

• Most recover within 1–3 weeks
• Respiratory tract recovery can take longer, often lost to competition for >3 months
• The prognosis is excellent if sufficient rest is provided
• Secondary bacterial pneumonia or pleuropneumonia results in worse prognosis, but most will recover with aggressive treatment and prolonged rest

MISCELLANEOUS

AGE-RELATED FACTORS

Foals without maternal antibodies against influenza can develop severe viral pneumonia, prognosis is generally guarded, even with intensive care.

ZOONOTIC POTENTIAL

EIV has not been shown to infect humans.

PREGNANCY/FERTILITY/BREEDING

• Pregnant mares that become infected may abort
• NSAIDs may help prevent abortion in exposed mares

SYNONYMS

Equine flu

ABBREVIATIONS

• AAEP = American Association of Equine Practitioners
• EHV = equine herpesvirus
• EI = equine influenza
• EIV = equine influenza virus
• ELISA = enzyme-linked immunosorbent assay
• EVA = equine viral arteritis
• FEI = Fédération Equestre Internationale
• HA = hemagglutinin
• NA = neuraminidase
• NSAID = nonsteroidal anti-inflammatory drug
• RT-PCR = reverse transcription–polymerase chain reaction
• OIE = Office International Epizooties/ World Organisation for Animal Health

Internet Resources
Animal Health Trust. Equiflunet. https:// www.aht.org.uk/disease-surveillance/ equiflunet

Suggested Reading
Cullinane A, Newton JR. Equine influenza— a global perspective. Vet Microbiol 2013;167:205–214.
Landolt GA. Equine influenza virus. Vet Clin North Am Equine Pract 2014;30:507–522.
Slater J, Borchers K, Chambers T, et al. Report of the international equine influenza roundtable expert meeting at Le Touquet, Normandy, February 2013. Equine Vet J 2014;46:645–650.

Author Imogen Johns
Consulting Editor Ashley G. Boyle

 Client Education Handout available online

BASICS

DEFINITION
IH is a variably pruritic summer seasonal dermatitis characterized by self-inflicted trauma and sometimes urticaria, resulting from a hypersensitivity response to biting insects such as midges (*Culicoides* spp.) and black flies (*Simulium* spp.).

PATHOPHYSIOLOGY
Susceptible animals become sensitized to arthropod antigens, principally salivary proteins, by producing allergen-specific IgE, which binds to receptor sites on mast cells; further allergen exposure leads to a type I hypersensitivity reaction with mast cell degranulation and the release of histamine and other inflammatory mediators with recruitment of eosinophils and basophils. Delayed type IV hypersensitivity is also commonly a component.

SYSTEMS AFFECTED
Skin

GENETICS
A familial tendency and heritability associated with certain equine leukocyte antigen haplotypes demonstrated. A genetic basis has been demonstrated in imported Icelandic horses.

INCIDENCE/PREVALENCE
• IH is the commonest allergic skin disease
• Reported incidence rates range from 2.8% in the UK to 32% in Australia
• In cooler climates, IH presents as recurrent and seasonal
• In warmer climates the incidence may present as a nonseasonal disease

GEOGRAPHIC DISTRIBUTION
• Worldwide. Limited to areas conducive to arthropod breeding.
• *Culicoides* spp. require still water or marshy areas that also support mosquito development
• *Simulium* spp. require moving water for larval development
• *Stomoxys calcitrans* breeds in decaying materials such as compost piles

SIGNALMENT
Breed Predilections
Any breed of horse or pony may be affected, but some breeds may be at increased risk in certain locations (Icelandic Ponies, Shire Horses in Germany, Friesians, Shetlands, Welsh Ponies, Arabs, Connemaras, Swiss Warmbloods, Quarter Horses).

Mean Age and Range
Typically seen in horses from 2 years of age onwards as previous sensitization is required. Can start later in life.

Predominant Sex
No known sex predilection.

SIGNS
General Comments
Lesions occur at the site of insect feeding, resulting in clinical signs in specific distribution patterns. Primary acute lesions are papules or crusted papules and rarely papular urticaria. Pruritus results in typical lesions of self-trauma such as excoriation, represented as erosions and ulcers, serous effusions, scale, crusts, exfoliation, lichenification, pigmentary disturbances, and various degrees of patchy alopecia represented by mild hypotrichosis to severe hair loss. The mane and tail are reduced to sparse, broken, and distorted hairs that give the appearance of a "roached mane" and "rat tail."

Historical Findings
• Note the age of onset of disease, seasonality, duration, locations of the initial disease, and how it has progressed
• Inquire if a response to strict insect control and/or administration of anti-inflammatory therapy has had an effect

Physical Examination Findings
• IH can have various clinical presentations based on the offending insect(s) and their preferred feeding sites
• In general, the appearance of 3 lesional distribution patterns can be recognized:
   1. Dorsal—involves the face, pinnae, poll, mane, withers, and tail-head; insects implicated are various *Culicoides* spp. and *Simulium* spp.
   2. Ventral—involves the intermandibular space, ventral thorax and abdomen, axillae, ventral midline, and groin; insects implicated are some *Culicoides* spp., *Simulium* spp., and *Haematobia irritans*
   3. A combination of 1 and 2—the caudal lateral aspects of both the front and hindlimbs are preferred feeding areas of *Aedes* and *S. calcitrans*, typically resulting in papulourticarial lesions
• Secondary moderate to severe bacterial dermatitis is common

CAUSES
Insect salivary protein, venom, excrement, or other proteinaceous body parts acting as allergens.

RISK FACTORS
• Proximity to insect habitat
• Concurrent pruritic dermatoses, such as AD or ectoparasitic disease (summation effect)

 DIAGNOSIS

DIFFERENTIAL DIAGNOSIS
• AD
• Cutaneous adverse reaction to food or supplements
• Onchocerciasis (uncommon with ivermectin use)
• Cutaneous drug reaction
• Contact hypersensitivity
• Oxyuriasis
• Ectoparasitic disease (acariosis, pediculosis, trombiculosis, strongyloidiasis)
• Dermatophytosis
• Dermatophilosis

CBC/BIOCHEMISTRY/URINALYSIS
NA

IMAGING
NA

OTHER DIAGNOSTIC PROCEDURES
• Tape strips and skin scrapings to rule out ectoparasites. Cytology from erosions or ulcers shows a neutrophilic exudate with cocci representative of a secondary folliculitis
• If suspected on examination and cytology perform dermatophyte cultures
• If significant bacterial infection present may need bacterial culture to determine species and antimicrobial susceptibility
• Diagnosis made on the basis of characteristic clinical presentation. Serum IgE tests are not reliable for the diagnosis of IH and although intradermal testing can be helpful both false-positive and false-negative results may occur since IgE reactions can develop as part of a normal immune response to biting insects without development of clinical hypersensitivity

PATHOLOGIC FINDINGS
• The histologic pattern of IH has variable degrees of orthokeratotic to parakeratotic hyperkeratosis, epidermal hyperplasia, eosinophilic and lymphocytic epidermal exocytosis, erosion, ulceration, and a predominantly eosinophilic superficial and deep perivascular to interstitial dermatitis and folliculitis
• Findings can support a diagnosis of IH but will not conclusively rule out differentials such as atopic disease, food allergy, or some ectoparasites

 TREATMENT

AIMS
• Resolve secondary infections
• Control pruritus
• Institute integrated pest management including the use of topical pesticides, protective fly wear, avoidance measures, and stable modifications

APPROPRIATE HEALTH CARE
Outpatient medical management.

NURSING CARE
• Use of fly repellents containing permethrins; frequency of application required may be more often than labeled. Alternatives include DEET, and products containing citronella oil may also be effective
• Frequent cool water bathing with antimicrobial, keratolytic, and keratoplastic

shampoos can remove surface irritants, bacteria, allergens, and pruritogenic substances and provide temporary soothing
• Application of topical antipruritics such as colloidal oatmeal help to raise the pruritic threshold by cooling and moisturizing dry skin
• Avoidance of bites by use of insect-proof blankets and rugs; permethrin-impregnated rugs, attachment of long-acting permethrin fly tags to rugs; attention to stable hygiene, locate horse away from muck heaps, fans to create light breezes to interfere with insect flight; use of insect traps and timed misters to emit pulses of insecticide fogs targeting the flying midges may be of benefit.

ACTIVITY
• Stable horse at the time the predominant insect is feeding. *Culicoides* spp. are night feeders, whereas *Simulium* spp. feed around dawn and in the mornings
• Relocation may be the best option but is often impractical
• Use of electric fencing to prevent rubbing and self-trauma is not an acceptable treatment for IH as it does nothing to address the underlying pruritus and inflammation

DIET
Essential fatty acid supplementation may be beneficial.

CLIENT EDUCATION
• Successful control of the disease may be represented by an 80% control of pruritus
• Discuss that therapeutic modifications over the life of the horse are to be expected
• Owing to the hereditary component, owners should be advised that affected animals should not be bred
• Advise disease is not curable, but rather manageable and lifelong therapy may be needed

MEDICATIONS
DRUG(S) OF CHOICE
Corticosteroids
• Prednisolone orally at 0.5–1.5 mg/kg every 24 h until control achieved; then reduce to lowest dose alternate-day regimen, e.g. 0.2–0.5 mg/kg every 48 h
• Prednisolone-refractory cases—try dexamethasone. Initial loading oral or IV dose of 0.02–0.1 mg/kg every 24 h for 3–5 days; then taper to 0.01–0.02 mg/kg every 48–72 h for maintenance
• Repository injectable corticosteroids should be avoided
• Localized use of topical steroids such as hydrocortisone aceponate spray can be useful for maintenance

Antihistamines
• Not useful for control of moderate to severe pruritus; rather use as a preventative either before the onset of pruritus or in a maintenance regimen to suppress pruritus once controlled
• Equine pharmacokinetic data for antihistamines is limited. Anecdotal reports suggest that H_1-receptor antagonist hydroxyzine hydrochloride/pamoate (0.5–1 mg/kg every 8 h), chlorpheniramine (chlorphenamine) (0.25 mg/kg every 12 h), diphenhydramine (0.75–1.0 mg/kg every 12 h), pyrilamine maleate (mepyramine) (1 mg/kg every 12 h) or cetirizine (0.2–0.4 mg/kg every 12 h) may decrease pruritus
• Give antihistamines at least 10–14 days to determine efficacy. If no response, select another class of antihistamine

CONTRAINDICATIONS
Antihistamines may thicken mucus in the respiratory tract. Extra caution should be used in horses with respiratory problems due to excess mucus.

PRECAUTIONS
• Corticosteroids—use judiciously to avoid laminitis, iatrogenic hyperglucocorticism, diabetes mellitus, polydipsia and polyuria, aggravation of bacterial folliculitis, decreased muscle mass, weight loss, and poor wound healing
• Antihistamines—can produce sedation and/or behavior changes, whole-body or fine tremors, or seizures
• Note drug withdrawal times pertaining to horse show or racing associations

POSSIBLE INTERACTIONS
None

ALTERNATIVE DRUGS
• Polyunsaturated omega 3 and 6 fatty acids—variable response in decreasing pruritus, provide support for epidermal barrier function, and anti-inflammatory properties. Exact dosing for horse is lacking.
• Allergen-specific immunotherapy—the benefit is unclear owing to the lack of appropriate long-term double-blind placebo-controlled studies

FOLLOW-UP
PATIENT MONITORING
Observe animals for evidence of pruritus or lesions indicating the onset of midge season.

PREVENTION/AVOIDANCE
Alter insect breeding habitat if possible; use fans to create light drafts over animals and fine mesh screen/netting doubled over in front of and over stalls. Use repellents on horses and/or misters with timers to emit fog of short-acting pyrethrins during insect feeding times. Use full coverage protective fly apparel, i.e. sheets with belly-bands, neck and face masks.

POSSIBLE COMPLICATIONS
Severe secondary infections and permanent scarring.

EXPECTED COURSE AND PROGNOSIS
Not life-threatening unless intractable pruritus persists.

MISCELLANEOUS
ASSOCIATED CONDITIONS
Often concurrent association with AD.

AGE-RELATED FACTORS
Severity of clinical signs may progress as the horse ages.

ZOONOTIC POTENTIAL
N/A

PREGNANCY/FERTILITY/BREEDING
None

SYNONYMS
• Sweet itch
• Queensland itch
• No-see-um hypersensitivity

SEE ALSO
• Atopic dermatitis
• Ectoparasites

ABBREVIATIONS
• AD = atopic dermatitis
• DEET = *N,N*-diethyl-meta-toluamide
• Ig = immunoglobulin
• IH = insect hypersensitivity

Suggested Reading
Lloyd DH, Littlewood JD, Craig JM, Thomsett LR. Practical Equine Dermatology. Oxford, UK: Blackwell, 2003:17.

Author Janet Littlewood
Consulting Editor Gwendolen Lorch
Acknowledgment The author and editor acknowledge the prior contribution of Cliff Monahan.

BASICS

DEFINITION
In animals, dyspnea is used to describe clinical signs associated with difficult, labored breathing or respiratory distress, which can be present throughout the respiratory cycle or be primarily associated with either inhalation (i.e. inspiratory dyspnea) or exhalation (i.e. expiratory dyspnea).

PATHOPHYSIOLOGY
• Generally a sign of impaired gas exchange, with the increased effort to inhale being associated with an increased need to ventilate the lung
• Primary causes—failure of delivery of air into the lung (i.e. alveolar hypoventilation) and of exchange between the lung and blood (i.e. ventilation, diffusion, or perfusion problem). The former can result from airway obstruction, pleural disease, chest wall or diaphragmatic injury, pneumothorax, intrusion of the abdomen on the thorax (e.g. advanced pregnancy, diaphragmatic hernia), or central nervous system disease. Relevant exchange problems primarily are those causing alveolar disease (e.g. pneumonia, pulmonary edema)
• Can also be a sign of decreased oxygen delivery to the tissues (e.g. cardiovascular disease, anemia) and of the need to eliminate more carbon dioxide to correct a metabolic acidosis
• The most severe cases usually result from obstruction of the extrathoracic airways because the negative pressure generated during inhalation tends to collapse these structures

SYSTEMS AFFECTED
• Respiratory
• Cardiovascular
• Hemic/lymphatic/immune
• Endocrine/metabolic—response to metabolic acidosis
• Nervous

INCIDENCE/PREVALENCE
Unknown

GEOGRAPHIC DISTRIBUTION
Worldwide

SIGNALMENT
Depends on the underlying cause.

SIGNS
• Inspiratory dyspnea is a sign, but associated signs can indicate the source of the dyspnea
• Inappetence can indicate inflammatory disease, or inability to eat as a consequence of severe dyspnea or pharyngeal dysfunction
• Cough indicates inflammation of the tracheobronchial tree or nasopharynx
• Bilateral nasal discharge usually indicates inflammation of the guttural pouches or

lower airways, or bilateral inflammation of the nasal cavities or sinuses
• Unilateral discharge suggests nasal or nasopharyngeal (including the sinuses and guttural pouches) disease
• Noisy breathing (stridor) indicates obstruction of the extrathoracic airways

Historical Findings
• Sudden onset of inspiratory dyspnea can indicate acute inflammatory disease of the lung or pleural space; trauma to the chest wall, diaphragm, or extrathoracic airway; or acute blood loss
• Dyspnea of slower onset may result from a space-occupying mass encroaching on the respiratory system

Physical Examination Findings
• Flared nostrils, increased excursions of the thorax, and retractions (i.e. "sinking in") of the intercostal spaces, particularly if laboring against an upper airway obstruction
• Exaggerated excursions of the diaphragm lead to increased movement of the anal sphincter
• Nasal obstruction—noisy breathing, decreased airflow
• Strangles—fever, nasal discharge, swollen or draining lymph nodes
• Guttural pouch tympany—fluctuant swelling of the parotid region (usually bilateral)
• Laryngeal paralysis—if severe or bilateral, severe inspiratory dyspnea and strident inspiratory noise
• Alar fold collapse, laryngeal hemiplegia, and epiglottic retroversion—no signs at rest but can lead to reduced exercise tolerance and inspiratory noise
• Pneumonia—fever, adventitious sounds
• Pulmonary edema—fine, inspiratory crackles
• Pneumothorax—lack of breath sounds and little air movement despite large effort
• Pleural effusion/pleuritis—lack of lung sounds ventrally, friction rubs, fever, depression, abducted elbows indicating pain
• Fractured ribs—signs of trauma, sounds of air entering and leaving wounds
• Diaphragmatic hernia—reduction in lung sounds, signs of colic, or borborygmi audible in chest
• Anemia—pallor
• Cardiac disease—murmurs, thrills, or arrhythmias

CAUSES
Respiratory
• Extrathoracic airway
  ◦ Paresis of the external nares, alar fold collapse
  ◦ Severe atheroma (rare)
  ◦ Congestion of the nasal mucosa—Horner syndrome; inflammatory disease, amyloidosis
  ◦ Deviation of the nasal septum

  ◦ Space-occupying lesion affecting the nasal cavity—foreign body, intraluminal mass, ethmoid hematoma, or extraluminal mass or swelling
  ◦ Congenital pharyngeal cysts
  ◦ Pharyngeal or laryngeal paresis, permanent DDSP
  ◦ Space-occupying masses protruding inside the pharynx—enlarged lymph nodes; guttural pouch enlargement, abscesses
  ◦ Trauma to the hyoid bone or larynx
  ◦ Laryngeal or pharyngeal paresis—degenerative nerve disease, lead poisoning, or trauma to recurrent laryngeal nerves (e.g. by jugular perivascular injection)
  ◦ Tracheal foreign body or collapse
• Intrathoracic respiratory tract
  ◦ Equine asthma (heaves, pasture asthma)—accompanied by expiratory dyspnea, which is predominant
  ◦ Pulmonary edema—cardiogenic or noncardiogenic
  ◦ Pneumonia—bacterial, viral, or fungal
  ◦ Pleuritis/pleuropneumonia
  ◦ Accumulation of pleural fluid
  ◦ Pneumothorax
  ◦ Diaphragmatic hernia
  ◦ Fractured ribs/flail chest
  ◦ Mediastinal masses
  ◦ EMPF
  ◦ Equine multisystemic eosinophilic epitheliotropic disease

Nonrespiratory
• Cardiovascular—congenital cardiac defect with right-to-left shunt, cardiac failure, or pulmonary embolus
• Hemic—anemia, methemoglobinemia, carbon monoxide or cyanide poisoning
• Endocrine/metabolic—severe metabolic acidosis; hyperthermia
• Nervous—trauma to recurrent laryngeal nerves or pharyngeal plexus, mediastinal masses, lead poisoning, phrenic nerve injury, or diaphragmatic paralysis
• Reproductive—advanced pregnancy; hydrops

DIAGNOSIS

DIFFERENTIAL DIAGNOSIS
Differentiating Similar Signs
• Expiratory dyspnea—enhanced abdominal component to exhalation, with a tucking up of the abdomen toward the end of exhalation
• Tachypnea—not accompanied by prolonged inhalation
• Deep breathing with a marked inspiratory effort also follows strenuous exercise

Differentiating Causes
• Upper airway obstructions can produce severe respiratory distress and often are accompanied by inspiratory noise

INSPIRATORY DYSPNEA (CONTINUED)

- Lung and pleural disease is often inflammatory and therefore accompanied by fever and inappetence
- Damage to the respiratory pump (i.e. chest and diaphragm) may result in strenuous efforts to breathe, with little movement of air
- Cardiac disease usually is accompanied by other signs—murmurs, arrhythmia, edema
- Metabolic acidosis is accompanied by signs of primary disease

CBC/BIOCHEMISTRY/URINALYSIS
Contingent on cause of dyspnea.

OTHER LABORATORY TESTS
- Arterial blood gas analysis identifies hypoventilation (increased $PaCO_2$) and hypoxemia
- Elevated $PaCO_2$ (>45 mmHg) accompanied by hypoxemia (PaO_2 < 85 mmHg) indicates severe upper airway obstruction, damage to the respiratory pump, or severe lung disease

IMAGING
Radiography
- Skull—nasal obstructions; sinus disease, factures
- Throat—guttural pouch tympany and empyema, abscesses, DDSP, laryngeal injury
- Neck—tracheal damage or collapse, foreign bodies
- Thorax—pleural fluid, pneumonia, pulmonary edema, pneumothorax, cardiac enlargement, fractured ribs, diaphragmatic hernia

Ultrasonography
- Thorax—pleural fluid, superficial masses (abscesses; neoplasia; EMPF nodules) or intestines in case of hernia
- Echocardiography—chamber enlargement, congenital defects, valvular disease

Endoscopy
- Essential for diagnosing space-occupying lesions
- Endoscopy during exercise may be necessary to determine the significance of pharyngeal or laryngeal collapse

OTHER DIAGNOSTIC PROCEDURES
- Cytology of lower airways
- Bacterial and fungal culture of tracheal exudate or pleural fluid
- Thoracocentesis determines the presence of air or fluid in the pleural space
- Transient suture of the alar folds during exercise can alleviate nasal obstruction and lead to diagnosis

TREATMENT

AIMS
Relieving Upper Airway Obstruction
- Relieve upper airway obstruction sufficient to cause panic or life-threatening hypoxemia by tracheotomy. Tracheotomy is not useful if

dyspnea originates from the lower airways or thorax
- Nasotracheal intubation can be used to bypass the obstruction, especially if that obstruction will be corrected surgically within a short time

Support Ventilation
- Animals with hypoventilation resulting from thoracic damage may need positive-pressure ventilation, which can be accomplished via a nasotracheal tube until the horse is anesthetized for correction of the injury
- Ventilation to maintain gas exchange in an animal with pulmonary disease is difficult

APPROPRIATE HEALTH CARE
In- or outpatient medical management.

NURSING CARE
Oxygen Therapy
- Supplemental oxygenation relieves hypoxemia and accompanying distress when dyspnea results from lung disease
- In cases of upper airway obstruction or thoracic trauma, oxygen can be life-saving until the problem is surgically corrected
- Severe anemia sufficient to cause dyspnea requires administration of blood

Thoracocentesis
Can be both diagnostic and therapeutic.

SURGICAL CONSIDERATIONS
Contingent on diagnosis.

MEDICATIONS
Contingent on diagnosis.

FOLLOW-UP

PATIENT MONITORING
- After surgery for upper airway obstruction, monitor for signs of further obstruction caused by postoperative swelling
- Tracheotomy tubes need to be cleaned regularly to prevent occlusion
- Rarely, strictures at the site of the tracheotomy may lead to further inspiratory dyspnea
- Monitor for recurrence of upper airway masses, pleural effusion, and pneumothorax
- Dysphagia can occur secondary to nerve damage or inflammation in the upper airways or guttural pouches

MISCELLANEOUS

PREGNANCY/FERTILITY/BREEDING
Fetal growth retardation and fetal death may be observed in mares with severely compromised respiratory function.

SEE ALSO
- Acute epiglottiditis
- Arytenoid chondropathy
- Aspiration pneumonia
- Diaphragmatic hernia
- Equine herpesvirus 5
- Expiratory dyspnea
- Guttural pouch tympany
- Pleuropneumonia
- Pneumothorax
- Thoracic trauma

ABBREVIATIONS
- DDSP = dorsal displacement of the soft palate
- EMPF = equine multinodular pulmonary fibrosis
- $PaCO_2$ = partial pressure of carbon dioxide in arterial blood
- PaO_2 = partial pressure of oxygen in arterial blood

Suggested Reading
Barakzai S. Treadmill endoscopy. In: McGorum BC, Dixon PM, Robinson NE, Schumacher J, eds. Equine Respiratory Medicine and Surgery. Philadelphia, PA: WB Saunders, 2006:235–247.
Laverty S. Thoracic trauma. In: Robinson NE, ed. Current Therapy in Equine Medicine, 4e. Philadelphia, PA: WB Saunders, 1997:463–465.
McGorum BC, Dixon PM. Clinical examination of the respiratory tract. In: McGorum BC, Dixon PM, Robinson NE, Schumacher J, eds. Equine Respiratory Medicine and Surgery. Philadelphia, PA: WB Saunders, 2006:103–117.
Parente EJ. Diagnostic techniques for upper airway obstruction. In: Robinson NE, ed. Current Therapy in Equine Medicine, 4e. Philadelphia, PA: WB Saunders, 1997:401–403.

Author Emmanuelle van Erck-Westergren
Consulting Editors Mathilde Leclère and Daniel Jean
Acknowledgment The author and editors acknowledge the prior contribution of N. Edward Robinson.

INSULIN LEVELS/INSULIN TOLERANCE TEST

BASICS

DEFINITION
- Blood insulin concentrations can be used to evaluate a horse's ability to regulate its blood glucose
- Insulin secretion is closely tied to blood glucose concentrations in normal horses. Insulin concentrations are low (<20 μU/mL) with fasting but increase rapidly when glucose or a meal high in soluble carbohydrates is consumed
- Blood insulin concentrations may be consistently elevated (>50 μU/mL) in horses with insulin dysregulation, which is commonly observed with EMS or PPID
- Insulin response or tolerance tests may better reflect a horse's endocrine status than a one-time measurement
- Insulin tolerance test—give 0.1 IU/kg IV regular insulin and determine blood glucose at baseline and 30 min. Blood glucose should decrease by 50% at 30 min
- Blood insulin response can also be measured after administering 0.5 g/kg IV dextrose. Insulin should be low when starting, increase within 5 min of the dextrose load, and then decrease rapidly once blood glucose levels begin to drop. Serum glucose should normalize within 1–2 h after dextrose administration. An elevated blood insulin 3 h after beginning the test is clear evidence of insulin resistance
- The combined glucose–insulin test—administer 150 mg/kg 50% solution dextrose IV, immediately followed by 0.10 U/kg regular insulin IV. Collect blood at 45 min. Insulin resistance is present if blood glucose is above baseline and/or insulin above 100 μU/mL
- The most common pathologic processes leading to abnormal insulin concentrations are EMS or PPID

PATHOPHYSIOLOGY
- Inappropriately low blood insulin—pancreatitis, leading to destruction of beta cells and development of type 1 diabetes mellitus
- Increased insulin levels in hypoglycemic horse—insulin-secreting tumor (i.e. insulinoma) or iatrogenic insulin administration
- Increased blood insulin levels in hyperglycemic horses—peripheral insulin resistance or an insulin antagonist (e.g. cortisol)
- Increased blood insulin with normal blood glucose concentration—insulin dysregulation associated with EMS or PPID
- Horses with hyperlipemia may also exhibit insulin resistance

SYSTEMS AFFECTED
The endocrine system is primarily affected by abnormal blood insulin and insulin response

tests—decreased insulin is diagnostic of diabetes mellitus; increased insulin is most commonly associated with insulin dysregulation.

SIGNALMENT
- Ponies tend to have higher blood insulin levels than horses and are more prone to hyperlipemia
- No sex difference
- Obese animals, particularly ponies, are more insulin resistant than are thinner animals
- PPID tends to occur in old horses (>18 years)

SIGNS
- The most common signs in horses with an abnormal insulin response test are those of equine insulin dysregulation/metabolic syndrome—obesity with abnormal fat distribution, infertility, and laminitis. However, prolonged fasting (>6 h) causes tissue insulin resistance in any horse
- The eyelids can look swollen, and the supraorbital fat pad may look bulged
- The horse may be dull or depressed
- Similar clinical signs, with the addition of hypertrichosis (previously referred to as hirsutism) or an abnormal haircoat, weight loss, polyuria and polydipsia, and chronic infections particularly sinusitis and hoof abscess, are seen in horses with PPID
- Clinical signs in horses with type 1 diabetes mellitus—weight loss, polyuria and polydipsia, lethargy, or depression
- Signs of excess insulin caused by exogenous overdose or insulinoma are those of hypoglycemia—muscle trembling, ataxia, nystagmus, depression, and facial twitching, leading to convulsions, coma, and death
- Signs of hyperlipemia include depression, anorexia, and icterus

CAUSES
- The primary cause of increased blood insulin, abnormal response to an insulin response test, or increased insulin after IV glucose is peripheral insulin resistance or the presence of insulin antagonists. Exogenous or endogenous corticosteroids are the most common insulin antagonists but other hormones (e.g. growth hormone, epinephrine) also have this effect
- The most common reason for increased blood insulin without insulin resistance is an insulin-secreting tumor
- The most common reason for type 1 diabetes mellitus is pancreatic damage presumably due to parasite migration

RISK FACTORS
- Obesity, particularly in ponies, is associated with insulin resistance, as is hyperlipidemia. PPID is associated with the development of abnormal insulin secretion
- Glucocorticoid administration or increased cortisol from a stress response may also lead to insulin resistance and hyperglycemia

DIAGNOSIS

DIFFERENTIAL DIAGNOSIS
- Polyuria, polydipsia, and glucosuria in horses with suspected endocrine disorders should alert the practitioner to a disorder in glucose homeostasis and, thus, in insulin levels
- Hypoglycemia from excess insulin—myositis, neurologic disease, and hepatic failure
- Determination of abnormally low blood glucose should cause the practitioner to suspect inappropriate insulin levels

LABORATORY FINDINGS
Drugs That May Alter Laboratory Results
- Corticosteroids
- α_2-Agonists (xylazine, detomidine)

Disorders That May Alter Laboratory Results
Delayed separation of serum or plasma from cells falsely lowers blood glucose values, making interpretation of insulin levels more difficult.

Valid if Run in a Human Laboratory?
Yes. It is important to have laboratory-specific reference ranges as insulin results can vary markedly depending on which assay is used.

CBC/BIOCHEMISTRY/URINALYSIS
- Horses with abnormal insulin levels caused by PPID may have a stress response with mature neutrophilia, lymphopenia, and eosinopenia. They may also have increased blood glucose and glucosuria
- Horses with type 1 or 2 diabetes mellitus have hyperglycemia
- Horses with insulinoma or exogenous insulin overdose have hypoglycemia
- Horses with hyperlipemia may have increased bilirubin. Increases in hepatic enzyme activity may be observed if hepatic lipidosis is present

OTHER LABORATORY TESTS
- Pituitary function—endogenous ACTH determination (fall), TRH stimulation test (winter, spring, summer)
- Increased resting ACTH and positive TRH response test are consistent with PPID

IMAGING
In cases of hyperglycemia associated with PPID, increased pituitary gland size may be depicted with specialized modalities—CT.

OTHER DIAGNOSTIC PROCEDURES
In cases of hyperglycemia associated with type 1 diabetes mellitus, findings from an exploratory laparotomy or abdominocentesis may be consistent with a damaged pancreas but should be considered extremely low-yield procedures because the pancreas is normally difficult to visualize and pancreatic tumors often are microscopic.

I

INSULIN LEVELS/INSULIN TOLERANCE TEST (CONTINUED)

TREATMENT

APPROPRIATE HEALTH CARE
• Horses with hypoglycemia require inpatient medical management if the disease is severe and IV dextrose to maintain blood glucose at adequate levels
• Horses with hyperlipemia also require inpatient medical management that includes IV dextrose, balanced electrolyte solutions, caloric replacement, heparin, and exogenous insulin
• All other horses with abnormal insulin levels may be treated as outpatients

NURSING CARE
• Carefully monitor hypoglycemic animals to prevent them from collapsing and injuring themselves
• Horses with laminitis need corrective hoof trimming and shoeing and an appropriate diet

ACTIVITY
• Limit the activity of horses with laminitis
• Increase the activity of sound, obese horses in an effort to lose weight

DIET
• Horses with laminitis generally benefit from a low-carbohydrate, high-fiber diet
• Keep any horse with insulin resistance on a low-carbohydrate diet
• Restrict or increase caloric intake until a condition score of 4–6 out of 10 is achieved
• Horses that are insulin resistant that are underconditioned should receive additional calories in the form of high-quality complex fiber or fat such as beet pulp or rice bran

CLIENT EDUCATION
• Horses with PPID may be managed with medication and nursing care, but their prognosis is quite variable. Owners need to understand that treatment of PPID is palliative and required for life
• Encourage clients to maintain their horses at condition scores of 4–6 out of 10 and to prevent obesity from developing

MEDICATIONS

DRUG(S) OF CHOICE
• The agent most commonly used to treat PPID is pergolide (0.5–2 mg/day)
• Insulin-deficient horses (i.e. type 1 diabetes mellitus) require insulin supplementation, with the dose being changed in response to the blood glucose level. Protamine zinc insulin (0.5 IU IM BID) normalized blood glucose in a case report of a pony with insulin deficiency
• Exogenous insulin for the treatment of hyperlipemia—protamine zinc insulin (0.075–0.4 IU/kg SC or IM BID or SID). Regular insulin (0.4 IU/kg) has also been used

PRECAUTIONS
• Dextrose for injection should always be available when administering insulin. If signs of hypoglycemia occur, treat immediately with IV dextrose. Horses that are being tested using the 2-step insulin test may be given IV dextrose after the 30 min sample is collected. This will prevent further decrease in blood glucose concentrations and minimize the chances of symptomatic hypoglycemia developing
• Horses that receive an overdose of pergolide may exhibit anorexia, lethargy, and ataxia

FOLLOW-UP

PATIENT MONITORING
• Retest horses with PPID every 4–6 weeks with endogenous ACTH determination or TRH response testing. Abnormal results indicate the need for an increased dose or a change in medication. If a horse has been stable for several months, testing can be performed less frequently
• Check the glucose level of horses with diabetes mellitus receiving insulin therapy at least twice a day. Insulin doses should be increased or decreased in response to blood glucose values outside the normal range.

MISCELLANEOUS

ASSOCIATED CONDITIONS
• Hypertrichosis, chronic infections, and laminitis are commonly associated with PPID
• Obesity, laminitis, and hyperlipemia are commonly associated with the insulin resistance that accompanies EMS

PREGNANCY/FERTILITY/BREEDING
Pregnant mares tend to have higher blood insulin levels than nonpregnant horses. This tendency is most profound during early gestation, but blood glucose levels remain normal.

SEE ALSO
• Equine metabolic syndrome (EMS)/insulin resistance (IR)
• Glucose, hyperglycemia
• Glucose, hypoglycemia
• Glucose tolerance tests
• Pituitary pars intermedia dysfunction

ABBREVIATIONS
• ACTH = adrenocorticotropic hormone
• CT = computed tomography
• EMS = equine metabolic syndrome
• PPID = pituitary pars intermedia dysfunction
• TRH = thyrotropin-releasing hormone

Suggested Reading
Bertin FR, Taylor SD, Bianco AW, Sojka-Kritchevsky JE. The effect of fasting duration on baseline blood glucose concentration, blood insulin concentration, glucose/insulin ratio, oral sugar test, and insulin response test results in horses. J Vet Intern Med 2016;30:1726–1731.
Dunbar LK, Mielnicki KA, Dembek KA, et al. Evaluation of four diagnostic tests for insulin dysregulation in adult light-breed horses. J Vet Intern Med 2016;30:885–891.

Authors Heidi Banse and Janice Kritchevsky
Consulting Editors Michel Levy and Heidi Banse

INTERNAL ABDOMINAL ABSCESSES

BASICS

DEFINITION
Internal abdominal abscesses are commonly associated with weight loss, chronic or recurrent colic signs, or fever, or any combination of these signs.

PATHOPHYSIOLOGY
• Internal abdominal abscesses are classified as primary or secondary depending on anatomic origin. Primary abscesses originate from systemic infection and secondary abscesses may occur due to abdominal trauma, ulceration, perforation, or surgery
• The pathogenesis of mesenteric abscesses has not been elucidated; however, it has been proposed that the development of the internal infection is associated with the inability of the animal to develop adequate immune response to the microorganisms involved, thereby allowing systemic spread of infection
• Given that abdominal abscesses are often caused by *Streptococcus equi* ssp. *equi,* it has been suggested that treatment with penicillin prior to abscess maturation and drainage may favor the hematogenous spread of the bacteria
• Once the internal abdominal abscess has developed, it can remain dormant or flare up and peritonitis may develop. This seems to be responsible for the different clinical presentations. Colic events may be due to tension on the mesentery or from acute or chronic obstruction secondary to intestinal adhesions

SYSTEMS AFFECTED
Gastrointestinal

INCIDENCE/PREVALENCE
There is no information regarding incidence or prevalence.

SIGNALMENT
All horses are at risk.

SIGNS
• Usually, horses with internal abdominal abscesses present with 1 of 2 chief complaints—a history of intermittent or prolonged colic. However, there are cases with a history of acute colic. These animals show depression, congested mucous membranes, increased rectal temperature (>38.6°C), increased and shallow respiratory rate, groaning on expiration, partial or complete anorexia, constipation, decreased peristaltic sounds, and dehydration. Dysuria can be noticed in some cases
• In the second form, the chief complaint is chronic ongoing weight loss. The body condition in these animals ranges from the cachectic horse to the thin horse that is unable to gain weight. Some animals are depressed, inconsistently anorexic, and have poor shaggy haircoats. The rectal temperature and heart and respiratory rates may be

elevated. Abdominal peristaltic sounds are usually normal. Combinations of the 2 forms can occur
• In some cases there is evidence of diarrhea, and this seems to be more commonly associated with abscesses caused by *Rhodococcus equi* infection in foals and in growing horses

CAUSES
• The infectious agents implicated are variable but most commonly involved are *S. equi* ssp. *equi, S. equi* ssp. *zooepidemicus, Corynebacterium pseudotuberculosis, Salmonella* spp., *Escherichia coli*
• Rarely *Serratia marcescens* and *R. equi* in foals, and obligate anaerobes (*Bacteroides* spp., *Clostridium novyi* type A, and *Fusobacterium necrophorum*)
• There has been a report of internal abdominal abscess in association with *Parascaris equorum* in a foal

RISK FACTORS
• Heavy parasitism, or a previous history of respiratory disease or lymphadenitis are believed to predispose to internal abdominal abscessation
• More common on farms where infections with *S. equi* ssp. *equi* and *R. equi* are present
• Abdominocentesis should be considered a risk factor when enterocentesis has occurred

DIAGNOSIS

DIFFERENTIAL DIAGNOSIS
• Other causes of chronic weight loss, such as pleuropneumonia, neoplasia, chronic hepatic disease, chronic intestinal malabsorption, chronic renal failure, severe parasitism, and dental problems
• Other causes of colic and peritonitis

CBC/BIOCHEMISTRY/URINALYSIS
• The CBC may indicate anemia of chronic inflammation
• The WBC count is variable and >40% of the affected horses may present a neutrophilic leukocytosis and a left shift
• Plasma fibrinogen concentration is frequently increased, with values >1000 mg/dL (10 g/L) in some cases
• Hyperproteinemia due to increased globulin fractions and hypoalbuminemia are common. The albumin to globulin ratio may be decreased, ranging from 0.17 to 0.63 (normal 0.65–1.46)

OTHER LABORATORY TESTS
Peritoneal fluid is usually determined to be an exudate based on specific gravity (>1.017), protein level (>2.5 g/dL (>25 g/L)), and WBC count (>10 000 cells/μL (>10⁹ cells/L)). The protein levels, WBC count, and fibrinogen can be as high as 8.5 g/dL (85 g/L), 400 000 cells/μL (365 × 10⁹ cells/L), and 500 mg/dL (5 g/L),

respectively. Intracellular bacteria (both cocci and bacilli) can be observed, but only on rare occasions are free bacteria observed.

IMAGING
Transrectal or percutaneous US can be useful in diagnosing these abscesses, especially when they can be located during rectal examination. Nuclear scintigraphy using technetium-99 m or indium-111-labeled WBCs can be potentially used to diagnose abscesses that are difficult to localize.

OTHER DIAGNOSTIC PROCEDURES
• Rectal palpation may be limited by the fact that some animals often show severe abdominal straining and rectal expulsive efforts during the colic episodes. In both clinical presentations, detailed rectal examination may allow the detection of an abdominal mass
• A Gram stain and anaerobic and aerobic bacterial culture of the peritoneal fluid should be carried out
• Abdominal laparoscopy/laparotomy may allow visualization of masses. Fine needle aspiration of the abscess could be done percutaneously with US guidance or by laparoscopy

PATHOLOGIC FINDINGS
Abdominal abscessation can involve the mesentery or intraabdominal organs, such as lymph nodes, intestines, spleen, liver, and kidneys. Rare cases involve umbilical remnants. When localized in the mesentery, adhesions to various organs might be present.

TREATMENT

APPROPRIATE HEALTH CARE
Most cases can be managed in a farm setting. However, hospitalization may be warranted in some cases.

ACTIVITY
Stall or pasture rest until the problem has resolved.

DIET
Normal diet when colic has been resolved.

CLIENT EDUCATION
Long-term antibiotic therapy may be required once discharged from hospital. Compliance can be a problem, particularly with parenteral therapy, as many horses rapidly become intolerant to IM injections.

SURGICAL CONSIDERATIONS
• The severity of the colic signs may warrant intensive care management and even surgical management in some cases
• Surgical treatment can be attempted in cases with a grave prognosis, but it is complicated by the need to drain the abscess without contaminating the abdominal cavity
• Abdominal lavage is indicated in cases where rupture of the abscess occurs. This procedure

I

INTERNAL ABDOMINAL ABSCESSES

is not without constraints and difficulties. There have been reports of successful outcomes following marsupialization of the abscesses when they are located close to the abdominal wall

MEDICATIONS

DRUG(S) OF CHOICE
• Medical treatment of abdominal internal abscesses is usually preferred. For the most part it is empirical, as the causative organism(s) is not usually positively identified. Farm history and clinical findings are the basis for antibiotic selection. Antimicrobials are usually administered for a minimum of 30 days and may extend up to 90 days in some cases, depending on the response to therapy
• Sodium or potassium penicillin have been used in a dose range of 20 000–40 000 IU/kg IV every 6 h. Procaine penicillin at 20 000–50 000 IU/kg every 12 h has been also recommended
• In the author's experience, the combination of rifampin (rifampicin) 10 mg/kg BID PO and trimethoprim–sulfamethoxazole 30 mg/kg BID PO has been successful
• Rifampin may alternatively be combined with erythromycin estolate 15 mg/kg BID to TID, or clarithromycin 7.5 mg/kg BID in foals
• Metronidazole 20–25 mg/kg TID could be added in the case of a suspected or isolated anaerobic pathogen

FOLLOW-UP

PATIENT MONITORING
In order to follow up the patient, repeated rectal examinations, CBC, abdominocentesis, and US examinations are necessary.

PREVENTION/AVOIDANCE
On problem farms, careful monitoring of all horses may lead to early detection of the problem. If *S. equi* ssp. *equi* is the etiologic agent, then consideration should be given for a vaccination program.

POSSIBLE COMPLICATIONS
• Peritonitis
• Purpura haemorrhagica
• Intestinal adhesions

EXPECTED COURSE AND PROGNOSIS
The prognosis is usually good to guarded when there is a favorable response within 2 weeks of treatment. The prognosis becomes grave if there is either intestinal involvement and obstruction or internal rupture of the abscess and evidence of intestinal adhesions. In a review of 61 cases only 24.6% survivability was reported.

MISCELLANEOUS

SEE ALSO
• Colic, chronic/recurrent

ABBREVIATIONS
• US = ultrasonography, ultrasound
• WBC = white blood cell

Suggested Reading
Arnold CE, Chaffin MK. Abdominal abscesses in adult horses: 61 cases (1993–2008). J Am Vet Med Assoc 2012;241:1659–1665.
Berlin D, Kelmer G, Steinman A, Sutton GA. Successful medical management of intra-abdominal abscesses in 4 adult horses. Can Vet J 2013;154:157–161.
Mair TS, Sherlock CE. Surgical drainage and postoperative lavage of large abdominal abscesses in six mature horses. Equine Vet J 2011;43(Suppl. 39):123–127.
Mogg TD, Rutherford DJ. Intra-abdominal abscess and peritonitis in an Appaloosa gelding. Vet Clin North Am Equine Pract 2006;22:e17–e25.
Pusterla N, Whitcomb MB, Wilson WD. Internal abdominal abscesses caused by *Streptococcus equi* subspecies *equi* in 10 horses in California between 1989 and 2004. Vet Rec 2007;160:589–592.

Author Olimpo Oliver-Espinosa
Consulting Editors Henry Stämpfli and Olimpo Oliver-Espinosa

BASICS

DEFINITION
These tests assess the absorptive integrity of the small intestine by measuring the efficiency of sugar absorption from the intestinal lumen. They are indicated in weight loss cases where an overt cause is not established and there is apparent adequate food intake.

PATHOPHYSIOLOGY
Weight loss can result from many different clinical conditions (see chapter Chronic weight loss).

SYSTEMS AFFECTED
Gastrointestinal—small intestine.

DIAGNOSIS

DIAGNOSTIC PROCEDURES

OGAT
Glucose is absorbed from the small intestine by specific transport processes and thus it can be used to assess small intestinal function. It provides empiric evidence of the absorptive capacity of the small intestine. The test is easily performed, inexpensive, and requires only readily available reagents.

Test Procedure
The horse is weighed as accurately as possible (e.g. scale or girth weight tape). It is fasted overnight (14–16 h) and kept on inedible bedding. Access to water is restricted during the firsts 2 h of the test. Anhydrous or monohydrate D-glucose (1 g/kg of body weight), mixed in warm water to form a 20% (20 g/dL) solution w/v, is administered via stomach tube. Since the test depends on the rapid entry of the given glucose solution into the small intestine, and because gastric emptying is delayed by excessive glucose concentration, the quantity of glucose and the concentration of the solution are paramount. Blood samples are collected by direct venipuncture into fluoride oxalate glass vacutainers immediately prior to glucose administration and 30, 60, 90, 120, 150, 180, 240, 300, and 360 min later. Samples are submitted to the laboratory for glucose measurements or analyzed by handheld glucometers. Access to food is denied until the end of the sampling; if the patient is not adequately fasted the presence of food in the stomach will mix with the solution and then interfere with the availability of the glucose in the small intestine, thus causing spurious results.

Curve Plotting
The glucose values at each time period are plotted arithmetically.

Test Interpretation
• The absorption curve in normal conditions has 2 phases. Glucose absorption from the small intestine occurs continuously during the first 2 h and the fasting plasma glucose concentration almost doubles (>85% increase in normal horses) during this period. This phase is dependent on mucosal integrity, the rate of gastric emptying, intestinal transit time, previous dietary history, and age. It has been reported that altering the diet, from pasture to hay and concentrate and vice versa, in the week previous to testing results in different oral glucose tolerance curves. The second phase (>2 h) is insulin dependent and is characterized by a progressive decline to resting levels by 6 h. A late but normal-sized glucose peak may occur in cases of delayed gastric emptying
• The interpretation of an abnormal curve is dependent on the characteristics of the curve. A flat line (<15% increase) is indicative of a total malabsorption state and is associated with progressive inflammatory or neoplastic cellular infiltration of the small intestinal wall; this constitutes generally a grave prognosis. The diseases include the different causes of inflammatory bowel diseases (IBD)—lymphosarcoma, granulomatous enteritis, eosinophilic gastroenteritis, and intestinal mycobacteriosis. The definitive diagnosis of these conditions is made by histopathologic examination of a small intestinal biopsy
• A curve positioned between these previous values or that takes longer to see increased plasma glucose levels indicates partial malabsorption. It may be caused by several reversible or nonspecific entities, such as villous atrophy, circulatory disturbances, and inflammatory reversible changes due to intestinal parasitism. Partial malabsorption, when associated with normal small intestinal histology, may result from delayed gastric emptying, rapid intestinal transit, intestinal bacterial overgrowth, or abnormalities in cellular uptake and metabolism as is believed to occur in equine motor neuron disease

D-Xylose Absorption Test
• D-Xylose is a pentose sugar that is absorbed in the small intestine by passive diffusion and active transport by a sodium-absorption carrier
• The oral D-xylose absorption test has been used widely as an index of the small intestine absorptive function. Since it is not a normal constituent of the plasma, its absorption curve is not affected by the endogenous metabolic events influencing blood glucose

concentration. Based on these characteristics, the D-xylose absorption test is considered to provide a more accurate assessment of absorption than the glucose absorption test

Test Procedure
The horse is weighed and fasted as for the OGAT. A commercial-grade xylose solution at 10% (10 g/dL) is prepared and administered at a dose of 0.5 g/kg via a nasogastric tube. The sampling protocol is started with a pretest sample (time 0) followed ideally by sampling at 30, 60, 90, 120, 180, 240, 300, and 360 min after dosing. However, a 2 h sampling period is considered adequate in a clinical practice. The samples are taken into potassium oxalate–sodium fluoride anticoagulant vacutainers. Ideally, the laboratory conducting the analysis of samples has established a laboratory-specific normal reference ranges for horses.

Test Interpretation
• Blood xylose concentration rises from zero to a peak concentration of 1.37–1.67 mmol/L or 0.68–0.85 mmol/L (Roberts and Norman 1979) 60–90 min after dosing. As with OGAT, it is easy to determine total malabsorption and normal absorption curves, but an intermediate curve is difficult to interpret
• The shape of the xylose plasma concentration curve can also be affected by a number of factors other than absorption per se. Factors identified include rate of gastric emptying, intestinal transit time, mucosal blood flow, renal clearance, bacterial overgrowth, cellular or intraluminal metabolism of sugar, and composition of previous diets
• Most commercial laboratories do not process these samples routinely. Thus, the OGAT is more commonly performed

OLTT
• The OLTT is an indirect assay used to determine if persistent maldigestion and diarrhea in a foal are secondary to milk intolerance associated with lactase deficiency. This may follow intestinal epithelial damage caused by enteric disease such as rotavirus infection and *Clostridium difficile* enterocolitis
• Lactase (neutral β-galactosidase), a disaccharidase produced by small intestine mucosal cells, hydrolyzes lactose to monosaccharide glucose and galactose. This hydrolytic process is essential for milk digestion

Test Procedure
The foal is weighed as accurately as possible. It is fasted for 4 h before lactose administration and for the duration of the test. The foal should not be allowed to have access to water especially in the first hour of the test, as it

INTESTINAL ABSORPTION TESTS (CONTINUED)

may dilute the lactose and alter its digestion. Then, 1 g/kg of body weight of a 20% (20 g/dL) solution of lactose monohydrate (in warm water) is administered via stomach tube. The sampling protocol is started with a pretest sample (time 0) and followed by samplings at 30, 60, 90, 120, 180, 240, and 300 min after dosing. The samples are taken into potassium oxalate–sodium fluoride anticoagulant vacutainers.

Test Interpretation
- The general shape of this curve is similar to those reported for sugar tolerance tests. The mean peak in glucose level occurs approximately 1 h after dosing, with a return to fasting values by 3 h. The initial increase in plasma glucose indicates that it is absorbed from the intestine at a faster rate than it is removed from blood. As blood glucose increases, it enters the cells (particularly hepatic cells that convert glucose to glycogen), facilitated by the insulin activity. An increase of >1.4 mmol/L within 30 min of lactose administration is indicative of normal digestion and absorption. There are some variations with age, with the absorption being higher in older foals
- When an appropriate increase in blood glucose is not observed, an oral glucose or xylose test should be performed and will help to differentiate maldigestion from malabsorption

IMAGING
Nuclear Scintigraphy
Nuclear scintigraphy with technetium-99m-labeled hexamethyl-propyleneamine oxime-labeled leukocytes has been used to evaluate small intestinal malabsorption. It has shown limitations given the requirements of specialized equipment and also the presence of some false-negative results in horses with intestinal pathology.

MISCELLANEOUS
ABBREVIATIONS
- IBD = inflammatory bowel disease
- OGAT = oral glucose absorption test
- OLTT = oral lactose tolerance test

Suggested Reading
Jacobs KA, Norman P, Hodgson DRG, Cymbaluk N. Effect of diet on the oral D-xylose absorption test in the horse. Am J Vet Res 1982;43:1856–1858.
Mair TS, Hillyer MH, Taylor FGR, Pearson GR. Small intestinal malabsorption in the horse: an assessment of the specificity of the oral glucose tolerance test. Equine Vet J 1991;23:344–346.
Mair TS, Perason GR, Divers TJ. Malabsorption syndromes in the horse. Equine Vet Educ 2006;8:383–394.
Martens RJ, Malone PS, Brust DM. Oral lactose tolerance test in foals: technique and normal values. Am J Vet Res 1985;46:2163–2165.
Menziers-Gow NJ, Weller R, Bowen IM, et al. Use of nuclear scintigraphy with 99mTc-HMPAO-labelled leucocytes to assess small intestinal malabsorption in 17 horse. Vet Rec 2003;153:457–462.
Murphy D, Reid SWJ, Love S. The effect of age and diet on the oral glucose tolerance test in ponies. Equine Vet J 1997;29:467–470.
Rice L, Ott EA, Beede DK, et al. Use of oral tolerance tests to investigate disaccharide digestion in neonatal foals. J Anim Sci 1992;70:1175–1181.
Roberts MC. Small intestinal malabsorption in horses. Equine Vet Educ 2000;2:269–274.
Roberts MC, Hill FWG. The oral glucose tolerance test in the horse. Equine Vet J 1973;5:171–173.
Roberts MC, Norman P. A re-evaluation of the D(+)xylose absorption test in the horse. Equine Vet J 1979;11:239–243.
Weese JS, Parsons DA, Staempfli HR. Association of *Clostridium difficile* with enterocolitis and lactose intolerance in a foal. J Am Vet Med Assoc 1999;214:229–231.

Author Olimpo Oliver-Espinosa
Consulting Editors Henry Stämpfli and Olimpo Oliver-Espinosa

INTRA-ABDOMINAL HEMORRHAGE IN HORSES

BASICS

DEFINITION
Free hemorrhage within the peritoneal cavity.

PATHOPHYSIOLOGY

Acute Abdominal Hemorrhage
Acute massive blood loss of 30% ($\approx$10–12 L) or more of TBV results in hypovolemic shock. Splenic contraction maintains initial PCV.

Chronic Abdominal Hemorrhage
More than 30% of TBV must be lost before clinical signs become evident. Redistribution of interstitial fluid intravascularly can take up to 24 h, and erythropoiesis is maximal within 1 week. Approximately two-thirds of the erythrocytes from the hemorrhage are autotransfused into the systemic circulation within 24–72 h.

SYSTEMS AFFECTED

Cardiovascular
Hypovolemic shock with massive blood loss.

Urinary
Urine output is decreased because of vasoconstriction.

GI
Colic possible.

INCIDENCE/PREVALENCE
Uncommon

SIGNALMENT

Breed Predilections
Arabians and Thoroughbreds.

Mean Age and Range, Predominant Sex
• Older horses (>13 years)
• Multiparous broodmares >11 years of age due to reproductive tract bleeding

SIGNS

General Comments
Frequently nonspecific. Abdominal discomfort.

Historical Findings
• Dullness, weakness, depression, and lethargy
• Anorexia
• Colic
• Shock

Physical Examination Findings
Tachycardia, tachypnea, weak peripheral pulses, pale mucous membranes, CRT >2 s, oliguria. Ileus and abdominal distention may be observed.

CAUSES
• Idiopathic
• Trauma
• DIC
• Hemorrhage from the female reproductive tract
  ∘ The ovaries, uterus, or utero-ovarian blood vessels inside or outside the broad ligament
  ∘ Rupture of granulosa cell tumors and from ovarian follicular hematomas
  ∘ Birth-related trauma to the uterine vessels or with uterine neoplasia (leiomyomas or leiomyosarcoma)
• Hemorrhage from the GI tract
  ∘ Ulcerations
  ∘ NSAID toxicity
  ∘ Rupture of the mesenteric arteries secondary to *Strongylus vulgaris* larval migration
  ∘ Small strongyles
  ∘ Granulomatous intestinal disease (histoplasmosis, tuberculosis, granulomatous enteritis)
  ∘ Splenic rupture secondary to blunt trauma or neoplasia
  ∘ Entrapment of the small intestine within the epiploic foramen
  ∘ GI vascular leakage secondary to neoplasia or abscessation, coagulopathies, surgery, renal trauma, and hepatic disease
  ∘ Diaphragmatic hernia
  ∘ Phenylephrine administration

RISK FACTORS

Age
• Periparturient hemorrhage most frequently observed in older broodmares (age-related degeneration of the vasculature)
• Rupture of the caudal vena cava in older horses with epiploic foramen entrapment

Pregnancy
Peripartum hemorrhage can occur before, during, or after foaling.

Blunt External Trauma
Splenic and renal rupture.

Parasitism
Infestation by *S. vulgaris,* small strongyles.

DIAGNOSIS

DIFFERENTIAL DIAGNOSIS
• All disorders resulting in colic (including other causes of peritonitis)
• Uterine torsion, uterine rupture, and dystocia in broodmares
• Disorders resulting in hypovolemic shock

CBC/BIOCHEMISTRY/URINALYSIS
• Hematologic abnormalities (decrease in PCV, total red blood cell count, and hemoglobin concentration and hypoproteinemia) will be seen after the initial 24 h due to the physiologic compensatory mechanisms and spleen contraction. Sequential measurement of PCV will be helpful in determining whether the blood loss and resulting anemia are progressive or controlled
• Coagulation profile reveals thrombocytopenia due to blood loss

OTHER LABORATORY TESTS

Abdominocentesis
• Hemoperitoneum is definitively diagnosed by abdominocentesis. On cytologic examination, platelets are not typically present unless the hemorrhage is peracute (<45 min) and clotting is not observed
• The PCV of hemoperitoneum is lower than that of venous blood. In an iatrogenic splenic sample, the PCV will be higher than that of the peripheral blood. On cytologic examination, hypersegmented pyknotic neutrophils and hemosiderophages are observed

Blood Lactate
Blood lactate levels are a more sensitive indicator of early blood loss than PCV. In 1 study, peak lactate concentration was 5.6 ± 7.1 mmol/L.

Blood Gas Analysis
Arterial blood gas analysis can provide useful information about cardiopulmonary function in hypovolemic shock states. It may reveal metabolic acidosis (decreased pH and $[HCO_3^-]$) with respiratory compensation (decreased PCO_2).

IMAGING

Abdominal US
US evaluation of the abdomen, performed transabdominally or transrectally, reveals homogeneous echogenic "swirling" cellular fluid within the abdomen. The kidneys, liver, and spleen should be examined to identify the origin of the hemorrhage.

OTHER DIAGNOSTIC PROCEDURES

Rectal Palpation
Fluid accumulation within the abdomen or broad ligament, abnormal (neoplastic) masses, abnormalities within the reproductive tract, or other lesions associated with the site of hemorrhage, and gas-distended intestine may be noted on rectal palpation.

Surgery
May confirm the diagnosis of hemoabdomen and the source of bleeding.

PATHOLOGIC FINDINGS
Necropsy may confirm hemoabdomen.

TREATMENT

AIMS
The primary aims are maintenance of tissue perfusion and oxygenation by restoration of blood volume and hemoglobin and controlling bleeding. The cause and severity of the hypovolemic state are important factors in fluid (crystalloid, colloid, blood products) selection and volume.

APPROPRIATE HEALTH CARE
Rapid action must often be taken to save the life of horses with hemoperitoneum. Most cases will respond favorably to aggressive medical treatment. However, exploratory laparotomy or standing laparoscopy may be needed in patients when the source of bleeding cannot be determined or effectively

I

INTRA-ABDOMINAL HEMORRHAGE IN HORSES   (CONTINUED)

controlled. Surgery should be performed only when patients are stabilized.

NURSING CARE

Fluid Therapy
• When hypovolemic shock is present, the condition is addressed by prompt IV therapy with isotonic crystalloid solutions (lactated Ringer's solution, 20–40 mL/kg/h). Replacement fluid volume necessary to maintain perfusion in hemorrhagic shock is usually 2–7 times greater than the actual blood loss. Monitoring is important. Improvement in mentation, jugular distensibility, and CRT, increased pulse strength, and decreased heart rate and increased urine production are indications of improved cardiovascular status
• Replacement of intravascular volume may also be accomplished with hypertonic saline (5–7.5%, 4 mL/kg) to expand vascular volume, to enhance vascular tone, and to restore intravascular pressure. Contraindicated when bleeding is not controlled
• Colloids provide volume expansion and oncotic pressure. Use in addition to other types of fluid therapy. Hydroxyethyl starch (hetastarch 6% solution) is given at 10 mL/kg/day infusion. Higher doses can cause coagulation problems

Blood Transfusion
• Administer when the PCV has rapidly decreased to 15% (0.15 L/L) or the hemoglobin concentration falls below 5 g/dL (50 g/L). Whole-blood transfusion is required to increase oncotic pressure and oxygen-carrying capacity. The volume of blood transfusion will depend on the rate and quantity of blood loss. Whole blood should be administered at 15–25 mL/kg of body weight and repeated if necessary. Balanced crystalloid solutions should be administered concurrently to maintain perfusion
• Autotransfusion of blood from the abdomen can be life-saving in an exsanguinating horse if no other source of hemoglobin is available. However, it does provide platelets and clotting factors

ACTIVITY
Horses should be strictly rested. Horses surviving a large blood loss should not be exercised for 90 days.

DIET
N/A

CLIENT EDUCATION
Inform the client that their horse is in danger of cardiac collapse and death.

SURGICAL CONSIDERATIONS
Patients not responding to medical treatment and requiring surgical exploration of the abdominal cavity have a low survival rate.

MEDICATIONS

DRUG(S) OF CHOICE
Use of procoagulant and antifibrinolytic agents in horses with bleeding disorders is empirical and their efficacy is not proven.
• Aminocaproic acid—loading dose of 70 mg/kg IV (diluted in 1 L of saline and given over 20 min) followed by a constant rate infusion at 15 mg/kg/h
• Opioid antagonist (naloxone, 1 treatment of 8 mg IV)
• 10–30 mL of 10% buffered neutral formalin added to 500 mL of 0.09% NaCl IV

CONTRAINDICATIONS
Phenothiazine tranquilizers (acepromazine) are contraindicated since they decrease blood pressure.

PRECAUTIONS
Use α_2-agonists (xylazine and detomidine) with extreme caution because they decrease the cardiac output.

ALTERNATIVE DRUGS
Broad-spectrum antimicrobials, conjugated estrogens, vitamin K, Chinese herb yunnan baiyao, and propranolol have been used anecdotally, but their efficacy has not been demonstrated.

FOLLOW-UP

PATIENT MONITORING
• Cardiovascular status should be assessed by monitoring mentation, heart rate, pulse strength, CRT, and jugular vein distensibility. From every 5 min to a few times a day depending on whether the hemorrhage is controlled or not
• Urine output to assess renal blood flow
• Serial blood lactate measurement can be useful. Lactate concentration should decrease over time if the treatment is successful

PREVENTION/AVOIDANCE
Prevention strategies aimed at the different primary causes.

POSSIBLE COMPLICATIONS
• Cardiovascular collapse and death
• Bacterial contamination can be a risk during abdominocentesis. US can be more useful to confirm the diagnosis since is a noninvasive method
• NSAIDs have antiplatelet activity and may lead to renal failure when hypovolemia is present

EXPECTED COURSE AND PROGNOSIS
• Overall survival rate is between 50% and 70%
• Horses with high respiratory rate (>30 breaths/min), neoplasia, mesenteric injury, or DIC are less likely to survive
• In postparturient broodmares with rupture of the utero-ovarian artery, 2 clinical outcomes are possible depending on whether the hemorrhage is confined in the uterine broad ligament. In the former, a large hematoma develops in the broad ligament and the mare survives. In the latter, death can occur within minutes to days after parturition
• Horses that survive in the short term have a good prognosis for long-term survival with few complications
• The prognosis is guarded for a postoperative hemoperitoneum after exploratory celiotomy because of the potential sequelae of septic peritonitis and adhesion formation

MISCELLANEOUS

AGE-RELATED FACTORS
Older animals are at risk.

PREGNANCY/FERTILITY/BREEDING
Reasonable prognosis for fertility (50%) for broodmares suffering peripartum hemorrhage.

SYNONYMS
Hemoperitoneum

ABBREVIATIONS
• CRT = capillary refill time
• DIC = disseminated intravascular coagulopathy
• GI = gastrointestinal
• NSAID = non-steroidal anti-inflammatory drug
• PCO_2 = partial pressure of carbon dioxide
• PCV = packed cell volume
• TBV = total blood volume
• US = ultrasonography, ultrasound

Suggested Reading
Conwell RC, Hillyer MH, Mair TS, et al. Haemoperitoneum in horses: a retrospective review of 54 cases. Vet Rec 2010;167: 514–518.

Author Albert Sole-Guitart
Consulting Editors Henry Stämpfli and Olimpo Oliver-Espinosa

Acknowledgment The author and editors acknowledge the prior contribution of Ludovic P. Bouré.

 Client Education Handout available online

INTRACAROTID INJECTIONS

 BASICS

DEFINITION
Accidental injection of drugs into the carotid artery associated with acute neurologic signs.

PATHOPHYSIOLOGY
• The proximity of the common carotid artery to the jugular vein and patient movement makes the accidental injection of drugs into the carotid artery a real hazard. The injected material often travels via the carotid artery and distributes to the ipsilateral forebrain supplied by the middle cerebral artery. This is associated with acute, and possibly severe, cerebral disturbances
• Marked cardiovascular changes, such as bradycardia, arrhythmias, and blood pressure fluctuations may accompany CNS signs
• Local cerebral pathology and clinical signs are dependent on the potential of the drug to induce tissue abnormalities, and the rate of and quantity injected (see Expected Course and Prognosis)

SYSTEMS AFFECTED
CNS—in addition signs may include arrhythmias, changes in blood pressure, "blowing" respiration.

SIGNALMENT
No breed, sex, or age predisposition.

SIGNS
Historical Findings
A very recent history of parenteral drug administration.

Physical Examination Findings
• A violent reaction typically occurs within 5–30 s from the time of initiating the injection
• Signs can be delayed by a few minutes and be preceded by apprehension, facial twitching, head-shaking, kicking, propulsive circling. This may lead to recumbency, loss of consciousness, and seizures.

CAUSES
Fractious animals and attempts at an IV injection.

RISK FACTORS
See Causes.

 DIAGNOSIS

History and onset of clinical signs.

DIFFERENTIAL DIAGNOSIS
The preacute onset after attempted injection should rule out other causes of encephalopathies.

PATHOLOGIC FINDINGS
• Most affected horses recover. However, in horses that have received oil-based injections, diffuse perivascular necrosis with marked edema, vascular endothelial damage, hemorrhage, and neuronal degeneration are evident on histopathology
• Ipsilateral retinopathy and blindness reported after intracarotid injection of phenylbutazone

 TREATMENT

Treatment is largely supportive and symptomatic. Padding and sedation are indicated for thrashing, delirious horses.

 MEDICATIONS

DRUG(S) OF CHOICE
• Dexamethasone 0.1–0.25 mg/kg IV, DMSO 1 g/kg diluted in physiologic saline 1:6 IV, and anticonvulsant therapy may be useful
• Hypertonic (7%) saline solution may useful
• Use of mannitol may be considered in horses that do not rapidly improve despite the risk of cerebral hemorrhage
• Status epilepticus may be treated with diazepam 0.01–0.4 mg IV

PRECAUTIONS
• It is surprisingly easy to inject the carotid artery by mistake
• It behooves clinicians, particularly those who are not highly experienced, to use a large-gauge needle (i.e. 18 gauge) and to take the needle off the hub after insertion, ensuring that the blood that flows out is slow dripping and dark colored

 FOLLOW-UP

PATIENT MONITORING
Regular detailed neurologic examinations.

PREVENTION/AVOIDANCE
Always use a large-bore needle and insert the needle into the vein before attaching the syringe.

POSSIBLE COMPLICATIONS
• Complications often arise from self-induced trauma if the horse falls or has seizures
• Unilateral blindness possible

EXPECTED COURSE AND PROGNOSIS
• Injection of water-soluble drugs (e.g. xylazine, butorphanol, acetylpromazine (acepromazine)) is usually associated with complete recovery within hours. Some horses may require up to 7 days to recover and, on rare occasion, some die
• Common signs during recovery are facial hypoalgesia, blindness, and poor menace response contralateral to the side of injection
• Intracarotid injection of procaine penicillin, phenylbutazone, and oil-based or poorly water-soluble drugs is associated with a poorer prognosis. Intracarotid injection of such drugs is often associated with prolonged intractable seizures, coma, or stupor

 MISCELLANEOUS

ABBREVIATIONS
• CNS = central nervous system
• DMSO = dimethylsulfoxide

Suggested Reading
Gabel AA, Koestner A. The effects of intracarotid artery injection of drugs in domestic animals. J Am Vet Med Assoc 1963;142:1397–1403.
Mayhew IG. Large Animal Neurology, 2e. Chichester, UK: Wiley Blackwell, 2008.

Author Caroline N. Hahn
Consulting Editor Caroline N. Hahn

I

IONOPHORE TOXICOSIS

 BASICS

DEFINITION
- Horses are exquisitely sensitive to ionophore toxicity
- Ingestion of ionophores can result in a physicochemical and/or pathologic disruption of cardiac muscle, skeletal muscle, nerves, liver, and kidney
- All ionophores should be considered toxic with similar clinical effects. The LD_{50} doses for monensin, lasalocid, and salinomycin are 2–3 mg/kg, 21.5 mg/kg, and 0.6 mg/kg body weight, respectively

PATHOPHYSIOLOGY
- Ionophores are used as growth promoters in cattle and coccidiostats for poultry
- Ionophores transport ions across the membrane, down concentration gradients, resulting in the loss of ionic gradients across the membranes of excitable cells (muscle and nervous) as well as across the mitochondrial membrane
- Monensin has a higher affinity for sodium than potassium ions, whereas salinomycin has higher affinity for potassium than sodium ions. Lasalocid binds to calcium and magnesium ions
- For each ion transported into a cell, another ion is transported out. Loss of the ion gradients across the mitochondrial membrane prevents oxidative metabolism
- Loss of intracellular potassium suppresses ATP production and decreases cell energy production; increases in intracellular sodium lead to water influx and mitochondrial swelling; ionophores potentiate intracellular calcium influx, and all of these effects contribute to cell death
- Clinical effects and fatality rates are influenced by the quantity of ionophore ingested:
  ◦ With large amounts, the progression can be extremely rapid with death ensuing within 1–15 h. Lesions may not be found in horses that experience SCD
  ◦ With lesser amounts, signs and pathologic abnormalities related to skeletal and cardiac myopathy are observed. Cardiomyopathy can occur weeks or months later

SYSTEMS AFFECTED
- Cardiovascular—mitochondrial damage results in myocardial necrosis. Loss of ion gradients alters the polarity of the excitable tissues. Cardiac function, including conductance through the heart muscle, is altered. Connective tissue replaces necrotic myocardial cells, resulting in permanent myocardial dysfunction
- Musculoskeletal—often similar but less severe damage to skeletal muscle. Muscle fibrosis can occur

- Nervous—nerve and muscle conduction can be altered, resulting in altered reflexes and muscle coordination
- Renal/urologic—renal tubular damage associated with myoglobin casts can be seen
- Hepatobiliary—hepatocellular necrosis and decreased function can occur
- GI—diarrhea often occurs

INCIDENCE/PREVALENCE
Ionophore poisoning still occurs, in spite of increased awareness.

SIGNALMENT
No breed, age, or sex predilections.

SIGNS
General Comments
The severity and speed of onset reflect the amount of ionophore ingested.

Historical Findings
- Multiple horses can be affected
- Feed refusal, colic, ataxia, weakness, and recumbency are early signs

Physical Examination Findings
- SCD
- Tachycardia
- Cardiac arrhythmias
- Tachypnea
- Muscle weakness and ataxia
- Profuse sweating
- Epistaxis
- Signs of CHF
- Exercise intolerance

CAUSES
Accidental contamination of feed at feed mills, in feed trucks, or when horses inadvertently gain access to cattle or poultry feed.

RISK FACTORS
Vitamin E and/or selenium deficiency can predispose to more severe tissue damage, but adequate concentrations do not prevent toxicosis.

 DIAGNOSIS

DIFFERENTIAL DIAGNOSIS
- Acute GI diseases
- Acute neurologic diseases
- Rhabdomyolysis
- Vitamin E/selenium deficiency
- Viral, bacterial, or other toxic forms of myocardial failure

CBC/BIOCHEMISTRY/URINALYSIS
- Increased serum activity of creatine kinase, aspartate aminotransferase, and lactate dehydrogenase
- Increased blood urea nitrogen and indirect bilirubin concentrations
- Hyperglycemia
- Hypocalcemia, hypokalemia, hypomagnesemia, and hypochloremia
- Myoglobinuria

OTHER LABORATORY TESTS
- Elevated cardiac troponin I or cardiac troponin T; if normal, does not rule out ionophore toxicosis
- Blood lactate can be increased

IMAGING
ECG
Paroxysmal or sustained supraventricular and/or ventricular arrhythmias can be present.

Echocardiography
Echocardiographic abnormalities range in severity and include:
- Dilation of the left and/or right ventricle with possible rounded apices
- Regional or generalized hypokinesis or dyskinesis
- Decreases in fractional shortening
- Marked spontaneous contrast
- Increases in the mitral E-point—septal separation
- Increased pre-ejection period and decreased left ventricular ejection period
- Flattening of the aortic root, reduced aortic root diameter
- Mild pericardial effusion

Thoracic Ultrasonography
With pulmonary edema, peripheral pulmonary irregularities (B-lines, previously known as comet-tail artifacts) are visible.

Thoracic Radiography
Possible pulmonary edema.

OTHER DIAGNOSTIC PROCEDURES
- Radiotelemetric ECG monitoring—for real-time ECG when unstable cardiac rhythms present
- Continuous 24 h Holter monitoring—for identifying intermittent or paroxysmal cardiac arrhythmias, quantifying numbers of premature complexes, and assessing response to therapy
- Exercising ECG—for characterization of exercise-induced cardiac arrhythmias and their clinical significance. This should be undertaken 4 months after exposure in horses that have shown minimal signs
- Toxicology—stomach contents and feedstuffs should be analyzed for ionophores. Monensin has been found in highest concentrations in the heart. Blood, serum, liver tissue, and urine can all be used to confirm exposure

PATHOLOGIC FINDINGS
- No lesions with SCD
- Heart and skeletal muscle—vacuolation, swollen mitochondria, lipid vesicles, hypereosinophilia, pyknosis, mineralization, and loss of fiber striation progressing to myocardial fibrosis and chamber dilation with chronicity
- Nervous system—polyneuropathy of peripheral nerves with axonal degeneration and neuronal vacuolation
- Additional findings—widespread petechial hemorrhages in the lungs, heart, GI tract, and

spleen. Pleural and peritoneal effusion, pulmonary edema, and peripheral edema can occur

TREATMENT

AIMS
- No specific antidote
- Prevent further toxin absorption
- Supportive therapy is aimed at restoration of cardiac output and improved tissue perfusion, stabilization of cell membranes, and antiarrhythmic therapy if unstable, life-threatening arrhythmias are present

APPROPRIATE HEALTH CARE
- Severely affected cases should be hospitalized
- Mildly affected cases should be rested and the degree of cardiac damage determined

NURSING CARE
- Continuous ECG monitoring if the cardiac rhythm is unstable
- Horses should be kept quiet and not moved if cardiac output is low
- Severely ataxic horses may benefit from head protectors, bandaging, and housing in a padded area

ACTIVITY
- Horses should be stall rested for up to 4 months, if possible. An echocardiogram and exercising ECG should then be performed to identify persistent cardiomyopathy
- Although caution is advised, if these tests are normal, the horse can be returned successfully to performance

DIET
Vitamin E and selenium have been effective as a pretreatment in cattle and pigs. However, their efficacy after exposure to ionophores has not been established.

CLIENT EDUCATION
- Ionophore toxicosis can have significant medicolegal implications. The client should make detailed records of events leading up to the onset of signs and to have these corroborated by third parties, if possible
- Horses that are clinically normal post exposure are at risk for developing cardiac compromise later. An echocardiogram performed at the time of diagnosis should identify the horses at risk. The horses should not be used for riding activities for 4 months. After this time, an echocardiogram and exercising ECG should be performed to identify persistent cardiomyopathy

MEDICATIONS

DRUG(S) OF CHOICE
- Gastric lavage with activated charcoal and a saline cathartic, administered by nasogastric tube, can reduce further absorption of the toxin
- IV fluid therapy should be used with care as it can exacerbate pulmonary edema if acute myocardial failure is present
- Thiamine (0.5–5.5 mg/kg IM), vitamin E (up to 20 IU/kg daily PO), and selenium (0.01 mg/kg IM) might promote stabilization of cell membranes
- Antiarrhythmic drugs—see chapters Supraventricular arrhythmias and Ventricular arrhythmias

CONTRAINDICATIONS
- Digoxin acts synergistically with ionophores through inhibition of Na^+,K^+-ATPase and increases in cellular calcium influx, promoting cell death
- Chloramphenicol, sulfonamides, and macrolides can also potentiate ionophore toxicity

PRECAUTIONS
All antiarrhythmic drugs can be proarrhythmic. The ECG should be monitored continuously during antiarrhythmic therapy.

POSSIBLE INTERACTIONS
See Contraindications.

FOLLOW-UP

PATIENT MONITORING
Acutely, frequent assessment of heart and respiratory rate, pulse quality, blood pressure, blood lactate concentrations, and continuous ECG monitoring are indicated.

PREVENTION/AVOIDANCE
Feed manufacturers must take every precaution to ensure that ionophores are not accidentally included in equine feeds.

POSSIBLE COMPLICATIONS
CHF can occur in horses that survive the initial stages.

EXPECTED COURSE AND PROGNOSIS
- Mortality varies widely. The amount of ionophore ingested varies markedly. The bitter taste may deter many horses, particularly if they have access to alternative feed sources
- Some asymptomatic horses develop CHF, whereas others may have decreased cardiac function that is performance limiting

MISCELLANEOUS

PREGNANCY/FERTILITY/BREEDING
There is a high risk of fetal compromise if mares develop low cardiac output during pregnancy.

SYNONYMS
- Monensin toxicosis
- Salinomycin toxicosis
- Lasalocid toxicosis

SEE ALSO
- Myocardial disease
- Supraventricular arrhythmias
- Ventricular arrhythmias

ABBREVIATIONS
- CHF = congestive heart failure
- GI = gastrointestinal
- LD_{50} = median lethal dose
- SCD = sudden cardiac death

Suggested Reading
Bautista AC, Tahara J, Mete A, et al. Diagnostic value of tissue monensin concentration in horses following toxicosis. J Vet Diagn Invest 2014;26:423–427.
Decloedt A, Verheyen T, De Clerq D, et al. Acute and long-term cardiomyopathy and delayed neurotoxicity after accidental lasalosid poisoning in horses. J Vet Intern Med 2012;26:1005–1011.
Hall JO. Feed-associated toxicants: ionophores. In: Plumless KH, ed. Clinical Veterinary Toxicology. St. Louis, MO: Mosby, 2004:120–127.
Hughes KJ, Hoffman KL, Hodgson DR. Long term assessment of horses and ponies post exposure to monensin sodium in commercial feed. Equine Vet J 2009;41: 47–52.
Peek SF, Marques FD, Morgan J, et al. Atypical acute monensin toxicosis and delayed cardiomyopathy in Belgian draft horses. J Vet Intern Med 2004;18:761–764.

Authors Virginia B. Reef and Jeffery O. Hall
Consulting Editors Celia M. Marr and Virginia B. Reef
Acknowledgment The authors acknowledge the prior contribution of Celia M. Marr.

I

IRIS PROLAPSE

BASICS

OVERVIEW
• IP follows ocular trauma, particularly sharp perforating corneal injuries, or blunt injuries causing rupture of the cornea, limbus, and/or sclera
• IP can also occur secondary to rapid enzymatic degradation of stromal collagen in progressive melting or infected corneal ulcerations

SIGNALMENT
All ages and breeds of horses are at risk.

SIGNS
• The eye may be cloudy or red. Blepharospasm and epiphora are present. Slight downward deviation of the upper eyelashes may be a subtle sign of corneal pain
• A brown to red structure protruding through a corneal defect is diagnostic
• The anterior chamber will be shallow or collapsed

CAUSES AND RISK FACTORS
Corneal perforation with IP may be a sequela to traumatic insult or to infectious and noninfectious corneal ulcerations.

DIAGNOSIS

DIFFERENTIAL DIAGNOSIS
Ocular pain may be found with corneal ulcers, uveitis, conjunctivitis, blepharitis, and dacryocystitis.

DIAGNOSTIC PROCEDURES
• Fluorescein dye will indicate the site of corneal perforation, and the dye may leak into the anterior chamber
• Seidel's test may indicate aqueous leakage through the corneal perforation

TREATMENT

• Most IPs are ideally addressed with surgical repair. The decision to pursue surgery is initially based upon the possibility of useful vision and survival of the globe. Replacement of the missing cornea with a corneal transplant is recommended. The transplant site should be covered with a CF or an amniotic membrane graft

• Key techniques in repairing an IP:
1. Remove necrotic cornea before placing the corneal graft. Replace missing cornea with a larger diameter frozen corneal graft and suture in place
2. Make CF thin before suturing it to the cornea atop the corneal graft. CF fibrosis and failure may be associated with aqueous leakage under the flap. Aqueous humor leakage induces fibroplasia such that the flap does not adhere well to the wound
3. CF bruising may indicate flap ischemia
4. A white CF has become avascular
5. CF bulging may indicate IP. Check for low intraocular pressure and positive Seidel's test
6. Continue anti-proteinase medications after flap placement or absorbable sutures may dissolve prematurely
7. Anchor CF with sutures at the limbus to reduce tension

MEDICATIONS

DRUG(S) OF CHOICE
• Topical antibiotics (every 1–4 h initially), atropine (1%; QID), and serum (every 1–4 h) are recommended. Systemic NSAIDs (flunixin meglumine 1 mg/kg BID PO, IV), and broad-spectrum parenteral antibiotics are indicated
• Intensive postoperative medical therapy, especially use of systemic NSAIDs, is critical for successful management of iridocyclitis

CONTRAINDICATIONS/POSSIBLE INTERACTIONS
Horses receiving topical atropine should be monitored for colic.

FOLLOW-UP

PATIENT MONITORING
• Horses with IP and secondary uveitis should be stall rested until the condition is healed. Intraocular hemorrhage and increased severity of uveitis are sequelae to overexertion
• The horse should be protected from self-trauma with a hard- or soft-cup hood
• Ocular pain should gradually diminish following surgical repair

POSSIBLE COMPLICATIONS
Infectious endophthalmitis is a complication that will require enucleation. Vision compromise may be minimal to complete.

EXPECTED COURSE AND PROGNOSIS
• Prognosis of perforating corneal lacerations is guarded. Perforating wounds caused by sharp insults are associated with a better prognosis than those caused by blunt insults. High-energy blunt trauma may result in hyphema and/or globe rupture, most often occurring at the limbus or equator where the sclera is the thinnest
• Iridocyclitis may predispose to fibropupillary membrane formation, posterior synechiae, and cataract development. Some of these eyes will become phthisical and permanently blind
• Traumatic perforating wounds <15 mm have a better prognosis than those >15 mm
• There is a direct relationship between a prolonged duration of ulcerative keratitis prior to IP and poor visual outcome. Eyes with IP due to ulcerative keratitis >2 weeks' duration, and melting or infected ulcers, tend to have a poor visual outcome or may require enucleation due to endophthalmitis

MISCELLANEOUS

ASSOCIATED CONDITIONS
Ulcerative keratitis in the horse frequently incites severe anterior uveitis.

ABBREVIATIONS
• CF = conjunctival flap
• IP = iris prolapse
• NSAID = nonsteroidal anti-inflammatory drug

Suggested Reading
Brooks DE. Ophthalmology for the Equine Practitioner, 2e. Jackson, WY: Teton NewMedia, 2008.
Brooks DE, Matthews AG. Equine ophthalmology. In: Gelatt KN, ed. Veterinary Ophthalmology, 4e. Ames, IA: Blackwell, 2007:1165–1274.
Gilger BC, ed. Equine Ophthalmology, 3e. Ames, IA: Wiley Blackwell, 2017.

Author Caryn E. Plummer
Consulting Editor Caryn E. Plummer
Acknowledgment The author/editor acknowledges the prior contribution of Dennis E. Brooks.

BASICS

OVERVIEW
• Caused by oral or parenteral iron salts supplementation
• Most documented cases occurring in neonates <3 days of age from oral administration of a nutritional supplement containing ferrous fumarate
• Toxicity depends on the amount of elemental iron present—ferrous sulfate is 20% elemental iron; ferrous gluconate is 12% elemental iron
• Causes corrosive damage to the GI mucosa, resulting in edema, ulceration, and hemorrhage
• After absorption, ferrous iron (Fe^{2+}) is converted to ferric iron (Fe^{3+}), releasing an unbuffered hydrogen ion and causing metabolic acidosis
• Iron disrupts oxidative phosphorylation and causes free-radical formation and lipid peroxidation, resulting in cell death
• Periportal hepatocytes are especially vulnerable to damage and necrosis
• Iron also can result in a coagulopathy from inhibition of thrombin
• Iron is cardiotoxic, resulting in decreased cardiac output
• Hypovolemia from GI fluid loss and decreased cardiac output contribute to circulatory shock

SIGNALMENT
• Most common in neonates because of their lower capacity to bind iron to transferrin and their increased oral absorption of iron
• Toxic doses for neonates are estimated to be 25-fold less than those for adults

SIGNS
• Early signs associated with oral ingestion include colic, diarrhea, and melena
• Anorexia, lethargy, and icterus are common
• Signs of hepatoencephalopathy (e.g. ataxia, head pressing, coma) may be seen

CAUSES AND RISK FACTORS
Iron is more toxic in selenium- or vitamin E-deficient individuals.

DIAGNOSIS

DIFFERENTIAL DIAGNOSIS
Adult Horses
• Other hepatotoxicants
• Theiler disease
• Causes of hemolytic anemia
• Immune-mediated thrombocytopenia
• Disseminated intravascular coagulation
• Bacterial cholangiohepatitis
• Lymphosarcoma

Foals
• Septicemia
• Neonatal isoerythrolysis
• Tyzzer disease
• Equine herpesvirus

CBC/BIOCHEMISTRY/URINALYSIS
• Thrombocytopenia, lymphopenia, and prolonged prothrombin time and activated partial thromboplastin time
• Increased serum γ-glutamyltransferase, alkaline phosphatase, total and conjugated bilirubin, bile acids, fibrinogen, fibrin degradation product, and ammonia
• Metabolic acidosis

OTHER LABORATORY TESTS
• High serum iron concentration, high saturation of iron binding, and high free iron in tissues
• Postmortem interpretation of high liver iron concentrations is difficult in the absence of compatible histopathologic lesions

PATHOLOGIC FINDINGS
Gross
Lesions include icterus, small liver with dark red areas or tan discoloration and uneven surfaces, GI hemorrhages, and thymic atrophy in foals.

Histopathologic
• Periportal or panlobular hepatocellular necrosis, bile duct and fibrous connective tissue proliferation, mixed inflammatory cell infiltration, and cholestasis
• Necrosis in the gastric glandular mucosa and in the lamina propria of the small intestine
• Mild to severe lymphoid lesions, including thymic lymphoid necrosis and necrosis in splenic lymphoid follicles
• Extensive hemosiderin deposits in liver, spleen, thyroid, and bone marrow

TREATMENT
• Stabilize the patient, paying particular attention to cardiovascular support and acid–base status
• GI decontamination is unlikely to be beneficial because of the inability of activated charcoal to bind iron

MEDICATIONS

DRUG(S) OF CHOICE
• Use of the specific iron-chelator deferoxamine mesylate is possible; but efficacy and safety studies in horses are lacking
• For mild intoxications, chelation therapy probably offers little advantage compared with supportive care

• A suggested deferoxamine dosage based on experience in humans and dogs is 15 mg/kg/h IV; if used, therapy probably should be limited to 24 h

CONTRAINDICATIONS/POSSIBLE INTERACTIONS
• Do not give deferoxamine to patients with renal impairment or to pregnant animals
• Rapid administration of deferoxamine can cause cardiac dysrhythmias and exacerbate existing hypotension
• Corticosteroids may increase serum free-iron concentrations

FOLLOW-UP

PATIENT MONITORING
Monitor serum iron concentrations, liver function, and cardiovascular status.

PREVENTION/AVOIDANCE
• Do not oversupplement iron in individuals without confirmed iron deficiency
• A normal dietary requirement of iron in adult horses is 40 ppm

EXPECTED COURSE AND PROGNOSIS
• Individuals with mild liver pathology have a good prognosis with good supportive care
• Individuals with severe liver pathology or hepatoencephalopathy have a guarded prognosis

MISCELLANEOUS

ABBREVIATIONS
GI = gastrointestinal

Suggested Reading
Edens LM, Robertson JL, Feldman BF. Cholestatic hepatopathy, thrombocytopenia and lymphopenia associated with iron toxicity in a Thoroughbred gelding. Equine Vet J 1993;25:81–84.
Mullaney TP, Brown CM. Iron toxicity in neonatal foals. Equine Vet J 1988;20: 119–124.

Authors Arya Sobhakumari and Robert H. Poppenga
Consulting Editors Wilson K. Rumbeiha and Steve Ensley

I

ISCHEMIC OPTIC NEUROPATHY

BASICS

OVERVIEW
• Atrophy of the optic nerve as a sequela to infarction or injury to the vascular supply to the optic nerve
• Systems affected—ophthalmic

SIGNALMENT
N/A

SIGNS
• Acute blindness
• Dilated pupil
• Absent pupillary light reflex
• Absence of ocular pain
• Following sudden loss of blood supply, the optic disk at first appears normal, but the eye is blind. Within 24 h, there is swelling and mild hyperemia of the optic disk. Focal white, raised lesions overlying the optic nerve and its margins are observed within 48 h, and may be associated with peripapillary hemorrhages. After several weeks, there are ophthalmoscopic signs of optic nerve atrophy with pallor and vascular attenuation of the optic disk
• Peripapillary depigmentation may be observed as the disease progresses, and represents early retinal atrophy. With time, there are increasing signs of retinal atrophy

CAUSES AND RISK FACTORS
Any condition that may result in sudden hypoxia of the optic nerve, such as:
• Acute hypovolemia
• Thromboembolic diseases
• Surgical ligation of the internal carotid, external carotid, and greater palatine arteries for treatment of epistaxis caused by guttural pouch mycosis

DIAGNOSIS

DIFFERENTIAL DIAGNOSIS
• Traumatic optic neuropathy
• Exudative optic neuropathy
• Proliferative optic neuropathy
• Optic nerve atrophy

CBC/BIOCHEMISTRY/URINALYSIS
N/A

OTHER LABORATORY TESTS
N/A

IMAGING
N/A

OTHER DIAGNOSTIC PROCEDURES
The electroretinogram will be normal initially but will be reduced to absent as the ischemia becomes prolonged.

PATHOLOGIC FINDINGS
Peripapillary retinal ischemia results in microinfarcts of the nerve fiber layer, which appear clinically as depigmentation. These are areas of a thickened nerve fiber layer consisting of aggregates of ruptured and swollen axons.

TREATMENT

There is no treatment for the condition itself; however, treatment of the underlying cause is recommended, if possible.

MEDICATIONS

CONTRAINDICATIONS/POSSIBLE INTERACTIONS
N/A

FOLLOW-UP

EXPECTED COURSE AND PROGNOSIS
Poor prognosis for return of vision.

MISCELLANEOUS

SEE ALSO
• Exudative optic neuropathy
• Optic nerve atrophy
• Proliferative optic neuropathy

Suggested Reading
Brooks DE. Retinopathies and ocular manifestations of systemic diseases in the horse. In: Brooks DE, ed. Ophthalmology for the Equine Practitioner, 2e. Jackson, WY: Teton NewMedia, 2008:207–225.
Gilger BC. Equine ophthalmology. In: Gelatt KN, Gilger BC, Kern TJ, eds. Veterinary Ophthalmology, 5e. Ames, IA: Wiley Blackwell, 2013:1560–1609.
Nell B, Walde I. Posterior segment diseases. Equine Vet J Suppl 2010;37:69–79.
Wilkie DA. Diseases of the ocular posterior segment. In: Gilger BC, ed. Equine Ophthalmology, 2e. Maryland Heights, MO: Elsevier Saunders, 2011:367–396.

Author Bianca C. Martins
Consulting Editor Caryn E. Plummer
Acknowledgment The author and editor acknowledge the prior contribution of Maria Källberg and Dennis E. Brooks.

ISOCOMA PLURIFLORA TOXICOSIS

BASICS

OVERVIEW
- *Isocoma pluriflora* (rayless goldenrod) was previously known as *Isocoma wrightii* or *Haplopappus heterophyllus*
- The plant is an erect, bushy, unbranching perennial shrub that grows 60–120 cm (2–4 feet) in height
- The leaves are alternate and linear and generally have a smooth margin but can be toothed; the leaves also may have a sticky feel to them
- The flowers are yellow, tubular, and terminal and number 7–15 per head
- The plant prefers the arid southwest and is found in dry rangelands of southern Colorado, through New Mexico and Arizona, western Texas, and into northern Mexico
- The plant grows well in river valleys, along drainage areas, and is abundant along the Pecos River
- Tremetone, a ketone, is reportedly the toxic agent

SIGNALMENT
N/A

SIGNS
- No cases of *I. pluriflora* intoxication have been documented in horses. However, cases of alkali disease were reported in the early 1900s in horses and is believed to be from *I. pluriflora*
- The toxin is the same as that found in *Eupatorium rugosum* (white snakeroot), and presumptive evidence exists that the same clinical signs could be expected—heart muscle degeneration, muscle tremors, ataxia, reluctance to walk, heavy sweating, myoglobinuria, and depression
- Horses that eat *E. rugosum* have an onset of clinical signs within 2–3 weeks after ingestion; generally, 2–3 days of ingestion is required. Generally this is believed to be approximately 1–2% of their body weight
- The disease has been documented in nursing young of horses, sheep, and cattle
- Affected horses stand with their legs wide apart and develop swelling near the thoracic inlet and along the ventral neck
- There may be a jugular pulse and associated tachycardia
- ECG changes—increased heat rate, ST elevation, and variable QRS complexes
- Cardiac arrhythmias often are present and detectable on auscultation

CAUSES AND RISK FACTORS
- Environmental conditions such as drought result in less desirable forages or weeds being consumed
- Hungry or thirsty horses that are unfamiliar with a given area are more likely to consume *I. pluriflora*

DIAGNOSIS

DIFFERENTIAL DIAGNOSIS
- Evidence of consumption and occurrence of compatible clinical signs remain the best way of diagnosing intoxication
- Examination of the pasture may reveal that the plant has been browsed
- Selenium/vitamin E deficiency (white muscle disease)—measurement of selenium and vitamin E in whole blood, serum, or liver
- Ionophore intoxication—detection of ionophore in feed or gastrointestinal contents

CBC/BIOCHEMISTRY/URINALYSIS
- Horses intoxicated with *E. rugosum* have elevated serum creatine kinase, aspartate aminotransferase, and alkaline phosphatase activities
- Presumably, horses consuming *I. pluriflora* have similar abnormalities

OTHER LABORATORY TESTS
- ECG changes may be noted as described above
- Detection of toxin may be possible

IMAGING
N/A

OTHER DIAGNOSTIC PROCEDURES
N/A

PATHOLOGIC FINDINGS
- Horses ingesting *E. rugosum* have nonspecific histopathologic lesions
- Lesions associated with suspected *I. pluriflora* intoxication—myocardial degeneration, necrosis, and fibrosis, renal tubular degeneration, and hepatic fatty changes
- The pericardial sac may contain straw-colored fluid, and the subendocardium may have extensive pale areas

TREATMENT

- Decontamination with AC and a saline cathartic may be helpful, especially to reduce enterohepatic circulation of the toxin
- Monitor ECG and treat arrhythmias accordingly
- Recovery may be protracted and high-quality forage is important to help alleviate the severe ketosis and acidosis
- Administration of parenteral carbohydrates for control of the low glucose levels in the blood
- Animals that survive may be left with a severely scarred heart and circulatory dysfunction; therefore, symptomatic and supportive care is always appropriate

MEDICATIONS

DRUG(S) OF CHOICE
- AC (1–4 g/kg PO in a water slurry (1 g of AC per 5 mL of water))
- Sodium or magnesium sulfate (250 mg/kg PO as a 20% solution)

CONTRAINDICATIONS/POSSIBLE INTERACTIONS
N/A

FOLLOW-UP

PATIENT MONITORING
N/A

PREVENTION/AVOIDANCE
- Preventing access to the plant is the best solution for avoiding intoxication
- Herbicides can be used to control plant growth

POSSIBLE COMPLICATIONS
N/A

EXPECTED COURSE AND PROGNOSIS
N/A

MISCELLANEOUS

ASSOCIATED CONDITIONS
N/A

AGE-RELATED FACTORS
N/A

ZOONOTIC POTENTIAL
N/A

PREGNANCY/FERTILITY/BREEDING
N/A

ABBREVIATIONS
AC = activated charcoal

Suggested Reading
Burrow GE, Tyrl RJ. Toxic Plants of North America. Ames, IA: Iowa State University Press, 2001:181–183.
Olson CT, Keller WC, Gerken DF, Reed SM. Suspected tremetol poisoning in horses. J Am Vet Med Assoc 1984;185:1001–1003.
Sanders M. White snakeroot poisoning in a foal: a case report. J Equine Vet Sci 1983;3: 128–131.

Author Tam Garland
Consulting Editors Wilson K. Rumbeiha and Steve Ensley

Client Education Handout available online

JUGLANS NIGRA (BLACK WALNUT) TOXICOSIS

BASICS

OVERVIEW
Juglans nigra (black walnut) is a large tree native to the eastern USA whose wood is prized for furniture and gun stocks. When fresh black walnut shavings are used as bedding, horses can develop laminitis and pyrexia within 12–24 h. It usually presents as a stable-wide outbreak, but not all horses in contact with black walnut-contaminated bedding will develop problems.

SIGNALMENT
No breed, age, or sex predilections.

SIGNS
• Laminitis (can be severe)
• Pyrexia
• Depression
• Limb edema
• Colic

CAUSES AND RISK FACTORS
• An unknown compound in fresh black walnut shavings
• Toxicity decreases with exposure of shavings to light and air
• Problems can occur when as little as 5–20% of bedding is black walnut

DIAGNOSIS

DIFFERENTIAL DIAGNOSIS
• Other causes of laminitis—history, no evidence of exposure to black walnut
• *Berteroa incana* (hoary alyssum) ingestion—evidence of exposure
• History will indicate that multiple horses bedded with black walnut shavings develop laminitis over a relatively short period of time

CBC/BIOCHEMISTRY/URINALYSIS
N/A

OTHER LABORATORY TESTS
• Black walnut shavings can be identified by their dark brown color (with a hint of purple)
• Samples can be submitted to diagnostic laboratories or forestry departments for positive identification by microscopy

IMAGING
N/A

OTHER DIAGNOSTIC PROCEDURES
N/A

PATHOLOGIC FINDINGS
Laminitis

TREATMENT
• Remove all animals from suspect bedding
• Wash legs with mild soap and water
• Treat for laminitis

MEDICATIONS

DRUG(S) OF CHOICE
• If ingested, administer oral activated charcoal at 1–4 g/kg body weight in a water slurry
• Treat for laminitis

CONTRAINDICATIONS/POSSIBLE INTERACTIONS
N/A

FOLLOW-UP

PATIENT MONITORING
N/A

PREVENTION/AVOIDANCE
Inspect bedding deliveries for black walnut contamination.

POSSIBLE COMPLICATIONS
Ventral rotation of the third phalanx.

EXPECTED COURSE AND PROGNOSIS
Good with no complications.

MISCELLANEOUS

ASSOCIATED CONDITIONS
N/A

AGE-RELATED FACTORS
N/A

ZOONOTIC POTENTIAL
N/A

PREGNANCY/FERTILITY/BREEDING
N/A

SEE ALSO
Laminitis

Suggested Reading
Belknap JK. Black walnut extract: an inflammatory model. Vet Clin North Am Equine Pract 2010;26(1):95–101.
Burrows GE, Tyrl RJ. Toxic Plants of North America. Ames, IA: Iowa State University Press, 2001:725–728.
Uhlinger C. Black walnut toxicosis in ten horses. J Am Vet Med Assoc 1989;195:343–344.

Author Larry J. Thompson
Consulting Editors Wilson K. Rumbeiha and Steve Ensley

BASICS

DEFINITION
Laminitis is failure of the hoof–distal phalanx attachment apparatus.

PATHOPHYSIOLOGY
• The lamellae suspend P3 within the hoof capsule—epidermal lamellae extend like sheets from the stratum medium of the inner hoof wall, interdigitating with dermal lamellae that are ultimately connected to P3. Each primary lamella has multiple secondary lamellae, increasing surface area and strength of attachment. The basement membrane separates the epidermal and dermal lamellae and is a key structural component. Collagen bundles, arranged in linear rows, connect the basement membrane to P3, forming the "suspensory apparatus of the distal phalanx"
• Although the pathophysiology remains unclear, loss of normal epidermal basal cell adhesions/cytoskeletal integrity appears to be a key early event regardless of cause. Altered growth factor signaling, inflammation, and changes in perfusion and/or energy balance appear to trigger these events, leading to loss of structural integrity, with the distractive forces of weight-bearing then contributing further to damage
• There are 3 distinct major forms of laminitis based on the underlying cause and mechanisms—laminitis associated with severe systemic disease (sepsis associated); laminitis associated with insulin dysregulation (endocrinopathic laminitis); and laminitis associated with excessive weight-bearing on a foot (supporting limb laminitis)
• Endocrinopathic laminitis is intrinsically linked to insulin dysregulation in horses/ponies and encompasses laminitis associated with EMS, PPID, and exogenous corticosteroid administration. Current evidence suggests that excess insulin overstimulates growth factor receptor IGF-1R, which triggers a response in lamellar epidermal cells that involves disruption of normal cell adhesions
• Sepsis-associated laminitis occurs with severe systemic inflammation, usually as a result of infection (e.g. pneumonia) or the absorption of bacterial products (particularly endotoxin) from the gastrointestinal tract (e.g. colitis, natural/experimental alimentary carbohydrate overload). Marked local inflammation including infiltration of the lamellae with neutrophils is characteristic
• Supporting limb laminitis appears to be the result of ischemia due to reduced lamellar perfusion due to both increased load and reduced unweighting/load cycling on a limb
• Pasture-associated laminitis may involve pathophysiologic elements of both endocrinopathic and sepsis-associated forms

• Once the lamellar attachments are weakened, the nature and severity of the resultant pathology are determined by the extent of lamellar damage. Severe, wholesale acute lamellar detachment can result in downward P3 "sinking" within the hoof capsule. In less severe cases, deep flexor tendon tension and lamellar epidermis proliferation result in palmar rotation of P3 away from dorsal hoof wall and formation of the "lamellar wedge." Loss of the suspensory function of the lamellae leads to compression of the sole corium by the distal surface of P3, a considerable source of pain in chronic cases. With displacement of P3, growth of the hoof wall becomes disrupted, and vascular structures may be compressed
• In many endocrinopathic cases chronic laminitis pathology is very slowly progressive and substantial pathology is often already present by the time clinical signs are first recognized
• In many acute cases damage is mild and there is no resultant detectable displacement of P3

SYSTEMS AFFECTED
Musculoskeletal—foot.

GENETICS
N/A

INCIDENCE/PREVALENCE
N/A

GEOGRAPHIC DISTRIBUTION
N/A

SIGNALMENT
• Rare (absent?) in foals or weanlings
• Pony breeds more susceptible to the endocrinopathic form
• Chronic laminitis is common in broodmares

SIGNS
General Comments
• Wide range of clinical presentations, from severe lameness and recumbency to poor performance in an athletic horse that is not overtly lame
• Laminitis is divided into 3 phases—developmental, acute, and chronic

Historical Findings
• Acute or recurrent lameness of variable severity in 1 or more limbs
• Reluctance to move ± more frequent recumbency
• Lameness worse when circling or on hard ground
• Recent systemic disease or access to excess grain or lush pasture
• ± Severe, prolonged contralateral limb lameness

Physical Examination Findings
• Developmental phase
  ○ No clinical signs; however, primary disease and pathologic processes that lead to lamellar damage are under way

• Acute laminitis
  ○ Increased digital pulse amplitude and hoof wall/coronary band temperature
  ○ ± Distal limb edema
  ○ Incessant shifting weight in fore- and hindlimbs
  ○ In mild cases, subtle lameness
  ○ With increasing severity, obvious lameness at the walk; worse circling on a hard surface
  ○ Most often, 1 or both front feet are affected; less severe in the hindlimbs
  ○ Characteristic stance—forelimbs extended forward and hindlimbs underneath the body
  ○ In severe cases, unwillingness to move and recumbency
  ○ ± Difficulty lifting limbs due to reluctance to bear weight on opposite limb
  ○ Tachycardia, tachypnea, and sweating may be profound
  ○ Highly variable response to hoof testing. ± Generalized hoof pain or focal pain in toe region. ± Reaction to tapping the hoof wall
• Chronic laminitis
  ○ Defined by ≥48 h of clinical laminitis and/or radiographic displacement of P3 within the hoof capsule
  ○ Increased digital pulse amplitude
  ○ Variable lameness
  ○ ± Prolonged periods in recumbency
  ○ Palpable coronary band cleft
  ○ Prolapse of the sole in the toe; ± P3 penetration through the sole
  ○ ± Uneven hoof growth rings, wider in quarters/heels, narrower in dorsal hoof wall
  ○ Characteristic "dished" appearance to dorsal hoof wall
  ○ ± White line separation, seedy toe, and abscess
  ○ ± Persistent tachycardia and hypertension
  ○ Weight loss in moderate to severe cases

CAUSES
• Systemic septic diseases including colitis (bacterial, Potomac horse fever, grain overload), anterior enteritis, colonic volvulus, septic peritonitis, pneumonia, metritis/retained fetal membranes
• Insulin dysregulation due to EMS or PPID
• Pastures rich in nonstructural carbohydrate, particularly in combination with EMS or PPID
• Excessive weight-bearing on a limb due to pain or dysfunction of the opposite limb
• Exertional rhabdomyolysis
• Exposure to black walnut (*Juglans nigra*) heartwood shavings
• Ingestion of the toxic plant hoary alyssum (*Berteroa incana*) in hay or pasture
• Excessive work on hard surfaces
• Corticosteroid administration
• Excessive intake of cold water (empirical reports only)

RISK FACTORS
See Causes.

L

DIAGNOSIS

DIFFERENTIAL DIAGNOSIS
• Other painful conditions such as rhabdomyolysis, tetanus, or pleurodynia secondary to pleuropneumonia. Rule out by absence of increased digital pulse amplitude and digital hyperthermia
• Unilateral limb laminitis or laminitis that is more severe in 1 digit must be differentiated from hoof abscess or P3 fracture. Rule out by hoof testing and radiographs

CBC/BIOCHEMISTRY/URINALYSIS
• Abnormalities due to inciting cause(s)
• ± Stress leukogram

OTHER LABORATORY TESTS
• Testing of the pituitary adrenal axis in cases of suspected PPID (Cushing disease). Baseline adrenocorticotropic hormone concentration or thyrotropin-releasing hormone response test preferred to dexamethasone suppression test
• Baseline insulin concentration or preferably dynamic testing (oral sugar test) for the diagnosis of insulin dysregulation of PPID or EMS.
• Plasma creatinine and albumin concentrations with NSAID use to monitor for toxicity

IMAGING
• Standard lateromedial radiographs to assess P3 position relative to the hoof capsule. Radiopaque marker placed on dorsal hoof wall at the coronary band aids in measurements. A steel rod of known length can be used to correct for magnification
• Radiographs obtained at onset of clinical signs to document progression
• P3 rotation, dorsal hoof wall to P3 distance, and coronary band to the extensor process of P3 distance can guide progression and prognosis
• Digital venograms may be useful in chronic cases to determine vascular compression or thrombosis. ± Guide hoof wall resection or coronary grooving. Adhere to published descriptions of this technique to avoid common artifacts

OTHER DIAGNOSTIC PROCEDURES
Avoid perineural anesthesia unless there is difficulty isolating lameness to the foot.

PATHOLOGIC FINDINGS
• Chronic—sagittal sectioning of the feet reveals characteristic formation of lamellar wedge and palmar rotation of P3
• Acute—lamellar histopathology recommended, gross changes may not be obvious

TREATMENT

AIMS
• Treat underlying cause(s)
• Acute—limit mechanical damage, control inflammation
• Chronic—provide mechanical support, encourage normal hoof growth
• Provide adequate analgesia and supportive care

APPROPRIATE HEALTH CARE
Developmental Phase
• Laminitis is irreversible; focus is prevention during the developmental phase and minimizing progression in the early acute phase
• With septic disease/endotoxemia, aggressive systemic treatment with anti-inflammatory and antiendotoxic therapy as well as continuous cooling of the feet. Ideally, an ice and water mixture is applied from the proximal metacarpal/metatarsal region to (and including) the hooves and is regularly replenished. Maintain ice boots for up to 7 days
• Preemptive shoe removal and application of frog/sole support

Acute Phase
• Once clinical signs are apparent, limit mechanical damage
• Strict stall confinement
• Continuous cooling of the feet after the onset of lameness in sepsis-associated cases
• Light sedation may encourage recumbency
• In less painful horses, shoe removal, excessive toe conservatively trimmed
• Bed on sand or apply silicone impression material or Styrofoam padding to the sole
• Styrofoam pads custom sized to the foot and taped on overnight. Once crushed down, remove pad and cut off the toe portion. Reapply pad with an additional second pad underneath to preferentially load the caudal foot
• ± Heel elevation (10–20°) to reduce deep flexor tendon tension and redistribute distracting forces from the dorsal wall to quarters/heels
• Judicial NSAID use; excessive analgesia may encourage locomotion and increase mechanical damage
• ± Sling support during standing periods especially with rapid P3 sinking

Chronic Phase
• Medical management of underlying endocrinopathy (EMS or PPID), diet management, restrict nonstructural carbohydrate consumption (soaked hay, commercially formulated feeds)

• Ongoing farriery and a close client–veterinarian–farrier relationship are required for successful management
• Avoid radical trimming or shoeing. Gradual changes over >1 shoeing interval to avoid destabilizing the foot and worsening of clinical signs
• Shoe/pad/trim or other farrier techniques that redistribute weight from hoof wall to frog and caudal sole, minimize breakover forces, and reduce deep flexor tendon tension
• Radiographs should be used as a guide for trimming and shoeing

NURSING CARE
• Deep bedding, particularly if recumbent for prolonged periods
• Sling support may facilitate trimming and shoeing

ACTIVITY
• In acute phase, absolute strict stall confinement
• Stall rest for at least 1 month, and up to ≥6 months, after an acute laminitis; depends on severity
• Very, very gradual reintroduction to exercise

DIET
• Avoid excessive carbohydrate in grain, hay, and pasture
• Obese and/or EMS horses benefit from controlled, gradual weight loss

CLIENT EDUCATION
• Clients should be made aware of the potentially life-threatening nature of the disease
• Client compliance with management of restricted turnout and diet (including access to pasture) is vitally important to treatment success

SURGICAL CONSIDERATIONS
• With significant P3 rotation (>15°) or where the dorsal tip of P3 is penetrating the sole or causing solar prolapse, deep flexor tenotomy may be beneficial
• In chronic cases, coronary grooving or dorsal hoof wall resection can relieve tension on the coronary band, reduce sublamellar venous compression, and facilitate better quality hoof wall regrowth

MEDICATIONS

DRUG(S) OF CHOICE
• NSAIDs—phenylbutazone (2.2–4.4 mg/kg every 12 h) tends to provide superior analgesia to flunixin meglumine (1 mg/kg every 12 h)
• Acepromazine (0.02–0.04 mg/kg IV or IM every 6 h) during the acute phase

CONTRAINDICATIONS
Avoid corticosteroid administration.

L

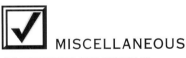

PRECAUTIONS
Monitor for signs of toxicity with long-term NSAID use.

POSSIBLE INTERACTIONS
N/A

ALTERNATIVE DRUGS
• Constant rate infusion of lidocaine, ketamine, and morphine, alone or in combination, can provide potent short-term analgesia
• Gabapentin (20 mg/kg orally every 12 h) in severe acute or chronic cases
• Metformin and pergolide should be restricted to patients with confirmed insulin dysregulation or PPID, respectively

FOLLOW-UP

PATIENT MONITORING
• Daily monitoring of acute cases
• Chronic cases require consistent monitoring; the frequency depends on the experience of the owner/trainer and disease severity
• Initially, repeat radiographs obtained at each trimming/shoeing interval (2 weeks) and subsequently at 4 week intervals
• Repeat endocrine testing for EMS and PPID as appropriate

PREVENTION/AVOIDANCE
• Aggressive and early treatment of primary disease in systemically ill horses
• Identify horses with EMS/PPID or insulin dysregulation and strict dietary control to avoid hay/grain and pasture high in soluble carbohydrate; maintain an ideal body weight
• For high-risk horses, avoid pasture turnout when nonstructural carbohydrate levels are likely to be highest—midmorning to late afternoon, spring and fall, during flowering and early seeding or after frosts
• Use a grazing muzzle during high-risk periods

POSSIBLE COMPLICATIONS
• Detachment and sloughing of hoof wall in severe acute/subacute cases
• Progressive rotation, sinking, and sole penetration of P3 followed by necrosis and osteomyelitis in chronic disease
• ± Persistent hypertension with cardiac hypertrophy in chronic disease
• ± Renal failure and right dorsal colitis from long-term NSAID use

EXPECTED COURSE AND PROGNOSIS
• Depends entirely on extent of the lamellar damage; however, lameness severity is always the most useful prognostic indicator regardless of other factors
• "Sinking" of P3 results in a poor prognosis for survival
• Sole penetration by P3 significantly worsens prognosis
• Chronic cases with >15° of P3 rotation have a guarded prognosis for survival and grave prognosis for soundness
• Return to athletic activity is highly variable; horses with >5° of P3 rotation or sinking of P3 are unlikely to return to athletic activity

✓ MISCELLANEOUS

ASSOCIATED CONDITIONS
N/A

AGE-RELATED FACTORS
N/A

ZOONOTIC POTENTIAL
N/A

PREGNANCY/FERTILITY/BREEDING
N/A

SYNONYMS
Founder

ABBREVIATIONS
• EMS = equine metabolic syndrome
• NSAID = nonsteroidal anti-inflammatory drug
• PPID = pituitary pars intermedia dysfunction
• P3 = third phalanx

Suggested Reading
Belknap JK, Geor R, eds. Equine Laminitis. Ames, IA: Wiley Blackwell, 2017.

Author Andrew W. van Eps
Consulting Editor Elizabeth J. Davidson

L

LANTANA CAMARA TOXICOSIS

BASICS

OVERVIEW
• *Lantana camara* (lantana or red sage) is a herbaceous, perennial, ornamental shrub
• It is erect or sprawling, clumped, stout, and hairy and grows to 210 cm tall, with several stems arising out of the base
• It has square twigs or stems that have small, scattered spines. The branches have an opposite arrangement which is characteristic even in the dormant phase
• The leaves are simple, opposite or whorled, and are oval shaped, with a petiole up to 1.5 cm long
• The net-veined leaf blade is aromatic when crushed; the blades are broadly lanceolate and between 5 and 11 cm long and 2.5 and 6 cm wide, with a wedge-shaped base and regularly spaced, toothed margins
• The flowers most often consist of 2 colors, ranging from white, yellow, or orange to red, blue, or even dark violet; the flowers are small and tubular in flat-topped clusters
• A green, immature, berry-like fruit also is found, with hard seeds that turn blue to black at maturity
• The plant is regarded as ornamental, but some varieties have escaped cultivation over most of the USA and Canada. It also grows widely in tropical and subtropical countries around the world
• The green berry apparently is the most toxic, although the entire plant is toxic
• There are numerous cultivars and hybrids, and toxicity seems to vary considerably among them. Common pink-flowered types are low in lantadene A and B, while the red-flowered type is high is lantadene A and B. Nevertheless caution is warranted not to rely only on flower color as judge of toxicity
• The toxins are polycyclic triterpenoid PAs—lantadene A and lantadene B
• Lantana toxins cause intrahepatic cholestasis, characterized by inhibition of bile secretion without extensive hepatocyte necrosis
• The toxins may cause kidney failure as well
• Horses are suspected of developing liver disease, but not photosensitization

SIGNALMENT
N/A

SIGNS
• Anecdotally, horses develop nonspecific liver and renal dysfunction that is evident on clinicopathologic tests and at necropsy
• Horses are not believed to develop photosensitization with lantana intoxication, but 1 report described associated crusty, contact-type lesions around the muzzles and light-skinned areas
• Some owners report icterus of the sclera and mucous membranes after ingestion

CAUSES AND RISK FACTORS
• Animals that are hungry or unfamiliar with the plants are more likely to consume *L. camara*
• Hepatic metabolism differences between species may account for the variable susceptibility to lantana toxins
• Injury to the liver cells could result from the action of the metabolite rather than the parent compound

DIAGNOSIS

The most valuable tool for the diagnosis is a good history.

DIFFERENTIAL DIAGNOSIS
• Consider other hepatotoxins—aflatoxin (detection in feed and histopathology), PAs (ingestion of alkaloid-containing plants and histopathology), and iron toxicosis (tissue iron concentrations and histopathology)
• In addition to PA-containing plants, consider exposure to other hepatotoxic plants—*Nolina texana*, *Agave lechuguilla*, *Panicum* spp., and *Trifolium hybridum*
• A nontoxic differential includes Theiler disease (history and histopathology)

CBC/BIOCHEMISTRY/URINALYSIS
Hyperbilirubinemia (conjugated) is the most consistent finding.

OTHER LABORATORY TESTS
• Lantadenes may be detected in stomach contents if death occurs close to the time of consumption
• Portions of the plant may be identified in the stomach contents by a competent microscopist

IMAGING
Ultrastructural studies have observed obstructive cholangitis.

OTHER DIAGNOSTIC PROCEDURES
N/A

PATHOLOGIC FINDINGS
• Liver lesions—cholestasis, pigmentation and degeneration of hepatocytes, and fibrosis
• Kidney lesions—vacuolation and degeneration of convoluted tubule epithelium and presence of various casts. Occasionally, multifocal, interstitial, mononuclear cell infiltration, and fibrosis may be evident

MEDICATIONS

DRUG(S) OF CHOICE
• AC (2–4 g/kg in a water slurry (1 g of AC per 5 mL of water))
• Sodium thiosulfate 0.5 g/kg body weight given IV

CONTRAINDICATIONS/POSSIBLE INTERACTIONS
N/A

FOLLOW-UP

PATIENT MONITORING
Monitor hepatic function.

PREVENTION/AVOIDANCE
• Preventing access to the plant is the best solution for avoiding toxicosis
• Herbicides can be used to control the plant
• The plant is quite susceptible to the herbicide 2,4-dichlorophenoxyacetic acid

POSSIBLE COMPLICATIONS
N/A

EXPECTED COURSE AND PROGNOSIS
N/A

MISCELLANEOUS

ASSOCIATED CONDITIONS
N/A

AGE-RELATED FACTORS
N/A

ZOONOTIC POTENTIAL
N/A

PREGNANCY/FERTILITY/BREEDING
N/A

ABBREVIATIONS
• AC = activated charcoal
• PA = pyrrolizidine alkaloid

Suggested Reading
Burrow GE, Tyrl RJ. Toxic Plants of North America. Ames, IA: Iowa State University Press, 2001:1170–1174.
Pass MA. Poisoning of livestock by lantana plants. In: Keeler RF, Tu AT, eds. Toxicology of Plant and Fungal Compounds: Handbook of Natural Toxins. New York, NY: Marcel Dekker, 1991:297–311.

Author Tam Garland
Consulting Editors Wilson K. Rumbeiha and Steve Ensley

 Client Education Handout available online

LARGE COLON TORSION

BASICS

DEFINITION
• Rotation of the large colon about the mesocolic axis in a dorsomedial or dorsolateral direction
• Most commonly located adjacent to the cecal base (less commonly involves the sternal and diaphragmatic flexures)
• Transverse colon or cecum may also be involved
• Most torsions are in an anticlockwise/dorsomedial direction
• Rotation of 90–270° will cause partial obstruction of lumen and passage of ingesta
• Rotation of 270–360° results in complete obstruction, and torsions ≥360° result in strangulating obstruction of the colon

PATHOPHYSIOLOGY
• Volvulus causes varying degrees of mechanical bowel obstruction which decreases normal colonic absorption and results in electrolyte imbalances and hypomotility, which in turn may contribute to further twisting of the colon
• Strangulation of the large colon is typically hemorrhagic rather than ischemic, i.e. venous drainage of the colon is compromised but arterial inflow is relatively intact
• With venous obstruction, blood eventually extravasates into the submucosa and colonic lumen. This causes the colonic epithelium to slough, and these phenomena produce increased gas and fluid accumulation within the colonic lumen
• Vascular damage results in degeneration of blood vessels and intraluminal hemorrhage
• With damage to the bowel wall, bacteria and endotoxins, as well as fluid and protein, leak into the peritoneal cavity, which results in endotoxemia, hypovolemia, and hypoproteinemia. Within 4–5 h, the colonic mucosa undergoes complete necrosis
• Severe systemic shock leads to cardiovascular collapse and death
• With complete arterial and venous obstruction, tissue perfusion decreases, with resultant hypoxia and ischemia that cause reduced absorption and hypomotility. Prolonged ischemia causes bowel necrosis, with leakage of bacteria and endotoxins into the peritoneal cavity
• Endotoxemia and hypovolemia result in severe systemic shock, cardiovascular collapse, and death

SYSTEMS AFFECTED
• GI
• Cardiovascular

GENETICS
No known genetic basis.

INCIDENCE/PREVALENCE
• Of horses that actually undergo surgical treatment for colic, 10–25% have large colon volvulus. 1 study reported 65% of horses undergoing surgery having a strangulating (>360°) volvulus
• Prevalence is increased in geographic areas that have a high population of broodmares

SIGNALMENT
Mature horses, especially broodmares in the postparturient period, are more commonly affected.

SIGNS

Historical Findings
History is reflective of how quickly and how fully a complete volvulus (i.e. >360°) occurs. Can be a chronic colic that suddenly worsens, or a sudden onset of severe abdominal pain.

Physical Examination Findings
• If large colon volvulus is strangulating, horses show severe uncontrollable abdominal pain
• Initially horses may have normal cardiovascular parameters, and rectal palpation can be unremarkable. As the condition progresses these parameters deteriorate. A heart rate >80 bpm is associated with poor survival
• Amount of gastric reflux depends on the degree of compression of the small intestine by the distended large colon
• Abdominal distention may be seen
• Normal gut sounds are reduced or absent in all GI quadrants
• Signs of shock become rapidly evident

CAUSES
• Exact cause is unknown
• Hypomotility and increased intraluminal gas accumulation are thought to initiate a rotation of the colon. Nonstrangulating obstructions may progress to strangulating obstructions by this mechanism
• Horses undergoing a sudden dietary change may be predisposed to increased gas production and altered GI motility
• Postparturient broodmares are thought to be predisposed because of increased space within the abdomen

RISK FACTORS
• Foaling within the past 90 days
• Change of feeding practice
• Feeding sugar beet
• A recent increase in the number of hours of stabling

DIAGNOSIS

DIFFERENTIAL DIAGNOSIS
• Nonstrangulating obstruction—torsion <360°
• Other abnormalities involving the large colon, including right or left dorsal colon displacement, impaction, tympany, enterolithiasis
• Other acute abdominal accidents—including those affecting the cecum, small intestine, stomach, and small colon

CBC/BIOCHEMISTRY/URINALYSIS
• A high packed cell volume (>50%) is associated with a poor prognosis, as is a low total protein
• Nonspecific hematologic changes such as leukopenia, neutropenia, with or without a left shift, lymphopenia, and thrombocytopenia are reflective of inflammation and/or endotoxemia
• Elevated lactate may reflect ischemic injury and a value of >6 mmol/L has been associated with a poor prognosis for survival in horses with large colon volvulus
• A metabolic acidosis may be apparent on venous blood gas analysis
• On urinalysis, isosthenuria, glucosuria, proteinuria, and casts or red blood cells may occur from prerenal or renal azotemia, caused by hypovolemia and shock

OTHER LABORATORY TESTS
Elevated protein concentration and lactate in the peritoneal fluid are useful indicators of a strangulating obstruction of the large colon. Visual assessment of peritoneal fluid is also useful—a turbid, red to brown appearance is indicative of a strangulating lesion.

IMAGING
• Ultrasonography is useful. The dorsal colon can be imaged in the ventral abdomen if a 180° or 540° volvulus is present
• A colonic wall thickness of >9 mm is suggestive of a large colon volvulus

OTHER DIAGNOSTIC PROCEDURES
• Nasogastric intubation is a necessary part of all colic examinations
• Rectal examination can be challenging in the severely painful horse and it is not always possible to complete a full examination. Chemical and physical restraint can facilitate the procedure
• Findings at rectal examination will vary depending on the progression of the volvulus
• Distended large colon and tight colonic bands can be palpated further on in the progression, and edema of the colon may be evident
• Sometimes, gas distention in the colon is so severe that a complete rectal examination cannot be performed

PATHOLOGIC FINDINGS
• The location and degree of the volvulus can be identified during surgery or at postmortem evaluation
• The level of devitalization of the large colon is dependent on the location and degree of the volvulus, and the duration

L

LARGE COLON TORSION (CONTINUED)

TREATMENT

APPROPRIATE HEALTH CARE
• Physical examination, nasogastric intubation, and rectal examination should be performed
• Surgery is necessary for chance of a successful outcome
• Rapid referral for surgery is of paramount importance for increasing the chance of survival
• Pain medication including flunixin meglumine, α_2-agonists and opioids may be required
• Withhold feed preoperatively

NURSING CARE
Refer affected horses to a surgical facility immediately after initial diagnosis.

ACTIVITY
• In the 4 weeks following surgery, stall rest with hand-walking daily is advised
• Following this time, horses can be turned out into a small paddock for limited exercise for a further 4 weeks
• A gradual return to exercise over weeks 9–12 following surgery is recommended

DIET
• Fasting prior to surgery
• Gradual feed reintroduction in the postoperative period

CLIENT EDUCATION
• Inform clients that prompt diagnosis and early surgical intervention are very important in the outcome for survival. A survival advantage is seen in horses with a colic duration of <2 h before surgical intervention
• Complications following surgery may affect outcome, including colic, ileus, peritonitis, incisional infection, jugular thrombophlebitis, and diarrhea
• 1 paper reports a recurrence of 5%
• Pregnant mares may abort

SURGICAL CONSIDERATIONS
• Surgical correction is performed via exploratory laparotomy
• Some surgeons advocate resection to prevent recurrence. The decision-making process for resection is complex. Removing the majority of diseased colon may reduce endotoxemia. However, the procedure has risks of complication and, depending on the location of the volvulus, it may not be possible to remove all of the diseased portion
• A colopexy technique is not often performed.

MEDICATIONS

DRUG(S) OF CHOICE
• Administer flunixin meglumine
• Further analgesics including α_2-agonists and opioids may be administered if necessary

CONTRAINDICATIONS
As described for other causes of colic.

PRECAUTIONS
• Deterioration in condition may be difficult to detect if repeated administration of analgesics
• Repeated dosing of long-acting α_2-agonists may affect cardiovascular hemodynamics

POSSIBLE INTERACTIONS
N/A

ALTERNATIVE DRUGS
N/A

FOLLOW-UP

PATIENT MONITORING
• Horses are usually hospitalized for up to 1–2 weeks following surgery, depending on occurrence of postoperative complications
• Once discharged from the hospital, routine daily monitoring should be performed

PREVENTION/AVOIDANCE
• Employ feeding practices that avoid large quantities of lush pasture, large amounts of grain, and sugar beet wherever possible
• Make all dietary changes gradually over a period of several days
• Allow as much turnout as possible because increased stabling may be a risk factor
• Provide dental care to prevent quidding
• Resection or colopexy of the large colon can prevent recurrence

POSSIBLE COMPLICATIONS
• Large colon necrosis and rupture may occur preoperatively as a result of the rapid progression of the disease
• Similarly, large colon rupture may occur intraoperatively as the volvulus is corrected
• Anesthetic death is possible as of result of the compromised preoperative cardiovascular status
• Complications following surgery may affect outcome, including ileus, peritonitis, incisional infection, jugular thrombophlebitis, and diarrhea

EXPECTED COURSE AND PROGNOSIS
• Surgery is required for strangulating volvulus. Without surgery, the horse will die
• >19–33% of horses with strangulating volvulus do not recover from anesthesia due to the severity of lesions
• Reported short-term (i.e. discharge from hospital) survival rates following surgery vary from 35% to 88%. Prognosis is improved substantially by early referral and prompt surgical treatment. Long-term survival may be low compared with other causes of colic treated surgically

MISCELLANEOUS

ASSOCIATED CONDITIONS
Endotoxemia

AGE-RELATED FACTORS
N/A

ZOONOTIC POTENTIAL
N/A

PREGNANCY/FERTILITY/BREEDING
• Broodmares that have foaled within the past 90 days appear to be at increased risk
• The combination of endotoxemia, hypovolemia, general anesthesia, and surgery all pose a risk to the viability of the fetus

SYNONYMS
Large colon torsion.

SEE ALSO
• Acute adult abdominal pain—acute colic
• Endotoxemia
• Right and left dorsal displacement of the colon

ABBREVIATIONS
GI = gastrointestinal

Suggested Reading
Hackett ES, Embertson RM, Hopper SA, et al. Duration of disease influences survival to discharge of Thoroughbred mares with surgically treated large colon volvulus. Equine Vet J 2015;47:650–654.

Author Nicola C. Cribb
Consulting Editors Henry Stämpfli and Olimpo Oliver-Espinosa

Client Education Handout available online

BASICS

DEFINITION
Includes normal/abnormal causes; 1 or both ovaries achieve a size significantly larger than considered normal, detected by TRP and/or US.

PATHOPHYSIOLOGY
Physiology
• Estrous cycles/ovulatory period normally occurs spring and summer
• Light duration is the predominant influence on ovarian activity
• Outside the optimal season for breeding activity, gonad size and activity waxes and wanes
• Reproductive activity initiated at puberty
  ○ GnRH increases in the springtime, increasing FSH/LH leading to ovarian activity
  ○ A lag time of 60–90 days follows the winter equinox for increasing light to be reflected in regular estrous cycles/ovulation
  ○ After the summer solstice, day length decreases, GnRH tapers, LH/FSH decrease, until levels are insufficient to complete maturation and/or induce ovulation
• *Persistent follicles in vernal (spring) transition*
  ○ Variable sizes through transition; late vernal (spring) transition follicles may regress after persisting for a month or more
  ○ May stimulate ovulation late in vernal transition by administration of hCG
• *Persistent follicles in fall (autumnal) transition*
  ○ Early in fall transition can induce additional ovulations, especially if identified early in fall transition and follicles ≥35 mm
  ○ All will eventually regress (decrease in size) as daylight wanes; mare enters into winter anestrus (bilateral small, inactive ovaries)

Normal Ovary, Persistent Follicles
• Most common LOS cause
• May be single or multiple, present on 1 or both ovaries
• Normal structures that will resolve if left alone

Normal Ovary, Hematoma
• Second most common LOS cause
• Enlargement resolves without assistance over time
• PGF treatment may stimulate earlier initiation of estrous cyclic activity. Often slower to luteinize than a normal-sized CH; often requires longer (6–14+ days) to become responsive
• Hematoma can harm ovarian stroma if repeated due to successive pressure inside ovarian tunic

Abnormal Ovary, Tumors, and Other Causes
• Hormone treatments fail to elicit desired response

• TRP/US—appearance inconsistent with normal ovarian structures
• Systemic illness
• Identify cell type on histopathologic examination of tissue following OVX

SYSTEMS AFFECTED
Reproductive

GENETICS
N/A

INCIDENCE/PREVALENCE
Persistent Follicles
• Potentially 80% of reproductively normal mares
• ≈20% of Northern Hemisphere mares experience year-round estrous cycle activity, albeit may be some variation from the "norm" of 21 days

Hematoma
Less common, a few cases a year will be recognized within a normal population of mares; ovulatory season.

Tumors
GCT/GTCT—most common ovarian tumor, but rare.

SIGNALMENT
• Females of breeding age
• All breeds

SIGNS
Persistent Follicles
• Seasonal component—during 1 of the 2 transition periods
• Usually extended periods (1+ month) of *teasing in* (receptive to stallion)
• Estrus behavior longer than during a normal estrous cycle (>12–14 days in the spring)
• TRP/US—presence of follicles, multiple, variable size; follicular appearance is normal
• May increase in size/diameter with time, the increase is slower than with dominant follicles (5–6 mm/day) during the ovulatory period

CAUSES
Persistent Follicles
Day length relationship: Vernal (spring) transition before sufficient LH; Autumnal (fall) transition after LH decreases.

DIAGNOSIS

DIFFERENTIAL DIAGNOSIS
Ovaries During Pregnancy (>37–40 Days' Gestation)
• Endometrial cups with subsequent equine chorionic gonadotropin production, secondary follicles luteinize to become secondary corpus lutea. Pregnant mare ovaries become bilaterally enlarged
• Mare's behavior may mimic aggression of some mares with a GCT/GTCT
  ○ Most likely related to increased circulating testosterone (fetal gonads), may be >100 pg/mL by 60–90 days gestation.

  ○ Testosterone peaks at ≈200 days' gestation; returns to basal levels by time of foaling

Ovarian Hematoma
• Occurs following ovulation; the CH increases to a size substantially larger than the follicle that preceded it
• Acute pain associated with rapid stretch of the ovarian tunic (short-term *colic*)
• Post ovulation (2–4 days), the mare's behavior is that of diestrus, i.e. normal (teases out; rejects the stallion's advances); blood P_4 rises (>1 ng/mL) by 5–6 days post ovulation, ovulation confirmation
• Contralateral ovary is normal
• US of hematoma—eventually similar to a CH, albeit a large one
• Resolution—time or PGF treatment. Complete luteinization may be slow; thus delayed response to PGF (>6 to 14+ days post ovulation)

GCT/GTCT
• TRP characterized by unilateral gonad enlargement (tumor growth rate varies significantly by case)
  ○ Surface of tumor remains smooth, may exhibit gentle lobulations
  ○ Ovulation fossa disappears (fills in) early in tumor's development
  ○ Over time, contralateral ovary shows evidence of suppression; the number/size of follicles decreases, then total volume/size of parenchyma decreases
  ○ Chronic GCT/GTCTs may have a contralateral ovary so small to be difficult for the novice to detect during TRP
  ○ Rare contralateral ovary will continue with follicular activity and ovulations
• Elevation of circulating levels of AMH and inhibin with GTCT
• Behavior
  ○ Mares typically exhibit 1 of 3 primary behaviors—chronic anestrus, increased aggression, persistent estrus, a reflection of the specific tumor cell type involved, with a possible steroid hormone component
  ○ Mares rarely exhibit pain (in contrast to a hematoma) due to more gradual stretch of ovarian tunic.
  ○ May exhibit discomfort at the trot or refuse to go over jumps due to painful stretching of the mesovarium; behavioral change (pain, anger, reticence to perform) possible

Teratoma/Dysgerminoma
• Rare, not hormonally active
• TRP of contralateral ovary is normal. Surface of teratoma may exhibit somewhat sharper protuberances reflective of its contents
• No effect on behavior or estrous cycle activity
• Teratoma is benign

Dysgerminoma
• Rare

LARGE OVARY SYNDROME

• Initial presentation for intermittent chronic colic, weight loss, stiff extremities
• Presence of tumor may only be discovered once mare's health deteriorates due to metastases
• Potentially highly malignant

Cystadenoma
• Unilateral, no effect on contralateral ovary
• No effect on behavior
• Appearance—large, cystic structures, may confuse early on with persistent follicles, remains nonresponsive to hCG
• Rare hormonal impact; elevated testosterone

Ovarian Abscess
• Rare
• Early reports may have been associated with attempts to reduce the size/number of persistent follicles via flank approach aspiration
• Contralateral ovary normal
• No effect on behavior or estrous cycle activity

CBC/BIOCHEMISTRY/URINALYSIS
N/A

OTHER LABORATORY TESTS
GCT/GTCT
Diagnostic tests and sensitivity of detection:
• Sensitivity for circulating inhibin levels (>0.7 ng/mL) in 80% of GCT/GTCTs
• Sensitivity for testosterone (>50–100 pg/mL) in 48% of affected mares
• Combining results of inhibin with testosterone levels raises the level of confidence to 84%
• Progesterone levels are usually <1 ng/mL in the absence of luteal tissue
• AMH—98% sensitivity of detection (greater than for inhibin or testosterone). AMH originates from the granulosa cells of normal ovaries (in both cycling and pregnant mares) as well as GCTs. The systemic levels of AMH in mares with GCTs are elevated above those produced by normal ovaries. Its normal reference range is ≤4.2 ng/mL

Ovarian Hematoma
Blood progesterone will increase by 5–7 days of hematoma formation.

Dysgerminoma
• Reports of hypertrophic pulmonary osteoarthropathy
• Radiography, biopsies for metastasis

IMAGING
US
Important adjunct tool to evaluate/differentiate cases of LOS
• *Persistent follicle*—except for larger size, appearance is similar to normal follicle
• *Hematoma*
  ◦ Recent—fluid-filled space
  ◦ By 2–10 days hyperechoic areas began to appear; ongoing clotting of blood, contraction of clot, invasion of luteal cells
  ◦ Eventually takes on uniform hyperechoic appearance of a large CH

Table 1

Blood hormone evaluations		
Hormone	*Normal range*	*GCT/GTCT*
Progesterone, estrus	<1 ng/mL	
Progesterone, diestrus	>1 ng/mL	
Progesterone		<1 ng/mL
Testosterone		>50–100 pg/mL
Inhibin	0.1–0.7 ng/mL	>0.7 ng/mL
AMH	<4.2 ng/mL	Often as much as 5× or more than the normal level

• *GCT/GTCT*
  ◦ Multicystic spaces, can appear quite irregular; fluid pockets range from a few millimeters to multiple centimeters
  ◦ Size/location of tumor during US scan can range from readily accessible off tip of uterine horn to very pendulous (dependent on weight stretch of mesovarium)
  ◦ Recorded weights ranged from <1 to 45+ kg
  ◦ When detected, majority will be <30 cm diameter
• *Teratoma*
  ◦ Variable echogenicity, reflecting the nature of its contents, i.e. soft tissue, fluid, hair, bone, teeth

OTHER DIAGNOSTIC PROCEDURES
Blood hormone evaluations are a valuable adjunct (Table 1).

PATHOLOGIC FINDINGS
• Neoplasms can potentially arise from any ovarian tissue type
• Classification based on the origin and surface epithelium—sex cord–stromal tissue, germ cell, mesenchymal tissue
• *GCT/GTCT*—sex cord–stromal tumor, endocrine effects, specific in mare: inhibin and AMH are produced by granulosa cells (GTCT)
• *Teratoma*—many tissue types, including germ cells, within the mass; can include hair, skin, respiratory epithelium, tooth, bone. Metastases not a routine concern in the mare
• *Cystadenoma*—from epithelium; forms cystic neoplastic masses
• *Dysgerminoma*—from germ cells, analogous to seminoma of the testis; cells are arranged in sheets and cords with a dense population of large pleomorphic cells; all malignant

 TREATMENT

NURSING CARE
• None specific to conditions
• General postoperative medical care recommended following an OVX

CLIENT EDUCATION
• Explain need for serial examinations (TRP/US) to reach accurate diagnosis of LOS; avoid unnecessary OVX
• Vast majority of LOS cases are due to persistent follicle(s) and hematoma
• GCT/GTCTs are the most common tumor causing ovarian enlargement, but are still rare
• *History*
  ◦ Season—during transitional periods, persistent follicle(s) is first to rule out
  ◦ Estrous activity—e.g. a mare recently showing estrus is now out of estrus, acutely painful, enlarged ovary is detected. Hematoma is the first to rule out
  ◦ Response to treatment—progesterone supplementation, prostaglandin, hCG
  ◦ Behavior changes—prolonged anestrus, increased aggression, nymphomania
• *Serial TRP*
  ◦ At interval of 7–10 days, may require 3–5 examinations (if not doing endocrine testing)
  ◦ Avoid too frequent examinations (if interval too short unlikely significant increase or decrease in size of affected ovary); avoid unnecessary cost/surgery
    ▪ Examine 2x within the span of a potential estrus period—(1) compare affected and contralateral ovary, (2) rate of size increase, (3) activity of opposite gonad
• US is a most effective tool to evaluate the internal characteristics of the enlarging gonad
• Circulating hormone levels
  ◦ Inhibin, testosterone, progesterone, AMH
  ◦ Ovarian tumor *endocrine panel*—evaluate most likely rule-outs

SURGICAL CONSIDERATIONS
OVX

 MEDICATIONS

DRUG(S) OF CHOICE
Hematoma
• No treatment, wait for ovary to regress in size and other follicular activity to develop, or
• $PGF_{2\alpha}$ 5–10 mg IM when >7–10 days post ovulation

- May be unresponsive to treatment within first 2+ weeks (may need to repeat PGF)
- Successful treatment is noted by the mare returning to estrus within 2–5 days

Persistent Follicles
- Can elect "no treatment, but for time," wait for estrous activity to begin (vernal transition) or cease (fall transition) on its own
- To shorten duration of spring transition
  ○ Regu-Mate- do not start treatment before significant follicular activity is present. In transition, mare experiences behavioral, not physiologic, estrus. See chapter Abnormal estrus intervals. Wear protective gloves. Dosed PO at 0.044 mg/kg (1 mL/50 kg (110 lb) body weight) daily for 15 days. Delivered by dose syringe PO or place on grain at feeding time
  ○ hCG 2500–3000 IU IV; may induce ovulation late in vernal transition. Wait until a follicle of ≥35 mm is present; ovulation within 36–44 h
  ○ Deslorelin (GnRH analog) injection. Ovulation within 38–60 h; a decapeptide, it does not stimulate antibody production as can hCG. A subset of mares will experience persistent anestrus if PGF is administered 1 week after deslorelin administration
  ○ P+ (150 mg P_4 + 10 mg estradiol-17β) —10 day treatment; results in more effective ovulation and follicular suppression than P_4 alone. Administered IM daily. PGF on the last day of treatment. Approximately 80% of mares will ovulate 8–10 days after PGF. hCG may be used once a ≥35 mm follicle is present (induce ovulation)
  ○ Other P_4 products are available—P_4 in oil (IM); Bio Release P+ LA (long-acting) and P+ in oil (50 mg/mL P_4 + 3.3 mg/mL estradiol-17β IM); P+ microspheres— 2 week interval of administration

PRECAUTIONS
- Some behavior changes can be dramatic; use caution around mares showing aggressive behavior; consider individual paddock, distance from other mares in estrus, separation from foals, stallions
- Large ovarian tumors develop extensive blood supplies. Intraoperative time can be increased due to time required to properly

ligate vessels supplying the tumor; increases surgical risks

 FOLLOW-UP

PATIENT MONITORING
Routine postoperative care for OVX.

PREVENTION/AVOIDANCE
N/A

POSSIBLE COMPLICATIONS
- Any operative procedure/anesthesia holds potential risk for death
- GCT/GTCT—time from OVX to resumption of estrous cycle activity is influenced by the time of year and length of suppression
  ○ Usually <1–3 years
  ○ Rare cases of permanent suppression
  ○ Rare case of remaining ovary developing into a GCT/GTCT
  ○ A few mares with GTCT will continue to develop follicles and ovulate on the contralateral ovary

EXPECTED COURSE AND PROGNOSIS
Prognosis, Poor
- *Dysgerminoma*—potential for metastasis
  ○ Usually advanced state of disease by the time of diagnosis

Prognosis for Future Reproduction, Good
- *Hematoma*—large size returns nearly to normal over 1–6 months
  ○ Rare hematoma will destroy remaining ovarian tissue secondary to pressure within the ovarian tunic.
  ○ Some mares develop a hematoma on subsequent cycles within a season
- *Persistent follicles*—100% resolution with time and season

Prognosis for Life, Good
- GCT/GTCT
- Abscess
- Cystadenoma
- Teratoma

Recommendation for OVX
- GCT/GTCT—removal of affected gonad for reproductive function to return, prognosis fair to good depending on size of tumor, surgical route, duration of suppression of contralateral ovary
- Cystadenoma—reported testosterone production
- Abscess, teratoma—dysfunctional ovary

 MISCELLANEOUS

ASSOCIATED CONDITIONS
- Dysgerminoma—hypertrophic osteoarthropathy developing secondary to metastatic dysgerminoma
- Behavior changes with GCT/GTCT

AGE-RELATED FACTORS
- Of breeding age
  ○ Hematoma
  ○ Persistent follicles
- Tumors
  ○ No age limitation

SEE ALSO
- Abnormal estrus intervals
- Anestrus
- Ovulation failure
- Pregnancy diagnosis
- Prolonged diestrus

ABBREVIATIONS
- AMH = anti-Müllerian hormone
- CH = corpus haemorrhagicum
- FSH = follicle-stimulating hormone
- GCT = granulosa cell tumor
- GnRH = gonadotropin releasing hormone
- GTCT = granulosa–theca cell tumor
- hCG = human chorionic gonadotropin
- LH = luteinizing hormone
- LOS = large ovary syndrome
- OVX = ovariectomy
- P_4 = progesterone
- PGF = prostaglandin F (natural prostaglandin)
- TRP = transrectal palpation
- US = ultrasonography, ultrasound

Author Carla L. Carleton
Consulting Editor Carla L. Carleton

L

LARYNGEAL HEMIPARESIS/HEMIPLEGIA (RECURRENT LARYNGEAL NEUROPATHY)

BASICS

DEFINITION
- This disease is a result of neuropathy of the recurrent laryngeal nerve
- Failure of an anatomically normal left (rarely right) arytenoid cartilage to abduct fully during inspiration results in inspiratory respiratory obstruction
- Genomic analysis establishes a correlation between growth and laryngeal neuropathy in Thoroughbreds

PATHOPHYSIOLOGY
- Although trauma to the left recurrent laryngeal nerve can produce the clinical condition, in most cases the underlying pathologic basis is a bilateral mononeuropathy characterized by distal loss of large myelinated fibers (i.e. distal axonopathy) predominantly in the left recurrent laryngeal nerves
- The right recurrent laryngeal nerve is also affected histologically. Lesions in the right nerves are far less severe, however, and clinical signs rarely, if ever, are associated with these abnormalities
- The peripheral neuropathy is progressive and accompanied by attempts at axonal regeneration such that both axonal degeneration and regeneration are observed histologically with their respective lesions in the laryngeal muscles
- The loss of abductory function associated with neurogenic atrophy of the CAD muscle causes the clinical signs. Impaired CAD function leads to inability of the left arytenoid cartilage to abduct and to (in a sustained way) resist pressure swings in the upper airway during exercise. As a result, negative pressure during inspiration leads to adduction of the left arytenoid cartilage, which obstructs the airway, leading to inspiratory stridor and diminished airflow during inspiration

SYSTEMS AFFECTED
Respiratory—upper respiratory tract.

GENETICS
Evidence beyond the tendency to have tall offspring suggests this is an inheritable defect. Genetic analysis is mixed—there is an association with height and RLN in Thoroughbreds and a protective haplotype in Warmbloods.

INCIDENCE/PREVALENCE
- Worldwide in horses
- Rarely affects ponies

GEOGRAPHIC DISTRIBUTION
Worldwide

SIGNALMENT
- Tall male horses, particularly Thoroughbreds, Warmbloods, and draft horses, are more commonly affected
- Approximately 5% (range 1.8–9.5%) of Thoroughbreds and up to 42% of draft breeds

are affected; far less common in Standardbreds and almost nonexistent in ponies
- In Thoroughbreds, the incidence is reported to increase from 6.5% in 2-year-old horses to 9.5% in 6-year-olds

SIGNS
- Horses are presented for upper respiratory noise, exercise intolerance, or both
- Laryngeal collapse significantly interferes with ventilation in horses that perform at high speed.
- In show horses, abnormal upper respiratory noise is the main owner concern

CAUSES
- Most commonly RLN of unknown cause
- Genetic predisposition correlated with height
- Any peripheral or central neural damage/neuropathy affecting the left (or right) recurrent laryngeal nerve can result in laryngeal hemiparesis/hemiplegia
- Viral neuritis
- Intoxications (e.g. organophosphate, lead) may cause bilateral paresis of the laryngeal nerves

RISK FACTORS
- Perivenous injection—look for damage to vagosympathetic trunk (e.g. Horner syndrome)
- Cervical trauma
- Surgical procedures near the left recurrent nerve

DIAGNOSIS

DIFFERENTIAL DIAGNOSIS
- Arytenoid chondritis
- Laryngeal collapse not associated with RLN
- Arytenoid subluxation
- Fourth branchial arch defect—be alert for congenital malformation of the muscular process of the arytenoid cartilage and/or of the thyroid lamina and/or cricoid cartilage in right-sided paresis/paralysis

CBC/BIOCHEMISTRY/URINALYSIS
Of no value.

OTHER LABORATORY TESTS
Arterial blood gases during exercise, with which hypoventilation can be evaluated—in affected horses at maximal exercise, $PaCO_2$ can be >55 mmHg and PaO_2 can be <65 mmHg.

IMAGING
- External laryngeal US allows identification of the increase in echogenicity and change in muscle fiber pattern in the ipsilateral CAL and vocalis muscle compared with the contralateral side
- Esophageal US, CT, and MRI yield various measurements of the geometry of the CAD muscle which have been shown to correlate

with presence or absence of laryngeal collapse at exercise

OTHER DIAGNOSTIC PROCEDURES
Videoendoscopy at Rest (see the Havemeyer Laryngeal Grade)
- The larynx is evaluated for morphologic abnormality and is "graded" based on its resting endoscopy in unsedated horses
- Statistically, horses with laryngeal grade I (complete and symmetrical abduction) and II (complete but asymmetrical abduction) are generally normal at exercise while most (but not all) horses with laryngeal grade III (incomplete or unstained abduction) have some form of collapse at exercise. Virtually all horses with grade IV (no significant abduction) have dynamic arytenoid collapse at exercise
- On external palpation, the left CAD muscle may be atrophied compared with the right

Examination at Exercise (Gold Standard)
- Endoscopy at exercise is the most accurate and precise test to identify and determine the degree of laryngeal collapse as well as recognizing additional structural collapse such as right aryepiglottic fold and right focal fold
- Arterial blood gases during exercise, with which hypoventilation can be evaluated

PATHOLOGIC FINDINGS
Gross
- Atrophy of the left CAL usually is most severe and is best detected by laryngeal US
- Atrophy of the CAD is most obvious clinically and can be estimated by manual palpation of the dorsal aspect of the cricoid and muscular process of the arytenoid cartilage

Histopathologic
- Distal loss of large, myelinated fibers in the left (and to a much less degree in the right) recurrent laryngeal nerves
- Left intrinsic laryngeal muscles exhibit angular fiber atrophy and fiber-type grouping (far milder lesion on the right)

TREATMENT

AIMS
- Reduce or eliminate abnormal upper respiratory sound associated with the collapsed vocal cord and resulting dilated ventricle
- Improve airway patency by preventing collapse (adduction) of the arytenoid cartilage during inhalation and by dynamically (i.e. nerve transplant) or fixed (i.e. laryngoplasty) increasing the cross-sectional diameter of the larynx by abduction of the arytenoid cartilage

APPROPRIATE HEALTH CARE
N/A

NURSING CARE
N/A

(CONTINUED) LARYNGEAL HEMIPARESIS/HEMIPLEGIA (RECURRENT LARYNGEAL NEUROPATHY)

ACTIVITY
N/A

CLIENT EDUCATION
Unless a traumatic or iatrogenic cause is identified, clients should be informed of the possible genetic basis for this disease and that breeding to affected horses may not be indicated.

SURGICAL CONSIDERATIONS
• Treatment is not necessary if exercise intolerance is not present and owners are willing to tolerate the upper respiratory noise
• Placement of a laryngeal prosthesis that fixes the left arytenoid cartilage in near-maximal abduction coupled with cordectomy or ventriculocordectomy is the treatment of choice in horses used for strenuous athletic activities. Chronic coughing during eating is seen in as many as 10–20% of horses after this surgery
• Unilateral or bilateral ventriculocordectomy is superior to laryngoplasty in reducing or eliminating the abnormal upper respiratory noise associated with this condition
• Unilateral or bilateral ventriculocordectomy can improve exercise tolerance in selected horses with laryngeal grade III, in which arytenoid abduction is adequate yet vocal cord collapse is present, and in sport horses where the exercise is less intense
• Laryngeal reinnervation of the CAD muscle by nerve implantation

MEDICATIONS

DRUG(S) OF CHOICE
None, other than routine, perioperative antimicrobial and anti-inflammatory agents.

CONTRAINDICATIONS
N/A

PRECAUTIONS
N/A

POSSIBLE INTERACTIONS
N/A

ALTERNATIVE DRUGS
N/A

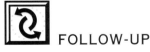

FOLLOW-UP

PATIENT MONITORING
• Upper airway endoscopy is required 4–6 weeks after surgery to monitor response to

fixed abduction surgery (laryngoplasty), and by dynamic endoscopy for laryngeal reinnervation at ~6 months
• Determining the final response to treatment or monitoring of affected horses is made on the basis of evaluating exercise tolerance and upper respiratory noise

PREVENTION/AVOIDANCE
N/A

POSSIBLE COMPLICATIONS
Horses undergoing laryngeal prosthesis may experience chronic coughing and, rarely, aspiration pneumonia.

EXPECTED COURSE AND PROGNOSIS
• Laryngeal hemiplegia—horses with grade IV will not exhibit any further deterioration of athletic activity or upper respiratory noise
• Laryngeal hemiparesis—horses with a varying degree of collapse may exhibit further deterioration of athletic activity or upper respiratory noise

MISCELLANEOUS

ASSOCIATED CONDITIONS
Untreated horses may be predisposed to exercise-induced pulmonary hemorrhage if submitted to strenuous exercise. In addition, it is likely that untreated horses are distressed or are at risk of orthopedic injury because of the marked hypoxia associated with this condition during intense exercise.

AGE-RELATED FACTORS
N/A

ZOONOTIC POTENTIAL
N/A

PREGNANCY/FERTILITY/BREEDING
N/A

SEE ALSO
• Dynamic collapse of the upper airways
• Exercise-induced pulmonary hemorrhage (EIPH)

ABBREVIATIONS
• CAD = dorsal cricoarytenoid muscle
• CAL = lateral cricoarytenoid muscle
• CT = computed tomography
• MRI = magnetic resonance imaging
• $PaCO_2$ = partial pressure of carbon dioxide in arterial blood
• PaO_2 = partial pressure of oxygen in arterial blood
• RLN = recurrent laryngeal neuropathy
• US = ultrasonography, ultrasound

Suggested Reading
Barakzai SZ, Dixon PM. Correlation of resting and exercising endoscopic findings for horses with dynamic laryngeal collapse and palatal dysfunction. Equine Vet J 2011;43:18–23.
Boyko AR, Brooks SA, Behan-Braman A, et al. Genomic analysis establishes correlation between growth and laryngeal neuropathy in Thoroughbreds. BMC Genomics 2014;15:259–267.
Brown DL, Derksen FJ, Stick JA, et al. Ventriculocordectomy reduces respiratory noise in horses with laryngeal hemiplegia. Equine Vet J 2003;35:570–574.
Chalmers HJ, Cheetham J, Yeager AE, Ducharme NG. Ultrasonography of the equine larynx. Vet Radiol Ultrasound 2006;47:476–481.
Duncan ID, Griffith IR, Madrid RE. A light and electron microscopic study of the neuropathy of equine idiopathic laryngeal hemiplegia. Neuropathol Appl Neurobiol 1978;4:483–501.
Robinson NE. Consensus statements on equine recurrent laryngeal neuropathy: conclusions of the Havemeyer Workshop. Equine Vet Educ 2004;16:333–336.
Shappel KK, Derksen FJ, Stick JA, Robinson NE. Effects of ventriculectomy, prosthetic laryngoplasty, and exercise on upper airway function in horses with induced left laryngeal hemiplegia. Am J Vet Res 1988;49:1760–1766.
Taylor SE, Barakzai SZ, Dixon P. Ventriculocordectomy as the sole treatment for recurrent laryngeal neuropathy: long-term results from ninety-two horses. Vet Surg 2006;35:653–657.

Author Norm G. Ducharme
Consulting Editors Daniel Jean and Mathilde Leclère
Acknowledgment The author and editors acknowledge the prior contribution of Richard P. Hackett.

L

LAVENDER FOAL SYNDROME

BASICS

OVERVIEW
LFS, or coat color dilution lethal, is a tetanic neurologic syndrome of neonatal foals of Egyptian Arabian breeding. The disease is rare and the outcome is uniformly fatal in affected individuals. The disease is genetic and appears to have an autosomal recessive mode of inheritance.

SIGNALMENT
• LFS affects neonatal Arabian foals of pure Egyptian lineage, with clinical signs of disease noted immediately after birth
• Cases involving other breeds have not been reported, and there is no apparent sex predilection

SIGNS
• Persistent seizure-like activity with pronounced extensor rigidity, opisthotonos, and frequent paddling
• Apparent blindness
• Failure to stand
• Preserved, often strong, suckle reflex
• Dilute coat color, classically silver-gray "lavender," but may also be dilute chestnut or pale slate gray
• Affected foals are not always of "lavender" coloration

CAUSES AND RISK FACTORS
A genetic basis has been documented with an autosomal recessive mode of inheritance. A single point mutation in the myosin Va gene has been associated with the condition.

DIAGNOSIS

DIFFERENTIAL DIAGNOSIS
• Neonatal maladjustment syndrome
• Neonatal septicemia
• Idiopathic epilepsy of Arabian foals—also noted in Arabian foals of Egyptian breeding, but affected foals are normal at birth and between episodes, and may "outgrow" the seizure disorder by 12–18 months of age
• Occipitoatlantoaxial malformation—also noted more commonly in Arabian foals. Palpation and diagnostic imaging (radiography) confirm this diagnosis
• Hydrocephalus—seizures are characteristic, and affected foals often display visible doming of the skull

CBC/BIOCHEMISTRY/URINALYSIS
The CBC is typically unremarkable, unless septicemia develops. Serum biochemistry analysis is usually normal, but it may display evidence that the foal has not nursed its dam or received colostrum (hypoproteinemia, hypoglobulinemia, hypogammaglobulinemia, and hypoglycemia).

OTHER LABORATORY TESTS
• Definitive diagnosis can be achieved through genetic testing of affected foals
• Serum/plasma immunoglobulin G will be low if there has been inadequate ingestion of colostrum

IMAGING
Skull and cervical spinal radiography may be performed to rule out congenital bony malformations in these regions, but imaging is not useful for supporting a diagnosis of LFS.

OTHER DIAGNOSTIC PROCEDURES
Histopathologic analysis of skin biopsy specimens may reveal melanin clumping and follicular dysplasia in affected individuals.

PATHOLOGIC FINDINGS
No gross or histologic lesions of the central nervous system have been noted during postmortem examination of affected foals. Evidence of self-trauma inflicted during paddling and changes associated with recumbency (dependent pulmonary atelectasis, decubital ulceration) are often the only gross postmortem findings. Melanin clumping in the dermal follicular bulbs and hair shafts may be noted histologically.

TREATMENT
Affected foals may be referred to a tertiary care facility for evaluation and treatment for neonatal maladjustment syndrome or sepsis. Failure to respond to conventional treatment for these diseases, as well as the characteristic signalment and appearance of these foals, is often sufficiently diagnostic. There is no treatment for LFS, and the prognosis is hopeless for affected individuals.

MEDICATIONS

DRUG(S) OF CHOICE
N/A

CONTRAINDICATIONS/POSSIBLE INTERACTIONS
N/A

FOLLOW-UP

PATIENT MONITORING
A lack of response to treatment and recognition of the likely diagnosis based on breed and color should prompt euthanasia in most cases. Genetic testing can confirm the diagnosis antemortem.

PREVENTION/AVOIDANCE
Based on the known genetic nature and mode of inheritance of the disorder, it is recommended that genetic testing of Egyptian Arabian breeding stock be performed and carriers removed from breeding programs in an attempt to prevent the disease.

EXPECTED COURSE AND PROGNOSIS
Affected foals do not recover and invariably die or are euthanized in the hours or days following birth.

MISCELLANEOUS

ASSOCIATED CONDITIONS
Mares and stallions that have produced affected foals have also produced foals with juvenile epilepsy. The relationship, if any, between these 2 syndromes is not clear, but they do not appear to occur concurrently.

SEE ALSO
• Seizures in foals
• Septicemia, neonate

ABBREVIATIONS
LFS = lavender foal syndrome

Suggested Reading
Brooks SA, Gabreski N, Miller D, et al. Whole-genome SNP association in the horse: identification of a deletion in myosin Va responsible for lavender foal syndrome. PLoS Genet 2010;6(4):e1000909.
Page P, Parker R, Harper C, et al. Clinical, clinicopathologic, postmortem examination findings and familial history of 3 Arabians with lavender foal syndrome. J Vet Intern Med 2006;20:1491–1494.

Author Teresa A. Burns
Consulting Editor Margaret C. Mudge

LAWSONIA INTRACELLULARIS INFECTIONS IN FOALS

BASICS

OVERVIEW
PE is a transmissible enteric disease caused by *Lawsonia intracellularis*, an obligate intracellular Gram-negative bacterium. It affects a number of animal species and has a worldwide distribution. A fecal–oral transmission and spread via drinking water and food are suspected. The incubation period of the disease is believed to be 2–3 weeks in foals. Isolated cases are most common but outbreaks do occur.

SIGNALMENT
• Foals 4–7 months of age are most susceptible, although it may also affect young adults
• No breed predisposition, but colts are possibly more commonly affected

SIGNS
• May be asymptomatic and self-limiting
• Growth retardation, lethargy, fever, anorexia, weight loss, ventral edema, diarrhea, and colic are common. Concomitant conditions such as upper or lower respiratory tract infection, intestinal parasitism, gastric ulcers, and dermatitis are common in severely affected foals

CAUSES AND RISK FACTORS
Weaning is a predisposing factor.

DIAGNOSIS

DIFFERENTIAL DIAGNOSIS
• Parasitism, gastroduodenal ulcers, sand impaction, acute intestinal obstruction, infiltrative bowel disease including neoplasia (lymphoma), eosinophilic gastroenteritis, and intoxication with plants and chemicals, including pharmacologic agents such as NSAIDs
• Infectious diarrhea caused by *Salmonella* spp., *Rhodococcus equi*, *Clostridium* spp., *Neorickettsia risticii*, *Campylobacter jejuni*, and rotavirus

CBC/BIOCHEMISTRY/URINALYSIS
• Hypoproteinemia/hypoalbuminemia
• Occasionally, leukocytosis, neutrophilia, hyperfibrinogenemia, increased creatine kinase, hypocalcemia, hyponatremia, azotemia, and anemia

OTHER LABORATORY TESTS
• Serology using immunofluorescence may help confirm exposure to the bacteria. Serology may be positive when the clinical signs are first detected, and foals may remain seropositive for more than 6 months
• Positive PCR on feces will confirm the presence of *L. intracellularis* in the intestine. However, fecal excretion of *L. intracellularis* detected by PCR ends soon (<4 days) after the beginning of an effective antimicrobial administration. Positive PCR on feces may be present in horses of all ages without EPE
• *L. intracellularis* does not grow on conventional bacteriologic media

IMAGING
Abdominal ultrasonography often reveals thickening of segments of the small intestinal wall.

OTHER DIAGNOSTIC PROCEDURES
N/A

PATHOLOGIC FINDINGS
• Marked thickening of the small intestinal mucosa, giving its surface an irregular and corrugated appearance
• Thickened mucosa and severe hyperplasia of crypt epithelium
• Silver-stained sections reveal numerous short and slightly curved bacterial rods in the apical cytoplasm of the immature epithelial cells.
• Diagnosis is confirmed by immunohistochemistry
• Ulcerative and necro-hemorrhagic enteritis may also be observed

TREATMENT
• Less severely affected foals may be treated as outpatients
• Transfusion of fresh or fresh-frozen plasma may be required in foals with severe hypoproteinemia
• Additional symptomatic treatment such as antiulcer therapy, IV crystalloid or colloid fluid therapy, and parenteral feeding are indicated in some cases

MEDICATIONS

DRUG(S) OF CHOICE
• Erythromycin estolate (15–25 mg/kg PO every 8 h), or azithromycin (10 mg/kg PO every 24 h), or clarithromycin (7.5 mg/kg PO every 12 h) alone or combined with rifampin (rifampicin) 10 mg/kg PO every 12–24 h), administered for 2–3 weeks
• Doxycycline (10 mg/kg PO every 12 h) and chloramphenicol (50 mg/kg PO every 6 h) may also be viable options
• Drugs should also target concurrent infections when present

CONTRAINDICATIONS/POSSIBLE INTERACTIONS
Rifampin may decrease the intestinal absorption of clarithromycin.

FOLLOW-UP

PATIENT MONITORING
• A rapid improvement in clinical signs is observed in most foals, following administration of appropriate antimicrobials
• Hypoproteinemia may take up to a month to resolve

PREVENTION/AVOIDANCE
• Passively acquired antibodies do not appear to be protective for EPE
• Environmental contamination by fecal shedding from infected foals is likely to be minimal once antimicrobial treatment is initiated

POSSIBLE COMPLICATIONS
N/A

EXPECTED COURSE AND PROGNOSIS
Prognosis is favorable with therapy unless necrotizing enteritis or severe concurrent medical complications are present.

MISCELLANEOUS

ASSOCIATED CONDITIONS
Marked hypoproteinemia may lead to thromboembolic diseases.

AGE-RELATED FACTORS
Weaning time is a predisposing factor, suggesting that ration changes, mixing, and transportation may contribute to EPE.

ZOONOTIC POTENTIAL
PE is not currently considered to be a zoonosis, although it affects nonhuman primates.

SEE ALSO
• Protein-losing enteropathy (PLE)

ABBREVIATIONS
• EPE = equine proliferative enteropathy
• NSAID = nonsteroidal anti-inflammatory drug
• PCR = polymerase chain reaction
• PE = proliferative enteropathy

Suggested Reading
Pusterla N, Gebhart CJ. Equine proliferative enteropathy—a review of recent developments. Equine Vet J 2013;45:403–409.

Author Jean-Pierre Lavoie
Consulting Editors Henry Stämpfli and Olimpo Oliver-Espinosa

L

LEAD (PB) TOXICOSIS

 BASICS

OVERVIEW
- Pb toxicosis (plumbism) affects the nervous, musculoskeletal, GI, hematopoietic, and renal systems
- Horses are less susceptible to plumbism than cattle or dogs. Lead intoxication in horses is relatively uncommon in the USA
- Acute (rare) and chronic forms result from exposures to Pb-contaminated forages in habitats adjacent to mines and smelters or environments with buildings or fences built prior to 1977 (with Pb pipes) and coated with Pb-based paints
- Ingestion of Pb from Pb-acid batteries, soil contaminated with Pb-containing products, or the ashes of combusted older buildings also poses a risk of Pb intoxication to horses
- Lead binds to sulfhydryl groups and mimics calcium, thereby disrupting heme synthesis, neurotransmission, and vitamin D metabolism

SIGNALMENT
- No breed predilections
- Young, growing foals are most susceptible as they absorb 10–20% of ingested Pb
- Pregnant and lactating mares also have enhanced GI absorption of Pb and transfer Pb to the fetus or neonate

SIGNS
- Peripheral neuropathies including abnormal lip and tongue movements, laryngeal hemiplegia ("roaring") or paralysis, dysphagia, esophageal obstruction ("choke"), aspiration pneumonia
- Anorexia
- Depression
- Weight loss
- Weakness
- Ataxia
- Muscle fasciculations
- Hyperesthesia
- Lameness and swollen joints (young, growing horses or Pb-containing foreign bodies near joint surfaces)
- Colic, diarrhea
- Anemia
- Seizures
- Death

CAUSES AND RISK FACTORS
- Acute exposures to >500–750 mg/kg
- Chronic exposures to 1.7–7 mg/kg/day
- Habitats near smelting or mining operations
- Housing in or around barns or fences built prior to 1977 that contain Pb-lined pipes and/or walls painted with Pb-based paints
- Premises contaminated with Pb-containing batteries, shot, solder, gasoline, oil, or ashes of combusted older buildings
- Diets deficient in calcium, zinc, iron, or vitamin D
- Trauma from Pb-containing objects

 DIAGNOSIS

DIFFERENTIAL DIAGNOSIS
- Laryngeal hemiplegia or paralysis ("roaring"), esophageal obstruction ("choke"), and EIPH not associated with plumbism—physical examination, endoscopy, radiography, no identified sources of Pb exposure, history of trauma
- Rabies and other viral encephalitides
- Equine motor neuron disease and equine degenerative myeloencephalopathy
- Fumonisin B_1 intoxication ("moldy corn poisoning" or equine leukoencephalomalacia)
- Botulism
- Intoxications by *Centaurea* sp.
- Arsenic toxicosis

CBC/BIOCHEMISTRY/URINALYSIS
- Anemia
- Nucleated red blood cells
- Basophilic stippling and Howell–Jolly bodies
- Proteinuria (uncommon)

OTHER LABORATORY TESTS
- Antemortem—whole-blood concentrations of Pb >0.35 ppm in the presence of appropriate clinical signs, alterations in erythrocyte ALAD activity (decreased), zinc protoporphyrin concentrations (increased), and increased urinary excretion of coproporphyrin and uroporphyrins (ALAD and porphyrin analyses not performed in many veterinary diagnostic laboratories)
- Postmortem—concentrations of Pb in liver or kidney >10 ppm on a wet-weight basis (>5 ppm in chronic cases), bone concentrations of Pb >40 ppm on a dry-matter basis in chronic cases

IMAGING
- Radiography to detect Pb-containing objects in the GI tract of small foals or around joints
- Radiographic visualization of "Pb lines" at epiphyseal plates of long bones in young, growing horses

OTHER DIAGNOSTIC PROCEDURES
- Endoscopy to diagnose laryngeal hemiplegia or to visualize Pb-containing foreign bodies in the stomach
- Measurement of 24 h urinary excretion of Pb following chelation therapy (logistically challenging)

PATHOLOGIC FINDINGS
- Gross—inconsistent gross pathologic changes in horses, aspiration pneumonia, and emaciation in chronic cases
- Histologic—peripheral neuropathy with segmental degeneration of axons and myelin in distal motor fibers, pulmonary changes consistent with aspiration pneumonia, reports of renal tubular disease in chronic cases

 TREATMENT

- Prevent further Pb exposure
- Administer sulfate-containing cathartics to bind Pb in GI tract (decrease absorption) and to increase elimination of Pb
- Enhance urinary Pb excretion with chelation
- Control pain and hyperexcitability
- Treat aspiration pneumonia with appropriate antibiotics and NSAIDs
- Provide supportive care for dehydration, circulatory shock, and dysphagia

 MEDICATIONS

DRUG(S) OF CHOICE
- Sodium or magnesium sulfate administered by nasogastric tube (250–500 mg/kg)
- Dimercaprol (British anti-Lewisite) to chelate intracellular and extracellular Pb at a dimercaprol loading dose of 4–5 mg/kg given by deep IM injection, followed by 2–3 mg/kg every 4 h for 24 h and then 1 mg/kg every 4 h for 2 days; adverse reactions include tremors, convulsions, and coma
- Ca-EDTA to chelate Pb at a dosage of 75 mg/kg/day divided into 2 or 3 equal treatments and administered for 5 days by slow IV infusion as a 6.6% solution in normal saline or 5% dextrose (1.1 mL of 6.6% EDTA solution/kg); if deemed necessary, retreatment with Ca-EDTA after a 2 day "rest"; adverse effects include depletion of zinc and essential electrolytes
- In cattle, thiamine hydrochloride at dosages of 2–10 mg/kg twice daily IM for 2 weeks is used; but dosage and efficacy not clearly established in horses
- Flunixin meglumine at 0.55–1.1 mg/kg IV every 12–24 h and/or butorphanol tartrate at 0.02–0.1 mg/kg IV every 3–4 h up to 48 h for abdominal discomfort
- Xylazine hydrochloride at 0.3–1.1 mg/kg IV alone (higher dosage) or with butorphanol at 0.01–0.02 mg/kg IV (lower dosage of xylazine) for sedation or control of severe pain
- Diazepam administered to adults (25–50 mg IV) or foals (0.05–0.4 mg/kg IV) for hyperesthesia, muscle tremors, and seizures (can repeat in 30 min)
- Appropriate fluid therapy as necessary

CONTRAINDICATIONS/POSSIBLE INTERACTIONS
- Chelators may deplete essential cations and electrolytes
- Sedatives in ataxic horses
- Cautious use of NSAIDs in GI and renal disease or dimercaprol if renal disease is present

FOLLOW-UP
• Identification and removal of Pb source
• Proper disposal of or limited access to Pb sources
• Recheck Pb concentration in whole blood 2 weeks after final chelation dose; repeat chelation if >0.35 ppm
• Monitor serum electrolytes and supplement as needed
• Provide supportive treatment as needed

PATIENT MONITORING
• Monitor hemogram and whole-blood Pb concentrations
• Periodic neurologic assessments

PREVENTION/AVOIDANCE
• Prevent exposure to habitats near smelters or mines
• Avoid use of Pb-containing paints
• Clean up Pb-contaminated pastures, paddocks, or soil

POSSIBLE COMPLICATIONS
• Aspiration pneumonia
• Concurrent exposure to other toxic metals

EXPECTED COURSE AND PROGNOSIS
Long-term neurologic deficits possible following removal from Pb source and partial recovery of neurologic function.

MISCELLANEOUS
ASSOCIATED CONDITIONS
• Other metal intoxications
• Laryngeal hemiplegia
• EIPH
• Esophageal obstruction

AGE-RELATED FACTORS
Young, growing horses.

ZOONOTIC POTENTIAL
N/A

PUBLIC HEALTH IMPORTANCE
Appropriate regulatory agencies should be notified of Pb-contaminated matrices that could potentially poison children, e.g. soil or water.

PREGNANCY/FERTILITY/BREEDING
Lead can cross the placenta and, potentially, have adverse effects on the fetus.

ABBREVIATIONS
• ALAD = D-aminolevulinic acid dehydratase
• Ca-EDTA = calcium disodium ethylenediaminetetraacetic acid
• EIPH = exercise-induced pulmonary hemorrhage
• GI = gastrointestinal
• NSAID = non-steroidal anti-inflammatory drug

Suggested Reading
Casteel SW. Metal toxicosis in horses. Vet Clin North Am Equine Pract 2001;17:517–527.
Gwaltney-Brant S. Lead. In: Plumlee KH, ed. Clinical Veterinary Toxicology. St. Louis, MO: Mosby, 2004:204–210.
Kruger K, Saulez MN, Nesser JA, Soldberg K. Acute lead intoxication in a pregnant mare. J S Afr Vet Assoc 2008;79(1):50–53.

Author Tim J. Evans
Consulting Editors Wilson K. Rumbeiha and Steve Ensley

LEARNING, TRAINING, AND BEHAVIOR PROBLEMS

 BASICS

DEFINITION
- Learning influences everything a horse does throughout its life. It is a consequence of the animal's experience with the environment and is one of the basic mechanisms of survival
- *Behavior modification* is the analysis and treatment of undesirable behavior using learning principles
- *Training* describes the process of teaching an animal to perform a new behavior or exhibit a species-typical behavior in designated circumstances
- Parallel and overlapping terminology have evolved within diverse groups of people in applied behavioral professions
- Training and behavior modification often require a delicate balance of modifying a specific segment in a sequence of behaviors without interfering with desirable components of a behavior pattern and without introducing new problems
- Familiarity with species-typical behaviors and principles of learning are fundamental to recognizing when a behavior is affected by pathophysiologic states, experience, or learning

PATHOPHYSIOLOGY
- Pain, anxiety, and fear are common causes of handling, training, and other behavioral problems
- Undesirable, learned behaviors may persist after medical or environmental etiologies are corrected
- Numerous physiologic states and pathologies can affect learning:
  - Chronic back pain and vision problems are often unrecognized in the riding horse
  - Endocrine states can affect temperament, motivation, and species-typical behaviors, which in turn can result in training and behavior problems

SYSTEMS AFFECTED
Fear, anxiety, and pain can affect almost all physiologic and behavior systems.

GENETICS
- Learned behaviors are genetically constrained by temperament, intelligence, and physical ability to perform specific behaviors. A practical way to gauge the influence of genetics on the behavior of an individual is to determine if closely related individuals (under different management) exhibit the same problems
- Often training problems stem from owners' unrealistic expectations of what a horse is capable

INCIDENCE/PREVALENCE
Unknown

GEOGRAPHIC DISTRIBUTION
Regional training practices may influence the type and frequency of specific training and learning problems.

SIGNALMENT

Breed Predilections
Breeds vary in temperament and physical abilities, which can influence performance and learning.

Mean Age and Range
Any age.

Predominant Sex
Intact males may pose more problems for handlers and thereby result in more training problems.

SIGNS

General Comments
- Behavioral signs may be similar whether the cause is pathophysiologic, learned, or a species-typical behavior. See chapter Fear
- Analysis of training and learning problems requires excellent observational skills and understanding of principles of learning
- Observation by the clinician is usually necessary. Sometimes the horse will exhibit the behavior when brought to the clinician. Audio/visual recordings can be helpful. Often a personal visit to where the horse exhibits the behavior is required. Observation of the horse's environment can provide details the owner has overlooked or when filming

Historical Findings
- Objective, detailed descriptions and history of development of the problem
- History of punitive training techniques or traumatic incidents
- Expectations of owners, handlers, and trainers

Physical Examination Findings
- Signs indicative of pain or fear
- Evidence of trauma
- Be aware that an aroused animal can override physical signs of pain
- Observe in a different environment or circumstances, e.g. different handler, rider, tack, location. This may help determine if the problem is related to the environment as opposed to a medical problem

CAUSES
- Normal, species-typical behaviors that interfere with management or training, such as defensive responses, play, social behaviors (e.g. greeting behaviors, separation distress responses, courtship behaviors, intermale aggression/displays)
- Fear
- Pain
- Common problematic training and handling techniques are inconsistent use of signals/cues, inadvertently rewarding unwanted behaviors, and/or inappropriate use of aversive stimuli

RISK FACTORS
- Trainers, handlers, or riders with poor psychomotor skills
- Personnel who base their training/handling philosophies on "showing the horse who is dominant" or believe that horses "are trying to get away with something or are willfully disobedient." People with such beliefs are less likely to analyze situations critically for the precise stimuli and conditions that cause undesirable behaviors and are more likely to be punitive
- Addressing learning and training problems requires the cooperation of open-minded, competent, and flexible rider/trainer/owners
- Sometimes it is not possible for a horse to perform specific tasks at the level an owner expects. Such a mismatch can lead to welfare problems for the horse and frustration for the owner
- Young animals are especially susceptible to experiences. Isolation, barren environments, and lack of exposure to novel environments and novel stimuli can affect the development of nervous and endocrine systems. In turn, these changes affect the animal's subsequent responses to the environment and learning processes

 DIAGNOSIS

DIFFERENTIAL DIAGNOSIS
- Identification of precise stimuli and conditions associated with behavior problems. If necessary, brief exposure to the stimulus or reduced intensity of the stimulus can confirm the eliciting stimuli
- If unwanted behaviors arise only during training sessions, the entire process should be carefully examined. If the methods adhere to sound principles of learning and the horse is not subject to abusive techniques, pathophysiologic conditions are more likely
- Pathophysiologic conditions can exist concurrently and independently with inappropriate training and riding techniques

CBC/BIOCHEMISTRY/URINALYSIS
Usually normal. Dependent on presenting signs.

OTHER LABORATORY TESTS
Dependent on presenting signs; may be indicated to rule out medical conditions.

IMAGING
See Other Laboratory Tests.

OTHER DIAGNOSTIC PROCEDURES
See Other Laboratory Tests.

PATHOLOGIC FINDINGS
Dependent on the problem.

L

TREATMENT

AIMS
• Identify and treat physical problems
• Recognize species-typical behaviors and implement management to alleviate, minimize, or accommodate these behaviors
• Realize that after physical problems are successfully treated and management/environmental conditions are changed, behavior problems may persist and still need to be addressed
• Treat or refer to an appropriate expert for treatment of learned aspects of the problems
• Educate, refer, or supply sources of information to owners, handlers, and trainers

PRINCIPLES OF LEARNING
• Even if a clinician does not assume responsibility for treating a behavior problem, knowledge of learning principles is helpful in making a differential diagnosis, assisting the owner, and assessing referral experts
• Animals learn in many ways. Learning can occur as a consequence of exposure to environmental situations or by direct interaction with stimuli in the environment. It may not be immediately apparent by the animal's behavior that it has learned something
• *Conditioning* refers to learning associations between stimuli or between a stimulus and a response. Conditioning processes allow the horse to anticipate, predict, and/or prepare for subsequent stimuli. Conditioning also provides the horse with responses for coping with the occurrence of specific stimuli
• Operant or instrumental conditioning is a process by which the frequency of a behavior is modified by the consequence of the animal's response to a stimulus
• Positive reinforcers increase the probability that an animal will repeat a behavior
• Behaviors acquired by intermittent positive reinforcement may persist for a prolonged time after reinforcement stops
• When positive reinforcement of unwanted behaviors stops, the behaviors may temporarily increase in intensity and/or frequency
• Negative reinforcers also increase the occurrence of behaviors. Horses perform behaviors to avoid or escape aversive stimuli. Horses learn to avoid aversive stimuli by throwing their heads back, bucking, fleeing, and engaging in other evasive maneuvers. To avoid detrimental consequences training aids must be of appropriate intensity and applied appropriately
• Successful escape and avoidance of aversive stimuli are highly reinforcing and difficult to extinguish by simply ceasing the aversive reinforcer. A counterconditioning program is usually necessary

• Punishment is the use of aversive stimuli to stop *and* reduce/prevent the future occurrence of a behavior. Considerable judgment and timing are required to appropriately implement punishment. A correctly used punisher (the aversive stimulus) should be of high enough intensity to interrupt a behavior but not so high as to cause side effects—such as anxiety, fear, and aggression. It should be applied immediately at the onset of the behavior and used every time the unwanted behavior is initiated. It helps many people to think of punishing the behavior, not punishing the horse. An effective punisher should work within a few applications. Attempts to use an aversive stimulus as a punisher without adhering to these guidelines are, at best, harassment and, at worse, abuse
• Aversive stimuli *always* carry the potential of inducing anxiety, fear, and defensive aggression. Even if an aversive stimulus achieves a specific result, the horse may also acquire detrimental behaviors as a consequence. Aversive stimuli are almost always contraindicated if fear is a component of an undesirable behavior
• The success of "natural horsemanship" and "positive training" techniques attest to the value of nonpunitive and positive reinforcement techniques in training and management of horses

APPROPRIATE HEALTH CARE
Adequate exercise and social interactions are integral parts of maintaining physical and mental health.

ACTIVITY
Meet the species-typical behavioral needs of the horse, e.g. exercise, opportunity to play, social contact, time spent foraging/grazing/chewing.

DIET
Investigation of the role of diet in learning and behavior is continuously ongoing.

CLIENT EDUCATION
Educate, refer, or supply sources of information regarding learning principles and normal behaviors of the horse.

SURGICAL CONSIDERATIONS
Castration or ovariectomy may be indicated.

MEDICATIONS

DRUG(S) OF CHOICE
See chapter Fear, Medications.
No drugs are approved for facilitation of training of horses. One study reported use of a combined analgesic/sedative medication, detomidine, that allowed pain-free therapeutic farriering of difficult horses and eventually safe handling without drug therapy.

CONTRAINDICATIONS
Off-label use of tranquilizers or sedatives may alter the visual perception, balance, proprioception, and musculoskeletal coordination of horses. These effects could be detrimental to horse, handler, bystanders, riders, and drivers.

PRECAUTIONS
Although use of medications may reduce excitability or fear and minimize or suppress unwanted behaviors, there is no guarantee that a horse will learn the desired behaviors while under the influence of the medications. Some medications, such as diazepam, can have animistic properties. Sometimes anxiolytics and tranquilizers, such as benzodiazepines, lower thresholds for aggression.
Owners should always be advised if a drug is being used off-label and what are the possible side effects and contraindications.

ALTERNATIVE DRUGS
• Modipher EQ is a commercially available synthetic pheromone reported to prevent/reduce anxiety and fearful reactions if administered before exposure to the anxiety/fear-eliciting situations
• Synthetic progestins are used off-label to sedate, calm, and lower libido to facilitate training and showing horses. This raises a question of ethics. Synthetic progestins are not disallowed when used to regulate the estrus cycle of performance mares. The drugs, however, are usually banned for use in other performance horses

FOLLOW-UP

PATIENT MONITORING
• Behavior modification programs frequently need to be adjusted
• Veterinarians assuming partial or full responsibility for treatment of a behavior problem should instruct clients to contact them immediately if the behavior gets worse. Otherwise, follow-up contact is recommended by 2 weeks after initiating treatment procedures. Thereafter, frequency of contact depends on the individual problem and treatment
• If medical problems have been ruled out or successfully treated and the horse continues to exhibit the problem behavior, the client should be advised to consult with a person qualified to deal with that specific problem
• If the veterinarian refers the client to a nonveterinarian, it is still beneficial to contact the owner. Signs of a previously subclinical medical problem may become apparent
• Follow-up information is valuable in assessing the success of treatment programs that the owner is using

L

PREVENTION/AVOIDANCE
- Gradually introduce horses to novel environments and new tasks
- Be cognizant of inadvertent reinforcement of unwanted behaviors
- Inappropriate use of aversive stimuli in attempts to change behavior
- Horses that have been successfully treated for fear-based behavior problems should periodically be exposed to the fear-eliciting stimulus to prevent "spontaneous recovery" of the fearful behaviors

POSSIBLE COMPLICATIONS
- Undetected underlying medical cause of the problem
- Persistence of behavior after successful treatment of initial medical cause

EXPECTED COURSE AND PROGNOSIS
Highly variable—dependent on recognition of underlying medical problems, diagnosis of the behavior problem, temperament of the horse, management strategies, and abilities of owner, handler, trainer, and behavior expert.

MISCELLANEOUS
ASSOCIATED CONDITIONS
- Medical problems, especially those causing pain
- Fearful behavior

SEE ALSO
- Fear
- Self-mutilation
- Stallion sexual behavior problems

Suggested Reading

Borchelt PL, Voith VL. Punishment. In: Voith VL, Borchelt PL, eds. Readings in Companion Animal Behavior. Trenton, NJ: Veterinary Learning Systems, 1996:72–80.

Domjan M. The Principles of Learning and Behavior: Active Learning Edition. Belmont, CA: Wadsworth, 2006.

Goolsby HA, Brady HA, Prien DS. The off-label use of altrenogest in stallions: a survey. J Equine Vet Sci 2004;24:72–75.

Mansmann RA, Currie MC, Correa MT, et al. Equine behavior problems round farriery: foot pain in 11 horses. J Equine Sci 2011;31:44–48.

McGreevy P. Equine Behaviour: A Guide for Veterinarians and Equine Scientists, 2e. Philadelphia, PA: WB Saunders, 2012.

Mills DS, McDonnell S. Domestic Horse: The Origins, Development, and Management of its Behaviour. New York, NY: Cambridge University Press, 2005.

Waring GH. Horse Behavior, 2e. Norwich, NY: Noyes Publications/William Andrew Publishing, 2003.

Author Victoria L. Voith
Consulting Editor Victoria L. Voith

LENS OPACITIES/CATARACTS

BASICS

DEFINITION
- The transparency of the lens is made possible by layers of perfectly aligned linear cells or lens fibers
- Disruption of the precise anatomic arrangement of these lens fibers results in opacification or cataract formation of the lens
- The basic mechanism of cataract formation is a decrease in soluble lens proteins, failure of the lens epithelial cell sodium pump, a decrease in lens glutathione, lens fiber swelling, and fiber membrane rupture
- These lens opacities or cataracts can vary in size depending on the number of lens fibers damaged. Very small incipient lens opacities are common and not associated with blindness
- As cataracts develop or mature, they become more opaque, and blindness develops
- Cataracts can be classified by the degree of lens involvement (incipient, immature, mature, hypermature, Morgagnian), lens location (capsular, nuclear, cortical, anterior/posterior) age of onset (congenital, juvenile, senile), and cause of cataract (e.g. inherited, traumatic)

INCIDENCE/PREVALENCE
- 5–7% of horses are reported to have cataracts as a primary ocular disease
- 33.6–35.3% of foals with congenital ocular anomalies are reported to have cataracts

SIGNALMENT
All ages and breeds of horses are at risk for cataract development. Cataracts are a frequent congenital ocular defect in foals.

SIGNS
- Horses manifest varying degrees of blindness as cataracts mature. The tapetal reflection is seen with incipient, immature, and hypermature cataracts but not with mature cataracts. The rate of cataract progression and development of blindness cannot be predicted in most instances
- Blepharospasm and lacrimation may accompany cataracts in horses due to associated ERU or lens-induced uveitis; the latter is seen less commonly in horses than in other species such as dogs
- Assessment of visual function can be made by observation of the horse walking, feeding, and interacting with other horses. Visually impaired horses may demonstrate a reluctance to run or even walk, although some horses with bilateral cataracts appear to do quite well in a familiar environment. Differences in head posture may be associated with cataracts, as a unilaterally blind horse may attempt to keep its sighted eye toward activity in its environment.

CAUSES
- Heritable, traumatic, toxic, nutritional, and postinflammatory etiologies have been proposed
- Congenital cataracts may be associated with other congenital defects such as microphthalmos, aniridia, persistent pupillary membranes, persistent fetal vasculature, colobomas, and anterior segment dysgenesis
- Cataracts secondary to ERU or trauma are frequently seen, while juvenile-onset cataracts are uncommon in horses. True senile cataracts that interfere with vision are found in horses older than 20 years

RISK FACTORS
- Congenital cataracts are reported in Thoroughbreds, Belgian draft horses, and Quarter Horses. Morgan horses can have congenital, nonprogressive, nuclear, bilaterally symmetrical cataracts that do not generally interfere with vision
- Rocky Mountain Horses can develop cataracts in association with multiple congenital ocular anomalies syndrome

DIAGNOSIS

DIFFERENTIAL DIAGNOSIS
- Increased cloudiness of the lens occurs with age and is called nuclear or lenticular sclerosis. It is common in older horses, but vision is clinically normal as nuclear sclerosis does not cause vision loss
- Older horses may develop brunescence in association with lenticular sclerosis, which gives the nucleus of the lens a yellow discoloration
- Lens luxation, fibrin associated with uveitis
- Blindness in horses can also occur secondary to ERU, glaucoma, and retinal disease

CBC/BIOCHEMISTRY/URINALYSIS
CBC, chemistry, and fibrinogen levels are recommended as part of the preoperative evaluation for cataract surgery.

OTHER LABORATORY TESTS
There are no tests currently available to screen for inherited cataracts in horses.

IMAGING
B-scan US is beneficial in assessing the anatomic status of the retina if a cataract is present.

OTHER DIAGNOSTIC PROCEDURES
Afferent pupillary defects in a cataractous eye cannot be attributed to the cataract alone, and normal pupillary light reflexes do not necessarily exclude some degree of retinal or optic nerve disease. ERG is beneficial in assessing the functional status of the retina if a cataract is present.

PATHOLOGIC FINDINGS
Epithelial cell dysplasia/metaplasia, migration of lens epithelial cells along the posterior lens capsule, liquefaction of lens material, Morgagnian globules, and lens fiber swelling is noted.

TREATMENT
- Most veterinary ophthalmologists recommend surgical removal of cataracts in foals <6 months of age if the foal is healthy, no uveitis or other ocular problems are present, and the foal's personality will tolerate aggressive topical therapy. Adult horses with visual impairment due to cataracts are also candidates for surgery
- Therapy for cataracts is necessarily surgical, although some degree of spontaneous cataract resorption may occur with hypermature cataracts. Horses considered for lens extraction should be in good physical condition. Complete ophthalmic and general physical examinations should be performed, and intraocular pressure should be measured. Preoperative CBCs and serum chemistries are important for evaluating systemic organ function
- Any signs of anterior uveitis should delay cataract surgery until the cause of the inflammation is diagnosed and has been successfully treated. Cataract surgery should also be delayed in the presence of active eyelid, conjunctival, or corneal disease
- Phacoemulsification is the recommended surgical technique for equine cataract surgery. Immature, mature, and hypermature cataracts have been successfully removed in horses with this technique
- Intraocular lenses of 18 diopters (D) are recommended in horses

MEDICATIONS

DRUG(S) OF CHOICE
- Subpalpebral lavage placement assists in the delivery of topical medications, particularly in a postoperative patient
- Topically applied corticosteroids, such as prednisolone acetate (1%), are beneficial in treating lens-induced uveitis as well as pre- and postoperative uveitis
- Topically administered NSAIDs, such as flurbiprofen and diclofenac, can be used TID to QID in treating lens-induced uveitis, as well as pre- and postoperative uveitis
- Topically applied 1% atropine is effective in stabilizing the blood–aqueous barrier, minimizing pain from ciliary muscle spasm, and causes pupillary dilation. Atropine may be used as often as every 6 h, with the frequency of administration reduced as soon as the pupil dilates. This can be used pre- and postoperatively as indicated based on the degree of uveitis present

L

LENS OPACITIES/CATARACTS   (CONTINUED)

• Systemically administered NSAIDs, such as flunixin meglumine (1.1 mg/kg IV or PO BID), are effective in reducing anterior uveitis in horses with cataracts, as well as treating postoperative intraocular inflammation
• Broad-spectrum topically applied antibiotics such as neomycin–polymyxin B–gramicidin ophthalmic solutions are used starting the day before surgery, and are continued postoperatively. These are typically administered every 4–6 h
• Systemically administered antibiotics are indicated peri- and postoperatively. Penicillin and gentamicin are typically administered IV perioperatively, followed by trimethoprim–sulfa PO postoperatively

PRECAUTIONS
Horses receiving topical atropine should be monitored for colic.

CONTRAINDICATIONS, POSSIBLE INTERACTIONS
• Cataract surgery is not recommended in any patient that has uncontrolled systemic disease
• Animals with poor retinal function, as determined by preoperative ERG and US, are not candidates for cataract surgery
• Animals with cataracts secondary to controlled ERU may be candidates for cataract surgery; however, horses with ERU may also be at higher risk for postoperative complications, particularly glaucoma

FOLLOW-UP

PATIENT MONITORING
• Horses with cataracts should be monitored for blepharospasm and lacrimation as cataracts can be associated with uveitis
• Blind horses should be monitored in their environment

• Horses that have had cataract surgery should be monitored for signs of ocular discomfort, self-trauma, recurrence of blindness, and colic

PREVENTION/AVOIDANCE
Breeding of horses with cataracts should be avoided.

POSSIBLE COMPLICATIONS
Postoperative complications can include persistent iridocyclitis and plasmoid aqueous, fibropupillary membranes, synechiae, iris bombé, corneal ulceration, corneal edema, posterior capsular opacification, wound leakage, glaucoma, vitreous presentation into anterior chamber, retinal degeneration, retinal detachment, and infectious endophthalmitis. General anesthesia with its attendant risks is required for cataract surgery.

EXPECTED COURSE AND PROGNOSIS
• Surgery is easiest to perform on foals because the globe size is small enough that the standard cataract surgical equipment is of a satisfactory size, general anesthesia is less of a risk in foals, and foals tend to heal quickly following cataract surgery. Early return of vision is paramount in foals for development of the higher visual centers
• Slight corneal edema is usually present from 24 to 72 h postoperatively; 1 week following surgery the pupil should be functional, any fibrin in the anterior chamber resorbing, and the fundus visible; 3 weeks following surgery the eye should be nonpainful, the patient visual, pupillary movement normal, and the ocular medium clear
• Most reliable reports of vision in successful cataract surgery in horses indicate that vision is functionally normal postoperatively. From an optical standpoint, the aphakic eye should be quite far-sighted or hyperopic postoperatively, and was +9.94 D in 1 study. Images close to the eye would be blurry and

appear magnified. Placement of an artificial intraocular lens should improve acuity

MISCELLANEOUS

ASSOCIATED CONDITIONS
• Retinal detachment
• ERU
• Microphthalmos
• Iridal hypoplasia

AGE-RELATED FACTORS
• Foals may present with congenital cataracts
• Older horses may present with senile cataracts

ZOONOTIC POTENTIAL
N/A

PREGNANCY/FERTILITY/BREEDING
N/A

ABBREVIATIONS
• ERG = electroretinography
• ERU = equine recurrent uveitis
• NSAID = nonsteroidal anti-inflammatory drug
• US = ultrasonography, ultrasound

Suggested Reading
Brooks DE. Ophthalmology for the Equine Practitioner, 2e. Jackson, WY: Teton NewMedia, 2008.
Gilger BC. Equine ophthalmology. In: Gelatt KN, Gilger BC, Kern TJ, eds. Veterinary Ophthalmology, 5e. Ames, IA: Wiley Blackwell, 2013:1560–1609.
Gilger BC, ed. Equine Ophthalmology, 3e. Ames, IA: Wiley Blackwell, 2017.

Author Shari M. Greenberg
Consulting Editor Caryn E. Plummer
Acknowledgment The author and editor acknowledge the prior contribution of Dennis E. Brooks.

L

BASICS

DEFINITION
An important waterborne disease caused by pathogenic members of the spirochetal genus *Leptospira*. It is a zoonotic disease that affects a number of species of domestic, peridomestic, and wild animals. Clinical infection in horses is primarily characterized by spontaneous abortions, neonatal disease, and recurrent uveitis. Recent studies suggest that it is widespread but the majority of animals remain asymptomatic.

PATHOPHYSIOLOGY
Animals that are natural reservoirs of *Leptospira*, such as rats and other small wild mammals, clear infections from their bodies but continue to harbor the bacteria in their kidneys. Colonization of the renal proximal tubules of reservoir animals results in shedding of leptospires in the urine. The bacteria can persist for prolonged periods in moist and alkaline environments. Naive animals get the infection when they come in contact with urine from infected animals or urine-contaminated water. Leptospires penetrate mucosal and skin surfaces and result in a bacteremia, followed by invasion of internal organs. Outcome of infection depends on the host's humoral response and the pathogenicity of the infecting serovar. Organisms multiply in organs and release metabolites that, combined with immune-mediated damage, cause the clinical signs associated with the disease. Leptospires evade the immune system in the proximal renal tubules, genital tract, central nervous system, and eyes.

SYSTEMS AFFECTED
- Reproductive—abortion, stillbirth
- Ophthalmic—recurrent uveitis
- Renal/urologic—renal disease and pyuria
- Neonatal disease—hepatic and renal disease, weakness, pulmonary hemorrhage
- Hepatobiliary—liver disease and jaundice

INCIDENCE/PREVALENCE
Recent data suggest that the infection is widespread, with the incidence and infecting serovars varying considerably in different geographic regions.

SIGNALMENT
Nonspecific

SIGNS
- Low-grade fever, listlessness, and anorexia are seen in the milder form of the disease
- Clinical presentation in more severe forms may include conjunctival suffusion, jaundice, anemia, petechial hemorrhages on the mucosa, and general depression
- Signs associated with organ invasion are indicative of the specific organ involved
- Leptospiral abortions occur late in the gestation, typically without any prior clinical signs. In a small number of cases, premature or full-term emaciated and icteric foals are born. Grossly, the placenta is edematous with nodular cystic allantoic masses and necrosis of the chorion
- Chronic disease is associated with recurrent uveitis

Physical Examination Findings
- Reproductive—abortion (usually late gestation), stillbirth, or premature birth or neonatal disease depending on stage of gestation and infection
- Neonatal disease—weakness, icterus, renal failure, hematuria. 1 outbreak also reported respiratory distress, pyrexia, and depression
- Ophthalmic—initially, blepharospasm, excessive tearing, photophobia, chemosis, miosis, aqueous flare, hypopyon, and corneal edema. Chronic sequelae include synechia formation, retinal detachment, chorioretinitis, cataracts, atrophy of corpora nigra, and phthisis bulbi
- Renal/urologic—azotemia, polyuria/polydipsia, pyuria, hematuria, pyrexia
- Hepatobiliary—jaundice, pyrexia, lethargy

CAUSES
- In North America, primarily *Leptospira interrogans* serovar pomona. Serovars grippotyphosa and hardjo are less frequently associated with equine leptospirosis
- In the northern parts of Ireland, the serovar Bratislava is identified most frequently

RISK FACTORS
- Direct transmission with host-to-host contact via infected urine, exposure to postabortion discharge, and aborted fetuses
- Indirect transmission via urine-contaminated water or soil. Skunk and raccoons are maintenance hosts for the major incriminating serovars
- Warm, moist environment; neutral to slightly alkaline soil pH; and a high density of carrier and susceptible animals

DIAGNOSIS

DIFFERENTIAL DIAGNOSIS
Recurrent Uveitis
- *Toxoplasma* spp., *Onchocerca cervicalis*, *Streptococcus* spp., viral agents, ocular trauma
- *Onchocerca* microfilariae and viral inclusion bodies are found in conjunctival scraping and biopsy
- Rising serum titers are associated with *Toxoplasma* spp.

Abortion
- Infectious causes—EHV-1 is differentiated by characteristic histologic lesion of intranuclear eosinophilic inclusion bodies and indirect immunofluorescent tests. Placentitis (bacterial and fungal) is differentiated by gross evidence of placentitis, isolation of organisms from the placenta and fetal organs, especially the stomach. Equine viral arteritis is differentiated by viral isolation from placental and fetal tissues
- Noninfectious causes—placental abnormalities, twinning, twisted umbilical cord, and maternal systemic disease

Renal/Urologic
- Bacterial pyelonephritis is identified by pyuria and the presence of bacteria in the urine
- Hemodynamic renal dysfunction is differentiated by other physical examination findings
- Nephrotoxicity is identified by exposure to a source

Neonatal Disease
- Neonatal isoerythrolysis is associated with hemolytic anemia
- Tyzzer disease is seen in older foals; organisms are seen in the liver with Warthin–Starry stain
- EHV-1 is differentiated from severe leukopenia and pneumonia
- Septicemia is differentiated by other physical examination findings, blood culture, and postmortem specimens

Hepatobiliary
- Hemolytic anemia, fasting, cholelithiasis, neoplasia, hepatic abscess, acute and chronic hepatitis
- Differentiated on ultrasonographic findings, hematology, and serum biochemistry

CBC/BIOCHEMISTRY/URINALYSIS
- Serum biochemistry profile reflects specific organ involvement; leukocytosis, hyperfibrinogenemia
- Urinalysis (if renal involvement) shows red and white blood cells and casts

OTHER LABORATORY TESTS
- Culture and identification of the infecting leptospiral isolate provides unequivocal diagnosis. However, culture of *Leptospira* has limited value due to fastidious growth requirements and length of time required for culture
- PCR-based assays can detect leptospiral DNA in a variety of clinical specimens and have capability of discriminating at the genus level
- For serologic diagnosis, MAT is the most widely used test. In leptospiral abortions, MAT on fetal fluids and maternal sera usually gives a very high titer and is diagnostic
- Leptospires can also be demonstrated in the placenta or fetal kidney by the fluorescent antibody test or silver staining

L

LEPTOSPIROSIS

IMAGING
Ultrasonography may assist in the evaluation of hepatic and renal disease.

PATHOLOGIC FINDINGS
Fetus and neonates—most common findings are icterus, generalized petechial and ecchymotic hemorrhages, and microabscesses of kidneys. Placenta is edematous with a necrotic chorion covered with mucous exudates. Allantoic membrane may contain cystic nodular masses.

TREATMENT

APPROPRIATE HEALTH CARE, NURSING CARE

Reproductive
Aborting mares should be isolated and the area they inhabited disinfected. Contaminated bedding and fetal and placental tissues should be rapidly removed and appropriately disposed. Mares can shed leptospires in urine for up to 4 months post abortion.

Renal/Urologic
Appropriate antimicrobials and supportive care to ensure adequate renal function should be administered.

Neonatal Disease
Appropriate antimicrobials and supportive care should be administered. Foals should be isolated as high numbers of leptospires are shed in urine.

Hepatobiliary
Appropriate antimicrobials and supportive care should be administered.

ACTIVITY
Activity should be restricted to decrease environmental contamination.

CLIENT EDUCATION
The client should be informed as to the zoonotic potential. Infection can occur through contact of mucous membranes or skin lesions with urine or tissue from an infected animal.

MEDICATIONS

DRUG(S) OF CHOICE
• Treatment regimens for horses mostly extrapolated from other species. Streptomycin (10 mg/kg) and/or penicillin (10 000–15 000 IU/kg) are the antibiotics of choice, with tetracyclines as an alternative

• The use of streptomycin in horses is on a decline owing to severe toxic side effects of this antibiotic

Ophthalmic
Therapy is aimed at reducing immune-mediated inflammation and providing mydriasis and analgesia. An intraocular device containing cyclosporine A (ciclosporin), which blocks the transcription of interleukin 2, and pars plana vitrectomy have been shown to be effective in long-term control of the disease. Usefulness of antibiotics in treating the infection is not clear.

Reproductive
If a mare has a high titer of leptospiral antibodies, a high dose of penicillin G (20×10^6 UI, twice daily) is recommended for preventing the intrauterine infection of the fetus.

CONTRAINDICATIONS
N/A

PRECAUTIONS
Avoid use of potentially nephrotoxic drugs if renal disease is suspected.

POSSIBLE INTERACTIONS
N/A

ALTERNATIVE DRUGS
Oxytetracycline (5–10 mg/kg) for 7 days.

FOLLOW-UP

PATIENT MONITORING

Ophthalmic
Recurrent episodes of uveitis.

Reproductive
Therapy should be instituted if fetal membranes are retained or if signs of systemic illness become evident. Monitor in-contact mares' serum titer levels and consider antibiotic therapy of in-contact pregnant mares.

Renal, Urologic, Neonatal Disease, Hepatobiliary
Monitor hepatic and renal function.

PREVENTION/AVOIDANCE
• In North America, a monovalent vaccine has recently been approved for use in broodmares in all 3 trimesters of pregnancy
• Limit access to wet environments, and avoid contamination with other domestic animals and wildlife

• Isolate affected animals, and consider antibiotic therapy for in-contact pregnant mares

POSSIBLE COMPLICATIONS
• Ophthalmic—blindness associated with recurrent uveitis
• Reproductive—abortion outbreak
• Neonatal disease—foals from infected dams may be born with clinical disease

EXPECTED COURSE AND PROGNOSIS
• Ophthalmic—inflammatory bouts interspersed with periods of no or low inflammation
• Reproductive—uneventful recovery of mare
• Neonatal disease, renal/urologic, and hepatobiliary—prognosis is guarded in severe acute disease and depends on the extent of organ invasion and the severity of tissue injury

MISCELLANEOUS

ASSOCIATED CONDITIONS
N/A

ZOONOTIC POTENTIAL
Clinical signs are variable from asymptomatic infection to sepsis and death. Most common complaints are flu-like symptoms and vomiting; however, neurologic, respiratory, cardiac, ocular, and gastrointestinal manifestations can occur.

PREGNANCY/FERTILITY/BREEDING
Abortion, stillbirths, and neonatal disease can be sequelae, depending on the stages of infection and gestation.

ABBREVIATIONS
• EHV = equine herpesvirus
• MAT = mixed agglutination test
• PCR = polymerase chain reaction

Suggested Reading
Bernard WV. Leptospirosis. Vet Clin North Am Equine Pract 1993;9:435–444.
Donahue JM, Williams NM. Emergent causes of placentitis and abortion. Vet Clin North Am Equine Pract 2000;16:443–456.

Author Ashutosh Verma
Consulting Editor Ashley G. Boyle
Acknowledgment The author and editor acknowledge the prior contribution of Jane E. Axon.

L

LETHAL WHITE FOAL SYNDROME

 BASICS

OVERVIEW
LWFS (ileocecocolonic aganglionosis) is a fatal heritable syndrome of horses with white patterning occurring most frequently in foals of overo–overo Paint crosses. Failure of proper development of neural crest-derived cells results in a lack of dermal melanocytes and myenteric ganglion cells in the caudal GI tract. Affected foals are completely white (or almost so) and show signs of colic within 24 h of birth. The syndrome is inherited as an autosomal recessive trait and is invariably fatal. A genetic test is available to identify heterozygous carriers.

SIGNALMENT
- Neonatal foals of overo–overo American Paint Horse cross-breeding
- Signs of colic usually noted by 12–24 h of age
- White coloration
- No sex predisposition

SIGNS
- White color, often with blue eyes
- Typically normal, vigorous foals that stand and nurse
- Failure to pass meconium
- Progressive signs of colic noted within 12–24 h of birth (exacerbated with enteral feeding)
- Progressive abdominal distention
- Death within 48–72 h of birth
- May also have congenital deafness

CAUSES AND RISK FACTORS
- LWFS is caused by a mutation in the *EDNRB* gene, which results in problems with migration of neural crest-derived cells, particularly melanocytes and the cells of many autonomic ganglia. Failure of neural crest cells to migrate and mature properly results in the characteristic phenotype (a nonpigmented foal with functional ileus due to an abnormal enteric nervous system)
- Affected foals are homozygous for the mutation, while their parents are heterozygous. The gene is likely involved, or linked closely, with white patterning and deafness in horses. The heterozygous carrier state appears to be highest among overo Paint horses, especially frame overos

 DIAGNOSIS

DIFFERENTIAL DIAGNOSIS
- Meconium retention/impaction
- Congenital atresia of the GI tract
- Intussusception
- Mesenteric volvulus
- Enterocolitis
- Neonatal maladjustment syndrome
- Rupture of the urinary bladder

CBC/BIOCHEMISTRY/URINALYSIS
Often within normal limits. Not diagnostic.

OTHER LABORATORY TESTS
Genetic testing to detect mutation (affected horses and carriers)—whole blood or hair (with roots) can be submitted.

IMAGING
Abdominal radiographs may reveal gas distention of the cranial GI tract, and barium contrast studies may be useful to rule out congenital atresia. Imaging studies are rarely required to make the diagnosis.

OTHER DIAGNOSTIC PROCEDURES
Exploratory laparotomy confirms the diagnosis but is rarely indicated. The diagnosis is usually made on the basis of clinical findings.

PATHOLOGIC FINDINGS
- Hypoplasia of the ileum, cecum, and the ascending and descending colons with transverse and descending colons most severely affected. Affected segments are very small and contain no ingesta. The more orad regions of the GI tract are grossly normal but may be distended with gas and/or ingesta
- Histologically, absence of myenteric and submucosal ganglia characterizes the abnormal intestine; the enteric nervous system is normal in the stomach and proximal small intestine

 TREATMENT

LWFS is inevitably fatal with no known viable treatment options. Humane euthanasia is recommended if the syndrome is strongly suspected.

 MEDICATIONS

None

 FOLLOW-UP

PREVENTION/AVOIDANCE
A genetic test is available for use in breeding stock. Any horse that is a product of white-patterned horses, or itself is a white-patterned horse, is a potential carrier (including solid-colored "breeding stock" Paint horses). As LWFS is inherited as an autosomal recessive trait, the offspring of 2 carriers has a 1:4 chance of being affected. Carriers should either not be bred or bred only to noncarriers to avoid the production of a lethal white foal.

EXPECTED COURSE AND PROGNOSIS
Affected foals inevitably die within 48–96 h of birth (most within 48 h). Although surgical intervention has been attempted, no reports of successfully treated foals exist. Humane euthanasia is recommended.

L

 MISCELLANEOUS

AGE-RELATED FACTORS
Congenital syndrome—signs are seen soon after birth.

SEE ALSO
- Colic in foals
- Meconium retention

ABBREVIATIONS
- EDNRB = endothelin-B receptor
- GI = gastrointestinal
- LWFS = lethal white foal syndrome

Suggested Reading
Parry NMA. Overo lethal white foal syndrome. Compend Contin Educ Pract Vet 2005;27:945–950.

Author Teresa A. Burns
Consulting Editor Margaret C. Mudge

LEUKOCYTOCLASTIC PASTERN VASCULITIS

BASICS

OVERVIEW
• Specific dermatitis that affects the lateral and medial aspects of nonpigmented lower limbs of horses at pasture
• The condition is most likely an immune-mediated disorder, although the exact etiology has not been clarified

SIGNALMENT
• No sex or breed predilections, but observed in adults and the majority of cases occur in horses with nonpigmented lower limbs; occurrence in pigmented limbs is rare
• There may be a genetic predisposition; in some farms with many related horses the incidence of this normally sporadic disease can be much higher

SIGNS
• Often multiple and reasonably well-demarcated skin lesions with oozing and erythema. Crusting erosions and superficial ulcerations develop almost exclusively on the lateral and medial aspects of the pastern, the fetlock, and the canon (Figure 1)

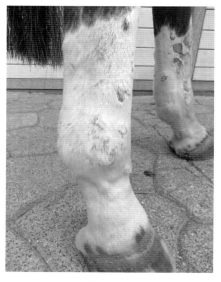

Figure 1.

Severe leucocytoclastic pastern vasculitis of both hind limbs.

• Lesions are (very) painful but not pruritic
• Sometimes the lesions coalesce and affect larger, less well-defined areas
• The affected limb(s) is often significantly edematous

CAUSES AND RISK FACTORS
• Horses at summer pasture; most likely, grass plays a significant etiologic role by either ingestion or direct contact
• Photoexacerbation may be a factor
• Restriction of the lesions to nonpigmented lower limbs suggests a role of direct sunlight (ultraviolet radiation) in the pathogenesis. However, horses with a known history of leukocytoclastic pastern vasculitis did not show lesions when kept in a paddock instead of at pasture

DIAGNOSIS

DIFFERENTIAL DIAGNOSIS
• Any inflammatory dermatosis of the nonpigmented lower limb including "scratches" or "greasy heel," although all of these disorders are almost always located on the palmar/plantar aspect of the lower limb
• Photosensitization mostly affects all white parts of the horse (limbs, nose, etc.); a careful history will eliminate plant etiology and a check on liver function is indicated
• Localised sarcoidosis, although this is mostly on all sides of the lower limb and may include coronary band

CBC/BIOCHEMISTRY/URINALYSIS
No significant abnormalities in blood or urine.

OTHER LABORATORY TESTS
None

IMAGING
None

OTHER DIAGNOSTIC PROCEDURES
Skin punch biopsy under local anesthesia; the lesions are often extremely painful and heavy sedation is necessary before local anesthesia can be administered (regional blocks can be effective, but sometimes disappointing).

PATHOLOGIC FINDINGS
Perivascular edema and (peri)vascular lymphohistiocytic inflammation in the superficial dermis with very localized vascular necrosis and thrombosis (Figure 2).

TREATMENT
• Remove from pasture and limit exposure to strong sunshine
• The use of white cotton stockinettes may make it possible to keep the horse at pasture (Figure 3)
• Topical treatment is of limited value and may be dangerous as these patients are very painful
• Clipping the affected areas may reveal the full extent of the disorder but is not advisable as secondary infections may occur as result of clipping; healing is probably no faster than without clipping

MEDICATIONS

DRUG(S) OF CHOICE
• Prednisolone (1 mg/kg PO every 24 h), to be given between 7:00 and 9:00AM
• In severely affected limbs with significant edema, antimicrobials (e.g. trimethoprim–sulfa 30 mg/kg PO every 12 h) may be helpful

CONTRAINDICATIONS/POSSIBLE INTERACTIONS
In cases with a history of laminitis, corticosteroids should be used with care.

FOLLOW-UP

PATIENT MONITORING
• If horses with lesions are not removed from pasture or protected from sunshine, lesions will deteriorate and the horse eventually will become lame
• Significant improvement occurs within 2 weeks following stabling/sun protection and treatment with corticosteroids

PREVENTION/AVOIDANCE
• Horses known to have this problem should preferably not be at pasture (at least during day time) in subsequent years or the skin should be protected
• Bandaging the horse or the use of white cotton stockinettes may prevent or limit the severity of the condition

POSSIBLE COMPLICATIONS
Lameness may occur in severe cases.

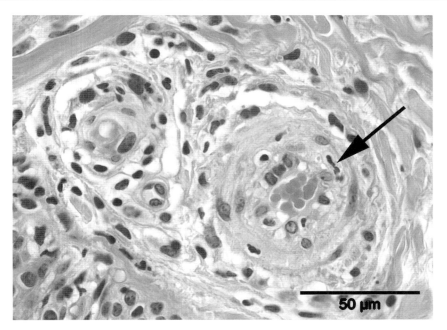

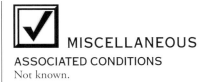

Figure 2.

Histology of a small superficial dermal vessel with thickening and degenerative changes of the vessel wall. Neutrophils are present within the vessel wall (arrow).

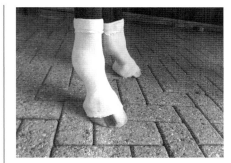

Figure 3.

Lower limbs are protected by a cotton elasticated surgical tubular stockinette.

EXPECTED COURSE AND PROGNOSIS

If vulnerable horses are not at pasture but stabled or in a paddock, they do not show the symptoms; this makes direct sunlight as a primary cause less likely.

☑ MISCELLANEOUS

ASSOCIATED CONDITIONS

Not known.

AGE-RELATED FACTORS

Only recognized in adult horses; very rarely in youngsters and never in foals

ZOONOTIC POTENTIAL

None

PREGNANCY/FERTILITY/BREEDING

Not known, although corticosteroids may be a risk.

SEE ALSO

• Pastern dermatitis
• Photosensitization

Suggested Reading

Stannard A. Pastern leucocytoclastic vasculitis. Vet Dermatol 2000;11:217–220.

Author Marianne M. Sloet van Oldruitenborgh-Oosterbaan
Consulting Editor Gwendolen Lorch

L

LEUKOENCEPHALOMALACIA

 BASICS

DEFINITION
A generally fatal, rapidly progressing neurologic disease caused by ingestion of fumonisin mycotoxin and characterized by liquefactive necrosis of subcortical white matter of the cerebral hemispheres. FB1 is the most abundant in corn naturally infected with *Fusarium verticillioides*; and has also been recently identified in contaminated rolls of hay.

PATHOPHYSIOLOGY
Fumonisin mycotoxins interfere with sphingolipid metabolism, resulting in damage to the vascular endothelium of the brain and, in some animals, hepatocellular necrosis and vacuolization.

SYSTEMS AFFECTED
• Nervous—damage to vascular endothelium of the central nervous system
• Hepatobiliary—pathogenesis not definitively known
• Cardiovascular—an association has been detected between experimentally induced fumonisin neurologic disease and decreased cardiovascular function in horses

GENETICS
N/A

INCIDENCE/PREVALENCE
• Sporadic but important equine toxicosis
• Worldwide, most often in humid climates after a dry summer and wet harvest season
• Outbreaks are seasonal, most occurring from fall through early spring
• Although variable, 15–25% or more of horses in a group can be affected
• There appears to be marked variation in the amount of toxin required to cause clinical disease, and individual susceptibility should be considered

SIGNALMENT
• Affects horses and other equids
• Mature horses appear most susceptible

SIGNS
Neurologic Syndrome
• Anorexia
• Depression, with little response to stimuli
• Frantic behavior such as head pressing, agitation, and hyperexcitability
• Progressive ataxia and proprioceptive defects
• Delirium
• Blindness, 1 or both eyes
• Aimless wandering, often in circles; tendency to lean to 1 side
• Eventual recumbency
• Seizures
• Coma
• Body temperature generally normal
• Death from 12 h to as long as 1 week after onset of signs

Hepatotoxic Syndrome
• Often occurs subclinically concurrent with leukoencephalomalacia
• Signs of liver failure are uncommon but may occur with or without signs of leukoencephalomalacia
• Icterus
• Swelling of the lips and nose
• Petechiae in mucous membranes
• Lowered head
• Reluctance to move
• Abdominal breathing
• Hemoglobinuria
• Death within hours to a few days

CAUSES
Ingestion of corn products contaminated (>5 ppm) with fumonisin mycotoxins, especially FB1, which are produced by *F. verticillioides* (synonym *Fusarium moniliforme*) and *Fusarium proliferatum* molds growing on corn. Intoxication following ingestion of contaminated baled hay reported, however this is rare.

RISK FACTORS
• Fumonisins are produced in corn during hot, dry weather at pollination, and increase when temperature and moisture remain high into harvest, resulting in contaminated corn products used for horse feed
• Corn screenings contain small, shrunken, and broken kernels—often heavily contaminated with fumonisin
• Development of disease depends on fumonisin concentration in feed and duration of exposure
• Death may result from the ingestion of 10 ppm for 30 days
• Onset of clinical disease generally occurs 2–9 weeks after start of continuous consumption of fumonisin-containing feeds
• Reported intoxication following ingestion of contaminated hay associated with rainy and cold weather. An additional contributing factor may be consumption of hay from hay rolls (versus square bales)

 DIAGNOSIS

DIFFERENTIAL DIAGNOSIS
• Rabies
• Eastern equine encephalomyelitis
• West Nile encephalomyelitis
• Hepatoencephalopathy (pyrrolizidine alkaloid hepatotoxicosis, aflatoxicosis, serum hepatitis)
• Head trauma
• Bacterial meningoencephalitis
• Equine protozoal myeloencephalitis

CBC/BIOCHEMISTRY/URINALYSIS
• Inconsistent values among affected horses
• Anemia
• High or low white blood cell count

• High total bilirubin, γ-glutamyltransferase, and aspartate aminotransferase with liver damage
• CSF may be normal but often has high protein and neutrophil count. Horses with experimentally induced leukoencephalomalacia had high CSF protein, albumin, immunoglobulin G concentrations, and albumin quotients

OTHER LABORATORY TESTS
• Feed analysis for FB1; >5 ppm of FB1 is significant; may contain 40–100 ppm
• Fumonisin contaminates hay inhomogeneously, therefore dosage found in sample may not correlate directly with dosage ingested by affected animal(s)
• High sphinganine to sphingosine ratio in serum or tissues—consistent with fumonisin ingestion

PATHOLOGIC FINDINGS
• The primary lesion is softening and liquefactive necrosis, chiefly of the white matter of the cerebrum
• Lesions may be markedly asymmetric
• Massive softening of the interior of the hemispheres may create large cavitations of liquefactive necrosis
• Microscopically, liquefaction and proliferation of macrophages in response to the necrosis are seen

 TREATMENT

APPROPRIATE HEALTH CARE
• Horses with neurologic signs usually die or are euthanized
• When clinical signs appear, significant and irreversible cerebral necrosis may be present; therapy may be an option in selected clinical cases

NURSING CARE
• Supportive therapy—tube feeding and PO and IV fluids for rehydration
• Sedation of demented/maniacal horses to prevent injury to themselves and caregivers
• Oral activated charcoal with saline cathartic may help to eliminate toxin already in gastrointestinal tract

DIET
Immediately *eliminate* feeds suspected of contamination with fumonisin.

CLIENT EDUCATION
• Inform clients of risk of using custom or home-grown corn-based feeds, specifically containing corn screenings or moldy feeds. Commercial feeds are subject to state regulations for fumonisin concentration and are seldom implicated
• Inform clients that there is some risk associated with feeding round-bale hay, as, although rare, toxic strains of *Fusarium* fungi have been isolated

• Inform clients of risk in years with drought or insect stress during growing season and periods of high moisture at harvest
• Feed containing corn and baled hay should be kept dry and protected from moisture when stored to prevent levels of fumonisins from increasing
• Corn and corn byproducts used in horse feed should contain <5 ppm fumonisins and constitute no more than 20% of the dry weight of the total ration
• Do not use corn screenings in horse feed
• Baled hay should be consumed rapidly, and inspected carefully prior to feeding

MEDICATIONS

DRUG(S) OF CHOICE
No specific antidote.

FOLLOW-UP

PATIENT MONITORING
• Continue supportive care
• Monitor for progression or remission of neurologic signs

PREVENTION/AVOIDANCE
See Client Education.

POSSIBLE COMPLICATIONS
Neurologic deficits may remain if horses recover.

EXPECTED COURSE AND PROGNOSIS
• Treatment of horses with significant neurologic signs is rarely successful; death generally occurs from 12 h to 1 week after onset of signs, regardless of treatment
• Euthanasia of advanced cases often is advised

MISCELLANEOUS

ASSOCIATED CONDITIONS
Corn infected with *Fusarium* spp. molds also may contain DON, but feeds with ≤14 ppm DON have no effect on horses.

SYNONYMS
• Corn stalk poisoning
• Fumonisin toxicosis
• Moldy corn poisoning
• Equine leukoencephalomalacia
• *Fusarium verticillioides* (synonym *F. moniliforme*)

SEE ALSO
• Eastern (EEE), western (WEE), and Venezuelan (VEE) equine encephalitides
• Equine protozoal myeloencephalitis (EPM)
• Head trauma
• Hepatic encephalopathy
• Seizure disorders

• Septic meningoencephalomyelitis
• West nile virus

ABBREVIATIONS
• CSF = cerebrospinal fluid
• DON = deoxynivalenol, vomitoxin
• FB1 = fumonisin B1

Suggested Reading
Foreman JH, Constable PD, Waggoner AL, et al. Neurologic abnormalities and cerebrospinal fluid changes in horses administered fumonisin B1 intravenously. J Vet Intern Med 2004;18:223–230.
McCue PM. Equine leukoencephalomalacia. Compend Contin Educ Pract Vet 1989;11:646.
Smith GW, Constable PD, Foreman JH, et al. Cardiovascular changes associated with intravenous administration of fumonisin B1 in horses. Am J Vet Res 2002;63:538–545.
Uhlinger C. Leukoencephalomalacia. Vet Clin North Am Equine Pract 1997;13:13.
Vendruscolo CP, Frias NC, de Carvalho CB, et al. Leukoencephalomalacia outbreak in horses due to consumption of contaminated hay. J Vet Intern Med 2016;30(6): 1879–1881.

Authors Demia J. de Tonnerre and Robert J. MacKay
Consulting Editor Caroline N. Hahn
Acknowledgment The authors and editor acknowledge the prior contribution Steven T. Grubbs.

L

LOCOMOTOR STEREOTYPIC BEHAVIORS

 BASICS

DEFINITION
- A stereotypic behavior is a relatively invariant, repetitive pattern of movement with no obvious purpose
- It arises from a thwarted normal maintenance behavior (walking), but is performed excessively and out of context to the exclusion of normal behaviors, and so is a welfare concern
- Equine locomotor stereotypic behaviors include stall/box-walking; weaving; fence running
- Weaving consists of an obvious lateral swaying movement of the head, neck, forequarters, and sometimes hindquarters, with the limbs typically tensing in the sequence of the walk or trot, even if the animal does not move forward (see Web Video 1). The horse may toss, nod, and shake its head at the same time, but this should not be confused with the separate condition of headshaking syndrome

PATHOPHYSIOLOGY
- Unclear but appears to relate to motivational conflict
- Proposed mechanisms implicate serotonergic and dopaminergic systems, but there is no evidence of dysfunction

SYSTEMS AFFECTED
- Behavioral—may interfere with expression of normal maintenance behaviors or with performance of learned responses
- Musculoskeletal—uneven hoof wear or muscle development
- Decreased performance if the behavior is performed to the point of fatigue or self-injury but this is rare

GENETICS
A genetic predisposition is suspected, but the precise nature of inheritance has not been determined.

INCIDENCE/PREVALENCE
Weaving occurs in about 3% of horses but the prevalence varies with circumstances (range 0–10%). For stall-walking average prevalence is around 2% (range 0–7%).

GEOGRAPHIC DISTRIBUTION
Worldwide

SIGNALMENT
- No age or sex predilection, but the occurrence of 1 locomotor stereotypic behavior increases the risk of another
- Warmbloods and Thoroughbreds are at a general increased risk of developing stereotypic behaviors
- More common among endurance horses and horses with reduced or restricted exercise (<1.5 ha), especially if kept in face-to-face stalls, where locomotion is likely to be frequently thwarted as they try to interact with horses opposite
- Median age of onset is 64 weeks for weaving and 60 weeks for box-walking

SIGNS
General Comments
- Time spent performing the behavior varies. The behaviors are often elicited by arousal associated with a desire to engage with stimuli outside the stall (e.g. food or other horses being led to and from barns or pastures, toward or away from herd mates; or in anticipation of pleasurable experiences outside the stall). The intensity of the behavior may increase at times of increased emotional arousal
- Stall-walking—circular pacing when confined to a stall. The horse may circle in 1 or both directions, repeatedly tracing its path, sometimes even placing its feet in exactly the same place during each circuit
- Weaving—rhythmic side-to-side swaying of the head and neck, often accompanied by an obvious alternate stepping in place with the front limbs and possibly all 4 limbs to the beat of the walk or trot
- Fence running—the horse walks, trots, or canters in a repetitive pattern along a fence line or before a gate, with the distance traveled and the location and features of the turns being the same each time
- Head nodding, tossing, and shaking as well as kicking out at the stall walls or door may also occur with any of these locomotor behaviors

Historical Findings
Owners may report a gradual onset or an inciting event after which the behavior was seen to become more obvious.

Physical Examination Findings
Unremarkable, except for possible lesions from rubbing on the stall door etc. or uneven shoe or hoof wear.

CAUSES
Environment and management practices that inhibit expression of locomotion or locomotor expectations (e.g. periods of extensive exercise followed by periods of enforced rest).

RISK FACTORS
- Endurance horses
- Abrupt box weaning
- Any bedding other than straw

 DIAGNOSIS

DIFFERENTIAL DIAGNOSIS
- Anxiety specific to separation from herd mates
- Bilateral foot-related lameness causing shifting from 1 limb to the other
- A learned response reinforced by a reward (e.g. a horse shakes its head and bangs the stall door at feeding time and is fed by the caretaker; thus reinforcing the behavior)

CBC/BIOCHEMISTRY/URINALYSIS
NA

OTHER LABORATORY TESTS
NA

IMAGING
N/A unless laminitis or similar foot lameness suspected.

OTHER DIAGNOSTIC PROCEDURES
N/A

 TREATMENT

AIMS
- Ethologically based approaches to address behavioral needs, especially the balance between exercise, diet, and confinement. Housing which allows greater social contact either directly or via a mirror should be encouraged if the horse is sociable
- Devices and management measures that focus on preventing performance of the behavior without addressing the psychologic aspects do not constitute humane treatment. Anti-weaving stall doors may reduce neck swaying during weaving, but can redirect the behavior into another form, e.g. box-walking
- Psychoactive medication is experimental and rarely justified in practice

APPROPRIATE HEALTH CARE
- Treatment plan focuses on management practices such as decreasing confinement, isolation, and emotional arousal
- Manage as an outpatient
- Recommended modifications in management practices—increased turnout time, preferably with a compatible companion; increased grazing time; increased opportunities for social contact within the confines of the stall
- Deep bedding, especially straw, which gives the horse something to investigate, decreases wear and tear on the horse's feet and extremities. Stalls may need protection from incidental damage caused by kicking
- Increasing time spent foraging using double or triple layers of hay net with small holes or toys that release food when moved about by the horse can help, but may increase oral frustration (see chapter Oral stereotypic behaviors). If using multiple hay nets, there should be some hay between the net layers. 2 or 3 nested nets can be hung at a safe height in different corners of the stall. Feeding forage from the floor in piles around the circuit traced by a stall-walker may encourage a more natural browsing pattern
- Increase contact between individuals when housed, if safe to do so, e.g. through bars between stalls if group housing deemed too risky. An unbreakable scratch-resistant mirror

(CONTINUED)

LOCOMOTOR STEREOTYPIC BEHAVIORS

(e.g. polished steel) may be provided to the side of the door where the horse weaves as an alternative to a companion and seems to serve as a distraction when the horse is at the front of the stable and about to weave. This is not suitable for unsociable horses

ACTIVITY

Maintain a consistent high level of grazing, turnout, and aerobic activity in accordance with the work of the horse.

DIET

Increased roughage, reduce/eliminate concentrate.

CLIENT EDUCATION

• Caution owners against reinforcing undesirable, repetitive behaviors
• Scientific evidence does not support that these behaviors cause unthriftiness

SURGICAL CONSIDERATIONS

N/A

MEDICATIONS

DRUG(S) OF CHOICE

• Medications are generally not justified on risk, welfare, cost, and feasibility grounds. Owners should be counseled accordingly
• Opioid antagonists, such as naltrexone and naloxone, have a short half-life, high cost, and require IV administration
• Tricyclic antidepressants and SSRIs such as amitriptyline, clomipramine, doxepin, fluoxetine, and imipramine might be theoretically useful for increasing inhibitory control, but few (if any) uses of these drugs in horses are reported. The risks generally outweigh any potential benefits. Paroxetine has been used to reduce weaving at a dose of 0.5 mg/kg PO every 24 h

CONTRAINDICATIONS

If medication is used, careful monitoring of serum chemistry values and clinical signs is essential.

PRECAUTIONS

• Owners should be aware that use of psychotropic medication constitutes experimental and off-label use and is not usually justifiable on welfare grounds
• Owners should sign an informed consent form and receive an explanation (preferably in writing) of the medication, selection rationale, expected benefits, and possible side effects
• CBC and serum chemistry panel are recommended before initiating drug therapy
• Laboratory diagnostics should be repeated 6 weeks after start of medication and whenever clinical signs warrant
• Cardiac conduction abnormalities are a contraindication for use of tricyclic antidepressants, which are arrhythmogenic in humans and may be so in horses

POSSIBLE INTERACTIONS

Combinations of tricyclics and SSRIs may be synergistic and should not be used.

ALTERNATIVE DRUGS

Acepromazine has been used experimentally, but is not justifiable in practice.

FOLLOW-UP

PATIENT MONITORING

• Drug dosages may need adjustment, so weekly follow-up is recommended. If long-term use of medication is intended, semiannual or annual monitoring of CBC and serum chemistry is recommended
• Monitor owner compliance regarding management recommendations. Intervals for follow-up vary depending on problem severity

PREVENTION/AVOIDANCE

Avoid abrupt weaning, and provide social contact when possible. Maintain a consistent exercise regime in accordance with the use of the horse, and avoid unnecessary concentrate, using forage in place wherever possible. Avoid inadvertent reinforcement through the provision of food and social contact when the horse shows these behaviors or other signs of high arousal.

POSSIBLE COMPLICATIONS

Situations of stress and especially frustration may exacerbate these problems.

EXPECTED COURSE AND PROGNOSIS

Treatment is aimed at improving welfare and minimizing the display of the behaviors; owners should be counseled about such management and to avoid measures which simply prevent the behavior and potentially increase frustration.

MISCELLANEOUS

ASSOCIATED CONDITIONS

• Lameness
• Impaired performance

AGE-RELATED FACTORS

Median age of onset is just over a year.

PREGNANCY/FERTILITY/BREEDING

Use of medication is contraindicated in pregnant individuals.

SYNONYMS

• Compulsive disorders
• Obsessive–compulsive disorders
• Stable vices
• Stereotypies

SEE ALSO

• Headshaking
• Oral stereotypic behaviors
• Self-mutilation

ABBREVIATIONS

SSRI = selective serotonin-reuptake inhibitor

Suggested Reading
Cooper JJ, McDonald L, Mills DS. The effect of increasing visual horizons on stereotypic weaving: implications for the social housing of stabled horses. Appl Anim Behav Sci 2000;69(1):67–83.
Crowell-Davis SL, Murray T. Veterinary Psychopharmacology. Ames, IA: Blackwell Publishing, 2006.
McGreevy P. Equine Behavior: A Guide for Veterinarians and Equine Scientists, 2e. Philadelphia, PA: WB Saunders, 2012.
Mills DS, McDonnell SM. The Domestic Horse: The Origins, Development and Management of its Behaviour. New York, NY: Cambridge University Press, 2005.
Mills DS, Taylor KD, Cooper JJ. Weaving, headshaking, cribbing, and other stereotypies. Proc Am Assoc Equine Pract 2005;51:220–230.

Author Daniel S. Mills
Consulting Editor Victoria L. Voith
Acknowledgment The author and editor acknowledge the prior contribution of Soraya V. Juarbe-Díaz.

L

LUNGWORM—PARASITIC BRONCHITIS AND PNEUMONIA

BASICS

OVERVIEW
The development of an inflammatory response in the airways and lung parenchyma due to an infection with the lungworm *Dictyocaulus arnfieldi.*

SIGNALMENT
• Donkeys and mules are most likely to harbor patent lungworm infections
• There is no breed or sex predilection
• All ages can be affected, but the prepatent period for *D. arnfieldi* is 6 weeks; therefore, disease is less likely in very young foals

SIGNS
• Chronic, nonprogressive cough that is unresponsive to antibiotic or anti-inflammatory therapy. More than 1 horse can be affected at the same time
• An elevated respiratory rate, and bilateral nasal discharge possible
• Audible wheezes and crackles may be evident during thoracic auscultation
• Donkeys and mules do not typically exhibit clinical signs of infection

CAUSES AND RISK FACTORS
• Ingestion of infective larvae of *D. arnfieldi* from contaminated pasture
• Horses kept on green or irrigated pastures that concurrently or previously contained donkeys or mules
• Infections usually occur during warm, wet weather in temperate climates

DIAGNOSIS

DIFFERENTIAL DIAGNOSIS
Equine asthma, tumor or polyp in the airway, tracheobronchial foreign body, chronic bacterial pneumonia, pulmonary abscess, postviral airway hyperreactivity. In an individual horse, signs are often indistinguishable from those associated with severe equine asthma (heaves).

CBC/BIOCHEMISTRY/URINALYSIS
• CBC—peripheral eosinophilia is variable but if present is strongly suggestive of a parasitic infection
• Routine biochemistry and urinalysis are unremarkable

OTHER LABORATORY TESTS
• The definitive diagnosis is established with the identification of larvae in a TTA or identification of larvae recovered from feces using the modified Baermann technique
• Horses will commonly be negative for larvae using the modified Baermann technique but co-pastured donkeys should be tested and will likely be positive
• The larvae in TTA fluid can be concentrated using centrifugation to improve the likelihood of discovery
• Cytologic examination of the TTA will reveal a mixed inflammatory response with eosinophilia

IMAGING
Thoracic radiography can be useful to rule out chronic bacterial pneumonia or pulmonary abscesses.

OTHER DIAGNOSTIC PROCEDURES
Endoscopy may reveal an increase in mucus production in the airways. Rarely, an adult worm may be seen.

TREATMENT
Lungworm infection in the horse can be successfully treated with anthelmintic therapy and removal of horses from the contaminated pasture.

MEDICATIONS

DRUG(S) OF CHOICE
• Ivermectin (0.20 mg/kg PO) and moxidectin (0.40 mg/kg PO) have been confirmed to be highly effective against the mature and larval forms of *D. arnfieldi.*

Moxidectin is highly lipophilic and persists in the tissues longer than ivermectin
• Eprinomectin (0.50 mg/kg) used as a pour-on is reported to be highly effective in treating *D. arnfieldi* in donkeys

CONTRAINDICATIONS/POSSIBLE INTERACTIONS
N/A

FOLLOW-UP

PATIENT MONITORING
• If donkeys are treated, then repeating the modified Baermann technique on feces will allow the efficacy of therapy to be monitored
• Horses can be monitored for the resolution of clinical signs

PREVENTION/AVOIDANCE
Do not pasture horses with donkeys that are not on a helminth control program.

EXPECTED COURSE AND PROGNOSIS
Lungworm infection in the horse has an excellent prognosis for full recovery post treatment. Resolution of clinical signs should be seen in 7–10 days after treatment.

MISCELLANEOUS

ABBREVIATIONS
TTA = transtracheal aspirate

Suggested Reading
Boyle AG, Houston R. Parasitic pneumonitis and treatment in horses. Clin Tech Equine Pract 2006;5:225–232
Veneziano V, Di Loria A, Masucci R, et al. Efficacy of eprinomectin pour-on against *Dictyocaulus arnfieldi* infection in donkeys (*Equus asinus*). Vet J 2011;190:414–415.

Author Johanna L. Watson
Consulting Editors Mathilde Leclère and Daniel Jean

BASICS

DEFINITION
• Usually caused by the spirochete *Borrelia burgdorferi* in the USA; *Borrelia afzelii* and *Borrelia garinii* in Europe. Most frequent tick-borne disease of humans in the USA. Only sporadic clinical cases in horses have been documented
• Definitive diagnosis is difficult and clinical diagnosis is usually presumptive, based on clinical signs, confirmed or potential tick exposure in an endemic region, supportive serology, PCR testing, elimination of other possible causes, ± response to treatment
• Well-documented syndromes include neuroborreliosis, uveitis, and dermatitis (pseudolymphoma). Other reported clinical signs include weight loss, behavior changes, hyperreactivity, lethargy, performance problems, fevers, lameness, joint effusion, muscle pain, and stiffness

PATHOPHYSIOLOGY
• Ticks become infected with *B. burgdorferi* with their first blood meal from an infected host. The spirochete penetrates the gut epithelium and invades the salivary gland, where it resides until transmission
• *B. burgdorferi* causes a localized skin infection after the tick has been feeding for 24 h. Transient bacteremia may follow, disseminating the spirochete
• Postmortem findings from experimentally infected ponies suggest a possible migration of the organism through connective, perineural, and perivascular tissues in the skin, fascia, muscle, and synovial membranes. *B. burgdorferi* induces a secondary inflammatory reaction. The differences in host reaction may explain the relatively few infected horses that develop clinical signs, thought to occur months after infection

SYSTEMS AFFECTED
• Musculoskeletal—polyarthritis, stiffness, lameness
• Ophthalmic—uveitis
• Nervous—encephalitis, meningitis, myelitis, radiculitis, neuritis
• Skin—dermatitis, pseudolymphoma

INCIDENCE/PREVALENCE
Worldwide distribution in humans, with reports of disease in horses limited to the USA, UK, and Europe. United States seroprevalence ranges from <1% in nonendemic areas to 75% in endemic areas.

SIGNS
• Neuroborreliosis—muscle atrophy or weight loss, cranial nerve deficits, ataxia, behavior changes, dysphagia, muscle fasciculations, neck stiffness, episodic respiratory distress. Uveitis, fever, joint effusion, and cardiac arrhythmias might accompany neurologic signs but are less common
• Uveitis—most commonly observed with neurologic signs, can be seen alone; blepharospasm, photophobia, aqueous flare, hypopyon, and miosis
• Dermatitis or pseudolymphoma—at the site of tick attachment, nonpainful dermal papules to nodules that histologically appear as a densely cellular lymphohistiocytic dermal infiltrate
• Other clinical findings often attributed include shifting lameness, behavioral changes, (poly)arthritis, stiffness, hyperesthesia, fever, distal limb edema, and lethargy. Fever and limb edema may be a result of *Anaplasma phagocytophilum* infection as many ticks are infected with both organisms

CAUSES
The 2 year life cycle for *B. burgdorferi* involves an *Ixodes* tick vector and a small mammal (white-footed mouse) intermediate host for the larval and nymph stages, with a deer as the final host for the adult. Principal vector—*Ixodes pacificus* (Western black-legged tick) in the western USA and *Ixodes scapularis* (black-legged or deer tick) in the upper midwestern and eastern USA.

RISK FACTORS
Contact with *Ixodes* ticks in Lyme endemic areas. Transmission between horses has not been reported.

DIAGNOSIS

DIFFERENTIAL DIAGNOSIS
• Neuroborreliosis—equine protozoal myeloencephalitis, viral encephalitides, equine herpesvirus 1 myeloencephalopathy, rabies, CNS nematodiasis, bacterial meningoencephalitis, cervical vertebral stenotic myelopathy, or botulism
• Uveitis—recurrent uveitis and other infectious uveitis (leptospirosis)
• Pseudolymphoma—cutaneous lymphoma, sarcoids, or granulomas
• Arthritis—other noninfectious and infectious causes of arthritis
• Muscle stiffness—polysaccharide storage myopathy, chronic intermittent rhabdomyolysis, and osteoarthritis of the axial skeleton

CBC/BIOCHEMISTRY/URINALYSIS
Usually unremarkable; leukocytosis, neutrophilia, and increased acute-phase protein levels (hyperfibrinogenemia, increased serum amyloid A) possible.

OTHER LABORATORY TESTS
• Culture and isolation of *B. burgdorferi* from blood, urine, CSF, skin, and ocular fluids
• The following have been used to detect anti-*B. burgdorferi* antibodies in serum, CSF, synovial fluid, and ocular fluids:
  ◦ Indirect fluorescent antibody test and ELISA—quantitative; positive results must be confirmed by WB
  ◦ WB—qualitative test, giving information regarding vaccination status and infection stage.
  ◦ SNAP® 3Dx and 4Dx tests—stall-side assays; qualitative; positive results indicate natural exposure, not vaccination
  ◦ Lyme Multiplex Assay—antibodies against 3 recombinant antigens: OspA, OspC, and OspF; quantitative; pattern thought to indicate stage of infection; can help differentiate vaccination response from natural exposure
  ◦ Positive serologic results indicate past or current infection; do not indicate clinical disease; false-negative results can occur in first few weeks of infection. Some horses with immune deficiencies or chronic infection localized to an immune-privileged site (CNS or eye) might be seronegative despite active infection and clinical disease. False-positive results might occur owing to cross-reactivity with other *Borrelia* or bacterial spp. Magnitude of antibody titer is not known to correlate with likelihood of clinical disease
  ◦ PCR detection of the organism DNA in the synovial membrane, joint fluid, CSF, skin, or ocular fluid is indicative of active infection

IMAGING
Radiographs are useful in assisting with the differential diagnosis of lameness and neurologic dysfunction.

OTHER DIAGNOSTIC PROCEDURES
• Synovial fluid analysis might show neutrophilic inflammation
• Synovial biopsy and histopathology with IHC or PCR
• CSF cytology might show neutrophilic and/or lymphocytic pleocytosis with increased total protein. Some horses with neuroborreliosis have normal CSF cytology. CSF PCR rarely positive
• Aqueocentesis with cytology, immunologic testing, and PCR
• Skin biopsy with histopathology, IHC, and/or PCR
• FISH on affected tissues

PATHOLOGIC FINDINGS
• Nervous system—gross lesions generally limited to the meninges: opacification, yellow discoloration, hyperemia, and edema; characteristic histologic finding is multifocal, predominantly lymphohistiocytic, pleocellular leptomeningitis and perivasculitis

L

LYME DISEASE

• Eyes—mixed inflammatory infiltrate within multiple ocular structures; demonstrate presence of spirochetes with silver stains
• Joints—arthritis with congested hyperplastic synovial membrane; may have lymphoplasmacytic infiltrate

TREATMENT

NURSING CARE
Tube feeding might be required for horses with dysphagia.

CLIENT EDUCATION
• Examine horse and remove ticks with tweezers or gloves
• Spirochetes are not transferred from the ticks until at least 24 h of feeding

MEDICATIONS

DRUG(S) OF CHOICE
• IV tetracycline (6.6 mg/kg IV every 12–24 h), oral doxycycline (10 mg/kg PO every 12 h), or oral minocycline (4 mg/kg PO every 12 h) for at least 4 weeks. Tetracycline for 1 week prior to starting doxycycline may provide a more rapid response. Tetracycline in experimentally infected animals resulted in elimination of the infection, but may differ in chronic infections
• Parenteral treatment with high-dose penicillin (44 000 U/kg IV every 4–6 h) or third generation cephalosporins (cefotaxime 25–50 mg/kg IV every 6–8 h; ceftazidime 20–40 mg/kg IV every 6–12 h) might be warranted for neuroborreliosis
• Tetracycline drugs have anti-inflammatory properties that may lead to nonspecific clinical improvement
• NSAID therapy may be used with antibiotic therapy
• Uveitis—reduce inflammation and provide mydriasis and analgesia

PRECAUTIONS
Colitis may occur secondary to antimicrobial therapy.

POSSIBLE INTERACTIONS
Jarisch–Herxheimer reaction (exacerbation of clinical signs with antibiotic therapy) has been reported in humans and is believed to be an immune-associated reaction caused by destruction of spirochetes. Pyrexia associated with the initiation of tetracycline therapy has been documented in 1 equine case.

ALTERNATIVE DRUGS
Corticosteroid therapy remains controversial and is not usually recommended.

FOLLOW-UP

PATIENT MONITORING
A marked improvement in clinical signs should be seen after antibiotic therapy.

PREVENTION/AVOIDANCE
• No commercially available equine vaccine; vaccine using recombinant OspA antigen is currently being investigated
• Avoid tick-infested areas endemic for Lyme disease; groom daily to remove ticks
• Use appropriate insecticide sprays (not amitraz) for horses. No adverse effects have been reported with the use of commercially available canine tick sprays (e.g. fipronil)

POSSIBLE COMPLICATIONS
• Death
• Chronic inflammatory arthritis
• Recurrent episodes of uveitis
• Persistence of neurologic signs

EXPECTED COURSE AND PROGNOSIS
• Prognosis is difficult to determine due to the difficulty in establishing a definitive diagnosis antemortem. Horses with neuroborreliosis often succumb to the disease despite appropriate treatment
• Horses with arthritis may be unable to return to previous athletic performance

MISCELLANEOUS

ZOONOTIC POTENTIAL
No zoonotic potential. Humans in contact with infected horses may have increased risk of infection due to increased exposure from animals bringing ticks into their environment.

PREGNANCY/FERTILITY/BREEDING
Intrauterine infection of foals with and without positive titers. The significance of the isolated organisms is questionable.

SYNONYMS
• Borreliosis
• Lyme arthritis
• Lyme borreliosis
• Neuroborreliosis

ABBREVIATIONS
• CNS = central nervous system
• CSF = cerebrospinal fluid
• ELISA = enzyme-linked immunosorbent assay
• FISH = fluorescent in situ hybridization
• IHC = immunohistochemistry
• NSAID = nonsteroidal anti-inflammatory drug
• Osp = outer surface protein
• PCR = polymerase chain reaction
• WB = western immunoblot

Suggested Reading
Chang Y-F, Novosol V, McDonough SP, et al. Experimental infection of ponies with *Borrelia burgdorferi* by exposure to ixodid ticks. Vet Pathol 2000;37:68–76.
Chang Y-F, Ku KW, Chang CF, et al. Antibiotic treatment of experimentally *Borrelia burgdorferi*-infected ponies. Vet Microbiol 2005;107:285–294.
Johnstone LK, Engiles JB, Aceto H, et al. Retrospective evaluation of horses diagnosed with neuroborreliosis on postmortem examination: 16 cases (2004-2015). J Vet Intern Med 2016;30:1305–1312.
Priest HL, Irby NL, Schlafer DH, et al. Diagnosis of *Borrelia*-associated uveitis in two horses. Vet Ophthalmol 2012;15:398–405.
Sears KP, Divers TJ, Neff RT, et al. A case of *Borrelia*-associated cutaneous pseudolymphoma in a horse. Vet Dermatol 2012;23:153–156.

Author Amy L. Johnson
Consulting Editor Ashley G. Boyle
Acknowledgment The author and editor acknowledge the prior contribution of Jane E. Axon.

LYMPHADENOPATHY

BASICS

OVERVIEW
• Disease of LNs that may be local, regional, or generalized; primary or secondary; and usually results in LN enlargement
• Enlargement can be due to benign (lymphoid hyperplasia, lymphadenitis) or malignant (primary or metastatic neoplasia) causes

SIGNALMENT
Lymphoid pharyngeal hyperplasia and enlarged LNs of the anorectal region are common in young horses.

SIGNS
• History and clinical signs depend on underlying cause and location of enlarged LNs
• History may include previous or current signs of infection, wounds, and vaccination for strangles
• Peripheral LNs most accessible for examination are mandibular and superficial cervical
• Infected LNs may be enlarged, warm, soft, painful on palpation, and draining purulent material
• Neoplastic LNs may be enlarged, firm, and often not warm or sensitive to palpation
• Mandibular and retropharyngeal lymphadenopathy may cause anorexia, dysphagia, and airway obstruction; enlarged internal LNs may cause obstruction of the pharynx, esophagus, trachea, bronchi, and intestine with dyspnea, anorexia, reflux, pleural effusion, ascites, diarrhea, or other signs of organ dysfunction; dyschezia, abdominal pain, and urinary dysfunction if anorectal LNs are involved
• Nonspecific signs include elevated rectal temperature, signs of depression, anorexia, weight loss, pale mucous membranes, tachypnea, and tachycardia

CAUSES AND RISK FACTORS
• *Lymphoid hyperplasia* is caused by immune stimulation associated with regional immunity of a nearby pathologic process; *lymphadenitis* by inflammation/infection within the LN itself (primary) or drainage of purulent site (secondary); *neoplasia* may be primary lymphoid neoplasia (lymphoma) or metastatic spread (e.g. melanoma, leukemia)
• Risk factors include lymphoid hyperplasia—intranasal modified-live strangle vaccines; lymphadenitis—recent introduction of new horses, exposing horses to infected animals (e.g. during competition), or transporting naive horses to areas with endemic disease
• Range of infectious agents associated with localized or generalized lymphadenitis

DIAGNOSIS

DIFFERENTIAL DIAGNOSIS
• If LN enlargement is primary presenting sign, lymphoid hyperplasia, lymphadenitis (primary or secondary), or neoplasia must be differentiated
• If nonspecific signs, due to involvement of other body systems, are primary presenting signs, appropriate and thorough investigation of these signs is warranted

CBC/BIOCHEMISTRY/URINALYSIS
• Variable depending on cause of LN enlargement and LNs involved
• Inflammatory leukogram if lymphoid hyperplasia and lymphadenitis
• Rarely, neoplastic lymphocytes in peripheral blood with lymphosarcoma cell leukemia or leukemic phase of lymphoma

OTHER LABORATORY TESTS
• Cytologic evaluation of LN aspirates, blood, bone marrow, or fluids; histologic evaluation of biopsies can confirm underlying cause if cytology is equivocal
• Culture of aspirate if lymphadenitis present
• Serology for infectious agents
• Serum protein electrophoresis if neoplastic LN and marked hyperglobulinemia

IMAGING
Ultrasonography to assess size, detect fluid and infiltrative disease, and allow for guided biopsy.

OTHER DIAGNOSTIC PROCEDURES
Rectal palpation to evaluate accessible internal LNs.

PATHOLOGIC FINDINGS
• *Lymphoid hyperplasia*—variable population of normal lymphocytes, including numerous germinal centers and plasma cells
• *Lymphadenitis*—increased proportions of inflammatory cells, including neutrophils, macrophages, or eosinophils depending on cause and chronicity of process
• *Lymphoid neoplasia* (lymphosarcoma)—abnormal lymphocytes among reactive normal lymphocytes; alternatively, the cells in metastatic neoplasia reflect the primary neoplasm

TREATMENT

Aimed at underlying disease process and supportive care.

MEDICATIONS

DRUG(S) OF CHOICE
• Appropriate antibiotics or antiparasitics
• Anti-inflammatory medication (e.g. flunixin meglumine 0.5–1 mg/kg)
• Treatment choice for neoplasia depends on type/distribution

FOLLOW-UP

PATIENT MONITORING
Monitor for systemic effects and airway obstruction.

EXPECTED COURSE AND PROGNOSIS
• Prognosis is good for lymphoid hyperplasia/lymphadenitis if treated promptly
• Prognosis poor for neoplasia

L

MISCELLANEOUS

ASSOCIATED CONDITIONS
Can be associated with underlying inflammatory processes, which warrant full evaluation to determine extent of disease.

ZOONOTIC POTENTIAL
Some infectious causes of lymphadenitis are zoonotic.

SEE ALSO
• *Corynebacterium pseudotuberculosis*
• Lymphosarcoma
• *Rhodococcus equi (Prescottella equi)*
• *Streptococcus equi* infection

ABBREVIATIONS
LN = lymph node

Suggested Reading
Cowell R, Tyler D, Dorsey K, Guglick M. Lymph nodes. In: Cowell R, Tyler D, eds. Diagnostic Cytology and Hematology of the Horse, 2e. St. Louis, MO: Mosby, 2001:99–106.

Author M. Julia B. Felippe
Consulting Editors David Hodgson, Harold C. McKenzie, and Jennifer L. Hodgson
Acknowledgment The author acknowledges the prior contribution of Jennifer L. Hodgson.

LYMPHOCYTIC–PLASMACYTIC ENTEROCOLITIS

BASICS

OVERVIEW
• LPE is a pathologic description of a type of infiltrative intestinal disease within the complex of idiopathic inflammatory bowel disease in the horse
• Malabsorption and protein-losing enteropathy result from the diffuse infiltration of well-differentiated lymphocytes and plasma cells into the lamina propria, between crypts, and sometimes in the submucosa of the small intestine and to a lesser extent the large intestine
• Lesions involving the small intestine are more common than lesions involving the large intestine. Normal fecal consistency indicates that the majority of the large intestine is functional
• LPE is an uncommon equine intestinal disease that is difficult to diagnose antemortem

SIGNALMENT
• No breed, age, or sex predisposition
• Median age 12 years (n = 14)

SIGNS
• Chronic weight loss (95%)
• Thin to emaciated
• Generalized weakness
• Lethargy (20%)
• Inappetence (50%)
• Normal feces consistency or diarrhea (35%). Diarrhea indicates that LPE involves the large intestine
• Normal vital signs
• Recurrent colic (20%)
• Per rectal examination—firm mass in the craniodorsal abdomen suggestive of mesenteric lymphadenopathy in the region of the cranial mesenteric artery possible (3/12)

CAUSES AND RISK FACTORS
Exact cause is unknown, although there is a strong probability that LPE is an immune-mediated disorder.

DIAGNOSIS

DIFFERENTIAL DIAGNOSIS
• Malnutrition
• Internal parasitism
• Granulomatous enteritis
• Alimentary lymphosarcoma
• Eosinophilic enteritis
• Multisystemic eosinophilic epitheliotropic disease
• Tuberculosis
• Histoplasmosis
• Basophilic enterocolitis

CBC/BIOCHEMISTRY/URINALYSIS
• Hypoalbuminemia (<30 g/L) (11/20)
• Hypoproteinemia (<60 g/L) (7/20)
• Hyperbilirubinemia if horse is inappetent
• Increased plasma fibrinogen (5/8)
• Normal urinalysis

OTHER LABORATORY TESTS
• D-Xylose absorption test/oral glucose tolerance test abnormal (14/17)
• Serum protein electrophoresis abnormal

IMAGING
N/A

OTHER DIAGNOSTIC PROCEDURES
• Rectal mucosal biopsy—abnormal (3/7). Moderate to large numbers of lymphocytes and plasma cells seen in the lamina propria. Unlikely to be diagnostic as lymphoid and plasma cells may also be found in rectal tissue of horses with granulomatous disease, cyathostomiasis, and malignant lymphoma
• Definitive diagnosis by small intestine biopsy—standing flank or laparoscopy; infiltration with lymphocytes and plasma cells

TREATMENT
Poor prognosis.

MEDICATIONS

DRUG(S) OF CHOICE
Corticosteroids (e.g. prednisolone 1 mg/kg PO every 12 h or dexamethasone 0.1 mg/kg IM every 24 h for 3 days, then 0.02 mg/kg IM). Anecdotal reports of brief resolution of diarrhea in some cases when given for several weeks.

CONTRAINDICATIONS/POSSIBLE INTERACTIONS
Corticosteroids at this dosage may be immunosuppressive and also may have significant metabolic side effects. Therapy should be withdrawn gradually.

FOLLOW-UP
N/A

MISCELLANEOUS

SYNONYMS
Lymphocytic–plasmacytic enteritis.

SEE ALSO
• Protein-losing enteropathy (PLE)

ABBREVIATIONS
LPE = lymphocytic–plasmacytic enterocolitis

Suggested Reading
Allen KJ, Pearson GR, Fews D, et al. *Lawsonia intracellularis* proliferative enteropathy in a weanling foal, with a tentative histological diagnosis of lymphocytic plasmacytic enteritis. Equine Vet Educ 2009;21:411–414.
Barr BS. Infiltrative intestinal disease. Vet Clin North Am Equine Pract 2006;22:e1–7.
Chandler K, McNeill PM, Murphy D. Small intestinal malabsorption in an aged mare. Equine Vet Educ 2000;12:166–171.
Clark ES, Morris DD, Allen D, Tyler DE. Lymphocytic enteritis in a filly. J Am Vet Med Assoc 1988;193:1281–1283.
Kemper DL, Perkins GA, Schumacher J, et al. Equine lymphocytic-plasmacytic enterocolitis: a retrospective study of 14 cases. Equine Vet J Suppl 2000;32:108–112.
MacAllister CG, Mosier D, Qualls Jr CW, Cowell RL. Lymphocytic-plasmacytic enteritis in two horses. J Am Vet Med Assoc 1990;196:1995–1998.
Schumacher J, Edwards JF, Cohen ND. Chronic idiopathic inflammatory bowel diseases of the horse. J Vet Intern Med 2000;14:258–265.

Author John D. Baird
Consulting Editors Henry Stämpfli and Olimpo Oliver-Espinosa

BASICS

DEFINITION

• Lymphocyte count in peripheral blood greater than the upper limit of the laboratory reference interval; usually >5500 cells/μL (5.5×10^9 cells/L)
• Lymphocytes constitute the second most common WBC in peripheral blood
• Lymphocytes are a heterogenous group of cells that have an essential role in adaptive immune responses and also contribute to innate immunity
• Broadly, lymphocytes are divided into T cells (responsible for cell-mediated immunity), B cells (responsible for humoral immunity), null cells (killer and natural killer cells), and newly recognized innate lymphoid cells; however, the functions of the different cell types are strongly interrelated
• Lymphocyte counts can change rapidly due to physiologic influences, antigenic stimulation, neoplasia, or due to vaccination or corticosteroid administration
• Young animals have higher lymphocyte counts than adults

PATHOPHYSIOLOGY

• Lymphopoiesis occurs in central (bone marrow and thymus) and peripheral (lymph nodes, spleen, and mucosa-associated lymphoid tissue) lymphoid tissues
• Bone marrow pluripotential stem cells provide lymphoid stem cells that populate central lymphoid organs to form 2 functionally different populations; these cells then migrate to the peripheral lymphoid organs to give rise to T and B lymphocytes and possibly null cells
• B cells are involved in antigen presentation and the production of antigen-specific immunoglobulins
• Immunoglobulins are secreted by terminally differentiated B cells called plasma cells
• T cells regulate immune responses and are responsible for cell-mediated immunity
• Most lymphocytes in blood originate from the peripheral lymphoid tissues; both B and T cells circulate, although T cells are predominant
• <5% of the total body lymphocyte pool is in blood
• B and T cells cannot be differentiated on examination of a blood smear without special immunohistochemical staining
• Among leukocytes, a unique feature of lymphocytes (principally T cells) is the ability to recirculate between the blood and tissues; recirculation facilitates exposure of T cells to antigens in tissues and distribution of sensitized cells throughout the body for appropriate adaptive immune responses
• Antigenic reexposure triggers memory T and B cells and subsequent clonal

proliferation of effector T and B cells of the adaptive immune response
• The lymphocyte count in blood is influenced by rates of production, recirculation, utilization, and destruction

SYSTEMS AFFECTED

• Hemic/lymphatic/immune
• Involvement of other body systems is dependent on the underlying cause of the lymphocytosis
• Lymphoma may occur in generalized, multicentric, alimentary, cutaneous, or mediastinal (thymic) forms
• Leukemia (the presence of neoplastic lymphocytes in the blood) may be a result of primary bone marrow neoplasia, or may be secondary to lymphoma that has infiltrated the bone marrow

GENETICS

N/A

INCIDENCE/PREVALENCE

N/A

GEOGRAPHIC DISTRIBUTION

N/A

SIGNALMENT

• Variable
• Physiologic and reactive lymphocytosis are more common in young horses

SIGNS

General Comments

Clinical signs depend on the cause of the lymphocytosis.

Historical Findings

• Physiologic causes may be a result of endogenous epinephrine release due to excitement or intense exercise
• Diseases that result in chronic antigenic stimulation and lymphoma may be associated with a history of weight loss, lethargy, or inappetence

Physical Examination Findings

• Physiologic cause; increased heart rate, alert mentation
• Chronic antigenic stimulation and lymphoproliferative disorders; signs of organ dysfunction, pyrexia, weight loss
• Enlargement of peripheral lymph nodes may or may not be associated with lymphocytosis; when present, lymph node enlargement may be localized or generalized; generalized lymph node enlargement is indicative of severe systemic disease

CAUSES

Physiologic Causes

• Fear, excitement, or intense exercise
• Lymphocytosis is transient (<30 min) and occurs more frequently in horses <2 years of age
• Blood lymphocyte count may reach 15 000 cells/μL (15×10^9 cells/L), and concurrent neutrophilia is common
• Results from release of epinephrine and mobilization of rapidly accessible pool of

lymphocytes due to increased blood flow in the microvasculature
• In addition, uptake of lymphocytes by lymphoid tissues may be reduced

Chronic Antigenic Stimulation (Reactive Lymphocytosis)

• Bacterial infection, e.g. pneumonia, peritonitis, abscess
• Viral infection, e.g. EIA, EVA
• Fungal infection; less common than bacterial or viral infections
• Vaccination
• Reactive lymphocytes may be observed in peripheral blood smears

Neoplasia

• Lymphoid neoplasia; lymphoma or lymphocytic leukemia
• Occasionally, marked lymphocytosis may be observed (up to 250 000 cells/μL (250×10^9 cells/L))
• Morphology of circulating lymphocytes is variable and ranges from atypical, immature, or blast cells to well-differentiated lymphocytes
• Lymphocytic leukemia may be due to primary bone marrow neoplasia or secondary invasion of the bone marrow by lymphoma

DIAGNOSIS

DIFFERENTIAL DIAGNOSIS

The underlying cause of lymphocytosis (physiologic vs. inflammatory vs. neoplastic) should be determined.

CBC/BIOCHEMISTRY/URINALYSIS

• Lymphocyte count >5500 cells/μL (>5.5×10^9 cells/L)
• If a mature neutrophilia is concurrently observed, consider physiologic response or chronic antigenic stimulation
• If a left shift ± morphologic (toxic) changes in neutrophils are observed, consider inflammatory condition, especially bacterial infections
• The presence of antigenically stimulated lymphocytes (immunocytes) suggests inflammatory lymphocytosis
• If atypical, blast, or poorly differentiated lymphocytes are observed, consider acute lymphocytic leukemia; however, reactive lymphocytosis needs to be excluded
• Examination of peripheral blood smears by a veterinary hematologist may facilitate diagnosis
• If anemia, thrombocytopenia, and granulocytopenia are noted, consider myelophthisis due to lymphocytic leukemia or lymphoma with bone marrow involvement
• If IMHA or IMTP is present, consider lymphoma
• If hypercalcemia is reported, consider lymphoma (paraneoplastic syndrome due to

L

LYMPHOCYTOSIS

release of parathyroid hormone-related peptide by neoplastic lymphocytes)
• If hyperglobulinemia is present, consider chronic antigenic stimulation or neoplasia

OTHER LABORATORY TESTS
• Serum protein electrophoresis to determine if a polyclonal or monoclonal gammopathy is present; if polyclonal, consider chronic antigenic stimulation or neoplasia; if monoclonal, consider lymphoma or multiple myeloma
• Flow cytometry to identify surface antibody deposition in cases of IMHA or IMTP
• Agar gel immunodiffusion/ELISA for EIA
• Serology for EVA or other viral, bacterial, or fungal infections
• Quantification of individual immunoglobulin classes; horses with lymphoma may have abnormal immunoglobulin levels

IMAGING
• Ultrasonography of the thorax and abdomen for detection of organomegaly, abscess, neoplasia, and cavitary effusion
• Radiography of the thorax for detection of pneumonia, abscess, or lymphoma
• Radiography of the skeleton for detection of inflammatory or neoplastic lesions
• Scintigraphy using radiolabeled autologous neutrophils for detection of occult abscesses

OTHER DIAGNOSTIC PROCEDURES
• Biopsy and histopathology of enlarged lymph nodes or organs deemed abnormal by diagnostic imaging; fine needle aspirates are rarely diagnostic for lymphoma
• Rectal or duodenal biopsy for detection of diffuse gastrointestinal lymphoma
• Abdominocentesis, thoracocentesis, or cerebrospinal fluid collection to determine if inflammatory or neoplastic processes are present; depending on localizing signs
• Bone marrow biopsy if lymphoma or myelophthisic disorders are suspected
• Laparoscopy/thoracoscopy for exploration and biopsy

PATHOLOGIC FINDINGS
• Dependent on the underlying cause
• Histopathology of lymphoma reveals sheets of round cells that replace the normal architecture of affected organs/tissues; round cells can be classified as B or T cells using immunophenotyping

TREATMENT
AIMS
Vary with the nature of the underlying cause and may include elimination of infection, resolution of inflammation, or treatment of neoplasia; medical and/or surgical treatment may be required.

APPROPRIATE HEALTH CARE
• Physiologic causes of lymphocytosis require no treatment
• Reactive lymphocytosis associated with vaccination requires no treatment
• Inpatient medical and/or surgical management of horses with reactive lymphocytosis (due to infection) or neoplasia may be required
• Radiation therapy can be used for treatment of solitary lymphoma

NURSING CARE
Dependent on the underlying cause.

ACTIVITY
Dependent on the underlying cause.

DIET
N/A

CLIENT EDUCATION
• Persistent lymphocytosis often denotes the presence of an underlying disease that will require appropriate diagnostic assessment and treatment
• Lymphoma has a poor long-term prognosis

SURGICAL CONSIDERATIONS
Dependent on the underlying cause.

MEDICATIONS
DRUG(S) OF CHOICE
• Bacterial or fungal infections require antimicrobial therapy based on culture and sensitivity testing
• Chemotherapy in the form of single or multidrug protocols may result in clinical remission of lymphoma for a period of time
• Corticosteroid therapy often results in palliation of clinical signs of lymphoma

CONTRAINDICATIONS
Avoid corticosteroids in cases with infectious disease or laminitis.

PRECAUTIONS
Use of cytotoxic drugs requires appropriate use of personal protection equipment during preparation, administration, and disposal to minimize exposure of personnel to the drugs

POSSIBLE INTERACTIONS
N/A

ALTERNATIVE DRUGS
N/A

FOLLOW-UP
PATIENT MONITORING
Serial monitoring of CBC and lymphocyte morphology.

PREVENTION/AVOIDANCE
N/A

POSSIBLE COMPLICATIONS
N/A

EXPECTED COURSE AND PROGNOSIS
• Depends on the underlying cause
• Reactive lymphocytosis resolves with removal of chronic antigenic stimulation
• Prognosis for lymphoproliferative disorders is poor for long-term survival

MISCELLANEOUS
ASSOCIATED CONDITIONS
N/A

AGE-RELATED FACTORS
• Lymphocyte counts increase gradually after birth over the first 3 months
• Physiologic lymphocytosis is more common in horses <2 years of age

ZOONOTIC POTENTIAL
None

PREGNANCY/FERTILITY/BREEDING
Mares that are suspected of having lymphoma should not be bred.

SEE ALSO
• Lymphadenopathy
• Lymphosarcoma
• Pancytopenia

ABBREVIATIONS
• EIA = equine infectious anemia
• EVA = equine viral arteritis
• IMHA = immune-mediated hemolytic anemia
• IMTP = immune-mediated thrombocytopenia
• WBC = while blood cell

Suggested Reading
Latimer KS. Diseases affecting leukocytes. In: Colahan PT, Merritt AM, Moore JN, eds. Equine Medicine and Surgery, 5e. St. Louis, MO: Mosby, 1999:2025–2034.
Latimer KS, Prasse KW. Leukocytes. In: Latimer KS, Mahaffey EA, Prasse KW, eds. Duncan & Prasse's Veterinary Laboratory Medicine Clinical Pathology, 4e. Ames, IA: Blackwell, 2003:54–79.
Author Krista Estell
Consulting Editors David Hodgson, Harold C. McKenzie, and Jennifer L. Hodgson
Acknowledgment The author and editors acknowledge the prior contribution of Kristopher Hughes.

BASICS

OVERVIEW
• Lymphocyte count in peripheral blood less than the lower limit of the laboratory reference interval; usually <1500 cells/µL
• Lymphocyte count can change rapidly owing to physiologic influences, disease, or administration of drugs
• Lymphopenia can be caused by corticosteroids, acute infectious disease, increased loss, or decreased production

SIGNALMENT
Hereditary (primary) immunodeficiencies have breed, age, and sex predilections but other causes of lymphopenia have none.

SIGNS
Dependent on cause.

CAUSES AND RISK FACTORS

Corticosteroid Induced
• Endogenous (stress) or exogenous corticosteroids predictably induce lymphopenia
• Mechanism involves redistribution of circulating lymphocytes (predominantly T cells) with transient sequestration in lymphoid tissues or bone marrow
• Prolonged high doses of corticosteroid administration may cause lympholysis of thymic cortical lymphocytes and uncommitted lymphocytes in lymph nodes; effector B and T cells are resistant

Acute Inflammation and Infection
• Viral infections, e.g. equine influenza, equine herpesvirus, equine coronavirus
• Bacterial diseases, e.g. bacteremia, peritonitis, pleuropneumonia; mechanisms may involve endogenous corticosteroid release (stress), sequestration of lymphocytes in lymphoid and other tissues, and trapping of recirculating lymphocytes in lymph nodes
• Rickettsial infections, e.g. *Anaplasma phagocytophilum*, *Neorickettsia risticii* (Potomac horse fever)
• Protozoal infections, e.g. equine piroplasmosis (*Theileria equi* and *Babesia caballi*)

Increased Loss
Loss of lymphocyte-rich lymph into the thorax (chylothorax); rare in horses.

Decreased Production
• Hereditary (primary) immunodeficiencies
• Cytotoxic chemotherapeutic agents (e.g. azathioprine, cyclophosphamide, cyclosporine (ciclosporin), and tacrolimus) suppress clonal lymphocyte proliferation
• Radiation kills rapidly dividing cells
• Copper and vitamin A deficiencies
• Iron toxicity is associated with multifocal lymphoid necrosis
• Protein-calorie malnutrition induces T-cell lymphopenia; B-lymphocyte function and humoral immunity unaffected
• Neoplasia (e.g. lymphoma) disrupting lymph node architecture

DIAGNOSIS

CBC/BIOCHEMISTRY/URINALYSIS
• Lymphocyte count <1500 cells/µL ($<1.5 \times 10^9$ cells/L)
• Concurrent neutrophilia and eosinopenia suggest endogenous (stress) or exogenous (iatrogenic) corticosteroids
• Presence of neutropenia/neutrophilia, increased band neutrophil count, toxic changes in neutrophils, and elevated acute-phase protein concentration (e.g. fibrinogen, serum amyloid A) are consistent with acute infection
• Persistent marked lymphopenia (<1000 cells/µL ($<1.0 \times 10^9$ cells/L)) consistent with SCID and common variable immunodeficiency

OTHER LABORATORY TESTS
• Genetic testing (PCR) for SCID
• Lymphocyte subtyping via flow cytometry; normally 18% B lymphocytes, 62% CD4+ T cells, and 18% CD8+ T cells

IMAGING
Ultrasonography and/or radiography of the thorax or abdomen.

OTHER DIAGNOSTIC PROCEDURES
Abdominocentesis, thoracocentesis, cerebrospinal fluid collection, or blood culture if infectious disease is suspected.

PATHOLOGIC FINDINGS
Dependent on underlying cause.

TREATMENT
• Corticosteroid-induced lymphopenia does not require treatment
• Lymphopenia associated with acute infection, increased loss, or decreased production usually require medical treatment until underlying condition is stabilized

MEDICATIONS

DRUG(S) OF CHOICE
Bacterial infections require antimicrobial therapy based on culture and sensitivity testing.

CONTRAINDICATIONS/POSSIBLE INTERACTIONS
N/A

FOLLOW-UP

PATIENT MONITORING
• Serial monitoring of the CBC and lymphocyte count
• Persistent marked lymphopenia without identification of an underling etiology consistent with a primary immunodeficiency

PREVENTION/AVOIDANCE
N/A

POSSIBLE COMPLICATIONS
Acquired secondary infections due to impaired immunologic function.

EXPECTED COURSE AND PROGNOSIS
• Dependent on underlying cause
• Corticosteroid-induced lymphopenia occurs within a few hours of corticosteroid exposure, is transient, and usually resolves within 24 h
• Persistent lymphopenia is a poor prognostic indicator while progressive increase in lymphocyte counts represent recovery
• Hereditary (primary) immunodeficiencies are invariably fatal

MISCELLANEOUS

ASSOCIATED CONDITIONS
Acute viral/bacterial infections.

AGE-RELATED FACTORS
Lymphocyte counts normally low in foals in first week of postnatal period, then increase gradually over next 3 months in normal foals.

ZOONOTIC POTENTIAL
None

PREGNANCY/FERTILITY/BREEDING
N/A

SEE ALSO
• Immunoglobulin deficiencies
• Severe combined immunodeficiency

ABBREVIATIONS
• PCR = polymerase chain reaction
• SCID = severe combined immunodeficiency

Suggested Reading
Latimer KS, Mahaffey EA, Prasse KW, eds. Duncan & Prasse's Veterinary Laboratory Medicine—Clinical Pathology, 4e. Ames, IA: Blackwell, 2003.

Author Jamie G. Wearn
Consulting Editors David Hodgson, Harold C. McKenzie, and Jennifer L. Hodgson
Acknowledgment The author and editors acknowledge the prior contribution of Kristopher Hughes.

LYMPHOSARCOMA

BASICS

DEFINITION
Malignant, neoplastic disorder of lymphoid tissue.

PATHOPHYSIOLOGY
• Neoplastic cells in equine lymphoid tumors are primarily of B or T cells
• Equine lymphoid tumors have been classified as T-cell-rich large B-cell lymphoma (most common), peripheral T-cell lymphoma, diffuse large B-cell lymphoma, cutaneous T-cell lymphoma, and anaplastic T-cell lymphoma

SYSTEMS AFFECTED
• 4 forms of equine lymphosarcoma described based on location of tumors—multicentric (generalized); intestinal (alimentary); mediastinal (thymic); and cutaneous
• Lymphocytic leukemia secondary to lymphosarcoma is rare and characterized by presence of mild to moderate numbers of atypical lymphocytes in blood
• Most common sites for tumors include peripheral and internal lymph nodes, skin/subcutis, spleen, liver, intestine, kidneys, mediastinum, heart, and lungs
• More rarely nervous, ocular, and reproductive

GENETICS
N/A

INCIDENCE/PREVALENCE
Most common tumor of equine hemolymphatic system, but prevalence is <5%.

GEOGRAPHIC DISTRIBUTION
Worldwide

SIGNALMENT
• Most common in horses 5–10 years of age, with range from aborted fetus to 25 years
• No sex predilections, but cutaneous lymphosarcoma more common in Thoroughbreds

SIGNS

General Comments
• Clinical signs may be caused by—organ and tissue dysfunction due to infiltration of tumor lymphocytes; physical obstruction from tumor masses; or cytokines released by tumor cells
• Space-occupying masses may cause compression and impairment of venous and lymphatic circulation, causing edema or intracavitary fluid collection
• Clinical signs are variable; depend on organ or system affected by neoplastic infiltrate; may have gradual or sudden onset, but often progress slowly over weeks to months
• Some horses with lymphosarcoma have compromised humoral or cellular immunity, which may predispose to secondary infection

Historical Findings
• Chief complaints include signs of dullness, weight loss, inappetence, and decreased performance
• History of weight loss in intestinal (alimentary) form due to poor absorption, loss of protein, colic, or diarrhea

Physical Examination Findings
• Most common findings include fever, poor body condition, pallor of mucous membranes, ventral edema, and enlarged lymph nodes, which may be internal, external, regional, or generalized
• Alimentary form may see ventral edema
• Mediastinal (thymic) form may cause tachypnea, dyspnea, dysphagia/esophageal reflux, distended jugular/pulse, and pleural effusion
• Cutaneous form may present with single or multiple dermal or subcutaneous nodules (1–20 cm diameter) covered with hair, not painful or warm to touch
• Nodules may appear suddenly, grow slowly, remain static, or regress and recur
• Local lymph nodes often enlarged, but metastasis to internal organs is rare

CAUSES
Viral association has been proposed, but cause and effect not been confirmed.

RISK FACTORS
Infection with viruses (e.g. equine herpesvirus) may predispose to lymphosarcoma.

DIAGNOSIS

DIFFERENTIAL DIAGNOSIS
• Chronic inflammatory diseases may present with signs of dullness, inappetence, weight loss, fever, pallor, and ventral edema
• Clinical presentation of inflammatory bowel disease is similar to intestinal lymphosarcoma due to loss of absorption and protein-losing enteropathy; histologic distinction between lymphocytic–plasmacytic enteritis and lymphosarcoma can be challenging
• Infectious diseases including equine infectious anemia and babesiosis (piroplasmosis) can cause fever, pallor, and weight loss
• Immune-mediated hemolytic anemia and immune-mediated thrombocytopenia may be associated with lymphosarcoma
• Borrelia-associated cutaneous pseudolymphoma resembles histologically cutaneous lymphosarcoma or lymphoid hyperplasia

CBC/BIOCHEMISTRY/URINALYSIS
• Laboratory findings are variable, often nonspecific, and usually indicate a chronic inflammatory condition
• CBC reveals neutrophilic leukocytosis, hyperfibrinogenemia, and anemia
• Lymphocyte counts are normal or mildly decreased; reactive lymphocytes on a peripheral blood smear are common, but lymphocytic leukemia with atypical and/or increased lymphocyte counts is rare
• Biochemistry reveals hypoalbuminemia and hyperglobulinemia; either inflammatory globulins, polyclonal gammopathy (common), or a monoclonal gammopathy (rare)
• Hypercalcemia associated with pseudohyperparathyroidism of malignancy occurs occasionally
• Low serum levels of immunoglobulin M reported, but in <50% of horses, and positive predictive value for lymphosarcoma is low
• Increased activities of liver-derived enzymes may be caused by neoplastic infiltration of liver

OTHER LABORATORY TESTS
• In cases of concomitant leukemia, aspiration of bone marrow may reveal myelophthisis characterized by decreased red and white blood cell precursors and infiltration by neoplastic lymphocytes
• Oral glucose or xylose absorption tests may be abnormal due to neoplastic infiltration of small intestine
• Coombs test verifies immune-mediated hemolytic anemia and platelet factor 3 test is an indirect test for immune-mediated thrombocytopenia

IMAGING
• Thoracic US examination for pleural effusion and enlargement of lymph nodes; thoracic radiographs may reveal metastasis but false-negative results are possible
• Abdominal US examination for ascites, enlargement/infiltration of lymph nodes, spleen, liver, and kidneys, and increased intestinal wall thickness

OTHER DIAGNOSTIC PROCEDURES
• Rectal palpation and thoracic radiographs may reveal intracavitary masses and enlarged lymph nodes
• Definitive diagnosis of lymphosarcoma based on observation of neoplastic lymphocytes in aspirate or biopsies from a lymph node or fluid collected from the thoracic or abdominal cavity, cerebrospinal fluid, or aqueous humor
• For intestinal lymphosarcoma, mucosal samples can be collected via duodenoscopy and rectal biopsies; chances of achieving a diagnosis increases in diffuse disease
• Histologic examination of biopsies is preferred as it may be difficult to differentiate neoplastic versus reactive lymphocytes in cytologic evaluation of aspirates; imprint smears of biopsies directly on glass slides improves diagnosis
• Immunophenotyping can be performed in cytologic and histologic samples in order to characterize type of tumor (e.g. B or T cell); these data can be used to determine tumor

severity, progression, treatment choices, and prognosis
• Laparoscopy, exploratory laparotomy, or postmortem examination may be required to make a definitive diagnosis

PATHOLOGIC FINDINGS
• Gross lesions include lymphadenomegaly and neoplastic masses in the spleen, liver, kidney, intestine, heart, lung, thymus, and/or skin
• Affected lymph nodes are white-gray and glisten on cut surface
• Cytologic and histologic findings reveal variably sized lymphocytes that are larger and darker staining (cytoplasmic basophilia) than normal, contain a variable nucleus to cytoplasm ratio, prominent or multiple nucleoli, clumping of nuclear chromatin, indented or binucleate nuclei, and mitotic figures
• Histologically, the neoplastic cellular morphology varies, but destruction of normal tissue architecture by a population of lymphoid cells aids diagnosis

TREATMENT

AIMS
To reduce the size of neoplastic tissue while minimizing normal tissue damage, systemic effects, toxicity, and acquired drug resistance of tumor cells.

APPROPRIATE HEALTH CARE
Combination therapy, such as surgical removal, chemotherapy, and/or radiation therapy, has been increasingly used for lymphosarcoma in horses.

NURSING CARE
In-house care may be required for horses undergoing chemotherapy and/or radiation therapy.

ACTIVITY
N/A

DIET
N/A

CLIENT EDUCATION
Caution owners about poor prognosis.

SURGICAL CONSIDERATIONS
Surgical removal of a solitary masses (e.g. cutaneous, intestinal, or splenic mass) may prolong life of horses without evidence of metastasis.

MEDICATIONS

DRUG(S) OF CHOICE
• Drug choice or treatment protocols based on type of tumor (phenotype) not yet available for horses

• Chemotherapeutic agents including cytarabine, cyclophosphamide, vincristine, doxorubicin, L-asparaginase, and lomustine, used in various combination protocols, and in conjunction with prednisolone administered orally daily
• Cutaneous form of lymphosarcoma is responsive to oral administration of dexamethasone or prednisolone, but cutaneous or subcutaneous masses may recur (potentially more aggressive and rapidly progressive) in horses treated with systemic glucocorticoids for inadequate periods
• Response to progestin (altrenogest) or progestogen (megestrol) treatment has shown variable results
• Intralesional cisplatin suspended in sesame oil has been used successfully to treat solitary cutaneous masses
• Glucocorticoids used to treat concomitant immune-mediated hemolytic anemia or immune-mediated thrombocytopenia

CONTRAINDICATIONS
N/A

PRECAUTIONS
• Prolonged glucocorticoid and/or combination chemotherapy may cause adverse reactions
• Horses should be monitored to assess side effects, such as infections, gastrointestinal ulcers, kidney disease, cardiotoxicity, bone marrow suppression, and other organ dysfunction

POSSIBLE INTERACTIONS
N/A

ALTERNATIVE DRUGS
N/A

FOLLOW-UP

PATIENT MONITORING
Reduction in size of lymph node(s) or mass(es) and improved attitude, appetite, and weight gain can indicate positive response to treatment.

PREVENTION/AVOIDANCE
N/A

POSSIBLE COMPLICATIONS
Infections due to immunosuppression, side effects, and organ failure due to drug toxicity, and resistance of tumoral cells to drugs (recurrence).

EXPECTED COURSE AND PROGNOSIS
• Prognosis for a horse with multicentric, intestinal, or mediastinal forms of lymphosarcoma is poor; most untreated horses do not live beyond 6 months after diagnosis
• Treatment of horses with these forms using combination chemotherapy may prolong the life by a few months

• Horses with the cutaneous form of lymphosarcoma have a better prognosis and a longer clinical course; lesions may regress spontaneously or with treatment and patients can survive beyond 6 months post diagnosis

MISCELLANEOUS

ASSOCIATED CONDITIONS
• Lymphocytic–plasmacytic inflammatory bowel disease
• Lymphadenopathy
• Immune-mediated hemolytic anemia
• Immune-mediated thrombocytopenia
• Immunosuppression

AGE-RELATED FACTORS
Alimentary form more common in younger horses.

ZOONOTIC POTENTIAL
None

PREGNANCY/FERTILITY/BREEDING
• Combination chemotherapy may pose a risk to the fetus, especially when administered during the first trimester
• Combination chemotherapy administered during months 6–11 of pregnancy and discontinued 1 week prior to foaling had no adverse effects on foal

SYNONYMS
Malignant lymphoma, lymphoma, lymphoid tumor.

SEE ALSO
• Immunoglobulin deficiencies
• Lymphadenopathy

ABBREVIATIONS
US = ultrasonography, ultrasound

Suggested Reading
Ness SA. Lymphoma. In: Felippe MJB, ed. Equine Clinical Immunology. Ames, IA: Wiley Blackwell, 2016:181–191.
Author M. Julia B. Felippe
Consulting Editors David Hodgson, Harold C. McKenzie, and Jennifer L. Hodgson
Acknowledgment The author and editors acknowledge the prior contribution of W. Kent Scarratt.

L

MAGNESIUM (MG^{2+})

BASICS

OVERVIEW
- Essential for cellular energy-dependent reactions involving ATP
- Important in the regulation of Ca^{2+} channel function
- Ionized Mg^{2+} is the active form
- Pathophysiology
  ◦ Approximately 99% of total Mg^{2+} is intracellular or bone deposited, with only 1% in extracellular fluid (serum)
  ◦ Approximately 60% of total Mg^{2+} is found in bone, 20% in muscle, and 20% in other soft tissues including the liver
  ◦ Approximately 70% of serum Mg^{2+} is ionized (active) while 30% is protein bound
  ◦ Extracellular Mg^{2+} depends on GI absorption renal excretion/reabsorption, and bone exchange, although Mg^{2+} is poorly mobilized from bone
  ◦ PTH increases Mg^{2+} absorption in the GI tract and resorption in the kidneys. Mg^{2+} renal reabsorption increases with activation of arginine vasopressin, β-adrenergic agonists, insulin, and PTH
  ◦ Renal reabsorption of Mg^{2+} decreases with hyperglycemia, hypercalcemia, hypermagnesemia, and hypophosphatemia
- Systems affected—neurologic; cardiovascular; gastrointestinal; musculoskeletal

SIGNALMENT
Dependent on the underlying cause.

SIGNS
Historical Findings
Dependent on the underlying cause.

Physical Examination Findings
- Clinical signs associated with hypomagnesemia are uncommon unless severe
- Clinical signs of hypermagnesemia are attributed to concurrent increases in other electrolytes
- Colic from ileus
- Weakness, muscle fasciculations, ataxia, seizures, and coma
- Severe hypomagnesemia can cause ventricular or supraventricular arrhythmias, or atrial fibrillation
- Hypomagnesemia and hypocalcemia can cause synchronous diaphragmatic flutter

CAUSES AND RISK FACTORS
Hypomagnesemia
- Anorexia
- Decreased GI absorption (e.g. infiltrative GI disease, enteritis)
- Renal loss (e.g. renal disease, diuretics, aminoglycoside administration)
- Prolonged exercise (i.e. loss through sweat)
- Sepsis/endotoxemia
- Lactation
- Hypersalivation

Hypermagnesemia
- Dehydration
- Iatrogenic

DIAGNOSIS

DIFFERENTIAL DIAGNOSIS
- Muscle fasciculations—hypocalcemia, West Nile virus, weakness
- Weakness—equine motor neuron disease, botulism
- Atrial fibrillation—exercise (high vagal tone), heart failure, atrioventricular valve insufficiency, electrolyte disturbance
- Ventricular arrhythmia—oleander toxicosis, heart failure, electrolyte disturbance

CBC/BIOCHEMISTRY/URINALYSIS
CBC
Dependent on the underlying cause.

Biochemistry
- Hypo- or hypermagnesemia, depending on the underlying cause
- Hypoalbuminemia leads to hypomagnesemia
- Hypomagnesemia contributes to hypokalemia due to hypomagnesemia-induced decreases in ATP
- Hypomagnesemia contributes to hypocalcemia, likely through decreased PTH
- Acidosis increases serum Ca^{2+} and Mg^{2+} concentrations due to displacement by H$^+$ on albumin-binding sites
- Alkalosis decreases serum Ca^{2+} and Mg^{2+} concentrations due to increased albumin binding

Urinalysis
Fractional clearance of Mg^{2+} can be assessed.

OTHER LABORATORY TESTS
N/A

IMAGING
N/A

OTHER DIAGNOSTIC PROCEDURES
ECG (Hypomagnesemia)
- Prolongation of PR interval
- Widening of QRS complex
- ST segment depression
- Peaked T waves
- Atrial fibrillation or ventricular arrhythmias might be present

TREATMENT
Directed at the underlying cause.

DIET
Provide adequate dietary Mg^{2+}.

MEDICATIONS

DRUG(S) OF CHOICE
- Recommended dose rates for MgSO$_4$ in adult horses are 25–150 mg/kg/day (0.05–0.3 mL/kg of a 50% solution) diluted to a 5% solution in isotonic fluids IV
- An IV constant rate infusion of 150 mg/kg/day of 50% MgSO$_4$ solution (0.3 mL/kg/day) provides daily requirements
- Mg^{2+} supplementation should be considered in horses with diarrhea or postoperative ileus
- MgSO$_4$ is used to treat ventricular arrhythmias, including those secondary to quinidine administration. For ventricular arrhythmias, IV administration of 2–6 mg/kg/min of MgSO$_4$ to effect is recommended

FOLLOW-UP

PATIENT MONITORING
Serial biochemical analyses to monitor disease process.

POSSIBLE COMPLICATIONS
Hypomagnesemia
- Colic (ileus)
- Cardiac arrest

MISCELLANEOUS

SEE ALSO
- Calcium, hypercalcemia
- Ileus
- Protein, hypoproteinemia
- Ptyalism

ABBREVIATIONS
- GI = gastrointestinal
- PTH = parathyroid hormone

Suggested Reading
Berlin D, Aroch I. Concentrations of ionized and total magnesium and calcium in healthy horses: effects of age, pregnancy, lactation, pH and sample type. Vet J 2009;181:305–311.
Stewart AJ. Magnesium disorders in horses. Vet Clin North Am Equine Pract 2011;27:149–163.
Toribio RE. Magnesium and disease. In: Reed SM, Bayly WM, Sellon DC, eds. Equine Internal Medicine, 3e. St. Louis, MO: WB Saunders, 2010:1291–1297.

Author Jenifer R. Gold
Consulting Editor Sandra D. Taylor

M

BASICS

OVERVIEW

• Serum magnesium concentration above or below the reference range. • Pathophysiology ○ Magnesium helps regulate calcium channels and is necessary for nerve conduction and ion transportation. ○ Since <1% of the magnesium is in the serum, serum concentration may not be a good measure of total body magnesium. ○ Free ionized magnesium is the physiologically active form and is the more sensitive test for hypomagnesemia. Ionized magnesium is becoming easier to measure with ion-sensitive electrodes. ○ Magnesium is present in many digestive secretions and could be lost in the feces if absorption does not keep up. ○ Magnesium is secreted into milk, which makes lactating mares more susceptible. ○ Hypomagnesemia results in increased neuromuscular activity, hyperirritability, tachycardia, and decreased release of parathyroid hormone. • Systems affected—neuromuscular; nervous; endocrine/metabolic; cardiovascular

SIGNALMENT

• Lactating mares. • Hard-working or transported draft horses. • Endurance horses. • Horses with blister beetle toxicosis. • Anorexic horses

SIGNS

• Muscle fasciculations. • Weakness. • Ventricular arrhythmias, atrial tachycardia, or atrial fibrillation. • Synchronous diaphragmatic flutter if ionized calcium is also low. • Tetany is less likely in horses than in cattle

CAUSES AND RISK FACTORS

• Insufficient intake due to anorexia along with continued loss in intestinal secretions. • IV fluid therapy with solutions without magnesium (i.e. lactated Ringer's solution). • Severe and painful gastrointestinal disturbances, may be related to increased endotoxins. • Lactation and loss of magnesium in the milk along with inadequate diet. • Exhaustion from endurance rides or long-term transportation with inadequate diet—the typical equine diet with green forage usually supplies adequate magnesium (13 mg/kg body weight/day); this makes anorexia an important factor

DIAGNOSIS

DIFFERENTIAL DIAGNOSIS

• Any condition manifesting neuromuscular abnormalities. • Other causes of cardiac arrhythmias. • Eclampsia in mares that have nursed a foal

LABORATORY FINDINGS

Valid if Run in a Human Laboratory?
Yes

CBC/BIOCHEMISTRY/URINALYSIS

• Low concentration of serum magnesium (e.g. total Mg <0.62 mmol/L, 1.5 mg/dL or ionized Mg^{2+} <0.42 mmol/L, 1.02 mg/dL in adults). • Normal values may vary slightly with age, pregnancy, and lactation. • Hemolysis may increase serum magnesium concentration. • Most laboratories will list their own normal range. • Calcium levels are related to magnesium—hypercalcemia reduces serum ionized magnesium levels; hypocalcemia may accentuate the signs of hypomagnesemia. • Total serum magnesium may be reduced if low serum albumin. • Increased pH will lower concentration of ionized magnesium

OTHER LABORATORY TESTS

• Low fractional excretion of magnesium indicates dietary deficiency or lack of absorption. • High fractional excretion of magnesium indicates renal loss. • Vitreous humor magnesium levels are accurate up to 2 days postmortem

DIAGNOSTIC PROCEDURES

An ECG will help detect or analyze any arrhythmias.

TREATMENT

Initiate treatment of the underlying cause or the condition will persist.

MEDICATIONS

DRUG(S) OF CHOICE

• If the serum magnesium level is low enough to cause clinical signs, administer 5% solution of $MgSO_4$ in water or glucose, IV slowly. • Up to 64 mg/kg body weight of $MgSO_4$ can be given safely IV over a 60 min period. • Total amount of $MgSO_4$ should be limited to 150 mg/kg body weight/day. • $MgSO_4$ at 4–16 mg/kg body weight can be added to each 5 L bag of IV fluids. • Up to 8 L of fluid containing $MgSO_4$ (Epsom salts) can be given by nasogastric tube every 30 min to a 500 kg horse; however, excess $MgSO_4$ could cause diarrhea and this volume could cause discomfort

CONTRAINDICATIONS/POSSIBLE INTERACTIONS

• Excess magnesium causes mild sedation and could further suppress an anesthetized horse.

• Do not give fluids by nasogastric tube if there is gastric reflux and the stomach is not emptying. • Magnesium can potentiate the toxic effect of aminoglycosides. • $MgSO_4$ is incompatible with sodium bicarbonate

FOLLOW-UP

PATIENT MONITORING

• Determine serum magnesium and calcium concentrations once or twice a day to detect overdosage or recurrence and 4–6 h after treatment. • ECG to monitor arrhythmias. • Monitor temperature, pulse and respiration and presenting physical signs during and after treatment

PREVENTION/AVOIDANCE

Include magnesium in IV fluids.

EXPECTED COURSE AND PROGNOSIS

Should recover with adequate supplementation.

MISCELLANEOUS

ASSOCIATED CONDITIONS

• Hypocalcemia. • Hypokalemia

Hypermagnesemia
Hypermagnesemia is usually iatrogenic and due to: • Magnesium-containing oral laxatives used in cases of impaction. • Excess magnesium-containing IV fluids

SYNONYMS

Transport tetany.

Suggested Reading
Borer KE, Corley KTT. Electrolyte disorders in horses with colic. Part 1: potassium and magnesium. Equine Vet Educ 2006;18:266–271.
Stewart AJ. Magnesium disorders in horses. Vet Clin North Am Equine Pract 2011;27:149–163.

Author Erwin G. Pearson
Consulting Editors Michel Levy and Heidi Banse

Client Education Handout available online

M

MALABSORPTION

 BASICS

DEFINITION
• Malabsorption or malassimilation from the intestine occurs when there is diffuse or localized intestinal disease that inhibits the transference of nutrients from the intestinal lumen to the vasculature
• Transient malabsorption occurs with enteritis caused by viral and bacterial agents
• Chronic malabsorption is caused by parasitism, infiltrative bowel diseases, amyloidosis, and neoplasia. Besides parasitism, the causes of chronic inflammatory bowel disease are uncommon
• The small intestine is usually affected in the chronic diseases; however, the large intestine may also be involved

PATHOPHYSIOLOGY
• Malabsorption is caused by loss of the intestinal absorptive area (villus atrophy), loss of absorptive villus epithelial cells, and enlargement of junctional areas between epithelial cells
• Thickening of the intestinal wall with edema, hypertrophy, inflammatory cells, or fibrous tissue inhibits the absorptive capacity
• Blockage of normal lymphatic drainage (lymphangiectasia) and decreased intestinal blood flow due to verminous arteritis may be involved
• Horses that have had extensive small intestinal resection may also suffer from malabsorption
• Viral and bacterial infections of the bowel wall can result in the temporary loss of the absorptive capacity of the small intestine
• Chronic malabsorption is caused by uncontrolled immune reactions (infiltrative bowel diseases, such as lymphocytic/plasmacytic enteritis, granulomatous enteritis, or eosinophilic granulomatous enteritis)
  ◦ The initiating factors in this group of diseases are unknown; however, allergens or infectious agents have been considered stimuli
  ◦ Chronic diseases include infections with *Mycobacterium avium, Mycobacterium avium* ssp. *paratuberculosis,* and fungi (*Aspergillus* spp., *Histoplasma* spp.)
  ◦ Alimentary neoplasia may also cause similar signs
• Transient malabsorption may result in short-term weight loss, delayed growth, and diarrhea. These problems should resolve once the infection and immune reaction subside and the intestines achieve normal structure and function
• The signs of chronic malabsorption persist; however, the progression and severity may vary. A hallmark of chronic disease is hypoproteinemia resulting from decreased protein intake (due to inappetence),

malabsorption of nutrients, and protein loss into the bowel. Decreased albumin production may occur due to negative feedback mechanisms in response to elevated globulin levels, thus maintaining plasma oncotic pressure. Other disease entities cause protein-losing enteropathy than malabsorptive diseases

SYSTEMS AFFECTED
GI
Normal feces or diarrhea if diffuse colonic involvement with weight loss.
Endocrine/Metabolic
Altered protein levels and ratios.
Hemic/Lymphatic/Immune
Lymphadenopathy with neoplasia or granulomatous disease.
Hepatobiliary
Decreased feed intake may cause mild increase in bilirubin; eosinophilic epitheliotropic disease may affect many organs, including the liver.
Musculoskeletal
• Weight loss
• Muscle atrophy
Skin/Exocrine
Owing to malnutrition, vasculitis, or inflammatory cell infiltration.
Behavioral
Mild depressed demeanor.

SIGNALMENT
Any breed or sex; younger horses usually involved (1–6 years).

SIGNS
• Colic
• Cutaneous lesions—alopecia; rough, dry haircoat
• Dermatitis
• Coronitis
• Depressed demeanor
• Diarrhea or normal feces
• Edema
• Lethargy
• Lymphadenopathy
• Pyrexia
• Weakness
• Weight loss

CAUSES
• Parasitic damage due to *Strongylus* spp. or cyathostomes. *Parascaris equorum* may cause disease in young horses
• Infiltrative diseases may be due to an allergic response or uncontrolled response to an infectious agent
• Proliferative enteropathy due to infection with *Lawsonia intracellularis* has been increasingly identified in the young horse (see chapter *Lawsonia intracellularis* infections in foals). This organism is occasionally identified as a cause of disease in the nonjuvenile horse. Familial occurrence has been reported
• The causes of alimentary neoplasia, such as lymphosarcoma, are unknown

 DIAGNOSIS

DIFFERENTIAL DIAGNOSIS
A detailed history and physical examination are required. Initially, common causes of weight loss should be considered, such as inadequate nutritional intake for metabolic demands (poor feed quality, bad dentition, competition for food). Many other diseases should be considered using a systematic approach.
Differential diagnoses for hypoproteinemia include:
• Decreased protein absorption (inadequate intake, gastroenteric disease), decreased production (liver failure), sequestration into third spaces (pleural cavity, peritoneal cavity, abscesses), or loss (alimentary or renal)
• Protein-losing enteropathy may be caused by acute/subacute colitis, parasitism, NSAID use, GI neoplasia (lymphosarcoma, adenocarcinoma), infiltrative bowel disease, tuberculosis, or congestive heart failure
• Chronic proliferative bowel disease is caused by *Lawsonia* infection and chronic infiltrative bowel disease is caused by lymphocytic/plasmacytic enteritis, eosinophilic granulomatous enteritis, and granulomatous enteritis

CBC/BIOCHEMISTRY/URINALYSIS
CBC
Common findings include neutrophilia, anemia (due to chronic inflammatory disease or blood loss from ulcerations), and hypoproteinemia. The neutrophil level can be high, normal, or low.
Biochemistry
• Hypoalbuminemia
• Globulin level—low, normal, or elevated
• Fibrinogen—mild elevation
• Hypocalcemia (due to loss of protein-bound calcium)
• Elevations of hepatobiliary parameters:
  ◦ γ-Glutamyltransferase
  ◦ Aspartate amino transferase
  ◦ Alkaline phosphatase
  ◦ Bilirubin (conjugated)
  ◦ Lactate dehydrogenase, glutamate dehydrogenase, inositol dehydrogenase (sorbitol dehydrogenase)
  ◦ Bile acids
  ◦ Serum amyloid A protein—normal to elevated
Urinalysis
Normal
Abdominal Fluid Analysis
Normal
Fecal Examination
Identification of large or small strongyles; if present, strongyles do not necessary pinpoint parasites as the cause of malabsorption.

 M

Ultrasonography
Determine thickness of wall of small intestine and the presence of masses.

Carbohydrate Absorption Tests
Horse should be fasted for at least 12 h but not >24 h. A blood sample should be collected before the administration of the sugar, then at 30 min intervals for up to 4 h. Water intake should be restricted for the initial 2 h of the test period. Low or no absorption levels are consistent with delayed gastric emptying, enteric disease, or delayed intestinal transit. In addition to absorption, distribution, metabolism, and excretion are important factors to consider.

D-Xylose Absorption Test
Give 0.5 g/kg as a 10% solution via nasogastric tube. Samples may be collected into heparinized tubes. A peak is expected at approximately 60 min.

Glucose Absorption Test
Give 1 g/kg as a 20% solution via nasogastric tube. Collect blood samples into tubes containing sodium fluoride to prevent cellular metabolism of glucose. Heparinized samples can be used if the glucose level is determined immediately after collection. Normal absorption is a 2-fold increase in the baseline glucose level within 90–120 min. Low levels may occur if there is metabolism of the glucose in the lumen. Levels also reflect the metabolic/endocrinologic status of the animal.

Rectal Mucosal Biopsy
Use uterine biopsy forceps or other instrument (bottle cap, syringe-case cap); collect mucosal sample from dorsal or lateral rectal wall in region of retroperitoneal space (30 cm orad to anus). Samples with infiltration of lymphocytes, plasmacytes, eosinophils, and/or histocytes may represent diffuse disease. Negative sample is nondiagnostic, necessitating intestinal biopsy.

Small Intestinal Biopsy
Requires general anesthesia, celiotomy, and full-thickness biopsies. Risks of anesthesia, surgery, and poor wound healing due to catabolic state with hypoalbuminemia. Laparoscopic techniques have been described.

TREATMENT
Symptomatic care or specific treatment for transient diseases.

DIET
Consider feeding highly digestible feed; high-protein feed; high-quality fiber should be fed for colonic digestion. Multiple small feedings should be given. Intestinal resection for localized small intestinal disease.

MEDICATIONS
DRUG(S) OF CHOICE
Anthelmintics
Treatment should be appropriate for the specific parasite; repeat treatment may be required for encysted stages of nematode:
• Ivermectin—0.2 mg/kg PO
• Moxidectin—0.4 mg/kg. Consider prior treatment with prednisolone or dexamethasone if treating for encysted cyathostomes
• Fenbendazole—10 mg/kg PO once daily for 5 days
• Pyrantel tartrate—2.2 mg/kg/day. Used as a preventative; other anthelmintics should be used to kill adult worms
• Note that anthelmintic resistance has become prevalent in some geographic areas. Treatment recommendations may be adjusted accordingly

Corticosteroids
• Infiltrative bowel disease
• Prednisolone—1–2 mg/kg PO, IM BID
• Dexamethasone—0.05–0.2 mg/kg PO SID or by parenteral administration

Antibiotics
Trimethoprim–sulfonamide 30 mg/kg PO or IV every 12 h.

CONTRAINDICATIONS
Corticosteroids have been associated with laminitis.

POSSIBLE INTERACTIONS
N/A

ALTERNATIVE DRUGS
N/A

FOLLOW-UP
PATIENT MONITORING
• Appetite
• Demeanor
• Feces
• Body condition

POSSIBLE COMPLICATIONS
Drug-associated (immunosuppression; laminitis; Cushing or Addison disease).

EXPECTED COURSE AND PROGNOSIS
• Parasitism—poor to good
• Infiltrative bowel disease—poor
• Neoplasia—poor

MISCELLANEOUS
ASSOCIATED CONDITIONS
N/A

AGE-RELATED FACTORS
N/A

ZOONOTIC POTENTIAL
May be possible if shedding mycobacterial organisms or *Salmonella* spp.

PREGNANCY/FERTILITY/BREEDING
Debilitation may lead to infertility, early embryonic death, or abortion.

SYNONYMS
• Chronic inflammatory bowel disease
• Granulomatous bowel disease
• Infiltrative bowel disease

SEE ALSO
Colic, chronic/recurrent

ABBREVIATIONS
• GI = gastrointestinal
• NSAID = nonsteroidal anti-inflammatory drug

Suggested Reading
Brown CM. The diagnostic value of the D-xylose absorption test in horses with unexplained chronic weight loss. Br Vet J 1992;148:41–44.
Kaikkonen R, Niinisto K, Sykes B, et al. Diagnostic evaluation and short-term outcome as indicators of long-term prognosis in horses with findings suggestive of inflammatory bowel disease treated with corticosteroid and anthelmintics. Acta Vet Scan 2014;56:35.
Kalck KA. Inflammatory bowel disease in horses. Vet Clin North Am Equine Pract 2009;25:303–315.
Lindberg R, Nygren A, Persson SG. Rectal biopsy diagnosis in horses with clinical signs of intestinal disorders: a retrospective study of 116 cases. Equine Vet J 1996;28:275–284.
MacAllister CG, Mosier D, Qualls Jr CW, Cowell RL. Lymphocytic-plasmacytic enteritis in two horses. J Am Vet Med Assoc 1990;196:1995–1998.
Schumacher J, Moll HD, Spano JS, et al. Effect of intestinal resection on two juvenile horses with granulomatous enteritis. J Vet Int Med 1990;4:153–156.
Sweeney RW. Laboratory evaluation of malassimilation in horses. Vet Clin North Am Equine Pract 1987;3:507–515.

Author Daniel G. Kenney
Consulting Editors Henry Stampfli and Olimpo Oliver-Espinosa

M

MALICIOUS INTOXICATION

BASICS

OVERVIEW
• Equine insurance mortality policies often contain exclusions, especially for death due to intoxication. It is critical to determine the cause and manner of death in order to substantiate claims and the ultimate liability of insurers
• A systematic postmortem examination to confirm death due to toxicant exposure, whether accidental or malicious
• Documentation of proper sample collection, storage, and laboratory submission is crucial

SIGNALMENT
N/A

SIGNS
• Signs vary considerably depending on the toxicant
• Toxicants used maliciously often causes rapid death, without specific postmortem lesions, and is difficult to detect in tissue or fluid samples
• Most toxicants that result in sudden death impair the central or peripheral nervous systems, cardiovascular system, or respiratory system
• Depending on the toxicant, there may be evidence of struggle before death
• Most malicious deaths follow a single administration of a highly toxic compound or mixture of compounds

CAUSES AND RISK FACTORS
• Potential toxicants include strychnine, phosphides, cholinesterase-inhibiting insecticides (organophosphates and carbamates), nicotine, metaldehyde, cyanide, fluoroacetate; illicit drugs such as amphetamines (amfetamines), cocaine, heroin, and morphine; metals such as mercury, arsenic, lead, selenium, and iron; drugs such as insulin, barbiturates, reserpine, and succinylcholine (suxamethonium); and electrolytes such as potassium or calcium
• Although less common, exposure to toxic plants such as *Nerium oleander*, *Taxus* spp., *Conium maculatum*, or *Cicuta* spp. should be considered, as should zootoxins such as cantharidin
• Mixtures of potent toxicants may be used

DIAGNOSIS

DIFFERENTIAL DIAGNOSIS
• Physical causes include trauma, electrocution, lightning strike, suffocation, heat stroke, and gunshot
• Natural or genetic causes include hyperkalemic periodic paralysis, cardiac conductive disturbances, acute myocardial necrosis, cerebral thromboembolism, aortic aneurysm or other vessel rupture, and neoplasia
• Infectious causes include acute clostridial diseases, salmonellosis, Tyzzer disease, anthrax, equine monocytic ehrlichiosis, foal actinobacillosis, and babesiosis
• Metabolic and nutritional causes include hypoglycemia, hypocalcemia, hypomagnesemia, and selenium deficiencies

CBC/BIOCHEMISTRY/URINALYSIS
Whole blood, serum, plasma, and urine should be collected prior to death if possible for clinical pathologic and toxicologic analysis.

OTHER LABORATORY TESTS
• Other samples for toxicologic analysis include stomach contents, urine, liver, kidney, brain, eye, and heart blood
• Tissue from around a suspected injection site
• Representative feed and water samples
• All samples should be handled under chain-of-custody procedures that identify all specimens, document their condition and container in which packaged, the time and date of transfer and receipt of samples, and all individuals involved in the handling, transferring, or receiving of samples
• Ancillary tests such as PCR and ELISA should be done to rule out infectious causes

DIAGNOSTIC PROCEDURES
Definitive analytical toxicology tests vary depending of the nature of the toxicant.

PATHOLOGIC FINDINGS
• Complete and thorough postmortem examination in a veterinary diagnostic facility. If not possible, a field postmortem should be conducted and any suspected abnormalities recorded and photographed
• Gastrointestinal contents should be examined carefully for evidence of toxic plant fragments or unexpected grain or forage ingestion
• Formalin-fixed samples should be collected from all major organ systems and any gross lesions and submitted to a veterinary pathologist for histopathologic examination

TREATMENT
Directed toward stabilization of vital organ systems. Once stabilized, oral and dermal decontamination procedures should be initiated if appropriate, including the administration of AC and a cathartic or washing skin. Antidotes are not available for many toxicants.

MEDICATIONS

DRUG(S) OF CHOICE
AC at 1–4 g/kg body weight in water slurry (1 g AC in 5 mL water) PO; 1 dose of cathartic PO with AC if no diarrhea or ileus (70% sorbitol at 3 mL/kg or sodium or $MgSO_4$ at 250–500 mg/kg). Administration of other drugs is dependent on each situation.

CONTRAINDICATIONS/POSSIBLE INTERACTIONS
N/A

FOLLOW-UP
Depends on the specific toxicant under suspicion or analytically confirmed.

PATIENT MONITORING
Dependent on the situation. Monitoring of vital functions is critical.

POSSIBLE COMPLICATIONS
Dependent on the toxicant involved.

EXPECTED COURSE AND PROGNOSIS
Dependent on the toxicant involved.

MISCELLANEOUS

ABBREVIATIONS
• AC = activated charcoal
• ELISA = enzyme-linked immunosorbent assay
• PCR = polymerase chain reaction

Suggested Reading
Haliburton JC, Edwards WC. Medicolegal investigation of the sudden or unexpected equine death: toxicologic implications. In: Robinson NE, ed. Current Therapy in Equine Medicine, 4e. Philadelphia, PA: WB Saunders, 1997:657.

Authors Arya Sobhakumari and Robert H. Poppenga
Consulting Editors Wilson K. Rumbeiha and Steve Ensley

BASICS

DEFINITION
Inflammation of the mammary gland most commonly caused by bacterial colonization within the gland; other causes may include neoplasia and mycotic infection.

PATHOPHYSIOLOGY
Initial infection may occur by hematogenous spread, adjacent dermatologic inflammation, or, most commonly, ascending infection via the teat canal. Bacterial colonization of the teat cistern does not always lead to mastitis, which suggests failure of the immune system locally or systemically. Inflammation may involve 1 or several lobes of 1 or both mammary glands. Cellular debris clogs the teat canal and leads to an increase in pressure within the gland, no effective drainage, and the infection may spread to surrounding tissues.

SYSTEMS AFFECTED
Reproductive

INCIDENCE/PREVALENCE
Incidence is low. Protective factors—frequent nursing by the foal, a short lactation period, and small teats.

SIGNALMENT
Most cases occur in lactating mares.

SIGNS
Historical Findings
Reluctance of the mare to allow the foal to nurse, depression, anorexia, and severe adverse behavior when udder is palpated.

Physical Examination Findings
- Enlarged or swollen mammary gland
- Heat or pain on palpation
- Abnormal mammary secretions
- Ventral edema
- Hindlimb lameness or gait change
- Signs of concurrent disease

CAUSES
Infectious
- Bacterial—most commonly *Streptococcus zooepidemicus;* others include *Staphylococcus, Actinobacillus, Pseudomonas, Klebsiella,* and *Escherichia coli*
- Fungal—*Aspergillus* spp. and *Coccidioides immitis*
- Other—aberrant parasitic migration

Noninfectious
Neoplasia—mammary adenocarcinoma.

RISK FACTORS
- Lactation, trauma, or manual manipulation of the teats
- Systemic disease that may spread to the mammary gland
- Local cellulitis, wounds, or *Culicoides* hypersensitivity
- Recent surgical incision
- Compromised foals or mares that require hand-milking

 DIAGNOSIS

DIFFERENTIAL DIAGNOSIS
Other Causes of Mammary Heat, Pain, or Abnormal Secretions
Abscess may be differentiated from diffuse mastitis by palpation or US. The udder may be painful if transiently distended, but this should resolve completely with stripping of the udder.

Other Causes of Abnormal Udder Development
Placentitis, impending parturition, or abortion.

CBC/BIOCHEMISTRY/URINALYSIS
Leukocytosis with neutrophilia, hyperfibrinogenemia, increased SAA, or anemia of chronic disease possible.

IMAGING
US

OTHER DIAGNOSTIC PROCEDURES
Samples from each teat cistern should be collected aseptically and submitted for aerobic culture and cytologic examination for definitive diagnosis. Gram-stain preparations of mammary secretions or milk may guide initial treatment. Anaerobes are not significant bacterial pathogens. Cytologic examination of milk—often acellular or contains rare neutrophils from normal, lactating mares; contains macrophages with vacuoles present (*foam cells*) and lymphocytes in the drying-off period; shows numerous intact and degenerated neutrophils and cellular debris, and may show large numbers of bacteria or fungal hyphae with mastitis. Mammary gland biopsy indicated if clinical signs are not responsive to initial treatment for bacterial infection, or if cytologic examination is not suggestive of infectious mastitis.

 TREATMENT

- Frequent stripping out of the affected lobes
- Hot packing
- Hydrotherapy
- Light exercise, to decrease edema formation
- Surgery to establish drainage from a mammary abscess, or mammectomy to remove suspected neoplasia

 MEDICATIONS

DRUG(S) OF CHOICE
- Antimicrobial agent is dictated by culture and sensitivity
- Trimethoprim–sulfadiazine (30 mg/kg every 12 h)—effective in 75% of cases; administer pending culture and sensitivity results. Penicillin with an aminoglycoside is effective in most cases (procaine penicillin 22 000 units/kg IM every 12 h, gentamicin 8.8 mg/kg IM every 24 h)

ALTERNATIVE DRUGS
Clean and disinfect teat orifice prior to local infusions with lactating cow intramammary treatments. Use caution—equine teat canal is smaller and shorter than the bovine.

 FOLLOW-UP

PATIENT MONITORING
Palpate udder and take rectal temperature daily. Treatment should continue for a minimum of 5–7 days or until 24 h after signs have resolved. If abnormalities in the peripheral blood exist, repeat CBC, fibrinogen, or SAA. Renal function should be monitored with long-term aminoglycoside and nonsteroidal administration.

POSSIBLE COMPLICATIONS
Sepsis, bacteremia, endotoxemia, laminitis, colitis, lymphadenopathy, lymphangitis, and fibrosis of the affected mammary glands with subsequent decreased milk production.

 MISCELLANEOUS

ABBREVIATIONS
- SAA = serum amyloid A
- US = ultrasonography, ultrasound

Suggested Reading
McCue PM, Wilson WD. Equine mastitis—a review of 28 cases. Equine Vet J 1989;2:351–353.

Author Jennifer K. Linton
Consulting Editor Ashley G. Boyle
Acknowledgment The author and editor acknowledge the prior contribution of Kerry Beckman.

M

MATERNAL FOAL REJECTION

BASICS

OVERVIEW
• 2 major forms—rejection of the foal's attempts to suckle and overt aggression toward the foal
• Because a mare's identification of her foal largely depends on smell, iatrogenic foal rejection can occur if the foal's odor changes because of extensive clinical treatments
• Can occur without any physical pathology; however, any painful condition (e.g. mastitis) may cause this behavior
• Systems affected—nervous: central nervous system; mechanism unknown.

SIGNALMENT
• More common in primiparous and Arabian mares but can occur in any breed at any age
• Most common immediately postpartum but can occur hours or months after initial acceptance

SIGNS
• Rejection of attempts to suckle—squealing by mare and signs of fear and avoidance, including repeatedly moving the hindquarters away from the foal or walking away from the foal, especially when the foal moves its head toward the teats
• Aggressive rejection—squealing by mare, head-threat (i.e. ears laid back against the neck), threatening to bite, biting, threatening to kick, kicking, threatening to strike, and striking

CAUSES AND RISK FACTORS
• Genetics may be a contributing factor; the problem has been identified as being more common in Arabians and in certain pedigrees
• Turgid udders and lack of experience in primiparous mares probably are the most relevant factors in failure to allow suckling with a first birth; the mare has not yet learned that allowing the foal to suckle relieves her discomfort
• First birth
• Arabians, especially if relatives have exhibited this behavior
• Previous foal rejection
• A highly disrupted environment or unusual circumstances at the time of birth

DIAGNOSIS

DIFFERENTIAL DIAGNOSIS
Any pathologic condition that might cause pain or discomfort (e.g. mastitis or musculoskeletal disease).

CBC/BIOCHEMISTRY/URINALYSIS
• Should be normal if the problem is purely behavioral

• Abnormalities supporting the diagnosis of a physical pathology suggest that rejecting behavior is secondary to pain

OTHER LABORATORY TESTS
N/A

IMAGING
N/A

OTHER DIAGNOSTIC PROCEDURES
N/A

TREATMENT

PRIMIPAROUS MARES
• Restraining the mare until the foal can suckle allows the mare to learn that suckling relieves the discomfort in her udder and familiarizes her with the process of standing for nursing
• Do not immediately remove the placenta and fluids from the area of birth, as odors from them stimulate normal maternal behavior
• Do not punish the mare. She is already fearful and punishment will exacerbate her fear

AGGRESSIVE MARES
• Restrain the mare to prevent injury of the foal. Cross-tying the mare still allows the mare to kick. Separating the foal and mare with a pole or partition allows the foal to reach under to suckle while the mare is held in place and reduces the likelihood she can kick the foal
• Provide close supervision for at least the first 24 h
• Restrain the mare during all interactions with the foal for at least 3 days; if the mare's behavior does not improve in 7 days, acceptance of the foal is unlikely
• If it is impossible for the foal to nurse during the first 8 h postpartum it must be given colostrum

MEDICATIONS

DRUG(S) OF CHOICE
• Acepromazine (0.02–0.06 mg/kg IV, IM, or SC every 2–4 h to effect)
• Butorphanol (0.05 mg/kg IV) to relieve pain from turgid udder; if no complicating painful conditions are present, do not repeat

CONTRAINDICATIONS/POSSIBLE INTERACTIONS
• Benzodiazepines (e.g. diazepam) are contraindicated in aggressive animals because these drugs may disinhibit aggression
• Administration of anxiolytics and progestins for foal rejection constitutes extra-label use, and owners should be so informed

• Review all side effects, and prepare an informed consent form for the owner to sign

ALTERNATIVE DRUGS
• Anxiolytics (e.g. diazepam) may help with fearful mares
• Progestins may help with aggressive mares

FOLLOW-UP

PATIENT MONITORING
Intensive monitoring until the mare consistently allows the foal to suckle and fails to show aggression for several hours.

POSSIBLE COMPLICATIONS
Inadequate supervision and restraint of an aggressive mare may result in injury to or death of the foal.

MISCELLANEOUS

ASSOCIATED CONDITIONS
Mastitis

AGE-RELATED FACTORS
Most common in primiparous mares.

ZOONOTIC POTENTIAL
N/A

PREGNANCY/FERTILITY/BREEDING
N/A

SYNONYMS
N/A

SEE ALSO
Aggression

Suggested Reading
Crowell-Davis SL, Houpt KA. Maternal behavior. Vet Clin North Am Equine Pract 1986;2:557–571.
Houpt KA. Foal rejection and other behavioral problems in the postpartum period. Compend Contin Educ Pract Vet 1984;6:S144–S148.
Houpt KA. Foal rejection—a review of 23 cases. Equine Pract 1984;6:38–40.
Houpt KA, Lieb S. A survey of foal rejecting mares. Appl Anim Behav Sci 1994;39:188.
Juarbe-Diaz SV, Houpt KA, Kusunose R. Prevalence and characteristics of foal rejection in Arabian mares. Equine Vet J 1998;30:424–428.
Tajik J, Kheirandish R. Aggression to a foal after 4 months of nursing. J Vet Behav 2014;9(3):136–139.

Author Sharon L. Crowell-Davis
Consulting Editor Victoria L. Voith

BASICS

DEFINITION
• Meconium refers to the fetal feces made up of cellular debris, amniotic fluid, intestinal secretions, and bile
• Meconium is normally passed within 3 h of birth, and is considered retained if the foal has not passed all meconium by 12 h after birth
• Most meconium impactions are in the small colon at the pelvic inlet, but they also occur in the right dorsal colon or transverse colon

PATHOPHYSIOLOGY
Delayed passage of meconium can create an obstruction in the distal small colon, resulting in discomfort and accumulation of gas orad to the obstruction. Colic pain and abdominal distention can lead to additional systemic effects secondary to hypoglycemia, ileus, and dehydration.

SYSTEMS AFFECTED
GI

GENETICS
N/A

INCIDENCE/PREVALENCE
Meconium impaction is the most common cause of colic in neonatal foals. No specific incidence rate has been reported.

GEOGRAPHIC DISTRIBUTION
N/A

SIGNALMENT
• All breeds
• Possible higher incidence in colts
• Neonatal foals, usually 6–36 h of age

SIGNS
• Abdominal pain (colic)—tail flagging, kicking at abdomen, rolling
• Straining to defecate; tenesmus—resulting in mild rectal prolapse and/or reopening of the urachus
• Failure to pass meconium. The foal may pass some meconium but retain enough meconium to cause an impaction
• Depression and decreased nursing
• More severe or advanced impactions can cause abdominal distention and severe signs of colic
• Initial signs are usually within 6–24 h of birth

CAUSES
• Narrow pelvic canal (more common in colts)
• Delayed colostrum ingestion
• Systemic disease, such as hypoxia or sepsis, can result in decreased intestinal motility
• Dehydration, prolonged recumbency, and drugs that slow GI motility may also contribute

RISK FACTORS
See Causes.

DIAGNOSIS

DIFFERENTIAL DIAGNOSIS
• Atresia coli—similar signs initially, but no meconium staining is seen after repeated enemas
• Intestinal aganglionosis (lethal white foal syndrome)—in white foals, offspring of overo Paint breeding; usually no meconium production
• Other GI causes of neonatal colic—enterocolitis, small intestinal volvulus, intussusception
• Uroperitoneum—foal may posture and strain in a similar manner; free fluid in abdomen and electrolyte abnormalities help to confirm uroabdomen. Excessive straining from meconium impaction causes bladder tears in some foals, and may also cause the umbilicus to reopen due to excessive abdominal pressure

CBC/BIOCHEMISTRY/URINALYSIS
• No consistent abnormalities
• Dehydration/hemoconcentration and hypoglycemia will occur in foals that have not been nursing adequately

OTHER LABORATORY TESTS
Foals with inadequate colostrum ingestion will have a low IgG concentration.

IMAGING
• Abdominal radiography—gas-filled large and small colon with radiodense fecal material in distal small colon; barium enema can help to confirm the site of obstruction and barium also acts as an osmotic agent in the enema
• Abdominal ultrasonography—dense fecal material in the small colon; can rule out enteritis, uroabdomen, or other causes of colic/abdominal distention

OTHER DIAGNOSTIC PROCEDURES
• Abdominal palpation—identify abdominal distention; firm fecal material/meconium may be recognized on deep abdominal palpation when there is not significant gas distention
• Digital rectal examination—use a well-lubricated, gloved finger; hard feces may be identified in the rectum; rule out atresia ani

TREATMENT

APPROPRIATE HEALTHCARE
• Foals with mild meconium impaction may be treated with enemas at the farm. Foals with more severe impactions or with concurrent medical problems should be admitted for inpatient medical care
• Enemas—administration of soapy water or sodium phosphate enemas is usually effective; 200–300 mL of warm, soapy water can be

administered gently by gravity or very gentle syringe pressure via a red rubber catheter advanced only into the caudal rectum. Acetylcysteine retention enemas are used for impactions that are refractory to soapy water or sodium phosphate enemas. Acetylcysteine (4%) will cleave disulfide bonds in the mucoprotein of the meconium, causing the surface to become slippery. Acetylcysteine retention enemas are administered via Foley catheter with an inflated bulb. Gravity flow is used to administer 100–200 mL of solution, and it is retained for approximately 30–40 min. Enemas will cause some rectal irritation, and continued straining due to irritation should not be confused with persistent meconium impaction. Use of phosphate enemas should be limited in order to avoid hyperphosphatemia
• Oral laxatives—mineral oil can be administered via nasogastric tube in order to encourage passage of feces. Colostrum also appears to have a laxative effect. In more refractory cases of impaction, osmotic agents such as sodium sulfate can be given via nasogastric tube; however, these can be irritating to the GI tract, and may place the foal at risk of sepsis secondary to bacterial translocation. Mineral oil and other laxatives should not be used in foals <24 h of age

NURSING CARE
The foal should be encouraged to rise and nurse every hour as long as enteral nutrition is tolerated. IV fluids are needed in more severe cases to hydrate the foal and prevent/treat hypoglycemia. Foals that have not nursed well or that have meconium retention secondary to lack of colostrum intake should be treated with hyperimmune plasma if indicated by low IgG.

ACTIVITY
Stall rest is useful for monitoring feces and colic signs, although strict rest is not necessary.

DIET
• Nutrition—if the foal is colicky and has a continued obstruction, supplementation with IV fluids and dextrose or with parenteral nutrition should be initiated
• Foals can be supplemented with mare's milk via feeding tube if not nursing adequately. Feed small volumes initially as the meconium retention can lead to colic and reflux

CLIENT EDUCATION
Clients should be instructed to monitor for passage of meconium and recognize normal neonatal feces. Any decrease in nursing or lethargy should prompt an examination by a veterinarian.

SURGICAL CONSIDERATIONS
Surgical treatment—very rarely necessary; ventral midline celiotomy with guided enema and bowel massage is usually sufficient to

M

MECONIUM RETENTION

resolve the impaction. Severe cases may require enterotomy to remove hard meconium or other obstructive material.

MEDICATIONS

DRUG(S) OF CHOICE
• NSAIDs such as flunixin meglumine (0.5–1.1 mg/kg IV or PO every 12–24 h) or ketoprofen (1.1–2.2 mg/kg IV every 12–24 h) can be given for analgesia
• Sedation and analgesia are often needed for administration of the enema—xylazine (0.5–1.1 mg/kg IV), butorphanol (0.02–0.1 mg/kg IV), or diazepam (0.1 mg/kg IV)

PRECAUTIONS
• NSAIDs should be used with caution in neonates, especially if there are signs of dehydration or renal compromise
• The foal should be monitored closely for changes in condition—analgesics and sedation may mask a more serious underlying condition

POSSIBLE INTERACTIONS
N/A

ALTERNATIVE DRUGS
Midazolam (0.1–0.2 mg/kg) can be used instead of diazepam. Butorphanol is preferred over an NSAID for pain control, especially if the foal is less than 24 h of age.

FOLLOW-UP

PATIENT MONITORING
• Progression of colic signs and abdominal distention—take serial measurements of the abdomen by marking a site on the dorsum and ventrum and using a tape measure or string to assess for increasing abdominal circumference
• Passage of fecal material—pasty yellow "milk" feces are passed after all meconium has been passed

PREVENTION/AVOIDANCE
• Ensure adequate colostrum intake
• Routine administration of a warm soapy water enema is recommended if the foal has not passed its meconium within 3 h of birth

POSSIBLE COMPLICATIONS
• Frequent enemas can cause rectal irritation and further signs of straining
• Rectal tear from overzealous enemas
• Secondary ileus
• Bacterial translocation and sepsis from irritated GI mucosa
• Foals that require surgical correction of the impaction are at risk of abdominal adhesions

EXPECTED COURSE AND PROGNOSIS
Meconium impactions have a very good prognosis, and rarely require surgery. Generally, 1 or 2 enemas will resolve mild meconium impactions.

MISCELLANEOUS

ASSOCIATED CONDITIONS
Neonatal hypoxia and sepsis can contribute to meconium retention.

AGE-RELATED FACTORS
This is a condition of neonatal foals.

SEE ALSO
• Colic in foals
• Lethal white foal syndrome
• Uroperitoneum, neonate

ABBREVIATIONS
• GI = gastrointestinal
• IgG = immunoglobulin G
• NSAID = nonsteroidal anti-inflammatory drug

Suggested Reading
Pusterla N, Magdesian KG, Maleski K, et al. Retrospective evaluation of the use of acetylcysteine enemas in the treatment of meconium retention in foals: 44 cases (1987-2002). Equine Vet Educ 2004;16:133–136.
Ryan CA, Sanchez LC. Nondiarrheal disorders of the gastrointestinal tract in neonatal foals. Vet Clin North Am Equine Pract 2005;21:313–332.

Author Margaret C. Mudge
Consulting Editor Margaret C. Mudge

M

BASICS

OVERVIEW
• Melanomas are tumors that arise from the transformation of melanocytes. In gray horses, the disease presents as a clinical continuum of benign and malignant tumors. The "melanocytic" disease process includes hyperpigmentation and infiltration of the dermis and epidermis, resulting in plaque-like lesions rather than true masses or tumors. Mutations within the *STX17* gene, MCR-1, and ASIP have been associated with changes in melanocyte-specific gene expression and increased melanoma susceptibility. These mutations lead to increased activity of melanocyte-specific signaling pathways, cellular proliferation, and tumor formation within gray horses; however, further changes are needed for malignant transformation
• Affected organ systems—skin, gastrointestinal, hepatobiliary, hemolymphatic, and neurologic
• Melanomas constitute 3.8–15% of all skin tumors, second only to sarcoids
• Prevalence rates as high as 80% are reported in older gray horses. Both benign and malignant variants are described in non-gray horses, although rare

SIGNALMENT
Marked predisposition present in gray horses with Lipizzaners, Paso Finos, Arabians, and Percherons overrepresented. Average age of onset is 6–8 years and incidence increases with age. Lipizzaners have a heritability estimate of 0.36 with *STX17* mutations responsible for the phenotypic variance.

SIGNS
• Progressive dermal hyperpigmentation leading to plaque-like thickenings, multifocal nodules, and slowly growing mass(es). Masses are often clinically silent but symptoms occur as disease burden increases and involves visceral sites
• Common sites are the perineum, along the ventral tail, the parotid region, or other locations in the head and neck. Multifocal sites are common. Rectal examination may identify intrapelvic extension or metastatic lymphomegaly

CAUSES AND RISK FACTORS
Risk factors are gray coat color, mutations within the ASIP and MCR-1 protein.

DIAGNOSIS

DIFFERENTIAL DIAGNOSIS
Cutaneous variants are easily diagnosed by heavily pigmented appearance. Subcutaneous and visceral locations require cytology and/or biopsy samples for histologic confirmation.

CBC/BIOCHEMISTRY/URINALYSIS
Heavy disease burdens are associated with low-grade anemia, inflammatory leukograms, and liver enzyme changes in cases of hepatic metastases.

IMAGING
Ultrasonography, CT, and rarely MRI are used to determine disease extent prior to surgical resections.

TREATMENT

• It is believed that melanomas should be treated with early aggressive surgical removal to prevent further local tumor progression and possible metastatic spread. There are no recommended restrictions in activity or diet
• Client education—disease progresses over years, resulting in reduced performance and poor cosmetic appearance. Functional impairment can also be seen pending location. Visceral tumor sites may result in severe symptoms. Early and effective treatment may delay/prevent this progression
• Surgical considerations—familiarity with the anatomy of the perineum, pelvic canal, retroperitoneum, and parotid area is important to ensure morbidity is minimized. Marginal resection is often sufficient and tumor beds can routinely be left to heal by second intention

MEDICATIONS

DRUG(S) OF CHOICE
• Cimetidine 2.5–5 mg/kg PO BID–TID—believed to modify biologic response, although evidence is limited
• Cisplatin or carboplatin aqueous or suspended in sesame oil (1:1 ratio) can be administered by intratumoral injection every 2–4 weeks until therapeutic effect

• DNA-based vaccination strategies, including targeting the melanocyte-specific protein tyrosinase, have demonstrated activity and are currently being investigated.
• Veterinarians administering chemotherapy should be familiar with potential hazards to personnel

FOLLOW-UP

PATIENT MONITORING
• Quarterly to biannual rechecks are recommended to ensure early detection of disease regrowth/progression
• For intratumoral cisplatin/carboplatin recheck every 2–4 weeks prior to injection and then 1 month following completion of injections—quarterly to biannual rechecks thereafter

POSSIBLE COMPLICATIONS
• Difficulties with parturition, urination, or defecation are possible with disease progression
• Effects of eventual metastasis depend on the body system involved

EXPECTED COURSE AND PROGNOSIS
• Short- to intermediate-term prognosis is excellent
• Development of metastatic disease or local disease progression leads to a poor quality of life or acute decompensation. Early and aggressive treatment of external disease sites may delay/prevent metastatic tumor progression

MISCELLANEOUS

PREGNANCY/FERTILITY/BREEDING
Avoid cisplatin and carboplatin during the first trimester of pregnancy.

SEE ALSO
Sarcoid

Author Jeffrey Phillips
Consulting Editor Gwendolen Lorch
Acknowledgment The author and editor acknowledge the prior contribution of Douglas Thamm.

Client Education Handout available online

M

MELENA AND HEMATOCHEZIA

BASICS

OVERVIEW
• Melena results from bleeding from the GI or respiratory tract. The dark, black, or tarry appearance of feces is caused by intestinal microbial digestion of iron bound to hemoglobin. Large quantities of blood are necessary for melena to be evident
• Hematochezia is the presence of undigested blood in the feces. The probable bleeding sites include the distal parts of the large colon, small colon, and rectum
• Pathophysiology
  ◦ GI bleeding may be occult, slow, and/or rapid
  ◦ Slow bleeding may eventually lead to hemodynamic instability or shock
  ◦ Rapid bleeding may lead to hypovolemic shock and death
  ◦ The loss of iron is of concern

SIGNALMENT
No age, breed, or sex predisposition.

SIGNS
Historical Findings
Dark or bloody feces is often observed. In cases of chronic or severe bleeding, exercise intolerance and/or pale mucous membranes may be present. Low-grade colic signs are possible.

Physical Examination Findings
Dark or tarry feces or frank blood in feces. Mucous membranes may become pale and capillary refill time extended if substantial blood loss has occurred. Other signs depend on the underlying disease.

CAUSES AND RISK FACTORS
History is helpful in establishing the diagnosis:
• Rectal examination—rectal tears
• Nasogastric intubation—upper GI tract trauma
• NSAID treatment—GI erosions, colitis
• Exposure to toxins (acorn, aflatoxin, arsenic, cantharidin, *Crotalaria* spp., mycotoxin, oak, organophosphate, warfarin)
Other causes/differential diagnoses include:
• Parasitism
• Enteritis/colitis syndrome
• Gastric neoplasia
• Small or large bowel neoplasia
• Lymphoma
• Colonic hematomas
• Swallowed blood from the respiratory tract
• Gastroduodenal ulcers
• Purpura haemorrhagica
• Thrombocytopenia
• Coagulopathies
• Vasculitis
• Mesenteric arterial aneurysm

DIAGNOSIS

DIFFERENTIAL DIAGNOSIS
Oral iron supplement may result in dark feces and positive fecal occult test.

CBC/BIOCHEMISTRY/URINALYSIS
• CBC may show anemia. Hypoproteinemia possible from loss of protein into the GI lumen. Thrombocytopenia may result in significant GI hemorrhage. Leukopenia is present in many bacterial enterocolitis cases. Electrolyte and acid–base abnormalities are often present. Dehydration may result in mild azotemia. Urine usually concentrated from fluid retention
• Anemia may be associated with decreased bone marrow iron. Serum iron may be decreased, whereas iron-binding capacity may increase. Eventually microcytic, hypochromic erythrocytes are seen on CBC

OTHER LABORATORY TESTS
• Fecal examination for parasites and bacterial cultures
• Coagulation profile may reveal primary or secondary clotting abnormality
• Commercial (fecal occult) tests for detection of fresh or digested blood in feces. Fecal occult blood tests are often negative because colonic microflora digest hemoglobin

DIAGNOSTIC PROCEDURES
Should aim at identifying location/source of bleeding.

Gastroscopic Examination
Identification of bleeding in the respiratory tract, esophagus, stomach, and duodenum. It is rare to have melena from bleeding gastric ulcers in the horse.

Proctoscopy
Useful in hematochezia.

TREATMENT
Some patients may require hospitalization. Restoration of normal blood volume is necessary in hypovolemic patients. Fluid electrolyte and acid–base abnormalities should be corrected.

MEDICATIONS
Blood transfusion should be considered if the PCV is <12% (0.12 L/L), or is low and rapidly falling. A 454 kg (1000 lb) horse with a PCV <12% should receive 5–8 L of whole blood.

DRUG(S) OF CHOICE
N/A

CONTRAINDICATIONS/POSSIBLE INTERACTIONS
• NSAIDs should not be administered to patients with suspected or proven NSAID toxicosis
• NSAIDs should not be administered, or should be used with caution, to patients diagnosed with GI mucosal lesions

FOLLOW-UP

PATIENT MONITORING
PCV should be monitored twice daily until stabilized.

POSSIBLE COMPLICATIONS
Anemia, hypovolemic shock.

MISCELLANEOUS

ASSOCIATED CONDITIONS
N/A

AGE-RELATED FACTORS
N/A

ZOONOTIC POTENTIAL
The zoonotic potential of *Salmonella* spp., *Clostridium difficile*, and *Cryptosporidium* (foals) should be considered.

PREGNANCY/FERTILITY/BREEDING
Mares receiving blood transfusions develop alloantibodies to the transfused red blood cells. The alloantibody may be transferred to neonatal foals via the colostrum and cause neonatal isoerythrolysis.

ABBREVIATIONS
• GI = gastrointestinal
• NSAID = nonsteroidal anti-inflammatory drug
• PCV = packed cell volume

Suggested Reading
Pearson EG, Smith BB, McKim JM. Fecal blood determinations and interpretations. Proc Am Assoc Equine Pract 1987;33:77–81.
Smith BP. Alterations in alimentary and hepatic function. In: Smith BP, ed. Large Animal Internal Medicine, 4e. St. Louis, MO: Mosby, 2009:106–107.
Wilson D. Hematemesis, melena, and hematochezia. In: Walker HK, Hall WD, Hurst JW, eds. Clinical Methods, 3e. Boston, MA: Butterworths, 1990:439–442.

Author Modest Vengust
Consulting Editors Henry Stämpfli and Olimpo Oliver-Espinosa

BASICS

OVERVIEW
Bacterial meningitis is an uncommon but serious sequela to septicemia in foals. Up to 5–10% of septic neonatal foals develop meningitis, resulting from hematogenous spread of bacteria to the central nervous system. The disease is rapidly fatal if untreated.

SIGNALMENT
Neonatal foals, usually <2 weeks of age.

SIGNS
Clinical signs vary widely but may include:
- Lethargy/depression
- Decreased nursing
- Fever
- Ataxia, weakness
- Cervical stiffness/splinting
- Hyperesthesia
- Opisthotonus
- Cranial nerve deficits
- Anisocoria, abnormal pupillary light responses
- Strabismus, nystagmus
- Recumbency
- Seizures, coma (late findings; poor prognostic indicators)
- Clinical signs are usually rapidly progressive. Signs of other concurrent septic foci are frequently present (e.g. enteritis, arthritis)

CAUSES AND RISK FACTORS
- Failure of transfer of passive immunity is the strongest risk factor
- Bacterial isolates are similar to those implicated in neonatal septicemia
- Infection may occur via the respiratory, gastrointestinal, cutaneous, or umbilical route

DIAGNOSIS

DIFFERENTIAL DIAGNOSIS
- Neonatal maladjustment syndrome
- Congenital anomaly—hydrocephalus, hydranencephaly, other brain anomalies
- Metabolic—hypoglycemia, hepatic encephalopathy, kernicterus, electrolyte and acid–base abnormalities
- Nutritional myodegeneration
- Tetanus
- Trauma—external evidence typically present

CBC/BIOCHEMISTRY/URINALYSIS
- CBC—normal, increased, or decreased segmented neutrophils; toxic changes
- Biochemistry—hyperfibrinogenemia, increased serum amyloid A; hypogammaglobulinemia

OTHER LABORATORY TESTS
Serum IgG concentration—usually <400 mg/dL, often <200 mg/dL.

IMAGING
Radiography of the skull to rule out fracture, congenital anomaly.

OTHER DIAGNOSTIC PROCEDURES
- CSF analysis—*diagnostic test of choice.* Fluid usually discolored (yellow, orange), turbid. Cytology—increased nucleated cell count (>6/μL, often >100/μL), predominantly degenerate neutrophils; intra- and extracellular bacteria often noted. Gram stain may identify the predominant bacterial population present
- Bacterial culture and susceptibility of CSF is diagnostic
- Blood cultures or cultures of other septic foci may be useful

PATHOLOGIC FINDINGS
- Thickened, discolored, opaque meninges over cerebrum, cerebellum, brainstem
- Meningeal vascular congestion

TREATMENT
- Inpatient medical care and emergency stabilization are often required
- Fluid therapy and nutrition
- Padding and supervision to prevent self-trauma
- Nasal oxygen or mechanical ventilation for respiratory failure

MEDICATIONS

DRUG(S) OF CHOICE
Antimicrobials
- Broad-spectrum, bactericidal antimicrobial drugs that penetrate the blood–brain barrier
- Third- and fourth-generation cephalosporins (cefotaxime 40 mg/kg IV every 6 h; ceftriaxone 25–50 mg/kg IV every 12 h; cefepime 11 mg/kg IV TID) are preferred
- Penicillin, tetracyclines, and aminoglycosides do not reliably penetrate CSF

Anti-inflammatory Medication
- Corticosteroids (dexamethasone 0.1 mg/kg IV or prednisolone 1–2 mg/kg IV)—recommend use early in the course of the disease, but no evidence that this treatment improves survival in horses
- DMSO (1 g/kg as a 5–10% solution IV once daily)
- NSAIDs (ketoprofen 1.1–2.2 mg/kg IV every 12–24 h or flunixin meglumine 0.5–1.1 mg/kg IV every 12–24 h) for analgesia

Seizure Control
- Diazepam (0.2–0.5 mg/kg IV as bolus, can be given every 15–20 min)
- Midazolam (0.06–0.1 mg/kg IV; 0.02–0.2 mg/kg/h as constant rate infusion)
- Phenobarbital (10–20 mg/kg IV over 20 min, then 2–10 mg/kg PO SID–BID)

CONTRAINDICATIONS/POSSIBLE INTERACTIONS
Immunocompromise secondary to steroid administration is a concern in septicemic foals.

FOLLOW-UP

PATIENT MONITORING
- Serial physical and neurologic examinations
- Recheck CBC, plasma fibrinogen concentration, ± repeated CSF

PREVENTION/AVOIDANCE
- Ensure adequate colostral intake and serum IgG >800 mg/dL within first 24 h of life
- Clean, hygienic environment

POSSIBLE COMPLICATIONS
Persistent neurologic deficits possible in recovered foals.

EXPECTED COURSE AND PROGNOSIS
- Rapidly fatal without treatment
- Guarded prognosis with treatment; poor if signs progress to seizures and/or coma
- At least 4–6 weeks of antimicrobial treatment recommended

MISCELLANEOUS

ASSOCIATED CONDITIONS
Concurrent septic foci (pneumonia, arthritis, enteritis, uveitis, omphalitis, etc.).

AGE-RELATED FACTORS
Failure of transfer of passive immunity predisposes.

ZOONOTIC POTENTIAL
Unlikely, but use caution if *Salmonella* spp. isolated from CSF, blood.

SEE ALSO
- Neonatal maladjustment syndrome
- Septicemia, neonate

ABBREVIATIONS
- CSF = cerebrospinal fluid
- DMSO = dimethylsulfoxide
- IgG = immunoglobulin G
- NSAID = nonsteroidal anti-inflammatory drug

Suggested Reading
MacKay RJ. Neurologic disorders of neonatal foals. Vet Clin North Am Equine Pract 2005;21:387–406.
Viu J, Monreal L, Jose-Cunilleras E, et al. Clinical findings in 10 foals with bacterial meningitis. Equine Vet J Suppl 2012;41:100–104.

Author Teresa A. Burns
Consulting Editor Margaret C. Mudge

M

MERCURY TOXICOSIS

BASICS

OVERVIEW
• A toxic syndrome involving the GI and renal systems, resulting primarily from the ingestion or dermal absorption of blistering agents containing inorganic mercury salts (e.g. mercuric iodide or mercuric chloride)
• Toxicosis from ingesting seeds treated with mercury-containing fungicides is unlikely, because such fungicides are no longer used
• Mercury binds to a variety of sulfhydryl-containing enzymes resulting in nonspecific cell injury and death

SIGNALMENT
No breed, age, or sex predilections.

SIGNS
• Depression
• Colic
• Diarrhea
• Weakness
• Skin erosions, ulcerations, and crusting
• Dehydration
• Oliguria
• Laminitis

CAUSES AND RISK FACTORS
• Excessive application of mercury-containing blistering agent
• Application of mercury-containing blistering agent to damaged skin
• Failure to prevent the animal from ingesting a dermally applied mercury-containing agent
• Application of mercury-containing blistering agent in combination with DMSO

DIAGNOSIS

DIFFERENTIAL DIAGNOSIS
• Lead toxicosis—likely evidence of neurologic dysfunction; measurement of whole-blood or tissue lead concentrations
• Arsenic toxicosis—measurement of whole-blood, urine, or tissue arsenic concentrations
• NSAID toxicosis—history of previous use; measurement of an NSAID in plasma or serum
• Cantharidin toxicosis—evidence of cystitis; detection of cantharidin in stomach contents or urine
• *Quercus* spp. (oak) toxicosis—detection of plant material in the GI tract; evidence of oak consumption
• Ethylene glycol
• Salmonellosis—fecal cultures
• Ehrlichial colitis—serology
• Acute cyathostomiasis—fecal egg counts
• Clostridial colitis—isolation of pathogenic clostridia; identification of toxins
• Antimicrobial-induced colitis (e.g. lincomycin, tetracycline)—history of drug use

CBC/BIOCHEMISTRY/URINALYSIS
• Increased packed cell volume
• Hyperfibrinogenemia
• Serum electrolyte changes—hyponatremia, hypochloremia, hyperphosphatemia, and hyperkalemia
• Hyperglycemia
• Azotemia
• Urinalysis—glycosuria, proteinuria, isosthenuria, hematuria, waxy or granular casts
• Occult blood in feces

OTHER LABORATORY TESTS
• Antemortem—measurement of mercury in urine or blood
• Postmortem—measurement of mercury in liver or kidney tissue

IMAGING
N/A

OTHER DIAGNOSTIC PROCEDURES
N/A

PATHOLOGIC FINDINGS
Gross
• Watery feces
• Intraluminal hemorrhage
• GI mucosal edema
• Mucosal ulcerations in the oral cavity, stomach, and colon
• Subcutaneous edema
• Pale, soft, and swollen kidneys

Histopathologic
• Acute, severe renal tubular necrosis
• Severe, extensive ulcerative colitis and enteritis

TREATMENT
• Remove source of mercury
• Treat for dehydration, circulatory shock, and renal failure
• Provide a bland diet containing reduced amounts of high-quality protein

MEDICATIONS
DRUG(S) OF CHOICE
• Enhance mercury elimination with a chelator:
  ◦ Dimercaprol (British anti-Lewisite) is a classic mercury chelator—loading dose of 4–5 mg/kg by deep IM injection followed by 2–3 mg/kg every 4 h for 24 h and then 1 mg/kg every 4 h for 2 days; adverse reactions include tremors, convulsions, and coma
  ◦ Succimer is a less toxic chelator—dose is not established for horses, but 10 mg/kg PO every 8 h is suggested
• Control abdominal pain:
  ◦ Flunixin meglumine (1.1 mg/kg IV every 12–24 h) or butorphanol tartrate (0.1 mg/kg IV every 3–4 h up to 48 h)
  ◦ Xylazine hydrochloride (1.1 mg/kg IV) may be used in conjunction with butorphanol (0.01–0.02 mg/kg IV)
• Demulcents—mineral oil; kaolin–pectin

CONTRAINDICATIONS/POSSIBLE INTERACTIONS
Use NSAIDs cautiously because of possible adverse GI and renal effects.

FOLLOW-UP
PATIENT MONITORING
Monitor renal function.

PREVENTION/AVOIDANCE
• Identify and properly dispose of the source of exposure
• Avoid use of mercury-containing blisters

POSSIBLE COMPLICATIONS
N/A

EXPECTED COURSE AND PROGNOSIS
• Dependent on the severity of clinical signs
• Renal impairment suggests a poor prognosis
• 1 equine case report described brain neuronal degeneration
• Long-term neurologic deficits are possible after recovery

MISCELLANEOUS
ASSOCIATED CONDITIONS
N/A

AGE-RELATED FACTORS
N/A

ZOONOTIC POTENTIAL
N/A

PREGNANCY/FERTILITY/BREEDING
• Most forms of mercury can cross the placenta
• The significance of fetal exposure after use of mercury salts on pregnant mares is unknown

ABBREVIATIONS
• DMSO = dimethylsulfoxide
• GI = gastrointestinal
• NSAID = nonsteroidal anti-inflammatory drug

Suggested Reading
Guglick MA, MacAllister CG, Chandra AM, et al. Mercury toxicosis caused by the ingestion of a blistering compound in a horse. J Am Vet Med Assoc 1995;206:210–213.

Authors Arya Sobhakumari and Robert H. Poppenga
Consulting Editors Wilson K. Rumbeiha and Steve Ensley

METABOLIC DISORDERS IN ENDURANCE HORSES

BASICS

DEFINITION
• Hypovolemia and dehydration are by far the most common problems seen and treated in endurance horses
• More seriously affected horses or those that do not receive appropriate care are at high risk for development of complications
• A variety of cases require referral to a secondary or tertiary care facility
• Arrangements for referral should be made before the need arises

PATHOPHYSIOLOGY
• Total body fluid losses due to profuse sweating for long periods
• Inadequate replacement fluid intake

SYSTEMS AFFECTED
• Cardiovascular
• Musculoskeletal
• GI
• Renal/urologic
• Nervous

GEOGRAPHIC DISTRIBUTION
Global

SIGNALMENT
• Arabian horses and Arab crosses are most commonly used for endurance competitions
• Most affected horses are 5–18 years old
• No sex predilection or genetic basis has been noted

SIGNS
• Affected horses appear dull, exhausted, and may be obtundent, stagger, or be reluctant to move. Severely hypovolemic, dehydrated horses often have heart rates ≥70–79 bpm
• Prolonged CRTs (>3 s), poor mucous membrane color, poor skin turgor
• Ileus—few or no gut sounds
• No interest in food or water
• Hypoglycemic horses may be lethargic and adopt a "sawhorse stance." Heart rate, CRT, and jugular refill time do not reflect the degree of compromise that one would expect in a hypovolemic horse showing similar clinical signs

CAUSES
• Inadequate conditioning
• Concurrent lameness
• Inexperienced, unbalanced riders
• Inability to pace the horse or recognize fatigue
• Riders not allowing horses to stop to drink
• Pushing horses beyond their physiologic limits

RISK FACTORS
See Causes.

DIAGNOSIS

DIFFERENTIAL DIAGNOSIS
• Fatigue
• Exertional rhabdomyolysis

CBC/BIOCHEMISTRY/URINALYSIS
• Hematocrit values are often 55–69 L/L
• Elevated total protein levels may reach as high as 14 mg/dL
• Serum creatinine levels are often markedly elevated
• Total protein and creatinine measurements provide a more accurate measure of fluid volume deficits than the hematocrit alone, and, along with the physical parameters, provide a helpful guide to the end-point for fluid therapy
• Hypocalcemia is often present (ionized calcium <1.2 mmol/L)
• Hypoglycemia may be present, with blood glucose levels of 30–50 g/dL (1.6–2.8 mmol/L)

IMAGING
N/A

OTHER DIAGNOSTIC PROCEDURES
Serial clinical examinations.

PATHOLOGIC FINDINGS
• Horses that fail to recover may have pathologic findings related to the organ system most affected
• Cardiomyopathy, renal tubular necrosis, laminar necrosis, cerebral edema, and pulmonary and GI infarcts have all been discovered at necropsy

TREATMENT

AIMS
• The primary aim of treatment is to restore fluid deficits and circulating plasma volume to minimize tissue hypoxia, protect organ function, and return homeostasis
• Most endurance horses with fluid deficits respond well to 10–20 L of IV fluids, administered through a 12 or 14-gauge jugular catheter
• 0.9% sodium chloride has traditionally been used for fluid replacement in endurance horses, but any isotonic fluid can be used
• Hypertonic saline should be avoided, except in cases where cerebral edema is suspected
• Longer catheters (14 cm (5.5 inches)) are preferred to short ones, since they are less likely to be dislodged in case of collapse. Catheters should be sutured in place
• Replacement fluids via nasogastric intubation are not routinely used because GI stasis is often present, and there is a risk of gastric rupture

MEDICATIONS
• Supplementation of calcium in horses with low ionized calcium (<1.2 mmol/L) or poor auscultable motility hastens recovery of GI motility (23% calcium gluconate, 120–240 mL in 3–5 L 0.9% NaCl IV to effect)
• Synchronous diaphragmatic flutter can occur without concurrent metabolic compromise, and may not require treatment. If treatment is deemed necessary, 23% calcium gluconate, 100–250 mL in 3–5 L 0.9% NaCl IV usually resolves clinical signs
• If the heart rate remains elevated (<50 bpm) and ileus is persistent, low-dose flunixin meglumine (0.3–0.6 mg/kg) can be administered, provided that fluid deficits have been replaced, and the horse does not have an elevated serum creatinine level
• Clinical improvement generally occurs within 30–40 min of flunixin meglumine administration
• All NSAIDs should be used judiciously and with extreme caution in the endurance horse due to their nephrotoxicity and the propensity for endurance horses to have renal compromise
• If hypoglycemia is present, 50–100 mL 50% glucose or dextrose diluted in a 3 or 5 L bag of normal saline is given to effect
• If colic is present and serum creatinine levels are high, butorphanol (0.01–0.02 mg/kg) combined with xylazine (0.3–0.5 mg/kg) or detomidine (0.01 mg/kg) can be used to provide analgesia while fluid therapy is administered

CONTRAINDICATIONS
Serious complications (renal failure) may occur if NSAIDs are used in endurance horses prior to volume expansion.

POSSIBLE INTERACTIONS
See Contraindications.

FOLLOW-UP

PATIENT MONITORING
Serial clinical examinations, monitoring heart rate, mucous membrane color, and return of intestinal borborygmi and interest in food and water are important is assessing response to therapy.

PREVENTION/AVOIDANCE
Rider education and familiarity with the horse is important in detection of impending metabolic compromise.

M

POSSIBLE COMPLICATIONS
- Laminitis
- Endotoxemia
- Multiple organ system compromise or failure

EXPECTED COURSE AND PROGNOSIS
- The vast majority of endurance horses with hypovolemia and dehydration, when treated promptly and appropriately, resolve without the need for further treatment or follow-up care
- Those that do not respond to treatment within 4–6 h of appropriate treatment often require referral for a longer period of therapy
- Horses with concurrent problems also require referral to a secondary or tertiary care facility
- If small intestinal volvulus is suspected (pain unresponsive to analgesia), referral should be immediate

MISCELLANEOUS

ASSOCIATED CONDITIONS
- Colic—most colic in endurance horses is due to nonstrangulated ileus, but small intestinal volvulus is a recognized postendurance phenomenon
- Synchronous diaphragmatic flutter
- Exertional rhabdomyolysis
- Cardiac arrhythmias
- Renal failure
- Heat stroke
- Enterocolitis
- Neurologic deficits

AGE-RELATED FACTORS
N/A

SEE ALSO
- Acute adult abdominal pain–acute colic
- Azotemia and uremia
- Calcium, hypocalcemia
- Exercise-associated arrhythmias
- Exertional rhabdomyolysis syndrome
- Glucose, hypoglycemia
- Ileus
- Polycythemia
- Synchronous diaphragmatic flutter

ABBREVIATIONS
- CRT = capillary refill time
- GI = gastrointestinal
- NSAID = nonsteroidal anti-inflammatory drug

Suggested Reading
Cunilleras EJ. Abnormalities of body fluids and electrolytes in athletic horses. In: Hinchcliffe KW, Kaneps AJ, Geor RJ, eds. Equine Sports Medicine and Surgery: Basic and Clinical Sciences of the Equine Athlete, 2e. Edinburgh, UK: Saunders, 2013:881–900.
Fielding CL, Magdesian GK, eds. Equine Fluid Therapy. Ames, IA: Wiley Blackwell, 2015.
Misheff MM. Diagnosis and treatment of metabolic conditions in the endurance horse. In: SIVA Proceedings, XXII International SIVE Congress, Italian Equine Veterinary Society, 2016.

Author Martha M. Misheff
Consulting Editor Jean-Pierre Lavoie

M

METACARPO- (METATARSO-)PHALANGEAL JOINT DISEASE

BASICS

OVERVIEW
- Any disease localized to the MCPJ/MTPJ
- The MCPJ/MTPJ has the greatest range of motion of any equine joint, which makes it susceptible to exercise-induced wear and tear. Hyperextension, high compressive, and torsional forces result in injury
- The term "osselets" is used to describe the thickening associated with synovitis and capsulitis of the joint
- Musculoskeletal—fetlock

SIGNALMENT
- All breeds and types of horses
- Most common in racehorses and elite performance horses

SIGNS
- Lameness is variable in onset, often bilateral with 1 limb more affected
- Pain, heat, synovial distention of the MCPJ/MTPJ
- Stiff gait and shortened stride
- Resentment and decreased range of motion during MCPJ/MTPJ flexion

CAUSES AND RISK FACTORS
- Sports that require intense exercise
- Poor conformation
- Specific diseases that may cause MCPJ/MTPJ synovitis or arthritis:
  ◦ Intra-articular osseous fragmentation(s)
  ◦ Articular fractures of the proximal first phalanx, proximal sesamoid bones, or distal metacarpus/metatarsus
  ◦ Osteochondrosis of the MCPJ/MTPJ
  ◦ Subchondral bone injury of distal palmar/plantar MCPJ/MTPJ
  ◦ Trauma, luxation of MCPJ/MTPJ

DIAGNOSIS

DIFFERENTIAL DIAGNOSIS
Joint distention and positive response to the lower limb flexion test may be a false localizing sign. Diagnostic analgesia and/or imaging will confirm or rule out MCPJ/MTPJ disease.

IMAGING
- Radiography—in early or acute disease, radiographic evaluation may be normal. Periarticular osteophyte formation, loss of joint space, and subchondral bone sclerosis are signs of chronic disease
- Nuclear scintigraphy—generalized increased radiopharmaceutical uptake of MCPJ/MTPJ. Focal increased radiopharmaceutical uptake of specific location(s) for corresponding fracture(s) and/or subchondral bone injury

- MRI/CT—excellent imaging modality for assessment of subchondral bone and articular cartilage

OTHER DIAGNOSTIC PROCEDURES
- Diagnostic analgesia—intra-articular MCPJ/MTPJ analgesia and low palmar/plantar analgesia
- Arthroscopy—global visualization of articular cartilage and articular lesions
- Synovial fluid analysis to rule out infectious arthritis

PATHOLOGIC FINDINGS
Periarticular osteophyte formation, thin cartilage, cartilaginous fibrillation, osteochondral fragmentation, enlarged dorsal synovial pad, subchondral sclerosis, and/or lysis.

TREATMENT
- Intra-articular anti-inflammatory(s)
- Rest for weeks to several months
- Reduce workload and athletic expectations
- Arthroscopic removal of osteochondral fragmentation(s)
- Surgical fixation of articular fracture(s) of the proximal first phalanx, distal third metacarpal/metatarsal bone, or proximal sesamoid bones
- Surgical arthrodesis of the MCPJ/MTPJ using dorsal bone plate and palmar/plantar tension band wiring in advanced disease as a salvage procedure

MEDICATIONS

DRUG(S) OF CHOICE
- NSAIDs—phenylbutazone (2.2 mg/kg every 12–24 h for 7–10 days)
- Intra-articular medications—methylprednisolone acetate (20–40 mg) or triamcinolone (3–6 mg), sodium hyaluronate (10–20 mg), platelet-rich plasma, interleukin receptor antagonist protein
- Polysulfated glycosaminoglycan (500 mg IM every 4 days for 7 treatments) or sodium hyaluronate (40 mg IV every 7 days for 3 treatments)
- Oral glucosamine/chondroitin sulfate powder (1 scoop (3.3 g) BID)

CONTRAINDICATIONS/POSSIBLE INTERACTIONS
Intra-articular corticosteroids are not recommended in horses with laminitis.

FOLLOW-UP

PATIENT MONITORING
- Resolution or decreased amount of joint distention is expected after treatment
- Periodic lameness evaluation as clinical signs dictate

PREVENTION/AVOIDANCE
- Appropriate training and conditioning for desired sport
- Recognition of acute disease and appropriate treatment in a timely manner
- Avoid the use of horseshoes with toe grabs
- Reduction in workload or alterative sport may prolong athletic career albeit at a lower level

POSSIBLE COMPLICATIONS
Inability to perform expected sport due to chronic lameness.

EXPECTED COURSE AND PROGNOSIS
- Early recognition and response to treatment may prolong the intended use of the horse
- Osteoarthritis of the MCPJ/MTPJ is progressive and a reduction in athletic soundness is expected over time
- In advanced disease or traumatic rupture of the suspensory apparatus, surgical arthrodesis is indicated. After arthrodesis, horses may be salvaged for breeding purposes or retired to pasture

MISCELLANEOUS

AGE-RELATED FACTORS
Uncommon in <2-year-olds unless associated with osteochondrosis.

SEE ALSO
- Osteoarthritis
- Osteochondrosis

ABBREVIATIONS
- CT = computed tomography
- MCPJ = metacarpophalangeal joint
- MRI = magnetic resonance imaging
- MTPJ = metatarsophalangeal joint
- NSAID = nonsteroidal anti-inflammatory drug

Suggested Reading
Richardson DW, Dyson SJ. The metacarpophalangeal joint. In: Ross MW, Dyson SJ, eds. Diagnosis and Management of Lameness in the Horse, 2e. St. Louis, MO: Elsevier Saunders, 2011:394–410.

Author Elizabeth J. Davidson

Consulting Editor Elizabeth J. Davidson

M

METALDEHYDE TOXICOSIS

BASICS

OVERVIEW
• Metaldehyde is primarily available in molluscicides; solid fuel metaldehyde is also a hazard
• Toxicosis is referred to as the "shake and bake" syndrome and involves adverse effects on the nervous and musculoskeletal systems ("classically" caudal-to-cranial progression of signs), GI tract, liver, and kidneys, as well as disrupted thermoregulation and coagulation
• Uncommon, but horses are particularly sensitive (onset from 15 min to 2 h); lethal dose is at least half of that in dogs and cats
• Usually results from mishandling of pelleted baits
• Associated with decreased brain concentrations of inhibitory neurotransmitters (e.g. GABA, norepinephrine, 5-hydroxytryptamine, and 5-hydroxyindoleacetic acid), as well as possibly increased concentrations of excitatory neurotransmitters

SIGNALMENT
No age, sex, or breed predilections.

SIGNS
• Salivation, agitation, anxiety, profuse sweating, hyperthermia
• Tachycardia and weak pulse, tachypnea, dyspnea
• Hyperesthesia and muscle fasciculations, tremors, ataxia, exaggerated leg movements, violent continuous convulsions
• Colic
• DIC
• Organ failure
• Death

CAUSES AND RISK FACTORS
• Acute exposures >60–100 mg/kg of metaldehyde is lethal
• Mishandling of pelleted baits or solid camp fuel
• Coastal or low-lying areas enzootic to snails and slugs

DIAGNOSIS

DIFFERENTIAL DIAGNOSIS
• Strychnine toxicosis
• Organochlorine insecticide toxicosis
• Acetylcholinesterase-inhibiting insecticides
• Zinc phosphide
• Bromethalin
• Anticoagulant rodenticides
• Plant intoxications with *Cicuta*, verticillate-leaved *Asclepias*, *Conium*, or *Nicotiana* spp.
• Cranial or cervical trauma
• Rabies
• Fumonisin B$_1$ intoxication
• Hepatic encephalopathy
• Tetanus

CBC/BIOCHEMISTRY/URINALYSIS
• Increased PCV and total protein
• Elevations in serum concentrations of liver and muscle enzymes, blood urea nitrogen, and creatinine
• Metabolic acidosis

OTHER LABORATORY TESTS
• Antemortem—analysis of metaldehyde in serum, plasma, urine, retrieved GI contents, feces (may not be completed until after death or resolution)
• Postmortem—analysis of metaldehyde in GI contents and feces

PATHOLOGIC FINDINGS
• Gross—generalized renal, hepatic, GI, and pulmonary congestion, petechial and ecchymotic hemorrhages throughout the body, subepicardial and subendothelial hemorrhages, hyperemia of the GI mucosa, and mild enteritis
• Histologic—swollen medullary axons and mild hepatic degeneration

TREATMENT
• Aggressive decontamination is best approach
• Gastric lavage immediately after exposure
• Administer AC soon after ingestion
• Administer mineral oil to enhance elimination of metaldehyde and acetaldehyde
• Provide supportive care for dehydration, hypovolemic shock, acidosis, and hyperthermia

MEDICATIONS

DRUG(S) OF CHOICE
• Xylazine hydrochloride alone or in conjunction with acepromazine maleate for sedation in the absence of convulsions
• AC (1–4 g/kg), possibly followed by 2–4 L of mineral oil via nasogastric tube
• Diazepam can be administered to adults (25–50 mg IV) or foals (0.05–0.4 mg/kg IV) for muscle tremors and convulsions (can repeat in 30 min)
• Phenobarbital (1–10 mg/kg IV) can be administered along with diazepam to control convulsions
• General anesthesia may be indicated to control convulsions
• Slow IV infusion of methocarbamol (15–25 mg/kg; up to 55 mg/kg recommended by manufacturer) for muscle relaxation
• Polyionic fluid therapy with or without sodium bicarbonate to control dehydration and acidosis

CONTRAINDICATIONS/POSSIBLE INTERACTIONS
• Sedatives and anesthetics should be used prudently in ataxic horses
• Acepromazine has been associated with lowered seizure thresholds and hypotension and should be avoided in the presence of convulsions or circulatory collapse

FOLLOW-UP
• Identification of source of metaldehyde
• Proper disposal of or limited access to metaldehyde-containing products

PATIENT MONITORING
• Monitor pulse rate, quality, and rhythm as well as capillary refill time and mucous membrane color continuously to assess the cardiovascular system
• Monitor body temperature, PCV, total protein, and acid–base status
• With severe hyperthermia, monitor liver and kidney function and blood clotting for several days

PREVENTION/AVOIDANCE
• Use molluscicides according to label instructions
• Properly store metaldehyde-containing products
• Use alternative products for control of populations of snails and slugs

POSSIBLE COMPLICATIONS
• DIC
• Multiorgan failure

EXPECTED COURSE AND PROGNOSIS
In the absence of hyperthermia-associated complications, the prognosis for long-term survival is good with immediate and aggressive therapy.

MISCELLANEOUS

AGE-RELATED FACTORS
N/A

ABBREVIATIONS
• AC = activated charcoal
• DIC = disseminated intravascular coagulation
• GABA = γ-aminobutyric acid
• GI = gastrointestinal
• PCV = packed cell volume

Suggested Reading
Talcott PA. Metaldehyde. In: Plumlee KH, ed. Clinical Veterinary Toxicology. St. Louis, MO: Mosby, 2004:182–183.

Author Tim J. Evans
Consulting Editors Wilson K. Rumbeiha and Steve Ensley

BASICS

DEFINITION
Methemoglobin is an abnormal form of hemoglobin where iron is in the ferric (Fe^{3+}) rather than the normal ferrous (Fe^{2+}) state. Methemoglobin reduces the oxygen-carrying capacity of blood, plus its presence shifts the oxyhemoglobin dissociation curve to the left (increases affinity of remaining hemoglobin for oxygen but releases oxygen to tissues less readily).

PATHOPHYSIOLOGY
• Small quantities of methemoglobin are normally formed during binding of oxygen to the RBC iron–hemoglobin molecule. Normal concentration is 1.77%
• Methemoglobin is usually continuously reduced back to hemoglobin by protective enzyme systems (major pathway via NADH-dependent methemoglobin reductase (cytochrome b_5 reductase); minor pathway via NADPH–methemoglobin reductase; ascorbic acid and glutathione enzyme systems also play a role)
• Methemoglobinemia is the presence of higher than normal concentrations of methemoglobin in the blood. It may be acquired or congenital and normally results when there is excessive production of methemoglobin and the body's regulatory mechanisms are overwhelmed
• Methemoglobinemia results in systemic hypoxia and can be fatal
• Many of the methemoglobin-producing oxidant toxins can also cause hemolysis by simultaneously oxidizing the sulfhydryl groups of the globin moiety in methemoglobin, resulting in denaturation and precipitation, Heinz body formation, and intravascular hemolysis

SYSTEMS AFFECTED
• Hemic/lymphatic/immune—decreased RBC oxygen-carrying capacity, cyanosis, and muddy brown mucous membranes
• Cardiovascular and respiratory—attempt to compensate for the decreased oxygen-carrying capacity, resulting in tachycardia and tachypnea
• Renal/urologic—pigment nephropathy (in cases with concurrent hemolysis) and renal hypoxic insult may result in dysfunction
• Hepatobiliary—hypoxia-induced centrilobular degeneration may occur
• Gastrointestinal—hypoxic damage to intestines may result in motility disorders, impaction, and colic
• Nervous—hypoxia may result in signs of lethargy and weakness
• Musculoskeletal—laminar hypoxia may result in laminitis

GENETICS
There is a report of familial methemoglobinemia caused by decreased erythrocyte glutathione reductase and glutathione.

INCIDENCE/PREVALENCE
No incidence/prevalence data available.

SIGNALMENT
• Any age, breed, or sex
• Familial methemoglobinemia and hemolytic anemia reported in 2 Trotter mares

SIGNS

Historical Findings
• Sudden onset of lethargy, inappetence, and signs of depression
• Exercise intolerance, tachycardia, and tachypnea may also be noted
• Cases with concurrent hemolysis may also have pigmenturia and icterus
• Exposure to wilted or dried leaves or bark of red maple (*Acer rubrum*) (fall), *Pistacia* leaves or seeds, or nitrate-containing plants. Absence of this information should not rule out this differential

Physical Examination Findings
• Findings depend on the severity of disease and organ systems involved
• Muddy brown cyanotic mucous membranes with brownish discoloration of the blood
• Clinical signs usually evident when methemoglobin concentrations are 30–40%, including weakness, lethargy, ataxia, tachycardia, tachypnea, exercise intolerance, colic, and laminitis
• Low-grade fevers, icterus, and pigmenturia associated with hemolysis
• Sudden death may occur

CAUSES
• Red maple (*A. rubrum*) toxicity
• *Pistacia* leaf/seed ingestion
• Other oxidant toxins, e.g. phenothiazine and onions (less severe)
• Nitrite/nitrate poisoning (rare)
• Deficiencies in protective RBC enzymes (glutathione reductase and flavin adenine dinucleotide deficiencies)

RISK FACTORS
• Access to dry/wilted red maple leaves/bark, or *Pistacia* leaves/seeds, often during fall
• Exposure to nitrate/nitrite sources (e.g. plants, forages, silages, fertilizer spills)
• Familial history of methemoglobinemia

DIAGNOSIS

DIFFERENTIAL DIAGNOSIS
• Immune-mediated hemolytic anemia can be differentiated by flow cytometry, RBC autoagglutination, hyperbilirubinemia, and bilirubinuria

• Infectious causes of anemia include equine infectious anemia (positive Coggins test or C-ELISA test), piroplasmosis (organisms observed in Giemsa-stained smears or positive serology), and anaplasmosis (*Anaplasma phagocytophilum*) (granular inclusions in neutrophils in Giemsa-stained smears or positive PCR)
• Hemolysis following administration of hypertonic or hypotonic solutions
• Other toxicities, including IV DMSO, heavy metal toxicosis, and snake envenomation
• Signs of depression and coma associated with endstage liver disease can be differentiated by increase in bile acids, liver enzymes, and chronic weight loss

CBC/BIOCHEMISTRY/URINALYSIS
• Horses may have concurrent Heinz body hemolytic anemia, hemoglobinemia, and neutrophilia
• There may be evidence of hypoxic injury to various organ systems with increases in blood urea nitrogen, creatinine, and bilirubin concentrations and/or liver enzymes
• Urinalysis may reveal hemoglobinuria, bilirubinuria, and proteinuria

OTHER LABORATORY TESTS
• Post-collection hemolysis of samples may falsely increase the methemoglobin value
• Co-oximeter analysis of blood samples should be performed quickly to determine methemoglobin concentration (concentrations decrease rapidly in vitro)
• The methemoglobin spot test consists of comparing a drop of patient blood, on absorbent paper, with that of a normal control horse. Methemoglobin content >10% results in a brown discoloration of patient blood compared with the red color of control blood
• Pulse oximetry reveals low saturations (does not correlate with methemoglobin concentration)
• Arterial PO_2 is normal, as this is a measure of oxygen dissolved in the plasma and not the carrying capacity of the hemoglobin; aids in differentiation from hypoxemia

IMAGING
N/A

OTHER DIAGNOSTIC PROCEDURES
• Blood smears stained with new methylene blue should be examined for Heinz bodies and Wright–Giemsa-stained smears for eccentrocytes and pyknocytosis
• Testing for RBC enzyme deficiencies can be performed at specialist laboratories

PATHOLOGIC FINDINGS
May include centrilobular hepatic degeneration, hemoglobinemic renal tubular nephrosis, icteric tissues, and erythrophagocytosis by splenic, adrenal, and hepatic phagocytes.

M

TREATMENT

APPROPRIATE HEALTH CARE
• In-hospital medical management may be necessary
• Fluid therapy (IV) with isotonic crystalloids should be initiated for increased tissue perfusion, dilution of red cell fragments that might trigger DIC, prevention of hemoglobin-induced nephropathy, and to promote diuresis
• Cross-matched blood or packed RBC transfusion may be considered if PCV falls to <11% over several days or to <18% in 1 day or less. Indication for blood transfusion can also include persistent tachycardia, tachypnea, weak pulse pressure, and poor response to isotonic fluids
• If renal function is adequate, judicious NSAID use may decrease inflammation and provide analgesia
• Administration of intranasal oxygen is of little benefit; low oxygen-carrying capacity of blood

NURSING CARE
Close monitoring of vital signs, fluid rates, urine output, and CBC/biochemistry is vital; and for signs of laminitis or colic.

ACTIVITY
Exercise or stress, which may increase oxygen demand, is contraindicated.

DIET
Palatable and nutritious diet should be provided to encourage voluntary feed intake.

CLIENT EDUCATION
Clients should be warned of the hazards of exposure to wilted red maple leaves (including hybrids), *Pistacia* leaves/seeds, and nitrate/nitrite-containing plants or fertilizer spills.

SURGICAL CONSIDERATIONS
• General anesthesia should be avoided due to hypoxia and associated risk
• Surgical hemorrhage also likely to exacerbate hypoxia

MEDICATIONS

DRUG(S) OF CHOICE
• If nitrate/nitrite poisoning is suspected, methylene blue (4.4 mg/kg) may be

administered slowly IV as a 1–2% solution in isotonic saline (repeat if necessary after 30 min) (see Precautions)
• If toxin ingestion is suspected, access should be eliminated and mineral oil and activated charcoal administered to reduce further absorption

CONTRAINDICATIONS
• Methylene blue treatment is contraindicated with diagnosed glucose-6-phosphate dehydrogenase deficiency because this enzyme is required for NADPH synthesis, which in turn is required for methemoglobin reductase to function. Furthermore, as methylene blue is not reduced, it can cause RBC oxidative stress, resulting in hemolysis
• Corticosteroids have been associated with decreased survival

PRECAUTIONS
Methylene blue is now rarely used in horses as it is considered ineffective and may exacerbate concurrent Heinz body hemolytic anemia. Use has been associated with decreased survival.

POSSIBLE INTERACTIONS
N/A

ALTERNATIVE DRUGS
• High doses of vitamin C (50–100 g IV daily) (not proven)
• Acetylcysteine at 50–140 mg/kg IV or PO for antioxidant support (not proven)

FOLLOW-UP

PATIENT MONITORING
• If methylene blue is administered, PCV should be monitored closely
• Clinical signs should be monitored for improvement/deterioration
• Renal function and urine output should be monitored

PREVENTION/AVOIDANCE
Limiting access to oxidant-containing plants and nitrate/nitrite sources.

POSSIBLE COMPLICATIONS
• Include colic, diarrhea, and laminitis; and cases with concurrent hemolysis are at risk of pigment nephropathy and acute anuric renal failure
• Coma and death if methemoglobin content of blood >80%

EXPECTED COURSE AND PROGNOSIS
• Cyanosis and the brown discoloration of blood should resolve if methemoglobin content falls below 10%
• Prognosis is generally guarded
• Mortality rates for cases of red maple toxicity can be around 60%

MISCELLANEOUS

ASSOCIATED CONDITIONS
Heinz body hemolytic anemia.

AGE-RELATED FACTORS
Diagnosis is more likely at a younger age with familial methemoglobinemia.

ZOONOTIC POTENTIAL
N/A

PREGNANCY/FERTILITY/BREEDING
N/A

SYNONYMS
N/A

SEE ALSO
• Anemia
• Anemia, Heinz body

ABBREVIATIONS
• DMSO = dimethylsulfoxide
• ELISA = enzyme-linked immunosorbent assay
• NSAID = nonsteroidal anti-inflammatory drug
• PCR = polymerase chain reaction
• PCV = packed cell volume
• PO$_2$ = partial pressure of oxygen
• RBC = red blood cell

Suggested Reading
Bozorgmanesh R, Magdesian KG, Rhodes DM, et al. Hemolytic anemia in horses associated with ingestion of *Pistacia* leaves. J Vet Intern Med 2015;29:410–413.

Author Rana Bozorgmanesh
Consulting Editors David Hodgson, Harold C. McKenzie, and Jennifer L. Hodgson
Acknowledgment The author and editors acknowledge the prior contribution of Nicholas Malikides.

METHYLXANTHINE TOXICOSIS

BASICS

OVERVIEW
• Methylxanthines include theobromine, caffeine, and theophylline
• Generally, they cause release of catecholamines (i.e. epinephrine, norepinephrine), increased muscular contractility, and stimulation of the central nervous system
• Theobromine (from cocoa bean hulls) and coffee husks have been associated with clinical intoxication in horses. Death has been associated with ingestion of theobromine in cocoa bean hulls. The diagnosis is established based on a history of ingestion and determination of theobromine or caffeine in serum, plasma, urine, or stomach contents
• Use and detection of methylxanthines in racehorses are of concern

SIGNALMENT
All Equidae are susceptible to theobromine or caffeine intoxication, but the few reported cases in horses do not allow for determination of breed or sex predilections.

SIGNS
• 1 case of theobromine ingestion by horses has been reported with "violent excitement" as the outstanding clinical sign
• Other reported cases of theobromine intoxication only described sudden death
• The clinical case of coffee husk poisoning and subsequent feeding trial report excitability, restlessness, involuntary muscle tremors, chewing movements/tremors of the lips and tongue, sweating, and increased respiration and heart rate. Similar clinical signs may be seen in foals administered caffeine as a respiratory stimulant
• Clinical signs of toxicosis reported in other species (primarily dogs)—hyperactivity, diarrhea, diuresis, muscle tremors, ataxia, cardiac arrhythmias, and death

CAUSES AND RISK FACTORS
• Theobromine is found in cocoa bean hulls, chocolate, and chocolate-containing bakery waste
• Caffeine is found in coffee husks, coffee beans and coffee, and some pharmaceuticals. It is also found in tea, chocolate, energy drinks, and other products
• Toxicoses and deaths have been reported through ingestion of cocoa bean hulls or coffee husks used as bedding or in feed
• Roughly, a dose of 100 mg/kg of theobromine given over 4 days as cocoa bean hulls in feed has been reported to cause death; the possibility of toxicosis at lower doses has not been investigated

• Cocoa bean hulls are reported to contain as much as 0.5% theobromine by weight
• Coffee husks have been reported to contain 0.9% caffeine. Ad libitum feeding resulted in the manifestation of clinical signs
• Theobromine and caffeine have been detected in the urine of racehorses fed small amounts of chocolate candy or incorporated into feed

DIAGNOSIS

DIFFERENTIAL DIAGNOSIS
Other causes of rapid/sudden death in horses from cardiac arrhythmias include accidental ingestion of ionophore feed supplements (test for ionophores in the feed), ingestion of *Eupatorium rugosum* or white snakeroot (history; evidence of ingestion and myocardial necrosis), or ingestion of bark and leaves of *Robinia pseudoacacia* or black locust (history; evidence of ingestion).

CBC/BIOCHEMISTRY/URINALYSIS
No abnormalities have been reported with theobromine toxicoses.

OTHER LABORATORY TESTS
N/A

IMAGING
N/A

OTHER DIAGNOSTIC PROCEDURES
• The diagnosis of theobromine or caffeine toxicosis is established based on clinical history, evidence of ingestion, and presence of theobromine in serum, plasma, urine, or stomach contents
• ECG can monitor for possible cardiac arrhythmias

TREATMENT
• Eliminate exposure
• Restrict activity because of possible cardiac arrhythmias

MEDICATIONS

DRUG(S) OF CHOICE
• Administer activated charcoal unless contraindicated (1–4 g/kg in a water slurry)
• Because of the limited number of reported cases, pharmacologic intervention in equine theobromine toxicosis has not been evaluated

CONTRAINDICATIONS/POSSIBLE INTERACTIONS
N/A

FOLLOW-UP

PATIENT MONITORING
Monitor ECG to evaluate cardiac status.

PREVENTION/AVOIDANCE
Do not allow horses to eat cocoa bean hulls, chocolate products, coffee husks, or products containing caffeine.

POSSIBLE COMPLICATIONS
N/A

EXPECTED COURSE AND PROGNOSIS
The rarity of theobromine toxicosis precludes generalization to all prospective equine cases; however, when less than toxic amounts are ingested and ECG abnormalities are not present, the prognosis is excellent.

MISCELLANEOUS

ASSOCIATED CONDITIONS
N/A

AGE-RELATED FACTORS
N/A

ZOONOTIC POTENTIAL
N/A

PREGNANCY/FERTILITY/BREEDING
N/A

SEE ALSO
N/A

Suggested Reading
Blakemore F, Shearer GD. The poisoning of livestock by cacao products. Vet Rec 1943;55:165.
Delfiol D, Oliveira-Filho J, Casalecchi F, et al. Equine poisoning by coffee husk (Coffea arabica L.). BMC Vet Res 2012;8:4.
Harkins JD, Rees WA, Mundy GD, et al. An overview of the methylxanthines and their regulation in the horse. Equine Pract 1998;20:10–16.
Machnik M, Kaiser S, Koppe S, et al. Control of methylxanthines in the competition horse: pharmacokinetic/pharmacodynamic studies on caffeine, theobromine, and theophylline for the assessment of irrelevant concentrations. Drug Test Anal 2017;9(9):1372–1384.

Author Stephen B. Hooser
Consulting Editors Wilson K. Rumbeiha and Steve Ensley

M

MITRAL REGURGITATION

 BASICS

DEFINITION
Occurs when the mitral valve allows blood to leak into the left atrium during systole and creates a systolic murmur with its point of maximal intensity over the heart base radiating caudodorsally.

PATHOPHYSIOLOGY
• Mitral regurgitation can occur with structurally normal valve cusps or when dysplastic, inflammatory, or degenerative disease, prolapse or rupture of a chorda tendinea is present
• Ventricular dilation, e.g. due to cardiomyopathy or severe aortic regurgitation, leads to mitral regurgitation
• During systole, blood regurgitates into the left atrium, causing increased left atrial pressure and a left atrial and ventricular volume overload
• As the regurgitation becomes more severe, increases in left atrial pressure produce pulmonary hypertension, pulmonary edema, and clinical signs of CHF
• Pulmonary artery dilation and rupture can be a sequela to pulmonary hypertension

SYSTEMS AFFECTED
Cardiovascular

GENETICS
N/A

INCIDENCE/PREVALENCE
The prevalence of mitral regurgitation murmurs in a middle-aged and older population of apparently healthy horses in the UK was 2.9% and in Thoroughbreds was 9% in flat and 19% in jump racing.

SIGNALMENT
Athletic breeds and older horses.

SIGNS
General Comments
Often an incidental finding. mitral regurgitation may not necessarily affect performance. The severity of signs is dependent on the nature and severity of valvular pathology.

Historical Findings
• Often poor performance
• Sometimes CHF

Physical Examination Findings
• Grade 2–6/6, band-shaped, crescendo or musical holosystolic or pansystolic murmur with point of maximal impulse in the mitral to aortic valve area (left fifth to fourth intercostal space) and radiating dorsally to the left heart base
• Other less common findings—supraventricular premature depolarizations, atrial fibrillation, accentuated third heart sounds, tachypnea, cough, and CHF

CAUSES
• Physiologic mitral regurgitation, often related to cardiac adaptation in response to athletic training
• Prolapse
• Degenerative changes of the mitral leaflets
• Nonvegetative valvulitis
• Ruptured chordae tendineae
• Infective endocarditis
• Congenital malformation

RISK FACTORS
• Athletes have a high prevalence of physiologic mitral regurgitation
• Increasing age
• Large ponies and horses had a higher prevalence of left-sided valvular regurgitation (i.e. mitral and/or aortic regurgitation) than small ponies

 DIAGNOSIS

DIFFERENTIAL DIAGNOSIS
Physiologic ejection murmur—this murmur is typically grade 1–3/6 and localized to the aortic valve.

CBC/BIOCHEMISTRY/URINALYSIS
May have leukocytosis and hyperfibrinogenemia and elevated SAA with infective endocarditis.

OTHER LABORATORY TESTS
• Increased concentrations of cardiac troponin I may be present with concurrent myocardial disease
• Positive blood culture may be obtained from horses with infective endocarditis

IMAGING
Echocardiography
• Diffuse or nodular thickened mitral valve leaflets
• Prolapse of a mitral leaflet (usually an accessory leaflet) into the left atrium
• Ruptured chorda tendinea, flail mitral leaflet, or bacterial endocarditis are detected infrequently
• Left atrium—enlarged and dilated, with a rounded appearance
• Left ventricle—enlarged and dilated, with a rounded apex
• Thinning of the left ventricular free wall and interventricular septum
• Subjective ventricular hyperkinesis, dilation, and increased fractional shortening suggest left ventricular volume overload
• Dilatation of the pulmonary veins and, later, the pulmonary artery in severely affected horses
• Doppler echocardiography reveals jet(s) of regurgitation in the left atrium. The size and extent of the jet semiquantitate severity

Thoracic Radiography
• Left-sided cardiac enlargement and dorsal displacement of the trachea
• Pulmonary edema with left-sided CHF

OTHER DIAGNOSTIC PROCEDURES
ECG
Ventricular and/or supraventricular premature depolarizations or atrial fibrillation may be present.

PATHOLOGIC FINDINGS
• Where the regurgitation is physiologic, no pathologic findings are expected
• Focal or diffuse thickening or distortion of 1 or more mitral leaflets may be present
• Ruptured chordae tendineae, flail mitral leaflets, infective endocarditis, or congenital malformations of the mitral valve infrequently are detected
• Jet lesions are detected in the left atrium
• Left atrial and ventricular enlargement in cases with significant regurgitation
• Dilatation of the pulmonary artery and veins with pulmonary hypertension
• In horses with CHF, peripheral edema, pleural effusion, pericardial effusion, chronic hepatic congestion, and, occasionally, ascites may be detected
• With acute severe left heart failure, frothy pulmonary edema may be found within the airways

 TREATMENT

AIMS
• Management by intermittent monitoring in horses with mitral regurgitation that is mild or moderate in severity
• Palliative care in horses with severe mitral regurgitation

APPROPRIATE HEALTH CARE
• Most affected horses require no treatment and can be monitored on an outpatient basis
• Horses with moderate to severe regurgitation may benefit from long-term vasodilator therapy, particularly with ACE inhibitors
• Treat horses with severe regurgitation and CHF with positive inotropic drugs, vasodilators, and diuretics on an inpatient basis, if possible, and monitor response to therapy

NURSING CARE
N/A

ACTIVITY
• Most horses with mitral regurgitation are safe to continue in full athletic work until the regurgitation becomes severe or ventricular arrhythmias develop
• Monitor horses with moderate to severe regurgitation by ECG during high-intensity exercise to ensure they are safe to continue in ridden work. These horses can be used for

lower level athletic activities until they begin to develop CHF
• Horses with significant ventricular arrhythmias or pulmonary artery dilatation are no longer safe to ride

CLIENT EDUCATION
• Regularly monitor the cardiac rhythm; any irregularities should prompt ECG
• Carefully monitor for exercise intolerance, respiratory distress, prolonged recovery after exercise, increased resting respiratory or heart rate, or cough; if detected, seek a cardiac reexamination

SURGICAL CONSIDERATIONS
N/A

MEDICATIONS

DRUG(S) OF CHOICE
• Treat affected horses in CHF with furosemide, torsemide vasodilators such as benazepril and quinapril, or the inodilator pimobendan
• Antimicrobials are indicated with infective endocarditis

CONTRAINDICATIONS
• ACE inhibitors are contraindicated in pregnancy
• Diuretics, ACE inhibitors, and other vasodilators must be withdrawn before competition to comply with the medication rules of the various governing bodies of equine sports

PRECAUTIONS
ACE inhibitors can cause hypotension; thus, do not give a large dose without time to accommodate to this treatment.

POSSIBLE INTERACTIONS
N/A

ALTERNATIVE DRUGS
N/A

FOLLOW-UP

PATIENT MONITORING
• Frequently monitor the intensity of the cardiac murmur, cardiac rhythm, and respiratory system
• Horses with moderate regurgitation should be reexamined echocardiographically every year. Mild cases should be reexamined every other year and horses with severe

regurgitation should be reexamined echocardiographically more frequently, particularly if the horse continues to be ridden
• Exercising ECG is indicated in horses with moderate to severe mitral regurgitation and should be repeated regularly and during exercise comparable with the horse's usual workload

PREVENTION/AVOIDANCE
N/A

POSSIBLE COMPLICATIONS
Chronic and/or severe regurgitation—atrial fibrillation; CHF, pulmonary artery rupture

EXPECTED COURSE AND PROGNOSIS
• Many affected horses have a normal performance life and life expectancy
• Prognosis for horses with mitral valve prolapse and mild regurgitation is excellent; in many, the amount of regurgitation remains unchanged for years
• Progression of regurgitation associated with degenerative valve disease usually is slow; if the regurgitation is mild, these horses also have a good prognosis
• Horses with ruptured chordae tendineae, flail mitral valve leaflets, infective endocarditis, or cardiomyopathy have a more guarded prognosis because regurgitation usually becomes more severe and results in shortened performance life and life expectancy
• Affected horses with CHF usually have severe underlying valvular heart and/or myocardial disease and a guarded to grave prognosis for life
• Most affected horses being treated for CHF respond to supportive therapy and improve. This improvement usually is short lived, however, and most are euthanized within 2–6 months of initiating treatment

MISCELLANEOUS

ASSOCIATED CONDITIONS
N/A

AGE-RELATED FACTORS
Old horses are more likely to be affected.

ZOONOTIC POTENTIAL
N/A

PREGNANCY/FERTILITY/BREEDING
• Affected mares should not experience any problems with pregnancy unless the regurgitation is severe

• The volume expansion of late pregnancy places an additional load on the already volume-loaded heart and may precipitate the onset of CHF in mares with severe regurgitation
• Pregnant mares affected with CHF should be treated for the underlying cardiac disease with positive inotropic drugs and diuretics; ACE inhibitors are contraindicated because of potential adverse effects on the fetus

SYNONYMS
Mitral insufficiency.

SEE ALSO
• Atrial fibrillation
• Endocarditis, infective

ABBREVIATIONS
• ACE = angiotensin-converting enzyme
• CHF = congestive heart failure
• SAA = serum amyloid A

Suggested Reading
Afonso T, Giguere S, Rapoport G, et al. Pharmacodynamic evaluation of 4 angiotensin-converting enzyme inhibitors in healthy adult horses. J Vet Intern Med 2013;27:1185–1192.
Afonso T, Giguere S, Rapoport G, et al. Cardiovascular effects of pimobendan in healthy mature horses. Equine Vet J 2016;48:352–356.
Reef VB, Bonagura J, Buhl R, et al. Recommendations for management of equine athletes with cardiovascular abnormalities. J Vet Intern Med 2014;28:749–761.
Stevens KB, Marr CM, Horn JN, et al. Effect of left-sided valvular regurgitation on mortality and causes of death among a population of middle-aged and older horses. Vet Rec 2009;164:6–10.
Young LE, Rogers K, Wood JL. Heart murmurs and valvular regurgitation in Thoroughbred racehorses: epidemiology and associations with athletic performance. J Vet Intern Med 2008;22:418–426.

Author Celia M. Marr
Consulting Editors Celia M. Marr and Virginia B. Reef
Acknowledgment The author acknowledges the prior contribution of Virginia B. Reef.

M

MONENSIN TOXICOSIS

BASICS

OVERVIEW
- Monensin is used as an anticoccidial agent and growth promotant in livestock species
- Horses are the most sensitive non-target species (LD$_{50}$ 2–3 mg/kg)
- Most affected organ systems are:
  - Cardiovascular—severe myocardial necrosis with secondary systemic congestion
  - Musculoskeletal—severe muscle necrosis

SIGNALMENT
No age, genetic, or sex predilection.

SIGNS
- Onset of clinical signs commonly occurs within 24 h but can be delayed for days to months
- Anorexia
- Ataxia
- Tremors
- Sweating
- Dyspnea
- Depression with hypoactivity or reluctance to move
- Weakness
- Recumbency with attempts to rise and thrashing of legs
- Sudden death

CAUSES AND RISK FACTORS
- Exposure to premix or feed containing monensin
- Feeding rations containing monensin, e.g. cattle, poultry, or swine feed
- Feed mixing errors in which monensin is inadvertently added to the ration
- Feed contamination at mills that mix cattle, poultry, or swine feed
- Gaining access to and consumption of bagged premix

DIAGNOSIS

DIFFERENTIAL DIAGNOSIS
- Other causes of myopathies including rhabdomyolysis, hyperkalemic periodic paralysis, vitamin E/selenium deficiency, seasonal pasture myopathy
- White snake root
- Cantharidin toxicosis
- Selenium toxicosis

CBC/BIOCHEMISTRY/URINALYSIS
- Often, there is minimal to no effect on hematopoietic parameters

- Owing to the potential delayed onset of clinical signs, serum chemistry abnormalities may not be observed as changes in serum chemistry typically occur within 24 h preceding death
- Creatine kinase and aspartate aminotransferase may be increased because of cardiac and skeletal myocyte damage
- Electrolyte abnormalities may be observed but typically occur late. Electrolyte changes include increased serum phosphorus and decreased serum calcium and potassium
- Urine glucose, protein, myoglobin, and hemoglobin can be increased, accompanied by a decrease in urine specific gravity and pH

OTHER LABORATORY TESTS
Cardiac troponins may be elevated.

IMAGING
N/A

OTHER DIAGNOSTIC PROCEDURES
- A quantitative analysis for monensin and other ionophores, which can cause similar clinical signs, in a representative feed sample through liquid chromatography mass spectrometry
- Feed samples may not be representative of what was consumed if the feed in question is gone, there is a delayed onset of clinical signs, or if the ration is hand-mixed for each feeding

PATHOLOGIC FINDINGS
- In cases of peracute death, gross and microscopic lesions may not be observed
- Gross findings include areas of pallor and streaking of cardiac and skeletal muscle along with epicardial and endocardial hemorrhage. Secondary lesions associated with heart failure include hydropericardium, pulmonary edema, hydrothorax, nutmeg liver, and ascites
- Microscopic findings include myocardial degeneration and necrosis characterized by vacuolization, loss of striation, and mineralization with chronic cases exhibiting myocardial fibrosis and lymphoplasmacytic infiltrate

TREATMENT
- There is no specific antidote for monensin toxicosis
- Remove suspect feed immediately to prevent further access and consumption
- Administration of vitamin E to minimize oxidative damage to tissues
- Gastric lavage or administration of activated charcoal immediately to minimize absorption.

- Administration of mineral oil to expedite gastrointestinal transit
- Restrict activity of affected horses for up to 3 months

FOLLOW-UP

PATIENT MONITORING
Echocardiograms can be used to monitor for cardiomyopathies in surviving individuals.

PREVENTION/AVOIDANCE
- Store feeds or premixes containing monensin away from horse feed and in an area inaccessible to horses
- Implementation of good feed-mixing practices

POSSIBLE COMPLICATIONS
May observe acute death months later without prior clinical signs.

EXPECTED COURSE AND PROGNOSIS
- The prognosis depends on the quantity of monensin ingested and the amount of damage to cardiac and skeletal muscle
- Poor to grave once clinical signs are observed
- Death is attributed to severe myocardial damage and decreased function

MISCELLANEOUS

ABBREVIATIONS
LD$_{50}$ = median lethal dose

Suggested Reading
Divers TJ, Kraus MS, Jesty SA, et al. Clinical findings and serum cardiac troponin I concentrations in horses after intragastric administration of sodium monensin. J Vet Diagn Invest 2009;21(3):338–343.
Hall JO. Ionophores. In: Plumlee KH, ed. Clinical Veterinary Toxicology. St. Louis, MO: Mosby, 2004:120–127.
Novilla NM. Ionophores. In: Gupta RC, ed. Veterinary Toxicology, 2e. San Diego, CA: Elsevier, 2012:1281–1299.
Poppenga RH. Feed additives. In: Smith BP, ed. Large Animal Internal Medicine, 5e. St. Louis, MO: Elsevier Mosby, 2015:1609–1610.

Author Scott L. Radke
Consulting Editors Wilson K. Rumbeiha and Steve Ensley

BASICS

OVERVIEW
• Monocyte count greater than the upper limit of laboratory reference interval: usually >600 cells/µL (>0.6 × 10^9/L). • Monopoiesis occurs in the bone marrow under the influence of interleukin 3, GM-CSF, and M-CSF. • GM-CSF and M-CSF are produced by endothelial cells, fibroblasts, lymphocytes, and cells of monocyte origin. • Monopoiesis is rapid: monocytes are released into blood within 6 days of initiation of stem cell division. • A bone marrow storage pool is absent for monocytes. • Monocytes have a circulating half-life of ≈3 days and account for ≈5% of peripheral blood leukocytes. • Monocytes migrate from blood to tissues and body cavities randomly or at specific sites of inflammation due to chemotactic factors (microbial products, chemokines) and undergo transformation into macrophages, accompanied by numerous morphologic, metabolic, and functional changes: they do not reenter the circulation. • Macrophages are free or fixed. Free macrophages are located in mesothelial and synovial cavities, alveoli, and inflammatory sites. Fixed macrophages are found in tissues, including the spleen, liver, bone, skin, connective tissue, lymph nodes, lung, brain, and gastrointestinal tract. • Monocytes and macrophages constitute the mononuclear phagocytic system, which is an integral component of the reticuloendothelial system. • Monocytes/macrophages have numerous functions—microbiocidal activity (including intracellular bacteria, fungi, protozoa, and viruses), phagocytosis, regulation of immune and inflammatory responses, cytotoxicity against tumor and foreign cells, hemostasis and tissue repair. • Monocytosis arises from an increased rate of monopoiesis and release of monocytes from the bone marrow and may be appropriate (increased tissue demand) or inappropriate (unassociated with tissue demand). • Hemic/lymphatic/immune systems are affected. • Other body systems can be involved due to underlying infections or monocytic myeloproliferative disease

SIGNALMENT
N/A

SIGNS
• Signs are dependent on the underlying disease causing monocytosis. • Inflammatory or myeloproliferative disorders may cause weight loss, inappetence, lethargy, and pyrexia. • Signs of specific organ involvement may occur

CAUSES AND RISK FACTORS
• Any inflammatory process stimulating a neutrophilia will cause monocytosis.

• Monocytic and myelomonocytic leukemias are rare in horses. Most cases are acute and progress rapidly. • Immunodeficiency syndromes in foals, e.g. FTPI or SCID, are risk factors

DIAGNOSIS

DIFFERENTIAL DIAGNOSIS
Underlying cause of monocytosis should be determined.

CBC/BIOCHEMISTRY/URINALYSIS
• Concurrent neutrophilia—consider inflammatory process. • Immature or bizarre monocytes/blast forms—myeloproliferative disease. • Marked monocytosis (>10 000 cells/µL (>10.0 × 10^9/L)), anemia, thrombocytopenia, and neutropenia—monocytic myeloproliferative disorder. • Biochemical analysis may reveal evidence of specific organ involvement

OTHER LABORATORY TESTS
• PCR for SCID. • Immunoglobulin G <400 mg/dL in neonates—FTPI. • Serology for viral or bacterial pathogens

IMAGING
• Thoracic and abdominal ultrasonography—inflammatory or neoplastic processes. • Thoracic radiography—pneumonia, lung abscess, neoplasia

OTHER DIAGNOSTIC PROCEDURES
• Abdominocentesis and/or thoracocentesis—inflammatory or neoplastic disease. • Endoscopy—inflammatory or neoplastic disease. • Bone marrow aspirate/biopsy—myeloproliferative disease. • Laparoscopy/thoracoscopy—abscess/tumor

PATHOLOGIC FINDINGS
Dependent on cause.

TREATMENT
• Elimination of underlying cause of monocytosis. • Often directed toward resolution of infectious disease. • Depends on cause and severity of underlying disease. • Often inpatient medical management is required. • Surgical management may be required to address specific infectious disease (e.g. abscess removal/drainage).

MEDICATIONS

DRUG(S) OF CHOICE
Bacterial infections require antimicrobial therapy based on culture and sensitivity testing.

CONTRAINDICATIONS/POSSIBLE INTERACTIONS
Corticosteroids should be avoided in horses with laminitis or infectious disease.

FOLLOW-UP

PATIENT MONITORING
Periodic monitoring of monocyte and neutrophil counts.

PREVENTION/AVOIDANCE
N/A

POSSIBLE COMPLICATIONS
N/A

EXPECTED COURSE AND PROGNOSIS
• Infectious/inflammatory disease—prognosis ranges from good to guarded/poor dependent on the etiology, severity, and response to treatment. • Myeloproliferative disorders—hopeless prognosis

MISCELLANEOUS

ASSOCIATED CONDITIONS
N/A

AGE-RELATED FACTORS
Monocyte counts are not affected by age.

ZOONOTIC POTENTIAL
Certain microorganisms that may stimulate monocytosis (e.g. *Mycobacterium* spp.) are zoonotic.

PREGNANCY/FERTILITY/BREEDING
N/A

SEE ALSO
Neutrophilia

ABBREVIATIONS
• FTPI = failure of transfer of passive immunity. • GM-CSF = granulocyte–macrophage colony-stimulating factor. • M-CSF = macrophage colony-stimulating factor. • SCID = severe combined immunodeficiency

Suggested Reading
Carrick JB, Begg AP. Peripheral blood leukocytes. Vet Clin North Am Equine Pract 2008;24:239–259.

Author Kristopher Hughes
Consulting Editors David Hodgson, Harold C. McKenzie, and Jennifer L. Hodgson

M

MULTIPLE ENDOCRINE NEOPLASIA SYNDROME

BASICS

OVERVIEW
• MEN syndrome defines a group of diseases characterized by the development of hyperplasia and/or neoplasia of 2 or more endocrine glands
• This rare syndrome is well described in humans and has been reported in dogs, cats, and cattle
• In humans, MEN syndrome is classified into 2 principal categories:
  ○ MEN type 1 (MEN 1)—usually the association of parathyroid, enterohepatic, endocrine, and pituitary neoplasia
  ○ MEN type 2 (MEN 2)—usually involves C-cell thyroid adenoma/carcinoma, pheochromocytoma, and parathyroid hyperplasia/adenomas. 2 subtypes of MEN 2 are identified
• A few equine cases have been reported at necropsy but it remains underrecognized
• The functional significance of these tumors in the horse is unclear at present
• Systems affected—endocrine/metabolic; other systems may be affected if the tumors compress or displace other organs (e.g. ocular globe)

SIGNALMENT
• No sex or breed predisposition reported
• Diagnosed in aged horses

SIGNS
• Signs are related to the different neoplasms present if active or to a mass effect
• Thyroid gland—usually no clinical signs other than enlargement of the gland. Weight loss may be present
• Pituitary gland—hypertrichosis, muscle atrophy, polyuria and polydipsia, weight loss, potbelly appearance, chronic laminitis
• Parathyroids—intermittent weakness, enlargement of facial bones, shifting lameness, weight loss possible
• Adrenals—sweating, tachycardia, tachypnea, abdominal pain, mydriasis, muscle tremors if the tumor is functional
• Exophthalmos in case of orbital neoplasm

CAUSES AND RISK FACTORS
Unknown

DIAGNOSIS

DIFFERENTIAL DIAGNOSIS
MEN should be suspected in horses presented with signs of pituitary pars intermedia dysfunction, thyroid enlargement, or when a mass of neuroendocrine origin is diagnosed.

CBC/BIOCHEMISTRY/URINALYSIS
Laboratory findings are variable and depend on the types of neoplasms present:
• With a pituitary adenoma—stress leukogram and/or hyperglycemia
• With a functional parathyroid neoplasm—hypercalcemia, hypophosphatemia, and hyperphosphaturia
• With a functional pheochromocytoma—hyponatremia, hyperkalemia, metabolic acidosis, hypocalcemia, hyperphosphatemia, azotemia, hyperglycemia, glucosuria, and occult hematuria

OTHER LABORATORY TESTS
Endocrine tests may help in the diagnosis of the different types of tumors:
• Serum triiodothyronine or thyroxine may be increased or decreased with a thyroid tumor
• Endogenous plasma adrenocorticotropic hormone levels or thyrotropin-releasing hormone stimulation test if suspicion of a pituitary adenoma
• Plasma or urinary catecholamine levels when suspecting a pheochromocytoma
• Serum PTH may be elevated in cases of a neoplastic parathyroid gland

IMAGING
• Thyroid tumors may be imaged via US
• Parathyroid neoplasia may be detected using nuclear scintigraphy or US

OTHER DIAGNOSTIC PROCEDURES
Fine needle aspirate may identify a thyroid tumor; a biopsy may help a definitive diagnosis on the type of tumor.

PATHOLOGIC FINDINGS
• MEN syndrome is mainly diagnosed at necropsy
• Most cases identified at necropsy had a combination of C-cell thyroid adenoma and pheochromocytoma. Pituitary pars intermedia adenoma and orbital paraganglioma have also been associated with these tumors

TREATMENT

Surgical excision when warranted. Medical treatment and management of clinical signs associated with primary tumors.

MEDICATIONS

DRUG(S) OF CHOICE
Indicated depending on the type of endocrine tumor diagnosed—pergolide if pituitary adenoma, diuretics and/or corticosteroids to promote urinary calcium excretion if hypercalcemia associated with a parathyroid gland adenoma or adenocarcinoma.

CONTRAINDICATIONS/POSSIBLE INTERACTIONS
Dependent on the tumor.

FOLLOW-UP

• Standard postoperative follow-up if a tumor is removed surgically
• Monitor endocrine testing, as indicated (e.g. PTH if involvement of the parathyroid)

MISCELLANEOUS

SEE ALSO
• Pituitary pars intermedia dysfunction
• Primary hyperparathyroidism
• Thyroid tumors

ABBREVIATIONS
• MEN = multiple endocrine neoplasia
• PTH = parathyroid hormone
• US = ultrasonography, ultrasound

Suggested Reading
De Cock HEV, MacLachlan NJ. Simultaneous occurrence of multiple neoplasms and hyperplasias in the adrenal and thyroid gland of the horse resembling multiple endocrine neoplasia syndrome: case report and retrospective identification of additional cases. Vet Pathol 1999;36:633–636.
Germann SE, Rutten M, Derungs SB, Fenge K. Multiple endocrine neoplasia-like syndrome in a horse. Vet Rec 2006;159:530–532.
Luethy D, Habeker P, Murphy B, Nolen-Watson R. Clinical and pathological features of pheochromocytoma in the horse: a multicenter retrospective study of 37 cases (2007-2014). J Vet Intern Med 2016;30:309–313.

Author Michel Levy
Consulting Editors Michel Levy and Heidi Banse

M

MULTIPLE MYELOMA

BASICS

OVERVIEW
• Rare neoplasm caused by the malignant proliferation of plasma cells
• Primarily arises from the bone marrow, but can originate from, or metastasize to, extramedullary organs

SIGNALMENT
• Quarter Horses are overrepresented
• Age range—3 months to 25 years

SIGNS
• Nonspecific signs; weight loss, peripheral edema, fever, and lymphadenopathy
• Other signs include anorexia, pneumonia, rear leg paresis/ataxia, epistaxis, bone pain, and soft feces

CAUSES AND RISK FACTORS
None identified.

DIAGNOSIS

• Diagnosis made if combination of 1 major and 1 minor criteria or 3 minor criteria are found
• *Major* criteria—bone marrow plasmacytosis >30%; biopsy diagnosis of a plasmacytoma with evidence of uncontrolled production of a monoclonal immunoglobulin or protein fragment (paraprotein or M-component)
• *Minor* criteria—bone marrow plasmacytosis <30%, serum or urine paraprotein present in lower concentrations; 50% decrease in other immunoglobulin classes; and osteolytic bone lesion(s)

DIFFERENTIAL DIAGNOSIS
• Lymphoma and lymphoid leukemia; differentiated by identification of neoplastic lymphocytic proliferation on tissue/bone marrow biopsy
• Single plasmacytoma; differentiated by lack of paraneoplastic syndromes, monoclonal gammopathy, or diffuse bone marrow involvement
• Other causes of monoclonal gammopathy, e.g. chronic bacterial or fungal infection; differentiated by response to treatment and diagnostic serology identifying causative agent
• Benign monoclonal gammopathy; diagnosis of exclusion

CBC/BIOCHEMISTRY/URINALYSIS
• Hyperproteinemia with hyperglobulinemia and hypoalbuminemia
• Hyperviscosity of serum
• Myelophthisic disease; anemia, thrombocytopenia, leukopenia
• Plasma cell leukemia
• Hypercalcemia due to PTHrP or renal failure
• Renal failure with proteinuria and azotemia
• Hyponatremia

OTHER LABORATORY TESTS
• Serum/urine electrophoresis indicative of a monoclonal gammopathy
• Bence Jones proteinuria
• Elevated PTHrP

IMAGING
• Radiography; focal, punctate bone lysis, periosteal reaction and sclerosis, diffuse osteoporosis, or pathologic fractures
• Ultrasonography; masses in the abdominal or thoracic cavities

OTHER DIAGNOSTIC PROCEDURES
• Bone marrow aspirate/biopsy; identification of plasmacytosis (>10%) and atypical plasma cells with nuclear–cytoplasmic asynchrony
• Repeat bone marrow aspirates at several sites if bone involvement is focal
• Biopsy of extraosseous tissues such as spleen, liver, lymph nodes, and kidney may reveal infiltration of neoplastic plasmacytoid cells
• Immunofluorescence/histochemical labeling of cytoplasmic or surface immunoglobulins can identify monoclonal plasma cell populations suggestive of malignant plasmacytosis

PATHOLOGIC FINDINGS
• Neoplastic plasma cell infiltration (>10%) of bone marrow
• Focal or diffuse bone lesions including osteoporosis, cortical erosion, pathologic fractures, and grossly visible tumor with normal to increased number of plasma cells or atypical plasma cells
• Plasma cell infiltration of tissues, particularly spleen, liver, lymph nodes, and kidney
• Immunoglobulin or amyloid deposition in the kidneys

TREATMENT

Inpatient care to provide supportive treatment to relieve associated clinical problems and side effects of chemotherapeutic agents.

MEDICATIONS

DRUG(S) OF CHOICE
• Short-term stabilization of disease (7–12 months) reported in horses treated with melphalan; cyclophosphamide and prednisolone also given to these horses; dose rates not reported
• Doxorubicin (70 mg/m² IV every 2 weeks) may result in clinical improvement
• Corticosteroid therapy (prednisolone 1 mg/kg PO every 24 h or dexamethasone 0.1 mg/kg every 24 h) may provide palliative relief

CONTRAINDICATIONS/POSSIBLE INTERACTIONS
• Cyclophosphamide—bone marrow suppression and hemorrhagic cystitis
• Doxorubicin—bone marrow suppression, hyperthermia, colic
• Corticosteroids—laminitis, iatrogenic Cushing syndrome

FOLLOW-UP

PATIENT MONITORING
• Progressive pancytopenia due to myelophthisis
• Serial monitoring of PTHrP and globulin concentrations in horses with unconfirmed multiple myeloma may be useful

PREVENTION/AVOIDANCE
N/A

POSSIBLE COMPLICATIONS
Acquired secondary infections, particularly pneumonia, due to impaired immunologic function.

EXPECTED COURSE AND PROGNOSIS
Median life expectancy after diagnosis is 3 months; range 1.5 months to 2 years.

M

MISCELLANEOUS

ASSOCIATED CONDITIONS
• Systemic light-chain amyloidosis (1 case)
• Idiopathic multifocal smooth muscle hypertrophy (1 case)

AGE-RELATED FACTORS
N/A

ZOONOTIC POTENTIAL
None

PREGNANCY/FERTILITY/BREEDING
Most chemotherapeutic agents have embryo lethal and teratogenic effects.

SEE ALSO
Lymphosarcoma

ABBREVIATIONS
PTHrP = parathyroid hormone-related protein

Suggested Reading
Munoz A, Riber C, Trigo P, Castejon F. Hematopoietic neoplasias in horses: myeloproliferative and lymphoproliferative disorders. J Equine Sci 2009;20:59–72.

Author Krista Estell
Consulting Editors David Hodgson, Harold C. McKenzie, and Jennifer L. Hodgson
Acknowledgment The author and editors acknowledge the prior contribution of Rachel Tan.

MULTISYSTEMIC EOSINOPHILIC EPITHELIOTROPIC DISEASE

BASICS

OVERVIEW
• A chronic, progressive condition of unclear etiology associated with weight loss, dermatitis, and the presence of eosinophilic infiltrates in multiple organs
• Similar conditions exist in humans, cats, and dogs. Parasitic, allergic, autoimmune, viral, and toxic causes have been implicated. The coexistence of T-cell lymphosarcoma and the syndrome in horses suggests that the production of cytokines (such as interleukin 5) by clonal neoplastic cells stimulates production and proliferation of eosinophils
• Skin, GI, hepatobiliary, and respiratory systems are affected

SIGNALMENT
• Standardbreds may be predisposed
• Horses 3–13 years of age

SIGNS
• Most horses present with weight loss of several weeks' or months' duration, although a few cases have presented acutely. Roughly half of these horses will have diarrhea concurrently
• Examination often shows concomitant crusting, pruritic and exfoliating dermatitis, and alopecia. Skin lesions are most commonly found on the distal limbs, coronary bands, and head, or are generalized

CAUSES AND RISK FACTORS
Multiple etiologies have been proposed, including parasitism, hypersensitivity, and T-cell lymphosarcoma. An underlying cause is often not identified and the pathogenesis is unknown.

DIAGNOSIS

DIFFERENTIAL DIAGNOSIS
Tissue biopsy and laboratory testing help differentiate this disease from other diseases that present with similar signs such as:
• Causes of chronic weight loss, including dental problems, poor nutrition, parasitism, and infiltrative bowel diseases, including alimentary lymphosarcoma
• Causes of dermatitis, including dermatophilosis, dermatophytosis, pyoderma, and autoimmune skin diseases
• Sarcoidosis (not to be confused with the common equine skin tumor) can cause weight loss and skin lesions, but may be differentiated by tissue biopsy

CBC/BIOCHEMISTRY/URINALYSIS
• Hypoproteinemia
• Hypoalbuminemia

• Hyperfibrinogenemia
• Hypereosinophilia
• Evidence of other organ involvement including increased γ-glutamyltransferase, alkaline phosphatase, or creatinine

OTHER LABORATORY TESTS
Abdominocentesis may reveal a modified transudate containing eosinophils.

IMAGING
• Thoracic radiographs may reveal patterns consistent with miliary or granulomatous infiltrates
• Ultrasonography of liver, spleen, or kidneys may show granulomatous changes

OTHER DIAGNOSTIC PROCEDURES
• Tissue biopsy (GI tract, liver, lungs)—multifocal or diffuse eosinophilic and lymphoplasmacytic infiltrates
• Bone marrow biopsy may have large clusters of proliferating eosinophils or precursors
• Skin biopsy for histopathology—ulceration and acanthosis with infiltrating neutrophilic and lymphocytic exudate and eosinophilic granulomas
• Glucose or xylose GI absorption test—may be abnormal
• Exploratory laparotomy findings may include multifocal nodules or diffuse thickening of the GI tract due to eosinophilic and lymphocytic infiltration. Focal or disseminated lymphosarcoma may be found

TREATMENT

• Outpatient medical treatment may be appropriate, although horses with severe diarrhea or other organ system dysfunction may require hospitalization with fluid therapy and supportive care for diarrhea and skin lesions. Rest affected horses
• Encourage appetite. The diet should be modified to optimize absorption, including increasing high-quality forage and caloric intake (by increasing both the amount of feed and caloric density through fat supplementation)
• Consider exploratory laparotomy to obtain tissue biopsies, to rule out other intestinal involvement, or to resect a primary alimentary lymphosarcoma

MEDICATIONS

DRUG(S) OF CHOICE
Attempt treatment with dexamethasone (0.05–0.1 mg/kg IV or PO daily, reducing over several weeks) or other

anti-inflammatory medications. In 1 report, the condition resolved with dexamethasone, trimethoprim–sulfamethoxazole, hydroxyzine hydrochloride, and fenbendazole.

CONTRAINDICATIONS/POSSIBLE INTERACTIONS
None

FOLLOW-UP

PATIENT MONITORING
• Monitor the horse's weight
• Monitor response to medication through examination, hematology, biochemistry, and/or imaging

EXPECTED COURSE AND PROGNOSIS
The disease is associated with a poor prognosis and low survival. Most horses require euthanasia after several months of poor response to treatment, although a few reported cases have responded well and survived longer than 8 months after diagnosis.

MISCELLANEOUS

ASSOCIATED CONDITIONS
Lymphosarcoma

SYNONYMS
• Hypereosinophilic syndrome
• Multisystemic eosinophilic epitheliotrophic disease

ABBREVIATIONS
GI = gastrointestinal

Suggested Reading
Bosseler L, Verryken K, Bauwens C, et al. Equine multisystemic eosinophilic epitheliotropic disease: a case report and review of literature. N Z Vet J 2013;61:177–182.

Author Laura K. Dunbar
Consulting Editor Gwendolen Lorch
Acknowledgment The author and editor acknowledge the prior contribution of Richard J. Piercy.

Client Education Handout available online

M

BASICS

OVERVIEW
- Rare tumors involving neoplastic myeloid hematopoietic cells (nonlymphoid) within bone marrow or extramedullary tissues
- Results in pathologic ablation of normal tissue architecture and ultimately loss of bone marrow elements and myelophthisis
- Malignant histiocytosis and myeloid leukemia are 2 forms of this disease
- Myeloid leukemia further classified into monocytic and myelomonocytic leukemia, granulocytic leukemia, megakaryocytic leukemia, and primary erythrocytosis; eosinophilic myeloproliferative disorder is the other single-cell leukemia reported in horses
- Malignant histiocytosis involves proliferation of mononuclear phagocytes intermediate in differentiation between monoblasts and tissue histiocytes
- Familial megakaryocytic hypoplasia reported in Standardbreds, but other forms of leukemia of megakaryocytes not described
- Primary erythrocytosis (polycythemia vera) is very rare

SIGNALMENT
- Age range for monocytic leukemia is 2–11 years
- Other myeloproliferative disorders 10 months to 16 years

SIGNS
- Most clinical signs are nonspecific and relate to destruction of tissue by invasive neoplastic cells; fever, weight loss, signs of depression, and exercise intolerance
- Dependent edema, lymphadenopathy, pallor of mucous membranes, petechial hemorrhages, and oral ulceration
- Occasionally epistaxis, dyspnea, and colic
- Icterus in cases with secondary immune-mediated hemolytic anemia

CAUSES AND RISK FACTORS
Remain undefined.

DIAGNOSIS

DIFFERENTIAL DIAGNOSIS
- Lymphoma and lymphocytic leukemia
- Anaplasmosis
- Acute enteritis/colitis, Potomac horse fever, salmonellosis, coronavirus
- Ventral and limb edema observed in vasculitis, impaired lymph drainage, hypoproteinemia, or purpura haemorrhagica
- Immune suppression and secondary infections may occur in horses with myeloproliferative disorders and may complicate diagnosis

CBC/BIOCHEMISTRY/URINALYSIS
- Anemia, thrombocytopenia, or pancytopenia
- Leukopenia, leukocytosis, or normal white cell count with or without abnormal circulating leukocytes depending on whether horse is leukemic, subleukemic, or aleukemic
- Immune-mediated hemolytic anemia and immune-mediated thrombocytopenia
- Gammopathy or mild hypoproteinemia

OTHER LABORATORY TESTS
Blood gas analysis and erythropoietin concentration for diagnosis of primary erythrocytosis; decreased concentrations of erythropoietin with a normal PaO_2 and elevated hematocrit are observed with or without thrombocytosis or leukocytosis.

IMAGING
- Abdominal US; lymphadenopathy, hepatomegaly, or splenomegaly
- Thoracic US and radiographs; respiratory infection or enlarged lymph nodes

OTHER DIAGNOSTIC PROCEDURES
- Bone marrow aspirates or biopsies; elevated myeloid to erythroid ratio (normal 0.5–3.75) and neoplastic cells as a monomorphic population
- Increased serum lysozyme (muramidase) concentrations; normally <5 μg/mL
- Cytochemistry; nonspecific myeloid markers include Sudan black B, PAS stain, alkaline phosphatase, peroxidase, and chloroacetate esterase; esterase stains (e.g. α-naphthyl-butyrate or -acetate) differentiate granulocytic cells from monocytic and megakaryocytic cells; megakaryocyte stain used to differentiate monocytic and megakaryocytic cells

PATHOLOGIC FINDINGS
- Gross findings include generalized lymphadenopathy, hepatomegaly, splenomegaly, and discoloration of myeloid tissue
- Extensive hemorrhage in severe cases
- Histopathology; immature myeloblastic cells in bone marrow, lymph nodes, spleen, liver, kidneys, lungs, and heart
- Leukostasis; white cell accumulation causing blood vessel occlusion

TREATMENT
- Limited response to therapy and timely euthanasia usually warranted
- Inpatient care is required if treatment attempted
- Client should be made aware of poor prognosis and limited treatments

MEDICATIONS

DRUG(S) OF CHOICE
- Most antineoplastic agents not effective and treatment options limited
- Available drugs expensive with little guarantee of success
- Cytarabine (10 mg/m² every 12 h for 3 weeks) shown most promise
- Antibiotics to treat any secondary infections during chemotherapy

CONTRAINDICATIONS/POSSIBLE INTERACTIONS
N/A

FOLLOW-UP

PATIENT MONITORING
CBC and biochemical profile performed periodically to assess side effects of chemotherapy such as bone marrow and organ dysfunction.

PREVENTION/AVOIDANCE
N/A

POSSIBLE COMPLICATIONS
Secondary infections due to immunosuppression.

EXPECTED COURSE AND PROGNOSIS
- Poor prognosis
- Rapid progression with most horses dying within weeks of initial presentation

MISCELLANEOUS

SEE ALSO
- Anemia
- Multiple myeloma
- Pancytopenia
- Thrombocytopenia

ABBREVIATIONS
- PaO_2 = partial pressure of oxygen in arterial blood
- PAS = periodic acid–Schiff
- US = ultrasonography, ultrasound

Suggested Reading
Munoz A, Riber C, Trigo P, Castejon F. Hematopoietic neoplasias in horses: myeloproliferative and lymphoproliferative disorders. J Equine Sci 2009;20:59–72.

Author Krista Estell
Consulting Editors David Hodgson, Harold C. McKenzie, and Jennifer L. Hodgson
Acknowledgment The author and editors acknowledge the prior contribution of Laura Lee.

M

MYOCARDIAL DISEASE

 BASICS

DEFINITION
• Myocardial disease includes myocardial degeneration, ischemia, necrosis, inflammation, fibrosis, fibrofatty infiltration, or a combination of these
• It may be focal or generalized; clinical signs are generally more severe when widespread

PATHOPHYSIOLOGY
• Focal myocardial disease often leads to arrhythmias, which, if rapid, reduce diastolic filling time and compromise cardiac output
• Generalized myocardial disease leads to decreased systolic function, reduced cardiac output, and poor perfusion of vital organs/tissues, including the myocardium
• Lack of forward flow can lead to pulmonary congestion, edema, and signs of acute left-sided heart failure

SYSTEMS AFFECTED
• Primary—cardiovascular
• Secondary—renal, gastrointestinal, hepatobiliary, musculoskeletal

GENETICS
N/A

INCIDENCE/PREVALENCE
Uncommon

GEOGRAPHIC DISTRIBUTION
N/A

SIGNALMENT
No specific breed, age, or sex predilections.

SIGNS
General Comments
The severity of clinical signs generally reflects the nature and extent of myocardial pathology.

Historical Findings
• Poor performance
• Collapse and distress
• Possible fever

Physical Examination Findings
• Tachycardia
• Arrhythmias
• Weakness
• Weak peripheral pulses
• Pale mucous membranes
• Pulse deficits
• Respiratory distress, tachypnea, cough, and frothy nasal discharge
• Moist crackles in the lungs

CAUSES
• Focal fibrosis/fibrofatty infiltrate—incidental or found in horses with persistent arrhythmias; etiology unknown
• Bacterial infection (localized to the myocardium or by extension from endocardial or pericardial lesions)
• Viral infection
• Fungal infection
• Aberrant parasite migration
• Immune-mediated disease
• Toxins (ionophores, snake venom, hypoglycin A, and others)
• Neoplastic infiltration, e.g. lymphosarcoma, hemangiosarcoma
• Myocardial failure occurs with MODS and SIRS, principally due to dysregulation of systemic vascular function and accompanied by microthrombosis. A direct myocardial depressant effect mechanism may also occur
• Streptococcal toxic shock
• Brain–heart syndrome
• White muscle disease (linked to selenium deficiency, primarily in young animals)
• Amyloidosis
• Coronary artery disease; not well documented but may occur

RISK FACTORS
Grazing seeds of *Acer pseudoplatanus* or *Acer negundo* during late fall or early spring or grazing marsh mallow weed.

 DIAGNOSIS

DIFFERENTIAL DIAGNOSIS
• Secondary causes of arrhythmias—hypoxia, toxemia, septicemia, or metabolic disturbances
• Valvular heart disease including infective endocarditis—murmurs usually present, differentiate echocardiographically
• Pericarditis—muffled heart sounds and/or friction rubs, differentiate echocardiographically
• Severe skeletal myopathies—increases in serum activities of creatine kinase and myoglobinuria
• Pneumonia—differentiate with thoracic US and radiography
• Hemoperitoneum or hemothorax—differentiate with US

CBC/BIOCHEMISTRY/URINALYSIS
• Increased serum creatinine concentration and blood urea nitrogen suggest prerenal or, if marked, concurrent renal dysfunction
• Neutrophilic leukocytosis and hyperfibrinogenemia may be present

OTHER LABORATORY TESTS
• Elevated cardiac troponin I or cardiac troponin T possible early but usually quickly returns to normal; often normal with focal myocardial disease. Marked increases indicative of myocardial disease; mild increases are nonspecific
• Blood lactate may be increased, reflecting poor tissue perfusion
• Blood culture and viral serology in selected cases
• Transtracheal aspirates for bacterial or fungal culture in selected cases
• Serum selenium and glutathione peroxidase concentrations if white muscle disease suspected

IMAGING
ECG
Paroxysmal or sustained supraventricular and/or ventricular arrhythmias may be present.

Echocardiography
• With focal myocardial disease, the echocardiogram may be normal or focal abnormalities are observed
• With generalized myocardial disease abnormalities could include:
  ○ Ventricular dilation (left and/or right); ventricular apices may be rounded
  ○ Regional or generalized hypokinesis or dyskinesis
  ○ Decreased fractional shortening
  ○ Marked spontaneous contrast
  ○ Increases in the mitral E point–septal separation
  ○ Increased preejection period and decreased left ventricular ejection period
  ○ Flattening of the aortic root, reduced aortic root diameter
  ○ Mild, usually anechoic, pericardial effusion
• With myocardial neoplasia, nodular masses with mixed echogenicity may be visible

Thoracic US
With pulmonary edema, peripheral pulmonary irregularities (B-lines—previously known as comet-tail artifacts) are visible.

Thoracic Radiography
Possible pulmonary edema.

OTHER DIAGNOSTIC PROCEDURES
Radiotelemetric ECG Monitoring
For real-time monitoring of unstable cardiac rhythms.

Continuous 24 h Holter Monitoring
For identifying intermittent or paroxysmal cardiac arrhythmias, quantifying numbers of isolated premature complexes, and assessing response to therapy.

Exercise ECG
For characterization of exercise-induced cardiac arrhythmias and their clinical significance.

Noninvasive Blood Pressure Measurement
For monitoring horses with generalized myocardial disease.

Toxicology
Analyze stomach contents, heart muscle, and feedstuffs for ionophores, particularly in group outbreaks of myocardial disease.

Endomyocardial Biopsy
Safety in clinical cases unknown.

PATHOLOGIC FINDINGS
• Grossly, there may be focal or diffuse areas of discolored, pale myocardium
• Histologically, there may be focal or diffuse myocardial degeneration, ischemia, necrosis, inflammation, fibrosis, and/or fibrofatty infiltrate

• Neoplastic infiltration is generally visible grossly, but must be confirmed histologically
• Evidence of poor perfusion may be evident on histologic examination of kidneys, liver, and intestine
• There may be accumulation of frothy pink-tinged fluid in the alveoli and small and large airways

TREATMENT

AIMS
• Restoration of cardiac output and improved tissue perfusion
• Specific therapy aimed at cause
• Antiarrhythmic therapy if unstable, life-threatening arrhythmias are present

APPROPRIATE HEALTH CARE
• Anti-inflammatories, antiarrhythmics, and, if necessary, pressor support may be useful in generalized myocardial disease, in addition to specific measures aimed at the cause, if known
• With focal myocardial disease, rest with or without corticosteroid therapy is helpful in some cases. If the problem persists, and exercising ECG is normal, the horse may still be able to be used for some level of ridden exercise

NURSING CARE
• Continuous ECG monitoring indicated if the cardiac rhythm is unstable
• Horses should be kept quiet and not moved if showing signs consistent with low cardiac output

ACTIVITY
Horses with active focal or generalized myocardial disease should be rested until there is significant improvement in their clinical status, echocardiogram, and ECG.

DIET
• In white muscle disease, selenium, vitamin E, and other antioxidants should be added to the diet
• If feed-derived toxins are suspected, the source of feed should be changed. If associated with grazing, horse should be removed from affected pasture

CLIENT EDUCATION
Clients must be warned of the grave prognosis with generalized myocardial disease.

SURGICAL CONSIDERATIONS
N/A

MEDICATIONS

DRUG(S) OF CHOICE
• Antiarrhythmic drugs—see chapters Supraventricular arrhythmias and Ventricular arrhythmias

• Broad-spectrum antimicrobials, such as penicillin and gentamicin, are indicated if bacterial myocarditis is diagnosed
• Furosemide (1 mg/kg IV every 8 h) may relieve pulmonary congestion or torsemide at 0.5–1 mg/kg POP every 12 hours
• Dobutamine (1–5 μg/kg/min constant rate infusion) may improve cardiac output, and digoxin (0.011 mg/kg PO every 12 h or 0.22 mg/100 kg IV every 12 h) has potentially beneficial positive inotropic and negative chronotropic effects
• Corticosteroids may be useful in horses with immune-mediated or other forms of inflammatory myocarditis; either prednisolone 1 mg/kg PO every 48 h or dexamethasone 0.05–0.1 mg/kg IV or 0.1 mg/kg PO every 24 h for 3 or 4 days and then continued every 3–4 days in decreasing dosages is recommended
• Vitamin E supplementation at up to 10 IU/kg PO every 24 h may be beneficial

CONTRAINDICATIONS
• Digoxin contraindicated if ionophore toxicity suspected
• Corticosteroids contraindicated with concurrent pituitary pars intermedia dysfunction

PRECAUTIONS
• Use potentially nephrotoxic drugs cautiously in horses with poor tissue perfusion
• Therapeutic drug monitoring is recommended

POSSIBLE INTERACTIONS
Monitor plasma concentrations of digoxin when used concurrently with other drugs with known interactions, such as quinidine.

ALTERNATIVE DRUGS
N/A

FOLLOW-UP

PATIENT MONITORING
• Monitor systemic blood pressure and blood lactate to assess early response to therapy
• If biomarkers are increased, monitor to follow resolution of the active myocardial disease
• Frequent echocardiographic and 24 h Holter ECG recordings should be obtained in the convalescent period

POSSIBLE COMPLICATIONS
Renal failure and congestive cardiac failure.

EXPECTED COURSE AND PROGNOSIS
• Focal myocardial disease can have limited clinical significance, although cardiac arrhythmias may persist
• Generalized myocardial disease is life-threatening with a grave prognosis. Horses can return to athletic activity if they survive the acute stages of myocardial failure.

Persistent echocardiographic evidence of significantly reduced ventricular function and exercising arrhythmias warrant retiring horses from ridden activities

MISCELLANEOUS

ASSOCIATED CONDITIONS
Myocardial disease can be associated with respiratory infection, SIRS, or MODS.

AGE-RELATED FACTORS
N/A

ZOONOTIC POTENTIAL
N/A

PREGNANCY/FERTILITY/BREEDING
High risk of fetal compromise if mares develop low cardiac output during pregnancy.

SEE ALSO
• Endocarditis, infective
• Ionophore toxicosis
• Supraventricular arrhythmias
• Ventricular arrhythmias

ABBREVIATIONS
• MODS = multiple organ dysfunction syndrome
• SIRS = systemic inflammatory response syndrome
• US = ultrasonography, ultrasound

Suggested Reading
Bauquier J, Stent A, Gibney J, et al. Evidence for marsh mallow (*Malva parviflora*) toxicosis causing myocardial disease and myopathy in four horses. Equine Vet J 2017;49(3):307–313.
Bonagura JD, Reef VB, Schwarzwald CC. Cardiovascular diseases. In: Reed SM, Bayly WM, Sellon DC, eds. Equine Internal Medicine, 3e. St. Louis, MO: WB Saunders, 2010:372–487.
Decloedt A, DeClerq D, Ven S, et al. Right atrial and right ventricular ultrasound-guided biopsy technique in standing horses. Equine Vet J 2015;48:346–351.
Gilliam LL, Holbrook TC, Ownby CL, et al. Cardiotoxicity, inflammation and immune response after rattlesnake envenomation in the horse. J Vet Intern Med 2012;26:1457–1463.
Verheyen T, Decloedt A, DeClerq D, van Loon G. Cardiac changes in horses with atypical myopathy. J Vet Intern Med 2012;26:1019–1026.

Author Virginia B. Reef
Consulting Editors Celia M. Marr and Virginia B. Reef
Acknowledgment The author acknowledges the prior contribution of Celia M. Marr.

M

NARCOLEPSY AND CATAPLEXY

BASICS

OVERVIEW
REM sleep disorders result in excessive daytime sleepiness and paroxysmal sleep attacks with REMs (narcolepsy) or complete loss of muscle tone and reflexes (cataplexy).

Pathophysiology
In laboratory species and dogs, it has been shown that the neuropeptide hypocretin (orexin) is central to the control of sleep and arousal. Hypocretin neurons project to areas involved in these processes, including the ascending reticular activating system; hypocretin levels fluctuate across the sleep–wake cycle and increase with sleep deprivation. Hypocretin neurons activate brainstem "REM-off" neurons and reduce the activity of "REM-on" neurons, acting as a gate to entry into REM sleep. Recent work suggests that an excess of a class of neurons containing histamine may be the cause of the loss of hypocretin cells in narcoleptics, and inhibiting histamine signaling could be a new way to treat narcolepsy. In humans, narcolepsy has been associated with reduced hypocretin levels, while in dogs narcoleptic lines that lack hypocretin receptors have been bred for narcolepsy research projects. Neither reduced hypocretin levels nor the lack of receptors has been demonstrated in horses, and animals with "sleep attacks" may simply be REM sleep deficient (i.e. not lying down enough).

Systems Affected
Central nervous system.

SIGNALMENT
Narcolepsy-like episodes can be seen transiently in foals, particularly in miniature horses, Fell Ponies, Shetland and Welsh Ponies, and Appaloosas. Usually, the episodes resolve with time. More commonly, it is seen in aged horses.

SIGNS

Foals
• An attack may progress from buckling at the knees without falling to sudden and total collapse and areflexia, usually with maintenance of some eye and facial responses and normal cardiorespiratory function
• Each recumbent episode may last up to hours if the foal is totally undisturbed, but the patient usually can be aroused from this state with varying degrees of difficulty

Adults
• Most commonly, this includes horses resting at the back of a field that can be seen to "buckle" at the knees, rarely resulting in collapse
• Excessive somnolence is easily noted by owners with the patient often resting the head or hindquarters on objects
• Most times the animal awakes with the (impending) fall to resume the somnolent state or revert to wakefulness
• Some horses have had relentless persistence of the syndrome to the point of severe knee and face trauma
• In some patients, episodes may be triggered by specific stimuli such as saddling, hosing down, or feeding, with no permanent consequences. Only occasionally do episodes occur with the excitement of being ridden

CAUSES AND RISK FACTORS
• No specific cause has been identified, but rigorous assessment of hypocretin levels has not been undertaken
• In some older horses, the cause may well be due to sleep deprivation, perhaps because the horse is unwilling to lie down as a result of joint pain or fear of enclosed spaces
• Risk factors have not been identified

DIAGNOSIS

Diagnosis by exclusion only. It is worthwhile getting the owner to set up 24 h video recording to assess how often these episodes occur, and whether the animal appears to go into normal REM sleep (~20 min/day total, in lateral recumbency).

DIFFERENTIAL DIAGNOSIS
Syncope, seizures.

CBC/BIOCHEMISTRY/URINALYSIS
No specific abnormalities.

PATHOLOGIC FINDINGS
No associated findings.

TREATMENT

Long-term therapy is inappropriate, although short-term responsiveness to the tricyclic antidepressant imipramine (1–2 mg/kg IM or IV every 6–12 h) and other drugs can alter the severity of the clinical syndrome.

MEDICATIONS

DRUG(S) OF CHOICE
See Treatment.

FOLLOW-UP

EXPECTED COURSE AND PROGNOSIS
Prognosis poor for the persistent form, and excellent for the neonatal form, although persistent signs have been noted in Shetland and Suffolk foals.

MISCELLANEOUS

SEE ALSO
Seizure disorders.

ABBREVIATIONS
REM = rapid eye movement

Suggested Reading
Lunn DP, Cuddon PA, Shaftoe S, Archer RM. Familial occurrence of narcolepsy in miniature horses. Equine Vet J 1993;25: 483–487.
Scammell TE. Narcolepsy. N Engl J Med 2015;373:2654–2662.
Swick TJ. Treatment paradigms for cataplexy in narcolepsy: past, present, and future. Nat Sci Sleep 2015;7:159–169.

Author Caroline N. Hahn
Consulting Editor Caroline N. Hahn

BASICS

OVERVIEW
• Palmar foot lameness due to injury of NB and/or NB apparatus (impar ligament, collateral suspensory ligament, distal DDFT, navicular bursa). • NB degeneration due to abnormal forces in heel (NB, surrounding ligaments, DDFT). • Faulty distal limb conformation, improper hoof balance, and poor shoeing lead to abnormal forces in navicular area. • Musculoskeletal system—foot

SIGNALMENT
• Middle age. • Quarter Horses primarily, Thoroughbreds, Warmbloods, mixed breeds. • Rare in ponies, donkeys, mules, Arabians, drafts

SIGNS
Historical Findings
• Initially intermittent, slowly progressive lameness. • Lameness worse on hard ground. • Bilateral forelimb lameness. • ± Unilateral forelimb lameness, rare in hindlimbs. • Short, choppy stride. • Stumbling. • Increased lameness right after shoeing. • ± Point affected limb. • With soft tissue injury, unilateral acute lameness

Physical Examination Findings
• Long toe–low heel conformation. • Heat in hoof capsule. • Increased digital pulses. • ± Hoof tester pain in frog or heels. • Atrophied frog. • Lameness, often bilateral, more lame in 1 limb

CAUSES AND RISK FACTORS
• Hoof imbalance. • Poor or inadequate shoeing. • Poor hoof conformation (long toe–low heel, excessive toe length, underrun heel). • Lack of heel support. • Quarter Horse breed. • Big horse with small feet. • Faulty distal limb conformation. • Mismatched front feet. • Excessive hard ground work

DIAGNOSIS

DIFFERENTIAL DIAGNOSIS
• Laminitis—acute, severe bilateral forelimb lameness. Hoof tester pain in toe. • Sheared heels. • Bruised feet

IMAGING
Radiography—Navicular Bone
• Variable sized synovial foramina. • Osteolysis or cyst formation. • Enthesophyte. • Flexor cortex erosion. • Medullary sclerosis. • DDFT calcification. • Distal bone fragments

Ultrasonography—Transcuneal Approach
• Distal DDFT tendonitis. • Impar desmitis. • Navicular bursitis

Nuclear Scintigraphy
Increased radiopharmaceutical uptake in palmar foot.

MRI
• Best imaging for soft tissue injury (distal DDFT, collateral suspensory ligament, impar ligament, distal annular ligament, navicular bursa). • NB edema

OTHER DIAGNOSTIC PROCEDURES
• Diagnostic analgesia—palmar digital, IA DIP, or navicular bursa. • Navicular bursoscopy. • Contrast radiography of navicular bursa

PATHOLOGIC FINDINGS
• NB cartilage erosion. • Linear or core DDFT lesions. • Adhesion between DDFT and NB

TREATMENT

• Rest. • Improve/restore hoof balance, shorten toe, ease foot breakover. • Heel support, secondary wedge shoe or pad, eggbar shoe. • IA medication (DIP, navicular bursa, or digital tendon sheath). • Reduce workload, expectations. • Palmar digital neurectomy • Biophospate therapy (Osphos IM)

MEDICATIONS

DRUG(S) OF CHOICE
• NSAIDs—phenylbutazone (2.2 mg/kg every 24 h for 7–10 days). • Isoxsuprine hydrochloride (1 mg/kg PO every 12 h for 3 weeks then 1 mg/kg every 24 h PO for 3 weeks, then 1 mg/kg PO every 48 h for 3 weeks). • IA corticosteroids—methylprednisolone acetate (20–40 mg) or triamcinolone (3–6 mg). • IA sodium hyaluronate (10–20 mg). • IA corticosteroids and sodium hyaluronate combination. • Systemic chondroprotective drugs—polysulfated glycosaminoglycan (500 mg IM every 4 days for 7 treatments) or sodium hyaluronate (40 mg IV every 7 days for 3 treatments). • Oral chondroprotective medications—glucosamine/chondroitin sulfate powder (1 scoop (3.3 g) every 12 h), bisphosphonate (Osphos; clodronate (clodronic acid) injection) (60 mg/mL, 15 mL IM divided into 2 sites; ± repeated >6 months)

CONTRAINDICATIONS/POSSIBLE INTERACTIONS
• IA corticosteroids *not* recommended with previous laminitis. • ± Mild abdominal discomfort <30 min after clodronate

FOLLOW-UP

PATIENT MONITORING
• Reassess lameness after medical therapy. • ± NSAIDs prior to excessive use. • ± IA DIP/navicular bursa medication, 2 or 3 times per year. • Therapeutic trim, shoe every 6 weeks

PREVENTION/AVOIDANCE
• Workload reduction, alterative sport. • Frequent, proper trimming and shoeing

POSSIBLE COMPLICATIONS
• Laminitis secondary to IA corticosteroids. • Gastric ulceration, right dorsal colitis, or kidney damage secondary to chronic NSAIDs. • Neuroma formation, nerve regrowth, DDFT rupture after palmar digital neurectomy

EXPECTED COURSE AND PROGNOSIS
• Early mild disease—return to athletic use with medical therapy. • Usually progressive—increased lameness, NB degeneration expected. • After neurectomy—sound for 2 years. Surgery as last resort owing to postoperative complications. • DDFT injury—poor for athletics

MISCELLANEOUS

ASSOCIATED CONDITIONS
• Sheared heels, chronic heel bruising in poorly conformed foot. • DIP disease or arthritis

AGE-RELATED FACTORS
• Uncommon <5 years. • Palmar digital neurectomy not recommended in younger horses

SYNONYMS
• Caudal heel pain. • Navicular disease. • Palmar foot pain

ABBREVIATIONS
• DDFT = deep digital flexor tendon. • DIP = distal interphalangeal joint. • NB = navicular bone. • IA = intra-articular. • MRI = magnetic resonance imaging. • NSAID = nonsteroidal anti-inflammatory drug

Suggested Reading
Dabareiner RM, Carter GK. Diagnosis, treatment, and farriery for horses with chronic heel pain. Vet Clin North Am Equine Pract 2003;19:417–441.

Author Robin M. Dabareiner
Consulting Editor Elizabeth J. Davidson

N

NEONATAL ISOERYTHROLYSIS

BASICS

DEFINITION
Alloimmune-mediated destruction of a neonatal foal's erythrocytes, caused by ingesting maternally (colostral) derived anti-foal erythrocyte antibodies.

PATHOPHYSIOLOGY
• Requires that a naive mare is sensitized to a new RBC antigenic sequence during blood transfusion or exposure to fetal RBCs that express the new antigenic sequence. Exposure may occur at parturition, or secondary to in utero disease such as placentitis
• During a subsequent pregnancy, the foal inherits the same stallion's RBC surface antigen
• At birth, the foal ingests antibody-rich colostrum and absorbs anti-foal RBC antibodies that cause destruction of RBCs
• Antibodies attach to the foal erythrocytes causing hemolysis and/or premature removal of damaged RBCs by the reticuloendothelial system
• Results in anemia

SYSTEMS AFFECTED
• Hemic/lymphatic/immune—intravascular and extravascular hemolysis leading to anemia, jaundice, and hemoglobinemia
• Renal/urologic—hemoglobinuria leading to pigment nephropathy, acute tubular necrosis, and acute kidney injury
• Cardiovascular—tachycardia from hypoxic anemia
• Nervous—hypoxic anemic shock causing weakness; hyperbilirubinemia causing basal ganglia dysfunction and seizures (kernicterus)
• Hepatic—liver failure development associated with high-volume blood transfusion

GENETICS
• There are many RBC surface antigen factors, and in theory any of these can be involved in NI development. However, Aa in the A system and Qa in the Q system represent the majority of cases
• In mules, the "donkey factor," which is unique to all donkeys and not horses, is commonly involved

INCIDENCE/PREVALENCE
• Among Thoroughbreds and Standardbreds, the prevalence of disease is ≈1–2%
• In mule foals, the prevalence is as high as 10–25%
• Breed variability reflects the frequency of specific genes involved in erythrocyte antigenicity or blood groups found in each breed
• Most horse mares bred to donkey jacks are at high risk (see Risk Factors)

GEOGRAPHIC DISTRIBUTION
Worldwide

SIGNALMENT

Breed Predilections
• The antigenic factors are not specific for, or limited to, any particular breed of horse
• Most mule pregnancies are incompatible regarding the blood group factor, "donkey factor," in which donkeys express and horses do not

Mean Age and Range
• Usually foals born to multiparous mares
• Most foals present during the first 4 days of life (mean range 0–8 days)

Predominant Sex
Both sexes are equally affected.

SIGNS

General Comments
The severity of clinical signs varies depending on the magnitude and rate of hemolysis.

Historical Findings
• Affected foals are generally healthy at birth and nurse appropriately
• Nonspecific signs such as lethargy begin within hours to days of colostral ingestion and immunoglobulin absorption. These signs may mimic other common neonatal disorders such as septicemia
• Icterus and generalized pallor soon develop
• Mare may have a history of producing jaundiced or NI-confirmed foals from previous pregnancies, especially if the same stallion had sired these foals
• Mare history of previous blood or other blood transfusion

Physical Examination Findings
• Lethargy, disinterest in suckling
• Tachypnea; tachycardia
• Pallor (acute stages) often progressing to jaundice
• Pigmenturia (hemoglobinuria)
• Recumbency
• Mild fever is often present
• Systemic signs of hypoxic insult and/or hyperbilirubinemia including colic, melena, and seizure activity (hypoxia; kernicterus)

CAUSES
Maternal production of anti-foal erythrocyte immunoglobulin from exposure of incompatible fetal blood.

RISK FACTORS
• Mares lacking erythrocyte factors Aa and/or Qa are at greater risk (>90%) of producing antibodies to these blood types
• *Donkey RBC antigen, "donkey factor"*—the risk of an incompatible mating between a horse and a donkey (or the chance of a mare becoming sensitized to this antigen) is 100%. Because clinical NI in mule foals only occurs ≈8–10% of the time, it is suggested that many mule foals may have subclinical NI

DIAGNOSIS

DIFFERENTIAL DIAGNOSIS
• Anemia due to blood loss
• Hepatopathy—icterus may be present but severe anemia is usually not present with hepatic disease
• Neonatal maladjustment syndrome—weakness, lethargy present; icterus and anemia should differentiate
• Neonatal septicemia—icterus, leukocytosis/leukopenia, and weakness may be present, but significant anemia is uncommon with septicemia
• In endemic areas, consider neonatal babesiosis (piroplasmosis)

CBC/BIOCHEMISTRY/URINALYSIS
• Anemia—decreased PCV (usually <20%), decreased hemoglobin concentration, and decreased erythrocyte number
• Hemoglobinemia
• Hemoglobinuria
• Hyperbilirubinemia (primarily indirect, unconjugated fraction); kernicterus is associated with total bilirubin >20 mg/dL
• Mild leukocytosis
• Mild thrombocytosis
• Hypoglycemia is often present

OTHER LABORATORY TESTS
• Coombs testing (direct antiglobulin test)—detects antierythrocyte factor in mare's serum and colostrum
• JFA test—this is a field screen test to detect NI. The foal's RBCs are exposed to the mare's colostrum or serum
• Saline agglutination or complement-mediated hemolytic test can be performed by some laboratories

DIAGNOSTIC PROCEDURES
Foal IgG determination—clinical evidence of jaundice with complete failure of transfer of passive immunity makes NI less likely.

PATHOLOGIC FINDINGS
• If the foal dies acutely, pallor and icterus may be observed throughout the body. If the foal dies later, the conversion of free hemoglobin to bilirubin leads to widespread jaundice of the body
• Splenomegaly
• Pigment nephropathy related to hemoglobinuric nephrosis
• Bone marrow hypoplasia

TREATMENT

AIMS
• Restore oxygen-carrying capacity with transfusion of whole blood, packed RBCs, or hemoglobin-based oxygen carrier
• Prevent further intake of maternal colostrum

APPROPRIATE HEALTH CARE

• If the foal is showing signs of icterus and lethargy/weakness, emergency inpatient intensive care management may be required, including blood transfusion
• If there is early recognition of the problem, withholding further maternal colostrum and providing supportive care in the field may be adequate

NURSING CARE

Blood Transfusion

• Blood transfusion with packed RBCs should be considered in foals where the PCV is <12–15% and/or the foal is showing clinical signs of decompensating anemic hypoxia. Transfusion is not essential to all cases of NI, only those where it is considered a life-saving measure
• Washed RBCs from the mare are ideal. The stallion is the most unsuitable blood donor
• A healthy gelding with no previous history of transfusion or a previously blood-typed animal negative for Aa or Qa antibodies is also a suitable blood donor
• For a 50 kg foal, give whole blood 2–4 L slowly over 1–2 h or packed erythrocytes 1–2 L slowly over 1–2 h

Intranasal Oxygen

Nasal insufflation with humidified oxygen (5–10 L/min) may be used although this is not a substitute for transfusion in severely anemic foals.

Additional Treatments

• Balanced polyionic crystalloid fluids to promote renal perfusion and diuresis (with or without diuretic medication) for pigment nephropathy
• Deferoxamine has been given to foals to help prevent hepatic iron accumulation. Plasma exchange has been reported as a treatment of life-threatening hyperbilirubinemia and kernicterus

ACTIVITY

Foals should not be stressed and exercise should be at a minimum to conserve oxygen.

DIET

• If recognized before 24 h of age, the foal should be muzzled to prevent further ingestion of colostral antibodies. The mare should be milked out and the milk discarded
• Affected foals should be supplemented with mare's milk replacer for the first 24–36 h from birth; then resume nursing from the mare

CLIENT EDUCATION

Mares of NI foals are likely to produce NI foals in subsequent pregnancies, especially if the same stallion is used. Preventative strategies should be exercised to minimize the chance of having an NI foal.

MEDICATIONS

DRUG(S) OF CHOICE

Seizure control where appropriate.

PRECAUTIONS

• Cautiously administer plasma transfusions when serum IgG concentrations are low. Frequent assessment for disease exacerbation (i.e. hemolytic crisis) is necessary
• Nephrotoxic drugs such as aminoglycoside antimicrobials and NSAIDs should be avoided

FOLLOW-UP

PATIENT MONITORING

• CBC, PCV, and lactate to monitor anemia. In acute cases, monitoring may be required every 4–8 h
• Heart rate, arterial oxygen levels, venous oxygen pressure, oxygen extraction ratio, and attitude are also useful for determining response to therapy
• Blood urea nitrogen and creatinine concentrations to monitor pigment nephropathy

PREVENTION/AVOIDANCE

• Blood type to identify broodmares that are negative for the Qa and/or Aa erythrocyte antigens and sires that are positive for the Qa and Aa antigens. Avoid breeding negative mares to positive stallions to reduce the chance of NI
• Determine the probability of NI in potentially incompatible matings. The mare's serum is collected 2 weeks prior to parturition and tested against known blood cell groups or against the sire's RBCs. The presence of hemolysis or agglutination suggests that NI will develop
• In high-risk cases, withhold the mare's colostrum from the foal and feed colostrum from another low-risk mare. The foal should be foster fed for 2–3 days until gut closure occurs
• Perform a JFA test. Positive reactions at 1:16 or greater suggest incompatibility and the risk of NI

POSSIBLE COMPLICATIONS

• Renal failure due to pigment nephropathy
• Cerebral hypoxia and/or kernicterus with neurologic sequelae
• Secondary septicemia
• Liver failure

EXPECTED COURSE AND PROGNOSIS

• Peracute cases—prognosis is grave due to the rapidity of onset and severity of disease
• Acute cases—prognosis is good providing early recognition and diagnosis are established and appropriate therapy is instituted
• Subacute cases—prognosis is excellent. Even without treatment, most foals are expected to survive. Prognosis is guarded if kernicterus, liver failure, or sepsis-related complications occur. Foals administered large volume blood products are at higher risk of liver failure

MISCELLANEOUS

ASSOCIATED CONDITIONS

• Neonatal immune-mediated thrombocytopenia
• Evans syndrome
• Alloimmune neonatal neutropenia

AGE-RELATED FACTORS

Affected foals are typically 2–3 days of age at the onset of clinical signs.

SYNONYMS

• Hemolysis of newborns
• Jaundiced foal disease

SEE ALSO

• Anemia
• Anemia, immune mediated
• Neonatal maladjustment syndrome
• Nutritional myodegeneration
• Piroplasmosis
• Septicemia, neonate
• Uroperitoneum, neonate

ABBREVIATIONS

• IgG = immunoglobulin G
• JFA = jaundice foal agglutination test
• NI = neonatal isoerythrolysis
• NSAID = nonsteroidal anti-inflammatory drug
• PCV = packed cell volume
• RBC = red blood cell

Suggested Reading

Boyle AG, Magdesian KG, Ruby RE. Neonatal isoerythrolysis in horse foals and a mule foal: 18 cases (1988–2003). J Am Vet Med Assoc 2005;227:1276–1283.

Polkes AC, Giguere S, Lester GD, Bain FT. Factors associated with outcome in foals with neonatal isoerythrolysis (72 cases, 1988-2003). J Vet Intern Med 2008;22: 1216–1222.

Traub-Dargatz JL, McClure JJ, Koch C, Schlipf Jr JW. Neonatal isoerythrolysis in mule foals. J Am Vet Med Assoc 1995;206: 67–70.

Author Samuel D.A. Hurcombe
Consulting Editor Margaret C. Mudge

N

NEONATAL MALADJUSTMENT SYNDROME

 BASICS

DEFINITION
Neurologic, GI, and renal dysfunction with or without other evidence of primary organ dysfunction that occurs secondary to hypoxic events in the periparturient period.

PATHOPHYSIOLOGY
• It is speculated that hypoxic events or limitations to uteroplacental blood flow initiate hypoxic–ischemic injury. Intrauterine infection may also contribute to a decrease in blood flow, oxygen delivery, and nutrient supply
• Foals affected at birth have likely suffered hypoxia secondary to placental insufficiency, placental blood flow, gas exchange, or other in utero compromise. Foals that have peripartum asphyxia may not show neurologic signs until 24 h after birth. The delay in clinical signs in these foals may be related to the secondary reperfusion injury due to reintroduction of adequate blood flow and oxygen delivery and the formation of reactive oxygen species
• The renal and GI systems can be affected when blood flow to the fetus is limited and redistributed to the brain and heart (away from kidneys and GI tract)

SYSTEMS AFFECTED
• Nervous—encephalopathy is commonly suspected, with signs generally limited to the cerebrum. Behavioral abnormalities are common
• GI—ischemic damage and reperfusion injury can lead to mucosal degeneration and subsequent ileus, bacterial translocation, and enterocolitis
• Renal—acute renal failure (acute tubular necrosis) can occur after an ischemic episode

INCIDENCE/PREVALENCE
• Relatively common in the neonate; exact incidence unknown
• NMS or HIE is the most common cause of acquired seizures in the neonatal foal

SIGNALMENT
Breed Predilections
All breeds can be affected.

Mean Age and Range
Foals may be abnormal at birth, but signs may develop at 24–48 h of age.

Predominant Sex
No sex predisposition.

SIGNS
General Comments
Signs vary from mild depression to severe centralized seizures and generalized organ failure.

Historical Findings
Dystocia, premature placental separation ("red bag"), placentitis, prepartum illness in the mare, induced labor, and prolonged

gestation are maternal factors that can put the foal at an increased risk of NMS.

Physical Examination Findings
• Lack of interest in the mare, inability to urinate, or disorientation and "star-gazing"
• Tongue protrusion
• Weak/absent suckle or misdirected suckling, lack of normal nursing behavior
• Hyperresponsiveness
• Focal or generalized seizures
• Diarrhea or colic may be present if there is hypoxic injury to the GI system

CAUSES
Maternal Factors
• Placental insufficiency or dysfunction (including twins, placentitis, fescue toxicity, premature placental separation)
• Compromised blood flow or oxygenation secondary to colic, endotoxemia, pulmonary disease, and anemia

Peripartum Factors
• Dystocia
• Cesarean section and general anesthesia
• Compression/torsion of the umbilical cord
• Induction of labor with oxytocin
• Uterine inertia

Foal Factors
• Congenital cardiac abnormalities
• Pulmonary disease
• Anemia
• Sepsis

RISK FACTORS
• Fescue toxicity in mare
• High-risk pregnancies

 DIAGNOSIS

DIFFERENTIAL DIAGNOSIS
• Sepsis—sepsis score, blood culture, and leukogram changes should differentiate. Foals can suffer concurrently from sepsis and NMS
• Meningitis—fever, ataxia, depression; CSF analysis and culture can confirm
• Trauma—historical and physical examination information may help to differentiate
• Congenital neurologic abnormality—lack of improvement in clinical signs; neurologic deficits may not be restricted to the cerebrum
• Kernicterus—can occur with NI and very high serum bilirubin levels

CBC/BIOCHEMISTRY/URINALYSIS
• CBC and biochemistry are usually normal when the primary disorder is neurologic
• If there are significant abnormalities (neutropenia, azotemia), sepsis and multiple organ dysfunction should be suspected
• Hypoglycemia is common if the foal has not been able to nurse adequately

OTHER LABORATORY TESTS
• Serum immunoglobulin G—low if foal has

not been able to consume adequate colostrum or foal's GI tract cannot adequately absorb immunoglobulins, or mare has not produced good quality colostrum
• Blood gas analysis—hypoventilation can occur as a result of central nervous system damage. Hypercapnia with or without hypoxemia may be seen

IMAGING
• Skull radiographs or CT scan to rule out traumatic fracture as a cause of neurologic dysfunction
• MRI—cerebral edema and necrosis with severe cases, although there may be no abnormalities seen in early or mild cases. There is limited information on the use of this imaging modality in foals with NMS

OTHER DIAGNOSTIC PROCEDURES
CSF aspirate—will usually be normal with NMS; rule out bacterial meningitis.

PATHOLOGIC FINDINGS
• Consistent cerebral abnormalities have not been reported, although cerebral necrosis, edema, and hemorrhage may be seen. Uncomplicated cases have a good prognosis, so postmortem information is limited
• Hypoxic–ischemic injury to the kidneys may result in tubular necrosis
• Hypoxia and/or ischemia to the GI tract may cause necrosis and hemorrhage

 TREATMENT

AIMS
• Supportive care—mildly affected foals may only need to have adequate nutrition and immunoglobulin provided until they can nurse effectively on their own, usually within 2–3 days
• Seizure control
• Reduce or prevent further brain injury—anti-inflammatory and antiedema drugs
• Prevent sepsis in recumbent or debilitated foals
• Respiratory support may be needed if there is hypoventilation related to NMS

APPROPRIATE HEALTH CARE
• Mildly affected foals may be managed with careful monitoring and tube feeding with colostrum and mare's milk, if needed
• The majority of affected foals require inpatient medical management

NURSING CARE
• Oxygen therapy when hypoxemia is present. Avoid overzealous use, especially in the presence of hypercapnia
• Fluid therapy—maintenance fluids for foals that are transiently unable to nurse. Correct hypovolemia to maintain cerebral perfusion pressure, renal blood flow, and intestinal perfusion
• Protect from self-trauma during seizures or struggling activity and monitor for the

development of corneal ulcers or abrasions
• Squeeze-induced somnolence using rope restraint is a potential treatment for NMS
• Hyperimmune plasma IV if the foal has not been able to ingest adequate colostrum within the first several hours of birth

ACTIVITY
Activity will be limited by the treatments required and by the neurologic and metabolic status of the foal.

DIET
• Feed via nasogastric feeding tube until a strong suckle reflex and coordinated nursing is achieved. See chapter Nutrition in foals
• Care should be taken if GI ischemia is suspected. Foals with GI injury or ileus may require parenteral nutrition until intestinal function returns

MEDICATIONS
DRUG(S) OF CHOICE
For Seizure Control
(For drug information and dosages, see chapter Seizures in foals)
• Midazolam
• Phenobarbital
• Phenytoin

For Treatment of Cerebral Asphyxia/Edema
• Magnesium sulfate (50 mg/kg/h loading dose, then 25 mg/kg/h constant rate infusion)—blocks NMDA production
• Mannitol (0.25–1.0 g/kg as a 20% solution IV)—osmotic diuretic to reduce cerebral edema
• DMSO (0.5–1.0 g/kg as a 10% solution IV)—given shortly after the initial insult to scavenge free radicals and mediate ischemia–reperfusion injury. There is no evidence of efficacy of DMSO
• Thiamine (5 mg/kg IV slowly or diluted in fluids every 24 h)—to support mitochondrial metabolism

For Treatment of Hypoventilation
Caffeine (10 mg/kg initial dose, then 2.5 mg/kg PRN, given PO or per rectum)—respiratory stimulant for centrally mediated hypoventilation.

Antioxidants
• Vitamin E (alpha-tocopherol)—500–1000 IU PO every 24 h
• Vitamin C (ascorbic acid)—50–100 mg/kg PO every 24 h

For Renal Failure
Furosemide (1–2 mg/kg IV PRN)—if signs of fluid overload are present.

For Prevention or Treatment of Sepsis
• Broad-spectrum parenteral antimicrobials. Penicillin (22 000 IU/kg IV every 6 h) and amikacin (25 mg/kg IV every 24 h) are commonly used
• Metronidazole (15 mg/kg PO every 12 h) may also be used if anaerobic infection is suspected or if necrotizing enterocolitis is present

CONTRAINDICATIONS
• Corticosteroids are not indicated for the treatment of NMS
• Ketamine and xylazine increase intracranial pressure, and should be avoided, if possible
• Mannitol is contraindicated with cerebral hemorrhage

PRECAUTIONS
Aminoglycoside antimicrobials and NSAIDs should be used with caution if renal damage is suspected.

ALTERNATIVE DRUGS
If renal compromise is suspected, a third-generation cephalosporin can be used in place of the penicillin–amikacin combination (e.g. ceftiofur 5–10 mg/kg IV every 6 h; ceftazidime 50 mg/kg IV every 6 h)

FOLLOW-UP
PATIENT MONITORING
• Reevaluate at least daily for ability to stand and nurse. An adequate suckle reflex and ability to remain standing are required for reintroduction to nursing the mare. The foal may require assistance to stand as it is initially reintroduced to nursing
• Monitor closely for signs of sepsis, as many of the risk factors for NMS also place the foal at risk of sepsis
• Blood pressure should be monitored in more severe cases and hypotension treated in order to maintain perfusion to vital organs

PREVENTION/AVOIDANCE
Any potential underlying causes such as placental insufficiency, ascending uterine infection, or prolonged gestation due to fescue toxicity should be investigated in order to help prevent NMS in future foals.

POSSIBLE COMPLICATIONS
• Septicemia
• Enterocolitis
• Ventilatory failure (hypoxemia and hypercarbia)

EXPECTED COURSE AND PROGNOSIS
• Prognosis is good to excellent (approximately 75% survival) for uncomplicated NMS. Mildly affected foals generally respond to treatment within several days. Foals with additional organ dysfunction require more intensive and prolonged care
• Delayed treatment can result in failure of transfer of passive immunity and sepsis. Concurrent diseases such as sepsis will decrease the prognosis

MISCELLANEOUS
ASSOCIATED CONDITIONS
• Sepsis
• Enterocolitis/diarrhea

AGE-RELATED FACTORS
This is a condition of neonatal foals, with initial signs seen typically within 48 h of age.

SYNONYMS
• Neonatal maladjustment syndrome
• HIE
• Dummy foal
• Barker foal
• Neonatal encephalopathy

SEE ALSO
• Prematurity/dysmaturity in foals
• Seizures in foals

ABBREVIATIONS
• CSF = cerebrospinal fluid
• CT = computed tomography
• DMSO = dimethylsulfoxide
• GI = gastrointestinal
• HIE = hypoxic–ischemic encephalopathy
• MRI = magnetic resonance imaging
• NMDA = N-methyl-D-aspartate
• NMS = neonatal maladjustment syndrome

Suggested Reading
MacKay RJ. Neurologic disorders of neonatal foals. Vet Clin North Am Equine Pract 2005;21:387–406.
Paradis MR. Neurologic dysfunctions. In: Paradis MR, ed. Equine Neonatal Medicine: A Case-Based Approach. Philadelphia, PA: Saunders, 2006:179–190.
Wilkins PA. Perinatal asphyxia syndrome. In: Reed SM, Bayly WM, Sellon DC, eds. Equine Internal Medicine, 3e. St. Louis, MO: WB Saunders, 2010:1324–1328.
Author Eric L. Schroeder
Consulting Editor Margaret C. Mudge
Acknowledgment The author acknowledges the prior contribution of Margaret C. Mudge.

N

NERIUM OLEANDER (OLEANDER) TOXICOSIS

BASICS

OVERVIEW
• *Nerium oleander* (oleander) is an evergreen shrub (family Apocynaceae) with leathery, dark, gray-green, sharply pointed leaves 10–30 cm (4–12 inches) long with a prominent midrib and parallel secondary veins
• Oleander is native to Asia but now is a common ornamental plant in the southern and western USA and other parts of the world. Oleander contains several cardiac glycosides and ingestion can cause severe cardiac abnormalities and sudden death. The plant remains toxic when dry

SIGNALMENT
All animals are susceptible.

SIGNS
• Onset usually several hours after ingestion
• Anorexia
• Colic
• Diarrhea
• Cardiac arrhythmias
• Tremors
• Seizure-like activity
• Coma
• Death

CAUSES AND RISK FACTORS
• Cardiac glycosides including oleandrin, oleandroside, nerioside, digitoxigenin, and others
• Cardiac glycosides inhibit Na^+/K^+-ATPase
• Ingestion of 0.005% of plant by body weight may be lethal

DIAGNOSIS

DIFFERENTIAL DIAGNOSIS
• *Taxus* (yew) toxicosis (evidence of consumption)

• Other cardiac glycoside-containing plants such as *Thevetia peruviana* (yellow oleander) (evidence of consumption)
• Other causes of sudden death

CBC/BIOCHEMISTRY/URINALYSIS
N/A

OTHER LABORATORY TESTS
• Identification of oleander leaves in ingesta
• Chemical analysis of ingesta or serum for oleandrin

IMAGING
N/A

OTHER DIAGNOSTIC PROCEDURES
ECG disturbances are supportive—widening of the QRS wave, ST-segment depression, enlarged P waves, and a variety of ventricular arrhythmias.

PATHOLOGIC FINDINGS
• Identification of oleander leaves in ingesta
• Often no lesions in peracute cases
• Endocardial hemorrhages
• Increased pericardial fluid
• Necrosis of subendocardium, most often involving the left ventricle
• Pulmonary edema or hepatic congestion may be present

TREATMENT
• Keep animal quiet
• Supportive care

MEDICATIONS

DRUG(S) OF CHOICE
• Evaluate cardiac function (ECG) and treat appropriately
• Activated charcoal at 1–4 g/kg body weight by nasogastric intubation as a water slurry

CONTRAINDICATIONS/POSSIBLE INTERACTIONS
N/A

FOLLOW-UP

PATIENT MONITORING
ECG evaluation.

PREVENTION/AVOIDANCE
Remove oleander from animal access.

POSSIBLE COMPLICATIONS
N/A

EXPECTED COURSE AND PROGNOSIS
N/A

MISCELLANEOUS

ASSOCIATED CONDITIONS
N/A

AGE-RELATED FACTORS
N/A

ZOONOTIC POTENTIAL
N/A

PREGNANCY/FERTILITY/BREEDING
N/A

SEE ALSO
Cardiotoxic plants

Suggested Reading
Bandara V, Weinstein SA, White J, Eddleston M. A review of the natural history, toxinology, diagnosis and clinical management of *Nerium oleander* (common oleander) and *Thevetia peruviana* (yellow oleander) poisoning. Toxicon 2010;56(3): 273–281.
Galey FD, Holstege DM, Plumlee KH, et al. Diagnosis of oleander poisoning in livestock. J Vet Diagn Invest 1996;8: 358–364.
Renier AC, Kass PH, Magdesian KG, et al. Oleander toxicosis in equids: 30 cases (1995-2010). J Am Vet Med Assoc 2013;242(4):540–549.

Author Larry J. Thompson
Consulting Editors Wilson K. Rumbeiha and Steve Ensley

N

NEUROAXONAL DYSTROPHY/EQUINE DEGENERATIVE MYELOENCEPHALOPATHY

BASICS

OVERVIEW
NAD/EDM is a degenerative neurologic disease of young growing equids resulting in severe and progressive ataxia.

Pathophysiology
• NAD/EDM is associated with temporal deficiency of α-tocopherol in genetically susceptible individuals. Although the pathogenesis of NAD/EDM remains unclear, it has been shown that low serum α-tocopherol concentrations have a causative role in the development of NAD/EDM and that prophylactic administration of α-tocopherol to foals at risk of NAD/EDM results in a decreased incidence of the disease
• In predisposed animals, inadequate amounts of α-tocopherol result in lipid peroxidation of cellular membranes. Histopathologic lesions of NAD/DEM include oxidative injuries leading to axonal degeneration of the spinal cord and the brainstem nuclei

Genetics
NAD/EDM is an inherited polygenic trait or a dominant disorder with variable expression depending on breeds and families. No specific gene has been clearly involved in the pathogeny of the disease yet.

Geographic Distribution
The disease is reported in North America and Europe.

SIGNALMENT
• Breed—common in Arabians, Quarter Horse-associated breeds, Thoroughbreds, Standardbreds, and Paso Finos
• Age—the onset of clinical signs can vary from birth to 12 years of age but very rarely occurs after 2 years

SIGNS
• Clinical signs are a progressive and symmetric ataxia of all 4 limbs
• The disease progresses from mild proprioceptive deficits to severe general ataxia
• A history of progressive lameness or traumatic injury is not uncommon
• Pelvic limbs are usually more severely affected than the thoracic limbs
• Severe cases can show hyporeflexia over the neck and trunk (local cervical, thoracolaryngeal, and cutaneous trunci responses)
• There has been no evidence of cranial nerve deficits or muscle atrophy in horses with NAD/EDM

CAUSES AND RISK FACTORS
• The disease is caused by a deficiency in α-tocopherol in genetically susceptible individuals

• Risk factors include being born from a mare with low serum α-tocopherol, having siblings diagnosed with NAD/EDM, and having limited access to pasture

DIAGNOSIS

DIFFERENTIAL DIAGNOSIS
• Equine cervical stenotic myelopathy—common in growing horses; ruled out with radiographs, myelogram, or advanced imaging
• Trauma—common in young horses; ruled out with radiographs, cervical ultrasonography, or advanced imaging
• Cervical vertebral malformation and occipital–atlantoaxial malformation—reported in young Arabians; ruled out with radiographs, myelogram, or advanced imaging
• Equine protozoal myelopathy—common in horses <4 years of age; ruled out with immunodiagnostic testing of serum and CSF to identify intrathecal antibody production against *Sarcocystis neurona* or *Neospora hughesi*
• Equine herpesvirus myeloencephalopathy—more common in older horses; ruled out with epidemiologic data and virus identification from nasopharyngeal swab and buffy coat samples

LABORATORY TESTS
• There is no antemortem diagnostic test for NAD/EDM. Low serum α-tocopherol values (<2 mg/L) are suggestive of the disease but poorly specific
• CSF analysis is unremarkable

IMAGING
Imaging techniques are helpful to rule out differential diagnoses.

OTHER DIAGNOSTIC PROCEDURES
Thorough and repeated neurologic examination.

PATHOLOGIC FINDINGS
Diagnosis is made at necropsy—axonal degeneration and myelin loss of ascending and descending fibers in the thoracic spinal cord, nucleus thoracicus, and lateral cuneate nuclei of the rostral medulla oblongata.

TREATMENT
Access to pasture and properly cured hay containing high amounts of α-tocopherol.

MEDICATIONS
Treatment focuses on prophylaxis in affected farms with limited improvement of individuals already showing clinical signs; however, signs of improvement can be seen within 4 weeks of treatment.
• Prophylaxis—oral administration of 1–2 IU/kg/day of α-tocopherol
• Treatment—6000 IU/day of α-tocopherol mixed in grain or 10 IU/kg/day of a water-dispersible formulation of α-tocopherol

CONTRAINDICATIONS/POSSIBLE INTERACTIONS
Toxic levels of α-tocopherol in horses have not been documented.

FOLLOW-UP
• Horses on α-tocopherol therapy should be monitored for serum α-tocopherol levels to ensure adequate absorption. If levels do not increase within 30 days, malabsorption of the fat-soluble vitamins should be investigated
• Repeated neurologic examinations should be performed to assess the horse's evolution

MISCELLANEOUS

ABBREVIATIONS
• CSF = cerebrospinal fluid
• NAD/EDM = neuroaxonal dystrophy/equine degenerative myeloencephalopathy

SEE ALSO
• Cervical vertebral malformation
• Equine herpesvirus myeloencephalopathy
• Equine protozoal myeloencephalitis (EPM)

Suggested Reading
Dill SG, Correa MT, Erb HN, et al. Factors associated with the development of equine degenerative myeloencephalopathy. Am J Vet Res 1990;51:1300–1305.
Finno CJ, Higgins RJ, Aleman M, et al. Equine degenerative myeloencephalopathy in Lusitano horses. J Vet Intern Med 2011;25:1436–1446.

Author François-René Bertin
Consulting Editor Caroline N. Hahn
Acknowledgment The author acknowledges the prior contribution of Caroline N. Hahn.

N

NEUTROPENIA

BASICS

DEFINITION
• Absolute neutrophil count in peripheral blood less than the lower limit of the laboratory reference interval; usually $<2.5 \times 10^9$ cells/L
• Neutrophils are the predominant white blood cells in peripheral blood of horses and neutropenia usually leads to leukopenia
• Often associated with acute severe infection or endotoxemia/SIRS and can predispose to secondary bacterial infection, especially when numbers are $<0.5 \times 10^9$ cells/L
• May be accompanied by a left shift and toxic change

PATHOPHYSIOLOGY
• Granulopoiesis occurs continuously in the bone marrow to maintain neutrophil numbers in blood and tissues
• G-CSF is a key mediator in stimulation of granulopoiesis, functional maturation of neutrophil precursors, and neutrophil mobilization from bone marrow reserves
• Bone marrow transit time for neutrophils is ~6 days, with shorter transit times in cases of increased peripheral demand
• Neutrophils in peripheral blood are distributed evenly between the CNP and the MNP; it is the CNP that is sampled during blood collection
• Circulating neutrophils have a half-life of ~10.5 h, after which they migrate randomly to tissues and body cavities to undertake physiologic functions or are recruited to sites of inflammation
• In tissues, neutrophils have a half-life of ~12 h, then undergo apoptosis and are phagocytized by mononuclear cells or are lost from the body via mucosal surfaces
• Severe inflammatory disease can rapidly deplete the storage pool of mature neutrophils and result in increased immature neutrophils (neutrophil bands ± metamyelocytes ± myelocytes) in the circulation; this is a *left shift*
• Left shifts may be accompanied by toxic change within the neutrophil
• A left shift with immature neutrophils < mature segmented neutrophils and neutrophilia is an appropriate response to tissue demand for neutrophils
• A *degenerative* or uncompensated left shift (immature neutrophils > mature segmented neutrophils without neutrophilia) indicates that tissue use is exceeding the capacity of the bone marrow
• A persistent degenerative left shift is a poor prognostic indicator
• Neutropenia may occur as part of pancytopenia (with concurrent nonregenerative anemia and thrombocytopenia) due to bone marrow disease

SYSTEMS AFFECTED
• Hemic/lymphatic/immune
• Others, depending on underlying cause and development of secondary infections

INCIDENCE/PREVALENCE
No specific data available.

SIGNALMENT
• Neutropenia is common in foals with sepsis or prematurity/dysmaturity
• No breed or sex predilection

SIGNS
General Comments
• Depend on the underlying disease
• Signs of localized or systemic infection may be present

Historical Findings
• A history of colic, diarrhea, or metritis may be associated with endotoxemia/SIRS
• Recent transportation may be associated with the development of pleuropneumonia
• Lethargy, inappetence, pyrexia, weight loss, exercise intolerance may be seen in pancytopenia cases
• Foals may be born prematurely or have FTPI; mares may have a history of placentitis

Physical Examination Findings
• Signs of endotoxemia/SIRS include congested or cyanotic mucous membranes, tachycardia, tachypnea, pyrexia, or hypothermia
• Pyrexia
• Signs of pancytopenia may include mucous membrane pallor, petechial hemorrhages, epistaxis, mucosal bleeding, blood in feces, hematomas, or prolonged bleeding from wounds

CAUSES
Increased Migration to Tissues (Increased Peripheral Usage)
• Most common cause of neutropenia
• Owing to increased peripheral demand that depletes the storage pool so that rate of tissue migration exceeds bone marrow production
• Total neutrophil pool is reduced and left shift is usually present
• Commonly due to endotoxemia/SIRS associated with GI disease (e.g. strangulating lesion, acute colitis) or bacterial diseases such as neonatal septicemia, pleuropneumonia, peritonitis, metritis, or EGA
• May be observed in acute viral diseases such as equine influenza, equine herpesvirus 1, or equine viral arteritis

Lack of or Ineffective Granulopoiesis
• Rare
• Myelophthisis may involve myeloproliferative disorders, infiltrative neoplasia, myelofibrosis, myelodysplasia, bone marrow necrosis
• Aplastic anemia may be due to toxins, drugs, chemicals, or radiation
• Pancytopenia is likely with conditions affecting all hematopoietic cell lines (e.g. myelophthisis)

Increased Margination
• Common and is due to a shift from the CNP to MNP
• Usually associated with endotoxemia/SIRS caused by acute GI disease, peritonitis, metritis, or pleuropneumonia
• Results from upregulation of adhesion molecules on neutrophils and endothelial cells ± increased migration into tissues
• Total neutrophil pool may be unchanged
• Left shift usually present

Reduced Survival
• Increased migration to tissues with subsequent rapid destruction in bacterial infections
• Immune-mediated neutropenia due to presence of alloantibodies to neutrophils in neonates
• Total neutrophil pool is reduced and left shift is usually present

RISK FACTORS
• Placentitis, umbilical infection, and FTPI are risk factors for bacterial sepsis in foals
• Induction of parturition is a risk factor for prematurity
• Protracted administration of sulfadiazine–pyrimethamine drugs is a risk factor for folate deficiency and bone marrow suppression

DIAGNOSIS

DIFFERENTIAL DIAGNOSIS
Laboratory Error
• Failure to mix blood sample properly before analysis
• Leukocyte aggregation or entrapment in a partially clotted sample
• Evaluation of blood >24 h after collection may result in underestimation of neutrophil numbers owing to degradation of leukocytes

Sampling Error
Collection through an IV catheter used for fluid administration with dilution of blood sample.

CBC/BIOCHEMISTRY/URINALYSIS
• Neutropenia ± left shift
• Toxic change may be present
• Additional hematologic and biochemical changes depend on underlying condition
• Pancytopenia may occur with EGA, aplastic anemia, and myelophthisis
• Neutrophil cytoplasmic inclusions (morulae) may be observed in EGA

OTHER LABORATORY TESTS
• Serology or PCR for suspected viral infections
• Quantification of blood immunoglobulin G for detection of FTPI
• Flow cytometry for detection of neutrophil surface-associated antibodies

IMAGING
• Abdominal, thoracic, and soft tissue ultrasonography for detection of effusion or space-occupying lesion
• Thoracic and skeletal radiography for detection of a space-occupying lesion

OTHER DIAGNOSTIC PROCEDURES
• Collection of fluid from suspected site of inflammation (e.g. abdominocentesis, thoracocentesis, arthrocentesis, transtracheal wash) for cytology, culture, and sensitivity
• Blood culture
• Bone marrow aspirate/biopsy to investigate unexplained neutropenia, pancytopenia, or abnormal circulating cells
• Fecal culture, ELISA, or PCR for enteric pathogens

PATHOLOGIC FINDINGS
Depends on underlying cause and presence of any secondary infection.

TREATMENT

AIMS
• Resolution of underlying condition and correction of neutropenia
• Resolution of any secondary infection

APPROPRIATE HEALTH CARE
• Inpatient medical management is usually ideal until the condition is stabilized
• Some cases require surgical management either as an emergency (e.g. strangulating GI lesion) or once the patient is stabilized (e.g. peritonitis)

NURSING CARE
• IV fluid therapy required if fluid, electrolyte, and acid–base deficits are present
• Peritonitis and pleuritis may require therapeutic drainage
• Foals with sepsis and/or prematurity/dysmaturity require aggressive supportive treatment (e.g. fluid, oxygen, and nutritional therapy, postural support, and climate control)

ACTIVITY
Foals with sepsis/prematurity and horses with systemic disease require confinement.

CLIENT EDUCATION
Neutropenia is often associated with diseases with a guarded to poor prognosis, especially if a degenerative left shift and toxic change are present.

DIET
Enteric or parenteral nutrition may be required for nutritional support.

SURGICAL CONSIDERATIONS
Neutropenia increases the risk of postoperative infections, including surgical incisions and sites of IV catheterization.

MEDICATIONS

DRUG(S) OF CHOICE
• Bacterial disease requires administration of appropriate antimicrobials based on culture and sensitivity testing
• Several drugs can be used in the treatment of endotoxemia/SIRS, including NSAIDs, hyperimmune plasma or serum, polymyxin B, heparin, and positive inotropes
• Corticosteroids are indicated if immune-mediated disease is diagnosed

CONTRAINDICATIONS
Avoid use of corticosteroids in cases with infectious disease or laminitis.

PRECAUTIONS
Use of NSAIDs, aminoglycosides, trimethoprim–sulfonamide drugs, and polymyxin B should be avoided until fluid deficits are corrected.

ALTERNATIVE DRUGS
• Poor response of confirmed bacterial infection to treatment may precipitate alteration of the antimicrobial regimen
• Canine recombinant G-CSF has been used successfully to increase blood neutrophil count of foals; expense may be limiting

FOLLOW-UP

PATIENT MONITORING
• Clinical monitoring important to document clinical improvement and response to treatment
• Daily leukograms recommended until condition has stabilized
• Leukocyte and neutrophil counts increasing to reference intervals and resolution of left shift and toxic change are indicative of improvement
• Rebound neutrophilia is common after recovery from neutropenia

POSSIBLE COMPLICATIONS
Secondary infections (mostly bacterial).

EXPECTED COURSE AND PROGNOSIS
• Depend on underlying condition and presence of secondary infections
• Endotoxemia/SIRS with evidence of failure of ≥1 organ is associated with a poor prognosis
• Marked leukopenia and neutropenia in foals with sepsis increase the risk of mortality
• Prognosis of myeloproliferative disorders is hopeless
• Presence of degenerative left shift and/or severe toxic change denotes a poor prognosis

• Resolution of neutropenia with disappearance of bands and toxic change indicate a more favorable prognosis

MISCELLANEOUS

ASSOCIATED CONDITIONS
Secondary infections (mostly bacterial).

AGE-RELATED FACTORS
• Premature foals have significantly lower neutrophil counts than term foals
• In healthy foals, absolute neutrophil counts may exceed adult reference intervals until 3–4 months of age

ZOONOTIC POTENTIAL
None

SYNONYMS
None

SEE ALSO
• Equine granulocytic anaplasmosis
• Myeloproliferative diseases
• Pancytopenia
• Salmonellosis
• Septicemia, neonate

ABBREVIATIONS
• CNP = circulating neutrophil pool
• EGA = equine granulocytic anaplasmosis
• ELISA = enzyme-linked immunosorbent assay
• FTPI = failure of transfer of passive immunity
• G-CSF = granulocyte colony-stimulating factor
• GI = gastrointestinal
• MNP = marginating neutrophil pool
• NSAID = nonsteroidal anti-inflammatory drug
• PCR = polymerase chain reaction
• SIRS = systemic inflammatory response syndrome

Internet Resources
Cornell University College of Veterinary Medicine, Leukogram changes. http://www.eclinpath.com/hematology/leukogram-changes

Suggested Reading
Walton RM. Equine hematology. In: Walton RM, ed. Equine Clinical Pathology. Ames, IA: Wiley Blackwell, 2014:15–36.

Authors Marie-France Roy and Nicole J. Fernandez
Consulting Editors David Hodgson, Harold C. McKenzie, and Jennifer L. Hodgson
Acknowledgment The authors and editors acknowledge the prior contribution of Kristopher Hughes.

N

NEUTROPHILIA

BASICS

DEFINITION
• Absolute numbers of mature neutrophils in peripheral blood above upper limit of laboratory reference interval; for example $>7 \times 10^9$ cells/L (7000 cells/µL)
• Neutrophils are the predominant white blood cell in peripheral blood and neutrophilia usually leads to leukocytosis
• In horses, neutrophilic response to inflammation is usually less marked than in dogs and cats and a neutrophil count within reference intervals does not preclude the presence of inflammation
• Blood neutrophil counts depend on rate of supply from the bone marrow, distribution between the CNP and MNP, and rate of efflux of neutrophils into tissues
• Neutrophils are a critical component of the innate immune system, forming the first line of cellular defense against pathogens and helping to modulate the adaptive immune response
• Neutrophils can contribute to host tissue damage and morbidity if the underlying insult is not resolved
• Neutrophilia can be mild (e.g. $7–14 \times 10^9$ cells/L), moderate (e.g. $14–20 \times 10^9$ cells/L), marked (e.g. $20–30 \times 10^9$ cells/L), or extreme (e.g. $>30 \times 10^9$ cells/L)

PATHOPHYSIOLOGY
• Granulopoiesis occurs continuously in the bone marrow to maintain neutrophil numbers in blood and tissues
• G-CSF is key mediator in stimulation of granulopoiesis, functional maturation of neutrophil precursors, and neutrophil mobilization from bone marrow reserves
• Bone marrow transit time for neutrophils is ~6 days with shorter transit times in cases of increased peripheral demand
• Neutrophils in peripheral blood distribute evenly between the CNP and the MNP; CNP is sampled during blood collection
• Circulating neutrophils have a half-life of ~10.5 h, then migrate randomly to tissues and body cavities to undertake physiologic functions or are recruited to sites of inflammation
• In tissues, neutrophils have a half-life of ~12 h, then undergo apoptosis and are phagocytized by mononuclear cells or are lost from the body via mucosal surfaces
• During inflammation mature neutrophils are released from the bone marrow storage pool in response to inflammatory cytokines
• Inflammatory mediators promote neutrophil margination, adhesion to vascular endothelium, and migration into tissues
• Severe inflammatory disease can rapidly deplete the storage pool of mature neutrophils and result in release of immature neutrophils (neutrophil bands ± metamyelocytes ±

myelocytes) from bone marrow; this is a *left shift*

SYSTEMS AFFECTED
• Hemic/lymphatic/immune
• Others, depending on underlying cause

SIGNALMENT
No breed, age, or sex predilection.

SIGNS

General Comments
• Vary with the cause of the neutrophilia
• Clinical abnormalities may assist in determining which body system(s) is/are affected

Historical Findings
• Inflammatory or myeloproliferative disorders may cause weight loss, inappetence, lethargy, and pyrexia
• Neutrophilia can occur without a history of illness

Physical Examination Findings
• Excitability may be associated with physiologic neutrophilia
• Pyrexia is common with inflammatory and myeloproliferative disorders
• Signs of specific organ involvement may be present

CAUSES
Causes of neutrophilia include catecholamine- or corticosteroid-induced changes, inflammation, and myeloproliferative disorders.

Physiologic (Excitement) Neutrophilia
• Fear, pain, excitement, and brief strenuous exercise can result in a transient (20–30 min) neutrophilia
• Neutrophils move from the MNP to the CNP owing to decreased adhesion to the endothelium and increased flow
• Because the MNP approximates the CNP, the absolute neutrophil count can double
• May be accompanied by lymphocytosis and erythrocytosis due to splenic contraction

Corticosteroid-Induced Neutrophilia
• Endogenous release of corticosteroids (stress response) or exogenous corticosteroids causes mild to moderate neutrophilia
• Characterized by neutrophilia usually without a left shift, lymphopenia, monocytosis, and eosinopenia, although monocytosis is variable and eosinopenia can be difficult to document
• Neutrophilia is caused by increased release of mature neutrophils (and occasionally low numbers of bands) from the bone marrow; decreased tissue migration and increased movement from MNP to CNP may contribute
• Corticosteroid-induced neutrophilia may add to the neutrophilia of inflammation

Inflammatory Neutrophilia
• The hallmark of inflammation is neutrophilia and a left shift

• Inflammation may be due to infections, tissue damage/necrosis, neoplasia, or immune-mediated responses
• Any body tissue or space can be affected; common conditions include abscess, pleuropneumonia, peritonitis, colitis, traumatic wounds, and immune-mediated disease (IMHA, vasculitis, pemphigus)
• A left shift occurs when peripheral demand exceeds the bone marrow storage pool of mature neutrophils
• Degree of neutrophilia, left shift, and toxic change depend on severity of the inflammatory insult and have prognostic relevance
• Mild inflammation may not incite a left shift while a left shift with immature neutrophils < mature neutrophils and neutrophilia is the appropriate response to increased tissue demand for neutrophils
• Marked neutrophilia with a left shift that includes metamyelocytes and myelocytes indicates intense inflammation
• A *degenerative* or *uncompensated* left shift (immature neutrophils > mature segmented neutrophils without neutrophilia) indicates tissue use is exceeding bone marrow production; a persistent degenerative left shift is a poor prognostic indicator
• Chronic or established inflammation may lack a left shift if increased granulopoiesis replenishes the bone marrow storage pool and only mature neutrophils are released
• Toxic change in neutrophils indicate severe local/systemic infection, endotoxemia/systemic inflammatory response syndrome, or severe noninfectious inflammatory disorders and can include cytoplasmic basophilia, foamy vacuolation, toxic granulation, or Döhle bodies
• Mild and clinically insignificant toxic change may be seen in horses with no clinical evidence of inflammatory disease
• Resolution of toxic change is a positive prognostic indicator
• Sustained neutrophilia occurs when the rate of neutrophil release from bone marrow is greater than the rate of efflux into the tissues; both total blood neutrophil pool and CNP are increased
• Rebound neutrophilia may be seen following neutropenia

Myeloproliferative Diseases
• Granulocytic or myelomonocytic leukemia are rare
• Acute leukemia has poorly differentiated cells/blasts in circulation
• Cytopenias (nonregenerative anemia, thrombocytopenia) may occur secondary to myelophthisis
• Neutrophilia may be paraneoplastic

Other
G-CSF administration.

RISK FACTORS
Dependent on underlying cause.

DIAGNOSIS

DIFFERENTIAL DIAGNOSIS
- Underlying cause of neutrophilia must be determined
- If inflammatory, site and cause of inflammatory process must be determined
- Physiologic neutrophilia in nervous horses is transient and should resolve within 20–30 min
- Stress neutrophilia in recently transported horses should resolve within 24 h

CBC/BIOCHEMISTRY/URINALYSIS
- Neutrophil count > upper limit of laboratory reference interval
- A left shift indicates inflammation; toxic change may be present
- Trends for increasing, persistent, or decreasing neutrophil counts and change in neutrophil morphology assist in establishing diagnosis and prognosis
- Physiologic neutrophilia is mature in nature
- Corticosteroids cause a mature neutrophilia and lymphopenia
- Myeloproliferative disorders may result in circulating blast cells; nonregenerative anemia and thrombocytopenia may be present due to myelophthisis
- Biochemical analysis for evidence of underlying organ involvement and/or dysfunction

OTHER LABORATORY TESTS
- Coombs test for suspected IMHA
- Serology for viral, bacterial, or rickettsial agents
- Immunophenotypic techniques for classification of leukemia

IMAGING
- Ultrasonography of the thorax, abdomen, soft tissues for detection of lesions, organomegaly, and effusions
- Radiography of the thorax or skeleton for detection of inflammatory or neoplastic lesions
- Scintigraphy using radiolabeled autologous neutrophils for detection of an occult abscess

OTHER DIAGNOSTIC PROCEDURES
- Collection of fluid from suspected site of inflammation for cytology, culture, and sensitivity
- Bone marrow aspirate and biopsy for myeloproliferative disorders
- Fine needle aspirate/biopsy of internal/external space-occupying lesion
- Endoscopy (airways, esophagus/stomach, bladder)

PATHOLOGIC FINDINGS
Dependent on the underlying cause.

TREATMENT

AIMS
- Elimination of the underlying cause
- Vary with the underlying cause and may include elimination of infection, resolution of inflammation, and correction of fluid, electrolyte, and acid–base derangements

APPROPRIATE HEALTH CARE
- Physiologic neutrophilia and stress neutrophilia do not require treatment
- Mild forms of inflammatory neutrophilia can often be addressed by outpatient medical care
- Inflammatory neutrophilia may require inpatient medical and/or surgical treatment and some forms (e.g. acute sepsis, IMHA) require emergency intensive care

NURSING CARE
Dependent on the underlying cause.

ACTIVITY
Dependent on the underlying cause.

CLIENT EDUCATION
Neutrophilia often denotes the presence of an underlying disease that is the focus of diagnostic assessment and treatment.

SURGICAL CONSIDERATIONS
Dependent on the underlying cause.

MEDICATIONS

DRUG(S) OF CHOICE
- Bacterial or fungal infections require antimicrobial therapy based on culture and sensitivity testing
- Parasitism requires the use of anthelmintics
- NSAIDs to reduce inflammation
- Corticosteroids for treatment of immune-mediated disease

CONTRAINDICATIONS
Avoid corticosteroids in cases with infectious disease or laminitis.

PRECAUTIONS
Use of NSAIDs, aminoglycosides, and trimethoprim–sulfonamide drugs should be avoided until fluid deficits are corrected.

FOLLOW-UP

PATIENT MONITORING
Horses with inflammatory neutrophilia may require daily leukograms until stable.

POSSIBLE COMPLICATIONS
Neutropenia develops if tissue demand exceeds the rate of bone marrow production.

EXPECTED COURSE AND PROGNOSIS
- Dependent on the underlying cause
- Prognosis for marked inflammation or severe tissue trauma is guarded
- Prognosis for myeloproliferative disorders is hopeless

MISCELLANEOUS

AGE-RELATED FACTORS
In healthy foals, absolute neutrophil counts may exceed adult reference intervals for 3–4 months.

ZOONOTIC POTENTIAL
None

SEE ALSO
Neutropenia

ABBREVIATIONS
- CNP = circulating neutrophil pool
- G-CSF = granulocyte colony-stimulating factor
- IMHA = immune-mediated hemolytic anemia
- MNP = marginating neutrophil pool
- NSAID = nonsteroidal anti-inflammatory drug

Internet Resources
Cornell University College of Veterinary Medicine, Leukogram changes. http://www.eclinpath.com/hematology/leukogram-changes/

Suggested Reading
Walton RM. Equine hematology. In: Walton RM, ed. Equine Clinical Pathology. Ames, IA: Wiley Blackwell, 2014:15–36.

Authors Marie-France Roy and Nicole J. Fernandez
Consulting Editors David Hodgson, Harold C. McKenzie, and Jennifer L. Hodgson
Acknowledgment The authors and editors acknowledge the prior contribution of Kristopher Hughes.

N

NIGROPALLIDAL ENCEPHALOMALACIA

BASICS

OVERVIEW
Yellow star thistle poisoning, also known as "chewing disease," is a devastating disease caused by prolonged ingestion of yellow star thistle or Russian knapweed, resulting in degeneration of specific basal nuclei and the extrapyramidal system

Pathophysiology
• Access to hay or pasture containing yellow star thistle (*Centaurea solstitialis*) or Russian knapweed (*Centaurea repens*) for at least a month
• Toxicity produced when horses eat 50–200% of their bodyweight of the thistles, resulting in necrosis of the substantia nigra and globus pallidus
• Repin is the most abundant constituent isolated from these plants, and is a leading suspect for causing equine nigropallidal encephalomalacia. It has been shown to reduce cellular glutathione and increase reactive oxygen species
• Dopaminergic neurons in the basal nuclei may be more susceptible to oxidative stress

Geographic Distribution
Predominantly in northwestern USA. *C. repens* also grows in Australia, where it is known as yellow burr.

SIGNALMENT
Horses of any age, sex, or breed can be affected.

SIGNS
• Clinical signs appear suddenly in horses once they have consumed 50–200% of their bodyweight of the poisonous plants
• Paralysis of the lips and tongue present early in the course of the disease result in the horse being unable to eat
• Reduced jaw tone, tongue protrusion, and hypertonicity of the facial and upper lip musculature are also frequently observed. Other reported clinical signs include severe depression, with affected horses carrying their heads low
• Ultimately, poisoned animals are unable to eat, become weak and emaciated, and eventually die of starvation

DIAGNOSIS

The diagnosis is based on signalment, history, and physical and neurologic findings, and can be confirmed by MRI.

DIFFERENTIAL DIAGNOSIS
Tetanus

TREATMENT

Horses can be maintained with feeding through a nasogastric tube, but no specific treatment exists.

FOLLOW-UP

EXPECTED COURSE AND PROGNOSIS
The outlook is grave and affected horses starve to death.

MISCELLANEOUS

SEE ALSO
Tetanus

ABBREVIATIONS
MRI = magnetic resonance imaging

Suggested Reading
Chang HT, Rumbeiha WK, Patterson JS, et al. Toxic equine parkinsonism: an immunohistochemical study of 10 horses with nigropallidal encephalomalacia. Vet Pathol 2012;49:398–402.
Elliott CR, McCowan CI. Nigropallidal encephalomalacia in horses grazing *Rhaponticum repens* (creeping knapweed). Aust Vet J 2012;90:151–154.
Author Caroline N. Hahn
Consulting Editor Caroline N. Hahn

BASICS

OVERVIEW
• Nitrate intoxication is primarily a problem in ruminants because of their efficient reduction of nitrate to nitrite within the rumen
• Monogastrics generally tolerate rather high concentrations of nitrate because it is not rapidly reduced to nitrite in the gastrointestinal tract
• Nitrite is approximately 3- and 10-fold more toxic than nitrate for ruminants and monogastrics, respectively
• Nitrate is found in plants, water, fertilizers, and animal wastes
• Horses are most likely to be intoxicated after exposure to high concentrations of nitrate or nitrite in fertilizers, but no cases of equine nitrate/nitrite intoxication have been published
• Nitrite converts Fe^{2+} in hemoglobin to Fe^{3+}, forming methemoglobin, which cannot bind and transport oxygen. In turn, this leads to generalized tissue hypoxia

SIGNALMENT
• No breed or sex predispositions
• Neonates may be more sensitive because of their more efficient reduction of nitrate to nitrite, but data are lacking

SIGNS
• Polypnea
• Dyspnea
• Cyanotic or muddy mucous membranes
• Weakness
• Muscle tremors
• Reluctance to move
• Terminal convulsions
• Death

CAUSES AND RISK FACTORS
The most likely cause is acute exposure to a concentrated source of nitrate or nitrite (e.g. fertilizers or contaminated water source); a horse is unlikely to be exposed to sufficient nitrate from other sources such as plants to cause intoxication.

DIAGNOSIS

DIFFERENTIAL DIAGNOSIS
Other causes of methemoglobin formation such as *Acer rubrum* (red maple) toxicosis (clinical signs of icterus and anemia) or chlorate toxicosis (identified source of exposure to a chlorate salt, e.g. potassium or sodium chlorate).

CBC/BIOCHEMISTRY/URINALYSIS
• Methemoglobin imparts a brown discoloration to blood
• All routinely measured parameters are normal

OTHER LABORATORY TESTS
• Significant methemoglobinemia (>30%)
• High plasma, serum, or ocular fluid nitrate or nitrite concentrations—diagnostic concentrations have not been determined for horses
• Measurement of high nitrate/nitrite in an environmental source has been associated with a suspected fertilizer spill

IMAGING
N/A

OTHER DIAGNOSTIC PROCEDURES
N/A

PATHOLOGIC FINDINGS
No specific postmortem findings except for a dark red to brown discoloration of the blood and muscle as a result of methemoglobin pigmentation.

TREATMENT
Treat acidosis and ischemia-induced ECG changes.

MEDICATIONS

DRUG(S) OF CHOICE
• Reduce methemoglobin to hemoglobin
• The standard treatment for methemoglobinemia is methylene blue, which is not believed to be efficacious in horses (although this conclusion is based on limited data)

• Ascorbic acid (30 mg/kg BID given in IV fluids) may be beneficial in reducing methemoglobin, but, as with methylene blue, studies of clinical efficacy are lacking

CONTRAINDICATIONS/POSSIBLE INTERACTIONS
N/A

FOLLOW-UP

PATIENT MONITORING
Monitor methemoglobin concentrations, acid–base status, and ECG.

PREVENTION/AVOIDANCE
N/A

POSSIBLE COMPLICATIONS
N/A

EXPECTED COURSE AND PROGNOSIS
Because methylene blue may not be efficacious, prognosis is guarded.

MISCELLANEOUS

ASSOCIATED CONDITIONS
N/A

AGE-RELATED FACTORS
More efficient reduction of nitrate to nitrite might occur in neonates.

ZOONOTIC POTENTIAL
N/A

PREGNANCY/FERTILITY/BREEDING
Fetal hypoxia is a concern in pregnant animals.

SEE ALSO
Acer rubrum (red maple) toxicosis

Suggested Reading
Osweiler GD, Carson TL, Buck WB, Van Gelder GA. Nitrates, nitrites, and related problems. In: Osweiler GD, ed. Clinical and Diagnostic Veterinary Toxicology, 3e. Dubuque, IA: Kendall Hunt Publishing, 1985:460–467.

Authors Arya Sobhakumari and Robert H. Poppenga
Consulting Editors Wilson K. Rumbeiha and Steve Ensley

N

NUTRITION IN FOALS

BASICS

DEFINITION
• Enteral nutrition is consumed orally or administered through an NG feeding tube
• PN is an IV solution of dextrose, protein (amino acids), lipid emulsion, electrolytes, and multivitamins. Partial PN can consist of only dextrose and amino acids in a balanced electrolyte solution

PATHOPHYSIOLOGY
• Neonatal foals have little energy reserves and can become rapidly dehydrated and hypoglycemic if they are unable to nurse regularly. Sepsis, musculoskeletal abnormalities, and neurologic disease may prevent the foal from nursing regularly. Foals that are unable to nurse, but that have functional GI tracts, may be fed enterally
• Foals with enterocolitis, colic, or ileus may be unable to tolerate enteral feeding until the underlying cause of GI dysfunction has been treated

SYSTEMS AFFECTED
GI

SIGNALMENT
There are no known breed or sex differences for nutritional requirements in foals. Most nutritional information in foals has been collected from Thoroughbred populations.

SIGNS
Historical Findings
• Decreased nursing
• Weight loss or failure to gain weight
• Agalactia in mare—foal may make frequent, short attempts to nurse
• Debilitation or feed restriction in the mare

Physical Examination Findings
• Dehydration, weakness/depression
• Angular/flexural limb deformity—difficulty rising or remaining in standing position
• Dried milk on head—milk streaming from dam's udder when foal does not adequately nurse
• Diarrhea, colic, or abdominal distention

CAUSES
Indications for Enteral Nutrition Supplementation
• Musculoskeletal abnormalities—severe angular or flexural limb deformity
• Neurologic dysfunction or dysphagia/neonatal maladjustment syndrome, botulism
• Orphan foals

Indications for PN Supplementation
• Enterocolitis
• Lactose intolerance, secondary to rotavirus or *Clostridium* infection
• Colic—GI obstruction, ileus, or intolerance of enteral feeding
• GI dysfunction—secondary to sepsis, ischemic damage (NMS)

RISK FACTORS
• NMS—neurologic dysfunction or GI hypoxia
• Septicemia—enterocolitis or poor GI perfusion

DIAGNOSIS

CBC/BIOCHEMISTRY/URINALYSIS
• Hypoglycemia (blood glucose <80 mg/dL) will occur quickly in neonates unable to nurse
• Hemoconcentration due to dehydration

OTHER LABORATORY TESTS
Low immunoglobulin G (<800 mg/dL).

DIAGNOSTIC PROCEDURES
Lactose tolerance test—oral milk or lactose feeding with serial blood glucose measurements.

TREATMENT

AIMS
• Provide adequate nutrition for growth
• GI rest for foals with malabsorption diarrhea, hypoxic GI injury, or GI obstruction or other dysfunction

APPROPRIATE HEALTH CARE
• Enteral nutrition via feeding tube, bottle, or bucket can be administered in a farm or hospital setting. Bottle and NG tube feedings must be given frequently (every 1–2 h); therefore, inpatient medical management may be more appropriate. The underlying disease (e.g. sepsis, NMS, musculoskeletal abnormality) may require management in a hospital setting
• PN requires inpatient medical management

NURSING CARE
Orphan Foal Options
• Nurse mare—may be expensive and limited in availability but provides ideal nutrition and companionship for an orphan foal
• Bottle feeding—very labor intensive and risk of aspiration pneumonia (especially in debilitated foals). Syringe feeding should never be performed due to the risk of aspiration and inability to deliver adequate volumes
• Bucket feeding—foal may be slower to accept this feeding method, but it is less labor intensive than bottle feeding and reduces the risk of behavioral problems and aspiration pneumonia associated with bottle feeding
• Initial frequency of feeding is every 2 h, although this can be increased to every 4 h as the foal reliably consumes the milk or milk replacer

Enteral Feeding via NG Tube
• Pliable enteral feeding tubes (14 Fr) can remain in place and are well tolerated by foals

• Placement should be confirmed by palpation, endoscopy, or radiography
• The tube should also be aspirated prior to feeding to check for gastric reflux
• The foal should be fed in the standing or sternal position to reduce the risk of aspiration
• Feeding requirements for normal foals are 20–30% of bodyweight in milk per day, but in sick foals enteral feeding may begin at 5–10% of bodyweight per day
• Frequency of feeding is every 1–2 h, although a CRI may be used if bolus feedings are not well tolerated

PN
• A jugular IV catheter should be placed with sterile technique for administration of PN. Over-the-wire polyurethane catheters are preferred
• Although energy requirements in normal foals are 120–140 kcal/kg/day, sick foals require far less (30–50 kcal/kg/day)
• Parenteral feeding should begin at 25% of the target rate, increasing to the target rate within 24 h as long as blood glucose concentration remains normal. If the foal becomes hyperglycemic, the infusion rate should be decreased. Multiple days may be required to reach the desired rate. Insulin therapy may be needed in foals that are persistently hyperglycemic
• When PN is discontinued (change to enteral nutrition), the foal should be "weaned off" over 12–24 h in order to avoid hypoglycemia
• Supplemental IV fluids are needed to supply the balance of the maintenance requirements of the foal
• The mare should be milked every 2–4 h so that lactation continues and the foal can be reintroduced to the mare

Trophic Feeding
• Small enteral feedings (20 mL every 2–6 h) are recommended in foals on PN unless all enteral feeding is contraindicated (i.e. intestinal obstruction)
• Trophic feedings are meant to assist with intestinal development and barrier function (reduce the risk of bacterial translocation)

ACTIVITY
• Foals receiving PN should be disconnected from the IV solution as infrequently as possible to avoid contamination and changes in blood glucose levels. Foals need to be separated from the mare while on a CRI
• Orphan foals should get adequate exercise and socialization

DIET
Enteral Nutrition Formulations
• Mare's milk—ideal nutrition if enteral feeding is tolerated. The mare can be milked, and this can be fed via NG tube or by use of a bucket

- Milk substitutes
  - Mare's milk replacer—should mimic mare's milk as closely as possible. Mare's milk has approximately 25% crude protein, 17% crude fat, 11% total solids, and 0.5 kcal/mL digestible energy. Milk replacers should be made fresh before each feeding (every 2–4 h). Proper dilution of the milk replacer is very important to help avoid diarrhea, constipation, or hypernatremia. Dilution of the milk replacer by 25% (beyond the manufacturer's instructions) is recommended to prevent adverse effects
  - Cow's milk and goat's milk—higher in fat, protein, total solids, and lactose. Cow's milk (2% fat) with 20 g/L dextrose added or unmodified goat's milk may be used, but can cause diarrhea or constipation
  - Lactose-free cow's milk—for foals with lactose intolerance
- Solid feeds—milk pellets can be introduced, although the majority of nutrition requirements will be provided by milk feedings initially. Small amounts of good quality hay and 16% protein grain may also be introduced to the foal. By 8 weeks of age, the foal may be weaned off milk replacer and onto solid feed

PN Formulations
- Total energy and nutrition requirements are usually not met, but total PN consists of dextrose, amino acids, lipid emulsion, vitamins, and electrolytes. Partial PN may be provided as dextrose and amino acids
- Dextrose—up to a 5% solution may initially be given alone (the first 12–24 h of treatment), but this is not appropriate for long-term nutritional needs
- Amino acids—approximately 4–6 g/100 kcal nonprotein should be added to the PN formulation; 8.5% amino acid solutions are commonly used and provide 0.34 kcal/mL
- Lipid emulsion—a 10% emulsion supplies 1 kcal/mL

CLIENT EDUCATION
Owners should be instructed on proper introduction of bucket or bottle feeding and warned of the risks of behavioral problems in orphan foals that do not have proper socialization.

 MEDICATIONS
DRUG(S) OF CHOICE
- Insulin may be needed to treat hyperglycemia secondary to PN. Administer

0.1–0.5 IU/kg SC or IV, or alternatively a CRI of 0.01–0.02 IU/kg/h. Preferable to decrease rate of glucose administration
- Lactase tablets may be used in foals with lactose intolerance—for a 50 kg foal, 3000–6000 U PO with each feeding. Relatively ineffective treatment
- Domperidone (1.1 mg/kg PO every 24 h) can be administered to mares with suspected fescue toxicity or poor milk production to help stimulate lactation

CONTRAINDICATIONS
N/A

PRECAUTIONS
Hypoglycemia can occur with the use of insulin. Use caution especially if administering a separate CRI of insulin.

 FOLLOW-UP
PATIENT MONITORING
- Daily weight measurements—foals should gain approximately 1.0–1.5 kg/day (<30 days of age)
- Glucose measurements should be performed frequently (every 2–4 h) when PN is started in order to prevent hyperglycemia. Electrolytes should be monitored every 24–48 h unless there have been significant abnormalities (check more frequently)
- NG tube placement should be confirmed prior to enteral feedings
- Sick or debilitated foals should be monitored for abdominal distention, colic, and NG reflux. Enteral feeding should be reduced or discontinued if these complications occur
- IV catheter should be monitored for signs of thrombophlebitis and other catheter site problems. The catheter should be removed if there are any concerns about thrombophlebitis

PREVENTION/AVOIDANCE
N/A

POSSIBLE COMPLICATIONS
- Enteral nutrition—aspiration can occur with bottle feeding but is also a risk with NG tube feeding in debilitated/recumbent foals. Transient diarrhea can occur when the foal is introduced to milk replacer
- PN—hyperglycemia, phlebitis, and hyperlipidemia. Complications occur more frequently in severely ill foals

EXPECTED COURSE AND PROGNOSIS
- The goal of supplemental nutrition is to act as a "bridge" until the foal can be reintroduced to nursing the mare
- Foals with uncomplicated diarrhea often show improvement with 24 h of parenteral feeding, although PN may need to be continued for 3–5 days
- The foal should continue to have contact with the mare to facilitate reintroduction after a period of NG or parenteral feeding

 MISCELLANEOUS
ASSOCIATED CONDITIONS
- Diarrhea
- Prematurity

AGE-RELATED FACTORS
Although solid feeds can be introduced early, these should not make up the majority of the diet until the foal is at least 8 weeks of age.

SYNONYMS
Feeding

SEE ALSO
Diarrhea, neonate

ABBREVIATIONS
- CRI = constant rate infusion
- GI = gastrointestinal
- NG = nasogastric
- NMS = neonatal maladjustment syndrome
- PN = parenteral nutrition

Suggested Reading
Buechner-Maxwell VA. Nutritional support for neonatal foals. Vet Clin North Am Equine Pract 2005;21:487–510.
Krause JB, McKenzie HC. Parenteral nutrition in foals: a retrospective study of 45 cases (2000–2004). Equine Vet J 2007;39:74–78.

Author Laura K. Dunbar
Consulting Editor Margaret C. Mudge
Acknowledgment The author acknowledges the prior contribution of Margaret C. Mudge.

 Client Education Handout available online

NUTRITIONAL MYODEGENERATION

BASICS

DEFINITION
Nutritional myodegeneration (nutritional muscular dystrophy, nutritional myopathy, dystrophic myodegeneration, WMD) is a noninflammatory degenerative disease of skeletal and cardiac muscle associated with dietary deficiency of Se and vitamin E.

PATHOPHYSIOLOGY
• Se is an important component of GPx, an enzyme found in all animal tissue (high concentrations in liver and erythrocytes) that functions to reduce highly reactive oxygen metabolites that are produced during normal cellular metabolism. Deficiency of GPx increases membrane lipid peroxidation by these metabolites, resulting in membrane degradation and destruction of cells. Severe oxidative damage to myocytes and subsequent rhabdomyolysis underlie the pathogenesis of WMD in Se-deficient foals
• While vitamin E deficiency may also play a role, deficiency of this nutrient alone is not sufficient to cause clinical disease in foals; vitamin E deficiency likely promotes disease in the setting of Se deficiency
• Foals born to mares with dietary deficiency of Se are affected; however, not all Se-deficient foals display clinical signs of disease
• Affected animals may present with acute fulminant disease with myocardial involvement or with subacute, insidious disease; in either case, mortality can be high and animals may not consistently respond to treatment. Comorbidity is common and may mask the underlying primary problem

SYSTEMS AFFECTED
• Neuromuscular
• Cardiovascular

GENETICS
There does not appear to be a genetic component.

INCIDENCE/PREVALENCE
Dependent on geographic region and diet.

GEOGRAPHIC DISTRIBUTION
The regional distribution of cases corresponds to areas where Se-deficient soils predominate. In the USA, the northwest, southeast, and Great Lakes areas tend to have Se-deficient soil. Soil and pasture analysis is recommended to determine whether Se supplementation is needed.

SIGNALMENT
• Young foals, with the majority of cases diagnosed within the first 60 days of life (most <30 days). Animals up to 1 year of age may be affected, and lesions have been noted in aborted fetuses
• No breed or sex predisposition

SIGNS

Acute Form
• Sudden death
• Circulatory collapse
• Cyanosis
• Tachycardia, arrhythmia, systolic cardiac murmur
• Respiratory distress (pulmonary edema, respiratory muscle failure)
• Inability to rise, often with violent struggling

Subacute Form
• Profound muscular weakness—hallmark sign
• Stiff, stilted gait
• Muscle fasciculation/trembling
• Inability to rise or stand unassisted
• Dysphagia and/or poor suckle reflex (milk at nares, ptyalism)
• Aspiration pneumonia
• Weight loss or failure to gain due to inadequate dietary intake
• Swollen, painful muscles—limbs, lumbar, cervical musculature

CAUSES
• Se deficiency

RISK FACTORS
• Geographic area with Se-deficient soil or low Se forage

DIAGNOSIS

DIFFERENTIAL DIAGNOSIS
• Dysphagia
  ○ Cleft palate
  ○ Pharyngitis/pharyngeal malformation
  ○ Botulism
  ○ Weakness, any cause (e.g. sepsis)
• Neuromuscular weakness
  ○ Botulism
  ○ Tick paralysis
  ○ Neurologic/neuromuscular disease
• Stiff gait
  ○ Tetanus
  ○ Septic (poly)arthritis
  ○ Bacterial meningitis
  ○ Trauma
• Pneumonia
• Congenital cardiac anomaly
• Polysaccharide storage myopathy
• Glycogen branching enzyme deficiency
• Neonatal isoerythrolysis
• Sepsis

CBC/BIOCHEMISTRY/URINALYSIS
• CBC—hematocrit normal or increased (helpful to differentiate from neonatal isoerythrolysis, which may also cause pigmenturia)
• Biochemistry—hyponatremia, hypochloremia, hyperkalemia, hyperphosphatemia, azotemia (prenatal or postrenal), significant increases in CK, AST, and LDH; hypogammaglobulinemia
• Urinalysis—pigmenturia (myoglobinuria)

OTHER LABORATORY TESTS
• Whole-blood Se concentration—documents recent Se deficiency; may be used to assess adequacy of supplementation; should be performed prior to supplementation
• GPx concentration (erythrocyte)—documents Se deficiency in past weeks to months (Se is incorporated during erythropoiesis); should be interpreted according to reference ranges of laboratory performing analysis
• Cardiac troponin I concentration—can be used to evaluate myocardial involvement

IMAGING
N/A

OTHER DIAGNOSTIC PROCEDURES
Muscle biopsy—may be helpful to diagnose myopathy in animals with normal whole-blood Se, GPx.

PATHOLOGIC FINDINGS
Pale streaking of major skeletal muscle groups and myocardium (especially left ventricle) seen at necropsy. Histologically, hyaline degeneration and myolysis are seen acutely; chronic cases may display fibrosis and calcification of lesions.

TREATMENT

APPROPRIATE HEALTH CARE
Inpatient medical treatment is needed for foals with moderate to severe neuromuscular weakness. Mildly affected foals may be treated and monitored on the farm.

NURSING CARE
Fluid therapy (avoid potassium-containing fluids in hyperkalemic foals) and plasma are often required.

ACTIVITY
Affected foals should be strictly rested to avoid additional undue muscle damage.

DIET
Important for prevention of Se deficiency (see Prevention/Avoidance). Feed should be analyzed to ensure appropriate levels of Se.

CLIENT EDUCATION
• Feed should be analyzed, and additional feed or supplements used to correct/prevent Se deficiency
• Prophylactic treatment of mares and foals in the same geographic area is recommended

SURGICAL CONSIDERATIONS
N/A

MEDICATIONS

DRUG(S) OF CHOICE
• Se—0.06 mg/kg deep IM divided into 2 sites (semimembranosus/semitendinosus

(CONTINUED)

NUTRITIONAL MYODEGENERATION

recommended; do not use cervical, gluteal muscles); can be repeated 3 days and 8–10 days later. This corresponds to 1 mL of a vitamin E/Se combination product containing 2.5 mg Se/mL for a 45–50 kg foal
• Vitamin E (oral)—500 IU vitamin E/mL; recommended dose is 1–2 IU/kg PO daily
• NSAIDs—flunixin meglumine (1 mg/kg IV SID–BID) or ketoprofen (2.2 mg/kg IV SID–BID) may be used to reduce muscle pain and swelling; associated with gastric ulcers in neonates
• Broad-spectrum antimicrobials—affected foals often have FTPI due to decreased colostral intake (recumbent/weak, dysphagia); concurrent aspiration pneumonia common (antimicrobial therapy best directed with results of bacterial culture of percutaneous transtracheal aspirate)

CONTRAINDICATIONS
Anaphylactoid reactions may occur with IV administration of commercial vitamin E/Se preparations; this is not recommended.

PRECAUTIONS
See Prevention/Avoidance.

POSSIBLE INTERACTIONS
N/A

ALTERNATIVE DRUGS
N/A

 FOLLOW-UP

PATIENT MONITORING
• Rapid decreases (24–48 h) in plasma CK concentration indicate cessation of muscle damage; AST and LDH decrease much more slowly (weeks)
• Monitoring of whole-blood Se and GPx concentrations is recommended to gauge efficacy of supplementation

PREVENTION/AVOIDANCE
• Prevention via monitoring of dietary and animal Se status and supplementation of

pregnant mares is effective and recommended in Se-deficient areas or on farms where cases have been documented.
• Since nutritional myodegeneration is associated with a high mortality rate (even with appropriate treatment), prevention of the disease is preferred
• Farms in known Se-deficient areas should practice routine feed analysis; all dietary components (forage and grain) should contain at least 0.10 ppm Se, preferably 0.30 ppm
• Pregnant mares should be supplemented with dietary Se at the rate of 1–3 mg Se/mare/day through provision of a trace mineral salt (15–30 ppm) or in the ration at 0.50 ppm. Supplementation of mares in this fashion has been shown to prevent myopathy in foals and is more effective than supplementation of foals at birth (as they may be born diseased). Alternatively, IM administration of commercial vitamin E/Se preparations may be used for prevention

POSSIBLE COMPLICATIONS
• Selenium toxicity may occur with overzealous supplementation; the toxic dose is 200 µg/kg in foals
• Concurrent aspiration pneumonia and FTPI/septicemia are common
• Fibrosis of severely affected muscle groups may result in permanent gait deficits in recovered animals

EXPECTED COURSE AND PROGNOSIS
• Guarded prognosis
• Acute form, >90% mortality; subacute form, 50–75%
• Animals that do not respond to therapy within 2–5 days have a poor prognosis for recovery

 MISCELLANEOUS

ASSOCIATED CONDITIONS
• Septicemia
• Aspiration pneumonia

AGE-RELATED FACTORS
N/A

ZOONOTIC POTENTIAL
N/A

PREGNANCY/FERTILITY/BREEDING
See Prevention/Avoidance.

SYNONYMS
WMD

SEE ALSO
• Botulism
• Glycogen branching enzyme deficiency
• Pneumonia, neonate
• Septicemia, neonate
• Tetanus

ABBREVIATIONS
• AST = aspartate aminotransferase
• CK = creatine kinase
• FTPI = failure of transfer of passive immunity
• GPx = glutathione peroxidase
• LDH = lactate dehydrogenase
• NSAID = nonsteroidal anti-inflammatory drug
• Se = selenium
• WMD = white muscle disease

Suggested Reading
Lofstedt J. White muscle disease of foals. Vet Clin North Am Equine Pract 1997;13(1): 169–185.
Streeter RM, Divers TJ, Mittel L, et al. Selenium deficiency associations with gender, breed, serum vitamin E and creatine kinase, clinical signs and diagnoses in horses of different age groups: a retrospective examination 1996-2011. Equine Vet J Suppl 2012;43:31–35.

Author Teresa A. Burns
Consulting Editor Margaret C. Mudge

N

NUTRITIONAL SECONDARY HYPERPARATHYROIDISM (NSHPT)

BASICS

OVERVIEW
• NSHPT is a skeletal disorder of equids fed a diet with excess of phytates or oxalates, or a diet with a P:Ca ratio of >3:1. Phosphate, phytates, and oxalates bind calcium in the intestines, reducing Ca absorption. Low plasma ionized Ca stimulates secretion of PTH, leading to hyperparathyroidism
• Also known as big head, bran disease, miller's disease, osteodystrophia fibrosa, osteitis fibrosa, equine osteoporosis
• Systems affected—musculoskeletal, endocrine

SIGNALMENT
• Any breed, age, and sex
• Signs are more evident in growing equids
• Multiple animals may be affected

SIGNS
Physical Examination Findings
• Weight shifting
• Intermittent lameness
• Fractures
• Facial swelling (advanced NSHPT)
• Stridor
• Epiphora
• Loose teeth, difficulty chewing, weight loss
• Neurologic signs (secondary to vertebral fractures or spinal cord compression)

CAUSES AND RISK FACTORS
• Rations with a P:Ca ratio >3:1 even with adequate Ca
• Access to high oxalate-containing plants, including *Setaria* grass, buffel grass, purple pigeon grass, kikuyu, dallis grass, panic grass, pangola, and pearl millet, soursob, shamrock, red-rooted pigweed, *Halogeton*, purslane, rhubarb, sorrel, others

DIAGNOSIS

DIFFERENTIAL DIAGNOSIS
• Primary hyperparathyroidism has increased PTH concentrations and increased calcium concentrations
• Humoral hypercalcemia of malignancy results in hypercalcemia, hypophosphatemia, low to normal PTH, and increased PTH-related protein concentrations
• Chronic renal failure may result in hypercalcemia. Renal secondary hyperparathyroidism has not been reported in horses

CBC/BIOCHEMISTRY/URINALYSIS
• Low to normal Ca
• Low, normal, or high P

OTHER LABORATORY TESTS
• Serum PTH may be normal or increased
• Increased urinary fractional excretion of P (reference range 0–0.5%). Urinary excretion of Ca may be low but is often difficult to interpret due to excessive Ca content in equine urine
• Analysis of dietary Ca and P
• Plant oxalate content
• Byproducts of bone resorption (CTX-1) may be increased in serum or urine

IMAGING
• Decreased bone density may be visualized in skull radiographs. A minimum decrease of 30% is necessary for detection
• Loss of laminae durae of the mandible
• Decreased cortical bone thickness and demineralization may be seen in chronic cases. Fractures may be detected

PATHOLOGIC FINDINGS
• Bone mineral is replaced by fibrous tissue
• Increased bone volume but decreased bone density, primarily of the cancellous bone of the skull, ribs, and metaphyses of long bones
• Parathyroid gland hypertrophy and hyperplasia may be evident

TREATMENT

ACTIVITY
• Confine to a stall or small paddock until bone density normalizes
• Remove oxalate-containing plants from the diet
• Supplement Ca and P ($CaCO_3$ or $CaHPO_4$) 100–300 g/day at a ratio of 1 part $CaCO_3$ to 2 parts $CaHPO_4$ for horses grazing oxalate-rich pastures. For treatment, diet should have a Ca:P ratio of 3–4:1. Molasses may improve palatability
• Feed alfalfa hay
• Reduce grain intake

MEDICATIONS
• Use NSAIDs with caution—decreasing pain may lead to increased activity and skeletal trauma
• Vitamin D may promote bone formation and reduce PTH secretion
• The value of drugs that reduce osteoclast activity (e.g. bisphosphonates) is unknown

FOLLOW-UP

PATIENT MONITORING
Radiography to assess bone density (ideally, compare with age-matched unaffected horses).

PREVENTION/AVOIDANCE
• Avoid a high-bran diet
• Horses on high-grain diets should be supplemented with Ca to ensure a Ca:P ratio >1.5:1
• Limit access to pastures containing oxalate-accumulating plants

POSSIBLE COMPLICATIONS
Horses may lose teeth, or develop fracture or periosteal avulsions.

EXPECTED COURSE AND PROGNOSIS
• Lameness usually resolves 4–6 weeks after diet correction, and before bone density normalizes
• Recovery of bone strength may take 9–12 months. Severely affected horses may not recover
• In most cases, enlarged skull bones do not resolve

MISCELLANEOUS

PREGNANCY/FERTILITY/BREEDING
• Mares in the last 3 months of pregnancy and early lactation are susceptible
• Mares may raise a healthy foal once their diet is corrected

SEE ALSO
Primary hyperparathyroidism

ABBREVIATIONS
• CTX-1 = collagen type 1 crosslinked C-telopeptide, C-terminal telopeptide
• NSAID = nonsteroidal anti-inflammatory drug
• NSHPT = nutritional secondary hyperparathyroidism
• PTH = parathyroid hormone

Suggested Reading
Joyce JR, Pierce KR, Romane WM, Baker JM. Clinical study of nutritional secondary hyperparathyroidism in horses. J Am Vet Med Assoc 1971;158:2033–2042.
Mendoza FJ, Toribio RE, Perez-Ecija A. Nutritional secondary hyperparathyroidism in equids: Overview and new insights. Equine Vet Educ 2017;29:558–563.
Toribio RE. Disorders of calcium and phosphate metabolism in horses. Vet Clin North Am Equine Pract 2011;27:129–147.

Author Ramiro Toribio
Consulting Editors Michel Levy and Heidi Banse
Acknowledgment The author and editors acknowledge the prior contribution of Laurent Couëtil.

OCULAR/ADNEXAL SQUAMOUS CELL CARCINOMA

BASICS

DEFINITION
A malignant epithelial tumor of the eyelids, nictitans, conjunctiva, cornea, or limbus that is locally invasive but typically slow to metastasize.

PATHOPHYSIOLOGY
Etiopathogenesis is multifactorial. Predisposing factors include solar radiation, reduced periocular pigmentation, viral agents, advanced age, and genetic and immunologic factors. UV radiation targets the tumor suppressor gene *p53*, which is altered in equine SCC. Malignant lesions are usually preceded by actinic keratosis, solar elastosis, and epithelial dysplasia.

SYSTEMS AFFECTED
• Ophthalmic—eyelids, nictitans, conjunctiva, cornea, limbus
• Other systems or tissues may be affected by local extension or by metastasis. Any squamous epithelial cell in the body may undergo malignant transformation; however, those exposed to higher levels of UV radiation or those with minimal pigment are most susceptible

GENETICS
• No proven genetic basis, but apparent breed predispositions suggest heritability, and affected horses have mutant forms of the tumor suppressor gene
• Reduced periocular pigmentation inherited in certain breeds may predispose to ocular SCC

INCIDENCE/PREVALENCE
• Most common equine ocular/adnexal tumor
• Nictitating membrane and medial canthus are the most common sites, followed by limbus and eyelid

GEOGRAPHIC DISTRIBUTION
Increased prevalence with increase in longitude, altitude, or mean annual solar radiation.

SIGNALMENT
Breed Predilections
• An increased prevalence for SCC has been reported in Belgians, Clydesdales, other draft horses, Haflingers, Appaloosas, and Paints, with the lowest prevalence found in Arabians, Thoroughbreds, and Quarter Horses.
• White, chestnut, and palomino animals affected more frequently than those with bay, brown, and black hair coats

Mean Age and Range
Prevalence increases with age. Mean age at presentation approximately 10 years.

Predominant Sex
No proven sex predilection.

SIGNS
Historical Findings
• Epiphora or ocular discharge, squinting, redness or cloudiness of the cornea, or redness or ulceration of the eyelid margins or nictitans
• In advanced cases, raised, ulcerated, or proliferative masses, sometimes resembling granulation tissue, may be noted

Physical Examination Findings
• Nonspecific findings include serous to mucopurulent ocular discharge, blepharospasm, nictitans prolapse, and conjunctival hyperemia
• Closer inspection may reveal red to white plaque-like, proliferative, or erosive lesions of the eyelids, nictitans, conjunctiva, or limbus. On the cornea, SCC may be associated with vascularization, cellular infiltration, edema, and fibrosis. Corneal SCC is typically limited to the superficial cornea, though chronic SCC may invade intraocular structures. Chronic SCC may invade the deep tissues of the eyelids and orbit. Thorough palpation, followed by diagnostic imaging (radiography, CT, or MRI) is essential to evaluate the extent of the lesion

CAUSES
Unknown

RISK FACTORS
• UV radiation
• Lack of periocular pigmentation
• Possible genetic risk factors

DIAGNOSIS

DIFFERENTIAL DIAGNOSIS
• Diagnosis is made on the basis of biopsy results; however, a characteristic clinical appearance is helpful in differentiating SCC from other periocular diseases
• Differentials include other tumors such as papilloma, sarcoid, fibrosarcoma, lymphoma, and liposarcoma; parasites such as *Habronema*, *Onchocerca*, and *Thelazia*; and inflammatory lesions such as abscesses, granulation tissue, eosinophilic keratoconjunctivitis, and foreign body reactions

CBC/BIOCHEMISTRY/URINALYSIS
Results usually normal.

IMAGING
• Skull radiographs may be required if orbital or other bony involvement is suspected
• Thoracic radiographs are indicated if metastasis is suspected
• Orbital ultrasonography and CT may be helpful in determining extent of orbital invasion

OTHER DIAGNOSTIC PROCEDURES
• Cytologic evaluation of cells obtained by scraping followed by Giemsa or Wright's staining may reveal abnormal epithelial cells suggestive of SCC. Histopathologic examination of a biopsy specimen of the lesion is confirmatory
• Histopathologic examination of biopsy specimens from regional lymph nodes may indicate presence of metastatic disease

PATHOLOGIC FINDINGS
• Gross appearance varies from erosive to proliferative. The outer surface may demonstrate inflammation secondary to trauma or bacterial infection, and the mass may be covered by purulent exudate
• Histologically, the tumor consists of nests or cords of epithelial cells with varying degrees of dermal infiltration. Mitotic figures are common, and intercellular bridges may be present. Well-differentiated tumors form keratin "pearls" consisting of rings with central areas of keratinization. Poorly differentiated tumors usually lack keratin pearls but may exhibit dyskeratosis

TREATMENT

INPATIENT VERSUS OUTPATIENT
• Very small, superficial lesions of the eyelids and nictitans may be removed standing with sedation and local anesthesia. Larger, more invasive lesions of the eyelids or nictitans, or lesions involving the conjunctiva or cornea, require hospitalization for surgery
• Alternatively, eyelid lesions may be treated with local anesthesia using intralesional chemotherapy or PDT

ACTIVITY
Restrict during immediate postoperative period. The eye should be protected from self-trauma with a soft- or hard-cup hood.

CLIENT EDUCATION
• If intralesional chemotherapy is used, the client should wear gloves when handling the periocular region for several days post injection
• The client should be aware of signs of recurrence, metastasis, or the development of new lesions
• The client should also be aware of the possible role of UV radiation in order to take appropriate steps to minimize exposure to solar radiation

O

OCULAR/ADNEXAL SQUAMOUS CELL CARCINOMA (CONTINUED)

SURGICAL CONSIDERATIONS

• Tumors may be removed by surgical excision alone if adequate margins can be obtained. However, adjunctive therapy is often necessary, especially with large or invasive tumors. Adjunctive therapies include PDT, cryotherapy, irradiation, radiofrequency hyperthermia, CO_2 laser ablation, and intralesional chemotherapy. Reconstructive eyelid surgery may be required when eyelid margins are lost following tumor excision, and conjunctival or amniotic membrane grafts may be required following keratectomy
• Cryosurgery with liquid nitrogen or nitrous oxide induces cryonecrosis of malignant cells (−20°C to −40°C, double freeze–thaw technique). Beta-irradiation (strontium-90) is most beneficial in SCC of the cornea and limbus following superficial keratectomy, with reported success rates approaching 80%. Brachytherapy may be used following surgical debulking of invasive eyelid tumors. Small, superficial tumors may be treated with radiofrequency hyperthermia (41–50°C) following surgical excision. Excision of corneal limbal SCC followed by CO_2 laser ablation has also been advocated. Debulking of eyelid tumors followed by PDT is showing great promise in early studies

MEDICATIONS

DRUG(S) AND FLUIDS

Topical and Intralesional Immunotherapy/Chemotherapy
• Immunotherapy with bacillus Calmette–Guérin (BCG) cell wall extract has been used successfully for some periocular SCCs in horses
• Chemotherapy with intralesional, slow-release cisplatin or carboplatin has also been used with variable success. At least 4 sessions (sometimes more until tumor-free biopsy results are obtained) at 1–2 week intervals using 1 mg/cm³ are necessary. Tumors up to 20 cm³ may be treated using 3.3 mg/mL cisplatin or carboplatin in purified medical-grade sesame oil. If this therapeutic modality is chosen, the owner must be committed to the entire course of therapy because if the injections are prematurely discontinued, the tumor that recurs often will be resistant to treatment thereafter

• PDT consists of intralesional injection of the affected site with a photoactive dye that causes tumor cell death when the appropriate wavelength of light is applied to the wound bed
• Piroxicam (150 mg PO daily) can be beneficial in some ocular SCCs. The drug is begun once a day and then reduced to every other day
• Topical 5-fluorouracil (1% TID) or mitomycin C (0.02% QID) may be effective for corneal SCC in situ

Supportive Therapy

Topical and systemic broad-spectrum antibiotics may be required to prevent infection following surgical and adjunctive therapy of ocular/adnexal SCC. Topical atropine (1%) is used following keratectomy of corneal SCC to treat reflex anterior uveitis. Systemic NSAIDs are indicated following surgical excision or intralesional chemotherapy.

FOLLOW-UP

PATIENT MONITORING

Patients should be observed closely for recurrence of lesions, new lesions, and signs of metastasis. Tumor recurrence has been reported months to years post treatment.

PREVENTION/AVOIDANCE

Reduction of solar radiation exposure, through either avoidance of light (stalling during daytime, nighttime turnout) or use of protective headgear (fly masks), may reduce the incidence of recurrence or new tumor growth. Early recognition and intervention are critical to a successful outcome.

POSSIBLE COMPLICATIONS

• Tumor progression may lead to orbital involvement with subsequent exophthalmos, necessitating orbital exenteration
• Local invasion usually occurs in the orbit, guttural pouch, or nasal cavity
• Limbal SCC may invade intraocular structures, necessitating enucleation
• Chronic ulceration or tissue necrosis may lead to secondary infection and possible septicemia
• Metastasis occurs in 10–15% of horses with SCC, with regional lymph nodes, parotid salivary glands, and thorax being the most frequently affected sites

EXPECTED COURSE AND PROGNOSIS

• Prognosis is better if treatment is started early in the course of disease and owners are committed to long-term follow-up therapy and monitoring
• Factors affecting prognosis include tumor location, degree of invasiveness, presence or absence of metastasis, and the number of tumors present at the time of diagnosis
• Recurrence rates following therapy range from 25% to 42%
• Third eyelid tumors and eyelid tumors tend to spread and metastasize more frequently than does limbal SCC

MISCELLANEOUS

ASSOCIATED CONDITIONS

Precancerous changes include actinic keratosis, solar elastosis, and epithelial dysplasia.

SEE ALSO

Periocular sarcoid

ABBREVIATIONS

• CT = computed tomography
• MRI = magnetic resonance imaging
• NSAID = nonsteroidal anti-inflammatory drug
• PDT = photodynamic therapy
• SCC = squamous cell carcinoma
• UV = ultraviolet

Suggested Reading
Brooks DE. Ophthalmology for the Equine Practitioner, 2e. Jackson, WY: Teton NewMedia, 2008.
Brooks DE, Matthews AG. Equine ophthalmology. In: Gelatt KN, ed. Veterinary Ophthalmology, 4e. Ames, IA: Blackwell, 2007:1165–1274.
Gilger BC, ed. Equine Ophthalmology, 3e. Ames, IA: Wiley Blackwell, 2017.

Author Caryn E. Plummer
Consulting Editor Caryn E. Plummer

BASICS

OVERVIEW

• Appropriate restraint, sedation, and local nerve blocks can greatly facilitate a detailed examination. A good focal light source, such as a Finoff transilluminator and a direct ophthalmoscope, are necessary
• Prior to sedation and nerve blocks, the examiner should stand in front of the horse to assess symmetry and to compare size, shape, and position of the globes, eyelids, and pupils. Pupil size and symmetry is best assessed in dim light using the tapetal reflection. Comfort can be assessed by comparing the angle of the upper eyelashes. Normally, the upper eyelashes are nearly perpendicular to the cornea. Lashes pointing downwards can be indicative of pain or abnormal globe or eyelid position
• Cranial nerve assessment should be performed on both eyes. The menace response is assessed by making a quick, threatening motion toward the eye to elicit a blink response and/or movement of the head. Care is taken not to create air currents toward the eye. The pupillary light reflex (direct and indirect) is assessed by shining a bright light into the eye. The normal equine pupil responds somewhat sluggishly and incompletely unless the stimulating light is particularly bright. The dazzle reflex consists of shining a bright light into the eye and watching for a quick blink response, and is useful in evaluating the potential for vision when the cornea is opaque. The palpebral reflex is tested by touching the medial or lateral canthus, and observing a blink response
• Vision can be further assessed with maze testing, with blinkers alternatively covering each eye
• The position, margins, and surfaces of the eyelids and nictitans should be examined. Nasolacrimal duct patency can be assessed by visualizing fluorescein dye pass from the eye to the distal puncta in the nares (positive Jones test). Patency can also be determined with normograde irrigation, using a lacrimal cannula in the upper puncta, or retrograde irrigation through the distal puncta using a catheter

• The anterior segment should be examined using a light source. A slit or other focused beam held at a 45° angle can be used to identify the location of lesions within the cornea or to identify flare in the aqueous humor. The cornea should be clear, smooth, and shiny. Applying fluorescein dye to the cornea should be routine in every equine eye examination. Small corneal ulcers will stain that might otherwise be undetected. Rose bengal can be used to evaluate tear film integrity. Cultures and cytology can also aid in the diagnosis of corneal disease. Normal Schirmer tear test value in horses is 22 ± 6 mm wetting/min
• In most horses, there is a gray line at the medial and lateral limbus, which represents the insertion of the pectinate ligaments into the posterior cornea. This area should have open spaces between the ligaments, which allow aqueous outflow to the iridocorneal angle
• IOP is measured in horses using applanation tonometry after the application of topical anesthetic or rebound tonometry. Normal equine IOP is 23.3 ± 6.9 mmHg. The horse's head should be held above its heart to avoid falsely elevated measurements
• Pupillary dilation is necessary to examine the lens and posterior segment in detail. Tropicamide 1% will facilitate mydriasis. Dilation takes 15–20 min in a normal horse, and lasts for 4–6 h. The lens and vitreous are evaluated using a light source held at a 45° angle to the eye. Retroillumination is also used to highlight lenticular opacities, using light that is reflected off the tapetum
• The fundus can be examined using a direct ophthalmoscope, or using indirect ophthalmoscopy. With indirect ophthalmoscopy, the examiner stands arm's distance away from the horse holding the light near his/her own eye. Once a tapetal reflection is visualized, the lens is held in front of the patient's eye to examine the retina and optic nerve. This technique provides a wider field of view to examine the fundus; note that the image achieved is reversed and inverted
• Systems affected—ophthalmic

DIAGNOSIS

IMAGING
Electroretinogram, ultrasound (B-scan).

OTHER DIAGNOSTIC PROCEDURES
• Fluorescein/rose bengal stain
• Schirmer tear test
• Cytology/culture
• Tonometry

MEDICATIONS

DRUG(S) OF CHOICE
• Tropicamide 1% for mydriasis.
• Topical anesthetic for applanation tonometry, cytology

MISCELLANEOUS

SEE ALSO
All other ocular topics.

ABBREVIATIONS
IOP = intraocular pressure

Suggested Reading
Brooks DE. Ophthalmology for the Equine Practitioner, 2e. Jackson, WY: Teton NewMedia, 2008.
Gilger BC. Equine ophthalmology. In: Gelatt KN, Gilger BC, Kern TJ, eds. Veterinary Ophthalmology, 5e. Ames, IA: Wiley Blackwell, 2013:1560–1609.
Gilger BC, ed. Equine Ophthalmology, 3e. Ames, IA: Wiley Blackwell, 2017.

Author Shari M. Greenberg
Consulting Editor Caryn E. Plummer
Acknowledgment The author and editor acknowledge the prior contribution of Maria Källberg and Dennis E. Brooks.

O

OCULAR PROBLEMS IN THE NEONATE

 BASICS

DEFINITION
The equine neonatal eye has many features of immaturity that over time resolve to yield a healthy adult eye. A newborn foal may exhibit lagophthalmos, low tear production, a rounded pupil, reduced corneal sensitivity, lack of a menace response for several weeks, a gray coloration to the iris, hyaloid artery remnants possibly containing blood for hours after birth, prominent lens Y sutures, and a round optic disc with smooth margins. Additionally, neonates commonly have mild ventronasal strabismus that resolves with age.

PATHOPHYSIOLOGY
Congenital, developmental, inherited, and acquired diseases have been identified.

SYSTEMS AFFECTED
- Ophthalmic
- Others, if ocular disease is a manifestation of systemic disease

GENETICS
- Appaloosas, Paso Finos—congenital stationary night blindness (autosomal recessive)
- Morgan horses, Thoroughbreds—congenital nuclear cataracts (autosomal dominant)
- Rocky Mountain horses, miniature horses, Mountain Pleasure horses, and Kentucky Saddle horses—multiple congenital ocular anomalies syndrome (semidominant)
- Belgian draft horse, Thoroughbred, Quarter Horse—aniridia or iris hypoplasia with cataract ± dermoid (suspect autosomal dominant)
- Quarter Horses—suspected to have a form of inherited optic nerve coloboma

INCIDENCE/PREVALENCE
- Microphthalmos—incidence of 7–14.7%
- Esotropia in mules—incidence of 0.5%

SIGNALMENT
Equine neonates.

Breed Predilections
- See Genetics
- Microphthalmos with cataract and entropion is more common in Thoroughbreds
- Superficial, irregular corneal epithelial opacities may be found in the eye(s) of Thoroughbred foals. These do not appear painful and resolve with age
- Congenital glaucoma is seen with more frequency in Thoroughbreds and Standardbreds

SIGNS
Dependent on the condition. Ocular discomfort (e.g. blepharospasm, epiphora) and abnormal vision are often observed.

Historical Findings
- The neonatal foal may have serious, life-threatening problems and can concurrently develop traumatic or inflammatory (peri)ocular disease
- Alternatively, the neonate may not be adjusting well, gazing off into space with little physical activity, or may be easily startled with reluctance to move. NMS should be a consideration
- The owner or trainer may notice an abnormal appearance to 1 or both eyes with or without visual or behavioral problems

Physical Examination Findings
- It is helpful to have people present to handle the mare and assist with restraint of the foal. Sedating a fractious foal can facilitate examination
- See chapter Ocular examination for a detailed description of the ophthalmic examination process

CAUSES
- Corneal ulcers
  - Trauma
  - Entropion
  - Lagophthalmos
  - Distichia or ectopic cilia (rare)
- Uveitis
  - Ulcerative keratitis
  - Sepsis, from immune-mediated causes or from *Rhodococcus equi, Escherichia coli, Streptococcus equi* ssp. *equi, Actinobacillus equuli,* adenovirus, and EVA
- Conjunctivitis and subconjunctival hemorrhage
  - Environmental irritants
  - Secondary to pneumonia caused by adenovirus, equine herpesvirus 1, EVA, influenza virus, *S. equi* ssp. *equi, R. equi,* and *Actinobacillus* spp.
  - Trauma during birth
  - NMS
- Glaucoma
  - Goniodysgenesis
  - Trauma
- Microphthalmos
  - Congenital
- Strabismus
  - Congenital
  - Post trauma
- Blepharitis
  - Fly strike
  - Dermatophytosis
  - *Dermatophilus*
  - Staphylococcal folliculitis
  - Trauma
- Entropion
  - Microphthalmia
  - Dehydration
  - Malnutrition
  - Prematurity/dysmaturity
  - Eyelid trauma
  - Cicatrices
- Dermoids
  - Congenital
- Nasolacrimal system atresia
  - Congenital
- Dacryocystitis
  - Nasolacrimal system atresia
  - Systemic illness
- Aniridia, iridal hypoplasia, enlarged corpora nigra, iridal colobomata
  - Congenital
- Persistent pupillary membranes
  - Congenital
- Lens luxation
  - Congenital
  - Post trauma
- Cataracts
  - Congenital
  - Uveitis
  - Penetrating trauma
- Retinal dysplasia
  - In utero inflammation
- Retinal hemorrhage
  - Birthing trauma
- Retinal detachments
  - Congenital
  - Inflammatory
  - Traumatic
- Chorioretinitis
  - Possibly maternal systemic disease
- Optic nerve head colobomas
  - Congenital
- Optic nerve hypoplasia and optic nerve atrophy
  - Congenital/developmental
  - Inflammation in utero

RISK FACTORS
- "Downer" foals may develop entropion, blepharitis, conjunctivitis, and corneal ulcers
- Risk factors include malnourishment, sepsis, contact with soiled shavings, and pressure and friction placed on the eyes/eyelids from recumbency
- Protection of the eyes in these neonates (padding, eye lubricant) is critical

 DIAGNOSIS

DIFFERENTIAL DIAGNOSIS
N/A

CBC/BIOCHEMISTRY/URINALYSIS
Usually normal in primary eye disorders.

OTHER LABORATORY TESTS
Cytology and microbial (bacterial and fungal) culture of infected tissue, especially melting corneas or purulent ocular or nasolacrimal discharge.

IMAGING
Dacryocystorhinography to identify nasolacrimal system atresia.

OTHER DIAGNOSTIC PROCEDURES
- Complete ophthalmic examination
- Fluorescein stain, corneal culture and cytology, and Schirmer tear test
- Topical anesthesia should be applied before corneal cytology is obtained
- Diagnostic tests for cataract surgery candidates include ocular ultrasonography, electroretinography, and chest radiographs

PATHOLOGIC FINDINGS
Septic ulcerative keratitis will yield a suppurative inflammation with or without bacterial or fungal organisms.

TREATMENT

APPROPRIATE HEALTH CARE
• Aggressive therapy is necessary to preserve vision and eliminate pain in cases of severe uveitis and corneal ulceration. Initially hourly or bihourly instillation of medication is required; subpalpebral lavage placement facilitates this. Lavage placement in the lower fornix is beneficial in nursing foals. These eyes need to be examined several times daily until the clinical signs improve
• Most other types of neonatal problems can be managed on an outpatient basis

NURSING CARE
• A "downer" foal with eye disease needs appropriate medical management, and may benefit from a protective eye hood and artificial tear ophthalmic ointment applied 4–6 times daily
• All hospitalized foals should be monitored daily for corneal ulceration

ACTIVITY
In general, activity is restricted until the ocular lesions are healed.

DIET
Good nutrition is essential for growth, wound healing, and recuperation.

CLIENT EDUCATION
• Depending on the severity of disease, hospitalization may be necessary to initiate aggressive therapy. Treatment can be over days to weeks, and surgery may be necessary to preserve vision
• Neonatal anesthesia of a sick foal is a high-risk event and must be weighed heavily against the benefits of surgery, especially if the newborn is debilitated
• Genetic information should be shared with clients as necessary

SURGICAL CONSIDERATIONS
• General anesthesia in the neonate is not without risk
• Conjunctival or amniotic membrane grafting is a common surgery to aid in the healing of severe corneal ulcers
• Magnification and proper ophthalmic instrumentation is essential to a successful outcome
• Corneal scarring is a sequela to surgery but may diminish as the foal matures
• Entropion is corrected by placing temporary vertical mattress sutures in the skin, 2–3 mm from the edge of the eyelid margin. These sutures remain in place until the cause of the entropion is gone. Hotz–Celsus procedures

should *not* be done on neonatal eyelids; the foal usually outgrows neonatal entropion
• Cataract surgery (phacofragmentation) is performed in foals if no other ocular pathology (e.g. retinal detachment) is discovered during the diagnostic workup
• Glaucoma can be surgically treated with valve implants or laser surgery when refractive to medical therapy
• Eyelid lacerations should be corrected with maximal preservation of eyelid tissue. A 2-layer closure of skin–orbicularis muscle and tarsal–conjunctival layers is recommended
• Keratectomy or blepharoplasty is indicated in the diagnosis and treatment of dermoids
• Restoration of atretic nasal or palpebral puncta is done by cannulating and flushing the duct through 1 opening, and, after creating a new opening at the other end, leaving the polyethylene or silicone tubing in the duct for several weeks to allow epithelialization of the new puncta and resolution of dacryocystitis
• Anterior lens luxation requires lens removal to prevent secondary glaucoma
• Persistent corneal ulcers in foals may need repeated debridement with topical anesthesia and a sterile cotton swab in addition to medical therapy

MEDICATIONS

DRUG(S) OF CHOICE
• Drugs for ulcerative keratitis, uveitis, and glaucoma have been thoroughly outlined in other chapters
• Intracameral tissue plasminogen activator may be useful in dissolving fibrin clots that develop in the anterior chamber with uveitis

CONTRAINDICATIONS
Topical steroids must *not* be used on eyes with ulcerative keratitis.

PRECAUTIONS
• Foals on topical atropine should be carefully watched for signs of colic
• Topical corticosteroids to reduce scarring on a cornea with prior infectious ulcerative keratitis may cause a relapse of the infection

POSSIBLE INTERACTIONS
N/A

ALTERNATIVE DRUGS
N/A

FOLLOW-UP

PATIENT MONITORING
• Rechecks are advised until the eye shows no sign of active disease. If infection or inflammation recurs, a thorough workup is recommended

• Disease recurrence may also be due to failure to correct the underlying cause (e.g. entropion-induced ulcers)

PREVENTION/AVOIDANCE
• A clean, well-ventilated stall will help prevent infectious or traumatic ocular problems
• Some congenital lesions such as retinal dysplasia may be less likely if the mare maintains good health during pregnancy

POSSIBLE COMPLICATIONS
Many ocular conditions can impair vision, even when successfully treated.

EXPECTED COURSE AND PROGNOSIS
• Most vision-threatening problems in the neonate can be successfully managed if treated accurately and promptly
• Aphakic foals who had cataracts removed will adjust to their environment but will remain permanently hyperopic
• Even with complete recovery from an inflammatory disease in the eye, the owner needs to be observant for and report any recurrence of ocular pain

MISCELLANEOUS

ASSOCIATED CONDITIONS
• Sepsis
• Pneumonia

AGE-RELATED FACTORS
N/A

SYNONYMS
N/A

SEE ALSO
• Chorioretinitis
• Equine recurrent uveitis
• Eyelid diseases
• Glaucoma
• Orbital disease
• Ulcerative keratomycosis

ABBREVIATIONS
• EVA = equine viral arteritis
• NMS = neonatal maladjustment syndrome

Suggested Reading
Brooks DE. Ophthalmology for the Equine Practitioner, 2e. Jackson, WY: Teton NewMedia, 2008.
Gilger BC. Equine ophthalmology. In: Gelatt KN, Gilger BC, Kern TJ, eds. Veterinary Ophthalmology, 5e. Ames, IA: Wiley Blackwell, 2013:1560–1609.
Gilger BC, ed. Equine Ophthalmology, 3e. Ames, IA: Wiley Blackwell, 2017.

Author Shari M. Greenberg
Consulting Editor Caryn E. Plummer
Acknowledgment The author and editor acknowledge the prior contribution of Dennis E. Brooks.

O

OMPHALOPHLEBITIS

 BASICS

OVERVIEW
• Omphalophlebitis, or "navel ill," is an infection of 1 or more of the umbilical structures. Omphalophlebitis technically refers to infection of the umbilical vein, and omphalitis refers to infection of any of the umbilical structures. The structures that comprise the umbilicus—the umbilical vein, umbilical arteries, and urachus—can become infected alone or in combination, with the urachus most commonly affected. Infection of the umbilicus can occur secondary to ascending bacterial invasion from open umbilical structures or from hematogenous seeding in a septicemic foal
• The normal umbilicus should not be patent beyond 24 h and should become dry and involute by 3–7 days. The umbilicus should be essentially nonexistent by 3–4 weeks of age. The bacteria most commonly associated with septic omphalophlebitis are similar to those associated with neonatal septicemia, such as β-hemolytic streptococci, *Escherichia coli*, and *Actinobacillus* sp.

SIGNALMENT
• Most commonly seen in neonatal foals, usually several days of age, although umbilical abscesses have been reported in older foals and horses (reported up to 16 months of age)
• No breed or sex predisposition

SIGNS
• External abnormalities are seen in approximately 50% of cases
• Swollen, warm, and painful umbilicus
• Ventral edema may be present in more chronic cases
• Purulent discharge may be seen, and urine may leak due to presence of a patent urachus
• Deeper palpation may reveal thickened umbilical arteries and/or vein
• Fever, lethargy, and poor nursing are often recognized first. Secondary complications such as septicemia, septic arthritis, septic physitis, and pneumonia may be the most obvious clinical signs—the umbilicus should be carefully examined in these cases

CAUSES AND RISK FACTORS
• FTPI
• Poor hygiene in the foaling environment
• Septicemia
• Contamination of the umbilical remnant or improper care of the umbilicus

 DIAGNOSIS

DIFFERENTIAL DIAGNOSIS
• Patent urachus—this may occur secondary to omphalophlebitis especially if it is an acquired patent urachus; can occur as a primary congenital condition in the absence of omphalophlebitis—history and US examination can help to differentiate
• Umbilical hernia—an uncomplicated hernia should not have palpable heat, drainage, or enlargement of external or internal umbilical remnant structures. Foals with uncomplicated hernias generally do not have signs of systemic illness such as fever or lethargy

CBC/BIOCHEMISTRY/URINALYSIS
• An increase in WBC count and fibrinogen is commonly seen
• If the urachus is involved, urinalysis may reveal WBCs and bacteria

OTHER LABORATORY TESTS
• IgG should be evaluated, as FTPI is a common risk factor for omphalophlebitis
• SAA may increase with omphalophlebitis

IMAGING
US
• US of umbilical remnants using a 7.5 MHz probe—the urachus, umbilical arteries, umbilical vein, and bladder should be evaluated. The examination can be performed with the foal standing or restrained in lateral recumbency. Saturate the hair with alcohol and use US coupling gel. Clipping is not necessary but will improve image quality
• Normal umbilical vein should measure <1 cm in diameter, and normal umbilical arteries should measure <1.3 cm. The combined umbilical arteries and urachus should measure <2.5 cm at the apex of the bladder
• Affected structures will generally be enlarged with a fluid-filled core, and often with gas shadowing

Abdominal Radiography
Positive-contrast radiographs of the urinary tract (retrograde via the urethra) can help to identify any urachal tears that may be present secondary to umbilical sepsis.

OTHER DIAGNOSTIC PROCEDURES
• Blood cultures in neonatal foals to confirm septicemia and guide antimicrobial therapy
• Culture of umbilical stump to guide antimicrobial therapy
• Additional imaging may be required to assess for pneumonia, enteritis, and septic physitis

 TREATMENT

• Surgical resection of umbilical remnants—indicated if there is not adequate response to medical treatment, the umbilicus is severely enlarged and unlikely to respond quickly to medical therapy, or there is leakage of urine from the urachus. Surgical marsupialization of the umbilical vein remnant has been reported in cases where complete resection of the infected remnant was not possible
• Nursing care—the foal should be supported systemically if there is concurrent septicemia, inappetence, or dehydration. Septicemic foals should be hospitalized and may require emergency medical care

 MEDICATIONS

DRUG(S) OF CHOICE
• Systemic antimicrobials—broad-spectrum antibiotics should be continued as required for resolution of the infection, often for at least 2 weeks. The choice of antimicrobials will be guided by culture results, but a common initial choice is a penicillin (22 000 IU/kg IV QID) and an aminoglycoside (amikacin 25 mg/kg IV every 24 h). If long-term antimicrobials are needed, the choice of an oral antimicrobial may be guided by culture results, and the foal should be monitored closely to ensure that there is not a recurrence of infection
• NSAIDs—as needed for treatment of umbilical inflammation, fever, and discomfort or postoperatively to reduce the risk of adhesion formation and to reduce incisional discomfort. Flunixin meglumine (0.25–1.1 mg/kg IV BID) or ketoprofen (0.5–1.1 mg/kg IV BID)

CONTRAINDICATIONS/POSSIBLE INTERACTIONS
• Aminoglycosides should be used with caution in dehydrated foals or foals with renal compromise. Alternatively, a cephalosporin such as ceftiofur (10 mg/kg IV QID) may be used
• Gastroduodenal ulcer prophylaxis may be needed when NSAIDs are used. NSAIDs should be used with caution in neonates and dehydrated foals of any age

FOLLOW-UP

PATIENT MONITORING
• Foals should be monitored closely with palpation and serial US examinations for response to therapy
• Twice-daily physical examinations should be performed to monitor for septic arthritis, septic physitis, and other possible complications
• Follow-up blood work should reveal a decrease in fibrinogen/SAA and normalization of the leukogram

PREVENTION/AVOIDANCE
• Provide good hygiene in the foaling environment
• Ensure adequate transfer of passive immunity—check IgG and administer plasma if IgG < 800 mg/dL
• Dipping of the umbilical stump with dilute chlorhexidine (0.5%) or dilute povidone–iodine (1.0%) may help to prevent ascending infection

POSSIBLE COMPLICATIONS
• Primary or secondary septicemia can occur in association with omphalophlebitis, with septic arthritis being the most common complication
• Septic physitis, osteomyelitis, and pneumonia may also occur in combination with omphalophlebitis
• Acquired patent urachus is a possible sequela
• Infection of the urachus can lead to necrosis and possible uroabdomen and/or subcutaneous leakage of urine
• Extension of venous abscess to the liver

EXPECTED COURSE AND PROGNOSIS
• Foals with small, focal umbilical remnant infections usually respond to medical therapy. In foals with more extensive infection of the umbilical structures, surgical resection of the umbilical remnants appears to improve survival due to the reduced incidence of secondary infections
• The presence of infected joints worsens the prognosis

MISCELLANEOUS

ASSOCIATED CONDITIONS
• Patent urachus
• Septicemia
• Septic arthritis

AGE-RELATED FACTORS
Umbilical remnant infection is most commonly a condition of neonatal foals, and this population should also be evaluated critically for signs of generalized septicemia or other foci of infection.

ZOONOTIC POTENTIAL
N/A

PREGNANCY/FERTILITY/BREEDING
N/A

SEE ALSO
• Septic arthritis, neonate
• Septicemia, neonate

ABBREVIATIONS
• FTPI = failure of transfer of passive immunity
• IgG = immunoglobulin G
• NSAID = nonsteroidal anti-inflammatory drug
• SAA = serum amyloid A
• US = ultrasonography, ultrasound
• WBC = white blood cell

Suggested Reading
Adams SB, Fessler JF. Umbilical cord remnant infections in foals: 16 cases (1975–1985). J Am Vet Med Assoc 1987;190:316–318.
Edwards RB, Fubini SL. A one-stage marsupialization procedure for management of infected umbilical vein remnants in calves and foals. Vet Surg 1995;24:32–35.
Reef VB, Collatos CA. Ultrasonography of umbilical structures in clinically normal foals. Am J Vet Res 1988;49:2143–2146.
Reef VB, Collatos CA, Spencer PA, et al. Clinical, ultrasonographic and surgical findings in foals with umbilical remnant infections. J Am Vet Med Assoc 1989;195:69–72.
Smith M. Management of umbilical disorders in the foal. In Pract 2006;28:280–287.

Author Margaret C. Mudge
Consulting Editor Margaret C. Mudge

O

OPTIC NERVE ATROPHY

 BASICS

OVERVIEW
Atrophy of the optic nerve due to inflammatory or noninflammatory causes. In the early stages, the ophthalmoscopic appearance of the optic nerve head may be normal although the eye is blind. With time, the optic disc becomes pale with profound vascular attenuation and an obvious granularity of the optic disc due to exposure of the scleral lamina cribrosa.

Systems Affected
Ophthalmic

SIGNALMENT
N/A

SIGNS
Common signs regardless of the cause:
• Blindness and pupil dilatation of the affected eye
• Optic nerve pallor
• Visualization of the lamina cribrosa
• Peripapillary vascular attenuation

CAUSES AND RISK FACTORS
• Inflammatory—optic neuritis, equine recurrent uveitis, chorioretinitis, sphenopalatine sinusitis
• Noninflammatory—trauma to head and orbit, glaucoma, toxins, pituitary neoplasia, retrobulbar neoplasia, compression, acute blood loss

 DIAGNOSIS

DIFFERENTIAL DIAGNOSIS
• Optic nerve hypoplasia
• Orbital trauma
• Retinal detachment
• Glaucoma
• Cataract

CBC/BIOCHEMISTRY/URINALYSIS
N/A

OTHER LABORATORY TESTS
N/A

IMAGING
Ocular ultrasonography, MRI, or CT scan may be of value in cases of head trauma, neoplasia, and sinusitis.

OTHER DIAGNOSTIC PROCEDURES
Electroretinogram

 TREATMENT

There is no therapy for this condition; however, treatment of the underlying cause is recommended, if possible.

 MEDICATIONS

N/A

 FOLLOW-UP

EXPECTED COURSE AND PROGNOSIS
Poor prognosis for vision.

 MISCELLANEOUS

ASSOCIATED CONDITIONS
See Causes and Risk Factors.

SEE ALSO
• Glaucoma
• Ischemic optic neuropathy

ABBREVIATIONS
• CT = computed tomography
• MRI = magnetic resonance imaging

Suggested Reading
Brooks DE. Retinopathies and ocular manifestations of systemic diseases in the horse. In: Brooks DE, ed. Ophthalmology for the Equine Practitioner, 2e. Jackson, WY: Teton NewMedia, 2008:207–225.
Gilger BC. Equine ophthalmology. In: Gelatt KN, Gilger BC, Kern TJ, eds. Veterinary Ophthalmology, 5e. Ames, IA: Wiley Blackwell, 2013:1560–1609.
Nell B, Walde I. Posterior segment diseases. Equine Vet J Suppl 2010;37:69–79.
Wilkie DA. Diseases of the ocular posterior segment. In: Gilger BC, ed. Equine Ophthalmology, 2e. Maryland Heights, MO: Elsevier Saunders, 2011:367–396.

Author Bianca C. Martins
Consulting Editor Caryn E. Plummer
Acknowledgment The author and editor acknowledge the prior contribution of Maria Källberg and Dennis E. Brooks.

O

BASICS

DEFINITION
Neoplasms of the oral cavity may originate from dental tissue (odontogenic), bone (osteogenic), and soft tissue (gums, tongue, lips, and oropharynx) and may extend into adjacent tissues.

Odontogenic
Odontogenesis begins with the ingrowth of oral ectoderm into the mesenchyme of the jaw.
• Tumors of odontogenic epithelium without odontogenic mesenchyme
  ○ Ameloblastoma (adamantinoma)—benign but locally invasive. More common in lower jaw and often interosseal, distorting the mandible
  ○ Keratinizing ameloblastoma—with an increased tendency toward keratin expression
• Tumors of odontogenic epithelium with odontogenic mesenchyme
  ○ Ameloblastic odontoma (odontoameloblastoma)—benign, slowly expanding, and locally invasive
• Complex odontoma—contains all the elements of a normal tooth but structure is disorganized
  ○ Compound odontoma—contains all the elements of a normal tooth. Forms a tooth-like structure—denticles. Often regarded as a malformation
• Tumors composed primarily of odontogenic ectomesenchyme
  ○ Cementoma—dense, mineralized structure
  ○ Cementifying fibroma—analogous to ossifying fibroma but the components have lines of cementum

Osteogenic
Osteogenic tumors are usually benign and have a predilection for the mandibular symphysis.
• Osteomas
• Osteosarcomas
• Fibro-osteoma
• Ossifying fibromas

Soft Tissue Neoplasia
• Hemangiosarcoma
• SCC—tongue, gingiva, pharynx, and hard palate
• Lymphosarcoma—horse palate
• Fibrosarcoma—tongue
• Myosarcoma
• Melanomas
• Adenomas

PATHOPHYSIOLOGY
N/A

SYSTEMS AFFECTED
The neoplasms affect most commonly the digestive system but may also invade the respiratory tract.

GENETICS
N/A

INCIDENCE/PREVALENCE
Neoplasia of the oral cavity or pharynx is uncommon. In 1 study of 141 cases with SCC, only 5% involved the oral or pharyngeal mucosa.

SIGNALMENT
• The age of the horse may suggest the type of neoplasm. There is a high incidence of ameloblastic odontomas in young animals (6 weeks to 1 year of age). Ameloblastomas occur in older horses whereas osteogenic neoplasms have no age predilection
• Horses with osteogenic tumors of the intramembranous bone of the head are young. SCC, which is by far the most common type of soft tissue tumor, occurs in older horses
• No breed or sex susceptibility has been suggested for any of the neoplasms

SIGNS

Historical Findings
• The clinical signs are dependent on the location and size of the neoplasm and may include dysphagia, difficulty in prehension or mastication, halitosis, oral discharge/hemosalivation, and submandibular lymphadenopathy. Nasal discharge may be evident if the tumor has invaded the nasal chamber or paranasal sinuses. Weight loss, recurrent fever, and depression may be observed
• Neoplasms in the oral region are usually well advanced with extensive local infiltration before clinical signs appear

Physical Examination Findings
• Odontogenic neoplasms present as slowly growing, firm, immobile swellings of the mandible or maxilla
• The most common presentation of osteogenic tumors is unilateral proliferation of bony tissue on the rostral mandible; they rarely develop in the maxilla. The syndrome is classified as equine juvenile mandibular ossifying fibroma, usually presenting as a rapidly growing subgingival mass of the rostral mandible or, much less commonly, the premaxilla. The proliferation can be symmetric or may only involve the rostral aspect of 1 hemimandible. On palpation, the teeth may be loose but the mass is usually nonpainful. Prehension and mastication are initially unaltered
• The typical appearance of SCC of the oral cavity is a partially ulcerated multilobular mass projecting from the mucosa. The tumor is slow growing and locally invasive into the nasal cavity and paranasal sinuses and metastasis can occur. Displacement and loosening of the teeth are present
• Although lesions of the rostral mandible are readily identified, those affecting the more caudal part of the oral cavity and pharynx require a more detailed examination. Sedation and the use of a Haussmann gag and

headlamp or pen flashlight allow visualization of the tumor or palpation and a biopsy to be taken in many cases. The regional lymph nodes should be examined.

CAUSES
N/A

RISK FACTORS
N/A

DIAGNOSIS

The definitive diagnosis depends on histologic examination of the biopsy or at necropsy.

DIFFERENTIAL DIAGNOSIS
• Swellings of the mandible or maxilla due to underlying dental disease, especially periapical abscessation
• Foreign bodies in the oropharynx causing dysphagia and halitosis

CBC/BIOCHEMISTRY/URINALYSIS
N/A

OTHER LABORATORY TESTS
N/A

IMAGING
• Radiography is of value to evaluate the nature and extent of the neoplasm and in differentiating it from a dental problem
• Ameloblastomas appear as radiolucent multiloculated masses often well marginated by thick, sclerotic bone with cortical expansion on the lingual and buccal surfaces
• Ameloblastic odontomas are radiopaque masses that may appear to fill the maxillary sinus, often obstructing the nasal passage of the affected side
• Radiographs of osteogenic tumors are characterized by a smooth, bony proliferation of the rostral mandible with or without osteolytic changes involving the roots of the teeth
• Horses with hard palate SCC show dental displacement and loss of alveolar bone. Extension into the paranasal sinuses results in loss of the normal radiolucent appearance. Radiographs of the pharynx may show its dorsal wall to be deformed and thickened, particularly when affected by lymphosarcoma
• Endoscopy is of value in determining the extent of palatine and nasal involvement. Oral endoscopy carried out under general anesthesia allows a more thorough examination

OTHER DIAGNOSTIC PROCEDURES
Biopsy
• Biopsies of masses involving the mandible or maxilla enable differentiation between odontogenic and osteogenic tumors
• Biopsy of SCC of the mouth can be obtained without difficulty by breaking off a piece of the proliferative tissue, whereas biopsies of pharyngeal or palatine tissues may be accomplished with a biopsy instrument

ORAL NEOPLASIA   (CONTINUED)

through an endoscope or using uterine biopsy forceps under general anesthesia. If lymph node enlargement is present, a fine needle aspirate or surgical biopsy is necessary to determine if metastasis has occurred

PATHOLOGIC FINDINGS

Histology

• Ameloblastomas contain odontogenic islands set in well-vascularized connective tissue. The periphery of the follicle is composed of a layer of columnar cells with distinct polarization of nuclei away from the basement membrane, resembling ameloblasts. Toward the center of the follicles the cells form a loose network similar to the stellate reticulum of the developing tooth
• Ameloblastic odontomas differ from ameloblastomas in that the islands of epithelium are smaller, the formation of cysts is less frequent, and the stellate reticulum is less extensive
• It should be noted, however, that these tumor classifications are subjective, and because of their rarity and difficulties in their histologic recognition, a degree of nomenclature inconsistency exists
• Histologic diagnosis of oral and pharyngeal neoplasms is much less challenging

TREATMENT

• Neoplasms of the mouth and pharynx, such as SCC and lymphosarcoma, are usually too advanced when diagnosed. Several therapies have been tried in SCC and include surgical removal, radiotherapy (gamma radiation), and chemotherapy
• In melanoma, radiotherapy and chemotherapy have been attempted but with limited success
• There have been several reports of attempted surgical removal of odontogenic and osteogenic tumors of the mandible and maxilla. The ease of surgical debridement is dependent on the size and location of the tumor. Surgical excision and curettage are often followed by recurrence. Because the growth of ameloblastic odontomas is by expansion rather than infiltration, theoretically they may represent a better prognosis than ameloblastomas. Radical tumor resection in conjunction with partial

mandibulectomy and stabilization of the resulting defect with internal or external orthopedic devices has met with greater success. Recurrence is more common when the neoplasm is in the maxilla. Cryosurgery has been used as an adjunct therapy. This has the advantage of destroying neoplastic cells at the surgical margins without removing additional bone. The amount of dead space is decreased, and scaffolding is provided for new bone development
• Many neoplasms of the oral cavity and oropharynx are advanced before detection; consequently, surgical removal often leads to poor success rates. Confirmation of malignancy by histologic examination in an extensive lesion may warrant euthanasia
• The use of laser surgery had been advocated for the ablation of certain soft tissue neoplasms of the oropharynx or nasopharynx, but success is largely dependent on early tumor recognition

NURSING CARE, ACTIVITY, DIET

• Horses that have undergone radical surgical excision, including mandibulectomy, may have difficulty prehending short grass
• Cosmetically, the postoperative appearance of the horses is acceptable, even though all horses will have some flaccidity of the lower lip
• Horses with a mandibulectomy have been able to return to their intended use

MEDICATIONS

CONTRAINDICATIONS
N/A

PRECAUTIONS
N/A

POSSIBLE INTERACTIONS
N/A

ALTERNATIVE DRUGS
N/A

FOLLOW-UP

PATIENT MONITORING
N/A

PREVENTION/AVOIDANCE
N/A

POSSIBLE COMPLICATIONS
N/A

EXPECTED COURSE AND PROGNOSIS
Successful treatment depends on complete removal/destruction of the neoplasm.

MISCELLANEOUS

ASSOCIATED CONDITIONS
N/A

AGE-RELATED FACTORS
N/A

ZOONOTIC POTENTIAL
N/A

PREGNANCY/FERTILITY/BREEDING
N/A

ABBREVIATIONS
SCC = squamous cell carcinoma

Suggested Reading
Head KW, Else RW, Dubielzig RR. Tumors of the alimentary tract. In: Meuten DJ, ed. Tumors in Domestic Animals, 4e. Ames, IA: Iowa State Press, 2002:401–481.
Knottembelt DC, Patterson-Kane JC, Snalune JC. Clinical Equine Oncology. Edinburgh, UK: Elsevier, 2015:429–479.
Pirie RC, Tremaine WH. Neoplasia of the mouth and surrounding structure. In: Robinson NE, ed. Current Therapy in Equine Medicine, 4e. Philadelphia, PA: WB Saunders, 1997:153–155.
Priester WA, Mantel N. Occurrence of tumors in domestic animals. Data from 12 United States and Canadian Veterinary Colleges. J Natl Cancer Inst 1971;47:1333–1345.
Richardson DW, Evans LH, Tulleners EP. Rostral mandibulectomy in five horses. J Am Vet Med Assoc 1991;174:734.

Author Olimpo Oliver-Espinosa
Consulting Editors Henry Stämpfli and Olimpo Oliver-Espinosa

ORAL STEREOTYPIC BEHAVIOR

BASICS

DEFINITION
• Repetitive, apparently functionless behavior that may be considered to be compulsive
• The predominant oral stereotypy is cribbing (grasping a horizontal surface with the incisors, flexing the neck, and making a grunting sound)

PATHOPHYSIOLOGY
• Cribbing is the only stereotypy in which the pathophysiologic mechanism has been elucidated with endoscopy and fluoroscopy. Air is usually not completely swallowed, but stays in the upper esophagus causing transient dilation. The grunting noise is produced when air rushes through the cricopharynx. Contraction of the ventral neck muscles produces negative pressure in the esophagus that allows air to move in; the air then is expelled from the pharynx rostrally, with only a small amount passing into the lower esophagus
• Endogenous opiates may be involved, because administration of an opiate blocker inhibits cribbing for several hours. Cribbing does not cause release of endogenous opiates and measurement of opiates in cribbers in comparison with noncribbers has yielded contradictory results, but opiates are necessary for cribbing to occur
• Young horses that crib have more severe gastric ulcers that those that do not crib; therefore cribbing may cause ulcers due to vagally stimulated gastric acid secretion resulting from either the chewing movements or stimulation of the lips and mouth

SYSTEMS AFFECTED
GI, Neurologic, and Musculoskeletal
• Behavioral cribbing is repetitive, apparently functionless behavior involving the head. Some horses exhibit gas colic and a few suffer from epiploic foramen entrapment. Tooth grinding can lead to wear of the molars. Wear of the upper incisors is another outcome of cribbing, as is temporomandibular arthropathy
• Affected horses may have an increased incidence of colic, and possibly an increased risk of developing an entrapment of the small intestine in the epiploic foramen
• A greater percentage of horses with neurologic problems such as equine motor neuron disease seems to be affected
• Musculoskeletal thickening of the neck muscles can be a cosmetic problem

GENETICS
There is a definite breed predilection; Thoroughbreds are the most affected.

INCIDENCE/PREVALENCE
The prevalence of cribbing is approximately 4%. The mortality rate is unknown.

GEOGRAPHIC DISTRIBUTION
Cribbing has been observed worldwide.

SIGNALMENT
Usually an adult horse confined in a stall, fed a high-concentrate diet, and used for activities such as flat racing, jumping, 3 day eventing, or dressage.

Breed Predilections
Thoroughbreds have a higher risk of cribbing. Standardbreds have a very low incidence.

Mean Age and Range
The age of onset is at weaning and the frequency of diagnosis increases with age.

Predominant Sex
Males are more likely to crib, especially young horses. Older mares are more likely to crib than old geldings or stallions.

SIGNS
General Comments
Cribbing—the horse grasps a horizontal surface with its incisors, flexes its neck, and allows air to pass into the upper esophagus. A few horses do not grasp a horizontal surface, but flex their neck and make a grunting sound. These are called wind suckers.

Historical Findings
Stereotypic behavior usually begins with an abrupt change in the environment; e.g. taking a horse from pasture and immediately limiting its access to hay can be the initiating factor to cribbing.

Physical Examination Findings
Well-developed neck muscles and wear of the upper incisors with cribbing. Occasionally a horse is very thin because it spends so much time cribbing that it does not have time to ingest the calories it needs.

CAUSES
• The cause of stereotypic behavior is unknown
• Boredom probably is not a cause, because providing stall toys usually does not help and an increase in exercise increases time spent cribbing
• The horse is thwarted in some goal, usually grazing, and the frustration leads to repetition of a behavior that is part of the appetitive portion of that behavior (e.g. cribbing as part of biting a mouthful of grass as the first step of ingestion)
• Feeding sweet feed or other highly palatable food stimulates cribbing

RISK FACTORS
• Genetic predisposition for Thoroughbreds
• Stall confinement with limited (<7 kg) forage, <40 L/day of water, bedding other than straw, and minimal visual or tactile contact with other horses
• Race, dressage, jumping, and eventing horses are at greater risk than endurance horses
• In only 10% of cases has another horse begun to crib after a cribber arrived in the barn or pasture. There is little evidence that horses learn to crib by observing other horses; however, if a horse has a genetic predisposition to crib and is in an environment conducive to cribbing with other cribbers, it may acquire the behavior without observational learning having occurred

DIAGNOSIS

DIFFERENTIAL DIAGNOSIS
Differentiate cribbing from wood chewing. The cribbing horse grasps wooden edges but does not ingest them; the wood-chewing horse does. The cribbing horse makes a loud noise when the air passes through the pharynx; the only sound made by the wood-chewing horse is that of wood being splintered.

CBC/BIOCHEMISTRY/URINALYSIS
Perform a physical examination, chemistry screen, and CBC to determine the presence of an underlying disease and to judge whether medication can be administered safely.

OTHER LABORATORY TESTS
N/A

IMAGING
Endoscopic examination should be performed to rule out GI tract problems as a cause of cribbing.

OTHER DIAGNOSTIC PROCEDURES
Endoscopy and to determine if ulcers are present.

O

TREATMENT

AIMS
The aims are to decrease the horse's motivation to crib or engage in other stereotypies. The secondary aim is to prevent GI problems that are associated with oral stereotypies.
• Diet change has the most impact, especially in horses that have just begun to crib. Feeding a hay diet with another source of forage and no sweet feed results in the lowest rate of cribbing. Substitution of fat (e.g. corn oil) for carbohydrates (e.g. molasses and grain) can be done for horses that expend more calories than hay provides
• Other treatments are aimed at creating a normal equine environment, which means the horse has physical contact with other horses and available forage at all times. The best environment for the horse is to remove it from the stall and put it in a compatible social group with access to pasture or hay free choice. When the use of the horse precludes keeping it in a group with a run-out housing situation, eliminating risk factors (e.g. limited forage, wood shavings as bedding) helps. Stall

ORAL STEREOTYPIC BEHAVIOR

toys generally are ineffective as are taste repellents. Punishment is not the preferred method of treatment, but clinicians should be aware of this option. Several types of collars (wide leather straps, a nutcracker or metal collar, or one on a headstall to prevent slipping) can pinch the horse when it cribs or mechanically prevent neck flexion. A metal muzzle prevents the horse from making contact with a horizontal surface
• Provide oral stimulation in the form of several types of forage, pasture, or a barrel the horse can turn to receive pelleted feed or grain. If the behavior occurs before feeding, the horse probably is frustrated by hunger (i.e. undernourishment); if it occurs after feeding, the horse probably is frustrated from the lack of a specific dietary component (i.e. malnourishment)

APPROPRIATE HEALTH CARE
Outpatient care should be sufficient.

NURSING CARE
NA

ACTIVITY
Forced exercise may increase cribbing behavior.

DIET
The diet should be high in roughage and low in carbohydrates and grains other than oats.

CLIENT EDUCATION
The owners should be told that cribbing is not a "vice" but rather a response to the unnatural environment in which we keep horses. Managers of broodmares should know that weaning on pasture greatly reduces the risk of the foal beginning to crib.

SURGICAL CONSIDERATIONS
Accessory neurectomy and strap muscle myectomy can be performed. Reserve these surgical approaches for horses that experience colic when they crib or are emaciated because they crib rather than eat. The side effect is that a stomach tube cannot be passed through the stricture created by the myectomies

MEDICATIONS

DRUG(S) OF CHOICE
Opiate blockers such as naloxone (0.02–0.04 mg/kg IV), naltrexone (0.04 mg/kg SC), or nalmefene (0.08 mg/kg IM) inhibit cribbing, but these drugs are too expensive and too short acting to be practical. IV dextromethorphan 1 mg/kg has been used to reduce cribbing.

CONTRAINDICATIONS
Mares during late pregnancy.

PRECAUTIONS
GI side effects, including diarrhea, inappetence, and behaviors indicative of colic, are seen after naloxone administration.

POSSIBLE INTERACTIONS
N/A

ALTERNATIVE DRUGS
Acupuncture

FOLLOW-UP

PATIENT MONITORING
Regular follow-up after 2 weeks of treatment to evaluate the owner's compliance and the success of the treatments given.

POSSIBLE COMPLICATIONS
N/A

MISCELLANEOUS

ASSOCIATED CONDITIONS
N/A

AGE-RELATED FACTORS
Usually a disease of mature horses.

ZOONOTIC POTENTIAL
N/A

PREGNANCY/FERTILITY/BREEDING
N/A

SYNONYMS
• Crib biting
• Wind sucking

SEE ALSO
• Locomotor stereotypic behaviors
• Pica

ABBREVIATIONS
GI = gastrointestinal

Suggested Reading
Albright JD, Mohammed HO, Heleski CR, et al. Crib-biting in US horses: breed predispositions and owner perceptions of aetiology. Equine Vet J 2009;41:455–458.
Albright JD, Witte TH, Rohrbach BW, et al. Efficacy and effects of various anti-crib devices on behaviour and physiology of crib-biting horses. Equine Vet J 2015;48(6):727–731.
Archer DC, Pinchbeck GK, French NP, Proudman CJ. Risk factors for epiploic foramen entrapment colic: an international study. Equine Vet J 2008;40:224–230.
Delacalle J, Burba DJ, Tetens J, Moore RM. Nd:YAG laser-assisted modified Forssell's procedure for treatment of cribbing (crib-biting) in horses. Vet Surg 2002;31:111–116.
McGreevy PD, Richardson JD, Nicol CJ, Lane JG. Radiographic and endoscopic study of horses performing an oral based stereotypy. Equine Vet J 1995;27:92–95.
Rendon RA, Shuster L, Dodman NH. The effect of the NMDA receptor blocker, dextromethorphan, on cribbing in horses. Pharmacol Biochem Behav 2001;68:49–51.
Whisher L, Raum M, Pina L, et al. Effects of environmental factors on cribbing activity by horses. Appl Anim Behav Sci 2011;135:63–69.
Wickens CL, McCall CA, Bursian S, et al. Assessment of gastric ulceration and gastrin response in horses with history of crib-biting. Equine Vet J 2013;33(9):739–745.

Author Katherine Albro Houpt
Consulting Editor Victoria L. Voith

BASICS

DEFINITION
Oral ulcers are disruptions in the integrity of the oral mucosa that may be preceded by stomatic lesions such as vesicles, bullae, crusts, or traumatic injury.

PATHOPHYSIOLOGY
• The pathophysiologic events that lead to oral ulceration are variable and depend on the inciting cause
• Vesicular stomatitis is caused by a vesiculovirus (VSV), with short incubation period of 24 h, and invasion of oral epithelial cells. VSV induces intercellular edema of the Malpighian layer causing separation of the cells by vacuolar cavities. Vesicles develop when edematous and necrotic mucosa is filled with cellular exudate due to separation at the basal layer. Epithelial cell lesions progress rapidly from blanched maculae to vesicles and soon rupture, leaving sloughed epithelium and ulcers
• Phenylbutazone inhibits prostaglandin synthesis resulting in depletion of PGE_1 and PGE_2, which is thought to cause vasoconstriction of the microvasculature of the mucosa, leading to ischemia and ulcer formation
• The mechanism of action of cantharidin to induce ulcers is not well understood, but acantholysis and vesicle formation occur as a result of damage to the cell membrane due to interference with oxidative enzymes bound to mitochondria
• The oral ulcers caused by facial paralysis and dental problems are due to impaction of food material between the teeth and the cheek, as well as direct traumatic damage by the teeth
• Coarse forage and plant awns may cause oral ulcers and erosions due to physical trauma
• In uremia, oral ulcers develop as a consequence of increased excretion of urea into the oral cavity, degradation of urea into ammonia by bacterial urease, and subsequent disruption of oral mucosa integrity

SYSTEMS AFFECTED
• The different systems affected vary depending on the initial cause. With VSV the locomotor system is usually affected. The vesicular lesions are present on the coronary bands, and lameness is observed
• In cases of phenylbutazone toxicity, several sections of the GI tract are affected, causing gastric and intestinal ulceration and colitis of the right dorsal colon. The kidney is also affected, causing renal medullary crest necrosis. Ventral and peripheral edema may also be observed
• Blister beetle toxicosis (cantharidin toxicosis), besides affecting the mucosal surface, also affects the GI tract, causing colic. There is hypocalcemia and hypoproteinemia, and the kidney is slightly affected. Myocardial

necrosis and myopathy are common in affected horses. Some horses show stilted gait, as seen in myositis
• In the uremic syndrome, weight loss is the most common affliction; there is PU/PD, gastric ulceration, coagulation disorders, and halitosis (urine odor). There is excessive dental tartar, and there is ventral edema because of a decrease in oncotic pressure, increased vascular permeability, and increased hydrostatic pressure. Bone marrow, the endocrine system, and the CNS might be affected
• The other causes of oral ulceration are local phenomena limited to the buccal mucosa

SIGNALMENT
Oral ulcers can occur at any age, and there is no sex or breed predisposition.

SIGNS
Historical Findings
The history of oral ulceration cases is quite variable and is dependent on the initial cause. In the cases of vesicular stomatitis, it starts as an outbreak. The owner usually reports that the affected animals have excessive salivation, inappetence, and lameness. In the cases where toxicity is involved, there is a history of ingestion of toxic material. With phenylbutazone toxicity, the history indicates that an excessive dosage for several days or accidental administration of large amounts has occurred. Facial nerve paralysis is usually preceded by some history of trauma or CNS disease. The main complaint with uremia is usually PU/PD. In cases of physical trauma by coarse forage and awns, there is evidence of the presence of these plants in the pasture.

Physical Examination Findings
• In the majority of the cases of oral ulcers regardless of the cause, there is ptyalism, different degrees of anorexia, and dysphagia due to pain. Halitosis is common
• Vesicular stomatitis starts with oral vesicles that with time coalesce and turn into ulcers. Lameness of different degrees is observed
• In phenylbutazone toxicity there are signs typical of oral ulcers, but also there may be ventral and peripheral edema, bruxism, diarrhea (see chapter Right dorsal colitis), melena, ulceration of the digestive tract, and weight loss
• In addition to oral ulcers, cantharidin toxicosis is also manifested by depression; colic, fever, profuse diarrhea, stranguria, synchronous diaphragmatic flutter, and a stiff gait (see chapter Cantharidin toxicosis). Oral ulcers in uremia are accompanied by all the signs that distinguish the uremic syndrome (see chapter Chronic kidney disease (CKD))
• Equine ulcerative stomatitis resembles very closely vesicular stomatitis

CAUSES
• Vesicular stomatitis
• Phenylbutazone toxicity
• Uremia

• Cantharidin toxicosis
• Chemical stomatitis
• Periodontal disease
• Foxtail (*Setaria*) and plant thorn stomatitis
• Oral foreign body
• Oral ulcers secondary to yellow star thistle grass
• Bedding derived wood savings (plants of Simaroubaceae family)
• Dermatologic-related conditions (pemphigus foliaceus, equine exfoliative eosinophilic dermatitis)
• Food impaction between molar teeth and cheek (facial nerve paralysis, dental problems)
• Equine herpesvirus 2, equine arteritis virus, Jamestown virus, caliciviruses, and adenoviruses
• *Actinobacillus lignieresii*
• Equine ulcerative stomatitis (unknown etiology)

RISK FACTORS
The risk factors involved in oral ulcers are related to the primary cause (see each clinical entity).

 DIAGNOSIS

DIFFERENTIAL DIAGNOSIS
See chapter Ptyalism.

CBC/BIOCHEMISTRY/URINALYSIS
No findings are specific to oral ulceration, but changes may reflect the underlying causes.

IMAGING
• Radiographic studies are indicated when there is suspicion of dental problems or trauma has caused facial paralysis
• US examination of the kidneys may help in determining the cause of chronic renal failure

OTHER DIAGNOSTIC PROCEDURES
• A thorough history and physical and oral examination is indicated to rule out the different causes of oral ulceration
• To diagnose vesicular stomatitis, virus isolation from biopsy of the vesicles is done. A complement fixation test, fluorescent antibody test, and virus neutralization test in tissue culture are used for virus identification. An indirect sandwich ELISA is the diagnostic method of choice
• Cantharidin toxicosis diagnosis is based on detecting cantharidin in stomach contents or in urine or finding blister beetles in the forage
• The diagnosis of phenylbutazone toxicity is suggested by a history of inappropriate drug administration and a clinical picture compatible with it
• The diagnosis of chronic renal failure is based on serum urea and creatinine measurement, US examination of the kidneys, urinalysis, sodium fractional excretion, and kidney biopsy. Biopsy and histologic examination of lesions may assist in

O

ORAL ULCERS

narrowing the differential diagnosis and to rule out associated neoplastic events
• To rule out trauma due to ingestion of pasture awns, the horse environment should be examined

TREATMENT
Specific therapy for particular conditions may be indicated. The treatment strategies for oral ulcers involve local therapy to relieve pain and irritation, such as mild antiseptic mouthwashes with potassium permanganate (2%), hydrogen peroxide (0.5%), a saturated solution of boric acid, or povidone–iodine solution (1% v/v). If present, thorns or any foreign body should be extracted. Remove any chemical irritant that may be causing oral ulceration. This also applies for all toxicoses. When dental problems are the cause, appropriate dental prophylactic measures are indicated.

MISCELLANEOUS
ZOONOTIC POTENTIAL
Among the causes of oral ulcers, only vesicular stomatitis has zoonotic potential.

SYNONYMS
• Vesicles
• Crusts
• Growths

SEE ALSO
• Cantharidin toxicosis
• Chronic kidney disease
• Oral ulcers
• Pemphigus Foliaceus
• Periodontal disease
• Vesicular stomatitis

ABBREVIATIONS
• CNS = central nervous system
• ELISA = enzyme-linked immunosorbent assay
• GI = gastrointestinal
• PGE = prostaglandin E
• PU/PD = polyuria/polydipsia
• US = ultrasonography, ultrasound
• VSV = vesicular stomatitis virus

Suggested Reading
Baun KH, Shin SJ, Rebhun WC, Patten VH. Isolation of *Actinobacillus lignieresii* from enlarged tongue of a horse. J Am Vet Med Assoc 1984;185:792–793.
McCluskey BJ, Munford EL. Vesicular stomatitis and other vesicular, erosive and ulcerative diseases of horses. Vet Clin North Am Equine Pract 2000;16:457–469.
Meschter CL, Gilbert M, Krook L, et al. The effects of phenylbutazone on the intestinal mucosa of the horse: a morphological, ultrastructural and biochemical study. Equine Vet J 1990;22:255–263.
Rodriguez LL. Emergence and re-emergence of vesicular stomatitis in the United States. Virus Res 2002;85:211–219.
Schmitz DG. Cantharidin toxicosis in horses. J Vet Intern Med 1989;3:208–215.
Scrutchfield WL, Schumacher J. Examination of the oral cavity and routine dental care. Vet Clin North Am Equine Pract 1993;9:123–131.
Tell A, Egenvall A, Lundström T, Wattle O. The prevalence of oral ulceration in Swedish horses when ridden with bit and bridle and when unridden. Vet J 2008;178:405–410.
White SD. Diseases of the lips and oral cavity of domestic animals. Clin Dermatol 1987;5:190–201.

Author Olimpo Oliver-Espinosa
Consulting Editors Henry Stämpfli and Olimpo Oliver-Espinosa

BASICS

DEFINITION
• The equine orbit houses the globe, and is composed of the frontal, lacrimal, zygomatic, and temporal bones, with the medial wall of the orbit formed by the palatine and sphenoid bones. The orbital rim is complete in horses. The orbit is a closed conical cavity with a broad opening anteriorly. There are numerous foramina that open into the orbit, allowing nerves and blood vessels to enter this space. The orbit also contains additional extraocular supportive structures, including muscle, glands, fat, and fascia. The canaliculi of the nasolacrimal duct pass through the lacrimal bone. Pathology of any of these extraocular tissues, including the bony orbit, broadly defines orbital disease
• As orbital disease progresses, tissue within or adjacent to the orbit loses its ability to function. Discomfort may develop, and vision may be compromised. Compression by a space-occupying lesion, anatomic rearrangement by trauma or disease, or invasion of a systemic illness into the orbit highlights the major mechanisms of orbital disease

SYSTEMS AFFECTED
Ophthalmic, musculoskeletal, vascular, nervous, and upper respiratory systems, including sinuses can be involved.

SIGNALMENT
Older horses tend to develop neoplasia, whereas foals and yearlings, as well as polo ponies, may be more prone to acute trauma.

SIGNS
• Variable according to disease process
• Exophthalmos, or anterior displacement of the globe, with decreased ability to retropulse the globe. May also be associated with nictitans protrusion, exposure keratitis, and lagophthalmos
• Enophthalmos, or posterior displacement of the globe, which can occur secondary to atrophy of tissue behind the globe, nerve damage, and following some orbital fractures. Concurrent nictitans protrusion is often seen
• Strabismus
• Swollen periorbita
• Orbital asymmetry from fractures, cellulitis, and orbital emphysema
• Blepharedema, chemosis, corneal edema
• Epiphora or other ocular discharge
• Vision loss (usually unilateral)
• Nasal discharge or epistaxis, decreased airflow through the ipsilateral nostril
• Abnormal sinus percussion possible with conditions affecting the upper airways and sinuses
• Phthisis bulbi (globe atrophy)
• Fever, pain

CAUSES
• Trauma causing orbital fractures, cellulitis, and/or proptosis
• Foreign bodies leading to orbital abscesses
• Orbital neoplasia—meningioma, neuroendocrine tumor, extra-adrenal paraganglioma, lipoma, adenocarcinoma, lymphoma, melanoma, sarcoid, squamous cell carcinoma, hemangiosarcoma, multilobular osteoma, anaplastic sarcoma, medulloepithelioma, schwannoma, rhabdoid neoplasia, angiosarcoma, and neurofibroma have all been found in the equine orbit
• (Pyo)granulomatous diseases such as *Cryptococcus neoformans*, *Actinomyces* spp. or epizootic lymphangitis
• Retro-orbital cysts, dermoid cysts, dentigerous cysts
• Guttural pouch disease
• Sinusitis involving frontal, maxillary, sphenopalatine sinuses
• Tooth root abscesses
• Sinus neoplasia
• Orbital fat prolapse
• Varices or abnormal distention of venules causing a displacement of normal tissue
• Parasitism as in hydatid cysts, *Halicephalobus gingivalis*, and *Strongylus edentatus*
• Nutritional myopathy

RISK FACTORS
See Causes.

DIAGNOSIS

DIFFERENTIAL DIAGNOSIS
• Any cause of ocular pain
• Exophthalmos, a sign of orbital disease, can be confused with buphthalmos, which is a marked increase in globe diameter associated with chronic glaucoma
• Primary extraorbital disease that is close to, but not affecting, the orbit—sinusitis, guttural pouch disorders, dental disease

CBC/BIOCHEMISTRY/URINALYSIS
CBC may show a leukocytosis and elevated fibrinogen or other nonspecific inflammatory indicators.

OTHER LABORATORY TESTS
Systemic illness should be considered.

IMAGING
• Very important diagnostic tool in evaluating orbital disease
• Skull radiographs, orbital ultrasonography, CT (ideal for evaluation of fractures), or MRI where available (foals and small ponies primarily)

OTHER DIAGNOSTIC PROCEDURES
• Aspiration of fluid or biopsy of tissue should be performed
• Cytology, microbial culture and susceptibility, and histopathology are recommended as part of an orbital disease workup

• Orbitotomy can be diagnostic and therapeutic; however, it is difficult surgery that may require orthopedic instruments
• Trephination into paranasal sinuses may be indicated for microbial culture, irrigation, and drainage
• In cases of proptosis, careful ophthalmic examination will dictate viability of the eye. Miosis with severe hypotony and hyphema indicates severe trauma and poor visual prognosis

PATHOLOGIC FINDINGS
Varies greatly depending on the particular disease.

TREATMENT

• Highly dependent on underlying cause
• Minor orbital trauma may be treated medically; however, surgical intervention may be indicated in some cases (e.g. fractures, orbital neoplasia) with short hospital stays recommended until the owner or trainer can monitor and treat the patient at home
• Activity is based on degree of visual impairment and comfort of the horse. Some of these diseases are very painful especially after invasive surgery. Stall rest may be indicated for the short term
• No change in diet is necessary unless malnutrition is a cause of the atrophy of orbital contents
• For primary orbital disease, prognosis for vision is guarded initially. In severe, painful orbital disease with irreversible blindness, and in some cases of orbital neoplasia, the best management may be orbital exenteration
• In a sighted eye, orbitotomy is best for discrete, solitary retrobulbar cysts or masses that do not invade the optic nerve
• Enucleation may be recommended to remove a painful, blind eye and its associated conjunctiva and nictitans. An intraorbital prosthesis may be placed in the orbit to replace the globe if risk of infection or tumor recurrence is low. In the absence of infection or neoplasia, intrascleral prostheses are an acceptable alternative to enucleation and can be placed in an eviscerated scleral shell as long as the cornea is not severely diseased and there is no residual lagophthalmos or exophthalmos. Orbital bleeding should be minimized by careful hemostasis
• Exenteration is indicated if a neoplastic condition extends beyond the confines of the globe or if disease affects both the globe and other orbital tissues
• Periorbital fractures should be repaired quickly as fibrous union can occur as soon as 1 week post trauma. Tarsorrhaphies are beneficial to proptosed eyes and should not be removed until most of the periorbital swelling has subsided, usually 1–2 weeks

O

ORBITAL DISEASE

• Temporary or permanent tarsorrhaphy is indicated in cases of facial nerve trauma, neurogenic keratoconjunctivitis sicca/keratitis, and lagophthalmos

MEDICATIONS

DRUG(S) OF CHOICE
• Systemic antibiotics should be administered in cases of trauma or suspected orbital infection/cellulitis
• Anthelmintics in cases of parasitic orbital disease
• The globe itself may benefit from topical ophthalmic lubricants or antibiotics
• Periorbital swelling can be alleviated by judicious use of anti-inflammatories
• Occasionally uveitis is seen with orbital trauma and should be treated with topical or systemic anti-inflammatories
• Flunixin meglumine at a dose of 1 mg/kg IV, IM, or PO BID or phenylbutazone at a dose of 2.2–4.4 mg/kg PO twice daily can be given for pain associated with the orbital disease

CONTRAINDICATIONS
Topical steroids are contraindicated when ulcerative keratitis is present.

PRECAUTIONS
Long-term flunixin meglumine or phenylbutazone use may lead to systemic complications such as renal dysfunction or protein loss from the gut.

POSSIBLE INTERACTIONS
N/A

ALTERNATIVE DRUGS
Intralesional iridium implants or cisplatin chemotherapy into the orbital tumor may be beneficial in some types of neoplasia. Chemotherapy and corticosteroids may be beneficial in the treatment of orbital lymphosarcoma.

FOLLOW-UP

• Recheck visits are indicated for more extensive diseases, especially if orbital surgery is performed as for an aggressive tumor
• Long-term damage may be sustained in orbital trauma, including eyelid paralysis, chronic keratitis, keratoconjunctivitis sicca, or intermittent nasal or ocular discharge, necessitating chronic therapy and monitoring
• Providing a safe environment with good training may decrease the opportunity for trauma
• Recurrence of tumor, reinfection of orbit, and persistent pain and swelling can all occur during and after the treatment period
• Blindness and loss of the eye are possible sequelae of severe orbital disease
• Highly variable outcomes are based on correct diagnosis and appropriate treatment. Some orbital diseases such as trauma are one-time events with possible long-term side effects. Other diseases such as tumors may never be cured, only treated palliatively

MISCELLANEOUS

SEE ALSO
• Guttural pouch mycosis
• Head trauma
• Ocular/adnexal squamous cell carcinoma

ABBREVIATIONS
• CT = computed tomography
• MRI = magnetic resonance imaging

Suggested Reading
Brooks DE. Ophthalmology for the Equine Practitioner. Jackson, WY: Teton NewMedia, 2002.
Gilger BC. Equine ophthalmology. In: Gelatt KN, Gilger BC, Kern TJ, eds. Veterinary Ophthalmology, 5e. Ames, IA: Wiley Blackwell, 2013:1560–1609.
Gilger BC, ed. Equine Ophthalmology, 3e. Ames, IA: Wiley Blackwell, 2017.

Author Shari M. Greenberg
Consulting Editor Caryn E. Plummer
Acknowledgment The author and editor acknowledge the prior contribution of Dennis E. Brooks.

ORGANOPHOSPHATE AND CARBAMATE TOXICOSIS

BASICS

DEFINITION
• Toxicosis caused by exposure to AChE-inhibiting OP or carbamate compounds
• These compounds are active ingredients in many animal oral and topical parasiticides, as well as in numerous household and agricultural pesticide products. There are dozens of different, but structurally similar, OP and carbamate compounds with hundreds of different formulations, containing varying concentrations of active ingredient
• The toxicity among individual compounds varies tremendously
• Oral ingestion is the most common form of exposure in horses, either from ingesting pasture grass or hay where pesticide spills or drift have occurred or from overdosing with oral parasiticide products. Inhalation or dermal exposure leading to poisoning is not common but can occur
• *Be careful*—not all pesticides labeled as "carbamates" inhibit AChE

PATHOPHYSIOLOGY
• Most OP and carbamate pesticides are rapidly absorbed by the respiratory and GI systems and dermally
• Some are direct-acting compounds; others require metabolic activation by the liver to a toxic metabolite. The underlying biochemical change responsible for the clinical syndrome is an inhibition of AChE activity in the nervous system, resulting in accumulation of acetylcholine at synapses and myoneural junctions. Inhibition of the enzyme by OPs is considered irreversible, particularly once covalent bonding or aging has occurred
• Inhibition of the enzyme by carbamates is reversible. In order to restore AChE activity following pesticide exposure, the enzyme must either be reactivated or synthesized

SYSTEMS AFFECTED
• Nervous and musculoskeletal—excess acetylcholine at synapses and myoneural junctions initially excites, then paralyzes, transmission in cholinergic synapses found in the CNS and at parasympathetic and a few sympathetic nerve endings (muscarinic effects) and somatic nerves and ganglionic synapses of autonomic ganglia (nicotinic effects)
• Respiratory—build-up of secretions from the muscarinic effects can lead to respiratory difficulties, perfusion problems, and secondary bacterial invaders

INCIDENCE/PREVALENCE
Poisonings with these compounds in horses seem to be not as common as observed in other species. However, most cases occur in the spring and summer when agricultural and household pesticide use is highest. Poisonings

can occur from eating hay that was baled several months previously; any pesticide spilled or drifted onto the hay and then baled will have a slower rate of degradation, and some pesticides have been known to persist in baled hay for up to 6 months.

SIGNALMENT
There are no breed, age, or sex predilections.

SIGNS

General Comments
There is considerable variation in clinical signs between different species of animals despite the fact that the mechanism of action is the same. In the horse, GI signs predominate and nervous signs may be absent altogether. The severity of the clinical syndrome and time to onset depend on exposure dose, route of exposure, and formulation of the pesticide product. Clinical signs can be immediate, following inhalation or oral exposure, or may be delayed by several hours (oral or dermal route).

Physical Examination Findings
• Abdominal pain, accompanied by restlessness, anxiety, and sweating
• Markedly increased intestinal sounds
• Watery diarrhea
• Weakness and depression
• Mild to severe muscle tremors (seizures uncommon)
• Tachycardia or bradycardia
• Miosis or mydriasis
• Dyspnea
• Excessive salivation can occur

CAUSES
Most cases of poisoning occur via ingestion of pesticide-contaminated grass or hay or from overdosing of oral parasiticide products. Horses also can be poisoned by accidental access to spilled or improperly used, stored, or discarded pesticides. Dermal and inhalation exposure can also occur.

RISK FACTORS
Some of these compounds are lipophilic and are slowly released, so animals with a lean body mass may exhibit more severe signs.

DIAGNOSIS

DIFFERENTIAL DIAGNOSIS
• Bacterial or viral gastroenteritis (physical examination, bacteriology, serology), intestinal compromise such as a twist, torsion, or intussusception (physical examination)
• Peritonitis (physical examination, abdominocentesis)
• Inorganic arsenic poisoning (urine, whole blood, or tissue arsenic determination)

OTHER LABORATORY TESTS
• Inhibition of blood, brain, or retinal AChE activity is suggestive of exposure, particularly if the activity is reduced to < 50% of what is

considered normal. Assessment of AChE activity can be done up to several days after the suspect exposure
• Carbamate binding can be reversed during sample transit to a laboratory facility so lack of enzyme inhibition does not necessarily rule out carbamate exposure. In peracute to acute high-dose exposures, an animal may die of respiratory compromise before sufficient brain enzyme activity can be inhibited. In addition, some OPs and carbamates poorly penetrate the CNS, so that lack of brain AChE inhibition cannot totally rule out exposure to these compounds
• Tissue residue testing (liver, kidney, stomach contents, skin, fat, urine) is readily available at most diagnostic facilities and can confirm exposure

PATHOLOGIC FINDINGS
Visible evidence of insecticide granules in the stomach contents. Most OP and carbamate pesticides have a strong sulfur or "chemical" odor. There are no specific gross or histopathologic changes—pulmonary edema and effusions are sometimes reported.

TREATMENT

APPROPRIATE HEALTH CARE
Prompt and aggressive treatment is essential to a favorable outcome. Samples of blood, urine, or stomach reflux should be saved for toxicologic analysis before any specific treatments are initiated.

NURSING CARE
• Administration of IV fluids is important to correct intestinal fluid and electrolyte losses and to assist in renal excretion of the parent compound or its metabolites. Fluids should be continued until the fluid losses are under control and the horse can eat and drink on its own
• Decontamination procedures following oral exposures include administration of AC and a laxative/cathartic via stomach tube (laxatives should only be given if diarrhea is *not* present). AC is administered at 2–5 g/kg bodyweight (1 g AC in 5 mL water). Leave in the stomach for 20–30 min and then give a laxative (e.g. mineral oil) to hasten removal of the toxicant. Alternatively, an osmotic cathartic can be given (70% sorbitol at 3 mL/kg or sodium or magnesium sulfate at 250–500 mg/kg, the last 2 given in a water slurry)
• Care should be used in administering laxatives or cathartics to patients who are severely dehydrated due to diarrhea, and possibly these should be avoided. For cases of dermal exposure, bathe the patient with warm soapy water and follow up with a thorough rinse

ORGANOPHOSPHATE AND CARBAMATE TOXICOSIS   (CONTINUED)

MEDICATIONS

DRUG(S) OF CHOICE
• Diazepam (adults 25–50 mg IV; foals 0.05–0.4 mg/kg IV) can be used in those patients that are overly anxious or restless or have muscle tremors or seizures
• Atropine sulfate (0.2 mg/kg; give 25% of the dose IV and the remainder IM or SC) can be used to control the muscarinic signs. Do not exceed 65 mg atropine total dose in horses because of the risk of developing ileus. Butylscopolamine has been used for the control of colic associated with spasmodic, flatulent colic and simple impaction if there are complications with using atropine. The recommended dosage of atropine is somewhat controversial, and no one standard dosage is accepted by all. One suggestion is to give 25% of the 0.22 mg/kg dose IV and the remainder IM or SQ. This can potentially result in ileus, causing serious complications in horses
• Xylazine (0.3–1.1 mg/kg IV, repeat as necessary) can be used as a sedative/analgesic to control signs associated with colic but should not be used in conjunction with tranquilizers
• Butorphanol (0.1 mg/kg of body weight IV every 3–4 h) is an alternative analgesic to relieve the pain associated with colic
• Pralidoxime chloride (20–35 mg/kg *slow* IV, repeat every 4–6 h as necessary) reactivates AChE that has been inactivated by phosphorylation secondary to most OP exposures and is most effective in controlling muscle fasciculations within the first 24 h of exposure. Cost can be an issue in treating adult horses, but most patients require no more than 1–3 treatments
• Bronchoconstriction, pulmonary edema, and respiratory muscle weakness may occur. In these cases, the use of a diuretic

(e.g. furosemide at 0.25–1.0 mg/kg IV), a bronchodilator (e.g. albuterol, oral syrup 0.05 mg/kg or inhalation 0.36–0.9 mg every 8 h), and mechanical respiratory support may be necessary

CONTRAINDICATIONS
Phenothiazine tranquilizers may potentiate the signs associated with some OP poisonings.

PRECAUTIONS
Avoid overzealous use of atropine.

POSSIBLE INTERACTIONS
The use of OP anthelmintics in the horse may potentiate the action of succinylcholine (suxamethonium) chloride for up to 1 month after administration of the OP.

FOLLOW-UP

PATIENT MONITORING
Continuously monitor heart rate and rhythm, respiratory system, urination, defecation, and hydration and electrolyte status.

PREVENTION/AVOIDANCE
Care should be taken to read the label carefully on all products containing OPs and carbamates. Make sure they are used, stored, and disposed of in the appropriate manner.

POSSIBLE COMPLICATIONS
An intermediate syndrome has been described in animals where muscle weakness occurs several days after the pesticide exposure. Delayed neuropathy may occur following some OP exposures but this is not common. Bilateral laryngeal paralysis has been reported to occur in foals after dosing with an OP anthelmintic.

EXPECTED COURSE AND PROGNOSIS
Good in horses that have received prompt and aggressive therapy. Most animals recover uneventfully over a period of 24–48 h.

MISCELLANEOUS

ASSOCIATED CONDITIONS
N/A

AGE-RELATED FACTORS
N/A

ZOONOTIC POTENTIAL
N/A

PREGNANCY/FERTILITY/BREEDING
N/A

ABBREVIATIONS
• AC = activated charcoal
• AChE = acetylcholinesterase
• CNS = central nervous system
• GI = gastrointestinal
• OP = organophosphate

Suggested Reading
Gupta RC, Milatovic D. Organophosphates and carbamates. In: Gupta RC, ed. Veterinary Toxicology, 2e. San Diego, CA: Elsevier, 2012:573–585.
Plumlee KH. Clinical Veterinary Toxicology. St. Louis, MO: Mosby, 2004:178–180.
Organophosphorus compounds and carbamates. In: Radostits OM, Blood DC, Gay CC, eds. Veterinary Medicine: A Textbook of the Diseases of Cattle, Sheep, Pigs, Goats and Horses, 7e. London, UK: Bailliere Tindall, 1994:1514–1517.

Author Steve Ensley
Consulting Editors Wilson K. Rumbeiha and Steve Ensley

Acknowledgment The author and editors acknowledge the prior contribution of Patricia A. Talcott.

BASICS

DEFINITIONS
- Osmolality represents the number of dissociated solute particles per kilogram of solvent and is expressed as mOsm/kg
- Osmolarity represents the number of dissociated solute particles per liter of solvent and is expressed as mOsm/L
- Osmolality is a thermodynamically more precise term than osmolarity, because osmolality is based on weight, which is temperature independent, whereas osmolarity is dependent on volume and is temperature dependent
- Osmotic pressure governs the movement of water across membranes because of differences in solute content
- Hyperosmolality and hyperosmolarity are defined in horses as serum concentrations of osmoles above the reference interval. Normal intervals are >270–300 mOsm/kg and >270–300 mOsm/L, respectively
- Osmolal or osmolar gap is the difference between the measured and the calculated estimate of osmolality (normal gap range –5 to 15 mOsm/L)
- 1 osmole is the gram molecular weight of a nondissociable substance and contains Avogadro's number of particles. Effective osmoles are particles in solution that cannot freely move across cell membranes and therefore create an osmotic effect
- Tonicity is the effective osmolality of a solution due to the concentration of solutes that can cause a fluid shift across semipermeable membranes
- A solvent is a liquid holding another substance in solution; for osmolality, this is water
- A solute is the dissolved substance in the solution
- A solution, in this discussion, contains solutes within a solvent

PATHOPHYSIOLOGY
- In serum/plasma, Na^+ is the principal cation balanced by many anions (Cl^-, HCO_3^-, protein, sulfate, phosphate). Na^+ is the most osmotically active particle, with some contribution from Cl^- and HCO_3^-, and lesser contributions from glucose and urea. Animals that are hypernatremic are hyperosmolal, and hyponatremia is associated with hypo-osmolality
- Water loss increases the concentrations of solutes in serum/plasma, thereby increasing blood osmolality
- Dissolved particles that cannot move between adjacent compartments exert osmotic pressure and cause water movement to equilibrate solute concentrations between compartments
- Hypertonicity causes water to shift from the ICF to the ECF, resulting in cell shrinkage.

Not all cases of hyperosmolality produce hypertonicity
- Serum osmolality is a measure of ECF osmolality. The ECF compartment comprises one-third of total body weight, with the remaining two-thirds in the ICF compartment
- The osmolalities of ECF and ICF are equal, but the ionic compositions differ. ECF solutes are primarily Na^+ and Cl^-, with small concentrations of HCO_3^-, K^+, phosphate, Ca^{2+}, and Mg^{2+}, whereas ICF is high in K^+ and phosphate, with lower concentrations of Na^+, Cl^-, and Ca^{2+}
- Blood volume, hydration status, and ADH are involved in controlling the ECF volume. Hypovolemia stimulates carotid and aortic baroreceptors to respond to changes in blood pressure, causing ADH secretion
- Hyperosmolality stimulates ADH secretion from the neurohypophysis. The kidney's ability to produce urine of various concentrations maintains body regulation of osmolality. The hypothalamic thirst center is stimulated and causes an increase in water consumption to counteract serum hyperosmolality
- Rapid increases in serum osmolality cause water movement along its concentration gradient, from ICF to ECF spaces, resulting in neuronal dehydration, cell shrinkage, and cell death

SYSTEMS AFFECTED
- Nervous—rapid fluid shifts can lead to brain swelling
- Cardiovascular—hypotension and depressed ventricular contractility (due to loss of circulatory fluid volume)
- Renal/urologic—decreases urine output
- Multiple systems can be affected by hypoxia secondary to hypovolemia

GENETICS
N/A

INCIDENCE/PREVALENCE
N/A

GEOGRAPHIC DISTRIBUTION
N/A

SIGNALMENT
Any breed, age, or sex.

SIGNS
General Comments
- Excessive thirst may be the first sign of hyperosmolality
- Signs are primarily neurologic and behavioral
- Severity of signs relates to how quickly hyperosmolality occurs rather than the absolute magnitude of change
- Signs are most likely to develop with serum osmolality >350 mOsm/kg

Historical Findings
- A history of water deprivation
- Improper reconstitution of milk replacer in orphan foals

- Owner might report signs such as anorexia, lethargy, incoordination, increased thirst

Physical Examination Findings
- Dependent on the underlying cause
- Dehydration—tacky mucous membranes, sunken eyes, prolonged skin tent
- Hypovolemia—tachycardia, weak pulse, decreased urine output, cool extremities
- Neurologic deficits (e.g. depression, ataxia, weakness, seizures)

CAUSES
- Increased solutes—hypernatremia, hyperglycemia, severe azotemia, ethylene glycol toxicosis, propylene glycol toxicosis, salt poisoning, hypovolemic or septic shock, administration of mannitol, radiographic contrast solution, parenteral nutrition solutions, and lactate in patients with lactic acidosis
- Decreased ECF volume—dehydration or hypovolemia (e.g. GI loss, renal loss, cutaneous loss, third-space loss, low water consumption) and polyuria without adequate compensatory polydipsia

RISK FACTORS
- Predisposing medical conditions—renal failure, diabetes insipidus, diabetes mellitus, pituitary pars intermedia dysfunction, equine metabolic syndrome, heat stroke
- Therapeutic hyperosmolar solutions—hypertonic saline (hypovolemic shock), $NaHCO_3$ (renal tubular acidosis, diarrhea), sodium iodide (antimicrobial), and mannitol (cerebral edema)
- Hyperthermia
- Limited access to water

DIAGNOSIS

DIFFERENTIAL DIAGNOSIS
- Primary central nervous system disease from a variety of causes including inflammation, trauma, or neoplasia; serum osmolality usually is normal
- Assess hydration status, and obtain information regarding previous treatment that may have included Na^+-containing fluids or hyperosmolar solutions

CBC/BIOCHEMISTRY/URINALYSIS
- High hematocrit, hemoglobin, and plasma proteins in dehydrated patients; serum electrolytes also may be above the reference intervals
- Hyperosmolality is an indication to evaluate serum Na^+, BUN, and glucose concentrations. Estimated serum osmolality can be calculated as mOsm/kg = 2(Na^+) + BUN/2.8 + glucose/18; Na^+ concentration provides an estimate of the total electrolyte concentrations (anions and cations) and is therefore multiplied by 2. The denominators for BUN (2.8) and glucose (18) are necessary

OSMOLALITY, HYPEROSMOLALITY

to convert mg/dL to the same units as Na^+ (mmol/L, mEq/L)

- Normally, measured osmolality should not exceed the calculated osmolality by more than 10 mOsm/kg. If it does, calculate the osmolar gap (i.e. measured osmolality minus calculated osmolality)
- A decreased osmolar gap may indicate laboratory error
- An increased osmolar gap is usually due to (1) a decrease in serum water from hyperlipidemia or hyperproteinemia or (2) the presence of additional low-molecular-weight substances in the serum (e.g. mannitol, ethanol, ethylene glycol, isopropanol)
- A high osmolar gap with high measured osmolality indicates the presence of unmeasured solutes
- A normal osmolar gap with high measured osmolality indicates hyperosmolality from measured solutes (Na^+, K^+, glucose, or BUN)
- Serum Na^+ concentration may be low in patients with severe hyperglycemia and hyperosmolality
- Numerous calcium oxalate crystals in urine may indicate ethylene glycol toxicosis (rare)
- Hyposthenuria may indicate diabetes insipidus
- Low urine osmolality less than serum osmolality suggests diabetes insipidus

OTHER LABORATORY TESTS
- Serum osmolality can be directly measured by an osmometer
- Toxin analysis if indicated
- Blood lactate concentration and blood gas analysis

IMAGING
Renal ultrasonography to evaluate kidney size and architecture if warranted.

OTHER DIAGNOSTIC PROCEDURES
Indirect blood pressure measurement.

PATHOLOGIC FINDINGS
Dependent on the underlying cause.

TREATMENT

APPROPRIATE HEALTH CARE
- Mild hyperosmolality without clinical signs may not warrant specific treatment; however, any underlying diseases should be diagnosed and treated
- Patients with moderate to high osmolality (>350 mOsm/kg) or exhibiting clinical signs should be hospitalized and their serum osmolality *gradually* lowered with IV fluid administration while a diagnosis is pursued

NURSING CARE
Initial fluid therapy to restore hemodynamics and to replace fluid deficits depend heavily on the serum Na^+ concentration. Isotonic, and sometimes even hypertonic, crystalloids should be administered to ensure that decreases in serum Na^+ concentration do not exceed 0.5 mEq/L/h.

ACTIVITY
N/A

DIET
N/A

CLIENT EDUCATION
Dependent on the underlying cause.

SURGICAL CONSIDERATIONS
N/A

MEDICATIONS

DRUG(S) OF CHOICE
Seizures can be controlled with anticonvulsants.

CONTRAINDICATIONS
N/A

PRECAUTIONS
- Isotonic crystalloids may be used initially, but rapid administration may worsen neurologic signs. Administration of hypertonic fluids might be necessary if serum Na^+ concentrations are markedly elevated to ensure that serum Na^+ levels do not normalize too quickly. Do not decrease serum Na^+ concentration faster than 0.5 mEq/L/h or cerebral edema and neurologic signs might result
- Fluid administration that induces hypo-osmolality can produce intravascular hemolysis

POSSIBLE INTERACTIONS
N/A

ALTERNATIVE DRUGS
N/A

FOLLOW-UP

PATIENT MONITORING
- Monitor hydration status; avoid overhydration
- Monitor urine output during and after IV fluid administration; anuria can indicate renal function deterioration
- Monitor respiration since hyperosmolality can lead to respiratory depression

PREVENTION/AVOIDANCE
N/A

POSSIBLE COMPLICATIONS
Altered consciousness and abnormal behavior.

EXPECTED COURSE AND PROGNOSIS
Dependent on the underlying cause.

MISCELLANEOUS

ASSOCIATED CONDITIONS
- Perinatal asphyxia (treated with mannitol)
- Azotemia
- Hyperglycemia
- Hypernatremia

AGE-RELATED FACTORS
N/A

ZOONOTIC POTENTIAL
N/A

PREGNANCY/FERTILITY/BREEDING
N/A

SYNONYMS
Hyperosmolarity in the ECF, since osmolality and osmolarity are approximately the same in the ECF.

SEE ALSO
- Equine metabolic syndrome (EMS)/insulin resistance (IR)
- Glucose, hyperglycemia
- Pituitary pars intermedia dysfunction
- Sodium, hypernatremia

ABBREVIATIONS
- ADH = antidiuretic hormone
- BUN = blood urea nitrogen
- ECF = extracellular fluid
- GI = gastrointestinal
- ICF = intracellular fluid

Internet Resources
Cornell University College of Veterinary Medicine, Osmolality. http://www.eclinpath.com/search/osmolality

Suggested Reading
George JW, Zabolotzky SM. Water, electrolytes, and acid base. In: Latimer KS, ed. Duncan & Prasse's Veterinary Laboratory Medicine Clinical Pathology, 5e. Hoboken, NJ: Wiley Blackwell, 2011:146–147.
Jose-Cunilleras E. Abnormalities of body fluids and electrolytes in athletic horses. In: Hinchcliff KW, Kaneps AJ, Geor RJ, eds. Equine Sports Medicine and Surgery, 2e. Edinburgh, UK: Saunders, 2013:881–885.

Author Claire B. Andreasen
Consulting Editor Sandra D. Taylor

BASICS

DEFINITION
Progressive physical and biochemical damage to articular cartilage and subchondral bone accompanied by nonseptic inflammation of the synovial membrane and joint capsule.

PATHOPHYSIOLOGY
• Abnormal forces, such as repetitive trauma, overwhelm the normal metabolic repair functions of the joint, leading to a net cartilage matrix loss and chondromalacia. Unchecked, this cycle creates further damage and loss of viscoelastic properties of the remaining cartilage
• Capsulitis and synovitis result from biomechanical damage and are often part of the disease process of OA. The inflamed synovium contributes many inflammatory mediators and degradative enzymes (prostaglandins such as prostaglandin E_2, cytokines such as interleukin 1, and matrix-degrading enzymes such as matrix metalloproteinases). The viscous shock-absorbing and lubricating synovial fluid, rich in hyaluronan, loses viscosity in this inflammatory milieu, reducing its protective abilities
• The subchondral bone plate provides shock absorption. It remodels and becomes less compliant if repetitive trauma overwhelms its ability to heal microdamage normally. Remodeled stiffer subchondral bone offers less shock absorption to articular cartilage, further traumatizing it
• In addition to cartilage thinning and joint capsule thickening, joint changes occur. Capsulitis can result in enthesophyte formation. Osteophytes are formed at the articular cartilage margins. These fibrocartilage-covered bony outgrowths can fracture, becoming osteochondral fragments (chip fractures). Loose articular fragments can increases the inflammatory process within the joint

SYSTEMS AFFECTED
Musculoskeletal—diarthrodial joints.

GENETICS
None elucidated.

INCIDENCE/PREVALENCE
Undefined lameness to joint disease is the most significant factor responsible for loss of racehorses' performance.

GEOGRAPHIC DISTRIBUTION
N/A

SIGNALMENT
• Athletic horses
• Repetitive training that overwhelms repair mechanisms, e.g. race training
• All ages and both sexes

SIGNS
General Comments
The hallmark of OA is articular cartilage degeneration, a process occurring in a tissue devoid of innervation. Lameness is attributed to the involvement of periarticular soft tissue structures. Pain originating from subchondral bone changes is controversial.

Historical Findings
• Intra-articular fractures, previous septic arthritis, osteochondrosis, dislocation, or ligamentous damage are predisposing factors
• Insidious OA-related lameness in low-motion joints (distal intertarsal, tarsometatarsal joints) possible. High-motion joints (fetlock) more likely to have acute-onset lameness
• Lameness may decrease after rest period

Physical Examination Findings
• Variable lameness (mild lameness during exercise to lameness at walk)
• Lameness is rarely acute and severe in onset
• Pain on flexion
• Synovial effusion in high-motion joints
• Acute synovitis, heat
• Chronic OA joints—thickened joint capsule, reduced range of motion, ± crepitation, grossly thickened, ± palpable bony abnormalities

CAUSES
Exact cause is unknown. It is a combination of traumatic events that involve the soft tissue, bone, and cartilage of diarthrodial joints.

RISK FACTORS
• Abnormal limb conformation that increases joint stress, collateral ligament strain, or weight-bearing (e.g. carpal varus, flexural tendon laxity, "back-at-the-knees")
• Intense high-speed and/or repetitive training

DIAGNOSIS

DIFFERENTIAL DIAGNOSIS
• Septic arthritis—ruled out with synovial fluid analysis
• Young horses with joint effusion, osteochondrosis—ruled out with radiography

CBC/BIOCHEMISTRY/URINALYSIS
For research purposes, urine excretion of various "joint markers." Clinical application uncertain.

OTHER LABORATORY TESTS
Joint viscosity may be reduced.

IMAGING
• Radiology—mainstay of diagnosis. Good quality, standard 4 views per joint, ± other views (flexed lateral, "skyline")
• Radiographic changes include:
  ◦ Narrowing or loss of joint space
  ◦ Osteophyte formation or fragmentation
  ◦ Periosteal bone proliferation
  ◦ Subchondral bone sclerosis
  ◦ Ankylosis possible
  ◦ Osteolysis in distal intertarsal or tarsometatarsal joints
  ◦ ± Additional diagnostics to determine clinical significance of radiologic OA
• Nuclear scintigraphy—increased radiopharmaceutical uptake of joint and/or subchondral bone. Assesses metabolically active OA. Diagnostic of choice for subchondral bone changes
• Diagnostic arthroscopy—direct visualization of joint, articular cartilage
• MRI—pathologic changes in articular cartilage, subchondral bone, and periarticular soft tissue structures. High-field magnets preferred for cartilage assessment

OTHER DIAGNOSTIC PROCEDURES
Perineural and/or intra-articular anesthesia to localize joint pain causing lameness.

PATHOLOGIC FINDINGS
• Articular cartilage thinning, erosion, fibrillation, and scoring
• Osteophyte and enthesophyte formation
• Reduced synovial fluid viscosity
• Subchondral bone sclerosis

TREATMENT

AIMS
Reduce joint inflammation and facilitate restoration of joint homeostasis.

APPROPRIATE HEALTH CARE
• Mainstay of treatment is early recognition and medical management
• Numerous medications and combinations of medications are used. Decisions regarding treatment are multifactorial (specific joint, stage of OA, performance type, treatment costs, response to therapy, competition regulations regarding medications)
• Cartilage resurfacing techniques are in advanced experimental stages and are available at certain university teaching hospitals for clinical cases. They may play a role in OA management in the future

NURSING CARE
• Local cryotherapy (ice, cold water) during acute inflammation and joint swelling
• Postoperatively—passive motion (flexion) may be used

ACTIVITY
• Reduce activity
• In well-trained horses, swimming (maintains cardiovascular fitness while sparing the joints). This is not a substitute and should be carefully considered and integrated into a horse's program by experienced professionals.

DIET
Diets for prevention of osteochondrosis, a predisposing factor for OA.

CLIENT EDUCATION

Condition is progress. Periodic lameness, performance assessment after diagnosis. Judicious use of intra-articular corticosteroids.

SURGICAL CONSIDERATIONS

• Arthroscopy—visualization of joint, osteochondral fragment(s) removal, removal of damaged cartilage, subchondral bone forage
• In end-stage OA, surgical arthrodesis

MEDICATIONS

DRUG(S) OF CHOICE

• Systemic NSAIDs—phenylbutazone (2.2 mg/kg every 12–24 h) or flunixin meglumine (0.5 mg/kg every 12–24 h). Daily oral phenylbutazone can be used long term. Side effects include gastric ulceration, right dorsal colitis, and renal papillary necrosis
• Intra-articular HA—10–20 mg of high molecular weight (>1×10^6 Daltons)
• IV HA—40 mg daily every 14–28 days, as needed
• Polysulfated glycosaminoglycan (500 mg IM every 4 days for 7 treatments) or sodium hyaluronate (40 mg IV every 7 days for 3 treatments)
• Intra-articular corticosteroids—methylprednisolone acetate (20–60 mg/joint), triamcinolone (3–18 mg/joint), betamethasone sulfate (3–18 mg/joint). They are powerful anti-inflammatory agents but have dose-dependent deleterious effects on articular cartilage. Judicial use recommended. In high-motion joints, short- to medium-acting drug (betamethasone, triamcinolone). In low-motion joints, longer acting drug (methylprednisolone acetate)
• Corticosteroids and HA are often injected intra-articularly simultaneously
• Autologous conditioned serum (or interleukin receptor antagonist protein)—3–6 mL/joint every 7 days for 3 or 4 treatments

CONTRAINDICATIONS

• Do not use NSAIDs in dehydrated horses
• In horses with laminitis, intra-articular corticosteroids may exacerbate laminitis

PRECAUTIONS

• Strict aseptic technique should be used for all joint injections
• ± 125 mg of amikacin sulfate added with intra-articular injection(s)
• Patient sedation and adequate restraint are critical for successful injection
• NSAID therapy and rest after joint injection
• ± Joints are bandaged after intra-articular medication
• Frequent, repeated use of intra-articular corticosteroid(s) can cause cartilage damage

ALTERNATIVE DRUGS

Oral nutraceuticals that contain chondroitin sulfate and glucosamine are marketed. There is limited to no objective evidence to suggest efficacy for equine OA.

FOLLOW-UP

PATIENT MONITORING

• After intra-articular injection, monitor for increased lameness, joint inflammation, and/or joint sepsis
• Periodic lameness and radiographic evaluations to assess progression of OA

POSSIBLE COMPLICATIONS

• "Joint flare" (transient joint inflammation and effusion) after intra-articular injections should be distinguished from iatrogenic joint sepsis and treated with ice and NSAID therapy. The use of high-quality HA can reduce this chance
• Corticosteroids can cause laminitis
• Do not use compounded products intra-articularly

EXPECTED COURSE AND PROGNOSIS

• In general, OA is progressive. Continued exercise, athletics, intra-articular corticosteroids exacerbate disease
• Prognosis is extremely variable and depends on the location and severity of OA, use of the horse, and duration of clinical signs. Mild OA in low-motion joint(s)—with therapy, good athletic prognosis for years. Severe OA in high-motion joint(s)—poor prognosis for athletics, ± arthrodesis for breeding and/or retirement

MISCELLANEOUS

ASSOCIATED CONDITIONS
N/A

ZOONOTIC POTENTIAL
None

PREGNANCY/FERTILITY/BREEDING
N/A

SYNONYMS
• Osteoarthrosis
• Degenerative joint disease
• Arthritis

SEE ALSO
• Infectious arthritis (nonhematogenous)
• Osteochondrosis

ABBREVIATIONS
• HA = hyaluronic acid
• MRI = magnetic resonance imaging
• NSAID = nonsteroidal anti-inflammatory drug
• OA = osteoarthritis

Suggested Reading
Caron JP. Osteoarthritis. In: Ross MW, Dyson SJ, eds. Diagnosis and Management of Lameness in the Horse, 2e. St. Louis, MO: Elsevier Saunders, 2011:655–667.
Frisbie DD. Synovial joint biology and pathobiology. In: Auer JA, Stick JA, eds. Equine Surgery, 4e. St. Louis, MO: WB Saunders, 2012:1096–1113.
McIlwraith CW. Traumatic arthritis and posttraumatic osteoarthritis in the horse. In: McIlwraith CW, Frisbie DD, Kawcak CP, van Weeren PR, eds. Joint Disease in the Horse, 2e. St. Louis, MO: Elsevier, 2016:33–48.

Author José M. García-López
Consulting Editor Elizabeth J. Davidson
Acknowledgment The author and editor acknowledge the prior contribution of Emma Adam.

BASICS

DEFINITION
- Developmental disorder of bone and cartilage of unspecified etiology resulting in failure of endochondral ossification
- The term *osteochondritis dissecans* or OCD is generally reserved for a detachment or "flap" of abnormal cartilage, or cartilage and bone, from the surrounding tissue. Some SBCs are also considered to be of OCD origin

PATHOPHYSIOLOGY
- Failure of normal endochondral ossification results in thickening and retention of the hypertrophic zone of the growth cartilage. When this affects articular–epiphyseal cartilage, the disorder manifests as a flap or fragment(s) of cartilage or cartilage and bone (OCD), or defective cartilage infolding and formation of periarticular SBCs
- These lesions may be precipitated by abnormal chondrocyte structure or function, abnormal extracellular matrix production, or a vascular disorder
- What determines whether osteochondrosis results in the development of OCD or SBC is not fully understood. High-motion areas may subject the articular surface to shear forces predisposing to OCD, whereas SBCs tend to be located in areas of maximal compressive loads (i.e. maximal weight-bearing)
- Trauma leading to subchondral bone microfracture and necrosis, followed by cystic resorption and collapse of overlying articular cartilage, may also be part of the pathogenesis of SBCs
- Full-thickness articular cartilage defects at the points of maximal weight-bearing can lead to SBC development

SYSTEMS AFFECTED
Musculoskeletal—epiphyseal cartilage and bone.

GENETICS
- Certain genetic lines have high heritability
- Specific genetic defect responsible for endochondral ossification alteration not identified
- In Scandinavian Standardbreds, tarsocrural osteochondrosis heritability ranges from 0.24 to 0.52

INCIDENCE/PREVALENCE
Unknown

GEOGRAPHIC DISTRIBUTION
Worldwide

SIGNALMENT
Breed Predilections
Any breed, common in Standardbreds, Thoroughbreds, and Warmbloods.

Mean Age and Range
Yearlings or weanlings (range neonates to 3 years of age) most common, although it can occur at any time during bone development.

Predominant Sex
None

SIGNS
General Comments
- Depends on location, variable clinical signs, and physical examination findings
- Frequently bilateral with reported incidences between 45% and 60%
- Type and location of osteochondrosis:
  ○ Tarsus (tarsocrural joint)—cranial distal intermediate ridge of tibia, lateral trochlear ridge of talus, medial malleolus of tibia, lateral malleolus of tibia, medial trochlear ridge of the talus
  ○ Stifle—lateral trochlear ridge of femur, medial distal femoral condyle (SBC)
  ○ Fetlock—distal dorsal sagittal ridge of MCIII/MTIII, proximal palmar/plantar eminence of P1, proximal dorsal P1, distal MCIII/MTIII (SBC)
  ○ Shoulder—humeral head (OCD or SBC), distal scapula (SBC)
  ○ Other locations include proximal and distal P1, proximal and distal P2, proximal and distal radius, distal humerus, and distal tibia. These are infrequent and usually SBCs
  ○ OCD also affects the cervical vertebral articular facets, recognized cause of cervical vertebral instability or stenosis ("wobbler syndrome")

Historical Findings
Variable findings depending on location; classically joint effusion without lameness.

Physical Examination Findings
- Variable findings depending on location
- Joint effusion without lameness
- SBCs more likely to cause lameness

CAUSES
Complex, multifactorial etiology that is incompletely understood. Several factors have a direct effect on its development.

Growth Rate
Rapid growth rate.

Dietary Factors
- High carbohydrate load
- Extremely low copper or excessive zinc levels
- ± Overfeeding phosphorus and calcium

Genetics
- Specific genetic defect responsible for alteration of endochondral ossification has not yet been identified, although highly suspected in certain breeding lines
- Heritability of a predisposition for fast growth and larger skeletal size might be the most important factor

Trauma
- Trauma in susceptible cartilage
- Time-dependent window of vulnerability to trauma for growth cartilages in specific locations

RISK FACTORS
See Causes.

 DIAGNOSIS

DIFFERENTIAL DIAGNOSIS
- Nonseptic synovitis—rule out with radiography
- Septic synovitis—rule out with radiography, synovial fluid analysis
- Osteomyelitis—rule out with serial radiography, culture
- Traumatic fracture—rule out with radiography, histology

IMAGING
Radiography
- Best modality for diagnosis
- Subchondral radiolucency along articular margin(s)
- Osseous fragment(s) separated from subchondral bone by a radiolucent area
- SBC—round subchondral radiolucency, often articular
- Important to image contralateral joint

Nuclear Scintigraphy
SBC—increased radiopharmaceutical uptake; OCD flaps—often normal.

CT/MRI
Occult SBC identification.

Ultrasonography
Loss of normal cartilaginous contour, ± at sites difficult to radiograph (cervical articular facet joint).

OTHER DIAGNOSTIC PROCEDURES
Synovial fluid analysis and culture—differentiate from septic arthritis.

PATHOLOGIC FINDINGS
Histology—chondrocytes in mid-to-late hypertrophic zone, with failure of vascular invasion and subsequent osteogenesis resulting in retained cartilage cores.

 TREATMENT

AIMS
- Reduce or eliminate joint effusion
- Avoid the development of or reduce or eliminate lameness
- Eliminate lesion as part of presale

APPROPRIATE HEALTH CARE
- No treatment if an incidental finding or without active clinical signs
- In young animals (foals, weanlings), conservative management via exercise restriction, anti-inflammatory(s), IM polysulfated glycosaminoglycans and diet modification for 6–10 months can be useful

NURSING CARE
Postoperative care—surgical incisions are kept clean and bandaged until suture removal 10–14 days after surgery. Bandages replaced daily and incisions inspected every 2–3 days

O

OSTEOCHONDROSIS

or more often if wet, soiled, or dislodged. In areas where bandaging is not possible, the incisions are maintained covered with adhesive iodinated dressings.

ACTIVITY
Restricted activity for conservative treatment and/or after surgery—stall confinement and controlled exercise program. Duration depends on severity and/or location of the lesion. In general, 2 weeks of strict stall rest followed by 4–8 weeks of stall rest with daily walking. Then, limited turnout in a small paddock for 4–6 weeks followed by another 4–6 weeks of regular paddock turnout. SBCs may require 6–12 months of restricted activity before resuming training.

DIET
- Do not overfeed foals and yearlings; prevent excessive energy (carbohydrate/protein) in dominant individuals
- In young horses (weanlings to 2 years of age) that are at risk of developing osteochondrosis, decrease or eliminate high-energy hay (alfalfa) and high-energy concentrate
- Mild to moderate caloric reduction of intake while stall confined or resting

CLIENT EDUCATION
- Avoid high-energy feeds
- Monitor sires and mares suspected of yielding offspring with osteochondrosis
- Any young horse with persistent joint effusion should be evaluated, including radiography. Early identification and treatment of OCD and SBC can be successful in maintaining the horse's athletic ability. If left unrecognized, secondary osteoarthritis and lameness may develop

SURGICAL CONSIDERATIONS
- OCD(s)—arthroscopic removal, debridement
- SBC(s)—arthroscopic debridement, mosaicplasty, intralesional corticosteroids, osteostixis (forage), intralesional/intra-articular therapy (stem cells, platelet-rich plasma, bone marrow aspirate concentrate, bone graft), transcortical screw

MEDICATIONS

DRUG(S) OF CHOICE
- NSAIDs—phenylbutazone (2.2–4.4 mg/kg PO or IV every 12–24 h) or flunixin meglumine (1.1 mg/kg PO or IV every 12–24 h) for medical management or after surgery
- For SBCs, intralesional corticosteroids—methylprednisolone acetate (40–80 mg) or triamcinolone (6–12 mg)

CONTRAINDICATIONS
In immature horses, fluoroquinolones contraindicated.

PRECAUTIONS
Monitor NSAID toxicity with long-term or young patient use.

FOLLOW-UP

PATIENT MONITORING
Radiographic Evaluation
Objective assessment and progression; 6–8 weeks for conservative therapy, 2 and 6 months after surgery.

Lameness Examination
- For conservative treatment, monthly evaluation
- For surgery, prior to controlled exercise then 3–12 months

PREVENTION/AVOIDANCE
- Diet restriction in young horses at risk
- Caution when selecting for certain breeding lines

POSSIBLE COMPLICATIONS
- Lameness
- Osteoarthritis
- ± Negatively affect sale

EXPECTED COURSE AND PROGNOSIS
- Clinical signs noted in 1–3-year-olds
- In general, arthroscopic removal of OCD(s) is favorable
- SBCs are less favorable prognosis and more likely to develop arthritis with or without treatment
- Joint effusion improves but may not resolve postoperatively
- Prognosis depends on lesion location and type:
  ○ Tarsus—favorable, large lateral trochlear ridge OCD has less favorable racing prognosis
  ○ Stifle—lateral trochlear ridge OCD—fair to good, less favorable with extensive and/or bilateral disease. Medial femur SBC—fair to good prognosis with surgery, guarded for older horses, fair to guarded for conservative treatment (± intra-articular corticosteroids)
  ○ Fetlock—fair to good for racehorses, very good to excellent in nonracehorses. Palmar/plantar eminence P1 (good), sagittal ridge (fair to good), SBCs (guarded to fair)
  ○ Shoulder—guarded for athletic use ± surgical management

MISCELLANEOUS

ASSOCIATED CONDITIONS
- Osteoarthritis
- Cervical vertebral malformation

AGE-RELATED FACTORS
Clinical signs apparent in a young animal.

PREGNANCY/FERTILITY/BREEDING
None

SYNONYMS
- Osteochondritis
- Osteochondritis dissecans

SEE ALSO
- Cervical vertebral malformation
- Equine protozoal myeloencephalitis (EPM)
- Infectious arthritis (nonhematogenous)
- Osteoarthritis

ABBREVIATIONS
- CT = computed tomography
- MCIII = third metacarpal bone
- MRI = magnetic resonance imaging
- MTIII = third metatarsal bone
- OCD = osteochondrosis dissecans
- P = phalanx
- SBC = subchondral bone cyst

Suggested Reading
Douglas J. Pathogenesis of osteochondrosis. In: Ross MW, Dyson SJ, eds. Diagnosis and Management of Lameness in the Horse, 2e. St. Louis, MO: Elsevier Saunders, 2011:617–624.
van Weeren PR. Osteochondrosis. In: Auer JA, Stick JA, eds. Equine Surgery, 4e. St. Louis, MO: WB Saunders, 2012:1239–1254.
van Weeren PR. Osteochondritis dissecans. In: McIlwraith CW, Frisbie DD, Kawcak CP, van Weeren PR, eds. Joint Disease in the Horse, 2e. St. Louis, MO: Elsevier, 2016:57–84.
Von Rechenberg B, Auer JA. Subchondral cystic lesions. In: Auer JA, Stick JA, eds. Equine Surgery, 4e. St. Louis, MO: WB Saunders, 2012:1255–1263.

Author José M. García-López
Consulting Editor Elizabeth J. Davidson

O

OVULATION FAILURE

BASICS

DEFINITION
The failure of a mature, dominant follicle to ovulate in the estrus mare.

Pathophysiology
• Normal development of 1 or 2 mature follicles during estrus
• Follicular estradiol initiates the LH surge that stimulates prostaglandin production required for ovulation
• Ovulation failure results when the follicle(s) fails to respond to the LH surge. The follicle(s) continues to enlarge, the antrum becomes hemorrhagic, and granulosa cells luteinize
• Such follicles are called HAFs, luteinized unruptured follicles, or autumn (fall) follicles

Systems Affected
Reproductive

Incidence/Prevalence
HAFs occur in both the transitional and ovulatory seasons. Incidence in the range 5–20%.

SIGNALMENT
Any breed and age.

SIGNS

Historical Findings
• Mares appear to exit estrus normally
• May result in enlarged ovarian structures causing pain on palpation, under saddle, or mild colic

Physical Examination Findings
• TRP and US—failure to ovulate. Follicle may regress or enlarge to form a HAF
• Failure to respond to ovulation induction with either deslorelin or human chorionic gonadotropin. If the mare ovulates normally in the ensuing days, this is considered failure of induction of ovulation, rather than ovulation failure.

CAUSES

HAFs
• Causes unknown and spontaneous cases cannot be predicted
• HAF is diagnosed as a dominant follicle in estrus that fails to ovulate, develops intrafollicular hemorrhage, and undergoes remodeling and luteinization over time
• Can be induced by administration of high doses of COX inhibitors and debatably by shortening diestrus with PGF$_{2\alpha}$

Luteinized Follicles
In the pregnant mare, eCG causes luteinization of all large follicles, forming accessory CL. In mares that undergo EED after 35 days of gestation, eCG will continue this effect for up to 150 days post ovulation. Mares will appear to enter estrus, the CL will form, but ovulation will not occur.

RISK FACTORS
• Administration of high doses of COX inhibitors in estrus
• Seasonality (particularly fall)

DIAGNOSIS

DIFFERENTIAL DIAGNOSIS

Differentiating Similar Signs
Mild colic signs from other causes.

Differentiating Causes
• Reproductive records should be reviewed
• The mare should be examined by TRP and US

LABORATORY TESTS
• Serum progesterone—concentrations >1 ng/mL indicate functional luteal tissue
• Serum eCG—positive assay can determine if EED occurred after endometrial cup formation

IMAGING
Transrectal US is standard of care for reproductive examinations.

TREATMENT
No treatment if related to seasonality.

MEDICATIONS

DRUG(S) OF CHOICE
PGF$_{2\alpha}$ (Lutalyse 10 mg IM) or its analogs (cloprostenol 250 µg IM) to induce luteolysis after sufficient luteinization of HAF.

CONTRAINDICATIONS
PGF$_{2\alpha}$ and its analogs are contraindicated in mares with equine asthma and other bronchoconstrictive disease.

PRECAUTIONS
• Horses
  ○ PGF$_{2\alpha}$ causes sweating/colic-like symptoms due to stimulation of smooth muscle. Institute symptomatic treatment if not resolved in 1–2 h
• Humans
  ○ PGF$_{2\alpha}$ should not be handled by pregnant women, or persons with asthma/bronchial disease. Any skin exposure should be washed off immediately

ALTERNATIVE DRUGS
Cloprostenol sodium (Estrumate; 250 µg/mL IM) is a PGF$_{2\alpha}$ analog. Associated with fewer side effects than natural PGF$_2$. Not currently approved for use in horses.

FOLLOW-UP

PATIENT MONITORING
Mares intended for breeding should be monitored by serial TRP and US.

POSSIBLE COMPLICATIONS
Individual mares may develop more than 1 HAF in a season.

MISCELLANEOUS

ASSOCIATED CONDITIONS
Infertility if bred on that cycle.

PREGNANCY/FERTILITY/BREEDING
PGF$_{2\alpha}$ administration to pregnant mares can cause luteolysis and abortion.

SYNONYMS
• Hemorrhagic anovulatory follicles
• Luteinized unruptured follicles
• Autumn follicles

SEE ALSO
• Abnormal estrus intervals
• Anestrus
• Large ovary syndrome

ABBREVIATIONS
• CL = corpus luteum, corpora lutea
• COX = cyclooxygenase
• eCG = equine chorionic gonadotropin
• EED = early embryonic death
• HAF = hemorrhagic anovulatory follicle
• LH = luteinizing hormone
• PGF$_{2\alpha}$ = prostaglandin F$_2$ alpha
• TRP = transrectal palpation
• US = ultrasonography, ultrasound

Suggested Reading
Cuervo-Arango J. The effect of treatment with flunixin meglumine at different times relative to hCG administration on ovulation failure and luteal function in mares. Anim Reprod Sci 2011;127:84–90.

Ginter OJ, Gastal EL, Gastal MO, et al. Incidence, endocrinology, vascularity, and morphology of hemorrhagic anovulatory follicles in mares. J Equine Vet Sci 2007;27:130–139.

Martinez-Bovi R, Cuervo-Arango J. Intrafollicular treatment with prostaglandins PGE$_2$ and PGF$_{2\alpha}$ inhibits the formation of luteinized unruptured follicles and restores normal ovulation in mares treated with flunixin-meglumine. Equine Vet J 2016;48:211–217.

Author Lisa K. Pearson
Consulting Editor Carla L. Carleton
Acknowledgment The author and editor acknowledge the prior contribution of Carole C. Miller.

O

PANCREATIC DISEASE

BASICS

OVERVIEW
• Clinical pancreatic disease is rarely recognized in the horse
• Disorders—inflammatory disease, chronic eosinophilic pancreatitis, endocrine or exocrine insufficiency, neoplasia
• Acute and chronic pancreatic disease reported
• Fibrosis induced by parasitic migration of *Strongylus equinus* probably most common cause
• Aberrant migration of *Strongylus edentatus, Strongylus vulgaris,* and *Parascaris equorum* may also occur
• Pancreatitis reported in cholelithiasis
• DM rare in the horse. Most cases secondary to a demonstrable cause of insulin resistance, such as elevated concentrations of hormones, which antagonize the action of insulin. Most common etiology for secondary DM is induced by PPID. Insulin-dependent DM, far less common in the horse, has been reported secondary to pancreatic fibrosis

SIGNALMENT
• No breed, or sex predisposition
• Most common in adult horses. Few reports in foals
• Pancreatic neoplasia reported in aged horses and donkeys (>11 years)

SIGNS
Nonspecific signs.
• Signs of acute pancreatitis may include:
  ◦ Abdominal pain (moderate to severe)
  ◦ Gastric reflux
  ◦ Hypovolemic shock
  ◦ Cardiovascular compromise (tachycardia, prolonged capillary refill time, congested mucous membranes)
• Signs of chronic pancreatitis may include:
  ◦ Anorexia
  ◦ Weight loss
  ◦ Mild to recurrent colic
  ◦ Icterus, ± fever
• Signs of DM may include:
  ◦ Polyuria, polydipsia
  ◦ Weight loss despite polyphagia
  ◦ Rough hair coat
• Signs of pancreatic neoplasia may include:
  ◦ Weight loss
  ◦ Pyrexia
  ◦ Depression
  ◦ Lethargy
  ◦ Icterus
  ◦ Ascites
  ◦ Per rectum abdominal palpation—may be able to palpate neoplastic pancreas/masses

CAUSES AND RISK FACTORS
Parasitic migration (*S. equinus, S. edentatus, S. vulgaris, P. equorum*); duodenal ileus and ascending bacterial infection of pancreas; hematogenous bacterial infection; viral infections; immune-mediated disease; pancreatic hypoperfusion from cardiovascular compromise; biliary or pancreatic duct inflammation; vitamin A and E deficiency, selenium and methionine deficiency, and vitamin D toxicity; pancreatic neoplasia.

DIAGNOSIS

DIFFERENTIAL DIAGNOSIS
• Intra-abdominal abscessation
• Neoplasia

CBC/BIOCHEMISTRY/URINALYSIS
No specific abnormalities, making diagnosis difficult.
• Elevated serum amylase (normal 5–50 U/L)
• Elevated serum lipase (normal 40–80 U/L)
• Elevated plasma trypsin (normal 28.5 ± 19.2 ng/mL)
• Elevated peritoneal fluid amylase (normal <14 U/L)
• Persistent hyperglycemia and glucosuria
• ± Elevated serum γ-glutamyltransferase
• Hyperfibrinogenemia (acute pancreatitis)

OTHER LABORATORY TESTS
• Resting plasma adrenocorticotropic hormone or α-melanocyte-stimulating hormone, or dexamethasone suppression test to rule out PPID
• Plasma insulin concentration—elevated in insulin resistance and reduced in insulin-dependent DM
• Oral glucose tolerance test
• Insulin-dependent (type 1) DM—increased blood glucose with normal insulin
• Insulin-resistance (type 2) DM—blood glucose remains elevated for a prolonged period of time after infusion, despite high blood insulin levels. Most common type of DM in horses and ponies is usually associated with PPID
• Abdominocentesis—cytology

IMAGING
• Abdominal US
• Laparoscopy of abdomen

OTHER DIAGNOSTIC PROCEDURES
US-guided biopsy of pancreas.

TREATMENT
• Symptomatic medical management
• Indwelling nasogastric tube

MEDICATIONS

DRUG(S) AND FLUIDS
Acute Pancreatitis
• IV balanced polyionic electrolyte fluids
• Analgesics (NSAIDs, e.g. flunixin meglumine 1.1 mg/kg IV every 24 h) or opiates (e.g. butorphanol 0.02 mg/kg IV every 4 h)
• Broad-spectrum antibiotics
• Plasma transfusion may be indicated
• Calcium-containing fluids

CONTRAINDICATIONS/POSSIBLE INTERACTIONS
N/A

FOLLOW-UP
• Monitor hydration, serum calcium
• Monitor abdominal pain
• Prognosis poor to grave for acute pancreatitis

MISCELLANEOUS

SEE ALSO
Acute adult Abdominal pain—Acute colic

ABBREVIATIONS
• DM = diabetes mellitus
• NSAID = nonsteroidal anti-inflammatory drug
• PPID = pituitary pars intermedia dysfunction
• US = ultrasonography, ultrasound

Suggested Reading
Johnson PJ, Wiedmeyer CE, Messer NT. Clinical conditions of the equine pancreas. Equine Vet Educ 2009;21:26–29.
Newman SJ. Equine pancreatic disease: a review and characterization of the lesions of four cases. J Vet Diagn Invest 2015;27:92–96.
Yamout SZ, Nieto JE, Anderson J, et al. Pathological evidence of pancreatitis in 43 horses (1986-2011). Equine Vet J Suppl 2012;43:45–50.

Author John D. Baird
Consulting Editors Henry Stämpfli and Olimpo Oliver-Espinosa

PANCYTOPENIA

BASICS

OVERVIEW
- Term used to describe concurrent decrease in circulating erythrocytes, leukocytes, and thrombocytes
- Rare in horses
- Usually associated with disrupted hematopoiesis due to either a failure of stem cells to undergo differentiation (aplastic anemia) or destruction of the bone marrow microenvironment by neoplastic, fibrous, or inflammatory diseases (myelophthisis)

SIGNALMENT
N/A

SIGNS
- Clinical signs reflect inadequate numbers of functional cells in blood or tissues and are usually nonspecific—weight loss, lethargy, poor performance, and intermittent pyrexia
- Onset is often insidious
- Hemorrhage due to thrombocytopenia—petechiae, epistaxis, mucosal bleeding, blood in feces, or prolonged bleeding from wounds
- Mucous membrane pallor, tachycardia, and systolic heart murmur with marked anemia
- Secondary infections due to leukopenia

CAUSES AND RISK FACTORS
- Aplastic anemia may be congenital or acquired and can result from intrinsic stem cell failure or disruption of stem cell interactions in the bone marrow. It is often idiopathic, but is rarely associated with administration of drugs (e.g. phenylbutazone, chloramphenicol, estrogens, trimethoprim, or pyrimethamine) or secondary to infectious disease (e.g. EIA virus or *Anaplasma phagocytophilum*)
- Myelophthisis has been associated with myelofibrosis, myelodysplasia, myeloproliferative disorders, or lymphoproliferative disorders

DIAGNOSIS

DIFFERENTIAL DIAGNOSIS
- See Causes and Risk Factors
- Hemorrhage from vasculitis or thrombocytopenia unassociated with bone marrow dysfunction
- Lethargy, pallor, petechiae, and edema may occur in piroplasmosis (*Babesia caballi* or *Theileria equi* infection)
- Familial megakaryocytic and myeloid hypoplasia in Standardbred horses
- Concurrent immune-mediated anemia and thrombocytopenia

CBC/BIOCHEMISTRY/URINALYSIS
- Anemia, thrombocytopenia, and leukopenia

- Leukopenia—primarily due to a neutropenia without a left shift
- Lymphocyte count may be normal
- Anemia occurs after other derangements due to longer lifespan of erythrocytes ($\approx$140 days) compared with thrombocytes ($\approx$5 days) and neutrophils ($\approx$12 h)
- Examination of blood smears for *A. phagocytophilum* morulae in neutrophils, erythrocyte parasites (*B. caballi, T. equi*), absence of platelets, or abnormal leukocytes in leukemia

OTHER LABORATORY TESTS
- Serology—*B. caballi, T. equi,* or *A. phagocytophilum*
- Coggins test—EIA
- Coombs test

IMAGING
- Radiography of the skeleton and thorax—multiple myeloma
- Abdominal and thoracic ultrasonography—lymphoproliferative disorders

OTHER DIAGNOSTIC PROCEDURES
- Bone marrow aspiration/biopsy
- Obtain from the sternum or proximal rib (adults) and sternum, rib, or tuber coxae (foals)
- Biopsies best for confirmation of bone marrow hypoplasia and myelofibrosis
- Normal myeloid to erythroid ratio is 0.5–1.5: <0.5 suggests a regenerative erythrocyte response or myeloid hypoplasia
- Urine protein electrophoresis for detection of Bence Jones proteins in multiple myeloma
- Serum protein electrophoresis—monoclonal gammopathy suggests lymphoproliferative neoplasia
- Immunophenotypic techniques for classification of leukemia

PATHOLOGIC FINDINGS
- Variable, dependent on the cause of pancytopenia
- Leukoproliferative disorders—neoplastic cells in bone marrow samples
- Myelofibrosis—replacement of bone marrow with fibrous tissue
- Aplastic anemia—hypocellularity and fat infiltration of bone marrow

TREATMENT
- Remove suspected causative medications
- Supportive care; avoid trauma, rest

MEDICATIONS

DRUG(S) OF CHOICE
- Immunosuppressive treatment (e.g. corticosteroids) if immune-mediated disease is present
- Antimicrobial therapy if secondary infections occur

- Blood or platelet-rich plasma transfusions provide only temporary improvement
- Androgens may stimulate erythropoiesis in remaining hematopoietic tissue
- No treatment for EIA exists
- Treatment for *A. phagocytophilum* (oxytetracycline) or piroplasmosis (imidocarb dipropionate)

CONTRAINDICATIONS/POSSIBLE INTERACTIONS
- Immune status may be compromised by corticosteroid treatment
- Imidocarb is potentially fatal in donkeys

FOLLOW-UP

PATIENT MONITORING
- Monitor for pyrexia, lethargy, pallor, hemorrhage
- Regular hematologic monitoring

PREVENTION/AVOIDANCE
N/A

POSSIBLE COMPLICATIONS
Hemorrhage, secondary infections.

EXPECTED COURSE AND PROGNOSIS
- Anaplastic anemia; unpredictable prognosis
- Myeloproliferative and lymphoproliferative disorders; hopeless prognosis

✓ MISCELLANEOUS

ASSOCIATED CONDITIONS
N/A

AGE-RELATED FACTORS
N/A

ZOONOTIC POTENTIAL
N/A

PREGNANCY/FERTILITY/BREEDING
N/A

SEE ALSO
- Anemia
- Equine granulocytic anaplasmosis
- Infectious anemia (EIA)
- Lymphosarcoma
- Multiple myeloma
- Myeloproliferative diseases
- Piroplasmosis

ABBREVIATIONS
EIA = equine infectious anemia

Suggested Reading
Sellon DC, Wise LN. Disorders of the hematopoietic system. In: Reed SM, Bayly WM, Sellon DC, eds. Equine Internal Medicine, 3e. St. Louis, MO: WB Saunders, 2010:730–776.

Author Kristopher Hughes
Consulting Editors David Hodgson, Harold C. McKenzie, and Jennifer L. Hodgson

P

PANICUM COLORATUM (KLEINGRASS) TOXICOSIS

BASICS

OVERVIEW
• *Panicum coloratum* (kleingrass, kleingrass 75) is a tufted, perennial grass with stems usually 60–135 cm in height from a firm, knotty base
• The blades are elongate, 2–8 mm in width, smooth or stiff, with bristly hairs on 1 or both surfaces
• Loosely branched, pyramidal flower clusters are mostly 8–25 cm in length, with spikelets on spreading branches; the spikelets are 2.8–3.2 mm in length and smooth
• The rootstock is hearty and easily develops rhizomes
• *Panicum* spp. grow in Australia, New Zealand, South Africa, South America, Afghanistan, India, and Texas. In Texas, they reach from the high plains to Edward's Plateau and the Trans-Pecos area
• *Panicum* spp. were introduced into the USA from South Africa during the 1950s; *P. coloratum* was developed by Texas A & M University during the early 1970s and prefers improved pastures
• Some native species found outside the USA generally are not toxic
• The toxin is a saponin (saponins are composed of sapogenins and a sugar moiety) that is probably the same as that found in *Tribulus, Nolina,* and *Agave* spp.
• Horses have developed liver disease while grazing kleingrass or eating kleingrass hay, but they have not developed photosensitization

SIGNALMENT
No known breed, sex, or age predispositions.

SIGNS
• Horses develop liver disease and become icteric
• Anorexia and weight loss
• Horses tend not to develop secondary or hepatogenous photosensitization, although hepatoencephalopathy with head pressing and violent behavior may occur

CAUSES AND RISK FACTORS
N/A

DIAGNOSIS

DIFFERENTIAL DIAGNOSIS
• History of grazing kleingrass; compatible clinical signs

• Other hepatotoxins—aflatoxin (detection in feed and histopathology), PAs (ingestion of alkaloid-containing plants and histopathology), and iron toxicosis (tissue iron concentrations and histopathology)
• In addition to PA-containing plants, exposure to other hepatotoxic plants—*Nolina texana, Agave lechuguilla, Panicum* spp., and *Trifolium hybridum* (identification in animal's environment, evidence of consumption)
• Nontoxic differential—Theiler disease (history, histopathology)

CBC/BIOCHEMISTRY/URINALYSIS
• Horses on kleingrass have markedly high serum γ-glutamyltransferase activity, total and direct bilirubin, blood ammonia
• Sulfobromophthalein (or bromsulphalein) clearance times are slowed several-fold
• Serum sorbitol dehydrogenase, aspartate aminotransferase, and alkaline phosphatase activities are variable

OTHER LABORATORY TESTS
N/A

IMAGING
N/A

OTHER DIAGNOSTIC PROCEDURES
N/A

PATHOLOGIC FINDINGS
• Histopathologically, chronic hepatitis with varying degrees of fibrosis, which is dependent on the length of exposure
• Characteristic lesions—bridging hepatic fibrosis, cholangitis, and hepatocellular regeneration

TREATMENT
• Remove animals from the kleingrass pastures or hay
• Although horses have not shown photosensitization, shade may be helpful
• Symptomatic and supportive care

MEDICATIONS

DRUG(S) OF CHOICE
No specific therapeutic interventions.

CONTRAINDICATIONS/POSSIBLE INTERACTIONS
Impaired hepatic function may prolong clearance of drugs metabolized by the liver.

FOLLOW-UP

PATIENT MONITORING
Monitor hepatic function.

PREVENTION/AVOIDANCE
Do not allow horses to graze *Panicum* spp. or ingest hays containing the grass.

POSSIBLE COMPLICATIONS
• Photosensitization
• Photosensitization was noted in other *Panicum* spp., but not *P. coloratum*

EXPECTED COURSE AND PROGNOSIS
Onset of clinical signs is associated with significant hepatic fibrosis, making the long-term prognosis guarded to poor.

MISCELLANEOUS

ASSOCIATED CONDITIONS
N/A

AGE-RELATED FACTORS
N/A

ZOONOTIC POTENTIAL
N/A

PREGNANCY/FERTILITY/BREEDING
N/A

ABBREVIATIONS
PA = pyrrolizidine alkaloid

Suggested Reading
Burrows GE, Tyrl RJ. Toxic Plants of North America. Ames, IA: Iowa State University Press, 2001:913–915.
Cornick JL, Carter GK, Bridges CH. Kleingrass-associated hepatotoxicosis in horses. J Am Vet Med Assoc 1988;193:932–935.

Author Tam Garland
Consulting Editors Wilson K. Rumbeiha and Steve Ensley

 Client Education Handout available online

BASICS

OVERVIEW

• Papillomas commence as benign proliferative epithelial neoplasms associated with the presence of EcPV and may occasionally progress to malignancy
• Third most common cutaneous equine neoplasm and most common tumor in horses between 1 and 3 years of age
• 3 forms include papillomas/papillomatosis (warts) of the skin, genital, and aural plaque
• Systems affected—skin

SIGNALMENT

• Any age, but is more common in younger horses (<3 years of age). Congenital papillomas reported in a small number of neonatal foals; however, lack a definitive EcPV isolate
• No apparent breed or sex predisposition

SIGNS

• Muzzle and lips; however, also found on the eyelids, external genitalia, distal legs, and axilla
• Lesions may be solitary or multiple (up to 100); can cause problems because of physical location and esthetics
• Papillomas in any location, except of the ear, are 0.2–2 cm in diameter, 0.5 cm in height, broad-based to pedunculated, gray, pink or white; surface is hyperkeratotic with numerous frond-like projections. Solitary lesions can be larger

CAUSES AND RISK FACTORS

• 7 confirmed EcPVs have been isolated from various lesions and the presence of 1 or more types may occur within a lesion. A putative novel virus has recently been identified
• EcPV (a DNA papillomavirus)—penetrates stratified squamous or mucosal epithelium via trauma, which may or may not culminate in infection
• Transmitted by direct and indirect contact (e.g. biting insects, contaminated tack or buckets). Skin barrier breakage is needed for infection to be established
• Transmission of the virus from the dam to the foal may occur transplacentally (not proven) or inoculation of the skin may occur in the foal from infected sites on the dam during parturition

 DIAGNOSIS

DIFFERENTIAL DIAGNOSIS

• The appearance and distribution of the lesions are strongly suggestive of a diagnosis of papillomatosis
• Verrucose sarcoid (extensive areas are usually affected with markedly thickened skin around and evidence of hypotrichosis at the periphery of the lesion)
• Squamous cell carcinoma (especially facial, genital, and vulval proliferative forms)

DIAGNOSTIC PROCEDURES

• Biopsy and histopathologic examination to establish definitive diagnosis
• Immunohistochemistry to detect viral antigen within the lesion
• Electron microscopy—while not normally necessary to establish the diagnosis, hexagonal viral particles can be found in all forms of equine papillomatosis (except congenital form)

 TREATMENT

• Papillomas (warts) typically regress spontaneously within 1–9 months; therefore, treatment may not be necessary. If lesions persist, look for underlying cause of immunosuppression
• Surgical excision is the treatment of choice
• Cryosurgery is also effective
• Secondary infections may require treatment with topical antibacterial products (e.g. creams, gels, washes)
• Efficacy of autogenous vaccines is not proved

 MEDICATIONS

• Generalized papillomatosis—imiquimod 5% cream applied in a thin film to cover the surface of the lesion every 48 h until resolution; alternatively 5% acyclovir (aciclovir) ointment may be an option but no studies have evaluated the efficacy
• Anecdotal treatment with immunostimulatory agents have been used for persistent papillomatosis and include intralesional injections of interferon alpha or interleukin 2, cisplatin, and bacillus Calmette–Guérin

 FOLLOW-UP

PREVENTION/AVOIDANCE

• Papillomaviruses are resistant to freezing or desiccation; however, formalin, detergents, or high temperatures may decrease infectivity
• Avoid transmission of the virus among horses that are stabled or pastured together by isolation of affected horses and prevention of immunologically susceptible horses from entering the contaminated premise
• Preventing insect bites (e.g. repellent sprays) may decrease irritation in the affected horse and limit spread of the virus among horses
• Regular genital sanitation may prevent disease development as poor hygiene has been suggested as a promoter of genital carcinoma or induction of genital papillomatosis

EXPECTED COURSE AND PROGNOSIS

• Spontaneous regression of warts is common within 1–9 months
• Genital papillomas do not spontaneously resolve and may transform into squamous cell carcinoma
• Surgical excision—excellent prognosis and recurrence should not occur

 MISCELLANEOUS

ASSOCIATED CONDITIONS

Congenital papillomas are a cauliflower-like, flattened wart from 5 mm to 20 cm in diameter on the skin of a new foal. The lesions are usually single and located on the head, neck, or trunk.

ZOONOTIC POTENTIAL

None

PREGNANCY/FERTILITY/BREEDING

EcPV may be transmitted from an infected mare to the foal transplacentally (not proven) or from infected skin lesions on the mare to the foal during parturition.

SEE ALSO

• Aural plaques
• Sarcoid

ABBREVIATIONS

EcPV = *Equus caballus* papillomavirus

Author Gwendolen Lorch
Consulting Editor Gwendolen Lorch
Acknowledgment The author/editor acknowledges the prior contribution of Beverly Kidney.

P

PARAPHIMOSIS

BASICS

DEFINITION
Inability to retract the penis into the preputial cavity, often due to extensive penile and preputial edema.

PATHOPHYSIOLOGY
• Paraphimosis is often a complication of a primary traumatic injury, penile paralysis, or priapism
• Penile prolapse occurs initially and is complicated by excessive swelling and edema
• Vascular and lymphatic drainage are impeded, leading to further edema accumulation
• Drainage is further restricted by the swelling of the internal preputial lamina and stricture at the level of the preputial ring
• The exposed tissue may become excoriated and slough because of pressure necrosis
• Chronic prolapse may lead to penile/preputial trauma, balanoposthitis, or penile paralysis (damage to the internal pudendal nerves)

SYSTEMS AFFECTED
• Reproductive—prolapse of the penis and prepuce exposes them to trauma. Chronic paraphimosis may result in penile paralysis, fibrosis of the CCP, and an inability to achieve an erection
• Urologic—urethral obstruction may be the inciting cause of paraphimosis, or it may occur secondary to edema

SIGNALMENT
• Predominantly stallions, but geldings can also be affected
• No breed predilection
• Unlikely to occur in the first month of life, when normal adhesions exist between the free penis and inner lamina of the preputial fold

SIGNS

Historical Findings
• Acute cases often present as traumatic injury to the penile or preputial area
• Chronic cases—delay in presentation for veterinary care may occur if owners believed an injury was minor and attempted care themselves or the injury may only recently have become obvious because of its slow increase in size, e.g. a slow developing enlargement of the penis or preputial area such as is seen with *Habronema* spp. infections or neoplastic growths

Physical Examination Findings
• Prolapse of the penis and prepuce with severe penile enlargement is readily apparent. Caudoventral displacement of the glans penis is common. A careful visual and digital examination is necessary to properly define the nature of the injury
• Balanitis, posthitis, or balanoposthitis may be present. Serous or hemorrhagic discharges on the surface of the penis and prepuce are common. Lacerations, excoriations, ulcerative lesions, or neoplastic masses may be evident
• Hematomas, when present, are generally located on the dorsal surface of the penis and usually arise from blood vessels superficial to the tunica albuginea
• Transrectal palpation may reveal an enlarged urinary bladder indicative of urethral blockage
• Chronic prolapse may result in penile paralysis

CAUSES

Noninfectious Causes
• Trauma—breeding injuries, fighting or kicks, improperly fitting stallion rings, falls, movement through brush or heavy ground cover, whips, or abuse
• Priapism, penile paralysis, posthitis, or balanoposthitis
• Postsurgical complication—castration or cryptorchid surgery
• Neoplasia of the penis or prepuce—sarcoids, squamous cell carcinoma, melanoma, mastocytoma, hemangioma, or papillomas
• Debilitation or starvation
• Spinal injury or myelitis
• Urolithiasis/urinary tract obstruction

Infectious Causes
• Bacterial—*Staphylococcus, Streptococcus*
• Viral—EHV-1, EHV-3, EIA, EVA
• Purpura haemorrhagica—vasculitis as a sequela to infection or vaccine administration
• Parasitic—*Habronema muscae, Habronema microstoma, Draschia megastoma, Onchocerca* spp., *Cochliomyia hominivorax* (screw worm)
• Fungal—phycomycosis due to *Hyphomyces destruens*
• Protozoal—*Trypanosoma equiperdum* (dourine)

RISK FACTORS
• Use of phenothiazine tranquilizers in stallions
• Increased risk during transport
• Open-range/pasture breeding, not in-hand, stud management
• More aggressive stallions
• Poor management, unsanitary conditions, or malnutrition

DIAGNOSIS

DIFFERENTIAL DIAGNOSIS
• History, clinical signs, and examination of the lesions may help identify the underlying cause
• Trauma—the presence of visible lacerations or hematomas, or a history of trauma, or surgical intervention
• The presence of ulcerative or proliferative lesions warrants investigation to determine if the origin of the lesion is neoplastic, parasitic, or infectious
• Systemic signs indicative of neurologic or systemic disease include ataxia, depression, lymph node enlargement, or increased rectal temperature

CBC/BIOCHEMISTRY/URINALYSIS
• Generally, there are no abnormal findings unless the causative factor is an infectious agent, neoplastic disease, or severe debilitation/starvation
• Urinalysis may indicate urolithiasis/cystitis

OTHER LABORATORY TESTS
• Bacterial causes—culture (swab) of affected tissues
• EHV-1—rising antibody titers (paired sera, collected at a 14–21 day interval); virus isolation from nasopharyngeal swabs and blood (buffy coat) during the acute stage
• EHV-3—rising antibody titer (paired sera, collected at a 14–21 day interval); eosinophilic intranuclear inclusion bodies in cytologic smears; virus isolation from lesions during the acute stage
• EIA—agar gel immunodiffusion (Coggins) test
• EVA—rising antibody titer (paired sera collected at a 14–21 day interval); virus isolation from nasopharyngeal swabs
• Protozoal—identification of the causative agent in urethral exudates; serology—complement fixation

IMAGING
Ultrasonography findings are generally unrewarding. In other species, fibrosis of the CCP has been visualized in chronic cases.

OTHER DIAGNOSTIC PROCEDURES
Cytology or biopsy of masses or lesions may provide a diagnosis in the case of parasitic, neoplastic, or fungal disease.

TREATMENT
• The primary goals—reduce the inflammation and edema and return the penis to the prepuce to improve venous and lymphatic drainage. The initial management of the patient is intensive and may require hospitalization to allow adequate physical restraint and patient access
• Ensure urethral patency—catheterize or perform a perineal urethrostomy, if necessary
• Methods of manual reduction of the prolapse:
  ○ Elastic or pneumatic bandaging may reduce edema prior to attempting reduction
  ○ Preputiotomy if the preputial ring is preventing successful reduction
  ○ Purse-string suture of umbilical tape around the preputial orifice, tightened to a 1-finger opening, to hold the penis within the prepuce; has the additional benefit of maintaining pressure on the penis for sustained reduction of edema

(CONTINUED)

○ Additional support can be gained by putting on a net sling, which covers the cranial aspect of the prepuce but allows urine to drain
• In cases that are resistant to manual reduction, support remains of primary importance. Wrap the exposed penis and prepuce to reduce edema. Support in the form of a sling is essential. Nylon slings raise and maintain the penis close to the ventral belly wall. Using netting with small perforations allows urine to drain
• Hydrotherapy—cold hydrotherapy for the first 4–7 days until edema and hemorrhage subside, then warm hydrotherapy. Generally applied for 15–30 min BID–QID
• Massage the penis and prepuce BID–QID to reduce edema
• Topical emollient ointment application—vitamin A and D ointment, lanolin, petroleum jelly, nitrofurazone
• Exercise—confinement and limited activity until after active hemorrhage and edema subside, then slowly increase; aids in resolution of dependent edema
• No sexual stimulation in the early stages of therapy. It may be necessary to prevent exposure to mares for up to 4–8 weeks
• Local surgical resection, cryosurgery, or radiation therapy of neoplastic or granulomatous lesions, once the edema is resolved
• Chronic refractory paraphimosis may require surgical intervention, including circumcision (reefing or posthioplasty), penile retraction (Bolz technique), or penile amputation (phallectomy)

MEDICATIONS

DRUG(S) OF CHOICE
• NSAIDs, including phenylbutazone (2–4 g/450 kg/day PO) or flunixin meglumine (1 mg/kg/day IV, IM, or PO), for symptomatic relief and to reduce inflammation
• Systemic or local antibiotics as indicated to treat local infection and prevent septicemia
• Diuretics—furosemide (1 mg/kg IV daily or BID) if indicated in the acute phase for reduction of edema
• Specific topical or systemic treatments for parasitic, fungal, or neoplastic conditions as indicated by results of diagnostic testing

CONTRAINDICATIONS
• Tranquilizers, particularly the phenothiazine tranquilizers, should be avoided in males to avoid drug-induced priapism
• Nitrofurazone should not be used on horses intended for food
• Avoid sexual stimulation in the early stages and usually for 4–8 weeks after treatment for paraphimosis has begun

PRECAUTIONS
Diuretics are contraindicated if urinary obstruction is present. Their effectiveness in treating localized edema is in doubt.

POSSIBLE INTERACTIONS
N/A

ALTERNATIVE DRUGS
DMSO has been used topically (50:50 mixture by volume with nitrofurazone ointment) or systemically (1 g/kg IV as a 10% solution in saline BID–TID for 3–5 days) to reduce inflammation and edema. Note that the parenteral administration of DMSO is not approved and is considered extra-label use.

FOLLOW-UP

PATIENT MONITORING
• Initial management is intensive. Frequent evaluation is essential
• Good prognostic indicators—reduction of edema, coupled with the horse's ability to retain penis in the prepuce

POSSIBLE COMPLICATIONS
• Excoriations/ulcerations or further trauma of exposed skin surfaces
• Fibrosis of tissues, leading to the inability to achieve erection or to a urethral obstruction
• Chronic paraphimosis
• Continued hematoma enlargement indicates that a rent may be present in the tunica albuginea. The hematoma should be surgically explored
• Penile paralysis
• Frostbite due to exposure
• Myiasis
• Infertility

MISCELLANEOUS

ASSOCIATED CONDITIONS
N/A

AGE-RELATED FACTORS
N/A

ZOONOTIC POTENTIAL
N/A

PREGNANCY/FERTILITY/BREEDING
N/A

SEE ALSO
• Penile lacerations
• Penile paralysis
• Penile vesicles, erosions, and tumors
• Priapism
• Purpura haemorrhagica

ABBREVIATIONS
• CCP = corpus cavernosum penis
• DMSO = dimethylsulfoxide
• EHV-1 = equine herpesvirus 1, equine rhinopneumonitis
• EHV-3 = equine herpesvirus 3, equine coital exanthema
• EIA = equine infectious anemia, swamp fever
• EVA = equine viral arteritis
• NSAID = nonsteroidal anti-inflammatory drug

Suggested Reading
Arnold CE, Brinsko SP, Love CC, Varner DD. Use of a modified Vinsot technique for partial phallectomy in 11 standing horses. J Am Vet Med Assoc 2010;237:82–86.
Brinsko SP, Blanchard TL, Varner DD. How to treat paraphimosis. Proc Am Assoc Equine Pract 2007;53:580–582.
Clem MF, DeBowes RM. Paraphimosis in horses. Part I. Compend Contin Educ 1989;11:72–75.
Clem MF, DeBowes RM. Paraphimosis in horses. Part II. Compend Contin Educ 1989;11:184–187.
Gunn AJ, Brookes VJ, Hodder ADJ, et al. Balanoposthitis and paraphimosis in the stallion. A novel support for an inflamed penis and prepuce. Clin Theriogenol 2013;5:45–55.

Author Ahmed Tibary
Consulting Editor Carla L. Carleton
Acknowledgment The author and editor acknowledge the prior contribution of Carole C. Miller.

P

PASTERN DERMATITIS

BASICS

DEFINITION
- A variety of inflammatory skin conditions of the horse's distal extremity. Considered as a "syndrome or cutaneous reaction pattern" of the plantar/palmar aspects of the pastern and bulbs of the heels but may extend proximally to the mid-cannon
- "Grease heel" is *not a specific disease entity*

PATHOPHYSIOLOGY
Dermatitis is preceded by mechanical injury to the stratum corneum. Mechanical irritants include chronic moisture; frictional injury from bedding, tack, arenas, and track soils; ectoparasites; and microorganisms. Inflammation of the epidermis, dermis, and adnexa gives rise to crusts, scale, erosion, ulceration, alopecia, lichenification, fibrosis, exuberant, verrucous masses representing granulation tissue, and scarring.

SYSTEMS AFFECTED
Skin/exocrine.

GENETICS
Genetics may play a role, as anatomic features correlate with disease severity in draft horses.

INCIDENCE/PREVALENCE
- The most prevalent form of the disease is mild
- True incidence is unknown

GEOGRAPHIC DISTRIBUTION
Worldwide

SIGNALMENT
- Occurs in all breeds but most common in heavy draft horses
- Mean age of onset is 9 years—range 2.5–26 years of age
- No reported sex predilection

SIGNS
- Variable and dependent on the etiology and the stage of disease
- Bilateral symmetrical involvement of the caudal pastern of the hind limb is the most common presentation. Can be unilateral
- Signs begin on the palmar and plantar aspects of the fetlocks up to the carpal and tarsal joints and may progress to the metatarsal regions. All surfaces of the limbs can be involved
- Earliest lesions are mild scale and crusts with erythema, edema, exudation, matted fur, and alopecia. Other features are hyperkeratosis with hyperplastic plaque lesions and scaling
- Verrucous masses, referred to as "grapes," have rugged surfaces with fissures, scale, crusts, excoriations, erosion, ulceration, and varying degree of greasiness, malodor, and exudate
- In advanced cases, removal of thick adherent scale and crusts can cause significant pain, erosion, and ulceration. Serosanguineous or suppurative exudate is associated with

erosion, ulceration, crusts, or the presence of vasculitis on nonpigmented limbs
- Distal limb edema, cellulitis, and fissuring of hyperplastic skin can cause reluctance to ambulate
- Varying degrees of pruritus are present in all stages depending on the etiology. Distal extremities with white stockings may be more affected

CAUSES
Pastern dermatitis has numerous potential causes.
1. *Factors that provide the basis for the* ***development*** *of pastern dermatitis*
- In heavy draft horses
  - Circumference of cannon
  - Prominence of fetlock tufts of hair, chestnuts, ergots, and, if present, prominent bulges in the fetlock region
  - Poor hoof condition
- Chronically moist conditions, abrasion from plants in the pasture or irritants in the soils of tracks or riding areas, sand, or beddings
- Poor stable hygiene
- Use of irritant topical products, training devices, or treated bedding
- Keratinization disorder
2. *Factors that* ***initiate*** *dermatitis are considered primary disease etiologies*
- Parasitic
  - *Chorioptes* spp.
  - Trombiculidiasis
  - *Pelodera strongyloides*
  - *Strongyloides westeri* larvae
  - Habronemiasis
- Infectious
  - Dermatophytosis
  - Mycetoma
  - Sporotrichosis
  - Spirochetosis
- Immune mediated
  - Contact hypersensitivity
  - Photoactivated vasculitis
  - Leukocytoclastic pastern vasculitis
  - Cutaneous drug reaction
  - Pemphigus complex
  - Bullous pemphigoid
- Iatrogenic
  - Blistering agents
  - Pin firing
  - Scald from urine or feces
  - Wire injury
- Neoplastic
  - Fibroblastic or verrucose sarcoid
  - Squamous cell carcinoma
  - Cutaneous lymphoma
3. *Features of the dermatitis that* ***maintain***, *reinforce, and strengthen the disease process*
- Bacterial
  - *Staphylococcus* spp., *Corynebacterium* spp., fusiform bacteria, botryomycosis infections
  - *Dermatophilus congolensis*
- Environmental
  - Overvigorous washing and scrubbing
  - Application of occlusive ointments and dressings over necrotic skin and crusts

  - UV light exposure
  - Insect bites
- Chronic pathologic changes

RISK FACTORS
Risk factors are predisposing factors that increase susceptibility:
- Environmental—climate (more common in the winter), moisture, and stable and pasture hygiene
- Iatrogenic—adverse reactions to topical medications, use of splint boots
- Genetic—excessive hair or feathering on pastern, keratinization defect

DIAGNOSIS

DIFFERENTIAL DIAGNOSIS
Diagnosis is based on history, physical examination, and findings from diagnostic tests.
Additional differentials:
- Chronic progressive lymphedema
- Exfoliative eosinophilic dermatitis and stomatitis

CBC/BIOCHEMISTRY/URINALYSIS
- Perform if photosensitization, hepatopathy, or vasculitis is suspected
- Use to screen for metabolic disorders

OTHER LABORATORY TESTS
- Surface cytology with Diff-Quik® stains collected from erosions or ulcers shows a neutrophilic exudate with intra- and/or extracellular cocci and represents secondary folliculitis
- Skin scrapings to rule out ectoparasites
- Bacterial and dermatophyte cultures to determine bacterial species and susceptibility and/or dermatophyte infections

IMAGING
Radiographs may rule out other causes of lameness.

OTHER DIAGNOSTIC PROCEDURES
Obtain skin biopsies by wedge resection or double-punch technique in horses with marked hyperkeratosis or nodular or proliferative changes. Biopsies are essential for confirmation of pastern dermatitis due to immune-mediated or neoplastic disease, keratinization disorders, vasculopathies, or contact hypersensitivities.

TREATMENT

AIMS
The primary goal is to establish and eliminate factors in the 3 categories of the disease process. No single therapy applies to all cases owing to the variability of cause and clinical consequences.

P

APPROPRIATE HEALTH CARE
Outpatient medical management is appropriate for most cases.

NURSING CARE
• Debridement—remove all necrotic and contaminated tissues, keep the skin dry and free of irritation during treatment. Debridement may require sedation as severe cases are usually painful. Remove excess hair. Simple hydrotherapy with the application of an antimicrobial, keratolytic, and keratoplastic shampoo is used in the initial debridement
• In mild cases, a conservative approach of cleansing lesions every 12 h for 7–10 days may be all that is needed
• In moderate to severe cases, debridement is performed using creams with benzoic or salicylic acids and propylene glycol applied to the lesions, covered with thin plastic film, and wrapped with a lightly padded clean stable bandage for 12 h. Remove the dressing and gently wash with a mild antimicrobial shampoo. If crusting is still present, repeat the process. Assess the degree and depth of ulceration. Severely ulcerated skin will not heal if exposed to repeated wetting and trauma
• For exudative lesions, astringent solutions, such as Burow's solution, can be applied to the area every 8–12 h for 10 min; alternatively, soak the leg in an astringent solution for 15–30 min. Before application of astringent, wash extremities with an antimicrobial shampoo
• If providing a dry environment is not possible, consider applying a light barrier cream, such as petroleum jelly or liquid bandages

ACTIVITY
• Rest from work. Avoid areas that are wet, muddy, sandy, or have an abundance of sharp protruding roughage that initiates epidermal microtrauma. Keep in clean dry stall during wet weather
• If predominantly white legs are affected—suggestive of solar or photoactivated dermatitis; keep out of UV light until a definitive diagnosis is made

DIET
N/A

CLIENT EDUCATION
• Warn owners and plan for recurrence
• Describe multifactorial nature of the disease

SURGICAL CONSIDERATIONS
Surgical or cryosurgical intervention of exuberant granulation tissue may be required.

MEDICATIONS
DRUG(S) OF CHOICE
• For localized bacterial dermatitis, consider topical antimicrobials that penetrate the epidermis such as silver sulfadiazine or 2% mupirocin ointment, applied every 12 h for 2 weeks past clinical cure. Other effective topicals include 2–4% chlorhexidine sprays and mousses, Mud Stop® (UK), and products containing *Kunzea* oil
• For mild to deep bacterial dermatitis involving all 4 legs, use systemic antimicrobials, such as trimethoprim-potentiated sulfonamides (sulfadiazine or sulfamethoxazole) 30 mg/kg PO every 12–24 h until 2 weeks past clinical cure. Use in conjunction with antimicrobial shampoos and sprays to hasten resolution
• Dermatophytosis—topical rinses, sprays, shampoos, leave-on mousses such as 2% lime sulfur, 2% miconazole/climbazole with 2–4% chlorhexidine and 2% enilconazole can be used.
• Ectoparasiticides—topical pyrethroids, 5% lime sulfur solution, and 0.25% fipronil spray. Fipronil spray may reduce chorioptic mange but may not eliminate it. Apply 125 mL of spray from elbow, stifles downward to each leg. Reapply in 3 weeks. Treat all animals in contact with the infected animal simultaneously. Infestation with *Chorioptes* requires environmental decontamination as mites live off the host for up to 70 days. Topical eprinomectin solution at 500 µg/kg once weekly for 4 weeks was shown to be effective for psoroptic mange
• Judicious use of systemic steroids is indicated to reduce inflammation especially in idiopathic, contact, pastern leukocytoclastic vasculitis and immune-mediated conditions. Topical steroids such as triamcinolone 0.015% or hydrocortisone 1% sprays, betamethasone 1%, or mometasone 0.1% creams could be used alone or in conjunction with systemic steroids to decrease the dose needed with systemic therapy alone

CONTRAINDICATIONS
Overzealous application of topical ointments on the surface of necrotic skin and crusts.

PRECAUTIONS
None

POSSIBLE INTERACTIONS
N/A

ALTERNATIVE DRUGS
None

FOLLOW-UP
PATIENT MONITORING
Dependent on disease severity.

PREVENTION/AVOIDANCE
• Prevention relies on avoidance. Wet grass in the early summer morning can macerate the epidermis. Recurrent cases benefit from stalls with clean, dry bedding. Simple avoidance of UV light may not be sufficient to prevent disease
• Application of a light barrier cream before exercise, combined with cleansing and drying after exercise, may prevent recurrence
• Asymptomatic carriers of dermatophytosis or *Chorioptes* need treatment

POSSIBLE COMPLICATIONS
Lameness

EXPECTED COURSE AND PROGNOSIS
Prognosis depends on the stage of the disease.

MISCELLANEOUS
ASSOCIATED CONDITIONS
N/A

AGE-RELATED FACTORS
Severity may worsen with age.

ZOONOTIC POTENTIAL
Dermatophilosis, dermatophytosis, and *Chorioptes* are zoonotic.

PREGNANCY/FERTILITY/BREEDING
N/A

SYNONYMS
• Grease heel—early form
• Scratches—early form; colloquial term

SEE ALSO
• Chronic progressive lymphedema
• Dermatophilosis
• Ectoparasites

Suggested Reading
Psalla D, Rufenacht S, Stoffel MH, et al. Equine pastern vasculitis: a clinical and histopathological study. Vet J 2013;198:524–530.

Author Gwendolen Lorch
Consulting Editor Gwendolen Lorch

P

PATENT DUCTUS ARTERIOSUS

 BASICS

DEFINITION
- A persistently patent vascular communication between the aorta and pulmonary artery
- The ductus arteriosus is a vessel that allows blood to shunt from the pulmonary artery to the aorta in the fetus
- The ductus arteriosus normally constricts after birth in response to increased local oxygen tension and prostaglandin inhibition, and closure should be complete within 4 days of birth

PATHOPHYSIOLOGY
- When the ductus arteriosus remains patent, blood shunts from the higher pressure aorta to the lower pressure pulmonary artery, creating left atrial and left ventricular volume overload
- Size of the PDA determines severity of the volume overload—with a large PDA, stretching of the mitral annulus occurs over time, and mitral regurgitation develops; as mitral regurgitation becomes more severe, left atrial pressure increases, resulting in increased pulmonary venous pressure and clinical signs of left-sided CHF
- PDA may also be a component of more complex congenital cardiac defects

SYSTEMS AFFECTED
Cardiovascular

GENETICS
- Not yet determined in horses
- The condition is heritable in other species but rare in horses

INCIDENCE/PREVALENCE
PDA is a very rare, isolated congenital defect, but it occurs more frequently in horses with complex congenital heart disease.

SIGNALMENT
- Arabian horses appear to be predisposed to complex congenital cardiac defects
- Murmurs usually are detectable at birth
- Diagnosed most frequently in neonates, foals, and young horses but can be found at any age

SIGNS
General Comments
May be an incidental finding but usually is part of a more complex congenital cardiac disorder.

Historical Findings
- Exercise intolerance—medium-sized to large PDA and those associated with complex congenital cardiac defects
- CHF—large PDA and those associated with complex congenital cardiac defects

Physical Examination Findings
- A grade 3–6/6 continuous machinery murmur with point of maximal intensity over the main pulmonary artery between the pulmonic and aortic valve area
- Additional loud murmurs may be detected in complex congenital cardiac defects, with characteristics dependent on the exact nature of the defects
- Bounding arterial pulses
- Premature beats or an irregularly irregular heart rhythm of atrial fibrillation may be present with larger PDA or those associated with complex congenital cardiac defects

CAUSES
Lack of constriction of the ductus arteriosus.

RISK FACTORS
- Premature foal
- Hypoxia
- Neonatal pulmonary hypertension
- Neonatal respiratory distress syndrome
- Mares treated with prostaglandin inhibitors during late gestation

 DIAGNOSIS

DIFFERENTIAL DIAGNOSIS
- Physiologic flow murmur—usually systolic rather than continuous murmur; differentiate echocardiographically
- Ventricular septal defect with aortic regurgitation—pansystolic and holodiastolic murmur and point of maximal intensity of pansystolic murmur, usually in the tricuspid valve area; differentiate echocardiographically
- Complex congenital cardiac disease—differentiate echocardiographically

CBC/BIOCHEMISTRY/URINALYSIS
N/A

OTHER LABORATORY TESTS
N/A

IMAGING
ECG
Atrial premature depolarizations or atrial fibrillation may be present in horses with left atrial enlargement.

Echocardiography
- Difficult to visualize
- The left atrium and ventricle are enlarged and dilated and have a rounded appearance
- Pulmonary artery dilatation in horses with a large shunt
- Color-flow Doppler may reveal the shunt from aorta to pulmonary artery through the PDA
- Continuous, high-velocity, turbulent flow is detected with continuous-wave Doppler toward the main pulmonary artery
- Retrograde, turbulent flow in the main pulmonary artery may be identified with color-flow and continuous-wave Doppler
- Additional cardiac defects such as great vessel anomalies, right atrioventricular valve atresia, or hypoplastic left ventricle syndrome may be present. A segmental approach where each structure is identified and its connection to other structures documented echocardiographically is required to differentiate complex congenital cardiac defects. Color-flow and contrast echocardiography may allow documentation of the path of blood flow in affected horses

Thoracic Radiography
- Increased pulmonary vascularity and cardiac enlargement may be detected
- Pulmonary edema may be detected in foals or horses with CHF

OTHER DIAGNOSTIC PROCEDURES
Cardiac Catheterization
- Right-sided cardiac catheterization to directly measure pulmonary arterial and capillary wedge pressures and to sample blood for oxygen content
- Elevated pulmonary arterial and capillary wedge pressures as well as increased oxygen saturation of pulmonary arterial blood are found in horses with PDA

24 h Holter Monitoring
Continuous monitoring is useful for establishing the diagnosis in horses with suspected atrial premature depolarizations.

PATHOLOGIC FINDINGS
- The PDA is present between the aorta and main pulmonary artery
- Left atrial and ventricular enlargement and thinning of the left atrial and ventricular free wall in horses with a significant shunt
- Dilatation of the main pulmonary artery and right and left pulmonary arteries in those horses with a large shunt and in those with pulmonary hypertension
- Thickened media of the pulmonary arterioles in horses with chronic pulmonary hypertension
- Pulmonary edema in horses with CHF
- PDA is often identified in conjunction with additional defects in a variety of complex congenital cardiac defects including hypoplastic left ventricle syndrome, transposition of the great arteries, critical pulmonic stenosis, and atresia of the right atrioventricular orifice

 TREATMENT

AIMS
- Management by intermittent monitoring in horses with small isolated PDA
- Palliative care in horses with large PDA and those in which there are multiple cardiac defects

APPROPRIATE HEALTH CARE
- Most newborn foals with PDA should have the underlying pulmonary disease or pulmonary hypertension treated if present
- Monitor affected horses on an annual basis
- Horse with PDA and CHF could be treated

for the CHF with positive inotropic drugs, vasodilators, and diuretics. Consider euthanasia, however, because only short-term, symptomatic improvement can be expected

NURSING CARE
N/A

ACTIVITY
• Horses with a small PDA may be able to perform successfully at lower levels of athletic activities, but they are unlikely to be able to perform satisfactorily at upper levels
• Monitor affected horses echocardiographically on an annual basis to ensure they are safe to ride. Dilatation of the pulmonary artery should prompt discontinuation of ridden activities as it can be a precursor to pulmonary artery rupture
• Affected horses that develop atrial fibrillation need a complete cardiovascular examination to determine if lower levels of athletic performance are safe

DIET
N/A

CLIENT EDUCATION
• Regularly monitor the horse's rhythm; any irregularities other than second-degree atrioventricular block should prompt ECG examination
• Carefully monitor the horse for exercise intolerance, respiratory distress, prolonged recovery after exercise, increased resting respiratory or heart rate, or cough; if detected, obtain a cardiac reexamination

SURGICAL CONSIDERATIONS
• Closure of the PDA is possible with a transvenous umbrella catheter or coil having a diameter large enough to close the defect
• Surgical closure is not financially feasible or practical for obtaining an equine athlete at this time

MEDICATIONS

DRUG(S) OF CHOICE
N/A

CONTRAINDICATIONS
N/A

ALTERNATIVE DRUGS
N/A

FOLLOW-UP

PATIENT MONITORING
Frequently monitor the horse's cardiac rate, rhythm, respiratory rate, and effort.

PREVENTION/AVOIDANCE
N/A

POSSIBLE COMPLICATIONS
Large PDA and those forming part of complex congenital cardiac defects—atrial fibrillation, CHF, and pulmonary artery rupture.

EXPECTED COURSE AND PROGNOSIS
• Horses with a small PDA may have a normal performance life for lower levels of athletic competition and a normal life expectancy
• Horses with a moderate to large PDA may develop atrial fibrillation and have a guarded prognosis; these horses should have a shortened performance life at lower levels of athletic competition and a shortened life expectancy
• Horses with pulmonary artery dilatation have a grave prognosis for life and are not safe to ride
• Horses with associated CHF usually have a guarded to grave prognosis for life. Most horses with a PDA being treated for CHF should respond to the supportive therapy and transiently improve, but once CHF develops euthanasia is recommended

MISCELLANEOUS

ASSOCIATED CONDITIONS
• Complex congenital cardiac disease is the rule, rather than the exception, in affected horses
• Mitral regurgitation can develop in horses with PDA associated with stretching of the mitral annulus secondary to significant left atrial and ventricular volume overload
• Pulmonary artery rupture can occur secondary to the pulmonary artery dilatation and elevated pulmonary arterial pressures

AGE-RELATED FACTORS
Young horses are more likely to be diagnosed with this defect.

ZOONOTIC POTENTIAL
N/A

PREGNANCY/FERTILITY/BREEDING
Breeding affected horses should be discouraged even though the condition is rare and the heritable nature of this defect is not known.

SYNONYMS
N/A

SEE ALSO
Atrial fibrillation

ABBREVIATIONS
• CHF = congestive heart failure
• PDA = patent ductus arteriosus

Suggested Reading
Buergelt CD, Carmichael JA, Tashjian RJ, Das KM. Spontaneous rupture of the left pulmonary artery in a horse with patent ductus arteriosus. J Am Vet Med Assoc 1970;157:313–320.
Marr CM. Cardiac murmurs: congenital heart disease. In: Marr CM, Bowen M, eds. Cardiology of the Horse, 2e. Edinburgh, UK: Saunders Elsevier, 2010:187–197.
Reef VB. Cardiovascular ultrasonography. In: Reef VB, ed. Equine Diagnostic Ultrasound. Philadelphia, PA: WB Saunders, 1998:215–272.
Schwarzwald CC. Sequential segmental analysis—a systemic approach to the diagnosis of congenital cardiac defects. Equine Vet Educ 2008;20:305–309.
Scott EA, Kneller SK, Witherspoon DM. Closure of ductus arteriosus determined by cardiac catheterization and angiography in newborn foals. Am J Vet Res 1975;36:1021–1023.

Author Virginia B. Reef
Consulting Editors Celia M. Marr and Virginia B. Reef

P

PATENT URACHUS

BASICS

OVERVIEW
The urachus is the umbilical structure that directs urine from the fetal bladder to the allantoic fluid. The urachus normally closes at the time of birth, but it can remain patent or reopen secondary to inflammation or infection. The urachus that fails to close within hours of birth (congenital) or that begins to leak urine after it has initially closed (acquired) is considered a patent urachus.

SIGNALMENT
- Neonatal foals are affected by this condition
- There does not appear to be a breed or sex predilection

SIGNS
- Urine is seen streaming or dripping from the umbilicus when the foal urinates, or the umbilicus may be moist from urine leakage
- When there is infection associated with a patent urachus, the umbilicus may also be enlarged, painful, or warm, and the foal may exhibit fever, lethargy, and poor appetite

CAUSES AND RISK FACTORS
- Congenital factors such as excessive traction or twisting of the umbilical cord in utero may be related to congenital or persistent patent urachus
- After parturition, omphalophlebitis can lead to reopening of the urachus

DIAGNOSIS

DIFFERENTIAL DIAGNOSIS
Omphalophlebitis

CBC/BIOCHEMISTRY/URINALYSIS
- When patent urachus is complicated with omphalophlebitis, leukocytosis and hyperfibrinogenemia are often present
- Occasionally, tears in the urachus can extend intra-abdominally and result in uroperitoneum. Azotemia, hyponatremia, and hyperkalemia may be seen in these cases

IMAGING
- Ultrasonography can confirm patency between the bladder and the urachus, and can determine whether omphalophlebitis or urachal abscess is present
- Positive-contrast radiography—contrast material delivered retrograde via the urethra can confirm patency between the bladder and the urachus and can also reveal any leakage from the urachus into the abdomen or subcutaneous tissues

OTHER DIAGNOSTIC PROCEDURES
- Bacterial culture of the aseptically prepared umbilical stump if omphalophlebitis is suspected
- Blood cultures should be performed in neonates to rule out septicemia

TREATMENT
- The umbilicus should be kept clean by dipping in dilute chlorhexidine (0.5%) or dilute iodine (1%) twice daily until the umbilicus is no longer patent. Topical application of cauterizing compounds such as silver nitrate or strong iodine can be used for congenital uncomplicated patent urachus; however, these should never be used in cases of acquired patent urachus with omphalophlebitis
- Nursing care should also include protection of the skin from urine scalding (e.g. with petroleum jelly)
- Surgical resection of the umbilical remnants if infection is present with patent urachus or if the urachus has not closed after 5–7 days of medical treatment

MEDICATIONS

DRUG(S) OF CHOICE
- Systemic antimicrobials are recommended for congenital and acquired patent urachus
- Broad-spectrum antimicrobials—usually a penicillin and an aminoglycoside (e.g. amikacin), and treatment should be guided by culture and sensitivity from umbilical or blood cultures

CONTRAINDICATIONS/POSSIBLE INTERACTIONS
- Aminoglycosides should be used with caution in foals with renal compromise or dehydration
- Other broad-spectrum parenteral antimicrobial choices include ceftiofur (5–10 mg/kg IV or IM BID)

FOLLOW-UP

PATIENT MONITORING
- Monitor for signs of systemic infection such as fever, lethargy, joint effusion, or lameness
- Palpate umbilicus to detect any changes in size, consistency, or persistent urine leakage
- Serial ultrasonographic examinations of the umbilical remnants can detect development of omphalophlebitis

PREVENTION/AVOIDANCE
- Adequate colostrum
- Clean environment
- Avoid traction on the umbilicus during parturition
- Umbilical disinfection

POSSIBLE COMPLICATIONS
- Ascending infection and bacteremia can lead to septic omphalophlebitis, septicemia, and septic arthritis
- Treatment with cauterizing agents can lead to significant inflammation of the umbilicus, and can cause scalding of the ventral abdomen and prepuce if used incorrectly

EXPECTED COURSE AND PROGNOSIS
- Most foals with congenital patent urachus will have resolution with medical management. If the urachus remains patent after 5–7 days of treatment or if there are signs of progressive infection, surgical removal of the umbilicus is recommended
- Prognosis for congenital patent urachus is excellent. Prognosis for acquired patent urachus is good provided there are no secondary complications with infection
- Septicemia and septic arthritis will greatly reduce the prognosis

MISCELLANEOUS

ASSOCIATED CONDITIONS
Omphalophlebitis

AGE-RELATED FACTORS
This is a condition of neonatal foals.

SEE ALSO
- Omphalophlebitis
- Septicemia, neonate

Suggested Reading
Nolen-Walston R. Umbilical and urinary disorders. In: Paradis MR, ed. Equine Neonatal Medicine: A Case-Based Approach. Philadelphia, PA: Saunders, 2006:231–245.

Author Margaret C. Mudge
Consulting Editor Margaret C. Mudge

P

BASICS

OVERVIEW
• An autoimmune skin disease and the most common cause in the author's practice for noninfectious crusts in the horse. It is also the most commonly seen autoimmune skin disease in the horse, after purpura haemorrhagica
• The exact pathomechanism has not been investigated in the horse, but it is presumed to be similar to that for humans and the dog—autoantibodies are produced that attack the intercellular connections between the skin's epidermal cells. This leads to formation of transient pustules or bullae and subsequent crusts
• Geographic distribution of the disease is presumably worldwide. The incidence is unknown but the disease is relatively uncommon. In California, 80% of the horses first exhibited signs between September and February. Skin and hemolymphatic system are affected.

SIGNALMENT
• Appaloosa were predisposed in 1 study
• No sex predilection
• The mean age of onset was 8.6 years with a range of 2.5 months to 25 years

SIGNS
• Crusts frequently start on the face and legs and become generalized
• Occasionally, crusts only on the coronary band
• Alopecia
• Pustules
• Urticaria
• Peripheral edema ("stocking up")
• Lethargy, anorexia, pyrexia

CAUSES AND RISK FACTORS
Unknown in most cases. 1 published case—possibly caused by penicillin.

DIAGNOSIS

DIFFERENTIAL DIAGNOSIS
• Severe superficial staphylococcal dermatitis
• Dermatophytosis
• Dermatophilosis
• Sarcoidosis (chronic granulomatous disease)

CBC/BIOCHEMISTRY/URINALYSIS
Low-grade anemia combined with a leukocytosis.

OTHER LABORATORY TESTS
N/A

IMAGING
N/A

OTHER DIAGNOSTIC PROCEDURES
• Skin biopsy for histopathology. Very important *not* to surgically prepare the area to be biopsied. It is acceptable to surgically prepare the site *after* taking the biopsy sample (i.e. before suturing the site) to limit chances of infection. Choose multiple sites, and include the crust. Provide the pathologist with the patient signalment, a brief history, descriptions and locations of the biopsied sites, as well as differential diagnosis
• Cytology of aspirates or impression smears from pustules and crusts may reveal acantholytic cells and neutrophils
• Bacteriologic and fungal (dermatophyte test medium) cultures will identify secondary bacterial folliculitis or dermatophytosis, respectively

PATHOLOGIC FINDINGS
• Subcorneal or intracorneal pustules with acantholytic cells
• Certain strains of the dermatophyte species *Trichophyton* may cause acantholysis; therefore, any histology suggestive of PF should have special stains for fungi performed

TREATMENT
• Control disease, reduce lesions, return horse to function
• May not be able to eliminate all lesions

MEDICATIONS

DRUG(S) OF CHOICE
• CS at immunosuppressive doses (prednisolone 1 mg/kg every 12 h PO, dexamethasone 0.05–0.1 mg/kg every 24 h IM, PO, IV) for 2 weeks, then taper to lowest effective dose
• Azathioprine in combination with the above CS at 1 mg/kg every 24 h PO for 1 month, then every 48 h. Expect 1 month for effect. Azathioprine is used as a steroid-sparing agent and is moderately expensive. As it takes effect, the CS dosage should be slowly reduced

CONTRAINDICATIONS/POSSIBLE INTERACTIONS
• Horses with a predisposition to laminitis, or with a previous history of laminitis, should be monitored very closely for recurrence, or possibly just treated with azathioprine, although this method of treatment has not been substantiated in equine PF
• Therapeutic precautions include the following—CS: laminitis; azathioprine: bone marrow suppression (rare)

FOLLOW-UP

PATIENT MONITORING
• Physical examinations, especially looking for resolution of lesions as well as laminitis caused by CS
• If initially anemic, monitor with hemogram
• If using azathioprine, monitor hemogram and platelets, once monthly.

PREVENTION/AVOIDANCE
N/A

POSSIBLE COMPLICATIONS
• CS-induced laminitis
• Immunosuppression can predispose animal to secondary cutaneous (pyoderma, dermatophytosis) and systemic infections, although rare

EXPECTED COURSE AND PROGNOSIS
• Guarded to good, depending on response to treatment and if CS-induced adverse effects occur
• Some horses need lifelong treatment, others may have treatment discontinued after complete resolution of lesions without the PF recurring
• Advise client of the controllable, rather than curable, nature of the disease
• In a minority of cases, it is possible to taper down and stop medication without relapse
• Advise client of the adverse effects of medications

MISCELLANEOUS

PREGNANCY/FERTILITY/BREEDING
• Anecdotal reports of affected mares giving birth to affected newborn foals
• 1 report describes a female donkey in which PF occurred, then regressed, during 2 of its 5 pregnancies

ABBREVIATIONS
• CS = corticosteroid
• PF = pemphigus foliaceus

Suggested Reading
Vandenabeele SIG, White SD, Kass P, et al. Pemphigus foliaceus in the horse: 20 cases. Vet Dermatol 2004;15:381–388.

Author Stephen D. White
Consulting Editor Gwendolen Lorch

PENETRATING INJURIES TO THE FOOT

BASICS

OVERVIEW
• Puncture to sole or frog by sharp object (nail, screw, etc.). Also known as "street nail"
• Penetrating object carries debris (manure, soil, rust) into deeper structures, initiating infection. Infection can be within the soft tissues, bones, or synovial structures of the foot/pastern
• Systems affected—musculoskeletal; foot
  ○ Soft tissues—deep digital flexor tendon, digital cushion
  ○ Bones—P3, navicular bone
  ○ Synovial structures—DIP, navicular bursa, digital flexor tendon sheath

SIGNS
Historical Findings
• Acute, severe lameness
• ± Penetrating object in foot
• Initially, wound discharge, ± increased comfort quickly
• Subsequently, superficial wound closes, causing build-up of purulent discharge within the deeper structures and leading to increased lameness

Physical Examination Findings
• Varying lameness—initially severe, may improve
• Chronic injuries (>1 week)—increasingly lame
• Increased digital pulses, heat
• ± Severe pain with hoof testers
• ± Penetrating foreign body
• Critical sole inspection may identify wound tract
• ± Discharge from wound tract
• ± DIP or digital flexor tendon sheath effusion
• ± Fever

CAUSES AND RISK FACTORS
Stepping on a sharp object.

DIAGNOSIS

DIFFERENTIAL DIAGNOSIS
• Subsolar abscess—no history of foreign body or puncture wound
• P3 fracture—rule out by radiography
• Deep digital flexor tendon injury—severely affected will flip toe up at a walk; ultrasonography and radiography (DIP subluxation)
• Navicular bone fracture—rule out by radiography

CBC/BIOCHEMISTRY/URINALYSIS
Injury >24 h—hyperfibrinogenemia and increased serum amyloid A possible.

IMAGING
Radiography—Plain Films
• If foreign body present—leave in place, radiograph foot, determine tissue(s) involvement
• If foreign body not present—aseptically prepare hoof and tract, insert sterile radiopaque probe into tract and radiograph
• Additional views to rule out P3 or navicular bone fracture or to define wound tract

Radiography—Contrast Radiography
Contrast material into the wound tract or, alternatively, inject synovial structures with contrast material. Radiography to determine synovial structure(s) involvement.

OTHER DIAGNOSTIC PROCEDURES
• Synovial fluid analysis
• Microbial culture and sensitivity from wound tract and/or synovial fluid—obtain before antibiotic use

TREATMENT

• ± Life-threatening consequences; treat as an emergency
• If suspect synovial involvement, refer for surgery. Prior to referral, remove foreign body (after radiography), bandage foot, provide analgesia ± antibiotic therapy. Surgical treatment includes arthroscopic wound debridement and generous lavage of synovial structure(s)
• If no synovial involvement, debride wound tract, bandage foot, and medical treatment
• Foot bandage with duct tape helps maintain a clean, dry sole
• ± Regional limb perfusions with antibiotics
• Stall rest until tract healed
• With severe lameness, contralateral foot sole support

MEDICATIONS

DRUG(S) OF CHOICE
• Tetanus toxoid and antitoxin
• NSAIDs (phenylbutazone 2.2–4.4 mg/kg every 12–24 h)
• Broad-spectrum antibiotics until tract healed. Initial choice(s) adjusted after culture and sensitivity results
• Include anaerobic antimicrobials (i.e. penicillin, metronidazole)
• Daily regional limb perfusions with antibiotics—aminoglycosides (amikacin 2 g per adult horse diluted to 60 mL with sterile saline)

CONTRAINDICATIONS/POSSIBLE INTERACTIONS
Monitor renal function in chronically treated horse.

FOLLOW-UP

PATIENT MONITORING
• Monitor lameness daily. If lameness does not improve quickly (within 3–5 days) or increases despite treatment, consider referral
• If P3 involved, repeat radiography for possible sequestrum or septic osteitis

PREVENTION/AVOIDANCE
Routine pasture maintenance/inspection.

POSSIBLE COMPLICATIONS
• Septic arthritis, septic tenosynovitis, deep digital flexor tendonitis sepsis and subsequent rupture, P3 osteitis ± sequestrum, navicular bone fracture
• Complications may cause severe lameness, loss of athletic soundness, contralateral limb laminitis
• If severe, may require euthanasia

EXPECTED COURSE AND PROGNOSIS
• Without synovial involvement and with prompt medical treatment, prognosis is good to excellent
• Synovial involvement with prompt (i.e. <48 h) surgical treatment has a fair to good prognosis for soundness
• Prolonged synovial (i.e. >7 days) involvement without prompt surgical treatment has a poor to grave prognosis for soundness and life

MISCELLANEOUS

ASSOCIATED CONDITIONS
Contralateral limb laminitis.

PREGNANCY/FERTILITY/BREEDING
In late gestation, increased weight may exacerbate lameness.

SEE ALSO
• Septic arthritis, neonate
• Solar abscess

ABBREVIATIONS
• DIP = distal interphalangeal joint
• NSAID = nonsteroidal anti-inflammatory drug
• P3 = third phalanx

Suggested Reading
Getman LM, Trumble TN. Musculoskeletal system. In: Southwood LL, Wilkins PA, eds. Equine Emergency and Critical Care Medicine. Boca Raton, FL: CRC Press, 2014:155–252.

Author Liberty M. Getman
Consulting Editor Elizabeth J. Davidson

Client Education Handout available online

P

BASICS

OVERVIEW
• Penile traumatic injuries, including lacerations, are common in stallions
• Lacerations to the penile surface or urethral process are often the result of trauma (jumping a barrier or during breeding), tail hair, poor handling during collection on a phantom, or a poorly prepared artificial vagina
• Laceration may compromise the breeding activity or normal micturition

SIGNALMENT
No age or breed predilection.

SIGNS
• Bleeding may be noticed from the prepuce
• Severe cases are accompanied by inflammatory edema, cellulitis, and paraphimosis

CAUSES AND RISK FACTORS
• Trauma—breeding accidents, improperly fitted stallion rings, kicks, jumping injuries, masturbation, and improper surgical technique
• Aggressive stallions/colts housed or handled in unsafe conditions are more likely to injure themselves and others

DIAGNOSIS

DIFFERENTIAL DIAGNOSIS
Differentiating Causes
• Visual inspection generally reveals the laceration
• Paraphimosis may be present, but may be secondary to the laceration
• Ulcerative lesions caused by neoplastic or parasitic diseases should not be considered lacerations for this discussion

CBC/BIOCHEMISTRY/URINALYSIS
May be indicated in complicated cases.

OTHER LABORATORY TESTS
N/A

IMAGING
N/A

OTHER DIAGNOSTIC PROCEDURES
N/A

TREATMENT
• Ensure urethral patency. Placement of a urinary catheter may be indicated
• Cleanse and debride the wound as dictated by location and severity
• Acute post-trauma lacerations can be sutured to achieve first intention healing

• Old or grossly contaminated lacerations may have to heal by second intention, or delayed closure can be considered
• Support the penis and prepuce with slings, hydrotherapy, and judicious exercise to prevent or eliminate extensive dependent edema
• Sexual stimulation is absolutely contraindicated until healing is complete

MEDICATIONS

DRUG(S) OF CHOICE
• NSAIDs including phenylbutazone (2–4 g/450 kg body weight/day PO) or flunixin meglumine (1.1 mg/kg/day IV, IM, or PO) for patient comfort and to decrease inflammation. High initial dosages should be titrated to the lowest effective dose if more than 5 successive days of therapy is required
• Systemic or local antibiotics for local infections and to prevent septicemia, if indicated
• Emollient application as required to the penile surface to prevent or address urine scalding, if indicated

CONTRAINDICATIONS/POSSIBLE INTERACTIONS
Phenothiazine tranquilizers should never be used in the intact male.

FOLLOW-UP

PATIENT MONITORING
• If the penis can be maintained within the prepuce without support, less frequent evaluation is necessary
• If retraction of the penis is not possible, hospitalization may be required for frequent evaluation and care of the exposed penis

POSSIBLE COMPLICATIONS
• Urine leakage with extensive tissue necrosis is possible if the penile urethra has been lacerated
• Wounds that cannot be treated surgically are usually complicated by suppuration and cellulitis
• Scar formation can result in phimosis, erectile dysfunction, impotence, or infertility
• Hematomas generally arise from blood vessels superficial to the tunica albuginea. A hematoma that continues to enlarge is more likely attributable to a rent in the tunica albuginea, and closure of that defect is a priority
• Paraphimosis is a common sequela to penile lacerations
• Penile paralysis is possible as a result of the injury itself or secondary to paraphimosis

MISCELLANEOUS

ASSOCIATED CONDITIONS
• Hemospermia
• Impotence
• Paraphimosis
• Penile paralysis
• Phimosis

AGE-RELATED FACTORS
N/A

ZOONOTIC POTENTIAL
N/A

PREGNANCY/FERTILITY/BREEDING
N/A

SEE ALSO
• Paraphimosis
• Penile paralysis
• Phimosis

ABBREVIATIONS
NSAID = nonsteroidal anti-inflammatory drug

Suggested Reading
Ley WB, Slusher SH. Infertility and diseases of the reproductive tract of stallions. In: Youngquist RS, Threlfall WR, eds. Current Therapy in Large Animal Theriogenology, 2e. St. Louis, MO: Saunders Elsevier, 2007:15–23.
Schumacher J, Varner DD. Surgical correction of abnormalities affecting the reproductive organs of stallions. In: Youngquist RS, Threlfall WR, eds. Current Therapy in Large Animal Theriogenology, 2e. St. Louis, MO: Saunders Elsevier, 2007:23–36.
Schumacher J, Vaughan JT. Surgery of the penis and prepuce. Vet Clin North Am Equine Pract 1988;4:443–449.
Vaughan JT. Penis and prepuce. In: McKinnon AO, Voss JL, eds. Equine Reproduction. Philadelphia, PA: Lea & Febiger, 1993:885–894.

Author Ahmed Tibary
Consulting Editor Carla L. Carleton

Acknowledgment The author and editor acknowledge the prior contribution of Carole C. Miller.

P

PENILE PARALYSIS

BASICS

OVERVIEW
• Protracted extension of the penis in a flaccid state
• Penile paralysis may result from a compromise of sacral nerves or a direct insult to the retractor penis muscle, leading to the inability to retract the penis into the prepuce

SIGNALMENT
Stallions (predominantly) or geldings of any age.

SIGNS
N/A

CAUSES AND RISK FACTORS
• Trauma—direct penile trauma, spinal cord injury, or disease
• Infectious disease—EHV-1, rabies, EIA, purpura haemorrhagica, dourine (*Trypanosoma equiperdum*)
• Drug-induced—propiopromazine, acepromazine maleate, reserpine
• Chronic paraphimosis or priapism
• Exhaustion or starvation
• Spinal cord lesion

DIAGNOSIS

DIFFERENTIAL DIAGNOSIS
Differentiating Similar Signs
• Paraphimosis results in prolapse of the penis and prepuce; dependent edema develops. The inability to retract the penis is generally due to the accumulated edema rather than true penile paralysis
• Penile paralysis can be a sequela to chronic, severe paraphimosis. Longstanding penile paralysis can present as paraphimosis due to the formation of extensive dependent edema
• Priapism, a persistent erection with engorgement of the corpus cavernosum penis, should not be confused with penile paralysis in which the penis is flaccid

Differentiating Causes
• The presence of neurologic deficits other than the penile paralysis may link the penile problem with infectious causes and/or spinal cord injury as the primary problem
• A recent history of respiratory disease (affected horse or on its farm) may implicate EHV-1 as a possible cause

CBC/BIOCHEMISTRY/URINALYSIS
N/A

OTHER LABORATORY TESTS
EHV-1
• Rising antibody titers from paired sera, collected at a 14–21 day intervals
• PCR testing or virus isolation from nasopharyngeal swabs and blood in the acute stage of the disease

EIA
Agar gel immunodiffusion (Coggins) test.

Dourine
• Identification of the causative agent in preputial or urethral exudates; serologic testing by complement fixation test
• Note that dourine has been eradicated from North America and some areas of Europe

IMAGING
N/A

OTHER DIAGNOSTIC PROCEDURES
N/A

PATHOLOGIC FINDINGS
N/A

TREATMENT
• Replace the penis in the prepuce as soon as possible to prevent accumulation of dependent edema, drying of exposed surfaces, and traumatic injury. If replacement is impossible due to swelling, slings can be used to support the penis against the ventral abdominal wall
• Lubricate the exposed mucosal surfaces with an emollient or antimicrobial ointment
• In cases of chronic, nonresponsive penile paralysis, surgical intervention, including penile amputation or penile retraction (Bolz technique), should be considered. Castration generally precedes these surgical techniques

MEDICATIONS

DRUG(S) OF CHOICE
Anti-inflammatory medication (phenylbutazone 2–4 g/450 kg body weight/day PO) may be useful for patient comfort and to decrease inflammation.

CONTRAINDICATIONS/POSSIBLE INTERACTIONS
Phenothiazine tranquilizers should be avoided.

FOLLOW-UP

PATIENT MONITORING
• Initial management is intensive
• Frequent evaluation is of paramount importance
• Return of the ability to maintain the penis in the prepuce is a good prognostic indicator

PREVENTION/AVOIDANCE
N/A

POSSIBLE COMPLICATIONS
• Libido is often maintained, but if erection is impossible live cover will not be possible without human intervention and assistance

• Some affected stallions can be trained to ejaculate into an artificial vagina
• Ejaculation can be obtained by manual stimulation (i.e. application of hot compresses to the gland and base of the penis) and/or administration of tricyclic antidepressant
• Possible secondary complications of paralysis:
  ○ Paraphimosis due to the accumulation of dependent edema
  ○ Frostbite due to exposure
  ○ Surface excoriations—ulcers, secondary bacterial contamination, necrosis

EXPECTED COURSE AND PROGNOSIS
N/A

MISCELLANEOUS

ASSOCIATED CONDITIONS
• Paraphimosis
• Balanoposthitis

AGE-RELATED FACTORS
N/A

ZOONOTIC POTENTIAL
N/A

PREGNANCY/FERTILITY/BREEDING
N/A

SYNONYMS
N/A

SEE ALSO
• Equine herpesvirus myeloencephalopathy
• Paraphimosis
• Priapism
• Stallion sexual behavior problems

ABBREVIATIONS
• EHV = equine herpesvirus
• EIA = equine infectious anemia
• PCR = polymerase chain reaction

Suggested Reading
McDonnell SM, Turner RM, Love CC, LeBlanc MM. How to manage the stallion with a paralyzed penis for return to natural service or artificial insemination. Proc Am Assoc Equine Pract 2003;49:291–292.
Memon MA, Usenik EA, Varner DD, Meyers PJ. Penile paralysis and paraphimosis associated with reserpine administration in a stallion. Theriogenology 1988;30:411–419.
Vaughan JT. Surgery of the penis and prepuce. In: Walker DF, Vaughan JT, eds. Bovine and Equine Urogenital Surgery. Philadelphia, PA: Lea & Febiger, 1980:125–144.

Author Ahmed Tibary
Consulting Editor Carla L. Carleton
Acknowledgment The author and editor acknowledge the prior contribution of Carole C. Miller.

P

PENILE VESICLES, EROSIONS, AND TUMORS

BASICS

DEFINITION
Any vesicular, ulcerative, or proliferative lesion associated with the penis or preputial folds.

PATHOPHYSIOLOGY
- The normal surface of the penis is smooth when cleaned of smegma
- Irregularities in the penile surface or urethral process may be due to infectious, traumatic, inflammatory, or neoplastic lesions
- Infectious balanitis may be nonspecific bacterial or specific viral (EHV-3) or parasitic (*Habronema*)
- EHV-3 is a self-limiting highly contagious venereal disease. Its common name is equine coital exanthema. The incubation period is typically 4–7 days. Lesions are characterized by small raised papules, vesicles, then pustules that later break and form ulcerative lesions that are painful.
  ◦ No proof of a non-clinically apparent carrier state exists, although shedding has been reported to occur immediately prior to vesicle formation
  ◦ As with other herpes infections, virus recrudescence and formation of a new population of vesicles (infective stage) are associated with stress
- Habronemiasis occurs when larvae of stomach nematodes are deposited on moist mucosal surfaces by stable flies. The larvae cause an influx of eosinophils to the affected tissues, resulting in granulomatous reactions and intense pruritus. Ulceration of the lesions is common
- The most common neoplasia of the penis and urethral process is SCC. The appearance and progression of the lesions vary

SYSTEMS AFFECTED
- Reproductive
- Urologic
- Lymphatic
- Skin

GENETICS
N/A

INCIDENCE/PREVALENCE
N/A

GEOGRAPHIC DISTRIBUTION
Worldwide

SIGNALMENT
Any age and breed can be affected.

SIGNS

Historical Findings
- Poor libido or inability to mate, painful
- Hemospermia or hematuria

Physical Examination Findings
- May include visible lesions on the penis, prepuce, urethral process, fossa glandis, and on other mucocutaneous junctions

- Evidence of a prior EHV-3 infection—healed vesicles leave characteristic lesions on the penis and prepuce consisting of gray (loss of dark pigmentation) irregular patches of penile/preputial skin (many prior vesicles may coalesce into larger patches); affected area of skin remains pliable (interim/inactive phase of EHV-3). Note that there is similar evidence on the vulva of a mare affected by EHV-3
- Phimosis due to stricture formation, adhesions, or tumor proliferation
- Paraphimosis due to secondary edema formation or mechanical impedance
- Hematuria or hemospermia
- Enlargement of local lymphatics or draining

CAUSES
- Viral infections—EHV-3
- Parasites—*Habronema* spp.
- Neoplasia—SCC, sarcoid, melanoma, papilloma, hemangioma
- Trauma—chronic wounds, local irritants, thermal injuries
- Bacteria—abscessation such as that associated with bastard strangles

RISK FACTORS
- Because equine coital exanthema is a venereal disease, natural breeding programs are more likely to have an outbreak than programs using artificial insemination. Similarly, unsanitary breeding practices can put patients at greater risk
- Unsanitary housing conditions or poor fly control can contribute to Habronemiasis. It is more often seen in hot, humid locations in the spring or summer seasons
- Gray-colored horses are the most likely to present with melanoma
- Lightly pigmented horses are more likely to have SCC, and geldings may be affected more than stallions

DIAGNOSIS

DIFFERENTIAL DIAGNOSIS

Differentiating Causes
- EHV-3 infection, typical presentation—multiple, circular, 1–2 mm nodules that progress into vesicles and pustules and ultimately rupture to form ulcerations 5–10 mm in diameter on the penile/preputial mucosa. Systemic involvement is rare, although lesions have been found on other mucocutaneous junctions in some cases
- Habronemiasis—Bollinger's granules, caseous masses in the exuberant granulation tissue, are diagnostic for habronemiasis. Lesions typically are extremely pruritic. *Summer sores,* the characteristic lesion, most often occur in the area of the urethral process or on the preputial ring
- Neoplastic lesions can be either ulcerative or proliferative—SCCs usually are only locally

invasive, although they can metastasize to regional lymph nodes and other body tissues
- Chronic traumatic lesions can mimic any other disease process. Diagnosis is established by history, exclusion, or response to therapy

CBC/BIOCHEMISTRY/URINALYSIS
N/A

OTHER LABORATORY TESTS
- Confirmation of EHV-3 by virus isolation from vesicular aspirates
- Rising antibody titers for EHV-3 from paired sera, at a 14–21 day interval

IMAGING
N/A

OTHER DIAGNOSTIC PROCEDURES
- Cytology—intranuclear, eosinophilic inclusion bodies are indicative of EHV-3
- Biopsy and histopathology can distinguish between the various tumor types and habronemiasis

PATHOLOGIC FINDINGS
N/A

TREATMENT

APPROPRIATE HEALTH CARE
- Coital exanthema is a self-limiting disease with a course of disease of 3–5 weeks. The lesions can be quite uncomfortable, and secondary bacterial infections can occur. Daily cleansing and the application of emollient or antimicrobial ointments may be indicated. Sexual rest while vesicles form, rupture, and heal prevents venereal transmission
- Therapy for habronemiasis includes eradicating the infective larvae as well as controlling the local hypersensitivity reaction. Surgical resection of residual scar tissue may be necessary
- Tumors may be surgically excised, or eliminated with cryosurgery, radiation therapy, hyperthermia, reefing, or phallectomy, dependent upon their size, location, invasiveness, and type
- Papillomas often regress spontaneously in 3–4 months
- Topical or intralesional injections of chemotherapeutic agents have been used to address equine sarcoids and penile SCC
- Chronic wounds should be cleansed, debrided, and closed, when possible. Local irritants (i.e. povidone–iodine scrub) should be thoroughly rinsed off after application, if used
- Streptococcal infections should be treated with systemic antibiotics

NURSING CARE
See Appropriate Health Care.

ACTIVITY
Depends on the extent of the lesion. Hospitalization may be required.

P

PENILE VESICLES, EROSIONS, AND TUMORS (CONTINUED)

DIET
N/A

CLIENT EDUCATION
• Importance of regular and proper cleaning of the penis and sheath
• Importance of regular examination of stallions used for breeding to detect early lesions
• Prebreeding examination and quarantine of mares if natural cover

SURGICAL CONSIDERATIONS
Surgical intervention may be the only course of action for some advanced cases of neoplasia.

MEDICATIONS

DRUG(S) OF CHOICE
• *Habronema* larvae can be eradicated using ivermectin (0.2 mg/kg PO). The use of prednisone to diminish localized pruritic reactions is in question because of questionable gastrointestinal absorption
• NSAIDs including phenylbutazone (2–4 g/ 450 kg body weight/day PO) or flunixin meglumine (1 mg/kg/day IV, IM, or PO) are useful for symptomatic treatment of discomfort and to reduce local inflammation
• Systemic (procaine penicillin G 20 000– 22 000 IU/kg IM BID) or local (0.2% nitrofurazone ointment) antibiotics are used to treat primary or secondary bacterial infection

PRECAUTIONS
• Chronic steroid use can result in iatrogenic Cushing disease and may predispose the patient to developing laminitis due to systemic vasoconstrictive action
• Phenothiazine tranquilizers should be used with caution, or not at all, owing to the possibility of their causing priapism in intact stallions

POSSIBLE INTERACTIONS
N/A

ALTERNATIVE DRUGS
• Trichlorfon (metrifonate) (22 mg/kg diluted in 1–2 L of 0.9% NaCl slow IV) has been used to eliminate *Habronema* larvae. There is a risk of clinical organophosphate toxicity
• Topical application of trichlorfon in 0.2% nitrofurazone (4.5 g trichlorfon in 115 mL (4 oz) of 0.2% nitrofurazone) once daily to

granulomatous lesions can be effective in the acute stage of habronemiasis
• Autogenous vaccines have been suggested to deter the spread of papillomatosis within a herd
• 5-Fluorouracil in sesame oil has been reported to have some use as a topical sarcoid treatment

FOLLOW-UP

PATIENT MONITORING
The frequency of reevaluation depends upon the inciting cause and severity of the lesion.

PREVENTION/AVOIDANCE
Avoid breeding activity in the presence of active EHV-3 lesions, but some shedding may occur prior to and immediately after the appearance of vesicles.

POSSIBLE COMPLICATIONS
• Chronic *Habronema* spp. infection involving the urethral process can result in periurethral fibrosis; if severe, it will necessitate amputation of the urethral process
• Paraphimosis
• Phimosis
• Metastatic lesions in local lymph, lung, or other body tissues
• Progression of squamous papillomatous lesions to SCC has been reported
• Urethral blockage due to either the pathologic condition or therapeutic intervention can occur; urethral patency should be closely monitored

EXPECTED COURSE AND PROGNOSIS
Prognosis depends on the etiology and extent of lesions.

MISCELLANEOUS
N/A

ASSOCIATED CONDITIONS
N/A

AGE-RELATED FACTORS
• Young horses are more likely to present with papillomatous lesions
• Melanomas are more typically found in aged animals

ZOONOTIC POTENTIAL
N/A

PREGNANCY/FERTILITY/BREEDING
Coital exanthema does not cause abortion.

SYNONYMS
• EHV-3
• Equine coital exanthema
• Equine venereal balanitis
• Esponja
• Genital bursatti
• Genital horse pox
• Habronemiasis
• Summer sores
• Swamp cancer
• Warts

SEE ALSO
• Paraphimosis
• Penile lacerations
• Phimosis

ABBREVIATIONS
• EHV = equine herpesvirus
• NSAID = nonsteroidal anti-inflammatory drug
• SCC = squamous cell carcinoma

Suggested Reading
Arnold CE, Brinsko SP, Love CC, Varner DD. Use of a modified Vinsot technique for partial phallectomy in 11 standing horses. J Am Vet Med Assoc 2010;237:82–86.
Barrandeguy M, Thiry E. Equine coital exanthema and its potential economic implications for the equine industry. Vet J 2012;191:35–40.
Fortier LA, McHarg MA. Topical use of 5-fluorouracil for treatment of squamous cell carcinoma of the external genitalia of horses: 11 cases (1988–1992). J Am Vet Med Assoc 1994;205:1183–1185.
May KA, Moll HD, Lucroy MD. Recognizing tumors of the equine external genitalia. Compend Contin Educ Pract Vet 2002;24:970–976.
Pugh DG, Hu XP, Blagburn B. Habronemiasis: biology, signs, and diagnosis, and treatment and prevention of the nematodes and vector flies. J Equine Vet Sci 2014;34:241–248.
Van den Top JGB, de Heer N, Klein WR, Ensink JM. Penile and preputial squamous cell carcinoma in the horse: a retrospective study of treatment of 77 affected horses. Equine Vet J 2008;40:533–537.

Author Ahmed Tibary
Consulting Editor Carla L. Carleton
Acknowledgment The author and editor acknowledge the prior contribution of Carole C. Miller.

PENTACHLOROPHENOL (PCP) TOXICOSIS

BASICS

OVERVIEW
• PCP is highly lipid soluble and volatile. Primarily used as a wood preservative, fungicide, and herbicide. Exposure occurs through inhalation of vapors, gastrointestinal absorption, or dermal absorption
• PCP causes uncoupling of oxidative phosphorylation and direct irritation to the skin and the respiratory tract
• Acute and chronic intoxication syndromes have been described in animals. The chronic syndrome may be due to PCDD and PCDF isomers found in PCP
• Restrictions on the use of PCP owing to environmental and toxicity concerns make exposure and toxicosis unlikely

SIGNALMENT
N/A

SIGNS
• Acute—hyperthermia, restlessness, tachypnea, increased gastrointestinal motility, weakness, seizures, and collapse
• Chronic—anorexia, weight loss, dependent edema, alopecia, skin cracks and fissures, colic, joint stiffness, recurrent hoof problems, conjunctivitis, hematuria, and secondary opportunistic infections

CAUSES AND RISK FACTORS
• Most likely sources of exposure are treated wood used for fences or feedbunks, bedding from treated wood, or contact with contaminated soil
• High ambient temperatures and poor body condition

DIAGNOSIS

DIFFERENTIAL DIAGNOSIS
• Acute—infectious causes of pyrexia (CBC, bacterial culture, serology)
• Chronic—*Vicia villosa* toxicosis (skin biopsy)

CBC/BIOCHEMISTRY/URINALYSIS
• Acute—not reported for horses
• Chronic—changes consistent with hepatic dysfunction, anemia, and thrombocytopenia

OTHER LABORATORY TESTS
• Acute—antemortem detection of PCP in blood, serum/plasma, or urine; PCP is rapidly cleared so measurement is useful only in acute intoxications; postmortem detection of PCP in skin, liver, or kidney
• Chronic—measurement of PCDD or PCDF isomers in plasma/serum or tissues

IMAGING
N/A

OTHER DIAGNOSTIC PROCEDURES
N/A

PATHOLOGIC FINDINGS
• Acute—not reported for horses
• Chronic

Gross
Emaciation; alopecia; crusty, scaly dermatitis; cracks or fissures of the skin that exude clear serum-like fluid; splenomegaly.

Histopathologic
Chronic nonsuppurative dermatitis; hepatic bile duct proliferation, inflammation, and focal necrosis; splenic hemosiderosis; multifocal renal tubular necrosis; nonregenerative bone marrow hypoplasia.

TREATMENT

• Acute—control hyperthermia; remove from source of exposure; if recent oral exposure, consider gastrointestinal decontamination; wash exposed skin
• Chronic—remove from source of exposure; provide symptomatic and supportive care

MEDICATIONS

DRUG(S) OF CHOICE
Acute—AC at 1–2 g/kg in water slurry (1 g AC in 5 mL water) PO and either magnesium sulfate at 250 mg/kg PO or sorbitol (70%) at 3 mL/kg PO, given once with AC.

CONTRAINDICATIONS/POSSIBLE INTERACTIONS
N/A

FOLLOW-UP

PATIENT MONITORING
N/A

PREVENTION/AVOIDANCE
Avoid use of treated wood where animal contact is possible.

POSSIBLE COMPLICATIONS
N/A

EXPECTED COURSE AND PROGNOSIS
Poor prognosis and prolonged recovery in chronic intoxication due to dioxin.

MISCELLANEOUS

Current environmental restrictions on the use of PCP make clinically significant exposure and toxicosis unlikely.

ASSOCIATED CONDITIONS
N/A

AGE-RELATED FACTORS
N/A

ZOONOTIC POTENTIAL
N/A

PREGNANCY/FERTILITY/BREEDING
Chronic intoxication of pregnant horses with PCDD and PCDF can result in birth of weak foals susceptible to opportunistic infections.

ABBREVIATIONS
• AC = activated charcoal
• PCDD = dibenzo-*p*-dioxin isomers
• PCDF = dibenzofuran isomers
• PCP = pentachlorophenol

Suggested Reading
Kerkvliet NI, Wagner SL, Schmotzer WB, et al. Dioxin intoxication from chronic exposure of horses to penta-chlorophenol-contaminated wood shavings. J Am Vet Med Assoc 1992;201:296–302.

Authors Arya Sobhakumari and Robert H. Poppenga
Consulting Editors Wilson K. Rumbeiha and Steve Ensley

P

PERICARDITIS

 BASICS

DEFINITION
Inflammation resulting in accumulation of fluid (transudate or exudate), fibrin, or both in the pericardial sac.

PATHOPHYSIOLOGY
Accumulation of pericardial fluid compromises right atrial and ventricular filling, followed by impaired left ventricular filling, decreased cardiac output, generalized venous distention, and ventral edema.

SYSTEMS AFFECTED
Cardiovascular

SIGNS
General Comments
Horse may present for colic.

Historical Findings
• Colic
• Fever
• Exercise intolerance

Physical Examination Findings
• Depression
• Lethargy
• Tachycardia
• Other, less common findings—anorexia; weight loss; fever; generalized venous distention; ventral, pectoral, or preputial edema; weak arterial pulse; pulsus paradoxus; arrhythmias; muffled heart sounds; pericardial friction rubs; and dull cranioventral lung field

CAUSES
• Septic—viral or bacterial
• Bacterial infections—most frequently streptococcal or *Actinobacillus* sp.
• Viral infections most frequently may result in immune-mediated pericarditis
• Idiopathic—many of these also may be immune mediated; also potentially associated with outbreaks of mare reproductive loss syndrome involving ingestion of eastern tent caterpillars
• Neoplastic—rare

RISK FACTORS
• Pericarditis may be secondary to pleuropneumonia and be septic or immune mediated
• Mare reproductive loss syndrome and exposure to eastern tent caterpillars

 DIAGNOSIS

DIFFERENTIAL DIAGNOSIS
• Endocarditis—murmurs often detected, heart sounds not muffled, and pericardial friction rubs absent; differentiate echocardiographically
• Congestive heart failure—murmurs usually detected; differentiate echocardiographically

• Cranial mediastinal abscess/mass—heart sounds usually not muffled; no venous distention caudally; differentiate echocardiographically and ultrasonographically

CBC/BIOCHEMISTRY/URINALYSIS
• Neutrophilic leukocytosis, hyperfibrinogenemia, and elevated SAA are common
• Anemia of chronic disease possible
• Prerenal azotemia possible

OTHER LABORATORY TESTS
• Virus isolation is indicated
• Paired serology may be performed, looking for a significant increase in titer to equine viruses
• Elevated cardiac troponin I or cardiac troponin T indicates concurrent myocardial disease
• Perform cytologic evaluation, along with culture and sensitivity testing, of pericardial fluid, along with pleural or transtracheal wash fluid (if concurrent pleuropneumonia)

IMAGING
ECG
• Diminished amplitude of complexes and electrical alternans with significant pericardial effusion
• Atrial or ventricular premature complexes occasionally occur

Echocardiography
• The pericardial sac is usually distended with fluid and fibrin lining the epicardial and pericardial surfaces
• Fibrinous loculations may be present, and the pericardial sac may be thickened
• Occasionally, horses have a noneffusive pericarditis, with only a small amount of fibrin
• Right atrial and ventricular diastolic collapse occurs early, along with excessive swinging of the right ventricular free wall
• An inspiratory increase in right ventricle diameter and decrease in left ventricle diameter also occur with cardiac tamponade
• Abrupt cessation of ventricular filling during early diastole with diastolic flattening of the left ventricular free wall indicates constrictive pericarditis—rare

Diagnostic Ultrasonography
• An anechoic pleural effusion present in most horses with pericarditis
• With concurrent pleuropneumonia, pulmonary consolidation, a pulmonary abscess, or a composite pleural effusion may be present

Thoracic Radiography
• A globoid cardiac silhouette is detected
• Increased ventral lung field opacity and a pleural fluid line may be detected

OTHER DIAGNOSTIC PROCEDURES
Cardiac Catheterization
• Elevated central venous pressure with cardiac tamponade

• Elevated right atrial pressure with a preserved systolic *x* descent and absence of or a diminutive diastolic *y* descent
• Right ventricular, pulmonary arterial systolic, and pulmonary capillary wedge pressures usually are elevated

Pericardiocentesis
• If possible, insert a large-bore chest tube (26–32 F) and, with ultrasonographic guidance, obtain a sample for cytology and culture and sensitivity testing; leave the tube in place
• Obtain a sample of pleural fluid, if present, for cytology and culture and sensitivity testing
• With suspected pneumonia, obtain a transtracheal aspirate for cytology and culture and sensitivity testing

PATHOLOGIC FINDINGS
• Fibrin coating the parietal and visceral pericardial surfaces along with the pericardial effusion
• Pleural effusion common
• Concurrent fibrinous pleuritis or pneumonia in some horses

 TREATMENT

AIMS
• Correct cardiac tamponade by establishing drainage
• Remove bacterial infection, if present, with appropriate broad-spectrum antimicrobials
• Control immune-mediated mechanisms, if present, using anti-inflammatory drugs

APPROPRIATE HEALTH CARE
• Insert a large-bore, indwelling pericardial tube for drainage and lavage and direct instillation of antimicrobials if there is adequate space to do so safely
• After drainage, instill 1–2 L of isotonic saline into the pericardial sac, leave in place for 30–60 min, drain, and then instill 1 L of isotonic saline with 10–20 million IU sodium penicillin and/or 1 g gentamicin. Leave in place for 12–24 h. Repeat until the initial drainage consistently recovers less fluid than what was left in situ, then remove the tube. Continue broad-spectrum antimicrobials or systemic corticosteroids, if a septic cause has been ruled out
• Occasionally, minimal fluid accumulates, and the pericarditis resolves without drainage

ACTIVITY
Stall rest and hand-walking during treatment and for several weeks thereafter.

CLIENT EDUCATION
Closely monitor for tachycardia, venous distention, or exercise intolerance; if detected, seek cardiac reevaluation.

(CONTINUED)   **PERICARDITIS**

SURGICAL CONSIDERATIONS
Subtotal pericardiectomy has been tried in a horse with constrictive pericarditis but was not successful in the long term.

MEDICATIONS
DRUG(S) OF CHOICE
• Base the selection of antimicrobials on culture and sensitivity results. Initially, IV bactericidal broad-spectrum drugs are recommended
• The most common causative bacterial organisms—*Streptococcus* sp., usually sensitive to penicillin; Gram-negative organisms (usually *Actinobacillus* sp.), usually are sensitive to gentamicin. The drugs can also be directly instilled into the pericardial sac after lavage and drainage, which increases the drug concentration locally
• Once septic pericarditis has been successfully treated or ruled out, systemic corticosteroids may be administered
• If septic pericarditis is diagnosed, antimicrobial treatment for 4 weeks is indicated

CONTRAINDICATIONS
Do *not* use long-term corticosteroids in horses with an active bacterial or viral cause of pericarditis.

PRECAUTIONS
• Place an IV catheter before pericardiocentesis or placement of an indwelling pericardial tube so that rapid antiarrhythmic treatment can be performed, if necessary
• Monitor for any arrhythmias during pericardiocentesis and while the indwelling pericardial tube is in place
• Evaluate creatinine and blood urea nitrogen before starting aminoglycoside antimicrobials and use therapeutic drug monitoring to individualize dosage regimens

ALTERNATIVE DRUGS
• Base use of alternative antimicrobial drugs on results of culture and sensitivity testing of the pericardial fluid
• In horses with suspected septic pericarditis and pleuropneumonia and no growth on pericardial fluid culture, the results obtained from a transtracheal wash or pleural fluid aspirate may be used, because the organisms are likely the same

• Suspect an anaerobic infection (rare) if free gas echoes imaged; treat with metronidazole

FOLLOW-UP
PATIENT MONITORING
• Heart rate, generalized venous distention, and ventral edema should gradually return to normal with resolution of the effusion
• Amplitude of ECG complexes should gradually increase with reduction in the pericardial effusion
• Respiratory rate and temperature should return to normal as the pericarditis and pleuropneumonia resolve
• Monitor white blood cell count, SAA, fibrinogen, and creatinine until normal

PREVENTION/AVOIDANCE
Aggressive treatment of horses with pleuropneumonia may prevent pericarditis secondary to pleuritis.

POSSIBLE COMPLICATIONS
Constrictive pericarditis may develop due to scarring of the pericardial and epicardial surfaces and subsequent restriction to ventricular filling during late diastole.

EXPECTED COURSE AND PROGNOSIS
• Most horses treated aggressively with pericardial lavage and drainage, direct instillation of appropriate antimicrobials, and systemic broad-spectrum antibiotics or corticosteroids (if indicated) have a good prognosis for life and return to performance
• Remove indwelling pericardial tube when less fluid is recovered than was left in place for the previous 12–24 h; usually after 3–5 days
• Broad-spectrum antimicrobials are continued until no evidence of bacterial infection, after which corticosteroid therapy is initiated
• With septic pericarditis, continue IV bactericidal antimicrobials for at least 7–14 days, then switch to appropriate oral antimicrobials for another 2–4 weeks. The total length of antimicrobial treatment is at least 4–6 weeks followed by 4 weeks of rest and cardiac reevaluation before returning to work
• In most horses, any echocardiographic evidence of pericarditis is difficult to detect 1 month after discontinuation of treatment

MISCELLANEOUS
ASSOCIATED CONDITIONS
• Pleuritis and pleuropneumonia may result in direct extension of infection into the pericardial sac
• The pericardium may be involved with cranial mediastinal lymphosarcoma, mesothelioma, and hemangiosarcoma

AGE-RELATED FACTORS
• Pericarditis can occur at any age
• In older horses, a neoplastic cause, although rare, must be considered

PREGNANCY/FERTILITY/BREEDING
• Pericarditis; rare in pregnant mares; however, if cardiac tamponade is present, it may result in fetal compromise
• Aim treatment at successful drainage of the pericardial sac and restoration of normal cardiac output and organ perfusion

SEE ALSO
Pleuropneumonia

ABBREVIATIONS
SAA = serum amyloid A

Suggested Reading
Bernard W, Reef VB, Clark ES, et al. Pericarditis in horses: six cases (1982–1986). J Am Vet Med Assoc 1990;196:468–471.
Hardy J, Robertson JT, Reed SM. Constrictive pericarditis in a mare: attempted treatment by partial pericardiectomy. Equine Vet J 1992;24:151–154.
Marr CM. Cardiovascular infections. In: Sellon DC, Long MT, eds. Equine Infectious Disease, 2e. St. Louis, MO: Elsevier, 2014:21–41.
Reef VB. Cardiovascular ultrasonography. In: Reef VB, ed. Equine Diagnostic Ultrasound. Philadelphia, PA: WB Saunders, 1998:215–272.
Worth LT, Reef VB. Pericarditis in horses: a review of 18 cases (1986–1995). J Am Vet Med Assoc 1998;212:248–253.

Author Virginia B. Reef
Consulting Editors Celia M. Marr and Virginia B. Reef

P

PERINEAL LACERATIONS/RECTO-VAGINAL-VESTIBULAR FISTULAS

 BASICS

DEFINITION
- A laceration of the perineal body
- First-degree laceration involves the mucosa of the vestibule and the skin of the dorsal commissure of the vulva
- Second-degree laceration involves both the mucosa and the submucosa of the dorsal vulva and part of the musculature of the perineal body (constrictor vulvae muscle)
- Third-degree laceration involves full-thickness tears through the perineal body, extending through the rectal wall and anal sphincter
- RVVFs are full-thickness tears through the rectal wall and, possibly, involving the perineal body, but not involving the anal sphincter or vulva
- Recto-vestibular fistulas are much more common than RVFs

PATHOPHYSIOLOGY
- Perineal lacerations occur at parturition because of abnormal posture or position of the fetus, which predisposes the fetal extremities to be pushed more dorsal than normal, thus forcing the fetus's feet into and/or through the wall of the vagina or vestibule
- Although rare, an oversized fetus may be a cause
- Lacerations of the rectum or vagina can occur at breeding, but perineal lacerations are rare at this time
- Recto-vestibular fistulas can result from an unsuccessful surgical repair of a third-degree perineal laceration
- Mares with perineal lacerations or an RVVF are predisposed to recurrent uterine infections due to destruction of the anatomic structures (physical barriers) preventing contamination of the vagina

SYSTEMS AFFECTED
Reproductive

GENETICS
N/A

INCIDENCE/PREVALENCE
- No statistics available regarding incidence
- Common lesions in broodmares

SIGNALMENT
- All breeds
- Maiden mares are more predisposed to these injuries during parturition

SIGNS
General Comments
- The condition is not an emergency
- Because of the tearing, bruising, and edema occurring at and after injury, surgical correction of these lacerations is delayed until

the initial inflammation has subsided and laceration has healed by second intention; generally at least 30 days

Historical Findings
- Dystocia is common but not necessary
- Because of the excessive force generated by the abdominal musculature (*active labor*), it is possible for a mare to deliver a live foal unassisted while creating a perineal laceration

Physical Examination Findings
- Careful physical examination of the perineum, perineal body, vagina, and rectum
- Transrectal palpation and vaginal examination

CAUSES
- Abnormal posture or position of the fetus at parturition
- Fetal extremities are pushed more dorsal than normal within the birth canal, such that they penetrate and damage maternal soft tissue structures within the vagina, vestibule, and/or rectum

RISK FACTORS
- Dystocia—abnormal fetal position or posture, fetal oversize
- Small vulva and tight vestibulo-vaginal sphincter
- Because fetal posture and position can change within minutes before parturition, examinations conducted much before parturition are of little value
- Failure to open the vulva (Caslick's vulvoplasty; an episioplasty) prior to foaling in mares

 DIAGNOSIS

DIFFERENTIAL DIAGNOSIS
Diagnosis is self-evident.

CBC/BIOCHEMISTRY/URINALYSIS
N/A

OTHER LABORATORY TESTS
N/A

IMAGING
N/A

OTHER DIAGNOSTIC PROCEDURES
N/A

PATHOLOGIC FINDINGS
- Partial to full-thickness lacerations of the vestibule, vagina, anal sphincter, and/or rectum
- Aspiration of air into the vagina and/or uterus secondary to damaged normal barrier tissues, e.g. vulvar lips; vestibular sphincter
- Fecal contamination of the vagina and vestibule, followed by inflammation of the vestibule, vagina, cervix, and, possibly, the endometrium

 TREATMENT

APPROPRIATE HEALTH CARE
- Confirm whether the laceration extends into the peritoneal cavity, a rare occurrence with perineal laceration or RVF
- Systemic antibiotics seldom are indicated or necessary to control infection in this area; client education is imperative
- Local medication rarely is indicated
- Repair lacerations before attempting to rebreed
- Boost tetanus vaccination, if not recent

NURSING CARE
N/A

ACTIVITY
No restrictions.

DIET
No restrictions.

CLIENT EDUCATION
- Advise regarding the importance of close/ frequent observation of foaling mares
- Many lacerations occur before a problem is detected, even in the presence of trained foaling attendants

SURGICAL CONSIDERATIONS
General Comments
- Surgical repair is delayed until local inflammation and bruising have subsided (generally 4–6 weeks)
- Imperative after surgery that feces remain soft until healing is complete. Mare should be given oral mineral oil prior to surgery
- Early in the spring (preoperative), place the mare on pasture, and return it to pasture immediately after surgery. Green grass has a high moisture content, which should soften stool
- Other methods of stool softening include bran and mineral oil
- Several surgical techniques have been described for repair of third-degree perineal lacerations and RVVF. The success rate is highly dependent on the surgeon's experience

2-Stage Repair
Stage 1
- Epidural anesthesia and sedation of the mare
- The tail is wrapped and elevated over the mare and attached to a support directly above the animal
- The rectum and vagina/vestibule are emptied of feces and thoroughly but gently cleaned. Use of irritating scrubs could stimulate postoperative straining and is contraindicated
- Reconstruction of the perineal body:
  ○ An incision is made into the remaining shelf ≅2–3 cm anterior to the cranial limit of the laceration

P

(CONTINUED) PERINEAL LACERATIONS/RECTO-VAGINAL-VESTIBULAR FISTULAS

○ The incision is continued posteriorly along the sides of the existing laceration in a plane approximately equal to the original location of the perineal body
○ The vestibular and vaginal mucosa is reflected ventrally ≅2 cm
○ Simple interrupted sutures are placed through the area of the perineal body so that the perineal body is reapposed and the submucosal vaginal or vestibular tissue is brought together in the same suture pattern
○ After placement of 1 or 2 of these sutures, a continuous suture pattern is begun in the reflected mucosal membrane to oppose the submucosal surfaces
○ This suture pattern continues cranial to caudal, as additional simple interrupted sutures are placed

Stage 2
• Completed after healing of stage 1
• Debride the anal sphincter and dorsal vulvar commissure, and place sutures in these tissues to reestablish the sphincters, if possible
• Optimal success is achieved if sphincter tone is regained after repair

1-Stage Repair
Similar to 2-stage repair, except that repairs of the anal sphincter and dorsal vulvar commissure are completed at the time of the initial surgery.

MEDICATIONS
DRUG(S) OF CHOICE
• Systemic antibiotics may be indicated immediately after laceration to prevent possible systemic involvement, but the laceration must be quite severe to warrant their use
• Medications specific to accomplish the surgical repair
• Ensure adequate tetanus prophylaxis

CONTRAINDICATIONS
N/A

PRECAUTIONS
N/A

POSSIBLE INTERACTIONS
N/A

ALTERNATIVE DRUGS
Any agent designed for sedation and analgesia can be used during surgical correction.

FOLLOW-UP
PATIENT MONITORING
• An immediate examination is indicated with the possibility or concern that a laceration has occurred
• If its presence is confirmed but it does not extend into the perineal cavity, reexamine the area in ≅2 weeks to assess the degree of inflammation and formation of granulation tissue at the laceration site

PREVENTION/AVOIDANCE
• Occurrence is difficult to predict
• Close monitoring of mares (particularly maiden mares) during parturition

POSSIBLE COMPLICATIONS
• Abscesses may develop in the laceration area, but this is uncommon, aided in part by the abundant surface area that facilitates drainage and formation of granulation tissue from the deeper layers outward
• If the laceration is sutured immediately after the occurrence, the potential for abscessation may actually increase

EXPECTED COURSE AND PROGNOSIS
• Without surgical correction, mares with third-degree lacerations and an RVF have a very low probability of conceiving and maintaining a pregnancy to term
• Therefore, surgical correction is strongly recommended before attempting breeding
• Dehiscence and recto-vestibular fistula are possible complications requiring a second intervention

MISCELLANEOUS
ASSOCIATED CONDITIONS
N/A

AGE-RELATED FACTORS
N/A

ZOONOTIC POTENTIAL
N/A

PREGNANCY/FERTILITY/BREEDING
Occurs at parturition.

SYNONYMS
N/A

SEE ALSO
• Delayed uterine involution
• Dystocia
• Prolonged pregnancy
• Urine pooling/urovagina

ABBREVIATIONS
• RVF = recto-vaginal fistula
• RVVF = recto-vaginal-vestibular fistula

Suggested Reading
Aanes WA. Surgical repair of third degree perineal lacerations and recto-vaginal fistulas in the mare. J Am Vet Med Assoc 1964;144:485–491.
Belknap JK, Nickels FA. A one-stage repair of third-degree perineal lacerations and rectovestibular fistula in 17 mares. Vet Surg 1992;21:378–381.
Climent F, Ribera T, Argulles D, et al. Modified technique for the repair of third-degree rectovaginal lacerations in mares. Vet Rec 2009;164:393–396.
Colbern GT, Aanes WA, Stashak TS. Surgical management of perineal lacerations and recto-vestibular fistulae in the mare: a retrospective study of 47 cases. J Am Vet Med Assoc 1985;186:265–269.
Heinze CD, Allen AR. Repair of third-degree perineal lacerations in the mare. Vet Scope 1966;11:12–15.
McKinnon AO, Jalin SL. Surgery of the caudal reproductive tract. In: McKinnon AO, Squires EL, Vaala WE, Varner DD, eds. Equine Reproduction, 2e. Ames, IA: Wiley Blackwell, 2011:2545–2558.

Author Ahmed Tibary
Consulting Editor Carla L. Carleton
Acknowledgment The author and editor acknowledge the prior contribution of Walter R. Threlfall.

P

PERIOCULAR SARCOID

BASICS

DEFINITION
A neoplasm of fibroblastic origin that generally has a low metastatic potential, yet is often locally aggressive. There are several clinical forms ranging from areas of alopecia and altered, flaky skin to more pronounced nodular lesions with or without overlying skin involvement or fleshy, proliferative masses with ulceration.

PATHOPHYSIOLOGY
• Etiopathogenesis is unknown, but BPV has been implicated as an inciting agent. Intradermal inoculation with extract from bovine skin tumors caused by BPV has caused lesions in horses resembling equine sarcoid
• Additionally, genetic susceptibility may exist with equine sarcoid. Horses that express certain MHC-encoded ELAs (MHC-I ELA W3 and B1 and MHC-II ELA W13 and A5) have increased incidence and higher recurrence rates after surgery. Flies have been implicated as vectors for transfer of infectious agents or sarcoid cells between animals

SYSTEMS AFFECTED
• Eyelids and periocular skin
• Equine sarcoid can affect any cutaneous area, but approximately 32% of the tumors are located on the head and neck. As many as 14% of all the equine sarcoids are periocular

GENETICS
• No proven genetic basis, but genes in or near MHC have been implicated
• There has also been demonstrated a correlation between the development of sarcoids and heterozygosity for the equine severe combined immunodeficiency allele

INCIDENCE/PREVALENCE
Sarcoids are the most commonly reported equine tumor overall and the second most common periocular tumor of the horse.

GEOGRAPHIC DISTRIBUTION
No reported geographic distribution.

SIGNALMENT
Species
Horses, donkeys, and mules.

Breed Predilections
Nearly all breeds have been reported to have sarcoids. However, Quarter Horses, Appaloosas, Arabians, and Thoroughbreds are reported to have the highest risk, while Standardbreds and Lipizzaners have the lowest.

Mean Age and Range
Mean age of affected animals is between 3 and 7 years, with a range of 1 to >15 years.

Predominant Sex
No proven sex predilection.

SIGNS

Historical Findings
• Single or multiple areas of dermal thickening or nodules in the eyelids or periocular region
• Lesions may be ulcerated, and those affecting the eyelid margins or canthi may cause tearing, squinting, or ocular discharge
• Ocular irritation often occurs because of either disruption of eyelid function or direct rubbing on the globe
• Growth rate and biologic behavior are highly variable

Physical Examination Findings
• Nonspecific findings may include serous to mucopurulent ocular discharge, blepharospasm, and conjunctival hyperemia
• Solitary or multiple areas of linear or focal dermal thickening in the eyelids or periocular skin can be found. Lesions may also appear as nodules or pedunculated masses. Cutaneous ulceration and infection may be present

CAUSES
• Viral etiologies have been suggested
• A predisposition associated with genes on or near the MHC has also been suggested

RISK FACTORS
• Possible breed predilections, possible genetic risk factors
• Epizootics in herds suggest an infectious risk, possibly associated with fly vectors

DIAGNOSIS

DIFFERENTIAL DIAGNOSIS
• Diagnosis depends on an index of clinical suspicion and histopathology
• Differentials include granulation tissue or scarring; granulomas caused by habronemiasis, onchocerciasis, or foreign body reactions; fungal dermatitis; dermatophilus; and other tumors such as squamous cell carcinoma, papilloma, fibroma, and fibrosarcoma

CBC/BIOCHEMISTRY/URINALYSIS
Results usually normal.

IMAGING
Skull radiographs may be required if orbital or other bony involvement is suspected.

PATHOLOGIC FINDINGS
Gross
• Several morphologic types of sarcoid have been described
• Occult lesions are those with alopecia, altered hair, and small miliary nodules or plaques
• The verrucous ("warty") sarcoid is usually <6 cm in diameter, often with cauliflower edges and extensive flakiness of the skin with or without some ulceration
• Nodular lesions may or may not have epidermal involvement (type A versus type B)

• Fibroblastic lesions may be sessile and pedunculated. They often have a fleshy, ulcerated appearance
• The mixed sarcoid is a combination of the previous types
• Malignant sarcoids are unusual

Histologic
• Moderate to high density of fusiform or spindle-shaped fibroblastic cells that form whorls, interlacing bundles, and haphazard arrays (fibroblastic proliferation)
• Cytoplasmic boundaries are ill defined, and the amount of collagen varies considerably
• The mitotic rate is low
• In many sarcoids, fibroblastic cells are oriented perpendicularly to the overlying epithelial basement membrane
• A histopathologic diagnosis requires sampling the overlying skin as well as the deeper lesion of interest for nodular forms

TREATMENT

INPATIENT VERSUS OUTPATIENT
• Small superficial lesions may be removed standing with sedation and local anesthesia
• Larger more invasive lesions, or lesions involving the eyelid margins or canthi, may require hospitalization for surgery
• Alternatively, lesions may be treated under sedation and local anesthesia using intralesional chemotherapy, immunotherapy, or photodynamic therapy

ACTIVITY
• Restrict during the immediate postoperative period
• The eye should be protected from self-trauma with a soft- or hard-cup hood

CLIENT EDUCATION
• If intralesional chemotherapy is used, the client should be instructed to wear gloves when handling the periocular region for several days post injection
• The client should be made aware of clinical signs suggesting tumor recurrence
• Small insults to a sarcoid lesion, such as self-trauma from rubbing or even biopsy for confirmation of the diagnosis, may result in rapid progression, expansion, or transformation of the sarcoid. A plan for therapy to quickly follow biopsy should be made

SURGICAL CONSIDERATIONS
• Complete surgical excision of periocular sarcoid can be difficult or impossible, and recurrence rates of 50–64% have been reported with surgical excision alone. When surgical excision is combined with adjunctive therapy, success rates range from 65% to 95%. Various adjunctive therapies include cryotherapy, hyperthermia, CO_2 laser photoablation, topical chemotherapy, radiotherapy, and intralesional chemotherapy,

immunotherapy, and photodynamic therapy. Reconstructive eyelid surgery may also be necessary following excision of periocular sarcoids
• Intralesional BCG injections require multiple injections (every 1–2 weeks) with success rates ranging from 69% to 100%. Intralesional chemotherapy with either cisplatin or 5-FU can produce cures in up to 80% of cases. Cryotherapy (–20° to –40°C, triple freeze–thaw cycle) induces cryonecrosis of sarcoid cells with success rates of up to 75%. Radiofrequency hyperthermia has been reported to induce tumor regression (50°C for 30 s, 2 MHz). Multiple treatments may be necessary to prevent recurrence. 1 study reported an 81% success rate using CO_2 laser photoablation. Advantages included a clean, dry surgical site and a lack of postoperative pain and swelling. Radiation therapy has the highest success rates, in many cases approaching 100%, depending upon the source of radiation used. Unfortunately, radiation therapy, while it is the gold standard, is a difficult modality to access due to hazards to involved personnel

MEDICATIONS
DRUG(S) AND FLUIDS
Topical and Intralesional Immunotherapy/Chemotherapy
• Daily applications of topical 5-FU (1% TID) have been used with inconsistent results
• Herbal pastes of blood root extracts can be used topically in some sarcoids (XXTerra; Larson Labs, Fort Collins, CO)
• Intralesional chemotherapeutics including 5-FU and cisplatin have been used with some success. Intralesional cisplatin or carboplatin in purified medical grade sesame oil is administered in 4 or more sessions at 2 week intervals using 1 mg/cm³ of tumor
• Immunotherapy includes autogenous vaccines or immunomodulators. Intralesional injections of BPV vaccine have been successful in horses with sarcoids, but

systemic side effects have been severe in a few horses. Immunomodulation using BCG-attenuated *Mycobacterium bovis* cell wall in oil, however, has produced remission rates approaching 100%—1 mL of BCG/cm² of tumor surface area is injected into the lesion. Therapy is repeated every 2–4 weeks for up to 9 injections. Anaphylaxis may occur and can be minimized with pretreatment using flunixin meglumine (1.1 mg/kg IV) and corticosteroids or diphenhydramine

Supportive Therapy
Topical and systemic broad-spectrum antibiotics may be required to prevent infection following surgical and adjunctive therapy of periocular sarcoid. Systemic NSAIDs may be indicated following surgical excision or adjunctive therapy. Flunixin meglumine (1.1 mg/kg) provides analgesic and anti-inflammatory effects, and it may reduce the severity of anaphylaxis associated with intralesional immunotherapy.

FOLLOW-UP
PATIENT MONITORING
• Patients should be observed for signs of anaphylaxis immediately post injection when immunomodulating agents are used
• Long-term follow-up includes monitoring for tumor recurrence or failure of tumor regression

PREVENTION/AVOIDANCE
Fly control may reduce the incidence of sarcoid in herds with affected animals.

POSSIBLE COMPLICATIONS
• Tumor progression may lead to eyelid deformation, possibly resulting in secondary keratitis and conjunctivitis. Tissue necrosis causing similar ocular problems may occur with blood root extracts and other topical and intralesional therapies
• Ulceration of lesions may lead to secondary bacterial or fungal infections and possible septicemia. With ulcerated lesions, myiasis may be a problem

EXPECTED COURSE AND PROGNOSIS
• Prognosis for life is generally good for animals with single sarcoids, as these tumors do not metastasize
• In animals with numerous sarcoids, seen rarely in the USA and more commonly seen in the UK, prognosis for life is poor
• Factors affecting prognosis include tumor size, location, degree of local invasiveness, and response to previous therapy
• Recurrence rates following therapy depend on the therapeutic modalities used

MISCELLANEOUS
ZOONOTIC POTENTIAL
No proven zoonotic potential, but multiple occurrences in some herds suggest that this is possible. If so, fly vectors may be involved, possibly necessitating fly control.

PREGNANCY/FERTILITY/BREEDING
N/A

SEE ALSO
Ocular/adnexal squamous cell carcinoma

ABBREVIATIONS
• 5-FU = 5-fluorouracil
• BCG = bacillus Calmette-Guérin
• BPV = bovine papillomavirus
• ELA = equine leukocyte antigen
• MHC = major histocompatibility complex
• NSAID = nonsteroidal anti-inflammatory drug

Suggested Reading
Brooks DE. Ophthalmology for the Equine Practitioner, 2e. Jackson, WY: Teton NewMedia, 2008.
Brooks DE, Matthews AG. Equine ophthalmology. In: Gelatt KN, ed. Veterinary Ophthalmology, 4e. Ames, IA: Blackwell, 2007:1165–1274.
Gilger BC, ed. Equine Ophthalmology, 3e. Ames, IA: Wiley Blackwell, 2017.

Author Caryn E. Plummer
Consulting Editor Caryn E. Plummer

P

PERIODONTAL DISEASE

BASICS

DEFINITION
PD is an equine oral disorder that compromises the structures supporting the teeth, namely the periodontal ligament, the gingiva, the alveolar bone, and the cementum.

PATHOPHYSIOLOGY
• The predisposing feature of PD is food sequestrating in the interproximal space
• Diastemata (valve/open) or abnormal gaps between cheek teeth (due to supernumerary, displaced, or rotated teeth) are commonly observed in conjunction with PD. Valve diastemata are more prevalent and are associated with more severe PD than open diastemata
• Food material that becomes impacted incites focal gingivitis, leading to the development of a gingival sulcus. Impacted feed undergoes decay and bacterial fermentation (*Prevotella* spp. and *Veillonella* spp.), causing progressive destruction of the periodontal ligament and the alveolar bone, providing space for the impacted food to travel more deeply, advancing tooth destruction, and decreasing tooth support. Apical migration of the infection may result in periapical infection, abscess formation, and tooth root necrosis
• Equine PD may be secondary to abnormalities in dental wear. These abnormalities include step, shear, or wave mouth; missing or unopposed teeth, and hooks and ramps, which generate unevenly distributed forces, resulting in separation of the normally tightly aligned adjacent teeth
• Horses with mandibular or maxillary fractures can develop PD as a result of exposure of the periodontium to food material and as a result of alterations to normal mastication
• Transient PD associated with emerging dentition may occur in the immature equine mouth if food gets trapped around improperly shed deciduous teeth. Gingivitis and periodontitis resolve when the permanent teeth come into wear

SYSTEMS AFFECTED
• Gastrointestinal
• Musculoskeletal
• Respiratory (sinusitis)

GENETICS
N/A

INCIDENCE/PREVALENCE
The prevalence in the general equine population is reported to be 50%. In horses >15 years a prevalence of up to 60% has been described.

SIGNALMENT
PD occurs more frequently in mature animals. Disease as a result of retained deciduous teeth usually occurs between 2.5 and 4 years of age.

SIGNS
Oral pain including slow eating, dysmastication, oral dysphagia (quidding), hypersalivation, halitosis, anorexia, and weight loss. In the very early stages of disease no clinical signs may be present; however, changes will be observed during routine dental prophylaxis. If secondary maxillary sinusitis is present owing to oro-sinus fistulation purulent, malodorous nasal discharge, epiphora, and facial swelling may also be noted. Subtler clinical signs indicating oral pain may include head shyness, harness resentment, and resistance to the rider.

RISK FACTORS
• Domestic feeding practices and processed feeds often lead to abnormal mastication and decreased salivary fluid production, with resultant abnormality of wear and lowered local mechanical defense function, respectively
• Various conformational abnormalities become more common in geriatric horses; in addition, as horses age, there is progressive exposure of the reserve crown and consequently a less secure apposition between adjacent teeth
• Cushing syndrome and other systemic conditions that may alter immune function

DIAGNOSIS

DIFFERENTIAL DIAGNOSIS
Numerous pathologies of the oral cavity may lead to the clinical signs observed in conjunction with PD, highlighting the need for a very thorough oral examination.

CBC/BIOCHEMISTRY/URINALYSIS
Nonspecific

OTHER LABORATORY TESTS
N/A

IMAGING
Oral radiographs, especially open-mouthed oblique views of the teeth, may identify changes. Changes include destruction of the periodontal ligament as a loss of definition of the radiolucent ligament. Changes to the alveolus include bone lysis and sclerosis extending apically as far as the tooth roots as well as clubbing of tooth roots in more advanced cases. Other radiographic abnormalities include soft tissue densities and fluid lines in the sinuses. Many cases will require CT to identify the affected cheek teeth.

OTHER DIAGNOSTIC PROCEDURES
• A general physical examination, a close examination of the head structures, and a thorough oral examination with the horse restrained in stocks well sedated using a full mouth speculum and a good light source is performed. Rinsing the oral cavity is recommended after initial examination with a gag in place; this will allow assessment of areas of impacted or pocketed feed prior to their displacement
• Use of a dental mirror is inevitable for the evaluation of the buccal, lingual, and interproximal spaces of the cheek teeth. Oral endoscopy greatly enhances the assessment of the disorder and may also be helpful in measuring periodontal pocket depth
• Palpation of the gingiva can identify areas of swelling, hyperemia, recession, and pain. A gingival probe may be used to measure the depth of the periodontal pocket and a dental pick to identify loose teeth

PATHOLOGIC FINDINGS
Histopathologically gingival erosion and ulceration, neutrophilic exudate, bacterial rods, cocci, and spirochetes were found. Interestingly changes of the periodontal ligament were only mild and not deemed irreversible, highlighting the potential of this ligament to recover from mild disease.

TREATMENT

APPROPRIATE HEALTH CARE
• Debridement of food from the periodontal pockets is necessary so the gingival inflammation can regress and healing can commence. This may be done using high-pressure water and air, dental picks, and forceps (initially every 2 weeks and depending on the course of disease may be repeated every 2–3 months). Deposition of subgingival antibiotics or padding of the periodontal pocket with dental filling material, even though not evidence based, is performed by some clinicians. Widening (odontoplasty) of valve diastemata or areas of close interproximal contact is beneficial when feed material cannot be freed. Following odontoplasty feed material may be cleared from widened spaces during normal mastication
• Abnormalities in dental wear are addressed by promoting normal masticatory activity. Appropriate crown reduction and thereby reduced occlusion of an affected tooth will reduce abnormal forces and diminish pain. In cases of severe PD a loose tooth may have to be extracted

NURSING CARE
N/A

ACTIVITY
N/A

DIET
Lateral excursion of the mandible, which is important for normal dental wear, is associated with fiber length. Adequate dietary roughage is therefore important for the prevention of PD.

CLIENT EDUCATION

PD is very common in older horses. Routine dental prophylaxis is the best method for preventing PD and should be performed annually or even biannually.

SURGICAL CONSIDERATIONS

Standing tooth extraction is the method of choice. Alternative approaches in cases of fractured crowns include a minimally invasive buccotomy with screw extraction, intraoral tooth segmentation, or minimally invasive trephination and repulsion using Steinmann pins. Retrograde repulsion was traditionally widely practiced, but owing to the damage to the dental alveolus the above-mentioned minimally invasive techniques should be used. Postoperative radiography and/or oral endoscopy, confirming complete tooth removal, is recommended. Following tooth extraction, the resulting defect can be packed with swabs, dental wax, or similar to prevent feed impaction in the alveolus. In cases of secondary sinusitis following oro-sinus fistulation, the fistula should be debrided; local treatment is clinician dependent (honey, antiseptics, platelet-rich plasma), and sealing the alveolus from the oral cavity is a crucial step in the healing process. Sinus trephination and lavage should be performed and treatment with systemic antimicrobials may be necessary.

MEDICATIONS

DRUG(S) OF CHOICE

• Sedatives either per bolus injections or by constant rate infusion are required to complete a thorough and safe oral examination. α_2-Agonists provide adequate sedation. Premedication with acepromazine and the addition of an opioid can increase the reliability of the sedation achieved
• NSAIDs administered prior to extensive dental work helps to minimize discomfort both during and after dental treatment
• Systemic antibiotics are unlikely to halt progression of PD without removal of the underlying cause. Some clinicians advocate the use of antimicrobials subgingivally in affected areas

CONTRAINDICATIONS

N/A

PRECAUTIONS

N/A

POSSIBLE INTERACTIONS

N/A

ALTERNATIVE DRUGS

N/A

FOLLOW-UP

PATIENT MONITORING

Weight gain in horses with ill thrift should be monitored and is often impressive following successful treatment of PD. Mastication and feed intake should be monitored.

PREVENTION/AVOIDANCE

Regular dental prophylaxis can prevent the formation of dental conformational abnormalities as a result of abnormal wear. Feeding diets with adequate roughage may decrease abnormal dental wear.

POSSIBLE COMPLICATIONS

Improper odontoplasty may lead to iatrogenic damage of pulp cavities. Following oral tooth extraction complications are few and may include sequestrum formation from a piece of alveolus, unextracted tooth fragments, or feed impaction in the vacated alveolus due to swab/dental wax dislodgment. There is mesial drift of the teeth distal to the vacated alveolus and supereruption of the opposing tooth demanding regular corrective dentistry (annually or biannually).

EXPECTED COURSE AND PROGNOSIS

Conservative treatment consisting of regular dental floating and a high-quality roughage diet may successfully manage PD. The condition is generally considered progressive. In 202 horses with associated severe PD odontoplasty led to permanent remission of clinical signs in 50%, temporary remission in 22% of the cases, and a partial response in 17% of the cases. Tooth extraction may be necessary in advanced cases (with loose teeth) to successfully resolve the disease. Often mild PD in younger horses, with malocclusion due to abnormalities of permanent tooth eruption or mild abnormalities of dental wear, is reversible following resolution of the underlying cause.

MISCELLANEOUS

ASSOCIATED CONDITIONS

Ill thrift and weight loss are commonly associated with PD.

AGE-RELATED FACTORS

As horses age, the reserve crown is exposed and the gap between adjacent teeth increases. This increases the potential for feed to become impacted between adjacent teeth.

SYNONYMS

• Gingivitis
• Periodontitis

SEE ALSO

Bacteremia/sepsis

ABBREVIATIONS

• CT = computed tomography
• NSAID = nonsteroidal anti-inflammatory drug
• PD = periodontal disease

Suggested Reading
Dixon PM, Ceen S, Barnett T, et al. A long-term study on the clinical effects of mechanical widening of cheek teeth diastemata for treatment of periodontitis in 202 horses (2008-2011). Equine Vet J 2014;46(1):76–80.

Authors Andrea S. Bischofberger and Felix Theiss
Consulting Editors Henry Stämpfli and Olimpo Oliver-Espinosa
Acknowledgment The authors and editors acknowledge the prior contribution of Hugo Hilton.

P

PERITONITIS

BASICS

OVERVIEW
Peritonitis is defined as inflammation of the peritoneal cavity. It may be primary or secondary, diffuse or localized, and acute or chronic. Inflammation involves the liberation of many immune system mediators, resulting in the decrease in vascular integrity and a flux of inflammatory cells, protein, red blood cells, and electrolytes into the peritoneal cavity. The disease may range from mild to severe, thereby causing hypovolemic and septic/toxic shock and, ultimately, death.

Systems Affected
• GI—altered GI motility.
• Cardiovascular—from mild dehydration to tachycardia to shock.
• Renal/urologic—primary disease, azotemia.
• Reproductive—primary disease

SIGNALMENT
Any age, breed, or sex.

SIGNS
Primary Disease
• Depression. • Inappetence. • Fever. • Altered GI motility. • Distended abdomen.
• Splinting of abdomen. • Mild colic.
• Distended viscus; serosal fibrin deposition palpated per rectum

Secondary Disease
• Signs as listed previously. • Colic. • Evidence of trauma. • Laminitis

CAUSES AND RISK FACTORS
Primary
Hematogenous spread of bacteria.

Secondary
• Loss of GI integrity. • Vascular compromise thrombosis or intestinal torsion/volvulus.
• Trauma. • Loss of reproductive tract integrity. • Breeding injury. • Foaling injury.
• Wounds—penetrating. • Abdominal surgery. • Castration. • Abscess rupture.
• Uroperitoneum. • Hemorrhage. • Neoplasia.
• Parasite migration

DIAGNOSIS

DIFFERENTIAL DIAGNOSIS
• Includes any pain-causing, inflammatory, or infectious disease involving the GI system specifically. • Ovulation, uterine torsion, urinary tract obstruction, cholelithiasis, and cholangitis. • Pleuropneumonia

CBC/BIOCHEMISTRY/URINALYSIS
CBC
• Neutropenia/neutrophilia.
• Hypoproteinemia/hyperproteinemia

Biochemistry
• Hypoproteinemia/hyperproteinemia. Albumin levels may be normal or decreased. Globulin levels variable. • Urinalysis—azotemia due to fluid loss. • Serum amyloid A protein—increase may be mild to severe.
• Plasma fibrinogen—may be elevated

OTHER LABORATORY TESTS
Abdominal Paracentesis
• Appearance—turbid fluid with elevated protein, nucleated cells, or foreign material; green or brown fluid likely contains feed or fecal material. • Cytology—there may be an elevated nucleated cell count ($>10^4$ nucleated cells/μL), increased proportion of neutrophils, and an elevated protein level (>25 g/L). Bacteria, feed material, and sperm possible.
• Culture and sensitivity—consider Gram stain and aerobic and anaerobic culture of fluid. False-negative results are frequent.
• Other peritoneal fluid—serum-to-peritoneal fluid glucose levels >50 mg/dL, decreased glucose level <30 mg/dL, pH <7.3, elevated fibrinogen level >200 mg/dL support septic peritonitis even if bacterial culture does not yield any growth

IMAGING
Radiographs
Helpful in assessing foals' abdomens or searching for foreign bodies in adult horses.

US
May be used to detect areas of focally increased peritoneal fluid to guide aspiration. Can also be used to assess presence of fibrin deposition and peripheral abscess formation.

TREATMENT
• Resolve primary problem. • Abdominal exploration and lavage. • Fluid therapy.
• Protein replacement. • Laminitis prophylaxis

MEDICATIONS
DRUG(S) OF CHOICE
Antibiotic Therapy
• Broad spectrum initially (consider parenteral penicillin, cephalosporin, and aminoglycoside); macrolides such as erythromycin, azithromycin, or clarithromycin with/without rifampin (rifampicin) may be indicated in cases of abdominal abscessation; metronidazole should be used if anaerobic bacteria suspected. • Antibiotic therapy—adjust to sensitivity pattern of organisms isolated in culture. • NSAIDs (analgesia, decrease effects of toxins)

Alternative Drugs
Trimethoprim–sulfonamide (enteral or parenteral); potentiated penicillins (amoxicillin/sulbactam) may be useful.

CONTRAINDICATIONS/POSSIBLE DRUG INTERACTIONS
• Corticosteroids are contraindicated in peritonitis because a bacterial infection is usually present. • Aminoglycoside antibiotics should be used with caution because of nephrotoxicity. • Macrolide antibiotics, especially erythromycin, may cause enterocolitis (potentially fatal)

FOLLOW-UP
PATIENT MONITORING
Periodic peritoneal fluid analysis (every 2–3 days or if the patient does not show any improvement).

POSSIBLE COMPLICATIONS
Laminitis and thrombophlebitis are the most common complications. Abscess and adhesion formation may also occur.

MISCELLANEOUS
AGE-RELATED FACTORS
Immunodeficiency in the neonate.

PREGNANCY/FERTILITY/BREEDING
Fetal loss may occur.

SEE ALSO
• Colic, chronic/recurrent
• Rectal tears

ABBREVIATIONS
• GI = gastrointestinal.
• NSAID = nonsteroidal anti-inflammatory drug.
• US = ultrasonography, ultrasound

Suggested Reading
Davis JL. Treatment of peritonitis. Vet Clin North Am Equine Pract 2003;19:765–778.
Furst A, Kummer M, Kuemmerle JM, et al. Potential complications in equine colic surgery. Pferdeheilkunde 2012;28:522–530.

Author Daniel G. Kenney
Consulting Editors Henry Stämpfli and Olimpo Oliver-Espinosa

PETECHIAE, ECCHYMOSES, AND HEMATOMAS

BASICS

OVERVIEW
• Petechiae, ecchymoses, and hematomas are forms of interstitial bleeding; the result of impaired hemostasis, vascular abnormalities, or trauma. • Petechiae occur with thrombocytopenia or vasculitis. • Ecchymoses and hematomas occur with defects in any aspect of hemostasis (primary, secondary, or fibrinolysis), vascular abnormalities, or trauma. • A bruise is an ecchymosis/hematoma where hemoglobin is converted to bilirubin and hemosiderin; result is blue/green discoloration. • The systemic nature of the many underlying causes can result in internal bleeding. • Clinical signs relate to disorders of the hemic/lymphatic/immune or cardiovascular systems, resulting in overt signs in the skin/exocrine system. Note that coagulation abnormalities and vasculitis are frequently secondary to other primary diseases

SIGNALMENT
• Acquired—no age, sex, or breed predilection. • Inherited—young purebred horses; autosomal recessive

SIGNS
Historical Findings
Bleeding from injection sites or with surgery.

Physical Examination Findings
• Petechiae are tiny, flat, round hemorrhages visible in the skin, mucous membranes, or serosal surfaces. • Ecchymoses are larger (1–2 cm); a hematoma is a large, localized collection of clotted/partially clotted blood. • Ecchymoses/larger hemorrhages occur in sites of minor trauma and pressure points. • With hemostatic deficits, signs of mucosal bleeding (epistaxis, melena, hematuria) and bleeding into body cavities (hemoabdomen, hemothorax) may occur. • Signs of anemia; acute or chronic hemorrhage. • Signs of the underlying disease

CAUSES AND RISK FACTORS
Blood Vessel Damage
• Immune-mediated vasculitis (e.g. purpura haemorrhagica). • Vasculitis caused by infectious agents. • Septicemia/bacteremia. • Trauma

Platelet Abnormalities
• Thrombocytopenia—decreased platelet production; increased platelet destruction and platelet consumption; platelet sequestration. • Platelet dysfunction—thrombocytopathia

Defects in Secondary Coagulation
• Acquired coagulation defects (e.g. vitamin K deficiency). • Inherited coagulation defects (e.g. von Willebrand disease, hemophilia A, prekallikrein deficiency). • Liver disease. • Neoplasia. • DIC

Multifactorial (Complex Vascular/Platelet/Coagulation Abnormalities)
• Infections (e.g. equine infectious anemia, equine granulocytic ehrlichiosis, equine monocytic ehrlichiosis, equine viral arteritis, Venezuelan equine encephalitis, African horse sickness, equine herpesvirus, equine influenza, babesiosis, trypanosomiasis). • Septicemia/endotoxemia/DIC. • Neoplasia

DIAGNOSIS

DIFFERENTIAL DIAGNOSIS
Petechiae, ecchymoses, and hematomas are easy to identify on physical examination.

CBC/BIOCHEMISTRY/URINALYSIS
• Variable depending on underlying cause. • Include anemia, thrombocytopenia, and abnormal liver enzymes or function assays

OTHER LABORATORY TESTS
• Coagulation evaluation—platelet count, platelet function, activated clotting time, prothrombin time, activated partial thromboplastin time, fibrinogen, antithrombin, quantification of specific factors, D-dimers, protein C concentrations, viscoelastic coagulation testing. • Cytology, culture, and serology for underlying disease

IMAGING
• US of the thorax, abdomen, or soft tissues may be helpful for diagnosis or US-guided centesis. • Radiographs; if bone trauma suspected

OTHER DIAGNOSTIC PROCEDURES
• Buccal mucosal/template bleeding time. • As indicated for primary disease

PATHOLOGIC FINDINGS
Dependent on underlying cause.

TREATMENT
• Fluids for volume expansion if blood loss has been significant and acute. • Hemostatic abnormalities may require blood products. • Minimize activity. • Treatment of underlying disease

MEDICATIONS

DRUG(S) OF CHOICE
Dependent on underlying disease.

CONTRAINDICATIONS/POSSIBLE INTERACTIONS
• Corticosteroids contraindicated with laminitis and most infectious diseases. • Aspirin; other NSAIDs; colloids may impair platelet function. • Antiplatelet and anticoagulant therapy; exacerbate bleeding

FOLLOW-UP

PATIENT MONITORING
• Monitor for continued hemorrhage/shock. • Repeated evaluation of coagulation function. • Based on underlying disease

PREVENTION/AVOIDANCE
N/A

POSSIBLE COMPLICATIONS
• Avoid invasive procedures in patients at risk of bleeding. • SC bleeding may indicate other sites of hemorrhage that may result in hypovolemic shock

EXPECTED COURSE AND PROGNOSIS
Dependent on underlying disease.

MISCELLANEOUS

ASSOCIATED CONDITIONS
N/A

AGE-RELATED FACTORS
N/A

ZOONOTIC POTENTIAL
N/A

PREGNANCY/FERTILITY/BREEDING
N/A

SEE ALSO
• Coagulation defects, acquired. • Coagulation defects, inherited. • Disseminated intravascular coagulation. • Purpura haemorrhagica. • Thrombocytopenia

ABBREVIATIONS
• DIC = disseminated intravascular coagulation. • NSAID = nonsteroidal anti-inflammatory drug. • US = ultrasonography, ultrasound

Suggested Reading
Sellon DC. Disorders of the hematopoietic system. In: Reed SM, Bayly WM, Sellon DC, eds. Equine Internal Medicine, 2e. St. Louis, MO: WB Saunders, 2004:721–768.
Author Kira L. Epstein
Consulting Editors David Hodgson, Harold C. McKenzie, and Jennifer L. Hodgson
Acknowledgment The author and editors acknowledge the prior contribution of Jennifer L. Hodgson.

P

PHARYNGEAL LYMPHOID HYPERPLASIA (PHARYNGITIS)

BASICS

OVERVIEW
• Acute and chronic forms of pharyngitis are recognized. Acute inflammation of the lymphoid tissues in the pharynx is termed pharyngitis and chronic inflammation of the pharynx is defined as a pharyngeal lymphoid hyperplasia
• Pharyngeal lymphoid hyperplasia is commonly recognized in young athletic horses
• It is not generally considered to be a specific disease entity but rather a response to other diseases
• The pharyngeal tonsil consists of discrete lymphoid follicles diffusely distributed in the dorsal and lateral walls of the pharynx

SIGNALMENT
Common in weaning to performance horses 2–3 years of age.

SIGNS
• This condition has little consequence for athletic ability unless severe
• In acute pharyngitis, signs may include pain (dysphagia), nasal discharge, regional lymphadenopathy (submandibular, retropharyngeal nodes), respiratory noise (often inspiratory), pharyngeal swelling, and cough

CAUSES AND RISK FACTORS
• The cause of chronic pharyngitis is not known but is probably multifactorial
• Pharyngeal lymphoid hyperplasia is probably related to a local immune response to inhaled or ingested antigens
• *Streptococcus* spp., influenza, herpesvirus, picornavirus (equine rhinitis A and B virus), and paramyxovirus (parainfluenza 3) have been incriminated as specific causes of pharyngitis
• Physical and chemical causes of pharyngitis have been identified

DIAGNOSIS

DIFFERENTIAL DIAGNOSIS
• Rhinitis and laryngitis
• Dysphagia—tongue foreign bodies, fractures of the hyoid apparatus or jaws, and disease of guttural pouches should be considered
• If exercise intolerance is the primary complaint, pharyngitis should only be considered after all other possible causes of impaired performance have been eliminated

CBC/BIOCHEMISTRY/URINALYSIS
Changes in the hemogram and the biochemical profile are likely to result from a concurrent respiratory disease (leukopenia or leukocytosis, hyperfibrinogenemia, anemia) or reflect abscess formation (neutrophilia, hyperfibrinogenemia) or dehydration and fasting associated with dysphagia.

OTHER LABORATORY TESTS
Microbial culture of nasopharynx swab samples is helpful for the identification of the causative organism in acute upper respiratory tract infections. The interpretation of results may be difficult because (1) the pharynx normally has a resident microflora and (2) many of the microorganisms isolated are capable of opportunistic infections.

IMAGING
• Endoscopy—hyperplasia of the lymphonodular follicles within the pharyngeal mucosa and single or multiple lymphonodular masses may be within, or protrude from, the pharyngeal mucosa
• Radiography of the pharynx—exclusion of radiodense foreign bodies, soft tissue masses, fractures, and in guttural pouch diseases
• Ultrasonography of the pharynx area may identify abnormal structures (masses, inflammation, abscesses)

OTHER DIAGNOSTIC PROCEDURES
N/A

TREATMENT
• Inappetence or dysphagia—administration of NSAIDs should be considered
• Dehydration and dysphagia should be managed by either parenteral or enteral fluid administration
• Soft feeds should be offered when available if pharyngeal discomfort to eat
• Infections secondary to foreign body injuries should be treated with antibiotics (broad aerobic and anaerobic spectrum)
• Daily lavage of any cavitary wounds, debridement, and removal of feed material may be necessary
• Topical antifungal and systemic fungal treatment is indicated in fungal infection cases
• Rest from training for up to 4–8 weeks when associated with clinical signs such as dysphagia, anorexia

MEDICATIONS

DRUG(S) OF CHOICE
Custom topical preparations, usually containing an antibiotic, an anti-inflammatory drug, and a hygroscopic agent (glycerin) or DMSO, are often used for palliation of clinical signs. These preparations are administered 2 or 3 times daily through a transnasal catheter and sprayed onto the pharyngeal surface. The effectiveness of this treatment has to be proved.

FOLLOW-UP

PATIENT MONITORING
• Repeat upper respiratory endoscopy at 3–4 weeks post treatment
• Reevaluation of CBC if necessary

PREVENTION/AVOIDANCE
Methods used to control and prevent most of the common viral (influenza and herpesvirus 1 and 4) and bacterial respiratory diseases should limit herd problems with acute pharyngitis. However, there are no substantive data to support this contention.

EXPECTED COURSE AND PROGNOSIS
Dependent on the cause.

MISCELLANEOUS

ABBREVIATIONS
• DMSO = dimethylsulfoxide
• NSAID = nonsteroidal anti-inflammatory drug

Suggested Reading
Ainsworth DM, Hackett RP. Pharyngeal and laryngeal disorders. In: Reed SM, Bayly WM, Sellon DC, eds. Equine Internal Medicine, 3e. St. Louis, MO: WB Saunders, 2010:302–303.

Pascoe JR. Pharyngitis. In: Smith BP, ed. Large Animal Internal Medicine, 3e. St. Louis, MO: Mosby, 2002:530–532.

Sullivan EK, Parente EJ. Disorders of the pharynx. Vet Clin North Am Equine Pract 2003;19:159–167.

Author Daniel Jean
Consulting Editors Daniel Jean and Mathilde Leclère

P

PHEOCHROMOCYTOMA

BASICS

OVERVIEW
- PCC is a tumor of the catecholamine-producing cells of the adrenal medulla
- The most common clinical presentation of pheochromocytoma is colic with hemoabdomen or retroperitoneal hemorrhage, secondary to tumor rupture
- PCC in horses is occasionally functional, causing intermittent tachycardia, mydriasis, muscle tremors, and hyperglycemia from the release of epinephrine and norepinephrine
- Most reported equine PCCs are unilateral, well-encapsulated, benign neoplasms, and almost half are incidental findings at necropsy

Systems Affected
- Endocrine
- Cardiovascular

SIGNALMENT
- Median age is 28 years (range 12–38 years). However, malignant PCC has been reported in a 6-month-old foal
- No breed or sex predilection is apparent

SIGNS

Historical Findings
Lethargy, anorexia, abdominal pain, sweating, tachycardia, diarrhea, or neurologic signs possible

Physical Examination Findings
- Colic
- Sweating
- Tachycardia
- Excitement
- Tachypnea
- Mydriasis
- Muscle tremors
- Ileus
- Diarrhea
- Many clinical signs associated with functional PCC are nonspecific and can be caused by other diseases, and many of the tumors do not result in clinically apparent catecholamine release
- A mass may be palpated per rectum medially to the left kidney

CAUSES AND RISK FACTORS
- PCC is a benign or malignant tumor of the chromaffin cells of the adrenal medulla

DIAGNOSIS

DIFFERENTIAL DIAGNOSIS
- More common causes of colic (many) and hemoabdomen (splenic rupture, splenic neoplasia, trauma, uterine artery disruption) should be considered
- Clinical signs and biochemical abnormalities similar to those reported with PCC may be observed with shock, renal disease, enteritis, colitis, or other causes of cardiovascular, pulmonary, and neurologic diseases

CBC/BIOCHEMISTRY/URINALYSIS
- Laboratory findings are variable and nonspecific, and are usually consistent with hemorrhagic shock or sympathetic stimulation. Findings may include:
  - Hyperlactatemia
  - Hyperglycemia
  - Increased packed cell volume
  - Leukocytosis
  - Electrolyte disturbances

OTHER LABORATORY TESTS
Assays for catecholamines and their metabolites in plasma or urine are technically difficult and few laboratories perform these tests. Interpretation of the results may be complicated by the intermittent nature of catecholamine release in horses with PCC. However, recently horses with PCC have been found to have elevated plasma metanephrine and normetanephrine concentrations and increased urine metanephrine to creatinine and normetanephrine to creatinine ratios.

IMAGING
Ultrasonography may reveal hemoperitoneum or retroperitoneal hemorrhage. A mass medial or cranial to the kidney can be seen. For small patients, abdominal CT may aid in diagnosis.

OTHER DIAGNOSTIC PROCEDURES
Arterial blood pressure measurements may document hypertension. Abdominocentesis may confirm hemoperitoneum.

PATHOLOGIC FINDINGS
- Usually unilateral (89%)
- Solitary or multiple nodular masses within the adrenal gland may vary in size from a few millimeters to>10 cm, and 22% are malignant. Metastases can be seen in the brain, spinal cord, and lung
- May invade the posterior vena cava and result in extensive hemorrhage. This can lead to retroperitoneal hematoma or hemoperitoneum
- Histologically, PCCs often are necrotic and hemorrhagic, which also may result in adrenocortical hemorrhage and necrosis
- Concurrent endocrine tumors are common, including lesions consistent with multiple endocrine neoplasia syndrome in humans

TREATMENT
- Rarely diagnosed antemortem, so treatment is rarely an option. They are sometimes discovered during exploratory celiotomy for colic or hemoperitoneum, and euthanasia is usually performed at this time
- Medical care should be aimed at controlling pain, using fluid therapy to normalize renal function and electrolyte abnormalities, and stabilizing the cardiovascular function
- Consider surgical resection in cases of localized nodular tumors. This procedure is difficult technically and the risk of a fatal complication is high (hemorrhage, cardiac arrhythmia, or rhabdomyolysis)

MEDICATIONS

DRUG(S) OF CHOICE
In humans and small animals, α- and β-adrenergic blocking agents can control the effects of excessive catecholamine secretion.

FOLLOW-UP

PATIENT MONITORING
Monitor tumor size ultrasonographically and assess for metastases as clinically indicated.

POSSIBLE COMPLICATIONS
- Renal failure
- Hemorrhage
- Cardiac arrhythmia

EXPECTED COURSE AND PROGNOSIS
There are no reports of successful treatment of functional PCC in horses.

MISCELLANEOUS

PREGNANCY/FERTILITY/BREEDING
Abortion during late gestation and fatal hemorrhage during parturition have been reported.

SEE ALSO
Multiple endocrine neoplasia

ABBREVIATIONS
- CT = computed tomography
- PCC = pheochromocytoma

Suggested Reading
Luethy D, Habecker P, Murphy B, Nolen-Walston R. Clinical and pathological features of pheochromocytoma in the horse: a multi-center retrospective study of 37 cases (2007-2014). J Vet Intern Med 2016;30(1):309–313.

Author Rose D. Nolen-Walston
Consulting Editors Michel Levy and Heidi Banse
Acknowledgment The author and editors acknowledge the prior contribution of Laurent Couëtil.

P

PHIMOSIS

BASICS

OVERVIEW
• Phimosis is the inability of the horse to protrude the penis from the preputial orifice
• It may be caused by congenital or acquired stenosis of the external preputial orifice or the preputial ring. Phimosis may be the result of a penile mass or swelling of the internal preputial lamina

SIGNALMENT
• Stallions or geldings of any age
• Neonates and young foals with congenital stenosis or persistent attachment

SIGNS

Historical Findings
Urination within the preputial cavity and/or dysuria.

Physical Examination Findings
• Visible or palpable thickening of the external preputial orifice or the preputial ring. Excoriations due to urine scalding may be apparent
• Longstanding cases may have a large accumulation of smegma and a nauseous odor

CAUSES AND RISK FACTORS

Congenital
• Stenosis of the preputial orifice
• Hermaphroditism
• Penile dysgenesis

Acquired
• Trauma—breeding injury, postsurgical edema, chronic posthitis
• Neoplasia—sarcoid, SCC, papilloma, melanoma, hemangioma
• Parasitism—habronemiasis
• Viral infections—EHV-3
• Poor hygiene; accumulation of excessive smegma can lead to posthitis and subsequent phimosis from the formation of scar tissue
• Light-colored skin is associated with an increased incidence of SCC
• Gray horses are more commonly diagnosed with melanomas

DIAGNOSIS

DIFFERENTIAL DIAGNOSIS

Differentiating Similar Signs
Phimosis during the first 30 days of life is normally due to fusion of the internal preputial lamina to the free portion of the penis.

CBC/BIOCHEMISTRY/URINALYSIS
N/A

OTHER LABORATORY TESTS
Virus isolation using fluid from vesicular lesions may be diagnostic for EHV-3.

IMAGING
N/A

OTHER DIAGNOSTIC PROCEDURES
Cytology or biopsy (histopathology) may distinguish and/or provide a definitive diagnosis for neoplastic, granulomatous, or herpesvirus lesions.

TREATMENT
If phimosis is due to:
• Postsurgical edema—hydrotherapy, massage, exercise, and diuretics are indicated. Cleansing and application of topical emollients or antibiotics may be indicated
• Neoplastic or granulomatous lesions—surgical excision, cryosurgery, chemotherapy, or radiation, as indicated by type, location, and size
• A stricture of the external preputial orifice—surgical removal of a triangular section of the external preputial lamina
• A stricture at the preputial ring—incise the internal preputial fold (preputiotomy). Circumcision (reefing) may be necessary to remove the constricting tissue in its entirety

MEDICATIONS

DRUG(S) OF CHOICE
• NSAIDs, including phenylbutazone (2–4 g/450 kg body weight/day PO) or flunixin meglumine (1.1 mg/kg/day IV, IM, or PO), for symptomatic relief or to decrease inflammation
• Systemic or local antibiotics if indicated to treat local infections or prevent septicemia
• Diuretics—furosemide (1–2 mg/kg IV every 6–12 h) may be indicated in the acute phase to reduce edema
• Specific topical or systemic treatments for parasitic, fungal, or neoplastic conditions as indicated by test results

CONTRAINDICATIONS POSSIBLE INTERACTIONS
Phenothiazine tranquilizers should be avoided/used with caution in male horses.

FOLLOW-UP

PATIENT MONITORING
• Initially, daily evaluations—ensure that secondary posthitis, balanitis, balanoposthitis, urine scald, or penile/preputial excoriations are not complicating the phimosis
• As the initial problem is effectively treated, less frequent examinations will be necessary

POSSIBLE COMPLICATIONS
• Urination within the preputial cavity may cause inflammation of the epithelium, leading to a more extensive inflammation (posthitis, balanoposthitis) and scarring
• Infertility or impotence can result if scarring becomes extensive

MISCELLANEOUS

ASSOCIATED CONDITIONS
N/A

AGE-RELATED FACTORS
• Papillomas are more frequently diagnosed in young animals
• SCCs and melanomas are more frequently diagnosed in middle-aged to aged horses

ZOONOTIC POTENTIAL
N/A

PREGNANCY/FERTILITY/BREEDING
N/A

SYNONYMS
N/A

SEE ALSO
• Paraphimosis
• Penile vesicles, erosions, and tumors

ABBREVIATIONS
• EHV = equine herpesvirus
• NSAID = nonsteroidal anti-inflammatory drug
• SCC = squamous cell carcinoma

Suggested Reading
Schumacher J, Varner DD. Surgical correction of abnormalities affecting the reproductive organs of stallions. In: Youngquist RS, Threlfall WR, eds. Current Therapy in Large Animal Theriogenology, 2e. St. Louis, MO: Saunders Elsevier, 2007:23–36.
Schumacher J, Varner DD. Abnormalities of the penis and prepuce. In: McKinnon AO, Squires EL, Vaala WE, Varner DD, eds. Equine Reproduction, 2e. Ames, IA: Wiley Blackwell, 2011:1130-1144.

Author Ahmed Tibary
Consulting Editor Carla L. Carleton
Acknowledgment The author and editor acknowledge the prior contribution of Carole C. Miller.

P

PHOSPHORUS, HYPERPHOSPHATEMIA

BASICS

OVERVIEW
Serum P concentration greater than the reference interval.

Pathophysiology
- Kidneys, intestine, and skeleton are involved in P homeostasis in conjunction with diet and hormonal factors including PTH, calcitonin, and bioactive vitamin D
- Decreased glomerular filtration, excessive intestinal absorption, dietary supplementation, overuse of phosphate enemas, excessive bone resorption, or significant tissue injury with cell lysis can result in hyperphosphatemia

Systems Affected
General
- P and Ca^{2+} metabolism and homeostatic mechanisms are closely linked
- Hyperphosphatemia frequently occurs with hypocalcemia
- Metastatic calcification may develop with hyperphosphatemia and concurrent hypercalcemia
Skeletal
In response to hypocalcemia, Ca^{2+} is mobilized from bone and may lead to abnormal bone formation, bone demineralization, and a skeleton prone to injury.
Endocrine
Hyperphosphatemia stimulates PTH secretion, which causes increased resorption of Ca^{2+} from bone, kidneys, and intestine and increased renal excretion of P.

SIGNALMENT
- Any breed, age, or sex
- Young, growing animals have increased serum P concentrations (4.5–9 mg/dL)

SIGNS
General Comments
- Acute hyperphosphatemia—signs due to concurrent hypocalcemia (e.g. tetany, hyperexcitability, muscle fasciculations arrhythmia, colic)
- Chronic hyperphosphatemia—lameness, abnormal bone and cartilage development, osteodystrophia fibrosa, fractures

Historical Findings
- Dependent on the underlying cause
- Exposure to vitamin D-containing plants
- High bran diet

Physical Examination Findings
- Dietary P excess or imbalance—shifting leg lameness, joint pain, or stilted gait; as the disease progresses, abnormal bone formation and enlarged facial bones (e.g. bighead in NHP)
- Hypervitaminosis D—limb stiffness with painful flexor tendons and suspensory ligaments

CAUSES AND RISK FACTORS
- Young, growing animals—due to rapid bone turnover
- Decreased glomerular filtration—prerenal, renal (AKI), or postrenal azotemia; chronic renal failure usually is accompanied by hypophosphatemia
- Hypervitaminosis D—hyperphosphatemia and hypercalcemia result from excessive dietary supplementation with vitamin D-containing products
- Excessive dietary P or P imbalance—excessive P intake or excessive supplementation with bran, which is high in P, inhibits absorption of Ca^{2+}, resulting in Ca^{2+} deficiency
- NHP occurs from excess P and low Ca^{2+} intake. Secretion of PTH increases to correct the disturbance in mineral homeostasis
- Hyperphosphatemia from cellular lysis and release of intracellular P can occur with significant tissue injury or necrosis (rhabdomyolysis, tumor necrosis) or hemolysis
- Increased potential for metastatic calcification with concurrent hyperphosphatemia and hypercalcemia

DIAGNOSIS

DIFFERENTIAL DIAGNOSIS
See Causes and Risk Factors.

CBC/BIOCHEMISTRY/URINALYSIS
- NHP—normal renal function, hypocalcemia, hyperphosphatemia, elevated ALP concentration
- Renal disease—azotemia, isosthenuria

OTHER LABORATORY TESTS
- Dietary deficiency or imbalance—review dietary history, inspect feed, and analyze chemically for Ca^{2+} and P content
- NHP—increased urinary P fractional excretion

IMAGING
Radiographs may detect loss of skeletal mineralization when losses >30%.

TREATMENT
- NHP—correction of dietary deficiency or imbalance by supplying the deficient nutrient; dietary Ca^{2+}/P ratio must not exceed 1.5–2:1
- Removal of vitamin D sources
- With suspected AKI, fluid replacement and correction of electrolyte imbalances
- With acute cell lysis or iatrogenic causes, fluid therapy and diuretics

MEDICATIONS

DRUG(S) OF CHOICE
Hypervitaminosis D—removal of source, fluid diuresis, corticosteroid administration, and low Ca^{2+} and P feeds.

FOLLOW-UP

EXPECTED COURSE AND PROGNOSIS
If soft tissue mineralization in the heart or kidney occurs, prognosis is poor.

MISCELLANEOUS

ASSOCIATED CONDITIONS
Hypocalcemia

AGE-RELATED FACTORS
- Hyperphosphatemia and elevated ALP activity are common in healthy, young, growing animals
- Young animals are more prone to skeletal abnormalities resulting from dietary excess or imbalances

SYNONYMS
- Bioactive vitamin D—1,25-dihydroxyvitamin D3, calcitriol
- Metastatic calcification—soft tissue mineralization
- NHP—bighead disease, bran disease, osteodystrophia fibrosa

SEE ALSO
- Calcium, hypercalcemia
- Calcium, hypocalcemia
- Nutritional secondary hyperparathyroidism (NHP)
- Phosphorus, hypophosphatemia

ABBREVIATIONS
- AKI = acute kidney injury
- ALP = alkaline phosphatase
- NHP = nutritional secondary hyperparathyroidism
- PTH = parathyroid hormone

Suggested Reading
Toribio RE. Phosphorus homeostasis and derangements. In: Fielding CL, Magdesian KG, eds. Equine Fluid Therapy. Ames, IA: Wiley Blackwell, 2015:88–100.
Toribio RE. Parathyroid gland, calcium and phosphorus regulation. In: Smith BP, ed. Large Animal Internal Medicine, 5e. St. Louis, MO: Elsevier Mosby, 2015:1244–1252.

Author Karen E. Russell
Consulting Editor Sandra D. Taylor

P

PHOSPHORUS, HYPOPHOSPHATEMIA

BASICS

OVERVIEW
Serum P concentration less than reference interval.

Pathophysiology
• P is one of the most abundant elements in the body, with >80% found in bone and complexed with Ca^{2+} in the form of hydroxyapatite
• P, the major intracellular anion, is an important component of nucleic acids, phospholipids, and phosphoproteins
• Maintenance of cellular integrity and metabolism depends on phosphate-containing, high-energy compounds (e.g. ATP) and enzyme systems that require P
• Skeletal-associated abnormalities (e.g. demineralization, deformation, poor growth) are potential consequences of hypophosphatemia
• Depletion of ATP can affect any cell with high-energy requirements; erythrocytes, skeletal muscle cells, and brain cells are especially susceptible

Systems Affected
• Musculoskeletal—abnormal bone formation, bone demineralization, skeleton more prone to injury
• Reproductive—anestrus, irregular estrus, reduced fertility
• Hemic—severe deficiency may predispose to hemolysis

SIGNALMENT
Any breed, age, or sex.

SIGNS
Historical Findings
• CRF—weight loss, PU/PD
• Dietary P deficiency—poor growth, lameness, anestrus, irregular estrus, reduced fertility

Physical Examination Findings
• CRF—poor body condition, PU/PD, excessive tartar, oral ulcers, diarrhea, edema
• Dietary P deficiency—lameness, stiff gait, pica

CAUSES AND RISK FACTORS
CRF
Serum P concentration in horses with CRF may be normal or low, depending on the presence and degree of hypercalcemia.

Dietary P Deficiency
P deficiency or starvation. When caloric intake is increased, malnourished horses may develop complications associated with refeeding syndrome owing to increasing requirements for P; this necessitates close monitoring of serum P concentrations.

Primary Hyperparathyroidism
Parathyroid adenoma, parathyroid hyperplasia, or carcinoma.

Rickets
• Young, growing animals with vitamin D deficiency may be hypophosphatemic, hypocalcemic, and have elevated ALP activity
• Vitamin D deficiency causes defective mineralization of new bone, resulting in painful swelling of long bones and costochondral junctions, bowed limbs, and stiff gait

Critical Illness
• Sepsis may lead to hypophosphatemia, probably owing to redistribution of P from the extracellular fluid compartment
• Respiratory alkalosis, insulin administration, and parenteral nutrition may cause hypophosphatemia

Halothane Anesthesia
Prolonged halothane anesthesia (>12 h) can cause transient hypophosphatemia that persists for a few days (unknown mechanism).

DIAGNOSIS

DIFFERENTIAL DIAGNOSIS
• CRF—azotemia, isosthenuria, hypercalcemia, and exposure to nephrotoxins
• Primary hyperparathyroidism—hypercalcemia, hyperphosphatemia, increased serum PTH concentration, increased fractional P excretion, and low to normal concentrations of vitamin D

CBC/BIOCHEMISTRY/URINALYSIS
• Intravascular hemolysis can occur secondary to severe hypophosphatemia
• CRF—azotemia, hypercalcemia, and isosthenuria are common; hypophosphatemia, mild hyponatremia, hypochloridemia, and normo- or hyperkalemia also may be present
• Moderate to marked proteinuria in cases of glomerulonephritis
• Primary hyperparathyroidism—hypercalcemia and increased fractional excretion of P; renal function should be normal
• Severe Ca^{2+} or P deficiency—elevated serum ALP activity

OTHER LABORATORY TESTS
If suspect primary hyperparathyroidism, measure serum PTH concentration (elevated).

IMAGING
Radiography has little benefit in detecting loss of skeletal mineralization until such losses exceed 30%.

OTHER DIAGNOSTIC PROCEDURES
With suspected dietary P and Ca^{2+} deficiencies, thorough review of dietary history, inspection of feeds, and chemical evaluation of P and Ca^{2+} content in feeds are necessary.

TREATMENT
Supplementation with mineral sources (defluorinated phosphate, bonemeal, dicalcium phosphate, monocalcium phosphate, or monosodium phosphate).

MEDICATIONS

PRECAUTIONS
• Dietary Ca^{2+}/P ratio must not exceed 1.5–2:1
• With horses in CRF that are hypercalcemic, do not feed legume hays (e.g. alfalfa, clover) or high-Ca^{2+} rations, and do not treat with Ca^{2+}-containing fluids

MISCELLANEOUS

SEE ALSO
• Calcium, hypercalcemia
• Calcium, hypocalcemia
• Chronic kidney disease (CKD)
• Phosphorus, hyperphosphatemia

ABBREVIATIONS
• ALP = alkaline phosphatase
• CRF = chronic renal failure
• PTH = parathyroid hormone
• PU/PD = polyuria, polydipsia

Suggested Reading
Toribio RE. Phosphorus homeostasis and derangements. In: Fielding CL, Magdesian KG, eds. Equine Fluid Therapy. Ames, IA: Wiley Blackwell, 2015:88–100.
Toribio RE. Parathyroid gland, calcium and phosphorus regulation. In: Smith BP, ed. Large Animal Internal Medicine, 5e. St. Louis, MO: Elsevier Mosby, 2015:1244–1252.

Author Karen E. Russell
Consulting Editor Sandra D. Taylor

BASICS

DEFINITION
Photic headshaking is a condition where, in the absence of any external stimuli other than light, a horse vigorously and violently shakes its head in horizontal, vertical, or rotary directions. Clinical signs are alleviated immediately upon reduction of light.

PATHOPHYSIOLOGY
• Photic headshaking is probably a form of optic–trigeminal nerve summation in which retina and optic nerve stimulation produces referred sensation to facial sensory branches of the trigeminal nerve in the nasal cavity, including the infraorbital and sphenopalatine nerve, with possible involvement of the trigeminal ganglion. The irritability in the nasal cavity causes the horse to shake its head
• Recent studies confirmed the involvement of the trigeminal nerve in headshaking. It has been shown that the threshold for activation of the infraorbital nerve (a branch of the maxillary division of the trigeminal nerve) is significantly lower in affected horses than in healthy controls
• This condition shares similarities with the photic sneeze syndrome in human patients, when sudden exposure to bright light immediately leads to a single or a series of sneezes. Convergence in the brainstem between trigeminal and optic nerves has been suggested as a possible mechanism in the photic sneeze and may also play a role in photic headshaking
• Extracranial vasodilation via release of vasoactive peptide as a result of stimulation of the trigeminal nerve or ganglion has also been suggested as a possible cause for this condition

SYSTEMS AFFECTED
• Ophthalmic
• Nervous

GENETICS
Heritability and genetic background in the horse are unknown; however, photic sneeze in human patients appears to be determined by innate and hereditary factors.

INCIDENCE/PREVALENCE
N/A

GEOGRAPHIC DISTRIBUTION
Worldwide

SIGNALMENT
This condition affects adult horses with a mean age of 9 years. In one study, Quarter Horses were overrepresented while Thoroughbreds were overrepresented in another. Geldings are more frequently affected than mares.

SIGNS
• Excessive and occasionally violent rubbing, sneezing, snorting, and flipping of the nose usually accompany the headshaking
• Although clinical signs may be seen at rest or during exercise, most horses show clinical signs shortly after the beginning of exercise
• This condition is seasonal, and the most common onset of clinical signs is during the spring and early summer; however, in some cases, headshaking can develop in the fall. Usually clinical signs regress spontaneously in the winter and recur in the spring/summer
• Low head position and active seeking of shade is seen occasionally

CAUSES
Sunlight may stimulate referred sensation via parasympathetic activity in branches of the trigeminal nerve, resulting in irritating nasal sensations with ensuing headshaking.

RISK FACTORS
• Bright daylight
• Spring, summer, and to a lesser extent, the fall season
• The triggering factor leading to long-term photoperiod-dependent headshaking is unknown

DIAGNOSIS

DIFFERENTIAL DIAGNOSIS
• Middle or inner ear disorders
• Ear mites
• Cranial nerve dysfunction
• Maxillary osteomas
• Premaxillary bone cysts
• Guttural pouch disease
• Upper respiratory tract disease
• Vasomotor rhinitis
• Allergic rhinitis or sinusitis
• Equine protozoal myelitis
• Cervical injury and pain
• Dental diseases
• Ocular disease
• Iris cysts
• Cystic corpora nigra
• Infraorbital neuritis
• Behavioral abnormalities

CBC/BIOCHEMISTRY/URINALYSIS
Usually normal

OTHER LABORATORY TESTS
N/A

IMAGING
N/A

OTHER DIAGNOSTIC PROCEDURES
Photic headshaking is diagnosed based on characteristic clinical signs seen on bright sunny days and with a decrease or cessation of clinical signs when light is reduced or eliminated (e.g. blindfolding, evaluation during the evening). Clinical signs should be evaluated at rest and during exercise. Other etiologies for headshaking (see Differential Diagnosis) should be ruled out utilizing the appropriate diagnostic testing.

PATHOLOGIC FINDINGS
N/A

TREATMENT

APPROPRIATE HEALTH CARE
The complete workup may require overnight hospitalization. The medical management can be done by the trainer/owner.

NURSING CARE
Riding affected horses only during times of dim light or darkness is impractical. However, alleviation of clinical signs can be achieved by lowering the amount of light entering the eye. This can be accomplished by the use of a face mask and gray lenses. Placement of two overlying face masks sprayed with black paint was also reported to improve the photic headshaking. In some cases, more than one layer of gray lenses was needed to improve clinical signs. one study utilized tinted contact lenses and reported only a partial and temporary positive effect; however, the lenses used were blue or green (and not gray). It is possible that dark gray contact lenses will provide improvement of clinical signs.

ACTIVITY
Headshaking can occur at rest or during exercise. Because most headshakers show signs shortly after the onset of activity, there may be unforeseen risks in working an uncontrolled photic head shaker.

DIET
Magnesium increases the threshold for nerve firing, hence increasing the stimulus needed for depolarization. As headshaking was found to be associated with a reduced activation threshold of the trigeminal nerve, magnesium seems to be a rational therapy for this condition. Daily oral supplementation with 10–20 g of magnesium led to improvement in headshaking in about 40% of the horses in one report. Nevertheless, optimal serum magnesium levels have not been established in the horse. Evaluating ionized magnesium serum concentration before and 14 days after the beginning of supplementation is recommended to avoid possible toxicity.

CLIENT EDUCATION
• Severely affected horses that do not respond to therapy may inflict considerable

P

PHOTIC HEADSHAKING   (CONTINUED)

self-trauma and may be dangerous to handle or ride
• Avoiding bright light, such as riding at night or in an indoor facility, may be helpful. However, this is impractical in many cases, especially for performance horses

SURGICAL CONSIDERATIONS
• Infraorbital neurectomy—the response to this procedure is poor with high complication rates and, therefore, is not recommended
• Sclerosis of the posterior ethmoidal nerve is associated with high rate of recurrence
• Compression of the caudal infraorbital nerve has been described for the treatment of headshaking, with a reported overall success rate of about 50%. However, recurrence of clinical signs was observed in some of the horses requiring additional surgery. A transient increase in severity of clinical signs was seen in 63% of the horses postoperatively, and 4/58 horses had to be euthanized due to the severity of clinical signs and/or nonresolution. As such, this procedure should be considered only for horses that did not respond to medical therapy and euthanasia is the only other option

MEDICATIONS
Medical therapy controls, but does not cure, the condition. If effective, medical treatment may only be needed during the season in which the horses exhibit headshaking behavior.

DRUG(S) OF CHOICE
• Cyproheptadine (H_1 blocker), a serotonin antagonist that alters proopiomelanocortin metabolism, has the potential to alleviate the clinical signs at a dose of 0.3 mg/kg PO BID
• Carbamazepine is an anticonvulsant that stabilizes voltage-gated sodium channels. A dose of 4 mg/kg PO TID–QID may be effective; however, such a frequent administration schedule could be problematic. In one case, a higher dose of 8 mg/kg was needed to alleviate clinical signs
• A combined treatment of cyproheptadine and carbamazepine may be synergistic

CONTRAINDICATIONS
N/A

PRECAUTIONS
• Treatment of performance horses should comply with the rules of the governing organization
• Mild lethargy, anorexia, and depression have been reported in horses treated with cyproheptadine
• Drug eruptions have also been reported with cyproheptadine

POSSIBLE INTERACTIONS
Additive central nervous system depression may be seen if cyproheptadine is combined with barbiturates or tranquilizers. Cyproheptadine has anticholinergic effects, which may be intensified by monoamine oxidase inhibitors (e.g. furazolidone).

ALTERNATIVE DRUGS
To mimic winter conditions physiologically, melatonin therapy at a dose of 12 mg PO on a sugar cube once between 17:00 and 18:00 daily may also be beneficial. For horses with seasonal headshaking, best results are achieved when melatonin therapy is started before the onset of spring.

FOLLOW-UP

PATIENT MONITORING
Although improvement or cessation of clinical signs may be seen within 3–4 days after initiation of medical therapy, a 7 day trial may be needed to determine whether the patient will respond favorably to medical management. Therapy can be stopped periodically and reinstated if the behavior recurs and there are no side effects.

PREVENTION/AVOIDANCE
Horses kept in a dark environment may not show severe clinical headshaking. Light-blocking protectors or a "nose net" may also help control the clinical signs for some horses. This type of management, however, may not be practical for the horse or its owner and trainer.

POSSIBLE COMPLICATIONS
A horse with uncontrolled headshaking may develop unwanted head trauma, and the owner or trainer may find it difficult for the horse to optimally work or perform.

EXPECTED COURSE AND PROGNOSIS
Long-term, seasonal medical therapy can control, but not cure, this disease. Infraorbital nerve blocks may relieve clinical signs in some horses. In some cases, cessation of clinical signs was seen for months to several years. The reasons for the resolution and recrudescence of clinical signs are unclear.

MISCELLANEOUS

ASSOCIATED CONDITIONS
Photic sneezing in humans.

AGE-RELATED FACTORS
N/A

ZOONOTIC POTENTIAL
N/A

PREGNANCY/FERTILITY/BREEDING
N/A

SYNONYMS
Head tossing

SEE ALSO
Headshaking

Suggested Reading
Brooks DE. Ophthalmology for the Equine Practitioner, 2e. Jackson, WY: Teton NewMedia, 2008.
Gilger BC. Equine ophthalmology. In: Gelatt KN, Gilger BC, Kern TJ, eds. Veterinary Ophthalmology, 5e. Ames, IA: Wiley Blackwell, 2013:1560–1609.
Gilger BC, ed. Equine Ophthalmology, 3e. Ames: Wiley Blackwell, 2017.

Author Gil Ben-Shlomo
Consulting Editor Caryn E. Plummer
Acknowledgment The author and editor acknowledge the prior contribution of Dennis E. Brooks.

P

BASICS

DEFINITION
• Photosensitization is defined as UV-induced dermatitis caused by a photodynamic agent in the skin which increases the sensitivity of the skin to sunlight
• Decreased skin pigmentation and hair cover facilitate cutaneous penetration of UV

PATHOPHYSIOLOGY
• Upon exposure to UV, molecules of the photodynamic agent enter an excited or high-energy state. These excited molecules may cause skin damage directly but damage occurs mostly through the production of reactive oxygen metabolites and free radicals
• Photosensitization in horses generally fits into 1 of 2 categories: (1) *primary photosensitization*, which is caused when a preformed or metabolically derived photodynamic agent (e.g. plant or fungal products or chemicals) reaches the skin by ingestion, injection, or contact; and (2) *secondary (hepatogenous) photosensitization*, which occurs in cases of liver disease when phylloerythrin acts as a photodynamic agent
• Phylloerythrin, a porphyrin compound formed by microbial degeneration of chlorophyll in the intestine, is normally conjugated in the liver and excreted in the bile. Liver dysfunction and/or biliary stasis may result in the accumulation of phylloerythrin in the blood and body tissues, including the skin. Some toxins derived from grasses are directly phototoxic and hepatotoxic, which makes the above classification of photosensitization less clear

SYSTEMS AFFECTED
• Skin/exocrine—lesions usually restricted to light-skinned, sparsely haired areas such as the coronary band, muzzle, ears, eyelids, tail, and vulva
• Hepatobiliary—secondary photosensitization can be associated with any cause of hepatic insufficiency. However, it appears to be more commonly associated with hepatic insufficiency caused by the ingestion of hepatotoxic plants

GENETICS
N/A

INCIDENCE/PREVALENCE
N/A

GEOGRAPHIC DISTRIBUTION
More common in sunny areas.

SIGNALMENT
• All ages and breeds are susceptible
• Light-skinned horses will have the most severe lesions

SIGNS

Historical Findings
• Initial signs noted are restlessness and scratching and rubbing of the ears, eyelids, and muzzle
• Shade-seeking behavior
• Demarcated skin lesions characterized by redness, blister formation; weeping, and crusting
• In cases of *secondary photosensitization* owners may notice signs suggestive of liver failure (e.g. altered mentation, weight loss, abdominal pain, diarrhea, etc.)

Physical Examination Findings (Web Figures 3 and 4)
Cutaneous Lesions (Primary and Secondary Photosensitization)
• Usually restricted to sparsely haired, light-skinned areas on the dorsal aspects of the body (e.g. face, muzzle, eyelids, ears, coronary bands, vulva, and tail), but in severe cases can extend to dark-skinned areas
• Demarcation between lesions and normal skin is quite clear, particularly in multicolored animals
• Acute signs include erythema, edema, serous exudation, and crust formation; lesions may be sensitive to touch and/or pruritic
• As lesions become more chronic, crust formation and sloughing of the skin is noted
• Conjunctivitis, keratitis, and corneal edema may be seen
Liver Failure Signs (May Accompany Cutaneous Lesions in Cases of Secondary Photosensitization)
• Icterus
• Pruritus
• Weight loss
• Diarrhea
• Abdominal pain
• Altered mentation

CAUSES

Causes of Primary Photosensitization
• Associated with ingestion, injection, or contact with a photodynamic agent
• Photodynamic plants (e.g. St. John's wort (*Hypericum perforatum*), buckwheat (*Fagopyrum esculentum*), perennial ryegrass (*Lolium perenne*), burr trefoil (*Medicago denticulata*), spring parsley (*Cymopterus watsoni*), bishop's weed (*Ammi majus*), oat grass (*Avena fatua*), rape (*Brassica* spp.), Dutchman's breeches (*Thamnosma texana*), alsike clover (*Trifolium hybridum*), alfalfa (*Medicago* spp.), vetches (*Vicia* spp.), hogweed (*Heracleum sphondylium*), gluten, etc.)
• Chemicals (e.g. phenothiazines, thiazides, acriflavines, methylene blue, sulfonamides, tetracyclines, coal tar derivatives, furosemide, promazine, chlorpromazine, quinidine, rose bengal, etc.)
• Mycotoxins (e.g. phycocyanin produced by blue-green algae and phytoalexins produced by celery and parsnip)

Causes of Secondary Photosensitization
• Associated most often with chronic liver failure or conditions that result in biliary obstruction
• Chronic active hepatitis
• Hepatic abscessation
• Neoplasia (cholangiocellular carcinoma, lymphosarcoma)
• Chronic megalocytic hepatopathy (*Senecio* spp., *Crotalaria* spp., *Heliotropium* spp.)
• Burning bush, fireweed (*Kochia scoparia*)
• Mycotoxicoses (blue-green algae (*Microcystis* spp.), *Phomopsis leptostromiformis* (on lupines))
• Cholelithiasis/cholangitis

RISK FACTORS
• Exposure to plants and chemicals that cause primary photosensitization
• Chronic liver failure or biliary obstruction
• Lack of skin pigment and/or sparse hair cover
• Exposure to sunlight

DIAGNOSIS

DIFFERENTIAL DIAGNOSIS
The clinical signs in cases of photosensitization are identical regardless of the etiology. History and clinical findings can aid in the differentiation of primary vs. secondary photosensitization.

Primary Photosensitization
A history of exposure to plants (e.g. St. John's wort, buckwheat) or chemicals (phenothiazines, tetracyclines) known to cause primary photosensitization, and absence of liver failure signs, will support a tentative diagnosis of primary photosensitization.

Secondary Photosensitization
Photodermatitis accompanied by liver failure signs (e.g. icterus, weight loss, diarrhea, abdominal pain, neurologic lesions) should prompt the clinician to consider secondary photosensitization.

CBC/BIOCHEMISTRY/URINALYSIS
Primary Photosensitization
Liver enzyme activities (SDH, GGT, AST, ALP), bilirubin, and bile acid concentration are usually normal.

Secondary Photosensitization
Increased liver enzyme activities (SDH, GGT, AST, ALP), hyperbilirubinemia, and/or bilirubinuria will support a diagnosis of secondary or hepatogenous photosensitization.

OTHER LABORATORY TESTS
Increased serum bile acid concentration, prolonged clearance of foreign dyes such as bromosulfophthalein, and abnormal findings on a liver biopsy indicate a diagnosis of secondary photosensitization.

P

PHOTOSENSITIZATION

IMAGING

US
May detect changes in liver size and abnormalities in the hepatic parenchyma (e.g. abscesses, neoplastic masses, dilated bile ducts, choleliths) in cases of secondary photosensitization.

OTHER DIAGNOSTIC PROCEDURES

Liver Biopsy
• May yield diagnostic, prognostic, and therapeutic information in cases of secondary photosensitization
• Samples obtained using US-guided or blind techniques; placed in formalin for histopathology, transport medium for microbiology
• Complications—hemorrhage, pneumothorax, spread of infectious hepatitis, peritonitis (e.g. bile or ingesta contamination)
• Complications minimized by performing hemostasis profile, using US guidance

PATHOLOGIC FINDINGS

Primary Photosensitization
Lesions are limited to the skin and include edema, serous exudate, scab formation, and skin necrosis.

Secondary Photosensitization
Dependent on primary disease process.

TREATMENT

APPROPRIATE HEALTH CARE
Dependent on primary disease process.

NURSING CARE
• Identify and eliminate source of photodynamic agent
• Administer laxatives (mineral oil) and/or adsorbents (activated charcoal) to prevent further toxin absorption from the gastrointestinal tract
• IV fluids may be required in severely affected animals

ACTIVITY
Restrict activity and avoid exposure to sunlight.

DIET
For secondary photosensitization, a diet that provides 40–50 kcal/kg body weight in the form of a low-protein, high-energy feed is recommended (e.g. milo, *Sorghum*, beet pulp).

CLIENT EDUCATION
• Identification and removal of any plants causing primary or secondary photosensitization
• Knowledge of drug sensitivities to prevent further occurrences
• Management of specific disease process(es) for secondary photosensitization

SURGICAL CONSIDERATIONS
Surgical debridement is indicated to manage skin necrosis.

MEDICATIONS

DRUG(S) OF CHOICE

Medications for Cutaneous Lesions
• Use anti-inflammatory drugs (prednisolone 1.1 mg/kg PO every 24 h or flunixin meglumine 1.1 mg/kg PO, IV every 12 h) to decrease severity of inflammation in early stages
• Topical antibiotic—corticosteroid creams may be applied to affected areas
• Systemic antibiotics are indicated to manage secondary bacterial infections

Treatment for Hepatic and Extracutaneous Disorders
Treat underlying liver disease.

CONTRAINDICATIONS, PRECAUTIONS, POSSIBLE INTERACTIONS

Primary Photosensitization
Avoid use of drugs that may promote further photosensitization (e.g. tetracyclines, sulfonamides, or phenothiazines).

Secondary Photosensitization
• Avoid use of drugs metabolized primarily by the liver (e.g. anesthetics, barbiturates, or chloramphenicol)
• Sedatives metabolized by the liver (e.g. xylazine or diazepam) may have to be used at reduced dosages

ALTERNATIVE DRUGS
N/A

FOLLOW-UP

PATIENT MONITORING

Primary Photosensitization
Evaluate skin lesions every few days and debride necrotic lesions as required.

Secondary Photosensitization
• Manage skin lesions as for primary photosensitization
• Monitor liver enzyme activities, serum bile acids, and bilirubin concentration weekly until improvement is noted
• Repeat liver biopsy in 4–6 weeks to monitor disease progression

PREVENTION/AVOIDANCE
Identify and eliminate photodynamic agent from environment.

POSSIBLE COMPLICATIONS
• Patients with secondary photosensitization often succumb to underlying liver disease

• Rubbing and biting of affected areas may cause secondary self-trauma and bacterial infections

EXPECTED COURSE AND PROGNOSIS
In general, prognosis is favorable for primary photosensitization and poor for secondary photosensitization.

MISCELLANEOUS

ASSOCIATED CONDITIONS
• Local edema of nostrils, lips, and eyelids can cause dyspnea, abnormal feed prehension, or lacrimation
• Mares with teat lesions may not allow their foals to nurse, causing starvation
• Secondary septicemia may develop in severe cases

AGE-RELATED FACTORS
Factors leading to secondary photosensitization are generally seen in adult horses.

SEE ALSO
• Cholelithiasis
• Hepatic abscess and septic cholangiohepatitis
• Icterus (prehepatic, hepatic, posthepatic)
• Pyrrolizidine alkaloid toxicosis
• Toxic hepatopathy

ABBREVIATIONS
• ALP = alkaline phosphatase
• ASP = aspartate aminotransferase
• GGT = γ-glutamyltransferase
• SDH = sorbitol dehydrogenase
• US = ultrasonography, ultrasound
• UV = ultraviolet

Suggested Reading
Peterson AD, Schott AC. Cutaneous markers of disorders affecting adult horses. Clin Tech Equine Pract 2005;4:234–388.
Rashmir-Raven A, McConnico RS. Photosensitization. In: Sprayberry KA, Robinson NE, eds. Robinson's Current Therapy in Equine Medicine, 7e. St. Louis, MO: WB Saunders, 2015:536–542.
Scott DW, Miller WH. Environmental skin diseases. In: Scott DW, Miller WH, eds. Equine Dermatology, 2e. Maryland Heights, MO: Elsevier Saunders, 2011:398–420.

Authors Emily E. John and Jeanne Lofstedt
Consulting Editors Michel Levy and Heidi Banse

 Client Education Handout available online

BASICS

OVERVIEW
In human medicine pica is defined as an abnormal craving and compulsive eating of substances not normally deemed as food. In horses, the assessment of cravings is subjective; therefore, pica is a sign suggestive of nutritional, mental health, or behavioral imbalances.

Although the pathophysiology of pica is not understood, it is likely a conserved mechanism of adaptation to nutritional deficiencies. Clinically, pica can occur with obesity, parasitism, malnutrition, and deficiencies in fiber, electrolytes (sodium, chloride, or phosphorus), protein, or trace minerals (iron, copper, zinc). In stabled horses, pica might occur owing to lack of external motivation for masticatory muscle exercise or possibly "boredom." Decreased dietary roughage has been associated with wood chewing, although it is questionable as horses kept on pastures may ingest trees and shrubs. Behavior-altering diseases, such as rabies, or repetitive stereotypies may result in pica.

SIGNALMENT
• Miniature horses and foals are more prone; no associations with a particular signalment have been documented
• Pica may be seen in stabled horses with reduced pasture time and low-roughage/high-concentrate diets
• Coprophagia in foals and adults is normal

SIGNS
• History of eating nonfood items
• Colic, choke, or diarrhea may be secondary to consumption of inappropriate substances
• Animals with pica exhibit no differences in body weight, or changes in external appearance
• Excessive or abnormal wearing of teeth might be observed

CAUSES AND RISK FACTORS
Pica may be nutritional or mental in nature. Among the minerals, studies in horses indicate that iron and copper deficiencies may correlate with pica. Inadequate housing, exercise, stimulus, or nutrition can lead to pica.

DIAGNOSIS

DIFFERENTIAL DIAGNOSIS
• Dietary deficiencies should be investigated before determining if pica is behavioral
• Behavioral stereotypies may also be secondary to neurologic disorders (e.g. rabies) or malnutrition
• Pica could also occur in horses as a drug side-effect behavior

CBC/BIOCHEMISTRY/URINALYSIS
• Urinalysis may be normal, but fractional excretion of relevant electrolytes may aid in diagnosing specific mineral deficiencies
• Hematologic and biochemistry blood parameters are uninformative
• Low serum iron and copper concentrations and low copper/zinc ratios may be important treatable deficiencies in horses with pica. However, as nutritional factors in feedstuff and pastures oscillate with weather impacting nutrient availability in feed, serum test abnormalities may be interpreted with caution. In addition to iron and copper mild deficiencies, mild deficiencies in cobalt, magnesium, selenium, zinc, and marked deficiencies in phosphorus need to be assessed

OTHER LABORATORY TESTS
• If complete neurologic examination is normal, pica is likely behavioral
• Fecal examination for parasites and any other tests indicated by prior testing; feed evaluations, especially for trace minerals such as copper, cobalt, phosphorus, and zinc, are not conclusive or diagnostic, unless consistently deficient diets are documented

IMAGING
N/A

OTHER DIAGNOSTIC PROCEDURES
N/A

TREATMENT

• Treatment of pica will depend on the suspected underlying disease or risk factor and type of material ingested
• Redirecting the behavior, providing appropriate feedstuff substitute, increasing roughage, altering the environment causing the stereotypy (see chapter Oral stereotypic behaviors), altering the desirability of nonfood item by using unpalatable repellents, and increasing exercise
• Consider potential complications from ingesting aberrant materials and monitor, prevent, or treat clinical complications, e.g. toxicity from toxic materials, or intestinal impaction or perforations

MEDICATIONS

DRUG(S) OF CHOICE
N/A

CONTRAINDICATIONS/POSSIBLE INTERACTIONS
N/A

FOLLOW-UP

• The extent of follow-up required depends on the primary disease. Assess owner compliance and response to treatment. Repeated serum mineral analysis in plasma, and testing other animals is desirable
• Monitor potential complications, i.e. intestinal obstruction, teeth wear

MISCELLANEOUS

ASSOCIATED CONDITIONS
N/A

AGE-RELATED FACTORS
N/A

ZOONOTIC POTENTIAL
N/A

SEE ALSO
• Learning, training, and behavior problems
• Oral stereotypic behaviors

Suggested Reading
Aytekin I, Onmaz AC, Aypak SU, et al. Changes in serum mineral concentrations, biochemical and hematological parameters in horses with pica. Biol Trace Elem Res 2011;139(3):301–307.
Husted L, Andersen MS, Borggaard OK, et al. Risk factors for faecal sand excretion in Icelandic horses. Equine Vet J 2005;37:351–355.
McGreevy P. Ingestive behavior. In: McGreevy P, ed. Equine Behavior. A Guide for Veterinarians and Equine Scientists. Philadelphia, PA: WB Saunders, 2004:200–206.
McGreevy PD, Hawson LA, Habermann TC, Cattle SR. Geophagia in horses: a short note on 13 cases. Appl Anim Behav Sci 2001;71:119–215.

Author Alexander Rodriguez-Palacios
Consulting Editors Henry Stämpfli and Olimpo Oliver-Espinosa
Acknowledgement The author and editors acknowledge the prior contribution of Debora A. Parsons.

P

PIGMENTURIA (HEMATURIA, HEMOGLOBINURIA, AND MYOGLOBINURIA)

BASICS

DEFINITION
Discoloration of urine, red to brown in color, from increased excretion of RBCs (hematuria), hemoglobin (hemoglobinuria), or myoglobin (myoglobinuria).

PATHOPHYSIOLOGY

Hematuria
- Normal urine contains ≅5000 RBCs/mL or <5 RBCs/hpf on sediment examination
- Microscopic hematuria (10 000–2 500 000 RBCs/mL) can be detected as 10–20 RBCs/hpf on sediment examination or a trace to + + + reaction on a reagent strip
- Macroscopic or gross hematuria can be observed with >2 500 000–5 000 000 RBCs/mL (≅0.5 mL of blood per 1 L of urine)
- Hemorrhage from kidneys, ureters, or bladder leads to hematuria throughout urination. Hematuria at the beginning of urination indicates lesions of the distal urethra, and at the end of urination indicates lesions in the proximal urethra or bladder neck

Hemoglobinuria
Hemoglobinuria is a consequence of intravascular hemolysis and hemoglobinemia, and is observed when hemoglobinemia has reached a concentration of 1 g/L, which induces a pink discoloration of plasma.

Myoglobinuria
- Myoglobinuria is secondary to myoglobinemia due to muscle damage. Myoglobin is excreted in urine when plasma concentration exceeds 0.2 g/L
- Both hemoglobin and myoglobin are toxic to renal tubules

SYSTEMS AFFECTED
- Renal/urologic—pigmenturia, especially hematuria
- Hemic/lymphatic/immune—hemolysis; hemoglobinuria
- Hepatobiliary—hemolysis; hemoglobinuria
- Musculoskeletal—rhabdomyolysis; myoglobinuria

GENETICS
PSSM, malignant hyperthermia, and glycogen branching enzyme deficiency are genetic diseases of Quarter Horse breeds. Recurrent ER may be a genetic disease of Thoroughbreds.

INCIDENCE/PREVALENCE
Incidence of PSSM and other myopathies is common, yet clinical rhabdomyolysis is less common.

GEOGRAPHIC DISTRIBUTION
N/A

SIGNALMENT

Breed Predilections
- PSSM is most common in Quarter Horses but may also affect draft and Warmblood breeds
- Recurrent ER appears more common in Thoroughbreds
- Proximal urethral defects most commonly are observed in Quarter Horses
- Arabians and part-Arabians appear predisposed to IRH

Mean Age and Range
- NI affects neonatal foals and mule foals
- Vascular malformations more common in foals

Predominant Sex
- Proximal urethral defects, habronemiasis, and neoplasia of the penis and distal urethra occur in geldings and stallions
- Recurrent ER is a more significant problem in young, female racehorses

SIGNS

General Comments
Clinical signs vary with the primary disease.

Historical Findings
- Horses with pigmenturia often have obvious historical evidence of a primary problem—"tying-up," toxin ingestion, dysuria from cystolithiasis or lower UTI, or penile neoplasia
- Observation of pigmenturia may be the presenting complaint—vascular anomalies, cystolithiasis, proximal urethral defects, renal or bladder neoplasia, IRH, or exercise-associated hematuria

Physical Examination Findings
- Findings with hematuria are consistent with the underlying disease processes (e.g. AKI/ARF, urolithiasis, UTI, neoplasia, toxin ingestion) or may be normal (e.g. vascular malformations, proximal urethral defects, exercise-associated hematuria, IRH)
- Findings with hemoglobinuria or myoglobinuria reflect the underlying disease processes

CAUSES

Hematuria
- AKI/ARF—microscopic hematuria is common due to glomerular and tubular damage
- Urolithiasis—postexercise hematuria is common with cystoliths
- UTI—infection anywhere in the urinary tract, including habronemiasis of the prepuce and distal penis
- Neoplasia—nephroblastoma, renal adenocarcinoma, hemangiosarcoma, squamous cell carcinoma of the lower urinary tract, transitional cell carcinoma, and other bladder tumors (e.g. leiomyoma, lymphosarcoma)
- Renal vascular anomalies—arteriovenous and arterioureteral malformations

- Proximal urethral defects—consistently found at the dorsocaudal aspect of the urethra near the ischial arch; likely from a "blowout" of the corpus spongiosum penis into the urethral lumen during contraction of the bulbospongiosus and urethralis muscles. It can produce hemospermia or hematuria at the end of urination
- Exercise-associated hematuria—microscopic hematuria can be a normal physiologic consequence of exercise due to increased blood pressure and filtration of RBCs across glomerular capillaries; its magnitude increases with exercise intensity; gross hematuria after exercise may develop, when the bladder mucosa becomes "bruised" by trauma against the brim of the pelvis; urination prior to exercise increases risk, as urine in the bladder cushions against injury
- Blister beetle (cantharidin) toxicity can lead to inflammation and bleeding of the urinary tract
- IRH—syndrome of recurrent, potentially life-threatening hematuria of renal origin

Hemoglobinuria
- Primary immune-mediated hemolytic anemia—NI; incompatible blood transfusions; idiopathic
- Secondary immune-mediated hemolytic anemia—hemolysis with infectious diseases (e.g. equine infectious anemia, piroplasmosis, *Clostridium perfringens*), neoplasia, or drug administration (e.g. penicillins)
- Exposure to toxins—red maple leaves; onions; phenothiazines; ionophores
- Secondary to reabsorption of RBCs from previous hemorrhage into a body cavity
- Liver disease

Myoglobinuria
- Rhabdomyolysis—associated with exercise or other genetic (e.g. PSSM-1) and infectious (e.g. *Streptococcus equi* myositis, clostridial myonecrosis) diseases
- Nutritional myodegeneration—selenium deficiency
- Postanesthetic myopathy—due to crush injury of muscle during anesthesia and other factors, especially hypotension
- Atypical myopathy (see chapter Seasonal pasture myopathy/atypical myopathy)

RISK FACTORS
- Similar to those for AKI/ARF, urolithiasis, or UTI
- See Causes

DIAGNOSIS

DIFFERENTIAL DIAGNOSIS
- Blood accumulation at the vulval margins in pregnant mares may be due to hemorrhage from varicosities in the vagina rather than bleeding from the urinary tract

P

(CONTINUED) PIGMENTURIA (HEMATURIA, HEMOGLOBINURIA, AND MYOGLOBINURIA)

• Factitious pigmenturia occurs when dehydrated horses pass concentrated urine that is dark or when porphyrins in urine are oxidized after being voided (red to brown discoloration of snow, wood shavings, or with storage of urine over time)
• Pigmenturia can be observed as a side effect of medication (e.g. orange with rifampin (rifampicin) or Pyridium (phenazopyridine) and dark brown to black with doxycycline)
• Stallions with proximal urethral defects may present for hemospermia rather than hematuria

CBC/BIOCHEMISTRY/URINALYSIS
Changes characteristic for AKI/ARF, urolithiasis, UTI, liver disease when these cause hematuria (see specific topics).

CBC
• Normal laboratory values—renal vascular anomalies with mild hematuria
• Mild to moderate anemia—neoplasia, proximal urethral defects, IRH, primary or secondary immune-mediated hemolytic anemia
• Moderate to severe anemia—any disease causing severe hematuria, vascular anomalies, or IRH
• Anemia tends to have evidence of regeneration with increased mean corpuscular volume and anisocytosis
• Hemoglobinemia (red discoloration of plasma after centrifugation) and hemoglobinuria—primary or secondary immune-mediated hemolytic anemia

Biochemistry
• Hypoproteinemia—severe hemorrhage secondary to hematuria (IRH, vascular anomalies)
• Hypergammaglobulinemia—neoplasia, chronic infection
• Azotemia—all related conditions
• Hyperbilirubinemia—primary or secondary immune-mediated hemolytic anemia (mostly indirect), liver disease (direct or indirect), any disease causing decreased feed intake
• Increased creatine kinase and AST—rhabdomyolysis
• Increased liver enzyme activities (AST, γ-glutamyltransferase, sorbitol dehydrogenase, alkaline phosphatase), serum bile acids, and coagulation times, hypoglycemia—liver disease

Urinalysis
• See Pathophysiology
• Proteinuria accompanies any hemorrhage into the urine
• Abnormal cytology—neoplasia, UTI

OTHER LABORATORY TESTS
• Centrifugation of urine—RBCs form a red to brown pellet with clear supernatant (hematuria), whereas urine remains discolored with hemoglobinuria or myoglobinuria
• Urine reagent strips impregnated with orthotoluidine—react with hemoglobin and myoglobin; RBCs produce scattered red spots as long as hematuria is <250 000 RBCs/mL
• Hemoglobin can be differentiated from myoglobin in urine by protein electrophoresis or specific tests (e.g. radioimmunoassays, ELISAs)
• Quantitative urine culture—perform in all cases of suspected hematuria to assess for concurrent UTI
• Methemoglobinemia (oxidant injury)—red maple leaf toxicity, onions

IMAGING
• Transabdominal and transrectal ultrasonography—size and echogenicity of the kidneys, ureters, bladder, and proximal urethra, in case of hematuria
• Urethroscopy/cystoscopy—to confirm source of hematuria; imaging modality of choice for identifying proximal urethral defects

OTHER DIAGNOSTIC PROCEDURES
• Liver biopsy—further evaluation of liver disease
• Muscle biopsy—for further evaluation of rhabdomyolysis and other myopathies
• Biopsy of abnormal tissue in bladder or distal urinary tract

TREATMENT
This discussion is limited to hematuria; for the treatment of other disorders causing hemoglobinuria and myoglobinuria, see the chapters listed in See Also.

APPROPRIATE HEALTH CARE
• Hospitalization may be needed to stabilize the patient, ensure adequate circulating blood volume, and halt further hemorrhage
• AKI/ARF, UTI—inpatient/outpatient medical management, depending on severity; see specific topics
• Urolithiasis, neoplasia, renal vascular abnormality, proximal urethral defects—surgical management if necessary, once patient is stabilized
• Exercise-associated hematuria—bladder mucosal lesions in the rare horse with gross hematuria heal without treatment, but a few days of rest may be advised
• IRH—inpatient frequent monitoring, supportive care for hemorrhagic shock, including repeated blood transfusions

ACTIVITY
If mild anemia only, exercise may continue. Horses with moderate to severe anemia should have restricted exercise. Mild exercise restriction is recommended for a few days following exercise-induced hematuria.

DIET
See chapters Acute kidney injury (AKI) and acute renal failure (ARF), Urinary tract infection (UTI), and Urolithiasis.

CLIENT EDUCATION
• Counsel patience to owners of horses with proximal urethral defects with a short duration of hematuria and exercise-associated bladder mucosal damage because spontaneous resolution may occur
• Although the cause of hematuria in Arabian and part-Arabian horses with IRH is unknown, owners of affected horses should be advised not to breed affected horses

SURGICAL CONSIDERATIONS
• Urolithiasis—surgical removal of cystoliths is treatment of choice
• Neoplasia—complete surgical excision (rarely possible) combined with topical, intralesional, or systemic antineoplastic agents for bladder and urethral cancer. For renal neoplasia, unilateral nephrectomy may correct hematuria but rarely produces long-term success; most neoplasms, especially renal adenocarcinoma, have metastasized prior to diagnosis
• Renal vascular malformation—proper diagnosis and, when hematuria persists, appropriate surgical intervention (nephrectomy or renal arteriolar embolization)
• Proximal urethral defect—because some lesions heal spontaneously, no treatment is initially indicated; surgery is recommended for hematuria causing anemia or lasting for >1 month. A perineal urethrotomy approach into the corpus spongiosum penis, but not extending into the urethral lumen. The procedure creates a "pressure relief valve" for the corpus spongiosum penis, allowing the urethral defect to heal
• IRH—nephrectomy in Arabian and part-Arabian horses is *contraindicated* as bleeding from the contralateral kidney may ensue

MEDICATIONS
DRUG(S) OF CHOICE
• 5-Fluorouracil and triethylenethiophosphoramide are antineoplastic agents that may be used topically (at weekly or more frequent intervals) for bladder or penile neoplasms
• Piroxicam, a cyclooxygenase 2 inhibitor, for squamous and transitional cell carcinomas
• Prophylactic antibiotics are recommended for horses undergoing nephrectomy (e.g. penicillin/gentamicin) or a perineal urethrotomy approach for correction of a proximal urethral defect (e.g. trimethoprim–sulfonamide combination)
• α-Aminocaproic acid (10 mg/kg IV every 6 h) to enhance blood clot stabilization may be used in horses with renal hematuria from neoplasia or IRH

P

PIGMENTURIA (HEMATURIA, HEMOGLOBINURIA, AND MYOGLOBINURIA)   (CONTINUED)

CONTRAINDICATIONS
Do not perform nephrectomy in patients with azotemia or IRH.

FOLLOW-UP

PATIENT MONITORING
See chapters Acute kidney injury (AKI) and acute renal failure (ARF), Urinary tract infection (UTI), and Urolithiasis.

POSSIBLE COMPLICATIONS
Dissemination of neoplasia.

EXPECTED COURSE AND PROGNOSIS
• Patients with neoplasia have a poor long-term prognosis, but treatment and supportive care may prolong life
• Horses with vascular malformations may have other developmental anomalies that may not be apparent until later in life. Vascular malformations that resolve by spontaneous formation of a thrombus may redevelop
• Prognosis for recovery after surgical correction of a proximal urethral defect generally is favorable, but the problem may recur
• Recurrent bouts of hematuria over several years may occur with IRH. Resolution may happen; however, some may suffer acute, fatal renal hemorrhage

MISCELLANEOUS

ZOONOTIC POTENTIAL
Leptospirosis, which may cause hematuria and ARF, has zoonotic potential; avoid direct contact with infective urine.

PREGNANCY/FERTILITY/BREEDING
• Multiparous mares are at greater risk of producing alloantibodies that may lead to NI in their foals
• Vulval hemorrhage from varicosities can be confused with hematuria

SYNONYMS
Azoturia (for ER).

SEE ALSO
• *Acer rubrum* (red maple) toxicosis
• Acute hepatitis in adult horses (Theiler disease)
• Acute kidney injury (AKI) and acute renal failure (ARF)
• Anemia, Heinz body
• Anemia, immune mediated
• Atypical myopathy
• Cantharidin toxicosis
• Cholelithiasis
• Clostridial myositis
• Exertional rhabdomyolysis syndrome
• Hepatic abscess and septic cholangiohepatitis
• Methemoglobin
• Nutritional myodegeneration
• Polysaccharide storage myopathy
• Toxic hepatopathy
• Urinary tract infection (UTI)
• Urolithiasis
• Urinalysis (U/A)

ABBREVIATIONS
• AKI = acute kidney injury
• ARF = acute renal failure
• AST = aspartate aminotransferase
• ELISA = enzyme-linked immunosorbent assay
• ER = exertional rhabdomyolysis
• hpf = high-power field
• IRH = idiopathic renal hematuria
• NI = neonatal isoerythrolysis
• PSSM = polysaccharide storage myopathy
• RBC = red blood cell
• UTI = urinary tract infection

Suggested Reading
Schott HC. Hematuria. In: Reed SM, Bayly WM, Sellon DC, eds. Equine Internal Medicine, 4e. St. Louis, MO: WB Saunders, 2017:957-961.
Schumacher J. Hematuria and pigmenturia of horses. Vet Clin North Am Equine Pract 2007;23:655–676.

Author Harold C. Schott II
Consulting Editor Valérie Picandet

P

BASICS

DEFINITION
A tick-borne, noncontagious disease caused by infection of erythrocytes by either of 2 distinct protozoan parasites, *Babesia caballi* and *Theileria equi.*

PATHOPHYSIOLOGY
• Infection with *B. caballi* or *T. equi* results in clinical signs referable to infection and lysis of erythrocytes; dual infections occur
• The erythrocytic stage of *T. equi* can lyse erythrocytes in the absence of specific immune responses; however, the precise role of immune responses to parasite antigens of *T. equi* and *B. caballi* in anemia is not known
• Occlusion of capillaries within the pulmonary, hepatic, and CNS occurs during acute infection with *B. caballi*
• Those surviving acute infection become persistently infected and represent a problem for the international movement of horses due to several countries, including the USA, restricting entry of horses based on their serologic status to *T. equi* and *B. caballi*
• Intrauterine transmission appears to occur with *T. equi* but is rare with *B. caballi* infections; abortions due to fetal infections have been reported for both parasites

SYSTEMS AFFECTED
• Hemic/lymphatic/immune—lysis of infected erythrocytes leads to anemia and icterus
• Nervous, hepatobiliary, respiratory—occlusion of capillaries by *B. caballi* can lead to dysfunction within these organ systems

GENETICS
N/A

INCIDENCE/PREVALENCE
• Infection and clinical disease occur when susceptible horses move into endemic areas or persistently infected horses move into a nonendemic area with tick vectors capable of transmission. Compounding concerns about movement of persistently infected horses is the lack of knowledge about the ability of tick species in nonendemic areas to transmit *T. equi* and *B. caballi*
• According to the OIE, disease and persistent infection have been reported in southern Florida, Texas, Asia, Africa, South America, Central America, the Middle East, and southern Europe. Some countries, however, refrain from reporting identified cases. Therefore, the actual global prevalence is unclear
• Tick vectors include species of *Amblyomma, Dermacentor, Haemaphysalis, Hyalomma,* and *Rhipicephalus*

SIGNALMENT
• Horses, donkeys, their cross-breeds, and zebras are susceptible to piroplasmosis
• No known breed, age, or sex predilections

SIGNS
General Comments
• Clinical signs depend on the immune status of the horse
• Horses that survive acute infection are immune to clinical disease on reinfection; however, an exception may be those infected with *B. caballi* and treated by chemotherapy
• In endemic areas, clinical piroplasmosis seldom is seen, except when nonimmune (i.e. uninfected) horses are introduced

Historical Findings
• Acute disease—lethargy, anorexia, fever, anemia, petechial hemorrhages of mucous membranes, and icterus
• Hemoglobinuria can be observed in more severe cases of *T. equi* infection
• Exercise intolerance (related to the degree of anemia) is common

Physical Examination Findings
• Signs are common only during the acute phase of infection
• During acute *B. caballi* infection, high fever, lethargy, hyperemia of mucous membranes with petechial hemorrhages, ventral edema, constipation, colic, dehydration, and icterus are seen
• Acute *T. equi* infection is similar, with hemoglobinuria and a more pronounced icterus

CAUSES
• Infection of erythrocytes with the hemoprotozoan parasites *B. caballi* or *T. equi*
• Anemia—result of hemolysis caused by replication of the erythrocyte-stage parasites
• *B. caballi* sequesters in the capillaries of organ systems, including the CNS, leading to occlusion of blood flow

RISK FACTORS
The primary risk factor is movement of uninfected (i.e. nonimmune) horses into endemic areas.

DIAGNOSIS

DIFFERENTIAL DIAGNOSIS
• Equine infectious anemia—infected horses are seropositive
• Purpura haemorrhagica—petechial hemorrhages and ventral edema are common; often a history of previous exposure to *Streptococcus equi* or other respiratory pathogens; hemolysis is uncommon
• Equine viral arteritis virus—hemolysis is uncommon; diagnosis can be confirmed serologically or by viral isolation
• Equine ehrlichiosis—hemolysis is uncommon

• Trypanosomiasis
• Leptospirosis
• Red maple-leaf poisoning—Heinz bodies and methemoglobinemia are common

CBC/BIOCHEMISTRY/URINALYSIS
• Anemia
• Thrombocytopenia
• Leukocytosis
• Hyperbilirubinemia
• Hypophosphatemia
• Hemoglobinuria (*T. equi*)

OTHER LABORATORY TESTS
• Definitive diagnosis currently depends on identification of *Babesia* or *Theileria* organisms in Giemsa-stained blood smears or serologic tests (cELISA and IFAT). PCR assays have been utilized for detection of both parasites within laboratory settings
• Direct parasitologic verification of chronic *B. caballi* infection is almost impossible but occasionally is successful with chronic *T. equi* infection. The USDA in 2005 adopted cELISA as the official serologic test for equine piroplasmosis; this test measures antibodies to an erythrocyte stage protein epitope of *T. equi* or *B. caballi.* Some countries also accept the IFAT for the international movement of horses
• Horses that test positive on cELISA are restricted from entry into the USA. Serum submitted to state diagnostic laboratories is forwarded to the National Veterinary Services Laboratory (Ames, IA) for testing
• *T. equi* and *B. caballi* can now be routinely cultured

IMAGING
N/A

OTHER DIAGNOSTIC PROCEDURES
N/A

PATHOLOGIC FINDINGS
• Horses that die of acute infection may demonstrate subcutaneous edema, serous exudates in the body cavities and pericardium, pronounced icterus, hepatomegaly, splenomegaly, glomerulonephropathy, and petechial hemorrhages of mucosal membranes
• Histologically, the spleen contains macrophages with intracellular erythrocytes (erythrophagocytosis), centrilobular necrosis of the liver, microthrombi within the liver and lungs, degeneration of the renal tubular epithelium, and hemoglobin casts in the renal tubules

TREATMENT

APPROPRIATE HEALTH CARE
Inpatient or outpatient, depending on the severity of clinical signs.

NURSING CARE
Routine care; intensive care usually not needed.

P

PIROPLASMOSIS (CONTINUED)

ACTIVITY
Restrict activity.

DIET
Normal diet.

CLIENT EDUCATION
Inform clients of the reportable nature of this infection and its significance regarding the international movement of horses.

SURGICAL CONSIDERATIONS
N/A

MEDICATIONS

DRUG(S) OF CHOICE
• Imidocarb dipropionate is the most effective and safest chemotherapy to date. Its ability to clear *B. caballi* persistent infection has been demonstrated and is effective in complete elimination of *T. equi* persistent infection in most cases. Recommended dosing of imidocarb dipropionate for complete chemotherapeutic clearance of either organism is 4 mg/kg every third day for a total of 4 treatments. Some horses may require more than 1 treatment regimen to achieve chemosterilization. Each dose is given IM and divided among at least 4 injection sites
• Colic, agitation, sweating, transient salivation, and diarrhea are common after imidocarb treatment
• Single doses of either glycopyrrolate (glycopyrronium) at 0.0025 mg/kg or atropine sulfate at 0.01 mg/kg have been administered IV to prevent the gastrointestinal symptoms associated with imidocarb treatment. Both, however, have potential negative side effects. Therefore, *N*-butylscopolamine is often used to mitigate the anticholinesterase activity of imidocarb dipropionate
• When treating *T. equi*-infected horses with imidocarb dipropionate, do not initiate retreatment for at least 30 days after the first treatment

CONTRAINDICATIONS
• In endemic regions, antibabesial therapy may lead to susceptibility on reinfection. This is especially true for *B. caballi* infections, in which chemotherapy (imidocarb dipropionate) clears persistent infections

• Donkeys appear very susceptible to the toxic side effects of imidocarb dipropionate and should not be treated with this drug

PRECAUTIONS
N/A

POSSIBLE INTERACTIONS
N/A

ALTERNATIVE DRUGS
• Several chemotherapies with antibabesial activity have been tested; these therapies include phenamidine, benenil, and diampron
• For *T. equi,* parvaquone and buparvaquone have been tested
• Imidocarb dipropionate is the most effective and safest of all therapies tested to date

FOLLOW-UP

PATIENT MONITORING
Monitor hydration status and percentage parasitemia in the peripheral blood.

PREVENTION/AVOIDANCE
Control in endemic areas is most effectively directed at tick vectors.

POSSIBLE COMPLICATIONS
N/A

EXPECTED COURSE AND PROGNOSIS
• Horses that survive acute infection usually, with appropriate supportive care, can return to normal activity. Owners should be advised that such animals are persistently infected and remain a potential source of parasite transmission to susceptible horses
• Although chemotherapy eliminates some strains of *B. caballi* and *T. equi* infection, chemotherapeutic clearance of horses dually infected with both organisms may not be achievable with currently available medications

MISCELLANEOUS

ASSOCIATED CONDITIONS
N/A

AGE-RELATED FACTORS
N/A

ZOONOTIC POTENTIAL
N/A

PREGNANCY/FERTILITY/BREEDING
Abortion (especially with *T. equi* infection) is a possible outcome.

SYNONYMS
Babesiosis

ABBREVIATIONS
• cELISA = competitive–enzyme-linked immunosorbent assay
• CNS = central nervous system
• IFAT = immunofluorescence antibody test
• OIE = Office International Epizooties/World Organisation for Animal Health
• PCR = polymerase chain reaction
• USDA = United States Department of Agriculture

Suggested Reading
Friedhoff KT. The piroplasms of equidae—significance for international commerce. Berl Munch Tierarztl Wochenschr 1982;95:368–374.
Holman PJ, Chieves L, Frerichs WM, et al. Culture confirmation of the carrier status of *Babesia caballi*—infected horses. J Clin Microbiol 1993;31:698–701.
Knowles DP. Control of *Babesia equi* parasitemia. Parasitol Today 1996;12:195–198.
Knowles DP. Equine babesiosis (piroplasmosis): a problem in the international movement of horses. Br Vet J 1996;152:123–126.
Wise LN, Kappmeyer LS, Mealey RH, Knowles DP. Review of equine piroplasmosis. J Vet Intern Med 2013;27:1334–1346.

Authors Kelly P. Sears and Don Knowles
Consulting Editor Ashley G. Boyle

P

PITUITARY PARS INTERMEDIA DYSFUNCTION

BASICS

DEFINITION
PPID or equine Cushing disease is the most commonly diagnosed endocrinopathy in horses. This slowly progressive disorder shows a characteristic clinical picture. It is associated with functional adenomas or adenomatous hyperplasia of the pars intermedia of the pituitary gland.

PATHOPHYSIOLOGY
• The pars distalis and pars intermedia of the pituitary gland secrete the same precursor molecule, POMC, but they process it into different hormones
• The corticotroph cells of the pars distalis cleave POMC into ACTH and β-endorphin-related peptides. In health, glucocorticoid levels are maintained by ACTH secretion from the corticotroph cells
• The melanotroph cells of the pars intermedia cleave POMC mainly into melanocyte-stimulating hormone and β-endorphin-related peptides, with relatively small amounts of ACTH.
• Control of the pars intermedia appears to be via tonic inhibition of melanotrophs by dopamine secreted from hypothalamic neurons. Horses with PPID show oxidant-induced injury and degeneration of dopaminergic neurons of the hypothalamus and, consequently, decreased inhibition of the melanotrophs. This results in hyperplasia of the melanotrophs, significantly increasing POMC-related peptide synthesis and secretion (including ACTH)

SYSTEMS AFFECTED
Skin/Exocrine
Clinical signs most often include hypertrichosis, delayed hair coat shedding pattern, and abnormal sweating (hyperhidrosis).

Endocrine/Metabolic
Polyuria/polydipsia—may be due to:
• Excess cortisol can increase the glomerular filtration rate and antagonize the effect of ADH on water reabsorption by the renal tubules
• Hyperglycemia can lead to an osmotic diuresis, although polyuria/polydipsia is also observed in euglycemic horses
• Compression or destruction of the pars nervosa by enlargement of the pars intermedia can decrease ADH secretion

Musculoskeletal
Laminitis appears to be associated with hyperinsulinemia.

Behavioral
The more docile behavior of some patients may result from increased β-endorphins.

GENETICS
N/A

INCIDENCE/PREVALENCE
Reported prevalence of PPID in horses >15 years of age between 15% and 30%.

SIGNALMENT
• All breeds—may be more prevalent in ponies and Morgans
• Old horses—mean age is approximately 20 years, rare in horses <10 years
• No sex predilection

SIGNS
Historical Findings
Affected horses may have various problems that do not necessarily appear directly related to PPID, e.g. lethargy, exercise intolerance, weight loss, recurrent laminitis, infertility, or chronic infections.

Physical Examination Findings
• Muscle atrophy (often most prominent along the epaxial musculature) and associated weight loss is common. A pot-bellied appearance may be observed
• Hypertrichosis is the most common sign in late disease. In earlier stages, this may be observed as retained hairs under the mandible, along the distal limbs, or across the trunk. In end-stage disease, generalized hypertrichosis characterized by a long, wavy hair coat may be observed
• In some, shedding of the winter coat is delayed; in others, hair grows earlier during the fall months
• Excessive sweating, primarily in horses with hypertrichosis
• Polyuria and polydipsia—may not be noticed if the horse is on pasture
• Less frequent signs—chronic laminitis, regional adiposity, chronic infections, delayed wound healing, infertility, lethargy, blindness, or seizures

CAUSES
Loss of dopaminergic innervation, may be due to oxidative stress.

RISK FACTORS
Increasing age.

DIAGNOSIS

DIFFERENTIAL DIAGNOSIS
• Hypertrichosis is pathognomonic, except in breeds with a long hair coat—Missouri Foxtrotter or Bashkin
• EMS—regional adiposity (cresty neck, tail-head fat pad, shoulder fat pads) or general obesity and insulin dysregulation are characteristic. EMS can affect horses of any age, but appears most common in middle-aged horses. EMS and PPID can occur concurrently
• Chronic weight loss—poor management, parasitism, poor dentition, other chronic systemic diseases, or neoplasia

• Polyuria/polydipsia—chronic renal failure, diabetes insipidus, or diabetes mellitus (rare in horses)

CBC/BIOCHEMISTRY/URINALYSIS
• No consistent changes in laboratory values—hyperglycemia reported
• Hyperlipidemia may be observed
• Serum liver enzyme activity may be elevated
• CBC may show a stress leukogram

OTHER LABORATORY TESTS
Endocrinologic testing of the pituitary–adrenal axis most often confirms the diagnosis.

Resting Plasma ACTH Level
• Measurement of plasma endogenous ACTH concentration recommended for fall testing. Normal values vary among laboratories. ACTH levels vary with time of the year and latitude. Increased ACTH production extends between July and November with a peak in September. The highest specificity and sensitivity of plasma ACTH for the diagnosis of PPID is in the fall
• The sample requires special handling—blood must be collected in disodium EDTA tubes, centrifuged and refrigerated within 3 h, and shipped overnight on ice. If delivery is delayed, plasma should be separated and kept frozen until assayed. Values in stressed normal horses and those with early PPID can overlap

TRH Stimulation Test
The TRH stimulation test is currently recommended for the diagnosis of PPID outside the fall period. Stimulation of thyroid receptors leads to increase in plasma ACTH in healthy and PPID horses although the response is higher in PPID horses. The test consists in the collection of a plasma sample for ACTH, followed by the administration of 1 mg of TRH IV and collection of plasma for ACTH determination 10 and/or 30 min later. ACTH concentrations above the cutoff values of 110 pg/mL (10 min) and 65 pg/mL (30 min) are suggestive of PPID.

Glucose Tolerance Test, Insulin Levels, and Insulin Tolerance Test
PPID horses may also be insulin dysregulated. In these cases:
• Basal insulin levels also may be persistently increased, with or without hyperglycemia
• Normal horses challenged with glucose (0.5 g/kg IV as a 50% solution) show an immediate rise in plasma glucose concentration and return to baseline level in 1.5 h
• Insulin dysregulated horses show a delayed return of plasma glucose concentration to baseline
• When subjected to an exogenous insulin tolerance test (0.4 IU/kg IV), insulin dysregulated horses show no significant decline in blood glucose

P

PITUITARY PARS INTERMEDIA DYSFUNCTION

• When undergoing an oral sugar test (0.15 mL/kg of Karo Light syrup PO), insulin dysregulated horses will have an increased insulin concentration 60–90 min following syrup administration

IMAGING
CT and MRI have been used.

OTHER DIAGNOSTIC PROCEDURES
N/A

PATHOLOGIC FINDINGS
• Necropsy reveals an enlarged pituitary gland (3–4-fold normal weight)
• Tumors are composed of large columnar or polyhedral cells with hyperchromatic nuclei
• No metastases. Multiple sites of infection may be present

TREATMENT

APPROPRIATE HEALTH CARE
Pay particular attention to regular deworming, vaccination, dental care, and foot trimming.

NURSING CARE
Body clipping and appropriate blanketing recommended for horses with heavy hair coat.

ACTIVITY
No need to decrease activity unless infections or laminitis.

DIET
Increase the energy content of the ration of horses showing signs of weight loss.

CLIENT EDUCATION
• Remind owners about the importance of husbandry
• Owners need to be vigilant for complications (secondary infections, laminitis, nonhealing wounds) to readily recognize signs of disease and seek veterinary help early

SURGICAL CONSIDERATIONS
Bilateral adrenalectomy has not been successful in the long term.

MEDICATIONS

DRUG(S) OF CHOICE
• Pergolide mesylate is the drug of choice for the treatment of PPID. Its activity on the dopaminergic (D_2) receptors of the melanotrophs of the pars intermedia decreases the secretion of hormones. Starting dose is 0.002 mg/kg (1 mg for an average-sized horse) PO once a day. Some ponies can be

successfully maintained on 0.25 mg/day. Clinical improvement should be noted within 4 weeks. If horses show no improvement at lower doses, the dose can be increased by 0.5–1 mg/day to a maximum of 0.01 mg/kg
• Anorexia is the most common adverse effect with pergolide and may be managed by stopping treatment until appetite returns, and then starting at a lower dose or splitting the dose into a morning and evening treatment. Abnormal weight loss, colic, diarrhea, and lethargy have also been observed
• A complete treatment plan should include symptomatic therapy such as NSAIDs for laminitis and/or antibiotics for focal bacterial infections

CONTRAINDICATIONS
N/A

PRECAUTIONS
• Pergolide mesylate has not been evaluated in breeding, pregnant, or lactating mares and should be used with caution in these horses
• Pergolide mesylate is on the list of prohibited substances in equine competitions overseen by the Fédération Equestre Internationale

POSSIBLE INTERACTIONS
Unknown

ALTERNATIVE DRUGS
• Cyproheptadine is a serotonin antagonist that has also been used to treat horses with PPID
• Information regarding the basic pharmacokinetic behavior and metabolism of cyproheptadine in horses is lacking
• Reports of clinical efficacy vary
• Initial recommended dose is 0.25 mg/kg PO every 12–24 h for 1 month
• If no clinical response occurs, the dose can be increased to 0.3–0.5 mg/kg
• Cases in which cyproheptadine is unsuccessful often respond to pergolide treatment

FOLLOW-UP

PATIENT MONITORING
• The first clinical improvements are often attitude and activity level (first month); subsequently, improvements in skeletal muscle mass, haircoat, laminitis, and a decrease in water consumption may be observed
• Reevaluation of endogenous ACTH levels (4–6 weeks after starting therapy)
• If starting treatment in the fall, seasonal influence may make control of ACTH levels

more challenging and a higher dose may be required

PREVENTION/AVOIDANCE
N/A

POSSIBLE COMPLICATIONS
N/A

EXPECTED COURSE AND PROGNOSIS
Prognosis depends on the severity of clinical signs.

MISCELLANEOUS

ASSOCIATED CONDITIONS
Some horses with PPID may have concurrent EMS.

AGE-RELATED FACTORS
N/A

ZOONOTIC POTENTIAL
N/A

SYNONYMS
• Equine Cushing's disease
• Hyperadrenocorticism
• Pituitary adenoma
• Pituitary-dependent hyperadrenocorticism

SEE ALSO
• Equine metabolic syndrome (EMS)/insulin resistance (IR)
• Glucose, hyperglycemia
• Glucose tolerance tests
• Insulin levels/insulin tolerance test
• Thyroid releasing hormone (TRH) and thyroid stimulating hormone (TSH) tests

ABBREVIATIONS
• ACTH = adrenocorticotropic hormone
• ADH = antidiuretic hormone
• CT = computed tomography
• EMS = equine metabolic syndrome
• MRI = magnetic resonance imaging
• NSAID = non-steroidal anti-inflammatory drug
• POMC = proopiomelanocortin
• PPID = pituitary pars intermedia dysfunction
• TRH = thyroid-releasing hormone

Suggested Reading
Durham AE. Endocrine diseases in aged horses. Vet Clin North Am Equine Pract 2016;32:301–315.

Authors Michel Levy and Heidi Banse
Consulting Editors Michel Levy and Heidi Banse

P

BASICS

OVERVIEW
• Shape—diffuse; normal placenta covers entire endometrial surface; see exceptions in section Villi
• Origin—allantochorionic; fusion of fetal allantois and chorion
• Degree of invasion—epitheliochorial; fetal tissue directly apposes maternal endometrium. Endometrial cups only fetal extensions into maternal tissue
• Vascular structure—microcotyledonary/villous; maternal and placental vessels in near apposition
• Degree of attachment—adeciduate; no loss of maternal tissue during placental formation or expulsion

CHRONOLOGY
• Conceptus mobile to day 16 post conception (day 0); spherical until ≈day 35; thereafter ellipsoid
• Endometrial cup formation by days 36–38
• Pregnancy maintenance by allantochorionic placentation experimentally from day 70
• Placenta contacts entire endometrial surface by ≈day 77; development complete by day 150

ENDOMETRIAL CUPS
• Fetal trophoblast invades endometrium—days 36–38; peak function ≈day 70
• Cups necrose day 120–150, slough and form allantochorionic pouches
• Produce equine chorionic gonadotropin; support formation/function of accessory corpus luteum

EXAMINATION
• Placenta ruptures at cervical star; allantochorion usually passed with allantois exposed
• Complete examination requires observing chorionic surface, amnion, and umbilical cord
• Identify body and uterine horns; lay out as capital F
  ○ Confirm horn tips are present
  ○ Where torn, match allantoic blood vessels
• Tip of nonpregnant horn most likely part retained—identify in all examinations
• Cervical star—site of fetal exit; examine remnants
  ○ Allantochorionic thickening/exudates should be sampled
• Assess amnion—uniformity, color, fecal staining
• Assess umbilical cord—length, degree of twisting, signs of vascular compromise
• Healthy Thoroughbred—placenta ≈11% of foal birth weight

VILLI
• Up to 5 normal chorionic avillous areas
  ○ Endometrial cup sites (may be absent at term)
  ○ Cervical star
  ○ Ostium (horn tips)
  ○ Site of umbilical cord attachment
  ○ Invaginated/redundant folds from umbilical cord traction
• *Pathologic avillous areas*
  ○ Placental apposition (twin pregnancy)
  ○ Placentitis—allantochorionic detachment from endometrium, cervical star (ascending placentitis), body, and pregnant horn (nocardioform sp.)
  ○ Endometrial fibrosis—degenerative change prevents villous formation
• Endometrial cysts—degenerative change prevents allantochorionic apposition to endometrium

ALLANTOCHORION
Normal
• Chorion has "red velvet" appearance due to diffuse microvilli over entire surface
• Tip of pregnant horn thick and edematous compared with nonpregnant horn

Abnormal
• Abnormal if:
  ○ Thickened
  ○ Edematous
  ○ Exudate
• Ascending placentitis
  ○ Cervical star, adjacent placental body
• Nocardioform placentitis
  ○ Localized changes—placental body, horn base
• Demarcation may be prominent.
• Other causes usually more diffuse inflammatory changes
• Gross edema or thickening—vascular disturbance, fescue toxicosis

AMNION
Normal
• Completely separate from allantochorion
• White; translucent; highly vascular
• Focal proliferative areas, small discrete plaques may occur

Abnormal
• Discolored/edematous—fetal distress (e.g. fetal diarrhea)
• Thickened—amnionitis
• Widespread edema/thickening may indicate fetal compromise—decreased nutrient and gaseous exchange; umbilical cord blood flow compromise

UMBILICAL CORD
Normal
• Allantoic and amniotic portions (60–83 cm in length)
• Normal twists—up to 4 reported

Abnormal
• Length
  ○ >100 cm—increased risk of fetal strangulation, torsion
  ○ <30 cm—excessive traction on fetal body wall; increased risk of fetal umbilical/urachal abnormalities, hemorrhage
• Torsion—hypoperfusion; congestion, thrombosis, mineralization of allantochorion
• Abortion—autolysis, vascular damage, thrombi (abnormal, excessive twisting), urachal tearing
• Neonate—patent urachus, elongated umbilical remnant from excessive traction in utero

ALLANTOIC FLUID
• Clear/amber—hypotonic urine; fetal excretions
• Hippomane (allantoic calculus)—concentric layers of cellular debris; rubbery; brown, green, tan

AMNIOTIC FLUID
Translucent—respiratory and buccal secretions.

MISCELLANEOUS

SEE ALSO
• Placental insufficiency
• Placentitis

Suggested Reading
Bucca S, Fogarty U, Collins A, Small V. Assessment of feto-placental well-being in the mare from mid-gestation to term—transrectal and transabdominal ultrasonographic features. Theriogenology 2005;64:542–557.
Klewitz J, Struebing C, Rohn K, et al. Effects of age, parity, and pregnancy abnormalities on foal birth weight and uterine blood flow in the mare. Theriogenology 2015;83:721–729.
Morresey PR. How to perform a field assessment of the equine placenta. Proc Am Assoc Equine Pract 2004;50:409–414.
Renaudin CD, Troedsson MH, Gillis CL, et al. Ultrasonographic evaluation of the equine placenta by transrectal and transabdominal approach in the normal pregnant mare. Theriogenology 1997;47:559–573.

Author Peter R. Morresey
Consulting Editor Carla L. Carleton

P

PLACENTAL INSUFFICIENCY

BASICS

OVERVIEW
• Fetoplacental unit cannot meet fetal demands. • Intrauterine growth retardation, malnutrition, prolonged gestation, preterm delivery, pregnancy loss

Pathophysiology
• Physical constrictions—body pregnancy; intraluminal adhesions, endometrial cysts, lymphatic stasis, endometrial fibrosis, glandular degeneration (endometrosis). • Placentitis—disruption of microcotyledonary attachments. • Histiotroph—nutrient exchange prior to placental formation, continues between microcotyledonary attachments. ○ Increased during pregnancy. ○ Production depends on endometrial gland competence, density

Systems Affected
Reproductive

SIGNALMENT
• Aged; multiparous. • History of endometritis, reproductive failure. • Twin pregnancy

SIGNS

General Comments
• Preterm delivery. • Prolonged gestation, term delivery of fetus inappropriate for gestational age. Dysmaturity—underweight, silky haircoat, erupted incisors, major organ dysfunction, sepsis. Post maturity—elongated hair coat, appropriate skeletal formation, decreased muscle mass

Historical Findings
• Previous episode. • Endometrial biopsy—loss of epithelial layer, fibrosis, glandular nesting, decreased gland number

Physical Examination Findings
• Uterus—intraluminal adhesions; segmental aplasia; cystic structures. • Placenta—localized or generalized poorly villous chorionic surface, pale appearance

CAUSES AND RISK FACTORS
• Placentitis. • Degenerative endometrial change. • Age. • Increased parity. • Chronic endometritis. • Poor vulvar conformation. • Uterine infection

DIAGNOSIS

DIFFERENTIAL DIAGNOSIS
• Infectious abortion. • Noninfectious abortion—systemic illness, uterine torsion, developmental anomalies, umbilical pathology, spontaneous fetal death. • Prolonged gestation—fescue toxicosis; fetal endocrine abnormalities. • Fetal malnutrition—maternal disease

CBC/BIOCHEMISTRY/URINALYSIS
• Systemic pathology, if any. • No changes directly attributable to placental insufficiency

IMAGING

Transabdominal US
• Placental detachment. • Intrauterine growth retardation—more pronounced later in gestation. • Asymmetrical development—disproportionate; little body fat or muscle

Transrectal US
Cervical placenta—thickness, detachment.

PATHOLOGIC FINDINGS

Gross
• Placenta—avillous areas. • Small placenta—normal 11% foal birth weight (Thoroughbred). • Multiple pregnancies—placental apposition prevents endometrial attachment, nutrient/gas/waste exchange. ○ Abortion of both fetuses, or 1 dead and/or mummified. ○ If pregnancy reaches term, remaining twin small for gestational age. • Placentitis, detachment, exudate

Histopathologic
• Placenta—reduced microcotyledon formation. • Endometrial biopsy—fibrosis, glandular nesting, reduced endometrial glands, lymphatic stasis, varying inflammation

TREATMENT
• Placental insufficiency—postpartum diagnosis suggested by neonatal and placental appearance. • Prepartum—oxygen supplementation in an effort to raise fetal oxygen. • Manage inflammatory/infectious conditions affecting placenta

MEDICATIONS

DRUG(S) OF CHOICE
• Progestagen supplementation—may boost endometrial histiotroph production. • Progesterone in oil. • Altrenogest

CONTRAINDICATIONS/POSSIBLE INTERACTIONS
Establish fetal viability before treating—transabdominal US; fetal heart rate.

FOLLOW-UP

PATIENT MONITORING
• US. • Fetus—viability, fetal heart rate. • Placenta—thickness, detachment

PREVENTION/AVOIDANCE
• Detect/repair anatomic defects—vulvar conformation, cervical competence. • Endometrial biopsy—evaluate density of endometrial glands, inflammation (acute—neutrophilia; chronic—plasmacytic, lymphocytic), degenerative changes (periglandular fibrosis, diffuse; lymphatic, dilation, stasis). • Endometrial cytology—eosinophilia; association with pneumovagina. • Early detection—placental thickness, areas of detachment

POSSIBLE COMPLICATIONS
• Abortion. • Undersized, weak neonate. • Premature placental separation

MISCELLANEOUS

ASSOCIATED CONDITIONS
• Perinatal asphyxia. • Placentitis. • Premature placental separation. • Sepsis

AGE-RELATED FACTORS
Endometrial competence declines with increasing age, parity.

PREGNANCY/FERTILITY/BREEDING
Abortion

SEE ALSO
• Placenta basics. • Placentitis

ABBREVIATIONS
US = ultrasonography, ultrasound

Suggested Reading
Bracher V, Mathias S, Allen WR. Influence of chronic degenerative endometritis (endometriosis) on placental development in the mare. Equine Vet J 1996;28(3): 180–188.
Bucca S, Fogarty U, Collins A, Small V. Assessment of feto-placental well-being in the mare from mid-gestation to term: transrectal and transabdominal ultrasonographic features. Theriogenology 2005;64:542–557.
Giles RC, Donahue JM, Hong CB, et al. Causes of abortion, stillbirth, and perinatal death in horses: 3,527 cases (1986–1991). J Am Vet Med Assoc 1993;203:1170–1175.
Pozor M. Equine placenta—a clinician's perspective. Part 2: abnormalities. Equine Vet Educ 2016;28:396–404.
Wilsher S, Allen WR. The effects of maternal age and parity on placental and fetal development in the mare. Equine Vet J 2003;35:476–483.

Author Peter R. Morresey
Consulting Editor Carla L. Carleton

BASICS

DEFINITION
Inflammation of the placenta. Single most important cause of late-term abortion, stillbirth, and premature delivery in the mare.

PATHOPHYSIOLOGY
- An infectious agent (e.g. bacterial, viral, mycotic) invades the placenta, leading to an inflammatory response
- Typically, initial location is in the area of the cervical star, when cause is ascending
- Placental detachment and thickening—may be localized or widespread
- Uterine motility is altered in response to local inflammation
- Modes of entry
  - Ascending via cervix (most common)
  - Hematogenous, as part of systemic illness
  - Inoculation
  - Recrudescence of preexisting focus of infection

SYSTEMS AFFECTED
Reproductive

GENETICS
N/A

INCIDENCE/PREVALENCE
Common if any of modes of entry are in play or if vulvar conformation is less than ideal (ascending route of infection).

SIGNALMENT
Pregnant mare typically during late gestation.

SIGNS
- Vulvar discharge—purulent; hemorrhagic
- Cervical incompetence—discharge; inflammation
- Mammary—swelling; discharge; prepartum lactation
- Relaxation of pelvic musculature—vulva; sacrosciatic ligament
- Restlessness; premonitory foaling behavior
- Placenta—thickening; edema; increased weight; discoloration; discharge; adenomatous hyperplasia; plaque formation, especially centered on cervical star

CAUSES
Bacterial
- Throughout gestation
- 2 presentations
  - Acute, focal or diffuse
  - Chronic, focal or extensive
- Acute, focal or diffuse
  - Neutrophil infiltration
  - Necrosis of chorionic villi
  - Primarily early to mid-gestation
- Chronic, focal or extensive
  - Centered around area of cervical star
  - Eosinophilic chorionic material
  - Necrosis of villi
  - Adenomatous hyperplasia
  - Mononuclear cell infiltration
  - Primarily mid- to late gestation
- Common pathogens
  - *Streptococcus equi* ssp. *zooepidemicus*
  - *Streptococcus equisimilis*
  - *Escherichia coli*
  - *Pseudomonas aeruginosa*
  - *Klebsiella pneumoniae*
- *Leptospira* spp.
  - Diffuse, spirochete invasion
  - Hematogenous spread only
- *Crossiella equi*
  - Other actinomycete species also occur; base of horns and body
  - Gram-positive filamentous bacillus infiltration
  - Chronic nature

Viral
- Equine viral arteritis
  - Thickening of allantochorion attributable to a longer incubation time before abortion
  - Compare/contrast with equine herpesvirus 1, with which there are either no or nonspecific placental changes

Fungal
- Usually 300 days of gestation or later
- *Aspergillus* spp.—chronic, focal placentitis at cervical star similar to chronic bacterial cases
- *Candida* spp.—diffuse; necrotizing; proliferative
- *Histoplasma* spp.—multifocal; granulomatous

Anatomic
- Cervical incompetence—laceration; age-induced degeneration. Bacterial invasion resulting in placentitis
- Vulvar and vestibular incompetence—aspiration of external irritants and debris
- Production of prostaglandin $F_{2\alpha}$ by endotoxin release, leading to cervical relaxation

RISK FACTORS

DIAGNOSIS

DIFFERENTIAL DIAGNOSIS
- Impending parturition
- Fescue toxicosis—placental edema; delayed parturition; decreased lactation
- Other causes of vulvar discharge
  - Vaginitis (speculum examination to assess cervical integrity/discharge)
  - Endometritis
  - Pyometra
  - Metritis
  - Vaginal varicosities
- Uterine trauma or hemorrhage
- Urinary tract infection
- Urine pooling
- Uterine or vaginal neoplasia
- Other causes of lactation—endocrine, seasonal
- Other causes of relaxation—impending parturition

CBC/BIOCHEMISTRY/URINALYSIS
- CBC may remain normal even with significant placental pathology
- Leukocytosis with neutrophilia
- Hyperfibrinogenemia
- Biochemistry, usually normal
- Urinalysis, normal

OTHER LABORATORY TESTS
Mares with placentitis have been demonstrated experimentally to have increased concentrations of either P_5 and/or progesterone P_4 along with a number of metabolites. This suggests increased fetal production of P_5 and/or P_4 and increased uteroplacental metabolism in response to chronic stress.

IMAGING
Transrectal US
- Marked increase in the CTUP measured by US, especially in the cervical region of the uteroplacental unit
- Good indicator of ascending placentitis
- Normal ranges for the area immediately cranial to the cervix have been established from 4 months of gestation to term in normal pregnant mares using transrectal US
- Mean CTUP is:
  - Approximately 4 mm between the fourth and ninth months of pregnancy
  - After which time it increases 1.5–2 mm each month until the end of gestation
  - Alternately, CTUP of up to 7 mm prior to day 300 has been considered normal
  - Obtain measurements from a consistent area on the ventral body of the uteroplacental unit
- This is aided by including regional vein in field of view
- Edema at cervical pole common in final month of gestation

Transabdominal US
- Range of CTUP 12.6 ± 0.33 mm
- Avoid areas of compression by fetus
- Observe for anechoic or particulate fluid between uterus and allantochorion
- Ensure vascular structures are not erroneously identified
- Areas of placental folding or detachment from endometrium
- Allantoic fluid debris

OTHER DIAGNOSTIC PROCEDURES
- Microbial culture of discharge from cervix
- Cytology—neutrophils, with or without intracellular bacteria; fungal elements

PATHOLOGIC FINDINGS
Examination of the allantochorion.
Gross
- Thickened; discolored
- Bright red chorion becomes gray/brown, with plaques; avillous areas; exudative
- Examine umbilical cord, fetus for inflammatory changes

Histopathologic
- Necessary to differentiate bacterial from mycotic

P

- Inflammatory infiltrate, fibrosis, thrombosis, edema; causative agent—bacteria or fungal elements

Microbiologic Examination
Bacterial/fungal/viral isolation.

TREATMENT

APPROPRIATE HEALTH CARE
- Remove inciting cause—control infectious agent (bacterial, fungal)
- Control placental, endometrial inflammation, e.g. Caslick's vulvoplasty, progesterone supplementation
- Clinical trials indicate that long-term treatment improves pregnancy outcome
- Maintain fetoplacental function
- Prevent fetal expulsion
  ◦ If mare carries to 300 days, chance of fetal survival increases
  ◦ Stress of intrauterine environment accelerates fetal maturity
- Maintain maternal health

NURSING CARE
Minimize maternal and fetal stress.

ACTIVITY
Stall rest the mare.

DIET
N/A

CLIENT EDUCATION
Monitor subsequent pregnancies.

SURGICAL CONSIDERATIONS
Repair of cervical and conformational defects, if present.

MEDICATIONS

DRUG(S) OF CHOICE

Antibiotics
- Penicillin G; gentamicin
- Trimethoprim–sulfa
- Selection based on sensitivities of most likely pathogen

Anti-inflammatories
- NSAIDs decrease endotoxin production
- Decrease luteolytic potential
- Decrease myometrial contractility
- Decrease incidence of laminitis

Anticytokine Therapies
- Pentoxifylline 8.5 mg/kg BID PO
- Decreases production of inflammatory mediators
- Has led to pregnancy maintenance in mouse endotoxemia model

Progestagen Supplementation
- Altrenogest (Regumate) 0.044 mg/kg PO once daily for routine administration may be given at 0.088 mg/kg daily for the last 20 ± 5 days of pregnancy; helps to decrease uterine excitability

- Maintains production of histiotroph, fetal nutrition
- Aids cervical competency

CONTRAINDICATIONS
If fetal death occurs:
- Discontinue progestagens
- Allow abortion to occur
- Avoid in utero fetal decomposition
- Continue antimicrobial and anti-inflammatory treatment of mare
- Monitor for laminitic changes

PRECAUTIONS
N/A

POSSIBLE INTERACTIONS
N/A

ALTERNATIVE DRUGS
N/A

FOLLOW-UP

PATIENT MONITORING

Mare
- Transrectal US of cervix and caudal uterine body to evaluate thickness and detachment of placenta
- Transabdominal US to monitor placental integrity, fetal viability
- Attend parturition
  ◦ Increased incidence of premature placental separation, and/or
  ◦ Decreased likelihood of thickened allantochorion to rupture readily at cervical star during delivery
  ◦ Either circumstance can lead to neonatal asphyxiation
- Preterm mammary development (especially if >30 days before parturition)
- Premature lactation—loss of colostral antibodies; potential failure of passive transfer of immunity
- Placental examination—to ensure no retained fetal membranes
- Diagnostic samples—microbiologic and histologic from placenta, fetus
- Vaginal speculum examination to monitor cervix—closure, relaxation, and discharge
  ◦ Use with caution
  ◦ This procedure disrupts existing vulvar and vestibular barriers to ascending uterine infection

Neonate
- Increased potential for sepsis
- Increased potential for neurologic compromise
- Possible intrauterine growth retardation
- Prepartum lactation may have depleted colostral antibodies
- Fetal ECG in late gestation (final trimester)

PREVENTION/AVOIDANCE
- Breeding soundness examination of the mare when not pregnant; include examination of cervical competence

  ◦ Best if in diestrus at time of examination
- Prebreeding preparation of mare and stallion—hygiene
- Keep environment and housing of pregnant mares as clean as possible

POSSIBLE COMPLICATIONS
- Abortion
- Dystocia
- Sick, weak neonate

EXPECTED COURSE AND PROGNOSIS
N/A

MISCELLANEOUS

ASSOCIATED CONDITIONS
- Premature placental separation
- Laminitis
- Fetal sepsis—bacterial; fungal
- Neonatal sepsis and compromise

AGE-RELATED FACTORS
Endometrial health and cervical competence decline with age and increasing parity of mares.

ZOONOTIC POTENTIAL
N/A

PREGNANCY/FERTILITY/BREEDING
Abortion

SEE ALSO
- Placenta basics
- Placental insufficiency

ABBREVIATIONS
- CTUP = combined thickness of the uterus and placenta
- NSAID = nonsteroidal anti-inflammatory drug
- P_4 = progesterone
- P_5 = pregnenolone
- US = ultrasound, ultrasonography

Suggested Reading
Bucca S, Fogarty U, Collins A, Small V. Assessment of feto-placental well-being in the mare from mid-gestation to term: transrectal and transabdominal ultrasonographic features. Theriogenology 2005;64:542–557.
Macpherson ML. Treatment strategies for mares with placentitis. Theriogenology 2005;64:528–534.
Ousey JC, Houghton E, Grainger L, et al. Progestagen profiles during the last trimester of gestation in Thoroughbred mares with normal or compromised pregnancies. Theriogenology 2005;63:1844–1856.
Renaudin CD, Troedsson MH, Gillis CL, et al. Ultrasonographic evaluation of the equine placenta by transrectal and transabdominal approach in the normal pregnant mare. Theriogenology 1997;47:559–573.

Author Peter R. Morresey
Consulting Editor Carla L. Carleton

BASICS

DEFINITION
• Comprised primarily of albumin, immunoglobulin (globulin), fibrinogen, and clotting factors
• Other proteins include hormones, enzymes, and regulatory proteins
• Albumin (69 kDa) accounts for 80% of plasma oncotic pressure
• Immunoglobulins (globulins) are antibodies, with IgG representing the most abundant antibody class present in plasma
• Fibrinogen (340 kDa) is a positive acute-phase protein produced by the liver; production is increased in response to inflammatory stimuli

PATHOPHYSIOLOGY
• Proteins serve a wide variety of vital roles including coagulation, host defense, transport of metabolites and hormones, and providing the bulk of oncotic pressure
• Apart from immunoglobulins, the vast majority of plasma proteins are synthesized in the liver by hepatocytes
• Immunoglobulins are produced by plasma cells

SYSTEMS AFFECTED
Dependent on the underlying cause.

GENETICS
SCID is an autosomal recessive disease of Arabian foals.

INCIDENCE/PREVALENCE
N/A

GEOGRAPHIC DISTRIBUTION
N/A

SIGNALMENT
• Plasma fibrinogen concentration may be increased in foals up to 6 months of age and during pregnancy in mares
• FPT is a disease of neonates
• Serum proteins increase with age
• Neoplastic diseases (e.g. myeloma) tend to occur in older animals and may cause hyperproteinemia

SIGNS
• Dependent on the underlying cause
• Severe hypoalbuminemia can result in edema, reduced perfusion to tissues, and organ dysfunction

CAUSES

Panhyperproteinemia (Increase in Albumin and Globulin)
Dehydration leads to fluid shifting from the intracellular and extracellular fluid into the intravascular spaces to maintain blood volume. As the process continues, hemoconcentration occurs, leading to panhyperproteinemia.

Panhypoproteinemia (Decrease in Albumin and Globulin)
Protein loss—acute severe hemorrhage, PLE (e.g. colitis [*Salmonella*, Potomac horse fever, NSAID toxicity, severe parasitism], granulomatous enteritis, gastrointestinal lymphoma), or vasculitis (increased vascular permeability [purpura haemorrhagica, equine viral arteritis]).

Selective Hyperalbuminemia
Always a relative change secondary to dehydration with subsequent hemoconcentration.

Selective Hypoalbuminemia
• Negative acute-phase protein that will mildly to moderately decrease during inflammation. Globulins often elevate at the same time, resulting in a TP within reference range, with a low A:G ratio
• PLN—e.g. glomerulonephritis, amyloidosis. Since albumin is one of the smallest proteins, it is readily lost early in renal disease, and although there can ultimately be a panhypoproteinemia, the A:G remains low
• Third-space loss (e.g. pleuropneumonia, peritonitis, uroperitoneum, heart failure)
• Decreased production (e.g. hepatic failure)

Selective Hyperglobulinemia
• Positive acute-phase proteins (e.g. α_1 and α_2 globulins, C-reactive proteins) increase in the first 2 days of an inflammatory process followed by the delayed response proteins (β- and γ-globulins such as IgM and IgG, respectively) 1–2 weeks after the onset of inflammation
• Positive acute-phase proteins cause mild to moderate increases in globulin, whereas the delayed response proteins can cause moderate to marked elevations of globulin
• Neoplasia (e.g. plasma cell myeloma, lymphocytic leukemia, lymphoma). These proteins include intact immunoglobulins, heavy chains, light chains, and abnormal fragments of proteins

Selective Hypoglobulinemia
• FPT in neonates
• SCID in Arabian foals
• Selective IgM deficiency (rare)

Hyperfibrinogenemia
• Inflammation; levels generally peak 72–96 h after the initiation of inflammation
• Dehydration
• The plasma protein to fibrinogen ratio may help interpret elevations in fibrinogen—[plasma protein]/[fibrinogen]. Care should be taken that units match. If the elevation of fibrinogen is secondary to dehydration, the ratio should be >21; if it is due to inflammation, the ratio should be <16. The ratio should not be used in foals or in adult horses with diseases that lower fibrinogen concentration.

Hypofibrinogenemia
• Hepatic failure
• Disseminated intravascular coagulation

RISK FACTORS
See Causes.

DIAGNOSIS

DIFFERENTIAL DIAGNOSIS
• A complete history may also aid in the localization of inflammatory diseases
• Hyperfibrinogenemia suspected to be due to inflammation should prompt a thorough physical examination with secondary testing as needed to localize the focus of inflammation
• Other diseases may be suspected based on historical or physical examination findings

LABORATORY FINDINGS
• Plasma protein is often indirectly assessed via refractometry that it measures total solids.
• Serum proteins are measured using the biuret method
• Albumin is determined using a dye binding technique
• Globulin and the A:G ratio are calculated using the measured TP and albumin
• Fibrinogen can be determined by the heat precipitation method
• Lipemia and high concentrations of Na^+, Cl^-, glucose, and blood urea nitrogen can falsely elevate plasma protein concentrations

CBC/BIOCHEMISTRY/URINALYSIS
CBC
• Inflammatory leukogram (leukopenia or leukocytosis, left shift, toxic neutrophils) and mild normocytic, normochromic anemia may be seen in cases of inflammation
• Significant anemia may be present in cases of hemorrhage, with accompanying fluid shifts

Biochemistry
• The protein panel can be used to determine which fraction(s) are moving and in which direction to categorize the protein dyscrasia (i.e. panhypoproteinemia, selective hypoproteinemia, panhyperproteinemia, or selective hyperproteinemia)
• Changes may reflect a focus of disease with enzymatic changes or electrolyte disturbances depending on organ system(s) involved

Urinalysis
• Urine should contain very little protein. Transient mild proteinuria may be seen with exercise, stress, and in neonates
• The dipstick test for protein is semiquantitative and essentially only recognizes albumin
• Significant proteinuria should be present if hypoalbuminemia is due to a PLN

OTHER LABORATORY TESTS
• Protein fractions can be separated and quantified using SPE. Albumin, α_1, α_2, β_1, β_2, and γ regions are the zones of an SPE. Immunoglobulins fall within the β and γ regions

P

PLASMA PROTEINS (CONTINUED)

- Blood lactate concentration may help determine the magnitude of poor perfusion secondary to hypovolemia
- COP can be measured in cases of hypoalbuminemia (requires colloid osmometer)
- Stall-side immunoassay for FPT (i.e. SNAP IgG test)
- Coagulation profile
- Urine protein to creatinine ratio may be helpful in quantifying protein loss in the urine

IMAGING
- Transabdominal US if suspect:
  - Colitis
  - Infiltrative bowel disease
  - Peritonitis
  - Liver disease
- Transthoracic US if suspect:
  - Pleuropneumonia
- Umbilical US if suspect sepsis secondary to FPT in neonatal foal

OTHER DIAGNOSTIC PROCEDURES
Dependent on the suspected condition.

TREATMENT
- The goal of treating an inflammatory disease should be aimed at the underlying disease process
- If dehydration is the source of a hyperproteinemia, the cause should be identified and eliminated. The severity of dehydration and electrolyte imbalances will dictate the route, volume, and composition of fluids used to resuscitate blood volume
- Hypoproteinemia should be addressed by eliminating the primary disease, if possible

MEDICATIONS
DRUG(S) OF CHOICE
- Drug choices are dictated based on a tentative or definitive diagnosis and reflect the primary disease
- FPT can be treated with oral colostrum administration in foals <12 h of age; IV plasma must be used in neonates >12 h of age due to "gut closure" (inability to absorb large IgG molecules)
- Plasma administered IV may be warranted in cases of marked hypoproteinemia to increase oncotic pressure. Plasma is preferred to whole blood, unless anemia is also present or if there are financial limitations

- Oncotic pressure can be transiently increased by using synthetic colloids IV (e.g. hydroxyethyl starch)

CONTRAINDICATIONS
N/A

PRECAUTIONS
- Anaphylactic reactions can occur during IV plasma administration; monitor closely during infusion
- Theiler's disease is associated with administration of equine biologics, including plasma

POSSIBLE INTERACTIONS
N/A

ALTERNATIVE DRUGS
N/A

FOLLOW-UP
PATIENT MONITORING
- Treatment efficacy for an inflammatory disease may be monitored using serial CBCs and plasma fibrinogen concentrations
- Hydration status can be monitored using physical examination findings (e.g. capillary refill time, heart rate, and pulse quality) and laboratory findings such as packed cell volume/TP, lactate concentration, and electrolyte concentrations

PREVENTION/AVOIDANCE
Ensure early and adequate colostrum ingestion in neonatal foals.

POSSIBLE COMPLICATIONS
- FPT can lead to sepsis in neonatal foals
- Hypoalbuminemia (decreased COP) can lead to hypotension and subsequent multiorgan dysfunction

EXPECTED COURSE AND PROGNOSIS
Dependent on the underlying cause.

MISCELLANEOUS
ASSOCIATED CONDITIONS
N/A

AGE-RELATED FACTORS
- Reference ranges for TP, albumin, and globulin concentrations for foals are lower than adults
- Plasma fibrinogen concentration increases in normal foals during the first 6 months of life
- Adult protein concentrations remain relatively stable, although albumin decreases slightly over time, while globulin progressively increases with age due to antigenic stimulation.

ZOONOTIC POTENTIAL
Salmonella spp. (e.g. colitis causing PLE).

PREGNANCY/FERTILITY/BREEDING
- Plasma fibrinogen concentration will increase during pregnancy, with another small spike immediately postpartum; concentrations return to normal 14 days after foaling
- Globulin concentrations tend to increase slightly and albumin concentration decreases slightly during pregnancy
- Serum immunoglobulin concentrations increase until one month before foaling, when they are secreted into the mammary gland during colostrum production
- Serum albumin and TP concentrations decrease during lactation

SYNONYMS
- Oncotic pressure—colloid osmotic pressure
- Immunoglobulin—globulin, antibody

SEE ALSO
- Acute hepatitis in adult horses (Theiler's disease)
- Failure of passive transfer (FPT)
- Pleuropneumonia
- Potomac horse fever (PHF)
- Protein-losing enteropathy (PLE)
- Salmonellosis

ABBREVIATIONS
- A:G = albumin to globulin ratio
- COP = colloid osmotic pressure
- FPT = failure of passive transfer
- Ig = immunoglobulin
- NSAID = nonsteroidal anti-inflammatory drug
- PLN = protein-losing nephropathy
- PLE = protein-losing enteropathy
- SCID = severe combined immunodeficiency
- SPE = serum protein electrophoresis
- TP = total protein
- US = ultrasonography, ultrasound

Suggested Reading
Crisman MV, Scarratt WK, Zimmerman KL. Blood proteins and inflammation in the horse. Vet Clin North Am Equine Pract 2008;24(2):285–297.
Eckersall PD. Proteins, proteomics and dysproteinemias. In: Kaneko JJ, Harvey JW, Bruss ML, eds. Clinical Biochemistry of Domestic Animals, 6e. Burlington, MA: Academic Press, 2008:117–156.
Stockham SL, Scott MA. Fundamentals of Veterinary Clinical Pathology, 2e. Ames, IA: Blackwell Publishing, 2008:369–414.
Uzal FA, Diab SS. Gastritis, enteritis and colitis in horses. Vet Clin North Am Equine Pract 2015;31(2):337–358.

Author Craig A. Thompson
Consulting Editor Sandra D. Taylor

BASICS

OVERVIEW
The development of an inflammatory response in the lung parenchyma to bacterial pathogens, with extension to the pleural space and subsequent pleural effusion.

SIGNALMENT
• No breed or sex predilection
• All ages but rare in foals

SIGNS
• Acute—fever, lethargy, anorexia, tachypnea, decreased bronchovesicular sounds ventrally, radiating heart sounds, pleural friction rubs, nasal discharge, pleurodynia, soft cough, ventral or limb edema
• Subacute or chronic—fever (may be intermittent), weight loss, exercise intolerance, ventral or limb edema, intermittent colic, tachypnea relative to the volume of pleural effusion

CAUSES AND RISK FACTORS
• Mixed infections are common. *Streptococcus equi* ssp. *zooepidemicus* is the primary Gram-positive pathogen. *Escherichia coli, Klebsiella pneumoniae, Actinobacillus* spp., and *Pasteurella* spp. are the most common Gram-negative pathogens. Anaerobic bacteria are isolated in about one-third of cases. Mycoplasma has been isolated in rare cases
• The most significant risk factor is long-distance transport. Also, aspiration pneumonia, thoracic trauma strenuous exercise, exposure to dust or gases, exercise-induced pulmonary hemorrhage, viral disease, general anesthesia, immunodeficiency, immunosuppressive drugs, and malnutrition

DIAGNOSIS

DIFFERENTIAL DIAGNOSIS
Pneumonia, neoplasia, hemothorax, cardiac disease, equine infectious anemia, diaphragmatic hernia.

CBC/BIOCHEMISTRY/URINALYSIS
• Neutrophilic leukocytosis and hyperfibrinogenemia. Neutropenia can be present in acute cases
• Monocytosis, anemia, and hypergammaglobulinemia (subacute or chronic)

IMAGING
• Thoracic US—fluid between the thoracic wall and the lung parenchyma. Fluid may be loculated if there is significant fibrin deposition. Pulmonary consolidation or atelectasis, and pulmonary abscesses (if superficial) can be detected. Small hyperechoic images are suggestive of anaerobic infection
• Thoracic radiography—may be helpful after pleural drainage to reveal the extent of the pneumonia

OTHER DIAGNOSTIC PROCEDURES
• Cytology (including Gram stain) and culture of TTA and pleural fluid. TTA is more reliable for the positive identification of pulmonary pathogens
• Pleural fluid glucose concentration of <40 mg/dL, pH <7.2, or lactate level higher than venous blood suggest septic effusion
• Arterial blood gas

TREATMENT

• Mild cases with minimal fluid accumulation can be treated as outpatients. Hospitalization is recommended for any patient with significant fluid accumulation
• Polyionic fluids and oxygen insufflation may be required
• Repeated thoracic drainage or placement of an indwelling thoracic drain may be necessary

MEDICATIONS

DRUG(S) OF CHOICE
• Optimally, antimicrobial therapy should be based on identification of the pathogens and in vitro sensitivity testing. However, therapy is usually begun prior to definitive results and broad-spectrum drugs should be used owing to the high number of mixed infections
• Penicillin, ampicillin, and cephalosporins are effective against *S. zooepidemicus*. Penicillin is effective against the great majority of anaerobes but not against *Bacteroides fragilis,* a common anaerobic isolate. Common initial treatment choices would include penicillin or ampicillin and gentamicin or amikacin (or enrofloxacin in adult patients with compromised renal function), and metronidazole. Ceftiofur and metronidazole can be an option in milder cases
• NSAIDs—to reduce inflammation and provide analgesia
• Antithrombotic drugs—heparin and aspirin have been used but their use is controversial

• Intrapleural fibrinolytics have been used in a limited number of cases. Recombinant tissue plasminogen activator is reported to improve drainage in cases with organizing fibrin

CONTRAINDICATIONS/POSSIBLE INTERACTIONS
The nephrotoxicity of aminoglycosides may be potentiated by dehydration and NSAIDs.

FOLLOW-UP

PATIENT MONITORING
Frequent auscultation and thoracic US examinations are the most sensitive indicators.

PREVENTION/AVOIDANCE
• Avoid risk factors
• Vaccination against upper respiratory viruses

POSSIBLE COMPLICATIONS
• Pulmonary or subpleural abscesses are not uncommon.
• Bronchopleural fistulas, pleural adhesions, and pericarditis
• Laminitis is a common serious sequela

EXPECTED COURSE AND PROGNOSIS
Guarded to good prognosis with early diagnosis and aggressive antibacterial and supportive treatment. Prognosis is guarded to poor in cases that reach the subacute to chronic stage prior to accurate diagnosis.

MISCELLANEOUS

ABBREVIATIONS
• NSAID = nonsteroidal anti-inflammatory drug
• TTA = transtracheal aspirate
• US = ultrasonography, ultrasound

Suggested Reading
Reuss SM, Giguere S. Update on bacterial pneumonia and pleuropneumonia in the adult horse. Vet Clin North Am Equine Pract 2015;31:105–120.
Tomlinson JE, Reef VB, Boston RC, Johnson AL. The association of fibrinous pleural effusion with survival and complications in horses with pleuropneumonia (2002–2012): 74 cases. J Vet Intern Med 2015;29: 1410–1417.

Author Johanna L. Watson
Consulting Editors Mathilde Leclère and Daniel Jean

P

PNEUMONIA, NEONATE

BASICS

DEFINITION
- Inflammation of pulmonary parenchyma occurring in foals <4 weeks of age
- One of the most common sites of infection in neonatal foals

PATHOPHYSIOLOGY

Bacterial Septicemia
- Most common cause of neonatal pneumonia, frequently as a sequel to bacterial septicemia
- Low serum IgG concentration is highly correlated with incidence of disease
- Pathogens implicated in neonatal septicemia are most frequently isolated, including *Escherichia coli*, *Klebsiella pneumoniae*, *Actinobacillus equuli*, *Salmonella* spp., *Streptococcus* spp.

Viral Infection
- Can cause severe, refractory pneumonia in neonatal period
  - Foals may be infected in utero or shortly after birth
- Most affected foals succumb quickly
- Foals may be born preterm or aborted as consequence of maternal viral infection
- Most common:
  - EHV-1 (less frequently EHV-4)
  - Equine arteritis virus
  - Equine influenza virus
  - Equine adenovirus (e.g. in Arabian foals with SCID)

Aspiration Pneumonia
- Aspiration of milk and oral secretions occurs as a result of neonatal pharyngeal dysfunction and weakness
- Risk factors include cleft palate, botulism, sepsis, nutritional myodegeneration, iatrogenic (syringe or bottle feeding), NMS

SYSTEMS AFFECTED
- Respiratory
- In foals with septicemic disease, other systems (e.g. musculoskeletal and gastrointestinal) may be concurrently affected

GENETICS
Arabian foals affected by SCID.

INCIDENCE/PREVALENCE
- Affects up to 50% of neonatal foals examined at referral institutions
- Case fatality rate is unknown but likely depends on timeliness of therapeutic intervention, etiologic agent, and immune status of foal, among other factors

GEOGRAPHIC DISTRIBUTION
No geographic distribution in incidence of disease; however, there may be geographic differences in bacterial isolates.

SIGNALMENT

Breed Predilections
- No breed predisposition

- Exception is Arabian foals with SCID

Mean Age and Range
- Neonatal foals (<14 days of age)
- Most cases are <7 days of age at the time of presentation

Predominant Sex
No sex predisposition.

SIGNS

General Comments
- Foals may have severe pulmonary disease without overt clinical signs referable to the respiratory tract
- Foals with pneumonia often display nonspecific signs of disease (lethargy, inappetence, fever, etc.)

Historical Findings
- See Risk Factors
- History of maternal disease
- Prematurity
- Inadequate colostral ingestion
- Lethargy, depression, decreased nursing behavior

Physical Examination Findings
- Often vague, nonlocalizing clinical signs
- Weak, often increasingly recumbent
- Decreased frequency of nursing
- Fever, although may have increased, normal, or decreased body temperatures
- Tachypnea/dyspnea
- Pulmonary auscultation may reveal increased bronchovesicular sounds or absence of auscultable sounds over regions of consolidated/atelectatic lung, or may be normal (even in severely affected foals)
- Cyanosis not common, and might not be noted in anemic foals
- Cough and/or nasal discharge are not common findings in early disease

RISK FACTORS
- Failure of transfer of passive immunity is likely the single most important risk factor
- Maternal risk factors:
  - Maternal illness (colic, respiratory disease, etc.)
  - Dystocia
  - Running colostrum/milk prior to parturition
  - Ascending cervicitis/placentitis
  - Maternal rejection of neonate
  - Agalactia/hypogalactia
  - Maternal age (very young or old mares—lower quality colostrum)
- Neonatal risk factors:
  - Dystocia
  - NMS
  - Musculoskeletal disease preventing rising to nurse
- Unhygienic environment in immediate neonatal period—ingested or inhaled pathogens
- Prolonged lateral recumbency—vascular congestion, atelectasis of dependent lung may predispose to infection

DIAGNOSIS

DIFFERENTIAL DIAGNOSIS
- Anemia
- Cardiac disease (e.g. congenital cardiac anomaly)
- Hyperthermia
- Idiopathic tachypnea
- Trauma (rib fracture, pulmonary contusion)
- Neurologic disease—abnormal respiratory patterns
- Botulism—fatigue of ventilatory muscles

LABORATORY TESTS

CBC
- Segmented neutrophil count may be increased, normal, or decreased
- Toxic granulation, vacuolation may be evident associated with sepsis
- Viral infection may induce profound lymphopenia, but this is inconsistent
- Elevated lymphocyte counts (greater than neutrophil count) in premature foals
- Plasma fibrinogen, serum amyloid A often increased

Arterial Blood Gas Analysis
- Ideal method to determine adequacy of gas exchange and pulmonary function
- Best sampling sites include great metatarsal artery, brachial artery, or transverse facial artery
- Patient should be standing or sternally recumbent for $\approx$5–10 min prior to sampling
- Useful for monitoring response to therapy and assessing changes in patient's status
- PaO_2—values between 60 and 80 mmHg (normal >80 mmHg) may be associated with pulmonary disease or lateral recumbency at time of sampling. Values <60 mmHg indicate hypoxemia and poor pulmonary function
- $PaCO_2$—values >60 mmHg with concurrent hypoxemia indicate respiratory failure. Significant elevation is an indication for mechanical ventilation

Blood Culture
Likely to be helpful in identification of etiologic agent and antimicrobial susceptibility in septicemic cases.

Culture and Cytology of Samples of Respiratory Tract Secretions
- Not recommended in dyspneic patients—patient should be stabilized first
- Bacteria readily cultured, antimicrobial sensitivity helpful to guide therapy
- Viral isolation may be performed on respiratory tract samples

Serum IgG Levels
Serum IgG level often <400 mg/dL in affected neonates.

IMAGING
- Thoracic radiography
  - Useful for documenting extent and severity of disease

○ Hematogenous bacterial pneumonia—diffuse disease with an alveolar or interstitial/alveolar pattern
○ Aspiration pneumonia—cranioventral/caudoventral pulmonary fields (alveolar pattern)
○ Useful for monitoring response to therapy, resolution of disease (radiographic disease will typically lag behind clinical status of patient)
• Thoracic US
○ Can visualize parietal abscessation, pulmonary consolidation, pleural effusion
○ Also useful for monitoring response to therapy
• Thoracic CT
○ More sensitive than radiography, US for documenting pulmonary lesions

OTHER DIAGNOSTIC PROCEDURES
• Endoscopy of the upper respiratory tract
○ May be useful for identifying cause in patients with aspiration pneumonia
• Pulse oximetry may be useful as a continuous, noninvasive estimate of PaO_2; results should be periodically calibrated against arterial blood gas measurements

TREATMENT
AIMS
• Resolve infection within pulmonary parenchyma
• Promote efficient gas exchange
• Minimize inflammatory changes that may promote acute respiratory distress syndrome, systemic inflammatory response syndrome, and subsequent death of the patient

APPROPRIATE HEALTH CARE
Inpatient intensive management for severe disease.

NURSING CARE
• Oxygen—humidified oxygen should be administered via nasal cannula(s) inserted to the level of the nasopharynx at a rate of 5–10 L/min
• Thoracic coupage to mobilize; patients should be examined carefully for thoracic trauma (e.g. rib fractures) prior to instituting this therapy
• Maintain sternal recumbency to minimize dependent lung atelectasis
• Mechanical ventilation for foals in respiratory failure (hypoxemia with severe hypercapnia)
• Judicious suctioning of respiratory secretions (use care—may cause pulmonary collapse and exacerbate hypoxemia); suction only as needed and for short periods (<2 s)
• Fluid therapy to correct dehydration, electrolyte and acid–base abnormalities

ACTIVITY
Should be minimized to decrease metabolic oxygen demands, especially in hypoxemic patients.

DIET
• Enteral nutrition via an indwelling nasogastric feeding tube, particularly in patients with pharyngeal dysfunction or weakness that has resulted in aspiration
• Parenteral nutrition for foals that do not tolerate enteral feeding

MEDICATIONS
DRUG(S) OF CHOICE
Antimicrobials
• Broad-spectrum bactericidal drugs should be administered prior to results of culture and sensitivity testing
• Aminoglycoside/beta-lactam combinations are good choices for empiric therapy (e.g. amikacin 25 mg/kg IV daily and penicillin 22 000 IU/kg IV every 6 h)
• Third-generation cephalosporins (e.g. ceftazidime 50 mg/kg IV every 6 h) are also good empiric choices, particularly if patient has renal compromise
• Therapy may be adjusted based on culture and sensitivity results and should continue for 2–5 weeks
• Antiviral therapy (acyclovir (aciclovir)) has been used for viral pneumonia; unlikely to affect clinical course

NSAIDs
• Useful to minimize fever, inflammation
• Ketoprofen (2.2 mg/kg IV every 12–24 h)
• Flunixin meglumine (1.1 mg/kg IV every 12–24 h)
• Use judiciously and with caution in neonates

Gastroprotectants
• May be useful in foals receiving nonsteroidal medications
• See chapter Gastric ulcers, neonate

CONTRAINDICATIONS
Aminoglycosides should not be used in azotemic patients.

PRECAUTIONS
Oxygen therapy may cause hypoventilation in hypercapnic patients.

ALTERNATIVE DRUGS
Depending on results of bacterial culture/sensitivity, alternative antimicrobial drugs may be needed.

FOLLOW-UP
PATIENT MONITORING
• Attitude, respiratory rate, and pattern should be observed frequently until stabilized
• Arterial blood gas analysis should be performed daily or when status of patient changes
• CBC, fibrinogen every 3–5 days; when status of patient changes; prior to discontinuation of antimicrobial therapy

• Thoracic radiography—weekly; when change in patient status; prior to discontinuation of antimicrobial therapy
• Thoracic US may be performed daily or every other day

PREVENTION/AVOIDANCE
Ensure adequate transfer of passive immunity within the first 18–24 h of life.

POSSIBLE COMPLICATIONS
• Pulmonary abscessation
• Pleural adhesions
• Other septic foci (e.g. septic arthritis)

EXPECTED COURSE AND PROGNOSIS
• Approximately two-thirds of foals with pneumonia survive to hospital discharge
• Viral pneumonia is usually fatal
• Effects on future athletic performance difficult to predict, but many go on to be performance animals as adults

MISCELLANEOUS
ASSOCIATED CONDITIONS
• Prematurity
• Septicemia

SEE ALSO
• Failure of transfer of passive immunity (FTPI)
• Septicemia, neonate

ABBREVIATIONS
• CT = computed tomography
• EHV = equine herpesvirus
• Ig = immunoglobulin
• NMS = neonatal maladjustment syndrome
• NSAID = nonsteroidal anti-inflammatory drug
• $PaCO_2$ = partial pressure of carbon dioxide in arterial blood
• PaO_2 = partial pressure of oxygen in arterial blood
• SCID = severe combined immunodeficiency
• US = ultrasonography, ultrasound

Suggested Reading
Bedenice D. Manifestations of septicemia: foal with septic pneumonia. In: Paradis MR, ed. Equine Neonatal Medicine: A Case-Based Approach. Philadelphia, PA: Saunders, 2006:99–111.
Bedenice D, Heuwieser W, Brawer R, et al. Clinical and prognostic significance of radiographic pattern, distribution, and severity of thoracic radiographic changes in neonatal foals. J Vet Intern Med 2003;17(6):876–886.
Reuss SM, Cohen ND. Update on bacterial pneumonia in the foal and weanling. Vet Clin North Am Eq Pract 2015;31:121–135.

Author Teresa A. Burns
Consulting Editor Margaret C. Mudge

P

PNEUMOTHORAX

BASICS

OVERVIEW
• Presence of air within the pleural space, resulting in lung collapse and inadequate ventilation
• Most common with penetrating thoracic wounds or birth trauma and affecting one or both hemithoraces
• Open/closed PTX—air freely enters and leaves the pleural cavity through a chest wound (open) or a breach in the visceral pleura or mediastinum (closed)
• Tension PTX—air accumulates in the pleural space with each breath and cannot escape

SIGNS
• Tachypnea, nasal flaring, and superficial breathing
• Dyspnea can occur in severe and bilateral cases, and can progress to distress and cyanosis
• Mild cases can be asymptomatic at rest
• Absence of lung sounds dorsally, and increased resonance on percussion
• Inspection and palpation may reveal a penetrating thoracic or axillary wound. Thoracic pain, subcutaneous emphysema, and instability of the thoracic wall are compatible with fractured ribs

CAUSES AND RISK FACTORS
• Trauma
• Bronchopleural fistulas from pleuropneumonia
• Distal tracheal or esophageal lacerations
• Transtracheal wash, bone marrow aspiration, lung biopsy

DIAGNOSIS

DIFFERENTIAL DIAGNOSIS
• Pain can cause rapid, shallow breathing
• Diaphragmatic hernia
• Pleural effusion

CBC/BIOCHEMISTRY/URINALYSIS
• Stress leukogram
• Leukocytosis with secondary bacterial infection

OTHER LABORATORY TESTS
Arterial blood gas analysis may reveal hypercapnia and hypoxemia.

IMAGING
Thoracic Ultrasonography
• Air accumulates dorsally in standing horses or laterally in recumbent foals
• In 2D mode, the pleural line appears as a hyperechoic line that twinkles with normal lung movement ("gliding lung sign"). Absence of the "gliding sign" is strong, but not absolute, evidence for the presence of PTX

• Determination of the "lung point" (the point where the gliding sign meets free gas) is useful to assess the severity and monitor change over time

Thoracic Radiography
Retraction of lung margins from the thoracic wall (dorsoventral projection in recumbent foals) or from the ventral aspect of the thoracic vertebrae (lateral projection in standing horses)

OTHER DIAGNOSTIC PROCEDURES
N/A

TREATMENT

• These animals may suffer from polytrauma. If IV fluids are indicated, keep in mind that contused lung is more susceptible to fluid overload
• Open PTX—temporarily close the wound using sterile gauze. Suture it whenever possible to achieve an airtight seal. For wounds that are not amenable to primary closure, apply a thin film dressing to provide an airtight seal
• Thoracocentesis—indicated when respiratory distress is present. The site is the dorsal thoracic cavity between the 12th and 15th ribs. Avoid intercostal vessels along the caudal border of the ribs. A teat cannula, a 14 G over-the-needle catheter, or a large-gauge needle attached to a three-way stopcock, extension set, and 60 mL syringe
• With severe or active PTX, a thoracostomy tube can be placed dorsally in the pleural cavity and attached to a Heimlich valve or, in the case of rapid reaccumulation of air, a continuous suction apparatus. When PTX has persisted for some time, it should be aspirated slowly to avoid reexpansion pulmonary edema
• Uncontrolled PTX or recurrence is an indication for thoracoscopy. It is also useful to evaluate concurrent pulmonary and diaphragmatic trauma, or identify foreign bodies
• Administer oxygen to dyspneic and hypoxemic patients
• In mild cases, PTX can resorb with confinement alone, over a few weeks. In people, 1.5% of the volume can be reabsorbed each day

MEDICATIONS

DRUG(S) OF CHOICE
Broad-spectrum antibiotics, NSAIDs, and tetanus prophylaxis.

CONTRAINDICATIONS/POSSIBLE INTERACTIONS
Avoid drugs such as xylazine or opioids, because they may reduce PaO_2.

FOLLOW-UP

PATIENT MONITORING
• Monitor hourly (including respiratory rate and pattern) for the first 24–48 h
• Serial blood gas analyses and ultrasonography or radiography to monitor progress and document reexpansion of the lungs
• Thoracostomy tubes may be removed if ≤50 mL of air is aspirated over 12 h

POSSIBLE COMPLICATIONS
• Recurrence
• Pyothorax with open PTX

EXPECTED COURSE AND PROGNOSIS
• Tension PTX is a serious life-threatening condition if left untreated
• Full recovery is expected if the injury is not severe and does not involve other thoracic structures

MISCELLANEOUS

ASSOCIATED CONDITIONS
• Thoracic trauma
• Fractured ribs
• Diaphragmatic hernia
• Ruptured trachea

SEE ALSO
• Expiratory dyspnea
• Inspiratory dyspnea
• Pleuropneumonia
• Thoracic trauma

ABBREVIATIONS
• NSAID = nonsteroidal anti-inflammatory drug
• PaO_2 = partial pressure of oxygen in arterial blood
• PTX = pneumothorax

Suggested Reading
Hassel MH. Thoracic trauma in horses. Vet Clin North Am Equine Pract 2007;23(1): 67–80.
Jean D, Laverty S, Halley J, et al. Thoracic trauma in newborn foals. Equine Vet J 1999;31(2):149–152.
Laverty S, Lavoie JP, Pascoe JR, Ducharme N. Penetrating wounds of the thorax in 15 horses. Equine Vet J 1996;28(3):220–224.
Partlow J, David F, Hunt LM, et al. Comparison of thoracic ultrasonography and radiography for the detection of induced small volume pneumothorax in the horse. Vet Radiol Ultrasound 2017;58(3): 354–360.

Authors Florent David and Sheila Laverty
Consulting Editors Mathilde Leclère and Daniel Jean

P

BASICS

DEFINITION
Air in the vagina or uterus. Usually results from VC defect.

PATHOPHYSIOLOGY
• Air accumulates subsequent to poor VC and relaxation of the vestibular sphincter
• Negative pressure within the genital tract's lumen aids movement of air into the vestibule, vagina, uterus; eliciting a "windsucking" sound
• With motion, air is forced back out; can hear a characteristic expulsive sound

SYSTEMS AFFECTED
Reproductive

GENETICS
Possibly influencing VC conformation.

INCIDENCE/PREVALENCE
Common

SIGNALMENT
• All breeds, but individuals with less perineal muscle more severely affected
• Older pluriparous mares most commonly affected

SIGNS
General Comments
Described in 1937 by Dr. Caslick and remains a major cause of infertility.

Historical Findings
• May exhibit signs of chronic pneumovagina coupled with abnormal VC
• Subfertility/infertility linked with uterine infections and/or inflammation

Physical Examination Findings
• Determine if VC is normal:
  ◦ Assess relationship of dorsal vulvar commissure to the pubic floor; should lie at or below the floor of the pubis
• Effect of poor VC on fertility is confirmed by the presence of vaginitis, pneumovagina, or pneumouterus
• As age/parity increases:
  ◦ Anus is pulled cranially; attached to related soft tissue structures
  ◦ The vulva is pulled in a cranial slant, up over the posterior brim of the pubis

CAUSES
Predisposing Factors
• Changes in general conformation, e.g. sway back
• Loss of vaginal fat
• Stretching of the supporting soft tissue structures in the perineal area

RISK FACTORS
• Repeated pregnancies
• Poor nutritional condition

DIAGNOSIS

IMAGING
Ultrasonography—unnecessary, unless to confirm pneumouterus.

PATHOLOGIC FINDINGS
• Evidence of vaginitis and endometritis
• Subfertility, infertility
• May predispose to abortion after vaginitis and cervicitis develop

TREATMENT

APPROPRIATE HEALTH CARE
Little justification to treat a mare for a uterine infection/inflammation if poor VC is left uncorrected.

CLIENT EDUCATION
Advise clients to critically evaluate the VC of all mares; perform a vulvoplasty if needed.

SURGICAL CONSIDERATIONS
• Wrap and tie the mare's tail and clean the perineal area
• Local anesthetic into the mucocutaneous junction of the vulva; ≅10–12 mL typically used to infiltrate each side of the vulva; the dorsal portion of the "U" is particularly sensitive
• The tissue edges are *freshened*/incised in an upside-down "U": left and right vulvar lip and connecting the 2 in an arc, across the dorsal commissure. 2 methods:
  ◦ *Strip removal*—very narrow strip of tissue is cut from the edge of each vulvar lip, or
  ◦ *Split-thickness technique*—incising at the mucocutaneous junction along the line dilated with local anesthetic, i.e. no tissue is removed. The latter results in less vulvar scarring; preferred for the long-term reproductive welfare of the mare
  ◦ Both techniques are in use and considered acceptable
• Nonabsorbable suture material (e.g. no. 1 Braunamid), Ford interlocking pattern allows tension adjustment along its length
  ◦ At the time of suture removal, evaluate surgical site for presence of small fistulas through which contamination may continue. If present, repair at that time
• *Pouret technique* for severe/extremely poor VC—dissect the perineal body in a caudal (widest) to cranial (point) pie-shaped wedge that permits the tubular genital tract, ventral to the rectum, to slide caudally and away from the anal sphincter. Only the skin is closed, i.e. no deep reconstruction of dissected tissue
• *Gadd procedure*, aka deep Caslick, is a technique to reconstruct a torn perineal body
• Check mare's tetanus toxoid vaccination status

MEDICATIONS

DRUG(S) OF CHOICE
No antibiotics are indicated.

FOLLOW-UP

PATIENT MONITORING
Remove sutures 10–14 days after surgery.

PREVENTION/AVOIDANCE
Select broodmares with excellent VC.

POSSIBLE COMPLICATIONS
Necessary to open the vulvar commissure ≅5–10 days prepartum to prevent perineal tearing at delivery. The Caslickls should be replaced, immediately after foaling, or breeding and confirmation of ovulation in the next season, depending on the severity of the mare's VC.

EXPECTED COURSE AND PROGNOSIS
Without surgical correction, mares may remain infertile or abort during pregnancy.

MISCELLANEOUS

AGE-RELATED FACTORS
High probability of VC worsening with age. Even if a mare is not to be bred, a Caslick's should be placed to protect her genital tract from her poor VC.

PREGNANCY/FERTILITY/BREEDING
Surgery may be necessary to obtain a pregnancy.

SYNONYMS
• Windsucker
• Windsucking

SEE ALSO
• Dystocia
• Endometrial biopsy
• Endometritis
• Perineal lacerations/recto-vaginal-vestibular fistulas
• Vulvar conformation

ABBREVIATIONS
VC = vulvar conformation

Suggested Reading
Colbern GT, Aanes WA, Stashak TS. Surgical management of perineal lacerations and recto-vestibular fistulae in the mare: a retrospective study of 47 cases. J Am Vet Med Assoc 1985;186:265–269.
Rothrock L, Ellerbrock R, Canisso IF. Outcomes on four mares undergoing perineal body reconstruction. Clin Theriogenol 2016;8(3):343.
Author Carla L. Carleton
Consulting Editor Carla L. Carleton
Acknowledgment The author/editor acknowledges the prior contribution of Walter R. Threlfall.

P

POISONING (INTOXICATION)—GENERAL PRINCIPLES

BASICS

DEFINITION
• A *poison* or *toxicant* is a natural or synthetic substance causing disease via its own inherent qualities
• A *toxin* is a toxicant of biologic origin—e.g. plants, bacteria, fungi, algae, or animals
• *Toxicosis* refers to the disease state caused by a toxicant
• *Toxicity* refers to the amount of a poison that causes disease; substances with high toxicity require a lower dose to cause disease than do substances with low toxicity

PATHOPHYSIOLOGY
Mechanisms of action vary with the different toxicants and are discussed in the specific chapters dealing with those toxicants. Briefly, toxicants can cause local or general systemic effects. Injury to one organ could potentially negatively impact other body systems. Effects could be acute or could be chronic depending on dose and duration of exposure.

SYSTEMS AFFECTED
• All systems have the potential to be affected by toxicants. Most common—the GI system including the liver, nervous, renal, and cardiovascular systems
• Target different systems depending on the inherent toxicity of the specific toxicant. A toxic outcome however can be modulated by animal factors, e.g. genetics, or by the dose or the route of exposure, or by environmental conditions such as season, among others
• Some toxicants affect more than 1 system. The effects can occur concurrently, sequentially, or independently of each other

GENETICS
Genetics rarely plays a significant factor in the occurrence of clinical toxicosis in equines.

INCIDENCE/PREVALENCE
The incidence, prevalence, case fatality rate, and mortality rate vary with each specific toxicant, dose, animal factors such as age, nutritional status, or concurrent disease, or exposure to other toxicants.

GEOGRAPHIC DISTRIBUTION
The occurrence of specific toxicants, especially toxins, can vary depending on geographic location and weather conditions, as well as agricultural and management practices.

SIGNALMENT
• Some toxicants can have an age predilection, most often related to eating habits (and, therefore, dose ingestion) or to management practices
• Some toxicants have breed or gender predispositions, e.g. reproductive toxicants

SIGNS

General Comments
• Establishing a conclusive diagnosis of poisoning is like assembling multiple pieces of a giant puzzle. The importance of a complete history, physical examination, and complementary diagnostic tests cannot be overstated
• Thorough record-keeping is necessary because cases may go to courts of law, especially if a poisoning results from a faulty product, the negligence of others, or intentional malice

Historical Findings
• Establishing the history of the problem may be difficult and can require finesse by the veterinarian
• The client may already be convinced that poisoning has occurred, even though the onset of clinical signs is only coincidental with exposure of the animal to a particular substance
• Clients may not be forthcoming with complete information if they feel guilty because poisoning resulted from their own mistakes. Conversely, clients may give biased information if they believe poisoning resulted from a faulty product, the negligence of others, or suspected malicious intent
• The clinician should determine how many animals are at risk of poisoning and how many are actually affected
• Current or past health problems and treatments may reveal factors that can affect toxicity and influence therapeutic outcomes
• Collect detailed information regarding the current poisoning situation—clinical signs, date of onset, time of onset, treatment given by the owner, number of dead animals
• Determine how and when the animal was exposed to the toxicant
• Record the full label name of the product, the manufacturer, the lot number, and the active ingredients, including their concentrations. If the product is a pesticide, record the Environmental Protection Agency registration number (USA)
• If a potential adverse reaction to a therapeutic agent is involved, record the lot or batch number, determine if the product was used according to the manufacturer's recommendations, and determine the amount of exposure to the product

Physical Examination Findings
• Clinical signs vary with the different toxicants
• Not all potential signs are seen in each affected animal
• Remember clinical signs can vary with disease progression and your current clinical observation is like a snapshot of the toxicosis

CAUSES
Common toxicants in equines are discussed in specific chapters.

RISK FACTORS
• Risk factors can be due to the toxicant, the individual, or the environment
• Toxicant-related risk factors include the toxicity of the substance, physical nature, e.g. solid, powdered, nanoparticle, dose, exposure route (e.g. dermal, oral, inhaled, injected)
• Individual risk factors may include age, breed, sex, reproductive status, nutrition, weight, previous health status, and current treatments
• Environmental factors include seasons, drought, ambient temperatures, tracking, etc.

DIAGNOSIS

DIFFERENTIAL DIAGNOSIS
• First, attempt to determine if the illness actually resulted from a poisoning rather than from an infectious, metabolic, or nutritional disease. The diagnosis may be obvious from a quick history and physical examination but usually requires more thorough investigation by the clinician
• The foremost consideration in confirming a diagnosis of poisoning is to establish that clinical signs or lesions are compatible with a toxic exposure to a specific toxicant. This requires appropriate selection and testing of specimens
• The list of differential diagnoses varies with different toxicants. Resources to assist veterinarians in diagnosing toxicoses include diagnostic laboratories and Animal Poison Control Centers

CBC/BIOCHEMISTRY/URINALYSIS
These tests are often helpful in defining the cause and severity of the toxicosis and in determining the course of treatment.

OTHER LABORATORY TESTS
• Laboratory confirmation can be made for many toxicants via sample submission to diagnostic laboratories
• At a minimum whole blood, serum, and urine from live animals or liver, kidney, brain, fat, urine, and GI contents from dead animals. Hair, feces, bone, in some cases
• Toxicologic testing can rarely be performed on samples preserved in formalin; thus, samples for toxicology testing (except whole blood) should be frozen. However, other samples should be collected and put in formalin for histologic examination to help narrow the differential list
• Collect samples of feed, water, and any suspected source material; other samples also

P

may be necessary to confirm a diagnosis, depending on the toxicant
• Always contact the laboratory for specific information regarding submission protocols, because incorrect samples, inadequate sample size, and improper sample storage are common causes of diagnostic testing failures

IMAGING
Radiographs, ultrasonography, and other modern imaging techniques may help identify foreign objects and/or assess the severity of toxicosis.

OTHER DIAGNOSTIC PROCEDURES
N/A

PATHOLOGIC FINDINGS
• Presence or absence of pathologic lesions can help narrow the differentials list
• Gross and histopathologic findings vary depending on the specific toxicant and degree and duration of exposure
• Some toxicants cause pathognomonic lesions

TREATMENT

AIMS
• Remove animal from source
• With a life-threatening situation, immediately provide life support by maintaining respiratory and cardiac function. Control seizures if they occur
• Once the animal is stabilized, institute symptomatic and supportive care
• Give specific antidote
• Decontaminate the animal as appropriate

APPROPRIATE HEALTH CARE
Most toxicants lack specific antidotes. The type, the duration, and the intensity of supportive care coupled with an ideal environment to heal will most times make the difference whether the animal lives or dies.

NURSING CARE
• Maintain adequate hydration and control acid–base imbalances if present
• Maintain proper body temperature. Seizures or tremors can result in elevated temperatures. Conversely, severely depressed or comatose animals may have low body temperatures
• With a dermal route of exposure, bathe the animal with mild dishwashing detergent. Use personal protective equipment (e.g. wearing gloves) to prevent self-exposure
• With an ocular route of exposure, lavage the eye with copious amounts of water or normal saline

ACTIVITY
Provide sufficient rest to the animal if necessary to allow healing to occur.

DIET
Dietary restrictions or additions vary with each toxic incident. Parenteral alimentation may be required in some cases.

CLIENT EDUCATION
This is an important component of management of intoxications. Client education is essential to prevent recurrent exposure and prevent new exposures as well as outcome of case management.

SURGICAL CONSIDERATIONS
N/A

MEDICATIONS

DRUG(S) OF CHOICE
• Few poisons have specific antidotes. If a toxicant has a specific antidote, use it
• Relevant medications and antidotes are discussed in those sections dealing with the specific toxicants
• Many toxicants are adsorbed by AC, thereby reducing the amount of toxicant absorbed from the GI tract. AC binds many organic compounds but is relatively ineffective against inorganic compounds (e.g. heavy metals), mineral acids, and alkali. Mix the AC (1–4 g/kg) with warm water to form a slurry. Follow the AC with a laxative to hasten removal of the toxicant from the intestinal tract. The efficacy of mineral oil for treating intoxicated patients has not been established and its use is discouraged for routine GI decontamination
• Cholestyramine (colestyramine) is an alternative to AC
• Some toxicants are eliminated primarily by the fecal route or undergo enterohepatic recirculation. AC/cholestyramine followed by a laxative is the most effective means for increasing elimination of these toxicants
• Many toxicants are eliminated by the kidneys, and, in some cases, renal excretion can be enhanced by increasing urine output via fluid administration. Diuretics can be used to increase urine flow—furosemide (1 mg/kg IV); mannitol (0.25–1.0 g/kg as 20% solution by slow IV infusion)
• Manipulating the urine pH also can increase the excretion of some toxicants in the urine via ion trapping. Weak acids are ionized in alkaline urine, whereas weak bases are ionized in acidic urine. The normal range of pH for urine in adult herbivores is alkaline (pH 7–9)

CONTRAINDICATIONS
Antidotes can be harmful; do not use unless you are certain of your diagnosis.

PRECAUTIONS
• Toxicants typically are metabolized and/or excreted by the liver, GI tract, and/or kidneys. Select medications that will minimally affect these systems
• Before administering oral products, determine that the horse is not exhibiting gastric reflux

• Cathartics can result in significant diarrhea; therefore, ensure that the horse is adequately hydrated

POSSIBLE INTERACTIONS
N/A

ALTERNATIVE DRUGS
• Magnesium sulfate (Epsom salts) is an osmotic laxative that draws water into the intestines. The recommended dose is 250–500 mg/kg mixed in several liters of water
• Sorbitol 70% (3 mL/kg) or sodium sulfate (250–500 mg/kg mixed in several liters of water) is an alternative cathartic

FOLLOW-UP

PATIENT MONITORING
Potential sequelae vary with the toxicant and severity of the poisoning and are discussed in those sections dealing with specific toxicants.

PREVENTION/AVOIDANCE
Minimize the risk of intoxication by using medications and pesticides according to the label directions, storing all chemicals safely, and identifying and removing all potentially toxic plants in the animal's environment.

POSSIBLE COMPLICATIONS
The type and severity of complications as well as potential sequelae will vary with each toxic incident.

EXPECTED COURSE AND PROGNOSIS
Prognosis will vary with the type of toxicant, dose received, and time of onset of treatment, as well as individual and environmental factors.

MISCELLANEOUS

ASSOCIATED CONDITIONS
Laminitis is a possible secondary condition to any severe disease in horses.

AGE-RELATED FACTORS
The effect of age will vary with the specific toxicant.

ZOONOTIC POTENTIAL
N/A

PREGNANCY/FERTILITY/BREEDING
• Abortion or teratogenic disease may be a concern in pregnant mares depending on the toxicant and stage of pregnancy at the time of exposure
• Some poisons can affect the fertility of mares or stallions

SYNONYMS
Discussed in those chapters dealing with specific toxicants.

P

POISONING (INTOXICATION)—GENERAL PRINCIPLES (CONTINUED)

SEE ALSO
Chapters dealing with specific toxicants.

ABBREVIATIONS
- AC = activated charcoal
- GI = gastrointestinal

Suggested Reading
Galey FD. Diagnostic toxicology. In: Plumlee KH, ed. Clinical Veterinary Toxicology. St. Louis, MO: Mosby, 2004:22–23.

Oehme FW. General principles in treatment of poisoning. In: Robinson NE, ed. Current Therapy in Equine Medicine, 2e. Philadelphia, PA: WB Saunders, 1987:653–656.
Poppenga RH. Treatment. In: Plumlee KH, ed. Clinical Veterinary Toxicology. St. Louis, MO: Mosby, 2004:13–21.

Author Wilson K. Rumbeiha
Consulting Editors Wilson K. Rumbeiha and Steve Ensley
Acknowledgment The editors acknowledge the prior contribution of Konnie H. Plumlee.

P

BASICS

DEFINITION
• An increase in the circulating RBC (erythrocyte) mass, reflected by increases in RBC count, hemoglobin concentration, and PCV
• Increase in circulating RBC mass may be relative or absolute

PATHOPHYSIOLOGY
Relative Polycythemia
• Caused by hemoconcentration or splenic contraction
• Hemoconcentration results from a reduction in the plasma volume without a change in circulating RBC numbers. It is associated with external water loss or internal fluid shifts
• Common causes of hemoconcentration include reduced water intake, diarrhea, renal failure, diuresis, or excessive sweating. Endotoxemia is a common cause of a shift in water from the plasma space
• Splenic contraction results in a transient release of stored RBCs into the circulation. Contraction may increase the PCV by up to 50% for several hours dependent on the stimulus

Absolute Polycythemia
• An increase in circulating RBC mass without change in the plasma volume
• May be primary or secondary
• Primary absolute polycythemia is a myeloproliferative disorder where increased RBC mass is associated with normal PO_2 and normal or reduced EPO concentration
• Secondary absolute polycythemia results from increased erythropoiesis due to an increased synthesis of EPO that may be appropriate (response to tissue hypoxia; low PO_2) or inappropriate (excessive EPO or other hormone production and normal PaO_2)

SYSTEMS AFFECTED
• Cardiovascular
• Hemic
• Respiratory
• Hepatobiliary
• Nervous
• Renal
• Gastrointestinal

GENETICS
N/A

INCIDENCE/PREVALENCE
• Relative polycythemia is common in animals with hemodynamic compromise and when blood is collected from horses that have been exercised or are excited
• Absolute polycythemia is rare

GEOGRAPHIC DISTRIBUTION
Horses kept at altitudes >2200 m (7200 feet) are likely to have appropriate secondary absolute polycythemia.

SIGNALMENT
Breed Predilections
• There are no breed predilections
• Reference values for RBC count, hemoglobin concentration, and PCV are greater for light horse (i.e. hot-blooded) breeds (Thoroughbreds, Standardbreds, Arabians, and Quarter Horses) than draft (i.e. cold-blooded), pony, and miniature breeds and donkeys

Mean Age and Range
Animals of any age can develop polycythemia.

Predominant Sex
N/A

SIGNS
General Comments
• Signs of relative polycythemia are associated with the primary disease process
• Signs of absolute polycythemia vary with the degree of increase in RBC mass and any underlying condition

Historical Findings
• Relative polycythemia from splenic contraction may include a history of excitement or exercise
• Relative polycythemia from fluid shifts is dependent on the underlying disease process
• Absolute polycythemia may include a history of weight loss, lethargy, and inappetence

Physical Examination Findings
• Prolonged CRT, dry mucous membranes, cool extremities, and dull mentation may be observed in horses with relative polycythemia from fluid shifts
• Mucosal hyperemia (dark red to purple in color), prolonged CRT, lethargy, epistaxis and melena may be observed in horses with absolute polycythemia
• Abnormal mentation, tachycardia, and tachypnea may occur when PCV >60%, as increased blood viscosity impairs tissue oxygenation
• Cardiac murmur, tachycardia, and other signs of cardiac disease may be observed with congenital cardiac defects
• Tachypnea, abnormal bronchovesicular sounds, and dyspnea may occur with chronic pulmonary disease

CAUSES
Relative Polycythemia
• Inadequate water consumption—e.g. dysphagia (altered prehension or swallowing—many causes), restricted access, or altered mentation
• Increased fluid losses—e.g. diarrhea, diuretic therapy, polyuric renal failure, diabetes insipidus, excessive sweating, anterior enteritis, peritoneal or pleural effusion, ileus, or endotoxemia
• Internal fluid shifts—e.g. endotoxemia/SIRS, trauma, hyponatremia, hypoalbuminemia

• Splenic contraction—exercise, excitement, administration of α_1-adrenergic agonists (epinephrine, phenylephrine)

Absolute Polycythemia
• Primary absolute polycythemia is a rare myeloproliferative disorder that occurs as a single cell disorder or as a component of polycythemia vera (concurrent thrombocytosis and leukocytosis)
• Appropriate secondary absolute polycythemia is associated with congenital cardiac defects with right to left shunting (e.g. tetralogy of Fallot, pulmonary atresia with ventricular septal defect, persistent truncus arteriosus, tricuspid atresia), chronic pulmonary disease, and residence at high altitude
• Inappropriate secondary absolute polycythemia is a rare paraneoplastic syndrome from inappropriate EPO, EPO-like protein, or androgenic hormone secretion (hepatocellular carcinoma, hepatoblastoma, metastatic carcinoma, or lymphoma) or administration of exogenous androgens, EPO, or cobalt. In other species, chronic nephropathies (tumors, cysts, or hydronephrosis) may result in increased EPO production

Miscellaneous
Syndrome of red cell hypervolemia in Swedish Standardbred trotters.

RISK FACTORS
See Causes.

DIAGNOSIS

DIFFERENTIAL DIAGNOSIS
• Primary polycythemia is diagnosed on exclusion of relative or secondary polycythemia
• Laboratory error—insufficient blood sample centrifugation can result in an artificially high PCV

CBC/BIOCHEMISTRY/URINALYSIS
• RBC count, hemoglobin concentration, and PCV greater than upper limit of laboratory reference ranges
• Hyperproteinemia usually accompanies relative polycythemia from hemoconcentration unless protein loss occurs concurrently (e.g. diarrhea, glomerulonephritis, peritonitis, or pleuritis) where normal or reduced protein concentrations may be present
• Mild thrombocytosis may accompany relative polycythemia from splenic contraction
• Neutropenia, left shift, and toxic changes in neutrophils may occur in response to endotoxemia/SIRS
• Increased hepatic enzymes may be present in cases of inappropriate secondary absolute

P

polycythemia associated with hepatic neoplasia

OTHER LABORATORY TESTS
• PaO_2 to differentiate between appropriate and inappropriate secondary absolute polycythemia
• Blood concentrations of EPO may assist in the diagnosis of inappropriate secondary absolute polycythemia
• α-Fetoprotein in blood is consistent with hepatic neoplasia (hepatocellular carcinoma or hepatoblastoma)

IMAGING
• Echocardiography to detect congenital cardiac defects
• Tracheal wash and aspiration, bronchoalveolar lavage, thoracic ultrasonography and radiography, and pulmonary function testing to detect lung disease
• Renal and hepatic ultrasonography

OTHER DIAGNOSTIC PROCEDURES
• Liver biopsy if evidence of hepatic disease
• Renal biopsy if evidence of renal disease
• Bone marrow aspirate/biopsy to detect myeloproliferative disorders

PATHOLOGIC FINDINGS
Dependent on cause of polycythemia.

TREATMENT

APPROPRIATE HEALTH CARE
• The aims of treatment are resolution of polycythemia and any underlying disorder
• Relative polycythemia from splenic contraction requires no treatment
• Relative polycythemia from fluid shifts requires inpatient medical management
• Absolute polycythemia requires inpatient medical management

NURSING CARE
• Relative polycythemia from hypovolemia requires IV fluid therapy. If protein loss is concurrent, colloid therapy may be necessary
• Appropriate secondary absolute polycythemia requires oxygen therapy
• Absolute polycythemia may require phlebotomy if PCV remains >60%—10–20 mL of blood/kg can be removed and replaced by equivalent volume of polyionic crystalloid fluid. Phlebotomy is repeated every 2–3 days until PCV <50% and then as required
• Phlebotomy is contraindicated in relative polycythemia
• Phlebotomy should be used with caution in polycythemia associated with hypoxia as the increased RBC mass is a compensatory mechanism for tissue hypoxia

ACTIVITY
In cases of absolute polycythemia, activity should be restricted as persistent

polycythemia can result in hypertension, tissue hypoxia, thrombosis, and hemorrhage.

DIET
N/A

CLIENT EDUCATION
Response to treatment is dependent on the underlying cause. Most cases of absolute polycythemia have a poor to hopeless prognosis.

SURGICAL CONSIDERATIONS
Increased blood viscosity associated with marked absolute polycythemia increases the risk of anesthesia-associated complications.

MEDICATIONS

DRUG(S) OF CHOICE
• Hydroxyurea causes reversible bone marrow suppression and has been used successfully to treat polycythemia is humans and dogs
• The appropriate dosage of hydroxyurea in horses is unknown
• A suggested protocol for dogs is 30 mg/kg PO once daily for 7–10 days, then 15 mg/kg PO once daily

CONTRAINDICATIONS
Exogenous EPO, androgens, and cobalt should be avoided.

PRECAUTIONS
The efficacy and safety of hydroxyurea in horses is unknown.

POSSIBLE INTERACTIONS
N/A

ALTERNATIVE DRUGS
N/A

FOLLOW-UP

PATIENT MONITORING
• Monitor PCV, total plasma protein, and clinical variables reflecting hydration status in hypovolemic animals to monitor response to fluid therapy
• In cases of absolute polycythemia, PCV should be monitored initially every 2–3 days, particularly if phlebotomy is performed. Thereafter, measure PCV as required

PREVENTION/AVOIDANCE
N/A

POSSIBLE COMPLICATIONS
• Absolute polycythemia can increase viscosity of blood, resulting in an increased risk of tissue hypoxia, thrombosis, hemorrhage, and hypertension
• Cobalt salt may cause severe side effects

EXPECTED COURSE AND PROGNOSIS
• Relative polycythemia from splenic contraction resolves within hours

• Most cases of relative polycythemia associated with fluid shifts resolve with appropriate IV fluid therapy; however, shock may be more refractory to treatment
• Primary absolute polycythemia has a poor prognosis
• Secondary absolute polycythemia has a poor to grave prognosis, except when it is the result of compensation to residency at high altitude
• Syndrome of red cell hypervolemia in Swedish Standardbred trotters is associated with poor performance; however, horses are otherwise healthy

MISCELLANEOUS

ASSOCIATED CONDITIONS
N/A

AGE-RELATED FACTORS
RBC count, hemoglobin concentration, and PCV in foals decrease rapidly after birth and take several months to increase to near adult values.

ZOONOTIC POTENTIAL
N/A

PREGNANCY/FERTILITY/BREEDING
RBC count, hemoglobin concentration, and PCV tend to increase during pregnancy.

SYNONYMS
Erythrocytosis

SEE ALSO
• Complex congenital cardiac disease
• Endotoxemia
• Myeloproliferative diseases

ABBREVIATIONS
• CRT = capillary refill time
• EPO = erythropoietin
• PaO_2 = partial pressure of oxygen in arterial blood
• PCV = packed cell volume
• PO_2 = partial pressure of oxygen in tissues
• RBC = red blood cell
• SIRS = systemic inflammatory response syndrome

Suggested Reading
Sellon DC, Wise LN. Disorders of the hematopoietic system. In: Reed SM, Bayly WM, Sellon DC, eds. Equine Internal Medicine, 3e. St. Louis, MO: WB Saunders, 2010:730–776.

Author Kristopher Hughes
Consulting Editors David Hodgson, Harold C. McKenzie, and Jennifer L. Hodgson

BASICS

OVERVIEW
• Granulomatous inflammatory condition involving the extradural nerve roots of the cauda equina and often cranial nerves
• Used to be known as "cauda equina neuritis"; however, it can present with cranial nerve signs so has been renamed PNE

SIGNALMENT
No age or sex predilection; not usually seen in the very young or very old.

SIGNS
• Clinical signs usually include retention of feces and urine, or incontinence, loss of tail and anal tone, and analgesia of the tail and perineum. Urine scalding often present in the perineal area in mares and on the distal hind limbs in males with urinary incontinence
• Abnormalities in the pelvic limb gait and muscle wasting are seen less often
• Analgesia of the perianal skin may be surrounded by a zone of hyperesthesia. For that reason some cases can present for tail rubbing
• Asymmetric and fluctuating cranial nerve signs on occasion precede cauda equina signs. The cranial nerves most often affected include the trigeminal (masseter muscle paresis), facial (paresis of muscles of facial expression), vestibular (head tilt), and hypoglossal nerves (tongue paresis)
• Clinical signs generally progress more slowly than in typical EHV-1 cases, and only rarely are horses ataxic
• Lesions may progress to involve lumbar plexus, leading to pelvic limb paresis (initially subtle and asymmetric)

CAUSES AND RISK FACTORS
The cause is unknown, but it is thought to be predominantly an immune-mediated event that may be initiated by viral and/or bacterial infections.

DIAGNOSIS

DIFFERENTIAL DIAGNOSIS
• Sacral fractures—far more common than PNE. Rule out using rectal palpation, radiography, and scintigraphy
• EHV-1 myeloencephalopathy—tends have a more acute onset, stabilizes more rapidly, and responds well to treatment. May need CSF tap cytology and viral titers to differentiate
• Equine protozoal myeloencephalitis

• Rabies
• *Sorghum* cystitis

CBC/BIOCHEMISTRY/URINALYSIS
Most often normal—may be reflective of any secondary disease or complications that may have occurred, such as dehydration due to impaction colic or urinary tract infection due to urinary retention.

OTHER LABORATORY TESTS
Lumbosacral CSF tap to rule out equine protozoal myeloencephalitis. CSF may be difficult to obtain from the lumbosacral area due to the space-occupying nature of the lesions and may be xanthochromic with elevated protein levels and cell counts.

IMAGING
• Scintigraphy and radiography to help rule out sacral fractures
• Rectal ultrasonography can be used to make an antemortem diagnosis based on enlarged and hypoechoic appearance of the extradural sacral nerve roots as they exit the ventral sacral foramina

PATHOLOGIC FINDINGS
• Necropsy is the only way to reach a definitive diagnosis
• Cauda equina and cranial nerves become thickened and covered with fibrous material
• Granulomatous inflammation includes infiltrates of inflammatory cells, including neutrophils, lymphocytes, and macrophages. Axonal degeneration and myelin degeneration in the cauda equina and cranial nerves. Inflammation classically stops abruptly at the central nervous system/peripheral nervous system border

TREATMENT
• Supportive
• If cranial nerve signs are present and animals are having difficulty eating then they may have to be fed a complete feed as a mash. If fecal retention is a problem then feeding bran mash is appropriate
• May have to evacuate feces manually
• Some horses can be maintained for a long time with supportive care, but the disease is relentlessly progressive

MEDICATIONS

DRUG(S) OF CHOICE
• Antibiotics for secondary urinary tract infections

• Anti-inflammatory drugs are ineffective in the long term

CONTRAINDICATIONS/POSSIBLE INTERACTIONS
N/A

FOLLOW-UP
Follow progress of hypoalgesia in the tail region.

PATIENT MONITORING
Monitor for choke, impaction colic, and fecal and urinary incontinence.

EXPECTED COURSE AND PROGNOSIS
Disease usually progresses, and long-term prognosis is poor.

MISCELLANEOUS

ASSOCIATED CONDITIONS
None

AGE-RELATED FACTORS
Adult horses.

ZOONOTIC POTENTIAL
None

PREGNANCY/FERTILITY/BREEDING
N/A

SEE ALSO
• Equine herpesvirus myeloencephalopathy
• Equine protozoal myeloencephalitis (EPM)

ABBREVIATIONS
• CSF = cerebrospinal fluid
• EHV-1 = equine herpesvirus 1
• PNE = polyneuritis equi

Suggested Reading
Aleman M, Katzman SA, Vaughan B, et al. Antemortem diagnosis of polyneuritis equi. J Vet Intern Med 2009;23:665–668.
Divers TJ, Mayhew IG. Neurology. Clin Tech Equine Pract 2006;5(1):1–80.
Hahn CN. Polyneuritis equi: the role of T-lymphocytes and importance of differential clinical signs. Equine Vet J 2008;40:100.
Mayhew IG. Large Animal Neurology, 2e. Ames, IA: Wiley Blackwell, 2008.

Author Caroline N. Hahn
Consulting Editor Caroline N. Hahn

P

POLYSACCHARIDE STORAGE MYOPATHY

BASICS

DEFINITION
• Myopathy causing chronic exertional rhabdomyolysis characterized by increased skeletal muscle glycogen and amylase-resistant polysaccharide inclusions. • Type 1 PSSM and type 2 PSSM recognized

PATHOPHYSIOLOGY
• PSSM1 has a genetic basis. • Unknown PSSM2 cause(s)

SYSTEMS AFFECTED
• Endocrine/metabolic. • Neuromuscular. • Renal

GENETICS
• PSSM1—autosomal dominant mutation in *GYS1* gene. • PSSM2—possibly heredity in Quarter Horses

INCIDENCE/PREVALENCE
PSSM1 breed prevalence—North American Belgian, Percheron (high); Shire, Clydesdale (low); Quarter Horses (6–10%); Paint, Appaloosa (6–8%); halter Quarter Horses (28%); racing Quarter Horses (low); Warmblood, Irish Draught, Cob, Connemara (low); Arabian, Standardbred, Thoroughbred (very low).

GEOGRAPHIC DISTRIBUTION
Worldwide

SIGNALMENT
• 2–4-year-old Quarter Horses. • ± Foal

SIGNS
Quarter Horses
• "Tying-up" episodes shortly after exercise characterized by muscle stiffness, sweating, reluctance to move. • Tachypnea, tachycardia, muscle fasciculations, tucked-up abdomen, camped-out stance, firm painful lumbar and gluteal muscles, gait asymmetry, hindlimb stiffness. • Subclinical to severe with recumbency and renal failure. • Pawing or rolling, ± resembles colic. • ± Rapid muscle atrophy after concurrent respiratory disease

Draft Horses
• Variable—normal to weakness, recumbency. • Muscle soreness. • Generalized muscle atrophy. • Exertional rhabdomyolysis. • Hindlimb weakness, difficulty rising

CAUSES
Hereditary ± environmental influence.

DIAGNOSIS

DIFFERENTIAL DIAGNOSIS
• Sporadic or chronic exertional rhabdomyolysis. • Non-exercise-associated rhabdomyolysis, e.g. infectious and immune-mediated myopathies (*Clostridium*, influenza, *Streptococcus equi* ssp. *equi*, *Sarcocystis*), nutritional myodegeneration, traumatic myopathy, idiopathic pasture myopathy, and toxic muscle damage, e.g. monensin, white snake root ingestion. • Colic. • Laminitis. • Pleuropneumonia. • Aortoiliac thrombosis. • Tetanus. • Hyperkalemic periodic paralysis. • Recumbent neuropathy

CBC/BIOCHEMISTRY/URINALYSIS
• CK, AST elevations (>10 000 U/L) after exercise. • Persistent CK elevation. • Myoglobinuria. • ± Azotemia. • ± High potassium and low sodium and chloride serum concentrations. • ± CK, AST elevation in draft horses

OTHER LABORATORY TESTS
• Serum vitamin E and whole-blood selenium to rule out deficiency. • Fractional excretion of urine electrolytes. • Genetic testing for *GYS1* mutation

OTHER DIAGNOSTIC PROCEDURES
• Muscle (semimembranosus/tendinosus) biopsy. • Submaximal exercise test—>3–4-fold increased CK 4–6 h after 15 min walk/trot

PATHOLOGIC FINDINGS
Skeletal muscle—subsarcolemmal vacuoles, increased glycogen staining, amylase-resistant polysaccharide accumulation.

TREATMENT

APPROPRIATE HEALTH CARE
• Acute episode—oral and/or IV balanced polyionic fluids ± electrolytes, analgesia, rest. • Appropriate diet and exercise

ACTIVITY
Daily turnout, gradual return to consistent exercise.

DIET
• Forage 1.5–2% of body weight. • Low-starch (<10% daily energy) diet. • Eliminate grain, replace with fat (corn or soy oil). • ± Commercial made low-starch, high-fat ration

CLIENT EDUCATION
Appropriate diet and exercise management to control clinical signs.

MEDICATIONS

DRUG(S) OF CHOICE
• NSAIDs—phenylbutazone (4.4 mg/kg IV or PO every 12 h for 1 day then 2.2 mg/kg PO every 12 h) or flunixin meglumine (0.5–1.1 mg/kg IV or PO every 12–24 h). Care if dehydrated or myoglobinuric • Acepromazine (0.04–0.11 mg/kg IV or IM every 8–12 h). • ± Detomidine (0.005–0.02 mg/kg IV or IM).

• ± Methocarbamol (40–60 mg/kg PO daily). • ± IV DMSO (<10% solution)

CONTRAINDICATIONS
• NSAIDs with dehydration or myoglobinuria. • Acepromazine with dehydration

FOLLOW-UP

PATIENT MONITORING
• Monitor signs, especially during abrupt training changes. • Serum CK (resting or 4 h post exercise) prior to restarting exercise. • If myoglobinuria, monitor renal parameters. • If depressed or inappetent after acute episode, suspect acute renal failure and treat promptly

PREVENTION/AVOIDANCE
• Low-starch, high-fat diet. • Daily exercise and turnout careful obesity does not occur

POSSIBLE COMPLICATIONS
• Severe rhabdomyolysis and muscle damage, recumbency, death. • Renal failure

EXPECTED COURSE AND PROGNOSIS
With proper diet and exercise, good prognosis for athletics.

MISCELLANEOUS

ASSOCIATED CONDITIONS
Severe rapid muscle atrophy after concurrent respiratory disease in Quarter Horses.

AGE-RELATED FACTORS
• ± Signs and rhabdomyolysis in 1-day-old foal. • Muscle biopsy abnormalities after 1 year of age

PREGNANCY/FERTILITY/BREEDING
Heritable disorder, counsel breeders.

SYNONYMS
• EPSM, EPSSM (equine polysaccharide storage myopathy). • Azoturia. • Monday morning disease

SEE ALSO
• Colic in foals. • Exertional rhabdomyolysis syndrome. • Hyperkalemic periodic paralysis

ABBREVIATIONS
• AST = aspartate aminotransferase. • CK = creatine phosphokinase. • DMSO = dimethylsulfoxide. • *GYS1* = glycogen synthase 1. • NSAID = nonsteroidal anti-inflammatory drug. • PSSM = polysaccharide storage myopathy

Suggested Reading
Valberg SJ. Diseases of muscle. In: Smith BP, ed. Large Animal Internal Medicine, 5e. St. Louis, MO: Elsevier Mosby, 2015:1299–1304.

Author Anna M. Firshman
Consulting Editor Elizabeth J. Davidson

POLYURIA (PU) AND POLYDIPSIA (PD)

BASICS

DEFINITION
- PU—urine output >50 mL/kg/day
- PD—fluid intake >100 mL/kg/day

PATHOPHYSIOLOGY
- Production of concentrated or dilute urine requires generation of the interstitial concentration gradient from the renal cortex to the inner medulla, dilution of tubular fluid in the thick ascending limb of the loop of Henle and distal tubule (diluting segment of the nephron that has low water permeability), and presence or absence of water channels in the collecting ducts (controlled by ADH activity)
- Modest increases in plasma tonicity ($\cong 3$ mOsm/kg) stimulate production and release of ADH by the posterior pituitary gland and insertion of aquaporins (water channels) in the luminal membrane of collecting duct epithelial cells, leading to increased water permeability and reabsorption
- Decreases in plasma tonicity inhibit ADH release and insertion of aquaporins. As a result, collecting ducts become less permeable to water, and dilute urine is produced
- Transient PU may be an effect of fluid or drug administration (e.g. furosemide and other diuretic agents) or a consequence of loss of the medullary concentration gradient—medullary washout
- Persistent PU is generally associated with a number of disease processes—CKD, PPID, DI, DM, and endotoxemia
- There are 2 important stimuli for thirst—an increase in plasma tonicity and hypovolemia
- PD may be a physiologic response to PU (to prevent dehydration), a consequence of drug administration (e.g. corticosteroids), or a primary problem of excessive water intake
- Urine production and water consumption vary with age, diet, workload, environmental temperature, and gastrointestinal water absorption

SYSTEMS AFFECTED
- Renal/urologic—excessive urine production
- Endocrine/metabolic—PPID; DM
- Nervous—central DI
- Behavioral—excessive water intake, excessive salt consumption

GENETICS
Unknown—familial nephrogenic DI in Thoroughbred colts.

INCIDENCE/PREVALENCE
PPID may affect up to 15% of horses >20 years of age.

SIGNALMENT
Breed Predilections
PPID appears to be more common in Morgan horses and ponies.

Mean Age and Range
PPID occurs in older horses and ponies.

Predominant Sex
Familial nephrogenic DI in Thoroughbred colts.

SIGNS
Historical Findings
- Horses with mild to moderate PU/PD often go undetected by owners, or the horse may stop to urinate while being ridden or have excessive thirst after exercise
- With more substantial PU/PD (e.g. with primary PD), the magnitude of PU typically is dramatic, with owners reporting that horses drink 2–3-fold more water and that stalls can be flooded with urine
- Horses with acquired DI may have a recent history of medical problems or treatment with a potentially nephrotoxic medication

Physical Examination Findings
Consistent with the underlying disease processes (e.g. CKD, PPID) or normal (e.g. primary PD, excessive salt ingestion).

CAUSES
Primary PD
- Primary or "psychogenic" PD probably is the most common cause of PU/PD in adults
- The cause is unknown; however, in some horses it appears to be a stable vice, while in others it may develop after a change in management (e.g. stabling, diet, interaction with other horses, or medication administration)

Excessive Salt Consumption
"Psychogenic salt eaters" appear to be less common than those with primary PD; salt intake may have to exceed 5–10% of dry matter intake before PU/PD becomes apparent.

Drug Administration
Administration of enteral or IV fluids, diuretics, α_2-agonists, and corticosteroids.

CKD
- These horses cannot concentrate urine beyond the isosthenuric range (specific gravity 1.008–1.014)
- The degree of PU is modest compared with primary PD or DI, so it is a client complaint only in $\cong 50\%$ of affected horses

PPID
- An osmotic diuresis when plasma glucose concentration exceeds the renal threshold, leading to glucosuria
- Antagonism of the action of ADH on collecting ducts by cortisol
- A primary dipsogenic effect of excessive cortisol
- Compression of the posterior pituitary by growth of an adenoma leading to central DI

DI
- May occur because of inadequate secretion of ADH (neurogenic or central DI) or

decreased sensitivity of the epithelial cells of the collecting ducts to circulating ADH (nephrogenic DI)
- An acquired form of central DI has been described in horses and is idiopathic or secondary to encephalitis or other diseases accompanied by dehydration, endotoxemia, or administration of potentially nephrotoxic medications

DM
A state of chronic hyperglycemia accompanied by glucosuria resulting in an osmotic diuresis.

Sepsis/Endotoxemia
PU/PD occasionally is observed in horses with sepsis or endotoxemia. The mechanism is unclear but may result from endotoxin-induced prostaglandin production. Prostaglandin E_2 is a potent renal vasodilating agent that also can antagonize the effects of ADH.

RISK FACTORS
See chapters listed in See Also.

DIAGNOSIS

CBC/BIOCHEMISTRY/URINALYSIS
- CKD, PPID, sepsis/endotoxemia—see chapters listed in See Also
- Primary PD and DI—CBC and serum chemistry results are normal, but USG typically is <1.005
- DM—hyperglycemia and glucosuria are present

OTHER LABORATORY TESTS
- Measurement of fractional sodium clearance in horses with primary PD. It is increased (>1%) when excessive salt intake is the cause
- Measurement of plasma ADH concentration would be useful in cases of DI to differentiate neurogenic (low ADH) from nephrogenic (high ADH when dehydrated) forms, but this assay is not commercially available

IMAGING
Transabdominal/transrectal ultrasonography—to assess kidney size and echogenicity (should be normal, except with CKD).

OTHER DIAGNOSTIC PROCEDURES
- Overnight water deprivation is the most useful test to determine ability to concentrate urine. Horses with primary PD should concentrate urine to a specific gravity of 1.020–1.025; horses with CKD and DI fail to concentrate urine
- Approach water deprivation cautiously in horses with suspected DI, and do not perform when azotemia is detected (CKD). Measure body weight before water deprivation; do not extend the test beyond the time needed to lose 5% of body weight (may be <12 h in horses with DI)

P

• Horses are suspected to have DI when they fail to concentrate urine during water deprivation. Administration of desmopressin acetate (DDAVP; 0.1 mg/mL solution diluted in sterile water and 0.05 mg/kg, can be administered IV for this purpose) can be used to differentiate neurogenic DI (will concentrate urine to >1.020) from nephrogenic DI (will not concentrate urine)

TREATMENT

APPROPRIATE HEALTH CARE
• CKD, PPID, sepsis/endotoxemia—see chapters listed in See Also
• Primary PD, DI, DM—mostly outpatient medical treatment

NURSING CARE
• Primary PD—gradual restriction of water intake (initially to 100 mL/kg/day, which is approximately twice maintenance needs in a temperate climate, followed by a decrease to 75 mL/kg/day after several days) with careful monitoring of body weight and hydration status along with "trial and error" management changes
• DI—mild water restriction (to 100 mL/kg/day with careful monitoring of body weight and hydration status) and use of medications may help in limiting PU/PD; discontinue water restriction if dehydration or >5% loss of body weight occurs
• CKD, PPID—see chapters listed in See Also

ACTIVITY
May increase activity to modify behavior of horses with psychogenic PD.

DIET
• CKD, PPID—see chapters listed in See Also
• Increasing the amount of forage in the diet may help to decrease excessive water intake by horses with primary PD
• Limit availability of supplemental salt to horses with excessive salt consumption

CLIENT EDUCATION
• Inform clients that provision of adequate fresh water at all times is imperative to prevent dehydration with all pathologic causes of PU/PD
• Horses with primary PD may need "trial and error" management changes (e.g. increasing turnout time, increasing exercise, provision of a stablemate or other diversions in the stall) along with gradual water restriction
• DM—inform owners of the indications for euthanasia, i.e. loss of appetite and body condition; progressive weakness

MEDICATIONS

DRUG(S) OF CHOICE
PPID
See chapter Pituitary pars intermedia dysfunction.

DI
• With neurogenic DI, hormone replacement therapy with desmopressin (a potent ADH analog administered as eye drops) has been successful in small-animal patients but has not been described in horses and may be cost prohibitive
• With nephrogenic DI, replacement hormone therapy is ineffective; the only practical treatment is to restrict sodium and water intake and to administer thiazide diuretics

DM
Insulin replacement therapy in horses with low serum insulin concentrations.

CONTRAINDICATIONS
Gradual water restriction is contraindicated in horses with CKD, PPID, DM, or sepsis/endotoxemia.

PRECAUTIONS
• Perform water restriction with caution in horses with primary PD and DI to avoid significant dehydration
• Insulin therapy in DM could result in hypoglycemia

FOLLOW-UP

PATIENT MONITORING
• Closely monitor water intake, urine output, USG in all patients with PU/PD to minimize the risk of dehydration; horses with DI are at greatest risk of developing significant dehydration, even during short periods (hours) of water deprivation
• CKD, PPID——see chapters listed in See Also

POSSIBLE COMPLICATIONS
Moderate to severe dehydration may develop when horses with CKD, DI, or DM are unintentionally deprived of water for short periods.

EXPECTED COURSE AND PROGNOSIS
• The course and prognosis depend on the underlying cause. Horses with primary PD or excessive salt consumption generally respond rapidly and favorably with management changes
• The magnitude of PU/PD with inherited forms of DI may be reduced with mild salt and water restriction and medical therapy. With acquired forms of DI, especially nephrogenic DI from reversible renal disease or drug treatment, PU/PD may last for weeks to months but often may resolve over time
• Horses with CKD, DI, and DM have a guarded to poor long-term prognosis
• Horses with PPID can be effectively managed for years with appropriate treatment and management

MISCELLANEOUS

AGE-RELATED FACTORS
Foals consuming a predominantly milk diet (<2 months old) normally are polyuric. Daily fluid intake may approach 250 mL/kg/day and a USG <1.008 is normal.

SEE ALSO
• Chronic kidney disease (CKD)
• Endotoxemia
• Pituitary pars intermedia dysfunction

ABBREVIATIONS
• ADH = antidiuretic hormone
• CKD = chronic kidney disease
• DI = diabetes insipidus
• DM = diabetes mellitus
• PD = polydipsia
• PPID = pituitary pars intermedia dysfunction
• PU = polyuria
• USG = urine specific gravity

Suggested Reading
Mckenzie EC. Polyuria and polydipsia in horses. Vet Clin North Am Equine Pract 2007;23:641–654.
Schott HC. Polyuria and polydipsia. In: Reed SM, Bayly WM, Sellon DC, eds. Equine Internal Medicine, 4e. St. Louis, MO: WB Saunders, 2017:961–966.

Author Harold C. Schott II
Consulting Editor Valérie Picandet

BASICS

DEFINITION
• A result of RFM or contamination of the uterus by bacteria after parturition or dystocia
• Marked by inflammation of the deep layers of the uterus, endotoxemia and/or septicemia, and laminitis

PATHOPHYSIOLOGY
• After foaling, RFM, or kept stall bound, trauma and bacterial contamination of the uterus causes an inflammatory response, with nitric oxide production that decreases uterine contractility so debris, bacteria, endotoxins, and inflammatory byproducts are not expelled
• Accumulation of fluid, bacterial growth, inflammation, and toxin absorption may lead to septicemia, endotoxemia, and laminitis

SYSTEMS AFFECTED
• Reproductive
• Hemic/lymphatic/immune
• Musculoskeletal

GENETICS
N/A

INCIDENCE/PREVALENCE
N/A

SIGNALMENT
• Most common after a dystocia, associated with RFM, or extensive intrapartum uterine contamination
• Can occur after a normal delivery if uterine contraction and involution does not occur

SIGNS
• Metritis may be evident by 12–24 h postpartum, characterized by depression, abdominal discomfort, and anorexia
• Pyrexia, elevated pulse and respiratory rate, congested or toxic mucous membranes with shock, endotoxemia, or septicemia
• Uterus is enlarged, flaccid, and pendulous from accumulation of fetid, thick tan to chocolate-colored fluid
• The RFM may either be composed of a large portion of the total placenta with a free portion seen hanging through the vulva or be limited to only a small piece of the remaining placenta usually in the nongravid horn
• Signs of laminitis may appear 12 h to 5 days postpartum

CAUSES
• A history of placentitis, RFM, dystocia, abortion, prolonged or assisted delivery, fetotomy, stall bound, or cesarean section increases risk of postpartum metritis
• Postpartum complications depend on the amount and type of bacteria in the reproductive tract and the ability of the mare to clear her uterus
• Aerobic Gram-negative and -positive bacteria such as *Escherichia coli*, *Streptococcus zooepidemicus*, and other β-hemolytic

Streptococci, *Staphylococcus* sp., *Pseudomonas aeruginosa*, and *Klebsiella pneumoniae* are frequently involved
• The Gram-positive anaerobe *Bacteroides fragilis* resides in the external genitalia of mares and stallions and mucosal breakdown and necrotic tissue create favorable conditions for this bacterium's overgrowth
• Autolytic RFM with bacterial contamination and delayed uterine clearance initially results in endometritis, which progresses to the deeper layers; resulting in metritis
• Metritis, left untreated, can have systemic consequences leading to endotoxemia, septicemia, and laminitis

RISK FACTORS
See Causes.

DIAGNOSIS

DIFFERENTIAL DIAGNOSIS
Other Causes of Postpartum Abdominal Pain/Depression
• Bruising of the uterus or GI tract with peritonitis
• Uterine tear with peritonitis
• Rupture of cecum or right ventral colon
• Uterine artery rupture, with or without intra-abdominal hemorrhage

Other Causes of Postpartum Vaginal Discharge
• Normal postpartum lochia (≤6 days postpartum)—odorless, dark red-brown vaginal discharge associated with a palpable, normally involuting uterus, uterine walls are thickening and rugae present
• Vesiculovaginal reflux postpartum and vulvar discharge (thick yellow with urine crystals)

CBC/BIOCHEMISTRY/URINALYSIS
• Marked leukopenia (<2000 cells/μL) with toxic polymorphonuclear leukocytes/WBCs and left shift are seen in metritis. Response to treatment is evaluated by the return of WBCs to normal values (5000–12 000 cells/μl)
• Fibrinogen may increase to >500 mg/dL during the acute phase, but usually returns to normal values (<400 mg/dL) 2–3 days after WBC count returns to the normal range

OTHER LABORATORY TESTS
• Aerobic and anaerobic uterine bacterial culture
• *Bacteroides fragilis*—assume that it may be contributory if cultured
• Large numbers of mixed flora are expected from the uterus of normal, early postpartum mares

IMAGING
US
• Large amounts of fluid in the uterus 24–48 h postpartum

• Degree of echogenicity relates to the amount of debris or inflammatory cells in the fluid
• Uterine wall appears thick and edematous
• RFM may be present

OTHER DIAGNOSTIC PROCEDURES
N/A

PATHOLOGIC FINDINGS
• Postpartum acute inflammatory response can extend from the endometrium to the deeper layers, i.e. stratum compactum, stratum spongiosum, including the myometrium
• In contrast, endometritis in the mare is limited to the endometrium and lumen

TREATMENT

APPROPRIATE HEALTH CARE
• The primary objective is removal of the inciting cause—RFM, bacteria, and endotoxins from the uterine lumen. This can be accomplished with a large volume uterine lavage. A saline lavage (field treatment—12 L warm water with 150 g (6 oz) of salt added; can mix in a sterilized bucket). Infusion of 3–6 L at each treatment through a sterile nasogastric tube; uterine contents are then siphoned off; lavage repeated until the recovered fluid is clear. Depending on the mare's systemic compromise and amount and cellularity of the fluid this procedure may need to be performed 1–3 times a day
• Intrauterine infusion with broad-spectrum antibiotics should be initiated depending on the culture and sensitivity results
• Oxytocin to aid in uterine clearance and involution should be used but not at the same time as the above procedures
• Systemic support can include IV fluids, antiendotoxic doses of flunixin meglumine, pentoxifylline and broad-spectrum antibiotics. Polymyxin B may be used to neutralize circulating endotoxins
• Finding a thickened, corrugated uterine wall on palpation indicates a positive response to treatment and uterine involution
• Unresponsive mares have flaccid, thin uterine walls and accumulate large amounts of fluid between treatments. Treatment is discontinued when intrauterine fluid is clear or normal lochia present
• If a uterine tear is suspected begin with a smaller volume (1 L)
• See chapter Laminitis. Icing the feet (*ice boots*) as a preventative measure

NURSING CARE
N/A

ACTIVITY
Exercise—turnout as long as signs of laminitis are not present.

DIET
N/A

P

POSTPARTUM METRITIS   (CONTINUED)

CLIENT EDUCATION
N/A

SURGICAL CONSIDERATIONS
N/A

MEDICATIONS

DRUG(S) OF CHOICE

Fluids
• Use polyionic solutions, e.g. Normosol
• Estimate dehydration based on clinical signs (e.g. skin turgor), hematocrit, and total protein
• Calcium gluconate (125 mL of 23% solution) and oxytocin (40 IU) may be added to every other 5 L bag of Normosol
• Mild colic or discomfort will result from uterine contractions stimulated by treatment
• Discontinue or slow the rate of administration if signs of severe colic occur

Systemic Antibiotics
• Potassium penicillin for Gram-positive organisms—loading dose of 44 000 IU IV, followed by 22 000 IU IV QID
• Combine with gentamicin for Gram-negative organisms—2.2 mg/kg IV QID or 6.6 mg/kg IV daily
• For oral administration, use 15 mg/kg of trimethoprim–sulfa BID
• Metronidazole, for anaerobes, should always be combined with IV or PO therapy—loading dose of 15 mg/kg PO, followed by 7.5 mg/kg PO QID or 15–25 mg/kg PO BID

Intrauterine Antibiotics
• Ticarcillin/clavulanate (clavulanic acid)—3.1 g
• Potassium penicillin (500 000 IU) plus gentamicin (2 g)
• Ceftiofur—1 g

Uterotonic Drugs
• Oxytocin—multiple protocols have been proposed and used
  ○ 10 IU IV or 20 IU IM after uterine lavage if no intrauterine antibiotics administered
  ○ 40 IU added to IV fluids
  ○ 10 IU IV QID

NSAIDs
• Flunixin meglumine—antiendotoxic dose, 0.25 mg/kg IV or IM TID; anti-inflammatory dose, 1.1 mg/kg IV or IM BID
• Phenylbutazone—4.4 mg/kg IV or PO BID; at the onset of laminitis, recommended loading dose is 8.8 mg/kg IV

• Polymyxin B—administer 6000 U/kg IV in 1 L of sterile saline over 30–60 min; recommended BID for 1–2 days

CONTRAINDICATIONS
N/A

PRECAUTIONS
• NSAIDs may cause GI ulceration and nephrotoxicity
• Aminoglycosides can be nephrotoxic and ototoxic; ensure good hydration during treatment
• Polymyxin B—potentially nephrotoxic at therapeutic doses
• Dehydration and NSAID administration may potentiate the nephrotoxicity associated with aminoglycosides and polymyxin B
• Metronidazole can decrease appetite in a number of circumstances. If it decreases appetite, then milk production in postpartum mares could be affected

POSSIBLE INTERACTIONS
N/A

ALTERNATIVE DRUGS
See chapter Laminitis.

FOLLOW-UP

PATIENT MONITORING
• Monitor CBC for signs of endotoxemia or response to treatment
• See chapter Laminitis
• Monitor for signs of laminitis by early and repeated evaluation of digital pulses, signs of weight shift, and radiographs of the distal phalanx, rotation or sinking of third phalanx

PREVENTION/AVOIDANCE
N/A

POSSIBLE COMPLICATIONS
• Delayed uterine involution
• Septicemia/endotoxemia
• Laminitis
• Death

EXPECTED COURSE AND PROGNOSIS
• Prognosis depends on severity, duration, and secondary complications caused by metritis
• Rapid response to therapy indicates a favorable prognosis
• Laminitis due to postpartum metritis carries a guarded to grave prognosis

MISCELLANEOUS

ASSOCIATED CONDITIONS
N/A

AGE-RELATED FACTORS
N/A

ZOONOTIC POTENTIAL
N/A

PREGNANCY/FERTILITY/BREEDING
N/A

SYNONYMS
• Metritis/laminitis/septicemia complex
• Toxic metritis

SEE ALSO
• Delayed uterine involution
• Dystocia
• Endometritis
• Laminitis
• Retained fetal membranes

ABBREVIATIONS
• GI = gastrointestinal
• NSAID = nonsteroidal anti-inflammatory drug
• RFM = retained fetal membranes
• WBC = white blood cell

Suggested Reading
Asbury AC. Care of the mare after foaling. In: MacKinnon AO, Voss JL, eds. Equine Reproduction. Philadelphia, PA: Lea & Febiger, 1993:976–980.
Canisso IF, Rodriguez JS, Sanz MG, Coutinho da Silva MA. A clinical approach to the diagnosis and treatment of retained fetal membranes with an emphasis placed on the critically ill mare. J Equine Vet Sci 2013;33:570–579.
Ricketts SW, Mackintosh ME. Role of anaerobic bacteria in equine endometritis. J Reprod Fertil Suppl 1987;35:343–351.
Threlfall WR, Carleton CL. Treatment of uterine infections in the mare. In: Morrow DA, ed. Current Therapy in Theriogenology. Philadelphia, PA: WB Saunders, 1986:730–737.

Author Karen Wolfsdorf
Consulting Editor Carla L. Carleton
Acknowledgment The author and editor acknowledge the prior contribution of Maria E. Cadario.

BASICS

OVERVIEW
- Hyperkalemia is defined as an elevated concentration of potassium in serum/plasma
- Potassium is the major intracellular cation in biologic systems
- Plays a major role in determining the resting membrane potential of excitable tissue
- Readily absorbed by the gastrointestinal tract in health
- Excretion of excess potassium is performed by the kidney
- The quantity of potassium in extracellular fluid is <2% of total body potassium; as such, serum potassium evaluation is a poor assessment of whole-body potassium status
- Changes in serum potassium concentration can have marked effects on muscle and nervous tissue
- The 2 largest clinically significant body potassium stores are erythrocytes and skeletal muscle

SIGNALMENT
- Any breed, age, or sex.
- Uroperitoneum in neonates
- HYPP in Quarter Horses

SIGNS
- Skeletal muscle weakness
  - Fasciculations
  - Stiffness, myotonia
  - Staggering gait
  - Collapse
- Bradycardia, other cardiac dysrhythmias
- Sweating, anxiety
- Sudden death

CAUSES AND RISK FACTORS
- Strenuous exercise—causes transient hyperkalemia
  - Likely reflects lactic acidemia that develops during exercise, but myocytes also release potassium
  - Potassium may be responsible for peripheral vasodilation during exercise, increasing blood flow to skeletal muscle
- Rhabdomyolysis (or any condition resulting in severe, diffuse cellular injury/necrosis, resulting in leakage of intracellular potassium)
- Intravascular hemolysis (severe)
- HYPP—major cause of intermittent hyperkalemia
- Poor sample handling—leakage of intracellular potassium from erythrocytes and/or platelets; samples should be spun and removed from clot as soon as possible after collection
- Acidemia—intracellular translocation of interstitial fluid hydrogen ion in exchange for intracellular potassium
  - Mild to moderate elevation in serum potassium

- Affected horses likely to have total-body potassium *depletion* due to primary disease
- Acute kidney injury or chronic renal failure
  - Inconsistent finding
  - Anuria/oliguria more likely to cause clinically significant hyperkalemia
- Iatrogenic—IV parenteral potassium supplementation
- Uroperitoneum—postrenal obstruction, decreased potassium clearance
- Hyperosmolality

 DIAGNOSIS

CBC/BIOCHEMISTRY/URINALYSIS
Biochemistry—increased potassium concentration (>5.0 mmol/L).

OTHER LABORATORY TESTS
Arterial blood gas analysis may reveal acidemia.

IMAGING
Dependent on the underlying cause (e.g. ultrasonography to detect free abdominal fluid in foals with uroperitoneum).

OTHER DIAGNOSTIC PROCEDURES
- ECG
  - Peaked, tented T waves
  - Decreased Q–T interval
  - Decreased amplitude of P waves
  - Widened QRS complexes
  - Sinus bradycardia
  - Changes may be seen when plasma potassium level >6 mEq/L
  - Changes may be marked with plasma potassium level >8 mEq/L
  - Plasma potassium level >9–10 mEq/L often fatal
    - Ventricular fibrillation
    - Asystole

 TREATMENT

- Dependent on the underlying cause
- Hyperkalemia should be addressed as an emergency
- Diuresis with potassium-free polyionic fluids may be helpful (e.g. 0.9% NaCl)
  - In mild cases, may be all that is required
  - More severe cases require additional emergency medical treatment (see Drug(s) of Choice)
  - Use caution in patients with renal disease
- Hyperkalemia should be corrected prior to induction of anesthesia to minimize cardiovascular and musculoskeletal complications
  - Hyperkalemic patients should be offered potassium-poor diets

 MEDICATIONS

DRUG(S) OF CHOICE
- Calcium gluconate
  - 0.2–0.4 mL/kg of 23% solution diluted in 1–2 L 5% dextrose, administered slowly IV
  - Calcium is cardioprotective
- Dextrose/insulin
  - Insulin causes rapid intracellular translocation of potassium
  - Dextrose induces endogenous insulin release
  - Oral glucose may be given in emergency (oats, light corn syrup) but is not appropriate alone for severe cases
  - IV dextrose preferred (5%, 4.4–6.6 mL/kg)
- Sodium bicarbonate
  - Use care—rapid alkalinization of patients with metabolic acidemia may result in acute, profound hypokalemia
  - 1–2 mEq/kg IV as isotonic solution
- Diuretics
  - Acetazolamide (2–4 mg/kg PO every 12 h) is a potassium-wasting, carbonic anhydrase inhibitor diuretic that may be effective for managing horses with HYPP

CONTRAINDICATIONS/POSSIBLE INTERACTIONS
Do not administer sodium bicarbonate with calcium-containing fluids.

 FOLLOW-UP

PATIENT MONITORING
- ECG monitoring
- Serial evaluation of serum potassium concentration

POSSIBLE COMPLICATIONS
- Cardiac dysrhythmias
- Sudden death

 MISCELLANEOUS

SEE ALSO
- Acidosis, metabolic
- Hyperkalemic periodic paralysis
- Potassium, hypokalemia
- Uroperitoneum, neonate

ABBREVIATIONS
HYPP = hyperkalemic periodic paralysis

Suggested Reading
Borer KE, Corley KTT. Electrolyte disorders in horses with colic. Part 1: potassium and magnesium. Equine Vet Educ 2006;18(5):266–271.

Author Teresa A. Burns
Consulting Editor Sandra D. Taylor

P

POTASSIUM, HYPOKALEMIA

BASICS

OVERVIEW
- Hypokalemia is defined as decreased potassium concentration in serum/plasma, usually <2.5 mEq/L (depends on reference values of laboratory performing the assay)
- Potassium is the major intracellular cation in biologic systems
- Plays a major role in determining the resting membrane potential of excitable tissue
- Readily absorbed by the GI tract in health (typically in excess of body need); the average equine diet is potassium-rich, easily providing the daily requirement of 23 g for an adult horse
  - Alfalfa hay—13 lb (6 kg) provides 145 g potassium
  - Grass hay (average)—16 lb (7 kg) provides 121 g potassium
  - Trace mineral salt—2 oz provides 145 g potassium
- Excretion of excess potassium from dietary intake is performed by the kidney, preventing potentially toxic hyperkalemia in health
- Renal conservation of potassium is nonspecific and inefficient, developing over the course of several days in horses with decreased dietary potassium intake and/or excessive potassium losses. This aspect of potassium physiology increases risk of clinically significant hypokalemia in horses with inappetence or potassium-wasting diseases
- The quantity of potassium in the ECF is <2% of the total body potassium; as such, plasma potassium evaluation is a poor assessment of whole-body potassium status
- The *ratio* of ICF to ECF potassium concentration is critical to determining the resting membrane potential; changes in plasma potassium concentration can have marked effects on excitable tissue (muscle and nervous tissue)
- May be due to total body potassium deficit, or, more likely, may reflect a shift in potassium distribution between ECF and ICF
- Hypokalemia is uncommon in horses with normal feed intake

SIGNALMENT
Any breed, age, or sex.

SIGNS
- Usually noted when serum potassium concentration falls below 1.8 mEq/L
- Weakness
- Collapse
- Arrhythmia (ventricular premature beats, ventricular tachycardia)
- Sudden death
- Ileus

CAUSES AND RISK FACTORS
- Alkalemia (any cause)—extracellular potassium is exchanged for intracellular

hydrogen ion in an attempt to restore acid–base equilibrium
- Profuse sweating (sweat contains high concentration of potassium)
- Renal tubular acidosis (types 1 and 2)
- Decreased dietary intake (inappetence for any reason)
- GI loss
  - Diarrhea
  - Nasogastric reflux
- Iatrogenic
  - Sodium bicarbonate
  - Dextrose-containing fluids
  - Insulin
  - Prolonged parenteral nutrition

DIAGNOSIS

DIFFERENTIAL DIAGNOSIS
- Muscular weakness—underlying myopathy, other electrolyte, acid–base abnormalities (e.g. hypocalcemia, hypomagnesemia)
- Cardiac arrhythmia—underlying cardiomyopathy, other electrolyte, acid–base abnormalities

CBC/BIOCHEMISTRY/URINALYSIS
- CBC—may be helpful for identification of underlying disease
- Biochemistry—evidence of underlying disease may be present; other electrolyte abnormalities, such as hypomagnesemia and hypocalcemia, may be noted and may exacerbate clinical signs of hypokalemia
- Urinalysis—fractional clearance of potassium is variably affected

OTHER LABORATORY TESTS
Arterial blood gas analysis may reveal alkalemia.

DIAGNOSTIC PROCEDURES
ECG
- Peaked P waves
- Decreased amplitude of T waves
- Increased QRS duration
- Ventricular ectopic rhythms (ventricular premature contractions, ventricular tachycardia)

TREATMENT
- Definitive treatment of underlying cause is required
- Potassium-rich diet should be offered (e.g. legume hay)
- Oral supplementation with potassium chloride is typically sufficient in mild cases
  - 25–40 g/day via nasogastric tube in divided doses
- Potassium chloride supplementation IV (20–40 mEq/L; no more than 0.5 mEq/kg/h to avoid potentially dangerous hyperkalemia)

MEDICATIONS

DRUG(S) OF CHOICE
Potassium chloride (see Treatment).

CONTRAINDICATIONS/POSSIBLE INTERACTIONS
- Supplemental potassium should be given with caution in patients with known renal insufficiency; careful monitoring of serum potassium concentration should be performed
- Medications that may exacerbate hypokalemia should be avoided:
  - Sodium bicarbonate
  - Glucose/dextrose, insulin
  - Diuretics (acetazolamide, furosemide)

FOLLOW-UP

PATIENT MONITORING
- Serial assessment of serum potassium concentration
- ECG monitoring should be continued until normal

POSSIBLE COMPLICATIONS
- Cardiac arrhythmias (especially idioventricular rhythms)
- Sudden death
- Ileus, colic
- Predisposition to exertional rhabdomyolysis/myopathy

MISCELLANEOUS

SEE ALSO
- Alkalosis, metabolic
- Duodenitis–proximal jejunitis (anterior enteritis, proximal enteritis)

ABBREVIATIONS
- ECF = extracellular fluid
- GI = gastrointestinal
- ICF = intracellular fluid

Suggested Reading
Johnson PJ. Electrolyte and acid-base disturbances in the horse. Vet Clin North Am Equine Pract 1995;11:491–514.
Stäempfli H, Oliver-Espinosa O. Serum potassium. In: Smith BP, ed. Large Animal Internal Medicine, 5e. St. Louis, MO: Elsevier Mosby, 2015:357–358.

Author Teresa A. Burns
Consulting Editor Sandra D. Taylor

POTOMAC HORSE FEVER (PHF)

BASICS

DEFINITION
PHF is an acute and potentially fatal enterotyphlocolitis of horses caused by infection with the monocytotropic rickettsia *Neorickettsia risticii* (formerly known as *Ehrlichia risticii*).

PATHOPHYSIOLOGY
• The pathophysiology of PHF is poorly understood
• *N. risticii* is a Gram-negative, obligate intracellular bacterium with a predilection for blood monocytes and tissue macrophages. Within days of infection, *N. risticii* can be found in blood monocytes. *N. risticii* survives within phagosomes in macrophages by inhibiting phagosome–lysosome fusion. The neoricketsemia persists throughout the disease
• The pathogen has a predilection for the large colon and cecum, but is occasionally found in the jejunum and small colon. Mild cases of PHF without diarrhea have evidence of colitis. It is possible that many pathophysiologic changes observed in horses with PHF are secondary to effects of altered colonic flora

SYSTEMS AFFECTED
• Gastrointestinal—cecum and large colon
• Cardiovascular—dehydration and shock may develop in severe cases
• Reproductive—occasional abortion

GENETICS
N/A

INCIDENCE/PREVALENCE
In Ohio, 13–20% of horses on racetracks had serologic evidence of exposure to *N. risticii*, although only 10–20% of them had clinical signs of the disease.

GEOGRAPHIC DISTRIBUTION
PHF has been reported in the USA, Canada, South America, Europe, and India.

SIGNALMENT
All breeds and all ages may be affected. Horses <1 year of age less commonly develop PHF than adult horses. Clinical cases of PHF occur sporadically, with rarely more than 5% of horses on any one affected farm. Only in a significant epizootic infection does the attack rate on individual farms become high (20–50%).

SIGNS
• The majority of clinical disease appears to be mild or subclinical. In overt clinical illness, the manifestation of colitis is common in all cases. Not all cases show colic or diarrhea
• Depression (90%)
• Anorexia (80%)
• Fever (70%)
• Ileus (70%)—signs of ileus are one of the most consistent clinical findings

• Diarrhea (≈ 60%)—mild to severe, watery, pipe-stream diarrhea present in 45–60% of cases. Course of diarrhea ranges from 1 to 10 days
• Mild colic (30%) may accompany diarrhea
• Congested mucous membranes (70%)
• Dehydration
• Laminitis (usually involving all 4 feet) develops in about 20–25%
• Mortality rate from PHF—5–30%
• Clinical course is usually 5–10 days without treatment
• Infrequent abortion may occur

CAUSES
• Infection with *N. risticii*, an obligate intracellular Gram-negative bacteria
• Different strains of *N. risticii* identified; not all pathogenic
• *N. risticii* DNA has been found in trematodes (virgulate cercariae) that parasitize freshwater snails in endemic areas
• During periods of warm water temperatures, cercariae infected with *N. risticii* are released from the snails, infecting and developing into metacercariae in the second intermediate host, aquatic insects, such as caddis flies, mayflies, damselflies, dragonflies, and stoneflies
• Horses grazing near rivers or creeks could conceivably be exposed to *N. risticii* through skin penetration by infected cercariae in water, or ingest metacercariae in a second intermediate host such as an aquatic insect along with grass, consume adult insects trapped on the water surface, or consume adult insects that are attracted by stable lights or accumulate in feed and water
• No evidence for the spread of PHF by arthropod vectors
• Seasonal pattern in temperate climates with most clinical cases of PHF occurring mid to late summer

RISK FACTORS
Endemic areas have been identified. *N. risticii* infection has been strongly associated with rivers, lakes, or other aquatic habitats. Increased risk of PHF is associated with horses grazing pastures bordering waterways; horses coming from an area with a high PHF prevalence or a farm with history of PHF; or travel to an area with a high incidence of PHF.

DIAGNOSIS

DIFFERENTIAL DIAGNOSIS
All other causes of enterocolitis—acute salmonellosis, clostridial colitis, cyathostomes, antibiotic-induced colitis, intestinal ileus secondary to displacement or obstruction, NSAID toxicity, cantharidin toxicity; peritonitis; dietary changes.

CBC/BIOCHEMISTRY/URINALYSIS
• Hematology highly variable
• Elevated packed cell volume and total plasma protein are common abnormalities. Hypoproteinemia may also be present
• Leukopenia with a neutropenia and lymphopenia may initially be present, and within a few days a marked leukocytosis may occur
• Hyponatremia
• Hypochloremia
• Hypokalemia
• Metabolic acidosis
• ± Prerenal azotemia

OTHER LABORATORY TESTS
N/A

IMAGING
N/A

OTHER DIAGNOSTIC PROCEDURES
• Definitive diagnosis should be based on isolation of *N. risticii* from blood culture or detection of the DNA of *N. risticii* from the blood or feces of an infected horse. Isolation of the organism requires collecting heparinized blood and harvesting buffy coat for cell culture
• *N. risticii*-specific PCR assays that detect the partial 16S rRNA gene of *N. risticii* have facilitated PHF diagnosis. In naturally infected horses, PCR on peripheral blood and feces is more sensitive than blood culture. PCR may also be used in the detection of *N. risticii* DNA in fresh or formalin-fixed and paraffin-embedded colon tissue
• Serologic tests—IFA or ELISA tests of limited diagnostic value in a clinical case. IFA test has been the most widely used diagnostic test for PHF; however, interpretation of results difficult. PHF diagnosed by demonstrating a ≥4-fold increase or decrease in titers between acute and convalescent serum samples
• Failure to seroconvert does not rule out PHF. Expected antibody titer of naturally affected horses is >1:80. Persistence of high antibody titers (1:2560) for more than 1 year has been noted in clinical and subclinical cases after natural infection

PATHOLOGIC FINDINGS
• Gross distention of large colon and cecum with fluid contents
• Histologically—lesions mild: superficial epithelial necrosis, erosion, and fibrin effusion
• Silver stains—*N. risticii* seen as small, brown to black, intracellular dots (0.4–0.9 μm) in the apical cytoplasm of crypt enterocytes and also in the cytoplasm of macrophages in the lamina propria

P

POTOMAC HORSE FEVER (PHF) (CONTINUED)

TREATMENT

APPROPRIATE HEALTH CARE
Mild cases can be managed on the farm. Severely affected animals may require intensive care. As other causes of some of the clinical signs are potentially highly infectious (e.g. salmonellosis), animals should be managed in isolation. Early, appropriate treatment gives the best chance for a successful outcome.

ACTIVITY
Stall rest during therapy is recommended.

DIET
Grass hay diet is recommended until fecal consistency is normal.

CLIENT EDUCATION
N/A

SURGICAL CONSIDERATIONS
N/A

MEDICATIONS

DRUG(S) OF CHOICE
• Oxytetracycline 6.6 mg/kg IV every 24 h for 5 days treatment of choice. A rapid recovery and dramatic decrease in fatality rate is observed when oxytetracycline therapy is commenced within 24 h after the development of fever
• NSAIDs, such as flunixin meglumine (1.1 mg/kg IV every 12 h), may be useful to treat endotoxemia

FLUIDS
IV isotonic crystalloid fluid replacement therapy is extremely important in the treatment of hypovolemia and shock.

CONTRAINDICATIONS
N/A

PRECAUTIONS
• Diarrhea may occur in horses receiving parenteral antibiotics
• Nephrotoxicity possible with oxytetracycline, especially in a dehydrated horse, or with the concurrent administration of NSAIDs

ALTERNATIVE DRUGS
N/A

FOLLOW-UP

PATIENT MONITORING
Relapses rare following cessation of IV oxytetracycline therapy. If relapse occurs, administer a second course of IV oxytetracycline.

PREVENTION/AVOIDANCE
• Contact with recovered or currently ill animals not associated with the development of PHF
• Natural infection with PHF induces a protective immunity for as long as 20 months
• Horses do not remain chronic carriers
• Access to freshwater streams and ponds should be limited in endemic areas
• Horses in endemic areas may be vaccinated with an inactivated cell vaccine between early spring and early summer. Require 2-dose primary series 3–4 weeks apart. Revaccination at 6–12 month intervals dependent on whether in highly endemic area. High rate of vaccination failure (up to 89%) reported in endemic areas attributed to extensive variability in the major surface antigens and lack of cross-protection between strains. Anecdotal reports of reduced severity of clinical signs in vaccinated horses

POSSIBLE COMPLICATIONS
• Acute or chronic laminitis in 20–25% of PHF cases
• Thrombophlebitis
• Disseminated intravascular coagulopathy

EXPECTED COURSE AND PROGNOSIS
Horses with mild signs treated early in the course of the disease show a dramatic response to therapy and can be clinically normal in 3–5 days. Horses with more severe and longstanding problems require a longer period of therapy; if secondary problems are present, the clinical course may be much longer and the outcome less favorable.

MISCELLANEOUS

SYNONYMS
• Equine monocytic ehrlichiosis
• Equine ehrlichial colitis
• Equine neorickettsiosis

SEE ALSO
• Acute adult abdominal pain—acute colic
• Clostridium *difficile* infection
• Cyathostominosis
• Large colon torsion
• Cantharidin toxicosis
• Periodontal disease
• Peritonitis
• Protein-losing enteropathy (PLE)
• Salmonellosis

ABBREVIATIONS
• ELISA = enzyme-limited immunosorbent assay
• IFA = indirect fluorescent antibody
• NSAID = nonsteroidal anti-inflammatory drug
• PCR = polymerase chain reaction
• PHF = Potomac horse fever

Suggested Reading
Bertin FR, Reising A, Slovis NM, et al. Clinical and clinicopathological factors associated with survival in 44 horses with equine neorickettsiosis (Potomac horse fever). J Vet Intern Med 2013;27:1528–1534.
Madigan JE, Pusterla N. Life cycle of Potomac horse fever—implications for diagnosis, treatment, and control: a review. Proc Am Assoc Equine Pract 2005;51:158–162.
Pusterla N, Leutenegger CM, Sigrist B, et al. Detection and quantitation of *Ehrlichia risticii* genomic DNA by real-time PCR in infected horses and snails. Vet Parasitol 2000;90:129–135.
Rikihisa Y. New findings on members of the family Anaplasmataceae of veterinary importance. Ann N Y Acad Sci 2006;1078:438–445.

Author John D. Baird
Consulting Editors Henry Stämpfli and Olimpo Oliver-Espinosa

PREGNANCY DIAGNOSIS

BASICS

DEFINITION
• *Pregnancy*—the condition post fertilization of an embryo or fetus developing and maturing in utero
• *Pregnancy diagnosis*—determining pregnant state based on clinical signs and laboratory and physical findings, including TRP and US

PATHOPHYSIOLOGY
N/A

SYSTEMS AFFECTED
• Reproductive
• Other systems may be affected in abnormal pregnancy

GENETICS
N/A

INCIDENCE/PREVALENCE
N/A

SIGNALMENT
• Nonspecific; puberty occurs between 12 and 24 months in females
• Pregnancy may occur any time after puberty until advanced age in mares

SIGNS
Historical Findings
Failure of a mare that has been bred to return to estrus 16–19 days post ovulation.

Physical Examination Findings
• Early in pregnancy, little physical change may be noted
• As pregnancy advances, most mares will develop recognizable abdominal distention and weight gain
• In the final 2–4 weeks prior to parturition, most mares will have increased development of the mammary gland with secretion of fluid from the nipples ranging from thin and straw-colored to sticky and creamy

CAUSES
Mating

RISK FACTORS
N/A

DIAGNOSIS

DIFFERENTIAL DIAGNOSIS
Other Causes of Failure to Cycle
• *Seasonal anestrus* TRP and US—little ovarian activity; uterine and cervical tone is flaccid
• *Behavioral anestrus* serial TRP and/or US—distinguish mares in estrus from those in diestrus or that are pregnant
• *Prolonged luteal life span*—evidence of a CL by US examination of the ovary or progesterone assay. Responds to prostaglandin $F_{2\alpha}$ treatment

• *Granulosa–theca cell tumor*—abnormally enlarged, multicystic ovary and small contralateral ovary. Confirm with elevated serum inhibin and/or anti-Müllerian hormone concentrations
• *Chromosomal abnormalities* (gonadal dysgenesis, testicular feminization)—confirm by karyotype determination

Other US Findings Resembling Early Pregnancy
• *Uterine/lymphatic cysts*—US examination of the mare prior to breeding and pregnancy; record presence, number, size, shape of uterine cysts; a *uterine map* (horns and body) on each mare's record is easily referenced at early pregnancy examinations
  ◦ This permanent record of cystic structures is beneficial in distinguishing uterine cysts from early embryonic vesicles
  ◦ Update *maps* at the start of each breeding season, note changing appearance, number of cysts with increasing age

CBC/BIOCHEMISTRY/URINALYSIS
N/A

OTHER LABORATORY TESTS
Progesterone Assay
• ELISA and RIA for serum or milk progesterone concentrations
  ◦ Elevated concentrations of progesterone at 18–21 days post ovulation imply that functional luteal tissue is present; a presumptive test for pregnancy
• A useful adjunct to other methods of early diagnosis (i.e. TRP without US)
• Confirmation of pregnancy, e.g. estrone sulfate or total estrogens, is advisable if early diagnosis was solely by a progesterone assay

eCG Assay
• eCG is a hormone secreted by endometrial cups in the pregnant mare uterus
• Endometrial cups form at ≈36–37 days of gestation, when fetal trophoblasts from the chorionic girdle actively invade the endometrial epithelium
  ◦ The cups attain maximum size and hormone output at 55–70 days of gestation
  ◦ Endometrial cups regress at 80–120 days of gestation; secretion of eCG ceases at that time
• eCG is measured using an ELISA
• *False positives* occur if fetal death occurs after formation of endometrial cups:
  ◦ The cups can persist up to 3–4 months after a mare has lost a pregnancy, either a nonviable fetus in utero or fetal loss (early abortions often not noted)
• *False negatives* occur in samples:
  ◦ Before the endometrial cups form (<36 days of gestation)
  ◦ After the regression of the cups (>120 days of gestation)

Estrogen Assay
• Estrogens are secreted by the fetoplacental unit

• Total estrogens or estrone sulfate (conjugated estrogen) can be measured from plasma or urine; diagnose pregnancy after day 60 using RIA
• Estrone sulfate concentrations in milk are diagnostic for pregnancy after day 90 in the mare
• Fetal death and/or compromise to the fetoplacental unit results in rapid decline in estrone sulfate concentration

IMAGING
Transrectal US
Pregnancy diagnosis can be determined as early as 9 days after ovulation, with a 5 MHz transducer and a high-quality US scanner.

Days 15–16 Post Ovulation
• The optimal time to scan for early pregnancy. The embryonic vesicle is an anechoic, spherical yolk sac, averaging 6–20 mm in height
• Detection of an embryonic vesicle is reliable during this period; twin embryonic vesicles can consistently be identified at this time
• Early diagnosis of twins increases the success of twin reduction to a singleton; manual reduction (crush) technique

Days 18–24 Post Ovulation
• The US appearance of the vesicle—more triangular by day 18 as the bilaminar wall of the embryonic vesicle becomes less turgid
• The embryo proper often can be visualized by day 20–21; its heartbeat is visible as early as 24 days, should be evident with most US machines by 25 days
• The allantoic sac is visible ventral to the embryo by day 24

Days 25–48 Post Ovulation
• As the allantois develops and the yolk sac regresses, the embryo appears (during US examinations) to lift from the ventral aspect of the vesicle to a dorsal location
• The embryo is visualized mid-vesicle by 28–30 days and is in the dorsal aspect of the vesicle by day 35
• The umbilical cord forms and attaches at the dorsal aspect of the vesicle around day 40
• As the cord elongates, with US, the fetus descends to a more ventral location in the vesicle of pregnancy, reaching near its ventral aspect by day 48

Fetal Sexing by US
Days 60–70 of Gestation
• Determination of fetal gender is very useful in both horses and cattle, but high-resolution US equipment and experience are necessary for accurate identification of fetal gender
• Fetal sex is determined by locating the position of the genital tubercle during its developmental migration
• The genital tubercle is the precursor to the clitoris in females and the penis in males
• The structure is located on the ventral midline and is imaged as a hyperechoic,

P

bilobed structure that is approximately 2 mm in diameter
• The tubercle migrates from between the rear legs caudally toward the tail in female fetuses and cranially toward the umbilicus in male fetuses. The location and orientation of the fetus must be determined—locate the mandible (points ventrally and caudally); the heart is imaged on the ventral midline of the thorax. Examine the fetus cranially to caudally, locate the abdominal attachment of the umbilicus. Immediately caudal to that attachment is the *male* genital tubercle. The *female* tubercle is best visualized at the caudal-most aspect of the fetus under the tail-head; its optimal image appears within a triangle formed by the tail-head and the distal tibias or hocks

Days 70–130 of Gestation
• Days 70–75—the fetus can be visualized using transrectal US. There will be some variation depending on the mare's age and parity. At this time, the weight of the developing pregnancy pulls the uterus over the brim of the pelvis
• At 95 days of gestation—the fetus may move more dorsally within the pregnant uterus and can be imaged to determine fetal gender
• From 95 to 130 days of gestation—gender can be determined by locating external genital structures:
  ○ Female—mammary gland, teats, clitoris
  ○ Male—penis, prepuce, scrotum

Days 120–210 of Gestation
• Combination of transrectal and transabdominal US; visualize fetal sex organs (up to 240 days)
• A wider diagnostic window, more parameters to evaluate, more fully developed sex organs for easier diagnosis

OTHER DIAGNOSTIC PROCEDURES
Behavioral Assessment
If not pregnant—a mare teased to a stallion should begin to show signs of behavioral estrus 16–18 days after ovulation; a nonspecific indicator of the absence of pregnancy; serves only as an adjunct to more reliable means (TRP, US).

False Positive
• Failure to show estrus even as she returns to heat (*silent heat*)
• Pregnancy loss occurs after formation of endometrial cups
• Prolonged luteal activity but not pregnant

False Negative
Mare continues to exhibit signs of behavioral estrus when pregnant.

Vaginal Speculum Examination
• Under the influence of progesterone, the cervix is tightly closed, pale, and dry; not diagnostic for pregnancy as a functional CL in a cycling mare has the same effect on the cervix

• Often used as an adjunct to TRP of the reproductive tract (nonspecific)

TRP of the Reproductive Tract

Days 15–18 Post Ovulation
• Tubular tract becomes toned, and the "T" shape of the uterine bifurcation is often distinctly palpable. Palpation of a vesicle in the uterine horn reported as early as day 15; however, palpation of a true bulge at this stage is difficult in all but maiden mares with small uterine horns; possible to crush vesicle with harsh TRP
• The cervix is generally tightly closed, narrow, and elongated
• Both ovaries are active producing follicles during early pregnancy
• False diagnosis of pregnancy based on TRP alone, may be due to early embryonic death or persistent/prolonged luteal activity

Days 25–30 of Gestation
• Uterine tone is very distinct (elevated); the cervix is narrow and elongated
• Follicular activity is present
• A bulge (size—small hen's egg) at the caudoventral aspect of a uterine horn, adjacent to the uterine bifurcation
• The uterine wall is slightly thinner over the fluid-filled, resilient vesicle

Days 35–40 of Gestation
• Uterus still demonstrates increased tone; cervix is closed and elongated; ovaries active
• A tennis ball-sized bulge noted at the base of the uterine horn on the side of pregnancy
• Uterine tone begins to drop at/around the enlarging bulge as the uterine wall *thins* around the enlargement. Greatly increased uterine tone remains in the nonpregnant horn

Days 45–50 of Gestation
Palpable bulge increases to softball size.

Days 60–65 of Gestation
• Vesicle begins to expand into the uterine body, and the palpable bulge resembles the shape of a child-sized football
• Wall of the uterine horn is distinctly thinner at this stage and the pregnancy begins to lose some of its resiliency. Good uterine tone often maintained in the nongravid horn and at the tip of the gravid horn
• The increasing size of the pregnancy begins to pull the uterus ventrally

Days 150–210 of Gestation
• Uterine descent into the ventral abdomen is complete; ovaries often located near the midline
• The fetus may consistently be balloted within the fluid-filled uterus

To Term
• Pregnancy continues to occupy more of the uterus and uterine tone diminishes. It expands dorsally and resembles the size of a basketball, eventually to a large, distended uterus. Near term the fetus can readily be palpated in the uterine body and its activity assessed, as well as fetal presentation and position.

• The pregnant uterus can be confused with a full urinary bladder
• To distinguish the 2, the fluid-filled uterus can be traced back to the closed cervix at the caudal aspect of the uterine body
• Additionally, as the uterus continues to drop deeper into the abdomen, the ovaries are drawn ventrally and toward the midline
• After 7 months, near term/late in gestation, the fetus is visible (US). The amnion (thin, *floating* membrane) and characterisitcs of both amniotic and allantoic fluids can be observed.

PATHOLOGIC FINDINGS
N/A

 ## TREATMENT
APPROPRIATE HEALTH CARE
N/A

NURSING CARE
N/A

ACTIVITY
N/A

DIET
N/A

CLIENT EDUCATION
N/A

SURGICAL CONSIDERATIONS
N/A

 ## MEDICATIONS
DRUG(S) OF CHOICE
N/A

CONTRAINDICATIONS
N/A

PRECAUTIONS
N/A

POSSIBLE INTERACTIONS
N/A

ALTERNATIVE DRUGS
N/A

 ## FOLLOW-UP
PATIENT MONITORING
• Pregnant mares are routinely examined in the last trimester of gestation to verify fetal viability. Can often determine presentation late in gestation (anterior, posterior, transverse)
• The most common method of pregnancy diagnosis as this stage is TRP with ballottement of the fetus
• Transabdominal US may be used to measure fetal parameters—heart rate, aortic diameter,

activity, nature of fluid surrounding the fetus (amniotic, allantoic); combined thickness of uterus and placenta to monitor for placentitis

PREVENTION/AVOIDANCE
N/A

POSSIBLE COMPLICATIONS
Embryonic/fetal loss/abortion, twins, placentitis, ruptured prepubic tendon, abdominal wall herniation, hydrallantois, hydramnion, uterine torsion, uterine rupture, prolonged gestation, dystocia.

EXPECTED COURSE AND PROGNOSIS
A normal, viable fetus born at term gestation.

 MISCELLANEOUS

ASSOCIATED CONDITIONS
N/A

AGE-RELATED FACTORS
N/A

ZOONOTIC POTENTIAL
N/A

PREGNANCY/FERTILITY/BREEDING
N/A

SEE ALSO
• Abortion, spontaneous, infectious
• Abortion, spontaneous, noninfectious
• Conception failure in mares
• Dystocia
• Early embryonic death
• Placental basics
• Twin pregnancy

ABBREVIATIONS
• CL = corpus luteum
• eCG = equine chorionic gonadotropin
• ELISA = enzyme-linked immunosorbent assay
• RIA = radioimmunoassay
• TRP = transrectal palpation
• US = ultrasonography, ultrasound

Suggested Reading
Bucca S. Equine fetal gender determination from mid- to advanced-gestation by ultrasound. Theriogenology 2005;64(3):568–571.

Ginther OJ. Reproductive Biology of the Mare, 2e. Cross Plains, WI: Equiservices, 1992.
McCue PM, McKinnon AO. Pregnancy examination. In: McKinnon AO, Squires EL, Vaala WE, Varner DD, eds. Equine Reproduction, 2e. Ames, IA: Wiley Blackwell, 2011:2245–2261.
Sitters S. Palpation of the pregnant mare per rectum. In: Dascanio J, McCue P, eds. Equine Reproductive Procedures. Ames, IA: Wiley Blackwell, 2014:185–187.

Author Carla L. Carleton
Consulting Editor Carla L. Carleton
Acknowledgment The author/editor acknowledges the prior contribution of Margo L. Macpherson.

P

PREMATURE PLACENTAL SEPARATION

BASICS

DEFINITION
• Premature detachment of the CA membrane from the endometrium before delivery of the term fetus. • The CA is responsible for supplying the fetus with oxygen and nutrients and for removing its waste products; with PPS (e.g. parturition late stage 1, early stage 2), the fetus may die unless immediate aid in delivery is provided

PATHOPHYSIOLOGY
• Proposed origins—alterations in the CA membrane in the area of the internal cervical os or abnormal attachment of the CA membrane to the endometrium, predisposing to PPS. • Occurs secondary to cervical relaxation (hormonal, ascending infection, cervical incompetency) and development of low-grade placentitis

INCIDENCE/PREVALENCE
• Incidence increases significantly with induction of parturition. • Incidence of <1% in medium-sized to large breeds of horses; higher in miniature horses

SIGNALMENT
All ages and breeds; increased occurrence in miniature horses.

SIGNS
• An emergency—abrupt reduction in O_2 delivery to the fetus, immediate delivery assistance is essential as soon as the CA membrane protrudes through the vulvar lips. • Often a history of PPS. • Physical examination findings are normal. • CA membrane, when presented at the vulva, may appear to be characteristically red, velvety, and roughened

CAUSES
• Miniature horses. • Induction of parturition. • Older mares. • Placentitis, high-risk pregnancy

RISK FACTORS
See Causes.

DIAGNOSIS

DIFFERENTIAL DIAGNOSIS
• Evagination of the vaginal wall. • Eversion of the urinary bladder. • Prolapse of the vaginal wall. • Lacerations of the vaginal wall and prolapse of the intestines

CBC/BIOCHEMISTRY/URINALYSIS
N/A

OTHER LABORATORY TESTS
N/A

IMAGING
US
• Prepartum examination may reveal an area of detachment cranial to the cervix (ventral aspect of the uterine body and its placental attachment), which also may indicate a mare at risk for placentitis; record combined thickness of uterus and placenta to assess the severity of placentitis. • Intrapartum appearance of the CA membrane protruding through the vulvar lips (i.e. "red velvet" or "red bagging") is diagnostic in itself.

OTHER DIAGNOSTIC PROCEDURES
Best diagnostic method—visual examination of the exposed tissue.

PATHOLOGIC FINDINGS
N/A

TREATMENT
When PPS is observed, tear the CA membrane, then the amniotic membrane (closest sac) surrounding the fetus and assist in its delivery.

APPROPRIATE HEALTH CARE
N/A

CLIENT EDUCATION
• Knowledge regarding the normal appearance of a placenta at term. • With normal parturition—CA first to break = *breaking water*, but it is internal. When it tears (following pressure by fetal extremities), allantoic fluid is observed in a *gush*, but not the membrane at that time. The first membrane observed at the vulva should be the amnion—smooth and white, opaque, or pale pink. • Any reddish or roughened protruding membrane indicates a problem requiring immediate action (it is the CA). • This is a true emergency. Because of fetal hypoxia, insufficient time is available to seek outside assistance and still deliver a live foal. • Examine the placenta when freshly delivered, serves as an excellent teaching tool to educate clients regarding what is normal vs. abnormal. • If PPS is observed and the client cannot/will not tear the CA and assist in delivery, instruct the client to walk the mare until the veterinarian arrives. ○ May reduce further/full abdominal contractions and thus decrease further/full placental separation (still only partial usefulness) for a few minutes until your arrival

MEDICATIONS

DRUG(S) OF CHOICE
N/A

CONTRAINDICATIONS/POSSIBLE INTERACTIONS
Oxytocin is contraindicated before fetus has been delivered.

FOLLOW-UP

PATIENT MONITORING
• Mares do well after delivery. • If alive when delivered, the neonate can suffer permanent damage due to O_2 deprivation during delivery

PREVENTION/AVOIDANCE
• No known method to prevent this condition. • Observe parturition for any mare with a history of PPS

POSSIBLE COMPLICATIONS
• Mare—none. • Fetus—this is a high-risk delivery; death caused by lack of oxygenation; dummy foal postpartum; prepare for neonatal intensive care.

EXPECTED COURSE AND PROGNOSIS
Delayed delivery results in hypoxia, and either a *dummy foal* and/or fetal death.

MISCELLANEOUS

ASSOCIATED CONDITIONS
N/A

AGE-RELATED FACTORS
N/A

ZOONOTIC POTENTIAL
N/A

PREGNANCY/FERTILITY/BREEDING
Only occurs at the end of gestation.

SYNONYMS
• Red bag.
• Red bagging

SEE ALSO
• Dystocia.
• Prolonged pregnancy

ABBREVIATIONS
• CA = chorioallantoic/chorioallantois.
• PPS = premature placental separation.
• US = ultrasound, ultrasonography

Suggested Reading
Bucca S, Fogarty U, Collins A, Small V. Assessment of feto-placental well-being in the mare from mid-gestation to term: transrectal and transabdominal ultrasonographic features. Theriogenology 2005;64:542–557.
Cheong SH, Lawlis SM, Gilbert RO. Parturition augmentation in mares—efficacy and safety. Clin Theriogenol 2015;7(3):303.
Roberts SJ. Veterinary Obstetrics and Genital Diseases (Theriogenology), 3e. Woodstock, VT: SJ Roberts, 1986:251–252.

Author Carla L. Carleton
Consulting Editor Carla L. Carleton
Acknowledgment The author/editor acknowledges the prior contribution of Walter R. Threlfall.

P

PREMATURITY/DYSMATURITY IN FOALS

BASICS

DEFINITION
• *Prematurity*—condition resulting from preterm birth (<320 days of gestation or less than a mare's normal gestational length). Normal 306–390 days in Thoroughbred mares
• *Dysmaturity*—condition in which foals are born after their expected gestational length, but are small and have some physical characteristics of premature foals. This definition typically includes foals with some degree of intrauterine growth retardation

PATHOPHYSIOLOGY
• Typically, prematurity/dysmaturity results from placental insufficiency, umbilical abnormalities, maternal infection, fetal disease, or iatrogenic induction of parturition
• Any cause of insufficiency of the uteroplacental unit can affect its functional ability; diffusion of substances between the maternal and fetal circulation is disrupted and nutrient delivery, oxygen supply, and waste removal are reduced
• The final maturation of the foal's HPA axis occurs during the later stages of pregnancy. Any stressors to the fetus, either fetal or maternal in origin, can induce premature maturation of the fetal HPA axis and can culminate in a premature or dysmature foal

SYSTEMS AFFECTED
• Renal/urologic—placental insufficiency may decrease creatinine clearance from the fetus
• Gastrointestinal—intestinal motility dysfunction, gas accumulation, fecal retention, and gastric distention. In severe cases may develop necrotizing enterocolitis
• Endocrine/metabolic—insulin and glucose dysregulation, ACTH and cortisol dysregulation, and thermoregulatory abnormalities (related to triiodothyronine levels)
• Neuromuscular—weak, sometimes display signs of PAS
• Musculoskeletal—failure of ossification of cuboidal bones
• Cardiovascular—cardiovascular collapse and inconsistent response to vasoactive therapy

GENETICS
No known genetic predilection.

INCIDENCE/PREVALENCE
Out of a large subset of hospitalized foals, the prevalence of prematurity was 11–15% (unpublished).

GEOGRAPHIC DISTRIBUTION
N/A

SIGNALMENT
Breed Predilections
No known breed predilection.

Mean Age and Range
Neonates

Predominant Sex
None known.

SIGNS
General Comments
Premature and dysmature foals are difficult to distinguish from one another from examination findings alone. Typically, foals are considered dysmature when signs of prematurity are present in a foal of normal gestational length.

Historical Findings
Born earlier or later than expected, smaller than expected gestational size, history of maternal illness.

Physical Examination Findings
• Affected foals often have a low birth weight and are small in size; they may be thin with poor body condition, muscle weakness, and poor muscular development
• They often display a weak or uncoordinated suckle, have a slower than normal righting reflex, are slow to stand and nurse, and have thermoregulatory abnormalities, GI tract dysfunction, renal dysfunction, and poor glucose regulation
• Other findings may include periarticular laxity, hypotonia, a highly compliant thoracic wall, ± low lung compliance ("stiff lung"), a short, silky haircoat, domed forehead, entropion ± corneal ulceration, soft, floppy ears, and occasionally meconium staining

CAUSES
• An underlying cause is often not specifically determined
• Placental insufficiency or infection—premature placental separation, placentitis, twins
• Maternal illness—placentitis, systemic disease (colic, endotoxemia, etc.), chronic malnourishment or debilitating disease, pelvic anatomic abnormalities, uterine torsion, mare reproductive loss syndrome
• Fetal abnormalities—sepsis (bacterial or viral), malformation, hydrops amnion, umbilical abnormalities, endophyte-infected fescue toxicosis, congenital hypothyroidism (related to nitrate consumption by mare or iodine imbalances)
• Iatrogenic—inappropriate induction of parturition with exogenous oxytocin or prostaglandins or premature cesarean section
• Unknown/idiopathic

RISK FACTORS
• Poor reproductive conformation
• Older age of the dam

DIAGNOSIS

DIFFERENTIAL DIAGNOSIS
• PAS
• Neonatal septicemia

CBC/BIOCHEMISTRY/URINALYSIS
• Neutrophil to lymphocyte ratio <1 predicts a poorer prognosis. If white blood cell count does not improve within 24–48 h, then prognosis is poorer
• Mean cell volume is higher in premature foals (>39 fL/cell)
• Difficulty regulating glucose and insulin levels within first 24–48 h
• Azotemia due to placental insufficiency

OTHER LABORATORY TESTS
Increased plasma fibrinogen levels suggest adequate HPA axis maturation and in utero fetal immune response. Increased fibrinogen is a good prognosticator.

IMAGING
Radiography
• Radiograph carpi and tarsi to assess for incomplete ossification of cuboidal bones
• Thoracic radiography may be useful (at 24 h and 3–5 days later) to monitor lung maturity
US
• Thoracic US can be difficult to interpret in neonatal foals due to recumbent lung atelectasis and/or mild fluid retention
• Abdominal US may help identify pneumatosis intestinalis or necrotizing enterocolitis

OTHER DIAGNOSTIC PROCEDURES
Additional tests such as echocardiography, ECG, blood pressure monitoring, and endoscopy (gastroscopy/duodenoscopy) may be indicated based on clinical signs.

PATHOLOGIC FINDINGS
There are no pathognomonic pathologic findings associated with these conditions.

TREATMENT

APPROPRIATE HEALTH CARE
Inpatient medical management at a referral hospital is typically indicated for premature or dysmature neonatal foals. If adequately mature for the gestational age, a foal may be managed in the field with intensive nursing care, appropriate environmental conditions, and veterinary oversight.

NURSING CARE
• Keep the neonate clean and dry and in a heavily bedded or padded environment. Maintain in sternal recumbency if recumbent
• Stand the recumbent foal frequently to help strengthen its muscles and tendons. If sufficient tendon laxity is present, light, protective bandages on the distal limbs can help prevent decubiti
• Closely monitor for decubiti and corneal ulcers if the foal is recumbent
• Warmed crystalloid fluids are typically necessary for the first several days of life for both hydration and nutritional support.

P

PREMATURITY/DYSMATURITY IN FOALS (CONTINUED)

Avoid overhydration as it may cause pulmonary edema in affected foals

ACTIVITY
Supervised, controlled exercise can benefit foals, especially if they have failure of ossification of cuboidal bones. Ossification is stimulated by weight-bearing, but the foal must be supervised to help ensure its limbs stay in a normal position to avoid crush syndrome.

DIET
• If the foal is not able to nurse independently or has an uncoordinated suckle, an indwelling nasogastric tube should be placed and the foal fed mare's milk every 2–3 h
• Fluids with dextrose or parenteral nutrition may be necessary depending on the physiologic state of the foal. See chapter Nutrition in foals.

CLIENT EDUCATION
Discuss overall prognosis with the owner. Performance-limiting problems may arise secondary to severe respiratory disease or failure of ossification of cuboidal bones.

SURGICAL CONSIDERATIONS
N/A

MEDICATIONS

DRUG(S) OF CHOICE
• General supportive care, adequate fluid, and nutritional and metabolic support are the mainstays of therapy for this condition. Oxygen and pressor therapy may also be necessary
• Medications should be used depending on the clinical problems in the premature/dysmature foal. Many premature and dysmature foals can have signs of PAS, septicemia, multiorgan dysfunction, or other conditions. Treatments for the aforementioned conditions are discussed in other chapters

CONTRAINDICATIONS
N/A

PRECAUTIONS
N/A

POSSIBLE INTERACTIONS
N/A

ALTERNATIVE DRUGS
N/A

FOLLOW-UP

PATIENT MONITORING
• Assess ability to stand and nurse and coordination of suckle, with attention to signs of aspiration

• Monitor body temperature; affected neonates may have difficulty thermoregulating for the first 24–48 h
• Daily (or more frequent) electrolyte, blood gas, urine output, urine specific gravity, and body weight measurements
• Monitor for secondary disease states such as septicemia, uroabdomen, pneumatosis intestinalis, and evidence of PAS
• Monitor fecal output and tolerance of feeding (e.g. signs of colic, gastric reflux) to assess GI function
• Cortisol response to exogenously administered ACTH may be useful for prognostication (typically poor response)

PREVENTION/AVOIDANCE
Any mare that gives birth to a premature or dysmature foal should be considered high risk for future pregnancies. The mare should have a reproductive soundness examination performed before rebreeding and future pregnancies should be closely monitored.

POSSIBLE COMPLICATIONS
Long-term complications of prematurity or dysmaturity may include:
• Organ dysfunction (renal, GI, neurologic)
• Respiratory distress syndrome (less likely if gestation >300 days)
• Angular or flexural limb deformities
• Neonatal septicemia
• Uroabdomen
• Meconium aspiration
• Acute death if severely affected

EXPECTED COURSE AND PROGNOSIS
• The clinical course of a premature or dysmature foal is largely dependent on its degree of endocrinologic maturity at birth, physical maturity, and the influence of other stresses such as asphyxia, septicemia, or meconium aspiration
• Fetuses exposed to chronic intrauterine stress (i.e. placentitis) may show improvement after 24 h of supportive care
• Foals with incomplete HPA axis maturation fail to improve and begin to progressively develop abnormalities including weakness, obtundation, seizures, respiratory difficulty or failure, feeding intolerance, and cardiovascular collapse
• Survival rate 80–85% with intensive care and lack of uncontrolled septicemia. Most of these foals have successful athletic careers

MISCELLANEOUS

ASSOCIATED CONDITIONS
• PAS
• Neonatal septicemia
• Pneumatosis intestinalis or necrotizing enterocolitis

• Incomplete ossification of cuboidal bones
• Neonatal equine respiratory distress syndrome
• Omphalophlebitis
• Uroabdomen
• Entropion and corneal ulceration

AGE-RELATED FACTORS
Gestational age at birth is not as important as once thought at predicting long-term outcome. Fetal readiness for birth can vary depending on underlying cause and rapidity of parturition following an adverse event.

ZOONOTIC POTENTIAL
N/A

PREGNANCY/FERTILITY/BREEDING
N/A

SYNONYMS
N/A

SEE ALSO
• Failure of transfer of passive immunity (FTPI)
• Nutrition in foals
• Septicemia, neonate

ABBREVIATIONS
• ACTH = adrenocorticotropic hormone
• GI = gastrointestinal
• HPA = hypothalamic–pituitary–adrenal
• PAS = perinatal asphyxia syndrome
• US = ultrasonography, ultrasound

Internet Resources
Palmer J, Prematurity, dysmaturity, and postmaturity in foals. http://nicuvet.com/nicuvet/Equine-Perinatoloy/NICU%20Lectures/Prematurity.pdf
Palmer J, Approach to fluid therapy in neonates. http://nicuvet.com/nicuvet/Equine-Perinatoloy/Web_slides_meetings/VECCS%202002/Practical%20Approach%20to%20Fluid%20Thera.pdf

Suggested Reading
Lester G. Maturity of the neonatal foal. Vet Clin North Am Equine Pract 2005;21(2):333–355.
McKenzie III H, Geor R. Feeding management of sick neonatal foals. Vet Clin North Am Equine Pract 2009;25(1):109–119.
Smith P. Prematurity and dysmaturity of foals. Resort Proc Am Assoc Equine Pract 2016;18:41–43.

Author Rachel S. Liepman
Consulting Editor Margaret C. Mudge

PREPUBIC TENDON RUPTURE

BASICS

DEFINITION
Prepubic tendon separates from its attachment to the cranial pubis.

PATHOPHYSIOLOGY
• Weight of the mare's abdomen, enlarging fetus, fetal fluids and membranes, and accumulating ventral abdominal edema place pressure on the prepubic tendon's pelvic attachment that surpasses the tendon's load limit. • Partial tear, half, or full rupture. • Abdominal wall falls ventrally as the tendon tears away from the pubis

SYSTEMS AFFECTED
• Musculoskeletal. • Reproductive

GENETICS
N/A

INCIDENCE/PREVALENCE
Extremely low.

SIGNALMENT
• All breeds; all of breeding age. • Older mares at increased risk. • Late/near-term pregnant mare. • Male prepubic tendon may rupture after severe trauma

SIGNS

General Comments
• Usually advanced pregnancy with twins, hydrops, or other cause for an enlarged uterus. • May occur after severe trauma

Historical Findings
• Mares usually present with a slowly enlarging, but very noticeably enlarged, abdomen. • Discomfort; difficulty breathing, or reluctance to lie recumbent

Physical Examination Findings
• Dependent edema of ventral abdomen may extend to/involve the legs. • Distinct profile viewed from the side—ventral abdominal line appears flat, no rise in the flank region by the udder. • Udder loses its normal orientation—its anterior aspect slants steeply down and lies at a lower point than its posterior aspect. • Definition between udder and abdominal wall is absent. • Transrectal palpation of the rupture may not be possible while the mare is pregnant. • Can identify intestines immediately below the skin, i.e. outside the abdominal musculature; indicates rupture of the tendon or abdominal wall

CAUSES
Excessive pressure/weight on the abdominal wall.

RISK FACTORS
• Twins or triplets pregnancy. • Excessive fluid accumulation—see Pathophysiology

DIAGNOSIS

• See Physical Examination Findings. • Determine degree of tear—partial, half (1 side), full

DIFFERENTIAL DIAGNOSIS
• Abdominal wall rupture. • Tearing of the muscles near the prepubic tendon; may be impossible to distinguish from actual tendon rupture

IMAGING
Abdominal ultrasonographic examination may confirm abdominal viscera immediately under the skin near the udder.

PATHOLOGIC FINDINGS
Tearing or rupture of the prepubic tendon.

TREATMENT

APPROPRIATE HEALTH CARE
• With complete rupture, the mare loses abdominal press needed for active labor, cannot expel the fetus at term. • Once *assisted delivery* is complete, a more accurate assessment can be made to determine if there are any realistic surgical options

NURSING CARE
• Keep mare off surfaces that could put her at risk of falling and/or further damage—slippery, angled, uneven. • Prevent rolling, if possible. • Close observation for intestinal obstruction or parturition, dystocia. • Consider use of trusses or supportive devices, but: ○ Problems may result from transferring all the abdominal weight and its contents onto the mare's back, plus increasing pressure on the ventral abdomen and its contents as they lose their normal orientation and position within the abdomen

ACTIVITY
Restrict exercise to hand-walking.

DIET
Changes in diet may be indicated; reduce additional abdominal cavity bulk.

CLIENT EDUCATION
Discuss the mare's impaired ability to participate in active labor if she loses her intact abdominal wall.

SURGICAL CONSIDERATIONS
• Dependent on degree of tissue damage as determined postpartum and the mare's value; incomplete tear—may survive well. • Reproductive life of the mare will be limited to embryo transfer if repair is possible. • The mare is not a candidate to be bred/carry a pregnancy ever again

MEDICATIONS

DRUG(S) OF CHOICE
Diuretics (e.g. furosemide) may reduce edema in dependent areas.

CONTRAINDICATIONS
Avoid any medications with detrimental fetal effects.

PRECAUTIONS
• Goal of mare care—medical stabilization. • Prepare and observe mare for an attended, induced, and assisted parturition

FOLLOW-UP

PATIENT MONITORING
Close observation is essential.

PREVENTION/AVOIDANCE
Terminate pregnancy in seriously at-risk mares before prepubic tendon ruptures.

POSSIBLE COMPLICATIONS
Mares may die prepartum or postpartum from gastrointestinal complications or rupture of the uterine or middle uterine arteries.

EXPECTED COURSE AND PROGNOSIS
• High probability of survival if managed properly. • Many do well after delivery without surgical repair if partial tendon rupture, if not rebred

MISCELLANEOUS

ASSOCIATED CONDITIONS
Any conditions that increase size and weight of the pregnant uterus.

PREGNANCY/FERTILITY/BREEDING
• Usually associated with the late-pregnant mare. • May occur in any horse that has suffered a severe, traumatic abdominal injury

SEE ALSO
• Dystocia.
• Prolonged pregnancy

Suggested Reading
Morrison MJW, Back B, McClure T, et al. Hydroallantois and prepubic tendon rupture in a Standardbred mare. Clin Theriogenol 2016;8(3):359.
Nahachewsky S, Card C, Manning S, et al. Prepubic tendon rupture in late term mares—a genetic link? Clin Theriogenol 2013;5(3):411.

Author Carla L. Carleton
Consulting Editor Carla L. Carleton
Acknowledgment The author/editor acknowledges the prior contribution of Walter R. Threlfall.

P

PRIAPISM

BASICS

OVERVIEW
- Persistent erection with engorgement of the CCP, in the absence of sexual arousal
- The pudendal nerves control the smooth muscles of the arteries that supply and the veins that drain the CCP
- *Parasympathetic* stimulation of the pudendal nerves causes arterial dilation and venous constriction to/from the CCP to promote erection
  - Allows relaxation of the retractor penis muscles (causing penile prolapse) and the smooth muscle cells (allows CCP to fill with blood)
- *Detumescence* is thought to be under sympathetic control
  - Agents/conditions interfering with sympathetic stimulation are thought to directly or indirectly block detumescence
  - When detumescence fails CO_2 tension in the CCP increases, causing increased blood viscosity and red blood cell sludging and further occlusion of venous outflow from the CCP

SIGNALMENT
Predominantly in stallions; geldings can be affected.

SIGNS
- Protruded, erect penis
- Distended CCP can be detected by digital palpation if partial
- Traumatic lesions may be present

CAUSES AND RISK FACTORS
- Most common—phenothiazine derivatives that block the α-adrenergic impulse to cause detumescence
  - Propiopromazine HCl, chlorpromazine HCl, acepromazine maleate
- Spinal cord injury or disease
- Other causes are rare and include general anesthesia, neoplasia, infectious diseases, postcastration complications, and nematodiasis of the spinal cord

DIAGNOSIS

DIFFERENTIAL DIAGNOSIS
Differentiating Similar Signs
- Paraphimosis is the prolapse of the penis and prepuce, with extensive edema of those tissues

- Penile paralysis is differentiated by a *flaccid* prolapsed penis

TREATMENT

- Massage, hydrotherapy, and application of an emollient dressing to the penis
- Elevate the penis in a sling to prevent further complications
- Physical replacement in the prepuce under general anesthesia if acute
- Flushing the CCP with heparinized saline (10 IU sodium heparin/mL 0.9% saline) using 12 G needles:
  - Proximal to the glans penis (ingress) and at the level of the ischium (egress)
  - When unresponsive to cholinergic blocking or α-adrenergic agents
- Vascular shunt created between the CCP and corpus spongiosum penis—efficacy unknown
- Chronic cases with detumescence may need surgery:
  - Circumcision (reefing)
  - Retraction (Bolz technique) to retain the penis within the prepuce
  - Penile amputation

MEDICATIONS

DRUG(S) OF CHOICE
- A cholinergic blocker (benztropine mesylate (benzatropine) 8 mg IV slow administration) for acute priapism caused by the administration of α-adrenergic blocking agents (e.g. phenothiazine TQ)
- Injection of 10 mg of 1% phenylephrine HCl (an α-adrenergic agent) directly into the CCP during the acute phase if unresponsive to cholinergic blocking agents
- Topical or systemic antibiotics for superficial or deep lacerations
- Anti-inflammatory medication if secondary paraphimosis or intractable inflammation exists

CONTRAINDICATIONS/POSSIBLE INTERACTIONS
- Phenothiazine TQ
- Avoid benztropine mesylate and phenylephrine HCl in patients with tachycardia or hypertension

ALTERNATIVE DRUGS
- β_2-agonist clenbuterol but efficacy is unknown

FOLLOW-UP

PATIENT MONITORING
- Hospitalization may be needed
- Pain and discomfort are managed with physical therapy
- Successful reduction of the erection and return of the penis to the prepuce are considered good prognostic indicators

PREVENTION/AVOIDANCE
Avoid use of phenothiazine TQ.

POSSIBLE COMPLICATIONS
- Chronic priapism may cause inflammation of the pudendal nerve, causing malfunction of the retractor penis muscles and permanent penile paralysis
- Secondary paraphimosis may develop as dependent edema accumulates
- Impotence can occur as a result of desensitization of the glans penis (nerve damage) or fibrosis of the CCP (nerve damage)

EXPECTED COURSE AND PROGNOSIS
- Prognosis for life is generally good. Return to fertility depends on extent of lesions and complications
- Erection and ejaculation can be stimulated by the use of topical testosterone cream and use of a tricyclic antidepressant in stallions with impotence

MISCELLANEOUS

ASSOCIATED CONDITIONS
- Paraphimosis
- Penile paralysis

SEE ALSO
- Paraphimosis
- Penile paralysis

ABBREVIATIONS
- CCP = corpus cavernosum penis
- TQ = tranquilizer

Internet Resources
Vet Folio, Priapism in horses. http://www.vetfolio.com/reproduction/update-on-equine-therapeutics-priapism-in-horses

Author Ahmed Tibary
Consulting Editor Carla L. Carleton
Acknowledgment The author and editor acknowledge the prior contribution of Carole C. Miller.

PRIMARY HYPERPARATHYROIDISM

BASICS

OVERVIEW
• PHPT is caused by excessive and autonomous secretion of PTH by hyperplastic or neoplastic parathyroid chief cells. Excessive PTH secretion originates from parathyroid hyperplasia, adenoma, or adenocarcinoma. This results in hypercalcemia (due to increased renal calcium reabsorption and excessive bone resorption), hypophosphatemia (due to decreased renal phosphorus reabsorption), and excessive bone loss
• Systems affected—endocrine and musculoskeletal

SIGNALMENT
• Any sex or breed
• Reported in aged equids

SIGNS
• Intermittent weakness
• Weight loss
• Anorexia
• Enlargement of facial bones
• Shifting lameness
• Difficult mastication

CAUSES AND RISK FACTORS
Excessive, uncontrolled secretion of PTH by chief cells of 1 or more parathyroid glands.

DIAGNOSIS

DIFFERENTIAL DIAGNOSIS
• Fibrous osteodystrophy may result from NSHPT in horses fed diets with excessive phosphorus, phytates, or oxalates, or low in calcium. However, depending on the cause, (phosphorus vs. oxalates), hypocalcemia (or normocalcemia) with variable phosphorus concentrations is consistent with NSHPT
• HHM from tumors (e.g. lymphoma, carcinomas) secreting PTHrP can lead to hypercalcemia and hypophosphatemia. PTHrP binds the PTH receptor. PTH is low and PTHrP high with HHM
• Other causes of hypercalcemia—chronic renal failure and hypervitaminosis D
• Normal serum blood urea nitrogen, creatinine concentration, and urine specific gravity rule out chronic renal failure
• Ingestion of oxalate-containing plants and vitamin D toxicosis can be eliminated based on history. In addition, vitamin D toxicosis is characterized by hyperphosphatemia

CBC/BIOCHEMISTRY/URINALYSIS
• Hypercalcemia, hypophosphatemia, and hyperphosphaturia are characteristic

• Hyperchloremic metabolic acidosis has been associated

OTHER LABORATORY TESTS
• Fractional excretion of phosphorus (reference range 0.0–0.5%) is increased
• PTH (increased) and PTHrP (normal)

IMAGING
• Decreased bone density of appendicular and axial bones, which becomes evident when >30% of bone mass is lost. Skull radiography may reveal radiolucency, fibrous proliferation of facial bones, and loss of the lamina dura surrounding premolars and molars
• Endoscopic examination may reveal narrowing of the nasal passages
• Nuclear scintigraphy using technetium (^{99m}Tc) sestamibi and ultrasonography may help identify adenomas

OTHER DIAGNOSTIC PROCEDURES
Horses have 2 pairs of parathyroid glands—the cranial pair is adjacent to the cranial pole of the thyroid gland and the caudal pair has variable location along the trachea to the thoracic inlet. Biopsy is indicated in any mass in these locations in a horse with signs of PHPT.

PATHOLOGIC FINDINGS
• Parathyroid gland chief cell hyperplasia, adenoma, or adenocarcinoma
• Equine parathyroid glands may be difficult to distinguish from surrounding tissues
• With parathyroid neoplasia, atrophy of the nonaffected parathyroid tissue is expected
• Single or multiple glands may be affected

TREATMENT
• Surgical removal of the affected parathyroid gland and medical treatment for hypercalcemia
• Hypocalcemia may develop after removal of affected parathyroid gland
• Reduce calcium intake in animals with hypercalcemia
• Long-term follow-up is recommended as adenomas may develop in other parathyroid glands, based on other species
• IV fluid therapy may promote calcium excretion

MEDICATIONS

DRUG(S) OF CHOICE
• Diuretics and corticosteroids may promote calcium excretion

• Vitamin D analogs may be considered to suppress parathyroid gland function. Drugs that reduce osteoclast activity/bone resorption (e.g. bisphosphonates) should be considered

FOLLOW-UP
• Monitor electrolytes, acid–base status, bone density, and PTH concentrations
• Possible complications—difficulty chewing because of loosening teeth and lameness secondary to osteopenia

MISCELLANEOUS

SEE ALSO
• Calcium, hypercalcemia
• Chronic kidney disease
• Lymphosarcoma
• Phosphorus, hypophosphatemia

ABBREVIATIONS
• HHM = humoral hypercalcemia of malignancy
• NSHPT = nutritional secondary hyperparathyroidism
• PHPT = primary hyperparathyroidism
• PTH = parathyroid hormone
• PTHrP = PTH-related protein

Suggested Reading
Frank N, Hawkins JF, Couëtil LL, Raymond JT. Primary hyperparathyroidism with osteodystrophia fibrosa of the facial bones in a pony. J Am Vet Med Assoc 1998;212: 84–86.
Tomlinson JE, Johnson AL, Ross MW, et al. Successful detection and removal of a functional parathyroid adenoma in a pony using technetium Tc-99 m sestamibi scintigraphy. J Vet Intern Med 2014;28:687–692.
Toribio RE. Disorders of calcium and phosphate metabolism in horses. Vet Clin North Am Equine Pract 2011;27:129–147.
Wong D, Sponseller B, Miles K, et al. Failure of technetium Tc99m sestamibi scanning to detect abnormal parathyroid tissue in a horse and a mule with primary hyperparathyroidism. J Vet Intern Med 2004;18:589–593.

Author Ramiro Toribio
Consulting Editors Michel Levy and Heidi Banse
Acknowledgment The author and editors acknowledge the prior contribution of Laurent Couëtil.

P

PROBIOTICS IN FOALS AND HORSES

 BASICS

DEFINITION
In 1908 Elie Metchnikoff, a Russian researcher, studied the longevity of Bulgarians. He attributed their longevity and health to consumption of large amounts of bacterially fermented milk. The bacterium responsible for milk fermentation was given the name *Bacillus bulgaricus* and he defined this "probiotic" as "live microorganisms, which exhibit a health promoting effect." The World Health Organization modified this initial definition in 2008 to "[l]ive microorganisms which when administered in adequate amounts confer a health benefit on the host."

BACTERIAL STRAINS USED
Potential probiotic strains should be able to survive the gastric environment, have antimicrobial properties, adhere to mucus and epithelial cells, and have properties to withstand the rigors of production. Both bacteria and yeast are used as microbial feed additives; the most common are *Saccharomyces* (yeast), *Lactobacillus*, *Escherichia coli*, *Enterococcus*, *Bacillus*, *Streptococcus*, and *Bifidobacterium*. These were initially selected based on knowledge from human medicine, as lactobacilli and bifidobacteria are particularly abundant in the human small intestine. Recent advances in knowledge of the microbiome have shown that the main species associated with GI health in horses are from the families Lachnospiraceae and Ruminococcaceae, of the order Clostridiales, which none of the above-described species belong to.

SURVIVAL IN THE GI TRACT
Colonization is superior to mere survival in the GI tract, as probiotics can act longer beyond the period of administration. Generally, host-specific strains are believed to be able to colonize the GI tract of the indigenous host for longer periods of time. Probiotic strains can be recovered from feces of adults for ≈ 1 week. In foals fecal recovery tends to be longer, up to 3 weeks.

MECHANISMS OF ACTION
There are 3 main mechanisms of action by which probiotics prevent colonization of the digestive tract by pathogenic strains or prevent disease:
• Modulation of the host innate and acquired immune system—the immune system constantly samples the antigens present in the GI lumen and reacts with local and systemic modifications to the immune system
• Antimicrobial action—some probiotics produce metabolites that are active against pathogenic bacteria and their toxins
• Competitive exclusion, also termed colonization resistance—probiotics compete with pathogens for nutrients and take up ecologic niches to prevent proliferation of pathogenic bacteria

Many reported mechanisms of action of probiotics are based on in vitro studies only, and extrapolation of these results to in vivo conditions is controversial. Some evidence also has been generated by in vivo studies performed in laboratory animals or humans.

REGULATION AND QUALITY CONTROL
In North America probiotics can be classified as dietary or feed supplements "generally regarded as safe" (GRAS). They do not need to go through the process of drug approval. The US Food and Drug Administration only requires that supplements be labeled in a truthful and not misleading manner; however, even this rule is not rigorously enforced. For example, probiotics are not allowed to contain the claim "health promoting" on the label, but many products with such a claim are on the market.

Manufacturers of over-the-counter products in North America have no obligation to perform quality control of their products. Consequently, in North America, there are numerous probiotic products for use in horses that can be obtained over the counter, and claim to benefit the horse in various ways. Studies have shown that quality control of the contents of probiotics is poor. Only 2/13 (15%) of veterinary and human probiotics contained the specified organism concentration indicated on the product label. Some were missing organisms entirely or contained too little or too much of an active ingredient. Actual bacterial concentrations ranged from 0% to 215% of claimed amounts. All veterinary products contained <2% of the listed concentrations. Additionally, peer-reviewed published studies proving the efficacy of these products are limited, and in most cases lacking. Based on these limitations currently the use of over-the-counter commercial probiotics cannot be recommended for research or in a clinical setting.

In Europe probiotics are marketed as feed additives and are regulated by the EU. Since 2010 new probiotic supplements can only be marketed if they adhere to EU legislation 1831/2003. Products are licensed for a specific species, indication, and for a maximum duration of 10 years. There are currently only 4 products for horses on the market.

EVIDENCE FOR USE
The scope of the current literature about equine probiotics use has focused mainly on GI disease application. Although some studies have shown beneficial effects of probiotics, other studies could not corroborate these results. Overall, few studies are available, and these cannot be compared easily because of differences in study design and formulations used.

Therapy for Acute Colitis
The results from 2 available studies are equivocal. In 1 study there was no beneficial effect of probiotic administration. In the second study probiotic-treated horses had a shorter duration of diarrhea; however, there was no effect on survival or duration of stay in the clinic. Both studies had low case numbers, making the results questionable.

Prevention of Neonatal Diarrhea
There is currently not enough evidence that probiotics had a beneficial effect on prevention of neonatal foal diarrhea from the 4 available studies—2 studies showed a potentially harmful effect on the foals, with increasing incidence of severe diarrhea, while 1 study showed no effect and only 1 study reported a decrease in incidence of neonatal foal diarrhea.

Salmonella *Shedding*
The effect of probiotic administration on fecal *Salmonella* shedding is questionable. Of the 3 available studies only 1 study showed a reduction in *Salmonella* shedding, albeit not significant.

Sand Clearance
Probiotics have also been studied as an adjunct therapy for sand excretion. In the only available study sand excretion was increased when administering a product containing psyllium and a probiotic. It is, however, unclear if this effect was due to the psyllium or the probiotic.

Effect on the Microbiota
In humans and other animals probiotic administration has been shown to have an effect on the composition and structure of the microbiota. In horses this has only been studied in foals and an effect could not be shown.

As commercial probiotics were used in some studies, the results of these should be considered with caution owing to the lack of quality control of the products. Consequently, the current overall evidence is weak.

SAFETY AND SIDE EFFECTS
Adverse effects of probiotic administration are rare. In adult horses, there are no published reports of enteric disease after probiotic administration. Even administration of up to 3 times the manufacturer's recommended dose to 18 healthy horses did not result in any adverse effects. Some adverse effects not related to enteric disease have been reported— 1 of the horses developed hives after administration of the probiotic; however other factors could also have been responsible for these signs. The effect of probiotics in foals is likely to be different from that in adult horses owing to major difference in GI microbiota composition; 2 clinical field trials have reported an increased incidence of severe diarrhea in foals when treated with different probiotics.

RECOMMENDATIONS

At this stage the use of commercial over-the-counter probiotics cannot be recommended. Currently there is no clear evidence that probiotics have beneficial effects but they actually might cause harm, particularly in foals, and potential side effects should always be considered.

FUTURE PERSPECTIVES

The GI microbiota of humans and animals consists of thousands of microbial species. All existing probiotics contain 1 or a few strains of bacteria, constituting only a very minor component of the total intestinal microbiota. Therefore, they might have limited ability to influence an individual's microbiota. Fecal microbial transplantation, the transfer of all microorganisms from a healthy donor to a diseased recipient, could be the future of probiotic research. Alternatively, selection of bacterial strain based on the current knowledge of the microbiota could be tried. Several bacteria now known to be associated with GI health could be selected and manufactured into a probiotic product.

TREATMENT

CLIENT EDUCATION

Clients often know superficially about probiotics and consider them a "natural treatment." Clients should be made aware that there are no regulations or safety standards behind commercial probiotics and that some harm has been shown in administration of probiotics to foals. They should also be educated about the current lack of evidence of effect.

MISCELLANEOUS

SEE ALSO

- Diarrhea, neonate
- Idiopathic colitis
- Salmonellosis
- Sand impaction and enteropathy

ABBREVIATIONS

- EU = European Union
- GI = gastrointestinal

Internet Resources
N/A

Suggested Reading

Schoster AS, Weese JS, Guardabassi LG. Probiotic use in horses—what is the evidence for their clinical efficacy. J Vet Intern Med 2014;28:1640–1652.

Schoster AS, Staempfli HR, Abrahams M, et al. Effect of a probiotic on prevention of diarrhea and *Clostridium difficile* and *Clostridium perfringens* shedding in foals. J Vet Intern Med 2015;29:925–931.

Weese JS, Martin H. Assessment of commercial probiotic bacterial contents and label accuracy. Can Vet J 2011;52:43–46.

Author Angelika Schoster
Consulting Editors Henry Stämpfli and Olimpo Oliver-Espinosa

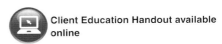

Client Education Handout available online

P

PROGRESSIVE ETHMOIDAL HEMATOMA (PEH)

BASICS

OVERVIEW
• An uncommon, slowly expanding, non-neoplastic mass originating in the submucosa of the ethmoturbinates that compresses and destroys adjacent tissue, causing signs of sinonasal disease
• May arise from the nasal or sinusal portion of the ethmoidal labyrinth; most arise from the sinusal portion
• Occasionally bilateral

SIGNALMENT
Affects horses of any age (median age, ≅10 years) or breed, affects males and females equally, and has a predilection for Arabians and Thoroughbreds. Standardbreds seem to be spared.

SIGNS
• Most common—intermittent, scanty, sanguineous nasal discharge
• Other signs—respiratory stridor, dyspnea, coughing, headshaking, and facial deformity
• May be visible at a nostril
• May cause no clinical signs, if small

CAUSES AND RISK FACTORS
None known.

DIAGNOSIS

DIFFERENTIAL DIAGNOSIS
• Other conditions that may cause sanguineous nasal discharge—sinonasal mycosis, including conidiobolomycosis; guttural pouch mycosis; facial trauma; neoplasia of any region of the respiratory tract; exercise-induced pulmonary hemorrhage; respiratory amyloidosis; and nasolacrimal duct infection
• Lesions of the nasal cavity that may resemble PEH endoscopically—polyp, fungal mass, and neoplasm

CBC/BIOCHEMISTRY/URINALYSIS
Usually normal but may reveal anemia.

IMAGING
• Radiographically, appears as an abnormal opacity of soft-tissue density, ventral and rostral to the ethmoidal labyrinth
• Positive-contrast sinusography or CT may allow more complete evaluation

OTHER DIAGNOSTIC PROCEDURES
• Rhinoscopic examination may reveal a yellow-red-green mass originating from the ethmoidal labyrinth; the origin of a large mass is often obscured

• A PEH originating from the sinusal portion of the ethmoidal labyrinth is not seen during rhinoscopy, unless it protrudes through the nasomaxillary aperture
• A PEH within the sinuses may distort the nasal passage
• Both nasal passages should be examined endoscopically because PEH may occur bilaterally
• Diagnosis is often based on clinical signs, location, and gross appearance of the lesion, but histological examination of a biopsy is confirmatory

PATHOLOGIC FINDINGS
Epithelium overlying submucosal fibrous tissue and old and recent hemorrhage, containing lymphocytes, multinucleated giant cells, and hemosiderin-filled macrophages.

TREATMENT
• Rarely resolve spontaneously
• Can be treated by ablating the PEH surgically or with a cryogen, a laser, or 10% formalin, injected into the lesion
• The PEH is ablated surgically through a frontonasal flap, with the horse anesthetized or standing. A lesion on the nasal portion of the ethmoidal labyrinth is exposed and removed by perforating the dorsal conchal sinus ventrally. Blood transfusion may be required. Surgery is accompanied by less hemorrhage when performed with the horse standing
• Can be ablated with a cryogen. This treatment causes minimal hemorrhage and can be performed with the horse sedated but is useful only if the lesion is small
• A small PEH can be ablated transendoscopically using a laser with the horse sedated. Multiple treatments are required

MEDICATIONS
• A PEH on the nasal portion of the ethmoidal labyrinth is destroyed most conveniently by injecting formalin into the lesion transendoscopically with the horse sedated. A lesion in the sinuses must be accessed for injection through a trephine hole into the maxillary or conchofrontal sinus
• The PEH is injected until it distends and begins to leak formalin
• The PEH should be injected at 3–4 week intervals until it is eliminated or is so small that injection is impossible; a small PEH may cause no clinical signs of disease

FOLLOW-UP

PATIENT MONITORING
• Recurrence possible years after apparent resolution
• Examining the horse's nasal passages and sinuses radiographically or endoscopically periodically for several years may help determine if a lesion has reappeared at the same or other sites

POSSIBLE COMPLICATIONS
• Complications of surgical ablation include severe hemorrhage; encephalitis, if the PEH has eroded the cribriform plate; dehiscence of the surgical wound; septic osteitis; and suture periostitis
• Injecting formalin into a PEH that has eroded the cribriform plate may result in death. Determining if the cribriform plate has been eroded may require CT or MRI. Erosion of the cribriform plate is rare
• Injecting formalin into a PEH that has eroded the orbit may blind the eye. Erosion of the orbit is rare

EXPECTED COURSE AND PROGNOSIS
Recurrence, regardless of the type of treatment, has been reported to range from 14% to 45% and is more likely if the horse is affected bilaterally.

MISCELLANEOUS

ABBREVIATIONS
• CT = computed tomography
• MRI = magnetic resonance imaging
• PEH = progressive ethmoidal hematoma

Suggested Reading
Schumacher J, Dixon P. Progressive ethmoidal haematoma. In: McGorum B, Dixon P, Robinson E, Schumacher J, eds. Equine Respiratory Medicine and Surgery. Philadelphia, PA: WB Saunders, 2006:409–417.

Author Jim Schumacher
Consulting Editor Mathilde Leclère and Daniel Jean

Client Education Handout available online

PROLIFERATIVE OPTIC NEUROPATHY

BASICS

OVERVIEW
• A slowly enlarging, well-defined white or gray mass protruding from the edge of the optic disk into the vitreal chamber. The lesion is generally "fixed" (i.e. it does not move when the eye moves). Can be associated with superficial vascularization and small hemorrhages
• Systems affected—ophthalmic

SIGNALMENT
Primarily horses >15 years of age.

SIGNS
• None, or minimal effect on vision
• Pupillary light reflex is normal
• Generally unilateral
• No signs of pain
• Usually incidental finding

CAUSES AND RISK FACTORS
Unknown

DIAGNOSIS

DIFFERENTIAL DIAGNOSIS
• Ischemic optic neuropathy
• Exudative optic neuropathy
  ○ Traumatic optic neuropathy
• Optic nerve neoplasia—glioma, astrocytoma, medulloepithelioma, and neuroepithelioma
• Granuloma
• Abscesses

CBC/BIOCHEMISTRY/URINALYSIS
N/A

OTHER LABORATORY TESTS
N/A

IMAGING
N/A

OTHER DIAGNOSTIC PROCEDURES
N/A

PATHOLOGIC FINDINGS
• Histologically it resembles a schwannoma in many cases but may also be similar to an astrocytoma or xanthoma
• Schwannomas are well-circumscribed masses attached to peripheral nerves, cranial nerves, or spinal nerve roots. They contain areas of densely packed spindle cells intermixed with looser, myxoid regions

TREATMENT
There is no therapy for this condition.

MEDICATIONS
N/A

FOLLOW-UP

PATIENT MONITORING
Observe for vision changes.

PREVENTION/AVOIDANCE
N/A

POSSIBLE COMPLICATIONS
None

EXPECTED COURSE AND PROGNOSIS
• Excellent prognosis for vision and life
• Slowly progressive in size

MISCELLANEOUS

ASSOCIATED CONDITIONS
N/A

AGE-RELATED FACTORS
Primarily horses >15 years of age.

SEE ALSO
• Exudative optic neuropathy
• Ischemic optic neuropathy

Suggested Reading
Brooks DE. Retinopathies and ocular manifestations of systemic diseases in the horse. In: Brooks DE, ed. Ophthalmology for the Equine Practitioner, 2e. Jackson, WY: Teton NewMedia, 2008:207–225.
Dubielzig RR, Ketring K, McLellan GJ, Albert DM. Veterinary Ocular Pathology. Philadelphia, PA: WB Saunders, 2010.
Gilger BC. Equine ophthalmology. In: Gelatt KN, Gilger BC, Kern TJ, eds. Veterinary Ophthalmology, 5e. Ames, IA: Wiley Blackwell, 2013:1560–1609.
Nell B, Walde I. Posterior segment diseases. Equine Vet J Suppl 2010;37:69–79.
Wilkie DA. Diseases of the ocular posterior segment. In: Gilger BC, ed. Equine Ophthalmology, 2e. Maryland Heights, MO: Elsevier Saunders, 2011:367–396.

Author Bianca C. Martins
Consulting Editor Caryn E. Plummer
Acknowledgment The author and editor acknowledge the prior contribution of Maria Källberg and Dennis E. Brooks.

P

PROLONGED DIESTRUS

 BASICS

DEFINITION
Persistence of a CL post ovulation such that the normal return to estrus is delayed.

PATHOPHYSIOLOGY
- Post ovulation, the CL forms and secretes P_4
- In mares, the CL is refractory to a single injection of $PGF_{2\alpha}$ to cause luteolysis until >5 days post ovulation; however, serial injections can cause luteolysis in <5 days
- In the absence of pregnancy, endogenous $PGF_{2\alpha}$ is produced and released by the endometrium approximately 14–15 days post ovulation to initiate luteolysis
- The lifespan of the CL is prolonged in idiopathic/spontaneous cases, or uteropathic cases (pyometra, EED) where $P_4 > 1$ ng/mL
  - The cause is likely failure of normal $PGF_{2\alpha}$ production, and not insensitivity of the CL to $PGF_{2\alpha}$
- Persistent CL can affect 8–10% of cycles during the season, and up to 25% of cycles in the fall transition period with a CL lifespan of approximately 2 months

SYSTEMS AFFECTED
- Reproductive
- Behavioral

GENETICS
N/A

SIGNALMENT
Postpubertal mares of any breed.

SIGNS

Historical Findings
Failure to return to estrus at the expected time interval in the cyclic mare.

Physical Examination Findings
- The physical examination is usually normal
- Transrectal palpation and US are used to assess the reproductive tract:
  - 1 or more CL can be visualized as a uniformly hyperechoic area within the ovary
  - If ovulation was recent, the CL may appear as a corpus haemorrhagicum, with a hypoechoic, blood-clot appearance to the center
  - In diestrus, the uterus and cervix should be toned
  - Pregnancy should be noted if present
  - Abnormal findings (uterine fluid, cysts) should be noted in the mare's examination record
- Vaginoscopy is used to examine the vaginal vault for abnormal content and the cervix for pathology

CAUSES

Diestrus Ovulation
Diestrus ovulations (after day 10 of the cycle) can occur spontaneously in mares, resulting in an immature CL being present at the time of normal luteolysis (day 14–15).

Pregnancy
CL function continues in the presence of a conceptus until placental progestogens take over pregnancy maintenance (100–120 days).

EED
- EED after maternal recognition of pregnancy will delay luteolysis (owing to lack of $PGF_{2\alpha}$ secretion)
- If EED occurs after endometrial cup formation (35–40 days post ovulation), cyclicity will not resume until endometrial cup regression and production of eCG ceases (120–150 days post ovulation)

Uterine Infections/Endometrial Degeneration
Pyometra, endometritis, and endometrial degeneration can affect endometrial function, inhibiting normal production/secretion of $PGF_{2\alpha}$.

Iatrogenic/Pharmaceutical
- Gonadotropin-releasing hormone agonist (deslorelin) implants (not available in the USA) to induce ovulation have been associated with prolonged interovulatory intervals in the absence of pregnancy if they are not removed after ovulation. These effects are not seen with injectable formulations
- Oxytocin can prolong CL function when administered 60 IU IM daily from day 7 to day 14 post ovulation or for 29 days at any time in the cycle
- Placement of intrauterine glass marbles has prolonged CL lifespan up to 90 days in some mares
  - This treatment is no longer recommended owing to risk of complications (some marbles have shattered; uterine reactions—endometritis) and variable efficacy
- Intrauterine infusion of plant oils has also prolonged CL function in some mares

Lactation
Persistent CL can develop following the first postpartum ovulation, particularly if mares foal during winter or are in poor body condition.

RISK FACTORS
N/A

 DIAGNOSIS

DIFFERENTIAL DIAGNOSIS

Differentiating Similar Signs
Diagnosis is based on finding a normal, nonpregnant, diestrus reproductive tract coupled with a history of failure to show estrus behavior >2 weeks post ovulation and a serum progesterone concentration of >1 ng/mL. Serial TRP and US (with or without teasing) are the cornerstones to proper interpretation of the reproductive cycle of an individual mare.

Differentiating Causes
- Pregnancy and/or EED can occur in any mare that had proximity to a stallion
  - Pregnancy should be ruled out prior to any invasive diagnostics or treatments
- Pyometra/endometritis are diagnosed by TRP, US, uterine culture, and cytology/biopsy
  - See chapters Endometritis and Pyometra
- History of a normal foal heat followed by reproductive quiescence can be due to either prolonged diestrus or lactational anestrus, particularly if foaling occurred in winter without artificial light supplementation
  - These can be differentiated by TRP and US
- Performance mares may have been treated with oxytocin or have had an intrauterine marble placed to suppress estrus
  - History, TRP, and US are used to diagnose; the marble may appear with a faint shadow outline with US
  - Hysteroscopy can identify marble fragments and facilitate removal
- All other cases of prolonged CL for which a cause cannot be identified are considered idiopathic/spontaneous

CBC/BIOCHEMISTRY/URINALYSIS
N/A

OTHER LABORATORY TESTS
- Serum P_4—concentrations >1 ng/mL indicate functional luteal tissue
- Serum eCG—positive assay can determine if EED occurred after endometrial cup formation

IMAGING
N/A

OTHER DIAGNOSTIC PROCEDURES
Uterine cytology, culture, and endometrial biopsy are useful to diagnose and treat pyometra and endometritis. See chapters Endometritis and Pyometra.

PATHOLOGIC FINDINGS
N/A

 TREATMENT

- Idiopathic/spontaneous prolonged CL is treated with $PGF_{2\alpha}$
- Pregnancy should be definitively ruled out prior to treatment
- Uteropathic causes of prolonged diestrus should be treated according to the inciting cause
- Endometrial biopsy may stimulate endogenous $PGF_{2\alpha}$ release

APPROPRIATE HEALTH CARE
N/A

NURSING CARE
N/A

ACTIVITY
N/A

(CONTINUED)   **PROLONGED DIESTRUS**

DIET
N/A

CLIENT EDUCATION
N/A

SURGICAL CONSIDERATIONS
N/A

 MEDICATIONS

DRUG(S) OF CHOICE
$PGF_{2\alpha}$ (Lutalyse (Pfizer) 10 mg IM) or its
analogs are used to stimulate luteolysis:
• Mares with a responsive CL at the time of
treatment typically exhibit estrus within
2–4 days and ovulate within 6–12 days,
depending on the status of the ovarian
follicular wave at the time of treatment
• 2 doses of $PGF_{2\alpha}$ given 5 days apart are
useful, if TRP and US cannot easily or safely
be accomplished. This regimen ensures that
immature/nonresponsive luteal tissue present
at the time of the first injection has time to
mature and is able to respond to the second
injection

CONTRAINDICATIONS
$PGF_{2\alpha}$ and its analogs are contraindicated in
mares with equine asthma/
bronchoconstrictive disease.

PRECAUTIONS
• Horses
  ◦ $PGF_{2\alpha}$ causes sweating/colic-like
  symptoms due to stimulation of smooth
  muscle
  ◦ Symptomatic treatment if not resolved in
  1–2 h
• Humans
  ◦ $PGF_{2\alpha}$ should not be handled by pregnant
  women, or persons with asthma/bronchial
  disease
  ◦ Any skin exposure should be washed off
  immediately

POSSIBLE INTERACTIONS
N/A

ALTERNATIVE DRUGS
Cloprostenol sodium (Estrumate
(Schering-Plough Animal Health) 250 µg/mL
IM) is a $PGF_{2\alpha}$ analog.
• This product is used in similar fashion to
natural $PGF_{2\alpha}$ and has been associated with
fewer side effects
• While it is not currently approved for use in
horses, it is in broad use in the absence of an
alternative

 FOLLOW-UP

PATIENT MONITORING
• Serial TRP and US (with or without
teasing) are recommended to monitor the
mare's reproductive tract function
• Serum progesterone concentrations can be
measured post treatment, but provide little
additional information than what US can
provide

PREVENTION/AVOIDANCE
N/A

POSSIBLE COMPLICATIONS
Prolonged nonpregnant periods and/or
infertility.

EXPECTED COURSE AND PROGNOSIS
N/A

 MISCELLANEOUS

ASSOCIATED CONDITIONS
N/A

AGE-RELATED FACTORS
N/A

ZOONOTIC POTENTIAL
N/A

PREGNANCY/FERTILITY/BREEDING
• $PGF_{2\alpha}$ administration to pregnant mares
can cause luteolysis and abortion

• Definitively rule out pregnancy before
administering this drug or its analogs

SYNONYMS
N/A

SEE ALSO
• Abnormal estrus intervals
• Anestrus
• Early embryonic death
• Endometritis
• Pyometra

ABBREVIATIONS
• CL = corpus luteum
• eCG = equine chorionic gonadotropin
• EED = early embryonic death
• P_4 = progesterone
• $PGF_{2\alpha}$ = prostaglandin $F_{2\alpha}$
• TRP = transrectal palpation
• US = ultrasonography, ultrasound

Suggested Reading
Coffman EA, Pinto CR. A review on the use
of prostaglandin F2α for controlling the
estrous cycle in mares. J Equine Vet Sci
2016;40:34–40.
Ginther OJ, Castro T, Baldrighi JM, et al.
Defective secretion of prostaglandin F2α
during development of idiopathic persistent
corpus luteum in mares. Domest Anim
Endocrinol 2016;55:60–65.
Ginther OJ, Baldrighi JM, Castro T, et al.
Concentrations of progesterone, a
metabolite of PGF2α, prolactin, and
luteinizing hormone during development of
idiopathic persistent corpus luteum in
mares. Domest Anim Endocrinol
2016;55:114–122.
Vanderwall DK, Parkinson KC, Rigas J. How
to use oxytocin treatment to prolong corpus
luteum function for suppressing estrus in
mares. J Equine Vet Sci 2016;36:1–4.

Author Lisa K. Pearson
Consulting Editor Carla L. Carleton
Acknowledgment The author and editor
acknowledge the prior contribution of Carole
C. Miller.

P

PROLONGED PREGNANCY

 BASICS

DEFINITION
• Gestation exceeding the normal range for the individual mare (can be significant variation between mares)
• Gestation that appears to be lengthened by abnormal characteristics of the fetus
• Normal range of gestation is 320–355 days, but it is not rare for gestational length to fall outside this range
• *Fescue toxicosis* may extend gestation length to >360 days

PATHOPHYSIOLOGY
Primary, Individual, Mare Variation
May be attributable to placental function or dysfunction, endocrine changes; may also involve damage to the endometrium, thus reducing the nutrient supply to the fetus; still able to sustain life, but resulting in fetal intrauterine growth retardation.

Fescue Toxicosis
• Fescue toxicity caused by an endophyte-infected perennial grass
• The endophyte *Neotyphodium coenophialum* produces multiple toxins (those affecting animal health—lolines, ergopeptine alkaloids)
• Ergot alkaloids act as dopamine D_2 receptor agonists on prolactin secretory cells of the anterior pituitary; results in decreased prolactin concentrations and hypogalactia or agalactia in the mare
• May block fetal corticotropin-releasing hormone, adrenocorticotropic hormone, and cortisol, resulting in a prolonged gestation, leads to a larger fetus
• Fetus suffers intrauterine hypoxemia
• Fetus may fail to properly position itself for parturition; resulting in an increased incidence of dystocia; dysmature, weak, or stillborn foals
• Placental compromise (thickened, edematous); increasingly difficult for membranes to tear during parturition (further fetal compromise)
• Prolonged gestation is but one manifestation attributed to infected fescue

SYSTEMS AFFECTED
Reproductive

GENETICS
N/A

INCIDENCE/PREVALENCE
• No statistics are available regarding incidence
• Other than fescue toxicosis, prolonged pregnancy is not a common reproductive problem

SIGNALMENT
• Females
• All breeds
• All of breeding age

SIGNS
General Comments
• Differs from other domestic species, in which prolonged pregnancy is linked with iodine deficiency, increased progesterone, and inherited factors
• May be caused by abnormal fetal pituitary and adrenal development or by lack of fetal hypothalamic maturity at term

Historical Findings
• *Individual mare*—usually appears to be a fetal problem, so historical information may have limited value
• *Fescue toxicosis*—has been grazing on endophyte-infected pasture within last 30+ days of gestation

Physical Examination Findings
Primary, Individual, Mare Causes
• Mare—no abnormalities unless excessive uterine fluid has accumulated
• Fetus—postpartum examination usually reveals a dead, dysmature or very weak fetus; smaller than normal; may appear undernourished
Fescue Toxicosis
• Pregnant mare >330 days of gestation, grazing endophyte-infected pasture; no signs of imminent foaling (failure of mammary development, no softening of tissues around tail-head and perineum in preparation for foaling)
• US may reveal thickened placental membranes:
  ○ Transrectal US of cervix and caudal uterine body to assess possible abnormalities—thickness, placental detachment
  ○ Transabdominal US to monitor placental integrity, fetal viability

CAUSES
Individual Mare
• Hormonal—the pituitary or adrenal glands are most commonly involved
• Not a mare problem; mares can be bred again with little concern for recurrence
• Fescue toxicosis
  ○ Grazing/being fed endophyte-infected pasture the last 30+ days before parturition

RISK FACTORS
See Causes.

 DIAGNOSIS

• Accurate history combined with transrectal palpation
• Outward gross appearance of the mare
• Appearance of the fetus—prepartum, postpartum, and/or necropsy

DIFFERENTIAL DIAGNOSIS
Hydrops
• Prolonged pregnancy with a hydrops is invariably shorter than the lengthened gestation associated with a fetus having a higher center defect
• Known breeding and ovulation dates facilitate differentiation

CBC/BIOCHEMISTRY/URINALYSIS
N/A

OTHER LABORATORY TESTS
Peritoneal Tap
To differentiate the location of excessive fluid accumulation between prolonged pregnancy and hydrops:
• If *hydrops amnii*—results from a fetal defect (segmental aplasia within GI tract, may be multiple affected loci; location(s) involved affect speed and volume of accumulation); excessive fluid is amniotic; failure of fetus to swallow and process amniotic fluid across GI tract as it is produced; excess fluid would normally be eliminated as waste into chorioallantoic fluid. Dam is not the cause
• If *hydrops allantois*—caused by a uteroplacental defect; excessive fluid is allantoic. The dam's uterus is incapable of normal placental function, not a good future prospect for breeding (rarely linked to a particular stallion)

IMAGING
US imaging, to determine:
• If excessive fluid is present
• If the endometrium is thickened
• If the approximate lengths of fetal extremities differ from what is normal for known gestational length
  ○ Evaluate the combined thickness of uterus and placenta, a measure of placentitis
  ○ Assess the appearance and approximate volumes of allantoic and amniotic fluids in relationship to the fetus for a known gestation length

OTHER DIAGNOSTIC PROCEDURES
When >30 days postpartum, perform an endometrial biopsy of the mare to determine her endometrial status before breeding again.

PATHOLOGIC FINDINGS
• The uterus may or may not be larger than normal
• If the fetus is dead or dies postpartum, a necropsy should be done to determine if its adrenal and pituitary glands and hypothalamus are normal

 TREATMENT

• Parturition induction is an option. However, it is essential that the breeding date is accurate, and that records can confirm its validity, to avoid inducing a preterm, nonviable foal
• Remind owners that fetal survival after a prolonged gestation will be in question. The actual circumstances of survival may not be known until after delivery

(CONTINUED)

PROLONGED PREGNANCY

• Routine care for the mare during the postpartum period
• With the exception of fescue toxicosis, emphasize to owners that prolonged pregnancies can occur and that most affected mares deliver normal foals
• Remind owners that gestational length may fall outside the normal range and still be normal for that individual

Fescue Toxicosis, Management/Treatments
• Remove mares from infected feed by 300 days of gestation
• If the sole source of feed is infected, institute treatment of the mare during the final 2–4 weeks of pregnancy
  ○ Domperidone—1.1 mg/kg/day PO. Can also treat post foaling, every 12 h for several days to increase milk production, but best to start treatment during the last month of pregnancy
  ○ Reserpine—0.01 mg/kg every 24 h PO; only effective in resolving postpartum agalactia
  ○ Sulpiride—3.3 mg/kg/day; to resolve postpartum agalactia, less effective than domperidone
• Monitor mammary gland development; plan for an observed parturition as delivery assistance will most likely be necessary, be prepared to assist neonate (treat as for a high-risk/critical care patient; likely FTPI so supplement immunoglobulin G, IV plasma, or other supplemental feeding)

APPROPRIATE HEALTH CARE
N/A

NURSING CARE
N/A

ACTIVITY
N/A

DIET
N/A

CLIENT EDUCATION
N/A

SURGICAL CONSIDERATIONS
N/A

 MEDICATIONS

DRUG(S) OF CHOICE
Refer to Fescue Toxicosis management/treatments, above.

CONTRAINDICATIONS
N/A

PRECAUTIONS
N/A

POSSIBLE INTERACTIONS
N/A

ALTERNATIVE DRUGS
N/A

 FOLLOW-UP

PATIENT MONITORING
• Monitor mares once they are suspected to be "overdue"
• Take no action unless pregnancy goes beyond the expected due date in the absence of external evidence of advancing gestation and approaching parturition
• A pluriparous mare should be close to a previous "term gestation" length in which she delivered a normal foal before considering inducing parturition
• Failure to show evidence of mammary development:
  ○ If there are intact horses (males) on the farm, must rule out every likelihood of the mare having been bred on a subsequent estrus, unobserved by owner/farm personnel
  ○ The suspected *prolonged gestation* may be of normal length, but the result of a later breeding
  ○ Delivery of a fetus 3 weeks early will be too immature to survive. Can determine parentage after the fact by DNA testing

PREVENTION/AVOIDANCE
• Unknown, because the major causes involve abnormal fetal pituitary, adrenals, or hypothalamus
• If grazing/being fed fescue-contaminated feed, remove from that source of feed during the last month of gestation

POSSIBLE COMPLICATIONS
• Prolonged pregnancy could result in dystocia
• Because the fetus usually is smaller than normal and has no ankylosis of joints, dystocia usually is not a problem

EXPECTED COURSE AND PROGNOSIS
Postpartum
• Normal postpartum examination of the mare
• The fetus is expected to be smaller than normal and has a low probability of survival
• Fescue toxicosis results in a dysmature foal (premature, mature; dysmature = overly long)
• The dysmature foal will be at high risk for FTPI
• Treat as would be done for other critical care neonates

 MISCELLANEOUS

ASSOCIATED CONDITIONS
N/A

AGE-RELATED FACTORS
N/A

ZOONOTIC POTENTIAL
N/A

PREGNANCY/FERTILITY/BREEDING
Occurs only during gestation.

SEE ALSO
Fescue toxicosis

ABBREVIATIONS
• FTPI = failure of transfer of passive immunity
• GI = gastrointestinal
• US = ultrasonography, ultrasound

Suggested Reading
Vandeplassche M. Obstetrician's view of the physiology of equine parturition and dystocia. Equine Vet J 1980;12:45–49.
Wolfsdorf KE. Fescue toxicosis. In: Carleton CL, ed. Blackwell's Five-Minute Veterinary Consult Clinical Companion, Equine Theriogenology. Ames, IA: Wiley Blackwell, 2011:259–265.

Author Carla L. Carleton
Consulting Editor Carla L. Carleton
Acknowledgment The author/editor acknowledges the prior contribution of Walter R. Threlfall.

P

PROTEIN, HYPERPROTEINEMIA

 BASICS

DEFINITION
• Occurs when the circulating protein concentration is >7.9 g/dL (>79 g/L)
• Increase may be due to higher than normal concentrations of all plasma proteins, i.e. panhyperproteinemia, or selective where specific protein concentrations are increased, e.g. hyperglobulinemia
• Predominant proteins present in blood—albumin, globulins, and fibrinogen. Globulins and albumin can be separated and quantified. Globulins further divided into α_1, α_2, β_1, β_2, and γ
• Paraproteins—immunoglobulins produced by neoplastic immune cells

PATHOPHYSIOLOGY
• Plasma proteins perform a nutritive function, exert colloidal osmotic pressure, and contribute to acid–base balance. Individual proteins serve as enzymes, antibodies, coagulation factors, hormones, and transporters
• Albumin and fibrinogen and ~80% of globulins formed in the liver; remainder formed in lymphoid tissue
• Filtration between intravascular and extravascular space, metabolic demands, hormonal balance, nutritional status, and water balance determine TP concentration
• TP in neonates is influenced by passive transfer of immunoglobulins. In adults TP remains stable unless influenced by pathologic processes

Panhyperproteinemia
• Result of relative water loss concentrating all plasma proteins proportionally
• Hypovolemia causes a shift of fluid into the intravascular space as body attempts to maintain blood volume. With tissue dehydration, intravascular fluid is lost, resulting in hemoconcentration and increase in TP. If renal function is adequate, urine output decreases
• Water loss may be due to decreased fluid intake or excessive losses
• There is usually an associated increase in PCV, though hemoconcentration with concurrent anemia results in hyperproteinemia with normal or decreased PCV

Hyperalbuminemia
Hyperalbuminemia represents a relative increase in albumin secondary to dehydration. Concurrent hyperglobulinemia is also present.

Hyperglobulinemia
• Increases may be relative (i.e. secondary to hemoconcentration) or absolute
• Absolute increases occur with inflammatory disease and immunostimulation; the result of synthesis of acute-phase proteins and immunoglobulins by plasma cells

• Changes in plasma proteins associated with inflammation:
  ◦ Hepatic production of *positive acute-phase proteins* (e.g. α_1 and α_2 globulins, fibrinogen, serum amyloid A, and C-reactive protein) during acute inflammation. Increased plasma or serum concentrations are usually detectable in ≈2 days
  ◦ Decreased hepatic production of *negative acute-phase proteins* (e.g. albumin, transferrin) in acute/chronic inflammation. Owing to the lifespan of these proteins, decreases may not be noted for >1 week, but persist for the duration of the response
  ◦ Increases in *delayed response proteins* (e.g. immunoglobulins, complement) during acute/chronic inflammation are detectable 1–3 weeks after onset. Predominantly IgG (γ globulins) are produced; also IgM and IgA (β globulins). Increased immunoglobulin synthesis by lymphocytes produces a polyclonal gammopathy
• Increases in acute-phase proteins may cause small increases in globulin concentration. Production of chronic-phase proteins (e.g. immunoglobulins) causes moderate to marked hyperglobulinemia/hyperproteinemia
• Absolute increase in globulins also may be caused by neoplasia:
  ◦ A neoplastic expansion of 1 type of B lymphocyte may result in production of a single immunoglobulin type; result—a monoclonal gammopathy. Neoplastic cells may produce intact immunoglobulins, free light chains (Bence Jones proteins), only heavy chains, or abnormal fragments
  ◦ Monoclonal gammopathies can be caused by multiple myeloma, lymphocytic leukemia, and lymphosarcoma
  ◦ Polyclonal gammopathies also occur with lymphosarcoma/other tumors
  ◦ Concentrations of immunoglobulins, other than the monoclonal protein, often decreased, resulting in mild/moderate hypoalbuminemia

SYSTEMS AFFECTED
See Pathophysiology.

SIGNALMENT
Hyperglobulinemia secondary to neoplasia more likely in older animals.

SIGNS
General Comments
Nonspecific physical findings associated with dehydration, inflammation, or neoplasia warrant further evaluation, which may demonstrate hyperproteinemia.

Historical Findings
Fever, decreased appetite, cough, nasal discharge, respiratory distress, exercise intolerance, poor performance, GI dysfunction, and weight loss may occur.

Physical Examination Findings
Signs of dehydration may include increased capillary refill time, decreased pulse pressure, tachycardia, and decreased urine output.

CAUSES
Panhyperproteinemia
• Associated with dehydration
• Decreased fluid intake may be due to:
  ◦ Dysphagia associated with pain (e.g. pharyngeal abscess, trauma), obstruction (e.g. esophageal obstruction/choke), or neurologic dysfunction (e.g. botulism, guttural pouch mycosis, yellow star thistle/Russian knapweed poisoning, lead toxicity, rabies)
  ◦ Lack of thirst, e.g. toxemia
  ◦ Lack of water
• Excessive fluid losses due to:
  ◦ GI disorders, e.g. diarrhea associated with acute colitis, salmonellosis, Potomac horse fever, intestinal clostridiosis, intestinal strangulating obstruction, proximal enteritis, endotoxemia
  ◦ Fluid sequestration—intestinal obstruction
  ◦ Polyuria—chronic renal failure
  ◦ Increased vascular permeability, e.g. purpura haemorrhagica, sepsis, endotoxemia
  ◦ Excessive sweating
  ◦ Exudation from extensive skin wounds, e.g. burns

Hyperglobulinemia
• Globulin concentrations may increase due to dehydration (relative increase), inflammation, in late stages of pregnancy, or neoplasia
• The inflammatory process is usually chronic:
  ◦ GI, e.g. peritonitis, parasitism, mesenteric abscessation, tooth root abscess
  ◦ Respiratory, e.g. pulmonary abscessation (*Rhodococcus equi*), guttural pouch empyema, pyothorax
  ◦ Hemic/lymphatic/immune, e.g. endocarditis, pericarditis, lymph node abscessation (*Streptococcus equi*, *Corynebacterium pseudotuberculosis*), immune-mediated vasculitis (purpura haemorrhagica)
  ◦ Urologic, e.g. glomerulonephritis, pyelonephritis
  ◦ Reproductive tract, e.g. pregnancy, endometritis
  ◦ Musculoskeletal, e.g. abscesses, septic arthritis, osteomyelitis
  ◦ Nervous, e.g. bacterial meningitis, abscess
  ◦ Hepatobiliary, e.g. cholangitis, chronic active hepatitis, hepatic abscess
  ◦ Skin, e.g. pemphigus foliaceus, chronic dermatitis, dermatophilosis
• Specific neoplastic disorders include multiple myeloma, lymphocytic leukemia, and lymphosarcoma
• Specific immune-mediated diseases, e.g. autoimmune hemolytic anemia and autoimmune thrombocytopenia

P

Hyperalbuminemia
Dehydration

Hyperfibrinogenemia
Most causes of hyperglobulinemia may result in increased fibrinogen (dehydration and inflammation).

RISK FACTORS
Age/sex.

DIAGNOSIS
DIFFERENTIAL DIAGNOSIS
• Selective vs. nonselective hyperproteinemia should be determined. Evidence of dehydration supports nonselective (relative) hyperproteinemia
• With selective hyperproteinemia infectious, inflammatory, and lymphoproliferative disorders should be differentiated and the cause of these processes determined

CBC/BIOCHEMISTRY/URINALYSIS
• Total protein concentration is commonly measured by refractometry, which is influenced by the concentration of solids within a sample. High concentrations of lipids, urea, Na$^+$, Cl$^-$ may increase refractive index and cause spurious effects on TP values
• Increased PCV, albumin, lactate, urine specific gravity, and prerenal azotemia support dehydration
• Laboratory findings associated with inflammation include anemia of chronic disease, neutrophilia/neutropenia, lymphocytosis/lymphopenia, monocytosis, and hypoalbuminemia
• Normal or decreased PCV with hyperproteinemia may indicate concomitant anemia with dehydration or infectious/inflammatory disease

OTHER LABORATORY TESTS
• Calculation of the A:G ratio may help interpretation of TP
• A:G ratio will remain normal if both fractions are increased uniformly, e.g. dehydration
• A:G ratio may be abnormal if an alteration of 1 fraction predominates; e.g. decreased A:G ratio with renal proteinuria and/or immunoglobulin production following antigenic stimulation; increased A:G ratio from poor immunoglobulin production in adults or lack of colostrum absorption in foals
• Serum protein electrophoresis can be used to quantitate individual protein fractions in hyperglobulinemia and to differentiate polyclonal from monoclonal gammopathies. Immunochemical and radioimmunologic methods allow specific identification and quantitation of individual proteins

• Additional tests for infectious or other inflammatory diseases to establish a diagnosis

IMAGING
Ultrasonography and radiography of the thorax, abdomen, or relevant soft tissues may help identify the cause of hyperglobulinemia.

OTHER DIAGNOSTIC PROCEDURES
Abdominocentesis, thoracocentesis, tracheal aspiration or bronchoalveolar lavage, endoscopy, laparoscopy, bone marrow aspiration, biopsy, and histopathology may determine location and etiology of infectious, inflammatory, or lymphoproliferative disorders.

PATHOLOGIC FINDINGS
Dependent on cause.

TREATMENT
APPROPRIATE HEALTH CARE
• With dehydration appropriate fluids
• Specific causes of dehydration, inflammation, or infection may require medical or surgical treatments

NURSING CARE
According to cause.

ACTIVITY
Limit according to cause.

DIET
Good quality.

CLIENT EDUCATION
As required based on cause.

SURGICAL CONSIDERATIONS
Based on cause.

MEDICATIONS
DRUG(S) OF CHOICE
Those indicated for treatment of the inciting cause.

CONTRAINDICATIONS
Steroids with infection.

FOLLOW-UP
PATIENT MONITORING
• Evaluation of hydration status using clinical and laboratory variables
• Frequency of monitoring depends on severity of signs and response to therapy

POSSIBLE COMPLICATIONS
Dependent on cause.

EXPECTED COURSE AND PROGNOSIS
Relative to cause and treatment.

MISCELLANEOUS
ASSOCIATED CONDITIONS
Dependent on cause.

AGE-RELATED FACTORS
• Serum TP is low at birth, increases after absorption of colostrum, declines over 1–5 weeks as antibodies in colostrum are metabolized, and then increases to adult concentrations over 6–12 months
• Adult TP remains relatively stable, although albumin decreases slightly over time, while globulins and acute-phase proteins progressively increase in old age

PREGNANCY/FERTILITY/BREEDING
• Fetal development in mares causes increased globulins with a concomitant decrease in albumin
• Serum immunoglobulins increase in the dam until ≈1 month before term, at which time they are secreted into the mammary gland (colostrum)
• Albumin and TP decrease during lactation

SYNONYMS
Gammopathy

SEE ALSO
• Acute phase response
• Anemia, chronic disease
• Lymphosarcoma
• Multiple myeloma
• Serum amyloid A (SAA)

ABBREVIATIONS
• A:G = albumin to globulin
• GI = gastrointestinal
• Ig = immunoglobulin
• PCV = packed cell volume
• TP = total protein

Suggested Reading
Sellon DC, Wise LN. Disorders of the hematopoietic system. In: Reed SM, Bayly WM, Sellon DC, eds. Equine Internal Medicine, 3e. St. Louis, MO: WB Saunders, 2010:730–776.
Author Nicola Menzies-Gow
Consulting Editors David Hodgson, Harold C. McKenzie, and Jennifer L. Hodgson
Acknowledgment The author and editors acknowledge the prior contribution of Jennifer L. Hodgson.

P

PROTEIN, HYPOPROTEINEMIA

BASICS

DEFINITION
• Occurs when plasma TP concentration <5.2 g/dL (<52 g/L)
• Decrease can be nonselective or selective
• Specific deficiencies can result in immune deficiency/defective hemostasis

PATHOPHYSIOLOGY
• Plasma contains numerous proteins that perform nutritive functions, maintain oncotic pressure, regulate immune function, aid acid–base balance, and affect hemostasis/fibrinolysis
• All albumin and fibrinogen and ~80% of globulins synthesized in the liver. Remaining globulins formed in lymphoid tissue
• TP is determined by filtration between the intravascular/extravascular spaces, metabolic demands, hormonal and water balance, nutritional status
• TP in neonates is influenced by passive transfer. In adults, TP remains relatively stable unless there is pathology
• Hypoproteinemia can:
  ○ Be nonselective—panhypoproteinemia
  ○ Be selective, i.e. hypoalbuminemia/hypoglobulinemia
  ○ Have normal TP with hypoalbuminemia and hyperglobulinemia
  ○ Have normal TP with hyperalbuminemia and hypoglobulinemia (rare)

Panhypoproteinemia
• Panhypoproteinemia—relative or absolute
• Relative panhypoproteinemia occurs when TP is decreased but absolute content of protein in vascular space is normal, e.g. dilution by excessive fluid therapy
• Absolute panhypoproteinemia occurs when there is a reduction in TP with a normal plasma volume due to impaired production/accelerated loss:
  ○ Reduced production—primarily as a result of malnutrition/starvation, possibly in the face of increased metabolic demand, e.g. growth, pregnancy, lactation. Liver disease—rare cause
  ○ Accelerated loss more common. Loss can be from the vascular into the extravascular compartment (increased capillary permeability) or from the body. These may cause panhypoproteinemia/selective protein loss. Hypoalbuminemia occurs first (small size and low molecular weight). If disease is severe/chronic, globulins also may be decreased
  ○ Severe/acute hemorrhage results in hypoproteinemia through direct loss of protein followed by dilution effect via movement of fluid from the extravascular to vascular space
  ○ Persistent, low-grade hemorrhage causes normovolemic anemia/hypoproteinemia

Selective Hypoproteinemia
Hypoalbuminemia
• Albumin—produced in liver; has the lowest molecular weight of plasma proteins; contributes 75% of osmotic pressure. Albumin binds/transports components lacking specific transport proteins
• Hypoalbuminemia may be accompanied by decreased/normal TP and normal/increased/decreased globulin concentrations. Hypoalbuminemia usually precedes hypoglobulinemia owing to preferential loss of albumin or synthesis of globulins
• Hypoalbuminemia usually the result of increased loss; decreased production and increased catabolism may occur
• Increased loss of albumin occurs with:
  ○ PLE—causes include ulceration, defective lymphatic drainage, increased mucosal permeability, and exudation. Most common
  ○ PLN—albumin is readily filtered through glomerular basement membrane defects. Glomerulopathies cause albuminuria/hypoalbuminemia
  ○ Congestive heart failure—retention of sodium and water forces fluid into the extravascular spaces with concomitant protein loss. Reduced food intake, inadequate protein absorption, and inadequate hepatic synthesis also contribute
  ○ Chronic inflammation—albumin lost via exudation, e.g. into thoracic/abdominal cavities
• Decreased production rarely due to liver disease; can occur with starvation, malnutrition, and chronic GI disorders. Inflammatory processes—albumin: decreased production; globulins: increased production. The half-life for albumin is ≈18 days; therefore, when decreased synthesis causes hypoalbuminemia, the underlying disease is usually chronic with increased globulins; results in normal/increased TP
• Albumin—catabolism may occur with increased metabolic demands/negative nitrogen balance. Chronic antigenic stimulation also increases albumin catabolism to provide amino acids for immunoglobulin production. Resulting hypoalbuminemia usually offset by hyperglobulinemia resulting in normal TP
• Hypoalbuminemia causes low plasma colloid oncotic pressure, allowing fluid movement from vascular to extravascular space, reducing plasma volume. May manifest as tissue edema and hypoperfusion and consequent organ dysfunction. Hypoalbuminemia also reduces transportation of molecules (and drugs) within plasma
Hypoglobulinemia
• Hypoglobulinemia with normal albumin is rare. Exception—FTPI
• Hypoglobulinemia with immunodeficiencies results in decreased gammaglobulins (lymphoid hypoplasia/aplasia). Compensatory increase in albumin
Hypofibrinogenemia
• Rare. May result from increased consumption/decreased synthesis; alone will not cause hypoproteinemia
• Severe, diffuse liver damage; decreased production
• Increased fibrinolysis (DIC); hypofibrinogenemia rare as inflammation masks increased consumption

SYSTEMS AFFECTED
Often with GI/renal disorders, hemorrhage, chronic hepatic disease.

GENETICS
• Specific immunodeficiencies
• Fell Ponies
• Purebred Arabs

INCIDENCE/PREVALENCE
Relatively common, depending on cause.

GEOGRAPHIC DISTRIBUTION
Fell pony immunodeficiency syndrome—Fell District, UK

SIGNALMENT
Neonates with hypoproteinemia, particularly hypoglobulinemia—FTPI and/or specific immunodeficiencies.

SIGNS
General Comments
No pathognomonic signs.

Historical Findings
Fever, lethargy, ventral edema, weight loss, GI dysfunction, dysuria, hemorrhage, or history of prolonged NSAID administration.

Physical Examination Findings
• Reflects underlying cause, e.g. weight loss, diarrhea, melena, polyuria
• Edema of distal extremities, ventral body wall, and head; usually TP <4 g/dL (40 g/L); albumin <1.5 g/dL (15 g/L)
• Pulmonary edema—hypoalbuminemic horses on IV fluids

CAUSES
Panhypoproteinemia
• Relative dilution, i.e. excessive fluid therapy/water intake
• Reduced production:
  ○ Malnutrition, starvation
  ○ Chronic liver disease, e.g. pyrrolizidine alkaloid toxicity
• Increased loss:
  ○ Endotoxemia/vasculitis, e.g. purpura haemorrhagica, African horse sickness
  ○ Acute/chronic hemorrhage, e.g. trauma, epistaxis, internal vascular rupture, coagulopathies; chronic blood loss
  ○ PLN, e.g. glomerulonephritis, amyloidosis, pyelonephritis
  ○ PLE, e.g. intestinal parasitism, salmonellosis, clostridiosis, Potomac horse fever, *Lawsonia intracellularis* infection, inflammatory bowel disease,

lymphosarcoma, NSAID toxicosis, exposure to caustic chemicals, strangulating GI obstructions/infarction
° Peritonitis/pleural effusion, e.g. bacterial pleuropneumonia
° Chronic heart failure

Hypoalbuminemia
• May occur in initial stages of diseases causing panhypoproteinemia
• Chronic antigenic stimulation/infections—increased catabolism, e.g. fever, trauma, surgery, neoplasia
• Chronic, diffuse/severe liver disease—decreased production, e.g. chronic hepatitis/fibrosis/neoplasia

Hypoglobulinemia
• FTPI
• Immunodeficiencies, e.g. SCID, selective immunoglobulin M deficiency, agammaglobulinemia, Fell Pony immunodeficiency syndrome
• Adult acquired immunodeficiency

Hypofibrinogenemia
• Impaired hepatic synthesis
• DIC
• Uncompensated loss—massive hemorrhage

RISK FACTORS
Certain breeds; age—neonate; underlying disease.

DIAGNOSIS
DIFFERENTIAL DIAGNOSIS
• Determine underlying cause
• Clinical signs referable to specific body systems: help localize source

CBC/BIOCHEMISTRY/URINALYSIS
• PCV and TP should be interpreted simultaneously to determine hemoconcentration or concurrent anemia
• A:G ratio may aid interpretation
• Hypoproteinemia with normal A:G ratio (i.e. absolute hypoproteinemia) reflects hemorrhage, starvation/malnutrition, or chronic disease
• Decreased A:G ratio occurs with inflammatory disease, B-lymphocyte neoplasia, and in selective hypoproteinemias due to hypoalbuminemia
• Increased A:G ratio is rare—reflects erroneous albumin measurement or decreased synthesis of gammaglobulins
• Fibrinogen—best measured by the heat precipitation or Clauss method. Falsely decreased values in samples containing clotted blood
• Proteinuria—abnormal finding. Transient slight proteinuria occurs with exercise/stress, and in neonates

OTHER LABORATORY TESTS
• Selective protein deficiencies—characterized by serum protein electrophoresis or measurement of specific proteins, e.g. immunoglobulins
• Characterization of immune system function indicated in cases of hypoglobulinemia (see chapters listed in See Also)
• Tests for specific infectious or inflammatory diseases may be indicated, e.g. *L. intracellularis*

IMAGING
Ultrasonography/radiography of thorax, abdomen, heart, or soft tissue may help define cause.

OTHER DIAGNOSTIC PROCEDURES
Abdominocentesis, thoracocentesis, tracheal aspiration, bronchoalveolar lavage, endoscopy, laparoscopy, bone marrow aspiration, cerebrospinal fluid evaluation, biopsy, and histopathology.

PATHOLOGIC FINDINGS
Variable; dependent on cause.

TREATMENT
APPROPRIATE HEALTH CARE
• Requires treatment of underlying disease and correction of hypoproteinemia
• Relative panhypoproteinemia will resolve with discontinuation of excessive fluid therapy or restriction of water intake

MEDICATIONS
DRUG(S) OF CHOICE
• FTPI requires administration of colostrum PO, or IV administration of hyperimmune plasma
• IV plasma in adult horses with marked hypoproteinemia; plasma preferred over blood
• Infuse plasma to increase albumin >2.0 g/dL (20 g/L)
• Increase plasma oncotic pressure by IV administration of synthetic colloids (e.g. hydroxyethyl starch/high molecular weight dextrans) (8–10 mL/kg or 6% solution IV over 6–12 h)

FOLLOW-UP
PATIENT MONITORING
• Laboratory variables: TP, albumin, globulins; hydration status: PCV, lactate, creatinine, urine specific gravity
• Monitoring frequency depends on severity/response to therapy

POSSIBLE COMPLICATIONS
• Complications depend on cause
• Dependent/pulmonary edema possible
• Upper airway obstruction may develop owing to pharyngeal and laryngeal edema and require tracheotomy
• Anaphylactic reactions during IV plasma administration

EXPECTED COURSE AND PROGNOSIS
Dependent on the underlying cause.

MISCELLANEOUS
ASSOCIATED CONDITIONS
Neoplasia

AGE-RELATED FACTORS
Values for TP, albumin, and globulins in foals lower than those in adults.

PREGNANCY/FERTILITY/BREEDING
TP falls in mare when producing colostrum.

SEE ALSO
• Anemia
• Failure of transfer of passive immunity (FTPI)
• Immunoglobulin deficiencies
• Severe combined immunodeficiency

ABBREVIATIONS
• A:G = albumin to globulin
• DIC = disseminated intravascular coagulation
• FTPI = failure of transfer of passive immunity
• GI = gastrointestinal
• NSAID = nonsteroidal anti-inflammatory drug
• PCV = packed cell volume
• PLE = protein-losing enteropathy
• PLN = protein-losing nephropathy
• SCID = severe combined immunodeficiency
• TP = total protein

Suggested Reading
Sellon DC. Disorders of the hematopoietic system. In: Reed SM, Bayly WM, Sellon DC, eds. Equine Internal Medicine, 2e. St. Louis, MO: WB Saunders, 2004:721–768.

Author Nicola Menzies-Gow
Consulting Editors David Hodgson, Harold C. McKenzie, and Jennifer L. Hodgson
Acknowledgment The author and editors acknowledge the prior contribution of Jennifer L. Hodgson.

P

PROTEIN-LOSING ENTEROPATHY (PLE)

BASICS

OVERVIEW
• GI protein loss may result from mucosal ulceration and plasma exudation, lymphatic obstruction with leakage and rupture of dilated lacteals, passive diffusion through intracellular spaces, active secretion by mucosal cells, intracellular loss, increased permeability of capillaries and venules, and disordered cell metabolism
• Excessive loss of proteins into the GI tract causes hypoproteinemia. The early intestinal protein loss in PLE involves relatively larger quantities of albumin than globulins. If severe, hypoalbuminemia may result in the development of subcutaneous edema. In the later stages of the disease, all protein fractions may be lost. If large colon function is not impaired, feces frequently normal
• PLE usually a progressive condition; however, accelerated protein leakage can occur in acute GI diseases

SIGNALMENT
• Eosinophilic gastroenteritis and GE most common in young adult horses. GE more common in Standardbreds
• Intestinal lymphosarcoma and intestinal parasitism occur in horses of all ages
• *Lawsonia intracellularis* in weanling foals
• Ponies and young animals are reportedly more susceptible to NSAID toxicity

SIGNS
Affected animals show some of the following:
• Chronic, progressive weight loss
• Dependent edema
• Depression
• Anorexia
• Reduced performance
• Lethargy
• Intermittent or chronic colic
• Diarrhea not present in PLE cases with lesions primarily in the small intestine
• ± Skin lesions
• ± Enlarged peripheral lymph nodes
• Acute colic and endotoxemia may occur in horses with intestinal parasitism or NSAID toxicity
• Per rectum examination—may palpate enlarged mesenteric lymph nodes; thickened bowel wall

CAUSES AND RISK FACTORS
Chronic inflammatory bowel diseases (lymphocytic–plasmacytic enterocolitis, GE, idiopathic eosinophilic enterocolitis, multisystemic eosinophilic epitheliotropic

disease), GI neoplasia, parasitic thrombosis of cranial mesenteric artery (*Strongylus vulgaris*), cyathostomiasis, NSAID toxicity, acute salmonellosis, other causes of acute enterocolitis, proliferative enteropathy due to *L. intracellularis*, congestive heart failure, amyloidosis.

DIAGNOSIS

DIFFERENTIAL DIAGNOSIS
Diagnosis of PLE usually made after protein loss through other routes and inability to synthesize protein ruled out.

CBC/BIOCHEMISTRY/URINALYSIS
• Hypoalbuminemia
• Decreased, normal, or increased plasma globulin concentrations
• Serum protein electrophoresis—preferred test for quantifying protein fractions
• Panhypoproteinemia
• Hypocalcemia may occur in conjunction with hypoalbuminemia because a large portion of serum calcium is protein bound
• Anemia

OTHER LABORATORY TESTS
• Coprology for parasitic ova and larvae
• Fecal PCR test for *L. intracellularis* in young foals and weanlings
• Ultrasonography—to determine intestinal wall thickness
• Oral D-xylose absorption test—preferable to oral glucose tolerance test
• Abdominocentesis—cytology to detect neoplasia. Normal abdominal fluid does not rule out neoplasia

DIAGNOSTIC PROCEDURES
• Immunoelectrophoresis
• Gastroduodenoscopy
• Rectal mucosal biopsy—histopathologic examination
• Exploratory laparotomy and intestinal biopsy—often necessary for definitive diagnosis

TREATMENT
• Treatment depends on the primary disease causing PLE or treating the hypoproteinemia
• Treatment frequently unrewarding
• Prognosis for recovery generally guarded to very poor

• Dietary management—provide palatable, easily assimilated, high-energy and -protein sources; electrolyte mixtures; zinc, copper, iron, fat- and water-soluble vitamins

MEDICATIONS

DRUG(S) OF CHOICE
• Plasma transfusion is usually indicated when total plasma protein concentration is or falls below 40 g/L (4 g/dL). The effect may be minimal owing to the continued protein losses
• If horse is receiving NSAIDs, therapy should be discontinued
• When internal parasites are suspected as the cause, administer larvicidal anthelmintics (moxidectin 0.4 mg/kg PO, ivermectin 0.2 mg/kg PO, or fenbendazole 10 mg/kg daily PO for 5 days)
• For *L. intracellularis* proliferative enteropathy—oral macrolides (azithromycin, clarithromycin, erythromycin) alone or in combination with or rifampin (rifampicin), or oral doxycycline for minimum of 21 days
• ± Total parenteral nutrition—in valuable horses
• Corticosteroid therapy often ineffective in treating chronic inflammatory bowel disease

FOLLOW-UP
• Monitor total serum protein and albumin concentrations
• Monitor body weight

MISCELLANEOUS

SEE ALSO
• Ascarid infestation
• Chronic weight loss
• *Lawsonia Intracellularis* infections in foals
• Lymphocytic plasmacytic enterocolitis
• Malabsorption
• Potomac horse fever (PHF)
• Right dorsal colitis

ABBREVIATIONS
• GE = granulomatous enteritis
• GI = gastrointestinal
• NSAID = nonsteroidal anti-inflammatory drug
• PCR = polymerase chain reaction
• PLE = protein-losing enteropathy
Author John D. Baird
Consulting Editors Henry Stämpfli and Olimpo Oliver-Espinosa

BASICS

DEFINITION
Ptyalism—excessive production and secretion of saliva. Pseudoptyalism—drooling saliva owing to the inability or reluctance to swallow.

PATHOPHYSIOLOGY
Results from hypersecretion of the salivary glands, but more commonly due to impaired neuromuscular control with dysfunctional voluntary oral and pharyngeal motor activity.

SYSTEMS AFFECTED
• Gastrointestinal. • Respiratory. • Nervous

GEOGRAPHIC DISTRIBUTION
• Slaframine toxicity—North America and Europe. • Vesicular stomatitis—North, Central, and South America

SIGNALMENT
Dependent on the primary problem.

Foals
• Pharyngeal and esophageal disorders—dysmaturity, septicemia, and congenital disorders. • Esophageal and gastroduodenal ulceration

Young Horses
Improper mastication—tooth eruption.

Aged Horses
• Neoplasia. • Improper mastication—tooth problems

SIGNS
• Salivation. • Quidding, refusal to eat hard food, preference for soft food. • Inability to close the mouth and dropped jaw (CN V), inability to move the lips (CN VII), loss of the gag reflex and inability to swallow (CN IX, CN X, CN XII). • Muscle atrophy—secondary to CN deficits, trauma, or myopathy. • Esophageal disorders—obstructions, diverticulum, neoplasia, foreign bodies. • Dysphagia—coughing during swallowing, frequent swallowing motions, extension of the neck. • Salivation following slaframine ingestion—occurs within 30–60 min and may persist for 24 h. Other signs—diarrhea, anorexia, polyuria, or abortion. Clinical signs resolve within 48–96 h of removing the contaminated feed. • Esophageal and gastroduodenal ulceration—bruxism, salivation, colic, and decreased appetite

CAUSES
• Hypersecretion—tranquilizers, anticonvulsants, and anticholinesterases. • Hypersecretion—parasympaticomimetics. Ingestion of forage or hay contaminated with *Rhizoctonia leguminicola* produces a mycotoxin, slaframine, which is a cholinergic agonist. • Cholinesterase inhibitor insecticides—organophosphates and carbamates. • Neurologic and neuromuscular

diseases—difficulties in oral and pharyngeal motor control. • Impairment of the oral phase of deglutition—secondary to trauma, oral pain, periodontal disease, mucosal penetration by a foreign body, or facial nerve paralysis. • Primary diseases of the salivary glands—uncommon: sialadenitis, salivary calculi, salivary mucocele, trauma, neoplasia, or infection (e.g. *Streptococcus equi*, rabies). • Stomatitis—vesicular stomatitis, irritants, caustic chemicals, yellow bristle grass, foxtails, NSAID toxicity, erosions secondary to point on teeth. • Lymphadenopathy—dysphagia. • Gastroesophageal reflux and ulceration. • Septicemia—neonates. • Esophageal intraluminal obstruction and esophageal rupture. • Heavy metal poisoning such as mercury and lead

RISK FACTORS
See Causes.

DIAGNOSIS

DIFFERENTIAL DIAGNOSIS
Determine the primary conditions.

CBC/BIOCHEMISTRY/URINALYSIS
• Results of the CBC are often normal, but may reflect the primary disease. • Stress leukogram. • Biochemical analysis—usually normal or consistent with the primary disease. • Prolonged ptyalism—metabolic alkalosis

OTHER LABORATORY TESTS
Fine needle aspiration and biopsy—oral masses or stomatitis.

IMAGING
• Radiographs of the skull—trauma; inability to close the mouth; to localize foreign bodies, retropharyngeal masses, or temporomandibular joint and periodontal diseases. • Ultrasonography—primary salivary gland or tongue diseases

OTHER DIAGNOSTIC PROCEDURES
• Oral examination. • Evaluate for primary central nervous system disease. • Nasogastric intubation. • Endoscopy—upper airway, esophagus, stomach, duodenum. • Examination of hay source or pasture—slaframine toxicity. • Immunofluorescent antibody testing on brain tissue—rabies

TREATMENT

APPROPRIATE HEALTH CARE
• Treat the primary condition. • Analgesic and anti-inflammatory—reduce pain and provide comfort. • Correct dehydration and acid–base disorders

DIET
Remove any feed material that may contain *R. leguminicola*.

CLIENT EDUCATION
Biannual dental examination should be part of a routine health maintenance program.

MEDICATIONS

DRUG(S) OF CHOICE
N/A

CONTRAINDICATIONS
N/A

POSSIBLE INTERACTIONS
N/A

FOLLOW-UP

PATIENT MONITORING
Monitor for signs of aspiration pneumonia, and pharyngeal and esophageal perforation.

PREVENTION/AVOIDANCE
Feeding practices and pica—increase likelihood of foreign body obstruction or choke.

POSSIBLE COMPLICATIONS
Aspiration pneumonia, dermatitis.

EXPECTED COURSE AND PROGNOSIS
Prognosis depends on the specific condition.

MISCELLANEOUS

ASSOCIATED CONDITIONS
N/A

AGE-RELATED FACTORS
N/A

ZOONOTIC POTENTIAL
Rabies is a possible cause—care should be taken to wear gloves when examining.

PREGNANCY/FERTILITY/BREEDING
N/A

SYNONYMS
Slaframine toxicity—slobbers

SEE ALSO
• Slaframine toxicosis. • Vesicular stomatitis

ABBREVIATIONS
• CN = cranial nerve. • NSAID = nonsteroidal anti-inflammatory drug

Suggested Reading
Easley KJ. Salivary glands and ducts. In: Smith BP, ed. Large Animal Internal Medicine, 2e. St Louis: Mosby, 1996:697.

Author Diego Gomez-Nieto
Consulting Editors Henry Stämpfli and Olimpo Oliver-Espinosa

P

PURPURA HAEMORRHAGICA

 BASICS

DEFINITION
Acute disease of horses characterized by immune-mediated vasculitis, edema of the head and limbs, petechial and ecchymotic hemorrhages in mucosae, musculature and viscera, and sometimes glomerulonephritis.

PATHOPHYSIOLOGY
• PH is an immune-mediated vasculitis associated with a type III hypersensitivity reaction
• Soluble immune complexes (mostly composed of IgA and SeM) are formed in moderate antigen excess
• Circulating complexes become deposited in the walls of small blood vessels with subsequent fixation and activation of complement to C5a, a potent chemotactic factor for neutrophils
• Release of proteolytic enzymes from localized neutrophils directly damages vessel walls, resulting in edema, hemorrhage, thrombosis, and ischemic changes in tissues
• Blood vessels of the skin are primarily affected
• Hydrostatic pressures within vessels in dependent areas of the body result in distribution of lesions in lower limbs and ventral abdomen

SYSTEMS AFFECTED
Hemic/lymphatic/immune/cardiovascular system/skin.

GENETICS
N/A

INCIDENCE/PREVALENCE
• Sporadic
• Reported incidence subsequent to *Streptococcus equi* ssp. *equi* varies from 0.5% to 5%
• Highest incidence reported in outbreaks of strangles, possibly because of reinfection of horses already sensitized by previous infection(s)

GEOGRAPHIC DISTRIBUTION
N/A

SIGNALMENT
There is no breed, sex, or age predilection.

SIGNS
General Comments
Clinical signs vary from a mild, transient reaction to a severe and fatal disease.

Historical Findings
• Exposure to, or infection with, respiratory pathogens frequently reported within previous 2–4 weeks
• Vaccination may precede disease

Physical Examination Findings
• Common signs include fever, depression, tachycardia, and tachypnea; reluctance to move; and reduced or absent appetite

• Subcutaneous edema is an early sign, with swelling beginning around the nostrils and muzzle then progressing to the entire head, distal limbs, and ventral abdomen
• Edema initially appears as well-demarcated areas of hot, sensitive swellings, which become cold and painless over time and merge into normal tissue without a line of demarcation
• Swellings can develop suddenly or gradually, are usually asymmetric and non-pruritic, and pit with gentle pressure
• Hyperemia and petechial and ecchymotic hemorrhages (purpura) may be observed in light-skinned areas and on mucous membranes
• Edema and hemorrhage may progress to skin infarction, necrosis, and exudation with large, distended areas oozing red-tinged serum. Skin of the distal limbs is most commonly and severely affected. These sites may slough and leave granulating wounds
• Mucosal surfaces may also ulcerate and slough
• If the larynx is involved, dysphagia and dyspnea may occur owing to swelling and pain
• Edema, hemorrhage, and necrosis can occur in other body systems resulting in lameness, colic, epistaxis, dyspnea, and ataxia
• Subclinical renal disease is common
• Secondary complications such as laminitis, thrombophlebitis, and localized infections are common
• Death may ensue as a result of pneumonia, cardiac arrhythmias, renal failure, or GI disorders
• An uncommon, more severe manifestation of PH (infarctive PH) is characterized by infarction of multiple tissues including the GI tract and muscle. Affected horses have colic and muscle swelling. The course of disease is 3–5 days, with death a common outcome due to severe colic and rapidly deteriorating metabolic status

CAUSES
• Antigens can be derived from infectious agents (bacteria, viruses) or drugs
• In 1 study, approximately 32% of horses had been infected with, or exposed to, *S. equi* ssp. *equi*; 9% had been vaccinated with SeM; 17% had been infected with *Corynebacterium pseudotuberculosis*; and 9% had a history of apparently infectious respiratory disease of unknown cause. A further 28% of horses had no history of recent infectious diseases
• Equine influenza virus, equine herpesviruses, equine viral arteritis, *S. equi* ssp. *zooepidemicus*, *Rhodococcus equi,* and prolonged drug administration have also been implicated
• Horses vaccinated excessively with modified live, killed whole-cell, or M protein-based *S. equi* ssp. *equi* vaccines may develop PH owing to high concentrations of antibody and antigen

• No inciting cause may be found in some cases (idiopathic vasculitis)

RISK FACTORS
• Role of vaccination in development of PH is contentious
• Streptococcal vaccines have not definitively been shown to be a risk factor for development of PH, but some authors recommend that horses with high serum antibody titers to streptococcal M protein should not be vaccinated for strangles
• Also not clear whether infected horses should be vaccinated during an outbreak of strangles owing to the potential association with development of PH

 DIAGNOSIS

DIFFERENTIAL DIAGNOSIS
Immune-mediated vasculitis must be differentiated from vasculitis directly caused by infectious agents, immune-mediated thrombocytopenia, and other causes of edema or petechial and ecchymotic hemorrhages.

CBC/BIOCHEMISTRY/URINALYSIS
• No characteristic abnormalities are associated with PH
• Length of illness, organ involvement, and secondary complications will influence changes observed
• Neutrophilic leukocytosis, hyperfibrinogenemia, hyperglobulinemia, and mild anemia are commonly observed due to chronic inflammation
• Moderate anemia occurs in some cases owing to increased red blood cell destruction
• Creatinine may be elevated and urinalysis may show traces of hematuria and/or proteinuria due to glomerulonephritis
• Elevations in creatine kinase and aspartate aminotransferase activities may be present owing to muscle lesions
• Horses with infarctive PH have marked elevations in muscle enzymes and neutrophilia, and in severely affected horses there is evidence of a consumptive coagulopathy, which will result in thrombocytopenia and decreased prothrombin and activated partial thromboplastin time

OTHER LABORATORY TESTS
Elevated IgA titers to *S. equi* ssp. *equi* and IgG–SeM titers >1:6400 are suggestive of PH.

IMAGING
N/A

OTHER DIAGNOSTIC PROCEDURES
• Diagnosis often based on history, clinical signs, exclusion of other causes of vasculitis, and response to therapy
• Documentation of leukoclastic vasculitis and/or presence of immune complexes support the diagnosis

• Full-thickness skin punch biopsies (≥6 mm diameter) should be obtained and preserved in 10% formalin and Michel's transport medium
• Multiple biopsies of early lesions (<24 h) are required as distribution of lesions is patchy and lesions >24 h may be nondiagnostic

PATHOLOGIC FINDINGS

• Subcutaneous edema and numerous, discrete, petechial and ecchymotic hemorrhages are seen in affected tissues
• Leukoclastic vasculitis (neutrophilic infiltration of small blood vessels with nuclear debris around involved vessels and fibrinoid necrosis) may be observed in the skin, lung, muscle, and GI tract
• Horses with infarctive PH have dark red to black, multifocal coalescing hemorrhages in skeletal muscles, lungs, and GI tract. Histologic examination reveals coagulative necrosis

TREATMENT

AIMS

Treatment involves removal of the inciting cause, reduction of inflammation, reduction of the immune response, and provision of supportive care.

APPROPRIATE HEALTH CARE

Administration of any drugs should be discontinued as PH could be caused by an adverse drug reaction.

NURSING CARE

• Horses with PH usually require immediate, aggressive nursing care
• Hydrotherapy can minimize edema, and pressure wraps are used to decrease limb swelling
• Isotonic fluid administration (IV or enteral) may be required to maintain hydration in animals with severe depression or dysphagia
• Sloughed areas of skin should receive topical wound therapy

ACTIVITY

Limited hand-walking may increase peripheral circulation, especially in cases with significant edema of the limbs.

DIET

Swelling of the head and pharynx may necessitate placement of a nasogastric feeding tube to permit enteral feeding of dysphagic horses.

CLIENT EDUCATION

N/A

SURGICAL CONSIDERATIONS

• Any accessible, mature abscesses should be drained

• Emergency tracheotomy may be required to relieve respiratory distress and prevent asphyxiation

MEDICATIONS

DRUG(S) OF CHOICE

• Corticosteroid use remains controversial and mild cases may resolve without immunosuppressive therapy
• Horses with life-threatening edema or organ dysfunction require early, aggressive corticosteroid treatment
• Dexamethasone (0.05–0.2 mg/kg IV SID) is initially administered until edema and inflammation are reduced
• Prednisolone (0.5–2.0 mg/kg PO BID–SID) can be used as a maintenance dose after initial dexamethasone treatment
• Once edema starts to resolve, the dosage of corticosteroids can be reduced (10–15% every 1–2 days) over 7–21 days while carefully monitoring for recurrence
• Some cases require >4–6 weeks of corticosteroid therapy, and relapse may occur if therapy is truncated or if dexamethasone is switched to prednisolone too early (<10 days)
• For horses suffering a relapse, the corticosteroid dose may need to be increased over the previously efficacious concentrations
• Antimicrobials should be used with corticosteroids to reduce the occurrence and severity of septic sequelae and to address suspected streptococcal infection. Penicillin should be given for 1–3 weeks or until clinical signs resolve
• Flunixin meglumine or phenylbutazone may help reduce vascular inflammation and edema and provide analgesia

CONTRAINDICATIONS

None

PRECAUTIONS

High-dose corticosteroid therapy may be associated with laminitis or secondary infections.

POSSIBLE INTERACTIONS

None

ALTERNATIVE DRUGS

None

FOLLOW-UP

PATIENT MONITORING

Glomerulonephritis can progress to chronic renal failure. Creatinine and urine protein should be monitored weekly.

PREVENTION/AVOIDANCE

• Control of strangles reduces incidence
• Caution should be given to the use of streptococcal vaccines in horses at low risk of developing strangles
• Horses with M protein antibody titers >1:32 000 should not be vaccinated

POSSIBLE COMPLICATIONS

• Skin sloughing may be followed by exuberant granulation tissue
• Laminitis and various infections such as cellulitis, pneumonia, colitis, and thrombophlebitis may occur due to long-term corticosteroid therapy

EXPECTED COURSE AND PROGNOSIS

• Most horses recover with early aggressive therapy and supportive care within 2–4 weeks; sequelae may prolong convalescence
• Prognosis depends on severity and extent of disease
• Extensive skin sloughing, evidence of internal organ involvement, development of secondary septic processes, or laminitis are poor prognostic indicators

MISCELLANEOUS

ASSOCIATED CONDITIONS

N/A

AGE-RELATED FACTORS

N/A

ZOONOTIC POTENTIAL

None

PREGNANCY/FERTILITY/BREEDING

N/A

SYNONYMS

None

SEE ALSO

Streptococcus equi infection

ABBREVIATIONS

• GI = gastrointerstinal tract
• Ig = immunoglobulin
• PH = purpura haemorrhagica
• SeM = *S. equi* ssp. *equi* M protein

Suggested Reading
Hunyadi LM, Pusterla N. Purpura hemorrhagica. In: Felippe MJB, ed. Equine Clinical Immunology. Ames, IA: Wiley Blackwell, 2016:31–38.

Author Jennifer L. Hodgson
Consulting Editors David Hodgson, Harold C. McKenzie, and Jennifer L. Hodgson

P

PURULENT NASAL DISCHARGE

 BASICS

DEFINITION
Fluid discharge of varying turbidity, color, amount, frequency, and odor from 1 or both nostrils.

PATHOPHYSIOLOGY
- Composed of combinations of leukocytes and varying amounts of fluid and mucus from any location in the respiratory tract
- Production originates from an inflammatory process incited by traumatic, immune, allergic, infectious, or noxious stimuli
- Discharge can be septic or nonseptic
- Color varies—white, yellow, green, reddish, or brown depending on the presence of bacteria, ingesta, blood, or necrotic tissue
- Unilateral discharge is most likely associated with a condition of the ipsilateral nasal cavity or paranasal sinus
- Bilateral discharge more likely originates caudal to the nasal septum, especially the lower airways
- Nasal discharge from the guttural pouches can be unilateral or bilateral depending on the volume of discharge
- Malodorous discharge is associated with anaerobic infections, foreign bodies, necrotic bone, and tooth root abscesses

SYSTEMS AFFECTED
- Respiratory—lower tract, consisting of alveoli, bronchioles, bronchi, and trachea; upper tract, consisting of nasopharynx, guttural pouches, larynx, turbinates, conchae, nasal passages, paranasal sinuses, and false nostrils
- Gastrointestinal—oropharynx and esophagus

INCIDENCE/PREVALENCE
Variable depending on underlying cause.

SIGNALMENT
- Foals and young horses or any immunocompromised animal more prone to infections
- Neonates with milk in the discharge may have cleft palate or selenium deficiency, and resulting aspiration pneumonia
- Older horses—tooth infections, sinusitis, neoplasia
- Any age horse can have trauma, or bacterial infection

SIGNS
Historical Findings
- Historical information should include whether nasal discharge is continuous or intermittent, spontaneous or occurs only during exercise or while eating, copious or scant, unilateral or bilateral, and whether discharge is accompanied by other signs such as coughing, fever, reluctance to eat, dyspnea, respiratory noise, odor, or exercise intolerance

- Response to previous treatments and management changes should also be documented
- Exposure to other animals with disease may indicate an infectious process
- Seasonal correlation with worsening or alleviation may indicate allergic disease
- Facial swelling or bony remodeling is indicative of a chronic sinus problem, trauma, or tooth disease

Physical Examination Findings
- Ongoing discharge or dried material at nares
- Normal or decreased airflow at the nares with airway compromise
- Fever—consistent with infectious agent
- Chronic dyspnea, tachypnea, nostril flaring, increased abdominal respiratory effort, and "heaves line" are suggestive of SEA (heaves, recurrent airway obstruction)
- Lymphadenopathy with swelling and inflammation of retropharyngeal or submandibular lymph nodes with *Streptococcus equi* ssp. *equi* (strangles) or, less commonly, *S. equi* ssp. *zooepidemicus* infection
- Guttural pouch distention with empyema, tympany, or chondroids
- Dull areas on percussion of paranasal sinuses indicate exudate or cystic structure
- Evidence of dental disease associated with sinusitis
- Foul odor occurs with tooth root infection, bony necrosis (i.e. neoplasia), foreign body, Gram-negative or anaerobic lung abscessation, or necrotizing pneumonia
- Abnormal lung sounds consistent with pneumonia, pleuropneumonia, or SEA; may be exacerbated or elicited with use of a rebreathing bag
- Percussion of lung field—dull areas are indicative of pleural fluid, abscess, or consolidated lung
- Auscultation of fluid in trachea with exudate in pneumonia or SEA
- Dysphagia with esophageal obstruction, guttural pouch disease (resulting in neuropathy), or episodes of HYPP
- Milk in discharge with cleft palate in neonates, severe depression, botulism, HYPP or nutritional myopathy
- Depression—severe illness with pneumonia or pleuropneumonia
- Plaque of edema between the front legs in cases of pleuropneumonia

CAUSES
- Common causes are bacterial infections, bacterial infections following initial viral infections, and SEA
- Bacterial infections—*S. equi* lymphadenitis, guttural pouch empyema, sinusitis, lung abscessation, pneumonia, and pleuropneumonia
- Mycotic rhinitis, guttural pouch infection, or sinusitis
- Foreign bodies or trauma with subsequent inflammation/infection

- Esophageal obstruction or pharyngeal dysfunction resulting in dysphagia and aspiration

RISK FACTORS
- Exposure to animals infected with upper respiratory virus or strangles. Lack of vaccination against respiratory pathogens
- Viral infections—influenza and equine herpesvirus especially with young animals and congregated housing
- Poor deworming history—migrating ascarids predispose foals and yearlings to secondary bacterial pneumonia
- Immunodeficiency and immunosuppression—FTPI, severe combined immunodeficiency syndrome, PPID, and steroid therapy
- Environmental—indoors, dust, molds, air pollutants, and smoke inhalation
- Transport—subsequent pleuropneumonia
- Dental disease
- Dysphagia and aspiration associated with esophageal choke, cranial nerve damage, guttural pouch disease (mycosis), botulism, HYPP episodes affecting pharyngeal muscles
- Selenium deficiency in foals resulting in dysphagia and aspiration

 DIAGNOSIS

DIFFERENTIAL DIAGNOSIS
Differentiating Similar Signs
Purulent or mucopurulent nasal discharge is not easily confused with other signs.

Differentiating Causes
See Historical Findings, Physical Examination Findings, Causes, and Risk Factors.

CBC/BIOCHEMISTRY/URINALYSIS
- May have an inflammatory leukogram with neutrophilia and hyperfibrinogenemia if localized or extensive
- Leukogram may be degenerative, with left shift and toxic cells depending on severity (especially with pneumonia)
- Anemia may be a feature if there is chronic hemorrhage or chronic inflammation

OTHER LABORATORY TESTS
- Serum immunoglobulin concentration for FTPI or immunodeficiency in neonates
- Serum/plasma for upper respiratory virus titers
- Culture or PCR detection of bacterial pathogens such as *Rhodococcus equi* and *S. equi*
- Arterial blood gases—PaO$_2$ for lower airway disease or pneumonia

IMAGING
- Endoscopy—nasal passages, sinuses (sinoscopy), pharynx, guttural pouches, trachea, and bronchi
- Radiography—sinuses, teeth, guttural pouches, pharynx, and lungs
- Ultrasonography—thorax

 P

- Scintigraphy, MRI, or CT scan may be available for further detailed imaging if the source of the discharge is elusive

OTHER DIAGNOSTIC PROCEDURES

- Culture and sensitivity of nasopharynx or guttural pouch to detect strangles
- Bronchoalveolar lavage—cytology in diffuse lower airway disorders
- Tracheal wash—culture and cytology
- Lymph node (if affected) aspiration—culture and cytology
- Sinus aspiration/trephination—culture and cytology
- Thoracocentesis—culture and cytology
- Respiratory function testing for inflammatory airway disease

PATHOLOGIC FINDINGS

Dependent on underlying disease.

TREATMENT

APPROPRIATE HEALTH CARE

- Institute isolation measures if infectious agents are suspected
- Routine vaccination of susceptible animals against infectious respiratory diseases
- Manage SEA through environmental modification, anti-inflammatories, and bronchodilators

NURSING CARE

Variable depending on underlying disease. Appropriate intensive care, nursing care, oxygen administration, and rest for pneumonia and pleuropneumonia patients.

ACTIVITY

Most respiratory infections require a period of rest to allow recovery. Insult to the airway mucociliary apparatus may take up to 7 weeks to repair.

DIET

- Appropriate for change in activity
- Decreased plane of nutrition for athletic animals during recovery period
- Adequate plane of nutrition for serious respiratory disease such as pleuropneumonia where animals may be in catabolic disease state

CLIENT EDUCATION

Contingent on the diagnosis. Infectious disease control, and environmental management control if appropriate.

SURGICAL CONSIDERATIONS

- May be required for sinus, guttural pouch, or dental conditions; removal of foreign body, trephination, drainage, flushing of the sinuses, surgical tooth expulsion
- Flushing of guttural pouches
- Drainage of abscesses
- Chest drainage may be indicated in pleuropneumonia
- Tetanus prophylaxis

MEDICATIONS

DRUG(S) OF CHOICE

- Antimicrobials based on culture and sensitivity results for bacterial infections
- NSAIDs such as flunixin meglumine
- Inhalant or systemic steroids and bronchodilators for SAE

CONTRAINDICATIONS, PRECAUTIONS

Dependent on underlying disease and treatment approach.

POSSIBLE INTERACTIONS

N/A

ALTERNATIVE DRUGS

N/A

FOLLOW-UP

Contingent on diagnosis.

PATIENT MONITORING

Contingent on diagnosis.

PREVENTION/AVOIDANCE

Contingent on diagnosis.

POSSIBLE COMPLICATIONS

- Aspiration pneumonia if dysphagia
- Recurrence if sinus infections
- Dysphagia and fatal hemorrhage if guttural pouch mycosis
- Purpura haemorrhagica if strangles

EXPECTED COURSE AND PROGNOSIS

Contingent on diagnosis.

MISCELLANEOUS

AGE-RELATED FACTORS

- Foals and young horses at risk of respiratory infections

- Foals with congenital cleft palate, selenium deficiency
- Young horses with congenital sinus cysts
- Older horses with PPID prone to recurring infections

PREGNANCY/FERTILITY/BREEDING

N/A

SEE ALSO

- Aspiration pneumonia
- Esophageal obstruction (choke)
- Guttural pouch empyema
- Heaves (severe equine asthma, RAO)
- Pleuropneumonia
- Pneumonia, neonate
- Sinusitis (paranasal)
- *Streptococcus equi* infection

ABBREVIATIONS

- CT = computed tomography
- FTPI = failure of transfer of passive immunity
- HYPP = hyperkalemic periodic paralysis
- MRI = magnetic resonance imaging
- NSAID = nonsteroidal anti-inflammatory drug
- PaO_2 = partial pressure of oxygen in arterial blood
- PCR = polymerase chain reaction
- PPID = pars pituitary intermedia dysfunction
- SEA = severe equine asthma

Suggested Reading

Ainsworth DM, Cheetham J. Disorders of the respiratory system. In: Reed SM, Bayley WM, Sellon DC, eds. Equine Internal Medicine, 3e. St. Louis: WB Saunders, 2010:290–371.

Wilson WD, Lakritz J. Alterations in respiratory function. In: Smith BS, ed. Large Animal Internal Medicine, 5e. St. Louis: Elsevier Mosby, 2015:48–53.

Author Ashley G. Boyle
Consulting Editors Mathilde Leclère and Daniel Jean
Acknowledgment The author and editors acknowledge the prior contribution of Wendy Duckett.

P

PYOMETRA

 BASICS

DEFINITION
Accumulation of a large volume of purulent exudate within the uterine lumen.

PATHOPHYSIOLOGY
• Impaired drainage of uterine fluids, often due to cervical incompetence subsequent to reproductive trauma, inflammation, and adhesion formation, and occasionally due to vaginal adhesion
• Associated with destruction of the endometrial epithelium, severe inflammation, and permanent gland atrophy
• Endometrial destruction decreases endogenous $PGF_{2\alpha}$ secretion, prolonging luteal progesterone production during diestrus, which further contributes to cervical closure
• Bacterial or yeast/fungal opportunistic endometritis occurs secondary to anatomic defects

SYSTEMS AFFECTED
Reproductive

GENETICS
N/A

INCIDENCE/PREVALENCE
N/A

SIGNALMENT
• Pluriparous or nulliparous mares
• Aging
• No breed predilections

SIGNS
General Comments
• The mare may cycle regularly or have a prolonged diestrus
• Signs of systemic disease, e.g. colic, anorexia, weight loss, and depression, are rare
• Can be an incidental finding on routine examination

Historical Findings
• Watery, milky, or purulent vaginal discharge may be continuous, intermittent, or absent depending on degree of cervical patency and stage of the estrous cycle
• Contact dermatitis of the inner thighs and hocks may be evident
• History of dystocia or foaling trauma
• Historical placement of intrauterine glass marble in an effort to suppress estrus

Physical Examination Findings
• External perineal conformation may be normal or abnormal due to prior reproductive trauma
• Chronic or intermittent purulent vaginal discharge may occur
• TRP reveals an enlarged, fluid-filled uterus that may be further described with US
  ◦ Large fluid volumes (0.5–80 L) may accumulate within the uterine lumen

• Manual digital cervical examination often reveals adhesions, stricture, or other abnormalities

CAUSES
• Physical obstruction of the cervical or vaginal canals, as from adhesion formation, inhibits uterine drainage
• Cervical laceration trauma as from foaling, dystocia, or cervical manipulations
• Intra-abdominal adhesions to the uterus may prevent the uterus from evacuating completely
• Chronic uterine distention impairs the ability of the uterus to contract and empty
• Chronic cervicitis, from reproductive procedures such as lavage for endometritis treatment or embryo retrieval, contributes to cervical fibrosis, stricture, and/or induration
• Chronic foreign body, such as intact or broken glass marbles, contributes to nidus of infection
• Aged mares with poor cervical dilation

Infectious
• Bacteria do not cause pyometra in the mare, they are opportunists
• Most common isolates: *Streptococcus equi* ssp. *zooepidemicus*, *Escherichia coli*, *Actinomyces* spp., *Pasteurella* spp., and *Pseudomonas* spp.

RISK FACTORS
See Causes.

 DIAGNOSIS

DIFFERENTIAL DIAGNOSIS
Pregnancy
• The uterus of a pregnant mare demonstrates a characteristic tone and responsiveness
• With a pyometra the uterine wall may become thickened and the uterus feels *doughy*
• US of uterine fluid of pyometra is almost always hyperechoic, flocculent, and echo dense

Placentitis
• May be characterized by purulent vaginal discharge in a pregnant mare
• Ascending placentitis occurs late in gestation and is localized at the cervical star
• Premature mammary development may be present

Pneumouterus/Pneumometra
• Poor tone of the vestibulovaginal sphincter allows air to pass through the open cervix and into the uterus, often occurring during estrus, or after use of sedatives
  ◦ Common name for pneumometra is wind-sucking

Mucometra/hydrometra
Mucoid exudate accumulation is rare.

Urometra
Urine accumulation in the uterus is more likely in the postpartum period, when the

uterus and cervix have not involuted adequately.

Distended Bladder
Distinguish the uterus from the bladder by the ability to follow the uterine horns to the ovaries during TRP.

OTHER CAUSES OF VAGINAL DISCHARGE
See chapter Endometritis.

CBC/BIOCHEMISTRY/URINALYSIS
• Mild normocytic, normochromic anemia, and/or neutropenia
• Increased fibrinogen or serum amyloid A

OTHER LABORATORY TESTS
• Culture and cytology of the uterine fluid are recommended
• When manually passing through an adhered, indurated cervix, avoid iatrogenic perforation of the adjacent vagina or uterus
  ◦ Its lumen may be severely compromised or tortuous
• Pass a guarded endometrial culturette (swab or brush) into the uterus or obtain fluid during drainage, by means of a sterile nasogastric or urinary tract-type tube

Cytology
• The swab for the cytology specimen is rolled onto a sterile glass slide; dried and stained with Diff-Quik
• Assess for the presence of neutrophils and for the presence of bacteria, yeast, or fungal hyphae, similar to those associated with infectious endometritis

Bacteria
• Bacterial isolation ranges from a mixed population of organisms to no bacterial growth
• Streak swab for culture on blood agar and MacConkey's plates, incubate at 37°C and examine at 24, 48, and 72 h

Yeasts/Fungi
• *Candida* and *Aspergillus* spp. organisms may grow on blood agar
• For fungal-specific culture, the sample is inoculated in Sabouraud agar and incubated for 4 days at 37°C

IMAGING
US
• Intrauterine fluid can be qualified by its presence, quantity, and quality
• The intraluminal uterine exudate of pyometra may be moderately to highly hyperechoic
• Glass marbles or shards may be identified as round or irregular hyperechoic structures

OTHER DIAGNOSTIC PROCEDURES
Endometrial Biopsy
• An important prognostic tool (see chapter Endometrial biopsy)
• Collect the initial sample before treatment
• Evacuate uterine content before performing the biopsy to lessen the risk of abdominal contamination

 P

(CONTINUED)

Endoscopy
- May reveal intrauterine adhesions that are precluding effective uterine drainage
- Purulent exudate may be attached to the walls and/or found free in the lumen
- Foreign bodies may be identified

PATHOLOGIC FINDINGS
- Endometrial biopsy may reveal severe inflammation and endometrial and glandular atrophy, depending on the severity and duration of the condition
- Atrophy may be permanent and confers an extremely poor prognosis for reproduction

TREATMENT
APPROPRIATE HEALTH CARE
- Drainage of uterine exudate, coupled with repeated uterine lavage (daily or alternate days) using a nasogastric tube and large volumes of warm saline. Several fillings and drainage may be required at each session, until the evacuated saline appears grossly free of exudate
- Infusion of N-acetylcysteine may assist with removal of exudate
- After lavage, administer either oxytocin or PGF$_{2\alpha}$
- Infuse the uterus with an antibiotic based on culture and sensitivity results (see chapter Endometritis)
- Antibiotics should be infused 45–60 min after oxytocin
- Administer a luteolytic dose of PGF$_{2\alpha}$ if a persistent corpus luteum is suspected

NURSING CARE
Manage contact dermatitis of the perineum and hindquarters with cleansing and emollient application.

ACTIVITY
Paddock turnout may facilitate uterine clearance of fluid, once the cervix is opened.

DIET
N/A

CLIENT EDUCATION
- Recurrence is possible and periodic retreatment may be necessary
- Poor fertility expected
- Endometrial biopsy is recommended—provides a more definitive prognosis of future fertility

SURGICAL CONSIDERATIONS
- Cervical wedge resection in the standing mare is a salvage technique to permanently open the cervix, so that drainage continues
  ○ Owing to the surgically created cervical defect, the mare will not be capable of carrying a foal
- Ovariohysterectomy is a major abdominal surgery, performed under general anesthesia
  ○ The uterus must be emptied before surgery

○ Life-threatening complications after hysterectomy have decreased significantly owing to improved techniques

MEDICATIONS
DRUG(S) OF CHOICE
- See chapter Endometritis
- PGF$_{2\alpha}$, dinoprost tromethamine (Lutalyse®) 5–10 mg total IM
- Oxytocin, 5–20 units IV or IM every 6–24 h
- N-Acetylcysteine, 30 mL of 20% solution, dilute to final volume of 60–150 mL with saline, infuse into uterus; lavage routinely the next day

CONTRAINDICATIONS
See chapter Endometritis.

PRECAUTIONS
To avoid iatrogenic laceration or rupture, use caution when passing the hand, instruments, or lavage tubing through the cervix and into the uterus. Infuse fluid for lavage carefully into the distended and friable uterus, beginning with relatively low volumes to avoid damage.

POSSIBLE INTERACTIONS
N/A

ALTERNATIVE DRUGS
N/A

FOLLOW-UP
PATIENT MONITORING
- TRP and US to evaluate response to treatment, by means of uterine size, tone, and amount of intrauterine fluid
- Endometrial biopsy and/or endoscopy after treatment for endometrial visualization, evaluation of response to treatment, and prognosis

PREVENTION/AVOIDANCE
N/A

POSSIBLE COMPLICATIONS
Iatrogenic abdominal contamination during reproductive procedures or surgery can cause peritonitis.

EXPECTED COURSE AND PROGNOSIS
- Recurrence is common
- Prognosis for fertility is poor to grave

MISCELLANEOUS
ASSOCIATED CONDITIONS
Cervical adhesions may obliterate the cervical lumen and keep it from opening and closing properly.

- With chronic irritation/infection/inflammation, the cells of the linear cervical folds are replaced by fibrous tissue. The cervix becomes uniformly firm/hard, precluding relaxation and active uterine clearance during estrus
- Opportunistic bacteria, yeast, fungi can accumulate in the uterine fluid and the process compounds itself, i.e. chronic endometritis occurs secondary to anatomic defects, leading to fluid pooling, opportunity for development of a chronic infection, and/or pyometra

AGE-RELATED FACTORS
Repeated uterine stretching associated with pregnancy results in a uterus suspended low in the abdomen, predisposing to fluid accumulation.

ZOONOTIC POTENTIAL
N/A

PREGNANCY/FERTILITY/BREEDING
- Pregnancy or embryo production only rarely achieved in mares after treatment for pyometra
- Obtaining offspring may be attempted by means of assisted reproductive techniques, such as oocyte collection or transfer and intracytoplasmic sperm injection

SEE ALSO
- Cervical lesions
- Endometritis
- Postpartum metritis
- Vulvar conformation

ABBREVIATIONS
- PGF$_{2\alpha}$ = prostaglandin F$_{2\alpha}$
- TRP = transrectal palpation
- US = ultrasonography, ultrasound

Suggested Reading
Arnold CE, Brinsko SP, Varner DD. Cervical wedge resection for treatment of pyometra secondary to transluminal cervical adhesions in six mares. J Am Vet Med Assoc 2015;246:1354–1357.
de Amorim MD, Chenier T, Nairn D, et al. Complications associated with intrauterine glass marbles in five mares. J Am Vet Med Assoc 2016;249:1196–1201.
Freeman DE, Rotting AK, Köllman M, et al. Ovariohysterectomy in mares: 17 cases (1988-2007). Proc Am Assoc Equine Pract 2007;53:370–373.
Hughes JP, Stabenfeldt GH, Kindahl H, et al. Pyometra in the mare. J Reprod Fertil Suppl 1979;27:321–329.
Lu K. Pyometra. In: McKinnon AO, Squires EL, Vaala WE, Varner DD, eds. Equine Reproduction, 2e. Ames, IA: Wiley Blackwell, 2011:2652–2654.
Tranquillo GG, Kelleman AA, Sertich PL. Theriogenology question of the month. J Am Vet Med Assoc 2009;235:1161–1164.

Authors Audrey A. Kelleman and Maria E. Cadario
Consulting Editor Carla L. Carleton

P

PYRROLIZIDINE ALKALOID TOXICOSIS

BASICS

DEFINITION
• Caused by the chronic ingestion of PA-containing plants; PAs are a distinct group of structurally similar molecules found in approximately 6000 plant species worldwide
• Hundreds of different alkaloids exist
• Alkaloid composition and concentration, as well as toxicity, vary tremendously among plants, within different parts of the plant, and with stage of plant maturity
• 3 plant families (Compositae, Leguminosae, and Boraginaceae) account for most PA-containing plants. Clinical disease in the USA most common with *Senecio, Amsinckia, Cynoglossum,* and *Crotalaria. Symphytum, Echium,* and *Heliotropium* also contain PAs
• Economic losses have decreased owing to widespread recognition of the problem and effective livestock management and biologic control measures (particularly with *Senecio jacobaea*)
• Intoxications usually occur when horses graze paddocks or pastures heavily contaminated with these plants or consume contaminated hay during a period of several weeks to months
• Acute intoxications are rare, primarily because of the large amount of plant material a horse would need to ingest at any 1 feeding or several feedings

PATHOPHYSIOLOGY
• PAs are rapidly absorbed from the gastrointestinal tract and undergo extensive hepatic metabolism by mixed-function oxidases
• Some are detoxified to harmless metabolites, which then are eliminated via the urine or bile. Others are activated by conversion to toxic metabolites, primarily by dehydrogenation, yielding highly toxic pyrrole derivatives
• Pyrroles alkylate double-stranded DNA, thus inhibiting cell mitosis. Nuclear and cytoplasmic cell masses expand because of the impaired ability to divide, thus forming megalocytes. As megalocytes die, they are replaced by fibrous connective tissue
• Pyrroles also bind to cellular constituents in lung and kidney tissues

SYSTEMS AFFECTED
• Hepatobiliary—interference with cell replication leads to hepatocytomegaly and necrosis with bile duct proliferation and fibrosis; endothelial proliferation in centrilobular and hepatic veins occurs
• Renal/urologic—pyrrole-bound molecules can lead to megalocytosis of the proximal convoluted tubules, atrophy of glomeruli, and tubular necrosis; this has not been described in horses
• Respiratory—pyrrole-bound molecules can lead to alveolar hemorrhage and edema,

progressive proliferation of alveolar walls, pulmonary arteritis, and hypertension; this is not commonly reported in horses
• Cardiovascular—right ventricular hypertrophy and cor pulmonale have been documented experimentally, most likely secondary to PA-induced lung damage

GENETICS
N/A

INCIDENCE/PREVALENCE
Most intoxications occur during the plant growing season; however, intoxications can occur at any time because of the persistent toxicity of these alkaloids in baled hay.

SIGNALMENT
N/A

SIGNS
General Comments
• Most affected horses suffer chronic weight loss and debilitation associated with hepatic insufficiency, which can be subtle in nature; this is referred to as the chronic-delayed form
• In the chronic-delayed form, clinical signs can appear quite suddenly, despite exposure and liver lesions having been chronic and progressive
• The extent of hepatic damage depends greatly on the daily amount of alkaloid consumption, degree of pyrrole conversion, age of the animal, and metabolic and mitotic status of the target cells
• Food intake and nutritional status also can modify the effects of PAs
• Most affected patients, particularly those with the chronic-delayed form, exhibit neurologic signs

Physical Examination Findings
• Loss of appetite
• Weight loss
• Weakness and sluggishness
• Photodermatitis
• Icterus
• Behavioral abnormalities—mania, derangement, yawning, aimless walking, head pressing, drowsiness, blindness, and ataxia
• Inspiratory dyspnea—related to paralysis of the pharynx and larynx
• Gastric impaction
• Ascites
• Diarrhea with tenesmus

CAUSES
• Plants commonly incriminated in the USA—*S. jacobaea* (tansy ragwort), *Senecio vulgaris* (common groundsel), *Senecio douglasii* var. *longilobus* (threadleaf groundsel), *Senecio riddellii* (Riddell's groundsel), and *Cynoglossum officinale* (hound's tongue)
• Most animals must ingest 1–5% of body weight in plant material daily before effects are observed. Sometimes as much as 50% is required before clinical signs become apparent
• With tansy ragwort, the chronic lethal dose for horses is 0.05–0.20 kg/kg (equivalent to 1

dried hound's tongue plant per day for 2 weeks)
• *Amsinckia* and *Crotalaria* spp. rarely cause problems, because the highest percentage of alkaloid is present in the seed. Intoxication can result from ingestion of contaminated grain, cakes, or rarely after chronic ingestion of *Amsinckia*-contaminated hay

RISK FACTORS
Intoxication occurs from grazing heavy stands of the plants or eating contaminated hay for extended periods of time (2–4 weeks to several months).

DIAGNOSIS

DIFFERENTIAL DIAGNOSIS
• Alsike clover (*Trifolium hybridum*) or red clover (*Trifolium pratense*) intoxication
• Other causes of liver diseases
• Viral encephalitis
• Nigropallidal encephalomalacia
• Leukoencephalomalacia
• Equine protozoal encephalomyelitis
• Miscellaneous hepatotoxic chemicals—more acute in nature; causing more necrosis (e.g. carbon tetrachloride, chlorinated hydrocarbons, pentachlorophenols, coal-tar pitch, phenol, iron, phosphorus)
• Aflatoxin poisoning—rare

CBC/BIOCHEMISTRY/URINALYSIS
• Elevations in γ-glutamyltransferase and alkaline phosphatase
• Hyperbilirubinemia
• Hypoalbuminemia
• Hypoproteinemia
• Inflammatory leukogram
• Hyperammonemia

OTHER LABORATORY TESTS
• Prolonged bromosulfophthalein clearance time
• Elevated bile acids
• Abnormal liver biopsy

IMAGING
Ultrasonography may detect extensive liver fibrosis.

OTHER DIAGNOSTIC PROCEDURES
• Detection of pyrrole metabolites in feed, stomach contents, blood, or hepatic tissue can be performed by some laboratories. This is more successful in the acute stages of the disease
• Identification of PA-containing plants on premise or in feed (less commonly stomach contents) is the preferred method of confirming exposure
• Liver biopsy to detect characteristic lesions is critical to the diagnosis
• Serum biomarkers of liver injury

PATHOLOGIC FINDINGS
• Poor body condition; loss of body fat
• Jaundice

P

- Ascites and generalized edema
- Small, pale, firm liver with a mottled, cut surface
- Megalocytosis, with mild necrosis
- Fibrosis—centrilobular and periportal
- Veno-occlusive lesions
- Biliary hyperplasia
- Pulmonary edema
- Interstitial pneumonia
- Brain status spongiosus
- Other, less recognized lesions—myocardial necrosis, cecal and colonic edema and hemorrhage, and adrenal cortical hypertrophy

TREATMENT

APPROPRIATE HEALTH CARE
- Primary goal—to provide supportive therapy until enough liver tissue can regenerate and function adequately for the intended use of the horse
- Most PA-poisoned patients respond poorly to treatment, because by the time the disease is diagnosed adequate liver regeneration is no longer possible

NURSING CARE
- IV fluids to correct dehydration
- Photodermatitis can be treated with appropriate combination of cleansing, hydrotherapy, and debridement, along with restricting exposure to sunlight

ACTIVITY
Rest and stress reduction.

DIET
- Replace contaminated feed with a high-nutrient diet (easily digestible, high caloric, low protein) divided into 4–6 daily feedings
- One suggested diet includes 1–2 parts beet pulp (or *Sorghum* or milo) and 0.25, 0.50, or 1 part cracked corn mixed with molasses and fed at a rate of 2.5 kg/45 kg
- Oat or grass hay
- Avoid alfalfa and other legumes because of their high protein content
- Consider weekly vitamin B_1, folic acid, and vitamin K_1 supplementation

CLIENT EDUCATION
- Recognize PA-containing plants of concern in the geographic area, and prevent access by the horse
- Provide adequate forage and prevent overgrazing to limit ingestion of toxic plants

SURGICAL CONSIDERATIONS
N/A

MEDICATIONS

DRUG(S) OF CHOICE
- Horses with neurologic signs may require diazepam (foals 0.05–0.4 mg/kg IV; adults 25–50 mg IV; may be necessary to repeat) or xylazine (1.1 mg/kg IV or 2.2 mg/kg IM)
- With low blood glucose, a continual 5% dextrose drip may be administered IV at a rate of 2 mL/kg/h. Dilute the 5% dextrose in normal saline or lactated Ringer's solution if the infusion will last longer than 24–48 h
- Oral neomycin, lactulose, or mineral oil have been used to decrease blood ammonia concentrations, but with varying results

CONTRAINDICATIONS
N/A

PRECAUTIONS
- Diarrhea is a common sequela after neomycin or lactulose therapy
- Exercise care when administering any medication that undergoes extensive hepatic metabolism

POSSIBLE INTERACTIONS
N/A

ALTERNATIVE DRUGS
N/A

FOLLOW-UP

PATIENT MONITORING
- Monitor appetite, weight, serum liver enzymes, and bile acids every 2–4 weeks
- Magnitude of the elevation of serum hepatic enzymes does not always correlate with degree of hepatic impairment

PREVENTION/AVOIDANCE
- Recognize PA-containing plants, both in the field and in feeds
- Use good management practices and appropriate herbicide control to avoid overexposure of horses to these plants
- Sheep and goats are relatively resistant and may be used to graze heavily contaminated land

POSSIBLE COMPLICATIONS
Pneumonia and chronic wasting are the most common sequelae.

EXPECTED COURSE AND PROGNOSIS
- Most affected horses are given a poor prognosis and are euthanized because of severe debilitation or nonresponsive neurologic signs
- Some animals can recover after several months of care but generally cannot regain their former fitness or activity level

MISCELLANEOUS

ASSOCIATED CONDITIONS
N/A

AGE-RELATED FACTORS
Foals or young ponies may be at greater risk because of their smaller body mass, less discriminating eating habits, higher metabolic activity, and higher susceptibility of tissues in which cells are rapidly dividing.

ZOONOTIC POTENTIAL
N/A

PREGNANCY/FERTILITY/BREEDING
- PAs have been detected in milk and are hepatotoxic and carcinogenic
- PAs cross the placenta, causing various fetotoxic effects

SYNONYMS
- Jaagsiekte
- Missouri bottom disease
- Pictou disease
- Sleepy staggers
- Walking disease
- Yawning disease

ABBREVIATIONS
PA = pyrrolizidine alkaloid

Suggested Reading
Craig AM, Pearson EG, Meyer C, Schmitz JA. Clinicopathologic studies of tansy ragwort toxicosis in ponies: sequential serum and histopathological changes. J Equine Vet Sci 1991;11:261.
Moore RE, Knottenbelt D, Mathews JB, et al. Biomarkers for ragwort poisoning in horses: identification of protein targets. BMC Vet Res 2008;4:30.
Pearson EG. Liver failure attributable to pyrrolizidine alkaloid toxicosis and associated with inspiratory dyspnea in ponies: three cases (1982–1988). J Am Vet Med Assoc 1991;198:1651.

Author Tina Wismer
Consulting Editors Wilson K. Rumbeiha and Steve Ensley
Acknowledgment The author and editors acknowledge the prior contribution of Patricia A. Talcott.

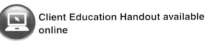
Client Education Handout available online

P

QUERCUS SPP. (OAK) TOXICOSIS

BASICS

OVERVIEW
• This genus of plants contains a variety of species, including trees and shrubs
• Species more commonly associated with poisoning include Gambel's oak (*Quercus gambelii*), Havard or shinnery oak (*Quercus havardii*), and white shin oak (*Quercus durandii* var. *breviloba*). Other species implicated in poisonings include wavyleaf oak (*Quercus undulata*), Emory oak (*Quercus emoryi*), shrub live oak (*Quercus turbinella*), and silverleaf oak (*Quercus hypoleucoides*)
• All *Quercus* spp. should be considered toxic. Ingestion of large quantities of leaves, leaf buds, or acorns results in a severe gastroenteritis/nephrotoxic syndrome
• Poisoning is most commonly associated with ingestion of acorns or new leaf buds, hence the common name "oak-bud poisoning"
• Gallotannins are the toxic principals. Ingested tannins react with dietary and tissue proteins, rendering them nonfunctional. Toxicosis generally occurs when oak is >50% of the diet
• Poisonings most commonly occur in early spring with ingestion of new leaf buds or in late fall with ingestion of acorns

SIGNALMENT
• Poisoning is rare in horses
• It can occur at any age
• Male and female equids are equally susceptible

SIGNS
• Abdominal pain, depression, anorexia, constipation (early) followed by hemorrhagic diarrhea
• Peripheral edema, diphtheritic membranes in feces
• Weakness, polydipsia, and polyuria
• Tachycardia
• Prostration and death

CAUSES AND RISK FACTORS
• Intoxication is often associated with a lack of available forage or dietary supplementation
• Drought or conditions that inhibit other forages from growing predisposes to ingestion of oak
• Most common in the early spring when leaf buds are developing or late fall when acorns are dropping

DIAGNOSIS

CBC/BIOCHEMISTRY/URINALYSIS
Increased serum blood urea nitrogen and creatinine, hyposthenuria, proteinuria, hematuria, hyperphosphatemia, hypocalcemia, hypomagnesemia, hypovolemia, hypoproteinemia, metabolic acidosis, increased aspartate aminotransferase.

OTHER LABORATORY TESTS
N/A

IMAGING
N/A

OTHER DIAGNOSTIC PROCEDURES
N/A

PATHOLOGIC FINDINGS
Gross
Subcutaneous edema, mucoid and/or hemorrhagic enteritis, pseudomembranous enteritis, edema of mesenteric lymph nodes, hydropericardium, perirenal edema, swollen and pale kidneys, ascites, petechial hemorrhage of kidneys, and hepatic congestion.

Histopathologic
• Kidneys—numerous pink to brown casts in the proximal tubules, proximal tubular necrosis, medullary congestion
• GI—pseudomembranous, necrotizing enteritis with hemorrhage and ulceration
• Other—vascular congestion of the liver and lungs, generalized tissue congestion

TREATMENT

• Prevent further exposure by removing horses from access to oaks
• Minimize further GI and renal damage with general decontamination and supportive care
• Decontamination may decrease the duration and severity of signs. AC should bind tannins in the GI tract, rendering them unabsorbable, but this has not been proven
• Decrease GI transit time with mineral oil or cathartics such as magnesium sulfate (Epsom salt). Use gastric demulcents or sucralfate for severe GI damage
• Administer IV normal saline to keep the horse hydrated and maintain urine flow

MEDICATIONS

DRUG(S) OF CHOICE
AC (1–4 g/kg PO once in a water slurry), magnesium sulfate (250–500 mg/kg as a 20% solution PO once), sucralfate (2 mg/kg PO TID).

CONTRAINDICATIONS/POSSIBLE INTERACTIONS
Do not give AC with mineral oil as the oil prevents binding of compounds to the charcoal. Do not give AC if there is evidence of severe GI mucosal damage, as the charcoal can imbed in mucosal erosions.

FOLLOW-UP

PATIENT MONITORING
Monitor renal function daily. Maintenance of renal function is a good indicator of treatment efficacy.

PREVENTION/AVOIDANCE
Avoid pasturing horses in areas containing oaks unless other adequate forage is unavailable. Supplementation with calcium hydroxide (15% pellet) to inactivate tannins has been beneficial in other species, but its effectiveness in horses is unknown.

POSSIBLE COMPLICATIONS
With severe GI ulceration and necrosis, scarring and strictures are possible.

EXPECTED COURSE AND PROGNOSIS
Recovery may require 2–3 weeks of intense care.

MISCELLANEOUS

ASSOCIATED CONDITIONS
N/A

AGE-RELATED FACTORS
N/A

ZOONOTIC POTENTIAL
N/A

PREGNANCY/FERTILITY/BREEDING
N/A

ABBREVIATIONS
• AC = activated charcoal
• GI = gastrointestinal

Suggested Reading
Harper KT, Ruyle GB, Rittenhouse LR. Toxicity problems associated with the grazing of oak in the intermountain and southwestern USA. In: James LF, Ralphs MH, Nielsen DB, eds. The Ecology and Economic Impact of Poisonous Plants on Livestock Production. Boulder, CO: Westview Press, 1988:197–206.

Author Jeffery O. Hall
Consulting Editors Wilson K. Rumbeiha and Steve Ensley

Q

BASICS

OVERVIEW
• A lethal encephalitis caused by a neurotropic, single-stranded RNA virus in the family Rhabdoviridae, genus *Lyssavirus*
• Rabies is usually transmitted via salivary contamination of a bite wound. Historically, an animal may have been bitten by a dog, racoon, skunk, fox, or bat several months prior to the onset of signs, although most bite wounds are healed by the onset of neurologic signs
• The virus amplifies in muscle tissue before invading the peripheral nervous system. It is not known how the virus enters the peripheral nerves
• The virus moves to the CNS by axoplasmic flow and passes along neurons within the nervous system
• Systems affected—nervous

SIGNALMENT
Any breed, sex, and age may be affected; however, smaller slower animals (donkeys) are at higher risk.

SIGNS
Historical Findings
Horses or donkeys where rabies is endemic.

Physical Examination Findings
• The presenting signs of rabies virus infection can be extremely varied; however, in practice, many of the symptoms are surprisingly characteristic of the disease, particularly in the more advanced stages
• Most animals appear alert and anxious with progressive ataxia and characteristic odd vocalizations. Automutilation or mutilation of surrounding objects is extremely common. Typically animals target a specific body site and hold the bite for several minutes
• Early signs of the disease are more subtle and varied. Animals can present with colic, which presents obvious risks to veterinary personnel
• Classically, the syndromes are divided into a cerebral or furious form, the brainstem or dumb form, and the spinal cord or paralytic form. In practice these syndromes may overlap and the "dumb" form seems to be rare in equids
• Forebrain signs often include aggressive behavior, hyperesthesia, vocalization, sialosis, tenesmus, and convulsions
• In the dumb form, somnolence, dementia, stupor, opisthotonos, facial hypoalgesia, pharyngeal paralysis, excessive drooling, and ataxia occur
• The paralytic form is characterized by progressive ascending paralysis; monoparesis/plegia; truncal, limb, and perineal hyporeflexia and hypoalgesia;

priapism; and altered frequency of miction; and urinary incontinence
• Self-mutilation is typical
• Once signs start, the clinical course is <14 days, but usually <5 days, and the animal dies in a mean period of 3 days
• Prodromal colic, lameness, anorexia, and hydrophobia may be recalled by owners
• Fever may occur independent of seizure activity
• Web Video 1 shows a donkey showing typical signs of the disease. Anxious alert expression, persistent automutilation usually of the same area, difficulty rising with ataxia evident on all four limbs.

CAUSES AND RISK FACTORS
• The disease is caused by serotype 1 rabies virus. This is a single-stranded RNA virus of the genus *Lyssavirus* and family Rhabdoviridae. There are 25 viruses in this family, but only serotype 1 is pathogenic
• Rabies has 2 cycles, which include canine (urban) and wildlife (sylvatic) rabies. Most wildlife vectors are small omnivores, such as skunks, raccoons, or foxes
• There is extension into domestic animals, which are essentially dead-end hosts
• Horses in enzootic areas are at risk

DIAGNOSIS

DIFFERENTIAL DIAGNOSIS
Togaviral encephalitides, heavy metal toxicity, Polyneuritis Equi, acute protozoal myeloencephalitis, *Sorghum*–sudangrass poisoning, hepatoencephalopathy, CNS trauma, moldy corn poisoning, and probably many other disorders. The presence of automutilation could rule out many of these differentials.

CBC/BIOCHEMISTRY/URINALYSIS
No specific abnormalities.

OTHER LABORATORY TESTS
Cerebrospinal fluid is often normal but may show moderate elevations in protein and mononuclear cell numbers.

PATHOLOGIC FINDINGS
• Premortem diagnosis is not currently possible although automutilation combined with ataxia is almost pathognomonic for rabies
• The animal should be evaluated for 10 days and, if euthanized, the head or $1/2$ fresh and $1/2$ formalin-fixed brain and fresh salivary gland should be sent to a veterinary diagnostic laboratory equipped to handle rabies virus-infected tissue. Direct and indirect immunofluorescent antibody testing for rabies virus may be done there, as well as mouse inoculation studies if indicated

TREATMENT

Only palliative treatment can be offered. A strong suspicion of rabies is an indication for euthanasia.

Prevention
• Horses in enzootic areas may be immunized with annual vaccination beginning at 6 months of age with commercial inactivated vaccine
• Horses previously immunized and bitten by suspect rabid animals can be given a 3-booster immunization series over 7 days. They should be quarantined for a minimum of 90 days

MEDICATIONS
N/A

FOLLOW-UP
N/A

MISCELLANEOUS

ZOONOTIC POTENTIAL
Horse-to-human transmission is rare but has been reported on 2 occasions in South America. Exposure to saliva, nervous, and other tissues from horses suspected to be rabid should be avoided.

SEE ALSO
• Eastern (EEE), western (WEE), and Venezuelan (VEE) equine encephalitides
• Equine protozoal myeloencephalitis (EPM)
• Head trauma
• Hepatic encephalopathy
• Leukoencephalomalacia
• Polyneuritis equi
• *Sorghum* spp. toxicosis

ABBREVIATIONS
CNS = central nervous system

Suggested Reading
Green SL. Rabies. Vet Clin North Am Equine Pract 1997;13:1–11.
Author Gigi Kay
Consulting Editor Caroline N. Hahn
Acknowledgment The author acknowledges the prior contribution Caroline N. Hahn.

R

RECTAL PROLAPSE

BASICS

DEFINITION
In rectal prolapse, tissue protrudes through the anus. Depending on the layers involved, it can be categorized into 4 types:
• Type 1 = rectal mucosa and submucosa protrude
• Type 2 = prolapse of all layers of the rectal ampulla
• Type 3 = in addition to a type 2 prolapse there is intussusception of peritoneal rectum or small colon into the rectum. The intussuscepted part does not protrude through the anus
• Type 4 = intussusception of the peritoneal rectum and varying lengths of the small colon through the anus

PATHOPHYSIOLOGY
Rectal prolapse results from an increase in pressure gradient between the abdominal cavity and the anus (i.e. straining), which causes the rectal mucosa and submucosa to glide backward over the muscularis layer. Unreduced prolapses become edematous and cyanotic owing to compromise of venous outflow. With type 3 and 4 prolapses, the entire rectum disengages from the perirectal tissues, resulting in complete displacement of the rectum as well as the distal small colon. Because the mesocolon of the distal small colon is relatively short, caudal displacement and tearing of the mesocolon during prolapse often result in avulsion of the colonic blood supply. If the blood supply to the small colon is disrupted, ischemic necrosis ensues.

SYSTEMS AFFECTED
• Gastrointestinal—rectal impaction, small colon necrosis, or peritonitis
• Behavioral—straining or mild to moderate abdominal pain
• Cardiovascular—circulatory shock may be evident in horses with thrombosis or rupture of the small colonic vasculature or as a result of endotoxemia caused by small colon necrosis

SIGNALMENT
More common in adult horses and mares. Type 4 rectal prolapse is seen with dystocia in mares.

SIGNS
Historical Findings
Prolonged straining due to diarrhea or colic; dystocia.

Physical Examination Findings
Palpation and inspection are simple means of differentiating between the 4 types of rectal prolapses. Types 1, 2, and 3 are continuous with the mucocutaneous junction of the anus. Characteristic findings include:
• Type 1—a circular, doughnut-shaped, edematous swelling at the anus that is usually most prominent ventrally

• Type 2—a larger, cauliflower-shaped swelling that is often thicker ventrally than dorsally
• Type 3—appears similar to type 2, but the invaginated peritoneal rectum or small colon can be palpated within the rectal lumen. This invaginated part (intussusceptum) does not protrude through the anus
• Type 4—a palpable trench exists between the prolapse and the anus, and can be appreciated by sliding a finger underneath the prolapse and past the normal mucocutaneous junction. Usually has a tube-like appearance

CAUSES
Rectal prolapse is most often associated with straining secondary to a variety of conditions:
• Parturition
• Dystocia
• Uterine prolapse
• Diarrhea
• Constipation
• Colitis
• Proctitis
• Rectal masses—neoplasms (leiomyoma, lipoma), foreign bodies, abscesses, polyps, hematomas
• Grade 2 rectal tears
• Intestinal parasitism
• Urethral obstruction—urolithiasis
In many cases, however, a cause cannot be identified.

RISK FACTORS
Any condition that induces straining. Poor body condition owing to loss of tone in the anal sphincter or decreased elasticity of the connective tissue may increase risk. Type 1 rectal prolapses are often seen in horses with severe diarrhea, and type 4 rectal prolapses are most often associated with dystocia in broodmares.

DIAGNOSIS

DIFFERENTIAL DIAGNOSIS
Prolapsed tissues may be mistaken for a neoplastic mass. Visual inspection and palpation can differentiate between the 2 conditions. Evaginated rectal tissues are obvious with a prolapse, whereas a neoplasm arises from a localized aspect of the rectal or perirectal tissues.

CBC/BIOCHEMISTRY/URINALYSIS
Systemic abnormalities corresponding to the inciting cause may be identified. Early in the course of type 3 and 4 prolapses, leukocytosis and neutrophilia with a left shift may be observed, as well as increases in packed cell volume, fibrinogen, TP, sodium, and potassium levels. With longer duration, leukopenia and neutropenia ensue. Chronicity may lead to decreases in potassium, sodium, and chloride levels and

increases in blood urea nitrogen, creatinine, and bilirubin.

OTHER LABORATORY TESTS
Abdominocentesis to assess if compromise to the small colon has occurred. Peritoneal fluid in horses with type 3 or 4 prolapse may have an increase in white blood cell count or TP level. These abnormal findings may not develop until necrosis of gut wall, leakage, and peritonitis have occurred.

IMAGING
Transabdominal ultrasonography may be used to identify possible free fluid in the abdomen and evaluate motility of the intestine.

OTHER DIAGNOSTIC PROCEDURES
A flank laparotomy, ventral midline celiotomy, or laparoscopy can be used to assess the degree of compromise to the mesocolon and small colon in type 3 and 4 prolapse; however, access to the terminal small colon can be challenging with a flank or ventral midline laparotomy. In the standing horse, laparoscopy provides superior visualization and selection of the most appropriate surgical procedure in a minimally invasive manner.

TREATMENT

• The first step in the treatment of rectal prolapse is to prevent straining. The specific cause of the prolapse should therefore be identified and addressed. Epidural anesthesia is an effective means of alleviating tenesmus. Alternatively, heavy sedation, use of lidocaine gel, or a lidocaine enema may provide some relief
• Early type 1 and 2 rectal prolapses without extensive edema, trauma, or contamination usually respond to conservative therapy aimed at reduction of tissue edema, manual reduction of the prolapse, and placement of a purse-string suture in the anus to prevent recurrence, and treatment of the primary cause for the prolapse:
  ◦ Reduction of edema—application of topical glycerin, or mannitol, or magnesium sulfate, and lidocaine jelly or lidocaine enema (12 mL of lidocaine in 50 mL of water)
  ◦ Reduce or prevent straining via epidural anesthesia
  ◦ Purse-string suture—use of a large (size 1–3), nonabsorbable (nylon, polypropylene, umbilical tape, caprolactam) material; placed using 4 wide bites located 1–2 cm from the anus. Following placement, the external anal sphincter should be dilatable to a diameter of 2–3 cm to permit defecation to some degree although normal defecation will be impaired. Therefore, suture opening every 2–4 h to allow defecation or manual removal of feces is recommended It is

usually advised to remove the suture within 48–72 h to minimize complications
○ The horse should be taken off feed for the first 24 h. Thereafter, mineral oil or other laxatives should be administered for at least 1 week and the horse should be fed a laxative diet for at least 2 weeks
○ Horses should be kept cross-tied in a box stall for the first week to prevent recumbency (increased abdominal pressure when recumbent)
• Type 1 and 2 prolapses that are chronic in nature or that have failed to respond to conservative therapy can be treated successfully by submucosal resection or by full-thickness partial rectal amputation. Both procedures can be performed in the standing, sedated horse using epidural anesthesia. Submucosal resection is preferred over full-thickness rectal amputation because the rectal vasculature and muscular layers are preserved, an aseptic peritoneal environment is maintained, there is decreased risk of postoperative perirectal abscess formation or of rectal stricture, and postoperative tenesmus is decreased
• Type 3 and 4 rectal prolapses require referral to a surgical facility as the damage to the mesocolon can be serious. Balanced polyionic IV fluid therapy may be required by horses with type 3 or 4 prolapses for treatment of hypovolemia or endotoxemic shock. The fluid rate should be based on the horse's hydration status and clinical condition

CLIENT EDUCATION
Horses with type 4 rectal prolapse have a serious condition carrying a guarded to poor prognosis for survival. Depending on the length of intussuscepted tissues, severity of small colon mesenteric damage, chronicity of the prolapse, the horse's medical status and value, and the owner's intentions for the horse, euthanasia may be warranted. If the owner wishes to pursue treatment, factors that require discussion include cost, the need for

extensive postoperative care, and multiple possible complications following resection/anastomosis or colostomy. Horses undergoing colostomy may require a second procedure for revision, although permanent colostomy after resecting the rectum and distal small colon involved in a type 4 rectal prolapse may be indicated.

SURGICAL CONSIDERATIONS
Notable hemorrhage may occur during submucosal resection or full-thickness rectal partial amputation, but can be controlled with electrocautery or ligation.

MEDICATIONS
DRUG(S) OF CHOICE
• Sedation may be achieved with xylazine (0.2–1.1 mg/kg IV) or detomidine (0.005–0.02 mg/kg IV). Both duration and quality of sedation may be enhanced by the coadministration of butorphanol tartrate (0.1 mg/kg IV)
• Epidural administration of a variety of agents may provide anesthesia for initial evaluation and treatment, as well as analgesia for prevention of postoperative straining (for details and dosages, see chapter Rectal tears)

FOLLOW-UP
PATIENT MONITORING
Following treatment, the patient should be observed regularly for evidence of tenesmus, rectal impaction, or relapse. Purse-string sutures should be removed within 24–48 h to minimize complications. In grade III and IV, serial abdominocentesis is advised.

PREVENTION/AVOIDANCE
Prompt recognition and treatment of factors predisposing to tenesmus reduce the likelihood of rectal prolapse.

POSSIBLE COMPLICATIONS
• Rectal impaction
• Re-prolapse
• Dehiscence of suture lines
• Perirectal abscess formation
• Rectal stricture
• Ischemic necrosis of the small colon
• Complications associated with colostomy, celiotomy, or resection/anastomosis procedures

EXPECTED COURSE AND PROGNOSIS
The prognosis for type 1 and 2 rectal prolapses is favorable, whereas the prognosis for type 3 and 4 prolapses is guarded to poor.

MISCELLANEOUS
ASSOCIATED CONDITIONS
• Endotoxemia
• Laminitis
• Uterine prolapse

SEE ALSO
• Dystocia
• Idiopathic colitis
• Perineal lacerations/recto-vaginal-vestibular fistulas
• Tenesmus
• Vaginal prolapse

ABBREVIATIONS
TP = total protein

Suggested Reading
Espinosa Buschiazzo CA, Cancela MCJ, Simian MV. Permanent colostomy after small colon prolapse in a parturient mare. Equine Vet Educ 2010;22:223–227.
Freeman DE. Rectum and anus. In: Auer JA, Stick JA, eds. Equine Surgery, 4e. St. Louis, MO: WB Saunders, 2012:494–505.

Author Luis M. Rubio-Martinez
Consulting Editors Henry Stämpfli and Olimpo Oliver-Espinosa
Acknowledgment The author and editors acknowledge the prior contribution of Judith B. Koenig and Annette M. Sysel.

R

RECTAL TEARS

BASICS

DEFINITION
A partial- to full-thickness tear in the wall of the retroperitoneal or peritoneal rectum.

PATHOPHYSIOLOGY
Rectal tears are usually a complication of manual palpation per rectum but can also be due to enema administration in foals, dystocia, and breeding accidents. Most tears are longitudinal and located dorsally and 15–55 cm from the anus. The following 4 grades have been described:
• Grade 1—tearing of the rectal mucosa and submucosa
• Grade 2—the muscular layer of the rectum is torn, and the intact mucosa and submucosa prolapse through the defect to create a diverticulum, which may act as a pocket for fecal impaction
• Grade 3a—disruption of the rectal mucosa, submucosa, and muscularis layers, with intact serosa resulting in a palpable void in the rectal wall that exposes the serosa
• Grade 3b—disruption of the rectal mucosa, submucosa, and muscularis layers, with intact mesorectum and retroperitoneal tissues. This tear is palpable as a defect in the rectal wall that exposes the fat-filled mesorectum. The presence of intact serosa or mesorectum prevents direct contamination of the abdominal cavity with fecal material; however, movement of bacteria through these tissues frequently induces peritonitis
• Grade 4—tearing of all layers of the rectum; as a result, direct communication exists between the rectum and the abdominal cavity

SYSTEMS AFFECTED
GI
Local and diffuse peritonitis may develop within 2 h of a rectal tear, especially in grade 3b and 4 tears. Ileus secondary to diffusion of bacteria and toxins may follow. Abdominal discomfort and straining may accompany rectal impactions, in horses with grade 2 rectal tears.

Behavioral
Signs of colic secondary to peritonitis and ileus initially that may progress to depression and endotoxic shock.

Cardiovascular
Vascular collapse secondary to endotoxemic shock

GENETICS
None

INCIDENCE/PREVALENCE
N/A

GEOGRAPHIC DISTRIBUTION
None

SIGNALMENT
Breed Predilections
• Arabians
• Miniature horses and other small breeds
• Ponies

Mean Age and Range
Any age but horses unaccustomed to rectal examination are at higher risk.

Predominant Sex
More often in mares.

SIGNS
General Comments
Tearing of the rectum during a rectal palpation may not be felt, but should be suspected if a significant amount of blood is evident on the rectal sleeve or in the feces following rectal examination.

Historical Findings
Horses with grade 1 or 2 rectal tears rarely show signs. Grade 2 tears are often not identified until signs of rectal impaction develop; grade 3 or 4 rectal tears are often associated with signs of colic, a splinted abdomen, or tachycardia within 2 h following rectal tear.

Physical Examination Findings
See Pathophysiology.

CAUSES
• Rectal palpation
• Misdirected intromission of a stallion's penis during breeding
• Enema
• Meconium extraction
• Dystocia
• External trauma
• Fractures of the pelvis or vertebrae
• Sodomy
• Ruptured small colon hematomas
• Spontaneous

RISK FACTORS
Repeated rectal examination.

DIAGNOSIS

DIFFERENTIAL DIAGNOSIS
Mucosal irritation may result in a few flecks of blood on the palpation sleeve. Colitis or conditions that compromise the vascular supply of the small colon may produce bloody or malodorous brown fluid on rectal examination.

CBC/BIOCHEMISTRY/URINALYSIS
Leukocytosis and neutrophilia with a left shift, as well as increases in packed cell volume, blood fibrinogen, TP, sodium, and potassium occur early in the course of grade 3 and 4 rectal tears, as well as leukopenia and neutropenia; decreases in blood potassium, sodium, and chloride levels; and increases in blood urea nitrogen, creatinine, and bilirubin may occur later.

OTHER LABORATORY TESTS
Increased peritoneal fluid, white blood cell count, or TP level are consistent with peritonitis. The presence of degenerate neutrophils, bacteria, or plant material on cytologic examination is indicative of septic peritonitis and is associated with a guarded to poor prognosis.

IMAGING
Abdominal ultrasonography may be useful in assessment of quantity and quality of peritoneal fluid.

OTHER DIAGNOSTIC PROCEDURES
• After administration of epidural lidocaine, careful evaluation of the rectum is performed using a bare-arm technique or a surgeon's glove. Buscopan (N-butylscopolammonium bromide) can be administered IV if the horse's systemic condition permits and lidocaine in an enema or jelly can be administered into the rectum. The veterinarian's arm should be lubricated copiously with a water-soluble gel and the feces gently removed from the rectum. The rectal tear should be assessed to determine the severity and distance from the anus
• A vaginal speculum may be used for visualization of the tear, but in-folding of the mucosa around the end of the speculum often hampers adequate assessment
• Rectal endoscopy can be useful to grade the tear
• Laparoscopy is indicated in horses with grade 3 or 4 tears to determine contamination of the abdominal cavity

PATHOLOGIC FINDINGS
See Pathophysiology.

TREATMENT

AIMS
• Reduce straining
• Reduce motility
• Decrease fecal contamination
• Prevent infection
• Prevent shock

APPROPRIATE HEALTH CARE
• Straining and rectal peristalsis should be reduced by sedation, epidural anesthesia, and/or parasympatholytic drugs. A lidocaine enema (12–25 mL of 2% lidocaine in 50 mL water) or lidocaine jelly may be used. Fecal softeners and a laxative diet are valuable in all rectal tear cases
• Grade 1 rectal tears usually respond well to a 3–5 day course of anti-inflammatory and broad-spectrum antibiotic therapy. Periodic cleaning may be needed to hasten healing and prevent abscess formation, a permanent diverticulum, or a rectal stricture
• Grade 2 rectal tears may be treated with a gentle lavage of the diverticulum

R

• Horses with grade 3a, 3b, or 4 rectal tears should be considered emergencies and referred to a surgical facility
• Prior to transport, the rectal tear should be packed with 7.5 cm (3 inch) wide stockinette filled with moistened roll cotton. This should be sprayed with povidone–iodine and lubricated with surgical gel and inserted to a point 10 cm proximal to the tear. The anus can be closed with towel clamps or a purse-string suture. Epidural anesthesia to prevent straining and parenteral anti-inflammatory and broad-spectrum antibiotic therapy should be initiated. IV fluids should be given to horses in shock. Feed should be withheld

NURSING CARE
See Appropriate Health Care.

ACTIVITY
Horses treated surgically should be confined to a stall for appropriate postoperative monitoring and management.

DIET
All horses with rectal tears should be fed a low-bulk laxative diet.

CLIENT EDUCATION
The owner should be informed of the presence of a rectal tear or a suspected tear immediately without acknowledging guilt or responsibility for payment. If treatment is pursued, the owner should be advised of the costs, care, and complications associated with surgical treatment.

SURGICAL CONSIDERATIONS
A grade 3 or 4 rectal tear may require surgical placement of a rectal liner, which may be sutured directly or under laparoscopic guidance, or may require a loop colostomy.

MEDICATIONS
DRUG(S) OF CHOICE
• Sedation may be achieved with xylazine 0.2–1.1 mg/kg IV or detomidine 0.005–0.02 mg/kg IV, which can be combined with butorphanol tartrate 0.1 mg/kg IV to enhance duration and sedation
• Epidural administration of a variety of agents (e.g. lidocaine, xylazine, detomidine) may provide anesthesia for initial evaluation and treatment as well as analgesia for prevention of postoperative straining. A caudal epidural catheter allows repeated drug administration
• Broad-spectrum antibiotic therapy is recommended for 3–10 days with grade 1 and 2 rectal tears. Extensive broad-spectrum antibiotic therapy is required for grade 3 and 4 tears
• Tetanus prophylaxis should be considered

• Flunixin meglumine therapy is recommended for inflammation and endotoxemia

CONTRAINDICATIONS
• Acepromazine is contraindicated for sedation of hypovolemic horses
• Indiscriminate use of atropine can result in GI complications, such as prolonged ileus with tympanic distention of the bowel, colic, and tachycardia

PRECAUTIONS
Administration of epidural lidocaine may be associated with ataxia.

POSSIBLE INTERACTIONS
If sedatives have been administered by the IM or IV route, the epidural dosage of xylazine or detomidine should be adjusted to avoid excessive cumulative sedation.

ALTERNATIVE DRUGS
N/A

FOLLOW-UP
PATIENT MONITORING
• Horses with grade 1 rectal tears should be monitored closely for 4–8 days
• Rectal palpation should be avoided for 30 days. Most grade 1 and 2 tears heal within 7–14 days
• Horses with grade 3 and 4 rectal tears should be monitored for complications associated with the surgical procedure(s) performed. These horses should be assessed with serial CBCs, fibrinogen levels, and peritoneal fluid analyses

PREVENTION/AVOIDANCE
• Rectal examination of horses should be reserved for veterinarians. Rectal examinations should be done only when necessary
• Appropriate restraint and careful technique should be used
• Appropriate supervision during breeding may reduce the likelihood of inadvertent tearing by the stallion

POSSIBLE COMPLICATIONS
• Progression of the tear
• Fecal contamination of the tear or of the abdomen
• Peritonitis
• Extensive cellulitis
• Abscess formation
• Rectoperitoneal fistula formation
• Rectal impaction or stricture
• Ileus
• Abdominal adhesions
• Complications associated with primary closure—excessive tissue trauma
• Complications associated with temporary liner placement
• Complications associated with colostomy—dehiscence; adhesions; abscessation; herniation/prolapse

EXPECTED COURSE AND PROGNOSIS
• Chances for survival improve with adequate and immediate first aid
• Grade 1 and 2 rectal tears have a good prognosis
• Grade 3a tears have a fair to guarded prognosis
• Grade 3b tears have a guarded to poor prognosis because of the likelihood of greater tissue damage and undermining
• Grade 4 tears have a poor to grave prognosis because gross fecal contamination of the abdomen predisposes to massive adhesion formation and fatal peritonitis

MISCELLANEOUS
ASSOCIATED CONDITIONS
• Peritonitis
• Endotoxemia
• Laminitis
• Abdominal adhesions

AGE-RELATED FACTORS
N/A

ZOONOTIC POTENTIAL
N/A

PREGNANCY/FERTILITY/BREEDING
Broodmares left with permanent colostomies are prone to intestinal herniation in advanced pregnancy and at parturition owing to unusual abdominal pressures placed against the colonic stoma.

SYNONYMS
None

SEE ALSO
• Acute adult abdominal pain—acute colic
• Endotoxemia
• Peritonitis
• Tenesmus

ABBREVIATIONS
• GI = gastrointestinal
• TP = total protein

Suggested Reading
Claes A, Ball BA, Brown JA, Kass PH. Evaluation of risk factors, management and outcome associated with rectal tears in horses: 99 cases (1985–2006). J Am Vet Med Assoc 2008;233:1605–1609.
Freeman DE. Rectum and anus. In: Auer JA, Stick JA, eds. Equine Surgery, 4e. St. Louis, MO: WB Saunders, 2012:494–505.
McMaster M, Caldwell F, Schumacher J, et al. A review of equine rectal tears and current methods of treatment. Equine Vet Educ 2015;27:200–208.

Author Luis M. Rubio-Martinez
Consulting Editors Henry Stämpfli and Olimpo Oliver-Espinosa

R

REGURGITATION/VOMITING/DYSPHAGIA

 BASICS

OVERVIEW
Regurgitation is a retrograde flow of esophageal or gastric contents through the nares or mouth. Vomiting (emesis) is a forceful expulsion of gastric contents. Neural pathways that control emesis are poorly developed in horses. Dysphagia is defined as difficult prehension, mastication, or swallowing.

Pathophysiology
• Regurgitation/vomiting in horses occurs from the nose rather than from the mouth, because of the specific anatomy of the soft palate
• Esophageal barriers (cranial esophageal sphincter, esophageal motor function, and cardia) must be breached to allow food to travel retrograde from the stomach
• Problems in the upper and/or lower GI system can cause dysphagia

Systems Affected
• The GI system is primarily affected
• Infectious or noninfectious diseases of the central or peripheral nervous system can cause regurgitation/vomiting
• Regurgitation secondary to a persistent right aortic arch is possible

SIGNALMENT
Predispositions are variable.

SIGNS
Historical Findings
The horse's age and diet, colic signs, prophylactic treatments, dental care, and possible exposures to poisonous plants, snakes, or other toxins should be communicated. The time of regurgitation in relation to feeding may further localize the anomaly. Regurgitation immediately following feeding is most often due to the esophageal obstruction (choke).

Physical Examination Findings
• Thorough physical examination is essential
• Nasal discharge consisting of feed and saliva. Cough, painful swallowing, and ptyalism may be evident
• Dysphagia is often associated with dropping feed from the mouth
• Variable colic signs may be present
• Nursing foals have a nasal discharge consisting of milk

CAUSES AND RISK FACTORS
• Causes may be congenital (i.e. persistent right aortic arch) or acquired (i.e. obstruction). They are physical (i.e. obstruction, persistent right aortic arch) or functional (i.e. disruption in the nervous or muscular control of swallowing)
• Risk factors depend on the underlying condition

 DIAGNOSIS

DIFFERENTIAL DIAGNOSIS
• Esophageal obstruction
• GI problems causing spontaneous nasogastric reflux
• Foreign body or mass, and/or inflammation in the oral cavity, pharynx, esophagus, stomach, thorax, and/or structures of the abdomen
• Congenital or acquired functional or physical GI disorders
• Gastric ulceration

CBC/BIOCHEMISTRY/URINALYSIS
The CBC and serum biochemistry profile may be normal or show evidence of dehydration. Hypochloremia and metabolic alkalosis secondary to loss of saliva may be evident.

OTHER LABORATORY TESTS
Variable, depending on the primary condition.

IMAGING
Radiography, ultrasonography, and/or fluoroscopy can assist in defining the problem.

OTHER DIAGNOSTIC PROCEDURES
Passage of a Stomach Tube
Passage of the stomach tube is essential. Care must be taken not to injure or perforate the esophagus during intubation.

Endoscopy
Endoscopic evaluation has a great value.

Esophageal Manometry
Of value in chronic choke cases.

 TREATMENT

Patients should be treated as an intensive care patient and kept off feed. Balanced polyionic fluids with or without chloride supplementation should be considered. Total or partial parenteral nutrition may be necessary in some patients. Surgical options exist for certain primary conditions.

 MEDICATIONS

DRUG(S) OF CHOICE
Drugs prescribed depend on the primary condition.

CONTRAINDICATIONS/POSSIBLE INTERACTIONS
N/A

 FOLLOW-UP

PATIENT MONITORING
It is variable depending on the primary condition.

POSSIBLE COMPLICATIONS
Esophageal penetration, aspiration pneumonia, dehydration, electrolyte abnormalities, and malnutrition.

 MISCELLANEOUS

ASSOCIATED CONDITIONS
• Gastric rupture
• Aspiration pneumonia
• Dehydration
• Colonic impaction
• Malnutrition
• Septicemia

AGE-RELATED FACTORS
The most likely differential diagnosis for an adult horse with regurgitation is an esophageal obstruction or a neurologic disorder, whereas congenital defects such as cleft palate or persistent right aortic arch are seen in foals.

ZOONOTIC POTENTIAL
Rabies must be ruled out.

PREGNANCY/FERTILITY/BREEDING
May affect gestation and fetal viability.

SEE ALSO
• Cleft palate
• Esophageal obstruction (choke)
• Gastric ulcers and erosions (equine gastric ulcer syndrome, EGUS)
• Lead (Pb) toxicosis
• *Nerium oleander* (oleander) toxicosis

ABBREVIATIONS
GI = gastrointestinal

Suggested Reading
Barton MH. Nasal regurgitation of milk in foals. Compend Contin Educ Pract Vet 1993;15:81–91.
Dougan VE, Bentz BG. Esophageal obstruction in horses. Compend Contin Educ Pract Vet 2004;11:877–884.
Smith BP. Regurgitation/vomiting. In: Smith BP, ed. Large Animal Internal Medicine, 5e. St. Louis, MO: Elsevier Mosby, 2015:100–101.
Smith BP. Dysphagia. In: Smith BP, ed. Large Animal Internal Medicine, 5e. St. Louis, MO: Elsevier Mosby, 2015:101–103.

Author Modest Vengust
Consulting Editors Henry Stämpfli and Olimpo Oliver-Espinosa

R

REMOVAL AND SHIPMENT OF OVARIES FOR POSTMORTEM ICSI

BASICS

DEFINITION
ICSI has become a clinically viable means of producing embryos in the horse. Embryos and foals can be produced from oocytes recovered from ovaries removed from mares peri- or postmortem. Using appropriate methods for ovary removal and shipment to ICSI laboratories increases the chance for owners to produce foals from mares, postmortem Information on removal and packaging of ovaries for shipment is provided in the section entitled Treatment.
2 important points of emphasis:
1. Equine oocytes do not tolerate temperatures less than about 13°C (55°F), therefore *do not place the ovaries on ice or in refrigeration*, and
2. Speed is of the essence; try to arrange a schedule so that the ovaries arrive at the ICSI laboratory within 12 h, preferably within 6 h, of the mare's death

INDICATIONS
Foal production from mares postmortem.

SIGNALMENT
• Can be performed on mares that have died; however, results are dependent upon the length of time the mare has been dead before ovaries are recovered
• Can be performed after euthanasia; however, the effects of the euthanasia method (barbiturates, KCl) on embryo production have not been critically evaluated
• For mares scheduled for euthanasia, ovary recovery under anesthesia immediately before euthanasia has been associated with good results, and this method is recommended

DIAGNOSIS
N/A

TREATMENT

MATERIALS NEEDED
• Drugs—ketamine, xylazine, and euthanasia solution (KCl or commercial solution)
• Syringes and needles for IV injection
• Clippers and surgical scrub materials
• Palpation sleeves
• Examination or surgical gloves
• Scalpel or sharp knife
• Clean palpation sleeve or plastic bag in which to place ovaries
• Styrofoam or other insulated container
• *Ballast at 37°C* (1 L bag of saline, coolant cans, water-filled double-bagged palpation sleeve, etc., warmed in an incubator), placed inside the insulated container

OVARY REMOVAL PROCEDURE
• If the mare is scheduled for euthanasia, necessary flight arrangements for ovary shipment should be made ahead of time, and the time of euthanasia coordinated to provide the shortest shipment time possible
• It is recommended that the mare be anesthetized with ketamine and xylazine, and the ovaries removed immediately prior to euthanasia
• Standard drug usage:
  ○ Xylazine 1–2 mg/kg IV (500–1000 mg/500 kg horse)
  ○ Followed in 5 min by:
    ▪ Ketamine HCl 2–3 mg/kg IV (1000–1500 mg/500 kg horse)
    ▪ Following ovary removal, KCl 1–2 mEq/kg, or a commercial euthanasia solution, is administered IV to effect euthanasia
    ▪ Euthanasia solution should be drawn up and ready to use prior to anesthetizing the mare; should the plane of anesthesia begin to lighten at any time during the ovary removal, immediate administration of euthanasia solution is recommended prior to completing ovary removal
• The mare may be placed on either side; both ovaries can be removed from an incision in 1 flank
• The site of ovary removal on the flank (the area of the flank between the tuber coxae and the last rib) should be made as clean as possible, ideally shaved (shaving can be done before anesthesia) and scrubbed as for surgery
• Don palpation sleeves on both arms, and don surgical or examination gloves over the sleeves
• Using a scalpel or sharp knife, make an incision through the abdominal muscles in the flank, beginning approximately 5 cm cranial to the tuber coxae and extending ventrally
• Extend the incision into the peritoneal cavity and insert the gloved hand into the peritoneum
• To locate the ipsilateral ovary, begin by identifying the uterine horn ipsilateral to the incision and follow the horn to the ovary. Alternatively, sweep along the dorsal body wall roughly level to the tuber coxae to identify the ovarian pedicle and follow it to the ovary
• Bring the ovary to the incision and pull to make the pedicle taut; cut the pedicle to remove the ovary
• The ovary should be placed into a palpation sleeve or plastic bag (no fluid is needed in the bag) and placed into the Styrofoam container that already contains the 37°C ballast, and the container covered
• The ovary contralateral to the incision is then similarly identified. Often this ovary is grasped through the mesentery; this is acceptable and the ovary can be removed effectively while covered in mesentery

• The contralateral ovary often cannot be brought completely to the incision site. To remove this ovary, put strong traction on the pedicle and cut the pedicle carefully within the peritoneal cavity—use extreme care not to cut the fingers holding the ovary
• Place this ovary in the same bag as the other ovary, close the bag (tie or seal) with a minimum of air in it, and return the bag to the insulated container
• Once both ovaries have been removed, administer the euthanasia solution to the mare
• *Do not place ovaries on ice or in refrigeration*

OVARY HANDLING AND SHIPMENT
• The purpose of the 37°C ballast in the Styrofoam container is to prevent the ovaries from initially cooling too rapidly
• For packaging for shipment, the bag containing the ovaries is removed from the Styrofoam container and placed in the isothermalizer of a passive insulated device (Equitainer, EquOcyte). Alternatively, more packaging may be added to the Styrofoam container and this container used for shipment, or a Styrofoam cooled semen shipment container used
• If using an Equitainer, place the bag of ovaries inside the isothermalizer. If the ovaries are too large to fit inside the isothermalizer, the bag of ovaries may be wrapped in protective padding, such as bubble wrap or foam padding, and this placed directly on top of the cans in the Equitainer
• If using the Styrofoam container, add more ballast (at temperatures as outlined below) to the container. Styrofoam containers or cooled semen shipment containers need to be enclosed in a cardboard box for counter-to-counter shipments
• The conditions of shipment are dependent upon the expected duration of shipment. All efforts should be made to get the ovaries to the ICSI laboratory within 12 h of the mare's death, and preferably within 6 h:
  ○ If shipment time is <4 h, ship with all materials starting at room temperature. Ballast immediately around the ovaries can be at body temperature; this will allow the ovaries to cool slowly to room temperature
  ○ If shipment time is expected to be >6 h, the goal is to slowly cool the ovaries to 13–18°C during shipment. This can be done in an Equitainer by using 1 frozen can on the *bottom* and 1 room temperature can on top of it, closest to the isothermalizer. If using a Styrofoam container, ballast cooled to ~13°C (55°F) can be used
• Package ovaries with additional padding (paper towels, etc.) if necessary, to minimize movement or damage during shipment

SHIPMENT REPORT
• Include the following mare-related information with the ovary shipment. This provides information about the factors affecting foal production postmortem:
  ○ Reason for euthanasia

R

REMOVAL AND SHIPMENT OF OVARIES FOR POSTMORTEM ICSI (CONTINUED)

- ○ Duration of illness before euthanasia
- ○ Treatments given for the illness leading up to euthanasia (general description and duration)
- ○ Drugs administered for ovary removal
- ○ Time of ovary removal
- Enclose communication information, including:
  - ○ Mare's name and age
  - ○ Owner's name, address, email, and primary contact phone number
  - ○ If possible, client-completed ICSI contract (contract is sent to the referring veterinarian or client by the ICSI laboratory)

CLIENT COMMUNICATION

- Decisions may be made hastily at the time of a valued mare's death, and owners need to understand what is involved in this procedure. Veterinarians should discuss expenses related to postmortem ICSI with owners *prior* to removing and shipping the ovaries. These include:
  - ○ The costs for anesthetizing the mare and removing the ovaries
  - ○ The costs for shipment of the ovaries to the ICSI laboratory
  - ○ The costs for shipment of semen to the ICSI laboratory
  - ○ The costs for ovary dissection, oocyte maturation, ICSI, and embryo production at the ICSI laboratory. In general, these could be estimated at US$2000–3000

- ○ The costs for embryo vitrification, if this is chosen (typically US$300–500)
- ○ The costs for shipment of the embryo(s) to the embryo transfer center
- ○ The costs levied by the embryo transfer center for transfer of the embryo, care of the recipient mare, and sale of the recipient mare
- ○ Costs and rules associated with enrolling the client's mare in breed-associated embryo transfer programs
- Clear communication with the ICSI laboratory is paramount in organization; the client should communicate directly with the ICSI laboratory to clarify any costs or procedural issues involving the laboratory
- Mare owners should be aware that they will be responsible for coordinating shipment of semen from their desired stallion to the ICSI laboratory
  - ○ Most ICSI laboratories request semen to arrive the day following ovary shipment, as ICSI usually occurs the second day after ovary shipment
- Mare owners will be responsible for identifying an embryo transfer facility for transfer of any embryos produced, or making the decision to vitrify the embryos for later transfer

EXPECTED RESULTS

- Based on results for postmortem ICSI at the Equine Embryo Laboratory at Texas A&M

University (2010–2015), an average of 1.3 blastocysts is expected per mare, with an average foal production of 0.54 foals per mare. Essentially, this means that *on average* the owner has a 50:50 chance of getting a foal from the procedure
- The likelihood of embryo and foal production is dependent on many factors, including the time of ovary removal (before or after death), the age of the mare, the mare's illness, medications received, and the time and conditions of ovary transport

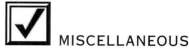

MISCELLANEOUS

ABBREVIATIONS

ICSI = intracytoplasmic sperm injection

Suggested Reading
Hinrichs K, Choi YH, Norris JD, et al. Evaluation of foal production following intracytoplasmic sperm injection and blastocyst culture of oocytes from ovaries collected immediately before euthanasia or after death of mares under field conditions. J Am Vet Med Assoc 2012;241:1070–1074.

Authors Kindra A. Rader and Katrin Hinrichs
Consulting Editor Carla L. Carleton

R

RESPIRATORY DISTRESS SYNDROME IN FOALS

BASICS

DEFINITION
• Sporadic, progressive, respiratory failure associated with pulmonary edema. • Acute onset, cyanosis, pulmonary hypertension without cardiac disease

PATHOPHYSIOLOGY
• A variety of insults that directly or indirectly injure the lung. • Inflammation, leading to permeability–pulmonary edema, and clinical respiratory failure. • Immunosuppressive disorders associated with acute respiratory distress syndrome/interstitial lung disease in foals. • Causal disease may progress to multiple organ dysfunction

SYSTEMS AFFECTED
• Primarily respiratory. • Renal, hepatic, and cardiovascular systems and clotting cascades

GENETICS
Not established.

INCIDENCE/PREVALENCE
Not established.

GEOGRAPHIC DISTRIBUTION
N/A

SIGNALMENT
Foals 1–8 months of age.

SIGNS
• Acute or peracute depression, lethargy, fever, labored breathing, tachypnea, nostril flaring, increased abdominal and intercostal effort with cyanosis. • Nasal discharge and cough—frequent

CAUSES
• Foals with subclinical respiratory disease. • Heat stress. • Erythromycin use in hot weather. • Viral and bacterial pneumonia

RISK FACTORS
• Antimicrobial or other drug use. • Heat stress, inhaled irritant gases, and pneumotoxicants. • Immunosuppression

DIAGNOSIS

DIFFERENTIAL DIAGNOSIS
• Viral pneumonia—equine influenza, viral arteritis, herpesviruses, paramyxovirus, and adenovirus. • Bacterial pneumonia. • Upper airway dysfunction. • Ingestion, inhalation, or exposure to xenobiotics

CBC/BIOCHEMISTRY/URINALYSIS
Common abnormalities—neutrophilic leukocytosis, elevated fibrinogen.

OTHER LABORATORY TESTS
• Arterial blood gas—hypoxemia, hypercapnia, and respiratory acidosis. • Blood samples; dehydration, disseminated

intravascular coagulation, and injury to other organs

IMAGING
Thoracic Radiography
• Lesions described include diffuse bronchointerstitial, coalescing interstitial to nodular, diffuse alveolar to coalescing alveolar infiltrates. • Pulmonary abscess

Transthoracic Ultrasonography
Consolidation, abscesses, in some foals.

OTHER DIAGNOSTIC PROCEDURES
• Culture and cytologic evaluation of transtracheal wash, bronchoalveolar fluid, or blood may provide valuable information. • Transthoracic lung biopsy may be useful diagnostically (except when bleeding or abscesses are evident)

TREATMENT

AIMS
• Improve oxygenation. • Reduce body temperature (in hyperthermic foals). • Reduce lung edema and inflammation. • Antimicrobial therapy

APPROPRIATE HEALTH CARE
Reduce body temperature of foals.

NURSING CARE
• Nasal oxygen insufflation (2–5 L/min) (nasal or transtracheal catheter). • Cold water enemas to reduce body temperature. • IV fluids to lower core temperature (balanced electrolyte solution). • Pulmonary edema may necessitate diuretics

CLIENT EDUCATION
• Education aimed at prevention. • Observe mares and foals on daily basis. • Possibility of hyperthermia when treating foals with erythromycin

MEDICATIONS

DRUG(S) OF CHOICE
• Drugs to address hypoxemia, hypercapnia, inflammation, and hyperthermia. • Modulation of pulmonary inflammation. • Appropriate antimicrobial therapy. • Use of corticosteroids in foals is controversial; limited use of short-acting corticosteroids (e.g. dexamethasone sodium phosphate 0.05–0.1 mg/kg IV, prednisolone sodium succinate 0.5–1 mg/kg IV) provide short-duration reduction of pulmonary inflammation. • NSAIDs (e.g. flunixin meglumine 0.25 mg/kg every 8 h) may lower body temperature and reduce discomfort associated with respiratory disease

CONTRAINDICATIONS
Discontinue any medications (especially erythromycin/rifampin (rifampicin)) that could produce significant interactions when used concurrently.

FOLLOW-UP

PATIENT MONITORING
• Arterial blood gases are the most sensitive indicator of progress. • Repeated thoracic radiography is useful to evaluate lungs

PREVENTION/AVOIDANCE
Avoid exposing foals with respiratory disease, and those being treated with macrolide antibiotics, to direct sun on hot days. This may necessitate indoor confinement.

POSSIBLE COMPLICATIONS
N/A

EXPECTED COURSE AND PROGNOSIS
• The mortality rate is high with or without intensive therapeutic intervention. • Long-term outcomes vary; however, full recovery has occurred in a few cases

MISCELLANEOUS

AGE-RELATED FACTORS
Can occur at all ages; however, foals 1–8 months of age are more commonly reported.

ZOONOTIC POTENTIAL
N/A

SYNONYMS
• Bronchointerstitial pneumonia. • Interstitial pneumonia. • Respiratory distress

SEE ALSO
• Expiratory dyspnea.
• Inspiratory dyspnea

ABBREVIATIONS
NSAID = nonsteroidal anti-inflammatory drug

Suggested Reading
Dunkel B, Dolente B, Boston RC. Acute lung injury/acute respiratory distress syndrome in 15 foals. Equine Vet J 2005;37:435–440.
Peek SF, Landolt G, Karasin AI, et al. Acute respiratory distress syndrome and fatal interstitial pneumonia associated with equine influenza in a neonatal foal. J Vet Intern Med 2004;18:132–134.
Wilkins PA, Seahorn T. Acute respiratory distress syndrome. Vet Clin North Am Equine Pract 2004;20:253–273.

Authors Jeffrey Lakritz and W. David Wilson
Consulting Editors Daniel Jean and Mathilde Leclère

R

RESUSCITATION, NEONATE

BASICS

DEFINITION
Resuscitation is required in cases of birth or during extreme illness that result in cardiac, respiratory, or cardiorespiratory insufficiency or failure to an extent that will not sustain life.

PATHOPHYSIOLOGY
• Maladaptation to extrauterine life can lead to respiratory arrest when the neonate fails to spontaneously breathe. Primary cardiac failure is uncommon in foals. Hypoxemia can lead to bradycardia followed by asystole and death. High-risk pregnancy conditions such as placentitis, premature placental separation, maternal illness, and twinning may predispose the newborn foal to a more challenging transition to extrauterine life
• Similarly, critical illness in the neonatal period may lead to cardiovascular collapse (i.e. septic shock) and cardiopulmonary arrest

SYSTEMS AFFECTED
• Respiratory
• Cardiovascular
• Secondary hypoxic injury to organs such as gastrointestinal tract and kidneys

GENETICS
N/A

INCIDENCE/PREVALENCE
There are no known data regarding incidence or prevalence for the need of resuscitation.

GEOGRAPHIC DISTRIBUTION
Worldwide distribution.

SIGNALMENT
Neonate. No breed or sex predisposition.

SIGNS
Decreased (<60 bpm) to absent heartbeat, slow/irregular breathing pattern to apnea, decreased to absent muscle tone, minimally responsive to absent response to nasal mucosal stimulation, lack of spontaneous motor activity, dark pink to cyanotic mucous membranes, and cold extremities.

CAUSES
See Risk Factors.

RISK FACTORS
• Any systemic disease leading to hypoxemia and/or acidosis
• Central respiratory center damage, primary lung/thorax disease, septic shock, hypovolemia, metabolic acidosis, hyperkalemia, vasovagal reflex, hypoglycemia, and hypothermia are risk factors
• Acidosis causes respiratory arrest and nonperfusing bradycardia, pulseless electrical activity, and asystole

DIAGNOSIS

DIFFERENTIAL DIAGNOSIS
Central neurologic disease (i.e. coma)—autonomic features of cardiopulmonary arrest (i.e. bradycardia/dysrhythmia) are generally not present.

CBC/BIOCHEMISTRY/URINALYSIS
Dependent on primary disease; e.g. sepsis (abnormal leukogram), congenital ruptured bladder, and uroabdomen (hyperkalemia, hyponatremia, hypochloremia).

OTHER LABORATORY TESTS
Arterial blood gas—increased L-lactate concentration, decreased pH, decreased bicarbonate concentration, increased base deficit, decreased PaO_2, increased $PaCO_2$.

IMAGING
Thoracic imaging (radiography or ultrasonography) may reveal primary thoracic disease, e.g. fractured ribs, pneumothorax, parenchymal disease. Echocardiography may show congenital heart defects.

OTHER DIAGNOSTIC PROCEDURES
• Capnography following nasotracheal or orotracheal intubation—used to detect impending failure, effectiveness of CPR, and/or ROSC. It also approximates the PaCO2
• ECG—essential to identify the cardiac rhythm. Pulseless cardiac arrest may be caused by ventricular fibrillation, pulseless ventricular tachycardia, pulseless electrical activity, or asystole

PATHOLOGIC FINDINGS
Findings reflect a primary disease process.

TREATMENT

APPROPRIATE HEALTH CARE
CPR
• Airway support—following recognition of arrest or impending arrest, establishing an airway and providing ventilatory support is essential. Options include mouth-to-nose breathing, muzzle mask with Ambu bag, naso- or orotracheal intubation (8–10 mm ID × 55 cm long)
   ◦ Initially clear the nares of mucus or fluid (a bulb syringe and/or postural drainage can facilitate this), then establish the airway. If available, 100% oxygen provision to the tube is recommended. Provide 8–10 breaths/min where inspiration time is ~1 s.

Watch chest excursion as a guide to tidal volume. Excessive ventilation with longer inspiratory pressures and bigger tidal volumes may worsen perfusion and be counterproductive
• Cardiac support—external compressions should be initiated immediately with minimal/no interruptions where a nonperfusing rhythm is present. With the foal in lateral recumbency on a firm surface, provide 100–120 compressions/min with complete chest recoil between compressions. Compression depth should be one-third to one-half the width of the chest. The operator kneels over the chest while placing 1 hand on top of the other with locked elbows, providing a piston-like compression over the heart. If rib fractures are present, place the side of the foal with the fractures down on the ground. Breaks from compressions should be minimized. Pupil size, capnography, ECG, and potentially palpation of a pulse can be used to determine effectiveness
   ◦ A "cycle" of CPR is considered to be 2 min. If only 1 operator is present, a chest compression to ventilation rate should be 30:2, where 30 compressions are given followed by 2 quick breaths and compressions resume

ACTIVITY
Activity following successful resuscitation depends on the inciting cause and response to treatment.

DIET
Largely dependent on the reasons for arrest and response to resuscitation. A septic neonate may be unable to handle much enteral feeding, therefore needing parenteral nutrition.

CLIENT EDUCATION
It is essential to set realistic expectations about a critically ill foal and the prognosis for both successful resuscitation and long-term outcome. If the foal is weak at birth but otherwise appropriate in terms of gestational and developmental age, rapid intervention and resuscitative support can be successful. If the arrest is secondary to critical illness, a prior conversation about the potential for arrest and whether resuscitation should be attempted, i.e. a "DNR" conversation, is helpful. If attempted, successful ROSC and survival is not common.

SURGICAL CONSIDERATIONS
Cardiac support (compressions)—internal cardiac compression may be considered in foals where external compressions are insufficient in establishing cardiac output. Foals must be intubated and ventilated as

R

pulmonary collapse occurs when opening the thorax. Open chest compressions are performed via thoracotomy and gently squeezing the heart from apex to base. This is considered a low-yield intervention with the potential for high morbidity.

 MEDICATIONS

Establish venous access as soon as possible, minimizing any breaks in compressions and ventilations. Central line catheters are preferred (i.e. jugular vein with tip in the distal jugular vein or cranial vena cava); however, even leaving a capped 20 G 38 mm (1.5 inch) needle in the jugular vein until catheter placement can be a useful temporary measure.

DRUG(S) OF CHOICE
• Cardiac arrest/nonperfusing rhythm—low-dose epinephrine (0.01–0.02 mg/kg) IV every 2 cycles (i.e. 4 min). Higher doses are not advised IV; however, intratracheal doses (0.05–0.15 mg/kg) can be given. Vasopressin (0.6 U/kg) IV every 2 cycles (i.e. 4 min) alternating with low-dose epinephrine can be provided
• Bradycardia—atropine (0.02 mg/kg IV) should be given only after attempting compressions and ventilations. Neonatal bradycardia is usually secondary to hypoxia, which should be treated with hyperventilation with 100% oxygen and epinephrine if it becomes pulseless
• Ventricular dysrhythmia—lidocaine (1 mg/kg IV) decreases ventricular automaticity. Magnesium sulfate (25–50 mg/kg diluted in 5% dextrose) for polymorphic ventricular tachycardia
• IV fluids—indicated if hypovolemia exists. During CPR, IV fluid volumes to essentially deliver drug therapy to the heart are all that are indicated. Cardiac arrest is an extreme form of backward/congestive heart failure. High IV fluid volumes exacerbate venous hypertension and impede coronary perfusion. Upon ROSC, IV fluids, often with glucose provision, may be necessary
• Respiratory support—doxapram, acting as a nonspecific central stimulant, has been advocated by some to stimulate respiration at 0.5 mg/kg IV
• Sodium bicarbonate—up to 1 mEq/kg IV is only indicated with life-threatening hyperkalemia, drug overdose (i.e.

phenobarbital), or with preexisting metabolic acidosis with pH <7.2
• Reversal drugs—if arrest is secondary to certain drug administration, reversal agents are indicated. For example, flumazenil for midazolam administration, naloxone for opioid administration, atipamezole for α_2-agonist administration

CONTRAINDICATIONS
High rates of IV fluid administration are contraindicated.

PRECAUTIONS
Vigorous chest compressions can fracture ribs.

 FOLLOW-UP

PATIENT MONITORING
• Ventilatory support should continue until the foal is consistently breathing >16 breaths/min. Careful monitoring for bradypnea and apnea should continue in case support is needed again
• In the hospital setting, ROSC is determined by capnography (ETCO$_2$ >20 mmHg) and ECG (sinus rhythm). In the field, the clinician relies on physical examination findings such as pupil responsiveness, spontaneous breathing, and palpable cardiac beat or arterial pulse. Thoracic compressions should continue until the heart rate is >60 bpm. Pauses in compressions to assess heart rate should be no longer than 10 s
• If CPR is unsuccessful after 12–15 min, the foal is unlikely to respond and survive

PREVENTION/AVOIDANCE
While arrest is unpreventable, careful monitoring of high-risk pregnancies is useful. Being physically present during foaling and proactively intervening early when unsuccessful stage 2 labor is evident is key. Being prepared with a resuscitation kit including supplies and drugs to perform basic life support/CPR is important. Annual review/refresher of CPR procedures prior to foaling season is recommended.

POSSIBLE COMPLICATIONS
Fractured ribs, infection (with open CPR), rearrest, death.

EXPECTED COURSE AND PROGNOSIS
• Prognosis often depends on the inciting cause for arrest
• ROSC is estimated to occur in 40–65% of all arrest patients. Foals with uncomplicated

bradycardia have a higher rate of ROSC (80%), while asystole is least likely to yield ROSC (7%)
• Overall survival following resuscitation is estimated around 20%, higher for at-birth resuscitation (31%) than after-birth resuscitation in critically ill foals (11%). Resuscitation for nonperfusing bradyarrhythmia likely yields the greatest chance for survival (42%). If successful, long-term neurologic sequelae appear to be uncommon in neonatal foals (~6%)

 MISCELLANEOUS

ASSOCIATED CONDITIONS
• Neonatal sepsis
• Dystocia
• Hypoxemia

AGE-RELATED FACTORS
N/A

ZOONOTIC POTENTIAL
None

PREGNANCY/FERTILITY/BREEDING
N/A

SYNONYMS
Stillborn, stillbirth, respiratory failure, cardiac failure, shock.

ABBREVIATIONS
• CPR = cardiopulmonary resuscitation
• DNR = do not resuscitate
• ETCO$_2$ = end-tidal CO$_2$
• ID = internal diameter
• PaCO$_2$ = partial pressure of carbon dioxide in arterial blood
• PaO$_2$ = partial pressure of oxygen in arterial blood
• ROSC = return of spontaneous circulation

Internet Resources
Palmer JE, VETTalks on cutting-edge research in critical care: CPR case series. http://nicuvet.com/nicuvet/Equine-Perinatoloy/Web_slides_meetings/IVECCS%202013/CPR.pdf

Suggested Reading
Palmer JE. Neonatal foal resuscitation. Vet Clin North Am Equine Pract 2007;23:159–182.

Author Samuel D.A. Hurcombe
Consulting Editor Margaret C. Mudge

R

RETAINED DECIDUOUS TEETH

BASICS

OVERVIEW
• Between the ages of 2.5 and 4.5 years, deciduous incisors (01s, 02s, 03s) and premolar cheek teeth (06s, 07s, 08s) are replaced with permanent dentition. Eruption of the permanent tooth, leading to resorption of the deciduous tooth roots and wear of the clinical crown, normally results in shedding of the deciduous tooth. Maleruption of a permanent tooth can lead to pathologic retention of a deciduous tooth. At the same time a retained deciduous tooth may lead to malalignment of the permanent tooth or retained dentition
• In cases of retained deciduous incisors the permanent incisor generally erupts lingual/palatinal and more rarely labial to or in between its deciduous precursor. This may result in malocclusion of the permanent incisor arcade and possibly periodontal disease as a narrow diastema may develop between the deciduous and erupted permanent tooth. Lingual displacement of 302s or 402s because of retained labially positioned deciduous incisors (702s or 802s) seems to be the most common sequela of retained deciduous incisors
• A certain amount of mild temporary oral discomfort (gingivitis and halitosis) may accompany normal shedding of deciduous cheek teeth (termed caps). Abnormal retention of deciduous cheek teeth or broken-off root slivers remaining in the subgingival space after the cap is shed may lead to prolonged and more severe oral discomfort as a result of gingivitis, periodontal disease, or lingual and buccal lacerations. Furthermore, retained caps may predispose to malocclusion and abnormal crown wear of permanent teeth
• The causal involvement of retained deciduous cheek teeth in the formation of enlarged eruption cysts (eruption pseudocysts, 3- or 4-year-old bumps) is unclear, because at this stage a retained premolar cap may play a role in vertical impaction of the erupting permanent tooth

SIGNALMENT
The deciduous incisors are shed approximately at 2.5 (01s), 3.5 (02s), and 4.5 (03s) years of age. The deciduous teeth of the second, third, and fourth premolars are shed at approximately 2.5 (06s), 3 (07s), and 4 (08s) years of age, respectively. Although there can be much individual variation in the timing of deciduous tooth shedding, these defined eruption times determine the age of affected horses. Breed and sex variations have not been reported, although horses with smaller heads and relative overcrowding of the teeth may be predisposed for this condition.

SIGNS
Clinical signs of discomfort because of retained deciduous teeth include head-shyness, head tossing during eating, rubbing the incisors on fixed objects, recurrent hemorrhage from the oral cavity, headshaking, quidding, and biting problems. Retained caps may also cause abnormal mastication, uneven dental wear, and occasionally weight loss.

CAUSES AND RISK FACTORS
Retained deciduous teeth are relatively common and may be caused by abnormalities of mastication as a result of either inadequate roughage in the diet or other causes of abnormal dental wear. Overcrowding of the dental arcades can also cause retention of deciduous teeth. Hooks or ramps in young animals may cause a displacement of the opposing dental arcade with a resultant overcrowding of the premolars. An excessively large first premolar (wolf tooth) or supernumerary teeth (polyodontia) may also lead to relative overcrowding.

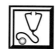

DIAGNOSIS

DIFFERENTIAL DIAGNOSIS
• The diagnosis of retained deciduous incisors or premolar caps is straightforward because of the typical age and presence of caps or malerupted teeth. Supernumerary incisors may be confused with retained deciduous incisors. Occasionally the premolar caps may not be easily distinguishable from the crown of a permanent tooth. Close evaluation of the occlusal surface is helpful to differentiate the newly erupted incisors with deep infundibula from worn deciduous crowns. The presence of 2 deep infundibular cups may help to identify permanent maxillary premolars. In uncertain cases radiographs are indicated
• Clinical signs are unspecific and may accompany a variety of painful conditions of the teeth and oral cavity

CBC/BIOCHEMISTRY/URINALYSIS
N/A

OTHER LABORATORY TESTS
N/A

IMAGING
• Radiography is the imaging modality of choice
• Incisor radiographs include intraoral and occasionally also laterolateral projections
• Retained premolar deciduous teeth are best radiographed with open-mouth lateral oblique projections, which allow evaluation of the deciduous teeth, permanent teeth, alveolar bone, and the adjacent teeth

OTHER DIAGNOSTIC PROCEDURES
A thorough visual and digital oral examination will usually detect loose or

displaced incisors or premolar caps or cap fragments. A small gap between the erupting permanent tooth and the deciduous premolar cap will help to identify a retained cap. As the deciduous premolar crown closely resembles the permanent tooth crown radiographs are used to identify them in uncertain cases.

TREATMENT

• Retained deciduous incisors can easily be extracted using dental elevators, under sedation and local anesthesia. After extraction of the retained deciduous incisor, the displaced permanent incisor tooth should gradually drift into proper alignment. Retained deciduous incisors on the lingual aspect or interposed between permanent incisors may be more difficult to extract and extra care should be taken to avoid damage to permanent incisors
• Deciduous premolar teeth can easily and safely be extracted when a line of demarcation is visible between the deciduous premolar and erupting permanent tooth. A 4-prong forceps ("cap extractors") or any long slim-bladed instrument may be used for this procedure
• Wolf tooth extraction forceps work well for the removal of premolars 3 and 4. Rolling the cap toward the lingual/palatinal surface will reduce the breakage of the buccal roots, which can leave slivers of the cap behind that may cause soft tissue damage and irritation. If 1 cap has been shed, some authors recommend all other caps in that corresponding quadruplet to be removed. This should only be done if the permanent teeth concerned have erupted completely through the gingiva and the premolar cap can be removed with moderate force. The practice of methodically removing deciduous teeth at set ages in an attempt to prevent the problems of retained caps will result in the premature removal of deciduous teeth in some horses and may predispose to cemental hypoplasia. Occasionally, caps may extend above the occlusal surface of the adjacent teeth but extraction is not possible without the use of excessive force. These caps should be floated down with the adjacent occlusal surface and evaluated for extraction 6–8 weeks later

MEDICATIONS

DRUG(S) OF CHOICE
In general, gingivitis, periodontal disease, or laceration of other soft tissue structures as a result of retained deciduous teeth do not require any anti-inflammatory or antimicrobial therapy. In cases of enlarged eruption cysts antimicrobial therapy may be

R

indicated to prevent anachoretic pulpitis and apical infection.

CONTRAINDICATIONS/POSSIBLE INTERACTIONS
• Removal of deciduous incisors interposed between permanent incisors may lead to iatrogenic damage of permanent teeth
• Premature removal of maxillary caps and thereby exposure and following destruction of the dental sac of the underlying permanent teeth will stop cementogenesis. Cemental hypoplasia may predispose to subsequent microbial fermentation, dissolution of cement (caries formation), and abnormal wear of the occlusal surface ("cubbing out"), which, if not corrected, can initiate an early wave mouth formation. Furthermore, changes of the occlusal surface may result in stress concentrations during mastication, predisposing the affected tooth to fracture

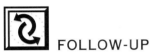

FOLLOW-UP
PREVENTION/AVOIDANCE
Adequate dental care for younger horses may decrease abnormal dental wear and resultant

overcrowding of the dental arcades. Regular dental care should also identify retained deciduous teeth prior to causing significant problems.

EXPECTED COURSE AND PROGNOSIS
Removal of retained deciduous teeth usually results in the normal alignment and development of the permanent teeth. When abnormal conformation of the arcades remains, this should be corrected.

MISCELLANEOUS
ASSOCIATED CONDITIONS
Associated conditions include abnormal dental wear and periapical abscessation.

AGE-RELATED FACTORS
Eruption of permanent teeth and shedding of deciduous teeth occur in the horse between 2.5 and 4 years of age. Even though there is interindividual variability and possibly some breed predilection, clinical signs of retained deciduous teeth typically appear around this age.

Suggested Reading
Baker GJ, Easley J. Equine Dentistry, 2e. Philadelphia, PA: Saunders, 2005.
Dixon PM. Developmental craniofacial abnormalities and disorders of development and eruption of the teeth. Proc Am Assoc Equine Pract 2011;57:85–92.
Dixon PM, Dacre I. A review of equine dental disorders. Vet J 2005;169:165–187.
Easley J. Deciduous tooth management. Proc Am Assoc Equine Pract 2011;57:141–146.

Authors Felix Theiss and Andrea S. Bischofberger
Consulting Editors Henry Stämpfli and Olimpo Oliver-Espinosa
Acknowledgment The authors and editors acknowledge the prior contribution of Hugo Hilton.

R

RETAINED FETAL MEMBRANES

 BASICS

DEFINITION
Fetal membranes not been passed by 3 h postpartum.

PATHOPHYSIOLOGY
Suggested Causes
• Pathologic adherence between the endometrium and chorion; possible recurrence with future pregnancies. • Infections between endometrium and chorion. • Any debilitating condition of the mare

SYSTEMS AFFECTED
Reproductive

INCIDENCE/PREVALENCE
• Most common postpartum condition, 2–10% incidence. • Increased incidence after dystocia or Caesarean section; in draft mares; a hydrops pregnancy; after prolonged pregnancy mares >15 years

SIGNALMENT
All females of breeding age.

SIGNS
General Comments
• RFM visible at vulvar lips—an unreliable indicator of the portion retained within the uterus. • With mare movement, portions of membranes tear free. • Search stall bedding for additional placental pieces
Historical Findings
• Previous history of RFM. • No effect—previous year's reproductive status, breeding method, sex of foal, birth of a weak foal or dead fetus
Physical Examination Findings
• Transrectal palpation—determine uterine size and tone, gauge fluid volume in the uterine lumen. • Vaginal examination not always essential—depends on mare's general health, condition of the placenta and uterus

CAUSES
See Pathophysiology.

RISK FACTORS
See Historical Findings.

 DIAGNOSIS

DIFFERENTIAL DIAGNOSIS
• Uterine infection. • Delay or failed postpartum involution

PATHOLOGIC FINDINGS
See Pathophysiology.

 TREATMENT

APPROPRIATE HEALTH CARE
• Oxytocin—best results. • Start oxytocin treatment ≤3 h postpartum if RFM ∘ Repeat every 60–120 min for the first 12–18 h postpartum. • If >12–18 h, consider treating with intrauterine irritants, antibiotics, or prostaglandins. • Systemic antibiotics if systemic disease. • Uterine lavage of value if a portion is retained. • Insufflation if membranes are largely intact. Place fluid (best—isotonic saline solution; alternatively lactated Ringer's solution or water) to dilate the uterine lumen within the innermost aspect of the fetal membranes; expand uterine lumen, stimulate uterine activity ∘ Gather exposed (external to the vulvae) portion of RFM; tie around it outside of the vulvae to maintain fluid within the uterus and placenta for a brief time; this maintains uterine expansion, stretches myometrium/endometrium to facilitate release of the microvilli. • Isolate a vessel of the umbilical cord of RFM at the vulvar lips; transect and place a 9 mm (or small diameter, if necessary) nasogastric tube into the incision; attach a low-pressure volume source of fluid for approximately 5 min; this induces edema and swelling of placental tissue; facilitates separation from the endometrium

NURSING CARE
• Administer oxytocin postpartum to all mares with a history of RFM. • Examine membranes after passage; confirm all portions are present

ACTIVITY
Normal exercise.

DIET
No changes are indicated.

CLIENT EDUCATION
• RFM is relatively common; treat if not passed within 3 h postpartum, regardless of the time of day or night when foaling occurred. • Advise owners to maintain a supply of oxytocin; begin treatment only after 3 h have passed; start by 2.5 h if a draft horse breed

 MEDICATIONS

DRUG(S) OF CHOICE
• Oxytocin (20 IU IV or 40 IU IM per injection), repeat injections at 60–120 min intervals. • After 18–24 h—can administer prostaglandin $F_{2\alpha}$ or analogs; antibiotics may be infused into uterus

CONTRAINDICATIONS
Higher doses of oxytocin may lead to uterine prolapse.

PRECAUTIONS
Oxytocin may induce uterine cramping, with potential to harm the foal.

ALTERNATIVE DRUGS
None as effective as oxytocin.

 FOLLOW-UP

PATIENT MONITORING
• Examine mare—determine if placenta has been expelled. • Evaluate uterine size (involution) and tone—determine if normal relative to the number of days postpartum

PREVENTION/AVOIDANCE
• Exercise and dietary supplementation with selenium may have value. • Avoid fescue pasture/hay near term

POSSIBLE COMPLICATIONS
• Septic metritis. • Laminitis

EXPECTED COURSE AND PROGNOSIS
• Of mares treated with oxytocin, >90% pass RFM with no other problems; excellent prognosis. • RFM passed without secondary involvement have no effect on foal heat breeding conception. • Affected mares treated with intrauterine antibiotics—higher rates of conception but higher rates of early pregnancy termination

 MISCELLANEOUS

ASSOCIATED CONDITIONS
See Historical Findings.

AGE-RELATED FACTORS
Old mares have a higher incidence on some farms.

PREGNANCY/FERTILITY/BREEDING
RFM incidence may increase with parturition induction.

SYNONYMS
Retained afterbirth

ABBREVIATIONS
RFM = retained fetal membranes

Suggested Reading
Blanchard TL, Varner DD. Postpartum septic/toxic metritis in the mare—observation & rationale for treatment. Clin Theriogenol 2011;3(3):3.
McNaughtyon JW, Meijer M, Macpherson ML. A novel approach to removing retained fetal membranes in the mare. Clin Theriogenol 2015;7(3):338.

Author Carla L. Carleton
Consulting Editor Carla L. Carleton
Acknowledgment The author/editor acknowledges the prior contribution of Walter R. Threlfall.

R

RHODOCOCCUS EQUI (PRESCOTTELLA EQUI)

BASICS

DEFINITION
An important cause of pneumonia in foals <6 months of age. Infection may also result in diarrhea, joint sepsis, intra-abdominal abscessation, and multifocal abscesses throughout the body. A proposed nomenclature change to *Prescottella equi* is currently under debate.

PATHOPHYSIOLOGY
• Gram-positive pleomorphic intracellular facultative organism that normally inhabits soil
• Inhalation of dust containing the organism thought to be the primary route of exposure for both the horse and humans
• Then resides within the alveolar macrophages, replicates, and can produce a severe, potentially life-threatening pyogranulomatous bronchopneumonia as necrosis and destruction of lung parenchyma occur
• Intestinal forms of the disease include ulcerative colitis and abdominal lymphadenitis. Associated GI infections likely arise from infected foals swallowing sputum containing the organism. Peyer's patches become infected and ulcerated significant mesenteric lymphadenitis can occur
• May disseminate to other body sites and produce septic arthritis, serositis, vertebral body abscesses, and cutaneous ulcerative lymphangitis
• Other extrathoracic manifestations—immune-mediated polysynovitis, uveitis/keratouveitis, immune-mediated hemolytic anemia, immune-mediated thrombocytopenia, hyperthermia associated with macrolide treatments, hyperlipemia, and telogen effluvium

SYSTEMS AFFECTED
• Respiratory
• GI
• Musculoskeletal
• Hemic/lymphatic/immune
• Ophthalmic
• Renal
• Skin
• Hepatobiliary
• Nervous

SIGNALMENT
• Foals 1–6 months of age, most show clinical signs before 4 months
• Immunocompromised adults or adults with concurrent illness

SIGNS
• Fever, cough, lethargy, depression, anorexia, poor weight gain, exercise intolerance, diarrhea, respiratory distress, joint distention, and sudden death

• May have abnormal thoracic auscultation and percussion findings, although severely affected foals may not have auscultable abnormalities

DIAGNOSIS

DIFFERENTIAL DIAGNOSIS
• Other causes of pneumonia (*Streptococcus equi* ssp. *equi, S. equi* ssp. *zooepidemicus,* parasite migration, and viral respiratory infections)
• Equine herpesvirus 2 infection may predispose foals
• *Definitive* diagnosis is based on culture of *Rhodococcus equi* although PCR techniques may be useful

CBC/BIOCHEMISTRY/URINALYSIS
• CBC—leukocytosis with a mature neutrophilia
• Increased fibrinogen and SAA
• Increased serum protein
• Severe disease—anemia and thrombocytopenia
• With diarrhea—may have electrolyte abnormalities (hyponatremia and hypochloremia)
• With dehydration—increased creatinine and blood urea nitrogen
• Renal and/or urinary tract involvement—abnormal urinalysis

OTHER LABORATORY TESTS
• PCR testing of tracheal fluid, bronchoalveolar lavage fluid, and aspirates from other sites for the presence of the VapA antigen, which is associated with virulence
• Testing for antibody directed against the VapA antigen is currently undergoing testing

IMAGING
Ultrasonography
Consolidation of lung parenchyma; pulmonary and intra-abdominal abscessation. Deep lesions will not be recognized.

Radiography
Thorax—increased interstitial density with dense patchy areas of alveolar pattern. Areas of consolidation and abscessation. Useful in monitoring response to therapy and determining the severity.

OTHER DIAGNOSTIC PROCEDURES
TTA
• Cytology—Gram-positive to Gram-variable pleomorphic ("Chinese character") intracellular rods
• Culture—positive *R. equi*
• PCR—*R. equi* and VapA antigen positive

Bronchoalveolar Lavage
• Results similar to TTA
• May recognize concurrent infection with *Pneumocystis carinii,* and requires specialized stain (silver stain)

• *Caution*—performing either TTA or bronchoalveolar lavage may be detrimental to a foal with significant respiratory disease and those in respiratory distress

PATHOLOGIC FINDINGS
• Related to the organ system involved
• Bilateral bronchopneumonia with severe coalescing abscess formation. Formation may be minimal in cases with associated acute respiratory distress syndrome. Ventral lung field involvement generally more severe. Abscesses range from a few millimeters to more than 10 cm. Generalized miliary abscess formation also common
• Pulmonary parenchyma surrounding pulmonary abscesses usually congested or consolidated
• Bronchial and mediastinal lymphadenopathy with abscessation
• Pleural empyema
• Pleural inflammation unusual unless empyema secondary to abscess rupture occurred
• GI lesions variable and may involve the entire GI tract. Mucosal villous atrophy, mucosal necrosis, diphtheritic membrane formation, ulcerative enterocolitis, and mesenteric lymphadenopathy with abscess formation
• Pulmonary histology—pyogranulomatous abscesses have a necrotic central core with surrounding degenerate neutrophils. Adjacent areas infiltrated with macrophages, lymphocytes, and occasional giant cells. Congestion, edema, and alveolar infiltration by macrophages and neutrophils, acute suppurative bronchitis, and peribronchitis
• GI histology—infiltration of phagocytic cells into the lamina propria. Necrosis of the villi and submucosa, mucosal ulceration, and pyogranulomatous lymphadenitis of the mesenteric or colonic lymph nodes
• Organisms identified using hematoxylin–eosin stain and/or Gram stains. Some organisms are acid fast
• Reports of concurrent infection with *P. carinii* identified via silver stains

TREATMENT

APPROPRIATE HEALTH CARE
• Affected foals may be treated at the farm
• Severely affected foals benefit from treatment at a referral facility with climate-controlled environments and oxygen supplementation
• Transport during cool times of the day and minimize stress
• Should not transfer from an endemic farm to a farm with no previous history

NURSING CARE
• Minimize stress

R

RHODOCOCCUS EQUI (PRESCOTTELLA EQUI) (CONTINUED)

• Climate-controlled environments, air conditioning, and good ventilation may improve the short-term prognosis with severely affected foals

ACTIVITY
Exercise should be restricted. Stall confinement is not necessary as long as turnout is in a small area only. Affected foals should be completely restricted from exercise during the hot periods of the day.

DIET
Parenteral nutrition for severely affected foals experiencing weight loss and anorexia.

CLIENT EDUCATION
• *R. equi* probably infects all horse farms to some degree. The difference in disease appearance is related to differences in environments, management techniques, and virulence of the isolate. On enzootic farms, infections result in huge economic losses associated with costs of prevention, treatment, and the death of some foals
• Most foals treated for *R. equi* infection recover. Severely affected foals are less likely to survive
• Severely immunocompromised humans have been diagnosed with *R. equi* infection

SURGICAL CONSIDERATIONS
Surgical drainage of easily accessible abscesses may be reasonable. Surgical removal of abdominal abscesses is unlikely to be rewarding.

MEDICATIONS

DRUG(S) OF CHOICE
• Erythromycin (10–37.5 mg/kg BID–QID PO) or rifampin (rifampicin) (5–10 mg/kg SID–BID PO) is the traditional standard therapy. Other macrolide antimicrobials azithromycin (10 mg/kg PO SID) and clarithromycin (7.5 mg/kg PO BID) are more commonly used today, have been efficacious, and may have reduced side effects
• Hyperthermia observed with macrolide therapy may be caused by decreased ability to sweat in affected foals, secondary to the treatment
• Treat until CBC, fibrinogen/SAA, and clinical presentation are normal and pneumonia resolved radiographically

CONTRAINDICATIONS, PRECAUTIONS, POSSIBLE INTERACTIONS, ALTERNATIVE DRUGS
• Some foals receiving the above-mentioned drug combinations may develop severe diarrhea. Decreasing dose may resolve the problem

• Mares housed with foals receiving erythromycin have developed severe fatal colitis, thought to be associated with *Clostridium difficile* infection secondary to ingestion of small amounts of erythromycin from the foal
• Idiosyncratic hyperthermia and tachypnea have been reported in foals receiving macrolides
• Aminophylline should not be used in combination with erythromycin owing to potential toxicity
• Foals diagnosed very early in the clinical course of infection may respond to trimethoprim–sulfa combinations, although this is not recommended
• Rifampin-resistant strains of *R. equi* have been identified. Rifampin should never be used alone owing to the rapidity of development of resistance

FOLLOW-UP

PATIENT MONITORING
Response to therapy can be monitored by resolution of clinical signs, normalization of CBC and fibrinogen, and radiographic improvement.

PREVENTION/AVOIDANCE
• Several strategies for prevention of *R. equi* infection exist. Decreasing the size of infective challenge by good housing and management practices and isolation of affected foals is important
• Early recognition of infection is important. This can be facilitated by daily temperature monitoring of foals, frequent routine physical examinations, and frequent thoracic ultrasonographic examinations
• Passive immunization by the IV administration of *R. equi* hyperimmune plasma has been used as a preventative technique, but its efficacy has been questioned. Timing of this treatment, if effective, is purportedly important and depends on expected exposure; it is typically administered during the first week of life and again at 30 days of age at many facilities
• To date, no active immunization protocol has been effective. However, experimental vaccination of mares with PNAG and the use of PNAG hyperimmune plasma appear promising for the prevention of *R. equi* infection in foals

EXPECTED COURSE AND PROGNOSIS
In well-established pulmonary cases, therapy may extend over 3–5 weeks.

MISCELLANEOUS

ABBREVIATIONS
• GI = gastrointestinal
• PCR = polymerase chain reaction
• PNAG = poly-*N*-acetyl glucosamine
• SAA = serum amyloid A
• TTA = transtracheal aspirate

Suggested Reading
Cohen ND. *Rhodococcus equi* foal pneumonia. Vet Clin North Am Equine Pract 2014;30:609–622.
Cywes-Bentley C, Rocha JN, Bordin AI, et al. Antibody to poly-N-acetyl glucosamine provides protection against intracellular pathogens: mechanism of action and validation in horse foals challenged with *Rhodococcus equi*. PLoS Pathog 2018;14:e1007160.
Giguère S, Berghaus LJ, Lee EA. Activity of 10 antimicrobial agents against intracellular *Rhodococcus equi*. Vet Microbiol 2015;178:275–278.
Giles C, Vanniasinkam T, Ndi S, Barton MD. *Rhodococcus equi* (*Prescottella equi*) vaccines; the future of vaccine development. Equine Vet J 2015;47:510–518.
Goodfellow M, Sangal V, Jones AL, et al. Charting stormy waters: a commentary on the nomenclature of the equine pathogen variously named *Prescottella equi*, *Rhodococcus equi* and *Rhodococcus hoagii*. Equine Vet J 2015;47:508–509.
Sanz MG, Oliveira AF, Loynachan A, et al. Validation and evaluation of VapA-specific IgG and IgG subclass enzyme-linked immunosorbent assays (ELISAs) to identify foals with *Rhodococcus equi* pneumonia. Equine Vet J 2016;48:103–108.

Author Pamela A. Wilkins
Consulting Editors Ashley G. Boyle

R

BASICS

OVERVIEW
• Rib fracture is the most commonly diagnosed fracture occurring within the first 24 h of life, typically due to trauma sustained during foaling
• Foals may present primarily with respiratory compromise secondary to the rib fracture or the rib fractures may be diagnosed as an additional finding during routine foal examination. Early recognition of life-threatening injury is necessary to implement appropriate therapeutic intervention
• Usually asymptomatic

SIGNALMENT
• Neonatal foals are most commonly affected as the injury is most often as a result of a dystocia
• Colts are affected 3 times as frequently as fillies

SIGNS
• Careful examination may reveal subcutaneous edema overlying injured ribs or along the ventrum. Subcutaneous emphysema rare but should alert the clinician to the high potential for rib fracture
• Audible or palpable crepitation over the fracture. The foal may groan or grunt when moving and flinch when the affected rib is palpated
• Tachypnea or dyspnea frequently present
• Abnormal thoracic auscultation may indicate the presence of hemothorax or pneumothorax
• Patients that have significant hemothorax may present in hemorrhagic shock owing to intracavitary blood loss

CAUSES AND RISK FACTORS
• Dystocia has been well documented as a significant risk factor for neonatal rib fractures
• Neither fetal thoracic diameter nor birth weight has been shown to play a role in occurrence of birth trauma
• Foals born to maiden mares and multiparous mares are thought to be equally affected

DIAGNOSIS

DIFFERENTIAL DIAGNOSIS
• Pleuropneumonia—thoracic radiography and US will help to rule out primary or concurrent pneumonia

• Rib osteomyelitis—has been reported in older foals, 3–6 weeks of age

CBC/BIOCHEMISTRY/URINALYSIS
• Anemia secondary to hemorrhage
• Septicemic foals may have abnormalities on CBC—leukopenia or leukocytosis are most common

OTHER LABORATORY TESTS
Routine immunoglobulin G testing recommended.

IMAGING
• Thoracic US—has been shown to be the most sensitive imaging modality for detecting rib fractures in foals. Fracture displacement, pneumothorax, hemothorax, and pulmonary contusion may be detected
• Thoracic radiographs—rib fractures, pneumothorax, hemothorax, and pulmonary contusion may be detected

OTHER DIAGNOSTIC PROCEDURES
• Palpation of the thoracic wall may reveal firm, focal swelling of 1 or more ribs, most typically at, or 5–7.5 cm (2–3 inches) dorsal to, the costochondral junction. Wetting the hair with alcohol allows the chest wall indentation or soft tissue swelling to be seen
• Thoracocentesis to evaluate for hemothorax

PATHOLOGIC FINDINGS
Pulmonary contusions, hemothorax, pneumothorax, diaphragmatic hernia and hemopericardium are significant consequences of rib fracture. Sudden death can result from fracture fragments lacerating the myocardium, pleural vessels, and pleura.

TREATMENT
• In patients with single nondisplaced rib fractures with minimal respiratory compromise, conservative management comprising severely restricted exercise for 4–6 weeks with weekly reevaluation is sufficient
• Encourage sternal or lateral recumbency with the affected side down to minimize ventilatory compromise to the undamaged lung
• Patients with hemorrhagic shock should be referred for fluid therapy, possible blood transfusion, and intranasal oxygen therapy
• Multiple (3 or more) displaced fractured ribs, a single displaced fragment in the vicinity of the heart, or a patient with flail chest warrants evaluation for internal fixation of the fracture fragments, and immediate referral is recommended

MEDICATIONS
Pain management with NSAIDs—ketoprofen (1.1 mg/kg IV every 12–24 h) or flunixin meglumine (0.5–1.1 mg/kg every 12 h) or butorphanol (0.04–1.0 mg/kg IV every 8–24 h).

CONTRAINDICATIONS/POSSIBLE INTERACTIONS
• Analgesia should be used judiciously as any sudden movement can cause rib fragments to lacerate internal vascular structures or the heart
• NSAIDs can have adverse renal and gastrointestinal effects—they should be used with caution in dehydrated or debilitated foals

FOLLOW-UP
Sequential thoracic US should be performed to assess fracture and pulmonary healing; 6 weeks is considered necessary for stabilization is most circumstances. The clients should be warned that sudden death is not an uncommon feature of this condition.

MISCELLANEOUS
The patient must be carefully evaluated for other common neonatal ailments associated with dystocia, including bladder rupture. As with any case, sepsis and failure of transfer of passive immunity must be ruled out.

SEE ALSO
• Pleuropneumonia
• Pneumonia, neonate
• Pneumothorax

ABBREVIATIONS
• NSAID = nonsteroidal anti-inflammatory drug
• US = ultrasonography, ultrasound

Suggested Reading
Jean D, Picandet V, Macieira S, et al. Detection of rib trauma in newborn foal in an equine critical care unit: a comparison of ultrasonography, radiography and physical examination. Equine Vet J 2007;39:158–163.

Authors Margaret C. Mudge and Katie J. Smith
Consulting Editor Margaret C. Mudge

R

RIGHT AND LEFT DORSAL DISPLACEMENT OF THE COLON

BASICS

DEFINITION
RDDLC
Anatomic relocation of the LC owing to migration of the pelvic flexure between the cecum and the right abdominal wall.

LDDLC
Anatomic relocation of the LC in a dorsal direction between the left body wall and the spleen towards the nephrosplenic space, where it can entrap.

PATHOPHYSIOLOGY
Speculative. Hypothetical factors:
• Lack of mesenteric attachment of the LC to the body wall makes it very mobile
• Excess soluble carbohydrate diet may cause increased fermentation and gas production in the LC
• Alteration of normal colonic motility patterns
• Rolling episodes
RDDLC
• Can occur in 2 directions—clockwise and counterclockwise (as viewed from the surgeon's perspective at surgery with horse in dorsal recumbency)
• Counterclockwise (most common)—the pelvic flexure moves craniad and then caudad between the cecum and the right body wall. The pelvic flexure often crosses the abdomen caudal to the cecum and continues in a cranial direction towards the diaphragm
• Clockwise (less common)—the pelvic flexure crosses the abdomen caudal to the cecum and displaces in a caudal-to-cranial direction between the cecum and the right abdominal wall
LDDLC
• The left colon ascends dorsally between the spleen and the body wall until entrapped in the nephrosplenic space
• The entrapped colon commonly rotates ventromedially 180°
• In type II LDDLC, the sternal and diaphragmatic flexures migrate cranially and dorsally to the stomach, which hampers nasogastric intubation
• Displaced colon may obstruct duodenum and therefore cause reflux

Vascular Compromise
Both displacements are non-strangulating; however vascular compromise can occur in:
• Volvulus of the LC at the root of the mesentery (RDDLC) or at the site of entrapment over the nephrosplenic ligament (LDDLC)
• Longstanding (>24 h) nephrosplenic entrapments causing colonic congestion, edema, and/or mural damage in the absence of volvulus

SYSTEMS AFFECTED
GI
• The LC is displaced, and this may lead to other abdominal GI tract displacements (cecum, small colon, and small intestine)
• Mechanical traction on the mesentery can result in considerable pain
• Although uncommon, vascular obstruction results in compromise, and potentially necrosis of the LC

Cardiovascular
With long duration or vascular compromise, dehydration and fluid shifts may cause circulatory compromise.

GENETICS
N/A

INCIDENCE/PREVALENCE
• In 1 study, 14% of exploratory celiotomies were nonstrangulating LC displacements
• In another study, 23% of all colic cases presented to a referral practice were LC displacements

SIGNALMENT
No particular signalment; foals can also be affected. Mares, particularly following parturition, may be predisposed to displacement of the LC.

SIGNS
• Referable to the amount of colonic distention and any vascular compromise
• Mild to moderate abdominal discomfort after 12–24 h
• Colic usually responds to analgesia or fasting initially but returns when the analgesic efficacy decreases and horse is re-fed
• Acute progression of signs is associated with increased bowel distention or compromise
• Gastric reflux is inconsistent but was present in up to 43% of horses with LDDLC. Nasogastric intubation may be difficult in horses with type II LDDLC
• Heart rate often is less than might be expected from the degree of pain displayed (LDDLC)

CAUSES
• Potentially, alteration to the intestinal motility and changes in the weight of the colon because of excess gas formation or mild impactions
• Changes in intra-abdominal volume and GI activity after parturition may predispose postpartum mares to LC displacement
• LDDLC—in addition to the above, gastric distention resulting in displacement of the spleen from the body wall, splenic contraction, and displacement of the spleen because of adhesions between the spleen and previous ventral midline celiotomy incisions

RISK FACTORS
• Adhesions of the spleen to midline (previous celiotomies), previous LC displacements, and other forms of colic may cause a horse to roll
• Sudden dietary changes

DIAGNOSIS

DIFFERENTIAL DIAGNOSIS
• Colonic/cecal tympany
• Retroflexion of the pelvic flexure
• Colonic impaction
• Colonic volvulus
• Enterolithiasis

CBC/BIOCHEMISTRY/URINALYSIS
• CBC and biochemistry most commonly normal, with mild alkalosis to mild acidosis in cases of nonstrangulating displacements
• Decreased hematocrit may result from sequestration of red blood cells in the spleen
• If strangulation of the colon occurs, significant dehydration, with a relatively decreased protein and metabolic acidosis, is common
• Horses with RDDLC showed higher serum γ-glutamyltransferase than horses with LDDLC

OTHER LABORATORY TESTS
• Peritoneal fluid usually normal, unless the bowel is compromised
• In LDDLC, splenocentesis may occur as the spleen is forced medially and ventrally

IMAGING
Ultrasonography
RDDLC
• Large intestine distended with gas and fluid
• Abnormally located colonic vessels along the right lateral abdomen are a good indicator of RDDLC and/or 180° LC volvulus
LDDLC
• Failure to visualize the left kidney because of gas in the LC and/or the dorsal border of the spleen partially obscured by colon or displaced ventrally
• A false-positive diagnosis can result from a gas-distended viscus near the left kidney, obstructing visualization of the kidney
• A false-negative diagnosis can result from lack of gas in the entrapped colon or angling the ultrasonography probe dorsoventrally
• 1 study reported a correct diagnosis in 88% of cases of nephrosplenic entrapment, with no false-positive results

OTHER DIAGNOSTIC PROCEDURES
RDDLC
Rectal examination—absence of pelvic flexure, LC lateral to cecum, colon bands coursing transversely in the caudal abdomen, gas distention or impaction of the LC, cecum may not be found or is distended.

LDDLC
Rectal examination—colon on the left, colon bands coursing craniodorsally toward the nephrosplenic space; medial or caudal displacement of the spleen; different grades of colon distention and sometimes impaction. The colon entrapped in the nephrosplenic space may be clearly palpable in some horses.

(CONTINUED) RIGHT AND LEFT DORSAL DISPLACEMENT OF THE COLON

Rectal palpation confirmed diagnosis of left dorsal displacement in 61–72% of cases. In other conditions the colon may adopt a dorsal position within the abdomen but continues cranially rather than into the nephrosplenic space.

PATHOLOGIC FINDINGS
Left dorsal displacement—some cases present another primary lesion involving another segment of the GI tract.

TREATMENT
APPROPRIATE HEALTH CARE
• RDDLC—medical treatment in patients with mild signs although close monitoring is required. Surgical correction is often required
• LDDLC—conservative management, administration of phenylephrine (with or without controlled exercise), rolling the horse under general anesthesia, surgical correction: 7.5% of horses were reported to have another concurrent lesion (i.e. small intestinal obstruction, 360° colon torsion, etc.)
• Choice of treatment depends on certainty of the diagnosis, degree of LC distention, and financial limitations
• If the diagnosis is not certain or colonic distention is marked, rolling and controlled exercise may be contraindicated
• Conservative treatment of both RDDLC and LDDLC is appropriate provided that diagnosis is accurate with no signs indicating surgical lesion or systemic compromise

NURSING CARE
• Vital
• Nasogastric intubation and gastric decompression are vital if mechanical obstruction of the small intestine
• Exploratory celiotomy—fluid volume deficits and acid–base and electrolyte imbalances need to be addressed
• Abdominal distention restricting respiratory tidal volume and requiring supplemental oxygen therapy is not common. Deflation of a markedly distended large intestine via percutaneous trocharization may be beneficial but may cause leakage of intestinal contents

ACTIVITY
• Controlled exercise may assist resolution of LDDLC
• Uncontrolled rolling may convert a nonstrangulating to a strangulating displacement

DIET
No food should be administered.

CLIENT EDUCATION
• Counsel owners on the decision of whether to treat LDDLC conservatively or surgically
• Stress that treatment without surgery has obvious benefits, but that risks are associated with conservative treatment—further compromise of a markedly distended entrapped viscus and less commonly rupture

SURGICAL CONSIDERATIONS
When the colon is not strangulated, the condition usually is straightforward to correct.

MEDICATIONS
DRUG(S) OF CHOICE
• Standard analgesia for colic—see chapter Acute adult abdominal pain—acute colic. Drug use and dosage depend on nature of the colic and the therapy chosen
• LDDLC—phenylephrine (10–20 mg diluted in 50 mL of saline injected IV slowly over 5–10 min) causes splenic contraction and may facilitate dislodging the LC from the nephrosplenic space

FOLLOW-UP
PATIENT MONITORING
• Routine postoperative monitoring after surgery or conservative therapy
• In 1 study horses with RDDLC were more likely to experience recurrent episodes of colic than other types of displacement
• Recurrence of nephrosplenic entrapment is 7.5–8.5%; however, horses that have a recurrence episode even higher

PREVENTION/AVOIDANCE
• The cause is poorly understood and avoidance is difficult
• Minimize management that may alter colonic activity, production of excess gas, and formation of impactions. Institute nutritional changes gradually
• Prevent horses from rolling when showing signs of mild colic
• Ablation of nephrosplenic space reduces risk of nephrosplenic entrapment although displacement of the LC to the lateral aspect of the spleen or other displacements may still occur
• Colopexy or colon resection is not routinely recommended

POSSIBLE COMPLICATIONS
• Displacement can progress such that the colon becomes strangulated secondary to volvulus of the displaced colon. Horses can then rapidly succumb to cardiovascular shock from endotoxemia and hypovolemia or to colonic rupture from devitalization of the colon
• Administration of phenylephrine has been associated with fatal internal hemorrhage in older horses

EXPECTED COURSE AND PROGNOSIS
• The prognosis is good, provided there has been no volvulus or significant vascular insult to the colon
• Long-term survival of horses with nonstrangulating displacements is excellent (>90%)

MISCELLANEOUS
ASSOCIATED CONDITIONS
• Cholestasis
• Colonic volvulus
• GI impaction
• Gastric distention

PREGNANCY/FERTILITY/BREEDING
• The colon is held in place largely by its association with surrounding organs. The empty abdomen in postpartum mares may predispose to displacement
• Volvulus rather than dorsal displacement is more commonly associated with postpartum mares

SYNONYMS
LDDLC—nephrosplenic ligament entrapment.

SEE ALSO
• Impaction
• Large colon torsion

ABBREVIATIONS
• GI = gastrointestinal
• LC = large colon
• LDDLC = left dorsal displacement of the large colon
• RDDLC = right dorsal displacement of the large colon

Author Luis M. Rubio-Martinez
Consulting Editors Henry Stämpfli and Olimpo Oliver-Espinosa
Acknowledgment The author and editors acknowledge the prior contribution of Judith B. Koenig and Simon G. Pearce.

R

RIGHT DORSAL COLITIS

BASICS

DEFINITION
Localized ulcerative inflammation of the right dorsal colon often associated with administration of NSAIDs, particularly phenylbutazone or flunixin meglumine; dehydration increases the risk of drug toxicity.

PATHOPHYSIOLOGY
• Nonspecific NSAIDs including phenylbutazone and flunixin meglumine inhibit COX activity (Web Figure 1) as a competitive antagonist for both constitutive COX-1, responsible for the production of PGs involved in physiologic homeostatic functions, and for inducible COX-2, upregulated with inflammation. Intestinal mucosal cell production of PGE_2 and $PGF_{2\alpha}$ is decreased by the inhibition of COX-1. This results in the loss of the PG-mediated protective effects on the intestinal mucosa. When the intestinal mucosa integrity is sufficiently compromised, local bacterial invasion of the mucosa, luminal endotoxin absorption, and plasma protein leakage into the intestinal lumen may occur
• NSAID toxicity is potentiated in dehydrated or hypovolemic horses because the normal protective vascular changes guarding from reduced blood flow are inhibited
• The development of RDC in absence of previous NSAID administration suggests that the condition may be multifactorial

SYSTEMS AFFECTED
Gastrointestinal Tract
• The right dorsal colon is primarily affected. Oral and gastric ulcerations may also develop from NSAID toxicity
• Histologically, lesions are characterized by multifocal to coalescing ulcerations in the wall of the right dorsal colon (Web Figure 2)
• Subacute lesions are characterized by a fibrinonecrotic ulcerative colitis
• In chronic cases, fibrous connective tissue is present in the lamina propria underlying the ulcerated mucosa. Colonic stenosis with ingesta impaction and subsequent necrosis and rupture of the colon can occur

GENETICS
N/A

INCIDENCE/PREVALENCE
RDC, now preferably called RDUC (U ulcerative), may be associated with the administration of phenylbutazone or other NSAID therapy at the manufacturer's recommended daily dose. The variable toxicity has been attributed to individual variation in response to NSAIDs, duration of treatment, diet composition, health status, age, and hydration status.

GEOGRAPHIC DISTRIBUTION
N/A

SIGNALMENT
Although there is no evidence to demonstrate overrepresentation for any particular age or breed, most reports involve miniature horses, ponies, and young performance horses.

SIGNS
General Comments
Most cases have a history of administration of oral or parenteral NSAIDs with phenylbutazone being the most commonly used. RDUC can also result following high-dose administration of flunixin meglumine or in combination with phenylbutazone. NSAID therapy is most commonly implemented for treatment of chronic or severe musculoskeletal conditions (i.e. laminitis).

Historical Findings
• NSAID toxicity cases commonly present with concurrent systemic dehydration, which may result from either systemic illness or an inability to maintain proper hydration
• Horses with acute disease commonly have clinical signs that include colic, depression, lethargy, partial or complete anorexia, fever, and diarrhea
• Horses with chronic disease may demonstrate intermittent colic, soft feces, weight loss, and ventral edema

Physical Examination Findings
• Acute disease is commonly associated with signs of colitis including watery diarrhea, severe dehydration, severe systemic illness, injected mucous membranes and/or marked endotoxemia
• Horses with chronic disease may have formed or soft "cow pie" feces, edema, and abnormal vital parameters that include often elevated heart rate

CAUSES
NSAID toxicity results from high-dose therapy, with individual horses having the ability to tolerate higher NSAID administration doses. It is not clear why ulcerative lesions are localized in the right dorsal colon.

RISK FACTORS
Dehydration in combination with NSAID administration are predisposing factors for RDUC.

DIAGNOSIS

DIFFERENTIAL DIAGNOSIS
• Other causes of infectious colitis including salmonellosis, *Clostridium difficile* infection, and Potomac horse fever should be considered
• Chronic NSAID toxicity may have similarities to other forms of PLE including cyathostomiasis, chronic inflammatory (infiltrative) bowel disease, alimentary lymphoma, *Lawsonia intracellularis*, chronic salmonellosis, gastric ulcers, or sand enteropathy. Definitive diagnosis is based on the history of NSAID administration, physical examination findings, and hematologic/biochemical evidence of marked PLE

CBC/BIOCHEMISTRY/URINALYSIS
CBC
With acute disease hematologic abnormalities often include neutropenia with mild to moderate toxic neutrophils in combination with a regenerative or a degenerative left shift. An increased packed cell volume is frequently observed. Patients that present with more chronic disease may have a less pronounced neutropenia, but neutrophil morphology may still reveal toxicity.

Biochemistry Profile
Serum biochemical abnormalities often include marked hypoproteinemia, hypochloremia, azotemia and metabolic acidosis. Hypoproteinemia may be observed despite hemoconcentration and will worsen with rehydration. Hypoalbuminemia is common, but when total protein concentration is <4.5 g/dL (45 g/L), panhypoproteinemia is typically observed.

OTHER LABORATORY TESTS
Abdominal Paracentesis
Elevation of total solids concentration and nucleated cell count may be observed.

Fecal Occult Blood Test
Generally positive—this should be performed before rectal examination to avoid any complications with interpretation of test result.

IMAGING
• Transabdominal ultrasonography at the right 10th to 13th intercostal spaces can be used in standing horses to image the right dorsal colon. Horses with RDUC have significantly greater colonic wall thickness than healthy horses ($N = 0.3–0.4$ cm). The right dorsal colon of affected horses also has a prominent hypoechoic layer associated with submucosal edema and inflammatory infiltrates (Web Figure 3)
• Gastroscopy—horses with RDUC commonly have concurrent gastric and potentially duodenal ulcers. Diagnosis of gastric ulceration will impact treatment protocols

OTHER DIAGNOSTIC PROCEDURES
Exploratory Celiotomy/Laparoscopy
Rarely indicated. Gross examination reveals marked edema, thickening, and/or when the reduced luminal diameter of the intestinal tract is restricted to right dorsal colon.

Intestinal Biopsy
Definitive diagnosis of the condition is made by histopathologic examination of a biopsy of the right dorsal colon obtained during celiotomy or at necropsy.

R

TREATMENT

AIMS
The treatment consists of discontinuation of NSAID therapy in combination with appropriate supportive therapy.

APPROPRIATE HEALTH CARE
The majority of patients with RDUC require hospitalization to receive appropriate medical supportive therapy.

NURSING CARE
Acute RDC
Horses with acute disease are treated with supportive treatment, including IV fluids (LRS), systemic broad-spectrum antibiotics, and analgesics. All NSAIDs should be discontinued. When hypoproteinemia is severe (albumin <1.5 g/dL; 15 g/L), plasma transfusion should be administered.

Chronic RDC
• Horses with chronic disease are managed with low-residue feeding and discontinuation of all NSAIDs
• Dietary management consists of frequent feeding (4–6 meals) of complete, pelleted (low residue) diet that contains 30% dietary fiber and 14% protein. Pelleted feed is advocated because it decreases the mechanical and physiologic load on the large colon. Long-stem roughage is eliminated or restricted to small amounts of fresh grass for at least 3 months. Low-residue diet is fed according to the manufacturer's recommendations. The diet change is gradually completed over a period of approximately a week.

ACTIVITY
Managements to decrease stress include discontinuing or decreasing or eliminating work such as strenuous exercise.

SURGICAL CONSIDERATIONS
Surgical intervention indicated when the RDUC cannot be controlled with medical treatment evidenced by recurrent colic episodes. Surgery requires either bypassing or resecting the diseased RDC. Side-to-side colo-colostomy, between the proximal intact part of the RDC and the small colon, can be performed to bypass the diseased part of the RDC. End-to-end colo-colostomy after resection of the diseased RDC can also be performed. The prognosis for horses that undergo surgery is guarded.

 MEDICATIONS

DRUG(S) OF CHOICE
Supportive treatment for horses with acute disease includes:
• LRS (60–120 mL/kg/24 h) for volume replacement
• Broad-spectrum systemic antibiotics (potassium penicillin G 22 000 IU/kg IV QID and gentamicin sulfate 6.6 mg/kg IV daily or ceftiofur 2.2 mg/kg IV BID)
• Analgesics such as butorphanol (0.02 mg/kg IV or as a constant rate infusion at 0.013 mg/kg/h IV in fluids) can be administered

PRECAUTIONS
• NSAIDs such as phenylbutazone or flunixin meglumine should be avoided because they are involved in the pathogenesis of the disease
• Aminoglycosides should be used with caution when clinical signs of severe dehydration (prerenal azotemia) are present owing to its potential nephrotoxicity

 FOLLOW-UP

PATIENT MONITORING
• Continual hematologic monitoring until resolution of hypoproteinemia
• Include overall vital parameters and during rehydration as well hematocrit and plasma protein concentrations. If plasma protein concentrations decrease below 4 g/dL (40 g/L) or albumin drops below 1.5 g/dL (15 g/L) plasma transfusion is indicated
• Continued monitoring of total protein concentrations will provide evidence of colonic healing. Once the total protein, specifically albumin concentration, is near or within normal ranges dietary restrictions can be gradually eliminated

• Colonic restitution and resolution of hypoproteinemia/hypoalbuminemia requires generally 3–6 months

POSSIBLE COMPLICATIONS
• Horses with acute disease can develop a severe diarrhea, endotoxemia with marked edema, laminitis, or renal disease
• Chronic disease may be associated with progressive weight loss, hypoproteinemia, colic, colonic stricture, and persistently loose feces

 MISCELLANEOUS

ABBREVIATIONS
• COX = cyclooxygenase
• LRS = lactated Ringer's solution
• NSAID = nonsteroidal anti-inflammatory drug
• PG = prostaglandin
• PLE = protein-losing enteropathy
• RDC = right dorsal colitis
• RDUC = right dorsal ulcerative colitis

Suggested Reading
Cook VL, Blikslager AT. The use of nonsteroidal anti-inflammatory drugs in critically ill horses. J Vet Emerg Crit Care 2015;25:76–88.
Jones SL, Davis J, Rowlingson K. Ultrasonographic findings in horses with right dorsal colitis: five cases (2000–2001). J Am Vet Med Assoc 2003;222:1248–1251.
Karcher LF, Dill SG, Anderson WI, King JM. Right dorsal colitis. J Vet Intern Med 1990;4:247–253.
McConnico RS, Morgan TW, Williams CC, et al. Pathophysiologic effects of phenylbutazone on the right dorsal colon in horses. Am J Vet Res 2008;69:1496–1505.
Moses VS, Bertone AL. Nonsteroidal anti-inflammatory drugs. Vet Clin North Am Equine Pract 2002;18:21–37.

Author Elizabeth Davis
Consulting Editors Henry Stämpfli and Olimpo Oliver-Espinosa
Acknowledgment The author and editors acknowledge the prior contribution of Ludovic Bouré.

ROBINIA PSEUDOACACIA (BLACK LOCUST) TOXICOSIS

BASICS

OVERVIEW
• *Robinia pseudoacacia* (black locust) toxicosis results from an unknown toxin found in all portions of the plant except the flowers
• A glycoprotein called robin is the putative toxin
• The tree is widely distributed east of the Mississippi River
• Signs relate to gastrointestinal and cardiovascular effects of the toxin
• Among domestic livestock species, horses may be the most susceptible
• Most cases involve horses eating the bark of the tree

SIGNALMENT
No known breed, age, or genetic susceptibilities.

SIGNS
• Depression
• Colic
• Diarrhea or constipation
• Decreased intestinal peristalsis
• Weakness
• Mydriasis
• Lack of menace response
• Cardiac dysrhythmias
• Hyperexcitability
• Dyspnea
• Laminitis

CAUSES AND RISK FACTORS
• Leaves are palatable and will be eaten if other forage is of poor quality or unavailable
• Clinical signs have been reported in horses ingesting as little as 70 g of bark
• Boredom and hunger predispose to ingestion

DIAGNOSIS

DIFFERENTIAL DIAGNOSIS
• Ionophore intoxication—differentiated by detection of an ionophore in feed
• *Eupatorium rugosum* (white snakeroot) intoxication—evidence of plant consumption
• Other causes of colic—appropriate physical examination and imaging (e.g. ultrasonography, radiography)

CBC/BIOCHEMISTRY/URINALYSIS
• Hypocalcemia was noted in 2 ill horses after leaf ingestion
• Recumbent horses have increased serum creatine kinase concentrations

OTHER LABORATORY TESTS
N/A

IMAGING
N/A

OTHER DIAGNOSTIC PROCEDURES
ECG may demonstrate cardiac dysrhythmias, but the types of dysrhythmias are not well documented.

PATHOLOGIC FINDINGS
Gross
• Plant material (e.g. bark, leaves, pods) in stomach contents
• Watery and hemorrhagic intestinal contents

Histopathologic
Enteritis characterized by diffuse villus-tip necrosis and hemorrhage.

TREATMENT

• Decontamination with AC and saline cathartic or mineral oil
• Balanced electrolyte fluids

MEDICATIONS

DRUG(S) OF CHOICE
• AC (1–2 g/kg PO in water slurry (1 g of AC in 5 mL of water))
• 1 dose of cathartic PO with AC if no diarrhea or ileus—70% sorbitol (3 mL/kg) or sodium or magnesium sulfate (250 mg/kg), with the latter 2 in a water slurry
• Treat cardiac dysrhythmias as appropriate; although dysrhythmias are reported to occur they are not well described
• Analgesics for abdominal discomfort—flunixin meglumine (1.1 mg/kg IV or IM as necessary)

CONTRAINDICATIONS/POSSIBLE INTERACTIONS
• Use NSAIDs with caution in dehydrated patients
• Do not give mineral oil concurrently with AC because of potential to impair binding ability of AC

FOLLOW-UP

PATIENT MONITORING
N/A

PREVENTION/AVOIDANCE
Prevent access to black locust; if not practical, provide good-quality diet in adequate amounts.

POSSIBLE COMPLICATIONS
N/A

EXPECTED COURSE AND PROGNOSIS
• Guarded prognosis in symptomatic animals
• No long-term sequelae are expected in recovered animals.

MISCELLANEOUS

ASSOCIATED CONDITIONS
N/A

AGE-RELATED FACTORS
N/A

ZOONOTIC POTENTIAL
N/A

PREGNANCY/FERTILITY/BREEDING
N/A

ABBREVIATIONS
• AC = activated charcoal
• NSAID = nonsteroidal anti-inflammatory drug

Suggested Reading
Burrows GE, Tyrl RJ. Toxic Plants of North America. Ames, IA: Iowa State University Press, 2001:602.

Authors Arya Sobhakumari and Robert H. Poppenga
Consulting Editors Wilson K. Rumbeiha and Steve Ensley

BASICS

DEFINITION
A non-enveloped RNA virus that is the most common infectious pathogen identified in foals with diarrhea.

PATHOPHYSIOLOGY
• Infection via the fecal–oral route
• Incubation period of 1–2 days
• Older immune foals may act as subclinical shedders
• Infects epithelial cells at the tips of the villi in the small intestine, leading to lysis and resulting in malabsorption and osmotic diarrhea (loss of lactase). Undigested lactose travels to the large intestine and undergoes fermentation, producing a hyperosmotic solution that attracts more fluid.
• Viral enterotoxin, the rotavirus nonstructural protein NSP4 —inhibits sodium–glucose transporter (impaired water uptake); reduces enzymatic breakdown of sugars (osmotic diarrhea); destruction of epithelial cell integrity

SYSTEMS AFFECTED
Gastrointestinal tract

INCIDENCE/PREVALENCE
Ubiquitous in horse population; can be responsible for outbreaks of foal diarrhea involving the majority of the foals on an individual farm.

GEOGRAPHIC DISTRIBUTION
Worldwide

SIGNALMENT
Clinical disease in foals <6 months, most commonly <3 months. Foals <1 month can have severe disease owing to limited ability to correct fluid and electrolyte loss.

SIGNS
Anorexia, dull mentation, diarrhea, abdominal distention, dehydration, fever, lethargy, recumbency.

RISK FACTORS
Exposure to infected foals, unvaccinated mares, FTPI, poor hygiene and biosecurity practices.

DIAGNOSIS

DIFFERENTIAL DIAGNOSIS
Equine coronavirus, *Clostridium difficile* A and B, *Clostridium perfringens*, *Lawsonia intracellularis*, *Rhodococcus equi*, *Salmonella* spp., *Neorickettsia risticii*. Coinfections can occur.

CBC/BIOCHEMISTRY/URINALYSIS
Dehydration (high packed cell volume, protein, creatinine, hyperlactatemia), and electrolyte loss (hyponatremia, hypochloremia, hypokalemia, acidosis).

OTHER LABORATORY TESTS
• ELISA
• Rapid antigen detection kits for humans have been evaluated for use in horses and are useful on the farm (less sensitive than ELISA)
• RT-PCR
• Reverse transcription loop-mediated isothermal amplification

IMAGING
Abdominal ultrasonography—nonspecific findings: fluid-filled bowel, hypo- or hypermotility, and small intestinal distention.

PATHOLOGIC FINDINGS
Pathology includes destruction of epithelial cells at the villi tips in the small intestine.

TREATMENT

Supportive care is aimed at maintaining hydration and electrolyte balance.

DIET
In severe cases, parenteral nutrition may be warranted.

CLIENT EDUCATION
Biosecurity measures owing to highly contagious nature of the virus. Quarantine infected foals. Vaccination of pregnant mares.

MEDICATIONS

DRUG(S) OF CHOICE
• Lactase 6000–9000 FCC lactase U/50 kg PO every 3–8 h for 10–14 days to improve digestion of lactose and reduce osmotic diarrhea/maldigestion
• Antidiarrheal therapy—Neonorm Foal (*Croton lechleri* tree extract): a chloride channel blocker that reduces water loss into the bowel lumen, 10 mL PO every 8–12 h for 3 days. Bismuth subsalicylate (1–3 mL/kg PO every 6–24 h). Biosponge paste (di-tri-octahedral smectite) 30–60 mL PO every 6–12 hours; discontinue as soon as diarrhea resolves
• Antimicrobial and IV plasma for foals at risk for or with evidence of sepsis

CONTRAINDICATIONS
Do not administer potentially nephrotoxic agents to dehydrated foals.

POSSIBLE INTERACTIONS
See Contraindications.

FOLLOW-UP

PATIENT MONITORING
• Signs of dehydration (need for IV fluids)
• Inappetence or anorexia, which may further contribute to dehydration and lethargy
• Prolonged episodes of diarrhea that may suggest coinfection with another pathogen
• Neurologic signs and abnormal behavior that suggests severe electrolyte imbalance, particularly hyponatremia. Careful fluid therapy and restoration of electrolyte balance is essential in these cases

PREVENTION/AVOIDANCE
• Inactivated rotavirus A vaccine is currently licensed in the USA. Administered to mares during each pregnancy at 8, 9, and 10 months of gestation. Shown to increase antibody in colostrum and reduce the incidence in foals. Foals may still develop diarrhea once colostral antibodies wane after 60 days. Severity and duration of diarrhea is shorter
• Good hygiene and use of phenolic disinfectants. Bleach is ineffective

EXPECTED COURSE AND PROGNOSIS
• Mortality is low; foals less than <14 days are at highest risk for death
• Usually self-limiting, with a typical course of 3–5 days
• Viral shedding can persist for up to 10 days. Chronic shedders exist and can shed the virus for up to 8 months

MISCELLANEOUS

ASSOCIATED CONDITIONS
May indicate failure to vaccinate, or FTPI via colostrum in foals <1 month. FTPI can be associated with potentially fatal infections (sepsis).

PREGNANCY/FERTILITY/BREEDING
Vaccination is safe in pregnant mares.

ABBREVIATIONS
• ELISA – enzyme-linked immunosorbent assay
• FCC = Food Chemicals Codex
• FTPI = failure of transfer of passive immunity
• RT-PCR = reverse transcription polymerase chain reaction

Suggested Reading
Bailey KE, Gilkerson JR, Browning GF. Equine rotavirus—current understanding and continuing challenges. Vet Microbiol 2013;167:135–144.

Author Michelle Abraham Linton
Consulting Editor Ashley G. Boyle

R

SALMONELLOSIS

 BASICS

DEFINITION
Salmonellosis refers to clinical disease resulting from infection with various serovars (aka serotypes) of *Salmonella enterica* ssp. *enterica*.

PATHOPHYSIOLOGY
Considered an opportunistic pathogen, *S. enterica* colonizes the small intestine, cecum, and colon of warm- and cold-blooded vertebrates. Organisms can be shed intermittently in feces and may be carried latently in mesenteric lymph nodes. Transmission occurs by the fecal–oral route. Once in the GI tract, bacteria can invade the mucosa (typically through M cells) and spread to lymphoid tissue. Virulence factors promote host tissue invasion, damage mucosa and epithelial cells, promote the inflammatory response and neutrophil recruitment, stimulate fluid secretion into the GI tract, and can lead to severe cardiovascular impairment and toxemia.

SYSTEMS AFFECTED
Primarily affects the GI tract, causing enterocolitis.

GENETICS
N/A

INCIDENCE/PREVALENCE
• Equine shedding prevalence varies markedly from an estimated 0.8% among the general population up to 13% among horses with GI illness
• Outbreaks have been recognized on farms, at boarding and sales facilities, and veterinary hospitals; and are commonly associated with inadequate environmental hygiene

SIGNALMENT
No breed or sex predilection has been reported.

SIGNS
• 4 clinical syndromes are classically reported in horses: (1) asymptomatic disease with intermittent shedding, (2) fever without diarrhea, (3) enterocolitis, and (4) sepsis
• *Salmonella* is often carried asymptomatically with intermittent shedding occurring at times of stress
• Signs are nonspecific and may include fever, diarrhea, colic, and leukopenia. In addition, cardiovascular function may be compromised owing to dehydration and systemic effects of endotoxemia. If infection results in severe intestinal inflammation, horses may have tachycardia, injected mucous membranes, delayed capillary refill time, hypoproteinemia, and peripheral edema
• Adult horses may have fever and colic signs without diarrhea

• Neonatal foals may develop septicemia and thus clinical signs may vary according to organ system(s) affected

CAUSES
The most common serotypes reported in horses in 2014 by the USDA National Veterinary Services Laboratory were *Salmonella* Typhimurium, *Salmonella* Javiana, *Salmonella* Newport, *Salmonella* Anatum, and *Salmonella* Rubislaw/Thompson.

RISK FACTORS
• Factors that may disrupt natural barriers can predispose to development of clinical salmonellosis; including antimicrobial therapy, sudden feed change, systemic illness, surgical intervention, and transportation
• Any horse with severe disease has an increased risk of shedding *Salmonella* in its feces

 DIAGNOSIS

DIFFERENTIAL DIAGNOSIS
• Other causes of acute diarrhea in adult horses may include Potomac horse fever, intestinal clostridiosis, antibiotic-associated diarrhea, sand enteropathy, NSAID toxicity, cyathostomiasis, arsenic toxicity, cantharidin toxicity, and idiopathic colitis
• Endotoxemia due to GI disorders and in mares with placental retention
• Signs of colic may be associated with other disorders
• Congestive heart failure and vasculitis

CBC/BIOCHEMISTRY/URINALYSIS
CBC
• Hemoconcentration
• Decreased to normal total solids
• Leukopenia due to neutropenia
• Leukocytosis in colitis of several days' duration
• White blood cells can have a highly reactive appearance
• ± Hyperfibrinogenemia

Serum Chemistries
• Azotemia
• Hypoalbuminemia
• Hyponatremia, hypochloremia, hypokalemia, hypocalcemia
• Metabolic acidosis
• Hyperglycemia

Urine Analysis
Isosthenuria, proteinuria, hematuria, cylindruria, and glucosuria.

OTHER LABORATORY TESTS
• Fecal culture (3–5 enriched cultures) or PCR testing with subsequent antimicrobial susceptibility testing and serotyping of isolates
• Abdominocentesis for animals with signs of colic

IMAGING
Transabdominal or transrectal ultrasonography may be used to detect bowel wall thickening or peritoneal fluid accumulation.

OTHER DIAGNOSTIC PROCEDURES
• Rectal palpation
• Exploratory laparotomy may be indicated to rule out other causes of colic; intestinal biopsy for culture of *Salmonella* may be done to confirm a suspected case. The risk vs. benefit of such a biopsy must be considered on a case-by-case basis

PATHOLOGIC FINDINGS
Lesions at necropsy include diffuse fibrinous or hemorrhagic inflammation of the cecum and colon. Mucosa may be thickened, have areas of necrosis, greyish pseudomembranes, and, in chronic cases, focal mucosal ulcers.

 TREATMENT

APPROPRIATE HEALTH CARE
N/A

NURSING CARE
• Correction of electrolyte deficits and restoration and maintenance of fluid volume are critical for patients with severe diarrhea
• If severe hypoproteinemia, colloidal fluids (e.g. plasma, hetastarch), with or without heparin, should be administered
• Separation of suspect or confirmed cases from other patients and personnel via isolation and/or use of contact precautions is recommended. To minimize bacterial transmission, ensure compliance with all environmental and personal hygiene policies
• Regular cleaning of soiled areas on the patient to reduce skin damage from fecal material

ACTIVITY
Restricted proportionate to severity of illness.

DIET
• Feeding small amounts of palatable feed frequently may improve food consumption. Low-bulk, low-soluble-carbohydrate feeds (e.g. complete pelleted rations, good quality grass hay) are ideal
• Fresh water should always be available. Some horses will consume electrolyte-containing fluids orally, which can reduce the need for IV electrolytes
• Patients with prolonged anorexia may benefit from parenteral nutrition

CLIENT EDUCATION
• In general, infected horses should be maintained separately from other horses including separate housing and cleaning utensils, and contact precautions should be used when managing these horses or their environments

S

(CONTINUED)

• *Salmonella* is a zoonotic pathogen that may cause GI illness in people, and, in particular, in immune-compromised individuals

SURGICAL CONSIDERATIONS
If shedding or suspect horses are taken to surgery, optimal biosecurity procedures should be used.

MEDICATIONS
DRUG(S) OF CHOICE
Antimicrobial Therapy
• Antimicrobial treatment of horses with subclinical infections has not been shown to eliminate the carrier state
• Opinions differ as to whether antimicrobial drugs should be given to adult horses with salmonellosis
• Foals with salmonellosis, particularly with concurrent septicemia, are routinely treated with antimicrobial drugs
• Use of an appropriate antimicrobial drug should be based on antimicrobial susceptibility testing or previous experience with *Salmonella* infections in a given geographic area. Antimicrobials used in salmonellosis include combinations of penicillin and gentamicin; ceftiofur and gentamicin; and fluoroquinolones such as enrofloxacin (contraindicated in foals owing to potential for cartilage damage)

Other Therapies
• Flunixin meglumine and ketoprofen to ameliorate effects of endotoxemia
• DMSO and products that contain antibody to LPS or that neutralize circulating LPS (e.g. polymyxin B) have been used with variable results
• Use of products to absorb bacterial toxins in the digestive tract (e.g. di-tri-octahedral smectite and/or bismuth subsalicylate) and those that may benefit enterocyte recovery (e.g. psyllium) may be indicated

CONTRAINDICATIONS
Use of NSAIDs, aminoglycosides, and polymyxin B in azotemic or dehydrated patients without ensuring rehydration and adequate urine production.

PRECAUTIONS
If glomerular filtration is impaired, administering drugs that depend on renal clearance should be done judiciously.

POSSIBLE INTERACTIONS
Concurrent use of NSAIDs along with aminoglycosides, particularly in dehydrated or azotemic patients, can potentiate nephrotoxicity of each drug.

ALTERNATIVE DRUGS
N/A

FOLLOW-UP
PATIENT MONITORING
• Clinical signs, CBC, and biochemistry abnormalities should resolve with appropriate therapy
• Fecal culture can be performed to determine cessation of shedding. To overcome low test sensitivity of fecal culture for the detection of *Salmonella*, 3–5 enriched cultures should be performed at 12–24 h intervals

PREVENTION/AVOIDANCE
• Practicing effective personal and environmental hygiene is critical for protecting patients and personnel
• Thorough cleaning and disinfection of areas where fecal contamination is likely, of common use equipment such as stomach tubes and buckets, and use of rigorous hand hygiene are key to effective risk mitigation
• Prompt detection of clinical and subclinical cases with subsequent contact precautions and separation or isolation from other horses and personnel is necessary to decrease the likelihood of transmission and environmental contamination

POSSIBLE COMPLICATIONS
• Laminitis
• Thrombophlebitis
• Colon infarction
• Disseminated bacterial infection
• Chronic diarrhea
• Chronic or recurrent colic
• Persistent poor body condition
• Persistent, intermittent fecal shedding of *Salmonella* spp.

EXPECTED COURSE AND PROGNOSIS
• Horses with fever and neutropenia without diarrhea have a good prognosis, often recovering within a few days
• Horses with profuse diarrhea and toxemia require intensive care and have a poor prognosis for survival. Horses that survive typically show substantial improvement within 7 days

MISCELLANEOUS
ASSOCIATED CONDITIONS
• Laminitis
• Venous thrombophlebitis
• Weight loss

AGE-RELATED FACTORS
Foals are predisposed to developing extraintestinal sites of infection such as joint and bone infections.

ZOONOTIC POTENTIAL
S. enterica is a zoonotic pathogen. Immunocompromised individuals (e.g. due to illness, medical therapy, young/old, or pregnancy) should take appropriate precautions.

PREGNANCY/FERTILITY/BREEDING
Abortion may occur with any serovar; however, *Salmonella* Abortusequi has been associated with abortion. *S.* Abortusequi has not been recognized in the USA in decades.

SEE ALSO
• *Clostridium difficile* enterocolitis
• Endotoxemia
• Idiopathic colitis
• Potomac horse fever (PHF)
• Protein-losing enteropathy (PLE)

ABBREVIATIONS
• DMSO = dimethylsulfoxide
• GI = gastrointestinal
• LPS = lipopolysaccharide
• NSAID = nonsteroidal anti-inflammatory drug
• PCR = polymerase chain reaction
• USDA = United States Department of Agriculture

Suggested Reading
Burgess BA, Morley PS. Managing *Salmonella* in equine populations. Vet Clin North Am Equine Pract 2014;30:623–640.
Burgess BA, Traub-Dargatz JL. Biosecurity and control of infectious disease outbreaks. In: Sellon DC, Long MT, eds. Equine Infectious Diseases, 2e. St. Louis, MO: Elsevier, 2014:530–543.
Dallap Schaer BL, Aceto H, Rankin SC. Outbreak of salmonellosis caused by *Salmonella enterica* serovar Newport MDR-AmpC in a large animal veterinary teaching hospital. J Vet Intern Med 2010;24:1138–1146.
Hernandez JA, Long MT, Traub-Dargatz JL, Besser TE. Salmonellosis. In: Sellon DC, Long MT, eds. Equine Infectious Diseases, 2e. St. Louis, MO: Elsevier, 2014:321–333.

Author Brandy A. Burgess
Consulting Editors Henry Stämpfli and Olimpo Oliver-Espinosa

S

SAND IMPACTION AND ENTEROPATHY

BASICS

DEFINITION
Gravitational sedimentation of ingested sand in the large intestine causing colonic impaction and mucosal irritation.

PATHOPHYSIOLOGY
Horses ingest sand while grazing on sandy soil or while eating from the ground in sandy stalls or paddocks. Some horses, particularly foals, develop pica and intentionally eat sand or fine grit contained in decomposed granite used for stall or paddock floors. Ingested sand sediments and accumulates in the large colon until impaction and partial or complete obstruction may occur. As the intestinal contents become dehydrated, the sand may dry out and take on a concrete-like consistency. Fine sand tends to accumulate in the ventral colon, whereas coarse sand or grit may also accumulate in the dorsal and transverse colons. Colonic displacement and/or volvulus is found in up to 54% of horses treated surgically for sand accumulation. The amount of accumulated sand required to induce clinical signs is not known and some horses may tolerate more sand than others. Abdominal pain is caused by colonic distention from the impaction or from ingesta and gas accumulating proximally owing to partial or complete obstruction, and by reflex intestinal spasms stimulated by distention. Chronic irritation of the bowel wall and reduction in the absorptive surface area may interfere with normal water absorption in the colon and give rise to diarrhea.

SYSTEMS AFFECTED
Gastrointestinal system only.

GENETICS
N/A

INCIDENCE/PREVALENCE
Worldwide, but more common in geographic locations with sandy soil or where horses are kept in sandy paddocks or stalls and fed on the ground.

SIGNALMENT
No breed or age predilection. Miniature horses may be more predisposed.

SIGNS

Historical Findings
Feeding hay and/or grain on the ground or grazing on pastures with sandy soil. Recurrent or chronic colic of mild to moderate severity, intermittent or chronic diarrhea, weight loss, and ill-thrift.

Physical Examination Findings
Colic, scant or absent feces, although watery to "cow pie" diarrhea, may accompany or precede the onset of colic and may be the major presenting sign. Other signs include anorexia, lethargy, depression, abdominal distention, prolonged capillary refill time, and tachypnea. Auscultation of the colon over the most dependent portion of the abdomen for 1–5 min reveals typical "sand sounds" from sand/sand and mucosal/sand friction. Sand sounds are sensitive and reliable indicators of sand accumulation.

In thin horses with massive accumulations of sand in the colon, external palpation and ballottement of the ventral and ventrolateral abdomen may reveal a firm, heavy viscus. Rectal examination usually reveals distinct distention of the large colon and/or cecum, but definitive diagnosis by rectal palpation is achieved in only about 15% of cases. Fecal sand may be detected as a "gritty" feeling during rectal examination and sand may sediment on the floor of the rectum in horses with concomitant diarrhea.

CAUSES
See Pathophysiology.

RISK FACTORS
See Pathophysiology.

DIAGNOSIS

DIFFERENTIAL DIAGNOSIS
• Large colon impaction, unless a concurrent large colon displacement or torsion is present
• All other causes of colic, but particularly those that are recurrent, including enterolithiasis, internal abdominal abscess, gastric ulcer, thromboembolic colic, peritonitis, abdominal neoplasia, cholelithiasis, and nephrolithiasis
• Chronic diarrhea and ill-thrift due to parasitism, inflammatory bowel disease with malabsorption, intestinal neoplasia, and abnormal fermentation associated with noninflammatory bowel disease or antibiotic use

CBC/BIOCHEMISTRY/URINALYSIS
Nonspecific

OTHER LABORATORY TESTS
• Feces may contain frank or occult blood
• Abdominocentesis should be performed with great care so as not to perforate the colon. Abdominal fluid may be normal in horses with sand accumulation, but if the colon is compromised the total protein concentration and white blood cell count may be elevated

IMAGING
• Abdominal radiography is diagnostic for presence of accumulated sand and serves to monitor the disappearance of sand with medical treatment, particularly in small horses, ponies, and foals. Sand may appear as a homogeneous or granular radiodense accumulation with a horizontal dorsal margin in 1 or more dependent portions of viscera
• Ultrasonographic evidence is less specific. Signs suggesting sand accumulation include increased contact of the large colon with the ventral abdominal wall, decreased gut motility and hyperechoic acoustic shadowing

OTHER DIAGNOSTIC PROCEDURES
• Observation of sand in the feces, abdominal auscultation, rectal palpation, abdominal radiography, abdominal ultrasonography, or sand palpated or obtained during abdominocentesis
• The sand sedimentation test is performed by breaking up 3 or 4 fecal balls in a rectal sleeve and mixing them with water to form a slurry. The sleeve is suspended to allow the sand to settle inside the fingertips. A sediment of more than 0.6 cm in the fingertips indicates that the horse is passing excessive quantities of sand in feces. In a more quantitative test, the finding of more than a teaspoon (5 g) of sand in the bottom of a bucket after suspending 6 fecal balls with water is considered abnormal
• Horses with sand impaction may not necessarily have sand in their feces at the time of examination

PATHOLOGIC FINDINGS
N/A

TREATMENT

• Horses with well-formed impactions or profuse diarrhea benefit from administration of balanced electrolyte solutions intragastrically or IV
• Analgesia is dictated by the degree of pain
• Fasting for 24 h or more and intragastric administration of mineral oil and water promotes lubrication and dissolution of the feed impaction
• Resuspension and removal of sand is best accomplished by intragastric administration of laxatives containing *Psyllium hydrophila* mucilloid (0.25–0.5 kg/500 kg) in combination with mineral oil and magnesium sulfate (500 g/500 kg horse). Because psyllium gels quickly when mixed with water, it is best administered mixed with 2 L of mineral oil, followed by 4 L of water
• Daily administration of 0.25–0.5 kg of psyllium orally mixed with grain or sweet feed for mild impactions or administered by nasogastric tube in combination with mineral oil and magnesium sulfate for 10–14 days for severe impactions is recommended

APPROPRIATE HEALTH CARE
• Initial treatment is handled on an outpatient basis
• Transportation to a referral center is usually necessary for radiographic confirmation of the diagnosis and surgical management of horses that do not respond to medical therapy

NURSING CARE
Prevention of rolling and self-induced trauma, provision of analgesia, and maintenance of hydration.

ACTIVITY

Horses should be stall-rested and hand-walked until the impaction has resolved.

DIET

Fasting during medical treatment is needed until the impaction has broken down, feces have been passed, and abdominal pain has abated.

CLIENT EDUCATION

Feeding practices must be modified to prevent further ingestion of sand.

SURGICAL CONSIDERATIONS

Affected horses with reduced or absent intestinal motility, with large accumulations of sand, and horses that fail to respond to medical treatment within 48–72 h have uncontrollable pain, abdominal distention, and sudden worsening of clinical signs. Prognosis for long-term survival is favorable if successful evacuation of the colon is achieved and is dependent on concurrent pathology identified at surgery.

MEDICATIONS

DRUG(S) OF CHOICE

See Treatment.

CONTRAINDICATIONS

Acepromazine is contraindicated in horses showing evidence of shock.

PRECAUTIONS

Repeated use of potent NSAID analgesics to control colic pain should be avoided unless appropriate diagnostic and therapeutic intervention is also pursued.

POSSIBLE INTERACTIONS

N/A

ALTERNATIVE DRUGS

N/A

FOLLOW-UP

PATIENT MONITORING

Repeat physical examinations, sand sedimentation—testing of feces at weekly intervals for 2–4 weeks. Abdominal radiographs to confirm the clearance of sand. Thereafter, abdominal auscultation and sand sedimentation tests should be performed at intervals of 3–6 months.

PREVENTION/AVOIDANCE

- Identification and evacuation of accumulated sand from the large colon and modification of feeding and management practices to minimize further ingestion of significant quantities of sand
- The source of sand and causes of pica should be identified, horses should not be fed on the ground, and pastures should not be grazed too short. Feeders should be placed above a solid, sand-free surface
- Horses should receive appropriate quantities of feed, including good quality roughage, on a regular schedule and fresh water should be freely available
- Avoiding sand as the flooring material for stalls and paddocks may also be necessary
- Intermittent "purge" treatments with psyllium-containing products is also recommended. Daily oral administration of 0.25 kg of psyllium for 7 consecutive days each month has proved to be effective

POSSIBLE COMPLICATIONS

Include chronic diarrhea, bowel perforation, peritonitis, bowel displacement, with or without strangulation.

EXPECTED COURSE AND PROGNOSIS

- Medical therapy is usually successful in resolving sand impaction and relieving signs of colic within 1–4 days. Prognosis is good for sand impactions diagnosed early
- A guarded prognosis is given in more chronic, high-volume sand impactions which are more likely to require surgical intervention, although survival after surgery is reported to be 75–90%
- The long-term prognosis depends on preventing sand ingestion and on the degree of mucosal injury and scarring resulting from the original episode

MISCELLANEOUS

ASSOCIATED CONDITIONS

Chronic diarrhea, ill-thrift, colonic displacement, colonic rupture, septic peritonitis, endotoxemia, and other postoperative complications listed above have been recognized in association with sand impaction.

AGE-RELATED FACTORS

Can occur in horses of any age, including young foals.

ZOONOTIC POTENTIAL

N/A

PREGNANCY/FERTILITY/BREEDING

Pregnant mares requiring surgical treatment for sand colic are at increased risk for abortion.

SYNONYMS

- Sand colic
- Sand enteritis
- Sand enteropathy
- Sand impaction

SEE ALSO

Colic, chronic/recurrent

ABBREVIATIONS

NSAID = nonsteroidal anti-inflammatory drug

Suggested Reading

Hart KA, Linnenkohl W, Mayer JR, et al. Medical management of sand enteropathy in 62 horses. Equine Vet J 2013;45(4):465–469.

Keppie NJ, Rosenstein DS, Holcombe SJ, Schott 2nd HC. Objective radiographic assessment of abdominal sand accumulation in horses. Vet Radiol Ultrasound 2008;49(2):122–128.

Authors Sarah S. le Jeune and W. David Wilson
Consulting Editors Henry Stämpfli and Olimpo Oliver-Espinosa

S

SARCOID

 BASICS

DEFINITION
Dermal fibroblast neoplasm with a minor epidermal component, with a variety of clinical forms. Often locally aggressive with a high propensity for recurrence after surgical excision, but does not metastasize.

PATHOPHYSIOLOGY
Incompletely characterized, complex, and multifactorial:
1. BPV infection
BPV infection potentially causal:
  ◦ BPV DNA detected within fibroblast nuclei in most sarcoids, and at low levels in epidermis in some sarcoids (BPV-1 most commonly, also BPV-2, BPV-13, and horse-specific BPV-1 variants)
  ◦ Viral proteins (e.g. oncoproteins E5, E7) consistently detected
However, viral involvement unconfirmed:
  ◦ BPV-1 DNA also detected in skin and blood of healthy horses
  ◦ PV virions not detected via electron microscopy or virus isolation in sarcoids
  ◦ BPV inoculation does not reproduce persistent disease
2. Environmental factors also implicated
  ◦ Epizootic disease outbreaks occur, with apparent transmission between horses
  ◦ Insect transmission likely (identical BPV-1 DNA in sarcoids and flies in same regions)
  ◦ Worldwide occurrence without seasonal or geographic predilection suggests other transmission routes (e.g. direct wound contact, indirect fomites)

SYSTEMS AFFECTED
Skin

GENETICS
Genetic susceptibility to sarcoids suspected, and a polygenic inheritance pattern proposed:
• Higher risk in some breeds and families
• Increased risk linked to MHC I genes (e.g. *ELA-A3*), MHC II genes (*ELA-W13*), and MHC II and non-MHC genes on *ECA-20, ECA-22* (involved in host immune response)

INCIDENCE/PREVALENCE
Most common neoplasm of horses, with a prevalence of 1–12% reported, and accounting for 15–65% of all neoplasms, ahead of SCC, melanoma, and papilloma.

GEOGRAPHIC DISTRIBUTION
Worldwide

SIGNALMENT

Breed Predilections
• Higher risk—Quarter Horses; possibly Appaloosas, Arabians, and Thoroughbreds
• Lower risk—Standardbreds

Mean Age and Range
• Mean age—variable, suggested 3–9 years
• Range—6 months to 15+ years

Predominant Sex
No gender predisposition.

SIGNS

Historical Findings
Single or multiple lesions in a variety of body regions; may occur at sites of previous injury. May progress into more aggressive forms spontaneously.

Physical Examination Findings
• Most frequent on the head (pinnae, lip margins, periocular), neck, lower limbs, and ventral body (inguinal, preputial, perineal)
• Clinical forms are variable, and often mixed, including:
  1. Occult—focal, roughly circular, non-raised areas of alopecia with foci of scaling, lichenification, or papules. May start with subtle hair color/quality change. May be more common in relatively hairless body areas. May remain static for years, slowly enlarge, or progress to verrucous forms
  2. Verrucous (warty)—irregular papillomatous and scaly plaques to peduncles, often surrounded by a zone of mild lichenification with altered coat quality. May be less common on the limbs except for coronary band areas. Slow growing
  3. Nodular—firm, well-defined dermal or subcutaneous nodules of variable size (≥0.5–20 cm). May be solitary, or in small to occasionally myriad clusters. Predilection sites include inguinal, preputial, and periocular areas
  4. Nodular and ulcerated ("fibroblastic")—irregularly nodular locally invasive lesions with prominent ulceration and exudation, often resembling exuberant granulation tissue ("proud flesh"). Fly worry, myiasis, and bacterial infections commonly complicate
  5. Malevolent—rare, invasive, irregularly nodular lesions that can infiltrate lymphatics and potentially local lymph nodes

CAUSES
Likely caused by a complex association between BPV and inheritable traits of the horse, with environmental influences.

RISK FACTORS
• Suspected genetic and familial predispositions
• Potential BPV transmission via flies, fomites, or direct wound contamination

 DIAGNOSIS

DIFFERENTIAL DIAGNOSIS
Wide variety of clinical presentations lends to numerous differentials. Accurate diagnosis cannot be based on clinical appearance alone (1 study of 345 cases determined 31% error in presumed diagnosis of sarcoid).

• Occult—infectious folliculitis (dermatophytosis, bacterial), dermatophilosis, pemphigus foliaceus
• Verrucous—papillomas, developmental hamartomas, SCC
• Nodular—infections (bacterial, fungal, habronemiasis, pythiosis, hypodermiasis), sterile inflammation (exuberant granulation tissue, foreign body reactions, eosinophilic granuloma), cysts (dermoid, follicular), and other neoplasms (fibroma/fibrosarcoma, melanoma, neurofibroma/sarcoma, cutaneous lymphoma, SCC, and mast cell tumor)

CBC/BIOCHEMISTRY/URINALYSIS
No specific findings.

OTHER LABORATORY TESTS
N/A

IMAGING
Radiography will reveal no involvement of underlying bone in facial or limb lesions.

OTHER DIAGNOSTIC PROCEDURES
• Surface skin cytology and potentially fungal culture are indicated for alopecic lesions to screen for other differentials
• Fine needle aspiration of nodular lesions may suggest or confirm alternate diagnoses
• Skin biopsy is needed for definitive diagnosis:
  ◦ Anecdotal reports suggest biopsy may transform occult, verrucous, or nodular forms into more aggressive types. Frequency of such exacerbation is undocumented
  ◦ Biopsy is recommended if treatment will be undertaken once diagnosis is confirmed, and to ensure margins clear for excisional biopsy
  ◦ Important to sample different depths of large lesions—multiple etiologic agents may be concurrent (e.g. exuberant granulation tissue, sarcoid, secondary infection)

PATHOLOGIC FINDINGS

Gross Changes
• Reflect clinical types, from alopecic to nodular and ulcerated
• May have smaller satellite lesions surrounding main tumor

Histologic Changes
• Dermal proliferation of transformed fibroblasts, often with associated epidermal changes
  ◦ Dermis—dominated by proliferation of immature fibroblasts and collagen fibers forming whorls, interlacing bundles, and disorganized arrays
    ▪ Alignment of neoplastic fibroblasts perpendicular to the epidermis in a "picket fence" pattern may occur
    ▪ Neoplastic fibroblasts are spindle-shaped or fusiform with pointed nuclei and large, irregular, pleomorphic nuclei
    ▪ The mitotic rate is usually low
  ◦ Epidermis—hyperkeratosis and acanthosis, with elongated truncated rete

S

ridge projections into dermis, and absence of classical PV changes
◦ Differentiation from fibroma or fibrosarcoma may be difficult; PCR testing for BPV may be helpful supportive evidence

 TREATMENT

APPROPRIATE HEALTH CARE
N/A

NURSING CARE
Good wound hygiene and fly control before and after surgery.

ACTIVITY
May need restricted activity post surgery depending on body site.

DIET
N/A

CLIENT EDUCATION
High propensity for recurrence after treatment, and for development of new tumors at new sites. Greatest success in treatment is achieved by close monitoring and prompt additional treatment as required. Observation without treatment is an option for small tumors; however, potential for aggressive growth remains.

SURGICAL CONSIDERATIONS
• Early and complete surgical excision appears optimal whenever possible
• Conventional surgery most effective (cure rates up to 82%; recurrence rates 50–70%)
◦ Tumor margins should be assessed histologically—extension of tumor beyond obvious clinical borders is common
◦ Incomplete excision should be promptly followed by reexcision and/or other treatment modalities
◦ Surgery combined with another treatment modality may have highest success
• Cryosurgery may be useful for lesions difficult to excise; however, accurately determining adequate depth of treatment is difficult
• Laser therapy may also be useful, but has limited availability

RADIATION
Intralesional radiation (brachytherapy) variably effective (cure rates 60–94%), but restricted to accredited institutions.

 MEDICATIONS

DRUG(S) OF CHOICE
A variety of medical treatments are described with varying success rates. Medical options may be best considered supplementary to surgical excision/debulking, but may have value as sole treatments for small superficial lesions.

Chemotherapy
• 5-FU
◦ Intralesional injections (each 2 weeks; up to 7 times) evaluated in 1 study of occult and verrucous sarcoids, with resolution in 9 of 13 horses; 3 year follow-up
• Topical cytotoxic agents have anecdotal success (safety and efficacy poorly evaluated)
◦ AW-3-LUDES (5-FU/thiouracil/heavy metal salts)
◦ XTERRA (Eastern bloodroot and zinc chloride)
◦ Animex (blood root extract)
• Cisplatin—intralesional injections effective (cure rates up to 80%), but exposure risks for administering veterinarians; use restricted to experienced clinicians with appropriate facilities

Immunostimulation
• Imiquimod 5% gel—applied 3 times weekly
◦ Used in small sarcoids (cure in 60% of lesions)
• Mycobacterial products (commercial whole-attenuated BCG)—intralesional injections (each 2–4 weeks; up to 6 times) with apparent success in periocular sarcoids
• Autologous vaccines—2 small studies (15 horses); cure rates of ~65%; complications in ~50% (swelling and rare abscessation at implantation sites)

Antiviral
• Acyclovir (aciclovir) 5% cream (daily for 2–6 months) in 22 horses (cure in 68% of sarcoids)
• Cidofovir 1% gel (daily for 1 month); effective in 2 sarcoids after surgical debulking

CONTRAINDICATIONS
N/A

PRECAUTIONS
• Severe inflammatory reactions may occur with immunomodulatory therapies. Treatment interruption or reduction in frequency may be needed
• Anaphylaxis reported with BCG immunotherapy; pretreatment with corticosteroids or diphenhydramine may minimize risk
• Exposure risks to operators/owners with cytotoxic therapies

POSSIBLE INTERACTIONS
None reported.

ALTERNATIVE DRUGS
N/A

 FOLLOW-UP

PATIENT MONITORING
Monitoring closely for recurrence is the prime need, with prompt additional treatment indicated if recurrence occurs.

PREVENTION/AVOIDANCE
Fly control/avoidance, good patient hygiene, and good management hygiene practices are anecdotally reported to reduce the incidence of transmission between horses.

POSSIBLE COMPLICATIONS
Related to surgical excision (wound breakdown, restricted movement, wound infections). Interference with performance and cost of treatments may result in requests for euthanasia.

EXPECTED COURSE AND PROGNOSIS
• Dependent on number, size, location and invasiveness of tumors—larger and more aggressive forms have a poorer prognosis; single sarcoids have a better prognosis
• Variable progression—may remain static for years, progress quickly or slowly into more aggressive forms, or spontaneously regress (rare)

 MISCELLANEOUS

ASSOCIATED CONDITIONS
N/A

AGE-RELATED FACTORS
N/A

ZOONOTIC POTENTIAL
None

PREGNANCY/FERTILITY/BREEDING
N/A

SYNONYMS
N/A

SEE ALSO
• Ocular/adnexal squamous cell carcinoma
• Papillomatosis

ABBREVIATIONS
• 5-FU = 5-fluorouracil
• BCG = bacillus Calmette–Guérin
• BPV = bovine papillomavirus
• ECA = equine chromosome
• ELA = equine leukocyte antigen
• MHC = major histocompatibility complex
• PCR = polymerase chain reaction
• PV = papillomavirus
• SCC = squamous cell carcinoma

Suggested Reading
Bergvall KE. Sarcoids. Vet Clin North Am Equine Pract 2013;29:657–671.
Author Linda J. Vogelnest
Consulting Editor Gwendolen Lorch
Acknowledgment The author and editor acknowledge the prior contribution of Sandra Nogueira Koch.

 Client Education Handout available online

S

SEASONAL PASTURE MYOPATHY/ATYPICAL MYOPATHY

BASICS

OVERVIEW
• Caused by hypoglycin A, a toxic amino acid found in seeds of the maple species *Acer negundo* (box elder) and *Acer pseudoplatanus* (sycamore maple)
• A highly fatal nonexertional rhabdomyolysis of horses at pasture termed SPM (North America) or AM (Europe)
• Methylenecyclopropylacetic acid, the toxic metabolite of hypoglycin A, inhibits various mitochondrial dehydrogenases, resulting in acquired MADD
• MADD causes disruption of fatty acid beta-oxidation and subsequent lipid accumulation and degeneration in muscle with high oxidative capacity, such as postural, respiratory, and cardiac muscles
• Large outbreaks in Europe. In North America only few horses on a given pasture are affected

SIGNALMENT
No breed, sex, or gender predilection.

SIGNS
• Lethargy, acute muscular weakness, muscle fasciculations, stiffness, reluctance to move, recumbency
• Congested mucous membranes, tachycardia, tachypnea, dyspnea
• Myoglobinuria, dysuria, distended bladder
• Sweating, colic signs
• Esophageal obstruction, dysphagia

CAUSES AND RISK FACTORS
• Typically occurs in the fall when seeds are abundant and pasture grass is sparse. Cases in the subsequent spring are common and may be caused by ingestion of seedlings
• Young horses and naive horses recently introduced to the pasture are at increased risk
• Lack of supplemental feed (hay, grain) encourages browsing and consumption of maple seeds
• Inclement weather (cold temperatures, strong wind) may lead to a negative energy balance and dispersal of the seeds
• Stress (exercise, transport, cold weather) may trigger clinical signs in subclinical cases

DIAGNOSIS

DIFFERENTIAL DIAGNOSIS
• *Eupatorium rugosum* (white snake root) toxicity caused by tremetone
• Other causes of rhabdomyolysis
• Ionophore toxicity
• Laminitis
• Other causes of colic

CBC/BIOCHEMISTRY/URINALYSIS
• Leukocytosis/neutrophilia
• Marked increase in CK and aspartate aminotransferase activities
• Hyperglycemia
• Hypocalcemia
• Lactic acidemia
• Increased liver enzymes
• Hyperlipemia
• Myoglobinuria

OTHER LABORATORY TESTS
• Metabolic defect of MADD—elevated short, medium, and less frequently long chain acylcarnitines in serum and urine. Increased urinary excretion of ethylmalonic acid, methylsuccinic acid, butyryl-, isovaleryl-, and hexanoylglycine. Testing may be available through human metabolic institutes
• Elevated cardiac troponin I possible
• Elevated Hypoglycin A and MCPA carnitine in serum

DIAGNOSTIC PROCEDURES
Muscle biopsy of postural or intercostal muscle shows Zenker's necrosis and neutral lipid accumulation (Oil red O or Sudan III stain) in type 1 muscle fibers.

PATHOLOGIC FINDINGS
• Multifocal areas of pallor or hemorrhage in postural and respiratory muscles and less frequently in myocardium
• Histopathology—severe acute myonecrosis and lipid storage myopathy

TREATMENT
• Require intensive care in a veterinary hospital
• IV fluid therapy for diuresis to prevent pigment nephropathy
• Frequent carbohydrate-rich meals or IV glucose to supply muscle energy from carbohydrate metabolism

MEDICATIONS

DRUG(S) OF CHOICE
• No antidote is available
• Insulin to combat hyperglycemia and stimulate insulin-mediated lipogenesis
• Riboflavin (vitamin B2) is a precursor of flavin adenine dinucleotide, a cofactor of all acyl-CoA dehydrogenases affected in MADD, and supplementation may enhance residual enzyme activity
• Antioxidants (vitamin C, vitamin E, selenium)
• NSAIDs or other analgesics

CONTRAINDICATIONS/POSSIBLE INTERACTIONS
Oral carnitine—lack of evidence of beneficial effects and possibly arrhythmogenic side effects in human MADD patients.

FOLLOW-UP

PATIENT MONITORING
Monitor electrolyte derangements, renal, respiratory, and cardiac function.

PREVENTION/AVOIDANCE
• Avoid exposure to box elder or sycamore maple seeds in fall and spring. If not possible, limit (<12 h/day) turnout on pasture and provide supplemental feeding
• Co-grazers of SPM/AM-affected horses should be removed from the pasture. Monitor serum CK activity and avoid stress

EXPECTED COURSE AND PROGNOSIS
• Case fatality rate is high (>70%)
• Rapid progression with death or euthanasia within 72 h

MISCELLANEOUS

ABBREVIATIONS
• AM = atypical myopathy
• CK = creatine kinase
• CoA = coenzyme A
• MADD = multiple acyl-CoA dehydrogenase deficiency
• NSAID = nonsteroidal anti-inflammatory drug
• MCPA = methylene cyclopropyl acetic acid
• SPM = seasonal pasture myopathy

Internet Resources
Michigan State University, Seasonal pasture myopathy.
https://cvm.msu.edu/research/faculty-research/comparative-medical-genetics/valberg-laboratory/seasonal-pasture-myopathy

Suggested Reading
Bochnia M, Scheidemann W, Ziegler J, et al. Predictive value of hypoglycin A and methylencyclopropylacetic acid conjugates in a horse with atypical myopathy in comparison to its cograzing partners. Equine Vet Educ 2016;30:24–28.
Sander J, Cavalleri JMV, Terhardt M, et al. Rapid diagnosis of hypoglycin A intoxication in atypical myopathy of horses. J Vet Diagn Invest 2016;28:98–104.
Votion DM. The story of equine atypical myopathy: a review from the beginning to a possible end. ISRN Vet Sci 2012;2012:281018.

Author Beatrice T. Sponseller
Consulting Editors Wilson K. Rumbeiha and Steve Ensley

S

SEIZURE DISORDERS

BASICS

DEFINITION
Seizures are paroxysmal, transient electrical disturbances of brain function that have a sudden onset, cease spontaneously, and tend to recur.

PATHOPHYSIOLOGY
• Seizures are caused by excessive neuronal excitation or loss of neuronal inhibition
• Horses almost always have a focal onset that may secondarily generalize. Often secondary to trauma (which can have occurred a long time previously) or diseases or toxins that have an effect on neuronal function
• Classic idiopathic epilepsy has not been reported in this species

SYSTEMS AFFECTED
CNS, trauma to other systems from seizure, systems affected by the initiating disease.

GENETICS
Juvenile epilepsy in Arabian foals is likely to have a genetic basis.

INCIDENCE/PREVALENCE
Low prevalence.

SIGNALMENT
More likely in adult horses. A benign form of juvenile epilepsy can occur in young growing Arabian foals of Egyptian lineage up to 12 months of age.

SIGNS

Historical Findings
A history of trauma or toxin exposure rarely reported.

Physical Examination Findings
• Seizures are classified as generalized, partial, or partial with secondary generalization
• In horses, the most common expression of a focal seizure is involuntary movement of facial muscles
• The onset of a generalized seizure is often preceded by a short period of restlessness and disorientation, as well as inappropriate chewing, teeth grinding, and other bizarre behaviors
• Subsequently generalized muscular rigidity, recumbency, tonic/clonic paddling movements, salivation, urination, and defecation are common features of a generalized seizure

CAUSES
• Trauma, neoplasm, cholesterol granuloma, hydrocephalus, cerebral abscess, thromboembolism, intracarotid injection, hypoxic–ischemic encephalopathy, hypoxemia, moldy corn poisoning, hepatoencephalopathy, hypoglycemia, hyposmolality, hyperosmolality, and bacterial, viral, verminous, and protozoal encephalitides have all been associated with seizures

• No other disease process is evident in juvenile epilepsy

RISK FACTORS
Exposure to infectious diseases and toxins, etc.

DIAGNOSIS
• Neuroanatomic diagnostic examination may help localize the site of a seizure focus
• Cerebrospinal fluid analysis may reveal an underlying infectious process
• Disease-specific tests may be useful. Advanced imaging may be useful to identify structural lesions

DIFFERENTIAL DIAGNOSIS
• Diseases causing abnormal movements and loss of consciousness, e.g. heart blocks and sleep disorders
• Hyperkalemic periodic paralysis and blood electrolyte abnormalities such as hypocalcemia may result in tremors and recumbency but are not associated with loss of consciousness

CBC/BIOCHEMISTRY/URINALYSIS
No pathognomonic abnormalities.

IMAGING
Advanced imaging is preferable; skull radiographs may reveal fracture lines.

PATHOLOGIC FINDINGS
Dependent on associated disease. Some CNS changes such as hippocampal sclerosis or ischemic neurons may be secondary to the seizures rather than due to the primary disease.

TREATMENT

TREATMENT OF STATUS EPILEPTICUS
Control of status epilepticus in adult horses—50 mg IV doses of diazepam. In foals start with a 5 mg diazepam dose. If no benzodiazepines available use standard doses of sedative drugs.

MAINTENANCE ANTICONVULSANT THERAPY
• Phenobarbitone at 5 mg/kg SID PO. If unacceptable sleepiness occurs and seizures are not controlled, reduce dose by 20% and add KBr at 25–90 mg/kg SID PO, with or without loading doses of 120–200 mg/kg SID PO for 1–5 days
• After control, monitor serum concentrations; phenobarbitone therapeutic range 15–40 μg/mL; bromide 1000–4000 μg/mL

• Long-term administration with anticonvulsants requires the adherence to demanding treatment protocols (see Suggested Reading) and should only be considered after careful discussions with the owner; an apparently stable horse is nevertheless unsafe to ride on medication as breakthrough seizures may occur

CLIENT EDUCATION AND PROGNOSIS
• Severity and frequency of seizure episodes may increase with time and the horse is a danger to himself and his handler during seizuring
• A horse in anticonvulsant treatment is not safe to be ridden, and a useful guide is that a horse that has had seizures should only be ridden once it has been off medication and seizure free for 6 months
• Most foals with juvenile epilepsy have a reduction in frequency to cessation of seizures

MEDICATIONS

CONTRAINDICATIONS
Drugs that reduce seizure threshold (e.g. acepromazine). Other drugs such as chloramphenicol or tetracyclines may inhibit hepatic enzymes and prolong the activity of barbiturates.

MISCELLANEOUS

SEE ALSO
• Calcium, hypocalcemia
• Hyperkalemic periodic paralysis
• Narcolepsy and cataplexy

ABBREVIATIONS
CNS = central nervous system

Suggested Reading
Lacombe VA, Furr M. Differential diagnosis and management of horses with seizures or alterations of consciousness. In: Furr M, Reed S, eds. Equine Neurology, 2e. Ames, IA: Wiley Blackwell, 2015:79–92.
Mayhew IG. Large Animal Neurology, 2e. Oxford, UK: Wiley Blackwell, 2009.

Author Caroline N. Hahn
Consulting Editor Caroline N. Hahn

S

SEIZURES IN FOALS

BASICS

DEFINITION
• Abnormal movement or loss of consciousness associated with abnormal electrical activity of the brain
• Partial seizures involve a focal area of the cerebral cortex. Partial seizure with secondary generalization occurs when partial seizures progress and spread throughout the cerebral cortex
• Complex partial seizures are partial seizures in which consciousness is impaired
• Generalized seizures involve the entire cerebral cortex, and result in generalized tonic–clonic activity and loss of consciousness
• Status epilepticus is rare, but appears as multiple generalized seizures in succession

PATHOPHYSIOLOGY
• Mechanisms of abnormal electrical activity in the brain include increased excitatory neurotransmitters and decreased inhibitory neurotransmitters
• Electrolyte abnormalities can cause abnormal electrical activity, leading to seizures. Hypoglycemia is a rare cause of seizures in foals
• NE is the most common cause of seizures in neonatal foals. It is proposed that periods of asphyxia may be associated with cerebral edema and necrosis. Hypoxia leads to a breakdown of cerebral energy metabolism, alterations in neurotransmitter metabolism (particularly glutamate), increase in cytosolic calcium concentration, and alterations in cerebral blood flow, leading to neuronal cell death. Alterations in neurosteroid metabolism may also represent a cause of NE distinct from perinatal asphyxia

SYSTEMS AFFECTED
Nervous

GENETICS
• Idiopathic epilepsy affects Arabians. A genetic link is suspected
• Lavender foal syndrome also affects primarily Egyptian Arabians—autosomal recessive; a genetic test is available
• Persistent hyperammonemia in Morgan foals—suspected inherited disorder

GEOGRAPHIC DISTRIBUTION
Locoweed is most commonly found in western USA, but is an uncommon cause of seizures in foals.

SIGNALMENT

Breed Predilections
• Idiopathic epilepsy in the Arabian breed
• Persistent seizures in Egyptian Arabian foals affected by lavender foal syndrome
• Hyperammonemia in weanling Morgan foals

Mean Age and Range
• Usually <2 days of age

• Foals with bacterial meningitis and systemic sepsis are generally <2 weeks of age
• Seizures secondary to congenital abnormalities usually occur within the first few days of birth
• Seizures secondary to intestinal hyperammonemia in Morgan foals occur shortly after weaning

Predominant Sex
None

SIGNS

General Comments
Generalized seizures are the most common form of seizure in foals, although partial and complex partial seizures may be seen. Status epilepticus is uncommon.

Historical Findings
A history of dystocia, placental insufficiency or placentitis, and maternal illness should raise the suspicion of NE as a cause of seizures.

Physical Examination Findings
• Partial seizures can appear as facial twitches, rapid eye movements, or compulsive chewing or suckling
• Generalized seizures result in tonic–clonic muscle contractions. Paddling of the limbs, jaw movements, extensor rigidity, and opisthotonos are common. Depression is seen after the seizure (postictal)
• Foals with HE or kernicterus will be icteric
• Signs of sepsis with seizure activity are suggestive of bacterial meningitis
• Abrasions and corneal ulcers may indicate a previous seizure

CAUSES

Neonatal Encephalopathy
• Dystocia
• Premature placental separation
• Maternal illness (colic, endotoxemia)

Congenital Neurologic Abnormalities
• Hydrocephalus
• Hydranencephaly
• Idiopathic epilepsy of Arabians

Traumatic
Brain trauma

Metabolic
• Electrolyte abnormalities—hyponatremia, hyperkalemia, hypocalcemia, hypomagnesemia, hypo- or hyperosmolality
• Hypoglycemia
• HE
• Intestinal hyperammonemia
• Kernicterus (secondary to neonatal isoerythrolysis)

Infectious
• Septicemia
• Bacterial meningitis
• Cerebral abscesses
• Viral meningitis (equine herpes virus 1)
• Severe pneumonia (hypoxia)

Toxic
• Moldy corn
• Locoweed

• Organophosphates
• Strychnine
• Metaldehyde
• Moxidectin

RISK FACTORS
• Dystocia, placental insufficiency, and maternal illness are associated with NE
• Failure of transfer of passive immunity, poor environmental hygiene, and early infections are associated with sepsis, which can lead to septic meningitis

DIAGNOSIS

DIFFERENTIAL DIAGNOSIS
• Septicemia—depression and weakness; seizures with septic meningitis
• Colic/pain—paddling/flailing may be seen, but the tonic–clonic contractions typical of seizures are not seen and mentation is generally normal
• Hyperkalemic periodic paralysis—muscle fasciculations and prolapsed nictitating membrane are typical but do not progress to tonic–clonic movements or loss of consciousness. Occurs in Quarter Horses and crosses
• Syncope secondary to cardiac abnormalities
• Narcolepsy—uncontrollable loss of muscle tone with gradual lowering of the head and collapse
• Tetanus—muscular rigidity may appear similar to seizure activity, but contractions are progressive and not "tonic–clonic" as with seizures. Usually occurs in foals >7 days

CBC/BIOCHEMISTRY/URINALYSIS
Dependent on the underlying cause.

OTHER LABORATORY TESTS
• Check IgG
• Blood culture to confirm septicemia in cases of septic meningitis
• Plasma ammonia concentrations if HE or intestinal hyperammonemia are suspected

IMAGING
• Skull radiographs to rule out fracture
• MRI or CT of brain/skull to rule out skull fracture, subdural hematoma, intracranial abscess, and cerebral edema

OTHER DIAGNOSTIC PROCEDURES
• Cerebrospinal fluid analysis—increased protein and white blood cell count can be indicative of meningitis. Increase in red blood cells may indicate trauma or disruption of the blood–brain barrier
• Electroencephalography can document abnormal electrical activity from the cerebral cortex

PATHOLOGIC FINDINGS
Postmortem examination of the brain may reveal edema, necrosis, or abscessation.

S

(CONTINUED)

 TREATMENT

AIMS
- Control and prevent seizure activity
- Prevent or decrease hypoxic–ischemic damage
- Antimicrobial coverage

APPROPRIATE HEALTH CARE
Any foal with signs of seizure activity should have further evaluation to address any underlying cause. Initial treatment and monitoring require emergency inpatient intensive care management.

NURSING CARE
- Soft bedding to prevent pressure sores or decubital ulcers in foals that are recumbent and paddling
- Eyes should be lubricated with artificial tears and examined for self-trauma/corneal ulcers
- Plasma should be given IV if serum IgG is <800 mg/dL
- Hypotension will lead to decreased cerebral perfusion and possible worsening of neurologic function. IV fluids and pressors may be needed to maintain perfusion
- If hypoglycemia is the suspected cause, dextrose should be administered immediately and blood glucose levels should be monitored closely
- Respiratory function should be monitored, and oxygen supplementation and ventilation started, if needed. Elevated $PaCO_2$ can worsen cerebral edema

ACTIVITY
Foals may need to be restrained to prevent trauma during seizure activity.

DIET
- Normal mentation, suckle reflex, and swallowing reflex should be confirmed before nursing from the mare is permitted. If the foal is unable to nurse but is able to sit sternally it may be fed via nasogastric feeding tube
- If the foal is minimally responsive or if intestinal function is uncertain, parenteral nutrition should be instituted

CLIENT EDUCATION
Owners should be informed of the possible genetic link in those conditions (see Genetics).

SURGICAL CONSIDERATIONS
Craniotomy for abscess drainage has been described in horses.

 MEDICATIONS

DRUG(S) OF CHOICE
For Seizure Control
- Diazepam—0.1–0.4 mg/kg IV

- Midazolam—0.04–0.1 mg/kg IV or IM, or constant rate infusion of 1–3 mg/h in a 50 kg foal for recurrent seizures
- Phenobarbital—2–10 mg/kg IV (maintenance 2–10 mg/kg PO every 12 h). Start with the lowest dosage and increase until desired effect is achieved. Phenobarbital has a long half-life in foals and therefore increases in dosing should be done with caution
- Phenytoin—1–5 mg/kg IV or PO

Antimicrobial Coverage
- Trimethoprim–sulfa—20–30 mg/kg PO every 12 h
- Cefotaxime (40 mg/kg IV every 6 h) or ceftazidime (50 mg/kg IV every 6 h)
- For septicemia without meningitis, penicillin (22 000 IU/kg IV every 6 h) and amikacin (25 mg/kg IV every 24 h)

Prevent Further Neurologic Damage
- Magnesium sulfate—50 mg/kg/h as a 1% solution for 1 h, then decrease to maintenance dose of 25 mg/kg/h
- DMSO—0.5–1.0 g/kg as a 10% solution IV every 12 h
- Mannitol—0.25–1.0 g/kg as a 20% solution IV, up to every 12 h to decrease cerebral edema
- Corticosteroids—dexamethasone 0.05–0.2 mg/kg IV every 12–24 h or methylprednisolone sodium succinate 1–2.5 mg/kg IV within 4 h of trauma. Use of corticosteroids is controversial
- Thiamine and antioxidants have also been used without evidence of effect

CONTRAINDICATIONS
- Acepromazine—may lower the seizure threshold
- Xylazine—may increase intracranial pressure and decrease cerebral blood flow, causing further cerebral hypoxia
- Corticosteroids—high doses are contraindicated with septicemia

PRECAUTIONS
- Higher or repeated doses of phenobarbital can cause hypotension, hypothermia, and decreased respiratory drive
- Mannitol should not be used if intracranial bleeding is suspected
- The use of corticosteroids with cerebral inflammation or trauma is controversial, and steroids should be used with caution if underlying septicemia is suspected
- Ketamine—increases intracranial pressure, which may exacerbate seizures, although may be beneficial in targeting NMDA receptors

 FOLLOW-UP

PATIENT MONITORING
24 h monitoring to detect further seizure activity and to prevent self-trauma.

POSSIBLE COMPLICATIONS
- Head trauma during seizures
- Pressure sores
- Corneal ulceration

EXPECTED COURSE AND PROGNOSIS
- Survival of foals with uncomplicated NE is 80%, and long-term neurologic deficits are rare. Athletic performance is not typically affected. Concurrent septicemia will decrease prognosis
- Foals with head trauma have variable prognosis, dependent on the severity and extent of injury
- Foals with septic meningitis have a guarded to poor prognosis
- Foals with lavender foal syndrome have a grave prognosis. Arabian foals with idiopathic juvenile epilepsy generally outgrow the seizure activity by 12 months of age

 MISCELLANEOUS

ASSOCIATED CONDITIONS
- Neonatal encephalopathy
- Septicemia

SYNONYMS
- Epilepsy
- Convulsions

SEE ALSO
- Lavender foal syndrome
- Meningitis, neonate
- Neonatal maladjustment syndrome

ABBREVIATIONS
- CT = computed tomography
- DMSO = dimethylsulfoxide
- HE = hepatoencephalopathy
- Ig = immunoglobulin G
- MRI = magnetic resonance imaging
- NE = neonatal encephalopathy
- NMDA = N-methyl-D-aspartate
- $PaCO_2$ = partial pressure of carbon dioxide in arterial blood

Suggested Reading
MacKay RJ. Neurologic disorders of neonatal foals. Vet Clin North Am Equine Pract 2005;21:387–406.
Wilkins PA. How to use midazolam to control equine neonatal seizures. Proc Am Assoc Equine Pract 2005;51:279–280.

Author Laura K. Dunbar
Consulting Editor Margaret C. Mudge
Acknowledgment The author acknowledges the prior contribution of Margaret C. Mudge.

 Client Education Handout available online

S

SELENIUM INTOXICATION

BASICS

OVERVIEW
• Acute selenosis results from oversupplementation via either treated feedstuffs or parenteral medications
• Clinical signs involve the respiratory, cardiovascular, hematologic, and GI systems
• Chronic selenosis is most often associated with naturally contaminated forages or hay; the most obvious clinical signs involve the hair or hoof
• The condition described as "blind staggers" is caused by other maladies mistakenly ascribed to selenium toxicosis

SIGNALMENT
• No known breed, age, or sex predilections
• Horses are somewhat more sensitive to chronic selenosis than ruminants and, thus, may be poisoned on pastures that do not affect cattle

SIGNS
Acute Selenosis
• Can present as sudden death with few, if any, clinical signs
• When present, clinical signs progress rapidly
• Muscular weakness, anorexia, and progressively worsening dyspnea beginning 1–24 h after exposure
• Colic and diarrhea may occur
• Heart rate and respiration are elevated, pulse is weak, and animals frequently are cyanotic
• Fever, polyuria, and hemolytic anemia have been reported in some cases
• Lethally poisoned animals usually become comatose and die within 12–48 h

Chronic Selenosis
• Also called alkali disease
• Requires chronic (30–90 days) exposure to seleniferous forages or pastures
• Bilaterally symmetric alopecia and dystrophic hoof growth are most obvious
• Alopecia of the mane and tail but, in severe cases, may involve other parts of the body
• Lameness, erythema, and swelling of the coronary bands followed by a circumferential crack parallel to and just distal to the coronet and subsequent hoof separation. Affected animals become so lame that they cannot eat or drink and, thus, starve

CAUSES AND RISK FACTORS
Selenium- or vitamin E-deficient animals are more susceptible to acute selenosis.

DIAGNOSIS

DIFFERENTIAL DIAGNOSIS
Acute Selenosis
• Heavy metal (e.g. arsenic) intoxication
• Endotoxemia
• Blister beetle intoxication

Chronic Selenosis
• *Leucaena leucocephala* intoxication
• Ergotism
• Laminitis (history, clinical signs, and physical examination)
• Thallium intoxication

CBC/BIOCHEMISTRY/URINALYSIS
• Changes suggest nonspecific damage to the heart, liver, and GI tract in acute selenosis
• Uncomplicated chronic selenosis is not generally associated with abnormalities

OTHER LABORATORY TESTS
• Tissue selenium concentrations are not reliably predictive of damage and are influenced by the form of selenium ingested (organic in forage vs. inorganic selenium salts)
• Blood and liver concentrations <1.0 ppm usually rule out selenosis except in chronic cases when samples are taken several weeks after the onset of signs. Higher concentrations may indicate excessive exposure but do not prove selenosis

PATHOLOGIC FINDINGS
Acute Selenosis
• The most obvious gross lesions in the thorax and GI tract
• The heart may be pale or mottled and flaccid and hydrothorax and ascites with congestive heart failure
• Petechial or ecchymotic hemorrhages within the myocardium and throughout the thoracic viscera
• The lungs are congested, with prominent septal edema and froth in the airways
• The intestinal tract may be hyperemic or hemorrhagic
• Hepatic centrilobular necrosis and renal proximal tubular necrosis often occur but seldom are recognizable grossly

Chronic Selenosis
• Alopecia of the mane and tail and separation of the hoof wall
• Histologically, atrophy of the primary hair follicles. Accessory follicular structures are unaffected
• Degeneration and necrosis of keratinocytes near the tips of the primary laminae

TREATMENT

• No proven effective therapies for acute selenosis. Supportive care for shock and antioxidants (vitamin E) may be helpful
• Uncomplicated chronic selenosis has been successfully treated with palliative measures

MEDICATIONS

DRUG(S) OF CHOICE
• No specific drugs for treating acute selenosis
• Analgesics and NSAIDs are essential in keeping a horse with chronic selenosis both mobile and eating

CONTRAINDICATIONS/POSSIBLE INTERACTIONS
N/A

FOLLOW-UP

PREVENTION/AVOIDANCE
• Prevention consists of avoiding excess selenium exposure
• Total dietary concentrations as low as 5 ppm of dry matter are potentially, but not always, toxic
• Avoid selenium-containing mineral supplements in seleniferous areas
• Low dietary protein levels potentiate selenium toxicity

EXPECTED COURSE AND PROGNOSIS
• Poor prognosis with acute selenosis
• Prolonged recovery with chronic selenosis

MISCELLANEOUS

PREGNANCY/FERTILITY/BREEDING
Selenium does not appear to be teratogenic in mammals.

ABBREVIATIONS
• GI = gastrointestinal
• NSAID = nonsteroidal anti-inflammatory drug

Suggested Reading
Davis TZ, Stegelmeier BL, Hall JO. Analysis in horse hair as a means of evaluating selenium toxicoses and long-term exposures. J Agric Food Chem 2014;62:793–797.
Desta B, Maldonado G, Reid H, et al. Acute selenium toxicosis in polo ponies. J Vet Diagn Invest 2011;23(3):623–628.
Raisbeck MF. Selenosis. Vet Clin North Am Food Anim Pract 2000;16:465–481.

Author Wilson K. Rumbeiha
Consulting Editors Wilson K. Rumbeiha and Steve Ensley

BASICS

OVERVIEW
• Biting at the flank, stifle, or chest
• May be a sign of underlying pathology or behavioral in origin
• In mild cases, only the hair is bitten; in more severe cases, the skin is torn

SIGNALMENT
• Almost always a male, usually an intact male
• The median age of onset is 18 months
• Arabians and American Saddlebreds are overrepresented

SIGNS
• Biting at the flank or, more rarely, the pectoral area, forelimbs, prepuce, or stifle. The biting may not break the skin, especially if the affected animal is a colt or a gelding, but a stallion may inflict severe injuries to his skin or even underlying tissue
• Geldings and mares are more apt to rub, roll, and spin than stallions
• Most horses self-mutilate on both sides, but those that have a side bias turn to the right significantly more often. The horses frequently vocalize and kick out
• The behavior may occur many times a day or as rarely as monthly. Bouts range from seconds to hours. The median duration is 1–10 min

CAUSES AND RISK FACTORS
• The cause is unknown, but it most often occurs in isolated stallions and sometimes in geldings living in social groups with mares
• Sometimes aggression is redirected to targets other than the eliciting stimuli. Self-mutilation may be aggressive behavior redirected to the horse itself
• Horses aroused by the presence of other horses or, in severe cases, by any environmental stimulation may self-mutilate
• Seasonal changes, excitement, and/or anticipation of food can lead to an increase in frequency

 DIAGNOSIS

DIFFERENTIAL DIAGNOSIS
• It is extremely important to eliminate discomfort as a cause of self-mutilation such as penile, testicular, or urethral lesions, gastrointestinal pain, limb pain, bladder disease, dermatologic problems
• Any pruritic condition such as external parasites or dermatitis must also be ruled out

CBC/BIOCHEMISTRY/URINALYSIS
If physical examination warrants.

OTHER LABORATORY TESTS
If physical examination warrants.

IMAGING
Ultrasonography examination of the pelvic area is recommended if the presenting signs and physical examination so warrant.

OTHER DIAGNOSTIC PROCEDURES
• A rectal examination and a neurologic examination should be done
• A skin scraping should be taken

 TREATMENT

• Castration of 10 horses was reported as curative in 3, substantially improved in 2, and slightly improved in 2
• Numerous suggestions have been made, albeit without robust evidence of efficacy:
  ○ Change in the social environment
  ○ Allowing a stallion to live with a mare and away from other stallions
  ○ Donkeys or goats as stall companions
  ○ Removing mares from a gelding's environment may be helpful
  ○ Removal of sources of olfactory stimuli such as feces (the stallion's own or another horse's) and skin secretions rubbed onto stall walls have been suggested to help
  ○ Modifications to the diet and increased exercise can help
  ○ Blanketing the horse or applying a cradle around the horse's neck can reduce damage to the hair coat and skin but is of questionable ethics. Also, the horse is still able to engage in other behaviors that usually accompany self-mutilation such as vigorous kicking, which can be dangerous to itself and people

 MEDICATIONS

• An opioid antagonist, nalmefene, has been reported to reduce self-mutilation in a dose-related manner when given IM at doses of 100–800 mg over a 4 day period to an Arabian stallion
• Amitriptyline, a tricyclic antidepressant, has been used successfully at a dose of 250 mg/day/horse orally to reduce self-mutilation. Its use is contraindicated in patients with cardiac conduction abnormalities, glaucoma, seizures, and urinary and fecal retention problems

• A wide variety of drugs have been tried therapeutically with mixed results. The sample size of horses treated in reports on the efficacy of medical therapy is small (1–12). Generally, the drugs are used in conjunction with other techniques; if there is a response to drug therapy, it is transitory. Medications reported to have some effect on the behavior are topical applications (antiseptics, shampoos, parasiticides, anti-inflammatory agents, and taste repellents), ulcer medication, antihistamines, steroids, phenylbutazone, flunixin meglumine, synthetic progesterone, acepromazine, and fluphenazine decanoate

FOLLOW-UP

• Environmental changes should reduce the self-mutilation within 2 weeks
• Drug therapy may take up to 3 weeks. If there is no improvement in 1 month, another treatment should be tried

Suggested Reading
Dodman NH, Normile JA, Shuster L, Rand W. Equine self-mutilation syndrome (57 cases). J Am Vet Med Assoc 1994;204:1219–1223.
Dodman NH, Shuster L, Patronek GJ, Kinney L. Pharmacologic treatment of equine self-mutilation syndrome. Intern J Appl Res Vet Med 2004;2:90–98.
McDonnell SM. Practical review of self-mutilation in horses. Anim Reprod Sci 2008;107:219–228.

Author Katherine Albro Houpt
Consulting Editor Victoria L. Voith

S

BASICS

DEFINITION
Septic arthritis is infection of the articular structures, usually bacterial in origin, resulting in inflammation, pain, and effusion.

PATHOPHYSIOLOGY
• Most commonly hematogenous seeding of the synovium and subsequent joint infection. Growing foals have increased blood flow through the transphyseal vessels and to the joint capsule
• Organisms involved are similar to those seen with systemic sepsis. *Enterobacter, Escherichia coli, Klebsiella, Salmonella,* and *Actinobacillus* are common Gram-negative isolates. *Streptococcus* spp. and *Staphylococcus* spp. are common Gram-positive isolates
• Increased production of cytokines and migration of neutrophils result in a painful, effusive joint. Synovial fluid has increased protein and WBCs, and the inflammatory and degradative enzymes in this fluid can eventually cause articular cartilage damage
• Traumatic joint penetration (wounds, lacerations, punctures) can also lead to joint sepsis, although this etiology is more common in adult horses than in neonates

SYSTEMS AFFECTED
• Musculoskeletal—synovium, cartilage, bone, and surrounding soft tissues can all be affected
• Neonates can have multiple systems (e.g. GI, pulmonary) affected if systemic sepsis is present

GENETICS
N/A

INCIDENCE/PREVALENCE
Approximately 25% of septic foals are affected with septic arthritis.

GEOGRAPHIC DISTRIBUTION
N/A

SIGNALMENT
Septic arthritis secondary to hematogenous spread is most common in foals ;<1 month of age. Foals can be affected as early as 1 day of age and foals with other systemic bacterial disease (e.g. pneumonia) may be affected at several months of age.

SIGNS

Historical Findings
• Frequent recumbency or reluctance to rise
• Inadequate ingestion of colostrum—mare leaking colostrum prior to foaling; delayed ingestion of colostrum

Physical Examination Findings
• Stilted gait or lameness; lameness may not be noted if the foal is mostly recumbent or if the lameness is bilateral
• Joint effusion ± heat, pain on manipulation
• Tarsocrural, stifle, and carpal and fetlock joints are most commonly affected
• Periarticular edema
• Fever
• Decubital ulcers owing to frequent or prolonged recumbency

CAUSES
• Septicemia
• Penetrating wounds
• Iatrogenic—joint injections (uncommon in foals)

RISK FACTORS
• Systemic sepsis is the most important risk factor in neonates. Pneumonia, enteritis, and omphalophlebitis are often associated with septic arthritis
• Failure of transfer of passive immunity
• Premature/dysmature foals can maintain increased blood flow through the transphyseal vessels for longer periods of time, keeping the physis and joint at higher risk of sepsis

DIAGNOSIS

DIFFERENTIAL DIAGNOSIS
• Septic physitis—can occur concurrently with septic arthritis; radiographs can identify septic physitis
• Osteomyelitis—can occur concurrently with septic arthritis; radiographic changes may not be evident for 10–14 days
• Trauma
• Foot abscess

CBC/BIOCHEMISTRY/URINALYSIS
Hyperfibrinogenemia is consistently seen. Leukocytosis or leukopenia may be found on CBC, but these changes are not specific for septic arthritis.

OTHER LABORATORY TESTS
Serum IgG concentration—often low (<800 mg/dL).

IMAGING
• Radiography—bony abnormalities are often not seen in the early stages of septic arthritis. Radiographic changes associated with osteomyelitis may not been seen for 1–2 weeks. Initial radiographs are useful for determining prognosis and as a baseline for identifying changes on follow-up radiographs
• CT and MRI—may detect early bone infection
• US of joints—joint effusions and bony irregularity can help to identify likely septic joints or areas of abscessation
• US of the umbilicus should be performed in neonates to rule out concurrent omphalophlebitis

OTHER DIAGNOSTIC PROCEDURES
• Joint aspirate cytology. WBCs >30 000/µL and often >100 000/µL, with 80–90% neutrophils and total protein >4 g/dL. Normal synovial fluid has total protein <2 g/dL and WBCs <500/µL with <10% neutrophils. Low pH is also found in the synovial fluid of septic structures
• Joint aspirate culture and sensitivity. Sample should ideally be taken before the foal is started on antibiotics. Do not discontinue antimicrobial therapy in order to obtain a culture if the foal is septicemic or has a septic synovial structure. Treatment with antimicrobials should begin immediately after culture is taken, but culture results can help to guide therapy if there is poor response to the initial treatment
• If septic physitis is suspected, needle aspirate of the abnormal physeal area can be performed
• Blood culture can be very useful for identifying the cause of septicemia

PATHOLOGIC FINDINGS
Early in the course of septic arthritis, there may not be significant gross lesions of bone or cartilage. Advanced septic arthritis can result in significant cartilage degradation and osteomyelitis/septic physitis.

TREATMENT

AIMS

Joint Lavage
• Primary treatment for any septic synovial structure
• Via 14 G needles or teat cannulas—through-and-through lavage with several liters of balanced electrolyte solution (volume depends on severity of sepsis and size of synovial structure). Multiple lavages (usually 48 h apart) are often needed

Local Antimicrobial Delivery
• Intra-articular injection delivers the highest concentration of antibiotics to the joint. Aminoglycosides such as amikacin (250–500 mg) or gentamicin are commonly used. Continuous infusion catheters have also been used successfully to deliver high concentrations of antibiotics to septic synovial structures
• Regional limb perfusion or intraosseous perfusion if a regional vein is not available

Systemic Antimicrobial Treatment
• Broad-spectrum, parenteral, bactericidal antimicrobials are initiated immediately after fluid is sampled for culture. The combination of beta-lactams and aminoglycosides provides good coverage in most cases
• Systemic antimicrobials are generally continued for approximately 2 weeks after resolution of the infection

Pain Management
• It is important for the foal to be comfortable enough to willingly rise and nurse
• NSAIDs are used for pain management and control of fever and inflammation related to the septic structure

• Opioids may be used if additional analgesia is needed or if there are contraindications to using NSAIDs

APPROPRIATE HEALTH CARE
Inpatient medical and surgical therapy.

NURSING CARE
• Stall should be deeply bedded to prevent decubital ulcers
• Foals are often reluctant to rise and should therefore be encouraged or assisted to rise in order to nurse, ideally every hour
• Immunologic support—plasma transfusion if IgG <800 mg/dL

ACTIVITY
Stall rest is necessary until the joint inflammation has resolved. Concurrent systemic disease may be the limiting factor in the foal's activity.

DIET
Foals should be encouraged or assisted to rise and nurse frequently (at least every 1–2 h). Debilitated foals or those unable to stand for long periods of time require supplemental feedings via nasogastric feeding tube.

CLIENT EDUCATION
Management practices of good hygiene and ensuring adequate colostrum intake should be emphasized.

SURGICAL CONSIDERATIONS
• Joint lavage—through-and-through needle lavage may be successful in the early treatment of septic arthritis. If there is significant fibrin or longstanding infection, arthroscopic lavage and visualization or arthrotomy should be performed
• Umbilical resection should be performed in cases of severe septic omphalophlebitis or when unresponsive to antimicrobials

MEDICATIONS
DRUG(S) OF CHOICE
Antimicrobials
• Initial broad-spectrum coverage often includes penicillin and amikacin, although third-generation cephalosporins may also be used
• Penicillin—22 000–44 000 IU/kg IV every 6 h
• Amikacin—25 mg/kg IV every 24 h
• Ceftiofur—5–10 mg/kg IV every 6–12 h
• Ceftazidime—50 mg/kg IV every 6 h
• Cefotaxime—40 mg/kg IV every 6 h

NSAIDs
• Ketoprofen (1.1–2.2 mg/kg IV every 12 h)
• Flunixin meglumine (0.5–1.1 mg/kg IV or PO up to every 12 h)

Antiulcer Medication
• Ranitidine 6.6 mg/kg PO every 8 h or omeprazole 4 mg/kg PO every 24 h
• May be needed for foals under stress, especially if treated with NSAIDs. Septicemic foals may actually have alkaline gastric pH, so antiulcer medications may not be indicated in this group

CONTRAINDICATIONS
Enrofloxacin should not be used as part of the antimicrobial regimen in foals.

PRECAUTIONS
• Aminoglycosides can cause renal compromise, especially in dehydrated or debilitated foals
• All NSAIDs can cause renal and GI damage, although ketoprofen is less ulcerogenic and has more renal safety than phenylbutazone

FOLLOW-UP
PATIENT MONITORING
• Foals should be monitored twice daily for development of additional sites of sepsis
• If lameness and joint effusion persist, repeat radiographs (at 7–10 days) are indicated to determine presence of septic physitis or osteomyelitis
• Repeat joint aspiration to help assess response to therapy

PREVENTION/AVOIDANCE
• Consumption of adequate amounts of high-quality colostrum
• Good hygiene in foaling area
• Routine measurement of IgG levels

POSSIBLE COMPLICATIONS
• Degenerative joint disease
• Osteomyelitis

EXPECTED COURSE AND PROGNOSIS
• Response to therapy depends upon the severity of infection and the presence of concurrent systemic disease
• Reported prognosis for survival ranges from approximately 40% to 86%
• Septic arthritis decreases the likelihood of racing for Thoroughbreds, and appears to prolong the period of time needed to start in their first race
• Multisystem disease decreases the prognosis for discharge from the hospital to approximately 50%
• Multiple joint involvement and infection with *Salmonella* spp. appear to further decrease the prognosis. Presence of concurrent osteomyelitis also decreases the prognosis (guarded)

MISCELLANEOUS
ASSOCIATED CONDITIONS
• Septic physitis
• Septicemia
• Diarrhea
• Omphalophlebitis
• Pneumonia

AGE-RELATED FACTORS
Physeal infections appear to be more common in older foals, whereas synovial sepsis alone is more common in younger foals.

ZOONOTIC POTENTIAL
N/A

PREGNANCY/FERTILITY/BREEDING
N/A

SYNONYMS
• Joint ill
• Septic joint

SEE ALSO
• Failure of transfer of passive immunity (FTPI)
• Septicemia, neonate

ABBREVIATIONS
• CT = computed tomography
• GI = gastrointestinal
• IgG = immunoglobulin G
• MRI = magnetic resonance imaging
• NSAID = nonsteroidal anti-inflammatory drug
• US = ultrasonography, ultrasound
• WBC = white blood cell

Suggested Reading
Glass K, Watts AE. Septic arthritis, physitis, and osteomyelitis in foals. Vet Clin North Am Eq Pract 2017;33:299–314.
Hepworth-Warren KL, Wong DM, Fulkerson CV, et al. Bacterial isolates, antimicrobial susceptibility patterns, and factors associated with infection and outcome in foals with septic arthritis: 83 cases (1998-2013). J Am Vet Med Assoc 2015;246:785–793.
Smith LJ, Marr CM, Payne RJ, et al. What is the likelihood that Thoroughbred foals treated for septic arthritis will race? Equine Vet J 2004;36:452–456.
Steel CM, Hunt AR, Adams PL, et al. Factors associated with prognosis for survival and athletic use in foals with septic arthritis: 93 cases (1987–1994). J Am Vet Med Assoc 1999;215:973–977.

Author Margaret C. Mudge
Consulting Editor Margaret C. Mudge

S

SEPTIC MENINGOENCEPHALOMYELITIS

BASICS

DEFINITION
Septic meningoencephalomyelitis is defined as bacteria-associated inflammation of the CNS.

PATHOPHYSIOLOGY
Microbial invasion of the CNS occurs with hematogenous spread, traumatic injury, or via an ascending infection. Hematogenous spread is the most common and is associated with immunosuppression/immunodeficiency and sepsis. Following bacterial invasion, inflammation leads to increased permeability of the BBB, vasculitis, cerebral edema, and, occasionally, hydrocephalus.

Systems Affected
CNS

SIGNALMENT
Young foals, but adult horses may be affected.

SIGNS
Historical Findings
• Inadequate passive transfer of maternal immunoglobulin, prematurity, and other illnesses are important historical factors in foals
• Infection within the head such as sinusitis and thrombophlebitis, bacteremia, or head trauma are other important historical factors

Physical Examination Findings
• Fever (not always present), lethargy, and behavioral changes (aimless walking, somnolence, abnormal vocalization, lack of affinity for the mare) characterize the early stages
• Later, tactile and auditory hyperesthesia over the entire body and a stiff and extended neck posture may be noted
• CNS pain is often manifested by reluctance to move the head or neck and trismus (spasms of the muscles of mastication)
• Signs progress to loss of the suckling reflex, cranial nerve abnormalities, ataxia, paresis, and blindness. Recumbency, coma, seizures, and death quickly follow

CAUSES
• The bacteria involved are those most commonly associated with neonatal sepsis including coliforms, *Salmonella* spp., and *Klebsiella* spp.
• Adult horse meningitis has been associated with a wide variety of organisms; however, *Streptococcus equi* and *Actinomyces* spp. predominate

RISK FACTORS
Include those that are associated with septic conditions of foals—maternal uterine infection, premature placental separation, poor hygiene during parturition, failure of passive transfer of maternal immunoglobulins, etc. A risk factor in adults is the hypogammaglobulinemia associated with CVID.

DIAGNOSIS

• Early diagnosis and aggressive treatment are essential
• A CBC may reveal a neutrophilic leukocytosis, but neonatal foals frequently have neutropenia with sepsis. Adults with CVID may have marked lymphopenia with hypoglobulinemia on chemistry profile. Additional testing is required to demonstrate low IgM and IgG
• In acute cases, CSF contains high neutrophils and protein. In protracted and treated cases mononuclear cells often predominate. Low glucose (compared with blood) and high lactate are consistent with CNS sepsis
• Blood and CSF culture and Gram stain

DIFFERENTIAL DIAGNOSIS
Viral encephalomyelitis, hepatic encephalopathy, intoxication.

TREATMENT
N/A

MEDICATIONS

DRUG(S) OF CHOICE
• Most antibiotics are likely to get into the CSF as the BBB is damaged
• Third-generation cephalosporins, such as cefotaxime and ceftriaxone, have good CNS penetration; however, they are expensive. Ceftiofur is a third-generation cephalosporin that is inexpensive; however, its penetration into the CNS is questionable
• The fluoroquinolones are efficacious but adverse effects on cartilage must be considered in foals
• Potentiated sulfonamides have good CNS penetration but resistance is common. Chloramphenicol has good CNS penetration, but is bacteriostatic and human health concerns such as aplastic anemia should be considered
• Antimicrobial administration *must* begin immediately and be broad spectrum. A combination of potassium penicillin G (22 000 U/kg IV every 6 h), ceftiofur (2.2–5.0 mg/kg IV every 12 h), or ampicillin (22 mg/kg IV every 8 h) *plus* amikacin (25 mg/kg IV every 24 h) or gentamicin (6.6 mg/kg IV every 24 h) provides a good initial regimen
• Additional therapy including caloric, fluid, electrolyte, respiratory, and thermic support is essential
• Seizures may be managed with diazepam (5–20 mg IV) and repeated as necessary in 50 kg foals. Intractable seizures may require phenobarbital (10–20 mg/kg diluted in saline and administered slowly over 15 min IV every 12 h)
• Corticosteroids (e.g. dexamethasone 0.1 mg/kg IV) may be given initially, preferably beginning 30 min before antimicrobials. NSAIDs should be administered to mitigate effects of inflammation and fever
• Drugs to resolve secondary problems should be considered (e.g. antiulcer medications, ocular medications)

FOLLOW-UP

PATIENT MONITORING
Foals will need to be continuously monitored and supported.

POSSIBLE COMPLICATIONS
The prognosis for foals or adults with septic meningitis is poor to grave. The prognosis of horses with CVID with meningitis is hopeless.

MISCELLANEOUS

AGE-RELATED FACTORS
Young foals are most often affected.

SEE ALSO
Seizure disorders

ABBREVIATIONS
• BBB = blood–brain barrier
• CNS = central nervous system
• CSF = cerebrospinal fluid
• CVID = common variable immunodeficiency
• Ig = immunoglobulin
• NSAID = nonsteroidal anti-inflammatory drug

Authors Liz Nelson and Robert J. MacKay
Consulting Editor Caroline N. Hahn
Acknowledgment The authors acknowledge the prior contribution Caroline N. Hahn.

S

BASICS

DEFINITION
• SIRS—characterized by at least 2 of the 4 following abnormalities: (1) hyperthermia or hypothermia, (2) tachycardia, (3) tachypnea/hypocapnia, and (4) leukopenia, leukocytosis, or left shift
• Sepsis—SIRS with a source of confirmed or suspected infection
• Septic shock—sepsis with hypotension refractory to fluid resuscitation
• Bacteremia—presence of bacteria in the bloodstream
• Septicemia—bacterial or bacterial toxin invasion into the bloodstream with SIRS

PATHOPHYSIOLOGY
• In utero infection and postnatal infections within the first week of life are the most common causes of neonatal septicemia. Bacteria can gain entry via placental infection, ingestion of organisms, or through umbilical structures or the respiratory tract
• Overwhelming bacterial infection or inadequate defense against invading pathogens can lead to sepsis. Gram-negative bacteria are most commonly involved, although the incidence of Gram-positive septicemia is high in some recent reports. *Actinobacillus* spp., *Escherichia coli*, *Enterobacter* spp., *Klebsiella* spp., *Salmonella* spp., *Streptococcus* spp. and *Enterococcus* spp. are common isolates

SYSTEMS AFFECTED
• Cardiovascular—may have an early increase in cardiac output that can rapidly progress to decompensated septic shock
• Endocrine/metabolic—relative adrenal insufficiency may occur with severe sepsis. Energy homeostasis (hypoglycemia), mineral metabolism (hypocalcemia, hypomagnesemia), and pressure regulation (renin–angiotensin aldosterone system) may be affected
• GI—the intestinal tract is often the primary site of infection (as with colitis and enteritis) or secondary ileus
• Hemic/lymphatic/immune—neutropenia and immune compromise; less common—thrombocytopenia with disseminated intravascular coagulation and coagulopathies
• Hepatobiliary—inflammatory cytokines can impair hepatocellular function
• Musculoskeletal—septic arthritis and septic physitis are common sequelae of septicemia
• Nervous—infection can localize as meningitis (rare)
• Ophthalmic—uveitis possible; entropion in severe dehydration; corneal ulcers
• Renal/urologic—renal insufficiency secondary to hypoperfusion and endotoxemia

• Respiratory—bacterial pneumonia secondary to sepsis occurs most often via hematogenous spread. May also occur through inhalation or aspiration

GENETICS
There does not appear to be a genetic predisposition to sepsis.

INCIDENCE/PREVALENCE
Sepsis is one of the most common reasons for neonatal foals to present to referral centers. It is the main cause of mortality in the first week of life. It is reported to cause approximately 25–30% of neonatal deaths.

GEOGRAPHIC DISTRIBUTION
Incidence of septicemia does not appear to have a specific geographic distribution, although bacterial isolates may vary by geographic location.

SIGNALMENT
Mean Age and Range
In utero infection can occur; it is most common within the first week of life.

Predominant Sex
None

SIGNS
Historical Findings
• Illness or stress in mare prior to parturition
• Placentitis, vulval discharge, milk leakage prior to parturition
• Premature delivery or prolonged gestation
• Dystocia
• Foal has never nursed or was slow to stand and nurse

Physical Examination Findings
• Lethargy/depression
• Decreased nursing; loss of suckle reflex
• Fever or hypothermia
• Tachycardia and tachypnea, can have bradycardia in late stages
• Injected mucous membranes; petechiation
• Late/decompensated sepsis—obtunded, cold extremities, cyanotic, weak pulses, hypothermia
• Localizing signs—diarrhea, joint effusion, respiratory distress, uveitis, omphalophlebitis

CAUSES
• In utero infection (transplacental)
• Bacterial inoculation via the GI tract or respiratory tract
• Entry of bacteria via umbilical structures or wounds

RISK FACTORS
• Maternal—short or prolonged gestation, placental disorders, dystocia, maternal diseases
• Foal—failure of transfer of passive immunity, prematurity/dysmaturity, NMS, hypoxia, immunosuppression, viral infections, severe combined immunodeficiency syndrome
• Environment—poor farm management, poor hygiene

DIAGNOSIS

DIFFERENTIAL DIAGNOSIS
• NMS
• Prematurity/dysmaturity
• White muscle disease
• Botulism
• Congenital neurologic or cardiac abnormalities

CBC/BIOCHEMISTRY/URINALYSIS
• Leukopenia (often neutropenia with left shift and toxic changes), although may have normal white blood cell count or leukocytosis
• Hyperfibrinogenemia or increased serum amyloid A concentration shortly after birth suggestive of in utero infection
• Hypoglycemia is common
• Azotemia and elevated liver and muscle enzymes may be present

OTHER LABORATORY TESTS
• Serum IgG concentrations—failure of transfer of passive immunity is common
• Blood cultures (aerobic and anaerobic) can confirm sepsis and help direct antimicrobial therapy
• Blood L-lactate—normal foals <12 h old have L-lactate concentrations up to 4 mmol/L; decreases to <2.5 mmol/L by 24 h of age
• Blood gas—mixed metabolic and respiratory acidosis is common
• Arthrocentesis with cytology and culture if septic arthritis suspected
• Cerebrospinal fluid aspirate with cytology and culture if bacterial meningitis suspected

IMAGING
Radiography
• Thoracic radiography—pneumonia may be seen
• Musculoskeletal radiography if septic arthritis/physitis suspected

US
• Abdominal US—detects signs of ileus and enterocolitis
• US of umbilical remnants—umbilicus may appear normal externally, but internal structures are commonly affected
• Thoracic US—detects pleural effusion, consolidation, or pleural roughening

OTHER DIAGNOSTIC PROCEDURES
Sepsis score—historical data, clinical examination, CBC, and other laboratory data are scored to give a prediction of sepsis. If in doubt, treat the foal for septicemia pending results of blood culture.

PATHOLOGIC FINDINGS
• Localized infection—pneumonia, septic arthritis, enterocolitis, etc.
• Generalized petechiation and adrenal hemorrhage are consistent with, but not specific to, neonatal septicemia

S

SEPTICEMIA, NEONATE (CONTINUED)

TREATMENT

APPROPRIATE HEALTH CARE
Inpatient medical management, and often emergency inpatient intensive care management.

NURSING CARE
- Fluid therapy—needed to maintain hydration and perfusion
- Dextrose supplementation for hypoglycemic foals
- Transfusion with hyperimmune plasma for foals with IgG <800 mg/dL. IgG levels should be rechecked in septic foals as they may consume IgG
- Oxygen therapy if PaO_2 is low
- Pressors/inotropes if IV fluids do not correct hypotension
- Prevention of pressure sores—padding and maintain sternal recumbency
- Eye lubrication

ACTIVITY
Activity is restricted (stall rest) in weak foals and those with musculoskeletal involvement.

DIET
- Enteral feeding via nasogastric feeding tube is needed in foals with a weak suckle reflex or inability to stand and nurse
- Parenteral feeding for foals that are unable to maintain sternal recumbency or do not tolerate enteral feeding (e.g. enterocolitis)

CLIENT EDUCATION
Sepsis with multisystem involvement can be very expensive to treat and has a guarded prognosis. Clients should be aware of the costs and potential complications.

SURGICAL CONSIDERATIONS
- Joint lavage for treatment of septic arthritis
- Umbilical resection for omphalophlebitis that does not respond to medical therapy

MEDICATIONS

DRUG(S) OF CHOICE
Antimicrobials
- Broad-spectrum antimicrobial combination based on penicillin (e.g. potassium penicillin 22 000 IU/kg IV every 6 h) in combination with an aminoglycoside (e.g. amikacin 20–25 mg/kg IV every 24 h) until results of blood culture are available or there is a lack of response to this combination. A third-generation cephalosporin (e.g. ceftazidime or cefotaxime 40–50 mg/kg IV every 6–8 h) may be indicated
- Metronidazole (for foals <10 days of age, 10 mg/kg q12 h; for foals >10 days of age, 15 mg/kg q12 h IV or PO) if there is suspicion of anaerobic sepsis. Chloramphenicol (40–50 mg/kg PO every

6–8 h) can be considered in foals that remain febrile or have umbilical abscess

Anti-inflammatories
- Flunixin meglumine (0.5–1.1 mg/kg IV every 12 h)
- Ketoprofen (1.1–2.2 mg/kg IV every 12 h)
- Corticosteroids—low-dose hydrocortisone may be used to treat relative adrenal insufficiency or refractory septic shock, but there is no clear evidence for its use in foals
- Carprofen
- Meloxicam (0.6 mg/kg PO every 12 h)

Antiendotoxin Therapy
Polymyxin B (3000–5000 IU/kg IV every 8–12 h).

Vasopressors/Inotropes
- Dobutamine (1–5 µg/kg/min IV CRI) for inotropic effects
- Norepinephrine (0.1–1.0 µg/kg/min IV CRI) for vasopressor effects
- Vasopressin (0.1–3 µg/kg/min IV CRI)

Gastroprotectants
Routine use of acid suppressors (e.g. omeprazole, ranitidine) to raise the gastric pH is discouraged in septic foals, as these foals tend to have an alkaline gastric pH, and further alkalinization may encourage bacterial overgrowth and translocation.

PRECAUTIONS
- Aminoglycosides, NSAIDs, and polymyxin B should be used with caution in hypotensive and hypovolemic foals owing to the risk of renal damage
- NSAIDs may contribute to development of renal damage and gastric ulcers

ALTERNATIVE DRUGS
Dopamine and vasopressin (argipressin) may also be used for treatment of septic shock.

FOLLOW-UP

PATIENT MONITORING
- Intensive monitoring with frequent checks of vital parameters (every 1–4 h). Advanced monitoring includes blood pressure, urine output, and cardiac output measurements
- L-Lactate, blood glucose, renal parameters, electrolytes, and CBC should be monitored to assess response to therapy. Localized infections (septic arthritis, pneumonia, etc.) may develop during hospitalization

PREVENTION/AVOIDANCE
- Clean foaling environment; reduce contamination of mare's udder and limbs
- Ensure adequate colostrum intake; administer IV plasma if IgG is not adequate
- Dip umbilicus with dilute chlorhexidine or povidone–iodine

POSSIBLE COMPLICATIONS
- Organ failure (renal, respiratory)
- Decreased athletic performance after septic arthritis

EXPECTED COURSE AND PROGNOSIS
Short-term survival is approximately 50%, with reported ranges from 30% to 70%. Gram-negative septicemia, multisystem disease, and high sepsis score have been correlated with higher mortality. The ability of the foal to stand and normal L-lactate concentration on admission are positively correlated with survival.

MISCELLANEOUS

ASSOCIATED CONDITIONS
- Septic arthritis
- Omphalophlebitis
- Diarrhea

AGE-RELATED FACTORS
Foals are most commonly affected in the first week of life.

SYNONYMS
Bacteremia

SEE ALSO
- Diarrhea, neonate
- Fluid therapy, neonate
- Gastric ulcers, neonate
- Meningitis, neonate
- Omphalophlebitis
- Pneumonia, neonate
- Septic arthritis, neonate

ABBREVIATIONS
- CRI = constant rate infusion
- GI = gastrointestinal
- IgG = immunoglobulin G
- NMS = neonatal maladjustment syndrome
- NSAID = nonsteroidal anti-inflammatory drug
- PaO_2 = partial pressure of oxygen in arterial blood
- SIRS = systemic inflammatory response syndrome
- US = ultrasonography, ultrasound

Suggested Reading
Corley KT, Donaldson LL, Furr MO. Arterial lactate concentration, hospital survival, sepsis, and SIRS in critically ill neonatal foals. Equine Vet J 2005;37:53–59.
Sanchez LC. Equine neonatal sepsis. Vet Clin North Am Equine Pract 2005;21:273–293.
Wong DM, Wilkins PA. Defining the systemic inflammatory response syndrome in equine neonates. Vet Clin North Am Equine Pract 2015;31:463–481.

Author Ramiro Toribio
Consulting Editor Margaret C. Mudge
Acknowledgment The author acknowledges the prior contribution of Margaret C. Mudge.

BASICS

DEFINITION
• SAA is a major APP, which is a highly sensitive but poorly specific indicator of inflammation in horses
• The laboratory reference range is 0–20 mg/L, with some healthy adult horses having undetectable levels
• Concentrations are thought to reflect the intensity and extent of inflammation based on the degree of increase
• Depending on the stimulus, concentrations rapidly rise (>100-fold) above the upper limit of the reference range within 24 h of an inflammatory stimulus, peak at 36–72 h, and usually return to normal within 7–14 days of resolution of the underlying cause (but can remain increased for up to 4 weeks in some cases)

PATHOPHYSIOLOGY
• SAA is an apolipoprotein produced primarily by the liver during the APR and is highly conserved across species. Three isoforms have been identified, one of which can be produced by extrahepatic synthesis in other tissues
• During the APR, proinflammatory cytokines are released and act on hepatocyte receptors, causing synthesis of APPs including SAA
• Rate of synthesis determines plasma concentration, and clearance is rapid (hepatic degradation within 30–120 min). As SAA has a short half-life, decreases in plasma concentrations occur rapidly after cessation of synthesis
• Functions of SAA include acting as an inflammatory and immunomodulatory protein, inducing inflammatory cytokine secretion, and inducing chemotaxis of neutrophils and mast cells

SYSTEMS AFFECTED
• Increased SAA in itself rarely has detrimental effects, except in cases of chronic inflammation where SAA fragments may be deposited in tissues (amyloidosis)
• Amyloid deposition can occur in single or multiple tissues, but in cases caused by chronic inflammation, it most commonly affects:
  ○ Hepatobiliary—deposits in the liver
  ○ Renal/urologic—deposits in the kidneys
  ○ Hemic/lymphatic—deposits in the spleen

GENETICS
N/A

INCIDENCE/PREVALENCE
N/A

GEOGRAPHIC DISTRIBUTION
N/A

SIGNALMENT
• Any breed, age, or sex
• Can be increased in neonatal foals and pregnant mares around parturition (see Age-Related Factors and Pregnancy/Fertility/Breeding)

SIGNS
Dependent on the underlying cause of inflammation.

CAUSES
• Acute or chronic inflammatory conditions affecting any organ system can result in increased SAA concentrations
• Gastrointestinal—enteritis, colitis, large colon volvulus, peritonitis, parasitism, endotoxemia, meconium retention, tooth root abscess, sialoadenitis, laparotomy, laparoscopy
• Respiratory—pneumonia (pleuro-, broncho-, aspiration, abscessation), sinusitis, upper respiratory tract infection (influenza, equine herpesvirus), guttural pouch empyema, airway surgery
• Musculoskeletal—lacerations, septic and nonseptic arthritis, osteomyelitis, cellulitis, abscesses, trauma, fractures, myositis, rhabdomyolysis, neoplasia, surgery
• Hepatobiliary—acute hepatitis (Theiler's disease), chronic active hepatitis, Tyzzer's disease, cholangitis, hepatic lipidosis, neoplasia
• Reproductive—endometritis, metritis, placentitis, castration, orchitis, abortion, early embryonic loss, parturition
• Renal/urologic—cystitis, nephritis (pyelo-, glomerulo-), urinary calculi, neoplasia
• Hemic/lymphatic/immune—sepsis, lymph node abscessation, lymphangitis, omphalophlebitis, leukemia, vaccination
• Skin—pyoderma, chronic dermatitis, pemphigus foliaceus
• Nervous—meningitis, encephalitis, perinatal asphyxia, neoplasia
• Ophthalmic—uveitis, trauma, neoplasia
• Cardiovascular—thrombophlebitis, endocarditis, pericarditis, vasculitis, arteritis
• Endocrine/metabolic—laminitis, hyperlipidemia

RISK FACTORS
See Causes.

DIAGNOSIS

DIFFERENTIAL DIAGNOSIS
• Increase in SAA concentration is a nonspecific marker of inflammation and, as such, gives no indication of etiology. Establishing the primary etiology of the underlying inflammatory process is paramount. Therefore, a thorough physical examination is warranted, and further diagnostic tests may also be indicated
• Localization of the site of inflammation may be challenging in some cases

CBC/BIOCHEMISTRY/URINALYSIS
• Horses may have concurrent WBC abnormalities (increased or decreased) as well as increased band neutrophils ± toxicity
• Hyperfibrinogenemia may be present in more chronic cases and there may also be hypoalbuminemia (negative APP) and hyperglobulinemia owing to chronic immune stimulation
• Other CBC and biochemistry changes relate to the underlying cause of inflammation
• Urinalysis is indicated in cases of suspected urinary tract disease

OTHER LABORATORY TESTS
• SAA can be measured in synovial fluid and colostrum as well as in peripheral blood
• Other APPs have been evaluated in horses for use as inflammatory markers including haptoglobin, C-reactive protein, and α_1-acid glycoprotein, but have been found to be less reliable, and assays are not yet as widely available as SAA and plasma fibrinogen concentration

IMAGING
Radiography, ultrasonography, gamma scintigraphy, or CT may help to elucidate the location of the inflammatory focus.

OTHER DIAGNOSTIC PROCEDURES
• Depending on the organ system affected, further diagnostic procedures may be indicated such as abdominocentesis, tracheal aspiration, pleural fluid drainage, nasal swab, guttural pouch lavage, and biopsy
• Samples should be submitted for cytology (or histopathology for biopsies) and culture or PCR if an infectious process is suspected
• Serology may also identify a specific pathogen in some cases

PATHOLOGIC FINDINGS
Dependent on the underlying cause.

TREATMENT

APPROPRIATE HEALTH CARE
Cases may be managed as inpatients or outpatients depending on the underlying cause of inflammation, severity of disease, and ease of drug administration.

NURSING CARE
Cases should be monitored closely for any deterioration or signs of concomitant disease.

ACTIVITY
Depending on the severity of disease, exercise should be limited to walking until the inflammation has resolved.

S

SERUM AMYLOID A (SAA)   (CONTINUED)

DIET
• Horses with inflammatory disease may be anorexic. Palatable and nutritious feed should be provided to encourage voluntary intake, unless this is contraindicated owing to the primary disease (e.g. enteritis with ileus)
• More specific diet recommendations depend on the underlying disease process

CLIENT EDUCATION
N/A

SURGICAL CONSIDERATIONS
• "Source control" may be warranted in some cases of infection and may involve drainage or debridement
• Cases requiring surgery should be stabilized medically first to decrease the risk of anesthetic complications

MEDICATIONS

DRUG(S) OF CHOICE
• Ideal drug therapy depends on the underlying cause of inflammation and the systemic state of the horse
• In cases of bacterial infection, empiric broad-spectrum antibiotic therapy may be indicated initially, followed by antimicrobial selection based on culture and sensitivity results
• Anti-inflammatory medications, such as NSAIDs, may be indicated to decrease inflammation and associated systemic signs
• Careful consideration of the overall systemic state of the horse should aid in drug selection (e.g. dehydrated or azotemic horses should not be treated with potentially nephrotoxic medications)

CONTRAINDICATIONS
N/A

PRECAUTIONS
N/A

POSSIBLE INTERACTIONS
N/A

ALTERNATIVE DRUGS
N/A

FOLLOW-UP

PATIENT MONITORING
• Daily measurement of SAA is useful for real-time monitoring of the course of inflammation and response to treatment, owing to the rapid onset of synthesis following an inflammatory stimulus and the short half-life

• Concentrations vary in parallel with the severity of inflammation, allowing inferences to be made regarding effectiveness of treatment
• Plasma fibrinogen concentration and WBC count can also be used in conjunction with SAA for monitoring; however, studies have shown SAA to be more sensitive and better for assessment of real-time inflammatory activity

PREVENTION/AVOIDANCE
Prevention of the underlying cause of inflammation will vary depending on the disease process.

POSSIBLE COMPLICATIONS
• Amyloidosis is a systemic or localized condition where amyloid (abnormally folded protein) is deposited in tissues. Chronic inflammation can result in secondary reactive amyloidosis where fragments of SAA are deposited
• Systemic amyloidosis is usually the AA type, occurs as a result of chronic immune stimulation, and has been reported in cases of chronic pleuropneumonia, peritonitis, parasitism, and in horses hyperimmunized for plasma donation. Amyloid is usually deposited in the liver, spleen, and kidneys and may cause no obvious clinical signs, or can result in organ dysfunction, failure, and eventually death

EXPECTED COURSE AND PROGNOSIS
Prognosis depends on the cause of inflammation, severity of disease, and response to therapy.

MISCELLANEOUS

ASSOCIATED CONDITIONS
N/A

AGE-RELATED FACTORS
• Neonates may have significantly increased SAA concentrations (noted at 72 h of age) associated with tissue trauma induced by the birthing process, as well as the release of cytokines from the maternal circulation during foaling
• Studies have also shown that SAA-3 (mammary-associated SAA) can be found in colostrum and, thus, increased levels in foals may be related to colostrum consumption

ZOONOTIC POTENTIAL
N/A

PREGNANCY/FERTILITY/BREEDING
• SAA concentrations remain within the normal range throughout normal pregnancy and begin to rise 2 days prepartum, reaching a modest peak (around 100 mg/L) 3 days postpartum, likely reflecting the inflammatory nature of the birthing process and associated tissue trauma. Levels usually normalize 1 month post-foaling
• Early embryonic death may cause an increase in SAA during early pregnancy

SYNONYMS
N/A

SEE ALSO
Plasma proteins

ABBREVIATIONS
• AA = amyloid A
• APP = acute-phase protein
• APR = acute-phase response
• CT = computed tomography
• NSAID = nonsteroidal anti-inflammatory drug
• PCR = polymerase chain reaction
• SAA = serum amyloid A
• WBC = white blood cell

Suggested Reading
Belgrave RL, Dickey MM, Arheart KL, Cray C. Assessment of serum amyloid A testing of horses and its clinical application in a specialized equine practice. J Am Vet Med Assoc 2013;243:113–119.
De Cozar M, Sherlock C, Knowles E, Mair T. Serum amyloid A and plasma fibrinogen concentrations in horses following emergency exploratory celiotomy. Equine Vet J 2019; DOI:10.1111/evj.13117.
Satué K, Calvo A, Gardón JC. Factors influencing serum amyloid type A (SAA) concentrations in horses. Open J Vet Med 2013;3:58–66.
Witkowska-Pilaszewicz OD, Zmigrodzka M, Winnicka A, Miskiewicz A, Strzelec K, Cywinska A. Serum amyloid A in equine health and disease. Equine Vet J 2018;DOI:10.1111/evj.13062

Author Rana Bozorgmanesh
Consulting Editor Sandra D. Taylor

S

SEVERE COMBINED IMMUNODEFICIENCY

BASICS

OVERVIEW
• Inheritable lethal disease of foals characterized by complete absence of functional B and T lymphocytes and lack of adapted immune system
• autosomal recessive trait; affected (homozygous) foals have no antigen-specific immune responses, heterozygous foals show no abnormalities
• ~8–15% of Arabian horses carriers; 0.18–4% of Arabian foals affected; decreasing numbers owing to genetic testing for breeding

SIGNALMENT
• Arabian or Arabian-cross foals
• Clinical signs develop by 1–2 months of age; most foals die by 5 months

SIGNS
• Affected foals physically normal at birth
• When circulating, colostrum-derived antibodies drop below protective levels (1–2 months), SCID foals become susceptible to infectious agents
• Clinical signs include cough, nasal discharge (pneumonia), recurrent pyrexia (bacteremia), diarrhea (enteritis), lameness (arthritis), colic (peritonitis), impaired growth, and weight loss
• Equine adenovirus most common pathogen isolated from affected foals; *Cryptosporidium parvum, Pneumocystis jirovecii*, and bacterial pathogens also isolated

CAUSES AND RISK FACTORS
• Mutation in gene encoding catalytic subunit of DNA-dependent protein kinase
• Loss of functional enzyme results in failure of gene rearrangement for T- and B-cell receptor variable region development, thus absence of T and B lymphocytes
• Risk factor is breeding of Arabian horses not tested for genetic mutation

DIAGNOSIS

DIFFERENTIAL DIAGNOSIS
• Total or partial FTPI; foals with FTPI have low serum IgG concentration on day 1 or 2 of life, normal absolute lymphocyte counts and lymphoid tissues; foals with SCID often have normal serum IgG values until 4–6 weeks, but low absolute lymphocytes counts and lymphoid tissues
• Foals with transient hypogammaglobinemia of the young have low IgM and IgG values and normal or low normal lymphocyte counts with normal lymphoid tissues
• Foals with selective IgM deficiency have persistently low serum IgM and normal lymphocyte counts and lymphoid tissues

• Agammaglobulinemia not reported in Arabian foals and is characterized by lack of immunoglobulins, B cells, plasma cells, and germinal centers in lymphoid tissues; absolute lymphocyte count often normal owing to presence of T lymphocytes

CBC/BIOCHEMISTRY/URINALYSIS
• Profound, *persistent* lymphopenia (<1000 lymphocytes/μL) over 1–2 weeks
• Total white blood cell and neutrophil counts can be low, normal, or high depending on infections
• Anemia may develop later in clinical course of disease
• Biochemistry and urinalysis usually normal or reflect organ system involved in infection

OTHER LABORATORY TESTS
• Quantitation of serum IgM; absent before colostrum consumption or after 3 weeks of age owing to catabolism of maternally derived antibodies
• Phytohemagglutinin intradermal test and/or in vitro leukocyte stimulation test are negative owing to absence of cell-mediated immune responses
• Definitive diagnosis based on positive genetic test for DNA-dependent protein kinase from blood or cheek swab (VetGen LLC, Ann Arbor, MI); test determines if foal is free, heterozygous (carrier), or homozygous (affected) for genetic mutation

IMAGING
Radiographs/ultrasonography may reveal sites of infection.

PATHOLOGIC FINDINGS
• Small thymus with fatty appearance and hypoplastic lymph nodes
• Severe lymphoid hypoplasia, lack of germinal centers, and periarteriolar lymphocytic sheaths

TREATMENT
• Medical management unrewarding as death is inevitable
• Therapy is supportive and aimed at infection control
• SCID can be corrected by transplanting histocompatible stem cells from a genetically matched donor, but technique is rarely performed

MEDICATIONS

DRUG(S) OF CHOICE
Antimicrobials for the treatment of infections.

FOLLOW-UP

PATIENT MONITORING
Affected animals may be monitored for development of infection.

PREVENTION/AVOIDANCE
• Avoid production of affected foals by genetic testing stallion and mare before breeding
• Breeding 2 carriers (heterozygous) will result in 25% of offspring with SCID, 50% carriers, and 25% normal
• Breeding a carrier with a normal horse will produce nonaffected foals but with 50% chance of being carrier
• All offspring should be tested and heterozygous animals used for nonreproductive pursuits

POSSIBLE COMPLICATIONS
Recurrent infections, septicemia, and organ dysfunction.

EXPECTED COURSE AND PROGNOSIS
Grave prognosis; foals die from acquired infections by 5 months.

MISCELLANEOUS

ASSOCIATED CONDITIONS
Infections with opportunistic organisms.

AGE-RELATED FACTORS
Only observed in young animals.

SEE ALSO
Immunoglobulin deficiencies

ABBREVIATIONS
• FTPI = failure of transfer of passive immunity
• Ig = immunoglobulin
• SCID = severe combined immunodeficiency

Suggested Reading
Felippe MJB. Immunodeficiencies. In: Felippe MJB, ed. Equine Clinical Immunology. Ames, IA: Wiley Blackwell, 2016:193–204.
Author M. Julia B. Felippe
Consulting Editors David Hodgson, Harold C. McKenzie, and Jennifer L. Hodgson
Acknowledgment The author and editors acknowledge prior contribution of Jennifer L. Hodgson.

S

SHIVERS (SHIVERING)

BASICS

OVERVIEW
Classic shivering is a chronic, often gradually progressive movement disorder characterized by involuntary flexion of the pelvic limbs and testicles, as well as extension of the tail.

SIGNALMENT
Most often seen in draft horses, but other breeds may be affected. It usually begins before 7 years of age and has a higher prevalence in tall, male horses.

SIGNS
• Mild cases may be difficult to detect because of clinical signs occurring at irregular intervals. However, in most cases the clinical signs are characteristic
• Clinical signs are usually noticed when an attempt is made to back or turn the horse, or force it to step over an object
• The affected limb is held off the ground in a flexed and abducted manner while muscles of the upper limb and tail may quiver. After a short time, the quivering ceases and the limb and tail return to a normal position
• The horse then appears to be normal, but clinical signs reappear if attempts are made to turn or back the affected horse
• The difficulties backing into traces historically made this a disease of significant morbidity when draft horses were used for agricultural work
• Even in well-developed shivering cases signs may not be seen when the horse is standing still. In some horses there is evidence of involvement of the muscles of the thoracic limbs, neck, or even trunk and face, but it is unclear whether these present severe cases of classical shivering or represent other myotonic syndromes

CAUSES AND RISK FACTORS
• The etiology is unknown but is likely to involve an alteration in the feedback loop between α_1-afferent and γ-efferent fibers

• Recent work has suggested that neuroaxonal degeneration in the deep cerebellar nuclei may be involved in the etiology
• Some other diseases that include shivering as a clinical sign are equine polysaccharide storage myopathy and "stiff-horse syndrome"

DIAGNOSIS

DIFFERENTIAL DIAGNOSIS
• Shivering should be distinguished from stringhalt, which also results in increased pelvic limb flexion but occurs during forward motion and has a more consistent, rapidly ascending, hyperflexed, adducted pelvic limb gait
• Equine polysaccharide storage myopathy cases generally show additional clinical signs including generalized paresis, mild to moderately increased serum creatine kinase levels, and abnormal polysaccharide accumulations in muscle fibers
• "Stiff-horse syndrome" is a recently recognized syndrome that is associated with generalized myotonia with severe muscle cramps. It appears to be related to a deficiency in the inhibitory neurotransmitter glutamic acid decarboxylase

DIAGNOSTIC PROCEDURES
Muscle biopsy to rule out equine polysaccharide storage disorder.

TREATMENT

No effective treatment is presently available.

MEDICATIONS

DRUG(S) OF CHOICE
None

FOLLOW-UP

EXPECTED COURSE AND PROGNOSIS
• Classically the condition is slowly progressive but there is no way of predicting if or when horses will deteriorate
• Polysaccharide storage myopathy may be reasonably well controlled with a consistent exercise program and a low-carbohydrate/high-fat diet
• Too little is currently known about stiff-horse syndrome to offer good treatment advice

MISCELLANEOUS

SEE ALSO
Polysaccharide storage myopathy

Suggested Reading
Firshman AM, Baird JD, Valberg SJ. Prevalences and clinical signs of polysaccharide storage myopathy and shivers in Belgian draft horses. J Am Vet Med Assoc 2005;227:1958–1964.
Valberg SJ, Lewis SS, Shivers JL, et al. The equine movement disorder "shivers" is associated with selective cerebellar Purkinje cell axonal degeneration. Vet Pathol 2015;52:1087–1098.
Valentine BA, Lahunta AD, Divers TJ, et al. Clinical and pathologic findings in two draft horses with progressive muscle atrophy, neuromuscular weakness, and abnormal gait characteristic of shivers syndrome. J Am Vet Med Assoc 1999;215:1661–1665.

Author Caroline N. Hahn
Consulting Editor Caroline N. Hahn

S

BASICS

DEFINITION
Inflammation of the paranasal sinuses, usually caused by primary or secondary bacterial infection but sometimes caused by mycotic infection.

PATHOPHYSIOLOGY
• May be primary, following transient, systemic bacterial infection (usually streptococcal)
• Bacterial sinusitis commonly occurs secondary to infection of 1 of the maxillary molars (dental sinusitis); the tooth most commonly infected is the first molar
• Bacterial sinusitis occurs less commonly secondary to necrosis caused by an expanding mass within the sinuses, such as a cyst, neoplasm, osteoma, or progressive ethmoidal hematoma
• Generally accompanied by empyema that, regardless of its cause, may become inspissated. Inspissated exudate is found most commonly in the VCS
• Mycosis of the sinuses is caused most commonly by *Aspergillus fumigatus*
• All compartments communicate with each other, so all may be involved

SYSTEMS AFFECTED
Respiratory

GENETICS
None

INCIDENCE/PREVALENCE
• Worldwide
• Primary and secondary bacterial sinusitis is common. Mycotic sinusitis is less common

GEOGRAPHIC DISTRIBUTION
• None for bacterial sinusitis
• Mycotic sinusitis is seen most commonly in cool, humid climates

SIGNALMENT
No age, sex, or breed predilections

SIGNS
General Comments
• The most common clinical sign, regardless of the cause, is purulent or mucopurulent nasal discharge from the affected side
• Mycotic infection sometimes results in a sanguineous discharge
• Horses may uncommonly be affected bilaterally
• Malodorous nasal exudate is characteristically associated with dental sinusitis, an expanding mass, or mycotic sinusitis, whereas odorless exudate is more characteristic of primary bacterial sinusitis; primary bacterial sinusitis may result in malodorous nasal exudate, especially if exudate becomes inspissated

Historical Findings
A common complication of strangles or may accompany signs of dental disease.

Physical Examination Findings
• Common signs include ipsilateral epiphora, conjunctivitis, and enlarged submandibular lymph nodes
• Facial distortion and obstructed airflow are sometimes features of horses with an expanding mass within the sinuses
• Oral examination may reveal evidence of disease of a maxillary molar or a diastema adjacent to a maxillary molar

CAUSES
A complication of strangles or dental disease.

RISK FACTORS
• Horses 1–5 years old are most susceptible to *Streptococcus equi* var. *equi* infection and, therefore, are most susceptible to primary bacterial sinusitis
• The incidence of infundibular caries and periodontal disease, both causes of dental infection, increases with age, as does the incidence of neoplasia
• Horses that are confined to a stable or have recently undergone sinonasal surgery are at most risk of developing sinonasal mycotic infection

 DIAGNOSIS

DIFFERENTIAL DIAGNOSIS
Bilateral nasal discharge may signal that the right and left sinuses are infected, but bilateral nasal discharge is more indicative of diseases caudal to the nasal septum.

CBC/BIOCHEMISTRY/URINALYSIS
Usually normal.

IMAGING
• The different radiodensities of teeth and sinuses necessitate acquisition of multiple radiographs taken at different exposures and positions of the tube head to demonstrate detail of the sinuses and dental structures. The cassette should be positioned on the affected side
• Radiographs usually show increased opacity of the affected sinuses. Horizontal fluid lines within the sinuses are usually visible on a lateral radiograph of the skull
• The VCS is the usual site of inspissated exudate. Identifying a soft-tissue density dorsal to the maxillary molars on a lateral radiograph and medial to those teeth on a dorsoventral radiograph is evidence of a mass within the VCS
• To examine the apices of the maxillary teeth, the cassette is positioned on the affected side, and the tube head is placed dorsally, angled 30° ventrally, and centered on the rostral end of the facial crest

• Disease of a tooth whose apex resides within the sinuses can be recognized radiographically, with confidence, in only half of the cases
• CT can often provide additional details of the structures involved but may require general anesthesia

OTHER DIAGNOSTIC PROCEDURES
• Percussion may identify loss of resonance within the sinuses
• The oral cavity should be examined for evidence of dental problems
• Rhinoscopy may reveal exudate discharging from the sinuses at the drainage angle in the middle meatus or distortion of 1 or both conchae caused by an expanding mass within the sinuses
• Sinoscopy, performed through a trephine hole, may reveal the presence of exudate, a mass, or mycotic plaques. The VCS can be examined through a portal into the conchofrontal or caudal maxillary sinus, after the bulla of the maxillary septum has been perforated

PATHOLOGIC FINDINGS
• Cytologic examination and culture of exudate obtained by sinocentesis may help to determine whether sinusitis is caused by primary infection or is secondary to other disease. Multiple bacterial colonies can be cultured if infection is caused by dental disease or a mass. Identifying a single bacterial organism, usually a β-hemolytic *Streptococcus* sp., during cytologic examination or culture indicates that infection is primary, but sometimes a mixed bacterial population is cultured, obscuring the bacterial agent responsible for initiating the primary infection
• The cause of sinusitis is determined to be mycotic based on histologic observation of fungal hyphae and conidiophores in plaques removed from the sinuses and on culture of a heavy, pure growth of a potentially pathogenic fungus from the plaques

 TREATMENT

AIMS
The aim of treatment for primary sinusitis is to resolve infection by administering appropriate antimicrobial therapy and by evacuating exudate. The aim of treatment for secondary sinusitis is to resolve the primary cause.

APPROPRIATE HEALTH CARE
• Lavage of the sinuses and parenteral administration of antimicrobial therapy to resolve non-inspissated empyema caused by primary bacterial infection. The bacterial organism commonly isolated is usually sensitive to penicillin and other β-lactam antibiotics
• The sinuses are usually lavaged through an ingress portal created in the conchofrontal or

S

caudal maxillary sinus; the rostral maxillary sinus and VCS are most effectively lavaged, however, through a portal created in the rostral maxillary sinus. The nasomaxillary aperture provides egress for lavage solution
• Inspissated exudate in the VCS should be suspected when primary bacterial sinusitis fails to resolve with lavage and parenterally administered antimicrobial therapy; inspissated exudate must be removed
• Mycotic sinusitis can usually be resolved by lavaging the affected sinuses with an antifungal agent (e.g. itraconazole, fluconazole, enilconazole, miconazole, ketoconazole, natamycin, or clotrimazole) for 1–2 weeks
• To resolve sinusitis secondary to another disease (e.g. dental disease or a mass within the sinuses), the cause of the sinusitis must be resolved, often surgically. Resolving sinusitis secondary to dental infection usually necessitates removing the infected tooth

NURSING CARE
NSAIDs to reduce discomfort.

ACTIVITY
Exercise should be restricted for at least several weeks after signs of sinusitis have resolved.

SURGICAL CONSIDERATIONS
• Inspissated exudate is most easily removed from the VCS through a frontonasal flap, which often can be created with the horse standing. The bulla of the maxillary septum must be perforated to expose the VCS
• A molar can be extracted or repelled through a trephine hole or maxillary flap. A maxillary molar cannot be removed by lateral buccotomy, and endodontic therapy is often ineffective in resolving dental infection
• Extracting an infected tooth is usually accompanied by few complications and can be accomplished with the horse standing, whereas repelling a tooth is often accompanied by serious complications and is most commonly accomplished with the horse anesthetized

 MEDICATIONS

DRUG(S) OF CHOICE
• Primary bacterial empyema—parenteral administration of an antibiotic to which streptococci are susceptible, usually a β-lactam

antibiotic (e.g. procaine penicillin 20 000–50 000 IU/kg IM every 12 h) in conjunction with lavage of the sinuses
• Sinusitis secondary to other disease—administration of an antimicrobial drug, either broad spectrum or based on results of sensitivity testing of cultured bacteria, in conjunction with removing the source of infection
• Ancillary treatment for mycotic infection includes systemic administration of sodium iodide (20–40 mg/kg IV once daily) for 2–5 days and then oral administration of organic iodide (ethylenediamine dihydroiodide), until clinical signs have resolved

CONTRAINDICATIONS
Sodium iodide and organic iodide should not be administered to pregnant mares.

PRECAUTIONS
Side effects of systemic treatment with sodium iodide or organic iodide include excessive lacrimation, generalized alopecia, cough, abortion, and birth of a hypothyroid foal.

 FOLLOW-UP

PATIENT MONITORING
• Continued resolution of abnormal nasal discharge after antimicrobial therapy has been discontinued indicates infection has resolved
• Distortion of the nasal passages caused by an expanding mass resolves within several weeks after the mass has been removed
• Increased opacity of the sinuses may be observed radiographically long after sinusitis has resolved

PREVENTION/AVOIDANCE
• Vaccination of susceptible horses against S. equi on farms where strangles is endemic may decrease the incidence of primary sinusitis
• Routine dental care may decrease the incidence of dental disease that leads to dental infection and associated dental sinusitis

POSSIBLE COMPLICATIONS
• Unsuccessful treatment for primary sinusitis can usually be attributed to retention of inspissated exudate within the VCS
• Unsuccessful treatment for dental sinusitis can usually be attributed to alveolar infection caused by retention of osseous or dental

sequestra within the alveolus or, less commonly, from the presence of inspissated exudate within the VCS

EXPECTED COURSE AND PROGNOSIS
The long-term prognosis for horses affected by primary or dental sinusitis is good, provided that the horse receives proper treatment.

 MISCELLANEOUS

ASSOCIATED CONDITIONS
Horses affected by primary sinusitis caused by S. equi infection may have other sites of infection, including the guttural pouch.

SEE ALSO
• Guttural pouch empyema
• Purulent nasal discharge

ABBREVIATIONS
• CT = computed tomography
• NSAID = nonsteroidal anti-inflammatory drug
• VCS = ventral conchal sinus

Suggested Reading
Tremaine H, Freeman DE. Disorders of the paranasal sinuses. In: McGorum B, Dixon P, Robinson E, Schumacher J, eds. Equine Respiratory Medicine and Surgery. Philadelphia, PA: WB Saunders, 2006:393–407.
Author Jim Schumacher
Consulting Editors Mathilde Leclère and Daniel Jean

 Client Education Handout available online

BASICS

OVERVIEW
• The indolizidine alkaloid slaframine, or "slobber factor," is a mycotoxin produced by the "blackpatch" fungus *Rhizoctonia leguminicola*
• Slaframine is a pathogen of legumes, usually red clover (*Trifolium pratense*)
• Recent research involving nucleic acid sequencing suggests that the blackpatch fungus should be reclassified into the phylum Ascomycota as a new genus of ascomycete
• Other, less common substrates include alfalfa (*Medicago sativa*) and ladino or white clover (*Trifolium repens*)
• Following ingestion, slaframine is converted to an active metabolite (a ketoimine) in the liver that has a high affinity for the muscarinic receptor subtype responsible for regulation of exocrine glands (salivary glands and pancreas)
• The "blackpatch" fungus produces another indolizidine alkaloid, swainsonine, that may lead to signs including stiffness, weight loss, and violent behavior

SIGNALMENT
There are no breed, age, or sex predilections.

SIGNS
• Onset of hypersalivation (drooling) within hours of ingestion is the hallmark of this condition. Polydipsia is a consequence of fluid loss
• Less commonly reported signs include anorexia, weight loss, excessive lacrimation, polyuria, pollakiuria, abortion, colic, and diarrhea. Neurologic signs including stiffness and violent behavior may occur in slobbering horses in which significant ingestion of swainsonine has occurred

CAUSES AND RISK FACTORS
• Blackpatch is the fungal disease of clover associated with slaframine production. The plant pathogen, *R. leguminicola*, is most likely to grow on clover during warm, wet, humid weather
• A moist, humid environment with a temperature range of 25–29°C (the fungus does not grow at temperatures below 25°C) and a substrate pH of 5.9–7.5 is necessary to support growth. The fungus appears as dark spots or concentric rings on infected leaves and stems. Contaminated seed spreads the fungus. Consumption of infected pastures or second-cutting forage is usually associated with intoxication
• Geographic locations in which blackpatch has been confirmed include the midwestern and southeastern USA, Canada, Brazil, Japan, and the Netherlands

DIAGNOSIS

DIFFERENTIAL DIAGNOSIS
• Excessive salivation (sialorrhea) may result from dental disease, stomatitis, or foreign objects lodged in the oral cavity or the pharynx
• Ptyalism may result from inflammation of the oral mucosa or salivary glands by penetrating wounds or plant awns such as foxtail
• Hypersalivation seen in organophosphate and carbamate poisoning is associated with more life-threatening signs of dyspnea, colic, and diarrhea
• Staggering, nervousness, and lack of coordination may also be seen in animals affected with swainsonine toxicosis associated with locoism

CBC/BIOCHEMISTRY/URINALYSIS
N/A

OTHER LABORATORY TESTS
• Diagnosis is usually based on recognition of rapid onset of profuse salivation associated with consumption of legume forage infected with *R. leguminicola*
• Chemical analysis of suspect forage will confirm the presence of slaframine
• Slaframine can be detected in plasma samples obtained from affected animals
• Plant pathologists can confirm blackpatch disease on suspect forages

IMAGING
N/A

OTHER DIAGNOSTIC PROCEDURES
N/A

PATHOLOGIC FINDINGS
N/A

TREATMENT
Although specific antidotes are not available or in most cases necessary, introduction of uncontaminated forage will resolve the condition in 1–3 days.

MEDICATIONS

DRUG(S) OF CHOICE
The administration of atropine has been suggested for severe cases. Empirical evidence suggests that atropine given prior to exposure will prevent hypersalivation, although administration after the onset of hypersalivation is not particularly effective. Atropine should be used cautiously in horses because the risk of gastrointestinal side effects is significant (ileus, colic, etc.).

CONTRAINDICATIONS/POSSIBLE INTERACTIONS
N/A

FOLLOW-UP
Resolution of the problem occurs when horses are provided with uncontaminated forage.

PATIENT MONITORING
N/A

PREVENTION/AVOIDANCE
Storage of contaminated hay for several months results in significant reduction in toxicity. Red clover hay containing 50–100 ppm slaframine contained only about 7 ppm after 10 months of storage. Reseeding with newer clover varieties that are resistant to *Rhizoctonia* infection can solve persistent problems on a specific premises.

POSSIBLE COMPLICATIONS
N/A

COURSE AND PROGNOSIS
Removal of contaminated forage results in uncomplicated recovery in 1–3 days.

MISCELLANEOUS

ASSOCIATED CONDITIONS
N/A

AGE-RELATED FACTORS
N/A

ZOONOTIC POTENTIAL
N/A

PREGNANCY/FERTILITY/BREEDING
N/A

Suggested Reading
Croom WJ, Hagler WM, Froetschel MA, Johnson AD. The involvement of slaframine and swainsonine in slobbers syndrome: a review. J Anim Sci 1995;73:1499–1508.
Kagan IA. Blackpatch of clover, cause of slobbers syndrome: a review of the disease and the pathogen, *Rhizoctonia leguminicola*. Front Vet Sci 2016;3:3.

Authors Stan W. Casteel and Philip J. Johnson
Consulting Editors Wilson K. Rumbeiha and Steve Ensley

S

SMALL INTESTINAL OBSTRUCTION

 BASICS

DEFINITION
Impaired aboral transit of ingesta between the stomach and cecum.

PATHOPHYSIOLOGY
Small intestinal obstruction can be classified according to its degree of vascular involvement as strangulating or nonstrangulating. Whatever the cause, intestinal obstruction leads to distention with gas, fluid, and ingesta; this can compress intramural vasculature, leading to an increase in venous and capillary pressures and resulting in edema and, with time, necrosis of the intestinal wall. Once a certain intraluminal pressure threshold is reached there is net secretion, and more fluid will be sequestered in the lumen. This exacerbates distention and hypovolemia. Additionally, distention produces vascular compromise of the intestinal wall, contributing to adhesion formation. Intestinal distention activates pain receptors. In cases of vascular obstruction, simultaneous occlusion of the intestinal lumen and its blood supply occurs, leading to ischemic injury and possibly necrosis of the affected segment. A combination of pain (sympathetic stimulation) and inflammation results in ileus, further exacerbating the clinical signs.

SYSTEMS AFFECTED
• *GI*—vascular obstruction results in congestive and/or ischemic damage of the intestinal wall. Failure to resolve the obstruction will lead to intestinal wall necrosis. Chronic nonvascular obstructions may lead to hypertrophy of the intestinal muscular layer, reducing the intestinal lumen
• *Behavioral*—activation of pain receptors is associated with clinical signs of colic
• *Cardiovascular*—shock occurs secondary to hypovolemia, endotoxemia, and altered electrolyte balance; with gastric distention, pressure on the vena cava decreases cardiac return, thus cardiac output
• *Respiratory*—decreased pulmonary function may be secondary to pressure on the diaphragm from gastric distention or diaphragmatic herniation
• *Endocrine/metabolic*—affected patients frequently demonstrate metabolic alkalosis secondary to loss of chloride in intestinal secretions; as the condition progresses and hypovolemia ensues, metabolic lactic acidosis develops
• *Hemic/lymphatic/immune*—once tissue pressures exceed venous portal pressures, the small veins, venules, and lymphatics that drain the affected intestine collapse, and net fluid secretion into the bowel is potentiated. Hypovolemia results when excessive fluid is sequestered into the intestinal lumen

• *Renal/urologic*—hypovolemia is associated with decreased glomerular filtration rate and renin, angiotensin II, and aldosterone production and secretion

GENETICS
Inflammatory bowel disease—granulomatous enteritis and eosinophilic gastroenteritis.

GEOGRAPHIC DISTRIBUTION
Southeastern USA—ileal impaction and proximal enteritis.

SIGNALMENT
• Any age, sex, or breed
• Ascarid jejunal impactions are seen most commonly in foals/weanlings/yearlings
• Small intestinal intussusception and volvulus occur most often in horses < 3 years of age
• Small intestinal volvulus is most common in foals 2–4 months of age
• Abdominal tumors usually are identified in older horses
• 47–71% of horses with epiploic foramen entrapment are < 11 years of age
• Incidence of strangulating lipoma is 5 times higher in horses > 15 years
• Inguinal hernias are observed in stallions
• Proximal enteritis may occur more commonly in stallions
• Gastrosplenic ligament incarceration of the small intestine has been described most often in male horses
• Mesoduodenal rents and diaphragmatic hernias can be seen in mares during late gestation
• Warmbloods, Standardbreds, Tennessee Walking Horses, and American Saddlebreds appear to be predisposed to inguinal herniation

SIGNS

Historical Findings
• Horses with partial obstruction may display subacute, intermittent signs of abdominal pain or vague signs of lethargy, weakness, or weight loss. Transient episodes of abdominal pain may recur over a period of weeks to months and may progress in severity with time
• Complete small intestinal obstruction is associated with signs of severe, persistent abdominal pain and ileus
• Recent anthelmintic treatment contributes to ascarid impaction
• Previous infection with *Streptococcus equi* can result in abscessation within the small intestinal mesentery ("bastard strangles")

Physical Examination Findings
• Clinical signs depend on the lesion present, its location, duration, and severity
• Most common signs—abdominal discomfort, tachycardia, discolored mucous membranes, prolonged capillary refill time, clinical dehydration, decreased to absent small intestinal borborygmi, gastric reflux from the small intestine (yellow-brown, fetid odor, pH 6–8), and distended loops of small

intestine and/or dehydrated colon contents contained within prominent colon haustra on rectal examination

CAUSES

Nonstrangulating, Intraluminal Obstruction
• Impaction—feed, trichobezoar, ascarids, or tapeworms
• Foreign body
• Healed duodenal ulcer, with scarring and stricture
• Granulomatous enteritis

Nonstrangulating, Extraluminal Obstruction
• Tension on duodenocolic ligament secondary to distention or displacement of the large colon
• Adhesions—ischemic bowel, peritonitis, prolonged distention, excessive or traumatic surgical manipulation, anastomotic leakage, tissue dehydration, and inappropriate suture or technique
• Ileal muscular hypertrophy
• Ileal neurogenic stenosis
• Ileocecal valve edema or infarction secondary to migrating strongyle larvae
• Diverticula—traction, pulsion, or Meckel's
• Mesenteric abscess
• Neoplasia—pedunculated lipoma, lymphosarcoma, leiomyosarcoma, or carcinoid
• Intramural hematoma

Strangulating Obstruction
• Volvulus
• Herniation—inguinal/scrotal, umbilical, diaphragmatic, epiploic foramen, gastrosplenic, nephrosplenic, or tears in mesentery/omentum/ligaments/fibrous bands/adhesions
• Intussusceptions
• Vaginal evisceration

Functional (Ileus)
• Intestinal distention and ischemia
• Intestinal inflammation—duodenitis/proximal jejunitis, enterocolitis, surgical manipulation, or resection/anastomosis
• Endotoxemia
• Peritonitis
• Pain—GI, musculoskeletal
• Drugs—α-adrenergic agonists, opioids
• General anesthesia
• Hypovolemia/hypotension
• Electrolyte imbalances
• Parasitism

RISK FACTORS

Diet
• Sudden changes in feed or feeding practices
• Moldy hay or grain
• Poor quality or low-grade roughage
• Decreased roughage intake over 24 h
• Coastal Bermuda hay—ileal impaction (regional)
• Pelleted feed—impaction

S

• Decreased water intake or availability—impaction

Management
Poor deworming program—ascarid impaction, large strongyle migration, and infarction.

Body Condition
Obesity—pedunculated lipoma.

DIAGNOSIS
DIFFERENTIAL DIAGNOSIS
Differentiating Similar Signs
GI reflux usually is pathognomonic for small intestinal obstruction.

Differentiating Causes
The ability to differentiate between causes depends on the severity of clinical findings, which may be influenced by location of the lesion, length of intestine involved, and stage of disease.

Abdominal Pain
• In affected horses, some degree of gastric distention usually is present, which contributes to signs of abdominal pain
• Abdominal pain may be absent in foals with umbilical or inguinal hernias
• Biphasic abdominal pain has been associated with ileal impaction
• Severe, acute abdominal pain usually is associated with strangulating lesions—volvulus
• Ileocecal intussusception is accompanied by severe, acute abdominal pain, which subsides in 8–12 h to mild, intermittent pain that can persist for weeks to months, until complete obstruction occurs

Clinical Findings
• Intestinal involvement in an umbilical hernia usually is evident on palpation—pain on palpation of the hernia may indicate a strangulating hernia
• Inguinal hernias may be accompanied by mild to severe scrotal swelling, palpable loops of intestine within the scrotum, and decreased scrotal temperature because of vascular obstruction

Palpation per Rectum
• Only the caudal 30–40% of the abdomen is palpable on rectal evaluation, but distention usually pushes affected intestinal segments backwards
• In cases of small intestinal strangulation, distended loops of small intestine were palpated in 50–98% of horses
• A thick, tubular structure palpable in the center of the abdomen may indicate ileal impaction, jejunal intussusception, or ileal intussusception
• Resentment to palpation of the ileocecal region often accompanies ileocecal intussusception

• Asymmetric inguinal rings, intestine or mesentery extending into an inguinal ring, or inability to identify 1 inguinal ring represent palpation findings in horses with inguinal herniation
• If ileum is involved in inguinal herniation, the edematous antimesenteric ileocecal band may be palpable entering the ring on the affected side

CBC/BIOCHEMISTRY/URINALYSIS
• The WBC count usually is not affected by acute intestinal strangulation or obstruction
• Leukocytosis/neutrophilia with a left shift may be observed with peritonitis, proximal enteritis, or mesenteric abscessation
• Leukopenia/neutropenia may develop secondary to intestinal necrosis or endotoxemia
• Most cases are accompanied by an increased packed cell volume and TP because of fluid sequestration within the bowel
• Hypoproteinemia may develop as the disease progresses
• Hypoalbuminemia may be observed with proximal enteritis or mesenteric abscessation
• Hypergammaglobulinemia may be found with mesenteric abscessation or lymphosarcoma—β- and γ-fractions
• Decreased potassium and chloride levels occur with intraluminal fluid loss, and decreased sodium and calcium levels occur secondary to extracellular fluid shifts
• Loss of hydrochloric acid with gastric reflux results in metabolic alkalosis
• Acute strangulating obstructions associated with release of endotoxin, increased production of lactic acid, and hypoperfusion result in metabolic acidosis
• If small intestinal obstruction occurs in the region of the hepatopancreatic ampulla, increases in total bilirubin, alkaline phosphatase, and γ-glutamyltransferase may be observed
• Serum amyloid A concentrations improve the ability to differentiate horses requiring surgical intervention

OTHER LABORATORY TESTS
N/A

IMAGING
• Abdominal ultrasonography should be used to assess small intestinal wall thickness and movement
• Edema of the wall of the small intestine (> 3 mm wall thickness), distention, and absence of motility are suggestive of strangulating obstruction
• Intestinal intussusception may display a characteristic concentric ring or "bull's eye" appearance
• Abdominal radiography may be useful in distinguishing small from large intestinal problems in foals
• Contrast radiography in foals may be used to demonstrate GI obstruction

OTHER DIAGNOSTIC PROCEDURES
Abdominocentesis
• Normal nucleated cell count for adults ranges from 5000 to 10 000 cells/μL; however, in foals a cell count > 1500 cells/μL is considered elevated
• As peritonitis and intestinal ischemia progress, the fluid becomes increasingly serosanguineous and cloudy as the cellularity and protein levels increase
• WBC to TP ratios < 3 and red blood cell to TP ratios < 15 represent nonstrangulating obstructions or proximal enteritis; ratios > 3 or 15, respectively, indicate strangulating lesions
• Peritoneal fluid may be evaluated cytologically for neoplastic cells
• Peritoneal lactate concentration higher than the simultaneously measured blood lactate concentration is indicative of intestinal strangulation and ischemia
• Horses with strangulating obstruction have a higher peritoneal lactate value (> 7 mmol/L) than those with nonstrangulating obstruction (< 3 mmol/L)

Endoscopy
• May be used to identify duodenal ulcers
• A 2.5–3.0 m endoscope is needed to visualize this region in adults

Laparoscopy and Celiotomy
May be performed to diagnose and correct the cause of obstruction or for intestinal biopsy.

TREATMENT
• Horses with strangulating lesions will require surgical intervention to correct the lesion
• Nasogastric decompression is vital. Horses may be transported with nasogastric tubes left in place
• Exploratory laparotomy is necessary if a surgical lesion can be identified during rectal palpation or abdominocentesis, if abdominal pain becomes uncontrollable, or if there is a lack of response to medical therapy
• IV fluid therapy is important to maintain hydration and tissue perfusion. Balanced polyionic IV solutions (e.g. lactated Ringer solution) are ideal; rate and quantity depend on the horse's status
• The decision whether to administer IV fluids before transport depends on the horse's condition. Often, rehydration increases the volume of gastric reflux, so gastric decompression may need to be performed more frequently
• Hyperimmune serum or polymyxin B (6000 U/kg body weight) may benefit horses with endotoxemia

S

SMALL INTESTINAL OBSTRUCTION

MEDICATIONS

DRUG(S) OF CHOICE
• Sedation and analgesia may be achieved with xylazine (0.2–1.1 mg/kg IV) or detomidine (0.005–0.02 mg/kg IV); both duration and quality of sedation or analgesia may be enhanced by coadministration of butorphanol tartrate (0.1 mg/kg IV)
• NSAIDs such as flunixin meglumine (1.1 mg/kg IM or IV BID) or phenylbutazone (2.2–4.4 mg/kg PO or IV BID) may be used for analgesic and anti-inflammatory effects as well as to mediate the effects of endotoxin
• Endotoxemia also may be treated with polymyxin B (6000 U/kg diluted in 0.5–1.0 L of saline IV BID) or pentoxifylline (8.5 mg/kg PO BID)
• Specific therapies for ileus, sepsis, gastric ulcers, and laminitis are discussed elsewhere

CONTRAINDICATIONS
Acepromazine for sedation in hypovolemic horses.

PRECAUTIONS
• Continued monitoring after administration of analgesics is important to ensure the drug is not masking signs of pain while the disease process progresses
• Certain drugs (e.g. xylazine, detomidine, opioids) decrease GI motility
• Gentamicin, amikacin, and polymyxin B are potential nephrotoxic drugs

POSSIBLE INTERACTIONS
N/A

ALTERNATIVE DRUGS
N/A

FOLLOW-UP

PATIENT MONITORING
Depends on cause of obstruction and method of treatment.

POSSIBLE COMPLICATIONS
• Gastric rupture
• Intestinal necrosis
• Abdominal adhesions
• Thrombophlebitis
• Laminitis
• Hypovolemic or endotoxic shock

MISCELLANEOUS

ASSOCIATED CONDITIONS
• Endotoxemia
• Ileus
• Impaction of the large or small colon secondary to dehydration
• Laminitis

AGE-RELATED FACTORS
N/A

ZOONOTIC POTENTIAL
N/A

PREGNANCY/FERTILITY/BREEDING
Outcome of pregnancy is determined more by the cardiovascular and metabolic status of the mare and fetus than by the specific cause of the condition.

SYNONYMS
N/A

SEE ALSO
• Acute adult abdominal pain—acute colic Duodenitis–proximal jejunitis (anterior enteritis, proximal enteritis)
• Endotoxemia
• Ileus

ABBREVIATIONS
• GI = gastrointestinal
• NSAID = nonsteroidal anti-inflammatory drug
• TP = total protein
• WBC = white blood cell

Suggested Reading
Desrochers A. White NA. Diagnostic approach to colic. In: Blikslager AT, White NA, Moore JN, Mair TS, eds. The Equine Acute Abdomen, Hoboken, NJ: Wiley-Blackwell, 2017:223–263.
Freeman DE. Small intestine. In: Auer JA, Stick JA, eds. Equine Surgery, 3e. St. Louis, MO: Saunders Elsevier, 2006:401–436.

Author Antonio M. Cruz
Consulting Editors Henry R. Stämpfli and Olimpo Oliver-Espinosa
Acknowledgment The author and editors acknowledge the prior contribution of Judith B. Keonig and Annette M Sysel.

S

SMOKE INHALATION

BASICS

OVERVIEW
• A mixture of hot air, solid particulates, gases, fumes, and vapors
• Composition depends on burning material(s) and fire environment
• Structural fires and wildfires may present different hazards
• Principal primary mechanisms that lead to injury are direct thermal and chemical injury to the respiratory tract, asphyxiation, and intoxication from toxic gases
• Secondary pathophysiologic mechanisms include cardiovascular dysfunction, immunosuppression, systemic inflammatory response, and delayed posthypoxic leukoencephalopathy
• Heat/flame denatures proteins from thermal injury
• Gaseous irritants and asphyxiants cause both local and systemic effects. Carbon monoxide, cyanide, hydrogen sulfide, and carbon dioxide are common asphyxiants
• Asphyxiants lead to hypoxia
• Water-soluble irritants such as ammonia cause irritation in the URT, leading to epithelial necrosis and edema
• Particulates ≤5 μm cause lung or respiratory tract injury depending on size
• Thermal burns to the skin are not covered in this book, but require attention
• There are 3 clinical phases of a severe smoke inhalation event—early phase (within 24 h), intermediate phase (12 h to 5 days), and late phase (>5–7 days):
  ◦ Clinical signs of early phase are caused mainly by carbon monoxide and cyanide; but also by thermal injury
  ◦ Clinical signs of the intermediate phase are caused by pulmonary edema and systemic inflammatory response
  ◦ Late phase is caused by bronchopneumonia—impaired mucociliary clearance and alveolar macrophage function, together with the effects of smoke inhalation, to predispose patients to Gram-negative bacterial infection
  ◦ Another late-phase sequela is delayed posthypoxic leukoencephalopathy characterized by laminar cortical necrosis and reactive gliosis caused by apoptotic die off triggered by CO
• Other systems affected include skin, cardiovascular, nervous, and renal systems

SIGNALMENT
N/A

SIGNS
• Depend on the composition of inhaled smoke, duration of exposure, and presence or absence of predisposing medical conditions
• Singed hair, URT inflammation, soot-stained nasal discharge, and the smell of smoke suggest smoke exposure; observe asymptomatic patients closely for 1 week after exposure
• In the early phase, clinical signs may reflect carbon monoxide and/or cyanide poisoning. Affected horses may show signs of severe hypoxemia, depression, irritable behavior, or be moribund to comatose. Horses may exhibit tachypnea and tachycardia
• Heat and chemical injuries may cause tachypnea, dyspnea, cough, drooling, or nasal discharge
• Cyanosis and dehydration may be observed
• Severe respiratory distress and signs of shock may be evident in the intermediate phase
• Upper airway edema may be progressive and lead to airway obstruction
• Thoracic auscultation may reveal decreased lung sounds, crackles, or wheezes
• Signs of multiple organ failure may be present in severe cases—acute renal failure, cardiac failure, and CNS effects such as ataxia, seizures, and coma
• In the late phase, clinical findings may be similar to bronchopneumonia
• In cases of secondary bacterial infection, fever will be present
• Worsening of clinical signs after initial improvement suggests secondary bacterial bronchopneumonia

CAUSES AND RISK FACTORS
• Confined/enclosed spaces
• Wild bush fires
• Preexisting conditions such as asthma, chronic obstructive pulmonary disease, and cardiovascular, CNS, or renal disease increase the risk of a severe outcome

DIAGNOSIS

DIFFERENTIAL DIAGNOSIS
• Inflammatory airway diseases—endoscopy, physical examination, tracheobronchial aspirates or lavage, clinical pathology
• Heaves (severe equine asthma, recurrent airway obstruction)—seasonal disorder associated with environmental changes, physical examination, endoscopy, radiography, bronchoalveolar lavage fluid cytology
• Acute respiratory distress syndrome—physical examination, history, radiographs, arterial blood gases
• Pneumonia (bacterial or fungal)—clinical signs, physical examination, clinical pathology, endoscopy, radiography, tracheobronchial aspirates or lavage, ultrasonography
• Exposure to poisonous gases or vapors—history of exposure, possible environmental gas measurement
• Pulmonary neoplasia—endoscopic examination, tracheobronchial aspirates or lavage, radiography, ultrasonography, biopsy

CBC/BIOCHEMISTRY/URINALYSIS
• Leukocytosis and hyperfibrinogenemia indicate an inflammatory process
• Severe cases may reveal increased creatinine and blood urea nitrogen, suggesting prerenal or renal failure
• Decreased oxygen saturation using pulse oximetry
• Carboxyhemoglobinemia
• Measurable blood cyanide
• Methemoglobinemia
• Lactic acidosis

OTHER LABORATORY TESTS
• Cytology of tracheal fluid may reveal carbon particles in phagocytic cells
• Bacterial culture and antibiotic sensitivity testing of transtracheal fluid to document bronchopneumonia and to determine appropriate antibiotic therapy

IMAGING
Thoracic Radiography
• Chest radiographs are a very important diagnostic aid. Expect diffuse bronchial and peribronchial lesions or diffuse, patchy interstitial infiltration, which are suggestive of edema
• Radiographic findings indicative of pneumothorax, pneumomediastinum, and emphysema may be found in severe cases
• Because the disease is progressive, take serial chest radiographs to monitor presence or lack of disease progression
• Radiographic lesions may not correlate with the severity of pulmonary dysfunction
• MRI for leukoencephalopathy

OTHER DIAGNOSTIC PROCEDURES
• Endoscopy may reveal airway edema and inflammation, mucosal necrosis, and soot deposits
• ECGs are recommended for animals with preexisting cardiovascular disease
• Other imaging procedures mentioned above

TREATMENT
• Remove animals from further exposure
• General supportive care should be aimed at providing a patent airway, reversing bronchospasms and hypoxemia, decreasing pulmonary inflammation and edema, and providing ventilatory support
• Nebulization
• Specific treatment for carbon monoxide and cyanide poisoning if indicated
• Supplemental humidified 100% oxygen may be needed if hypoxemia is severe
• Suction the URT to clear mucus and fluid, soot, and cell debris
• Perform a tracheotomy if signs suggest upper airway obstruction; patients maintained with tracheal tubes require careful and frequent nursing care to prevent obstruction of the tube by secretions

S

• IV fluid administration is indicated in most horses, because dehydration and renal failure often are present. Administer with caution, however, to prevent exacerbation of pulmonary edema and overhydration. Fluid selection is based on serum electrolyte disturbances and acid–base status
• Antibiotics to treat bronchopneumonia

MEDICATIONS
DRUG(S) OF CHOICE
• Early use of bronchodilators to control bronchospasm and airway obstruction—β_2-adrenergic agonists (e.g. clenbuterol 0.8–3.2 µg/kg PO every 12 h or albuterol (salbutamol) 0.8–1.5 µg/kg by inhalation) may be administered safely to most horses; aminophylline (5–10 mg/kg PO or IV every 12 h) may be associated with toxic side effects (e.g. tachycardia, hyperesthesia, and excitement)
• Furosemide (1–2 mg/kg IM or IV) may be given for treatment of upper airway or pulmonary tract edema
• DMSO (1.0 g/kg in a 20% solution IV (slowly) every 24 h or 12 h) may be potentially effective
• Antibiotic prophylaxis in affected horses is controversial because it may lead to development of bacterial resistance. In severe cases, however, early antibiotic treatment with broad-spectrum activity may be justified. In cases of confirmed secondary bacterial infection, use specific antibiotics as determined by culture and sensitivity tests

• NSAIDs (e.g. phenylbutazone 4.4 mg/kg PO or IV daily) may be beneficial in decreasing mediator release and controlling fever

CONTRAINDICATIONS/POSSIBLE INTERACTIONS
• Concurrent treatment with aminophylline may potentiate the diuretic effect of furosemide
• Corticosteroid therapy is controversial and associated with increased septic complications (e.g. bacterial bronchopneumonia); avoid such therapy if possible

FOLLOW-UP
• Horses with no or minimal respiratory tract edema have a favorable prognosis and those with bronchopneumonia have a guarded prognosis
• Horses should preferably be hospitalized for at least 12 h post exposure and monitored closely for 1 week. Sudden deterioration can occur
• The time required for complete recovery varies with the severity of the injury; several months may be needed before the animal can return to work
• Modify the environment to reduce dust, molds, and other irritants to avoid development of airway hypersensitivity
• Serial chest radiographs over several days or weeks should be helpful in assessing recovery
• Possible complications are heaves, bronchopneumonia, or permanent neural complications (e.g. seizures)

MISCELLANEOUS
ASSOCIATED CONDITIONS
N/A
AGE-RELATED FACTORS
N/A
ZOONOTIC POTENTIAL
N/A
PREGNANCY/FERTILITY/BREEDING
N/A
SEE ALSO
• Inspiratory dyspnea
• Pleuropneumonia
• Pneumothorax
ABBREVIATIONS
• CNS = central nervous system
• DMSO = dimethylsulfoxide
• MRI = magnetic resonance imaging
• NSAID = nonsteroidal anti-inflammatory drug
• URT = upper respiratory tract

Suggested Reading
Geor RJ, Ames TR. Smoke inhalation injury in horses. Compend Contin Educ Pract Vet 1991;13:1162–1169.
Kemper T, Spiers S, Barratt-Boyes SM, Hoffman R. Treatment of smoke inhalation in five horses. J Am Vet Med Assoc 1993;202:91–94.
Marsh PS. Fire and smoke inhalation injury in horses. Vet Clin North Am Equine Pract 2007;23:19–30.

Author Wilson K. Rumbeiha
Consulting Editors Wilson K. Rumbeiha and Steve Ensley

S

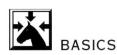

BASICS

DEFINITION
Condition associated with bite from a venomous snake.

PATHOPHYSIOLOGY
• Pit viper venoms are complex mixtures of enzymes (including myotoxins, proteases, hyaluronidase, bradykinin-releasing enzyme, phospholipase A_2, hemorrhagins) that are responsible for causing significant local tissue destruction, including myonecrosis, edema, hemorrhage, and inflammation. Systemically, venom enzymes and nonenzymatic peptides can alter capillary permeability with subsequent loss of plasma volume that can result in decreased cardiac output, hypoproteinemia, hypotension, and metabolic acidosis leading to respiratory and circulatory collapse. Other venom toxins induce hemolysis, platelet aggregation, thrombocytopenia, and alterations in the coagulation cascade. Mojave toxin, present in some rattlesnake subpopulations, is a neurotoxin that interrupts transmission at the neuromuscular junction, resulting in paralysis
• Coral snake venom consists mostly of neurotoxins; phospholipase A, which causes hemolysis, may also be present

SYSTEMS AFFECTED
Pit Vipers
• Skin, musculoskeletal—local skin and soft tissue necrosis and hemorrhage that advances outward from the bite; sloughing of skin and underlying tissue
• Respiratory—upper airway obstruction (head and neck bites), direct damage to alveolar membranes, hemorrhage of pulmonary capillary bed
• Hemic—alteration of vascular endothelial cell integrity, red blood cell lysis, vasodilation, stimulation of coagulation cascade via factor X activation, enhanced production of fibrin degradation products, enhanced platelet aggregation
• Neuromuscular—neuromuscular junction dysfunction causing loss of skeletal muscle control
• Cardiovascular—arrhythmia, myocardial necrosis ± fibrosis by unknown mechanism
• Renal/urologic—nephrotoxic effects of myoglobinuria, hemoglobinuria, defibrination syndrome, disseminated intravascular coagulopathy, direct toxic effect, and hypovolemic shock

Coral Snakes
• Nervous—neurotoxins cause irreversible decrease in neurotransmission at neuromuscular junctions. Possible sequelae include bulbar paralysis and respiratory arrest from diaphragmatic paralysis
• Hemic—hemolysis
• Musculoskeletal—rhabdomyolysis

GENETICS
N/A

INCIDENCE/PREVALENCE
• Most bites occur from April to October
• Several hundred horses are bitten each year by pit vipers, mostly by rattlesnakes in western USA; bites from coral snakes are rare

GEOGRAPHIC DISTRIBUTION
• Pit vipers—widely dispersed throughout the USA
• Coral snakes—restricted to southern edges of the USA

SIGNALMENT
N/A

SIGNS
General Comments
• Most horses are bitten on or near the muzzle, fewer are bitten on the lower limbs, and bites to the trunk are uncommon
• Less than 50% of bitten horses develop multiple or severe manifestations of envenomation
• Most pit viper envenomations elicit local swelling within 60 min. Onset of systemic signs may be delayed for up to 6 h, so patients should be monitored for at least that duration. Lack of local signs does not indicate that life-threatening problems will not occur, particularly with bites from pit vipers with neurotoxic venom
• Coral snake envenomations may have latent periods of up to 18 h between bite and onset of clinical signs

Physical Examination Findings
Pit Vipers
• Marked skin discoloration and painful soft tissue swelling with hemorrhage at bite location. Fang marks may be obscured by tissue edema
• Swelling of head/neck may lead to airway obstruction, causing dyspnea and tachypnea. With severe systemic toxicosis, dyspnea may occur owing to pulmonary edema or hemorrhage
• Hemolysis and/or coagulopathy may develop
• Cardiac abnormalities (tachycardia, dysrhythmias) may occur in severe cases
• Neurotoxic envenomations may lead to muscle fasciculation, weakness, flaccid paralysis, and/or respiratory failure
• Other possible signs include fever, epistaxis, lethargy, diarrhea, salivation, dysphagia, incontinence, laminitis, colic, shock, and coma

Coral Snakes
• Fang wounds are usually small and without hemorrhage
• Neurotoxic effects include dysphagia, salivation, muscle fasciculations, bulbar paralysis, flaccid paralysis, and respiratory paralysis

CAUSES
• In the USA 2 venomous snake families exist—Crotalidae (pit vipers), including *Agkistrodon* (copperheads and cottonmouth water moccasins), *Crotalus* (rattlesnakes), and *Sistrurus* (pygmy and massasauga rattlesnakes); and Elapidae, including eastern coral snakes (*Micrurus fulvius fulvius*) and Texas coral snakes (*Micrurus fulvius tenere*)
• Pit vipers have bilateral pits between nostrils and eyes, elliptical pupils, and well-developed and retractable maxillary fangs that are hollow, hinged, and rotate forward for striking and delivering venom
• Coral snakes have small heads, black snouts, round pupils, and banded red, yellow, and black color patterns. Coral snakes are shy, nocturnal, and have small, fixed, front maxillary fangs, all of which makes them less of a threat to large livestock

RISK FACTORS
• Because of their large body mass, adult horses have some innate protection from envenomations, but fatalities do occur
• Severity of venomous snake bites is based on species of snake, age of the snake, circumstances of the bite, and venom composition
• Snakes control the amount of venom delivered—defensive bites tend to be less severe than agonistic bites
• Venom from young snakes tends to contain a high peptide fraction, causing less severe local injury, but more severe systemic effects. Additionally, venom in early spring may contain higher peptide fraction concentrations
• Bite location, victim size, and activity level after envenomation influence the speed and extent of venom systemic circulation and severity of toxicosis

DIAGNOSIS

DIFFERENTIAL DIAGNOSIS
• Insect sting/bite
• Trauma
• Foreign body/abscess
• Clostridial myositis
• Purpura haemorrhagica
• Botulism

CBC/BIOCHEMISTRY/URINALYSIS
• Echinocytosis
• Elevated creatine phosphokinase, aspartate aminotransferase, sorbitol dehydrogenase, lactate
• Initial hemoconcentration
• Hemolysis, anemia
• Leukocytosis, inflammatory leukogram
• Hypoproteinemia
• Thrombocytopenia

S

SNAKE ENVENOMATION   (CONTINUED)

OTHER LABORATORY TESTS
• Coagulopathy—prolonged activated clotting time, prothrombin time, and partial thromboplastin time
• High fibrin degradation products
• Metabolic acidosis

IMAGING
N/A

OTHER DIAGNOSTIC PROCEDURES
ECG if dysrhythmias occur.

PATHOLOGIC FINDINGS
• Extensive soft tissue edema, hemorrhage, and necrosis at/around bite
• Generalized congestion, petechiation of major organs
• ± Myocardial inflammation/fibrosis with effusion
• Laminitis, pneumonia, secondary infections

TREATMENT

APPROPRIATE HEALTH CARE
• Goals include maintaining patent airway, preventing/controlling shock, neutralizing venom, reducing swelling, and alleviating pain
• Rigid tubing can be sutured into nostrils to maintain patent nasal passages. In 1 report, 57% of rattlesnake-envenomated horses required tracheotomy
• IV crystalloids to enhance tissue perfusion, maintain hydration, and combat shock and hypotension

NURSING CARE
• Whole blood or blood products to correct anemia, thrombocytopenia, and clotting abnormalities
• Local wound management—continuous cleansing, hydrotherapy, and debridement
• Administer tetanus antitoxin or toxoid as appropriate
• Swelling may affect food prehension or drinking—ensure adequate intake

ACTIVITY
Minimize activity to decrease distribution of venom.

CLIENT EDUCATION
• Size and condition of the wound site may not correlate with severity of the systemic signs
• Avoid first aid techniques such as tourniquets, cryotherapy, lancing, suction, and electroshock
• Systemic signs may be delayed by several hours, so immediate treatment is essential
• Delay in seeking medical intervention can significantly worsen prognosis

SURGICAL CONSIDERATIONS
Rarely, fasciotomy may be indicated to manage compartment syndrome.

MEDICATIONS

DRUG(S) OF CHOICE
• Specific antivenins:
  ○ *M. fulvius*—immune globulin, equine origin (Wyeth)
  ○ Crotalidae—polyvalent, equine origin (Boehringer Ingelheim); polyvalent F(ab), sheep origin (BTG International); polyvalent F(ab)$_2$, horse origin (Bioveteria, Instituto Bioclon, and MT Venom Co.)
  ○ Most effective when administered shortly after envenomation, especially when combating local tissue necrosis and neurologic sequelae
  ○ Initial dose is 5 vials IV; however, clinical improvement has been seen when 1 or 2 vials were administered to horses
• NSAIDs (e.g. flunixin meglumine) can be used 24 h after the bite for control of pain and swelling. Use caution when using NSAIDs in patients with coagulopathy or thrombocytopenia. Consider opioids in cases where NSAIDs are ineffective
• Broad-spectrum antibiotic may be indicated, especially for horses with distal leg wounds
• Tetanus toxoid administration as needed

CONTRAINDICATIONS
• Heparin
• DMSO

PRECAUTIONS
• Corticosteroid use is controversial. Single dose dexamethasone administered within hours of envenomation may help reduce swelling, inflammation, and pain. Long-term, high-dose corticosteroids may depress immune responses against venom, foster secondary infection, or alter laboratory parameters used in monitoring disease progression
• Antihistamines are of little benefit

POSSIBLE INTERACTIONS
N/A

ALTERNATIVE DRUGS
N/A

FOLLOW-UP

PATIENT MONITORING
• Assess CBC, serum chemistry panel, clotting panel, and fibrinogen at least every 12–24 h (more often if patient is deteriorating)

• Close monitoring of respiratory and cardiovascular systems is recommended
• Cardiac troponin levels in cases where cardiac dysfunction has occurred; peak troponin levels have occurred as late as 30 days post envenomation

PREVENTION/AVOIDANCE
N/A

POSSIBLE COMPLICATIONS
Cardiac dysfunction, liver disease, serum sickness (from antivenin), pneumonia, colitis, laminitis, pharyngeal paralysis, various wound complications (slough, infection, etc.).

EXPECTED COURSE AND PROGNOSIS
• Clinical signs may last up to 2 weeks
• Use of a modified rattlesnake bite severity score similar to that used in humans and dogs may be helpful in determining prognosis
• Equine mortality rate after rattlesnake bites in range 9–25%
• Coral snake envenomations with neuromuscular signs warrant guarded prognosis

MISCELLANEOUS

ASSOCIATED CONDITIONS
N/A

AGE-RELATED FACTORS
Young foals or ponies are at higher risk because of their small body mass.

SEE ALSO
N/A

ABBREVIATIONS
• DMSO = dimethylsulfoxide
• NSAID = nonsteroidal anti-inflammatory drug

Suggested Reading
Fielding CL, Pusterla N, Magdesian KG, et al. Rattlesnake envenomation in horses: 58 cases (1992–2009). J Am Vet Med Assoc 2011;238:631–635.
Gilliam LL, Holbrook TC, Ownby CL, et al. Cardiotoxicity, inflammation, and immune response after rattlesnake envenomation in the horse. J Vet Intern Med 2012;26:1457–1563.

Author Sharon Gwaltney-Brant
Consulting Editors Wilson K. Rumbeiha and Steve Ensley
Acknowledgment The author and editors acknowledge the prior contribution of Patricia A. Talcott and Michael Peterson.

S

BASICS

OVERVIEW
• A serum sodium concentration greater than the upper limit in normal horses is generally >144 mEq/L
• Sodium is the major extracellular cation in the body, and therefore, is critical for maintenance of the extracellular space
• Serum sodium concentration reflects the ratio of whole-body sodium to whole-body water; therefore, knowledge of the hydration state is important for accurate interpretation of serum sodium concentrations
• Hypernatremia usually reflects an absolute or relative water deficiency
• Systems affected—nervous: hypernatremia may lead to hyperosmolality and intracellular water loss from neurons, in turn leading to central nervous system shrinkage

SIGNALMENT
Any breed, age, or sex.

SIGNS
• Lethargy
• Weakness
• Seizures
• Coma
• Death
• Severity of signs depends on the duration and degree of hypernatremia
• Other signs depend on the underlying cause

CAUSES AND RISK FACTORS
• Normal whole-body sodium with pure water loss—water deprivation because of unavailable water source or physical abnormality causing decreased ingestion (e.g. botulism or dysphagia); prolonged hyperventilation; central and nephrogenic DI; evaporative loss from extensive burns; exhausted horse syndrome
• Low whole-body sodium with hypotonic fluid loss—urinary loss (osmotic diuresis, e.g., osmotic diuretic administration such as mannitol); gastrointestinal loss (early stages of diarrhea, before the point of compensatory water intake occurs)
• High whole-body sodium—excessive sodium chloride intake (i.e. salt poisoning) with water restriction; IV or oral administration of hypertonic saline or sodium bicarbonate solutions

DIAGNOSIS

DIFFERENTIAL DIAGNOSIS
• History or physical examination to detect decreased water intake or excessive water loss resulting in (hypertonic) dehydration
• See Causes and Risk Factors

CBC/BIOCHEMISTRY/URINALYSIS
• High serum sodium concentration
• Hyposthenuria—consider DI
• Decreased potassium, chloride, calcium, and magnesium; stress neutrophilia and lymphopenia, occasionally leukopenia—consider exhausted horse syndrome

OTHER LABORATORY TESTS
• Urinary FE_{Na}—a single urine sample can be used for sodium and creatinine measurements, which are compared with serum sodium and creatinine concentrations determined at the same time ($[Na^+_u/Na^+_s]/[Cr_u/Cr_s]$; normal <1%); suspect extrarenal water loss if urine volume with FE_{Na} <1% and clinical signs of dehydration; suspect osmotic diuresis if urine volume is increased with an FE_{Na} >1% and clinical signs of dehydration.
• Plasma osmolality—should be high with hypernatremia
• Other laboratory tests depend on the underlying cause:
  ○ ADH (vasopressin) blood concentration in conjunction with water deprivation—nephrogenic DI if vasopressin ≥3; neurogenic DI or not DI if vasopressin is normal
  ○ The ADH response test with vasopressin administered IV, and urine osmolality measured at 2 h intervals—neurogenic DI if urine osmolality/urine specific gravity increases to ≥1.025

IMAGING
N/A

OTHER DIAGNOSTIC PROCEDURES
N/A

TREATMENT
• Treatment depends on the severity of hypernatremia and the underlying disorder
• If increases in sodium and chloride are proportional, administer IV fluids such that decreases in serum sodium concentration do not exceed 0.5 mEq/L/h
• If chloride is increased disproportionately compared with sodium, evaluate and treat the acid–base imbalance

MEDICATIONS

DRUG(S) OF CHOICE
Treat the underlying disorder.

CONTRAINDICATIONS/POSSIBLE INTERACTIONS
The combination of hypernatremia and dehydration is a therapeutic dilemma because rapid reduction of serum sodium concentrations can lead to cerebral and pulmonary edema. Decreases in serum sodium concentration should not exceed 0.5 mEq/L/h.

FOLLOW-UP

PATIENT MONITORING
Electrolytes, acid–base status, urine output, water intake, and body weight.

POSSIBLE COMPLICATIONS
Seizures, convulsions, and probable permanent neurologic damage in severe, longstanding cases, or with rapid correction of serum sodium concentrations.

MISCELLANEOUS

SEE ALSO
• Chloride, hyperchloremia
• Osmolality, hyperosmolality

ABBREVIATIONS
• ADH = antidiuretic hormone
• DI = diabetes insipidus
• FE_{Na} = fractional excretion of sodium

Suggested Reading
George JW, Zabolotzky SM. Water, electrolytes, and acid base. In: Latimer KS, ed. Duncan & Prasse's Veterinary Laboratory Medicine Clinical Pathology, 5e. Hoboken, NJ: Wiley Blackwell, 2011:146–147.
Jose-Cunilleras E. Abnormalities of body fluids and electrolytes in athletic horses. In: Hinchcliff KW, Kaneps AJ, Geor RJ, eds. Equine Sports Medicine and Surgery, 2e. Philadelphia, PA: Saunders, 2013:881–885.

Authors Wendy S. Sprague and Martin David
Consulting Editor Sandra D. Taylor

S

SODIUM, HYPONATREMIA

 BASICS

OVERVIEW
• A serum sodium concentration less than the lower limit of normal horses is generally <132 mEq/L.
• Sodium is the major extracellular cation in the body, and therefore, is critical for maintenance of the extracellular space
• Serum sodium concentration reflects the ratio of the whole-body sodium to whole-body water; therefore, knowledge of the hydration state is important for accurate interpretation of serum sodium concentrations
• Hyponatremia usually results from relative water excess and is usually not clinically significant until serum sodium concentrations are <122 mEq/L
• Systems affected
  ○ Nervous—cerebral edema (also seen with rapid correction of severe hyponatremia)
  ○ Renal/urologic—medullary washout
  ○ Hemic/lymphatic/immune—intravascular hemolysis

SIGNALMENT
Any breed, age, or sex.

SIGNS
• Lethargy
• Tremors
• Abnormal gait
• Central blindness
• Seizures
• Severity of signs depends on the rapidity and degree of hyponatremia

CAUSES AND RISK FACTORS
• Loss of sodium-containing fluid—diarrhea, pronounced sweating, hemorrhage, excessive gastrointestinal fluid drainage by nasogastric intubation, excessive pleural fluid drainage, saliva loss, sustained exercise, protein-losing enteropathies, colitis, and acute kidney injury (usually in foals)
• Adrenal insufficiency (e.g. iatrogenic) or adrenal exhaustion
• Sequestration of fluid (third spacing)—peritonitis, ascites, uroperitoneum (usually in foals), and gut torsion, volvulus, obstruction, or ileus
• Iatrogenic—administration of hypotonic fluids or diuretics
• Inappropriate water retention—psychogenic polydipsia, renal disease, inappropriate antidiuretic hormone secretion, heart failure, hepatic fibrosis, and severe hypoalbuminemia
• Prolonged diuresis secondary to hyperglycemia and glucosuria may result in medullary washout and subsequent hyponatremia and hypochloremia

 DIAGNOSIS

DIFFERENTIAL DIAGNOSIS
• Dependent on the underlying cause
• Azotemia and hyperkalemia in foals—consider renal disease and uroperitoneum

CBC/BIOCHEMISTRY/URINALYSIS
• Low serum sodium concentration
• Other abnormalities depend on the underlying cause

OTHER LABORATORY TESTS
• Urinary FE_{Na}—a single urine sample can be used for sodium and creatinine measurements, which are compared with serum sodium and creatinine concentrations determined at the same time $([Na^+_u/Na^+_s]/[Cr_u/Cr_s]$; normal <1%); suspect renal disease if FE_{Na} >1%
• Plasma osmolality—should be low with hyponatremia; if in the normal or high range, rule out renal failure and causes of pseudohyponatremia

IMAGING
N/A

OTHER DIAGNOSTIC PROCEDURES
N/A

 TREATMENT

• Treatment depends on the severity of hyponatremia and the underlying disorder
• Correct acute, rapid hyponatremia and chronic hyponatremia (≅48 h) gradually
• Moderate hyponatremia (122–132 mEq/L)—treatment probably not critical, but depends on clinical signs
• Treat severe hyponatremia; therapy depends on acuteness of the disorder
• Acute hyponatremia—elevate serum sodium to 125 mEq/L over 6 h, then gradually increase to normal. The amount of Na^+ needed to elevate serum Na^+ to a concentration of 125 mEq/L = (125 – measured serum Na^+ (mEq/L) × 0.67 × body weight (kg)). Isotonic or hypertonic (3%) saline is suggested for states of volume contraction
• Chronic hyponatremia—not well-defined in horses; appropriate fluid would be 0.45% NaCl in 2.5% dextrose; use the formula above to calculate the amount of Na^+ needed
• If chloride is decreased disproportionately compared with sodium, evaluate and treat the acid–base imbalance

 MEDICATIONS

DRUG(S) OF CHOICE
• Sodium bicarbonate—if indicated for severe metabolic acidosis, calculate the dose carefully to avoid correcting sodium too rapidly
• DMSO and NSAIDs (e.g. phenylbutazone, flunixin meglumine) can be used for treatment of cerebral ischemia and inflammation
• Corticosteroids can be used with caution for cerebral edema
• Mannitol for cerebral edema; not recommended with suspected cerebral hemorrhage or chronic hyponatremia

CONTRAINDICATIONS/POSSIBLE INTERACTIONS
• Rapid correction of serum sodium in cases of chronic hyponatremia has led to osmotic cerebral demyelination in humans, but this has not been reported in horses
• Mannitol is hyperosmolar

 FOLLOW-UP

PATIENT MONITORING
Electrolytes, acid–base status, urine output, and body weight.

POSSIBLE COMPLICATIONS
Dependent on the underlying cause.

 MISCELLANEOUS

ASSOCIATED CONDITIONS
Other acid–base and electrolyte abnormalities.

SEE ALSO
• Acute kidney injury (AKI) and acute renal failure (ARF)
• Chloride, hypochloremia
• Diarrhea, neonate
• Potassium, hyperkalemia

ABBREVIATIONS
• DMSO = dimethylsulfoxide
• FE_{Na} = fractional excretion of sodium
• NSAID = nonsteroidal anti-inflammatory drug

Suggested Reading
Staempfli H, Oliver-Espinosa O. Clinical chemistry tests. In: Smith BP, ed. Large Animal Internal Medicine, 5e. St. Louis, MO: Elsevier Mosby, 2015:356–361.

Authors Wendy S. Sprague and Martin David
Consulting Editor Sandra D. Taylor

S

SOLANUM SPP. (NIGHTSHADE) TOXICOSIS

BASICS

OVERVIEW
• Numerous *Solanum* spp. (nightshade family) are potentially toxic to animals—*Solanum nigrum* (black nightshade), *Solanum dulcamara* (bittersweet nightshade), *Solanum carolinense* (horsenettle), *Solanum rostratum* (buffalo burr), *Solanum tuberosum* (potato), and others
• Plants in this genus are widely distributed
• Toxicity is attributed primarily to tropane alkaloids and steroidal glycoalkaloids (e.g. solanine), but few equine data are available
• Anticholinergic, muscarinic, and GI irritant effects have been described in intoxicated animals
• Muscarinic effects may result from cholinesterase inhibition, but this has not been verified clinically
• GI irritation is believed to result from a saponin-like effect of the steroidal glycoalkaloids
• Toxicity varies with environment, plant part ingested, and time of year
• Unripe berries contain the highest glycoalkaloid concentration, which declines with maturity
• Green portions of potato contain the highest toxin concentration
• Documented cases of equine intoxication are rare, and those in the literature do not provide significant information concerning pathophysiologic effects

SIGNALMENT
No known breed, age, or sex predilections.

SIGNS
• GI signs predominate—anorexia, nausea, salivation, colic, and diarrhea with or without blood
• Nervous system signs—apathy, drowsiness, trembling, progressive weakness or paralysis, recumbency, and coma

CAUSES AND RISK FACTORS
• Contamination of hay with *Solanum* spp.
• Unavailability of alternative desirable forage
• Access to old potatoes or potato refuse

DIAGNOSIS

DIFFERENTIAL DIAGNOSIS
• Establishing the diagnosis relies on evidence of consumption of *Solanum* spp.
• Detection of alkaloids in GI contents is possible but not commonly performed
• Other causes of colic—physical examination, lack of exposure to *Solanum* spp.

CBC/BIOCHEMISTRY/URINALYSIS
N/A

OTHER LABORATORY TESTS
N/A

IMAGING
N/A

OTHER DIAGNOSTIC PROCEDURES
N/A

PATHOLOGIC FINDINGS
• Evidence of plant in the stomach
• Grossly, there may be evidence of GI irritation and diarrhea with or without hemorrhage
• Histopathologically, there is congestion, inflammation, hemorrhage, and ulceration of the GI mucosa

TREATMENT
• Remove animal from source of exposure
• If soon after ingestion, consider GI decontamination
• Symptomatic and supportive care

MEDICATIONS

DRUG(S) OF CHOICE
• AC (1–2 g/kg PO in water slurry (1 g of AC in 5 mL of water))
• 1 dose of cathartic (70% sorbitol at 3 mL/kg PO or sodium or magnesium sulfate at 250 mg/kg PO, the last 2 being administered in a water slurry) with AC if no diarrhea or ileus
• NSAIDs—flunixin meglumine (0.1 mg/kg IV or IM as necessary)

CONTRAINDICATIONS/POSSIBLE INTERACTIONS
N/A

FOLLOW-UP

PATIENT MONITORING
N/A

PREVENTION/AVOIDANCE
• Limit or prevent access to *Solanum* spp.
• Do not feed potatoes or potato refuse

POSSIBLE COMPLICATIONS
N/A

EXPECTED COURSE AND PROGNOSIS
• With early intervention and appropriate symptomatic and supportive care, prospects for recovery are good
• With severe clinical signs, prognosis is guarded

MISCELLANEOUS

ASSOCIATED CONDITIONS
N/A

AGE-RELATED FACTORS
N/A

ZOONOTIC POTENTIAL
N/A

PREGNANCY/FERTILITY/BREEDING
Congenital craniofacial malformations have been induced in fetuses of pregnant laboratory animals fed *Solanum* spp. glycoalkaloids. The significance of this finding for horses is unknown, but do prevent pregnant mares from ingesting any *Solanum* spp.

ABBREVIATIONS
• AC = activated charcoal
• GI = gastrointestinal
• NSAID = nonsteroidal anti-inflammatory drug

Suggested Reading
Burrows GE, Tyrl RJ. Toxic Plants of North America. Ames, IA: Iowa State University Press, 2001:1127.
Dalvi RR, Bowie WC. Toxicology of solanine: an overview. Vet Hum Toxicol 1983;25:13–15.

Authors Arya Sobhakumari and Robert H. Poppenga
Consulting Editors Wilson K. Rumbeiha and Steve Ensley

S

SOLAR ABSCESS

BASICS

OVERVIEW
- Infection in the superficial subsolar aspect of the foot due to penetration of the sole with a sharp object followed by premature closure of the entrance hole, resulting in abscess formation
- Subsolar hematoma in a severely bruised foot may become secondarily infected through small cracks, allowing bacterial penetration
- Systems affected—musculoskeletal, foot

SIGNALMENT
No breed, sex, age, or sport predilection.

SIGNS
- Sudden acute severe lameness, pointing of the toe of the affected foot
- Heat in the hoof capsule and pounding digital pulses
- Swelling of the heel bulb or at the coronary band may indicate proximal migration of infection. Just before drainage, a painful soft focal area may be appreciated
- Focal sensitivity to hoof tester application or generalized solar pain
- Distal limb swelling may be noted, especially with deep or severe infections
- Malodorous fluid leakage from the tract once the abscess breaks open

CAUSES AND RISK FACTORS
- Penetration of the bottom of the foot with a sharp object (e.g. horseshoe nail, rock)
- Risk factors include laminitis, thin soles, and equine Cushing disease

DIAGNOSIS

DIFFERENTIAL DIAGNOSIS
- Severe solar bruising—no drainage will rule out
- Improper horseshoe nail placement—focal sensitivity around a nail after shoeing
- Laminitis—rule out with radiography
- Deep penetrating wound through the sole—rule out with contrast radiography
- Coffin bone fracture—rule out with radiography
- Navicular bone fracture—rule out with radiography

CBC/BIOCHEMISTRY/URINALYSIS
Usually normal; hyperfibrinogenemia and increased serum amyloid A in chronic cases.

OTHER LABORATORY TESTS
None

IMAGING
- Radiography—radiolucent gas or fluid within subsolar regions may be noted. Radiology is also useful to rule out other causes of foot lameness and identify possible complications

- Radiographic evaluation should be repeated in 2–3 weeks in chronic cases and/or if infectious osteitis is suspected. Bone lysis and bone sequestrum formation may be noted

OTHER DIAGNOSTIC PROCEDURES
- Hoof tester application
- Foot poultice or foot soaks often help to moisten sole and localize the abscess
- Conscientious and directed paring of the sole and frog with a hoof knife to encourage drainage
- Microbial culture and sensitivity of exudate is not necessary

TREATMENT
- The objective of treatment is to open and drain the abscess, remove diseased tissue, and protect the site from contamination
- Drainage is established by paring the sole with a sharp hoof knife. The hole should be just large enough for adequate drainage. Aggressive or overzealous debridement is discouraged
- For superficial, localized infection, antiseptic dressing and foot protection are all that is needed
- For deep infection, perineural analgesia of the foot may be necessary to facilitate extensive debridement
- The affected foot may be periodically soaked in hot or warm Epsom salt and povidone–iodine solutions until drainage and infection subside
- Foot protection is accomplished with bandages, bandages with duct tape, a waterproof foot boot, and, in some cases, a shoe with a hospital treatment plate
- Horses are stall confined or limited to small paddock turnout. Bedding should be dry and clean
- Long term, horses may be shod with pads until the solar defect fills in

MEDICATIONS

DRUG(S) OF CHOICE
- Tetanus toxoid and antitoxin
- NSAIDs—phenylbutazone 2.2–4.4 mg/kg every 12–24 h as needed
- Tincture of iodine can be applied to the wound
- Systemic broad-spectrum antimicrobials are indicated for horses with infectious osteitis and severe infections
- Regional limb antimicrobial perfusion is rarely necessary

CONTRAINDICATIONS/POSSIBLE INTERACTIONS
Systemic broad-spectrum antimicrobials may be contraindicated in mild cases since they prolong the clinical signs.

FOLLOW-UP

PATIENT MONITORING
Significant improvement in lameness and other clinical signs is apparent once drainage is established.

PREVENTION/AVOIDANCE
Horseshoes with pads are indicated in flat or thin-soled horses and in horses ridden on rocky or uneven terrain.

POSSIBLE COMPLICATIONS
- Infectious osteitis and bone sequestrum formation
- Contralateral limb laminitis in horses with prolonged non-weight-bearing lameness

EXPECTED COURSE AND PROGNOSIS
- For horses with superficial uncomplicated infections, disease course is short and prognosis is excellent
- Horses with complicated infections require longer and aggressive treatment. Prognosis is fair to good

MISCELLANEOUS

ASSOCIATED CONDITIONS
- Laminitis
- Older horses with pituitary pars intermedia dysfunction

AGE-RELATED FACTORS
None

ZOONOTIC POTENTIAL
None

PREGNANCY/FERTILITY/BREEDING
N/A

SEE ALSO
- Laminitis
- Penetrating injuries to the foot
- Pituitary pars intermedia dysfunction

ABBREVIATIONS
NSAID = nonsteroidal anti-inflammatory drug

Suggested Reading
Baxter GM, Stashak TS, Belknap JK. Penetrating wounds of the foot. In: Baxter GM, ed. Adams and Stashak's Lameness in Horses, 6e. Ames, IA: Wiley Blackwell, 2011:523–525.

Author Elizabeth J. Davidson
Consulting Editor Elizabeth J. Davidson

SOLUBLE OXALATE TOXICOSIS

BASICS

OVERVIEW
- Ingestion of plants containing oxalic acid or soluble sodium and potassium oxalates
- Oxalate concentrations in plant material vary widely between different parts of the plant, along with seasonal, environmental, and geographic factors
- Green leaves and fruiting structures tend to contain higher oxalate concentrations.
- *Halogeton* spp. are an exception—concentrations may increase as the plant matures and are often highest when the plant is dead and dry
- Plants potentially containing dangerous amounts of soluble oxalates include—*Agave americana, Amaranthus* spp., *Anagallis arvensis, Beta vulgaris,* some *Brassica* spp., *Chenopodium* spp., *Galenias* spp., *Halogeton glomeratus, Kochia scoparia, Mesembryanthemum* spp., *Oxalis* spp., *Phytolacca americana, Portulaca oleracea, Rheum rhaponticum, Rumex* spp., *Salsola* spp., *Sarcobatus vermiculatus, Setaria* spp., *Tetragonia* spp., and *Trianthema* spp.; most of these plants are considered unpalatable when the oxalate content is high
- Most common in the summer and fall months, when other forage is unavailable and large amounts of plant material are ingested over a short period of time
- Ingestion of excess soluble oxalates causes GI discomfort along with muscular weakness and paralysis owing to hypocalcemia; and acute renal injury
- Nephrosclerosis and osteodystrophia fibrosa have been recorded in horses after chronic ingestion of oxalates, though uncommon

SIGNALMENT
N/A

SIGNS
- Acute signs relate predominantly to hypocalcemia
- Within 2–6 h of ingestion—depression, colic, and muscular weakness
- Possible recumbency, convulsions, unconsciousness, and death
- Chronic signs may relate to renal disease, including polydipsia, polyuria, and generalized weight loss

CAUSES AND RISK FACTORS
- Overgrazing areas highly contaminated with oxalate-containing plants
- Inadequate supplemental feed
- Low-calcium diets enhance soluble oxalate absorption; calcium binds oxalate in the GI tract to form insoluble calcium oxalate

DIAGNOSIS

DIFFERENTIAL DIAGNOSIS
- Hypocalcemia—poor diet and starvation and lactation tetany
- Acute renal disease—vitamin K3, NSAIDs, vitamin D, heavy metal, aminoglycoside, and acorn toxicoses
- Chronic renal failure—glomerulonephritis, chronic interstitial nephritis, pyelonephritis, amyloidosis, and neoplasia

CBC/BIOCHEMISTRY/URINALYSIS
- Hypocalcemia most consistent
- In cattle and sheep—modest elevations in serum liver enzymes, hyperglycemia, azotemia, hyperphosphatemia, and hyperkalemia; proteinuria and hematuria

OTHER LABORATORY TESTS
Oxalate content of suspect plant material.

PATHOLOGIC FINDINGS
- Erythema and edema of the GI mucosa are most commonly seen
- Necrosis of the proximal renal tubules and collecting ducts, with birefringent crystals; crystals also may be seen within vascular spaces

TREATMENT
- Hospitalize patients for initial medical workup and management
- Fluid replacement therapy for any volume deficits and correction of any electrolyte and acid–base abnormalities are critical in patients with GI distress or possible renal failure
- Fluid therapy also tends to slow precipitation of calcium oxalate crystals within the renal tubule lumen

MEDICATIONS

DRUG(S) OF CHOICE
- IV infusion of calcium gluconate, e.g. 250–500 mL of 23% calcium gluconate diluted in fluids; alternatively 150–250 mg/kg calcium gluconate IV (slowly to effect) for hypocalcemia
- Acute or chronic renal failure should be treated accordingly; treatment options vary depending on whether oliguria or polyuria is present

CONTRAINDICATIONS/POSSIBLE INTERACTIONS
N/A

FOLLOW-UP

PATIENT MONITORING
- Monitor respiration and cardiac rate and rhythm during administration of calcium gluconate
- Monitor serum concentrations of calcium, sodium, chloride, potassium, bicarbonate, urea nitrogen, creatinine, packed cell volume, total protein, phosphorus, and central venous pressure in patients with severe GI distress or impaired renal function

PREVENTION/AVOIDANCE
- Prevent access to soluble oxalate-containing plants through pasture management—animal rotation; herbicide treatment
- Do not allow hungry animals access to highly contaminated areas
- Make adequate supplemental forage available to animals grazing contaminated areas
- Oral dicalcium phosphate prevents this disease in cattle and sheep

EXPECTED COURSE AND PROGNOSIS
- Clinically affected horses may not recover
- Animals that survive acute intoxication may suffer renal failure, which carries a poor prognosis
- Horses, being relatively resistant to the renal effects of soluble oxalates, may have a somewhat better prognosis than do affected cattle and sheep

MISCELLANEOUS

ABBREVIATIONS
- GI = gastrointestinal
- NSAID = nonsteroidal anti-inflammatory drug

Suggested Reading
Radostits OM, Gay CC, Blood DC, Hinchcliff KW, eds. Veterinary Medicine: A Textbook of the Diseases of Cattle, Sheep, Pigs, Goats and Horses, 9e. Philadelphia, PA: WB Saunders, 2000:1636–1639.

Author Steve Ensley
Consulting Editors Wilson K. Rumbeiha and Steve Ensley

Acknowledgment The editors acknowledge the prior contribution of Patricia A. Talcott.

S

SORBITOL DEHYDROGENASE (SDH)

BASICS

DEFINITION
• SDH catalyzes the reversible oxidation of D-sorbitol to D-fructose with the help of NAD
• The rate of oxidation of NADH is directly proportional to the rate of conversion of D-fructose to D-sorbitol
• SDH is present in high concentrations in hepatocytes, kidneys, and testes, but serum activity is attributed exclusively to hepatocyte origin
• Alanine aminotransferase activity is low in hepatocytes of horses; therefore, SDH is the enzyme of choice for detection of hepatocellular injury/necrosis

PATHOPHYSIOLOGY
• SDH is free within the cytoplasm of hepatocytes and is more specific than AST or glutamate dehydrogenase in detecting hepatocellular damage
• The half-life is less than 12 h, so serum concentrations can return to reference concentrations within days after a single insult
• SDH is a specific indicator of acute and ongoing hepatocellular injury because of its short half-life and tissue specificity
• The degree of elevation generally is proportional to the number of hepatocytes affected, not to the severity of a particular insult
• Activity of SDH may increase within 4 h of a single incident of hepatocellular injury and return to the reference range within 2–3 days. In comparison, AST (which is also an indicator of hepatocellular injury) takes longer to peak after injury and the half-life is 7–8 days
• When hepatocellular injury occurs, SDH increases rapidly, before AST. Elevated SDH concentrations with normal or increased AST concentrations are indicative of acute or ongoing hepatocellular injury
• If serial serum biochemistry profiles reveal continuously or progressively increased SDH concentrations, ongoing hepatocellular injury is likely
When treating hepatic disease, liver-specific enzymes can be used to monitor cessation of insult. If recent hepatocellular injury has been documented, and serial serum biochemistry panels reveal elevated AST and progressively decreasing or normal SDH activity, it is likely that the initial insult has ceased

SYSTEMS AFFECTED
Hepatobiliary

GENETICS
N/A

INCIDENCE/PREVALENCE
N/A

GEOGRAPHIC DISTRIBUTION
N/A

SIGNALMENT
• Any breed, age, or sex
• Tyzzer's disease occurs in neonatal foals

SIGNS
General Comments
Signs of hepatic failure do not appear until at least 75% of the hepatic functional mass is lost.

Historical Findings
• Exposure to hepatotoxins
• Weight loss

Physical Examination Findings
Icterus, poor body condition, bilirubinuria, neurologic deficits (hepatic encephalopathy), photosensitization, fever with liver diseases.

CAUSES
• Anomaly, congenital diseases—portosystemic shunts, biliary atresia
• Degenerative conditions—cirrhosis, cholelithiasis
• Infectious and immune-mediated disease—hepatitis (e.g. viral, bacterial, protozoal, fungal, parasitic), Theiler's disease, amyloidosis, sepsis, endotoxemia, chronic active hepatitis
• Metabolic diseases—shock, hypovolemia, hypoxia caused by severe GI disease, anesthesia or severe anemia
• Neoplastic or nutritional diseases—primary neoplasia, metastatic neoplasia, hepatic lipidosis
• Toxic or trauma—pyrrolizidine alkaloid-containing plants, cottonseed, castor bean, oak, alsike clover, fungal toxins (e.g. aflatoxins, cyclopiazonic acid, fumonisin, phalloidin [mushrooms]) and chemical compounds/elements such as ethanol, chlorinated hydrocarbons, carbon tetrachloride, monensin, copper, iron, and petroleum

RISK FACTORS
• Obesity
• Exposure to toxic compound or plants
• Halothane anesthesia, particularly of prolonged duration

DIAGNOSIS

DIFFERENTIAL DIAGNOSIS
See Causes.

CBC/BIOCHEMISTRY/URINALYSIS
CBC
• Liver disease may cause a nonregenerative anemia and morphologic changes (e.g. acanthosis, target cells, nonspecific poikilocytosis, normochromic microcytosis in portosystemic vascular shunts)
• Leukocytosis or leukopenia with or without a left shift may be seen with inflammation; neutrophil toxicity may also be observed

Biochemistry
• Glucose—decreased in end-stage liver disease and sepsis/endotoxemia
• Blood urea nitrogen—decreased in liver insufficiency and end-stage liver disease because of decreased conversion of ammonia to urea
• Albumin—decreased in end-stage liver disease because of decreased production; minimally to mildly decreased in inflammation
• Globulins—generally increased in end-stage liver disease and/or chronic antigenic stimulation
• AST—increased with injury to striated muscle and/or hepatocytes. Marked increases in serum AST and SDH concentrations are suggestive of acute or active hepatocellular injury. Marked increases in serum AST concentration with mild to moderate changes in SDH concentration suggest chronic hepatic injury or recovery from acute injury
• ALP—increased with concurrent cholestatic disease; the highest concentrations of serum ALP concentration are associated with cholangitis, biliary cirrhosis, or extrahepatic bile duct obstruction
• γ-Glutamyltransferase—increased with cholestatic disease or hepatocellular injury
• Conjugated bilirubin—increases in cholestatic disease
• Unconjugated bilirubin—increases with anorexia and hemolysis
• Triglycerides—may be increased in association with hepatic lipidosis
• SDH is unstable at room temperature or when refrigerated and may lose as much as 25% of its activity during freezing after 1 week, unlike other enzymes which are far more stable. If sample is not analyzed within 8–12 h, then storage in a freezer is highly recommended

Urinalysis
Bilirubinuria—conjugated bilirubin, detected by the commonly used "dipstick" and the diazo tablet methods indicates cholestatic disease and should not be elevated if only hepatocellular injury is present.

OTHER LABORATORY TESTS
SBAs
• Sensitive test for hepatobiliary disease but not specific for type of liver disease
• May be increased with cell injury, cholestasis, or hepatic insufficiency/decreased functional mass
• One advantage of SBA compared with plasma ammonia concentration (which is a more specific test for hepatic insufficiency/decreased functional mass) is that SBAs are not labile, so immediate analysis of the sample is not necessary

Plasma Ammonia Concentration
• Hepatic insufficiency/decreased functional mass is indicated by increased fasting or challenged concentration of ammonia

• A sensitive and specific test, because it is not affected by other factors (e.g. cholestasis); however, ammonia measurement requires special handling, which limits its general availability
• Consultation with the reference laboratory for specific submission requirements is needed

Coagulation Tests and Plasma Fibrinogen Concentration
• The liver synthesizes many coagulation factors, and significant decreases in liver function may lead to deficiencies in these factors and to coagulation abnormalities
• Activated partial thromboplastin time and prothrombin time—decreases in these parameters occur when <30% of the activity of the factors is present

Toxicology
Analysis of tissue biopsy, feed, ingesta, serum/plasma, or other body fluids may indicate presence of a toxin.

Bacterial, Fungal, or Viral Culture
• May establish a definitive diagnosis regarding the infectious agent and help guide treatment
• Request bacterial antibiotic sensitivity to determine appropriate antibiotic therapy

IMAGING

Transabdominal Ultrasonography
• Evaluate size, echogenicity, shape, and position of liver
• Useful for guidance when obtaining liver biopsy for cytology, histopathology, and microbiology

OTHER DIAGNOSTIC PROCEDURES
Liver biopsy for cytology (impression smear) and histopathology of formalin-fixed tissue.

PATHOLOGIC FINDINGS
Dependent on the underlying cause.

 TREATMENT
• Avoid negative energy balance, especially in ponies and donkeys, to avoid/treat hyperlipemia and hepatic lipidosis
• A high-carbohydrate, low-protein diet reduces ammonia production
• Specific therapy depends on the underlying cause

 MEDICATIONS

DRUG(S) OF CHOICE
• Fluid and nutritional support may be needed
• Anorexic and hypoglycemic cases may benefit from IV 5% dextrose (2 mL/kg/h); otherwise, fluid support depends on specific electrolyte and acid–base abnormalities
• Lactulose (333 mg/kg PO every 8 h) by nasogastric tube is suggested to combat GI ammonia production/absorption but may cause diarrhea

CONTRAINDICATIONS
N/A

PRECAUTIONS
With suspected hepatic insufficiency, assess coagulation profiles before performing invasive procedures.

POSSIBLE INTERACTIONS
Dependent on the underlying cause.

ALTERNATIVE DRUGS
N/A

 FOLLOW-UP

PATIENT MONITORING
Serial serum biochemical analyses to monitor progression or improvement of the disease process.

PREVENTION/AVOIDANCE
Dependent on the underlying cause.

EXPECTED COURSE AND PROGNOSIS
• Dependent on the underlying cause
• Hypoglycemia and hemolysis associated with liver disease indicate a poor prognosis

 MISCELLANEOUS

ASSOCIATED CONDITIONS
Dependent on the underlying cause.

AGE-RELATED FACTORS
See Signalment.

ZOONOTIC POTENTIAL
N/A

PREGNANCY/FERTILITY/BREEDING
N/A

SEE ALSO
• Ammonia, hyperammonemia
• Aspartate aminotransferase (AST)
• Bile acids
• Gamma-glutamyltransferase (GGT)

ABBREVIATIONS
• ALP = alkaline phosphatase
• AST = aspartate aminotransferase
• GI = gastrointestinal
• SBA = serum bile acid
• SDH = sorbitol dehydrogenase

Suggested Reading
Barton MH. Disorders of the liver. In: Reed SM, Bayly WM, Sellon DC, eds. Equine Internal Medicine, 3e. St. Louis, MO: WB Saunders, 2010:939–975.
Helene A, Perron MF, Sandersen C, et al. Prognostic value of clinical signs and blood parameters in equids suffering from hepatic diseases. J Equine Vet Sci 2005;25:18–25.
Meyer DJ, Walton RM. The liver. In: Walton RM, ed. Equine Clinical Pathology. Ames, IA: Wiley Blackwell, 2014:71–86.
Peek SF. Icterus. In: Robinson NE, Sprayberry KA, eds. Current Therapy in Equine Medicine, 6e. St. Louis, MO: WB Saunders, 2009:489–493.
Smith GW. Diseases of the hepatobiliary system. In: Smith BP, ed. Large Animal Internal Medicine, 5e. St. Louis, MO: Elsevier Mosby, 2015:843–872.

Author Jenifer R. Gold
Consulting Editor Sandra D. Taylor
Acknowledgment The author and editor acknowledge the prior contribution of Armando R. Irizarry-Rovira.

S

SORGHUM SPP. TOXICOSIS

BASICS

OVERVIEW
• Chronic ingestion of *Sorghum vulgare* var. *sudanense* (sudangrass or hybrid sudangrass) causes cystitis, ataxia, and teratogenesis in horses. Grazing of sudan pastures and ingestion of freshly cut hay are associated with the syndrome but feeding of cured hay is not
• Generally, intoxication occurs during periods of high rainfall and rapid plant growth. Fertilization has no effect on toxicity
• The toxin is believed to be a lathyrogenic agent, γ-glutamyl-β-cyanoalanine. Onset of clinical signs is after weeks to months (average of 8 weeks) of grazing a sudangrass pasture
• Geographically, sudangrass is most commonly used as a forage in the southwestern and central USA. Ingestion of *Sorghum* spp. is also associated with cyanide and nitrate toxicoses (see chapters Cyanide toxicosis and Nitrate/nitrite toxicosis for more in-depth discussion of these intoxications)

SIGNALMENT
Sorghum cystitis—ataxia is more common in mares but can occur in geldings or studs. All ages are susceptible.

SIGNS
• Posterior ataxia and incoordination
• Forced movement enhances ataxia
• Falling when backed up
• Recumbency
• Constant urine dribbling from a full bladder
• Urine scalding
• Cystitis
• Frequent opening and closing of vulva (winking)
• Mares may appear to be in constant estrus
• Fetal malformations (extreme flexion of joint or ankylosis) when mares graze sudangrass between days 20 and 50 of gestation
• Secondary complications of urinary tract and kidney infection

CAUSES AND RISK FACTORS
• Grazing sudangrass is the primary risk
• Johnson grass has also been implicated

DIAGNOSIS

DIFFERENTIAL DIAGNOSIS
• Polyneuritis equi (cauda equina neuritis)
• Cystitis of other causes
• Trauma
• Abscess
• Neoplasia
• Equine herpesvirus 1 myeloencephalitis
• Equine protozoal encephalitis
• Equine viral encephalitis
• Rabies

CBC/BIOCHEMISTRY/URINALYSIS
• Leukocytosis

• Lymphocytosis
• Sediment—large numbers of red blood cells, white blood cells, epithelial cells, bacteria, hyaline casts, and granular casts
• Normal pH and specific gravity
• Proteinuria

OTHER LABORATORY TESTS
Urine bacterial cultures generally isolate opportunistic bacteria such as *Escherichia coli*, *Proteus vulgaris*, *Staphylococcus* spp., *Pseudomonas aeruginosa,* or *Corynebacterium* spp.

IMAGING
N/A

OTHER DIAGNOSTIC PROCEDURES
N/A

PATHOLOGIC FINDINGS
• Gross pathology—cystitis with marked thickening of the bladder wall
  ○ Full bladder
  ○ Hyperemic ureters
  ○ Hyperemic urethra
  ○ Vaginal hyperemia
  ○ Ulcerations of the bladder mucosa
  ○ External abrasions from falling
  ○ Areas of urine-scalded skin
  ○ Pyelonephritis
• Histopathology—necrotizing cystitis
  ○ Pyelonephritis
  ○ Inflammation of the ureters, urethra, bladder, and vagina
  ○ Axonal degeneration of the spinal cord and cerebellum
  ○ Myelomalacia of the spinal cord and cerebellum

TREATMENT
• Treatment can be managed on an outpatient basis
• Generally, treatment is unsuccessful in horses that exhibit incoordination and/or urine dribbling
• Temporary cure of cystitis/pyelonephritis can be achieved but recurrence 2–3 weeks after therapy is stopped is common
• Prevent further exposure by removing horses from access to sudangrass
• Treat urine-scalded areas
• Antimicrobial treatment of cystitis/pyelonephritis should be based upon culture and sensitivity tests

MEDICATIONS

DRUG(S) OF CHOICE
Antibiotics should be chosen based on culture and sensitivity tests.

CONTRAINDICATIONS/POSSIBLE INTERACTIONS
Avoid use of potentially nephrotoxic antibiotics.

FOLLOW-UP

PATIENT MONITORING
Monitor urine for evidence of bacteria/cystitis twice weekly during and after antibiotic therapy.

PREVENTION/AVOIDANCE
Avoid exposure to sudangrass pastures.

POSSIBLE COMPLICATIONS
With severe ulceration and necrosis, scarring and strictures are possible.

EXPECTED COURSE AND PROGNOSIS
• Recovery of clinically effected horses is extremely rare
• Horses that do not continue to have recurrent cystitis should not be used for work or riding owing to residual nervous system damage
• Horses may still be used for breeding, but cystitis, vaginitis, or urethritis can complicate breeding efforts

MISCELLANEOUS

ASSOCIATED CONDITIONS
N/A

AGE-RELATED FACTORS
N/A

ZOONOTIC POTENTIAL
N/A

PREGNANCY/FERTILITY/BREEDING
Fetal malformations (extreme flexion of joints or ankylosis) occur when mares graze sudangrass between days 20 and 50 of gestation.

SEE ALSO
• Cyanide toxicosis
• Nitrate/nitrite toxicosis
• Polyneuritis equi
• Urinary incontinence
• Urinary tract infection (UTI)

Suggested Reading
Burrows GE, Tyrl RJ. Toxic Plants of North America. Ames, IA: Iowa State University Press, 2001:929.
Knight AP, Walter RG. A Guide to Plant Poisoning in North America. Jackson, WY: Teton NewMedia, 2001:242–243.
Van Kampen KR. Sudan grass and sorghum poisoning of horses: a possible lathyrogenic disease. J Am Vet Med Assoc 1970;156:629–630.

Author Jeffery O. Hall
Consulting Editors Wilson K. Rumbeiha and Steve Ensley

SPERMATOGENESIS AND FACTORS AFFECTING SPERM PRODUCTION

BASICS

DEFINITION
- *Spermatogenesis* occurs in testicular seminiferous tubules and is the process of:
  - Mitotic proliferation of spermatogonia
  - Meiotic divisions of primary (first meiotic division) and secondary (second meiotic division) spermatocytes to form spermatids
  - Maturation of spermatids into spermatozoa capable of motility and fertilization
  - Equids—sequence takes approximately 55–57 days
- *Spermiogenesis* is the portion of spermatogenesis that involves maturation of round spermatids into spermatozoa
- *Epididymal matura* or passage of sperm through the epididymis takes 9 days and is thought to be necessary for spermatozoa to achieve normal motility and fertilizing ability

PATHOPHYSIOLOGY

Endocrine Considerations
- Testosterone concentrations in the testis seem to be positively associated with spermatogenic activity:
  - Tissue concentrations of testosterone are related to blood concentrations
  - Difficult to assess testosterone activity in the testis or circulating levels with a single blood sample
- Modulation of spermatogenesis involves LH, FSH, GnRH, testosterone, estrogen, inhibin, prolactin, and other paracrine/autocrine factors not completely characterized

Seasonal Patterns
- Some studies report a higher testicular concentration of testosterone during the breeding season
- Sperm production during the winter months may be half of that observed during the maximum photoperiod
- Normal stallions potentially fertile year-round with little variation in sperm motility and percent of normal morphology

Age Related
- At puberty, positive correlation of testis weight with:
  - Potential DSO based on histologic evaluation of seminiferous tubules
  - Quantitative measures of spermatogenesis
- In 1–3-year-old horses, spermatogenic efficiency does not attain normal adult levels of 14–18 million spermatozoa/g of testicular tissue/day until the individual testis weight reaches 70–80 g, or a combined testicular volume of 133–152 mL (or cm^3)
  - Some 3-year-olds may reach this testicular volume without producing sufficient spermatozoa to rank them as *satisfactory* during a BSE

- After puberty, sperm production may continue to increase for years. Sperm production can continue to increase past 12 years of age. Full maturity of stallions (sperm production) is often considered to be 6 years
- Intratesticular testosterone (produced/g of testicular tissue) increases with age; related to sperm production
  - Differences between stallions may explain differences in sperm production
- In general:
  - Testicular size increases with age
  - Sperm production and sperm output increase with testicular size

Nutrition
Supplementation with omega-3 and omega-6 fatty acids, as well as their precursors (e.g. docosahexaenoic acid), especially when semen is to be frozen or cooled

SIGNS

Historical Findings
1 or more of the following:
- Abnormal or changes in sexual behavior
- Appearance and/or size changes
- Sperm numbers decrease
- Sperm motility or morphology changes
- Conception or foaling rates decrease

Physical Examination Findings
- Azoospermia or the absence of spermatozoa
- Oligospermia or oligozoospermia
- Small testes
- Abnormally large testes, especially with neoplasia or following trauma
- Softening or increased firmness of the testes
- Possibly altered sexual behavior
- Poor semen characteristics:
  - Reduced motility
  - Increased morphologic defects
  - Reduced total sperm numbers per ejaculate or DSO

CAUSES OF ARRESTED OR DISRUPTED SPERMATOGENESIS

Congenital
- Testicular hypoplasia due to hypogonadotropic hypogonadism
  - Abnormally low GnRH, LH, and FSH result in low testosterone
  - Probably rare
- Primary testicular degeneration
  - Unknown if part of a congenital lesion or acquired
- Chromosomal anomalies such as XXY
- Intersex conditions
- Cryptorchidism

Acquired
- Rare, testicular neoplasia
- Testicular heating due to inflammation/infection, fever, hydrocoele, ventral edema, trauma, exercise at elevated environmental temperatures
- Testicular degeneration associated with testicular metabolic changes is incompletely characterized; might be associated with either:

- Anabolic steroid or medications with steroid-like effects, i.e. androgens, estrogens, or progestins for behavioral or medical conditions; interfere with normal endocrine feedback loops, decreasing GnRH and LH
- Interference with normal metabolism by nutritional deficiencies, or exposure to toxic substances. Challenging diagnosis; few cases have been specifically documented in the stallion

DIAGNOSIS

DIFFERENTIAL DIAGNOSIS
- Failure to ejaculate
- Abnormal ejaculation
- Excurrent duct system blockage
- Behavioral disturbances

LABORATORY TESTS

Assessment of Overall Health and Wellbeing
- Complete physical examination including lameness
- CBC, serum biochemistry

Semen Evaluation
- Evaluate a set of *2 ejaculates* collected at a 1 h interval:
  - Minimum sample size to assess fertility and/or sperm production
  - Evaluate spermatozoid numbers, motility (total, progressive), and morphology. Spermatozoid numbers and motility—by spectrophotometer (concentration); or computer-assisted semen analysis—concentration, motility (including velocity, direction), and morphology
  - Differential interference contrast or phase contrast microscopy—much superior to normal bright-field light microscopy to evaluate motility and morphology
- DSO—daily collections until sperm numbers stabilize
- Rule out:
  - Bilateral blockage of the excurrent duct system
  - Ejaculatory disturbances
  - Behavioral abnormalities that cause failure of normal ejaculation
- If azoospermia or oligospermia is thought to be transient, reevaluate the stallion's semen no less than 60 days after cessation of the insult or disease

IMAGING

Ultrasonography
- Testicular dimensions, volume, texture, presence of fluid within the space between the parietal and visceral vaginal tunics
- Evaluate ampullae for blockage or sperm accumulation

S

OTHER DIAGNOSTIC PROCEDURES
- Measure serum/plasma concentrations of FSH, LH, estrogen, inhibin, and testosterone
  - Daily blood samples for 3 days
- GnRH stimulation test:
  - Single dose of 25 µg GnRH given IV at 9:00AM
  - Blood collected—baseline and 30 min intervals (i.e. 0, 30, 60, 90, 120 min)
  - Assay serum/plasma LH and testosterone
- Triple pulse GnRH stimulation test (nonbreeding season):
  - 3 IV doses of 5 µg of GnRH given 1 h apart
  - Samples taken 1 h before and 6 h after GnRH administration
  - Assay LH
- hCG stimulation test
  - Give 10 000 IU hCG IV
  - Blood samples 1 h before and 6 h after hCG
  - Assay testosterone and estrogen
- Anti-Müllerian hormone
  - Testicular biopsy—3 tissue samples: 1 sample fixed in Bouin's fluid or modified Davidson's solution for histopathologic evaluation and 2 placed in phosphate-buffered saline and snap-frozen for assay of paracrine/autocrine factors
- Flow cytometric procedures such as the sperm chromatin structure assay or sperm ubiquitin tag immunoassay
  - Detect alterations in sperm integrity
  - Available in some specialized research centers

PATHOLOGIC FINDINGS
Azoospermia in the Ejaculate
- Absence of germ cells in the seminiferous tubules (rare)
- Arrested spermatogenesis
- Bilateral blockage of the epididymis or ductus deferens
- Stallions with congenital absence of spermatogenesis or arrested spermatogenesis will have smaller testes than normal

Oligospermia in the Ejaculate
- Small testicular volume, reduced sperm-producing tissue
- Congenital malformations
- Testicular degeneration/disruption of spermatogenesis owing to toxicants, metabolic disorders, or testicular heating
- Trauma
- Neoplasia
- Inflammation of the testes or epididymides
- Partial blockage of the duct system
- Typically, stallions with chronic oligospermia have smaller than normal testes

Poor Fertility Following Cryopreservation and/or Cooling
- Ability to tolerate these special procedures varies by stallion

- Causes susceptibility of spermatozoa to damage during cryopreservation and/or cooling best described as *idiopathic*
  - Subtle disruptions in spermatogenesis cannot be ruled out
  - Further diagnostics might be indicated

TREATMENT
- Resolve underlying disease condition, if identified
- Hemicastration indicated if 1 testis is irreversibly affected by trauma, inflammation, infection, or neoplasia
- Treatments of infertility due to abnormal spermatogenesis are speculative at best, if the etiology and underlying pathologic process remain unidentified
- Use centrifugation strategies to manage semen from selected stallions, especially when semen is being frozen or cooled

NURSING CARE
Indicated in instances of systemic disease or hemicastration.

ACTIVITY
- Stallions need exercise in a stress-free environment
- Can be transient reproductive impairment while actively involved in competitions, especially with elevated environmental temperatures

DIET
Ensure proper levels of energy, protein, vitamins, and minerals.

CLIENT EDUCATION
Knowledge of spermatogenic cycle length; recovery may require 60–70 days.

FOLLOW-UP
PATIENT MONITORING
BSE of an injured or affected stallion—approximately 60 days from date of correction of underlying process.

PREVENTION/AVOIDANCE
- Control fever
- Manage minor scrotal edema and underlying etiology
- No anabolic steroids or progestins and caution in medications or supplements and to stallions currently or eventually used for breeding
- Controversial—avoid exposure of breeding stallions to endophyte-infected fescue, especially during the breeding season

MISCELLANEOUS
SYNONYMS
- Infertility
- Oligozoospermia
- Shooting blanks
- Sterility
- Subfertility

SEE ALSO
- Abnormal scrotal enlargement
- Abnormal testicular size
- Castration, Henderson castration instrument
- Castration, routine
- Cryptorchidism
- Disorders of sexual development
- Hernias (umbilical and inguinal)

ABBREVIATIONS
- BSE = breeding soundness examination
- DSO = daily sperm output
- FSH = follicle-stimulating hormone
- GnRH = gonadotropin-releasing hormone
- hCG = human chorionic gonadotropin
- LH = luteinizing hormone

Suggested Reading
Amann RP, Graham JK. Spermatozoal function. In: McKinnon AO, Squires EL, Vaala WE, Varner DD, eds. Equine Reproduction, 2e. Ames, IA: Wiley Blackwell, 2011:1053–1084.
Ball BA, Applications of anti-Mullerian hormone (AMH) in equine reproduction. Proc of hte Society for Theriogenology, July 2016 (Asheville, NC).
Johnson L, Griffin CE, Martin MT. Spermatogenesis. In: McKinnon AO, Squires EL, Vaala WE, Varner DD, eds. Equine Reproduction, 2e. Ames, IA: Wiley Blackwell, 2011:1026–1052.
Love CC. Modern techniques for semen evaluation. Vet Clin North Am Equine Pract 2016;32(3):531–546.

Author Tim J. Evans
Consulting Editor Carla L. Carleton
Acknowledgment The author and editor acknowledge the prior contribution of Rolf E. Larson.

BASICS

OVERVIEW
- Uncommon but can be life-threatening
- Diagnosis is difficult because of a lack of specific biomarkers
- The 2 most common venomous spiders in the USA are the black widow, *Latrodectus* spp., and the brown recluse (fiddleback), *Loxosceles reclusa*
- Venomous female black widow spiders are black with a red hourglass or other red shape on the ventral abdomen. They prefer to live outside all over the USA, under old woodpiles or in dark places. Their adult leg span is approximately 2–2.5 cm long
- Black widow venom contains neuroactive proteins and proteolytic enzymes and is neurotoxic. The principal toxin is α-latrotoxin, which causes an initial large release of acetylcholine and norepinephrine at postganglionic sympathetic synapses followed by depletion of the neurotransmitters
- Brown recluse spiders are brown with a dark brown violin shape on their back. They have delicate legs that span 2–3 cm as adults. They are nocturnal and are often found in closets and attics in south central USA
- Brown recluse venom contains hyaluronidase, esterases, alkaline phosphatases, and 32 kDa sphingomyelinase and causes localized necrosis

SIGNALMENT
N/A

SIGNS
Black Widow
- Most sensitive to *Latrodectus mactans* or *Latrodectus hesperus*
- Signs 15 min to 6 h after envenomation
- Subcutaneous edema and pain at the bite site are the main clinical signs
- Generalized hypertension and pain associated with regional lymph nodes and extremities as it spreads
- Muscle fasciculations and rigidity are major presentations
- Colic
- Ataxia
- Flaccid paralysis progressing to ascending paralysis possible
- Dyspnea possible

Brown Recluse
- Local and systemic signs
- Little or no pain from initial bite
- It starts as a central vesicle that becomes an ulcer with tissue around the site becoming red, swollen, and painful
- Tissue will slough over a period of weeks. Severity depends on site of bite
- Systemic signs are less common

CAUSES AND RISK FACTORS
- Garbage, sheds, old tarpaulins, and discarded furniture or farm equipment are good black widow spider habitats
- Old buildings, clothes, old newspapers, attics, and undisturbed places are good brown recluse habitats
- Many modern houses and barns have problems with brown recluse spider infestation

DIAGNOSIS

DIFFERENTIAL DIAGNOSIS
- Actually observing a spider on a horse is probably the only way to associate a bite wound with a spider
- Colic resulting from other causes
- Ionophore toxicosis
- Ascending paralysis is also a symptom of botulism (black spider)
- Nonhealing ulcerative lesions
- Red maple toxicosis (brown recluse)

CBC/BIOCHEMISTRY/URINALYSIS
- A serum chemistry and CBC may show evidence of a Coomb's negative hemolytic anemia
- Elevation of enzymes indicating skeletal muscle damage (creatine kinase, aspartate aminotransferase) may occur after a black widow bite
- Hemolytic anemia with hemoglobinuria associated with brown recluse

OTHER LABORATORY TESTS
N/A

PATHOLOGIC FINDINGS
- Swelling and erythema around the bite may be the only pathology noted with a black widow spider bite
- Tissue necrosis resulting in targetoid lesions is the primary lesion with brown recluse spider bites

TREATMENT
- Depends on the type of spider
- Supportive and symptomatic for both brown recluse and black widow
- Both types should be treated as emergencies, but usually time of bite is not known

MEDICATIONS

DRUG(S) OF CHOICE
Black Widow
- Diazepam for muscle rigidity
- Methocarbamol for muscle rigidity
- Opioids for pain

- A black widow antivenin exists but should be used only if necessary, because it is of equine origin and can result in anaphylaxis. If used, give undiluted (1 vial/horse) and administer IV

Brown Recluse
- There is no specific antidote
- Chlorhexidine diacetate topical 1% every 6 h
- Dapsone at 1 mg/kg every 12 h for 10 days (human treatment); efficacy questionable
- Analgesics such as flunixin meglumine at 0.5–1.1 mg/kg IV, IM, or PO every 8–12 h
- Antibiotics
- Wound care

CONTRAINDICATIONS/POSSIBLE INTERACTIONS
Watch the animal closely for signs of anaphylaxis if antivenin is administered.

FOLLOW-UP

PATIENT MONITORING
- The course of a black widow bite will generally occur much faster than a brown recluse bite unless systemic signs occur
- Brown recluse spider bites must be monitored at least twice a day to determine severity and secondary complications

PREVENTION/AVOIDANCE
Clean up potential spider habitats.

POSSIBLE COMPLICATIONS
Secondary wound infection may follow brown recluse bites.

EXPECTED COURSE AND PROGNOSIS
Recovery from a spider bite generally is within 7–14 days.

Suggested Reading
Gwaltney-Brant SM, Dunayer EK, Youssef HY. Terrestrial zootoxins. In: Gupta RC, ed. Veterinary Toxicology: Basic and Clinical Principles, 2e. San Diego, CA: Elsevier, 2012:969–992.
Roder JD. Spiders. In: Plumblee KH, ed. Clinical Veterinary Toxicology. St. Louis, MO: Mosby, 2004:111.

Author Wilson K. Rumbeiha
Consulting Editors Wilson K. Rumbeiha and Steve Ensley
Acknowledgment The editors acknowledge the prior contribution of Sandra E. Morgan.

S

SPLENOMEGALY

BASICS

OVERVIEW
• The spleen—stores blood cells; is the source of extramedullary erythropoiesis; is a major component of the MPS (also known as the reticuloendothelial system)
• Splenomegaly is a diffuse enlargement of the spleen, usually secondary to other diseases
• Splenomegaly can be caused by increased workload (hypersplenism), inflammation (splenitis), neoplastic infiltration, venous congestion, infarction, or hematoma

SIGNS
• Generally clinical signs are restricted to splenomegaly impinging on other organs
• Splenic abscesses may be associated with signs of depression, colic, fever, anorexia, weight loss, tachycardia/tachypnea
• Peritonitis is often coexistent with splenic abscess and produces signs of mild, recurrent abdominal pain and reluctance to move
• Acute hematoma or splenic rupture results in pooling of blood within the spleen or abdomen. Signs may include colic, tachycardia, cold extremities, and pallor of the mucous membranes

CAUSES AND RISK FACTORS
Hypersplenism
• Hypersplenism is caused by destruction of abnormal blood cells in the spleen and may be associated with disseminated intravascular coagulation, immune-mediated hemolytic anemia, immune-mediated thrombocytopenia, and purpura haemorrhagica
• Hypersplenism can be associated with hyperplasia of the MPS, giant cell formation, and marked hemosiderin accumulation

Infectious
• Acute splenitis or splenic abscess(es) results from infections with blood-borne pathogens and may result when a septic embolus lodges in the spleen (metastatic spread), or, more commonly, is due to extension of infection from a neighboring organ
• Cellular infiltrates vary from neutrophilic, pyogranulomatous, to granulomatous, depending on the infectious agent
• Splenic abscess due to metastatic spread has been reported as a result of infection with *Streptococcus equi* ssp. *equi, Corynebacterium pseudotuberculosis*, and *Rhodococcus equi*
• Moderate splenomegaly may occur in response to salmonellosis, anthrax, babesiosis, equine infectious anemia, equine ehrlichiosis, trypanosomiasis, and echinococcosis

Infiltrative
• Accumulations of neoplastic cells, or intracellular accumulations of abnormal lipid
• Primary neoplasia is rare—lymphoma and hemangiosarcoma. Splenomegaly also with leukemia (e.g. myelocytic) or metastatic neoplasia (e.g. melanoma)

Congestive States
• Right-sided heart failure or, more rarely, portal hypertension may cause splenomegaly
• Portal or splenic vascular occlusion secondary to parasites
• Lightning strike, electrocution, and euthanasia (barbiturate) may be associated with moderate splenomegaly

Miscellaneous
Splenic hematoma or in more severe cases splenic rupture—usually result from trauma.

DIAGNOSIS

DIFFERENTIAL DIAGNOSIS
• Differentiate from primary intestinal lesions
• Left dorsal displacement of colon/nephrosplenic entrapment causes splenic displacement medially
• Hepatomegaly may be differentiated by evaluation of liver enzymes, abdominal US, or liver biopsy
• Abdominal abscesses in other organs can be differentiated from splenic abscess with US
• Abdominal tumor—similar to that for abdominal abscess

CBC/BIOCHEMISTRY/URINALYSIS
• Variable depending on underlying cause
• Hypersplenism may cause anemia, thrombocytopenia, leukopenia, neutropenia, lymphopenia, hyperfibrinogenemia, increased hepatic enzyme activity, and hematuria
• Chronic splenic abscesses may cause leukocytosis/neutrophilia, hyperglobulinemia, hyperfibrinogenemia, anemia; marked leukocytosis (left shift)

OTHER LABORATORY TESTS
Blood culture/serology.

IMAGING
Transabdominal US to assess splenic size, detect infiltrative disease, altered echogenicity, and homogeneity, and allow for guided biopsy.

OTHER DIAGNOSTIC PROCEDURES
• Enlarged spleen—palpable per rectum; not consistent owing to marked normal variations in size
• Abdominocentesis—indicates chronic peritonitis with splenic abscess
• Splenic aspiration/biopsy; cytology/histopathology

TREATMENT
• Level of care and specific treatment depend on cause and severity of primary underlying disease
• Splenic abscess may be treated with splenectomy if adhesions and associated peritonitis are absent; often unrewarding owing to extensive nature of lesions before clinical signs appear

MEDICATIONS

DRUG(S) OF CHOICE
Appropriate antimicrobials/antiparasitics depending on the causative agent.

FOLLOW-UP

PATIENT MONITORING
• Monitor primary disease process
• Monitor splenic size by rectal palpation or US

POSSIBLE COMPLICATIONS
Splenic rupture of a grossly enlarged spleen may cause sudden death owing to internal hemorrhage.

EXPECTED COURSE AND PROGNOSIS
Variable depending on cause.

MISCELLANEOUS

SEE ALSO
• Anemia
• Infectious anemia (EIA)

ABBREVIATIONS
• MPS = mononuclear phagocyte system
• US = ultrasonography, ultrasound

Suggested Reading
Sellon DC. Disorders of the hematopoietic system. In: Reed SM, Bayly WM, Sellon DC, eds. Equine Internal Medicine, 4e. St. Louis, MO: WB Saunders, 2017: 798–838.

Authors David Hodgson and Jennifer L. Hodgson

Consulting Editors David Hodgson, Harold C. McKenzie, and Jennifer L. Hodgson

S

STALLION SEXUAL BEHAVIOR PROBLEMS

BASICS

DEFINITION
• Includes slow or variably inadequate precopulatory behaviors, sexual arousal, erection, or copulatory behavior
• Particular preferences and aversions for mares, handlers, breeding locations, procedures, or equipment have also been demonstrated; can also be general or specific to certain conditions
• In stallions, can be chronic or intermittent and can include certain aberrant precopulatory or copulatory behaviors—excessive biting or licking, savaging the mare or handler, or premature dismount

PATHOPHYSIOLOGY
In stallions, can be the result of single or multiple factors—genetic predisposition, inadequate social maturation, simple inexperience, suboptimal breeding stimuli, or aversive experience associated with sexual behavior, breeding, or general handling.

SYSTEMS AFFECTED
• Behavior—other behavior problems, including aggression stereotypies, can follow unresolved or ill-handled sexual behavior dysfunction; it is not uncommon for managers to physically abuse stallions for failure to perform sexually
• Reproduction—subfertility or infertility

SIGNALMENT
Novice and experienced breeders of any age, breed, or performance type.

SIGNS

Historical Findings
• Current and past general health, attitude, and temperament? Early socialization experience?
• Training and performance history?
• What is the stallion fed, including supplements?
• Any current medications?
• Current work and performance schedule?
• How is the stallion housed?
• Breeding experience?
• Age of first use?
• Libido and temperament?
• General behavior in stall and at pasture?
• Step-by-step details of behavior in sexual situation?
• Past and current breeding schedules and results?
• Natural cover or collection of semen?
• Stimulus and mount mares used?
• How is the stallion handled for breeding?
• Experience of personnel?
• Behavior of any other stallions at same facility?

Physical Examination Findings
Usually normal, but may yield evidence of current or possible past sources of discomfort (e.g. stallion ring, other scars).

CAUSES
• Inexperience
• Pain associated with breeding—legs, feet, chest, shoulder, stifle, back, penis, testicles, cord torsion, or inguinal testicle
• Punishment associated with sexual behavior
• Antimasturbatory devices or practices
• Injudicious punishment or rough or inconsistent handling during breeding, particularly intolerance of normal sexual behavior or overhandling of the head
• Breeding accidents—slipping during breeding, hitting the head on a low ceiling when mounting, or being kicked by a mare
• Overuse as a breeding stallion or overwork in performance
• Abuse
• Suboptimal stimulus mare
• Innate mare preferences
• Suboptimal breeding environment—poor footing, low ceilings, or noise and distractions
• Suboptimal artificial vagina or dummy mount conditions or techniques
• Too rigid or too flexible breeding organization

RISK FACTORS
• Age <2 years
• Novice breeders >5 years
• Sire with low or temperamental libido
• Heavy training or work
• Exposure to anabolic steroids and other performance-enhancing medications and feed supplements
• Discipline for showing normal sexual behavior
• Heavy breeding schedule
• Poor general health
• Physical abuse
• Hand-rearing, particularly if isolated from other horses during development
• Housing conditions—deliberate or inadvertent sensory, exercise, and social deprivation
• Injudicious, rough, or inconsistent handling during breeding
• Any musculoskeletal or genital pain, discomfort, or instability
• Fear of people or a particular person
• Obesity
• Severely underweight
• Extreme hot or cold environmental temperatures
• Change in environment, housing conditions, or management, which can suppress sexual response
• Self-serve dummy mounts

DIAGNOSIS

DIFFERENTIAL DIAGNOSIS
Medical differentials must be ruled out before a primary psychogenic diagnosis can be established.

CBC/BIOCHEMISTRY/URINALYSIS
Should be normal.

OTHER LABORATORY TESTS
• Endocrinology—stallion panel (i.e. testosterone, estradiol, luteinizing hormone, follicle-stimulating hormone, triiodothyronine, thyroxine, insulin, and cortisol) should be normal. For old stallions or those with suspected testicular degeneration, human chorionic gonadotropin and GnRH challenge tests may be useful. Use challenge and sampling protocols of an equine endocrine laboratory with a large stallion database and knowledge regarding interpretation of their protocol results
• Semen—can be evaluated for signs of infection or hemospermia that might suggest urogenital lesions causing discomfort

IMAGING
To rule out sources of present or past musculoskeletal or urogenital pain.

OTHER DIAGNOSTIC PROCEDURES
• Cardiovascular examination to rule out aortic iliac disease that may affect breeding ability
• Musculoskeletal and neurologic examinations on the ground and during breeding
• Video surveillance in the stall to observe erection and penile movement during normal, spontaneous erections
• Video surveillance of the stallion in the stall next to a mare or turned out at liberty with or near a mare to determine stallion-like behavior under less controlled conditions
• Video or direct observation of breeding procedures and stallion handling

TREATMENT

Management and Environment
• To the extent possible, correct obvious housing, handling, and breeding environment deficiencies, providing optimal stimulus mares, and physical facilities for breeding—excellent footing, ample head room, and plenty of space
• Establish a feeding and exercise program to maximize fitness for breeding and to minimize fatigue and pain
• Establish a breeding schedule to maximize libido and breeding performance; for stallions

S

with low or variable libido, a breeding schedule of 2 or 3 times weekly usually maximizes arousal and performance
• To the extent possible, identify and abide any specific preferences or aversions of the animal

Behavior Modification
• Provide as much uncontrolled access to mares as possible; this likely will increase endogenous male hormones and build confidence in responding to mares
• For slow-starting, novice breeders, continue daily exposure to breeding, with patient and gentle handling and a variety of stimulus mares; pasture breeding opportunities can build confidence and naturally train a stallion to breed
• When people are present, they can encourage and positively reinforce sexual arousal and response
• Educate handlers to use positive reinforcement-based stallion-handling procedures to encourage spontaneous erection and masturbation

MEDICATIONS

DRUG(S) OF CHOICE
• Analgesics or other therapies for management of any potential sources of physical discomfort or instability during breeding
• Anxiolytics as a training aid to overcome past, negative breeding experiences—diazepam (0.05 mg/kg (to maximum of 20 mg) slow IV 5–7 min before breeding; extralabel use)
• Unless androgen levels are greater than the normal range, administer GnRH (50 µg SC 2 h and again 1 h before breeding; extralabel use) to boost endogenous androgens, which often increases sexual interest and arousal and appears to make genital tissues more sensitive to stimulation
• If quick results are needed, short-term treatment with aqueous testosterone (50–80 mg SC every other day for at least 1 week; extralabel use) can effectively increase circulating testosterone and boost libido; the greatest improvement in libido typically occurs after 4–7 days of treatment
• Imipramine hydrochloride (500–800 mg for each 450 kg (1000 lb) PO 2–3 h before breeding; extralabel use) to lower the ejaculatory threshold and reduce the amount of work needed to breed

• Drug-induced ejaculation regimens (extralabel use) are available as substitutes for in copula breeding or collection of semen

PRECAUTIONS
• Caution handlers that benzodiazepine anxiolytics can lower the threshold of aggressive as well as sexual behaviors
• Increasing male hormone levels with GnRH or androgens also likely increases aggressive behavior. If the aggression is not skillfully directed or abided, mare or handler interaction with the stallion can be counterproductive
• Increasing the dose of testosterone often is tempting, but possible adverse side effects on pituitary gonadal function are a concern
• At certain levels, imipramine hydrochloride can inhibit rather than enhance ejaculation, disturb bladder neck function, and cause premature flaring of the glans penis. Should these occur, a lower dose usually is more effective at enhancing ejaculation without these side effects

FOLLOW-UP

PATIENT MONITORING
• Once- to twice-weekly follow-up for at least 1 month, with monthly follow-up thereafter during the current breeding season to monitor and fine-tune improvements and medications
• Reexamination near the end of the current breeding season and near the beginning of the next breeding season, or with change in environment or health status

POSSIBLE COMPLICATIONS
• Best results occur if everyone involved with the care and handling of the horse communicates openly among each other and with the clinician toward a positive outcome for the stallion
• Counterproductive blaming or failure of all to cooperate or comply with the treatment plan

MISCELLANEOUS

ASSOCIATED CONDITIONS
• Some stallions become "sour" if continually failing at breeding and may develop self-mutilation or tendencies to savage the mare or handlers
• Many stallions with low libido actually began as high-energy, unruly stallions that, in

association with discipline, became uninterested or slow to respond
• Subclinical lameness, neurologic disease, or aortic iliac disease that may specifically disturb pelvic circulation or cause hindlimb pain or weakness during copulation

AGE-RELATED FACTORS
• Inadequate sexual interest and response in young novice stallions is more likely to be psychogenic than a physiologic problem
• Most healthy, sound stallions maintain stable libido through their mature years and into old age. However, with advancing age and accumulated minor physical deterioration, once tolerable musculoskeletal discomfort or disabilities may become more problematic for breeding stallions
• Cardiac pathology, particularly with advancing age, often is associated with reduced libido, apparent anxiety on exertion during breeding, and delayed or urgent dismount

ZOONOTIC POTENTIAL
N/A

PREGNANCY/FERTILITY/BREEDING
N/A

SYNONYMS
• Libido problem
• Erection dysfunction
• Breeding dysfunction
• Sexual behavior dysfunction
• Poor breeding performance

SEE ALSO
• Aggression
• Fear
• Self-mutilation

ABBREVIATIONS
GnRH = gonadotropin-releasing hormone

Suggested Reading
McDonnell SM. Sexual behavior dysfunction of stallions. In: Robinson NE, ed. Current Therapy in Equine Medicine, 3e. Philadelphia, PA: WB Saunders, 1992:633–637.
McGreevy P. Equine Behaviour: A Guide for Veterinarians and Equine Scientists, 2e. Philadelphia, PA: WB Saunders, 2012:248–252.
Mills DS, McDonnell S. Domestic Horse: The Origins, Development, and Management of its Behaviour. New York, NY: Cambridge University Press, 2005.

Author Sue M. McDonnell
Consulting Editor Victoria L. Voith

S

STATIONARY NIGHT BLINDNESS

BASICS

OVERVIEW
• Congenital stationary night blindness is a hereditary disease that affects night (scotopic) vision and in severe cases, may also affect day (photopic) vision. It is nonprogressive, and persists throughout the horse's life. No morphologic abnormalities are seen ophthalmoscopically or by means of light and electron microscopy
• Systems affected—ophthalmic

SIGNALMENT
• Most common in the Appaloosa, but also described in the Miniature horse, the Thoroughbred, and the Paso Fino
• In Appaloosas and Miniature horses, CSNB is associated with the LP and it is likely that other horse breeds where LP spotting is present may be affected as well
• No sex predilection is known
• Disease is present at birth and persists throughout life

SIGNS
• Visual impairment in dim light and dark conditions, leading to behavioral uneasiness and unpredictability, despite a normal ophthalmoscopic examination
• Vision is usually normal in daylight. However, photopic visual impairment has been reported in some cases, and is believed to be a severe form of the disease
• Dorsomedial strabismus ("star gazing") and nystagmus may also be present in severely affected animals. Strabismus is not an obvious clinical sign in most cases
• Unlike CSNB in humans, affected horses have refractive error similar to unaffected horses, and do not suffer from severe myopia (nearsightedness)
• Owners may report repeated injuries to the horse during the evening hours
• Most affected horses function very well, and owners may be unaware that their horse is visually impaired. Clinical signs such as apprehension and anxiety in dim light are attributed to behavior and temperament rather than visual impairment

CAUSES AND RISK FACTORS
• A defect in the neural transmission between rod photoreceptors and bipolar cells in the mid-retina is responsible for this disease
• The rod photoreceptors are responsible for night vision. *TRPM1* is important for rod bipolar cells' depolarization. Decreased expression of *TRPM1* in the retina of affected Appaloosas and Miniature horses prevents the

depolarization of the rod bipolar cells, which in turn prevents the propagation of the signal to the optic nerve, resulting in night blindness
• Appaloosas and Miniature horses are affected by CSNB in association with homozygosity of the LP allele (autosomal recessive inheritance)
• Thoroughbreds and Paso Finos are likely affected by a different genetic mechanism

DIAGNOSIS

DIFFERENTIAL DIAGNOSIS
Other congenital and acquired blinding disorders of the retina, optic nerve, and brain have to be ruled out, such as colobomas, retinal detachments, and chorioretinitis. In the latter diseases, the visual impairment is not strictly limited to dim light.

CBC/BIOCHEMISTRY/URINALYSIS
N/A

OTHER LABORATORY TESTS
N/A

IMAGING
N/A

OTHER DIAGNOSTIC PROCEDURES
• The ocular fundi of affected horses appear normal
• Although there has been advancement in the understanding of the genetic mechanism of CSNB in recent years, the ERG is the only method for definitive diagnosis of the disease. A large negative a-wave potential and absence of b-wave amplitude in the scotopic full-field ERG are the hallmark of this disease and confirm the presence of night blindness. The photopic full-field ERG shows reduced amplitude and increased implicit time of the b-wave. In addition, the ERG oscillatory potentials in horses with CSNB are attenuated when compared with normal controls
• Genetic testing for the LP gene in Appaloosas is commercially available

PATHOLOGIC FINDINGS
Histologic and electron microscopic examination of the affected retinas are normal.

TREATMENT
None

MEDICATIONS
N/A

FOLLOW-UP

PREVENTION/AVOIDANCE
Affected horses should not be used for breeding. However, since owners of most horses affected with CSNB are unaware of the disease, and owing to the recessive inheritance, genetic exclusion of the disease is unlikely.

EXPECTED COURSE AND PROGNOSIS
Horses can undergo training and perform well during the day. Training and handling of these horses should be performed in a well-lit environment to assure the safety of horses and handlers.

MISCELLANEOUS

SEE ALSO
• Chorioretinitis
• Ocular problems in the neonate
• Optic nerve atrophy

ABBREVIATIONS
• CSNB = congenital stationary night blindness
• ERG = electroretinogram
• LP = leopard printing (leopard complex spotting pattern gene)
• *TRPM1* = transient receptor potential cation channel subfamily M member 1

Internet Resources
Animal Genetics, Appaloosa Coat Pattern—Leopard Print and Congenital Stationary Night Blindness (CSNB). http://www.animalgenetics.us/Equine/Coat_Color/Appaloosa.asp The Appaloosa Project. http://www.appaloosaproject.co

Suggested Reading
Sandmeyer LS, Bellone RR, Archer S, et al. Congenital stationary night blindness is associated with the leopard complex in the Miniature horse. Vet Ophthalmol 2012;15:18–22.

Author Gil Ben-Shlomo
Consulting Editor Caryn E. Plummer
Acknowledgment The author and editor acknowledge the prior contribution of Andras M. Komaromy and Dennis E. Brooks.

S

STREPTOCOCCUS EQUI INFECTION

 BASICS

DEFINITION
Acute upper respiratory tract infection characterized by fever, lethargy, purulent rhinitis, and regional lymph node abscessation.

PATHOPHYSIOLOGY
• *Streptococcus equi* ssp. *equi* is inhaled or ingested after direct contact with mucopurulent discharge from infected horses or contaminated equipment
• Adheres to the epithelial cells of the buccal and nasal mucosa
• Spreads to the regional lymph nodes, such as the submandibular, submaxillary, and retropharyngeal lymph nodes (with likely rupture into the GPs)
• Fever occurs 3–14 days after exposure
• Nasal shedding occurs 1–2 days after the onset of fever, persisting for at least 2–3 weeks
• Asymptomatic carrier horses are responsible for maintaining the infection in affected herds and can shed from GPs for many years

SYSTEMS AFFECTED
• Respiratory
• Hemic/lymphatic/immune

INCIDENCE/PREVALENCE
Disease occurs sporadically on farms. Morbidity rates will depend on age (range 32–100%). Mortality rates are considered low in uncomplicated cases (<2%).

GEOGRAPHIC DISTRIBUTION
Occurs worldwide.

SIGNALMENT
Any age group, 1–5 years are predisposed. No breed or sex predilection.

SIGNS
• Fever of >39.5°C (>103°F)
• Depression and listlessness
• Lymphadenopathy and abscessation of retropharyngeal and submandibular lymph nodes (rarely parotid and cranial cervical lymph nodes)
• Bilateral mucopurulent nasal discharge
• GP empyema
• Respiratory stridor
• Dysphagia, anorexia, cough, and neck extension
• Ocular discharge

CAUSES
S. equi ssp. *equi*, a Gram-positive coccus.

RISK FACTORS
The immunologically naive, young equine population housed in highly concentrated and transient populations.

 DIAGNOSIS

DIFFERENTIAL DIAGNOSIS
For Nasal Discharge
• Influenza
• EHV-1 and EHV-4
• Equine rhinitis virus
• Adenovirus
• Reovirus
• EHV-2
• Pharyngitis
• Chronic pharyngeal lymphoid hyperplasia
• Nasal/paranasal sinus infection/cysts/polyps/tumors
• Early bacterial pneumonia/pleuritis
• GP infection/mycosis
• Overflow of nasolacrimal ducts
• Severe equine asthma (heaves)

For Fever
Any disease that causes inflammation.

For Lymphadenopathy and Abscessation
• Lymphoma
• Upper respiratory tract infection
• *Corynebacterium pseudotuberculosis* lymphadenitis
• Bacterial endocarditis
• Ulcerative/epizootic/sporadic lymphadenitis
• Glanders
• Plasma cell myeloma
• Tuberculosis
• Hemolytic/uremic-like syndrome

CBC/BIOCHEMISTRY/URINALYSIS
• Hyperfibrinogenemia, leukocytosis characterized by a neutrophilia, and possibly anemia
• Serum biochemistry and urinalysis abnormalities may indicate complications

OTHER LABORATORY TESTS
• Samples—obtain from mature abscess aspirates, nasopharyngeal washes (have been shown to be higher yield than swabs), and GP washes. Rostral nasal swabs are not recommended
• Testing:
  ◦ Cytology—Gram-positive extracellular cocci in long chains support suspicion
  ◦ Culture—useful in animals with active disease, but sensitivity is very low in animals with low numbers of bacteria (early in disease, convalescent horses, and long-term carriers)
  ◦ PCR—fast (2 h) and high sensitivity with ability to detect small numbers of bacteria
  ◦ Serology—(1) SeM ELISA: may detect recent but not current infection, need for vaccination (do not vaccinate if ≥1:3200 owing to risk of PH), and support clinical diagnosis of *S. equi* PH and metastatic abscessation; (2) combined SeM and

SEQ2190 serology (currently available in Europe) can help detect infection as recent as 2 weeks and used to screen new horses for further testing via GP endoscopy and PCR

IMAGING
• GP/pharyngeal endoscopy—determine the severity of upper airway obstruction and the presence of GP empyema/chondroids in both active cases and asymptomatic carriers
• GP radiographs—presence of chondroids
• Abdominal ultrasonography or per rectum—detection of intra-abdominal abscessation

PATHOLOGIC FINDINGS
Hyperplastic lymph nodes—increased numbers of neutrophils, monocytes, and macrophages with Gram-positive cocci. Nasal lesions—edematous, hyperemic, and occasionally ulcerated mucosa with a variable amount of creamy yellow exudate. Complicated strangles—the pathologic findings are variable, depending on the organ system involved.

 TREATMENT

AIMS
To control transmission of *S. equi* and to eliminate infection while providing future, effective immunity to the disease.

APPROPRIATE HEALTH CARE
• Acute phase of the fever and depression—supportive care. Hot packing or topical treatment with 20% ichthammol to encourage maturation of the abscess and drainage, followed by flushing with 3–5% povidone–iodine solution once opened. Judicious use of nonsteroidal drugs can decrease swelling and promote eating. Treatment with antibiotics may prevent the formation of abscess. This practice is considered controversial
• Horses with complications benefit from systemic antibiotic therapy (22 000–44 000 IU/kg IM every 12 h of procaine penicillin or IV every 6 h of aqueous potassium penicillin) for 7–10 days
• If nasal discharge persists >2 weeks, GP examination is indicated to identify horses that may have empyema and require additional treatment
• Horses with GP empyema/chondroids require copious lavage with or without 20% acetylcysteine solution and systemic antibiotics. Local infusion of antibiotics once gross contamination is removed

NURSING CARE
Minimal unless respiratory obstruction or complications occur.

ACTIVITY

Horses and stables should be quarantined until there are no clinical signs and cases and in-contacts have been tested for carrier status.

DIET

Soft, moist, palatable food.

CLIENT EDUCATION

Segregation and preventing cross-contamination. Stables that housed infected animals should be rested for 2 weeks after cleaning and disinfecting.

SURGICAL CONSIDERATIONS

Tracheostomy for horses in severe respiratory distress. Surgical removal of chondroids from the GP is rarely necessary.

MEDICATIONS

DRUG(S) OF CHOICE

See Appropriate Health Care.

ALTERNATIVE DRUGS

Chloramphenicol; ceftiofur; treatment failures have been observed with trimethoprim–sulfa combinations.

FOLLOW-UP

PATIENT MONITORING

• Clinical and in-contact horses should be tested for carrier status no sooner than 3 weeks after resolution of clinical signs or potential exposure via GP endoscopy and PCR
• Wait at least 3 weeks from cessation of antibiotic treatment prior to testing
• Endoscopically guided GP lavage PCR to screen for carriers in cases and their contacts provides increased efficiency and sensitivity over 3 nasopharyngeal washes. Disinfect equipment between horses
• Continual positive tests despite endoscopically normal GP should be considered infections. Consider treatment with systemic antibiotics and sinus radiography

PREVENTION/AVOIDANCE

• Isolation of new horses for 3 weeks, with close observation for signs of strangles or any disease. Monitor temperature twice daily
• Persistent carriers of *S. equi* with the GP are a potential source of new infections on a farm. Negative GP PCR prior to entering the resident population
• If not treated with antibiotics, approximately 75% of horses develop a waning convalescent immunity to strangles as a result of individual immune response as well as natural exposure to disease over time contributing to reboosting and herd immunity

During an Outbreak

• Affected or suspect horses should be quarantined immediately
• Make 3 groups—affected, in-contacts, and healthy with designated equipment and caretakers
• Observe all horses closely for signs of disease and monitor temperatures twice daily. Move febrile horses to affected group as soon as identified
• Clean and disinfect—appropriate disinfectants include phenols, iodophors, and chlorhexidine compounds
• Exposure to air is essential for disinfection

Vaccination

Does not guarantee prevention. Currently, the following systemic vaccines are available:
• Strepvax II (concentrated M-protein extract of *S. equi*)—IM vaccine; adverse reactions include soreness or abscesses at injection sites and occasional cases of PH
• Pinnacle IN—intranasal vaccine contains an attenuated live strain of *S. equi* that is antigenic but has low pathogenicity. Live vaccine should be administered only to healthy animals >1 year of age with no known exposure to disease
• Equilis StrepE—intermittently available in Europe for administration submucosally on the inside of the upper lip. Immunity to experimental challenge persists for about 3 months. Painful reaction at injection site can occur and veterinarians have accidentally injected themselves
• Strangvac—a multicomponent vaccine in development in Sweden which has differentiation of infected from vaccinated animals capability

POSSIBLE COMPLICATIONS

• Reported in about 20% of cases
• Bastard strangles—*S. equi* metastasize to other lymph nodes or body systems (lungs, mesentery, liver, spleen, kidney, and brain); low occurrence 2–10%
• Upper respiratory tract obstruction from retropharyngeal lymph node abscessation, suppurative necrotic bronchopneumonia
• Myocarditis and myositis
• PH—aseptic vasculitis reported in mature horses after second natural exposure to infection or vaccination of animals that previously had strangles. Clinical signs—mild to life-threatening. Typical signs—pitting edema of dependent areas of the head, trunk, and extremities; petechiation and ecchymoses of mucous membranes.
Therapy—antimicrobials, corticosteroids, and supportive care
• Septicemia and the development of infectious arthritis, pneumonia, and encephalitis

EXPECTED COURSE AND PROGNOSIS

Prognosis is good for full recovery in cases of uncomplicated strangles. The course of the disease depends on the phase of the infection.

MISCELLANEOUS

AGE-RELATED FACTORS

Horses between the ages of 1 and 5 years are immunologically naive are most prone to developing the disease. Older horses may develop a mild form of strangles owing to previous exposure.

ZOONOTIC POTENTIAL

Cases in debilitated humans and a dog have been reported.

PREGNANCY/FERTILITY/BREEDING

Avoid infection in a pregnant mare. Suckling foals benefit from the protective effects of IgGb and IgA in milk from mares that recovered from strangles or were vaccinated IM.

SYNONYMS

• Distemper
• Strangles

ABBREVIATIONS

• EHV = equine herpesvirus
• ELISA = enzyme-linked immunosorbent assay
• GP = guttural pouch
• Ig = immunoglobulin
• PCR = polymerase chain reaction
• PH = purpura haemorrhagica
• SeM = *S. equi* M protein

Suggested Reading
Boyle AG. Strangles and its complications. Equine Vet Educ 2016;29:149–157.
Boyle AG, Stefanovski D, Rankin SC. Determining optimal sampling site for *Streptococcus equi* subsp *equi* carriers using loop-mediated isothermal amplification. BMC Vet Res 2017;13:75.
Boyle AG, Timoney JF, Newton JR, et al. *Streptococcus equi* Infections in Horses: Guidelines for Treatment, Control and Prevention of Strangles-Revised Consensus Statement. J Vet Intern Med. 2018;32:633–647.
Waller AS. New perspectives for the diagnosis, control, treatment, and prevention of strangles in horses. Vet Clin North Am Equine Pract 2014;30:591–607.
Durham AE, Hall YS, Kulp L, et al. A study of the environmental survival of *Streptococcus equi* subspecies *equi*. 2018;50:861–864.

Author Ashley G. Boyle
Consulting Editor Ashley G. Boyle

S

STRESS FRACTURES

BASICS

DEFINITION
Repetitive overuse bone injury.

PATHOPHYSIOLOGY
• Exercise-induced, repetitive mechanical loading of bone resulting in incomplete remodeling
• Under normal stresses, bone changes shape and structure in response to use (Wolff's law); bone resorption and replacement is balanced. Cortical bone responds by forming new bone (modeling) via periosteal callus and remodeling of existing bone. Subchondral bone responds by remodeling with sclerosis and lysis
• With excessive or intense training, resorption exceeds replacement, resulting in transient bone weakness. With continued stress, focal weakness functions as a stress riser, allowing stress fracture to occur under otherwise physiologic conditions
• Catastrophic fractures are severe manifestations of milder stress-related injury; postmortem findings confirm preexisting stress-related bony remodeling at stress fracture sites

SYSTEMS AFFECTED
Musculoskeletal—long bones (MCIII/MTIII, humerus, scapula, tibia), C3, ilium, P3.

INCIDENCE/PREVALENCE
• Exact incidence is unknown
• Musculoskeletal injuries prevent 45–63% of Thoroughbreds from racing
• Catastrophic fractures result in 1.1 deaths to 1.8 injuries per 1000 starts
• Type of racing affects location and injury type
• Thoroughbreds are 8.6 times more likely than Standardbreds to develop dorsal metacarpal bone disease

GEOGRAPHIC DISTRIBUTION
Horse-racing countries (North America, Europe, Japan, Australia).

SIGNALMENT

Breed Predilections
• Racehorses (Thoroughbreds, Standardbreds, Quarter Horses, Arabians)
• Site-specific breed predilections:
  ◦ P3—Standardbred overrepresented
  ◦ Dorsal MCIII—Thoroughbred, Quarter Horse
  ◦ Distal palmar/plantar MCPJ/MTPJ—Thoroughbred (forelimb), Standardbred (hindlimb)
  ◦ Subchondral C3—Standardbred, Thoroughbred
  ◦ Humerus, scapula, ilium—Thoroughbred
  ◦ Tibia—Thoroughbred, Standardbred, Quarter Horse

Mean Age and Range
2–5-year-old racehorses.

SIGNS

General Comments
• Clinical recognition is challenging
• Lameness is variable and physical examination findings are subtle or absent

Historical Findings
• Acute transient lameness after racing or training
• Poor performance
• Intermittent unilateral or multilimb lameness

Physical Examination Findings
• Cortical bone stress fractures—± periosteal thickening, variable pain during palpation
• Subchondral bone stress injury—± joint effusion, pain during flexion with chronic injury
• Examination findings specific to site:
  ◦ P3—unilateral lameness, distal interphalangeal joint distention, variable response to hoof tester application
  ◦ Palmar/plantar MCPJ/MTPJ—short, chopping, shifting limb lameness, joint distention, painful flexion in chronic disease
  ◦ Dorsal MCIII—"bucked shins": periosteal thickening, pain on palpation; "saucer fracture": focal bony bump, focal pain
  ◦ Proximal palmar MCIII—± pain, heat, swelling
  ◦ Subchondral C3—joint effusion, ± painful carpal flexion, limb abduction when trotting
  ◦ Humerus—± pain during upper forelimb manipulation
  ◦ Scapula—equivocal findings
  ◦ Tibia—painful to firm pressure of medial diaphysis, painful upper hindlimb flexion or with tibial torsion
  ◦ Ilium—plaiting, poor hindlimb action, tuber sacrale sore to palpation

CAUSES
• Repetitive, intense high-speed exercise
• Maladaptive or nonadaptive bone remodeling

RISK FACTORS
• Racing or race training
• Race training after lay-up
• Inconsistent racetrack surfaces
• Poor hoof conformation—long toe, underrun heel
• Horseshoe with toe grab
• Previous injury

DIAGNOSIS

DIFFERENTIAL DIAGNOSIS
• Complete bone fracture at sites of stress injury (i.e. MCIII/MTIII condylar fracture, C3 slab fracture)—severe or non-weight-bearing lameness, joint distention. Rule out with imaging
• Osteoarthritis—joint effusion, painful joint flexion. Rule out with imaging

• Suspensory desmitis—rule out with ultrasonography

IMAGING
• Nuclear scintigraphy—focal, moderate to intense IRU is the hallmark of a stress fracture. Specific sites of IRU stress fracture/reaction include:
  ◦ P3—lateral left front, medial right front
  ◦ Palmar/plantar MCPJ/MTPJ—distal palmar/plantar MCIII/MTIII. Flexed lateral images differentiate proximal sesamoid IRU
  ◦ Dorsal MCIII—"bucked shins": diffuse; "saucer fracture": focal
  ◦ Palmar proximal MCIII—palmar proximal MCIII
  ◦ Subchondral C3—medial middle carpal joint, C3
  ◦ Humerus—caudoproximal, craniodistal, or medial diaphysis
  ◦ Scapula—caudal distal
  ◦ Tibia—caudolateral, middle third
  ◦ Ilium—10–15 cm lateral to tuber sacrale. Dorsal oblique views enhance identification
• Radiography—often normal; periosteal reaction, callus formation, unicortical incomplete fracture; subchondral sclerosis and/or lysis; ± supplement views. Specific sites and potential radiographic findings:
  ◦ P3—lateral or medial wing fracture, usually nonarticular
  ◦ Palmar/plantar MCPJ/MTPJ—subchondral lucency and/or sclerosis; down-angled oblique views enhance identification
  ◦ Dorsal MCIII—"bucked shins": periosteal roughening, thickening; "saucer fracture": unicortical fracture
  ◦ Proximal palmar MCIII—crescent-shaped radiolucency (avulsion fracture), incomplete longitudinal fracture, subchondral sclerosis
  ◦ Subchondral C3—sclerosis of radial facet
  ◦ Humerus—callus formation, ± fracture line
  ◦ Scapula—equivocal
  ◦ Tibia—cortical thickening, callus formation, unicortical oblique fracture line
  ◦ Ilium—limited in standing horse
• Ultrasonography
  ◦ Proximal palmar MCIII—bony irregularity, suspensory avulsion, accompanying suspensory desmitis
  ◦ Ilium—irregular bony surface, discontinuity of bone contour, hematoma in acute injury

OTHER DIAGNOSTIC PROCEDURES
• Diagnostic analgesia—upper limb stress fracture suspected when lameness does not "block out" with distal limb analgesia. Intra-articular analgesia may incompletely alleviate pain in subchondral bone injury. Specifics:
  ◦ P3—abaxial analgesia, intra-articular distal interphalangeal analgesia
  ◦ Palmar/plantar MCPJ/MTPJ—low palmar/plantar or lateral palmar/plantar

metacarpal/metatarsal analgesia, incomplete analgesia with intra-articular MCPJ/MTPJ
○ Dorsal MCIII—high palmar and dorsal ring block
○ Proximal palmar MCIII—high palmar or lateral palmar analgesia, intra-articular middle carpal analgesia
○ Subchondral C3—intra-articular middle carpal analgesia
○ Humerus, scapula, tibia, ilium—pain not alleviated with distal forelimb analgesia
• Rectal examination (ilium)—± crepitus or hematoma

PATHOLOGIC FINDINGS
Periosteal callus, cortical remodeling, microfractures, subchondral sclerosis, and lysis.

TREATMENT
AIMS
• Halt or alter the continuum of bone stress
• Prevent stress fracture becoming catastrophic fracture
• Prevent subchondral bone injury progressing to osteoarthritis or osteochondral fragmentation

APPROPRIATE HEALTH CARE
• Early recognition via nuclear scintigraphy and/or radiography
• Once identified, most respond well to rest
• ± Extracorporeal shockwave therapy (single treatment, 2000 shocks)
• Restore or improve hoof balance, flat shoe
• Bar shoe for P3 fracture

ACTIVITY
• For stress fractures—1 month stall rest, then 1 month stall rest with hand-walking, then 2 months of small paddock turnout
• For subchondral injury—controlled exercise program and gradual return to exercise, i.e. 3 weeks hand-walking, then 3 weeks walking under saddle, then 3 weeks trotting. For severe injury, 3–4 months of rest. Intra-articular therapy for osteoarthritis

DIET
Caloric reduction while stall confined or resting.

CLIENT EDUCATION
Stress-related bone injuries are a continuum. If not recognized and treated or treated inappropriately, catastrophic fracture and/or osteoarthritis will ensue.

SURGICAL CONSIDERATIONS
• "Saucer fracture"—osteostixis, screw fixation, both
• Subchondral injury—arthroscopy

MEDICATIONS
DRUG(S) OF CHOICE
• For subchondral injury:
○ NSAIDs—phenylbutazone (2.2–4.4 mg/kg every 12 h)
○ Polysulfated glycosaminoglycan (500 mg IM every 4 days for 7 treatments) or sodium hyaluronate (40 mg IV every 7 days for 3 treatments)
○ Isoxsuprine hydrochloride (1 mg/kg PO every 12 h)
○ Intra-articular methylprednisolone acetate (20–40 mg), triamcinolone (3–6 mg), ± sodium hyaluronate (10–20 mg)

CONTRAINDICATIONS
Long-term NSAIDs are contraindicated owing to their ability to impair bone healing and risk of catastrophic fracture.

FOLLOW-UP
PATIENT MONITORING
• Decreased or absent IRU before resuming race training
• Periodic lameness and imaging examination after each exercise increment

PREVENTION/AVOIDANCE
• Allow bone to adapt (remodel) before increasing exercise intensity, suggest 1 month increments
• Fully investigate lameness in young racehorses. Nuclear scintigraphy is vital for diagnosis

POSSIBLE COMPLICATIONS
• Catastrophic bone fracture
• Reduced or poor performance
• Osteoarthritis

EXPECTED COURSE AND PROGNOSIS
After recognition and treatment, stress fractures have an excellent prognosis for racing; subchondral injury prognosis is less favorable. Unrecognized, stress-related bone injuries may result in fatal fracture or career-ending osteoarthritis.

MISCELLANEOUS
AGE-RELATED FACTORS
Occurs in young naive racehorses.

SYNONYMS
• Fatigue fracture
• Incomplete fracture
• Stress-related bone injury
• Stress reaction
• Maladaptive or nonadaptive bone disease

SEE ALSO
• Dorsal metacarpal bone disease
• Osteoarthritis
• Suspensory desmitis

ABBREVIATIONS
• C3 = third carpal bone
• IRU = increased radiopharmaceutical uptake
• MCIII = third metacarpus
• MCPJ = metacarpophalangeal joint
• MTIII = third metatarsus
• MTPJ = metatarsophalangeal joint
• NSAID = nonsteroidal anti-inflammatory drug
• P3 = distal phalanx

Suggested Reading
Davidson EJ. Pathophysiology and clinical diagnosis of cortical and subchondral bone injury. In: Ross MW, Dyson SJ, eds. Diagnosis and Management of Lameness in the Horse, 2e. St. Louis, MO: Elsevier Saunders, 2011:935–946.
Davidson EJ, Moss MW. Clinical recognition of stress-related bone injury in racehorses. Clin Tech Equine Pract 2003;2:296–311.
Stover SM. The epidemiology of Thoroughbred racehorse injuries. Clin Tech Equine Pract 2003;2:312–322.

Author Elizabeth J. Davidson
Consulting Editor Elizabeth J. Davidson

S

STRINGHALT

BASICS

OVERVIEW
Stringhalt ("springhalt") is a movement disorder characterized by a sudden, apparently involuntary, exaggerated flexion of 1 or both hindlimbs during attempted movement. There are 2 types of stringhalt—plant associated and sporadic.

SIGNALMENT
Usually adult horses are affected.

SIGNS
• Varying degrees of hyperflexion with delayed protraction can occur, ranging from mild, spasmodic lifting and grounding of the foot when the horse is backed or stopped suddenly to extreme cases during which the foot can contact the abdomen, thorax, and occasionally the elbow, leading to a peculiar bunny-hopping gait. The lateral digital extensor muscle is predominantly affected, but owing to the action of the reciprocal apparatus the whole pelvic limb is involved
• In the plant-associated stringhalt thoracic limbs can be involved and present as intermittent thoracic limb hypertonia with stumbling

CAUSES AND RISK FACTORS
Plant-Associated Stringhalt
• Plant-associated or "Australian" stringhalt is a syndrome most often recognized in Australia but has also been reported in New Zealand, North America, Chile, and Japan; it is likely to occur infrequently in other countries
• Outbreaks have been associated with the ingestion of the related plants dandelion (*Taraxacum officinale*), flatweed (*Hypochaeris radicata*), and cheeseweed (*Malva parviflora*). A recent study has identified cytotoxic activity in leaf exudates of *H. radicata*, which was upregulated when the plant was stressed—this explains why outbreaks are often associated with drier than normal summers
• Older, taller horses are predisposed, and cases are often more severe than seen in classical stringhalt

Sporadic Stringhalt
• This form occurs worldwide and usually only affects 1 pelvic limb
• The onset can be preceded by trauma to the dorsal tarsal region or the dorsoproximal metatarsus some weeks previously
• Etiologies are speculated to include tendon adhesions enhancing tarsocrural joint flexion or abnormalities in the myotatic reflex caused by tendon injury, possibly due to Golgi tendon organ damage

DIAGNOSIS

DIFFERENTIAL DIAGNOSIS
• Shivers (shivering) can look remarkably similar to acquired bilateral stringhalt during backward walking; however, stringhalt should occur more during forward walking and have a more consistent, rapidly ascending, hyperflexed, adducted pelvic limb gait at a walk
• Horses affected with polysaccharide storage myopathy can have gait changes that mimic shivering; in bilateral cases rule out EPSSM by submitting a muscle biopsy

PATHOLOGIC FINDINGS
Plant-Associated Stringhalt
Changes on postmortem examination are consistent with those of a distal axonopathy preferentially affecting large axons.

Sporadic Stringhalt
There has been no systematic survey of postmortem lesions in sporadic stringhalt cases, but some severely affected animals have had extensive examinations with no evidence of histologic lesions in the central nervous system or motor unit.

TREATMENT

Plant-Associated Stringhalt
Remove horses from affected pastures.

Sporadic Stringhalt
• Examine the affected limb using ultrasonography, radiographs, and scintigraphy as appropriate, in order to rule out and treat any underlying orthopedic lesions
• Surgical removal of a section of the myotendinous region, containing the Golgi tendon organs, of the lateral digital extensor muscle relieves the syndrome quite spectacularly in many cases; however, a retrospective study of a limited number of cases suggested that there appears to be no real difference in the follow-up outcomes between 4 conservatively treated cases and 6 treated by extensive myotenectomy

FOLLOW-UP

EXPECTED COURSE AND PROGNOSIS
Plant-Associated Stringhalt
The majority of animals recover in a few days to up to 18 months (average 6–12 months) when removed from the affected pasture.

Sporadic Stringhalt
Recovery is variable, presumably depending on the severity of the original injury—some cases remain unchanged, some improve, and a few show resolution of sign.

SEE ALSO
• Polysaccharide storage myopathy
• Shivers (Shivering)

Suggested Reading
Cahill JI, Goulden BE. Stringhalt—current thoughts on aetiology and pathogenesis. Equine Vet J 1992;24:161–162.
Crabill MR, Honnas CM, Taylor DS, et al. Stringhalt secondary to trauma to the dorsoproximal region of the metatarsus in horses: 10 cases (1986-1991). J Am Vet Med Assoc 1994;205:867–869.
MacKay RJ, Wyer S, Gilmour A, et al. Cytotoxic activity of extracts from *Hypochaeris radicata.* Toxicon 2013;70:194–203.

Author Caroline N. Hahn
Consulting Editor Caroline N. Hahn

S

SUMMER PASTURE-ASSOCIATED EQUINE ASTHMA (PASTURE ASTHMA)

 BASICS

DEFINITION
Seasonally recurring progressive lower airway disease. Exposure to inhaled particulates in pasture during hot months elicits inflammation, mucus hypersecretion, and bronchoconstriction. Available treatments are palliative. Removal from the pasture environment is necessary. SPA-EA is similar to asthma associated with barn dust, but differs in its specific association with pasture exposure during hot humid conditions.

PATHOPHYSIOLOGY
• SPA-EA exhibits key facets of human asthma including airway hyperresponsiveness, airway inflammation, and reversible bronchoconstriction. Exacerbations are elicited by particulates inhaled while grazing, especially during high heat and humidity. Mold spores and grass pollen are suspected triggering agents.
• Airway obstruction results from bronchoconstriction, mucus hypersecretion, decreased mucociliary clearance, and inflammatory exudate. Disease chronicity elicits progressive airway remodeling that limits reversibility of airway obstruction. Profound ventilation–perfusion inequalities and hypoxemia are common

SYSTEMS AFFECTED
Respiratory

GENETICS
Uncharacterized, likely a complex polygenic trait.

INCIDENCE/PREVALENCE
Unknown; unpublished survey reported 5% prevalence in Louisiana.

GEOGRAPHIC DISTRIBUTION
• Prevalent in the southeastern USA
• More recently described in the UK
• Anecdotal reports in other places

SIGNALMENT
• Overrepresentation of Quarter Horse-type breeds and ponies may reflect regional disparities in breed distribution and extensive pasture exposure
• Mature horses—12 ± 6 years
• No sex predilection

SIGNS
• Clinical exacerbations predictably occur during hot humid conditions, worsen annually, and remit during cooler months
• Initial signs are exercise intolerance and occasional cough
• With progression, prominent signs include hyperpnea, dyspnea, increased expiratory effort, flared nostrils, and coughing
• Vital signs may be increased, especially respiratory rate. Mildly increased (<39°C (<102.5°F)) body temperature is not uncommon; higher temperatures suggest alternate or intercurrent disease
• Severely affected horses stand with the neck extended, become anorexic, and may become emaciated. They can develop a "heaves line" (hypertrophy of the external abdominal oblique muscles)
• Thoracic auscultation reveals increased bronchovesicular sounds, expiratory wheezes (sometimes inspiratory), and crackles. In mild cases, auscultation is abnormal only during forced breathing

CAUSES
Airborne particulates inhaled during grazing in hot humid conditions are incriminated.

RISK FACTORS
• Extensive pasture exposure (>12 h/day) increases disease risk in the southeastern USA.

 DIAGNOSIS

DIFFERENTIAL DIAGNOSIS
• Viral, bacterial, fungal respiratory infections
• Anhidrosis often occurs in similar (hot and humid) environmental conditions. Associated tachypnea can be mistakenly interpreted as a respiratory condition

CBC/BIOCHEMISTRY/URINALYSIS
• Mild neutrophilia is common
• Mildly increased fibrinogen may occur

OTHER LABORATORY TESTS
• BALF cytology, the preferred diagnostic, identifies increased neutrophils (>10%, often >20%)
• Tracheal aspirate identifies mucopurulent inflammation with nondegenerate neutrophils. Bacterial and fungal elements reflect impaired mucociliary clearance, not necessarily infection. Intracellular bacteria and bacterial growth increase likelihood of active infection
• Arterial blood gases often identify hypoxemia (PaO_2 <80 mmHg). Hypocapnia ($PaCO_2$ <40 mmHg) progresses to hypercapnia ($PaCO_2$ >40 mmHg) in severe disease
• Transcutaneous lung biopsy carries a rare risk of fatal bleeding, outweighing its diagnostic utility

IMAGING
• Tracheal endoscopy reveals mucopurulent exudate. Carina thickening with disease chronicity
• Thoracic radiography may reveal increased bronchointerstitial pattern

OTHER DIAGNOSTIC PROCEDURES
• Tentative diagnosis from historical, signalment, and clinical findings is confirmed by neutrophilic BALF inflammation, exclusion of other diseases, and improvement following environmental modification
• Airway hyperresponsiveness to methacholine bronchoprovocation is identified in exacerbation and remission

PATHOLOGIC FINDINGS
• Chronicity causes airway remodeling with increases in airway smooth muscle mass, peribronchiolar inflammatory infiltrate, fibrosis, intraluminal mucus and inflammatory cells, epithelial hyperplasia with goblet cell hyperplasia/metaplasia, peribronchiolar fibers of the elastic network, and complex cellular disorganization of the terminal bronchiole (terminal bronchiolar remodeling)
• Areas of alveolar overinflation (air trapping) are common; true emphysema is rare

 TREATMENT

AIMS
Remove the inciting cause. Cases with overt distress or that improve slowly despite strict environmental management warrant therapeutic intervention to improve oxygen delivery, reverse airway obstruction due to bronchoconstriction and mucus accumulation, and limit airway inflammation.

APPROPRIATE HEALTH CARE
In- or outpatient medical management.

NURSING CARE
• Exacerbations are reversible with adequate quarantine from the pasture environment in a dust-free indoor environment during warm months of the year. Severely affected horses are stalled on rubber mats without bedding, or using low-dust bedding (pellets, shredded cardboard). Less severe disease may initially be managed on pasture that is cut very short (necessitating an alternate complete diet)
• During seasonal disease exacerbation, reexposure to inciting pasture elicits disease within days

ACTIVITY
Activity is dictated by disease severity and response to therapy; horses in clinical remission may be exercised normally.

DIET
• To minimize dust, a complete pelleted feed that addresses 100% of the forage requirement is preferred, even during cool season remission
• Cubed forage or haylage are preferred to hay (also during remission). When hay is fed, it should be fully submersed in water immediately prior to feeding
• Round hay bales should not be offered, even during remission

CLIENT EDUCATION
• During clinical remission, affected horses should be kept in a low-dust environment when stabled, and pasture should be relatively

S

SUMMER PASTURE-ASSOCIATED EQUINE ASTHMA (PASTURE ASTHMA) (CONTINUED)

short (a few centimeters high), necessitating an alternate complete diet
• Disease recurs predictably in successive years, allowing removal of affected horses from offending pasture prior to seasonal disease onset

MEDICATIONS

DRUG(S) OF CHOICE
Medications recommended for treating heaves are indicated for treating SPA-EA.

Oxygen
Animals with profound dyspnea, hyperpnea should receive inhaled oxygen supplementation (≥10 L/min).

Corticosteroids
• In severe cases, use parenteral dexamethasone 0.05 mg/kg every 24 h for 3 days; decrease dose and increase interval. Disease recrudescence after treatment should direct improved environmental management. Caution in horses with endocrinopathies
• Inhaled formulations (nebulization, pMDIs) are administered using equine spacers and decrease systemic side effects
• Effects of beclomethasone (beclomethasone) dipropionate (≥1 μg/kg every 12 h) or fluticasone propionate (4 μg/kg every 12 h) are delayed, but useful for chronic management

Bronchodilators
• Bronchodilators may be life-saving. Long-term administration must be combined with corticosteroids and environmental control
• Several inhaled β$_2$-adrenergic agonists are effective and available as pMDI or for nebulization. Fast-acting/short-lasting—levalbuterol (levosalbutamol) (1.25 mg/horse (author's recommendation, higher than published dosage)), albuterol (salbutamol) (1–2 μg/kg)
• Oral β$_2$-adrenergic agonists (clenbuterol and albuterol syrup; albuterol tablets; terbutaline sulfate) have low efficacy
• Due to the adverse gastrointestinal effects, systemic parasympatholytic bronchodilators should be limited to the short-acting muscarinic antagonist hyoscine butylbromide (Buscopan) at a dose of 0.3 mg/kg, IV, during asthmatic crisis
• Ipratropium bromide pMDI (1–4 μg/kg) is effective but can excessively dry respiratory secretions

Expectorant, Mucolytic, and Mucokinetic Agents
• Limited anecdotal reports of efficacy
• β$_2$-adrenergic agonists also improve mucociliary clearance

CONTRAINDICATIONS, POSSIBLE INTERACTIONS
• Corticosteroids are contraindicated with infection
• Oral mucokinetic agents that stimulate the gastropulmonary mucokinetic vagal reflex, such as iodides, can exacerbate bronchospasm

ALTERNATIVE DRUGS
• Horses with poor response to bronchodilators may benefit from IV magnesium sulfate administration (40 mg/kg given over 20 min). The effect is limited to the duration of the infusion. Concurrent doses have not been evaluated and have potential for toxicity
• Mast cell stabilizers have been advocated for limiting seasonal exacerbations

FOLLOW-UP

PATIENT MONITORING
• Monitor expiratory effort and pulmonary adventitial sounds
• Some horses with extreme small airway obstruction fail to respond to inhaled bronchodilators due to the severe hypoxic vasoconstriction and bronchoconstriction; they require prolonged inhaled oxygen therapy for improvement. These horses typically present with decreased lung sounds, lack adventitious lung sounds such as wheezes and crackles, and have a paradoxical breathing pattern
• Severely hypoxemic horses should be monitored by serial PaO$_2$ measurements

PREVENTION/AVOIDANCE
Dust-free environment, away from pasture during the warm months of the year.

POSSIBLE COMPLICATIONS
• SPA-EA is debilitating and fatal in severe cases without proper environmental control and medical treatment
• Chronic hypoxic vasoconstriction can lead to pulmonary hypertension and right heart failure

EXPECTED COURSE AND PROGNOSIS
• Though episodic dyspnea is reversible with environmental control and medical therapy, complete isolation from offending pasture particulates is impractical. Thus, affected horses worsen annually at a rate that is influenced by their management
• Neutrophilic airway inflammation often persists during seasonal disease remission
• The onset of disease in horses with SPA-EA is specifically associated with pasture in the summer, and the signs of disease tend to worsen over subsequent seasons. Advance cases may eventually develop clinical signs in response to barn dust, reflecting a progressive airway hyper-responsiveness

MISCELLANEOUS

PREGNANCY/FERTILITY/BREEDING
Fetal growth retardation and death may occur with hypoxic mares.

SYNONYMS
• Summer pasture heaves
• Summer pasture-associated equine asthma (SPA-EA)
• Summer pasture-associated recurrent airway obstruction

SEE ALSO
• Cough, acute/chronic
• Equine asthma
• Expiratory dyspnea
• Heaves (severe equine asthma, RAO)

ABBREVIATIONS
• BALF = bronchoalveolar lavage fluid
• PaCO$_2$ = partial pressure of carbon dioxide in arterial blood
• PaO$_2$ = partial pressure of oxygen in arterial blood
• pMDI = pressurized metered dose inhaler
• SPA-EA = summer pasture-associated equine asthma

Suggested Reading
Beadle RE. Summer pasture-associated obstructive pulmonary disease In: Robinson NE, ed. Current Therapy in Equine Medicine. New York, NY: WB Saunders, 1983:512–516.
Costa LRR, Seajorn TL, Moore RM, et al. Correlation of clinical score, intrapleural pressure, cytologic findings of bronchoalveolar fluid, and histopathologic lesions of pulmonary tissue in horses with summer pasture associated recurrent airway obstruction. Am J Vet Res 2000;61:167–173.
Costa LRR, Johnson JR, Baur ME, Beadle RE. Temporal clinical exacerbation of summer pasture associated recurrent airway obstruction and relationship with climate and aeroallergens in horses. Am J Vet Res 2006;67:1635–1642.

Authors Lais R.R. Costa and Cyprianna Swiderski
Consulting Editors Daniel Jean and Mathilde Leclère

Client Education Handout available online

S

SUPERFICIAL NON-HEALING ULCERS

BASICS

OVERVIEW
• Superficial non-healing or refractory ulcers are injuries of the corneal epithelium that do not penetrate the basement membrane. These ulcers can progress to become deeper ulcers once the basement membrane is injured. In the horse, superficial ulcers are commonly seen associated with protein deposits in the anterior stroma
• Systems affected—ophthalmic

SIGNALMENT
All ages and breeds affected.

SIGNS
• Chronic superficial corneal erosions have an opalescent grayish color, display faint retention of fluorescein dye, and have thin, undulating, acellular, stromal surface membranes
• Erosions are surrounded by a loose lip of migrating, nonattached epithelium, corneal vascularization, and crystalline stromal deposits
• Minimal uveitis is noted

CAUSES AND RISK FACTORS
Unknown; possible primary corneal disease with chronic secondary irritation. For example, this may be secondary to acute corneal ulceration from rubbing of a silicone subpalpebral lavage system. Aged horses, or those that are immunocompromised, are more commonly diagnosed with refractory superficial ulcers than other populations.

DIAGNOSIS

DIFFERENTIAL DIAGNOSIS
• Lid abnormalities such as distichiasis, trichiasis, and entropion; neuroparalytic and neurotrophic keratitis; keratoconjunctivitis sicca; corneal dystrophies; and corneal foreign bodies
• Inappropriate topical corticosteroid therapy causing delayed corneal healing

CBC/BIOCHEMISTRY/URINALYSIS
N/A

OTHER LABORATORY TESTS
Rule out infectious causes (bacterial or fungal) with corneal scrapings for cytology and culture.

IMAGING
N/A

OTHER DIAGNOSTIC PROCEDURES
N/A

PATHOLOGIC FINDINGS
• Histologically, ulceration with a thin membrane of altered corneal stroma, representing corneal stromal sequestration
• Lack of epithelial migration and/or attachment onto the ulcerated surface is present

TREATMENT
• Epithelial debridement of the loose lip of epithelium
• Debridement of the ulcer and disruption of the superficial membrane with a diamond burr
• Grid keratotomies may be used with caution on eyes that have been confirmed to be free of infection
• Superficial keratectomy
• Contact lenses act as bandages. A partial temporary tarsorrhaphy may improve retention of the contact lens
• Prevent self-trauma with a hard- or soft-cupped hood

MEDICATIONS

DRUG(S) OF CHOICE
• Topical broad-spectrum antibiotics (e.g. chloramphenicol, neomycin–polymyxin–gramicidin)
• Topical serum every 2–4 h or topical polysulfated glycosaminoglycans TID (Adequan; diluted with artificial tears solution to 50 mg/mL) may be beneficial

CONTRAINDICATIONS/POSSIBLE INTERACTIONS
• Gentamicin and the fluoroquinolone antibiotics topically may slow corneal healing

• If an infection of the corneal defect is not ruled out first by culture and/or cytology, a grid keratotomy can potentially lead to an infection of the deep corneal stroma with loss of vision or globe
• Solutions, rather than ointments, are the preferred formulation for refractory superficial ulcers

FOLLOW-UP

EXPECTED COURSE AND PROGNOSIS
• Lavage system-induced ulcers are notoriously slow to heal
• Infection is a risk owing to epithelial loss
• Scarring of the cornea may result

MISCELLANEOUS

ASSOCIATED CONDITIONS
• Infection
• Uveitis

SEE ALSO
• Burdock pappus bristle keratopathy
• Calcific band keratopathy
• Corneal/scleral lacerations
• Corneal stromal abscesses
• Corneal ulceration
• Eosinophilic keratitis
• Equine recurrent uveitis
• Glaucoma
• Ulcerative keratomycosis
• Viral (herpes) keratitis (putative)

Suggested Reading
Brooks DE. Ophthalmology for the Equine Practitioner, 2e. Jackson, WY: Teton NewMedia, 2008.
Brooks DE, Matthews AG. Equine ophthalmology. In: Gelatt KN, ed. Veterinary Ophthalmology, 4e. Ames, IA: Blackwell, 2007:1165–1274.
Gilger BC, ed. Equine Ophthalmology, 3e. Ames, IA: Wiley Blackwell, 2017.

Author Caryn E. Plummer
Consulting Editor Caryn E. Plummer
Acknowledgment The author/editor acknowledges the prior contribution of Andras M. Komaromy and Dennis E. Brooks.

S

SUPRAVENTRICULAR ARRHYTHMIAS

BASICS

DEFINITION
• Supraventricular arrhythmias originate in the atria or atrioventricular junction
• The term *supraventricular premature depolarization* refers to isolated premature complexes. More than 4 SVPDs in succession is SVT, and this can be paroxysmal or sustained
• AF is also a supraventricular arrhythmia but is described elsewhere (see chapter Atrial fibrillation)

PATHOPHYSIOLOGY
• Reentry, enhanced automaticity, and accelerated conduction can lead to supraventricular arrhythmias
• Primary myocardial disease is an infrequent cause
• Horses are often able to block conduction of SVPD into the ventricles at the atrioventricular node, a vagal effect, and there is rarely a rapid ventricular rate in the presence of supraventricular arrhythmias

SYSTEMS AFFECTED
Cardiovascular

SIGNALMENT
There are no specific predilections.

SIGNS
General Comments
• SVPDs are common but often incidental during routine examinations
• SVPDs occurring during or after strenuous exercise are rarely of any immediate clinical significance, but may be a risk factor for AF
• SVT is uncommon, but may be associated with poor performance

Historical Findings
Poor performance.

Physical Examination Findings
Individual premature beats or runs of rapid rhythm, usually with a rapid onset and offset.

CAUSES
• Hypoxia
• Sepsis
• Toxemia
• Drugs such as quinidine sulfate
• Autonomic imbalance
• Metabolic and electrolyte imbalance
• Primary myocardial disease

RISK FACTORS
• Mitral or tricuspid valvular disease and congenital cardiac disease leading to atrial enlargement
• Infective endocarditis

DIAGNOSIS

DIFFERENTIAL DIAGNOSIS
• Ventricular premature depolarizations—differentiate with ECG
• Sinus tachycardia—usually speeds up and slows down more subtly with sinus tachycardia than with SVT; differentiate with ECG

CBC/BIOCHEMISTRY/URINALYSIS
Electrolyte or metabolic abnormalities may be present.

OTHER LABORATORY TESTS
• Increased serum concentration of cardiac troponin I may be present
• Blood culture may be indicated in some cases

IMAGING
Echocardiography
• The echocardiogram is most often normal, or there may be a slightly low shortening fraction, particularly with SVT
• With primary myocardial disease, there are more profound decreases in fractional shortening and abnormalities of myocardial wall motion (dyskinesis or akinesis) and mitral and aortic valve motion
• Foci of increased or decreased echogenicity are occasionally seen within the myocardium
• Echocardiography may reveal evidence of other cardiac diseases such as infective endocarditis or severe valvular disease

OTHER DIAGNOSTIC PROCEDURES
ECG
• SVPDs are represented by a premature P wave, which may (conducted) or may not (unconducted) be followed by a QRS-T complex (Figure 1)
• The shape of the premature P wave is different from those of sinus origin, but the configurations of the premature QRS complex and T wave are the same as those of sinus origin as conduction through the ventricle is not affected
• The premature P wave may not be visible if it occurs sufficiently early that it is buried in the preceding T wave
• Junctional complexes do not have a P wave but do have the same QRS configuration as those of sinus origin
• Occasionally, SVPDs have QRS complexes that are of slightly larger duration and morphology compared to the sinus QRS complexes
• Characterizing the frequency with an ambulatory ECG over prolonged periods and presence or absence during exercise are invaluable for assessing the clinical significance and assessing response to therapy
• It can be helpful to examine multiple leads to differentiate premature P waves and confirm that all premature QRS complexes have a configuration that is identical to those of sinus origin

PATHOLOGIC FINDINGS
• There is often no underlying cardiac disease
• Focal or diffuse myocardial necrosis, inflammation, or fibrosis may be present
• Atrial enlargement and valvular pathology may be identified

TREATMENT

AIMS
• Address any predisposing causes
• Antiarrhythmic therapy in selected cases

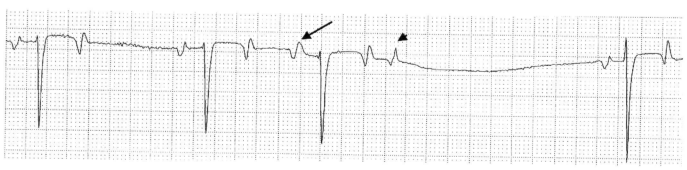

Figure 1.

Conducted (arrow) and unconducted (arrowhead) SVPDs—the premature P waves differ slightly from those of sinus origin whereas all QRS are the same; base–apex lead, 25 mm/s, 5 mm = 1 mV

APPROPRIATE HEALTH CARE

• Emergency antiarrhythmic therapy is restricted to cases in which the rhythm is unstable and life-threatening. This is very rarely necessary except in cases in which the rapid SVT is due to drug treatment such as quinidine sulfate
• Oral antiarrhythmic therapy is occasionally used for frequent SVPDs and/or SVT

NURSING CARE

Continuous ECG monitoring is indicated and horses should be kept quiet and not moved during the antiarrhythmic therapy.

ACTIVITY

• SVPDs are not an important cause of collapse during exercise; and if there is no poor performance, horses with SVPDs can be exercised normally
• Horses with poor performance may benefit from rest
• Horses with SVT during exercise should not be exercised

DIET

N/A

CLIENT EDUCATION

Clients should be counseled that the main risk associated with SVPD is that it may predispose the horse to developing AF in the future. Normal exercise can be performed in most horses with SVPD providing there is no poor performance.

SURGICAL CONSIDERATIONS

Surgical ablation techniques have been performed successfully in horses with supraventricular arrhythmias.

 MEDICATIONS

DRUG(S) OF CHOICE

• In the absence of any predisposing causes precluding their use, such as infective endocarditis, corticosteroids are often used in horses with SVPD. Either prednisolone 1 mg/kg PO every 48 h or dexamethasone 0.05–0.1 mg/kg IV, or 0.1 mg/kg PO every 24 h for 3 or 4 days and then continued every 3–4 days in decreasing dosages, is recommended. Vitamin C (20 mg/kg PO every 24 h) and vitamin E (10 IU/kg PO every 24 h) may also be beneficial owing to their antioxidant effect
• Phenytoin given orally at doses of 5–15 mg/kg every 12 h may be effective in suppressing SVPD, but the arrhythmia may recur on discontinuation of therapy
• Digoxin is given IV at 0.0022 mg/kg for emergency treatment of rapid SVT, particularly when it is associated with quinidine administration. For less rapid SVT during quinidine therapy, digoxin can be given at 0.011 mg/kg PO every 12 h. Digoxin is less likely to be effective against SVPDs,

although occasionally favorable responses have been observed when it is used orally
• Propranolol given IV at 0.03–2 mg/kg can be used for emergency treatment of rapid SVT, particularly if digoxin is unsuccessful
• Quinidine sulfate (single dose of up to 22 mg/kg PO) and quinidine gluconate (0.5–2.2 mg/kg IV boluses to a maximum of 12 mg/kg) are indicated for treating rare cases of rapid SVT when it is not associated with quinidine administration

CONTRAINDICATIONS

Corticosteroids should *not* be used in horses with concurrent pituitary pars intermedia dysfunction or active laminitis.

PRECAUTIONS

• Horses should be monitored for signs of laminitis if receiving corticosteroid therapy
• Adverse effects of digoxin include anorexia, depression, abdominal pain, and ventricular arrhythmias. Ideally, therapeutic drug monitoring should be used to ensure that plasma digoxin concentrations remain at therapeutic levels (1–2 µg/mL)
• Adverse effects of phenytoin include excitement, sedation, and other neurologic signs. Ideally, therapeutic drug monitoring should be used to ensure that plasma phenytoin concentrations remain at therapeutic levels (5–10 ug/ml)
• Adverse effects of quinidine include myocardial depression, colic, diarrhea, and ventricular arrhythmias. Ideally, therapeutic drug monitoring should be used to ensure that plasma phenytoin concentrations remain at therapeutic levels (3–5 µg/mL)

POSSIBLE INTERACTIONS

There is interaction between quinidine and digoxin.

ALTERNATIVE DRUGS

Other drugs used in humans for treatment of SVT may be beneficial in horses, but protocols for their use have yet to be defined. Sotalol is often prescribed for long-term oral antiarrhythmic therapy in humans and has intermediate bioavailability in horses. Doses of 1–4 mg/kg sotalol PO every 12 hours have been used, gradually increasing the dose. Sweating can occur with larger doses.

 FOLLOW-UP

PATIENT MONITORING

24 h Holter monitoring and exercise ECG are the most useful tools to assess the success of therapy and, when no treatment has been recommended, to monitor for any progression of the supraventricular arrhythmia.

POSSIBLE COMPLICATIONS

• The main risk associated with SVPD is that it may predispose the horse to developing AF in the future. However, the magnitude of this risk in horses that have not previously had

paroxysmal or sustained AF has not been quantified. Horses that have previously had AF are more likely to have recurrences if SVPDs are detected after treatment of the AF or SVT occurs during treatment. AF is also more likely to develop if there is underlying heart disease
• Horses that develop SVPDs in association with atrial enlargement and severe underlying cardiac disease are at particular risk of developing AF and this often marks the onset of declining clinical status and congestive heart failure. In these cases, the SVPDs can be regarded as a complication of the underlying condition rather than a cause of AF

EXPECTED COURSE AND PROGNOSIS

Horses in which SVPDs are detected as an incidental finding may frequently remain asymptomatic in work for prolonged periods.

 MISCELLANEOUS

ASSOCIATED CONDITIONS

• Tricuspid and mitral regurgitation
• Atrial septal defect
• Infective endocarditis

SEE ALSO

• Atrial fibrillation
• Atrial septal defect
• Endocarditis infective
• Ionophore toxicosis
• Myocardial disease
• Ventricular arrhythmias

ABBREVIATIONS

• AF = atrial fibrillation
• SVPD = supraventricular premature depolarization
• SVT = supraventricular tachycardia

Suggested Reading
Broux B, De Clercq D, Decloedt A, et al. Pharmacokinetics of intravenously and orally administered sotalol hydrochloride in horses and effects on surface electrocardiogram and left ventricular systolic function. Vet J 2016;208:60–64.
Dembek KA, Hurcombe SD, Schober KE, Toribio RE. Sudden death of a horse with supraventricular tachycardia following oral administration of flecainide acetate. J Vet Emerg Crit Care 2014;24:759–763.
Reef VB, Marr CM. Dysrhythmias: assessment and medical management. In: Marr CM, Bowen M, eds. Cardiology of the Horse, 2e. Edinburgh, UK: Saunders Elsevier, 2010:159–178.
Sage A, Mogg TD. Pharmacology of drugs used to treat cardiac disease. In: Marr CM, Bowen M, eds. Cardiology of the Horse, 2e. Edinburgh, UK: Saunders Elsevier, 2010:75–87.

Author Celia M. Marr
Consulting Editors Celia M. Marr and Virginia B. Reef

S

SUSPENSORY DESMITIS

BASICS

OVERVIEW
• SLD is acute or chronic SL injury of the proximal, body, and/or branches. • DSLD is a progressive, debilitating disorder resulting in continuous SL enlargement owing to ineffective collagen fiber repair and generalized interstitial and periligamentous fibrosis. • Systems affected—musculoskeletal: palmar/plantar MCIII/MTIII

SIGNALMENT
SLD
• Performance horses. • Hind SLD—Standardbreds, upper level dressage.
• Thoroughbred racers—SL rupture in catastrophic breakdown

DSLD
Peruvian Paso most common.

SIGNS
SLD
• Acute, insidious, mild to moderate lameness. • Lameness resolves with rest; recurs with exercise. • ± Forelimb lameness worse on outside of circle. • Subtle hindlimb lameness, worse when ridden. • ± Localized heat, swelling, pain. • ± Palpable thickening, positive limb flexions. • ± Fetlock effusion with branch injury. • Complete rupture—dropped fetlock, severe lameness

DSLD
• Acute—stiffness, reluctance to work, back pain. • Subtle, chronic intermittent or persistent unilateral to quadrilateral lameness.
• End-stage—reluctant to move, lie down often. • Palpable thickening, pain.
• Progressive fetlock drop

CAUSES AND RISK FACTORS
SLD
• Foot imbalance, long pasterns, fetlock hyperextension. • Back at the knee or tied-in below the knee, straight hock. • Axial splint exostosis ("blind splint")

DSLD
• Peruvian Paso heritage. • Abnormal proteoglycan deposition in connective tissues

DIAGNOSIS

DIFFERENTIAL DIAGNOSIS
SLD
• Proximal front—middle carpal or carpometacarpal joint pain, avulsion/stress MCIII fracture, carpal sheath/retinaculum pain. • Proximal hind—tarsometatarsal joint pain, avulsion/stress MTIII fracture

DSLD
Injury-mediated SLD.

IMAGING
US
• Acute—focal isoechoic/anechoic core lesion.
• Chronic—decreased echogenicity, abnormal fiber pattern. • Increased cross-sectional area.
• ± Periligamentous thickening, adhesions.
• Unweighted and "off-incidence" images enhance diagnosis. • Dystrophic calcification.
• DSLD—progressive enlargement, loss of echogenicity and fiber pattern, primarily in branches

MRI
• Superior to US. • SL changes, osseous involvement. • Indicated if lameness localized to SL and other imaging normal

Radiography
• ± Normal. • Proximal MCIII/MTIII—subchondral sclerosis, avulsion fracture.
• Sesamoiditis, sesamoid fracture. • Splint bone exostosis or fracture

Nuclear Scintigraphy
SLD often negative; proximal palmar/plantar MCIII/MTIII uptake with bony injury.

OTHER DIAGNOSTIC PROCEDURES
SLD
• Diagnostic analgesia—high palmar/plantar, lateral palmar, subtarsal, SL local infiltration.
• ± Diffusion of intra-articular middle carpal and tarsometatarsal analgesia into proximal SL

DSLD
• Diagnostic analgesia as for SLD. • ± Nuchal ligament biopsy

PATHOLOGIC FINDINGS
DSLD—histopathology: large proteoglycan accumulations in SL(s).

TREATMENT

SLD
• Acute—local and/or systemic analgesics and anti-inflammatory(s). • Controlled exercise program—stall rest and hand-walking for weeks to months then gradual return to exercise. • Hoof balance, heel support, eggbar shoes. • Ancillary therapies: ○ Extracorporeal shockwave therapy. ○ Percutaneous SL splitting (desmoplasty). ○ Palmar/plantar metacarpal/metatarsal fasciotomy.
○ Neurectomy of deep branch of lateral plantar nerve. ○ Intralesional injections (stem cells, platelet-rich plasma, bioscaffold material)

DSLD
• Local and/or systemic analgesics and anti-inflammatory(s). • Controlled exercise program. • Stall confinement. • Extended heel support, eggbar shoes

MEDICATIONS

DRUG(S) OF CHOICE
• NSAIDs—phenylbutazone 2.2–4.4 mg/kg SID–BID. • Systemic chondroprotective drugs—polysulfated glycosaminoglycan (500 mg IM every 4 days for 7 treatments) or sodium hyaluronate (40 mg IV every 7 days for 3 treatments). • Oral glucosamine/ chondroitin sulfate powder (1 scoop (3.3 g) BID)

CONTRAINDICATIONS/POSSIBLE INTERACTIONS
Intralesional corticosteroids.

FOLLOW-UP

PATIENT MONITORING
• US and lameness every 8–12 weeks.
• Recurrence of lameness, heat, swelling during rehabilitation prompts stall rest and reexamination

POSSIBLE COMPLICATIONS
Chronic lameness despite treatment.

EXPECTED COURSE AND PROGNOSIS
• Convalescence 6–12 months depending on lesion severity. • Good athletic prognosis for front proximal SLD; poor for hind proximal SLD. • High recurrence in inadequately rested horses. • DSLD—poor prognosis

MISCELLANEOUS

ASSOCIATED CONDITIONS
SLD
• MCIII/MTIII avulsion fracture. • Splint bone fracture, exostosis. • Sesamoid fracture, sesamoiditis

SEE ALSO
Tendonitis

ABBREVIATIONS
• DSLD = degenerative suspensory ligament disease. • MCIII = third metacarpus.
• MRI = magnetic resonance imaging.
• MTIII = third metatarsus. • SL = suspensory ligament. • SLD = suspensory ligament desmitis. • US = ultrasonography, ultrasound

Suggested Reading
Dyson SJ. The suspensory apparatus. In: Ross MW, Dyson SJ, eds. Diagnosis and Management of Lameness in the Horse. St. Louis, MO: Saunders, 2003:654–666.
Werpy NM, Denoix JM. Imaging of the equine proximal suspensory ligament. Vet Clin North Am Equine Pract 2012;28(3):507–525.

Author JoAnn Slack
Consulting Editor Elizabeth J. Davidson

SYNCHRONOUS DIAPHRAGMATIC FLUTTER

BASICS

OVERVIEW
• SDF ("thumps") is a rhythmic contraction of the diaphragm that is synchronous with the heartbeat
• Results from hyperexcitability of the phrenic nerve secondary to acid–base (alkalosis) and/or electrolyte (hypocalcemia, hypomagnesemia) imbalances; the electric impulse from atrial depolarization stimulates the phrenic nerve, causing diaphragmatic contractions synchronic with the heartbeat
• Pathophysiology
  ∘ Electrolyte and acid–base imbalances may increase phrenic nerve excitability
  ∘ The phrenic nerve is stimulated by atrial depolarizations where it passes over the right atrium
  ∘ Decreased calcium, potassium, and magnesium concentrations increase nerve excitability
  ∘ Alkalosis (respiratory or metabolic) increases calcium and magnesium binding to albumin, leading to ionized hypocalcemia and hypomagnesemia
• Systems affected—nervous, cardiac, and muscular

SIGNALMENT
Any breed, age, or sex. Rare in young animals.

SIGNS
Historical Findings
• Prolonged exercise accompanied by intense sweating (endurance horses, Thoroughbred or Standardbred racehorses)
• Also associated with GI disease, blister beetle toxicosis, lactation tetany, transportation, and trauma

Physical Examination Findings
• Pathognomonic sign—a spasmodic contraction of the flank that is synchronous with the first heartbeat (atrial depolarization) and independent of the respiratory cycle
• Flank twitching may not occur with every heartbeat
• Strong contractions may produce a thumping noise, which has led to the name "thumps"

CAUSES AND RISK FACTORS
• Electrolyte-deficient diets, diuretic use, excessive sweating (metabolic alkalosis), hyperventilation (respiratory alkalosis), GI disease, transportation, lactation tetany, and hypoparathyroidism
• Hypocalcemia, hypomagnesemia, hypokalemia, hypochloremia, and alkalosis, either individually or in combination

DIAGNOSIS

DIFFERENTIAL DIAGNOSIS
• Hiccups and nonsynchronous diaphragmatic flutter have been observed. In these cases, diaphragmatic twitching is not synchronous with cardiac contraction
• Forceful contractions of the abdominal muscles may accompany severe respiratory disease. Affected horses present with signs of respiratory disease, and abdominal contractions are associated with expiration, not a heartbeat

CBC/BIOCHEMISTRY/URINALYSIS
• Hypocalcemia, hypokalemia, hypochloremia, hypomagnesemia, and alkalosis (metabolic or respiratory) are common laboratory abnormalities
• Serum ionized calcium is more accurate than total calcium to diagnose hypocalcemia
• Serum ionized magnesium is more accurate than total magnesium to diagnose hypomagnesemia

OTHER LABORATORY TESTS
Blood gas analysis for acid–base status.

DIAGNOSTIC PROCEDURES
Simultaneously record the ECG and the diaphragmatic contractions, either manually or with electromyography or phonocardiography.

TREATMENT
• Correction of underlying condition and restoring electrolyte and acid–base abnormalities
• Oral or parenteral administration of balanced electrolyte solutions
• Hypocalcemia may be corrected by IV administration of 23% calcium gluconate solution (21.4 mg/mL calcium; add 50–100 ml/L of isotonic fluids). If SDF does not resolve, increase calcium dose or supplement fluids with $MgSO_4$ (1–2 g/L) or KCl (10–20 mEq/L), depending on laboratory abnormalities
• Rapid administration of calcium gluconate (e.g. 100 mL over 15–30 min) may be indicated if there are other signs of hypocalcemia (e.g. muscle fasciculations, excitability)
• Administration of 0.9% NaCl helps correct metabolic alkalosis and hypokalemia

MEDICATIONS

CONTRAINDICATIONS/POSSIBLE INTERACTIONS
Administration of alkalinizing solutions (e.g. bicarbonate) may worsen clinical signs by

decreasing available free calcium and free magnesium.

FOLLOW-UP

PATIENT MONITORING
Monitor electrolytes, acid–base status, and clinical signs.

PREVENTION/AVOIDANCE
• When large electrolyte losses are anticipated (e.g. endurance ride), administer electrolytes before, during, and after losses occur
• Avoid chronic calcium supplementation because it reduces parathyroid hormone secretion and may impair mobilization of calcium from bone when needed

POSSIBLE COMPLICATIONS
Electrolyte abnormalities may lead to ileus, muscle weakness, and cardiac arrhythmias.

EXPECTED COURSE AND PROGNOSIS
SDF is not life-threatening; in most cases; it is a transient condition that resolves either spontaneously or in response to treatment of the underlying problem. In horses with primary hypoparathyroidism SDF could last for days, is often recurrent after calcium therapy, and the prognosis for recovery is guarded.

MISCELLANEOUS

ASSOCIATED CONDITIONS
• Prolonged exercise in hot, humid conditions
• Lactation
• GI disease

SEE ALSO
• Calcium, hypocalcemia
• Magnesium (Mg^2)

ABBREVIATIONS
• GI = gastrointestinal
• SDF = synchronous diaphragmatic flutter

Suggested Reading
Toribio RE. Disorders of calcium and phosphorus. In: Reed SM, Bayly WM, Sellon DC, eds. Equine Internal Medicine, 4e. St. Louis, MO: Elsevier, 2018: 1029–1052.
Toribio RE. Magnesium and Disease. In: Reed SM, Bayly WM, Sellon DC, eds. Equine Internal Medicine, 4e. St. Louis, MO: Elsevier, 2018:1052–1058.
Toribio RE. Disorders of calcium and phosphate metabolism in horses. Vet Clin North Am Equine Pract 2011;27:129–147.

Author Ramiro Toribio
Consulting Editors Michel Levy and Heidi Banse
Acknowledgment The author and editors acknowledge the prior contribution of Laurent Couëtil.

S

SYNOVIAL FLUID

 BASICS

DEFINITION
• A dialysate of plasma with the addition of hyaluronan and certain glycoproteins
• Normal synovial fluid is light yellow, clear, free of particulate material, and viscous, producing a strand ≅2.5 cm in length. It is found in joints, tendons sheaths, and bursae
• Smears from normal synovial fluid have low cellularity—<1000 cells/µL (1×10^9/mL), consisting primarily of a mixture of small lymphocytes, macrophages, and synovial lining cells. Many laboratories report these cells collectively as mononuclear cells
• A consistent feature of normal synovial fluid is that neutrophils should constitute <10% of the cells. Few (if any) erythrocytes should be present
• Normal values for equine synovial fluid protein vary between author and method. Upper limits of normal, as reported by various authors, are generally in the range 1–3 g/dL
• Synovial fluid functions as a biologic lubricant and as a medium for transfer of nutrients and cytokines to avascular cartilage

PATHOPHYSIOLOGY
• Synovial fluid evaluation alone does not establish a specific diagnosis, but reflects the degree and type of inflammation of the synovial lining (synovitis)
• Damage to articular cartilage often is not reflected in routine synovial fluid analysis
• Synovial fluid analysis is most useful in the diagnosis of sepsis in synovial structures and, with currently available tests, has little value in differentiating the causes of degenerative and traumatic joint conditions
• Gross appearance is insensitive

SYSTEMS AFFECTED
Musculoskeletal

SIGNALMENT
Any breed, age, or sex.

SIGNS
Historical Findings
Lameness

Physical Examination Findings
• Lameness
• Swollen joint(s) or synovial structures

CAUSES
Septic Arthritis/Synovitis
• A clinical emergency that causes marked changes in synovial fluid
• Routine synovial fluid examination usually provides sufficient information to establish a presumptive diagnosis
• Depending on the cell count, fluid color may range from a slightly cloudy, dark yellow to an opaque cream. Red to red-brown is common with inflammation-induced hemorrhage

• Flocculent material may be apparent
• Fluid viscosity is markedly reduced
• Cytology usually shows >90% neutrophils
• Total nucleated cell count >10000 cells/µL (10×10^9/L), often much higher
• Total protein concentrations are markedly elevated, typically >4.0 g/dL
• In many cases, bacteria are not seen on cytologic examination. Lack of identifiable bacteria, however, should not diminish consideration of sepsis in fluids with markedly elevated neutrophil counts
• Culture of bacteria from the synovial fluid from septic joints can be expected to be positive in only about 50% of cases
• Many times, neutrophils do not show marked degenerative changes with septic arthritis
• Synovial fluid should be considered infected if total nucleated cell counts are >30000 cells/µL (30×10^9/L) with >80% neutrophils and/or total protein >4.0 g/L. However, immune-mediated synovitis may yield similar results

Resolving Synovial Disease or Chronic Synovitis
• Synovial disease that is resolving, especially from previous joint sepsis, may appear similar to traumatic or degenerative joint disease
• Mononuclear component with vacuolated macrophages and variable numbers of synovial cells and lymphocytes
• Neutrophils are <10% of the cell component
• Cell counts are within normal limits to slightly increased
• Chronic synovitis may have a predominance of macrophages/monocytes or lymphocytes
• Lymphocytic synovial fluid reflects lymphocytic inflammation within the synovial membrane and, rarely, may contain plasma cells
• Lymphocytic synovitis has been attributed to proliferative synovitis and infectious agents

Degenerative/Traumatic Joint Disease
• Many conditions result in traumatic or degenerative joint injury. Associated inflammation is variable and often mild
• Synovial fluid usually is clear, unless there is associated hemorrhage, in which case it may be red-tinged
• Viscosity may be decreased proportionately to the amount of effusion
• Cell counts vary from normal to moderately increased, usually being <10000 cells/µL (10×10^9/L) and consisting of >90% mononuclear cells
• Macrophages may be large and vacuolated, sometimes containing phagocytized debris
• An increased percentage of neutrophils (>10%) may occur in some cases of acute trauma or with hemorrhage into the joint that adds peripheral blood neutrophils to the joint fluid. The total nucleated cell count is much less than typically seen with septic arthritis

• Traumatic injury is typically associated with a mild <5000 cells/µL (5×10^9/L), predominantly mononuclear cell response
• Cartilage fragments may be seen in synovial fluid associated with trauma or degenerative joint disease (uncommon)

Other Non-Septic Joint Disease
Immune-mediated, chemical, and idiopathic synovitis are usually associated with systemic disease, intrasynovial injection, or may occur spontaneously and need to be differentiated from septic synovitis.

RISK FACTORS
• Septic arthritis—FPT in neonates
• Penetrating injuries or wounds near synovial structures
• Performance horses

 DIAGNOSIS

DIFFERENTIAL DIAGNOSIS
See Causes.

LABORATORY FINDINGS
General
• Place samples in an EDTA tube for the most important parameters—cell counts, cytology, and protein concentration
• If only a small amount (<0.25 mL) of fluid can be retrieved, make and submit air-dried direct smears
• Placing extremely small quantities of fluid in an EDTA tube results in excessive dilution of the sample and, possibly, in a falsely increased total protein concentration
• Fluid should be collected aseptically and placed in a dry sterile tube for bacteriology or, alternatively, in blood culture bottles

OTHER LABORATORY TESTS
Joint Fluid Analysis
Physical Characteristics
• Color, clarity, and an estimate of viscosity are noted
• Viscosity may be estimated by placing a drop of synovial fluid between the thumb and forefinger, slowly pulling the fingers apart, and evaluating the strand length before breaking. Alternatively, strand length before breaking can be noted as synovial fluid is expelled through the tip of a needle
Leukocyte Count (White Blood Cells)
• Leukocyte counts may be done manually using a hemocytometer or using electronic cell counters
• Cell counts often are too low to be accurately determined with an electronic cell counter
• Leukocyte counts are subject to sources of analytic error and must not be interpreted too strictly when comparing serial counts
• Markedly exudative samples (e.g. from septic joints) with dramatically elevated leukocyte counts >50000 cells/µL

$(5 \times 10^{10}/L)$ often contain numerous cell clumps that preclude an accurate cell count
• Samples of low cellularity are subject to a different source of error. In samples with normal viscosity, cell counts may be falsely low because the sample fails to mix evenly with the diluent
Erythrocyte Count
• Erythrocyte counts are obtained from electronic cell counters or hemocytometers if a diluent that does not lyse erythrocytes is used
• Erythrocytes indicate contamination during sample collection or hemorrhage secondary to hemostatic abnormalities, traumatic injury, or inflammatory disease. This is best differentiated at sample collection because hemorrhage during collection is usually apparent as a non-uniformly red-tinged fluid
• Marked blood contamination increases the nucleated cell count and alters the differential leukocyte count, usually increasing the percentage of neutrophils
Cytology
• Along with a nucleated cell count, probably the most diagnostically important parameter of synovial fluid evaluation
• With a limited sample, direct smears, from which the cell count an be estimated, should be made first
• Blood contamination, in additional to adding RBCs, can add various leukocytes in proportions typical of peripheral blood (i.e. predominantly neutrophils)
• Predominance of neutrophils, rather than of mononuclear cells, indicates inflammation of the synovial lining
• In most species, neutrophilic inflammation is seen with septic and immune-mediated joint diseases
• Because immune-mediated arthritis has not been well documented in horses, the main consideration for neutrophilic inflammation is septic arthritis, but traumatic injury and chemical synovitis should be considered
• Gram stain may demonstrate bacteria, although often bacteria are not seen even with sepsis. If bacteria are seen, it may be useful to direct antibiotic choice
• Erythrocytes indicate blood contamination during sample collection or hemorrhage from hemostatic defects, trauma, or inflammatory disease. Differentiating these conditions based on cytology is difficult. Macrophages containing phagocytized RBCs (i.e. erythrophagocytosis) indicate intra-articular hemorrhage if the slides were made soon after collection. Phagocytosis of erythrocytes by macrophages can occur in vitro during

prolonged transport (i.e. several hours). Platelets suggest blood contamination during sample collection
Total Protein Concentration
• Some laboratories measure protein concentration using a dye-binding method; others use a refractometer
• Protein measurements may help to indicate the presence of inflammation but are not useful in differentiating between types of inflammation
• Increased protein concentrations are seen with synovial inflammation. Concentrations of >2.5 g/dL are abnormal
• Nonseptic inflammatory conditions usually result in protein concentrations of <4.0 g/dL
Bacteriology
Bacterial culture and sensitivity of joint fluid when septic synovitis is suspected.

IMAGING
Radiography, ultrasonography, nuclear scintigraphy, CT, and MRI all may be useful for establishing a diagnosis.

OTHER DIAGNOSTIC PROCEDURES
Arthroscopy

PATHOLOGIC FINDINGS
• Cartilage degeneration, synovitis
• Dependent on the underlying cause

 TREATMENT
Directed at the underlying cause.

SURGICAL CONSIDERATIONS
Joint lavage.

 MEDICATIONS
DRUG(S) OF CHOICE
• Specific for the underlying cause
• Intra-articular antibiotics in some cases

PRECAUTIONS
Samples must be collected aseptically.

 FOLLOW-UP
Serial monitoring of synovial fluid often useful diagnostically and to monitor response to treatment.

PATIENT MONITORING
Dependent on the underlying disease.

✓ MISCELLANEOUS
ASSOCIATED CONDITIONS
Support-limb laminitis.

AGE-RELATED FACTORS
Neonates with FPT can develop sepsis and septic joints.

SYNONYMS
Joint fluid.

SEE ALSO
• Failure of transfer of passive immunity
• Osteoarthritis

ABBREVIATIONS
• CT = computed tomography
• FTPI = failure of transfer of passive immunity
• MRI = magnetic resonance imaging
• RBC = red blood cell

Suggested Reading
Adkins AR. Establishing a diagnosis of septic arthritis/osteomyelitis—a challenging process. Equine Vet Educ 2012;24: 615–617.
Cousty M, David Stack J, Tricaud C, David F. Effect of arthroscopic lavage and repeated intra-articular administrations of antibiotic in adult horses and foals with septic arthritis. Vet Surg 2017;46(7):1008–1016.
McIwraith CW. Use of synovial fluid and serum biomarkers in equine bone and joint disease: a review. Equine Vet J 2005;37:473–482.
Steel CM. Equine synovial fluid analysis. Vet Clin North Am Equine Pract 2008;24(2):437–454.
Trotter GW, McIlwraith CW. Clinical features and diagnosis of equine joint disease. In: McIlwraith CW, Trotter GW, eds. Joint Disease in the Horse. Philadelphia, PA: WB Saunders, 1996:137–141.

Author Tias Muurlink
Consulting Editor Sandra D. Taylor

S

TEMPOROHYOID OSTEOARTHROPATHY

BASICS

OVERVIEW
THO is a disorder of the joint formed by the stylohyoid and the petrous temporal bones. The condition can result in several clinical signs and in a dysfunction of the vestibulocochlear and facial nerves that can acutely worsen if a fracture of the adjacent bones occurs.

Pathophysiology
The exact etiology of THO is unknown. It is postulated that osteoarthritis of the temporohyoid joint precedes other changes and that involvement of the osseous bulla and proximal stylohyoid bone occurs by extension of the degenerative joint disease. The fused joint may fracture during normal movements of the tongue such as mastication or phonation, leading to impingement of the facial and vestibular nerve. In some cases, bone reaction might be secondary to otitis or guttural pouch disease; however, rarely has an infectious process been shown.

Systems Affected
Peripheral nervous system.

SIGNALMENT
The disease is most common in middle-aged horses, but clinical signs (ear rubbing and shyness) starting at a few months of age have been reported.

SIGNS
• Non-neurological clinical signs include difficulty chewing, pain over the periauricular area, headshaking, aural discharge, and behavioral problems
• Acute signs of vestibular disease are common and include a head tilt and nystagmus with the fast phase away from the side of the lesion. Severely affected horses can circle towards the side of the lesion or end up recumbent with the affected side down
• Damage to the facial nerve leads to ptosis and a dropped ear on the side of the lesion, and muzzle deviation away from the side of the lesion
• Facial nerve paresis can cause exposure keratitis

CAUSES AND RISK FACTORS
• Quarter Horses are overrepresented in some case series and crib-biters might be predisposed
• Veterinary procedures (nasogastric intubation, dental work) might precipitate the condition

DIAGNOSIS

DIFFERENTIAL DIAGNOSIS
Trauma, equine protozoal myeloencephalitis, otitis media and interna.

CBC/BIOCHEMISTRY/URINALYSIS
No specific abnormalities.

OTHER LABORATORY TESTS
N/A

IMAGING
• Radiographs are not as sensitive as endoscopy. A ventrodorsal view can be useful
• CT provides an excellent assessment of the bony abnormalities. MRI and scintigraphy are potentially useful to detect early lesions

OTHER DIAGNOSTIC PROCEDURES
• Endoscopic changes of temporohyoid bone ankylosis and enlargement of the proximal stylohyoid bone are pathognomonic
• A CSF tap when acute vestibular signs develop. Most cases have xanthochromia with elevated protein and nondegenerate inflammatory cells. A CSF culture is indicated when meningitis is suspected
• An otoscopy when an underlying otitis is suspected. A tympanocentesis (general anesthesia) may help to identify an infectious cause
• Brainstem auditory-evoked response can assess auditory function and help identify cases with bilateral disease
• Schirmer's tear test may reveal reduced tear production (damage to the parasympathetic lacrimal branch of the facial nerve)

TREATMENT
• Vestibular dysfunction may improve regardless of therapy owing to visual compensation
• Supportive care is essential. Provide soft feed to reduce risks of fracture displacement
• Partial stylohyoidectomy and ceratohyoidectomy reduce stresses on the temporohyoid joint with the latter procedure being currently considered the standard surgical approach
• A partial tarsorrhaphy may be necessary to manage palpebral dysfunction

MEDICATIONS

DRUG(S) OF CHOICE
• Broad-spectrum antibiotics are recommended for 2–4 weeks (e.g.

trimethoprim–sulfa 30 mg/kg PO twice daily)
• NSAIDs (phenylbutazone 2.2 mg/kg PO once or twice daily) may improve comfort and reduce inflammation
• Severe vestibular disease may benefit from corticosteroids (beginning at 0.04–0.08 mg/kg dexamethasone)

CONTRAINDICATIONS/POSSIBLE INTERACTIONS
The acute nature of the fracture and subsequent vestibular disease can make these horses dangerous to ride. Even horses that appear healed can look profoundly worse when blindfolded.

FOLLOW-UP

PREVENTION/AVOIDANCE
In horses with THO, reducing stress on the hyoid apparatus includes cautious dental procedures and use of a bitless bridle.

POSSIBLE COMPLICATIONS
• Meningitis can result from a fracture extending to the cranial vault. CSF leaking from the affected ear can be noted
• Dysphagia may occur if pain impairs mastication or if the fracture extends to the foramen lacerum where the glossopharyngeal and vagal nerves exit the skull

EXPECTED COURSE AND PROGNOSIS
Fair for long-term resolution even with surgery.

MISCELLANEOUS

SEE ALSO
• Equine protozoal myeloencephalitis (EPM)
• Head trauma

ABBREVIATIONS
• CSF = cerebrospinal fluid
• CT = computed tomography
• MRI = magnetic resonance imaging
• NSAID = nonsteroidal anti-inflammatory drug
• THO = temporohyoid osteoarthropathy

Suggested Reading
Koch C, Witte T. Temporohyoid osteoarthropathy in the horse. Equine Vet Educ 2014;26(3):121–125.

Author Sophie Mainguy-Seers
Consulting Editor Caroline N. Hahn
Acknowledgment The author acknowledges the prior contribution of Caroline N. Hahn.

BASICS

DEFINITION
Acute or chronic injury of tendon and/or musculotendinous junction; most commonly refers to SDFT and DDFT injury.

PATHOPHYSIOLOGY
- Normal SDFT of galloping Thoroughbreds elongates by up to 16% of its original length. SDFT failure occurs with elongations (strains) of ≥20%. This small safety margin is probably a major factor in the high incidence of SDFT injury in Thoroughbred racehorses
- Excessive tendon loading results in disruption of collagen fibrils and extracellular matrix. Intratendinous hemorrhage and hematoma occurs. Fibrin and inflammatory cells are released in proportion to injury size
- Scar formation begins type III collagen production, which provides early stability but little tensile strength. Type III collagen predominates in the first 6–8 weeks of healing
- Remodeling begins after 6–8 weeks. Type I collagen slowly replaces type III collagen. The tendon is resized and reshaped. Collagen fibers become aligned in the direction of stress and tendon tensile strength improves. Remodeling continues for many months
- Abnormal type III collagen quantities, small collagen fibrils, and lack of linear fiber arrangement can persist for up to 14 months. This slow rate of healing contributes to the high rate of reinjury

SYSTEMS AFFECTED
Musculoskeletal—tendons, musculotendinous junctions, areas of tendon insertion, tendon sheaths.

GENETICS
Unknown

INCIDENCE/PREVALENCE
- SDFT injury—Thoroughbred racehorses: 8–43%; event horse: CCI competitors higher than 1 day eventers; show jumpers: unusual except international competitors or >15 years of age
- SDFT injury front >hindlimb. Bilateral injury common
- DDFT—most common in hindlimb of dressage and show jumpers

SIGNALMENT
- SDFT—Thoroughbred racehorses, upper level eventers, Grand Prix jumpers. Infrequent in Standardbreds, racing Arabians and Quarter Horses, polo ponies, fox hunters, cutting horses, barrel racers
- DDFT—most common in jumpers or dressage >10 years of age

SIGNS

Historical Findings
- Acute unilateral lameness that responds to rest

- Swelling, focal sensitivity, and/or heat along palmar/plantar metacarpus/metatarsus
- Tendon enlargement with chronic injury

Physical Examination Findings—SDF Tendonitis
- Bowed (convex) tendon profile when standing
- ± Digital sheath effusion
- "Curb" if injury to tarsus
- Variable lameness depending on severity, location, and chronicity; ± lame in mild and/or chronic injury; acute transient lameness in moderate or moderately severe injury
- Carpal canal injury—carpal sheath distention, lameness, worse with carpal flexion, ± stands with carpus slightly flexed
- Pastern branch lesions often lame
- Complete rupture—severe lameness, dropped fetlock

Physical Examination—DDF Tendonitis
- Mild to moderate lameness
- ± Positive distal limb flexion
- Distal injury (within the foot)—unilateral lameness with no physical abnormalities
- Digital tendon sheath effusion
- Tarsal sheath distention with penetrating or blunt trauma to hock
- ± Carpal sheath effusion with injury to radial head of deep digital flexure muscle near musculotendinous junction

CAUSES
- Excessive biomechanical load
- Direct blunt or penetrating trauma
- Sepsis owing to penetrating wound of tendon sheath
- Encircling bandages ("bandage bow")

RISK FACTORS
- Speed
- Jumping
- Increased age
- Abnormal conformation—long pasterns, tied-in behind the knee, long toe/low heel, hoof imbalance
- Rough, uneven ground; wet slippery surfaces; deep footing
- Palmar digital neurectomy for distal DDFT rupture

DIAGNOSIS

DIFFERENTIAL DIAGNOSIS
- Suspensory desmitis
- Inferior check desmitis
- Long plantar desmitis or other causes of curb
- Primary/noninfectious tenosynovitis
- Manica flexoria tears
- Palmar/plantar annular ligament syndrome
- Rule out with US

IMAGING
- US—both transverse and longitudinal plane images. Lesion length and cross-sectional

measurements determines severity— mild = <15%, moderate = 15–25%, severe = >25% of total cross-sectional area
- US abnormalities:
  ○ Acute—focal anechoic core lesions, complete fiber loss, ± hematoma
  ○ Chronic—decreased echogenicity, abnormal fiber pattern, ± dystrophic calcification
  ○ Increased cross-sectional area
  ○ Adhesions noted during dynamic scan
  ○ Increased fluid, ± fibrin within carpal/tarsal or digital sheath
  ○ Careful assessment of DDFT margins— lateral injury is common, easily missed
- MRI (DDFT injury in foot)—core lesion, sagittal tear, dorsal border injury, insertional injury, combination injury
- Radiography—dystrophic mineralization, bony irregularity at insertion, osteochondroma of distal radius

OTHER DIAGNOSTIC PROCEDURES
- Diagnostic analgesia—high palmar/plantar, intrathecal digital sheath
- Tenoscopic exploration of tendon sheath— DDFT marginal tears, injury to radial head of DDFT muscle in carpal sheath

PATHOLOGIC FINDINGS
- <2 weeks—fragmented collagen fibers surrounded by fibrin strands and edema, polymorphonuclear cells, and macrophages; intratendinous, peritendinous hemorrhage
- 1–5 months—numerous fibroblasts, granulation tissue, immature fibrous tissue; paratenon, endotenon proliferation
- ≥6 months—variable fibrosis characterized by irregular collagen arrangement, widespread scar formation, prominent endotendinous tissue, paratenon fibrosis
- >14 months—hypercellular scar with little subdivision into bundles

TREATMENT

AIMS
- Limit inflammatory process, control pain, prevent further injury
- Optimize tendon repair quality
- Performance return with lowest reinjury risk

APPROPRIATE HEALTH CARE
- Rest and controlled exercise program essential
- Exercise intensity based on lameness and sonography every 8–12 weeks

NURSING CARE
- Cold water hydrotherapy
- Poultice
- Support wrap

ACTIVITY
- Controlled exercise program (rest, confinement, gradual exercise) is mainstay of treatment

TENDONITIS

- Duration determined by location, severity, response to treatment
- Stall rest initially
- Small paddock no sooner than 4 months after mild injury; no sooner than 6 months if moderate to severe injury
- Daily controlled exercise program (example):
  ○ Level 1—walk 30 min every day for 4 weeks then 45 min day for every 4 weeks
  ○ Level 2—trot 5 min every day for 4 weeks then 10 min every day for 4 weeks
  ○ Level 3—trot 15 min every day for 4 weeks then 20 min every day for 4 weeks
  ○ Level 4 (moderate to severe injury; mild go to level 5)—trot 25 min every day for 4 weeks then 30 min every day for 4 weeks
  ○ Level 5—canter/slow gallop 1 mile every day for 4 weeks then 2 miles every day for 4 weeks
  ○ Level 6—breeze every day for 4 weeks
  ○ Level 7—race
- Walking exercise in hand, on walker, or with a rider
- US and lameness evaluations repeated between each exercise level. Decreased exercise with continued lameness, US abnormalities

DIET
Caloric reduction while stall confined or resting.

CLIENT EDUCATION
- Early recognition and strict adherence to a controlled exercise program are essential for healing and return to athletic performance
- Risk of reinjury is high, especially during early healing phases and inappropriate exercise

SURGICAL CONSIDERATIONS
- Superior check desmotomy—for SDFT injury, improved outcome in Standardbreds, recommended for moderate to severe lesions, ± suspensory desmitis postoperatively
- Percutaneous tendon splitting—for acute core lesions to decompress hemorrhage ± promote vascularization
- Fetlock palmar/plantar annular desmotomy—for distal metacarpal/metatarsal tendonitis with impaired tendon gliding
- Proximal metacarpal fasciotomy and carpal retinacular release—for proximal SDF tendonitis
- Tenoscopy of digital flexor tendon sheath—debridement, adhesionolysis, foreign material removal (penetrating injuries); ± adhesion formation postoperatively

MEDICATIONS
DRUG(S) OF CHOICE
- Systemic NSAIDs—phenylbutazone (4.4 mg/kg/day) for 7–10 days
- Intrathecal sodium hyaluronan (10–20 mg)
- Intrathecal corticosteroids—methylprednisolone acetate (40 mg) or triamcinolone (6 mg)

CONTRAINDICATIONS
Intralesional or perilesional corticosteroids.

ALTERNATIVE DRUGS
- Intralesional stem cells, platelet-rich plasma
- Extracorporeal shock wave therapy
- Appropriate hoof care and shoeing
- Therapeutic US
- Counterirritation (iodine-based liniments, internal peritendinous injection of 2% iodine in almond oil, pin firing)

FOLLOW-UP
PATIENT MONITORING
- Quality of healing (via US) determines exercise level
- Lameness and US every 8 weeks until adequate healing in the face of exercise
- Lameness, heat, or swelling prompts exercise discontinuation and US reevaluation

PREVENTION/AVOIDANCE
- Avoid dangerous work surfaces
- Proper shoeing
- Prevent reinjury via controlled exercise, periodic US

POSSIBLE COMPLICATIONS
- Adhesion between tendon and peritendinous tissue or digital sheath
- Tendon rupture with severe tendonitis and continued exercise

EXPECTED COURSE AND PROGNOSIS
- 8–12 months rehabilitation regardless of treatment

- SDF tendonitis—guarded prognosis high-speed sports (race, elite eventers); high recurrence rate; Standardbred prognosis better than Thoroughbred; 50% of event horses and most show jumpers return to full athletic function
- DDF tendonitis—prognosis for soundness is guarded

MISCELLANEOUS
ASSOCIATED CONDITIONS
- Digital sheath tenosynovitis
- Navicular syndrome
- Desmitis of DDFT accessory ligament
- Annular ligament constriction
- Osteochondroma of distal radius

AGE-RELATED FACTORS
- Older horses—injury without significant athletic activity, heal slowly, require longer rehabilitation
- Carpal canal injury more frequent in older horses

SYNONYMS
Bowed tendon.

SEE ALSO
- Navicular syndrome
- Suspensory desmitis

ABBREVIATIONS
- CCI = Concours Complet International
- DDF = deep digital flexor
- DDFT = deep digital flexor tendon
- MRI = magnetic resonance imaging
- NSAID = nonsteroidal anti-inflammatory drug
- SDF = superficial digital flexor
- SDFT = superficial digital flexor tendon
- US = ultrasonography, ultrasound

Suggested Reading
Dyson SJ. The deep digital flexor tendon. In: Ross MW, Dyson SJ, eds. Diagnosis and Management of Lameness in the Horse. St. Louis, MO: Saunders, 2003:644–650.
Jorgensen JS, Genovese RL. Superficial digital flexor tendinitis. In: Ross MW, Dyson SJ, eds. Diagnosis and Management of Lameness in the Horse. St. Louis, MO: Saunders, 2003:628–643.

Author JoAnn Slack
Consulting Editor Elizabeth J. Davidson

T

BASICS

OVERVIEW
• Tenesmus is a repeated, uncontrollable sensation or need of straining to evacuate primarily the rectum, or bladder, with passage of small amounts of fecal matter or urine, or nothing at all. It is likely induced by constant stimulation of the sacral nerves owing to inflammation or physical stimulation of the organs (rectum, uterus, urinary bladder) that gives the horse a continual sensation of the need to defecate or urinate. Because tenesmus is pathologic, the repeated attempts to evacuate the bowel or bladder persist as the nervous stimulation remain unrelieved by the defecation/urination attempts
• Stimulation may result from intrinsic disease of the organ involved (e.g. rectal inflammation); therefore, tenesmus may be seen with diarrhea, colitis, or rectal laceration. Stimulation also may result from physical pressure on the organ from within (e.g. constipated feces) or from the pelvic space (e.g. pararectal abscess, pelvic masses, impactions). Tenesmus may lead to rectal prolapse, or in females it may lead to uterine prolapse through the vagina and bladder prolapse through the urethra

SIGNALMENT
More common in adult females.

SIGNS
• Repeated straining in attempts to defecate or urinate
• Prolapsed rectum, and uterus, or bladder secondary to tenesmus

CAUSES AND RISK FACTORS
• Rectal causes of tenesmus—internal stimulation (pressure) in case of constipation (meconium impaction in foals) or foreign bodies; external pressure on the rectum as in pararectal abscess or neoplasm; intramural stimulation of the rectum in the case of inflammation in proctitis, colitis/diarrhea or rectal tear
• Uterine causes—more likely during peripartum. Metritis, vaginitis, and retained placenta
• Urinary causes—ureteritis or urethritis as in lower urinary tract infections or obstruction in cystitis or calculi. Uroperitoneum
• Neurologic origin—central nervous system diseases such as central hepatic encephalopathy or rabies or peripheral nerve trauma caused by rabies, parturition, or dystocia

DIAGNOSIS

DIFFERENTIAL DIAGNOSIS
• Tenesmus is a clinical sign that may reflect various underlying diseases or causal

conditions that trigger stimuli for defecation/urination
• Dysuria (painful urination) and stranguria (straining to urinate) are the most important clinical differential diagnoses of tenesmus, which is especially difficult to distinguish in colts
• Clinical examination should be aimed at identifying which of 4 potential organs/systems (digestive, urinary, uterine, or neurologic) are affected and promote tenesmus
• Differential diagnoses to consider include colitis (including uncommon severe colonic infarction owing to salmonellosis), proctitis, rectal tears, strictures, polyps, neoplasms, small colon intussusceptions, and, in neonates, meconium impaction or uroperitoneum (ruptured bladder/urachus). Pelvic abscess, lymphadenopathy, neoplasias. Vaginitis or retained placenta. Urolithiasis or lower urinary tract infection. Neurologic origin includes hepatic encephalopathy, leukoencephalomalacia, and rabies (cerebral disease signs), or dietary toxicosis (oak acorn, *Psilocybe* magic mushroom, or lolitrem B/perennial ryegrass)

CBC/BIOCHEMISTRY/URINALYSIS
• Tenesmus is the clinical manifestation of a persistent arc reflex and as such no paraclinical tests are needed to confirm it. Paraclinical analyses are useful to identify potential differential diagnoses
• CBC may show neutropenia and thrombocytopenia with severe acute inflammatory conditions (rectal tear, retained placenta, colitis, intussusception), or neutrophilia with subacute–chronic inflammation (urolithiasis, colitis). Eosinophilia has been reported in tenesmus owing to eosinophilic proctitis
• Biochemistry is informative with liver diseases (hepatic encephalopathy; increased bile acids and blood ammonia) and uroperitoneum, or in foals with meconium impaction if repeated water enemas have been administered (hyperkalemia; hyponatremia, hypochloremia)
• Urinalysis may be abnormal with urinary tract diseases

OTHER LABORATORY TESTS
• Abdominocentesis for uroperitoneum and rectal tears
• Serum or urinary phenolic content using gallic acid standards to determine hydrolyzed tanin concentration in acute acorn toxicosis

IMAGING
• Abdominal radiography for meconium impaction
• Abdominal ultrasonography for uroperitoneum, intussusception, and pararectal abscess, or lymphadenopathy
• Bladder ultrasonography for urolithiasis or neoplasia

OTHER DIAGNOSTIC PROCEDURES
Diagnostic procedures should be aimed at identifying the underlying pathology, or the severity and prognosis of medical complications due to prolapse of pelvic organs. Basic procedures include vaginal and rectal examination to assess organ wall integrity (rectal endoscopy/vaginoscopy for tears, polyps, neoplasia, strictures, proctitis/colitis, or intussusception), and endoscopy of the urethra and bladder for lower urinary tract diseases. Tissue biopsy for proctitis, polyps, or neoplasia.

TREATMENT

• Tenesmus has to be addressed in an expedited manner as it may result in pelvic organ prolapse. If signs of colic are present, refer to appropriate management protocols
• Treatment depends on the inciting cause and whether organ prolapse has occurred or seems to be imminent. The goal is to eliminate the cause and relieve the tenesmus urgency, and to stabilize the animal (stop the straining, alleviate stress and pain, and prevent violent sudden colic-like behavior) to allow safe treatment of organ prolapse, if present. Prevent recumbence to minimize further tissue trauma of prolapsed organs
• As diagnostic or therapeutic interventions, local epidural analgesia and/or rectal infusions with local anesthetics can result in the transient cessation of tenesmus and perineal and perianal pain. Unlike other species (e.g. cattle), epidural anesthesia in the horse was earlier perceived as more difficult to perform because of handling-associated risks, and slightly different sacrococcygeal anatomy. However, safer approaches exist; infection and other risks are similar to those in other species
• Sedation is recommended to facilitate epidural anesthesia procedures, and/or to alleviate uncontrollable tenesmus, or to treat organ prolapse
• α_2-Agonists, opioids, and dissociative drugs have been studied as epidural anesthetics with great safety margins. Although the addition of xylazine to epidural injection reduces the dose of local anesthetic required to avoid postepidural hindlimb ataxia and paresis, morphine-like opioids for spinal use have the safest margin as they produce long-lasting analgesia without motor side effects
• Use of laxatives and stool softeners in the diet to facilitate fecal bolus passage and defecation. Transition of soft diets rich in fiber to the horse-accustomed regular diet may be considered
• Surgical management by permanent colostomy if untreatable neoplasia of the perianal region
• Retention enema in meconium impaction

T

MEDICATIONS

DRUG(S) OF CHOICE
No specific medication; treatment depends on the inciting cause. In humans, diltiazem (calcium channel blocker, potent inhibitor of intestinal smooth muscle contraction) and tolterodine (antimuscarinic/anticholinergic, reduces bladder smooth muscle contraction) have been shown preliminarily to partially alleviate pain and tenesmus in cancer or overreactive bladder patients. No evidence yet exists to support their use in equine tenesmus.

FOLLOW-UP

PATIENT MONITORING
Follow-up frequency depends on the inciting cause. Tenesmus has to be addressed in an expedited manner and monitored several times a day until it is resolved because it may result in organ prolapse. Short- and long-term monitoring is desirable in cases of prolapse, as prolapse can recur.

POSSIBLE COMPLICATIONS
Pelvic organ prolapse. Severe septicemia or septic shock if advanced tissue damage originates from repositioning a severely affected prolapsed organ.

EXPECTED COURSE AND PROGNOSIS
Prognosis depends on the cause, and, if present, prolapse severity.

MISCELLANEOUS

ASSOCIATED CONDITIONS
N/A

AGE-RELATED FACTORS
Given the wide range of conditions that induce tenesmus, it can be seen at any age depending on the inciting cause.

PREGNANCY/FERTILITY/BREEDING
Tenesmus is more likely to be observed as a consequence of dystocia or retained placenta.

SYNONYMS
• Urgency (human)
• Dyschezia (painful defecation)

SEE ALSO
• Impaction
• Meconium retention
• Rectal prolapse
• Rectal tears
• Uroperitoneum, neonatal neonate
• Vaginal prolapse

Suggested Reading
Anderson GA, Mount ME, Vrins AA, Ziemer EL. Fatal acorn poisoning in a horse: pathologic findings and diagnostic considerations. J Am Vet Med Assoc 1983;182(10):1105–1110.
Choo MS, Doo CK, Lee KS. Satisfaction with tolterodine: assessing symptom-specific patient-reported goal achievement in the treatment of overactive bladder in female patients (STARGATE study). Int J Clin Pract 2008;62(2):191–196.
Colbourne CM, Bolton JB, Yovich JV, Genovese L. Hamartomatous polyp causing intestinal obstruction and tenesmus in a neonatal foal. Aust Equine Vet 1996;14:78–80.
Duesterdieck-Zellmer KF. Equine urolithiasis. Vet Clin North Am Equine Pract 2007;23(3):613–629.
Frazer GS. Post partum complications in the mare. Part 2: fetal membrane retention and conditions of the gastrointestinal tract, bladder and vagina. Equine Vet Educ 2003;5:118–128.
Gibson K, O'Hara A, Huxtable C. Focal eosinophilic proctitis with associated rectal prolapse in a pony. Aust Vet J 2001;79(10):679–681.
Hubbell JA, Saville WJ, Bednarski RM. The use of sedatives, analgesic and anaesthetic drugs in the horse: an electronic survey of members of the American Association of Equine Practitioners (AAEP). Equine Vet J 2010;42(6):487–493.
Johnstone LK, Mayhew IG, Fletcher LR. Clinical expression of lolitrem B (perennial ryegrass) intoxication in horses. Equine Vet J 2012;44(3):304–309.
Jones J. "Magic mushroom" (*Psilocybe*) poisoning in a colt. Vet Rec 1990;127:603.
Munday BL, Monkhouse IM, Gallagher RT. Intoxication of horses by lolitrem B in ryegrass seed cleanings. Aust Vet J 1985;62:207.
Natalini CC. Spinal anesthetics and analgesics in the horse. Vet Clin North Am Equine Pract 2010;26(3):551–564.
Stowers KH, Hartman AD, Gustin J. Diltiazem for the management of malignancy-associated perineal pain and tenesmus. J Palliat Med 2014;17(9):1075–1077.
Vigani A, Garcia-Pereira FL. Anesthesia and analgesia for standing equine surgery. Vet Clin North Am Equine Pract 2014;30(1):1–17.

Author Alexander Rodriguez-Palacios
Consulting Editors Henry Stämpfli and Olimpo Oliver-Espinosa
Acknowledgment The author and editors acknowledge the prior contribution of Gail Abells Sutton.

T

BASICS

DEFINITION
• Germ cell tumor of the gonad; neoplastic transformation into multiple germinal cell types. • Generally benign, but can become malignant and metastasize into the abdominal cavity. • Contains mixture of mature and poorly differentiated structures. • Characterized by multiple tissue types within the tumor. • Contains somatic structures derived from all embryonic germ cell layers arranged randomly throughout the tumor: ◦ Ectoderm (hair, teeth). ◦ Neuroectoderm (nerves, melanocytes). ◦ Endoderm (salivary gland, lung). ◦ Mesoderm (fibrous, adipose, bone, cartilage, muscle). ◦ Nervous and adipose tissue (nearly always present). • Has been referred to as dermoid cyst owing to the presence of hair

PATHOPHYSIOLOGY
• Generally a benign, incidental finding. • Hormonally inactive, does not preclude pregnancy or normal cyclicity in female

SYSTEMS AFFECTED
• Reproductive—gonad, placenta also reported. • Rarely a systemic effect, unless metastasis occurs

GENETICS
See Causes.

INCIDENCE/PREVALENCE
• Female—rare, although second most common ovarian neoplasm following GTCT. • Male—rare, although most common testicular tumor; also most common tumor in retained testes

SIGNALMENT
• Horses of any age may display signs resulting from physical presence of teratoma, e.g. colic. • Young males—usual presenting age 1–2 years. • Cryptorchid testes—presence of a teratoma in the fetus can prevent testicular descent. • Females—discovered during routine reproductive examination

SIGNS
• Effects from physical presence of a teratoma if of high mass/weight: ◦ May lead to discomfort and extramural intestinal obstruction (if intraabdominal). • Has been associated with small colon torsion in a foal, colic in mares, and testicular cyst formation. • Females—palpably abnormal ovarian mass, altered consistency of ovarian tissue ◦ Generally unilateral. ◦ Solid and cystic areas, replacing normal tissue. • Males—scrotal mass ◦ Most often a cryptorchid testicle. ◦ May decrease spermatogenesis or induce tubular atrophy of adjacent testicular tissue

CAUSES
Congenital

RISK FACTORS
May be concurrent with other gonadal neoplasia—carcinoma; GTCT.

DIAGNOSIS

DIFFERENTIAL DIAGNOSIS
• Females—ovarian hematoma; GTCT; dysgerminoma; carcinoma; fibroma; abscess, lymphosarcoma, cystadenoma. • Males—seminoma; Sertoli cell tumor; interstitial cell tumor; carcinoma; testicular hematoma; fibroma, abscess

CBC/BIOCHEMISTRY/URINALYSIS
N/A

OTHER LABORATORY TESTS
Lack of endocrinologic abnormality consistent with other causes of gonadal enlargement.

IMAGING
US
• Couple with transrectal palpation in female. • Abnormal paraovarian mass—solid; multilocular. • May have hyperechoic structures present (mineralized bone, teeth). • Compatible testicular mass, heterogenous echogenicity, mineralized structures

OTHER DIAGNOSTIC PROCEDURES
N/A

PATHOLOGIC FINDINGS
• Histopathologic findings—multiple tissue types may be present within neoplasm (adipose, bone, cartilage, hair, nervous elements, and teeth). • Gross findings—solid, cystic multilocular form; yellow-white

TREATMENT

APPROPRIATE HEALTH CARE
Surgical removal.

NURSING CARE
N/A

ACTIVITY
N/A

DIET
N/A

CLIENT EDUCATION
N/A

SURGICAL CONSIDERATIONS
May necessitate concurrent gonadectomy.

MEDICATIONS

DRUG(S) OF CHOICE
N/A

FOLLOW-UP

PATIENT MONITORING
N/A

PREVENTION/AVOIDANCE
N/A

POSSIBLE COMPLICATIONS
N/A

EXPECTED COURSE AND PROGNOSIS
N/A

MISCELLANEOUS

ASSOCIATED CONDITIONS
N/A

AGE-RELATED FACTORS
N/A

ZOONOTIC POTENTIAL
N/A

SEE ALSO
• Abnormal testicular size. • Large ovary syndrome

ABBREVIATIONS
• GTCT = granulosa–theca cell tumor. • US = ultrasonography, ultrasound

Suggested Reading
Allison N, Moeller Jr RB, Duncan R. Placental teratocarcinoma in a mare with possible metastasis to the foal. J Vet Diagn Invest 2004;2:160–163.
Arensburg L, Olivier S, Boussauw B, De Cock H. An abdominal teratoma in a yearling Irish Cob with a strangulating obstruction of the small intestine. Equine Vet Educ 2012;9:433–436.
Binanti D, Livini M, Riccaboni P, Sironi G. A case of umbilical cord teratoma in an aborted foal. J Vet Diagn Invest 2013;25:173–175.
Buergelt CD. Color Atlas of Reproductive Pathology of Domestic Animals. St. Louis, MO: Mosby, 1997.
Catone G, Marino G, Mancuso R, Zanghi A. Clinicopathological features of an equine ovarian teratoma. Reprod Domest Anim 2004;39:65–69.
Gurfield N, Benirschke K. Equine placental teratoma. Vet Pathol 2003;40:586–588.
Jubb KVC, Kennedy PC, Palmer N. Pathology of Domestic Animals, 4e. San Diego, CA: Academic Press, 1993.
Lefebvre R, Theoret C, Dore M, et al. Ovarian teratoma and endometritis in a mare. Can Vet J 2005;46:1029–1033.
Prange T. Small colon obstructions in foals. Equine Vet Educ 2013;25:293–296.
Sassot LN, Ragle CA, Farnsworth KD, et al. Dermoid cyst in the intermandibular space of a 3-year-old Thoroughbred gelding: a case report. J Equine Vet Sci 2016;43:72–76.

Author Peter R. Morresey
Consulting Editor Carla L. Carleton

T

TETANUS

BASICS

DEFINITION
Tetanus is a disease characterized by muscular spasm, caused by a neurotoxin produced by *Clostridium tetani*.

PATHOPHYSIOLOGY
• *C. tetani* is a Gram-positive, spore-forming bacillus. The spores are widespread in the environment, particularly in soil and mammalian feces
• They typically gain access to the animal via a wound. The oxygen tension within the wound must be low to allow germination. Concurrent infection with other bacteria and the presence of foreign bodies or necrosis within the wound can help produce a favorable anaerobic tissue environment. Under such conditions, *C. tetani* organisms proliferate locally
• Death and lysis of the organisms within the wound result in liberation of tetanospasmin, a neurotoxin responsible for the characteristic clinical signs. Tetanospasmin travels to the CNS via the hemolymphatic system and via peripheral motor nerves. The toxin exerts its effect on presynaptic inhibitory interneurons in the ventral horn of the spinal cord. There it cleaves synaptobrevin, a vesicle-associated membrane protein necessary for release of the neurotransmitters glycine and γ-aminobutyric acid. This results in a loss of motor neuron inhibition, and the subsequent hypertonia and muscular spasm
• 2 other exotoxins are produced by *C. tetani*. Tetanolysin is thought to increase local tissue necrosis, promoting proliferation within the wound. Another nonspasmogenic toxin may have a sympathomimetic effect
• The incubation period is highly variable, but it is usually 1–3 weeks. The spores can survive in tissue and germinate after wound healing if conditions then become favorable. Castration wounds and injection sites have also been associated with the development of tetanus.

SYSTEMS AFFECTED
• Neuromuscular
• Secondary effects on other systems (respiratory, skeletal, etc.) depending on the presence of complications

GENETICS
N/A

INCIDENCE/PREVALENCE
• Horses are exquisitely sensitive to the toxin, and the disease has a worldwide distribution
• A higher incidence may be associated with poor husbandry
• There may be a higher incidence in warmer areas

SIGNALMENT
No sex, age, or breed predilections.

SIGNS
• There is usually a history of a wound 1–4 weeks earlier
• There may be lack of vaccination, although tetanus may occur in the face of vaccination
• The first signs may be vague (local stiffness, lameness, colic)
• The progression of signs depends on the extent of the infection, the vaccination status, and the age and size of the horse
• Generally, the signs progress within 24 h, with the horse beginning to exhibit a stiff/spastic gait
• Trembling, a raised tail-head, flared nostrils, and erect ears are seen
• Preferential effects on postural muscles result in the characteristic "sawhorse stance"
• Retraction of the eyes and protrusion of the third eyelids occur following a stimulus (noise or menace)
• Spasm of the masseter muscles can cause inability to open the mouth ("lockjaw")
• Dysphagia results in accumulation of saliva in the mouth and aspiration of feed material
• Increased rectal temperature and profuse sweating occur in response to prolonged muscular spasm
• All signs are exacerbated by stimulation and excitement
• Recumbency, with difficulty or inability to rise, occurs as the disease progresses. This can be accompanied by severe extensor rigidity
• Horses may exhibit difficulty urinating and defecating
• Respiratory failure occurs in fulminant cases

CAUSES
Infection of a necrotic wound with *C. tetani*.

RISK FACTORS
Unvaccinated horses that have sustained a contaminated soft tissue wound or penetrating wound to the foot are most at risk.

DIAGNOSIS

DIFFERENTIAL DIAGNOSIS
• Laminitis
• Hypocalcemia
• Rhabdomyolysis
• Rabies
• Myotonia

CBC/BIOCHEMISTRY/URINALYSIS
• Nonspecific
• Hemoconcentration and a stress leukogram may present
• May see hyperfibrinogenemia and leukocytosis with secondary aspiration pneumonia

OTHER LABORATORY TESTS
Anaerobic culture of *C. tetani* may be attempted from a wound.

IMAGING
• No specific diagnostic indications

• Thoracic radiography or ultrasonography if aspiration pneumonia is suspected
• Ultrasonography of wound sites may help confirm anaerobic infection

OTHER DIAGNOSTIC PROCEDURES
No specific diagnostic procedures—diagnosis is made based on clinical signs coupled with the history of a recent wound.

PATHOLOGIC FINDINGS
• Nonspecific
• May demonstrate a *C. tetani*-infected wound
• Secondary traumatic injury or aspiration pneumonia may be present

TREATMENT

APPROPRIATE HEALTH CARE
• Initial treatment is aimed at neutralizing unbound toxin and preventing further release by eliminating the infection
• Appropriate nursing care, particularly if the horse is recumbent, is vital to maximize the chances of a successful outcome
• Fluid therapy may be required to maintain hydration. Nasogastric fluids have the added benefit of hydrating colonic content; however, IV or rectal administration of fluids may be necessary in horses where a nasogastric tube cannot be maintained

NURSING CARE
• Confine to a quiet, dark stall with deep bedding
• Minimize auditory stimulation with ear plugs
• Padded walls and/or a padded helmet to minimize injury
• Frequent turning of recumbent horses (every 2–4 h)
• Recumbent horses that are unable to rise may benefit from slinging
• Manual rectal evacuation and/or urinary catheterization may be necessary

ACTIVITY
Restrict activity as much as possible through confinement and sedation.

DIET
• High-quality feed and free-choice water should be made easily accessible
• If the horse is dysphagic, a nasogastric tube can be placed for the administration of feed, water, and electrolytes. The tube can be left in place to avoid the stress of repeated passage
• In some cases, the passage of a nasogastric tube is not possible and feeding via esophagostomy or gastrostomy, or parenteral nutrition, may be required

CLIENT EDUCATION
Appropriate tetanus prophylaxis should be discussed.

SURGICAL CONSIDERATIONS
• Debride the wound and maximize exposure to air

T

- Esophagotomy or gastrostomy may facilitate feeding in severely dysphagic cases
- Tracheostomy may be necessary if laryngeal spasm and respiratory obstruction has occurred

MEDICATIONS

DRUG(S) OF CHOICE
- Tetanus antitoxin—100–200 U/kg IV or IM (single dose) will bind circulating toxin
- Acepromazine—0.05–0.08 mg/kg IV or IM every 3–6 h or as required
- Phenobarbital 6–12 mg/kg slow IV followed by 6–12 mg/kg PO every 12 h alone or in combination with acepromazine
- Penicillin G (potassium or sodium)— 22 000–44 000 IU/kg IV every 6 h for 7–10 days
- Consider intrathecal administration of 50 mL TAT (20–30 mL in foals) after removal of an equal amount of cerebrospinal fluid from the atlanto-occipital space (requires general anesthesia), or via lumbosacral puncture in the standing horse. This is thought to be most beneficial early in the disease process. There is evidence of improved survival in human patients when TAT is administered intrathecally
- Local infiltration of the wound with procaine penicillin and/or tetanus antitoxin (3000–9000 IU). This may help eliminate the infection and neutralize toxin present at the site
- Vaccination with tetanus toxoid—clinical disease does not result in a sufficient immune response. Use separate injection site for antitoxin

CONTRAINDICATIONS
N/A

PRECAUTIONS
- TAT has been associated with the development of Theiler disease (serum hepatitis)
- General anesthesia and intrathecal TAT administration can result in significant complications (meningitis, seizures). A significant improvement in outcome has not been definitively demonstrated with this procedure

POSSIBLE INTERACTIONS
- TAT will bind tetanus toxoid. These agents should be administered at different sites
- Phenothiazine drugs (acepromazine) may potentiate barbiturates, causing more profound CNS depression if used together

ALTERNATIVE DRUGS
- Magnesium, administered as $MgSO_4$ via IV constant rate infusion, has many potentially useful effects, including muscle relaxation, and reduces the requirement for other muscle relaxants and sedatives in human tetanus patients. Monitoring of serum Mg levels as well as the ECG for signs of toxicity (widening of the QRS) is recommended during therapy
- Haloperidol 0.01 mg/kg IM every 7 days for long-acting sedation
- Diazepam 0.01–0.4 mg/kg IV every 2–4 h
- Macrolides (in foals only), tetracyclines, and metronidazole are alternatives to penicillin that may also be effective in eliminating vegetative *C. tetani* at the infection site

FOLLOW-UP

PATIENT MONITORING
- Regular physical examination
- Serial monitoring of packed cell volume, total protein concentration, and/or urine specific gravity to monitor hydration

PREVENTION/AVOIDANCE
- Initial vaccination with 2 doses of tetanus toxoid 3–4 weeks apart
- Annual toxoid booster thereafter is the current recommendation (although new evidence suggests horses may have protective antibody titers for at least 3 years after the initial vaccine course)
- Tetanus toxoid should be administered in the case of a wound if there has not been vaccination within the past 6 months
- Pregnant mares should be given a toxoid booster 4–6 weeks prior to expected parturition
- Experimental studies indicate that immunity to tetanus challenge is present 8 days after administration of toxoid in horses

POSSIBLE COMPLICATIONS
- Myopathy
- Aspiration pneumonia
- Trauma (fractures, decubital ulcers)
- Idiopathic acute hepatic disease (Theiler disease) is a rare complication of TAT administration

EXPECTED COURSE AND PROGNOSIS
- Horses that are recumbent and unable to rise have a grave prognosis, particularly if progression has been rapid
- The presence of dyspnea and dysphagia may also negatively influence survival

- Horses that retain the ability to stand and ambulate have a fair prognosis
- The clinical signs may persist for weeks; however, survivors will generally stabilize after 7 days and begin to show improvement after 2 weeks
- Recovery may take as long as 6 weeks but is usually complete
- The attitude of the individual horse and the ability to provide ideal nursing care are important factors affecting outcome
- The overall mortality rate in horses is reported to be 50–80%

MISCELLANEOUS

ASSOCIATED CONDITIONS
N/A

AGE-RELATED FACTORS
N/A

ZOONOTIC POTENTIAL
N/A

PREGNANCY/FERTILITY/BREEDING
N/A

SYNONYMS
Lockjaw

ABBREVIATIONS
- CNS = central nervous system
- TAT = tetanus antitoxin

Suggested Reading
Green SL, Little CB, Baird JD, et al. Tetanus in the horse: a review of 20 cases (1970–1990). J Vet Intern Med 1994;8:128–132.
Mackay RJ. Tetanus. In: Smith BP, ed. Large Animal Internal Medicine, 5e. St. Louis, MO: Mosby, 2015:996–998.
Morresey PR. Tetanus. In: Reed SM, Bayly WM, Sellon DC, eds. Equine Internal Medicine, 3e. St. Louis, MO: WB Saunders, 2010:637–641.
Steinman A, Haik R, Elad D, Sutton GA. Intrathecal administration of tetanus antitoxin in three cases of tetanus in horses. Equine Vet Educ 2000;12:237–240.

Author Andrew W. van Eps
Consulting Editor Ashley G. Boyle

 Client Education Handout available online

T

THORACIC TRAUMA

BASICS

DEFINITION
- May be penetrating or blunt
- Penetrating trauma usually results from collision with an object
- Blunt trauma often occurs in neonatal foals at parturition

PATHOPHYSIOLOGY
Fracture of bones of the thoracic cage, lung injury, air in the pleural space and mediastinum, diaphragmatic injury, and heart or large vessel injury may occur. Concurrent trauma to the abdomen is also possible.
- Axillary laceration—often the result of a horse running into a fence or barbed wire. Can be accompanied by severe subcutaneous emphysema, pneumomediastinum, PTX
- Pulmonary contusion—occurs when the chest wall is compressed against the lung parenchyma. May cause hemorrhage into the alveolar spaces and induce respiratory distress, and pneumonia
- Pulmonary laceration—a traumatic disruption of the lung that causes PTX or HTX. Caused by a sudden compression of the thoracic wall or direct puncture of the lung. Complications such as pulmonary abscess or bronchopleural fistula may arise
- PTX causes varying degrees of lung collapse and inadequate ventilation
- Fractured ribs cause pain and may lead to hypoventilation. When combined with pulmonary contusions, can lead to pneumonia
- Pericardial effusion may result from hemopericardium, septic pericarditis, or hydropericardium, and potentially lead to cardiac tamponade
- Transdiaphragmatic perforation can cause viscus rupture, septic peritonitis, and herniation of abdominal organs

SYSTEMS AFFECTED
- Respiratory—PTX, rib fracture, and pulmonary contusions or lacerations
- Cardiovascular—cardiac tamponade, large vessel, and intercostal artery or pulmonary parenchymal vessel
- Gastrointestinal—foreign body penetration of the abdominal cavity

INCIDENCE/PREVALENCE
- Penetrating trauma is rare
- Blunt trauma occurs in 20% of newborn foals (primiparous and dystocia) at birth but clinical signs are rare
- In foals referred to neonatal intensive care units, fractured ribs were identified in 65%; mortality attributable to rib fractures may be as high as 25%

SIGNALMENT
Neonatal foals are predisposed to rib fracture and costochondral fracture/dislocation.

SIGNS

Historical Findings
- History of penetrating or blunt trauma
- History of dystocia or birth from a primiparous mare

Physical Examination Findings
- Palpation of the thoracic cage and axillary area to detect penetrating wound, edema, fractured ribs, subcutaneous emphysema, or thoracic wall instability and asymmetry
- Cyanotic or pale mucous membranes
- Absence of lung sounds—suggestive of PTX
- Reduced lung sounds ventrally—suggestive of HTX

CAUSES
- Collision with an object, particularly fences, is the most common cause of penetrating thoracic wounds
- Birth trauma most likely results from compression of the thorax during passage through the dam's pelvic canal

RISK FACTORS
- Horses at pasture, horse getting loose
- Dystocia and foals from primiparous mares

DIAGNOSIS

As these horses may suffer from polytrauma, an approach consisting of a first look, shock and emergency treatment, recheck, and then diagnosis is suitable.

DIFFERENTIAL DIAGNOSIS
- Pain can cause rapid shallow breathing
- Diaphragmatic hernia
- Pneumonia
- HTX, pleural septic effusion, or hydrothorax

CBC/BIOCHEMISTRY/URINALYSIS
Stress leukogram may be observed. Leukocytosis and increased acute-phase proteins are common with secondary bacterial infection; anemia caused by blood loss.

OTHER LABORATORY TESTS
Arterial blood gas analysis.

IMAGING

Thoracic US
- T-FAST to quickly detect PTX (see chapter Pneumothorax) and accumulation of pericardial or pleural fluid. Otherwise a complete examination of the entire thorax is recommended to detect fractured ribs or diaphragmatic hernia
- Foreign bodies or lung contusion may also be identified

Thoracic Radiography
PTX, radiopaque foreign objects, effusion, fractured ribs, or diaphragmatic hernia may be seen. However, radiographs are less sensitive than US for the detection of rib fractures.

OTHER DIAGNOSTIC PROCEDURES
- Thoracocentesis confirms a diagnosis of tension PTX or HTX (see Treatment)
- Thoracoscopy to evaluate the pleural space, potential non-radiopaque foreign bodies, and pulmonary pathology
- Abdominal US and paracentesis when abdominal cavity perforation is suspected

PATHOLOGIC FINDINGS
- HTX
- Rib fracture and flail chest
- Pulmonary contusion or laceration
- Large vessel injury, hemopericardium, and cardiac laceration
- Diaphragmatic laceration
- Intestinal or abdominal organ injury
- Septic pleuritis or peritonitis
- Extrathoracic trauma

TREATMENT

AIMS
- Support and restore respiratory function
- Treat shock if necessary
- Close wound whenever possible
- Administer broad-spectrum antibiotics, anti-inflammatory and analgesic drugs

APPROPRIATE HEALTH CARE
- Emergency care and continuous monitoring for severe cases
- Inpatient care until stabilized

NURSING CARE
- Oxygen by nasal insufflation to hypoxemic patients
- Control of external hemorrhage and shock treatment with IV fluids (hypertonic/isotonic) during the acute period. Blood or plasma transfusions should be considered in cases of severe blood loss. Contused lungs are extremely sensitive to crystalloid fluid overload
- Temporarily close penetrating wounds
- Decision to decompress the pleural cavity (air or blood) should be based on:
  ○ Exacerbation of clinical signs when the wound is sealed
  ○ Presence of a tension PTX or an increase in PTX size
  ○ Presence of a large accumulation of blood in the pleural space
  ○ Presence of HTX combined with a penetrating thoracic wound
- The site for air evacuation is the dorsal thoracic cavity just in front of the 12th to 15th ribs. The site for fluid evacuation is the ventral thoracic cavity and is best evaluated by US (usually, the fifth to eighth intercostal spaces). Avoid intercostal vessels along the caudal border of the ribs
- Perform thoracocentesis using a 14 G over-the-needle catheter, a teat cannula, or a large-gauge needle attached to a 3-way stop cock, extension set, and 60 mL syringe

- For severe or active PTX or HTX, place a thoracostomy tube in the pleural cavity, and attach to a Heimlich valve, a "home-made tip-truncated unlubricated condom," or continuous-suction apparatus in cases of rapid reaccumulation. Evacuation pressures ≤20 cmH$_2$O should be used, and the air or fluid should be removed from the thorax slowly
- Drain pericardial effusions when cardiac tamponade is detected. Ideally, a 14 G over-the-needle catheter is inserted through the pericardium under US guidance. ECG monitoring is recommended
- Fractured ribs are usually not stabilized, but rough edges may be rongeured and fragments removed in cases of open fracture. Indications for internal fixation are:
  ○ Displaced fractures of the third to sixth ribs at the costochondral junction on the left side, with lower fragment pressing in towards myocardium
  ○ Fractures of caudal ribs resulting in laceration of diaphragm or diaphragmatic hernia
  ○ Foals with existing extensive internal thoracic trauma
  ○ Presence of flail chest (3 or more consecutive ribs that are each fractured in at least 2 sites, resulting in a free-floating segment of the chest wall and paradoxical associated respiration) with severe respiratory dysfunction

ACTIVITY
- Box stall rest
- Confine foals with fractured ribs for a minimum of 2–3 weeks, and, if possible, avoid manipulations

CLIENT EDUCATION
- Discuss clinical signs of PTX, and advise immediate return with recurrence
- Inform of potential complications. Reevaluation is recommended if wound drainage occurs

SURGICAL CONSIDERATIONS
- Standing surgery when possible
- Stabilization of the patient, decompression of the PTX, and positive-pressure ventilation are mandatory for surgery under general anesthesia
- Suture wounds whenever possible to rapidly achieve an airtight seal. Conservative debridement is advised to permit primary closure. If impossible, apply an occlusive bandage

- Consider thoracoscopy for severe or recurrent PTX or when a foreign body is suspected
- Certain types of rib fractures may be successfully reduced and stabilized in foals using reconstruction plates, self-tapping screws, and cerclage wire or nylon strand suture
- Wound or thoracic exploration is indicated for uncontrolled hemorrhage

MEDICATIONS

DRUG(S) OF CHOICE
- Broad-spectrum antibiotics for patients with penetrating wounds
- NSAIDs to avoid splinting and hypoventilation because of pain from fractured ribs. If pain is not controlled, long-lasting intercostal blocks (bupivacaine) or opioid analgesics may be indicated

PRECAUTIONS
Drugs such as xylazine or opioids may reduce PaO$_2$.

FOLLOW-UP

PATIENT MONITORING
- Respiratory rate and effort, heart rate, auscultation, hematocrit, and total solids during the first 48 h
- Blood gas analyses for signs of hypoventilation
- Thoracic US and radiography can be repeated every 24–48 h until the condition is stable

POSSIBLE COMPLICATIONS
- Recurrence of PTX or HTX
- Pyothorax
- Bacterial pneumonia in young foals
- Septic peritonitis and shock when intestinal viscus penetration has occurred
- Rib and sternal fistulae
- Diaphragmatic hernia

EXPECTED COURSE AND PROGNOSIS
- Tension PTX and cardiac tamponade are serious life-threatening conditions
- Cardiac or large vessel laceration carries a poor prognosis
- Full recovery is expected if the injury is not severe and does not involve the large vessels, heart, or abdominal cavity

MISCELLANEOUS

ASSOCIATED CONDITIONS
- Fractured ribs
- Diaphragmatic hernia
- Ruptured trachea
- Thoracic and abdominal organ lacerations
- Other complications of trauma

SEE ALSO
- Diaphragmatic hernia
- Expiratory dyspnea
- Inspiratory dyspnea
- Pleuropneumonia
- Pneumothorax

ABBREVIATIONS
- HTX = hemothorax
- PaO$_2$ = partial pressure of oxygen in arterial blood
- PTX = pneumothorax
- T-FAST = thoracic focused assessment with sonography for trauma
- US = ultrasonography, ultrasound

Suggested Reading
Bellezzo F, Hunt RJ, Provost R, et al. Surgical repair of rib fractures in 14 neonatal foals: case selection, surgical technique and results. Equine Vet J 2004;36(7):557–562.
Jean D, Laverty S, Halley J, et al. Thoracic trauma in newborn foals. Equine Vet J 1999;31(2):149–152.
Jean D, Picandet V, Macieira S, et al. Detection of rib trauma in newborn foals in an equine critical care unit: a comparison of ultrasonography, radiography and physical examination. Equine Vet J 2007;39(2):158–163.
Laverty S, Lavoie JP, Pascoe JR, Ducharme N. Penetrating wounds of the thorax in 15 horses. Equine Vet J 1996;28(3):220–224.
Radcliffe RM. Thoracic injury in horses. In: Orsini JA, Divers TJ, eds. Equine Emergencies: Treatment and Procedures, 4e. St. Louis, MO: Elsevier Saunders, 2014:728–732.
Schambourg MA, Laverty S, Mullim S, et al. Thoracic trauma in foals: post mortem findings. Equine Vet J 2003;35(1):78–81.
Sprayberry KA, Barrett EJ. Thoracic trauma in horses. Vet Clin North Am Equine Pract 2015;31(1):199–219.

Authors Florent David and Sheila Laverty
Consulting Editors Mathilde Leclère and Daniel Jean

THROMBOCYTOPENIA

 BASICS

DEFINITION
A peripheral platelet (thrombocyte) count <100 000/μL (<100 × 10⁹/L).

PATHOPHYSIOLOGY
• Platelets are bone marrow-derived anucleate fragments of megakaryocytes; the smallest cellular particles in blood. • Platelets are integral to primary hemostasis via the formation of a platelet plug. They contribute to secondary hemostasis by localizing coagulation factors and providing cofactors. • Lifespan in circulation is ≈3–5 days. • Thrombopoiesis is stimulated by IL-3, IL-6, granulocyte–macrophage colony-stimulating factor, thrombopoietin. • 30–50% of mature platelets stored in the spleen. • In health, numbers are balanced between removal (circulation) and replacement (bone marrow). • Thrombocytopenia results from decreased production, increased consumption, increased destruction, or increased sequestration

Decreased Platelet Production
Causes include myelophthisis or aplastic anemia (intrinsic stem cell failure or disruption of interactions with other cells).

Increased Platelet Destruction
• IMTPs are most common. • Nonimmune-mediated destruction may occur in response to infections and after exposure to various toxins and drugs. • Primary IMTP is associated with production of autoantibodies directed against normal platelet surface antigens or against novel platelet antigens that develop in response to a primary disease. • Neonatal alloimmune thrombocytopenia develops when a foal inherits a platelet alloantigen from the sire, the mare produces alloantibodies, and these are ingested by the foal. • Secondary IMTP occurs when either circulating immune complexes (against neoplasms, drugs, or infection) attach to platelets nonspecifically. Antibodies directed against antigens attach to platelets; or via molecular mimicry. • Platelets coated with antibody are removed from circulation by the reticuloendothelial system

Increased Platelet Consumption
• DIC is the most common cause of thrombocytopenia. • Can also occur with localized activation of coagulation, trauma, severe hemorrhage

Platelet Sequestration
Caused by splenomegaly and vascular neoplasms.

Other
Pseudothrombocytopenia with collection of blood into EDTA or heparin tubes.

SYSTEMS AFFECTED
• Hemic/lymphatic/immune. • Hemorrhage can occur when the platelet count is <30 000/μL (<30.0 × 10⁹/L). Lesions mostly occur in the skin, renal/urologic, GI, and respiratory systems

GENETICS
• Genetic basis to neonatal alloimmune thrombocytopenia. • Genetic basis of familial megakaryocytic and myeloid hypoplasia in Standardbreds is suspected

INCIDENCE/PREVALENCE
Unknown, but rare.

SIGNALMENT
Breed Predilections
• Standardbred horses may be at increased risk. • Mules at increased risk for neonatal alloimmune thrombocytopenia

Mean Age and Range
• Neonatal alloimmune thrombocytopenia occurs in foals <7 days of age. • No age predilection for other forms

Predominant Sex
N/A

SIGNS
General Comments
Signs of spontaneous hemorrhage are most common with platelet counts <10 000/μL (<10.0 × 10⁹/L) or after trauma/surgery/venipuncture if platelet count is <30 000/μL (<30.0 × 10⁹/L).

Historical Findings
• Spontaneous or post-traumatic hemorrhage involving mucous membranes, skin, nasal cavity, GI, and urogenital tract. • Other signs related to primary disease

Physical Examination Findings
• Petechial and ecchymotic hemorrhages of oral, ocular, vaginal, and nasal mucous membranes. • Mucosal hemorrhage from respiratory (epistaxis), GI (melena), or urinary (hematuria) tract. • Prolonged hemorrhage from venipuncture or surgical sites. • Hyphema

CAUSES
Decreased Platelet Production
• Myelophthisis—including myelofibrosis, myelodysplasia, leukoproliferative disorders, or lymphoproliferative disorders. • Aplastic anemia due to idiopathic pancytopenia, drugs (e.g. phenylbutazone, estrogens, chloramphenicol), infectious or immune-mediated disease. • Megakaryocytic and myeloid hypoplasia in Standardbreds

Increased Platelet Destruction
• Primary IMTP—autoimmune or idiopathic. • Neonatal alloimmune thrombocytopenia. • Secondary IMTP due to neoplasia (e.g. lymphosarcoma), bacterial infection (sepsis), viral infection (e.g. EIA), drugs (e.g. heparin), or concurrent immune-mediated hemolysis. • Snake envenomation. • Toxin- or drug-induced platelet damage

Increased Platelet Consumption
• DIC/systemic inflammatory response syndrome. • Localized intravascular coagulation due to hemangioma/hemangiosarcoma, hemolytic uremic syndrome, thrombosis. • Excessive hemorrhage. • Severe trauma. • Vasculitis

Platelet Sequestration
• Splenomegaly. • Vascular neoplasms

Pseudothrombocytopenia
Collection of blood into EDTA.

Miscellaneous with Complex Mechanisms
• Viral—including EIA, equine herpesvirus, equine viral arteritis, VEE, African horse sickness. • Bacterial—neonatal septicemia, EGE (*Anaplasma phagocytophilum*), equine monocytic ehrlichiosis (*Neorickettsia risticii*). • Neoplastic—lymphosarcoma. • Endotoxemia. • Fell Pony syndrome

RISK FACTORS
• Any drug may potentially precipitate IMTP. Most common with heparin and myelosuppressive drugs. • Certain viral and bacterial infections. • Neoplasia. • Immune-mediated diseases. • Systemic diseases triggering DIC

 DIAGNOSIS

DIFFERENTIAL DIAGNOSIS
• Platelet dysfunction is a differential for abnormalities in primary hemostasis. This does not cause petechiae. • Vasculitis is a differential for petechiae. • Coagulopathy may also be associated with secondary deficits in hemostasis (e.g. anticoagulant therapy, vitamin K deficiency, hepatic failure, or congenital deficiencies)

CBC/BIOCHEMISTRY/URINALYSIS
• Platelet count <100 000/μL (<100 × 10⁹/L). • Equine platelets are smaller than human platelets and laboratory equipment must be calibrated accordingly. • Decreased platelet production frequently has concurrent decreases in granulocytes, monocytes, and RBCs. • Concurrent anemia may occur with chronic disease, EIA, immune-mediated hemolysis, and hemorrhage. • Changes in RBC morphology. • Inclusions in neutrophils in EGE. • Inflammatory leukogram (neutrophilia or neutropenia ± left shift) may be seen with DIC. • Pseudothrombocytopenia (platelet clumping in EDTA)—rule out with manual platelet count and microscopic examination of smear or repeat platelet count on citrated blood sample. • Various biochemical derangements may be present with underlying conditions

OTHER LABORATORY TESTS
• Coggins test for EIA. • Serology for *A. phagocytophilum, N. risticii,* and various viral agents. • Coagulation panel (prothrombin time, activated partial thromboplastin time, D-dimer, fibrinogen) for diagnosis of DIC/consumptive coagulopathies. • Blood culture for septicemia. • Immunophenotypic techniques to classify leukemia. • Flow cytometry for detection of platelet-bound antibody. • Platelet factor 3 test as indirect test for IMTP. • Cytologic evaluation of fluid and aspirate samples in underlying disease

IMAGING
Ultrasonography and radiography of thorax and abdomen as indicated for identification of underlying disease.

OTHER DIAGNOSTIC PROCEDURES
• Abdominocentesis. • Thoracocentesis. • Bone marrow biopsy to determine megakaryocyte numbers and evidence of myelophthisis or bone marrow hypoplasia. • Fine needle aspirate/biopsy of internal/external space-occupying lesion

PATHOLOGIC FINDINGS
• Petechial and ecchymotic hemorrhages in various tissues. • Other findings dependent on specific underlying disease

TREATMENT
APPROPRIATE HEALTH CARE
• Severe thrombocytopenia necessitates hospitalization. • If severe hemorrhage has occurred, resuscitation will likely be required. • Less severe disease may respond to treatment on an outpatient basis

NURSING CARE
• Minimize invasive procedures to limit potential for hemorrhage. • Apply prolonged pressure to venipuncture sites. • Prevent trauma. • Discontinue medications if IMTP is suspected. • Severe hemorrhage may be life-threatening—hypovolemic and/or anemic shock. Resuscitation with crystalloids for volume expansion and/or fresh whole blood. • Platelet replacement with fresh whole blood or platelet-rich plasma. Blood collection and processing should be in plastic containers to avoid activation associated with glass bottles

ACTIVITY
Restricted

CLIENT EDUCATION
Thrombocytopenia indicates the presence of an underlying disease that requires diagnostic management.

SURGICAL CONSIDERATIONS
• Elective surgery should be avoided until platelet counts are normal. • Emergency surgery may require concomitant administration of fresh whole blood/platelet-rich plasma

MEDICATIONS
DRUG(S) OF CHOICE
• For IMTP, initially dexamethasone (0.1 mg/kg IV or IM every 24 h, then reduce dose by 0.01 mg/kg/day when platelet count >100 000/μL. Longer term therapy with oral prednisolone (1–2 mg/kg PO or IM every 24 h). • EGE and equine monocytic ehrlichiosis—oxytetracycline (7 mg/kg IV every 12–24 h for 7 days). • Bacterial infection—appropriate antimicrobial therapy. • DIC—treatment of underlying disease

CONTRAINDICATIONS
• Corticosteroids—preexistent laminitis or infectious disease. • NSAIDs (especially aspirin) in most circumstances owing to impairment of platelet function

POSSIBLE INTERACTIONS
Avoid concurrent use of corticosteroids and NSAIDs—possible increased risk of GI damage

ALTERNATIVE DRUGS
For refractory IMTP, azathioprine (3 mg/kg PO every 24 h) or vincristine (0.01–0.025 mg/kg IV every 7 days)

FOLLOW-UP
PATIENT MONITORING
• Monitor for hemorrhagic diathesis. • Daily platelet count until stabilized, thereafter weekly until >100 000/μL

PREVENTION/AVOIDANCE
Avoid use of drugs suspected in development of IMTP.

POSSIBLE COMPLICATIONS
Excessive hemorrhage.

EXPECTED COURSE AND PROGNOSIS
• Variable, dependent on cause. • Most cases of secondary IMTP (drugs/infection) respond with withdrawal of the drug or successful treatment of the underlying infection. • Many cases recover in 3–4 weeks. • Myeloproliferative disorders have a grave prognosis. • EIA and neoplasia have a poor/grave prognosis. • Some cases are recurrent—require intermittent corticosteroid therapy. • Response to therapy is a useful prognostic indicator

MISCELLANEOUS
ASSOCIATED CONDITIONS
• Immune-mediated hemolysis. • Bacterial, viral, or fungal infection. • Neoplasia. • DIC

AGE-RELATED FACTORS
Platelet counts in young animals (<3 years) are often higher than those in older animals.

ZOONOTIC POTENTIAL
VEE

SEE ALSO
• Anemia, immune mediated.
• Coagulation defects, acquired.
• Coagulation defects, inherited.
• Disseminated intravascular coagulation.
• Equine granulocytic anaplasmosis.
• Hemangiosarcoma.
• Lymphosarcoma.
• Myeloproliferative diseases.
• Pancytopenia.
• Petechiae, ecchymoses, and hematomas.
• Thrombocytosis

ABBREVIATIONS
• DIC = disseminated intravascular coagulation.
• EGE = equine granulocytic ehrlichiosis.
• EIA = equine infectious anemia.
• GI = gastrointestinal.
• IL = interleukin.
• IMTP = immune-mediated thrombocytopenia.
• NSAID = nonsteroidal anti-inflammatory drugs.
• RBC = red blood cell.
• VEE = Venezuelan equine encephalomyelitis

Suggested Reading
Sellon DC. Disorders of the hematopoietic system. In: Reed SM, Bayly WM, Sellon DC, eds. Equine Internal Medicine, 2e. St. Louis, MO: WB Saunders, 2004:721–768.

Author Kira L. Epstein
Consulting Editors David Hodgson, Harold C. McKenzie, and Jennifer L. Hodgson
Acknowledgment The author and editors acknowledge the prior contribution of Kristopher Hughes.

T

THROMBOCYTOSIS

BASICS

OVERVIEW
- Increased peripheral platelet (thrombocyte) count usually >350 000/μL (>350 × 10⁹/L)
- Usually secondary reactive thrombocytosis associated with chronic inflammatory/infectious diseases. Cytokines produced during an inflammatory response may stimulate megakaryopoiesis
- Organ systems affected are associated with underlying cause
- Primary thrombocytosis with myeloproliferative disorders
- Physiologic thrombocytosis possible

SIGNALMENT
Although not pathologic, stallions and horses <3 years of age have higher platelet counts.

SIGNS
- Specific signs are seldom observed and hemostatic function is usually normal. Hemorrhagic diathesis can occur if platelet function is abnormal (thrombocytopathia). Thrombosis may occur with platelet counts >1 000 000/μL
- Signs will most likely relate to the primary underlying disease

CAUSES AND RISK FACTORS
Primary Thrombocytosis
- Occurs as a primary myeloproliferative disorder or associated with polycythemia vera
- Yet to be diagnosed definitively in horses

Secondary (Reactive) Thrombocytosis
- Physiologic causes include exercise/excitement (release of splenic platelet reserves)
- Rebound phenomenon occurs after thrombocytopenia or hemorrhage
- Immune-mediated hemolysis, including neonatal isoerythrolysis
- Iron-deficiency anemia
- Corticosteroid therapy
- Chronic inflammatory/infectious conditions
- Neoplasia
- Musculoskeletal trauma
- Splenectomy

DIAGNOSIS

DIFFERENTIAL DIAGNOSIS
Accurate history and complete physical examination should be used to localize (body system affected) and characterize (inflammatory, infectious, autoimmune, neoplastic, traumatic, physiologic).

CBC/BIOCHEMISTRY/URINALYSIS
- Platelet counts of 401 000 to >1 000 000/μL (401–1000 × 10⁹/L) have been recorded
- Other abnormalities related to underlying cause
- Leukogram in combination with fibrinogen and globulins can help diagnose infectious, inflammatory, immune-mediated, and/or neoplastic (including myeloproliferative) diseases and changes associated with corticosteroid administration
- Red blood cell morphology can help diagnose causes of anemia including chronic disease, iron deficiency, and hemolytic
- Polycythemia may occur with splenic contraction, hemoconcentration, organ disease, or polycythemia vera
- Changes in muscle enzymes, liver enzyme and function tests, and azotemia may occur related to primary disease
- Hypoproteinemia/hypoalbuminemia may be associated with protein-losing enteropathy/nephropathy or effusive disorders

OTHER LABORATORY TESTS
- Platelet function tests (automated platelet function analyzer; aggregometry; flow cytometry) for thrombocytopathia
- Viscoelastic coagulation testing for hypercoagulability
- Other abnormalities related to underlying disease
- Further diagnostics for anemia include Coomb's testing and iron assays (blood and bone marrow)
- Bone marrow aspirate cytology and immunophenotypic testing for myeloproliferative disorders

IMAGING
Ultrasonography/radiography of the abdomen, thorax, and/or musculoskeletal system to identify/characterize underlying disease.

OTHER DIAGNOSTIC PROCEDURES
- Template or buccal mucosal bleeding time for thrombocytopathia
- Cytology and culture of abdominal, thoracic, synovial fluid, and tracheal or bronchial samples
- Percutaneous, rectal, or surgical aspirates/biopsies as indicated for underlying disease
- Oral glucose absorption test for small intestinal malabsorption
- Endoscopy of the airway/gastrointestinal tract

PATHOLOGIC FINDINGS
Dependent on the underlying disorder.

TREATMENT
- Specific treatment to reduce platelet count (i.e. plasmapheresis) is seldom indicated
- The underlying disease process should be treated

MEDICATIONS

DRUG(S) OF CHOICE
- Aspirin or clopidogrel antithrombotic therapy for hypercoagulability
- In thrombocytopathia/bleeding tendencies fresh whole-blood or platelet-rich plasma transfusions may be indicated
- Treatment of any underlying disease process

CONTRAINDICATIONS/POSSIBLE INTERACTIONS
Avoid use of NSAIDs, especially aspirin, if there is evidence of platelet dysfunction.

FOLLOW-UP

PATIENT MONITORING
- Hematologic monitoring as needed
- Monitor response of underlying disease to treatment

PREVENTION/AVOIDANCE
N/A

POSSIBLE COMPLICATIONS
- Hemorrhagic diathesis with platelet dysfunction
- Thrombosis and possible ischemic tissue damage (e.g. laminitis, organ dysfunction)

EXPECTED COURSE AND PROGNOSIS
Dependent on successful treatment of underlying condition.

MISCELLANEOUS

ASSOCIATED CONDITIONS
N/A

AGE-RELATED FACTORS
Young horses at increased risk.

ZOONOTIC POTENTIAL
N/A

PREGNANCY/FERTILITY/BREEDING
N/A

SEE ALSO
- Coagulation defects, acquired
- Coagulation defects, inherited
- Thrombocytopenia

ABBREVIATIONS
NSAID = nonsteroidal anti-inflammatory drug

Suggested Reading
Sellon DC, Levine JF, Plamer K, et al. Thrombocytosis in 24 horses (1989–1994). J Vet Intern Med 1997;11:24–29

Author Kira L. Epstein
Consulting Editors David Hodgson, Harold C. McKenzie, and Jennifer L. Hodgson
Acknowledgment The author and editors acknowledge the prior contribution of Kristopher Hughes.

BASICS

OVERVIEW
• Thrombophlebitis is usually the consequence of IV injection or catheterization and therefore occurs most commonly in the jugular vein, although any vein can be affected. Both nonseptic and septic forms occur
• Systems affected—cardiovascular

SIGNALMENT
Any age group can be affected and there are no breed or sex predilections.

SIGNS
• The affected vein will be enlarged and firm
• Depending on the degree of occlusion of the vessel, venous distention and proximal swelling may be present and this is often most obvious around the cheek and supraorbital area
• Bilateral jugular thrombosis may cause sufficient swelling to compromise the airway
• With sepsis, the thrombus will be hot and painful on palpation

CAUSES AND RISK FACTORS
• Horses with severe gastrointestinal disease commonly have coagulopathy, which increases the risk of thrombophlebitis
• Use of hyperosmotic or homemade fluids and drugs that irritate the vascular endothelium such as oxytetracycline and phenylbutazone are also risk factors
• Flexible polyurethane over-the-wire catheters are less likely to be associated with thrombophlebitis than more rigid materials and over-the-needle types. Meticulous catheter care protocols will also reduce risk

DIAGNOSIS

DIFFERENTIAL DIAGNOSIS
Thrombophlebitis must be distinguished from perivenous reactions.

CBC/BIOCHEMISTRY/URINALYSIS
• With sepsis there will be leukocytosis and increases in plasma fibrinogen and serum amyloid A concentrations
• Assessment of clotting function is indicated, particularly in horses with other risk factors such as systemic infection or gastrointestinal disease

OTHER LABORATORY TESTS
Blood culture or culture of an aspirate from the thrombus can help identify specific bacteria and inform the choice of antimicrobials.

IMAGING
• Diagnostic ultrasonography is helpful to characterize the extent of the thrombus and determine the degree of vascular occlusion
• With sepsis, gas or fluid pockets produce a heterogeneous appearance whereas a nonseptic thrombus is typically more uniform. Layers may be visible within the thrombus

TREATMENT

• The IV catheter should be removed and topical hot packs applied
• If there is head swelling, the horse should be encouraged to keep its head up, such as feeding in hay nets

MEDICATIONS

DRUG(S) OF CHOICE
• Local application of anti-inflammatories such as hydroxyethyl salicylate may be helpful
• With confirmed or suspected sepsis, antimicrobials are indicated, ideally given IM or orally
• Aspirin (18 mg/kg PO every 48 h) and low-molecular-weight heparin (50 IU/kg SC SID for 3 days) may be useful. Clopidogrel at 2 mg/kg PO every 24 hours may also be useful

• In severe cases, thrombectomy or drainage of abscess cavities may be necessary. Reconstructive surgery using saphenous vein grafts or a synthetic vessel prosthesis have been reported

FOLLOW-UP

PATIENT MONITORING
Clinical signs and ultrasonographic appearance should be monitored while the condition is treated.

POSSIBLE COMPLICATIONS
• Horses with septic jugular thrombosis are at risk of infective endocarditis
• Damage to the recurrent laryngeal nerve with consequent laryngeal paralysis is also possible
• Generally, collateral circulation will develop, allowing a return to normal exercise activity. However, with obstruction to the venous return from the head, exercise-associated airway swelling can occur and compromise performance
• Platelet count should be monitored every 2–4 weeks in horses receiving long-term aspirin therapy

EXPECTED COURSE AND PROGNOSIS
The majority of patients with thrombophlebitis will recover and, even if the vein is permanently occluded, collateral circulation will develop within a few weeks.

Suggested Reading
Marr CM. Cardiovascular infections. In: Sellon DC, Long MT, eds. Equine Infectious Disease, 2e. St. Louis, MO: Elsevier, 2014:21–41.
Moreau P, Lavoie JP. Evaluation of athletic performance in horses with jugular vein thrombophlebitis: 91 cases (1988-2005). J Am Vet Med Assoc 2009;235:1073–1078.
Author Celia M. Marr
Consulting Editors Celia M. Marr and Virginia B. Reef

T

THYROID-RELEASING HORMONE (TRH) AND THYROID-STIMULATING HORMONE (TSH) TESTS

BASICS

DEFINITION
• TRH and TSH stimulation tests are performed to evaluate the ability of the thyroid gland to secrete T_3 and T_4. TRH may also be used to test horses with suspected PPID
• TRH test to evaluate thyroid function—give TRH (1 mg IV) and measure T_3 and T_4 levels at 0, 2, and 4 h. In normal horses baseline T_3 and T_4 are in the reference range. T_3 concentration doubles at 2 h, and T_4 concentration doubles at 4 h after TRH or TSH administration
• TSH test (5 IU IV) is performed in the same manner, with the same expected endpoints
• TRH test to evaluate pituitary function—give TRH (1 mg IV), and measure blood ACTH at 0 and at 10 min. In normal horses, ACTH concentrations do not change; however, an ACTH concentration >1.5 times baseline 10 minutes after TRH administration suggests that PPID is present

PATHOPHYSIOLOGY
• Thyroid hormone levels in blood are regulated by the thyroid–pituitary–hypothalamic axis. Endogenous TRH is released from the hypothalamus and travels to the pituitary gland. The pituitary gland then secretes TSH, which stimulates release of T_4 and T_3 from the thyroid gland
• When exogenous TSH is given, the thyroid gland's ability to secrete hormone is tested
• When TRH is given, the pituitary gland's ability to respond to this by secreting TSH and then the thyroid gland's ability to respond to the endogenous TSH are tested
• In equine medicine, test selection is based primarily on availability of the reagents. Presently, TSH is not available for clinical use but TRH can be obtained from compounding pharmacies at reasonable cost
• The inappropriate response of pituitary tumor cells to TRH is not completely understood. Tumor cells are hypothesized to have an alteration in the receptor/adenylate cyclase system that allows for a paradoxical response to specific and nonspecific challenges

SYSTEMS AFFECTED
The endocrine system is affected by abnormal results of the TSH or TRH stimulation tests—decreased thyroid hormone response to the stimulation test is diagnostic of hypothyroidism while increased ACTH in response to TRH suggests, but is not diagnostic, of PPID. The TRH stimulation to diagnose PPID should not be performed in the fall as the seasonally adjusted normal ranges have not been established.

SIGNALMENT
• No sex or breed predilections
• Hypothyroidism can occur at any age

• PPID occurs in older horses (>15 years)

SIGNS
• Signs associated with an abnormal TRH/TSH stimulation test are those of hypothyroidism or PPID
• Clinical signs of congenital hypothyroidism in foals—prognathism, ruptured common digital extensor tendon, forelimb contracture, retarded ossification, crushing of the carpal and tarsal bones, weakness, and poor suckle reflex
• Less common signs of congenital hypothyroidism in foals—goiter, angular limb deformities, respiratory distress, abdominal hernia, poor muscle development, and osteoporosis
• Hypothermia and bradycardia are consistent findings in adults with hypothyroidism. Other signs include poor hair coat and poor growth
• Clinical signs of PPID include hypertrichosis (previously termed hirsutism) and failure to shed. Also common are abnormal fat distribution, pendulous abdomen, weight loss, polyuria and polydipsia, laminitis, and chronic infections

CAUSES
• The primary cause for lack of response in a TSH/TRH stimulation test is primary hypothyroidism. Many factors can cause low T_3 and T_4 concentrations in blood; however, the horse cannot be diagnosed as truly hypothyroid unless it fails to respond to TSH/TRH stimulation testing
• The primary cause for increased ACTH after TRH administration is inappropriate response of a pituitary tumor to TRH

RISK FACTORS
• Known risk factors for thyroid abnormalities are dietary. Intake of excess or inadequate iodine or ingestion of goitrogens can lead to hypothyroidism
• In old populations, thyroid tumor is a risk factor for development of thyroid abnormalities
• PPID is a risk factor for development of abnormal ACTH secretion in response to TRH

DIAGNOSIS

DIFFERENTIAL DIAGNOSIS
The primary differential diagnosis for increased ACTH after TRH administration is stress response. Psychic stress from handling, receiving injections, and blood sample collections may result in increased blood ACTH.

LABORATORY FINDINGS
Drugs That May Alter Laboratory Results
N/A

Disorders That May Alter Laboratory Results
N/A

Valid if Run in a Human Laboratory?
Laboratory determination of ACTH, T_3, free T_3, T_4, and free T_4 is valid if run in a human laboratory. Use equine reference ranges to interpret results. Free T_3 and T_4 should be determined by equilibrium dialysis method.

CBC/BIOCHEMISTRY/URINALYSIS
• Hypothyroidism—anemia, leukopenia, and hypercholesterolemia
• PPID—stress response with a mature neutrophilia, lymphopenia, and eosinopenia; possibly increased blood glucose and glucosuria

OTHER LABORATORY TESTS
Pituitary function—endogenous ACTH determination, dexamethasone suppression testing, and domperidone response test; if results are consistent with PPID, this would support a positive TRH test.

IMAGING
• Ultrasonography—rarely useful in hypothyroidism, but an enlarged thyroid gland caused by tumor or goiter could be visualized
• Radiography—an enlarged thyroid gland caused by tumor or goiter might be seen as an increased soft tissue density in the throat-latch area
• Increased pituitary gland size may be visualized with specialized modalities—CT or venous contrast

OTHER DIAGNOSTIC PROCEDURES
Fine needle aspiration or biopsy may assist in assessing the thyroid gland.

TREATMENT

APPROPRIATE HEALTH CARE
• Foals with congenital hypothyroidism may require inpatient medical management as they often suffer from severe musculoskeletal disease
• All other horses with abnormal TRH/TSH tests can be treated as outpatients

NURSING CARE
• Foals may need assistance standing and milk administered via nasogastric tube if they are too weak to suckle
• Foals may need mechanical ventilation if they cannot breathe on their own
• Animals with a poor haircoat may need blanketing
• Horses with laminitis need corrective hoof trimming and shoeing. They may also require a low-carbohydrate diet if they evidence insulin dysregulation

(CONTINUED) THYROID-RELEASING HORMONE (TRH) AND THYROID-STIMULATING HORMONE (TSH) TESTS

ACTIVITY
• Limit activity of foals with musculoskeletal deformities—incomplete ossification of the carpal or tarsal bones
• Limit activity of horses with laminitis

DIET
• Examine the diet of any horse with hypothyroidism and of dams with foals born with hypothyroidism to ensure that the proper amount of iodine is being fed
• Pregnant mares should not receive endophyte-infected fescue hay or iodine supplementation, particularly during the last months of gestation
• Horses with laminitis generally benefit from a low-carbohydrate diet

CLIENT EDUCATION
• The prognosis is poor in most foals with congenital hypothyroidism and, thus, should be discussed with owners before expensive treatments begin
• Adult horses with hypothyroidism respond well to exogenous replacement hormone. Their prognosis generally is good.
• Mares in the northwestern portions of North America should not be fed green feed or irrigated pastures that are high in nitrates and should receive mineral supplementation including adequate amounts of iodine
• Horses with PPID may be managed via medication (pergolide) and nursing care, but their prognosis is quite variable. Some do well for several years; others are refractory to treatment. Owners need to understand that treatment is palliative and required for life

SURGICAL CONSIDERATIONS
If the abnormal TRH/TSH response test results from a tumor of the thyroid gland, surgical removal of the affected thyroid lobe should be curative.

MEDICATIONS

DRUG(S) OF CHOICE
• For decreased T_3 and T_4 caused by hypothyroidism, replacement therapy with synthetic T_4 is the drug of choice—20 µg/kg maintains T_4 and T_3 levels in the normal range for 24 h; this constitutes a dose of 10 mg in a 450 kg (1000 lb) horse
• The agent most commonly used to alter symptoms of PPID is pergolide (0.5–2 mg/day)

CONTRAINDICATIONS
If the horse has low resting T_3 and T_4 values because of some other severe disease (e.g. euthyroid sick syndrome), thyroid replacement therapies may cause further deterioration. Perform provocative testing before administering medication in any horse with suspected hypothyroidism that is debilitated or exhibits signs of any other disease.

PRECAUTIONS
• Exogenous thyroid hormone causes downregulation and, potentially, atrophy of the thyroid gland. Discontinue the supplement gradually over the course of several weeks
• Horses that receive overdoses of pergolide may exhibit anorexia, lethargy, and ataxia

POSSIBLE INTERACTIONS
N/A

ALTERNATIVE DRUGS
Other sources of thyroid hormone include iodinated casein (5.0 g/day) and concentrated bovine thyroid extract (10 g/day).

FOLLOW-UP

PATIENT MONITORING
• Monitor horses on thyroid supplement by retesting serum T_4 and T_3 levels every 30–60 days. If the serum level is low, increase the dosage until the normal range is achieved. If the serum level is too high or at the higher end of the normal range, decrease the dosage and retest the horse
• Failure to respond clinically after 6 weeks of therapy should prompt reconsideration of the original diagnosis of thyroid disease
• Retest horses with PPID every 12–20 weeks by endogenous ACTH determination. Abnormal results indicate the need for an increased dose of pergolide

MISCELLANEOUS

ASSOCIATED CONDITIONS
• Angular limb deformities, hypognathism, weakness, and respiratory distress often are associated with congenital hypothyroidism

• Skin problems and myositis have been associated with hypothyroidism in adults
• Hypertrichosis (previously termed hirsutism), chronic infections, and laminitis are commonly associated with PPID

AGE-RELATED FACTORS
On the first day of life, foals have little T_3 response to TRH/TSH administration. Only a T_4 response should be evaluated in neonatal foals.

ZOONOTIC POTENTIAL
N/A

PREGNANCY/FERTILITY/BREEDING
N/A

SEE ALSO
• Disorders of the thyroid, hypo- and hyperthyroidism
• Pituitary pars intermedia dysfunction

ABBREVIATIONS
• ACTH = adrenocorticotropic hormone
• CT = computed tomography
• PPID = pituitary pars intermedia dysfunction
• T_3 = triiodothyronine
• T_4 = thyroxine
• TRH = thyroid-releasing hormone
• TSH = thyroid-stimulating hormone

Suggested Reading
Beech J, Boston R, Lindborg S, Russell GE. Adrenocorticotropin concentration following administration of thyrotropin-releasing hormone in healthy horses and those with pituitary pars intermedia dysfunction and pituitary gland hyperplasia. J Am Vet Med Assoc 2007;231:417–426.
Durham AE, McGowan CM, Fey K, et al. Pituitary pars intermedia dysfunction: diagnosis and treatment. Equine Vet Educ 2014;26:216–223.
Frank N, Sojka J, Messer 4th NT. Equine thyroid dysfunction. Vet Clin North Am Equine Pract 2002;18:305–319.

Author Janice Kritchevsky
Consulting Editors Michel Levy and Heidi Banse

T

THYROID TUMORS

BASICS

OVERVIEW
• Thyroid adenoma, adenocarcinoma, and C-cell (parafollicular) tumors have been reported in horses
• Adenomatous change is quite common in older horses. In a postmortem survey of 100 horses, 34 had normal thyroids, 20 had hyperplastic changes, 9 had colloid tumors, and 37 had adenomas
• Tumors are usually incidental findings. Rarely, they may be present along with tumors of other endocrine organs in horses with multiple endocrine neoplasm syndrome

SIGNALMENT
• Common in older horses—over 17 years of age. No reported sex or breed predilections
• No known genetic basis for thyroid tumors

SIGNS
• Typically, there are no clinical signs associated with thyroid tumors. They are detected on physical examination by palpation. In rare cases, the tumors become so large they prevent normal esophageal function or compress the trachea
• Signs are more commonly associated with adenocarcinoma and C-cell tumors than with adenomas. These signs may be associated with either hypothyroidism or hyperthyroidism. The most frequently reported physical sign is weight loss. Other signs associated with thyroid tumors include nervousness, work intolerance, respiratory embarrassment, and cold intolerance. Behavioral disturbances include pacing and difficulty when being handled. Tachypnea and tachycardia may also be present
• Alterations in both total and ionized blood calcium can occur with C-cell tumors. Although levels outside the normal range may be detected on chemistry panels, clinical signs associated with alterations in blood calcium are not typically observed

CAUSES AND RISK FACTORS
No known risk factors for development of thyroid tumors.

DIAGNOSIS

• Diagnosis is usually made by a combination of physical examination and diagnostic tests

• Thyroid adenoma should be suspected in any older horse with an enlarged thyroid gland

DIFFERENTIAL DIAGNOSIS
• Goiter without neoplasia
• Retropharyngeal lymph node enlargement
• Hematoma
• Guttural pouch distention

CBC/BIOCHEMISTRY/URINALYSIS
Generally normal in horses with thyroid tumors.

OTHER LABORATORY TESTS
Blood total and free T_4 and T_3 levels may be increased or decreased if the tumor leads to either hypothyroidism or hyperthyroidism. In the 1 horse described with hyperthyroidism due to an adenocarcinoma, free T_4 concentrations were elevated above the normal range although the total T_4 levels were not increased. In horses with hypothyroidism, T_3 and T_4 serum concentrations will be below reference ranges and will not increase appropriately after evocative testing with thyroid-releasing hormone or thyroid-stimulating hormone.

IMAGING
A thyroid tumor can be imaged via ultrasonography as 1 or more nodules within the thyroid gland. If it is so large that the entire gland is enlarged, this may be seen on radiographs of the cervical region as a soft tissue density.

OTHER DIAGNOSTIC PROCEDURES
• A fine needle aspirate will allow one to identify the tumor as being thyroid in origin but will not often allow one to differentiate between an adenoma and adenocarcinoma
• A biopsy of the thyroid gland mass will provide the definitive diagnosis, though results are often equivocal and the organ is highly vascular and even a small sample may cause excessive hemorrhage

PATHOLOGIC FINDINGS
Most tumors are adenomas. Other tumor types and tumors in other endocrine organs occur infrequently but have been reported.

TREATMENT

If a discrete noninvasive thyroid tumor is found, surgical removal of the affected thyroid lobe is curative. If metastatic disease has occurred, prognosis is reduced. C-cell tumors

and adenocarcinoma spread slowly, however, and surgical removal is generally curative despite histopathologic evidence of malignancy.

MEDICATIONS

DRUG(S) OF CHOICE
Propylthiouracil has been used to induce hypothyroidism experimentally, but has not been reported as a treatment for clinical cases. Its use could be considered if local invasion or metastasis precludes complete surgical removal. If bilateral tumors occur and the complete gland is removed, then thyroxine supplement (20 μg/kg/day) is indicated. Calcium supplementation is not necessary as horses have parathyroid tissue spread diffusely in the cervical area.

FOLLOW-UP

Anesthetic complications have been reported following the removal of thyroid tumors. For this reason, surgery on hyperthyroid horses should be done in a controlled manner. Once the tumor is removed, clinical signs should gradually resolve.

MISCELLANEOUS

AGE-RELATED FACTORS
Horses with thyroid tumors tend to be older, >17 years of age.

SEE ALSO
Disorders of the thyroid, hypo- and hyperthyroidism

ABBREVIATIONS
• T_3 = triiodothyronine
• T_4 = thyroxine

Suggested Reading
Dalefield RR, Palmer DN. The frequent occurrence of thyroid tumours in aged horses. J Comp Pathol 1994;110:57–64.
Ramirex S, McClure JJ, Moore RM, et al. Hyperthyroidism associated with a thyroid adenocarcinoma in a 21-year-old gelding. J Vet Intern Med 1998;12:475–477.
Author Janice Kritchevsky
Consulting Editors Michel Levy and Heidi Banse

BASICS

OVERVIEW
• Many toxins can cause liver disease (i.e. toxic hepatopathy) in horses, with plant toxins being the most common
• The pathophysiology of the hepatic disease will vary depending upon the specific toxin. PAs are known to inhibit mitosis and to cause progressive fibrosis. Some plant hepatotoxins such as those produced by alsike clover and panicum as well as mycotoxins and iron toxicosis may cause mostly periportal inflammation/apoptosis, vacuolization, biliary proliferation, and fibrosis
• Drug-associated hepatopathy in the horse can occur with the coadministration of rifampin (rifampicin) and doxycycline in nursing foals being treated for *Rhodococcus equi*
• Regardless of the initial site and mechanism of disease, prolonged injury and activation of hepatic stellate cells will often result in hepatic fibrosis. Proliferation of hepatocytes, beginning in the periportal region and moving in towards perivenous zones, will occur in many toxic hepatopathies as an attempt to repair the injury. Once severe hepatic fibrosis and/or prolonged attempts of proliferative repair are established microscopic examination of the liver may be of little help in identifying the initial type of injury or specific toxin
• Treatment is primarily aimed at removing the source of the toxin and providing supportive care

SIGNALMENT
Any age, breed, or sex.

SIGNS
• Mostly those of hepatoencephalopathy—head pressing, circling, blindness, maniacal behavior or depression, and excessive yawning
• Photosensitization may occur on white-haired parts of the body or mucous membranes. A more generalized dermatitis may occur in association with liver disease. This more generalized disease may be caused by the adverse dermatologic effects of elevated serum bile acids, nutrient deficiencies caused by intestinal malabsorption, or from immune-mediated dermatitis. Uveitis may also occur from immune mechanisms
• Icterus and discolored urine may be noted
• Colic may occur because of gastric impaction, changes in liver size, or generalized discomfort
• Weight loss occurs in many but not all cases of chronic poisoning

CAUSES AND RISK FACTORS
Numerous, but the most common include the following.

PA-Containing Plants
• *Senecio* spp. (i.e. groundsel and ragwort), *Amsinckia intermedia* (i.e. fiddleneck), *Cynoglossum officinale* (hound's tongue), *Heliotropium europaeum* (heliotrope), and *Echium plantagineum* (Patterson's curse) are common in parts of North America
• Usually ingested when mixed in "first cutting" alfalfa hay
• Plants tend to be bitter with low palatability, but in drought conditions with sparse grasses may also be ingested in the pasture
• Estimated that horses must ingest 2% or more of body weight to develop hepatic failure

Alsike Clover
• One of the most common pasture-associated hepatopathies (northeastern USA and Canada)
• Increased incidence of disease in wet seasons when clover grows well
• Also causes disease when a large amount of clover is present in hay
• Unknown if the toxic principle is the plant itself or mycotoxin produced by fungus living on the plant

Panicum
• *Panicum coloratum* (kleingrass), *Panicum virgatum* (switchgrass), *Panicum dichotomiflorum* (fall *Panicum*)
• Ingestion of pasture or hay can lead to disease, environmental variables may play a role—several cases of toxicity in horses fed fall *Panicum* hay in the late fall/early winter which was harvested in the same year
• The toxic principle is thought to be saponin

Iron
• Generally a result of overzealous oral iron administration or chronic ingestion of very high iron contaminated water
• In newborn foals, even small amounts of iron given orally before colostrum may be fatal
• In adult horses, very large amounts of iron given orally are necessary to produce toxicity

Mycotoxins
• *Fusarium moniliformis* in horses fed contaminated grains
• Most horses with *Fusarium* spp. poisoning have clinical signs associated with leukoencephalomalacia rather than hepatic failure
• Horses have variable response to aflatoxins, ranging from no/minimal disease to death
• A horse with presumptive microcystin-associated liver failure has been described

Drug Induced
• Rare in the horse
• Severe toxic hepatopathy reported in nursing foals treated for *R. equi* with rifampin and doxycycline; recommended to use caution with this combination of antibiotics in foals
• No current reports of NSAID hepatopathy in horses

• Imidocarb use in donkeys linked to severe hepatic disease, but not in horses
• Age, species, genetic profiles affect hepatic metabolism and body elimination—generally, donkeys (especially miniatures) have increased hepatic metabolism, newborn foals have decreased hepatic metabolism

DIAGNOSIS

DIFFERENTIAL DIAGNOSIS
• Primary hyperammonemia seen in adult horses with intestinal disease, Morgan foals, and foals with portosystemic shunts and in horses with encephalitis, central nervous system trauma, and selected metabolic disorders (e.g. severe acidosis)
• Disorders leading to primary hyperammonemia generally involve only a mild increase in hepatic enzymes and do not have abnormalities in liver function tests (e.g. direct bilirubin, bile acids)

CBC/BIOCHEMISTRY/URINALYSIS
• CBC abnormalities most often involve neutrophilia and sometimes erythrocytosis
• Liver enzymes, both hepatocellular (i.e. AST, SDH, glutamate dehydrogenase) and biliary (i.e. GGT, ALP), are markedly elevated in acute toxic hepatopathy, although AST and ALP are not liver specific. SDH has a short half-life and repeated measurements can be used to determine progression of disease. In chronic toxicities (e.g. PA poisoning), enzymes may not be markedly elevated, although GGT remains elevated in most cases, even with chronic fibrosis
• Serum bile acids will be elevated in most cases if there is moderate loss of liver function
  ○ In horses with chronic liver disease values >25 mmol/L are indicative of a poor prognosis
• Blood urea nitrogen and fibrinogen generally are abnormally low
• Albumin, because of its long half-life, may remain normal or slightly low
• Both conjugated and unconjugated bilirubin levels are increased with liver failure. In most cases, the greatest increase involves unconjugated bilirubin. With severe cholestasis, the conjugated bilirubin concentration may be ≥25% of the total bilirubin
• Urine may be discolored (dark brown to orange) and, when shaken, the foam may appear green
• Urine dipstick examination usually is positive for bilirubin

OTHER LABORATORY TESTS
• Prothrombin and partial thromboplastin times are prolonged, but platelet numbers and function remain normal so clinically significant bleeding is unusual
• Blood ammonia may be high or normal

T

• Urinary and/or hepatic concentrations of specific toxins may be found
• Serum ferritin and measurement of hepatic iron may help to confirm the diagnosis of iron hepatopathy. Serum iron is frequently and secondarily elevated with a variety of liver diseases in the horse

IMAGING
Ultrasonography is the procedure of choice.

OTHER DIAGNOSTIC PROCEDURES
Liver biopsy is most commonly performed for microscopic diagnosis of either hepatocellular necrosis (e.g. acute iron poisoning), periportal or diffuse fibrosis from chronic toxicosis, and/or megalocytosis (e.g. PAs). Specific etiologies or etiopathogeneses are rarely found in cases of chronic hepatopathy, but the liver biopsy does allow for refining of the differential diagnosis list, treatment plan, or prognosis.

TREATMENT
• In some cases, such as with hepatoencephalopathy, horses may need hospitalization to control abnormal behavior and supply supportive therapy (see chapter Icterus (prehepatic, hepatic, posthepatic))
• Avoid activity, sunlight, and high-protein feeds but feed moderate amounts of protein to help prevent muscle catabolism and muscle aminogenesis

MEDICATIONS
DRUG(S) OF CHOICE
• Detomidine (5–10 µg/kg IV) may be required to control maniacal behavior and propofol (2 mg/kg IV) can be used to control seizure/maniacal behavior in foals; it is important to avoid oversedation

• Long-term sedation can be provided with pregabalin (3 mg/kg every 12 h PO) or gabapentin (5–12 mg/kg every 12 h PO)
• For horses with hepatic failure, anorexia, and neurologic signs, IV fluids should be used—acetated Ringer's solution supplemented with 20–40 mEq KCl/L and dextrose (50 g/L)
• In cases of hepatoencephalopathy, neomycin (10–20 mg/kg every 8 h PO for 1–3 days) to decrease ammonia produced by gastrointestinal bacteria. Lactulose (0.3–0.5 mL/kg every 8 h PO) can be administered concurrently to further decrease the chance of hyperammonemia and also soften stool in order to prevent constipation. Prebiotics or probiotics can also be given
• Pentoxifylline (8.4 mg/kg BID) can be used for anti-inflammatory/antifibrosis treatment
• S-adenosylmethionine (10 mg/kg daily), vitamin E (5 IU/kg daily PO), and milk thistle extract supplements can be used for antioxidant therapy
• Colchicine (0.03 mg/kg daily PO) may be administered in hopes of decreasing fibrosis

CONTRAINDICATIONS/POSSIBLE INTERACTIONS
Colchicine should not be used to treat PA toxicosis as both colchicine and PA pyrroles inhibit mitosis.

FOLLOW-UP
• Prevent toxin exposure to all horses in the future
• Feed a moderate-protein/high-energy feed, protect from sunlight
• Avoid stress
• Monitor serum enzymes and bile acids for progression of hepatic disease
• Prognosis depends on toxin, degree of fibrosis, and progression of disease

• All cases with moderate to extreme fibrosis have a guarded to poor prognosis for life >1 year

MISCELLANEOUS
SEE ALSO
• Ammonia, hyperammonemia
• Hepatic encephalopathy
• Icterus (prehepatic, hepatic, posthepatic)
• Photosensitization

ABBREVIATIONS
• ALP = alkaline phosphatase
• AST = aspartate aminotransferase
• GGT = γ-glutamyltransferase
• NSAID = nonsteroidal anti-inflammatory drug
• PA = pyrrolizidine alkaloid
• SDH = sorbitol dehydrogenase

Suggested Reading
Caloni F, Cortinovis C. Effects of fusariotoxins in the equine species. Vet J 2010;186:157–161.
Divers TJ. The equine liver in health and disease. Proc Am Assoc Equine Pract 2015;61:66–103.
Durham AE, Newton JR, Smith KC, et al. Retrospective analysis of historical, clinical, ultrasonographic, serum biochemical and haematological data in prognostic evaluation of equine liver disease. Equine Vet J 2003;35:542–547.
Smith MR, Stevens KB, Durham AE, Marr CM. Equine hepatic disease: the effect of patient- and case-specific variables on risk and prognosis. Equine Vet J 2003;35:549–552.

Authors Thomas J. Divers and Nikhita P. De Bernardis
Consulting Editors Henry Stämpfli and Olimpo Oliver-Espinosa

T

TREMORGENIC MYCOTOXIN TOXICOSES

BASICS

OVERVIEW
- Tremorgenic mycotoxins are the lolitrems (lolitrems A, B, C, and D), produced by *Neotyphodium lolii* and causing perennial ryegrass (*Lolium perenne*) staggers, and paspalitrems (paspalinine, paspalitrem A, B and C), produced by *Claviceps paspali* and causing dallis grass or paspalum staggers (associated with dallis grass (*Paspalum dilatatum*) and bahia grass (*Bahia oppositifolia*))
- The specific tremorgen associated with Bermuda grass (*Cynodon dactylon*) has not been isolated
- *N. lolii* is an endophytic fungus of ryegrass and propagates via seed
- *C. paspali* is a soil fungus that invades dallis and bahia grass under favorable environmental conditions
- Some tremorgens competitively inhibit CNS postsynaptic GABA receptors and cause chloride influx; GABA receptor antagonism leads to increased nerve discharge and neurologic signs
- Lolitrem B inhibits calcium-activated potassium channels, thereby perturbing motor function
- Annual ryegrass toxicosis, the clinical presentation of which is similar to that of tremorgenic mycotoxins, can result when the bacterium *Clavibacter toxicus* is carried into annual ryegrass seedheads by the nematode *Anguina funesta*. *C. toxicus* produces the neurotoxin corynetoxin, a glycolipid that inhibits the synthesis of lipid-linked oligosaccharides and blocks protein glycosylation

SIGNALMENT
No breed, sex, or age predispositions.

SIGNS

Perennial Ryegrass and Annual Ryegrass Staggers
- Signs occur 5–10 days after grazing highly toxic pastures
- Signs include head tremors and muscle fasciculations of the neck and legs, which progress to head nodding and swaying while standing

- Animals that are forced to move develop dysmetria and leg stiffening, leading to collapse and tetanic spasms; if left alone, animals recover in a few minutes and walk away with a relatively normal gait
- Affected animals rarely die unless they injure themselves during a tetanic spasm
- Affected animals may lose weight and are difficult to handle or move because of inducible spasms

Paspalum Staggers
Signs are identical to those above but often less severe.

CAUSES AND RISK FACTORS

Perennial Ryegrass Staggers
- Incidence is greater during the late summer and fall and on ryegrass pastures that have been heavily grazed
- Environmental temperatures are generally >23°C
- Frequency of intoxication relates to the degree of fungal infection of the ryegrass. Infection rates <25% are associated with sporadic outbreaks, whereas rates >90% are associated with large outbreaks

Paspalum Staggers
Toxin production is greatest during a warm and wet period following seedhead formation.

Annual Ryegrass Staggers
- Toxin concentration increases in seedheads during the summer and is greatest as the plant dries and seeds ripen
- Annual ryegrass occurs in patches, and alterations in grazing patterns may predispose to ingestion
- Newly introduced animals may ingest more ryegrass

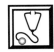

DIAGNOSIS

DIFFERENTIAL DIAGNOSIS
- Other plant intoxications such as locoism (*Astragalus* spp.) and white snakeroot (*Eupatorium rugosum*)—evidence of plant consumption, characteristic histopathologic lesions, detection of tremetol in white snakeroot toxicosis
- Viral or bacterial encephalopathy

CBC/BIOCHEMISTRY/URINALYSIS
N/A

OTHER LABORATORY TESTS

Perennial Ryegrass Staggers
- Positive identification of perennial ryegrass
- Microscopic detection of fungus in ryegrass
- Mouse bioassay of methanol extracts from ryegrass to produce characteristic clinical signs
- Detection of lolitrems in ryegrass—concentrations of lolitrem B >2 ppm are associated with effects in sheep and cattle
- ELISA for detection of lolitrem B

Paspalum Staggers
- Positive identification of dallis or bahia grass and associated fungal sclerotia on grass seedheads
- Detection of tremorgen

Annual Ryegrass Staggers
- Positive identification of annual ryegrass
- Identification of galls associated with nematode infestation
- ELISA for detection of corynetoxin

IMAGING
N/A

OTHER DIAGNOSTIC PROCEDURES
N/A

PATHOLOGIC FINDINGS
- Gross lesions generally are absent
- Animals with chronic ryegrass staggers may have loss of Purkinje cells in the cerebellum, which is believed to be secondary to hypoxia and hypoglycemia
- Histopathologic changes associated with annual ryegrass staggers include cerebellar, hepatic, and splenic hemorrhages that may be secondary to endothelial cell damage

TREATMENT
Remove animals from affected grass pastures.

MEDICATIONS

DRUG(S) OF CHOICE
N/A

T

TREMORGENIC MYCOTOXIN TOXICOSES

FOLLOW-UP

PATIENT MONITORING
Attempt to prevent self-injury during tetanic spasms.

PREVENTION/AVOIDANCE
Perennial Ryegrass Staggers
• Reduce overgrazing of pastures
• Remove animals from pastures during critical periods—late summer and fall for endophyte-infested ryegrass pastures
• Use endophyte-free ryegrass seed
• Use fungicides—reduces seed viability

Paspalum Staggers
• Inspect pastures for ergotized seedheads
• Mow pastures to remove toxic seedheads

Annual Ryegrass Staggers
• Break nematode life cycle by killing ryegrass for 2 or 3 growing seasons
• Integrated control measures—herbicide use in the spring, seeding pastures with legumes, burning infested pastures in the early fall, applying herbicides to selectively kill ryegrass during the summer, and heavy winter grazing

POSSIBLE COMPLICATIONS
• Traumatic injury
• Bloating or drowning during tetanic spasm

EXPECTED COURSE AND PROGNOSIS
• Once removed from affected pastures, animals generally recover within several weeks without treatment
• Degenerative CNS lesions associated with chronic perennial ryegrass staggers likely prevent full recovery

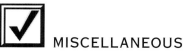

MISCELLANEOUS

ABBREVIATIONS
• CNS = central nervous system
• ELISA = enzyme-linked immunosorbent assay
• GABA = γ-aminobutyric acid

Suggested Reading
Cawdell-Smith AJ, Scrivener CJ, Bryden WL. Staggers in horses grazing paspalum infected with *Claviceps paspali.* Aust Vet J 2010;88(10):393–395.
Plumlee KH, Galey FD. Neurotoxic mycotoxins: a review of fungal toxins that cause neurologic disease in large animals. J Vet Intern Med 1994;8:49–54.

Authors Arya Sobhakumari and Robert H. Poppenga
Consulting Editors Wilson K. Rumbeiha and Steve Ensley

T

BASICS

DEFINITION
Occurs when the tricuspid (right atrioventricular) valve allows blood to leak backward into the right atrium and creates a systolic murmur with its point of maximal intensity in the tricuspid valve area radiating dorsally or cranially.

PATHOPHYSIOLOGY
• Tricuspid regurgitation can occur with structurally normal valve cusps or when dysplastic, inflammatory, or degenerative disease or rupture of a chorda tendinea is present
• During systole, blood regurgitates into the right atrium, and, if severe, increases right atrial pressure and leads to right atrial and ventricular volume overload
• As the regurgitation becomes more severe, increases in right atrial pressure produce increased central venous pressure, hepatic congestion, and right-sided CHF

SYSTEMS AFFECTED
Cardiovascular

GENETICS
N/A

INCIDENCE/PREVALENCE
The prevalence of murmurs characteristic of tricuspid regurgitation in a middle-aged and older population of apparently healthy horses in the UK was 1.1%, and in Thoroughbreds was 22% in flat and 43% in jump racing.

SIGNALMENT
Reported most frequently in athletes.

SIGNS
General Comments
Usually an incidental finding with no effect on performance. The severity of signs is dependent on the nature and severity of valvular pathology.

Historical Findings
• Sometimes poor performance
• Sometimes CHF

Physical Examination Findings
• Grade 2–6/6, band-shaped to crescendo or crescendo–decrescendo holosystolic murmur with its point of maximal intensity in the tricuspid valve area (right fourth intercostal space) radiating to the right heart base
• Approximately 30% of horses with tricuspid infective endocarditis do not have cardiac murmurs
• Other, less common findings—AF, jugular pulsations, generalized venous distention, and ventral edema

CAUSES
• Physiologic tricuspid regurgitation, a response to athletic training
• Degenerative, inflammatory, or congenital valvular disease

• Pulmonary hypertension
• Ruptured chordae tendineae
• Infective endocarditis

RISK FACTORS
• Infective endocarditis can be a sequela of septic jugular thrombophlebitis
• Athletes have a high prevalence of physiologic tricuspid regurgitation

 DIAGNOSIS

DIFFERENTIAL DIAGNOSIS
Ventricular septal defect—there is a loud murmur over the right hemithorax accompanied by the murmur of pulmonic stenosis over the pulmonic valve area (left third intercostal space); differentiate echocardiographically.

CBC/BIOCHEMISTRY/URINALYSIS
Leukocytosis and hyperfibrinogenemia and elevated SAA with infective endocarditis.

OTHER LABORATORY TESTS
• Increased concentrations of cardiac troponin I with concurrent myocardial disease
• Positive blood culture with infective endocarditis

IMAGING
Echocardiography
• Most affected horses have normal tricuspid valve leaflets
• Prolapse of a tricuspid leaflet into the right atrium frequently is detected in affected horses
• Thickening of the valve leaflets is not seen often but diffuse thickening of the free edge of the leaflets is more common than nodular thickening of the leaflets' free edge
• Ruptured chordae tendineae, flail tricuspid leaflets, or vegetations associated with infective endocarditis are detected infrequently
• Right atrium—enlarged and dilated, with a rounded appearance
• Right ventricle—enlarged and dilated, with a rounded apex and thinning of the right ventricular free wall and interventricular septum
• A pattern of right ventricular volume overload, including paradoxic septal motion, in severe cases
• Dilatation of the cranial and caudal vena cava and hepatic veins in severe cases
• Pulsed-wave or color-flow Doppler reveals a jet (or jets) of tricuspid regurgitation in the right atrium. In most horses with mild to moderate regurgitation, the jet is directed toward the aortic root. The size and extent of the jet are used to semiquantitate severity

Thoracic Radiography
Cardiac enlargement may be detected, with increased contact between the heart and the sternum.

OTHER DIAGNOSTIC PROCEDURES
ECG
Supraventricular premature depolarizations or AF may be present at rest and/or during exercise in horses with right atrial enlargement.

Ultrasonography
With a thrombosed jugular vein, detection of a cavitated thrombus is consistent with septic jugular vein thrombophlebitis.

PATHOLOGIC FINDINGS
• Where the regurgitation relates to physiologic adaptation to athletic training, no pathologic findings are expected
• Most horses have relatively normal-appearing tricuspid valve leaflets at postmortem examination
• Focal or diffuse thickening or distortion of 1 or more tricuspid leaflets may be present
• Ruptured chordae tendineae, flail tricuspid leaflets, vegetations due to infective endocarditis, or congenital malformations of the tricuspid valve are infrequent
• Jet lesions may be detected in the right atrium
• Right atrial and ventricular enlargement in cases with significant regurgitation
• Dilatation of the cranial and caudal vena cava and hepatic veins in horses with severe regurgitation
• Pale areas may be seen in the atrial myocardium, with areas of atrial fibrosis detected histopathologically
• Inflammatory cell infiltrate and/or myocardial necrosis occasionally is detected in affected horses with primary myocardial disease
• In horses with CHF, ventral and peripheral edema, pleural effusion, pericardial effusion, chronic hepatic congestion, and, occasionally, ascites may be detected

 TREATMENT

AIMS
• Management by intermittent monitoring in horses with tricuspid regurgitation that is mild or moderate in severity
• Palliative care in horses with severe tricuspid regurgitation and signs of right-sided or CHF

APPROPRIATE HEALTH CARE
• Most affected horses require no treatment and can be monitored on an outpatient basis
• Treat horses with severe regurgitation and CHF with positive inotropic drugs, vasodilators, and diuretics on an inpatient basis, if possible, and monitor response to therapy

NURSING CARE
N/A

TRICUSPID REGURGITATION (CONTINUED)

ACTIVITY
• Most horses with tricuspid regurgitation are safe to continue in full athletic work unless the regurgitation is severe or the horse develops exercise intolerance or CHF
• Horses with significant right ventricular dysfunction and exercise intolerance are no longer safe to ride

DIET
N/A

CLIENT EDUCATION
• Monitor the cardiac rhythm regularly; any irregularities should prompt ECG
• Carefully monitor for exercise intolerance, jugular or generalized venous distention, jugular pulses, ventral edema, prolonged recovery after exercise, increased resting heart rate or increase in the intensity of the murmur of tricuspid regurgitation; if detected, perform a cardiac reexamination

SURGICAL CONSIDERATIONS
N/A

MEDICATIONS

DRUG(S) OF CHOICE
Treat affected horses in CHF with furosemide, torsemide, vasodilators such as benazepril or quinapril, or the inodilator pimobendan. Antimicrobials are indicated with infective endocarditis.

CONTRAINDICATIONS
• ACE inhibitors are contraindicated in pregnancy
• Diuretics, ACE inhibitors, and other vasodilators must be withdrawn before competition to comply with the medication rules of the various governing bodies of equine sports

PRECAUTIONS
N/A

POSSIBLE INTERACTIONS
N/A

ALTERNATIVE DRUGS
N/A

FOLLOW-UP

PATIENT MONITORING
• Frequently monitor cardiac rhythm and respiratory system

• Annual echocardiographic reexaminations are recommended in moderate to severe cases

PREVENTION/AVOIDANCE
N/A

POSSIBLE COMPLICATIONS
Chronic cases—AF; CHF.

EXPECTED COURSE AND PROGNOSIS
• Many affected horses have normal performance and life expectancy
• Prognosis for horses with tricuspid valve prolapse and mild regurgitation is excellent, and, in many, the amount of regurgitation remains unchanged for years
• Progression of regurgitation associated with degenerative valve disease usually is slow. If regurgitation is mild, these horses have a good to excellent prognosis
• Horses with ruptured chordae tendineae, flail tricuspid valve leaflets, or infective endocarditis have a more guarded prognosis, because the regurgitation usually becomes more severe and may result in a shortened performance and life expectancy
• Affected horses with CHF usually have severe underlying valvular heart and myocardial disease and a guarded to grave prognosis for life
• Most affected horses being treated for CHF respond to supportive therapy and improve. Such improvement usually is short lived, however. Most of these horses are euthanized within 2–6 months of initiation of treatment

MISCELLANEOUS

ASSOCIATED CONDITIONS
Mitral regurgitation.

AGE-RELATED FACTORS
Physiologic regurgitation due to cardiac adaptation to athletic training is the most common form and is usually diagnosed in horses of racing age.

ZOONOTIC POTENTIAL
N/A

PREGNANCY/FERTILITY/BREEDING
• Affected mares should not experience any problems with the pregnancy unless regurgitation is severe

• The volume expansion of late pregnancy places an additional load on the already volume-loaded heart, which may precipitate CHF in mares with severe regurgitation
• Pregnant mares with CHF should be treated for the underlying cardiac disease with positive inotropic drugs and diuretics
• ACE inhibitors are contraindicated because of potential adverse effects on the fetus

SYNONYMS
Tricuspid insufficiency.

SEE ALSO
• Atrial fibrillation
• Endocarditis, infective
• Mitral regurgitation

ABBREVIATIONS
• ACE = angiotensin-converting enzyme
• AF = atrial fibrillation
• CHF = congestive heart failure
• SAA = serum amyloid A

Suggested Reading
Leroux AA, Detilleux J, Sandersen CF, et al. Prevalence and risk factors for cardiac diseases in a hospital-based population of 3,434 horses (1994-2011). J Vet Intern Med 2013;27:1563–1570.
Reef VB. Heart murmurs in horses: determining their significance with echocardiography. Equine Vet J Suppl 1995;19:71–80.
Reef VB, Bonagura J, Buhl R, et al. Recommendations for management of equine athletes with cardiovascular abnormalities. J Vet Intern Med 2014;28:749–761.
Stevens KB, Marr CM, Horn JN, et al. Effect of left-sided valvular regurgitation on mortality and causes of death among a population of middle-aged and older horses. Vet Rec 2009;164:6–10.
Young LE, Rogers K, Wood JL. Heart murmurs and valvular regurgitation in thoroughbred racehorses: epidemiology and associations with athletic performance. J Vet Intern Med 2008;22:418–426.

Author Celia M. Marr
Consulting Editors Celia M. Marr and Virginia B. Reef
Acknowledgment The author acknowledges the prior contribution of Virginia B. Reef.

T

BASICS

OVERVIEW
- *Trifolium hybridum* (alsike clover) has been implicated as the cause of equine hepatic failure and neurologic impairment
- Clinical manifestations of intoxication are acute and neurologic or chronic and cachectic
- Postmortem histopathologic lesions consistently are found in the liver and include biliary fibrosis and marked bile duct proliferation
- Occurrence of the 2 syndromes is associated with ingestion of alsike clover, but a specific toxin has not been identified
- Photosensitization can occur in conjunction with both syndromes but is uncommon
- Morbidity varies, but mortality is high
- A reversible, alsike clover-induced photosensitization has been described and is considered by some to be unrelated to the other 2 syndromes

SIGNALMENT
- When both syndromes are considered together, there are no apparent breed, age, or sex predispositions; however, a retrospective study of alsike clover-associated disease suggested the nervous form occurs more commonly in old, female horses
- Not all horses in an exposed group develop clinical signs

SIGNS
- Acute and neurologic—alternating depression and excitement, head pressing, aimless walking, incoordination, yawning and bruxism, coma, and death
- Chronic and cachectic—variable appetite, progressive loss of body condition, weakness, sluggishness, dry and rough haircoat, icterus, yawning, head pressing, and periodic excitement preceding sudden death
- Photosensitization—skin erythema and swelling, pruritus, exudation of serum, hair matting, skin exfoliation, lacrimation, conjunctivitis, photophobia, and keratitis

CAUSES AND RISK FACTORS
- The disease is associated with ingestion of alsike clover-containing pasture or hay
- Alsike clover is believed to be less palatable than other forages and horses on pasture may eat less if alternative plants are available
- The ability of horses to avoid alsike clover in hay is less than on pasture; thus, horses fed alsike clover-containing hay may ingest more of the plant

DIAGNOSIS

DIFFERENTIAL DIAGNOSIS
- Ingestion of plants containing pyrrolizidine alkaloids
- Locoism (*Astragalus* spp.)
- *Equisetum arvense* (horsetail) or *Pteridium aquilinum* (bracken fern)
- Fumonisin mycotoxins
- Rabies
- Equine protozoal myelitis
- Viral encephalitis
- Brain abscesses or meningitis
- Narcolepsy
- Other causes of liver disease, with or without hepatoencephalopathy

CBC/BIOCHEMISTRY/URINALYSIS
Clinicopathologic changes have not been described in most suspected cases, but 1 had elevated serum liver enzymes and blood ammonia concentrations.

OTHER LABORATORY TESTS
- Cerebrospinal fluid—normal
- Serology—normal

IMAGING
Ultrasonography—enlarged and irregular liver.

OTHER DIAGNOSTIC PROCEDURES
Liver biopsy can be useful in differentiating alsike clover toxicosis from other liver diseases.

PATHOLOGIC FINDINGS
Gross
- Enlarged and irregular liver
- Some fibrosis may be evident
- Icterus is variable

Histopathologic
- Hepatic lesions include fibrosis of portal triads and around proliferating biliary epithelium
- Inflammatory changes—uncommon

TREATMENT
- Treat photosensitivity by preventing sun exposure
- Remove animal from the source of the plant
- Treatment of the hepatic and nervous syndromes commonly is unrewarding
- Supportive care including sedation for nervous syndrome, balanced electrolyte fluid administration, correction of hypoglycemia if present, and treatment of liver failure and hyperammonemia
- Small meals given frequently are suggested
- Diet should provide adequate energy and limited protein, primarily as branched-chain amino acids

MEDICATIONS

DRUG(S) OF CHOICE
- Sedation—xylazine (0.3–0.5 mg/kg IV as needed)
- Hyperammonemia—neomycin (15 mg/kg PO every 6 h) or lactulose (90–120 mL PO every 6–8 h)
- Energy provision—continuous 5% or 10% dextrose drip (2 or 1 mL/kg/h IV, respectively)

CONTRAINDICATIONS/POSSIBLE INTERACTIONS
- Diazepam is contraindicated in hepatoencephalopathy
- Use care when administering drugs requiring hepatic metabolism for activity or elimination

FOLLOW-UP

PATIENT MONITORING
Monitor hepatic function.

PREVENTION/AVOIDANCE
Because the conditions under which animals are intoxicated are poorly defined, the best specific recommendation is to prevent horses from ingesting alsike clover.

POSSIBLE COMPLICATIONS
N/A

EXPECTED COURSE AND PROGNOSIS
- Recovery from hepatic and neurologic syndromes is unlikely
- Recovery from uncomplicated photosensitization is expected with appropriate treatment

MISCELLANEOUS

ASSOCIATED CONDITIONS
N/A

AGE-RELATED FACTORS
N/A

ZOONOTIC POTENTIAL
N/A

PREGNANCY/FERTILITY/BREEDING
N/A

SEE ALSO
N/A

Suggested Reading
Nation PN. Hepatic disease in Alberta horses: a retrospective study of "alsike clover poisoning" (1973–1988). Can Vet J 1991;32:602–607.

Authors Arya Sobhakumari and Robert H. Poppenga
Consulting Editors Wilson K. Rumbeiha and Steve Ensley

T

TROPANE ALKALOIDS TOXICOSIS

BASICS

OVERVIEW
- Tropane alkaloids include hyoscyamine, hyoscine, atropine, and scopolamine
- Tropane alkaloids act as competitive antagonists to acetylcholine at the muscarinic receptors (antimuscarinic)
- Tropane alkaloid-containing plants include *Datura stramonium* (jimsonweed or thornapple), *Atropa belladonna* (belladonna, or deadly nightshade), and *Hyoscyamus niger* (henbane)
- All parts of the plant should be considered toxic, especially the seeds, which accumulate higher amounts of the toxins
- Horses have been poisoned through ingestion of *Datura* seeds or *Datura*-contaminated hay
- These plants are not palatable, and poisoning rarely occurs if more palatable forage is available
- The toxic effects include gastrointestinal and neurologic signs, teratogenesis, and death

SIGNALMENT
No known breed, age, or sex predilections.

SIGNS
- Major presentation is colic, with signs of abdominal pain, anxiety, and increased borborygmi
- Mildly elevated rectal temperature
- Tachypnea (shallow breathing, nostrils wide open)
- Tachycardia (may have a weak pulse) owing to removal of the parasympathetic tone
- Mydriasis and diffusely reddened conjunctiva
- Anorexia, lack of thirst, defecation, and urination
- Dry mucosae (oral, nasal, vaginal, and rectal)
- Hyperesthesia and/or ataxia
- Intestinal gas accumulation due to ileus
In more severe cases:
- Lateral recumbency accompanied by kicking
- Sweating
- Bruxism
- Seizures
- Respiratory failure
- Death

CAUSES AND RISK FACTORS
- Toxic dose is estimated to be about 0.75 mg seeds/kg body weight, equivalent to 0.5% of *Datura* seeds in the feed, over a period of 10 days
- Contamination of feed with about 25% by volume of *Datura* can be sufficient to induce peracute signs of poisoning and death in horses

DIAGNOSIS

DIFFERENTIAL DIAGNOSIS
- Causes of colic
- Parenteral atropine overdose

CBC/BIOCHEMISTRY/URINALYSIS
N/A

OTHER LABORATORY TESTS
Performance horses may be tested for scopolamine (L-hyoscine), and even inadvertent environmental exposures can cause a positive test.

IMAGING
N/A

OTHER DIAGNOSTIC PROCEDURES
Analysis of gastrointestinal contents or urine for tropane alkaloids.

PATHOLOGIC FINDINGS
Gross
- Gastrointestinal irritation and diarrhea with or without hemorrhages
- Ruptured diaphragm
- Ruptured stomach
- Intestinal and gastric gas accumulation
- Plant parts in stomach

Microscopic
- Hyperemic mesenteric blood vessels
- Petechial hemorrhages on mesenteric and intestinal serosa

TREATMENT
- Remove the source of exposure
- Gastric lavage in cases of acute exposure
- Activated charcoal through nasogastric intubation
- Symptomatic and supportive care

MEDICATIONS

DRUG(S) OF CHOICE
- Activated charcoal 1–4 g/kg by nasogastric intubation in water slurry (1 g of activated charcoal in 5 mL of water)
- If no diarrhea or ileus, then 1 dose of cathartic should be given orally (70% sorbitol at 3 mL/kg or sodium or magnesium sulfate at 250–500 mg/kg as a 20% solution in water)
- Flunixin meglumine (1.1 mg/kg IV, preferred route for colic)
- Diazepam (0.05–0.4 mg/kg IV for foals; 25–50 mg IV for adult horses) for controlling seizures. Repeat in 30 min if necessary
- Phenobarbital—for seizures or mania, loading dose of 12 mg/kg once IV, then 6.6 mg/kg IV every 12 h if needed

CONTRAINDICATIONS/POSSIBLE INTERACTIONS
- Avoid stressing or stimulating the horse
- Do not give activated charcoal with mineral oil because oil can potentially prevent binding of the alkaloids to the activated charcoal
- Atropine is contraindicated

FOLLOW-UP

PATIENT MONITORING
Monitor hydration status and behavior.

PREVENTION/AVOIDANCE
Avoid exposure of the horses to tropane alkaloid-containing plants.

POSSIBLE COMPLICATIONS
- Colic
- Intestinal or diaphragmatic rupture
- Ileus

EXPECTED COURSE AND PROGNOSIS
- Course of the disease may be as short as minutes or hours and is usually less than 2–5 days (unless there is continuing exposure)
- The prognosis is favorable if, during the recovery from intoxication, polydipsia, polyuria, and frequent defecation are observed
- With severe clinical signs, the prognosis is guarded

MISCELLANEOUS

ASSOCIATED CONDITIONS
N/A

AGE-RELATED FACTORS
N/A

ZOONOTIC POTENTIAL
N/A

PREGNANCY/FERTILITY/BREEDING
Plants containing high amounts of scopolamine are potentially teratogenic.

SEE ALSO
N/A

Suggested Reading
Burrows GE, Tyrl RJ. Toxic Plants of North America, 2e. Ames, IA: Wiley Blackwell, 2013:1141–1148.

Author Charlotte Means
Consulting Editors Wilson K. Rumbeiha and Steve Ensley
Acknowledgment The author and editors acknowledge the prior contribution of Asheesh K. Tiwary.

BASICS

OVERVIEW
- Blood-borne parasitic disease, subtropical and tropical climates
- Several species of trypanosomes, differentiated by clinical disease, morphology, and country of origin
- Genetic techniques will likely reorganize these parasites
- *Trypanosoma congolense, Trypanosoma evansi, Trypanosoma vivax,* and *Trypanosoma brucei brucei* all infect horses
- Disease organized into New (South and Central America) or Old World animal trypanosomiasis (Africa and Asia), by disease presentation (surra, dourine, and African animal trypanosomiasis), or by parasite–vector relationships
- *T. evansi, T. equinum*—surra, mal de caderas
- *T. congolense, T. vivax, T. brucei brucei*—tsetse fly disease, African animal trypanosomiasis, nagana, sleeping sickness
- *Trypanosoma equiperdum*—dourine, quite possibly a strain or subspecies of either *T. evansi* or *T. brucei brucei*
- Hemic/lymphatic/immune system disease and secondary effects on hepatobiliary, nervous, ophthalmic, renal, and reproductive systems. Some species directly infect reproductive tract

SIGNALMENT
- Horses (more severe), mules, and donkey
- For venereal disease—donkeys are likely reservoir
  - Light breeds develop more severe disease
  - Indigenous breeds less susceptible
- Females have less mortality

SIGNS
General Comments
- Icterus, mucous membrane pallor, lymphadenopathy, splenomegaly
- Direct ocular infection—edema, hyperemia, and petechiation of conjunctiva
- Cyclical

Surra (Mal de Caderas)
- Inapparent to overt clinical signs
- Onset varies from acute to chronic and insidious
- Primarily fever, progressive anemia, weight loss, despite good appetite
- Urticaria with edematous plaques on ventral abdomen, distal limb edema, and petechial hemorrhages

- Neurologic signs—weakness and ataxia
- Stillbirth and abortion

African Animal Trypanosomiasis
- Initial infection of skin with chancre
- Anemia, intermittent fever, edema, weight loss
- Neurologic signs—common with *T. brucei brucei*
- Abortion, infertility

CAUSES AND RISK FACTORS
Surra
- *T. evansi*—host adapted with acute to chronic forms
- Disease present in horses and camels, also seen in cattle, buffalo, llamas, dogs, cats, sheep, goats, pigs, and elephants
- South America, northern Africa, Middle East, Asia, Indonesia, Philippines
- Transmitted by biting flies (*Tabanus* and *Stomoxys*)
- Likely transmitted by vampire bats (*Desmodus rotundus, Diphylla ecaudata, Diaemus youngi*)
- New emergence has high mortality
- *T. equiperdum* (dourine)—indistinguishable by diagnostic testing from *T. evansi*

African Animal Trypanosomiasis
- Can be infected with several trypanosomes at once. *T. congolense* has most deleterious effect on PCV while concomitant infection with *T. vivax* has ameliorating effect on *T. congolense*
- *T. vivax*—moderate to severe disease
- *T. congolense*—mild, peripheral edema
- *T. brucei brucei*—peripheral and scrotal edema; relapse with CNS infection common despite treatment
- Risk—tsetse fly-infected areas of Africa extending from the southern edge of the Sahara to Angola, Zimbabwe, and Mozambique
- Severe in horses; chronic in donkeys
- Cattle likely reservoir
- Biologic vector *Glossina* spp. (tsetse fly)
- Mechanical vectors—*Tabanus, Haematopota, Lyperosia, Stomoxys, Chrysops*
- Hippoboscid flies implicated in spread of *T. brucei* beyond tsetse fly range
- Incubation varies between species but generally 4–14 days
- Transmitted transplacentally, not colostrally
- Foals seropositive after suckling, but seronegative by 4–5 months of age if not infected

DIAGNOSIS

DIFFERENTIAL DIAGNOSIS
Trypanosomiasis, Anemia, Vasculitis, Edema
- Equine infectious anemia virus
- Equine viral arteritis
- African horse sickness
- *Babesia caballi, Babesia equi* (equine piroplasmosis)
- *Leptospira interrogans*
- *Anaplasma phagocytophilum*
- Systemic clostridial infections
- Immune-mediated hemolytic anemia (extravascular)
- Heinz body anemia
- Purpura haemorrhagica

CNS Disease
- West Nile virus
- Japanese encephalitis virus
- Eastern, Western, Venezuelan equine encephalitis virus
- Ross River virus
- Getah virus

Dourine
- Vesicular exanthema
- Equine herpesvirus 3

CBC/BIOCHEMISTRY/URINALYSIS
- Anemia
- Leukopenia, neutropenia, lymphocytosis, monocytosis
- Thrombocytopenia
- Metabolic acidosis
- Hyperbilirubinemia
- Hyperglobulinemia
- Hypoalbuminemia
- Azotemia

OTHER LABORATORY TESTS
- Crystal violet or new methylene blue stain for Heinz bodies
- Clotting profile

DIAGNOSTIC PROCEDURES
Direct Parasite Identification
- Thick/thin smears of Giemsa- or Leish-stained blood smears or lymph nodes aspirates
- Hematocrit centrifuge technique for detection of trypanosomes—better for chronic infection
- Mouse inoculation—parasitemia detected within 48–72 hours

T

TRYPANOSOMIASIS

- Organism detected within tissues
- Stained smears of exudates from skin lesions
- Stained cytospins of cerebrospinal fluid
- Stained impression smears of lungs, liver, and kidney

Antigen/Antibody Formats
- Lack of serologic and molecular markers that differentiate *T. evansi* from *T. equiperdum*
- Antigen and antibody-based ELISAs—newer ELISAs may differentiate between species
- Card agglutination tests specific for *T. evansi*
- Complement fixation test cannot differentiate *T. equiperdum* from *T. evansi*, *T. brucei gambiense*, or *T. brucei*. Will confirm clinical infection with trypanosomes
- For many tests, sensitivity and specificity for equine infection not established

Molecular Detection
- Real-time PCR developed to differentiate *T. brucei* from *T. congolense*—no OIE real-time protocol recommended
- PCR has improved sensitivity over blood smears
- *T. evansi* and *T equiperdum*—limited species-specific testing. Very short window of PCR detection in blood for *T. equiperdum*—tissues and exudates are more reliable

 TREATMENT

- Supportive care
- Blood transfusion
- Intravenous fluids

 MEDICATIONS

- Suramin (Germanin®)—polysulfonated naphthylurea receptor antagonist with antiparasitic and antitumor activity
- Quinapyramine sulfate—acute and chronic infections, but many adverse local reactions
- Isometamidium chloride
- Melarsen oxide—CNS infection
- Diminazene—side effects common

 FOLLOW-UP

- Reinfection common; limited long-term immunity
- Monitor PCV, appetite/weight loss, rectal temperature

PREVENTION/AVOIDANCE
- Prevention only with continuous chemotherapy
  - Quinapyramine salt
  - Combination suramin and diminazene
- Segregation, quarantine, vector control

 MISCELLANEOUS

ZOONOTIC POTENTIAL
None known for animal trypanosomiasis.

PREGNANCY/FERTILITY/BREEDING
Abortion

ABBREVIATIONS
- CNS = central nervous system
- ELISA = enzyme-linked immunosorbent assay
- OIE = Office International des Epizooties/World Organisation for Animal Health
- PCR = polymerase chain reaction
- PCV = packed cell volume

Internet Resources
http://www.oie.int/fileadmin/Home/eng/Health_standards/tahm/3.01.21_TRYPANO_SURRA.pdf
http://www.oie.int/fileadmin/Home/eng/Health_standards/tahm/3.04.16_TRYPANOSOMOSIS.pdf

Author Maureen T. Long
Consulting Editor Ashley G. Boyle

T

BASICS

OVERVIEW
Any infectious disease caused by *Mycobacterium* spp. is referred to as tuberculosis. Tuberculosis is very rare in horses and experimental studies have suggested that horses may be naturally resistant. Control measures for *Mycobacterium bovis* in cattle have caused a significant decrease in the incidence of this disease in horses. *Mycobacterium avium*, *M. bovis*, and *Mycobacterium tuberculosis* infections have all been described in horses, but no specific syndromes have been reported.

SIGNALMENT
There is no apparent age or breed predilection.

SIGNS
Signs are variable and vague. The disease involves formation of focal granulomas, and signs relate to the system or systems involved. Chronic weight loss, weakness, and lethargy are the most common presenting complaints. Fever, dyspnea, cough, and nasal discharge may be seen. The infections are chronic and slowly progressive. Other organ systems, including the gastrointestinal tract, liver, and vertebrae, may be affected, with clinical signs associated with these organ systems. In some horses with granulomatous enteritis, *M. avium* has been identified in the feces or the intestinal tissues. These latter horses have clinical signs of malabsorption, protein-losing enteropathy, or both.

CAUSES AND RISK FACTORS
Cases are rare and sporadic, therefore no specific risk factors have been identified. Ingestion is the most common route of transmission in horses, with subsequent hematogenous spread of the organism, but respiratory transmission is also possible.

DIAGNOSIS

DIFFERENTIAL DIAGNOSIS
Tuberculosis can be considered as a differential diagnosis for any granulomatous disease in horses; however, it is extremely rare and should therefore be low on the list. Additional differential diagnoses for equine granulomatous disease include *Rhodococcus equi*, *Burkholderia mallei*, fungal infections, and toxins.

CBC/BIOCHEMISTRY/URINALYSIS
There are no specific clinical pathology data typical for this disease in horses. Hematology may be consistent with a chronic inflammatory process (i.e. neutrophilia, hyperfibrinogenemia, and anemia). Other laboratory abnormalities may be observed depending on the organ system(s) involved.

OTHER LABORATORY TESTS
The intradermal tuberculin skin test in horses is unreliable, with a high incidence of false-positive results in normal horses. In addition, the tuberculin may induce an anaphylactic response. Identification of the organism in aspirates or biopsies using acid-fast staining is strongly supportive of a diagnosis of equine tuberculosis. Definitive diagnosis is usually made postmortem.

IMAGING
Depending on the region of the body affected, radiography or ultrasonography may demonstrate the nature and extent of the infection.

OTHER DIAGNOSTIC PROCEDURES
Biopsies of affected organs may be indicated to determine the nature of the lesions, and collection of exudate (e.g. by transtracheal aspiration or bronchoalveolar lavage) is indicated in specific cases.

PATHOLOGIC FINDINGS
Multiple lesions are often present in a variety of organs. The organism frequently establishes itself in the lymph nodes and spleen, and these are therefore common sites of lesions. Involvement of bone is said to be more frequent in horses than in cattle. Caseous necrosis of lymph nodes is a common finding. Lesions tend to be firm in all tissues, and may appear to be neoplastic. Histopathologic evaluation is needed to confirm the diagnosis.

TREATMENT
Owing to public health concerns, treatment is often not undertaken and prognosis is poor. If treatment is attempted, the horse should be isolated and public health officials should be consulted.

MEDICATIONS

DRUG(S) OF CHOICE
Rifampin (rifampicin), isoniazid, and streptomycin have been considered for treatment. Oral enrofloxacin has been used to treat a horse with pulmonary tuberculosis in South Africa. Based on experiences in human medicine it would be expected that therapy, if attempted in an equine case, would have to be given for several months or even a year or more.

CONTRAINDICATIONS/POSSIBLE INTERACTIONS
N/A

FOLLOW-UP
N/A

EXPECTED COURSE AND PROGNOSIS
As treatment is usually not a viable option, the prognosis for established cases is poor, and a recommendation for euthanasia would be appropriate.

MISCELLANEOUS

ZOONOTIC POTENTIAL
Tuberculosis is a potential zoonotic disease, especially for immunocompromised individuals, and is a reportable disease in other animal species. If a horse with confirmed disease is not euthanized, precautions should be taken to minimize the risk of zoonosis. Public health officials and appropriate health care workers should be consulted.

Suggested Reading
Pesciaroli M, Alvarez J, Boniotti MB, et al. Tuberculosis in domestic animal species. Res Vet Sci 2014;97:S78–S85.

Author Daniela Luethy
Consulting Editor Ashley G. Boyle
Acknowledgment The author and editor acknowledge the prior contribution of Christopher M. Brown.

T

TUMORS OF THE RESPIRATORY SYSTEM

BASICS

OVERVIEW
- Tumors of the respiratory system are most commonly located in the thoracic or sinusal/parasinusal structures
- Incidence is very low—thoracic cavity neoplasia was reported in 35 of 5629 necropsies. Primary lung tumors—7.9% of thoracic neoplasia
- The most frequent primary lung tumor is the granular cell tumor (or myoblastoma). They may be accompanied by osteoproliferative abnormalities of carpal, tarsal, and fetlock joints
- Lung is a relative frequent site for secondary metastases from other organs
- 50–68% of nasal passage tumors are malignant with SCC being the most frequent. SCC originates from mucosal or alveolar teeth epithelium and starts invading locally before metastasizing regionally

SIGNALMENT
- Nasal/paranasal tumors—SCC (most frequent); mature adults, more frequent in aged horses. Mean age 8–12.4 years
- Primary pulmonary tumors—>7 years. Pulmonary granular cell tumor (most frequent); mean age 13 years, range 8–22 years
- Lung metastases from distant primary tumors—mean age 8 years, range 3 months to 14 years
- Sex predilection—majority of females for pulmonary granular cell tumors and males for intrathoracic metastatic adenocarcinoma.

SIGNS

Historical Findings
- Weight loss
- Dullness
- Exercise intolerance
- Intermittent fever

Physical Examination Findings
- Thoracic respiratory tumors;
  - Underweight
  - Signs of pleural effusion and ventral edema
  - Tachypnea
  - Coughing
  - Dyspnea
  - Hemoptysis
  - Abnormal lung auscultation sounds
  - Pallor, icterus, and intermittent epistaxis in cases of hemangiosarcoma
  - Proliferative osteopathy of carpal, tarsal, fetlock joints rarely seen
- Nasal/parasinusal tumors:
  - Nasal discharge (frequent); foul smelling
  - Facial deformity for large tumors

CAUSES AND RISK FACTORS
Undetermined

DIAGNOSIS

DIFFERENTIAL DIAGNOSIS
- Thoracic respiratory tumors—equine asthma and inflammatory conditions, equine multinodular fibrosis, other neoplasia, idiopathic pleuritis, mycotic pneumonia
- Nasal/paranasal tumors; primary sinusitis, nasal inflammatory polyps, progressive ethmoidal hematoma

CBC/BIOCHEMISTRY/URINALYSIS
- CBC—results depend on the invasiveness of the primary tumor: often an inflammatory hemogram is present
- Chemistry—no abnormalities unless a specific organ is showing functional insufficiency

OTHER LABORATORY TESTS
- Thoracocentesis—neoplastic cells can be observed in the pleural fluid
- Lung biopsy—preferentially US-guided to sample a mass, or through an endoscope if a mass is visible in the airways
- Transtracheal aspiration cytology may reveal neoplastic cells
- For nasal/paranasal tumors—biopsy samples obtained deep within the mass. Superficial samples obtained by endoscopy are often nondiagnostic

IMAGING
- Head radiography—nasal/paranasal SCC; dorsoventral view is useful to assess sinuses
- Thorax radiography—pulmonary tumors; single or several soft tissue density
- Thorax US—pleural effusion, masses in the lung parenchyma
- Upper/lower airway endoscopy (including sinusoscopy)—nasal/paranasal SCC; often ulcerated. Pulmonary tumor; masses in the main bronchi occasionally seen

OTHER DIAGNOSTIC PROCEDURES
Thoracoscopy—to visualize and biopsy masses affecting the lung surface.

PATHOLOGIC FINDINGS
- Nasal/paranasal SCC—classified as well, moderately, or poorly differentiated. Degrees of differentiation not correlated with the presence of metastasis
- Pulmonary granular cell tumor—most frequent primary pulmonary tumor. Usually unilateral. Local metastases frequently reported
- Pulmonary carcinoma—usually unilateral, caudal lung. Pleomorphic epithelial cells. Rarely metastasize

- Metastatic hemangiosarcoma—primary tumor more frequently in skeletal muscle or skin
- Metastatic SCC—primary tumor more frequently in the stomach, but also penis, vulva, and eye

TREATMENT
- Lung neoplasm—mass and lung resection have been attempted
- Granular cell tumor removal by transendoscopic electrosurgery and ablation with a diode laser have been described. Nasal/paranasal mass removal—often malignant with risks of recurrence and metastasis

MEDICATIONS
None

FOLLOW-UP

PATIENT MONITORING
Improvement in attitude, clinical signs, and weight gain can be observed when nasal/paranasal mass is removed successfully.

EXPECTED COURSE AND PROGNOSIS
Grave for lung tumors and malignant nasal passage tumors; short life expectancy after diagnosis.

MISCELLANEOUS

ASSOCIATED CONDITIONS
- Primary neoplasms when lung metastases are present
- Rare cases of proliferative osteopathy of carpal, tarsal, fetlock joints

ABBREVIATIONS
- SCC = squamous cell carcinoma
- US = ultrasonography, ultrasound

Suggested Reading
Scarratt KW, Crisman MV. Neoplasia of the respiratory tract. Vet Clin North Am Equine Pract 1998;143:451–473.
Sweeney CR, Gillette DM. Thoracic neoplasia in equids: 35 cases (1967-1987). J Am Vet Med Assoc 1989;195:374–377.

Author Renaud Leguillette
Consulting Editors Daniel Jean and Mathilde Leclère

T

BASICS

DEFINITION
The intrauterine production of 2 or more embryos/fetuses.

PATHOPHYSIOLOGY
• The majority of multiple pregnancies are twins
  ◦ Most twins are dizygotic; result from double ovulations
  ◦ Early twin vesicles behave similarly to a singleton conceptus
  ◦ The vesicles undergo TUM until 15 days of gestation; fixation occurs in 1 or both uterine horns at ≈ day 16 gestation
  ◦ ≈ 75% of twin vesicles fix in the same horn (unicornual)
• ≈ 75% of *unicornual* twin pregnancies <40 days of age undergo natural reduction to 1 embryo
  ◦ The remaining embryo develops normally to term as a singleton
  ◦ If natural reduction of 1 embryo fails to occur by day 40, there is a strong probability that twin development will continue, only to abort later in gestation
• *Bicornual* twins do not undergo natural reduction; the twins usually develop through the last trimester of gestation, at which time abortion is common

SYSTEMS AFFECTED
Reproductive

GENETICS
Higher incidence of double ovulations in some horse breeds.

INCIDENCE/PREVALENCE
• Occurs more frequently in older and barren mares, Thoroughbreds, draft breeds
• Lower incidence in Arabians, Quarter Horses, ponies, primitive breeds

SIGNALMENT
Mares that develop twin pregnancies tend to have twins in subsequent pregnancies.

SIGNS
N/A

CAUSES
• Ovulation and fertilization of multiple ova, in most cases
• Rare incidences of monozygotic multiple pregnancies have been reported

RISK FACTORS
Breed, age, and reproductive status.

DIAGNOSIS

DIFFERENTIAL DIAGNOSIS
Differentiating Similar Signs
• Uterine cysts can be confused with developing embryonic vesicles, causing an improper diagnosis of twin pregnancy

• Recording location, size, and shape of lymphatic cysts prior to breeding (a *cyst map*) makes it easier to distinguish cysts from embryonic vesicles
• If prior season records are unavailable, reexamine the mare in 2 days. The vesicle of pregnancy will demonstrate a noticeable increase in diameter by US; the uterine/lymphatic cyst will not increase in that period of time
• A lymphatic cyst is also distinguished from an embryonic vesicle in which an embryo and an embryonic heartbeat will be observed at 24+ days of gestation

CBC/BIOCHEMISTRY/URINALYSIS
N/A

OTHER LABORATORY TESTS
N/A

IMAGING
Transrectal US
• For prompt diagnosis and treatment of twin pregnancies
• Twins may be detected as early as day 9 of gestation; however, twin pregnancies may differ in age by as much as 2 days. Because of the possible differences in age and size of early twins, US diagnosis, if a double ovulation is confirmed, is recommended between 14 and 15 days of gestation
• The embryonic vesicles at this time are an anechoic, spherical yolk sac; average 14–20 mm in height
• Twin vesicles are highly mobile for the first 15–16 days; they may be located adjacent to one another or in different locations within the uterus within a brief time frame
• It is critical to scan both uterine horns and the uterine body to the cervix, sequentially, with at least 2 full sweeps across the tract

Transabdominal US
For diagnosing twin pregnancies at >75–100 days of gestation (generally by identifying 2 fetal heartbeats).

OTHER DIAGNOSTIC PROCEDURES
TRP of the Reproductive Tract
• Pregnancy characteristics at days 25–30 by TRP—distinct uterine tone; a narrow, elongated cervix. A bulge the size of a small hen's egg at the caudoventral aspect of a uterine horn, adjacent to the uterine bifurcation
  ◦ If twin vesicles are bicornual in location—may be possible to diagnose twin pregnancies by TRP
  ◦ If twin vesicles are unicornual in location—it is impossible to diagnose twins by TRP alone. An experienced practitioner may note the bulge of pregnancy feels larger than anticipated

PATHOLOGIC FINDINGS
N/A

TREATMENT

Management of Twins Prior to Day 40 of Gestation
• Twins detected during TUM of the conceptus (days 9–15) are best managed by crushing 1 embryonic vesicle. 1 vesicle may be manipulated transrectally to the tip of a uterine horn, pressure placed on the vesicle, and it is crushed. Alternatively, its location/distance from the bifurcation of the uterine horns is confirmed by US, trapping the vesicle at that location between 3 fingers on its ventral aspect and thumb on top, increasing pressure on the sphere until the crush is felt. The success of a crush should always be confirmed by a follow-up US examination; dispersed fluid will be evident
• The remaining vesicle survives in approximately 90% of cases
• The crush technique is useful for twins in the mobility phase and bilateral twins prior to 30 days of gestation
• After 30 days of gestation, fluid released from the crushed vesicle tends to disrupt the remaining pregnancy. The increased pressure required to disrupt a larger vesicle may also result in prostaglandin release from the endometrium, leading to loss of the second vesicle
• Unicornual twins are usually both destroyed when crushing of 1 is attempted

Management of Twins After Day 40 of Gestation
Craniocervical Dislocation
• Technique of dislocating the first cervical vertebra from the cranium—involves a rocking motion applied to the head with pressure at the back of the skull to sever the spinal cord and disrupt the ligamentous attachments. Can be performed between 50 and 150 days of gestation; either transrectally, by laparotomy, or potentially via colpotomy
• Management of twin pregnancies in the fetal period (≥day 40) is further complicated by the formation of endometrial cups
• Pregnancy loss once endometrial cups have formed has been shown to cause irregular estrous cycles, and/or a delayed return to fertile cycles
• Consequently, maintenance of a singleton pregnancy following a >40 day reduction procedure is critical to the reproductive success of the mare

Alternate Methods of Twin Management That Have Been Attempted
• *Dietary restriction*—in 1 study, mares with twin pregnancies (diagnosed by TRP) were limited to poor quality grass hay early in gestation (day 21–49 of gestation)
  ◦ 1 viable foal was delivered in 56% (23 of 41) of the cases examined, i.e. reduction had occurred

T

• *Surgical removal of 1 twin*—was attempted in 7 unicornual and 8 bicornual twins at 41–62 days of gestation
  ◦ None of the unicornual twins survived
  ◦ 5 of 8 bicornual twin pregnancies were successfully reduced to a singleton
• *Intracardiac injection of potassium chloride (KCl)*—using transcutaneous US, 1 fetal heart is located and fetal death is caused by intracardiac injection of KCl
  ◦ The technique has been successful in approximately 50% of the cases attempted
  ◦ This procedure is most useful during 115–130 days of gestation
• *Transvaginal allantocentesis*—transvaginal US has been used to aid in identification of the allantoic sac of 1 twin fetus, a needle is passed into the allantois, allantoic fluid is aspirated
  ◦ Fluid aspiration collapses the vesicle, leading to fetal death
  ◦ To date, this technique has been successful in approximately 30% of attempted cases
  ◦ Most applicable for bicornual twins

APPROPRIATE HEALTH CARE
N/A

NURSING CARE
N/A

ACTIVITY
N/A

DIET
See Methods of Twin Management That Have Been Attempted.

CLIENT EDUCATION
• Importance of TRP in the periovulatory period (before and after breeding and insemination), and noting >1 ovulation during an estrus
• Emphasis of early (latest 16 days following ovulation), serial evaluations of a high-risk mare:
  ◦ Multiple ovulations
  ◦ Prior history of twinning
  ◦ Breeds with higher incidence of twinning
  ◦ Suspicious appearance of vesicle of pregnancy at initial examination warrants follow-up US within 2–4 days
• Earlier reduction of twins (<16 days, prior to fixation) increases likelihood of success, continuation of remaining embryo/fetus to term

MEDICATIONS
• Flunixin meglumine 1 mg/kg IV is often administered at the time of attempted twin

reduction to prevent prostaglandin release from the uterus and subsequent lysis of the corpus luteum
• Exogenous progestins (altrenogest 1 mL/50 kg body weight (0.044 mg altrenogest/kg body weight) PO daily) at double the recommended dose (2 mL/50 kg) may be administered when twin reduction is attempted to maintain uterine and cervical tone following uterine manipulation; to counter the effects of possible fetal fluid release into the uterine lumen

DRUG(S) OF CHOICE
N/A

CONTRAINDICATIONS
Twinning is undesirable in the mare and routinely ends in abortion.

PRECAUTIONS
N/A

POSSIBLE INTERACTIONS
N/A

ALTERNATIVE DRUGS
N/A

FOLLOW-UP

PATIENT MONITORING
• After any method of twin reduction is performed, it is useful to monitor the progress and viability of the remaining embryo/fetus using US
• It is critical to monitor the mare for embryo/fetal death if the mare is being treated with exogenous progestins
• Once weekly US examinations are warranted for the first 3 weeks following the procedure
• Less frequent examinations, i.e. once monthly, after the initial examinations are useful to monitor fetal progress
• The mare can also be monitored for signs of abortion such as mammary development, vulvar discharge, or fetal expulsion

PREVENTION/AVOIDANCE
• Serial, complete TRP, and maintenance of individual records for broodmares
• Record sizes of all follicles >30 mm on both ovaries during estrus (average growth is 5–6 mm/day) to account for ovulation or regression
• Double ovulation is the earliest indicator of mares at higher risk for developing twins
• Early diagnosis of pregnancy in mares from families with a history of twinning, or one known to have twinned in a prior pregnancy (same season or prior years)
• Earlier reduction is associated with greater success in achieving a singleton pregnancy

POSSIBLE COMPLICATIONS
Embryonic or fetal loss, abortion, dystocia.

EXPECTED COURSE AND PROGNOSIS
Success Associated With Each Reduction Technique
• 90% success with early crush of a bicornual twin
• 50% with KCl intracardiac injection during days 115–130 of gestation
• 20–30% with transvaginal aspiration of allantoic fluid from 1 of bicornual twins

MISCELLANEOUS

ASSOCIATED CONDITIONS
N/A

AGE-RELATED FACTORS
N/A

ZOONOTIC POTENTIAL
N/A

PREGNANCY/FERTILITY/BREEDING
N/A

SEE ALSO
• Abortion, spontaneous, noninfectious
• Dystocia
• Early embryonic death
• Placenta basics
• Placentitis

ABBREVIATIONS
• TRP = transrectal palpation
• TUM = transuterine migration
• US = ultrasonography, ultrasound

Suggested Reading
Ginther OJ. Ultrasonic Imaging and Reproductive Events in the Mare. Cross Plains, WI: Equiservices, 1986.
Ginther OJ. Reproductive Biology of the Mare, 2e. Cross Plains, WI: Equiservices, 1992.
Putt E, Christensen BW, Wimmer A. Transrectal cranio-cervical dislocation of a twin fetus in a mare. Clin Theriogenol 2014;6(3):356.
Schnobrich MTR, Riddle WT, Stromberg AJ, LeBlanc MM. Factors affecting live foal rates of Thoroughbred mares that undergo manual twin elimination. Equine Vet J 2013;45(6):676–680.
Sitters S, Wolfsdorf K. Twin reduction: cranio-cervical dislocation. In: Dascanio JJ, McCue PM, eds. Equine Reproductive Procedures. Ames, IA: Wiley Blackwell, 2014:222–225.

Author Carla L. Carleton
Consulting Editor Carla L. Carleton
Acknowledgment The author/editor acknowledges the prior contribution of Margo L. Macpherson.

T

TYZZER DISEASE (*CLOSTRIDIUM PILIFORME*)

BASICS

OVERVIEW
• A rapidly progressive, highly fatal disease of foals caused by *Clostridium piliforme* (previously *Bacillus piliformis*) characterized by peracute progressive hepatitis
• Worldwide distribution

SIGNALMENT
• Can be sporadic or occur in outbreaks
• Foals of any breed and sex are affected
• Age ranges from 5 days to 6 weeks old; average age 20 days

SIGNS
• Usually normal at birth and then develop rapidly progressive signs including lethargy, loss of suckle reflex, diarrhea, tachycardia, and dehydration
• Icterus, fever, seizures
• Foals are usually found dead without significant premonitory signs

CAUSES AND RISK FACTORS
• Ingestion of spore-containing feces with subsequent colonization of the intestine and liver via the portal circulation
• *C. piliforme*, a Gram-negative, endospore-forming, obligate intracellular bacterium found in soil and feces
• Foals born to nonresident mares and/or mares <6 years of age are more likely to develop disease, possibly owing to differences in colostral quality and specific protective immunoglobulin

DIAGNOSIS

Presumptive diagnosis may be made on history, physical examination, diagnostic imaging, and clinicopathologic data. Definitive antemortem diagnosis requires demonstration of *C. piliforme* on liver biopsy.

DIFFERENTIAL DIAGNOSIS
• Neonatal septicemia
• Neonatal isoerythrolysis
• Viral hepatitis
• Toxic hepatopathy (rare)

CBC/BIOCHEMISTRY/URINALYSIS
• CBC—hemoconcentration, hyperfibrinogenemia, and normal to low leukocyte count
• Biochemistry—hypoglycemia, metabolic acidosis. Elevated serum sorbitol dehydrogenase, γ-glutamyltransferase, alkaline phosphatase, bilirubin

OTHER LABORATORY TESTS
• PCR testing on samples of liver and/or cecum
• Coagulation profiles—prolonged prothrombin time/activated partial thromboplastin time, increases in fibrin degradation products, decreases in antithrombin

IMAGING
• Abdominal radiography may reveal hepatomegaly
• Transabdominal ultrasonography may reveal hepatomegaly with diffuse hyperechogenicity

OTHER DIAGNOSTIC PROCEDURES
• Percutaneous liver biopsy and demonstration of characteristic histopathologic findings (see Pathologic Findings)
• *C. piliforme* is extremely difficult to culture in vitro

PATHOLOGIC FINDINGS
• Hepatomegaly with coagulative necrosis surrounded by degenerate hepatocytes and neutrophilic (suppurative) inflammatory cell migration
• Confirmation of Tyzzer disease is achieved by histologic demonstration of intracellular interlacing bundles of filamentous bacilli (*C. piliforme*) at the periphery of the lesions within the liver

TREATMENT

• Limited reports exist of successful treatment in confirmed cases
• Fluid therapy is essential. Volume resuscitation, glucose provision, and electrolytes to assist in correcting metabolic acidosis

MEDICATIONS

DRUG(S) OF CHOICE
• Broad-spectrum antimicrobials, including Gram-negative anaerobic coverage such as penicillin (22 000 IU/kg IV every 6 h), tetracycline (10 mg/kg IV every 12 h), erythromycin (25 mg/kg PO every 6 h), sulfamethoxazole–trimethoprim (15–25 mg/kg PO every 12 h), and metronidazole (10 mg/kg PO every 12 h)
• Seizure management using diazepam (0.1–0.4 mg/kg IV) or midazolam (0.02–0.06 mg/kg/h constant rate infusion)
• Anti-inflammatory drugs, e.g. ketoprofen (1.1–2.2 mg/kg IV every 12 h)
• Lactulose (0.1–0.25 mL/kg PO every 6–8 h) to help reduce intestinal ammonia production

CONTRAINDICATIONS/POSSIBLE INTERACTIONS
• Barbiturates should be given with caution for seizure management given their extensive hepatic metabolism. Benzodiazepines have the potential to worsen hepatoencephalopathy owing to potentiation of GABA-induced sedation
• Metronidazole is given at a lower dose owing to reduced hepatic metabolism

FOLLOW-UP

PATIENT MONITORING
• Monitor plasma ammonia, acid–base status, and glucose frequently during therapy
• Consider decreasing doses of any medication that undergoes hepatic metabolism

PREVENTION/AVOIDANCE
None specific. Ensure adequate transfer of passive immunity.

EXPECTED COURSE AND PROGNOSIS
• Grave prognosis. Most foals die within 24 h from the onset of clinical signs. Early recognition, referral to an intensive care facility, and therapeutic intervention are required to have any chance of clinical resolution.

MISCELLANEOUS

ZOONOTIC POTENTIAL
Unknown

PREGNANCY/FERTILITY/BREEDING
N/A

SEE ALSO
• Septicemia, neonate
• Neonatal isoerythrolysis
• Hepatic encephalopathy

ABBREVIATIONS
• GABA = γ-aminobutyric acid
• PCR = polymerase chain reaction

Suggested Reading
Borchers A, Magdesian KG, Halland S, et al. Successful treatment and polymerase chain reaction (PCR) confirmation of Tyzzer's disease in a foal and clinical and pathologic characteristics of 6 additional foals (1986–2005). J Vet Intern Med 2006;20:1212–1218.
Fosgate GT, Hird DW, Read DH, et al. Risk factors for *Clostridium piliforme* infection in foals. J Am Vet Med Assoc 2002;220:785–790.
Swerczek TW. Tyzzer's disease in foals: retrospective studies from 1969 to 2010. Can Vet J 2013;54:876–880.

Author Samuel D.A. Hurcombe
Consulting Editor Margaret C. Mudge

T

ULCERATIVE KERATOMYCOSIS

BASICS

DEFINITION
Keratomycosis may present clinically in the horse as superficial keratitis, ulcerative keratitis (to varying degrees and appearances), or stromal abscess. Ulcerative keratitis refers to a disruption of the corneal epithelium with varying amounts of stromal loss, which may have concurrent bacterial and/or fungal infection. Ulcers infected with fungi range from minor corneal epithelial abrasions/erosions, to superficial plaques, to deep and severe interstitial keratitis.

PATHOPHYSIOLOGY
• Fungi are normal inhabitants of the equine conjunctival microflora, but can become opportunistically pathogenic following corneal injury. Fungal organisms are ubiquitous in the equine environment, although regional geographic differences exist to account for variation in the presence of particular fungal species to specific regions. Exposure to vegetative material (hay, grasses, shavings, straw) and dust in the horse environment may influence exposure to fungi
• The pathogenesis of ulcerative fungal keratitis commonly begins with corneal trauma, resulting in an epithelial defect and stromal invasion by the commensal fungal organism or seeding of fungi from a foreign body of organic origin. Tear film instability also predisposes to fungal keratitis or is induced by the fungi prior to fungal attachment and invasion. Stromal destruction results from the release of proteases and other enzymes from the fungi, leukocytes, and keratocytes. Fungi appear to have an affinity for Descemet's membrane, with hyphae frequently found deep in the equine cornea. Deeper corneal invasion by the fungi can lead to sterile or infectious endophthalmitis

SYSTEMS AFFECTED
Ophthalmic

GENETICS
N/A

INCIDENCE/PREVALENCE
Keratomycosis is more common and more aggressive in warm climates.

SIGNALMENT
All ages and breeds of horses may be affected.

SIGNS
• Clinical signs associated with ulcerative keratomycosis include blepharospasm, epiphora, photophobia, corneal opacity (edema, infiltrate, fibrosis, vascularization), and signs of anterior uveitis (miosis, aqueous flare)
• Slight downward deviation of the upper eyelashes may be a subtle sign of ocular pain
• The cornea can be dry in appearance, or display cellular invasion with varying amounts of vascularization or cellular infiltrate

CAUSES
Septate filamentous fungi associated with ulcerative keratomycosis include several species common to the equine eye (*Fusarium, Aspergillus, Penicillium* spp.). Yeasts (*Candida* spp.) may also contribute to keratomycosis.

RISK FACTORS
• Horses may be more susceptible to fungal invasion and infection of the cornea owing to the large surface area and prominence of the equine eye and some weakness in the corneal immune system
• Topical antibiotic and/or corticosteroid therapy of a noninfected corneal ulcer may predispose to fungal colony invasion and colonization

DIAGNOSIS

DIFFERENTIAL DIAGNOSIS
Ocular pain may also be found with bacterial corneal ulcers, uveitis, conjunctivitis, blepharitis, and dacryocystitis.

CBC/BIOCHEMISTRY/URINALYSIS
N/A

OTHER LABORATORY TESTS
N/A

IMAGING
N/A

OTHER DIAGNOSTIC PROCEDURES
The diagnosis of keratomycosis is based on finding fungal hyphae, mold, or yeast on at least 1 of the following: (1) cytologic examination of a corneal scraping, (2) culture of the corneal lesion, (3) PCR of corneal cytologic specimens, or (4) surgical histopathologic examination of a keratectomy specimen.

PATHOLOGIC FINDINGS
• Fungi show marked affinity for the deep corneal stroma and Descemet's membrane
• Hyphae are often found with neutrophils in the stroma and are rarely found free in the anterior chamber

TREATMENT

ACTIVITY
• Horses with keratomycosis and secondary uveitis should be stall-rested until the condition is healed
• Intraocular hemorrhage and increased severity of uveitis are sequelae to overexertion

DIET
Diet should be consistent with the activity and training level of the horse.

CLIENT EDUCATION
• Ulcerative keratomycosis is a serious sight- and globe-threatening disease in the horse
• Long duration of antifungal drug exposure (minimum of 4 weeks, often longer) is required for complete fungal destruction and resolution of the clinical signs

SURGICAL CONSIDERATIONS
• Combined medical and surgical therapy is indicated if ulcers are deep, if they are not responding to medical treatment, or if they worsen despite medical treatment
• Surgeries for keratomycosis include conjunctival grafts and full- and split-thickness penetrating keratoplasty. While surgical treatment may leave the horse with a larger scar, conjunctival grafts usually prevent corneal rupture and allow for physical support, a regional blood supply, and a supply of endogenous antiproteases to the ulcer site

MEDICATIONS

DRUG(S) OF CHOICE
• Treatment must be directed against the fungi, as well as against the corneal and intraocular inflammatory responses that occur following fungal replication and hyphal death
• Miconazole (1%) has been used successfully and frequently as a topical antifungal agent. The IV form is preferred, but human vaginal products may be used
• Natamycin 3.33–5% is the only FDA-approved topical antifungal agent. It is effective against many ocular fungal pathogens
• Voriconazole 1% is an effective broad-spectrum antifungal agent and has reasonably good corneal penetration
• Amphotericin B (1.5 mg/mL) may be administered topically
• Silver sulfadiazine (dermatologic preparation) is a topical antimicrobial agent with both antifungal and antibacterial activity that is believed to be fungicidal
• Dilute (1:50) povidone–iodine is effective topically against some fungal isolates. It can be irritating if used too frequently
• Itraconazole and fluconazole are used successfully topically for keratomycosis in horses in some cases
• Topically administered antifungal therapy for equine keratomycosis is administered 4–6 times per day

U

• Corneal ulcerations result in massive increases in tear film protease activity. Topical serum and topical EDTA are critical to speed healing. They should be administered as many times a day as possible. EDTA is believed to have a synergistic effect with antifungal agents when used together for keratomycosis
• Iridocyclitis is present any time a horse has a corneal ulcer, and can escalate in intensity following hyphal death after antifungal therapy is initiated. Flunixin meglumine (1 mg/kg BID IV, IM, PO) is the most frequently used NSAID in horses for systemic treatment of iridocyclitis. It may also reduce the speed of corneal vascularization
• 1% atropine sulfate, a parasympatholytic agent, is used in all cases for its mydriatic and cycloplegic effects to dilate the pupil and diminish ciliary body muscle spasms associated with the axon reflex uveitis that occurs with corneal ulceration in the horse. It may be administered every 4–6 h until the pupil is dilated, and then the frequency of administration reduced

CONTRAINDICATIONS
N/A

PRECAUTIONS
N/A

POSSIBLE INTERACTIONS
N/A

ALTERNATIVE DRUGS
N/A

 FOLLOW-UP

PATIENT MONITORING
• The eye should be protected from self-trauma with hard- or soft-cup hoods
• Patients should be monitored for colic and persistent signs of eye pain

PREVENTION/AVOIDANCE
N/A

POSSIBLE COMPLICATIONS
• Persistent pain, uveitis, endophthalmitis, globe rupture, iris prolapse, and blindness are complications
• Topically administered atropine must be used cautiously in horses as it may alter gastrointestinal motility

EXPECTED COURSE AND PROGNOSIS
• Vision following keratomycosis in horses may be retained in as few as 50% of eyes if treatment is not aggressive
• Aggressive medical and surgical therapy for ulcerative keratomycosis in horses should, however, result in a positive visual outcome and ocular survival in >90% of eyes. Despite this success, therapy is prolonged and scarring of the cornea may be prominent
• Enucleation may be necessary in horses that become blind and continue to experience ocular pain

 MISCELLANEOUS

ASSOCIATED CONDITIONS
Severe uveitis.

AGE-RELATED FACTORS
N/A

ZOONOTIC POTENTIAL
N/A

PREGNANCY/FERTILITY/BREEDING
N/A

SYNONYMS
N/A

SEE ALSO
Corneal ulceration

ABBREVIATIONS
• FDA = US Food and Drug Administration
• NSAID = nonsteroidal anti-inflammatory drug
• PCR = polymerase chain reaction

Suggested Reading
Brooks DE. Ophthalmology for the Equine Practitioner, 2e. Jackson, WY: Teton NewMedia, 2008.
Brooks DE, Matthews AG. Equine ophthalmology. In: Gelatt KN, ed. Veterinary Ophthalmology, 4e. Ames, IA: Blackwell, 2007:1165–1274.
Gilger BC, ed. Equine Ophthalmology, 3e. Ames, IA: Wiley Blackwell, 2017.

Author Caryn E. Plummer
Consulting Editor Caryn E. Plummer

UPWARD FIXATION OF THE PATELLA

BASICS

OVERVIEW
• Hindlimb gait abnormality characterized by the stifle (and hock) locked in extension and toe dragging
• Caused by failure of the patella to unlock from the medial trochlear ridge of the femur, which effectively locks the reciprocal apparatus
• Systems affected—musculoskeletal: stifle

SIGNALMENT
• Most common in young horses
• Ponies, Warmbloods, Thoroughbred, Standardbreds

SIGNS
• In cases of delayed patellar release, the patella briefly "catches," followed immediately by exaggerated hyperflexion of the stifle. The gait is more pronounced during downward transitions or going downhill
• When the patella is locked in position, the stifle (and hock) is held in rigid extension, the fetlock is flexed, and the horse drags the toe
• Femoropatellar joint distention infrequent
• Mild lameness may be noted in chronic intermittent cases

CAUSES AND RISK FACTORS
• Straight hindlimb conformation
• Poor muscle mass
• Stall confinement or abrupt decline in fitness level

DIAGNOSIS

DIFFERENTIAL DIAGNOSIS
• Coxofemoral joint luxation—differentiating signs include outward rotation of stifle and foot, inward rotation of tarsus, and inability to extend hindlimb caudally
• Luxation of the patella—this term has been incorrectly used to describe upward fixation of the patella. True patella luxation occurs primarily in foals and most commonly in miniature horses. Severely affected horses stand in a crouched position and are unable to extend the stifle. Mildly affected horses resist stifle flexion and are stiff gaited. Hypoplasia of the lateral trochlear ridge may be noted
• Stringhalt—exaggerated hock flexion when walking; absent or less apparent when trotting
• Shivers—episodic hindlimb hyperflexion and limb abduction when standing, walking, or backing

CBC/BIOCHEMISTRY/URINALYSIS
None

OTHER LABORATORY TESTS
None

IMAGING
• Radiography—osseous fragmentation and/or osteophyte formation along the distal aspect of the patella may be noted in chronically affected horses. Evaluate for concurrent osteochondrosis
• Ultrasonography—evaluate the periarticular and articular soft tissue structures for potential concurrent injury

OTHER DIAGNOSTIC PROCEDURES
Diagnostic testing for neuromuscular diseases such as polysaccharide storage disease, equine protozoal myelitis, shivers, or equine lower motor neuron disease may be warranted.

TREATMENT
• For mild cases, a conditioning program to improve muscle strength of the quadriceps is indicated. Consistent daily exercise in good footing and uphill work should be encouraged. Stall confinement is contradicted
• Wedged heel pads or eggbar shoes may be beneficial
• For horses with a locked patella, manually push the patella medially and distally while backing the horse
• Transection or ultrasonography-guided splitting of the medial patellar ligament in horses that do not respond to conservative management or severely affected horses

MEDICATIONS

DRUG(S) OF CHOICE
• Counterirritants (2% iodine, volatile salts, Sarapin)—SC injections along the medial and middle patellar ligaments
• Estrone sulfate—series of IM injections

CONTRAINDICATIONS/POSSIBLE INTERACTIONS
Swelling after counterirritant injection is expected.

FOLLOW-UP

PATIENT MONITORING
• Immediate resolution after surgery in horses with a locked patella
• Gradational elimination of clinical signs after treatment in horses with mild, intermittent gait abnormality

• Immature horses may outgrow the problem
• Recurrence in ponies

PREVENTION/AVOIDANCE
• Stall confinement or abrupt declines in exercise regimen should be avoided
• Consistent exercise program of adequate rigor for affected horses

POSSIBLE COMPLICATIONS
• Fibrous thickening at the surgical site
• Osteoarthritis, distal patellar fragmentation, chondromalacia of the patella, and patella fracture can occur following desmotomy

EXPECTED COURSE AND PROGNOSIS
• Most horses respond favorably to conservative management
• Horses with concurrent stifle osteochondrosis or soft tissue injury are more likely to be lame
• Surgical treatment is reserved for severely affected horses and horses in which the patella remains locked despite manipulation. Approximately 30% of horses will develop patellar lesions after medial patellar desmotomy. Arthroscopic removal of minor patella fragmentation is often successful

MISCELLANEOUS

ASSOCIATED CONDITIONS
None

AGE-RELATED FACTORS
Gait abnormality commonly seen in young horses and ponies.

ZOONOTIC POTENTIAL
None

PREGNANCY/FERTILITY/BREEDING
N/A

Suggested Reading
Dyson SJ, Ross MW. Mechanical and neurological lameness in forelimbs and hindlimbs. In: Ross MW, Dyson SJ, eds. Diagnosis and Management of Lameness in the Horse, 2e. St. Louis, MO: Elsevier Saunders, 2011:555–563.

Author Elizabeth J. Davidson
Consulting Editor Elizabeth J. Davidson

BASICS

DEFINITION
• Analysis of urine as an aid in the diagnosis of disease via visual inspection, dipstick analysis, refractometry or osmometry, and microscopy of sediment
• Urine is collected by free catch during voiding or by urethral catheterization
• Cystocentesis is not a method of urine collection in horses. Voided urine samples are easily contaminated. Catheterization is preferred for bacteriologic examination
• Urine appearance changes during urination, especially toward the end of micturition (more crystals)
• Urine volume and composition influenced by feed and water intake, salt supplementation, environmental factors, exercise stress, systemic disease, and drug administration

Normal Urine
• Visual inspection—color ranges from pale yellow to dark tan (may turn brown/red color after prolonged storage or exposure to air). Cloudy/turbid from large quantities of calcium carbonate (some calcium oxalate and phosphate). Viscous from the presence of mucus. Urine often appears red on snow or shavings
• Dipstick—alkaline pH, typically 7.0–9.0 (foals pH 5.0–7.0). Negative glucose; negative/trace protein; negative ketones; negative bilirubin; positive urobilinogen
• Osmometry—osmolality is the most accurate determinate of solute concentration of urine; typically 1500 mOsm/kg
• Refractometry—USG measured with a refractometer estimates solute concentrations
• Urine concentration classified as hyposthenuric (USG <1.008; osmolality <269 mOsm/kg); isosthenuric (USG 1.008–1.014; osmolality 260–300 mOsm/kg); hypersthenuric (USG >1.014; osmolality >300 mOsm/kg)
• Microscopy of sediment—refrigerate sample; must be evaluated within 1 h or cells/casts deteriorate, crystals dissolve/form. Method of collection can affect analysis; catheterization may result in mild trauma, increasing urine protein and RBCs
• Abundant calcium carbonate crystals, small numbers of calcium oxalate and phosphate crystals
• No epithelial casts
• RBCs <5 cells/hpf, WBCs <5 cells/hpf, small numbers of bacteria on voided sample (contamination)
• USG of foal urine should be <1.008 with osmolality <250 mOsm/kg. This reflects a normal high-volume milk diet

PATHOPHYSIOLOGY
• Kidneys determine body water content and ion composition
• Important components of this regulation include renal blood flow, glomerular filtration, tubular modification of glomerular filtrate
• Blood is filtered by the glomeruli in the kidneys. Small solutes are freely filtered at the glomerulus. The renal tubules extensively modify the ultrafiltrate by reabsorbing or secreting solutes
• Urinary bladder stores urine for elimination through the urethra

SYSTEMS AFFECTED
Renal/urologic

GENETICS
N/A

INCIDENCE/PREVALENCE
N/A

GEOGRAPHIC DISTRIBUTION
N/A

SIGNALMENT
• Any breed, age, or sex
• Idiopathic renal hematuria in Arabians

SIGNS
Dependent on the underlying cause.

CAUSES

Hyposthenuria
• Milk diet (foals)
• Psychogenic polydipsia
• Diabetes insipidus

Isosthenuria
• AKI—nephrotoxic drugs (e.g. NSAID, aminoglycosides, tetracycline), prolonged hypoperfusion, pigment nephropathy, toxicities (e.g. cantharidin, red maple leaf), leptospirosis, neoplasia, glomerulonephritis
• CRF—prolonged AKI

Hypersthenuria
Dehydration

Discolored urine
• Myoglobin (e.g. polysaccharide storage myopathy, exertional rhabdomyolysis, immune-mediated myositis)
• Hemoglobin (intravascular hemolysis, e.g. piroplasmosis, neonatal isoerythrolysis in foals, immune-mediated hemolytic anemia)
• RBCs (e.g. idiopathic renal hematuria, pyelonephritis, cystitis, neoplasia, trauma)
• Methemoglobin (e.g. toxicities—red maple leaf, onion, turnip, kale, garlic)
• Bilirubin (e.g. hepatic disease, cholestasis)

DIAGNOSIS

DIFFERENTIAL DIAGNOSIS
See Causes.

CBC/BIOCHEMISTRY/URINALYSIS

CBC
• Dependent on the underlying cause.
• CRF—mild anemia, due to decreased erythropoietin production

Biochemistry
• Prerenal azotemia in cases of dehydration (hypersthenuria)
• AKI—hyponatremia, hypochloremia; possibly hyperkalemia, hypocalcemia, hyperphosphatemia
• CRF—hypercalcemia, hypermagnesemia, hypophosphatemia, hypoalbuminemia
• Hypoalbuminemia if protein-losing nephropathy
• Myopathy/pigmenturia—elevated creatine kinase and aspartate aminotransferase

Urinalysis
Visual Inspection
Change in color—pigmenturia, bacteriuria, spermuria, excessive crystalluria. Dilute urine—polyuria. Pigmenturia throughout micturition—bladder or renal lesion. Pigmenturia at the beginning or end of micturition—urethral or accessory gland lesion.
Dipstick Analysis
• Decreased pH—vigorous exercise, high-concentrate diet, dehydration, anorexia, metabolic acidosis, hypochloremic metabolic alkalosis, bacteriuria
• Positive protein—false positive (alkaline or hemoglobinuria). More sensitive methods—sulfosalicylic acid precipitation test or by specific quantification with colorimetric assay
• Proteinuria and absence of WBCs, RBCs, bacteria, or casts—glomerulonephritis or amyloidosis
• Positive glucose—severe hyperglycemia above renal threshold (serum glucose concentration >180 mg/dL). Systemic disease such as equine metabolic syndrome or pituitary pars intermedia dysfunction. Elevated catecholamines or cortisol with corticosteroid therapy, intense exercise, pain, stress, or shock. Transiently after α_2-agonist. Glucosuria without hyperglycemia—renal tubular damage
• Positive blood—false positive (extremely alkaline urine). Dipstick cannot differentiate hemoglobin, myoglobin, or RBC. Proteinuria generally present. Hematuria—hemorrhage in urogenital tract. Hemoglobinuria—intravascular hemolysis
• Myoglobinuria—severe myopathy. Differentiate by centrifugation
• Positive bilirubin—increased circulation of conjugated bilirubin; consider myopathy, hepatic disease, posthepatic obstruction
• Positive urobilinogen—indicates patent bile duct. Increases—hemolytic, hepatic disease, posthepatic disease
Changes in Sediment
• Casts—indicates renal tubular abnormality. Can consist of RBCs, WBCs, or tubular epithelial cells
• Increased WBCs (>5 cells/hpf) with bacteriuria—cystitis, pyelonephritis.
• Increased RBCs (>5 cells/hpf)—hematuria, trauma, hemorrhage, urolithiasis,

URINALYSIS (U/A)

inflammation, infection, toxemia, neoplasia, coagulopathy, exercise, fulminant liver failure
• Bacteria—contamination in voided sample. If associated with pyuria—infection. Primary cystitis is rare

OTHER LABORATORY TESTS
• GGT to creatinine ratio—GGT is released into the urine from damaged proximal tubules
• Fractional clearance/excretion—evaluates tubular function. Damaged renal tubules fail to adequately reabsorb electrolytes, resulting in excessive loss in the urine
• Urine protein to creatinine ratio—quantifies protein loss in urine
• Culture and sensitivity—collect urine aseptically through catheter
• Water deprivation test—for patients with hyposthenuria to differentiate psychogenic polydipsia or diabetes insipidus

IMAGING
Ultrasonography of kidneys, ureters, and bladder may assist in diagnosing underlying disorder.

OTHER DIAGNOSTIC PROCEDURES
• Rectal palpation of kidneys, ureters, and bladder
• Cystoscopy if abnormal urination or hematuria. Allows examination of urethra, bladder, and occasionally ureters. May sample urine from individual ureters to assess individual kidneys
• Renal biopsy

PATHOLOGIC FINDINGS
Dependent on the underlying cause.

TREATMENT
• Dependent on the underlying cause
• Correct fluid, electrolyte, and acid–base abnormalities

MEDICATIONS
DRUG(S) OF CHOICE
Dependent on the underlying cause.

CONTRAINDICATIONS
Avoid nephrotoxic drugs if AKI or CRF.

PRECAUTIONS
Do not perform water deprivation test in horses with renal disease.

POSSIBLE INTERACTIONS
N/A

ALTERNATIVE DRUGS
N/A

FOLLOW-UP
PATIENT MONITORING
Dependent on the underlying cause.

PREVENTION/AVOIDANCE
Dependent on the underlying cause.

POSSIBLE COMPLICATIONS
• Pigmenturia can result in permanent renal tubular damage
• Uncorrected dehydration can result in permanent renal compromise
• Uroliths/cystoliths can result in urethral obstruction

EXPECTED COURSE AND PROGNOSIS
Dependent on the underlying cause.

MISCELLANEOUS
ASSOCIATED CONDITIONS
Dependent on the underlying cause.

AGE-RELATED FACTORS
N/A

ZOONOTIC POTENTIAL
N/A

PREGNANCY/FERTILITY/BREEDING
N/A

SYNONYMS
N/A

SEE ALSO
• Acute kidney injury (AKI) and acute renal failure (ARF)
• Azotemia and uremia
• Chronic kidney disease
• Exertional rhabdomyolysis
• Osmolality, hyperosmolality
• Pigmenturia
• Polyuria (PU) and polydipsia (PD)

ABBREVIATIONS
• AKI = acute kidney injury
• CRF = chronic renal failure
• GGT = γ-glutamyltransferase
• hpf = high-power field
• NSAID = nonsteroidal anti-inflammatory drug
• RBC = red blood cell
• USG = urine specific gravity
• WBC = white blood cell

Suggested Reading
Bohn AA. Laboratory evaluation of equine renal system. In: Walton RM, ed. Equine Clinical Pathology. Ames, IA: Wiley Blackwell, 2014:87–101.
Kisthardt KK, Schumacher J, Finn-Bodner ST, Carson-Dunkerley S, Williams MA. Severe renal hemorrhage caused by pyelonephritis in 7 horses: clinical and ultrasonographic evaluation. Can Vet J 1999;40(8):571–576.
Schott HC. Examination of the urinary system. In: Reed SM, Bayly WM, Sellon DC, eds. Equine Internal Medicine, 3e. St. Louis, MO: WB Saunders, 2010:1162–1176.
Schumacher J. Hematuria and pigmenturia of horses. Vet Clin North Am Equine Pract 2007;23(3):655–675.
Toribio RE. Essentials of equine renal and urinary tract physiology. Vet Clin North Am Equine Pract 2007;23(3):533–561.

Author Jenifer R. Gold
Consulting Editor Sandra D. Taylor
Acknowledgment The author and editor acknowledge the prior contribution of Grace Forbes.

BASICS

DEFINITION
• Inability to control urination with the involuntary passage of urine
• Incontinence develops when intravesical pressure exceeds resting urethral sphincter pressure

PATHOPHYSIOLOGY
• 3 types of bladder paralysis: (1) reflex or UMN bladder (also known as spastic or autonomic bladder); (2) paralytic or LMN bladder; and (3) myogenic or non-neurogenic bladder
  ○ Initially, a UMN bladder is characterized by increased urethral resistance, leading to increased intravesical pressure before voiding can occur. Voiding may occur as short bursts of urine passage with incomplete bladder emptying, and rectal examination will reveal a turgid bladder, small to increased in size
  ○ In contrast, LMN and myogenic bladder paresis result in chronic bladder distention due to decreased or absent detrusor activity. Rectal palpation reveals a large, flaccid bladder and urine can usually be expressed by placing pressure on the bladder
  ○ Although signs of a UMN bladder are initially different from those of the other 2 types, this type of problem is usually not recognized in horses until more significant incontinence develops in association with progressive loss of detrusor function
  ○ LMN disease limited to the external urethral sphincter with normal detrusor function has not been well documented in horses but may be related to hypoestrogenism in an occasional mare
  ○ By the time incontinence develops into a clinically important problem, the inciting cause can often not be determined
• In young horses, ectopic ureter; affected horses also posture and urinate normally when ectopic ureter is a unilateral problem

SYSTEMS AFFECTED
• Renal/urologic
• Nervous
• Musculoskeletal

GENETICS
N/A

INCIDENCE/PREVALENCE
Low

SIGNALMENT
Breed Predilections
None documented.

Mean Age and Range
Ectopic ureter is an anomaly of development and results in incontinence from birth.

Predominant Sex
• Bladder paralysis appears to be more common in male horses owing to the longer urethra
• Postpartum mares may also be at greater risk for incontinence because of trauma sustained during parturition
• An occasional mare may also develop incontinence consequent to hypoestrogenism

SIGNS
• Urinary incontinence and scalding of the perineal area (mares) and inner aspect of the hindlimbs in both sexes
• Horses may appear painful while posturing to urinate or may not assume a normal voiding posture. Horses may also pass urine involuntary and appear unaware of voiding
• Incontinence may be more apparent during exercise
• Weakness, ataxia, etc., if incontinence is due to an underlying neurologic disease
• Fever, partial anorexia, weight loss may be observed if complicated by pyelonephritis

CAUSES
• *Neurologic disease*—equine herpes myelopathy, EPM, spinal cord compression, cauda equina neuritis
• *Intoxication*—grazing *Sorghum* hybrids (sudangrass and Johnson grass) that contain hydrocyanic acid
• *Trauma*—postbreeding or postpartum in mares; direct injury to the urethral sphincter may occur and lead to urinary incontinence (and infertility)
• *Hypoestrogenism*—a suspected cause of incontinence in an occasional mare
• *Ectopic ureter*—young horses
• *Idiopathic*—possibly a consequence of lumbar pain/orthopedic disease resulting in posturing difficulty and incomplete bladder emptying, perhaps more common in male horses, which would lead to accumulation of crystalline sludge in the ventral aspect of the bladder (sabulous urolithiasis), progressive bladder distention, loss of detrusor function, and paralysis (myogenic bladder)

DIAGNOSIS

DIFFERENTIAL DIAGNOSIS
Normal estrous behavior in mares.

CBC/BIOCHEMISTRY/URINALYSIS
• CBC normal unless UTI extends to upper urinary tract, leading to variable leukocytosis
• Blood urea nitrogen and creatinine normal unless complicated by moderate to severe bilateral pyelonephritis
• Urine specific gravity usually normal (1.020–1.035) but increased numbers of red blood cells, white blood cells, and bacteria on urine sediment examination if complicated by UTI

OTHER LABORATORY TESTS
Quantitative urine culture should be performed in all cases of incontinence.

IMAGING
• *Transabdominal ultrasonography*—renal parenchymal architecture may be abnormal if complicated by pyelonephritis (see chapter Urinary tract infection (UTI))
• *Transrectal ultrasonography*—allows assessment of bladder size and wall thickness and may demonstrate accumulation of sabulous material
• *Abdominal radiography*—IV pyelography may confirm ectopic ureter in foals with incontinence; intrarenal pyelography (contrast injected transabdominally directly into renal pelvis) has a greater likelihood of outlining the ectopia
• *Urethroscopy/cystoscopy*—useful to assess bladder mucosa for inflammation, accumulation of sabulous material, and integrity of ureteral orifices (they may be wide open with chronic bladder paralysis supporting vesiculoureteral reflux and probable ascending pyelonephritis)
• *Lumbar radiographs ± nuclear scintigraphy*—to evaluate possible thoracolumbar musculoskeletal disease

OTHER DIAGNOSTIC PROCEDURES
• *Bulbocavernosus reflex* (male horses)—when normal, contraction of the urethral sphincter can be palpated per rectum when the glans penis is gently squeezed by an assistant
• *Cystometry*—continuous recording of intravesical pressure during saline infusion to assess detrusor muscle function; threshold for onset of detrusor contraction in normal horses is 90 ± 20 cmH$_2$O
• *Urethral pressure profile*—after passage of a balloon-tipped catheter into the bladder, the pressure in the balloon is continuously recorded as the catheter is withdrawn through the urethral sphincter to assess external sphincter muscle function; the pressure in normal horses typically exceeds 100 cmH$_2$O and waves of contractions can be appreciated on the tracing
• *Neurologic examination*—document additional neurologic deficits
• *Collection and analysis of cerebrospinal fluid*—cytologic analysis and appropriate testing for EPM
• *Electromyography*—assess perineal and tail muscles for evidence of denervation (LMN disease)

PATHOLOGIC FINDINGS
• The bladder often contains a concretion of chalky/sabulous material
• The bladder mucosa may be thickened and hemorrhagic with a neutrophilic or lymphocytic infiltrate
• Attempts to investigate the neurologic component of the urinary incontinence are often challenging (no lesions may be identifiable)

URINARY INCONTINENCE

TREATMENT

NURSING CARE
• Daily cleaning of perineum and hindlimbs to minimize skin irritation from incontinence; application of petrolatum to scalded areas
• In cases of myogenic bladder and sabulous urolithiasis, manual lavage of the bladder with saline may provide temporary relief of distention and can remove accumulated urine sediment
• Proper recognition and treatment of all underlying primary neurologic disease processes

ACTIVITY
• In cases of neurologic disease, advise not to ride the horse until resolution of ataxia or other underlying conditions
• If gait is normal and the horse is outwardly healthy, mild to moderate exercise may be continued

DIET
• Removal from exposure to cyanogenic grasses
• Grass hay is preferable to alfalfa or other legumes (higher in calcium)
• Urine acidifying agents can be supplemented (NH_4Cl or (NH_4SO_4) or an anionic diet can be fed in an attempt to limit urine crystal formation; however, no currently available products are palatable enough to be efficacious
• NaCl 28–56 g (1–2 ounces) BID added to feed or mixed with water and administered as an oral slurry will increase urine flow and decrease sedimentation of crystalloid material in the ventral aspect of the bladder

CLIENT EDUCATION
Urinary incontinence can be managed but requires dedication and repeated examinations and treatments for UTI.

SURGICAL CONSIDERATIONS
Surgical correction of ectopic ureter by unilateral nephrectomy or attachment of the distal ureter to the bladder neck.

MEDICATIONS

DRUG(S) OF CHOICE
• Bethanechol 0.25–0.75 mg/kg SC or PO every 8 h—parasympathomimetic agent selective on smooth muscle of the GI tract

and bladder; response to treatment is usually poor because of longstanding detrusor paresis/paralysis before the problem is clinically recognized (except perhaps with acute herpes myelopathy or EPM). If no improvement is noted within 3–5 days of treatment, therapy should be discontinued
• Phenoxybenzamine 0.7 mg/kg PO every 6 h—α-adrenergic blocker that can be used to decrease urethral sphincter tone in cases of UMN bladder
• Estradiol cypionate 4 µg/kg IM every other day—may improve urethral sphincter tone in mares with hypoestrogenism-associated incontinence
• Antimicrobials—trimethoprim–sulfonamide combination (sulfadiazine preferable to sulfamethoxazole because of less hepatic metabolism) 20 mg/kg PO every 12 h or 24 h; is the most practical long-term treatment; can be used prophylactically or therapeutically for established UTI (see chapter Urinary tract infection (UTI))

CONTRAINDICATIONS
N/A

PRECAUTIONS
Bethanechol—must be used cautiously as it may increase GI motility and lead to colic signs.

FOLLOW-UP

PATIENT MONITORING
• Patient monitoring in cases of neurogenic bladder should include regular repeat physical and neurologic examination, cystometry, and urethral pressure profiles could be repeated at 2–4 week intervals if clinical improvement is uncertain
• Monitoring of patients with longstanding idiopathic incontinence should include regular (weekly or monthly) assessment of overall condition (attitude, appetite, body weight, etc.)

POSSIBLE COMPLICATIONS
• Moderate to severe dermatitis consequent to urine scald
• Sabulous urolithiasis
• UTI—cystitis, possibly complicated by ascending pyelonephritis

EXPECTED COURSE AND PROGNOSIS
• The prognosis for recovery of cases of bladder paresis/paralysis and associated

incontinence due to neurologic disease is guarded and will depend on response to treatment of the underlying disease and duration of paresis/incontinence (generally more favorable if <2 weeks in duration); evidence of some detrusor function on cystometry and a normal urethral pressure profile improve the prognosis and such horses warrant aggressive treatment
• The prognosis for recovery of cases of longstanding "idiopathic" bladder paralysis and associated incontinence is *poor*; owner frustration often leads to a decision for euthanasia within a few months after the problem is first recognized

MISCELLANEOUS

ASSOCIATED CONDITIONS
Infertility (mares).

AGE-RELATED FACTORS
Hypoestrogenism would be more likely in older mares, and ectopic ureter is a problem recognized in young horses.

ZOONOTIC POTENTIAL
None

PREGNANCY/FERTILITY/BREEDING
N/A

SYNONYMS
Enzootic ataxia and cystitis (herd outbreaks associated with intoxication).

SEE ALSO
• Urinary tract infection (UTI)
• Urolithiasis

ABBREVIATIONS
• EPM = equine protozoal myeloencephalitis
• GI = gastrointestinal
• LMN = lower motor neuron
• UMN = upper motor neuron
• UTI = urinary tract infection

Suggested Reading
Bayly WM. Urinary Incontinence and Bladder Dysfunction. In: Reed SM, Bayly WM, Sellon DC, eds. Equine Internal Medicine, 4e. St. Louis, MO: WB Saunders, 2017:973–976.

Author Harold C. Schott II
Consulting Editor Valérie Picandet

U

URINARY TRACT INFECTION (UTI)

BASICS

DEFINITION
• 2 categories—those affecting the upper urinary tract (i.e. kidneys, ureters) and those affecting the lower urinary tract (i.e. bladder)
• Bacterial infection is most common, but yeast, protozoa, and other parasites may also cause UTI

PATHOPHYSIOLOGY
Bacterial Upper UTI
• Most commonly ascending infections secondary to stasis of urine flow (as with bladder paralysis) and vesiculoureteral reflux (retrograde flow of urine into ureters) or damage to renal parenchyma (i.e. polycystic disease and medullary necrosis)
• Less commonly a result of neonatal septicemia

Bacterial Lower UTI
• Usually a consequence of abnormal urine flow (anatomic or functional), especially bladder paralysis
• Frequently accompanied by urolithiasis

Parasitic Infection
• *Halicephalobus gingivalis (deletrix)* infection (rare) can be life-threatening owing to central nervous system involvement. Large granulomatous lesions full of rhabditiform nematodes usually are found in the kidneys. Renal involvement typically is inapparent but may cause hematuria
• *Dioctophyma renale.* Typical hosts are carnivorous species, but horses can ingest the intermediate host (annelid worm) while grazing or drinking natural water. The parasite may live 1–3 years in the kidney, shedding eggs in the urine. The renal parenchyma is completely destroyed, and death of the parasite leads to fibrosis of the kidney
• Occasionally, hydronephrosis or renal hemorrhage may be a serious complication of parasitic infection
• Infection with the coccidian parasite *Klossiella equi* is common, but clinically benign, and thus an incidental finding

Yeast Infection
Recumbent foals on broad-spectrum antibiotics may develop secondary *Candida* spp. cystitis.

SYSTEMS AFFECTED
• Renal/urologic—infection and failure (with bilateral upper UTI)
• Nervous—with *H. gingivalis* infection
• Dermatologic—urine scalding of hindlimbs

GENETICS
None documented.

INCIDENCE/PREVALENCE
• Bacterial UTIs are uncommon
• Clinically significant renal nematode infections are rare, despite necropsy surveys

revealing that up to 20% of equine kidneys have evidence of *Strongylus vulgaris* migration
• One necropsy survey found *K. equi* in 12% of horses examined

GEOGRAPHIC DISTRIBUTION
N/A

SIGNALMENT
Breed Predilections
None documented.

Mean Age and Range
• Foals <30 days of age are at greater risk for septic nephritis associated with septicemia
• Critically ill neonates receiving broad-spectrum antibiotic treatment may develop ascending UTI with *Candida* spp.

Predominant Sex
• A shorter urethra increases risk of UTI in females; however, UTI is still rare in mares
• Injury to the lower urinary tract during breeding and parturition increase risk of urethral damage (leading to incontinence), bladder paresis, and UTI, especially after dystocia

SIGNS
Historical Findings
• Upper UTI—usually weight loss or fever of undetermined origin; less commonly, hematuria or pyuria. Occasionally, recurrent colic when associated with urolithiasis
• Lower UTI—dysuria (e.g. pollakiuria, stranguria, hematuria). Urinary incontinence and skin scalding may be observed with either bladder paresis or pollakiuria

Physical Examination Findings
Upper UTI
• Lethargy, fever, partial anorexia, intermittent colic, and mild dehydration
• Rectal examination may reveal enlarged ureters and kidneys
• Occasionally, obstructing ureteroliths can be palpated
Lower UTI
• Dysuria with or without urine scalding, but general health usually is good
• Rectal examination—thickened bladder wall; cystoliths or other bladder masses may be detected if bladder is not full. Assess for bladder paresis (i.e. large atonic bladder with incontinence produced by compressing bladder) versus a small bladder usually present with pollakiuria

CAUSES
Upper UTI
• Bacterial ascending infections—*Escherichia coli, Proteus mirabilis, Klebsiella* spp., *Staphylococcus* spp., *Enterobacter* spp., *Corynebacterium* spp., and *Pseudomonas aeruginosa.* Mixed infections may be seen
• Less commonly, hematogenous infection—*Rhodococcus equi, Actinobacillus equuli,* and other Gram-negative bacteria
• Parasitic infection (see Pathophysiology)

Lower UTI
• Ascending infections
• Organisms similar to those causing upper UTIs
• Chronic antibiotic treatment or instrumentation of the urinary tract (indwelling bladder catheters, ureteral stents) may cause UTI with *Enterococcus* spp. or other antibiotic-resistant microbes
• Yeast infection (see Pathophysiology)
• Outbreaks of cystitis described with eating hybrids of *Sorghum* spp. (Johnson grass, sudangrass) in the southwestern USA, likely a complication of bladder paralysis
• Outbreak of cystitis, manifested by hematuria more than UTI or incontinence, in western Australia. A fungal toxin produced by *Pithomyces chartarum* was suspected

RISK FACTORS
• Vesiculoureteral reflux, which may develop with bladder paresis or partial obstruction, predisposing for ascending upper UTI
• Abnormal urine flow, especially with bladder paralysis, increases risk for lower UTI
• Use of indwelling catheters is a significant risk factor, but routine instrumentation of the urinary tract (bladder catheterization, cystoscopy) is relatively low risk
• Dystocia and subsequent trauma to the lower urinary tract may allow ascending infections

DIAGNOSIS

DIFFERENTIAL DIAGNOSIS
• Upper UTI—disease processes that lead to lethargy, partial anorexia, weight loss, fever, recurrent colic, or hematuria
• Lower UTI—normal estrus activity in mares, ectopic ureter, and other causes of dysuria (urolithiasis, neoplasia)

CBC/BIOCHEMISTRY/URINALYSIS
• Usually normal CBC, leukocytosis with upper UTI
• Azotemia when bilateral pyelonephritis results in CKD
• Urinary specific gravity—isosthenuria (1.008–1.014) when UTI is associated with CKD
• Urinalysis generally reveals microscopic or macroscopic hematuria and pyuria; bacteria, yeast, and protozoa may be seen on sediment examination

OTHER LABORATORY TESTS
• Perform quantitative urine culture and antimicrobial sensitivity testing in all suspected cases; recovery of >10 000 CFU/mL is diagnostic
• Consider bacterial culture of the center of uroliths accompanying UTIs, because many have positive results despite negative urine culture

URINARY TRACT INFECTION (UTI) (CONTINUED)

IMAGING

Transabdominal Ultrasonography
• Kidneys may be shrunken or enlarged, have loss of the corticomedullary junction, or areas of decreased echogenicity, particularly with pyelonephritis
• Nephroliths (diameter >1 cm) should be readily detected

Transrectal Ultrasonography
For evaluation of the left kidney, ureters, bladder.

Urethroscopy/Cystoscopy
To assess defects of the lower urinary tract, uroepithelial damage, and urine flow from the ureteral orifices.

OTHER DIAGNOSTIC PROCEDURES
• Urethral pressure profile measurements
• Ureteral catheterization—during cystoscopy (or by a manual transurethral approach in mares) collect urine from each ureter when unilateral pyelonephritis is suspected

PATHOLOGIC FINDINGS
• Pyelonephritis—deformation of renal architecture, with complete loss in severe unilateral infection, nephroliths, ureteroliths, and ureteral dilation
• Lower UTI—diffusely thickened bladder wall, inflamed mucosa with areas of erosion/ulceration, adhesion of crystalloid material, and possible cystolithiasis

TREATMENT

APPROPRIATE HEALTH CARE
• Mostly outpatient medical therapy
• Surgical intervention if necessary

NURSING CARE
Regular cleaning of perineum and hindlimbs and petrolatum.

ACTIVITY
Normal, unless systemically ill from upper UTI.

DIET
Sodium chloride (28 g PO BID–QID) to increase urine flow.

CLIENT EDUCATION
Primary UTIs are rare; further diagnostics needed to rule out predisposing causes.

SURGICAL CONSIDERATIONS
• Nephrectomy to remove unilaterally infected kidney. Ensure appropriate renal function in contralateral kidney
• Surgical removal of uroliths in the lower urinary tract
• Surgical repair of anatomic abnormalities of the lower urinary tract

MEDICATIONS

DRUG(S) OF CHOICE
• Trimethoprim–sulfonamide combinations (20–40 mg/kg PO every 12 h)—sulfadiazine, excreted largely unchanged in urine, may be preferred over sulfamethoxazole, largely inactivated before urinary excretion
• Procaine penicillin G (22 000 IU/kg IM every 12 h) and sodium ampicillin (10–20 mg/kg IV or IM every 6–8 h) for upper or lower UTI caused by susceptible *Corynebacterium* spp., *Streptococcus* spp., and some *Staphylococcus* spp. Many isolates of the Enterobacteriaceae family demonstrate resistance to ampicillin in vitro, but this drug is highly concentrated in urine and may be effective against many of these organisms
• Ceftiofur (4.4 mg/kg IV or IM every 12 h) or enrofloxacin (2.5 mg/kg PO every 12 h) when other antibiotic resistance demonstrated
• Reserve gentamicin (6.6 mg/kg IV every 24 h) and amikacin (15 mg/kg IV every 24 h) for lower UTI caused by highly resistant organisms or acute, life-threatening upper UTI caused by Gram-negative organisms
• NSAIDs—phenylbutazone (2.2 mg/kg PO every 12–24 h) or flunixin meglumine (0.5–1.0 mg/kg PO every 12–24 h) may be useful with pollakiuria or dysuria

CONTRAINDICATIONS
N/A

PRECAUTIONS
• Enrofloxacin—consider potential cartilage damage in young horses
• Administration of long-term antibiotics without correcting underlying cause (i.e. bladder paralysis) may lead to resistant bacterial growth
• Aminoglycoside antibiotics and NSAIDs—avoid or used sparingly in cases with renal compromise or azotemia

POSSIBLE INTERACTIONS
N/A

FOLLOW-UP

PATIENT MONITORING
• Institute antibiotic treatment for at least 1 week for simple (i.e. no apparent underlying cause) lower UTI, and for 4–6 weeks for upper UTI
• Follow-up with a quantitative urine culture the week after treatment is discontinued
• Assess renal function of patients with azotemia at regular intervals (i.e. monthly or longer) during the early stages of CKD

• Discontinuation of broad-spectrum antibiotics usually is sufficient for treating lower UTI caused by *Candida* spp. in neonates

PREVENTION/AVOIDANCE
Salt supplementation may increase urine flow and decrease risk of recurrence.

POSSIBLE COMPLICATIONS
• Urolithiasis
• CKD

EXPECTED COURSE AND PROGNOSIS
• Favorable prognosis for simple lower UTI
• Guarded prognosis in patients with upper UTI and recurrent lower UTI where the underlying cause remains (e.g. bladder paralysis)
• Guarded prognosis in patients with bilateral pyelonephritis accompanied by azotemia; typically progresses to CKD

MISCELLANEOUS

ASSOCIATED CONDITIONS
Urolithiasis—single large cystoliths predispose to UTI; however, it is difficult to determine if uroliths are a predisposing cause or a consequence of UTI.

AGE-RELATED FACTORS
N/A

ZOONOTIC POTENTIAL
N/A

PREGNANCY/FERTILITY/BREEDING
N/A

SYNONYMS
• Cystitis
• Pyelonephritis

SEE ALSO
• Chronic kidney disease (CKD)
• Urinary incontinence
• Urolithiasis

ABBREVIATIONS
• CFU = colony-forming unit
• CKD = chronic kidney disease
• NSAID = nonsteroidal anti-inflammatory drug
• UTI = urinary tract infection

Suggested Reading
Schott HC. Urinary Tract Infections. In: Reed SM, Bayly WM, Sellon DC, eds. Equine Internal Medicine, 4e. St. Louis, MO: WB Saunders, 2017:946–949.

Author Harold C. Schott II
Consulting Editor Valérie Picandet

BASICS

DEFINITION
• Urine reflux from urethral orifice into the vagina
• Urine may then enter the uterus during estrus (relaxed cervix) or with cervical irritation
• May cause infertility

PATHOPHYSIOLOGY
Altered position of the urethra in relationship to the vulvar cleft and vestibular sphincter; resulting in incomplete voiding or retention of urine in the vestibule/vagina.

SYSTEMS AFFECTED
• Reproductive
• Urologic

GENETICS
Inherited predisposition for VC and, thus, the location of the urethral orifice.

INCIDENCE/PREVALENCE
Incidence may increase with age, parity, worsening VC.

SIGNALMENT
• All breeds, but most common in those with less perineal muscle
• Greater problem in old pluriparous mares

SIGNS
• Few to no outward signs
• Sole complaint may be infertility
• On dismount, stallion may have urine evident on his penis
• Transrectal examination and ultrasonography may disclose fluid within the uterus
• Speculum examination may reveal pooled urine and increased hyperemia and ulcers (from urine scalding)—vaginal wall, external cervical os

CAUSES AND RISK FACTORS
• With increasing age, dorsal vulvar commissure can shift cranially and/or dorsally (inward slant) coupled with a more cranial urethral opening and/or relaxation of the vestibule, urine refluxes into the cranial vagina
• Inherited conformational traits
• Multiparous

DIAGNOSIS

DIFFERENTIAL DIAGNOSIS
• Vaginitis
• Pneumovagina

IMAGING
Ultrasonography showing liquid (urine) in the uterus.

PATHOLOGIC FINDINGS
• Uterine/vaginal urine results in endometritis/vaginitis

• Dorsal displacement of the external urethral os, cranial slant of the vulvae, and cranioventral/downward slant from the vagina to the cervix

TREATMENT

SURGICAL CONSIDERATIONS
Surgical repair—only permanent means of correction.

Pouret
Correction of inadequate VC by a caudal-to-cranial transection of the perineal body, separates the rectum from the tubular genital tract, allows the position of the vulva to lie more posterior and ventral, in tandem with posterior placement of the urethral orifice.

Urethral Extension
Posterior relocation of the urethral orifice by transverse splitting of the urethral fold—ventral shelf of the split tissue is brought to the midline and sutured, creates an extension of the urethra.

Monin Vaginoplasty
• Ventral tissue dam of, or immediately cranial to, the vestibular sphincter to reduce the likelihood of urine entering the vagina
• Limited success
• May require repair after parturition

MEDICATIONS
None

FOLLOW-UP

PREVENTION/AVOIDANCE
• None
• VC is inherited

POSSIBLE COMPLICATIONS
• Infertility
• Vaginitis

EXPECTED COURSE AND PROGNOSIS
• Early recognition and treatment to avoid permanent vaginal/endometrial damage
• Absent surgical correction, pooling continues
• Until corrected, both inflammation and pooling continue

MISCELLANEOUS
• In the absence of systemic signs, no systemic therapy is justified and/or necessary
• Flushing the uterus and vagina before insemination may increase the likelihood of

conception but does not prevent subsequent urine accumulation and pregnancy loss
• Pooling increases as uterine weight increases later in gestation; the vestibule is pulled more cranial and dorsal
• If poor vulvar and vestibular conformation are secondary to loss of vaginal fat (e.g. mare that is cachectic, thin, poor conditioning), urine pooling may resolve as the mare gains weight:
  ○ Increasing fat within the pelvic cavity may elevate the vestibular floor in relationship to the ventral vulvar opening
  ○ This is considered to be a temporary solution, however, because the condition most likely will recur with age, parity, or subsequent weight loss

ASSOCIATED CONDITIONS
• Thin mares may be more predisposed to urine pooling
• Usually most severe when the mare is in estrus and vestibular tissues are relaxed
• Increased inflammation and fibrosis of the endometrium

AGE-RELATED FACTORS
• Possible tendency for soft tissue supporting structures of the vestibule to decrease their tonicity with age
• Increased incidence in older mares

PREGNANCY/FERTILITY/BREEDING
May observe infertility or loss of pregnancy secondary to urine pooling.

SYNONYMS
Vesicovaginal reflux

SEE ALSO
Vulvar conformation

ABBREVIATIONS
VC = vulvar conformation

Suggested Reading
McKinnon AO, Beldon JO. Urethral extension technique to correct urine pooling (vesicovaginal reflux) in mares. J Am Vet Med Assoc 1988;192:647–650.
Schofield WA. Use of acupuncture in equine reproduction. Theriogenology 2008;70(3):430–434.
Shires GM, Kaneps AJ. A practical and simple surgical technique for repair of urine pooling in the mare. Proc Am Assoc Equine Pract 1986;27:51–56.

Author Carla L. Carleton
Consulting Editor Carla L. Carleton
Acknowledgment The author/editor acknowledges the prior contribution of Walter R. Threlfall.

UROLITHIASIS

 BASICS

DEFINITION
• Urolithiasis—macroscopic concretions of urine crystals (calculus or stone) in any portion of the urinary tract that may occur separately or together
• Sabulous urolithiasis—accumulation of a large mass of urine sediment in the ventral aspect of the bladder

PATHOPHYSIOLOGY
• Despite the large amount of calcium carbonate crystals in normal equine urine, urolithiasis is rare compared with small animals, possibly because of protective lubricating mucus produced by glands in the renal pelvis and proximal ureter
• The main component of equine uroliths is calcium carbonate along with inorganic elements (magnesium ammonium phosphate, calcium oxalate, or calcium sulfate) and organic matrix (mucoproteins)
• Urolith formation usually requires damage to the renal parenchyma or the uroepithelium of the ureters, bladder, or urethra that allows for adherence of calcium carbonate crystals, which serve as a nidus for stone formation
• Most spontaneously occurring bladder stones are disk-shaped, mildly spiculated, and porous

SYSTEMS AFFECTED
Renal/urologic

GENETICS
None documented.

INCIDENCE/PREVALENCE
• Urolithiasis is uncommon (0.11% of equine admissions to 22 teaching hospitals, accounting for ≅8% of all urinary tract disorders)
• In the same study, cystoliths were most common (60% of all urinary stones) followed by urethroliths (24%), nephroliths (12%), and ureteroliths (4%); ≅10% of affected horses had multiple calculi at different sites

SIGNALMENT

Breed Predilections
None documented.

Mean Age and Range
Adult horses (mean age ≅10 years) with wide age range with horses <1 year also being possibly affected

Predominant Sex
• ≅75% of all reports are in males—stallions and geldings
• A longer and less distensible urethra increases the risk of cystolithiasis and urethrolithiasis in males, but development of calculi at other sites is similar in both sexes

SIGNS

Historical Findings
• Nephrolithiasis and ureterolithiasis—weight loss or fever of undetermined origin, with hematuria or pyuria less common. Occasionally, recurrent colic may be reported
• Cystolithiasis—lower urinary tract signs (e.g. pollakiuria, stranguria, hematuria) predominate, and hematuria after exercise is common. Sometimes, behavior changes during exercise
• Sabulous urolithiasis—urinary incontinence
• Urethrolithiasis—may cause severe renal colic signs with partial to complete obstruction (e.g. pollakiuria, stranguria, anuria)

Physical Examination Findings
• Nephrolithiasis and ureterolithiasis—lethargy, fever, partial anorexia, intermittent colic, and mild dehydration
• Cystolithiasis—dysuria and possibly urine scalding, but general health usually good
• Urethrolithiasis—a distended, sometimes pulsating urethra may be found below the anus, and careful palpation may allow location of the obstructing urolith. Unlike colic signs arising from the gastrointestinal tract, the penis is often dropped in horses with urethral obstruction
• Rectal examination. Nephroliths—may palpate abnormal-shaped left kidney owing to hydronephrosis. Ureteroliths—enlarged, turgid ureters with focal concretions. Cystoliths—the calculi can be palpable in the neck of the bladder at the level of the pelvic canal if the bladder is not distended. The bladder wall is thickened. Sabulous urolithiasis—unlike cystoliths, this urolith often indents with firm digital pressure. Large atonic bladder with incontinence produced by compressing bladder indicates bladder paresis. Urethrolithiasis—markedly distended bladder when obstructed

CAUSES
• Nephrolithiasis—developmental anomalies, pyelonephritis, acute tubular necrosis, renal medullary necrosis due to NSAID use, and neoplasms can cause parenchymal damage that may serve as a nidus for nephrolithiasis. Ureterolithiasis most commonly is due to passage of small nephroliths into the ureters
• Cystolithiasis—may develop from ascending infections, anatomic or functional causes of abnormal urine flow (or stasis), or with damage to the bladder uroepithelium
• Sabulous urolithiasis—bladder paresis (see chapter Urinary incontinence)
• Urethrolithiasis—may develop at sites of damaged uroepithelium (e.g. site of previous perineal urethrotomy) but more commonly results from passage of small uroliths into the urethra

RISK FACTORS
Although poorly documented, high-calcium diets (e.g. alfalfa and other legume hays) are likely risk factors for calculi along the entire urinary tract.

 DIAGNOSIS

DIFFERENTIAL DIAGNOSIS
• Upper tract lithiasis—broad list of disease processes that may lead to lethargy, partial anorexia, weight loss, fever, recurrent colic, dysuria, or hematuria
• Lower tract lithiasis—normal estrus activity in mares and other causes of hematuria or dysuria (e.g. UTI, neoplasia)

CBC/BIOCHEMISTRY/URINALYSIS
• Normal to low packed cell volume (with severe hematuria), normal white blood cell count or leukocytosis (with concurrent upper tract infection), and normal to mildly decreased platelets (with hematuria)
• Azotemia—usually not present unless lower tract obstruction develops (i.e. postrenal azotemia) or bilateral nephrolithiasis/ureterolithiasis is associated with CKD
• Urine specific gravity—usually normal (>1.020) unless lithiasis is associated with CKD and isosthenuria (1.008–1.014)
• Urinalysis—generally reveals microscopic or macroscopic hematuria and pyuria; bacteria may be detected on sediment examination with concurrent UTI

OTHER LABORATORY TESTS
• Perform quantitative urine culture along with antimicrobial sensitivity in all cases of suspected urolithiasis to assess for concurrent UTI
• Consider bacterial culture of the urolith center after surgical removal, as many will culture positive despite negative urine culture results

IMAGING

Transabdominal Ultrasonography
• Nephroliths (diameter >1 cm) should be readily detected as echogenic structures producing acoustic shadows, possible increased echogenicity in adjacent renal tissue
• Dilation of the renal pelvis and proximal ureter (hydronephrosis) may be detected with obstructive ureterolithiasis

Transrectal Ultrasonography
Useful in evaluating the left kidney, ureters, bladder, and proximal urethra. Calculi can be visualized, along with sabulous urolithiasis and a thickened bladder wall.

Urethroscopy/Cystoscopy
To assess uroepithelial damage and urine flow from each side of the upper urinary tract.

PATHOLOGIC FINDINGS

• Nephroliths and ureteroliths may be incidental findings at necropsy
• Small, irregularly shaped kidneys are found with chronic renal failure, but nephroliths and ureteroliths occasionally may produce hydronephrosis when obstruction is present
• Cystolithiasis leads to bladder wall thickening
• Extensive bladder and urethral mucosal damage can accompany cystolithiasis and urethrolithiasis

 TREATMENT

APPROPRIATE HEALTH CARE
N/A

NURSING CARE
Regular cleaning of the perineum and hindlimbs to minimize skin irritation from incontinence or after perineal urethrotomy; application of petrolatum to scalded areas.

ACTIVITY
N/A

DIET
• Decrease dietary calcium intake by limiting legume hay. Changing from alfalfa to grass hay likely will decrease the amount of calcium carbonate crystals more effectively than adding acidifying agents to a legume-based diet
• Oral electrolyte supplementation—sodium chloride (28 g) can be administered in concentrate feed or as an oral slurry/paste BID–QID to encourage increased drinking and urine output (to decrease risk of further urolith formation)
• Feeding an anionic diet (i.e. low cation–anion balance) will reduce urine pH; however, it requires testing of hay and addition of necessary supplements

CLIENT EDUCATION
• Urolithiasis may recur in as many as 40% of patients
• Avoid use of NSAIDs in horses with upper tract lithiasis
• With sabulous urolithiasis, prognosis for recovery is guarded to poor because of underlying bladder paralysis

SURGICAL CONSIDERATIONS
• Nephrotomy for removal of obstructing nephroliths or possible unilateral nephrectomy for nephroliths accompanied by pyelonephritis and limited function of the affected kidney
• Elective surgical removal of cystoliths via parainguinal laparocystotomy, laparoscopic cystotomy, or perineal urethrotomy; manual removal of small cystoliths may be accomplished in mares
• Possible emergency perineal urethrotomy for relief of urethral obstruction in males or repair of ruptured bladder—after initial stabilization of electrolyte (i.e. hyperkalemia with uroperitoneum) and acid–base alterations
• Fragmentation using electrohydraulic or laser lithotripsy is the treatment of choice for ureteroliths when equipment is available; not useful for cystoliths owing to the larger size of bladder stones
• Placement of a bladder catheter and aggressive lavage and rectal manipulation of the bladder may allow removal of sabulous uroliths

 MEDICATIONS

DRUG(S) OF CHOICE
• Appropriate antibiotic agents for prophylaxis or treatment of UTI—see chapter Urinary tract infection (UTI)
• Urinary acidifying agents—ammonium chloride (50–200 mg/kg/day PO) and ammonium sulfate (200–300 mg/kg/day PO): may help decrease the amount of calcium carbonate crystals in urine; however, they are unpalatable

CONTRAINDICATIONS
N/A

PRECAUTIONS
Passing a urinary catheter or performing cystoscopy can complicate UTI in horses with sabulous urolithiasis, and/or bladder paresis.

 FOLLOW-UP

PATIENT MONITORING
• Surgical patients—assess clinical status at least twice daily during the 2–4 days after surgery, emphasizing urine output and signs of dysuria
• Nephrolithiasis or ureterolithiasis—assess renal function at regular intervals (monthly or longer) during the early stages of CKD
• Recurrent cystolithiasis or urethrolithiasis—carefully examine the entire urinary tract for predisposing causes such as anatomic defects or pyelonephritis
• Evaluate horses with recurrent urethral obstruction for upper tract lithiasis and infection

PREVENTION/AVOIDANCE
• Dietary modifications
• Use of urinary acidifying agents

POSSIBLE COMPLICATIONS
• Recurrent urolithiasis
• CKD
• Bladder rupture and uroperitoneum
• Urethral stricture
• UTI

EXPECTED COURSE AND PROGNOSIS
• Prognosis for recovery after surgical correction of cystolithiasis and urethrolithiasis generally is favorable, unless the problem is recurrent (guarded long-term prognosis)
• Issue a guarded long-term prognosis for patients with nephrolithiasis or ureterolithiasis; these problems usually are accompanied by loss of renal function (CKD)
• Poor prognosis for sabulous urolithiasis where underlying cause of bladder paresis cannot be resolved

 MISCELLANEOUS

ASSOCIATED CONDITIONS
UTI

AGE-RELATED FACTORS
N/A

PREGNANCY/FERTILITY/BREEDING
N/A

SYNONYMS
• Lithiasis
• Calculus formation
• Urinary tract stones

SEE ALSO
• Chronic kidney disease (CKD)
• Urinary incontinence
• Urinary tract infection (UTI)

ABBREVIATIONS
• CKD = chronic kidney disease
• NSAID = nonsteroidal anti-inflammatory drug
• UTI = urinary tract infection

Suggested Reading
Duesterdieck-Zellmer KF. Equine urolithiasis. Vet Clin North Am Equine Pract 2007;23(3):613–629.

Author Harold C. Schott II
Consulting Editor Valérie Picandet

UROPERITONEUM, NEONATE

BASICS

DEFINITION
Uroperitoneum is an accumulation of urine in the peritoneal cavity caused by rupture of the bladder or urachus, ureteral tear, or avulsion of the bladder from its urachal attachment.

PATHOPHYSIOLOGY
• Urine has a high concentration of potassium, low concentrations of sodium and chloride, and variable concentrations of urea, creatinine, and water
• Uroabdomen can result in urea, creatinine, and electrolytes moving across the semipermeable peritoneal membrane to equilibrate with plasma, leading to azotemia, hypochloremia, hyponatremia, and hyperkalemia
• Creatinine is less permeable than other solutes and may remain disproportionately elevated in the abdomen
• Pathologic abnormalities may not be apparent for several days following urine leakage
• Hyperkalemia is the most serious of the electrolyte derangements, where profound ECG dysfunction can occur
• Restrictive respiratory failure and colic may be observed in foals with progressive abdominal distention, and ventilation may become impaired

SYSTEMS AFFECTED
Urinary
• Rupture of 1 or more structures of the urinary tract; bladder most common
• Septic foci may predispose to bladder rupture

Gastrointestinal
• Colic and ileus associated with pain and progressive abdominal distention
• Inappetence
• Sterile peritonitis

Cardiovascular
Hyperkalemic dysrhythmias—atrial standstill, cardiac arrest, complete third-degree atrioventricular blockade, ventricular fibrillation.

Respiratory
Tachypnea associated with progressive abdominal distention and restrictive lung expansion.

Nervous
Depression associated with hyponatremia, progressing to seizure activity.

GENETICS
N/A

INCIDENCE/PREVALENCE
Sporadic event; greatest incidence in newborn foals.

GEOGRAPHIC DISTRIBUTION
Worldwide

SIGNALMENT
Breed Predilections
No known breed predilection.

Mean Age and Range
Congenital uroperitoneum tends to occur during vigorous parturition and in the immediate postpartum period. Most cases are recognized within 3–5 days of age. Acquired or secondary uroperitoneum occurs in foals from 1 to 60 days, with most cases diagnosed within the first 2 weeks of life.

Predominant Sex
• Congenital uroperitoneum occurs more commonly in colt foals (>80%). Dorsal urinary bladder tears can occur during parturition. Colts may be predisposed owing to the relatively long urethra, high tone of the urethral sphincter, and high intravesicular pressure of a distended bladder contributing to an increased resistance to emptying
• Congenital ureteral defects occur more commonly in fillies
• Acquired uroperitoneum occurs equally among colts and fillies

SIGNS
Historical Findings
• Foals usually are born normal
• Foals may be observed to still void some urine
• Clinical signs are usually evident by 24–72 h of age, yet can occur as late as 3–4 weeks

Physical Examination Findings
• Frequent attempts to urinate that may be partially successful and void a small stream. Often no urine is passed
• Progressive inappetence, dehydration, depression, lying down
• Progressive abdominal distention and the development of colic and/or tachypnea. Fluid ballottement may be possible
• Ventral edema may be present
• As electrolytes become more deranged, weakness and recumbency become a prominent feature
• Bradycardia or tachycardia

CAUSES
• Congenital rupture during and/or shortly after parturition
• Acquired urachal or bladder rupture associated with sepsis and/or local septic focus (e.g. omphalophlebitis)
• Rarely, embryologic failure of the halves of the bladder to unite (schistocystitis) or ureteral defects can cause uroperitoneum
• Iatrogenic rupture associated with catheters
• Traumatic rupture

RISK FACTORS
• Males for congenital rupture
• Age <4 days
• Septicemia
• Prematurity
• Abdominal trauma

• Omphalophlebitis
• Patent urachus

DIAGNOSIS

DIFFERENTIAL DIAGNOSIS
• Colic for various gastrointestinal reasons
• Meconium impaction should be differentiated from ruptured bladder. Generally, foals that strain to urinate adopt a base-wide stance with ventroflexion of the back whereas foals straining to defecate often show dorsiflexion in their back

CBC/BIOCHEMISTRY/URINALYSIS
• Hematologic abnormalities may reflect concurrent disease such as septicemia
• Electrolyte derangements include hyperkalemia, hyponatremia, hypochloremia. Foals receiving parenteral fluids are less likely to develop classic electrolyte changes
• Acid–base evaluation often reveals metabolic acidosis
• Azotemia

OTHER LABORATORY TESTS
Abdominocentesis may yield copious volumes of clear yellow fluid of low cellularity with a uriniferous odor. Peritoneal fluid creatinine concentration is at least twice the serum creatinine concentration. Occasionally, calcium carbonate crystals may be present in peritoneal fluid.

IMAGING
Abdominal Ultrasonography
• Increased hypoechoic fluid with abdominal viscera floating within this fluid
• A flaccid collapsed urinary bladder may be visualized
• Urachal examination may show the margins of a tear
• Note that the thorax should be evaluated as pleural fluid often accumulates and detection is important when considering anesthesia for surgical repair

Abdominal Radiography
• Loss of serosal detail of abdominal viscera
• Standing films may show obvious fluid line
• Positive contrast cystography using water-soluble contrast agent (e.g. 10% iohexol) should be considered to evaluate the position of a urogenital tear

OTHER DIAGNOSTIC PROCEDURES
ECG is indicated to assess potassium-related dysrhythmias, especially when potassium >6 mEq/L.

PATHOLOGIC FINDINGS
Presence of uroperitoneum and the structural urinary tract defect. Bladder defects tend to be dorsal. Ureteral defects lead to an accumulation of retroperitoneal urine.

U

TREATMENT

AIMS
• Correct hypovolemia, electrolyte, and acid–base disturbances
• Effective abdominal drainage
• Correct structural defects

APPROPRIATE HEALTH CARE
• Immediate referral to a surgical facility is recommended
• Surgery should be performed after metabolic stabilization

NURSING CARE

Stabilization
• Correction of hydration, electrolyte abnormalities, and acid–base derangements should be initiated before surgery
• Note that, when profound hyponatremia exists, correction should be done slowly to avoid hyponatremic encephalopathy ($\leq$1 mEq/L/h)
• When profound metabolic acidosis exists, isotonic sodium bicarbonate solutions are indicated
• Plasma transfusion if failure of transfer of passive immunity is evident
• Abdominal drainage via placement of an abdominal catheter. A balloon-tip Foley catheter or peritoneal dialysis catheter is ideal and can be placed through a small (5 mm) incision under local anesthesia
• Placement of a urinary catheter and bladder decompression should be done before surgery and may be useful for small defects in the bladder, when these may heal without surgery

Hyperkalemia
• Isotonic saline solutions with dextrose (2.5–5%) administered IV
• For unresponsive hyperkalemia, regular insulin can be administered with a continuous infusion of dextrose. Regular assessment of serum glucose should be performed
• Calcium gluconate may be administered for cardioprotective effects

ACTIVITY
Restricted movement is recommended before and after surgery for at least 14 days.

DIET
Allow the foal to continue to nurse until shortly before surgery.

CLIENT EDUCATION
• Clients will need to know about correct care for the abdominal incision
• Careful observation for recurrence suggesting surgical failure

SURGICAL CONSIDERATIONS
• Emergency surgery is not indicated until the foal is medically stable

• Before surgery, place a urethral catheter (e.g. Foley)
• Constant ECG monitoring and acid–base assessment should be performed during surgery
• Ventral midline celiotomy and laparoscopic techniques are described
• Thorough inspection and assessment of structural defects should identify any necrotic/infected tissue
• Conservative treatment is placement of urinary catheter (via urethra) for 3–5 days to allow constant drainage of bladder without surgical correction of tear. It is useful when surgical repair is not available (cost, expertise) and the defect is small

MEDICATIONS

DRUG(S) OF CHOICE
• Broad-spectrum antimicrobial coverage, especially neonates with presumed sepsis and acquired rupture, e.g. sodium penicillin (25 000–40 000 IU/kg IV every 6 h) and amikacin sulfate (25 mg/kg IV every 24 h)
• NSAIDs may be given to control pain and inflammation related to surgery
• Insulin (0.1–0.2 IU/kg SC or IV) may be given with dextrose infusions to help reduce the extracellular potassium concentration

CONTRAINDICATIONS
Avoid potassium-containing IV fluids or medications composed of potassium salts, e.g. potassium penicillin.

PRECAUTIONS
In hypovolemic patients, aminoglycosides and NSAIDs should be used with caution and at judicious dosages. Where possible, amikacin is the preferred aminoglycoside and ketoprofen is the preferred NSAID.

POSSIBLE INTERACTIONS
N/A

ALTERNATIVE DRUGS
For broad-spectrum antimicrobial coverage, third-generation cephalosporins may be used.

FOLLOW-UP

PATIENT MONITORING
• Serum electrolytes (especially potassium and sodium) and urea/creatinine concentrations should be performed every 2–6 h to assess response to stabilization
• Monitoring of urine output postoperatively—should be $\geq$1 mL/kg/h
• Postoperative indwelling urinary catheter use is controversial—reduces distinction on

the surgical site, but has a risk of ascending infection, and may lead to increased intravesical pressure if occluded

PREVENTION/AVOIDANCE
N/A

POSSIBLE COMPLICATIONS
• Significant anesthetic risk occurs where electrolyte derangements exist
• Surgical dehiscence and re-rupture of the bladder
• Incisional complications include infection, dehiscence, hernia, although uncommon
• Peritonitis

EXPECTED COURSE AND PROGNOSIS
• Congenital uroperitoneum associated with ruptured bladder and/or urachus carries a favorable prognosis, >80%, provided timely medical and surgical therapy is administered
• The prognosis for rupture of the ureter carries a poorer prognosis
• The prognosis for secondary uroperitoneum is considered less favorable, 50–60%, largely influenced by the primary disease process, such as septicemia

MISCELLANEOUS

SYNONYMS
• Uroabdomen
• Ruptured bladder

SEE ALSO
• Colic in foals
• Meconium retention
• Patent urachus

ABBREVIATIONS
NSAID = non-steroidal anti-inflammatory drug

Suggested Reading
Bryant JE, Gaughan EM. Abdominal surgery in neonatal foals. Vet Clin North Am Equine Pract 2005;21:511–535.
Dunkel B, Palmer JE, Olson KN, et al. Uroperitoneum in 32 foals: influence of intravenous fluid therapy, infection, and sepsis. J Vet Intern Med 2005;19:889–893.
Kablack KA, Embertson RM, Bernard WV, et al. Uroperitoneum in the hospitalised equine neonate: retrospective study of 31 cases, 1988–1997. Equine Vet J 2000;32:505–508.

Author Samuel D.A. Hurcombe
Consulting Editor Margaret C. Mudge

U

URTICARIA

BASICS

DEFINITION
Urticaria and AG are common inflammatory reaction patterns resulting from mast cell and, to a lesser extent, basophil degranulation. AG is a focal or diffuse excessive accumulation of tissue fluid within the interstitium, often at gravitative surfaces, that presents as edematous swellings, which may exhibit serum leakage through the skin or hemorrhage. Urticarial reactions vary in severity from inconsequential to problems of a life-threatening nature.

PATHOPHYSIOLOGY
The release of cellular inflammatory mediators such as histamine, platelet-activating factor, and prostaglandins contributes to increased vascular smooth muscle relaxation and endothelial cell retraction, causing plasma to extravasate and cause turgid edematous wheals. Urticaria is classified as immunologic, immediate immunoglobulin E-mediated (type I), immune complex-mediated (type III), or delayed cell-mediated (type IV) hypersensitivities, or nonimmunologic.

SYSTEMS AFFECTED
• Skin/exocrine
• Respiratory

GENETICS
Genetic predisposition is suspected.

INCIDENCE/PREVALENCE
Urticaria is within the top 10 most common equine dermatoses.

GEOGRAPHIC DISTRIBUTION
Worldwide

SIGNALMENT
Suspected Breed Predilections
Arabians, Thoroughbreds, Quarter Horses, and Warmbloods may be predisposed because of their propensity to develop allergic dermatitis. Larger cohorts must be compared with general hospital populations to confirm breed predispositions.

Mean Age and Range
Mean age of onset is unknown.

Predominant Sex
Equal distribution exists between males and females.

SIGNS
General Comments
• Onset of lesions can be acute or peracute episodes occurring 15 min to hours post challenge. Chronic urticaria is a relapsing presentation that persists for at least 6–8 weeks. The characteristic lesion is a wheal—a flat-topped papule/nodule with steep-walled sides resulting from localized transient edema within the dermis. Pitting edema is a key clinical feature of urticaria or

AG, although gyrate urticaria often does not pit. Clinical classification of urticaria relies on size and appearance
• Conventional—wheal size varies from 2–3 mm to 3–5 cm in diameter
• Papular—wheal size is uniform and small, ≈3–6 mm in diameter
• Gyrate (polycyclic)—wheals have unusual shapes such as annular, doughnut, serpiginous, aciform and can persist for months
• Giant—single or multiple wheals that range from 20 to 40 cm in diameter
• Exudative—severe dermal edema oozes from the skin, mats the hair, and causes alopecia, often mistaken for pyoderma, dermatophytosis, and pemphigus foliaceus
• Linear—firm, multiple, parallel contiguous banding patterns that can be present on the sides of trunk, shoulders, forearms, flanks, gaskins, and the cranial aspects of hocks. Often permanent and nonresponsive to steroid and antihistamine therapy. Multiple horses on farm may be affected
• AG (angioneurotic edema)—diffuse SC edema, affecting head, thorax, ventral abdomen, and/or gravity-dependent extremities

CAUSES
Causes are either immunologic or nonimmunologic, with the former the most common.
• Immunologic causes include:
  ○ Insect hypersensitivity (stinging and biting insects), atopy (pollens, molds, and epidermals), food allergy
  ○ Drugs (including vaccines, anthelmintics)
  ○ Various others such as penicillin, tetracycline, sulfonamides, neomycin, ciprofloxacin, phenylbutazone, flunixin, phenothiazines, guaifenesin, ivermectin, moxidectin, iron, dextrans, hormones, and vitamin B complex
  ○ Infections—bacterial (e.g. strangles, salmonellosis, botulinum,), pyoderma, cellulitis, lymphangitis, abscess, dermatophytosis, parasitic protozoal (e.g. *Trypanosoma equiperdum*)
  ○ Vasculitis (immune-mediated or photo-activated)
  ○ Contact with substance (e.g. leather soaps, conditioners, or rubber tack)
  ○ Snakebite
  ○ Plants (e.g. nettle and buttercup)
  ○ Mast cell or lymphoreticular neoplasia
  ○ Autogenous sweat
• Nonimmunologic factors include psychologic stresses, genetic abnormalities, temperature (heat, cold, or sunlight), physical (pressure or dermatographism), exercise, cholinergic, and administration of radiocontrast media and opiates
• Idiopathic—the likelihood of documenting a specific etiology of chronic urticaria is low, thus the diagnosis of "idiopathic" is common

RISK FACTORS
• Temperate environments with long allergy seasons
• Concurrent pruritic dermatoses, such as insect hypersensitivity (summation effect)
• Treatment by polypharmacy

DIAGNOSIS

DIFFERENTIAL DIAGNOSIS
Differential diagnoses for urticaria vary with the morphologic presentation.
• Conventional—vasculitis
• Papular—infectious and sterile folliculitis, frequently associated with biting insects, in particular mosquitoes and *Culicoides* spp.
• Giant—vasculitis
• Gyrate—erythema multiforme, drug reactions

CBC/BIOCHEMISTRY/URINALYSIS
• Leukocytosis suggests inflammatory or infectious disease
• Thrombocytopenia may be secondary to vasculitis.

OTHER LABORATORY TESTS
Relevance equated to etiology.

DIAGNOSTIC PROCEDURES
• Biopsy—used to differentiate urticaria, pyoderma, pemphigus, dermatophytosis, or vasculitis
• Dermatographism test—scratch the skin with blunt object and observe for reaction within 10–15 min. A positive reaction is an edematous wheal that follows the path of the scratch
• Heat- or cold-induced urticaria is confirmed by applying a reusable hand warmer or ice cube to the skin for a few minutes with the formation of a wheal within 15 min
• Exercise-induced urticaria requires a period of active exercise to occur, whereas cholinergic urticaria results from an active (exercise) or a passive (hot bath) increase in core body temperature
• Sweat-induced urticaria can be induced at work or with α_2-adrenoreceptor agonist drugs such as detomidine hydrochloride or xylazine. An IDT with purified sweat dilutions can be used to confirm diagnosis
• An IDT is used to identify causative allergens (pollens, molds, epidermals) for inclusion into allergen-specific immunotherapy
• Horses with a suspected adverse reaction to food should undergo a food exclusion trial. Start with a 4–8 week trial of a novel food source such as single-source hay (alfalfa, orchard, timothy, or coastal Bermuda grass). Single-source grains include rolled oats, beet pulp, or barley. Commence food trial by eliminating all grains, supplements, and drugs, and feed single-source hay. After resolution of urticaria, confirm food allergy

by rechallenging with the introduction of 1 item each week
• A patch test is used to identify contact reactions. Clip a small area on the lateral aspect of the neck with a no. 40 blade. Place a small amount of the test substance on a piece of gauze and affix it so that the substance is in contact with the clipped area. Remove the gauze and observe for urticaria 24–48 h after application
• Skin scrapings, fungal and bacterial cultures, and impression smears should be performed if infectious causes are suspected

 TREATMENT

AIMS
Identify and eliminate the primary cause.

APPROPRIATE HEALTH CARE
Depends on etiology.

NURSING CARE
Frequent bathing using cool water (antimicrobial shampoos, chlorhexidine, sulfur/salicylic acid, ± colloidal oatmeal rinses, antimicrobial sprays with 1% hydrocortisone or leave-on conditioners) removes allergens, crusts, bacteria, and debris, controls secondary infections, hydrates skin, and counters pruritus.

ACTIVITY
Determined by severity and cause.

DIET
Essential fatty acid supplementation may be beneficial. Omega 3 fatty acids provide EPA and DHA for anti-inflammatory and skin barrier support.

CLIENT EDUCATION
Depends on etiology.

 MEDICATIONS

DRUG(S) OF CHOICE
• Glucocorticoids are indicated to break the cycle of mediator-induced inflammation. Use a rapid-acting glucocorticoid such as prednisolone sodium succinate (0.25–10.0 mg/kg IV)
• If refractory to antihistamine therapy, use oral prednisolone at 0.5–1.5 mg/kg every 24 h until control achieved; then reduce to lowest dose alternate-day regimen, e.g. 0.2–0.5 mg/kg every 48 h

• If refractory to prednisolone, try dexamethasone at initial loading oral or IV dose of 0.02–0.1 mg/kg PO every 24 h for 2–4 days followed by oral maintenance dose of 0.01–0.02 mg/kg every 48–72 h for maintenance
• Repository injectable corticosteroids should be avoided as withdrawal upon an adverse reaction is not possible
• Antihistamines—hydroxyzine hydrochloride or pamoate at 1–2 mg/kg PO every 8–12 h or cetirizine hydrochloride at 0.4 mg/kg PO every 12 h or chlorpheniramine (chlorphenamine) at 0.25–0.5 mg/kg PO every 12 h may be effective

CONTRAINDICATIONS
• Because of the anticholinergic properties of antihistamines and tricyclic antidepressants, do not use in patients with a history of cardiac arrhythmias, colic, glaucoma, or urinary retention disorders. Antihistamines may thicken mucus in the respiratory tract. Use extra caution in horses with respiratory problems owing to excess mucus
• Administration of ivermectin with cetirizine can prolong cetirizine elimination half-life through P-glycoprotein inhibition

PRECAUTIONS
• Epinephrine may cause excitement in horses; if administered SC, its potent vasoconstriction activity leads to poor absorption and local tissue necrosis
• Adverse effects of epinephrine therapy are tachyarrhythmia and myocardial ischemia
• The use of epinephrine should be avoided with the use of α_2-adrenoreceptor agonists such as xylazine or detomidine HCl as they potentate α_2-agonist effects
• Taper patients on long-term steroid therapy so endogenous steroid production resumes
• Transient sedation may occur with antihistamines

POSSIBLE INTERACTIONS
Antihistamines have an additive effect with other CNS-depressant drugs.

 FOLLOW-UP

PATIENT MONITORING
Horses with respiratory and/or GI involvement should be monitored at a facility with an intensive care unit.

PREVENTION/AVOIDANCE
Depends on the etiology.

POSSIBLE COMPLICATIONS
• Most serious complication of AG is respiratory compromise
• AG may involve the GI tract, leading to intestinal wall edema and clinical signs of colic and/or diarrhea
• CNS signs may occur secondary to focal cerebral edema

EXPECTED COURSE AND PROGNOSIS
• Prognosis is generally good to excellent for control of urticaria
• Linear urticaria may be more difficult to control or resolve
• Spontaneous remission occurs

 MISCELLANEOUS

ASSOCIATED CONDITIONS
AG—pleural or peritoneal effusion.

AGE-RELATED FACTORS
Severity may worsen with age.

PREGNANCY/FERTILITY/BREEDING
Antihistamines—no information on teratogenicity is available for horses.

SYNONYMS
Hives

SEE ALSO
• Atopic dermatitis
• Insect hypersensitivity

ABBREVIATIONS
• AG = angioedema
• CNS = central nervous system
• DHA = docosahexaenoic acid
• EPA = eicosapentaenoic acid
• GI = gastrointestinal
• IDT = intradermal test

Suggested Reading
Fadok VA. Equine urticaria. In: Noli E, Foster A, Rosenkrantz W, eds. Veterinary Allergy. Chichester, UK: Wiley Blackwell, 2014:338–343.

Author Gwendolen Lorch
Consulting Editor Gwendolen Lorch

 U

UTERINE INERTIA

BASICS

DEFINITION

Primary Uterine Inertia

• Lack of myometrial contractions. • May result in RFM. • Associated/related conditions—lack of exercise, overconditioning, chronic illnesses, twinning, uterine disease, and aging

Secondary Uterine Inertia

• Usually follows prolonged labor without expulsion of the fetus and exhaustion of the myometrium. • More common than primary uterine inertia. • To increase the likelihood of delivering a live fetus, assist mares with uterine inertia, once the condition is diagnosed

PATHOPHYSIOLOGY

• *Primary inertia*—may result from failure of the myometrium to respond to hormonal stimulation; lack of hormonal release; or deficiency of hormonal receptors for oxytocin, estrogen, and/or $PGF_{2\alpha}$. • *Secondary inertia*—exhaustion of the muscle fibers occurs with prolonged labor

SYSTEMS AFFECTED

Reproductive

GENETICS

N/A

INCIDENCE/PREVALENCE

Secondary inertia—<1% of foaling mares.

SIGNALMENT

• All breeds. • All females of breeding age

SIGNS

• Mares in dystocia frequently are affected. • Often a history of prolonged labor, then signs/evidence of labor cessation

CAUSES

The major cause is dystocia

RISK FACTORS

• Restricted or lack of exercise during pregnancy has repeatedly been incriminated. • Limited exercise can also be linked with overconditioning and overweight mares. • Older mares may experience an increased incidence. • Benefits of exercise (fit mares) include less fatigue with/during delivery, shortened time for parturition, and improved body tone and abdominal strength

DIAGNOSIS

DIFFERENTIAL DIAGNOSIS

Dystocia from any cause.

CBC/BIOCHEMISTRY/URINALYSIS

N/A

OTHER LABORATORY TESTS

N/A

IMAGING

N/A

OTHER DIAGNOSTIC PROCEDURES

Observe the mare's expulsive efforts and examine the uterus to determine if purposeful contractions are occurring.

PATHOLOGIC FINDINGS

None specific.

TREATMENT

Primary Uterine Inertia

• First assist with delivery of the fetus, then administer oxytocin. • Foaling mares need assistance if normal delivery times for stages 1 and 2 are exceeded. • The window of time for successful delivery (i.e. to deliver a live foal) is very short in the mare

Secondary Uterine Inertia

• When diagnosed, no correction is possible before the dystocia is resolved. • If oxytocin is administered before fetal delivery, the uterus will contract around the fetus and compound delivery problems

APPROPRIATE HEALTH CARE

N/A

NURSING CARE

N/A

ACTIVITY

N/A

DIET

N/A

CLIENT EDUCATION

N/A

SURGICAL CONSIDERATIONS

N/A

MEDICATIONS

DRUG(S) OF CHOICE

After removal/delivery of the fetus, oxytocin 10 IU IM is the treatment and hormone of choice.

CONTRAINDICATIONS

N/A

PRECAUTIONS

N/A

POSSIBLE INTERACTIONS

• Avoid high doses of oxytocin, which are unnecessary and may cause excessive contractions and impact the likelihood of uterine prolapse. • $PGF_{2\alpha}$ enhances uterine contractions, but the clinical significance of these contractions has been questioned. • Do not attempt correction of uterine inertia before the fetus is delivered, and only then treat with low doses (10 IU IM) of oxytocin

ALTERNATIVE DRUGS

N/A

FOLLOW-UP

PATIENT MONITORING

Postpartum uterine examinations:
• Determine if involution is proceeding normally after oxytocin administration.
• Determine if all of the fetal membranes have passed

PREVENTION/AVOIDANCE

• Exercise and proper nutrition play important roles in preventing primary uterine inertia. • Secondary uterine inertia occurs most frequently, but may be impossible to prevent unless parturition is observed and assistance is rendered as soon as dystocia is observed

POSSIBLE COMPLICATIONS

• RFM. • Delayed uterine involution. • Both RFM and delayed uterine involution may result in uterine infection and/or inflammation, which can delay rebreeding or result in infertility

EXPECTED COURSE AND PROGNOSIS

• Excellent prognosis with proper treatment. • May be warranted to skip breeding on foal heat. • The final decision regarding feasibility of breeding on foal heat can be reserved until examination of the uterus near/at the time of breeding, to assess adequacy of the mare's recovery

MISCELLANEOUS

ASSOCIATED CONDITIONS

• Dystocia, especially if prolonged, can lead to secondary uterine inertia. • RFM can occur after uterine inertia

AGE-RELATED FACTORS

Incidence increases with age.

ZOONOTIC POTENTIAL

N/A

PREGNANCY/FERTILITY/BREEDING

Occurs only at parturition and shortly thereafter.

SEE ALSO

• Dystocia. • Postpartum metritis. • Uterine torsion

ABBREVIATIONS

• $PGF_{2\alpha}$ = prostaglandin $F_{2\alpha}$
• RFM = retained fetal membranes

Suggested Reading

Miller CD. Dystocia management in equine practice. Clin Theriogenol 2010;2(3):338–343.

Roberts SJ. Veterinary Obstetrics and Genital Diseases (Theriogenology), 3e. Woodstock, VT: SJ Roberts, 1986:347–352.

Author Carla L. Carleton

Consulting Editor Carla L. Carleton

U

BASICS

DEFINITION
Torsion or twisting of the uterus at its body, less often extending caudally to involve the cervix.

PATHOPHYSIOLOGY
• Stretching or lengthening of the broad ligament, which permits the uterus additional leeway to twist on itself
• This may result from repeated stretching during previous gestations, rapid movement of the fetus; rolling or falling and turning of the mare, faster than the speed with which the fetus and uterus can rotate (differential rate of rotation)

SYSTEMS AFFECTED
Reproductive

GENETICS
• No hereditary predisposition for uterine torsion
• If the supporting tissue (i.e. broad ligament) were longer in some animals because of genetics, it would support the theory of hereditary predisposition

INCIDENCE/PREVALENCE
• Infrequent occurrence; anytime during the last 6 months of pregnancy
• It is frequently found at 6–9 months and should be corrected when diagnosed
• The later in gestation torsion occurs, the more serious are the consequences

SIGNALMENT
• Females; all breeds
• Most affected are mares with deeper bodies or larger abdomens
• All mares of breeding age
• Increased occurrence in pluriparae

SIGNS
General Comments
The mare exhibits a variety of clinical signs, depending on the stage of gestation when torsion occurs.

Historical Findings
May present with signs of slight to mild colic, inappetence, depression, or general decrease or increase in activity, sweating, and increased urination.

Physical Examination Findings
• Depending on the stage of gestation, the mare may exhibit a tense abdomen, increased heart rate on auscultation, and increased respiratory rate
• TRP reveals twisting of the broad ligament and body of the uterus and/or cervix
• Vaginal examinations are less valuable in mares (compared with cows), because involvement of the vagina in the torsion is uncommon
• At term, mares fail to show signs of labor, because the fetus is unable to enter the pelvic canal and cervix (i.e. absence of Ferguson's reflex). Therefore, fetal death may occur from placental separation without the owner's knowledge

CAUSES
• Cause unknown
• There appears to be a causal relationship with either excessive relaxation of the broad ligament or an inadequate suspension provided by the broad ligament
• Fetal movement, or secondary to a mare falling or rolling, can affect the probability of developing uterine torsion

RISK FACTORS
• Dam with a large abdomen
• Multiple pregnancies
• Primiparae may be affected

 DIAGNOSIS

DIFFERENTIAL DIAGNOSIS
• Intestinal colic—rule out by TRP to determine if the broad ligament twists to the left or right
• Normal labor—rule out by the absence of membrane rupture and/or release of chorioallantoic fluid, etc.; assessment of normal uterine suspension between the left and right mesometria

CBC/BIOCHEMISTRY/URINALYSIS
N/A

OTHER LABORATORY TESTS
N/A

IMAGING
Transabdominal ultrasonography examination, if necessary, to determine fetal viability.

OTHER DIAGNOSTIC PROCEDURES
N/A

PATHOLOGIC FINDINGS
• The uterus may be turned clockwise or counterclockwise, placing increased tension on the broad ligament. The uterine wall may have increased tone
• Counterclockwise torsion is more common than clockwise torsion in the mare

 TREATMENT

APPROPRIATE HEALTH CARE
• Accurate diagnosis is important to correct torsion before the fetus dies
• If left untreated, a torsion of >180° compromises the blood supply to the fetus and uterus; fetal death may occur, especially if the mare is near term gestation

Rolling
• Usually not indicated, unless sufficient help is available and the mare is not near term (<9 months of gestation)
• Mare must be anesthetized. Multiple people are needed to rapidly roll the mare in the direction of the torsion:
  ○ Lay the mare down on the side toward which the torsion is turning
  ○ Clockwise torsion, on the mare's right side
  ○ Counterclockwise torsion, on the mare's left side
  ○ Then roll the mare over on its back to the other side—safety is critical
  ○ Advisable to place ropes on the mare's legs to lift and turn,; remain slightly distant from the legs and possible mishaps
• Contraindications as the mare approaches term pregnancy—uterine artery rupture or uterine wall tears (more common than when this same procedure is used to relieve torsion in cows)
• Assistance is required to remain available after the procedure until the mare recovers from anesthesia and stands

Laparotomy
• Excellent technique, because minimal assistance is necessary and repositioning is very successful, especially if <9 months of gestation
• As the mare approaches term, additional help may be required, including the possibility of a second incision in the opposite flank; 1 person to push from 1 side, rock and pull upwards to *unflip* on the opposite side, the 2 surgeons work as a team
• If 1 incision is to be used:
  ○ Must be adequate to allow the surgeon to pull the ventral aspect of the uterus into the proper position
  ○ It is easier to pull the uterus than it is to push the uterus and fetus
• If an additional incision is necessary, the second surgeon pulls/applies lift on the dorsal aspect, as the primary surgeon applies traction to the ventral aspect of the uterus

Caesarean Section
• Can be performed in cases of uterine torsion, but correcting the torsion before incising the uterus makes it easier to extract the fetus and to suture the uterus
• Usually only necessary when the fetus is at term and delivery must be immediate, or if the fetus is dead and vaginal delivery is not possible
• Usually unnecessary, because most torsions occur before the onset of labor

NURSING CARE
Implement care by:
• Bedding changes in the stall
• Cross-tying, or
• Other managerial options that may discourage the mare from rolling in the stall

ACTIVITY
• After correction of the torsion, stall rest the mare
• Hand-walk the mare until parturition, if possible

UTERINE TORSION (CONTINUED)

• Prevent the mare from running or having the opportunity to roll

DIET
• Permit access to free-choice hay
• Quality is not as important as quantity, keep the abdomen as full as possible

CLIENT EDUCATION
Remind owners that, with any condition of pregnant mares, subtle changes in her demeanor or behavior may indicate an abnormal gestation; seek immediate assistance.

SURGICAL CONSIDERATIONS
• A grid incision usually fails to provide sufficient area for manipulation, and incision of the abdominal muscles is necessary
• A hand is moved ventrally under the uterus, and a fetal hock or other extremity is grasped and pulled toward the incision
• At first, the uterus will be difficult to move, but as it begins returning to its normal position, movement will become easier
• Once uterine detorsion passes the halfway point, it will easily move the remainder of the distance
• If 1 person cannot return the uterus to its normal position, a second incision can be made on the opposite side of the mare, and both surgeons can pull the uterus to return it to its normal position

MEDICATIONS

DRUG(S) OF CHOICE
• Xylazine IV, followed 5–10 min later with IV morphine, detomidine, or drug of choice
• Infiltrate the area for incision with 2% mepivacaine (Carbocaine), to effect

CONTRAINDICATIONS
N/A

PRECAUTIONS
• Confirm the diagnosis as rapidly as possible, especially if the mare is near term, to save the fetus
• Administration of the previously mentioned agents should not be detrimental to fetal viability at any stage of gestation

POSSIBLE INTERACTIONS
N/A

ALTERNATIVE DRUGS
N/A

FOLLOW-UP

PATIENT MONITORING
• Frequent after correction of uterine torsion
• Close daily observation and TRP examination of the uterus at 1–2 week intervals until it appears that recurrence is unlikely
• Progesterone supplementation (altrenogest (ReguMate), 0.044 mg/kg once daily PO for 1–2 weeks) may provide some benefit; maintaining cervical tone and preventing ascending contamination of the genital tract after the stress of the procedure
• For mares at term and in labor, recurrence of this condition after delivery has not been reported

PREVENTION/AVOIDANCE
• Limiting exercise is 1 possible method to reduce the likelihood of the mare falling or rolling, but rarely is indicated or warranted
• Limited exercise may result in an increase in difficult deliveries
• Free-choice hay is advisable and it may reduce the occurrence of abdominal colic

POSSIBLE COMPLICATIONS
Uterine torsion can result in prolonged delivery and fetal death.

EXPECTED COURSE AND PROGNOSIS
Correction before term requires follow-up examinations; recurrence is possible.

MISCELLANEOUS
N/A

ASSOCIATED CONDITIONS
N/A

AGE-RELATED FACTORS
Old mares may have increased occurrence because of previous broad ligament stretching.

ZOONOTIC POTENTIAL
N/A

PREGNANCY/FERTILITY/BREEDING
Only occurs in pregnant animals.

SYNONYMS
N/A

SEE ALSO
• Dystocia
• Premature placental separation

ABBREVIATIONS
TRP = transrectal palpation

Suggested Reading
Blanchard TL, Taylor TS, Varner DD, Brinsko SP. Uterine torsion in the mare. Clin Theriogenol 2010;2(2):123–125.
Perkins NR, Robertson JT, Colon LA. Uterine torsion and uterine tear in a mare. J Am Vet Med Assoc 1992;201:92–94.
Wichtel JJ, Reinertson EL, Clark TL. Nonsurgical treatment of uterine torsion in seven mares. J Am Vet Med Assoc 1988;193:337–338.
Author Carla L. Carleton
Consulting Editor Carla L. Carleton
Acknowledgment The author/editor acknowledges the prior contribution of Walter R. Threlfall.

BASICS

Numerous factors must be considered when determining the need for vaccination of horses. The efficacy of the vaccine must be weighed against the risk and consequences of infection and the adverse effects and cost of the vaccine. The timing of the primary series may be influenced by the effect of passively acquired maternal antibodies on the foal's response to vaccination. The timing of subsequent vaccination is influenced by the duration of immunity provided by the vaccine and time of anticipated risk of exposure. The guidelines that follow have evolved with the consideration of these factors.

BOTULISM

Clostridium botulinum produces several different toxins. In North America, horses are most frequently affected by type B. Types A and C also occur in the USA, but they are rare compared with type B. Although all 3 forms cause severe neuromuscular paralysis, the currently available toxoid only protects against type B. Vaccination is effective and is not associated with side effects; thus, it is highly recommended for horses in endemic areas (most commonly the mid-Atlantic states and provinces)
• Horses in endemic areas should receive an initial series of 3 vaccinations 1 month apart and then an annual booster
• Broodmares—8, 9, 10 months of gestation to prevent toxicoinfectious botulism in foals. Thereafter, a single yearly booster is given 4 weeks prepartum
• Foals from vaccinated mares—3, 4, and 5 months age
• Foals from unvaccinated mares—2, 6, and 10 weeks of age (no maternal antibody interference)

ENCEPHALOMYELITIS

• In North America, EEE is restricted to the eastern and southeastern USA and Canada. WEE occurs primarily in the western USA and western Canada (although cases of WEE have been reported on the east coast)
• All commercially available encephalomyelitis vaccines are inactivated and provide protection against both EEE and WEE
• Venezuelan equine encephalitis has been reported in Mexico—horses residing in states on the Mexican border are frequently vaccinated
• Should be given in the spring prior to the emergence of the insect vector in cool climates
• Warm climates—vector is present throughout the year; biannual vaccination
• Pregnant mares—vaccinate 4–6 weeks prior to the anticipated foaling date
• Foals that receive adequate colostral antibody are protected for the first 6 months of life in cool climates

• Foals from vaccinated mares—first dose at 4–6 months of age, second 4–6 weeks after first, third dose at 10–12 months of age. Foals in southeastern USA should receive additional dose at 2–3 months of age.
• Foals from unvaccinated mares—first dose at 3–4 months of age, second 4 weeks later, third dose 8 weeks after second. Start at 3 months if in southeastern USA

EQUINE VIRAL ARTERITIS

• Causes abortion in mares and severe respiratory disease in neonates; fever, anorexia, limb and ventral edema, and nasal and ocular discharge in adult horses
• Frequently spread by aerosolized respiratory secretions during outbreaks of respiratory disease
• Chronically infected carrier stallions act as a reservoir and may infect mares by the venereal route
• Modified live vaccine has been effective in controlling outbreaks of respiratory disease, protecting mares that are to be bred to infected stallions, and preventing stallions from becoming chronically infected
• Some states/countries have developed programs aimed at controlling spread of the virus, and officials and breed associations should be consulted prior to vaccination
• Seropositive horses may be ineligible for export to some countries; therefore, horses should be tested for antibodies to this virus prior to vaccination to confirm that they are seronegative
• At-risk breeding stallions/teasers—4 weeks prior to the breeding season
• Open mares to be bred to infected stallions—not <3 weeks prior to breeding
• Pregnant mares should not be vaccinated
• Colts—single dose at 6–12 months

INFLUENZA

• Vaccination for influenza provides immunity that is short in duration and incomplete in protection
• Pathogen is ubiquitous and causes explosive outbreaks; regular vaccination is especially beneficial for horses entering high-risk environments, such as shows, training centers, and breeding farms
• Inactivated, modified live, and canary pox vector vaccines
• Foals from vaccinated and unvaccinated mares:
  ○ Inactivated—3-dose initial series— 6 months, 7 months, and 10–12 months of age; booster at 6 month intervals
  ○ Modified live vaccine (intranasal) and canary pox—6 months and 7 months; booster at 6 month intervals
  ○ Increased risk may warrant vaccination in younger foals, but a complete initial series should still be given after 6 months owing to maternal antibody interference
• Broodmares—modified live is not recommend; inactivated or canary pox vaccines—4–6 weeks prepartum

• Unvaccinated adults need 3-dose initial series for inactivated; 2-dose initial series for modified live and canary pox vaccines
• Semiannual vaccination for at-risk horses, annual for low-risk horses

POTOMAC HORSE FEVER

• Caused by *Neorickettsia risticii* and is characterized by fever, diarrhea, depression, anorexia, laminitis, colic, and death
• Documented in most of North America, risk factors include environments with access to water in the form of rivers, creeks, and irrigation ditches
• Inhabits fluke-infested snails, caddisflies, and mayflies
• Vaccination is generally limited to areas with a high prevalence
• Duration of immunity is short and protection is incomplete; may be due to heterogeneity of the organism
• Vaccine is safe and should be given prior to the disease season
• In the eastern and midwestern USA—occurs from mid-summer to fall; in California it occurs from fall to spring. Revaccination may be necessary 3–4 months later
• Broodmares—4–6 weeks prepartum
• Foals in endemic areas—3 doses 1 month apart, beginning at 3–5 months of age

RABIES

• Fatal zoonosis—all horses in endemic areas should be vaccinated
• Foals from nonvaccinated mares— 1 vaccination at 6 months of age +1 month later
• Foals from vaccinated mares—initial vaccination at 6 months of age or older +1 month later
• Annual vaccination
• Vaccination with the inactivated product can be given to pregnant mares prepartum or prior to prior to breeding

RHINOPNEUMONITIS

• EHV-1 and EHV-4 vaccination is short-lived and incomplete protection against abortion and respiratory disease
• Both modified live and inactivated vaccines are available
• Specifically labeled for protection against only respiratory disease or abortion
• No vaccine licensed to protect against the neurologic strain of EHV-1
• Foals should be vaccinated with inactivated or modified live—first dose 4–6 months of age, second dose 4 weeks later, third dose at 10–12 months of age
• Unvaccinated adult should receive initial 3-dose series
• Consider 6 month revaccination interval in horses <5 years of age, in contact with pregnant mares or on breeding farms, performance horses, or those in frequent contact with new horses
• Broodmares—prevention of abortion: vaccinate during the fifth, seventh, and ninth

VACCINATION PROTOCOLS   (CONTINUED)

months of gestation, with an optional dose at the third month with product labeled for EHV abortion. Vaccinate with product labeled for EHV-1 and EHV-4 respiratory disease at 4–6 weeks prepartum

ROTAVIRUS
• Can cause outbreaks of infectious diarrhea in the majority of a foal crop on individual farms during the first few weeks of life
• Inactivated rotavirus A vaccine containing the G3 (H-2) serotype is conditionally licensed in the USA for use in pregnant mares on endemic farms as an aid to preventing diarrhea in their foals caused by rotaviruses of serogroup A
• Safe and there is evidence of partial efficacy
• Vaccinate mare during months 8, 9, and 10 of gestation; repeat during each at-risk pregnancy

STRANGLES
• Caused by *Streptococcus equi* ssp. *equi*
• Vaccination is generally limited to horses at risk; horses residing on farms with previous outbreaks or horses entering these farms are candidates for vaccination. Although vaccination is not indicated for horses already infected, uninfected and unexposed horses may benefit from vaccination during an outbreak
• Purpura haemorrhagica is a rare adverse reaction to vaccination
• M-protein antigen extract vaccine (killed):
  ◦ Naive horses—3 doses at an interval of 3 weeks, booster doses are given once annually
  ◦ Additional booster at 6 months of age for foals when the initial series is started at <3 months of age
  ◦ Pregnant mares—1 month prepartum booster

• Modified live intranasal vaccine:
  ◦ Initial 2 doses at 2–3 week intervals. Annual booster
  ◦ Ideally no other vaccinations are given concurrently and invasive procedures such as joint injections, dental prophylaxis, and castrations should not be performed simultaneously owing to risk of abscess formation at these locations as a result of accidental contamination with live *S. equi*
  ◦ Not recommended in foals <1 year of age owing to risk of significant clinical disease (fevers and lymph node enlargement) and increased shedding of the vaccine strain

TETANUS
• Horses have high sensitivity to the toxin and it is ubiquitous in the environment
• Vaccination beginning at 6 months of age, with an initial series of 3 doses of toxoid 4 weeks apart
• Thereafter, yearly boosters
• Although vaccination confers long-lasting immunity, it is an accepted practice to booster horses that incur lacerations more than 6 months since the last vaccination
• Broodmares 4–6 weeks prior to the anticipated foaling date
• Unvaccinated horses or horses with an uncertain vaccination history should receive tetanus antitoxin and tetanus toxoid given at separate sites if wounded
• Foals born to unvaccinated mares should receive tetanus antitoxin and toxoid shortly after birth. Tetanus antitoxin is rarely associated with fatal acute hepatic necrosis

WEST NILE VIRUS
• Transmitted by infected mosquitos and results in meningoencephalitis
• Infection most commonly occurs from July to October; can be seen all year in southeastern USA

• Adult initial series—2–3 doses 4 weeks apart depending on brand
• Broodmares—4–6 weeks prepartum
• Annual vaccination prior to onset of vector season
• Consider 6 month revaccination interval for endemic areas, horses <5 years, geriatrics, immunocompromised horses
• Foals from both vaccinated and unvaccinated mares—vaccinate at 3–4 months of age with an initial series of 3 vaccines 1 month apart (maternal antibodies have been shown to not interfere with foal vaccination). Start at 3 months in endemic areas

 MISCELLANEOUS

ABBREVIATIONS
• EEE = Eastern equine encephalitis
• EHV = equine herpesvirus
• WEE = Western equine encephalitis

Internet Resources
American Association of Equine Practitioners, Vaccination Guidelines 2015. https://aaep.org/guidelines/vaccination-guidelines

Suggested Reading
Wilson WD. Strategies for vaccinating mares, foals, and weanlings. Proc Am Assoc Equine Pract 2005;51:421–438.

Author Ashley G. Boyle
Consulting Editor Ashley G. Boyle
Acknowledgment The author/editor acknowledges the prior contribution of Kerry E. Beckman.

BASICS

OVERVIEW
• Displacement of all or part of the vaginal wall posteriorly through the vulva
• The condition is primarily seen in the postpartum period in mares and is thought to be due to relaxation of the vaginal wall and vulvar lips, allowing eversion of the vagina
• Increased abdominal pressure (i.e. straining) places additional pressure on the vaginal wall
• Rarely, straining may be associated with the presence of pelvic or cervical masses

SIGNALMENT
• All breeds
• All females of breeding age

SIGNS
• The vaginal wall protrudes through the vulva
• The vaginal wall may become damaged and permit paravaginal fat to protrude through the prolapsed wall
  ○ This protruded fat may cause additional straining and further prolapse
• The protruding tissue has a characteristic pink to red color, depending on the length of time it has been outside the body
• Essential to differentiate vagina from bladder, intestines, uterus, cervix, and vestibule before initiating treatment

CAUSES AND RISK FACTORS
• Generally secondary to dystocia or other abnormalities that initially predispose mares to everting part of the vaginal wall
• This may cause straining and additional tissue protrusion and injury

 DIAGNOSIS

DIFFERENTIAL DIAGNOSIS
• Persistent hymen and hematocolpometra
• Eversion of the bladder, uterus, or cervix
• Vaginal tears through which paravaginal fat or intestines may be protruding
• Eversion of the vestibular wall

CBC/BIOCHEMISTRY/URINALYSIS
N/A

OTHER LABORATORY TESTS
N/A

IMAGING
Ultrasonography may be indicated to examine the prolapsed tissue, which may contain other structures.

OTHER DIAGNOSTIC PROCEDURES
Careful visual and digital examination to differentiate the vaginal wall from other prolapsed tissues.

PATHOLOGIC FINDINGS
Protrusion of the vaginal wall through the vestibule and vulvar lips.

 TREATMENT

• Reduction of prolapse, i.e. return tissues to their normal anatomic location, and terminate subsequent expulsive efforts; critical to permanent resolution
• Reduction of inflammation, if present, is advisable
• No restriction of activity, unless the activity increases abdominal pressure
• Any protrusion of tissue through the vulvar lips requires immediate attention
• Caslick's vulvoplasty may help prevent further vaginal irritation and, thus, decrease the likelihood of additional straining and tissue damage. Vulvoplasty, however, does not prevent recurrent prolapse from straining

 MEDICATIONS

DRUG(S) OF CHOICE
• Epidural anesthetic may be indicated to reduce straining
• Application of local, nonirritating antibiotics may aid in recovery

CONTRAINDICATIONS/POSSIBLE INTERACTIONS
N/A

 FOLLOW-UP

PATIENT MONITORING
At reexamination, careful and gentle assessment of previously affected tissues to prevent renewed irritation and reinitiation of straining.

PREVENTION/AVOIDANCE
• Treat any conditions, e.g. vaginal damage or irritation, that may initiate straining and result in eventual prolapse of the vaginal wall
• Once recognized, initiate treatment of prolapsed vaginal tissue as quickly as possible; limit tissue trauma

POSSIBLE COMPLICATIONS
Vaginitis, vaginal adhesions, vaginal tears.

EXPECTED COURSE AND PROGNOSIS
• Rapid recovery if the inciting cause is removed
• Satisfactory recovery if further damage can be avoided

 MISCELLANEOUS

ASSOCIATED CONDITIONS
N/A

AGE-RELATED FACTORS
N/A

ZOONOTIC POTENTIAL
N/A

PREGNANCY/FERTILITY/BREEDING
Usually occurs after parturition.

SEE ALSO
• Dystocia
• Vaginitis and vaginal discharge

Suggested Reading
Cox JE. Surgery of the Reproductive Tract in Large Animals, 3e. Liverpool, UK: Liverpool University Press, 1987:127–143.

Author Ahmed Tibary
Consulting Editor Carla L. Carleton
Acknowledgment The author and editor acknowledge the prior contribution of Walter R. Threlfall.

V

VAGINITIS AND VAGINAL DISCHARGE

BASICS

OVERVIEW
• Vaginitis is inflammation of the vagina, which can be infectious. • Vaginal/vulvar discharge can occur as a result of vestibulovaginitis, breeding injury, cervicitis, metritis, or abnormalities of the vagina or the urinary system (ectopic ureters).
• Pneumovagina—one of the major causes of vestibular and vaginal inflammation; caused by abnormal VC. • Also may occur in fillies or mares in training or racing because of incomplete vulvar development. • Breed differences—increased incidence in mares with poor body condition (i.e. little fat) or less muscle in the perineal area (e.g. contrast Thoroughbreds and Standardbreds with Quarter Horses). • Severe postpartum vaginitis (often necrotic) is observed following dystocia and lengthy obstetrical manipulations or fetotomy

Genetics
Possible inheritance of poor VC, which results in vaginitis.

SIGNALMENT
• All females of breeding age. • Occurs more often in old mares

SIGNS

Normal Discharge
• Urine, especially the characteristic appearance of calcium carbonate crystals that may accumulate at/on the ventral vulvar commissure during estrus. • This occurs secondary to frequent urination and evacuation of sediment common in equine urine, especially during estrus

Abnormal Discharge
• Consistency—mucoid or fluid, may be odiferous. • Color ranges—white to yellow to brown. • Note that mares may have vaginitis without external discharge. • Bloody vaginal discharge may be observed following breeding trauma

Historical Findings
• Infertility or subfertility. • Periodic discharge throughout the cycle. • Dystocia

Physical Examination Findings
When secondary to infection or inflammation, there may be: • Discharge on the tail and perineum. • Fluid in the vagina or uterus

CAUSES AND RISK FACTORS
• Poor VC. • Trauma at parturition. • Vaginal breeding injury. • Pneumovagina.
• Multiparous broodmares are highest risk.
• Less frequent in young maidens (not broodmares). • Congenital abnormalities of the vagina (double vagina) and urinary system (ectopic ureters)

DIAGNOSIS

DIFFERENTIAL DIAGNOSIS
• Uterine disease/infection. • Urinary tract infection

CBC/BIOCHEMISTRY/URINALYSIS
N/A

OTHER LABORATORY TESTS
N/A

IMAGING
N/A

OTHER DIAGNOSTIC PROCEDURES
Careful speculum examination per vagina is the best means to establish a definitive diagnosis.

PATHOLOGIC FINDINGS
• Hyperemia of the vaginal mucosa. • Fluid accumulation may be observed. • Abrasions, ulcerations, and lacerations may be present:
∘ Recent or chronic—adhesions or fibrin deposition. • Vulvar discharge does not always accompany vaginitis. • Large amounts of discharge may be adhered to the tail or attract flies during summer months.
• Discharge may be evident only when the mare is more excitable, being ridden, or otherwise worked

TREATMENT
• Exact cause must be determined before treatment is initiated. • If only vaginitis (i.e. not secondary to injury), treatment needs only to halt additional contamination, and inflammation should subside. • Systemic antibiotics—no value. • Local therapy if antibiotics are indicated and used.
• Postpartum application of antibiotic-containing emollient cream.
• Caslick's vulvoplasty—repair deficits in VC, if present

MEDICATIONS

DRUG(S) OF CHOICE
• If indicated after vulvoplasty, nonirritating, local application of antibiotics may reduce the mare's discomfort. • This is usually unnecessary, as inflammation decreases rapidly once the source of irritation is resolved

FOLLOW-UP

PATIENT MONITORING
Reexamination 1–2 weeks after vulvoplasty.

PREVENTION/AVOIDANCE
Caslick's vulvoplasty or other cosmetic repair of vulvae and vestibular sphincter: • Mares born with poor VC have an increased likelihood of vaginitis; breed or individual mare predisposition. • Postpartum, if injured at foaling

POSSIBLE COMPLICATIONS
If left untreated, may result in infertility, endometrial damage, and/or vaginal adhesions.

EXPECTED COURSE AND PROGNOSIS
• If treated early in the course of disease, excellent resolution and normal fertility.
• Postpartum necrotic vaginitis may result in vaginal adhesions

MISCELLANEOUS

ASSOCIATED CONDITIONS
Linked with chronic vaginitis and uterine contamination: • Metritis. • Endometritis.
• Pyometra

AGE-RELATED FACTORS
• Prevalence increases with age.
• Conformation problems and/or damage to the caudal genital tract increase with age and parity

ZOONOTIC POTENTIAL
N/A

PREGNANCY/FERTILITY/BREEDING
May prevent pregnancy or cause abortion.

SEE ALSO
• Contagious equine metritis (CEM).
• Dystocia. • Endometritis. • Postpartum metritis. • Pneumovagina/pneumouterus.
• Vulvar conformation

ABBREVIATIONS
VC = vulvar conformation

Suggested Reading
Threlfall WR, Carleton CL. Vaginitis and vaginal discharge. In: Carleton CL, ed. Blackwell's Five-Minute Veterinary Consult Clinical Companion, Equine Theriogenology. Ames, IA: Wiley Blackwell, 2011:576–584.

Author Ahmed Tibary
Consulting Editor Carla L. Carleton
Acknowledgment The author and editor acknowledge the prior contribution of Walter R. Threlfall.

BASICS

DEFINITION
Ventricular arrhythmias originate in the ventricle and the term *ventricular premature depolarization* refers to isolated premature complexes. VPD can occur singly, or in pairs or triplets. More than 4 VPDs in succession is VT and can be either paroxysmal or sustained. Complexes that have a uniform appearance are termed monomorphic, whereas if there are more than 2 configurations the VT is described as polymorphic.

PATHOPHYSIOLOGY
• A number of different electrophysiologic mechanisms are responsible for the development of ventricular arrhythmias, including reentry, enhanced automaticity, and accelerated conduction
• Ventricular arrhythmias often occur in association with other systemic illness
• Primary myocardial disease is an infrequent cause.

SYSTEMS AFFECTED
Cardiovascular

SIGNS
General Comments
• VPDs may be found incidentally when they are infrequent
• VT is often associated with what is perceived to be abdominal pain

Historical Findings
• Acute onset
• Poor performance
• Weakness and collapse
• Congestive heart failure

Physical Examination Findings
• Individual premature beats or runs of rapid, regular, or irregular rhythm
• Loud booming heart sounds
• Jugular pulses
• Respiratory distress

• Generalized venous distention and congestive heart failure

CAUSES
• Hypoxia
• Sepsis
• Toxemia
• Drugs such as inhalation anesthetics, digoxin, and quinidine sulfate
• Autonomic imbalance
• Metabolic and electrolyte imbalance
• Primary myocardial disease

RISK FACTORS
• Gastrointestinal and renal disease
• Endotoxemia
• Infective endocarditis
• Aortic regurgitation
• Aortic root rupture

DIAGNOSIS

DIFFERENTIAL DIAGNOSIS
• Supraventricular arrhythmias—differentiate with ECG
• Sinus tachycardia—differentiate with ECG

CBC/BIOCHEMISTRY/URINALYSIS
Electrolyte or metabolic abnormalities may be present.

OTHER LABORATORY TESTS
• Increased serum concentration of cardiac troponin I may be present
• Blood culture may be indicated in some cases

IMAGING
ECG
• VPDs are represented by a QRS–T complex that occurs prematurely and is different in configuration from those arising in the ventricle. The QRS complex usually appears widened and bizarre, with a T wave oriented in the opposite direction to the QRS complex. It is not preceded by a P wave

• With VT, there is a rapid ventricular rate with QRS and T complexes that are abnormal for the lead. P waves are present but occur less frequently than the ventricular depolarizations and are buried in the other complexes. The R–R interval may be regular or irregular. All ventricular QRS complexes and T waves may look identical (monomorphic; Figure 1 or vary in appearance (polymorphic; Figure 2)

Echocardiography
• With isolated VPD and monomorphic VT and no underlying cardiac disease, the echocardiogram is often normal or there may be a slightly low shortening fraction
• With polymorphic VT and primary myocardial disease, there are more profound decreases in fractional shortening and abnormalities of myocardial wall motion (dyskinesis or akinesis) and mitral and aortic valve motion
• Foci of increased or decreased echogenicity are occasionally seen within the myocardium
• Echocardiography may reveal evidence of other cardiac diseases such as infective endocarditis, severe valvular disease, pericarditis, or aortic root rupture

Thoracic Radiology
Pulmonary edema may be detected in horses with VT.

OTHER DIAGNOSTIC PROCEDURES
Continuous 24 h Holter Monitoring
This is particularly helpful in identifying intermittent or paroxysmal ventricular arrhythmias, in quantifying numbers of isolated VPDs, and in assessing response to therapy.

Exercise ECG
Characterization of the effect of exercise on ventricular arrhythmias is important in assessing their clinical significance.

PATHOLOGIC FINDINGS
• The heart may be normal, grossly and histopathologically, in horses with no underlying cardiac disease

V

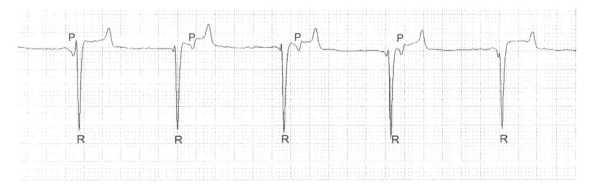

Figure 1.

Monomorphic ventricular tachycardia or accelerated idioventricular rhythm (AIVR)—the VPDs (R) have the same configuration and have no relationship to the P wave; base–apex lead 25 mm/s, 5 mm = 1 mV.

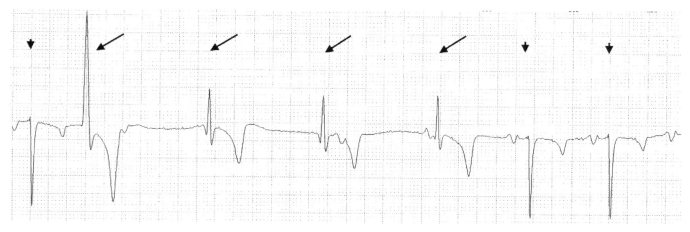

Figure 2.

Polymorphic ventricular tachycardia—4 VPDs (arrows) with 2 configurations that differ from those of sinus origin (arrowheads); base–apex lead 25 mm/s, 5 mm = 1 mV.

- Focal or diffuse myocardial necrosis, inflammation, or fibrosis may be present

 TREATMENT

AIMS
- Address any predisposing causes
- Antiarrhythmic therapy is restricted to cases in which the rhythm is unstable and life-threatening

APPROPRIATE HEALTH CARE
Antiarrhythmic therapy is considered if the horse shows signs of low cardiac output, the ventricular rate exceeds 100 bpm, an R-on-T phenomenon is present (QRS complexes come immediately after the preceding T wave), and/or the VT is polymorphic.

NURSING CARE
- Continuous ECG monitoring should be performed during antiarrhythmic therapy
- Horses should be kept quiet and not moved during the antiarrhythmic therapy

ACTIVITY
Horses with VT or frequent isolated VPDs during exercise should not be exercised.

CLIENT EDUCATION
The risks associated with the treatment need to be discussed with the owner (see Possible Complications).

 MEDICATIONS

DRUG(S) OF CHOICE
- VPDs are not usually treated with antiarrhythmics but may respond to corticosteroids if due to primary myocarditis
- Treatment of VT is usually an emergency and requires the use of IV preparations. The choice of the first drug used depends on the severity of the ventricular arrhythmia present and the onset of action of the drug selected, as well as the other side effects that the drug may have such as being a negative inotrope
- IV magnesium sulfate (25 g/450 kg slowly IV over 20–30 min) is occasionally successful in correcting sustained ventricular tachycardia in both hypomagnesemic and normomagnesemic horses and has no negative inotropic effect
- Lidocaine hydrochloride is very rapidly acting but has central nervous system side effects that limit the dose that can be administered to an awake horse (0.25 mg/kg IV as a bolus)
- Quinidine gluconate is one of the most successful antiarrhythmic drugs for horses with sustained ventricular tachycardia. Quinidine has a negative inotropic effect that is thought to be present only at high dosages but that may be a problem in horses with severe myocardial dysfunction. Quinidine gluconate is administered is small boluses of 0.5–1 mg/kg every 5–10 min up to a total dose of 12 mg/kg. Quinidine sulfate is rarely indicated in horses with sustained ventricular tachycardia because it must be administered via nasogastric intubation
- Procainamide 1 mg/kg/min to a total dose of 20 mg/kg IV has also been successful and its negative inotropic effect is thought to be less than that of quinidine
- Vitamin C (20 mg/kg PO every 24 h) and vitamin E (10 IU/kg PO every 24 h) may also be beneficial owing to their antioxidant effect

CONTRAINDICATIONS
- Antidysrhythmic drugs can have proarrhythmic effects and their effects must be monitored carefully
- Quinidine gluconate should be administered carefully to horses with VT and severe myocardial dysfunction

PRECAUTIONS
- See Possible Complications
- IV lidocaine can cause seizures that may last for 5–10 min
- The QRS duration should be measured prior to each quinidine treatment. A prolongation of the QRS duration >25% of the pretreatment duration should prompt discontinuation of quinidine treatment. The development of colic, ataxia, convulsions, or bizarre behavior is a sign of quinidine toxicity and should prompt discontinuation of treatment

POSSIBLE INTERACTIONS
Antiarrhythmic drugs with different mechanisms of action can be used in combination, but specific guidelines are lacking and interactions are possible.

ALTERNATIVE DRUGS
- Most other drugs with efficacy against ventricular arrhythmias may be beneficial in converting horses with VT but have been less effective
- Phenytoin has been effective in VT refractory to other antiarrhythmics and is given orally at a starting dose of up to 20–22 mg/kg every 12 h PO and then modified to keep the drug in the target range (usually 10–15 mg/kg). Side effects include excitement, sedation, and other neurologic signs
- IV propafenone at a dose of 0.5–1 mg/kg in 5% dextrose given slowly to effect over 5–8 min has been successful in converting 1 horse with ventricular tachycardia but is not available in the USA in the IV formulation. Oral propafenone in conjunction with IV procainamide may have been helpful in achieving conversion in several horses
- Propranolol can be tried at 0.03–0.1 mg/kg IV but is not as successful in correcting VT as many of the other antiarrhythmic drugs

V

FOLLOW-UP

PATIENT MONITORING
• Continuous ECG monitoring should be performed in all horses being treated for VT, as the antiarrhythmic drugs administered are also arrhythmogenic
• Following treatment of VT or VPD, continuous 24 h Holter ECGs are useful in assessing whether complete resolution has occurred. Before returning to athletic activities, an exercise ECG should be obtained
• Owners and trainers should regularly monitor their horse's cardiac rhythm before high-intensity exercise. Any irregularities in the cardiac rhythm or poor performance should prompt a cardiac reexamination

PREVENTION/AVOIDANCE
The possibility of ventricular arrhythmias should be considered in horses with systemic illness, particularly if the heart rate is unexpectedly high.

POSSIBLE COMPLICATIONS
• With sustained VT, congestive heart failure or sudden death may ensue
• There are a myriad of complications that have been reported in horses treated for VT that can be broken down into cardiovascular and neurologic categories

Cardiovascular
• Other ventricular arrhythmias—may need to be treated with an antiarrhythmic unless ventricular rhythm is slow (<100 bpm) and uniform and no R-on-T detected
• Hypotension—needs to be monitored and treated with IV polyionic fluids and, if severe, with IV phenylephrine at 0.1–0.2 μg/kg/min to effect
• Congestive heart failure—treat with digoxin at 0.0022 mg/kg IV and furosemide at 1–2 mg/kg IV, if needed

• Sudden death—try to prevent it with continuous ECG monitoring and treatment of arrhythmias that do occur

Neurologic
• Indicative of quinidine, phenytoin, or lidocaine toxicity
• Ataxia—resolves upon return of plasma quinidine concentration to negligible levels
• Convulsions—administer anticonvulsants
• Sedation and bizarre behavior—resolves upon return of plasma drug concentrations to negligible levels
• Colic—indicative of quinidine toxicity, treat with analgesics as needed; has also been seen in several horses with magnesium sulfate and severe multiform ventricular tachycardia and congestive heart failure

EXPECTED COURSE AND PROGNOSIS
• The majority of horses with monomorphic VT convert to sinus rhythm with antiarrhythmic therapy if there is little or no underlying cardiac disease. Recurrences of VT can occur as the antiarrhythmic medication wears off
• Horses with sustained polymorphic VT are more difficult to convert and are more likely to have underlying myocardial disease

 MISCELLANEOUS

AGE-RELATED FACTORS
Older horses that develop ventricular tachycardia are more likely to have significant underlying cardiac disease.

PREGNANCY/FERTILITY/BREEDING
VT leading to low cardiac output is likely to lead to fetal compromise.

SYNONYMS
VTach

SEE ALSO
• Aortic rupture
• Bacteremia/sepsis
• Endocarditis, infective
• Endotoxemia
• Ionophore toxicosis
• Mitral regurgitation
• Myocardial disease
• Septicemia, neonate

ABBREVIATIONS
• VPD = ventricular premature depolarization
• VT = ventricular tachycardia

Suggested Reading
Reef VB, Marr CM. Dysrhythmias: assessment and medical management. In: Marr CM, Bowen M, eds. Cardiology of the Horse, 2e. Edinburgh, UK: Saunders Elsevier, 2010:159–178.
Reef VB, Bonagura J, Buhl R, et al. Recommendations for management of equine athletes with cardiovascular abnormalities. J Vet Intern Med 2014;28:749–761.
Reimer JM, Reef VB, Sweeney RW. Ventricular arrhythmias in the horse: twenty-one cases (1984–1989). J Am Vet Med Assoc 1992;201:1237–1243.
Sage A, Mogg TD. Pharmacology of drugs used to treat cardiac disease. In: Marr CM, Bowen M, eds. Cardiology of the Horse, 2e. Edinburgh, UK: Saunders Elsevier, 2010:75–87.
Wijnberg ID, Ververs FF. Phenytoin sodium as a treatment for ventricular dysrhythmia in horses. J Vet Intern Med 2004;18:350–353.

Author Celia M. Marr
Consulting Editors Celia M. Marr and Virginia B. Reef
Acknowledgment The author acknowledges the prior contribution of Virginia B. Reef.

VENTRICULAR SEPTAL DEFECT (VSD)

BASICS

DEFINITION
• A congenital defect (i.e. hole) in the interventricular septum, resulting in communication between the right and left ventricles
• Can be located in any portion of the interventricular septum—membranous (most common)

PATHOPHYSIOLOGY
• Blood shunts from the higher pressure left ventricle to the lower pressure right ventricle, then returns to the left atrium and ventricle via the lungs, creating primarily a left atrial and ventricular volume overload and, to a lesser degree, a right ventricular volume overload
• The size and location of the VSD determine the severity of the volume overload and the degree of right ventricular involvement
• With a large, membranous VSD, the left atrial and ventricular volume overload is severe. Over time, stretching of the mitral annulus occurs, and MR develops. As the MR becomes more severe, increases in left atrial pressure cause increased pulmonary venous pressure, increased pulmonary capillary pressure, pulmonary edema, pulmonary hypertension, and clinical signs of left-sided CHF. As pulmonary hypertension becomes more severe, clinical signs of right-sided CHF appear
• With a large, muscular VSD, the left atrial and ventricular volume overload and right ventricular volume overload are severe, and clinical signs of right-sided heart failure may predominate
• When a large VSD is located immediately below the aortic valve, the aortic valve may become incompetent, which further exacerbates left ventricular volume overload

SYSTEMS AFFECTED
Cardiovascular

GENETICS
Not yet determined in horses, but likely heritable.

INCIDENCE/PREVALENCE
Welsh Mountain ponies, Arabians, and Standardbreds at higher risk.

SIGNALMENT
• Murmurs present at birth
• Diagnosed most frequently in foals and young horses but may be found at any age

SIGNS
General Comments
Often detected as an incidental finding in mature horses if the VSD is small.

Historical Findings
• Medium to large VSDs—poor performance
• Large VSDs—CHF

Physical Examination Findings
• Grade 3–6/6, coarse, band-shaped, pansystolic murmur with PMI in the tricuspid valve area; membranous defect has loudest murmur here
• Grade 3–6/6, coarse, band or crescendo–decrescendo, ejection shaped, holosystolic or pansystolic murmur with PMI in the pulmonic valve area; outflow defect has loudest murmur here. With membranous VSD, pulmonic murmur is usually 1 grade quieter than the right-sided murmur owing to relative pulmonic stenosis
• Other less common findings—accentuated third heart sound, grade 1–6/6 holodiastolic decrescendo murmur with PMI in the aortic valve area, and AF

CAUSES
Congenital malformation of the interventricular septum.

RISK FACTORS
N/A

DIAGNOSIS

DIFFERENTIAL DIAGNOSIS
• Tricuspid regurgitation—no pulmonic murmur; differentiate echocardiographically
• VSD with pulmonic stenosis or bicuspid pulmonic valve—loudest murmur usually in the pulmonic valve area; differentiate echocardiographically
• Tetralogy of Fallot—foals are often stunted and may be tachycardic and hypoxemic; loudest murmur usually in the pulmonic valve area; differentiate echocardiographically

CBC/BIOCHEMISTRY/URINALYSIS
N/A

IMAGING
ECG
Atrial premature complexes or AF may be present with left atrial enlargement. Ventricular premature complexes also occur in some cases.

Echocardiography
• The most common location is the membranous portion of the interventricular septum, immediately beneath the septal leaflet of the tricuspid valve and right or noncoronary leaflet of the aortic valve. VSDs that are <2.5 cm in 2 mutually perpendicular planes or with a ratio of the VSD to the aortic root of <1:3 are generally restrictive with little hemodynamic impact
• Outflow VSD is less common and more difficult to detect echocardiographically because of its location ventral to the aortic and pulmonic valves
• Muscular VSD in other portions of the interventricular septum is less common; however, the entire ventricular septum should be examined

• More than 1 defect may be present
• Left atrium and ventricle—enlarged, dilated, and rounded in appearance
• Left ventricular free wall and interventricular septum—thinner than normal; pattern of left ventricular volume overload if the ventricle is coping well with the left-to-right shunt
• Normal or decreased fractional shortening with left ventricular enlargement is consistent with myocardial dysfunction
• Pulmonary artery dilatation with a large shunt fraction
• Pulsed-wave or color-flow Doppler reveals left-to-right shunt through the VSD
• Hemodynamic significance determined by the peak velocity of the shunt through the VSD—a peak velocity >4 m/s is consistent with a restrictive defect; a peak shunt velocity ≤3 m/s indicates a very hemodynamically significant shunt and a large VSD
• MR may be present with a large VSD and marked left atrial and ventricular volume overload

Thoracic Radiography
• An enlarged cardiac silhouette, tracheal elevation, and increased pulmonary vascularity may be detected with a large VSD
• Pulmonary edema may be present in affected horses with CHF

OTHER DIAGNOSTIC PROCEDURES
Cardiac Catheterization
• Right-sided catheterization can be performed to directly measure right atrial, right ventricular, and pulmonary arterial pressures and to sample blood for oxygen content
• Elevated right ventricular pressure should be detected with an increased oxygen saturation of blood obtained from the right ventricle and pulmonary artery if the shunt is left to right

Continuous 24 h Holter Monitoring
Useful in the diagnosis of suspected arrhythmias.

PATHOLOGIC FINDINGS
• Most frequently found in the membranous septum underneath the septal leaflet of the tricuspid valve and the right or noncoronary leaflet of the aortic valve but also can be present in any portion of the interventricular septum
• Associated jet lesions along the margins of the defect and on the adjacent right ventricular endocardium
• Left atrial and ventricular enlargement and thinning of the left atrial and ventricular myocardium and interventricular septum with a large shunt
• Right ventricular enlargement and thinning of the right ventricular free wall with a VSD that is large or in a muscular location
• Pulmonary artery dilatation with a large shunt fraction and in those with pulmonary hypertension

TREATMENT

AIMS
• Management by intermittent monitoring in horses with small- or medium-sized membranous VSD
• Palliative care in horses with large membranous or muscular VSD and CHF

APPROPRIATE HEALTH CARE
• Most affected horses require no treatment
• Monitor horses echocardiographically on an annual basis
• Affected horses with CHF can be treated with positive inotropic drugs, vasodilators, and diuretics. Consider humane destruction if CHF progresses because only short-term, symptomatic improvement can be expected

NURSING CARE
N/A

ACTIVITY
• Horses with small VSDs are safe to continue in unrestricted athletic work provided there is no significant arrhythmias or pulmonary artery dilation
• Monitor horses with hemodynamically significant VSDs echocardiographically on an annual basis to ensure they are safe to ride and compete. These horses can be used for lower level athletic work
• Horses with significant pulmonary artery dilatation are no longer safe to ride
• Affected horses that develop significant arrhythmias often decompensate and are no longer safe to use for athletic performance

DIET
N/A

CLIENT EDUCATION
• Regularly monitor cardiac rhythm; any irregularities other than second-degree atrioventricular block should prompt ECG
• Carefully monitor for exercise intolerance, respiratory distress, prolonged recovery after exercise, increased resting respiratory or heart rate, or cough; if detected, perform a cardiac reexamination
• Because the defect most likely is heritable, do not breed affected horses

SURGICAL CONSIDERATIONS
• Closure of the VSD would be possible with transvenous umbrella catheters if the umbrella diameter was large enough to close the defect. There are no published reports of this technique being successfully performed in horses to date

• Surgical closure would require rib resection for the thoracotomy and cardiac bypass, which are not financially feasible or practical for obtaining an equine athlete

MEDICATIONS

DRUG(S) OF CHOICE
N/A

CONTRAINDICATIONS
N/A

PRECAUTIONS
N/A

POSSIBLE INTERACTIONS
N/A

ALTERNATIVE DRUGS
N/A

FOLLOW-UP

PATIENT MONITORING
• Frequently monitor cardiac rate and rhythm and respiratory rate and effort
• With defects >2.5 cm in 2 mutually perpendicular planes or peak shunt velocity <4.5 m/s, annual echocardiographic reexaminations are recommended

PREVENTION/AVOIDANCE
N/A

POSSIBLE COMPLICATIONS
Large VSD—AF; CHF.

EXPECTED COURSE AND PROGNOSIS
• Horses with small (≤2.5 cm), restrictive (peak shunt velocity >4.5 m/s), membranous VSDs should have normal performance and life expectancy; they can even race successfully, although not at the top levels
• Progression of MR in horses with moderate VSDs usually is slow. These horses have normal life expectancy, but usually perform successfully only in less demanding disciplines
• Horses with large (>4 cm) VSDs that are hemodynamically significant (peak flow velocity ≤3 m/s) have a guarded prognosis; they usually have shortened performance and life expectancy
• Affected horses with CHF and MR have a guarded to grave prognosis for life. Most affected horses being treated for CHF respond to supportive therapy and transiently improve, but once CHF develops euthanasia of the horse is recommended

MISCELLANEOUS

ASSOCIATED CONDITIONS
• Aortic regurgitation can develop in horses with VSDs and aortic valve prolapse, caused by the lack of aortic root support owing to the location of the VSD
• MR can develop in horses with significant left atrial and ventricular volume overload secondary to stretching of the mitral annulus, further contributing to left atrial and ventricular volume overload

AGE-RELATED FACTORS
Young horses are more likely to be diagnosed.

PREGNANCY/FERTILITY/BREEDING
Do not breed affected horses because of the possibly heritable nature of these defects.

SYNONYMS
• Septal defect
• Interventricular septal defect

SEE ALSO
Aortic regurgitation

ABBREVIATIONS
• AF = atrial fibrillation
• CHF = congestive heart failure
• MR = mitral regurgitation
• PMI = point of maximal intensity
• VSD = ventricular septal defect

Suggested Reading
Hall TL, Magdesian KG, Kittleson MD. Congenital cardiac defects in neonatal foals: 18 cases (1992–2007). J Vet Intern Med 2010;24:206–212.
Reef VB. Heart murmurs in horses: determining their significance with echocardiography. Equine Vet J Suppl 1995;19:71–80.
Reef VB. Evaluation of ventricular septal defects in horses using 2 dimensional and Doppler echocardiography. Equine Vet J Suppl 1995;19:86–95.
Reef VB, Bonagura J, Buhl R, et al. Recommendations for management of equine athletes with cardiovascular abnormalities. J Vet Intern Med 2014;28:749–761.

Author Virginia B. Reef
Consulting Editors Celia M. Marr and Virginia B. Reef

VERMINOUS MENINGOENCEPHALOMYELITIS

BASICS

DEFINITION
Meningoencephalomyelitis associated with aberrant and unusual helminth and insect parasitic invasion of nervous tissues.

PATHOPHYSIOLOGY
• Aberrant migration of parasitic organisms of other species or organ systems
• Helminth and arthropod parasites identified from the equine CNS include nematodes (*Strongylus vulgaris, Strongylus equinus, Angiostrongylus cantonensis, Halicephalobus gingivalis, Setaria* spp., and *Draschia megastoma*) and fly larvae (*Hypoderma* spp.)
• The clinical signs result from physical tissue destruction, hemorrhage, and inflammation, or a space-occupying effect, depending on the parasite. *S. vulgaris* is the most pathogenic of the large strongyles and can form fibrinoparasitic emboli that directly block cerebral vasculature
• An additional immune-associated inflammatory response may contribute to the pathophysiologic picture

SYSTEMS AFFECTED
CNS and other specific tissues associated with the more common parasitic migration pattern.

INCIDENCE/PREVALENCE
Much decreased with the introduction of modern anthelmintics.

SIGNALMENT
• Not specific
• No breed, sex, or age predisposition

SIGNS
Multifocal neurologic signs that can be attributed to brainstem, cerebellum, or spinal cord involvement. History and physical examination signs are associated with the migratory pattern in each specific case and can include progressive:
• Ataxia
• Ascending paresis
• Decreased perineal tone
• Cranial nerve deficits variable, e.g. decreased menace response, ptosis, dropped lips
• Intention head tremor
• Muscle wasting
• Pyrexia

CAUSES
Many parasites have been implicated and identified and depend on geographic location.

RISK FACTORS
Horses may be under good deworming management schemes.

DIAGNOSIS

Most commonly, the diagnosis is made histologically on necropsy specimens. Verminous involvement should be suspected in any case of acute CNS disease without a history of trauma or intracarotid injection.

DIFFERENTIAL DIAGNOSIS
• Any central nervous system dysfunction
• Equine protozoal myeloencephalitis in the Americas

CBC/BIOCHEMISTRY/URINALYSIS
None specific to the disease.

OTHER LABORATORY TESTS
Good diagnostic evidence of cerebrospinal helminthiasis and myiasis would be an eosinophilic or neutrophilic, aseptic pleocytosis in cerebrospinal fluid with varying numbers of macrophages and RBCs. Inflammatory or hemorrhagic cytologic findings (e.g. xanthochromia, elevated protein concentration, RBCs), however, are more common.

IMAGING
Cervical vertebral radiographs if horse is ataxic—cervical vertebral malformation is a far more common disease.

PATHOLOGIC FINDINGS
Parasitic lesions with typical eosinophilic and other inflammatory infiltrates.

TREATMENT

CLIENT EDUCATION
Appropriate anthelmintic schedule.

MEDICATIONS

DRUG(S) OF CHOICE
• Anti-inflammatory therapy (e.g. flunixin meglumine 1.1 mg/kg every 12–24 h; dexamethasone 0.05–0.1 mg/kg every 6–24 h) may be useful
• Suggested larvicidal doses of antiparasitic drugs should be administered

• Treatment of suspect horses with fenbendazole (60 mg/kg) given once is justified
• Avermectins may be useful
• Others may become available

PRECAUTIONS
Regular anthelmintic treatment.

FOLLOW-UP

Regular detailed neurologic examination to assess response to therapy.

PREVENTION/AVOIDANCE
Regular anthelmintic treatment.

POSSIBLE COMPLICATIONS
Trauma associated with the primary neurologic deficits.

EXPECTED COURSE AND PROGNOSIS
Depends on severity of initial neurologic signs.

MISCELLANEOUS

ASSOCIATED CONDITIONS
N/A

AGE-RELATED FACTORS
N/A

ZOONOTIC POTENTIAL
N/A

PREGNANCY/FERTILITY/BREEDING
N/A

SEE ALSO
• Cerebellar abiotrophy
• Eastern (EEE), western (WEE), and Venezuelan (VEE) equine encephalitides
• Equine herpesvirus myeloencephalopathy
• Equine motor neuron disease
• Equine protozoal myeloencephalitis (EPM)
• West nile virus

ABBREVIATIONS
• CNS = central nervous system
• RBC = red blood cell

Suggested Reading
Lester G. Parasitic encephalomyelitis in horses. Compend Contin Educ Pract Vet 1992;14:1624–1630.
Mayhew IG. Large Animal Neurology, 2e. Ames, IA: Wiley Blackwell, 2008.

Author Caroline N. Hahn
Consulting Editor Caroline N. Hahn

BASICS

OVERVIEW
• RNA viral disease (*Vesiculovirus*, Rhabdoviridae) that primarily affects horses, cattle, and swine and occasionally sheep, goats, camelids, and wildlife
• 2 primary serotypes (New Jersey and Indiana)
• Epidemic or only a few animals
• Clinically indistinguishable from foot-and-mouth disease in ruminants and swine
• Transmission via arthropod vectors, aerosol or contact exposure to saliva or fluid from ruptured vesicles
• Incubation period is typically 2–8 days
• Suspected cases reportable in many other countries, including the USA

SIGNALMENT
Any age, sex, or breed of susceptible species.

SIGNS
• Vesicles or ulcers (includes mucocutaneous junction)—oral cavity (most common), nares, coronary bands, mammary glands, or external genitalia
• Transient fever
• Ptyalism
• Anorexia
• Weight loss
• Coronitis resulting in lameness and/or hoof wall deformation/laminitis/hoof wall sloughing
• Epistaxis
• Nasal edema, laryngitis, or pharyngitis
• Drop in milk production

CAUSES AND RISK FACTORS
• Virus spread via insect vectors (black flies, sand flies, and *Culicoides* spp.), mechanical transmission, and movement of animals
• Moving streams/creeks

DIAGNOSIS

DIFFERENTIAL DIAGNOSIS
• NSAID toxicosis
• Candidiasis
• Blister beetle (cantharidin) toxicosis
• Organophosphate paste dewormers (i.e. trichlorfon, dichlorvos)
• Plant awn stomatitis ulcerations
• Equine coital exanthema (equine herpesvirus 3)
• Autoimmune diseases, such as bullous pemphigoid or paraneoplastic bullous stomatitis
• Uremia
• Mechanical trauma or chemical contact

CBC/BIOCHEMISTRY/URINALYSIS
• Often within normal limits
• Stress leukogram may be present

• Electrolyte abnormalities and hemoconcentration secondary to dysphagia or anorexia

OTHER LABORATORY TESTS
• Significant antibody levels via complement fixation, VN, and/or ELISA (capture ELISA for immunoglobulin M or competitive ELISA) tests in the presence of active lesions (ELISA and VN maintain antibody titers many years after exposure)
• Virus isolation or real-time reverse transcriptase polymerase chain reaction performed on vesicular fluid, epithelial tissue, or direct swabs from recently ruptured vesicles

DIAGNOSTIC PROCEDURES
Cytologic and histopathologic examination of lesions may be useful in differentiating VS from other diseases.

PATHOLOGIC FINDINGS
Biopsy of acute lesions reveals nonspecific neutrophilic dermatitis, edema, epidermal necrosis, and reticular degeneration.

TREATMENT
Supportive care. Softened feeds may decrease cachexia due to anorexia. Cleanse lesions with mild antiseptics to avoid secondary bacterial infections. IV fluids in older animals to maintain hydration.

MEDICATIONS
Oral or IV NSAIDs may be indicated to control painful lesions. Studies suggest recombinant equine interferon-β1 given at a dose of 0.3–1.0 µg/kg IM every 2 days may be useful as a prophylactic treatment for animals at high risk, or animals showing the initial signs of the disease.

FOLLOW-UP

EXPECTED COURSE AND PROGNOSIS
• Self-limiting; lesions often heal within 2 weeks
• Months may be required for complete regression, especially in the case of an immunocompromised or metabolically deranged animal
• Scarring or depigmentation may occur
• Prognosis is excellent for recovery unless laminitis or secondary bacterial infections are present
• Immunity hypothesized to be short lived
• Reinfection during subsequent outbreaks is observed
• No cross-strain immunity

EPIDEMIOLOGY/PREVENTION
• High morbidity and low mortality
• Endemic in northern South America, Central America, and Mexico
• Sporadic outbreaks occur in southwestern USA
• Highly contagious for the first few days after rupture of the vesicles
• Quarantine for at least 14 days from the onset of lesions in the last affected animal on the premises
• Disinfect facilities and fomites with chlorine, iodine, or a quaternary ammonium compound
• Institute insect control measures
• No commercially available vaccine in the USA

COMPLICATIONS
• Secondary bacterial infections
• Laminitis
• Dehydration and weight loss secondary to anorexia

MISCELLANEOUS

ZOONOTIC POTENTIAL
• Humans have rarely contracted VS (influenza-like illness) when handling infected animals and under laboratory conditions. Wear protective measures (gloves, eyewear, and frequent handwashing)
• OIE removed VS from its list of internationally reportable animal diseases in 2015
• Still reportable in the USA; regulatory quarantine action is required on premises

PREGNANCY/FERTILITY/BREEDING
No known effects on pregnancy are documented.

ABBREVIATIONS
• ELISA = enzyme-linked immunosorbent assay
• NSAID = nonsteroidal anti-inflammatory drug
• OIE = Office International des Épizooties/World Organisation for Animal Health
• VN = virus neutralization
• VS = vesicular stomatitis

Suggested Reading
Kim L, Morley P, McCluskey B, et al. Oral vesicular lesions in horses without evidence of vesicular stomatitis virus infection. J Am Vet Med Assoc 2000;216(9):1399–1404.

Author Angela M. Pelzel-McCluskey
Consulting Editor Ashley G. Boyle
Acknowledgment The author and editor acknowledge the prior contribution of Kerry E. Beckman.

VICIA VILLOSA (HAIRY VETCH) TOXICOSIS

BASICS

OVERVIEW
• A systemic granulomatous disease of horses grazing green *Vicia villosa* (hairy vetch) and hypothesized to result from an unknown immunogen
• Other *Vicia* spp. (e.g. *Vicia dasycarpa, Vicia benghalensis*) also have been implicated
• *Vicia* spp. are legumes found throughout temperate regions of the USA and used as pasturage, hay, and silage
• There are no reports of disease in animals fed hay or silage
• Low morbidity, but high mortality in affected individuals

SIGNALMENT
No reported breed, age, or sex predispositions.

SIGNS
• Listlessness
• Welts on the skin
• Alopecia
• Dermatitis
• Skin peeling around the nares
• Lymphadenomegaly
• Dependent-limb edema
• Low-grade, persistent fever
• Wasting
• Diarrhea

CAUSES AND RISK FACTORS
• The specific toxin responsible is unknown
• The condition is hypothesized to be a type IV hypersensitivity reaction
• Associated with ingestion of the green plant
• Outbreaks are more common at the peak of plant growth during the spring
• Not all individuals grazing hairy vetch are affected, so unknown factors (e.g. growth stage of plant, dietary or environmental factors, or individual susceptibility) may be involved

DIAGNOSIS

DIFFERENTIAL DIAGNOSIS
• Systemic granulomatous disease caused by other unidentified causes—no known exposure to *Vicia* spp.

• Dermatophytosis—negative fungal cultures
• Bacterial dermatitis—negative cultures for dermatopathogens
• Pemphigus foliaceus—skin biopsy
• Drug eruption—history of recent drug administration
• Chronic urticaria—skin lesions pit with pressure

CBC/BIOCHEMISTRY/URINALYSIS
• Lymphocytosis
• Hyperproteinemia

OTHER LABORATORY TESTS
N/A

IMAGING
N/A

OTHER DIAGNOSTIC PROCEDURES
Skin biopsy.

PATHOLOGIC FINDINGS
Gross
• Thickened skin with scaling and alopecia
• Paleness of organs—heart, kidney, adrenal, and lymphoid tissues
• Lymphadenomegaly

Histopathologic
• Cellular infiltrations of monocytes, lymphocytes, plasma cells, eosinophils, and multinucleated giant cells in multiple organs
• Lesions are especially prominent perivascularly

TREATMENT
Generally unrewarding.

MEDICATIONS

DRUG(S) OF CHOICE
Glucocorticoids—prednisolone (0.2–4.4 mg/kg PO daily or BID) or dexamethasone (0.02–0.2 mg/kg PO daily).

CONTRAINDICATIONS/POSSIBLE INTERACTIONS
N/A

FOLLOW-UP

PATIENT MONITORING
N/A

PREVENTION/AVOIDANCE
Avoid reintroduction to pastures containing *Vicia* spp.

POSSIBLE COMPLICATIONS
N/A

EXPECTED COURSE AND PROGNOSIS
Mortality is high in affected animals.

MISCELLANEOUS

ASSOCIATED CONDITIONS
N/A

AGE-RELATED FACTORS
N/A

ZOONOTIC POTENTIAL
N/A

PREGNANCY/FERTILITY/BREEDING
N/A

Suggested Reading
Knight AP, Walter RG. A Guide to Plant Poisoning in North America. Jackson, WY: Teton NewMedia, 2001:169–170.
Woods LW, Johnson B, Hietala SK, et al. Systemic granulomatous disease in a horse grazing pasture containing hairy vetch (*Vicia* sp). J Vet Diagn Invest 1992;4:356–360.

Authors Arya Sobhakumari and Robert H. Poppenga
Consulting Editors Wilson K. Rumbeiha and Steve Ensley

BASICS

DEFINITION
Panvasculitis leading to edema, hemorrhage, and abortion in mares; respiratory disease and edema in other adults; severe illness or death in the neonate.

PATHOPHYSIOLOGY
• Small, enveloped, positive-stranded RNA virus, resistant to freezing, drying, and long storage at − 70°C. Reliably destroyed by a 1:32 dilution of commercially available sodium hypochlorite solution
• 1 serotype—Bucyrus. Evidence of antigenic variation among different isolates and variation in the degree of clinical signs produced
• Incidence, determined seroconversion, varies considerably by population and geographic location
• Highly contagious. Spread by direct contact with infected horses and their bodily secretions, including urine and milk, nasal droplet spray among racehorses, and venereal route at breeding farms. Isolated from the urine for up to 3 weeks post infection
• High morbidity and low mortality in adults—high mortality in neonates
• Carrier stallions harbor the virus in their accessory sex glands and shed virus in their semen. Carrier state is testosterone dependent. Virus may be present in frozen or cooled semen from carrier stallions. Seronegative mares bred to either short- or long-term carrier stallions are primary source of virus spread
• Seropositive mares bred to a carrier stallion may shed virus for a short period. Abortion due to infection secondary to myometrial necrosis and edema, resulting in failure of the uteroplacental unit
• Foals born to seropositive dams acquire passive immunity through the colostrum and become seronegative after passive immunity wanes. Foals may also acquire the virus through colostrum and milk; at least 2 foals are thought to have acquired a fatal form of the disease in this manner
• Nasal challenge—virus first replicates within alveolar macrophages and then appears in the bronchial lymph nodes; virus spreads throughout the body via the circulation. Vascular lesions develop associated with virus present in the tunica media of myocytes and within the endothelium. Arterial damage may persist for weeks after infection. The kidney is a site of virus localization, as is the placenta, bronchiolar epithelium, thymic tissue, and enterocytes in foals

SYSTEMS AFFECTED
• Whole body, except central nervous system
• Predominant systems affected—respiratory system in young horses, foals; urogenital system in pregnant broodmares and intact males

SIGNALMENT
• Any age or breed. Standardbreds have the highest seroconversion rates in the USA
• Immediate perinatal period foals; young racehorses, and broodmares at farms with a carrier stallion have the highest rates of incidence

SIGNS
From clinically silent and recognizable only by seroconversion to acute-onset severe disease resulting in abortion and neonatal death.

Historical Findings
• Abortion and neonatal death—possible exposure by residing on a farm where a carrier stallion is present
• Seronegative mare returning to the farm after being bred by a carrier stallion
• Young horses in training—association with an outbreak of respiratory disease ranging from mild to severe
• Neonates born to seronegative mares or that have failure of passive transfer of maternal antibody when born to seropositive mares

Physical Examination Findings
• Young adults and broodmares that develop clinical signs typically are febrile for 5–9 days
• Distal limb (often hindlimbs), conjunctival, periorbital, scrotal, and preputial edema
• Epiphora and nasal discharge associated with rhinitis and conjunctivitis
• Urticarial skin rash
• Cough, lethargy, anorexia, lameness, and exercise intolerance
• Abortion and stillbirth
• Rare sudden death in adults with particularly virulent isolates
• Foals—born normal or weak, edema, lethargy; sudden death or period similar to hypoxic–ischemic asphyxia syndrome before progressing to respiratory failure and death; can survive for more than 2 weeks prior to death

DIAGNOSIS

DIFFERENTIAL DIAGNOSIS
In young adults, differential diagnoses for EVA include all other infectious causes of respiratory disease, including, but not limited to:
• Equine influenza
• EHV-1 and -4
• Equine rhinitis virus
• Equine infectious anemia
• Equine adenovirus
• Hendra virus
Differentials for edema due to vasculitis include:
• Equine infectious anemia
• EHV-1
• Equine anaplasmosis

• Purpura haemorrhagica
The primary differential in an abortion storm is EHV-1. Differentials for affected neonates include:
• EHV-1
• Bacterial sepsis
• Severe hypoxic–ischemic asphyxial or inflammatory perinatal insult

CBC/BIOCHEMISTRY/URINALYSIS
• Lymphopenia and thrombocytopenia possible
• Urinalysis—renal tubular inflammation with or without casts possible

OTHER LABORATORY TESTS
Virus Isolation
Can be diagnostic antemortem. Acute cases have positive virus isolation from nasopharyngeal swabs or buffy coats from EDTA or citrated whole-blood samples. Virus can be isolated from the urine in more chronic cases. EVA is isolated from the placenta or fetal tissues in the case of abortion, although maternal blood and urine may also be submitted.

Serology
CF and VN tests can be used. CF is best in acute cases and will show a rise in titer 2–4 weeks after infection. This titer becomes undetectable after about 8 months. VN titers develop along with CF titers, peak at 2–4 months, and remain increased for years.

IMAGING
Thoracic radiographs—possible increased bronchiolar and interstitial pattern with areas of consolidation.

OTHER DIAGNOSTIC PROCEDURES
Immunoperoxidase histochemistry or PCR performed on postmortem or biopsy tissues can provide an accurate diagnosis in cases where EVA is suspected but has not been confirmed or as an adjunct to virus isolation and serology.

PATHOLOGIC FINDINGS
• Aborted and stillborn fetuses seldom have gross or histologic lesions, although EVA antigen may be identified in the fetus and/or placenta
• Adults and foals that die of fulminant EVA infection have a bronchointerstitial pneumonia. The lungs are heavy, wet, and congested grossly. The pneumonia is characterized by hypertrophy and hyperplasia of type II pneumocytes and the presence of eosinophilic laminar to granular material scattered within the alveolar lumen. Histologically, the pneumonia may appear similar to morbillivirus (Hendra virus) infection in adults. Lymphocytic arteritis and periarteritis with varying degrees of tunica media fibrinoid necrosis may also be observed
• Some infected foals are also reported to have pronounced gastrointestinal lesions

VIRAL ARTERITIS (EVA) (CONTINUED)

- Renal tubular epithelial necrosis and interstitial nephritis are present in most chronic cases
- Areas of edema are characterized by a lymphocytic vasculitis and perivasculitis

TREATMENT

APPROPRIATE HEALTH CARE
- Most horses with clinical disease recover with only supportive care. Horses may be best managed at home
- In the case of an outbreak, all affected horses should be kept isolated for a period of 40 days following the appearance of the last case
- Affected neonates need intensive medical management and should be hospitalized, although kept isolated from the rest of the hospital population, particularly pregnant mares

NURSING CARE
- Nursing care is minimal for adults
- Animals should be encouraged to eat and have stalls with good ventilation
- Hydrotherapy and support wraps may benefit those patients with distal limb edema
- Affected foals require intensive nursing, including IV fluid administration, frequent turning, feeding by nasogastric tube or by IV parenteral nutrition if anorexic, and respiratory management, up to and including assisted ventilation

ACTIVITY
- Activity should be minimal
- Racehorses should be out of training until they are no longer shedding virus, a period of about 40 days
- Hand-walking is permissible, and may benefit those with edema, but contact with other horses should be minimal while the horse continues to shed virus
- Acutely affected colts and stallions should have a prolonged period of sexual rest to decrease their chance of being chronic carriers
- Affected foals are incapable of activity

DIET
No dietary changes are required.

CLIENT EDUCATION
- Owners of affected foals should be informed of the poor prognosis for survival
- Owners of affected colts and stallions should be informed of the risk of their horse becoming a carrier
- All owners should be informed of the potential economic implications of seroconversion to EVA regarding import and export
- It is important that clients be educated regarding control of EVA. Many states have regulations surrounding the use of EVA carrier stallions, notably New York and Kentucky. These programs have significantly decreased the incidence of the disease in those states

MEDICATIONS

DRUG(S) OF CHOICE
- There is no specific treatment for EVA
- NSAIDs may be used to treat fever in adults
- Affected neonates may be treated with broad-spectrum antimicrobial drugs to combat secondary bacterial infection. Anecdotally, treatment of foals with plasma harvested from a donor with high EVA titers has been attempted with apparent success

FOLLOW-UP

PATIENT MONITORING
Patients should be monitored for continued fever and potential secondary bacterial invaders.

PREVENTION/AVOIDANCE
- Vaccination against EVA is available but is tightly controlled in some states. It is a modified live vaccine and control programs usually involve vaccination of all noncarrier stallions and seronegative mares served by carrier stallions. Carrier stallions are evaluated periodically by breeding to seronegative mares and performing virus isolation on semen samples
- Although international rules are loosening, seroconversion of a horse post vaccination may result in problems regarding import and export to certain countries

MISCELLANEOUS

ABBREVIATIONS
- CF = complement fixation
- EHV = equine herpesvirus
- EVA = equine viral arteritis
- NSAID = nonsteroidal anti-inflammatory drug
- PCR = polymerase chain reaction
- VN = virus neutralization

Suggested Reading
Balasuriya UB. Equine viral arteritis. Vet Clin North Am Equine Pract 2014;3:543–560.
Brunner KR, Santschi E, Gerber V, et al. Development of PCR methods for detection of EAV infection. [In German.] Schweiz Arch Tierheilkd 2014;156:527–538.
Del Piero F, Wilkins PA, Lopez JW, et al. Equine viral arteritis in newborn foals: clinical, pathological, serological, microbiological and immunohistochemical observations. Equine Vet J 1997;29:178–185.
Doll ER, Knappenberger RE, Bryans JT. An outbreak of abortion caused by the equine arteritis virus. Cornell Vet 1957;47:69–75.
Gilkerson JR, Bailey KE, Diaz-Méndez A, et al. Update on viral diseases of the equine respiratory tract. Vet Clin North Am Equine Pract 2015;31:91–104.
McCollum WH, Swerczek TW. Studies on an epizootic of equine viral arteritis in racehorses. Equine Vet J 1978;2:293–297.

Author Pamela A. Wilkins
Consulting Editor Ashley G. Boyle

VIRAL (HERPES) KERATITIS (PUTATIVE)

 BASICS

OVERVIEW
• Keratopathy or keratitis with associated conjunctivitis and epiphora putatively caused by EHV-2
• Systems affected—ophthalmic

SIGNALMENT
All ages and breeds affected; may be seen in herds.

SIGNS
• Multiple, superficial epithelial to subepithelial anterior stromal, whitish, punctate (organized in a grid-like manner), or linear opacities of the cornea, which may become confluent with chronicity, leading to the formation of a geographic corneal opacification (leukoma), with or without fluorescein and/or rose bengal dye retention
• Varying amount of ocular pain, conjunctivitis, corneal edema, epiphora, corneal vascularization, and iridocyclitis
• Drooping of upper lid eyelashes may occur, and is associated with discomfort

CAUSES AND RISK FACTORS
EHV-2 and, to a lesser degree, EHV-5 are the suspected agents, but equal prevalence of positive PCR assays for EHV-2 and EHV-5 have been found in normal control horses.

 DIAGNOSIS

DIFFERENTIAL DIAGNOSIS
• IMMK
• Superficial keratomycosis
• Superficial corneal ulcers
• Equine recurrent uveitis
• Conjunctivitis
• Glaucoma
• Blepharitis
• Dacryocystitis

CBC/BIOCHEMISTRY/URINALYSIS
N/A

OTHER LABORATORY TESTS
• Rule out other infectious causes (bacterial or fungal) of keratitis with corneal scrapings for cytology and culture
• Culturing virus from ocular specimens, and identification of viral isolates by use of PCR or electron microscopy

IMAGING, OTHER DIAGNOSTIC PROCEDURES, PATHOLOGIC FINDINGS
Conjunctival and/or corneal biopsy and identification of viral isolates by use of PCR or electron microscopy.

 TREATMENT

• Outpatient treatment may not lead to acceptable control of the associated signs of disease because owner compliance and cooperation from the horse is necessary for extended duration
• Treatment may lead to amelioration of signs; however, recurrences or a waxing and waning pattern of progression is often observed in affected horses
• Affected horses may present with aggressive behavioral issues that may reveal ocular discomfort. Such behavior will generally disappear once the disease has been controlled
• Activity should be reduced during periods of active inflammation, especially if accompanied by discomfort

 MEDICATIONS

DRUG(S) OF CHOICE
• Topical idoxuridine, trifluorothymidine, or acyclovir (aciclovir)—initially every 2 h, then 4–6 times per day
• Topical NSAIDs (diclofenamic acid, flurbiprofen, or bromfenac every 12 h) may be beneficial in reducing the effects of active inflammation
• Topical antiproteases, such as serum, may aid healing if a corneal ulcer is present

CONTRAINDICATIONS/POSSIBLE INTERACTIONS
• Topical corticosteroids are contraindicated as they may result in exacerbation of an underlying bacterial or fungal infection (which may be extremely difficult to completely rule out) and may ultimately lead to pseudo-recurrence
• Horses presenting with only punctate epithelial/subepithelial anterior stromal corneal opacification without ocular discomfort, conjunctival hyperemia, chemosis, or corneal vascularization may be self-limiting or without clinical significance. In these cases, initiation of aggressive medical therapy should be considered carefully, as this may lead to an exacerbation of clinical signs and the development of pseudo-recurrent inflammation

 FOLLOW-UP

EXPECTED COURSE AND PROGNOSIS
Treatment is often successful in the short term, but recurrence is common.

 MISCELLANEOUS

ASSOCIATED CONDITIONS
Superficial keratomycosis, superficial forms of IMMK, secondary bacterial infection.

AGE-RELATED FACTORS
Multiple foals or adults in a herd may be affected.

SEE ALSO
• Burdock pappus bristle keratopathy
• Calcific band keratopathy
• Corneal ulceration
• Eosinophilic keratitis
• Equine recurrent uveitis
• Glaucoma
• Superficial nonhealing ulcers
• Ulcerative keratomycosis

ABBREVIATIONS
• EHV = equine herpesvirus
• IMMK = immune-mediated keratitis
• NSAID = nonsteroidal anti-inflammatory drug
• PCR = polymerase chain reaction

Suggested Reading
Brooks DE. Ophthalmology for the Equine Practitioner, 2e. Jackson, WY: Teton NewMedia, 2008.
Hollingsworth SR, Pusterla N, Kass PH, et al. Detection of equine herpesvirus in horses with idiopathic keratoconjunctivitis and comparison of three sampling techniques. Vet Ophthalmol 2015;18(5):416–421.
Matthews AG, Brooks DE, Clode AB. Diseases of the equine cornea. In: Gilger BC, ed. Equine Ophthalmology, 3e. Ames, IA: Wiley Blackwell, 2017:252–368.

Author Richard J. McMullen Jr.
Consulting Editor Caryn E. Plummer
Acknowledgment The author and editor acknowledge the prior contribution of Andras M. Komaromy and Dennis E. Brooks.

 V

VISION

BASICS

OVERVIEW

- Equine vision has been a topic of great interest for both scientists and the horse industry. Research in equine vision and visual perception leads to better understanding of horse behavior. In turn, training and handling methods can be developed to improve the safety of the horse and handler
- Horses are a primarily open-range, prey species, with arrhythmic (diurnal and nocturnal) activity. Hence, good visual acuity throughout a wide, panoramic field is crucial for survival and allows recognition of conspecifics, predators, food items, and navigational landmarks
- The equine eye has developed a number of unique anatomic and physiologic features to suit its special visual needs. Important adaptations to avoid predators include a large visual field and improved detection of motion. These adaptations, however, limit the ability to detect fine visual details and color perception
- The anterolaterally positioned large eyes of the horse, combined with a horizontally elongated pupil and horizontal visual streak on the retina, provide a wide visual field of about 350°
- Anatomic studies reported a uniocular visual field of 190–195° on average, and up to 228°. In addition, the vertical visual field has been reported to be approximately 178°. The binocular overlap is approximately 55–65°, with a relatively large area of 75° overlap below the horse's head. Hence, overall, horses have an almost spherical field of view when their head is held level, with blind spots

perpendicular to the forehead, below the nose, and directly behind the horse. Further behavioral investigation of the equine visual perception showed, under study conditions, that horses can detect the appearance of objects within an almost fully encompassing circle. They can detect objects at both ground level and about 0.9 m above ground. These findings are consistent with anatomic studies. This panoramic vision of the horse can lead to misunderstanding of the horse's behavior, such as when the horse startles from something not apparent to the frontally focused handler/rider
- Behavioral studies have also shown that horses can identify objects within most of their panoramic field of view. They can detect objects within a nearly full circle of horizontal vision, and discriminate objects in their lateral field of view (i.e. monocular vision). Moreover, horses are capable of recognizing the same object placed in different orientations (e.g. rotated or upside down). However, although horses can see an object anteriorly, they need to turn their head, even if partially, to identify the object
- Horses, with laterally placed eyes and large monocular vision, may have poor binocular vision (stereopsis). However, research shows that horses can use stereoscopic information and are capable of utilizing monocular depth cues in judging distance. Nevertheless, the binocular threshold for depth perception in horses is 5 times better than the monocular threshold
- The presence of a horizontal retinal streak suggests that the horse should have good visual acuity not only frontally, but also laterally, as supported by behavioral studies in which horses demonstrated the ability to

discriminate objects on the lateral visual field. Moreover, a study has shown that, following unilateral enucleation, 85% of horses returned to work in their previous discipline, including racing and jumping at high level. The duration of vision loss (i.e. acute vs. chronic) did not seem to affect whether horses returned to work or not. Nevertheless, the functional impact of unilateral loss of vision is unknown
- The horse has 0.6 times the visual acuity of humans, 1.5 times that of dogs, and 3 times that of cats. That would mean a Snellen acuity of 20/33 (i.e. a horse viewing an object at a distance of 6 m has approximately the visual acuity of a person viewing the object at 10 m)
- A large-scale study of 333 horses in the UK found that about 85% of them were emmetropic (normal, with no refractive error), in agreement with other studies, and with no overall trend towards myopia (near sighted) or hyperopia (far sighted). Only 2.7% of the horses were found to have a refractive error of more than +1.5 D or −1.5 D (hyperopia or myopia, respectively). Interestingly, Thoroughbred crosses showed a tendency toward myopia, and Warmbloods/Shires toward hyperopia
- The aphakic equine globe is +9.9 D hyperopic (20/1200 Snellen equivalent). Although aphakic horses seem to perform well visually after cataract surgery, the potential impact of refractive error on the horse's visual function, performance, and safety is unclear
- The retina of the horse contains both rod and cone photoreceptors with rods outnumbering cones. Rods are most sensitive to dim light and are useful for motion detection. Cones are most sensitive to bright light, are responsible for color vision, and provide good visual resolution

• Like most mammals, horses have only 2 cone pigments and dichromatic color vision, whereas most humans typically have 3 cones and trichromatic vision. Each cone pigment responds to certain wavelengths better than others. In vivo evaluation of the equine spectral sensitivity has shown a primary peak at 539 nm (green-yellow), in reasonable agreement with molecular methods measuring the peak around 545 nm. A second peak was found at 428 nm, the far blue end of the color spectrum. The horse thus sees blue and yellow colors, but not red, and its visual perception of colors is believed to be similar to red–green blind humans, with a significant reduction in the number of different colors seen compared with trichromatic vision. Since the cones are primarily located in the central retina, color vision is largely restricted to the central retina, and the ability of the peripheral retina to detect color is substantially reduced

• Based on a behavioral study, the horse can discriminate colors even under a very low light intensity of 0.02 cd/m^2 (light intensity similar to moonlight), like humans. This is consistent with calculation of the sensitivity of cone vision in horses

• Cone photoreceptors and retinal ganglion cell density in the retina of the horse is highest in the area centralis, which provides the area of maximal visual acuity. The equine area centralis is divided into 2 areas—(1) area centralis rotunda: a small, circular region temporal and dorsal to the optic disk and (2) the visual streak: a horizontal, narrow band above the optic nerve

• In the past, it was suggested that the horse cannot see directly in front when the nose is lowered owing to the horizontally oval shape of the pupil. However, this suggestion is unlikely to be true as the horse is a prey animal and would be vulnerable to predators while grazing with a lowered head. Horses have 6 extraocular muscles (4 rectus and 2 oblique muscles), allowing them to adjust the position of the eyeball. Recently, it has been shown that horses indeed keep the optimal horizontal eyeball position regardless of head position (i.e. lowered or raised). By doing so, the horse maintains its ability to scan the lateral horizon for potential danger, even while grazing

• The equine eyes are among the largest terrestrial eyes. The large cornea together with the very mobile pupil that can dilate to a great extent increase the chance of catching a photon of light at night. Moreover, the fibrous tapetum lucidum of the dorsal fundus increases the chance of a nonabsorbed photon being absorbed by the photoreceptors, hence, enhancing night vision. However, by scattering light, the tapetum lucidum degrades photoreceptor image resolution

• The optic nerve of the horse is unique in that it contains a substantial proportion of axons of large diameter. Large retinal ganglion cells possess large diameter axons and are involved in motion detection, stereopsis, and sensitivity to dim light, suggesting that the horse has strong retinal adaptations for these visual characteristics

• The equine eye also shows diurnal adaptations, such as the corpora nigra (protects the ventral retina during grazing), occludable pupils, and yellow pigment in the lens (limits transmittance of very short wavelengths, which helps protect the photoreceptors in the retina)

• Systems affected—ophthalmic

MISCELLANEOUS

SEE ALSO
Stationary night blindness

ABBREVIATIONS
• cd = candela
• D = diopter

Suggested Reading
Carroll J, Murphy CJ, Neitz M, et al. Photopigment basis for dichromatic color vision in the horse. J Vis 2001;1:80–87.
Gilger BC, ed. Equine Ophthalmology, 3e. Ames, IA: Wiley Blackwell, 2017.
Hanggi EB. Rotated object recognition in four domestic horses (*Equus caballus*). J Equine Vet Sci 2010;30:175–186.
Hanggi EB, Ingersoll JF. Lateral vision in horses: a behavioral investigation. Behav Processes 2012;91:70–76.
Utter ME, Wotman KL, Covert KR. Return to work following unilateral enucleation in 34 horses (2000–2008). Equine Vet J 2010;42:156–160.

Author Gil Ben-Shlomo
Consulting Editor Caryn E. Plummer
Acknowledgment The author and editor acknowledge the prior contribution of Maria Källberg.

VITRIFICATION OF EQUINE EMBRYOS

BASICS

DEFINITION
- Vitrification is cryopreservation using:
  - High concentrations of cryoprotectants
  - Low volumes of medium
  - Ultrarapid freezing (plunging in liquid nitrogen)
- Vitrification does not require step-wise cooling or seeding
- The vitrification procedure is faster and simpler than standard slow freezing

APPLICATIONS
- Embryo vitrification can be used to hold embryos in order to allow scheduling of the time of transfer so that the resulting foal is born at the desired time of year
- Mares may be flushed for embryo recovery to produce embryos regardless of season
- Embryos may be produced from ICSI programs regardless of season
- Embryos produced postmortem by ICSI, owing to a mare's untimely death, may be transferred when the foals produced will be most valuable
- Biopsied embryos may be vitrified to hold them while genetic diagnosis is conducted
- When recipient numbers are small, embryos may be vitrified to simplify scheduling of transfer; the embryo is warmed and transferred when the recipient mare is the correct number of days after ovulation:
  - Use of vitrification could decrease the number of recipient mares that are needed in an embryo transfer program
- In procedures such as ICSI, from live mares or postmortem, vitrification can be used to preserve embryos in excess of the number of recipients immediately available, or in excess of the number of foals desired for that year
- Embryo vitrification provides a method of shipment of valuable genetics nationally or internationally
- Preserving embryos by vitrification provides a method of genetic conservation; theoretically the half-life in liquid nitrogen is 50 000 years

CONSIDERATIONS
- Both vitrification and slow freezing are successful with small VVR embryos (<300 μm in diameter) and with IVP embryos
- Collection of small embryos in vivo requires flushing of the uterus at day 6.5 after ovulation, which may be associated with lower embryo recovery rates
- Mares are typically flushed for embryo recovery on day 7 or 8 after ovulation, and the embryo recovered is an expanded blastocyst

- Expanded blastocysts (>300 μm in diameter) have low pregnancy rates after standard slow freezing or vitrification
- Collapse of the blastocele, using micromanipulation, allows successful vitrification of expanded blastocysts, with normal pregnancy rates after warming and transfer

METHODS

Embryo Collection
Mares are managed as for standard embryo collection:
- Insemination during estrus
- Ultrasonography per rectum to determine the day of ovulation
- Uterine flush for embryo recovery on day 6.5 after ovulation, if small embryos are desired
- Uterine flush for embryo recovery day 7 or 8 after ovulation, if small embryos are not desired

Embryo Vitrification by the Practitioner
- Use when small embryos are recovered
- Equine embryo vitrification kits are available from several companies
- Kits provide vitrification and warming solutions and instructions
- Requires standard embryo transfer supplies including stereomicroscope, Petri dishes, pipets, and embryo straws
- Requires liquid nitrogen and a Styrofoam container to hold it, and a liquid nitrogen tank
- Open vitrification devices such as the Cryotop or Cryolock can be used successfully with the equine kits, instead of straws:
  - Open devices, which are associated with low volume of medium and rapid temperature change, improve embryo viability upon warming in many applications
  - Open devices have been used successfully for equine embryo vitrification, but have not directly been compared with straws for vitrification of horse embryos
- Embryos are placed in the different solutions for the instructed period of time, then loaded into the straw or onto the open device, and plunged in liquid nitrogen
- If a straw is used:
  - The embryo is loaded in the straw with dilution solution so that the embryo can be warmed in the straw and transferred directly to a recipient
  - Some kits recommend placing straws in nitrogen vapor for a period before plunging to limit the possibility of the straw cracking
  - Use of nonirradiated polyvinyl chloride straws may limit the possibility of the straw cracking

- On warming, the straw is typically held in the air for a few seconds before being placed in the warm bath to allow evaporation of liquid nitrogen from the surface
- If an open vitrification device is used:
  - The medium around the embryo should be aspirated away until only a film of medium is present around the embryo
  - To warm, the device is immersed in warming solution. The embryo is located and placed in the holding medium and loaded for transfer
  - Straw cracking and other failures are avoided
- Success of vitrification both in straws and on open devices is technician-dependent and may be poor until the practitioner gains experience

Packaging Embryos for Shipment to a Laboratory for Vitrification
- Used when embryos >300 μm diameter are recovered, that need to be collapsed before vitrification, or when the practitioner does not have the expertise or supplies to vitrify embryos
- Notify the receiving laboratory that the embryo has been collected and will be shipped, and ascertain that the person performing the micromanipulation and vitrification will be there to receive and process it
- Embryos are packaged in Equitainers or EquOcyte containers, with all packaging material, isothermalizer, and ballast at room temperature (~22°C)
- The coolant cans are also at room temperature (~22°C)
- Embryos may be shipped by courier, by air, or by overnight delivery
- Currently because of lack of familiarity of many practitioners with methods for embryo warming, warming is done at the vitrification laboratory and the warmed embryos are shipped back to the practitioner for transfer

Collapse and Vitrification of Expanded Embryos (>300 μm in Diameter)
- Embryos are placed on an inverted microscope with micromanipulators
- The embryo is held by a holding pipet
- An injection pipet is inserted through the capsule and into the blastocele
  - If a Piezo drill is used, the capsule is breached by placing the pipet against it and using multiple pulses with the Piezo drill at a high setting (speed 6, intensity 7)
  - Conventional micromanipulation can be used, with a standard pointed human ICSI pipet. The pipet is inserted through the capsule into the blastocele

○ Use of a coaxial system, in which the small diameter aspiration pipet is extruded through a larger holding pipet, has also been successful
• The blastocele fluid is aspirated gently, with the injection pipet held at the periphery of the blastocele cavity. As much fluid as possible is removed without trauma to the embryo
• The embryo is then vitrified using the methods above, or methods specific to the embryo laboratory performing the vitrification:
  ○ A vitrification device used successfully in our laboratory is the microloader pipet tip, which has a small diameter that limits the volume of medium around the embryo
• One drawback to blastocele collapse is the possibility of loss of the capsule upon warming; this currently happens in about 10% of embryos and renders the embryo nonviable

TREATMENT

CLIENT EDUCATION
See Expected Course and Prognosis.

FOLLOW-UP

EXPECTED COURSE AND PROGNOSIS
• Embryo vitrification is not approved by all breed registries
• Vitrification of IVP embryos can provide the same foaling rate as does fresh transfer
• Smaller VVR embryos have high success after vitrification (75% pregnancy rate)
• Vitrification of expanded VVR embryos after blastocele collapse is also effective. We obtained over a 70% pregnancy rate with research embryos using this method, and a 55% pregnancy rate for client embryos. Client embryos are shipped to the laboratory for collapse and vitrification, then warmed and shipped back for transfer

MISCELLANEOUS

SEE ALSO
• Embryo transfer
• Equine oocytes and intracytoplasmic sperm injection (ICSI)

ABBREVIATIONS
• ICSI = intracytoplasmic sperm injection
• IVP = in vitro produced
• VVR = in vivo recovered

Suggested Reading
Carnevale EM, Eldridge-Panuska WD, di Brienza VC. How to collect and vitrify equine embryos for transfer. Proc Am Assoc Equine Pract 2004;50:402–405.
Choi YH, Hinrichs K. Vitrification of in vitro-produced and in vivo-recovered equine blastocysts in a clinical program. Theriogenology 2017;87:48–54.
Choi YH, Velez IC, Riera FL, et al. Successful cryopreservation of expanded equine blastocysts. Theriogenology 2011;76:143–152.
Diaz F, Bondiolli K, Paccamonti D, Gentry GT. Cryopreservation of day 8 equine embryos after blastocyst micromanipulation and vitrification. Theriogenology 2016;85:894–903.
Eldridge-Panuska WD, Caracciolo di Brienza VC, Seidel Jr GE, et al. Establishment of pregnancies after serial dilution or direct transfer by vitrified equine embryos. Theriogenology 2005;63:1308–1319.

Authors Young-Ho Choi and Katrin Hinrichs
Consulting Editor Carla L. Carleton

V

VULVAR CONFORMATION

BASICS

DEFINITION
• The quality/grade of VC is determined by the anatomic orientation of the anal sphincter to the vulva and pubis. This orientation impacts directly on the mare's reproductive health and affects her ability to maintain a healthy uterus and to carry pregnancies to term
• *Good VC*—the dorsal commissure of the vulva is at or below the level of the floor of the pubic bone. This generally is coupled with vulvae that exhibit an efficient side-to-side seal and with no cranial slant, effectively protecting the genital tract from manure contamination or aspiration of air
• *Fair VC*—the dorsal vulvar commissure is elevated above the floor of the pubis and/or the vulvar lips slope anteriorly, permitting pneumovagina or manure contamination of the vestibule
• *Poor VC*—the dorsal vulvar commissure is elevated above the floor of the pubis. This usually is accompanied by an obvious anterior slant of the vulva. Manure contamination of the vestibule occurs frequently to continuously
• Problems with VC are major contributors to equine subfertility and infertility

PATHOPHYSIOLOGY
Additional factors predisposing mares to poor VC—breeds/individuals with less muscle in the perineal area; perineal lacerations, and being underweight.

SYSTEMS AFFECTED
Reproductive

GENETICS
• Influences VC (mother/daughter) and should be considered when selecting broodmares. This is particularly important if farm-born fillies are kept for replacement stock
• Mares with good VC have fewer reproductive problems

INCIDENCE/PREVALENCE
• Abnormal VC can affect all breeds, but is especially common in racing breeds, e.g. Thoroughbreds and Standardbreds
• More muscular breeds or certain families within breeds have less of a problem with compromised VC

SIGNALMENT
• All breeds and any stock of breeding age
• Incidence of poor VC increases in old, pluriparous mares

SIGNS

General Comments
• The condition is fairly easy to evaluate. Assessment of each broodmare's VC should be noted on her record at the start of each breeding season
• Can worsen with age

Historical Findings
• History of subfertility or infertility because of failure to conceive or termination of pregnancy
• In addition to endometritis, vaginitis or cervicitis may be present

Physical Examination Findings
• Less than ideal VC may result in gross/histopathologic changes of the tubular genital tract, e.g. endometritis, acute or chronic
• Transrectal palpation—enlargement of uterine horns, increased uterine size, intraluminal fluid accumulation, and aspiration of air (e.g. pneumovagina, pneumouterus); if severe, echogenicities identified at ultrasonography may be caused by manure aspiration into the uterus
• Vaginal examination using sterile lubricant and a sterile vaginal speculum may reveal inflammation, discharge (e.g. endometritis, cervicitis, vaginitis), urine pooling, and/or adhesions (if chronic)
• Other physical parameters usually are normal

CAUSES
• Inherited poor VC
• Perineal laceration resulting from abnormal posture or fetal position at parturition
• Vaginal or vestibular intrapartum injuries caused by the fetus' feet (extremities) penetrating the dam's tract, e.g. causing tears/damage to the wall of her caudal tubular tract

RISK FACTORS
• Inherited
• No specific risk factors other than compromising the mare's ability to carry a healthy pregnancy to term
• Posterior presentation of a fetus, hindlimbs extended, has the potential to cause perineal lacerations
• Fetal posture and position can change within minutes of birth, so previous examinations for fetal position and posture have little predictive value

DIAGNOSIS

DIFFERENTIAL DIAGNOSIS
N/A

CBC/BIOCHEMISTRY/URINALYSIS
N/A

OTHER LABORATORY TESTS
N/A

IMAGING
N/A

OTHER DIAGNOSTIC PROCEDURES
• Determine the location of the dorsal vulvar commissure in relation to the pubis
• Careful palpation of the vestibule, vagina, and rectum to identify lacerations
• Rectovaginal fistulas may be small and not readily identified but result in sufficient contamination of the uterus to affect fertility

PATHOLOGIC FINDINGS
• Partial- to full-thickness lacerations of the vestibule and/or vagina
• Aspiration of air into the vagina and/or uterus
• Fecal contamination of the vagina and vestibule, with resulting inflammation of the vestibule, vagina, and cervix, and, possibly, the endometrium

TREATMENT

APPROPRIATE HEALTH CARE
• Determine that a laceration does not extend into the peritoneal cavity; rare with perineal laceration or rectovaginal fistula
• Systemic antibiotics seldom are indicated
• Local medication is rarely indicated
• Repair lacerations before attempting rebreeding
• Boost tetanus toxoid vaccination, if status is not current or is unknown

NURSING CARE
N/A

ACTIVITY
Normal activity, no restrictions.

DIET
Normal; no restrictions.

CLIENT EDUCATION
• Review importance of closely observing foaling
• Many lacerations occur before a foaling problem is noticed, even with trained attendants

SURGICAL CONSIDERATIONS
• Surgical correction for poor VC (episioplasty) was first described by Caslick in 1937, i.e. Caslick's vulvoplasty
• First, wrap and tie the mare's tail away from the field of surgery, and thoroughly clean the perineal area with cotton and soap

• Mepivacaine (Carbocaine) or another local anesthetic is infiltrated into the mucocutaneous junction of the vulva; ≅10–12 mL can be used to infiltrate both sides of the vulvar lips
• The tissue edges are freshened before suturing, either by removing a very narrow strip of tissue from the edge or by incising the mucocutaneous junction with a no. 10 scalpel blade in a upside down "U" shape:
  ◦ The edges of the vulvar lip that have been dilated with local anesthetic open into a nice, approximately 1 cm wide incision
  ◦ The split-thickness technique results in no tissue removal, i.e. it is tissue sparing, in that it helps to retain the normal elasticity of the vulva during labor
It minimizes damage that can be attributed to an annual vulvoplasty. Both described techniques can be used, however, and are acceptable
• Use nonabsorbable suture material, e.g. no. 1 Braunamid, or staples (increase likelihood of fistula formation), with removal in no less than 10 days
• Mares will often have sutures left in until they are examined for pregnancy at 15–16 days to avoid 1 extra trip to the barn
• Ensure adequate mare's tetanus toxoid vaccination status
• Pouret technique—in cases of severe/extremely poor VC, it may be necessary to dissect the perineal body in a caudal (widest) to cranial (point), pie-shaped wedge to permit the genital tract that lies ventral to the rectum to slide caudally and away from manure contamination, as well as aspiration of air. Only the skin is closed (i.e. no deep reconstruction of dissected tissue)
• Vestibuloplasty is described as creating an artificial vestibular valve; some success reported in resolving chronic, persistent pneumovagina. The repair is constructed within 2 days following breeding and ovulation. Using either a 1- or 2-step procedure, an upside down U-shaped incision is made, beginning at the dorsum of the vestibule, dissecting subcutaneous tissue sufficiently to suture together the edges from the left and right, leaving at least a 2 cm opening for urination

MEDICATIONS

DRUG(S) OF CHOICE
• No antibiotics are indicated
• Selection of local anesthetic is at the discretion of the surgeon

CONTRAINDICATIONS
N/A

PRECAUTIONS
N/A

POSSIBLE INTERACTIONS
N/A

ALTERNATIVE DRUGS
N/A

FOLLOW-UP

PATIENT MONITORING
Suture removal 10–15 days after surgery to prevent the possibility of stitch abscesses at the suture site.

PREVENTION/AVOIDANCE
Select broodmares with excellent VC.

POSSIBLE COMPLICATIONS
• Primary contraindication for vulvoplasty is the necessity of reopening the vulvar commissure ≅5–10 days before parturition to prevent the perineum from tearing at delivery
• Failure to place a vulvoplasty after breeding and a confirmed ovulation, if it is necessary, may preclude the mare conceiving or carrying a pregnancy to term
• Caslick's vulvoplasty should be replaced (i.e. incised and sutured) immediately after foaling, or breeding and confirmation of ovulation in the next season, depending on the severity of VC

EXPECTED COURSE AND PROGNOSIS
Without surgical correction, mares may remain infertile or abort during pregnancy.

MISCELLANEOUS

ASSOCIATED CONDITIONS
N/A

AGE-RELATED FACTORS
High probability of this condition worsening with age.

ZOONOTIC POTENTIAL
N/A

PREGNANCY/FERTILITY/BREEDING
Surgery may be necessary to obtain a pregnancy

SYNONYMS
Wind sucker

SEE ALSO
• Dystocia
• Endometrial biopsy
• Endometritis
• Perineal lacerations/recto-vaginal-vestibular fistulas
• Pneumovagina/pneumouterus
• Urine pooling/urovagina

ABBREVIATIONS
VC = vulvar conformation

Suggested Reading
Caslick EA. The vulva and vulvo-vaginal orifice and its relationship to genital health of the Thoroughbred mare. Cornell Vet 1937;27:178–186.
Inoue Y, Sekiguchi M. Vestibuloplasty for persistent pneumovagina in mares. J Equine Vet Sci 2017;48:9–14.
Stickle RL, Fessler JF, Adams SB, et al. A single stage technique for repair of rectovestibular lacerations in the mare. J Vet Surg 1979;8:25–27.

Author Carla L. Carleton
Consulting Editor Carla L. Carleton
Acknowledgment The author/editor acknowledges the prior contribution of Walter R. Threlfall.

WEANING SEPARATION STRESS

BASICS

DEFINITION
Weaning separation stress includes any of a number of reactions of the foal to separation from the dam and/or cessation of nutrition from the dam. Foals that are weaned naturally by the dam or that are weaned artificially but kept physically near or with the dam are rarely stressed as long as nutritional needs are met.

PATHOPHYSIOLOGY
• Under natural social conditions, cessation of nursing of foals occurs gradually over a period of months to years within the first 1–3 years of life. Significant nutrition from nursing at regular intervals usually ends at about 7–10 months of age. Separation of the young from the dam typically does not occur until maturity. Long after nutritional dependence on regular nursing, offspring as old as 3 years or greater appear to gain social comfort by return to the dam and from nuzzling of the udder at moments of fear or threat, sometimes briefly latching on and apparently ingesting a small amount of milk
• Under most traditional equine industry protocols, weaning is imposed at 2–6 months of age by physical separation of the foal and dam. Abrupt separation from the nutritional and psychosocial support of the dam typically results in signs of physical and/or psychologic stress reaction for the foal

SYSTEMS AFFECTED
• Nervous (behavior)—frantic locomotor activity, calling vocalizations, and interruption of foraging
• Gastrointestinal—frequent defecation; gastric ulcers are common
• Immune—compromised immune function
• Musculoskeletal—physical injuries may be incurred during panic, usually related to attempts to breech barriers; reduced rate of weight gain
• Respiratory—increased respiratory disease
• Skin—loss of coat and body condition

GENETICS
Inherited temperament likely affects maturational readiness and the behavioral and physical response to separation from the dam.

INCIDENCE/PREVALENCE
• Incidence of weaning separation stress varies in direct association with the methods and management
• Abrupt permanent separation with relocation and without preweaning adaptation to alternative nutrition and hydration results in nearly all foals showing mild to moderate stress, loss of condition, and gastric ulcers
• With gradual separation and careful nutritional preparation, the incidence of weaning and eventual separation stress or complications is very low

GEOGRAPHIC DISTRIBUTION
May vary regionally with prevalent breeds and management practices, including weaning protocols and facilities.

SIGNALMENT
Breed Predilection
More easily excitable breeds, such as Egyptian Arabians or Thoroughbreds, and lines within breeds appear to have greater separation stress response than less excitable breeds and lines.

Mean Age and Range
Very early weaned foals of 1–3 months of age are believed to be at greater risk than more mature foals of 5–12 months of age.

Predominant Sex
1 study of 10 foals weaned at 6 months of age resulted in the suggestion that female foals have greater locomotion response to weaning separation than males.

SIGNS
• Behaviors suggesting nonpathologic stress of social separation include occasional whinny vocalization, increased level of alertness, calm walking, increased frequency of defecation, loose stool, mildly increased heart rate, and less recumbent rest but eating well
• Signs of distress of social separation include frequent whinny vocalization, pawing, pacing, nervous walking or trotting, frequent defecation, watery stool, increased heart and respiratory rate, little standing or recumbent rest, and interrupted or poor eating
• Signs of severe distress include reduced locomotion, depression, standing with lowered head, apathy, and not eating

General Comments
• Locomotor and vocalization behavior of separation stress is adaptive for finding the dam or family group. In domestic confinement, it is the physical barriers and thwarted locomotion that typically lead to injuries
• Groups of foals weaned and separated simultaneously often appear to suffer prolonged stress. Removal of only 1 or 2 dams at a time from a group of foals usually results in less stress for each foal than removing multiple or all dams at once. It is also useful to remove the dams of the most mature and behaviorally independent foals first

Historical Findings
Signs and observations often reported by the owner.

RISK FACTORS
• Abrupt weaning
• Weaning <3 months old
• Age at weaning
• Change of environment

DIAGNOSIS

DIFFERENTIAL DIAGNOSIS
• Temporal association of behavioral distress responses and separation from the dam usually make the diagnosis clear
• Weaning separation stress appears to be immediately evident
• If a foal is calm within the minutes and hours after separation, a delayed onset is not expected without further social change, relocation, or other stressor

CBC/BIOCHEMISTRY/URINALYSIS
As indicated to diagnose complications, e.g. gastric ulcers, dehydration, nutrition.

OTHER LABORATORY TESTS
Cortisol will be elevated, as it is in many circumstances, so it is not diagnostic for separation stress.

IMAGING
Gastroscopy can be used to evaluate for gastric ulcers.

OTHER DIAGNOSTIC PROCEDURES
None

PATHOLOGIC FINDINGS
Gastric ulcers.

TREATMENT

AIMS
• Physical safety, social comfort, adequate nutrition, and distraction
• Diagnosis and treatment of related injuries or illnesses. Specifically, gastric ulcers should be addressed and treated
• In cases of injury or frenetic distress, it may be advisable to reunite the mare and foal and undertake separation at a much more mature age

APPROPRIATE HEALTH CARE
Provide adequate nutrition, physical safety.

NURSING CARE
• Ensure hydration and nutrition
• If the dam is available, return the foal to the fence line—direct access to the dam may be considered
• If the dam still has milk, udder covers are commercially available to block nursing
• If return to the dam is not an option, companion horses, ponies, donkeys, goats, or chickens can provide social comfort and distraction. Also, human contact can be distracting and ameliorative
• A simultaneously weaned foal may not be the best companion owing to a tendency for interfoal aggression, which appears to emerge in foals stressed by separation from the dam

W

(CONTINUED)   **WEANING SEPARATION STRESS**

ACTIVITY
• Depending on the particular locomotor response, and the facilities, injuries may be greater with stall confinement than in a paddock
• Foals that have been started in training or have had interactions with people before weaning/separation may be distracted and calmed by engaging in those activities

DIET
• A preweaning diet high in fat and fiber compared with a high-sugar and -starch diet has been associated with less severe stress response to weaning separation
• Milk from the dam (milked at the time or from a frozen bank) for 1 to a few days after separation can appear to provide some comfort

CLIENT EDUCATION
See Patient Monitoring and Prevention/Avoidance.

 MEDICATIONS

DRUG(S) OF CHOICE
• Anxiolytics and other psychotropic medications have not been systematically evaluated for relieving weaning stress
• For the frenetically active foal, tranquilization may be useful. Effectiveness varies with the level of panic

CONTRAINDICATIONS
Some animals have paradoxical reactions to tranquilizers.

PRECAUTIONS
If tranquilizers are used, the foal should be watched carefully for at least an hour. Great care must be used to avoid incoordination, ataxia, or impaired judgment by the foal.

ALTERNATIVE DRUGS
A synthetic pheromone, Modipher EQ, is marketed as a calming agent for horses and specifically lists mare–foal separation as an indication for use. The effectiveness has not been critically evaluated in controlled studies.

 FOLLOW-UP

PATIENT MONITORING
• The foal should be observed for a return to a normal 24 h time budget of behaviors. For a 4–6-month-old foal, this would include at least 50% of time foraging, 25% standing or recumbent rest, minimal vocalization, at least 10% of time playing or playfully investigating the environment and interacting socially, with no stereotypic pawing, cribbing, perimeter walking, or running
• The activity pattern of a nonstressed foal includes alternating periods of foraging, play, and rest, with each foraging and rest period lasting ≈ 30–60 min

PREVENTION/AVOIDANCE
Preventive measures to reduce weaning stress and associated injury and illness include:
• Introducing the independent diet high in fat and fiber well before separation from the dam, including a balanced mineral supplement and salt
• Separating/weaning only healthy, thriving foals of at least 4 months of age
• Removing the dam from the established social group, rather than removing the foal to a new group
• Allowing the foal to establish play groups of foals and/or yearlings with which it can remain when the dam is removed
• Including in the foal group a familiar adult herd mate(s) (e.g. mare or gelding) before weaning that can remain with the foal(s) after separation from the dam as an adult guardian(s)
• Employing gradual weaning/separation protocols versus abrupt separation
• In mare and foal groups, removing 1 mare at a time, leaving foals and remaining mares together and in familiar surroundings
• Separating/weaning older (4–6 months) versus younger (2–4 months) foals
• Observing behavior of foals to determine readiness for weaning

• Minimizing additional stress at the time of separation from the dam (e.g. new social groups, new location, transportation, immunization, deworming, intense human interaction, or stressful handling or training)
• Ensuring a familiar, healthy, and safe environment for the foal at the time of separation (the most recent environment, good soft slip-free footing, safe fencing, free of obstacles, free of dust that can be stirred up with increased activity). Evidence indicates that foals confined indoors in stalls at the time of separation, whether alone or in weanling pairs, are at greater risk of behavior and health problems related to weaning and separation stress than when kept at pasture. Respiratory complications are higher with the increased activity with greater dust and poorer ventilation in stalls. Injuries are greater in pair-stalled weanlings in association with interfoal aggression

POSSIBLE COMPLICATIONS
• Long-term effects related to injury and interference with weight gain
• Affected foals are believed to be at a greater risk of developing abnormal behavior, including separation anxiety, isolation panic, cribbing, and other stereotypies

EXPECTED COURSE AND PROGNOSIS
Separation stress has a variable duration, usually from a few hours to several days.

Suggested Reading
McGreevy P. Equine Behavior: A Guide for Veterinarians and Equine Scientists, 2e. Philadelphia, PA: WB Saunders, 2012:270–272.
Moons C, Laughlin K, Zanella A. Effects of short-term maternal separations on weaning stress in foals. Appl Anim Behav Sci 2005;91(3–4):321–335.
Nicol CJ, Badnell-Waters AJ, Bice R, et al. The effects of diet and weaning method on the behaviour of young horses. Appl Anim Behav Sci 2005;95(3–4):205–221.

Author Sue M. McDonnell
Consulting Editor Victoria L. Voith

W

WEST NILE VIRUS

BASICS

OVERVIEW
• WNV is a seasonal and potentially fatal neurotropic disease that has expanded worldwide since 1999 when the lineage 2 neurotropic virus emerged in the USA. Since 2006, WNV lineage 1 has been expanding into Eurasia as a neurotropic infection causing outbreaks in horses. • At least 11 times more horses develop asymptomatic infection and all horses are dead-end hosts. • WNV is carried and transmitted by a wide variety of mosquitos, and in North America is principally spread by the very common *Culex* spp. • Wild birds are the principal reservoir for WNV. • WNV enters the body through the bite of an infected mosquito and then multiplies in the hemolymphatics, with multiplication observed in endothelial cells and infection in peripheral blood mononuclear cells. If it crosses the blood–brain barrier, it causes a multifocal poliencephalitis and sometimes death

SIGNALMENT
• Any age, breed, or sex. • Primarily horses, humans, and birds. • Older horses have increased risk of severe neurotropic infection.

SIGNS
• Incubation period 9–15 days. • Signs range from asymptomatic through acutely neurologic. • Presenting clinical signs are often insidious. Fever is common but is often missed. 1–2 days before presentation, colic, lameness, inappetence, and depression can occur. • Neurologic signs not pathognomonic. • Fasciculation is common early disease. • Ataxia and dysmetria can be present. Spinal deficits primarily lower motor neuron, with symmetric to asymmetric weakness. • About 30–40% of horses will progress to recumbence. • Brain signs include a variety of behavioral changes—hyperexcitation, severe obtundation. • Cranial nerve abnormalities with decreased tongue retraction, vestibular and balance abnormalities, and lack of menace. These can be symmetrical or asymmetrical

CAUSES AND RISK FACTORS
• WNV is a member of the genus *Flavivirus*, family Flaviviridae. • Risk factor—exposure to infected mosquitos. • Lack of vaccination

DIAGNOSIS

DIFFERENTIAL DIAGNOSIS
Other causes of equine neurologic disease include, but are not limited to:
• Viral encephalitis. • Equine protozoal myeloencephalitis. • Poisoning—moldy corn; lead. • Equine degenerative myelopathy. • Aberrant strongyles migration. • Cervical vertebral malformation. • Head trauma

CBC/BIOCHEMISTRY/URINALYSIS
• Typical of viral infection—absolute lymphopenia observed. • Cerebrospinal fluid analysis—during acute phase mononuclear pleocytosis with elevations in total protein. May be normal late in the course of the disease

OTHER LABORATORY TESTS
• Serum immunoglobulin M ELISA—the most reliable test available, particularly in horses previously vaccinated or of unknown vaccination status. Plaque reduction neutralization test in horses never vaccinated before. • Brain tissue—hindbrain preferable. • RT-PCR—virus load is low in horses. • Virus isolation useful if RT-PCR does not yield results. Some horses may be low positive on anticoagulated whole blood at time of clinical disease

PATHOLOGIC FINDINGS
Lesions of the brain and spinal cord consistent with encephalomyelitis.

TREATMENT
• No specific treatment. • Supportive care

MEDICATIONS
• No specific antivirals. • High titer anti-WNV plasma of questionable efficacy after clinical signs apparent. • Supportive therapy and anti-inflammatory medications. • Corticosteroids of questionable value. • Diazepam not recommended. • α_2-Adrenergic receptor agonists may reduce fasciculations and hyperexcitability

FOLLOW-UP

PREVENTION/AVOIDANCE

Vaccination
Vaccines are currently licensed for horses and foals, but none is currently labeled for pregnant mares.

Avoidance
Most important—minimize the standing water in which mosquitos breed.

POSSIBLE COMPLICATIONS
In 1 large study, 80% of horses that recovered did so fully; the remainder had residual effects.

EXPECTED COURSE AND PROGNOSIS
• Mortality rates 20–44%. • More severely affected horses have poorer prognoses. Horses are more likely to die if they develop caudal paresis or recumbency. • A recurrence of mild to moderate clinical signs noted in some horses within 5 days after signs significantly improve. • Most long-term behavioral or movement deficits abated by 6 months. • Vaccination appears to reduce severity of clinical signs and the risk of death from WNV

MISCELLANEOUS

AGE-RELATED FACTORS
Mortality increases with age.

ZOONOTIC POTENTIAL
• Horses do not seem to transmit WNV to other horses or humans. • Humans exposed to potentially infected horse brain and spinal cord tissue should wear appropriate personal protective equipment

PREGNANCY/FERTILITY/BREEDING
It is recommended that mares be fully vaccinated before breeding.

SEE ALSO
• Eastern (EEE), western (WEE), and Venezuelan (VEE) equine encephalitides
• Equine herpesvirus myeloencephalopathy
• Equine protozoal myeloencephalitis (EPM)
• Leukoencephalomalacia
• Lead (Pb) toxicosis
• Neuroaxonal dystrophy/equine degenerative myeloencephalopathy
• Verminous meningoencephalomyelitis
• West nile virus
• Cervical vertebral malformation
• Head trauma

ABBREVIATIONS
• ELISA = enzyme-linked immunosorbent assay. • RT-PCR = reverse transcription–polymerase chain reaction. • WNV = West Nile virus

Internet Resources
American Association of Equine Practitioners, West Nile Virus Vaccination Guidelines 2005. https://aaep.org/guidelines/vaccination-guidelines/core-vaccination-guidelines/west-nile-virus

Author Maureen T. Long
Consulting Editor Caroline N. Hahn
Acknowledgment The author and editor acknowledge the prior contribution of Jennifer Jacobs Fowler, Susan C. Trock, and Brianne Gustafson.

W

INDEX

Text in **boldface** denotes chapter discussions.

Osteotomy, corrective, 68
Otoacariosis, 246
Otobius megnini-associated muscle
    cramping, 240
Ovarian abscess, 440
Ovarian disorders
    anestrus, 65, 66
    large ovary syndrome, 439–441
Ovarian follicles
    hemorrhagic anovulatory (HAFs), 545
    luteinized unruptured, 545
    persistent, 439, 440–441
Ovarian hematoma, 439, 440, 441
Ovarian tumors
    anestrus, 66
    large ovary syndrome, 439–441
Ovariectomy
    for aggression, 40
    for ovarian disorders, 441
Ovaries, removal and shipment for
    postmortem ICSI, 655–656
Overo-overo Paint crosses
    colic in foals, 170
    lethal white foal syndrome, 455
Ovulation
    diestrus, 630
    failure, 545
    prediction, 83
Ovulation induction agents (OIA)
    for abnormal estrus intervals, 8
    for anestrus, 66
    for artificial insemination, 83, 85
Oxalate toxicosis
    hypocalcemia, 132–133
    soluble, 707
Oxfendazole, for cyathostominosis, 202
Oxygen therapy
    for anaphylaxis, 55
    for endotoxemia, 259
    for expiratory dyspnea, 297
    for Heinz body anemia, 61
    for hypoxemia, 388
    for inspiratory dyspnea, 416
    for neonatal isoerythrolysis, 505
    for neonatal maladjustment syndrome,
        506
    for neonatal pneumonia, 599
    for summer pasture-associated equine
        asthma (pasture asthma), 724
Oxygen toxicity, 23, 389
Oxytetracycline
    for anaerobic bacterial infections, 54
    for anthrax, 72
    for *Bordetella bronchiseptica,* 120
    for clostridial myositis, 160
    for equine granulocytic anaplasmosis,
        270
    for equine recurrent uveitis, 285
    for flexural limb deformity, 316
    induced hypocalcemia, 133

for leptospirosis, 454
for Potomac horse fever, 616
for thrombocytopenia, 743
Oxytocin
    for abnormal estrus intervals, 8
    for artificial insemination, 83, 84
    for conception failure, 176
    for delayed uterine involution, 209
    for dystocia, 239
    for endometritis, 256, 257
    for esophageal obstruction, 288
    for fescue toxicosis, 307
    for hydrops allantois/amnion, 380,
        381
    for postpartum metritis, 611, 612
    prolonged diestrus due to, 630
    for pyometra, 645
    for retained fetal membranes, 662
    for uterine inertia, 780

P

Pain
    abdominal. (*See* Colic)
    aggression and, 39
    back, 105
    bruxism, 126–127
    headshaking, 354
Paint
    chronic kidney disease, 153
    exertional rhabdomyolysis, 294
    gastric neoplasia, 332
    glycogen branching enzyme deficiency,
        346
    guttural pouch tympany, 353
    hereditary equine regional dermal
        asthenia, 369
    ocular/adnexal squamous cell
        carcinoma, 220, 521
    polysaccharide storage myopathy, 89,
        193, 608
Palatoschisis. (*See* Cleft palate)
Palmar foot pain. (*See* Navicular
    syndrome)
Pamidronate, for *Cestrum diurnum*
    toxicosis, 146
Pancreatic disease, 546
    amylase, lipase and trypsin levels, 52
Pancytopenia, 547
Panhyperproteinemia, 595, 634
Panhypoproteinemia, 595, 636–637
***Panicum coloratum* (kleingrass)
    toxicosis,** 548, 749
Panniculitis, 52
Papillomatosis, 549
Paranasal sinusitis, 693–694
Paranasal tumors, 760
Paraphimosis, 550–551
Paraproteins, 634
Parascaris equorum, 88

Parasitic diseases. (*See also* Protozoal
    infections)
    abdominocentesis, 5
    alopecia, 46
    ascarid infestation, 88
    conjunctivitis, 181–182
    cyathostominosis, 201–202
    cytology of bronchoalveolar lavage
        fluid, 203
    dourine, 232–233
    ear tick-associated muscle cramping,
        240
    ectoparasites, 246–247
    eosinophilia, 262
    lungworms, 462
    neonatal diarrhea, 217–218
    trypanosomiasis, 757–758
    urinary tract infection, 771–772
    verminous meningoencephalomyelitis,
        792
Parathyroid hormone (PTH), 625
Parenteral nutrition
    in foals, 516–517
    for hyperlipidemia/hyperlipemia, 385
    metabolic acidosis complicating, 20
    in neonatal septicemia, 687
Paroxetine, for locomotor stereotypic
    behaviors, 461
Parturition. (*See also* Pregnancy)
    broad ligament hematoma, 124
    cervical lesions, 142–143
    dystocia, 238–239
    fetal stress/distress/viability, 308–310
    high-risk pregnancy, 376
    neonatal resuscitation, 658–659
    perineal lacerations/recto-vaginal-
        vestibular fistulas, 566–567
    postpartum metritis, 611–612
    premature placental separation, 620
    retained fetal membranes, 662
    rib fractures in foals, 665
    uterine inertia, 780
Paso Fino
    equine metabolic syndrome/insulin
        dysregulation, 273
    melanoma, 481
    neuroaxonal dystrophy, 509
    ocular problems, 339, 524, 717
Paspalum staggers, 751–752
Pastern dermatitis, 552–553
    Chorioptes equi, 246
    dermatophilosis, 215
Pastern vasculitis, leukocytoclastic,
    456–457
Pasture asthma, 723–724
Patella, upward fixation of, 766
Patent ductus arteriosus, 178–179,
    554–555
Patent foramen ovale (PFO), 178–179
Patent urachus, 556

Sweet clover, moldy, 219
Sweet itch. (*See* Insect hypersensitivity)
Sycamore maple (*Acer pseudoplatanus*), 101, 678
Synchronous diaphragmatic flutter (SDF), 729
  endurance horses, 485
  hypocalcemia, 132–133
Synovial fluid, 730–731
Systemic inflammatory response syndrome (SIRS), 258, 686

T

T-2 toxin, 325
Tambora, 349
Tansy ragwort (*Senecio jacobaea*), 646
Tarsitis, distal, 229
Tarsocrural osteochondrosis, 543
Taxus spp. (yew), 136–137
Taylorella equigenitalis
  breeding shed biosecurity, 113–114
  contagious equine metritis, 183–184
Tea tree oil/sweet almond oil mixture, for superficial dermatomycoses, 214
Teeth. (*See also* Dental problems)
  extraction, 571, 660
  grinding. (*See* Bruxism)
  retained deciduous, 660–661
Telogen effluvium, 47, 48
Temporohyoid osteoarthropathy, 732
Tendonitis, 733–734
Tenesmus, 735–736
Tennessee Walking Horse
  cryptorchidism, 195
  equine metabolic syndrome/insulin dysregulation, 273
  hemophilia A, 165
  inguinal hernia, 370, 696
Teratoma, 737
  ovarian, 439, 440
Terbinafine, for dermatophytoses, 214
Testicular atrophy, 11
Testicular biopsy, 712
Testicular degeneration, 11, 12, 711
Testicular feminization, 222
Testicular hypoplasia, 11, 12, 711
Testicular neoplasia, 11, 12
Testicular rupture, 9
Testicular size, abnormal, 11–12
Testicular torsion, 9, 10
Testosterone
  serum, 195, 223
  for stallion sexual behavior problems, 716
Tetanus, 738–739
  nictitans protrusion, 220–221
  vaccination, 739, 784
Tetanus antitoxin, 739, 784

Tetany
  hypocalcemic, 132–133
  lactation. (*See* Eclampsia)
Tetracyclines. (*See also* Doxycycline; Oxytetracycline)
  for anaerobic bacterial infections, 54
  for Lyme disease, 464
  for Tyzzer disease, 763
Tetralogy of Fallot, 173–174, 178–179
Theiler disease, 28–29
Theiler disease-associated virus (TDAV), 28
Theileria equi, 587–588
Thelazia lacrimalis, 299
Theobromine toxicosis, 491
Theophylline toxicosis, 491
Theriogenology
  abnormal estrus intervals, 7–8
  abnormal scrotal enlargement, 9–10
  abnormal testicular size, 11–12
  abortion, spontaneous, infectious, 13–15
  abortion, spontaneous, noninfectious, 16–18
  agalactia/hypogalactia, 37–38
  anestrus, 65–66
  artificial insemination, 83–85
  biosecurity, disinfectants in the breeding shed, 113–114
  broad ligament hematoma, 124
  castration, Henderson castration instrument, 138
  castration, routine, 139
  cervical lesions, 142–144
  clitoral enlargement, 158
  conception failure in mares, 175–177
  contagious equine metritis, 183–184
  cryptorchidism, 195–196
  delayed uterine involution, 209
  disorders of sexual development, 222–223
  dourine, 232–233
  dystocia, 238–239
  early embryonic death, 241–242
  eclampsia, 245
  embryo transfer, 248–249
  endometrial biopsy, 252–253
  endometritis, 254–257
  equine oocytes and intracytoplasmic sperm injection, 279–280
  fetal stress/distress/viability, 308–310
  hemospermia, 364
  high-risk pregnancy, 375–378
  hydrops allantois/amnion, 380–381
  large ovary syndrome, 439–441
  mastitis, 477
  ovulation failure, 545
  paraphimosis, 550–551
  penile lacerations, 559
  penile paralysis, 560

penile vesicles, erosions and tumors, 561–562
perineal lacerations/recto-vaginal-vestibular fistulas, 566–567
phimosis, 576
placenta basics, 591
placental insufficiency, 592
placentitis, 593–594
pneumovagina/pneumouterus, 601
postpartum metritis, 611–612
pregnancy diagnosis, 617–619
premature placental separation, 620
prepubic tendon rupture, 623
priapism, 624
prolonged diestrus, 630–631
prolonged pregnancy, 632–633
pyometra, 644–645
removal and shipment of ovaries for postmortem ICSI, 655–656
retained fetal membranes, 662
spermatogenesis and factors affecting sperm production, 711–712
teratoma, 737
twin pregnancy, 761–762
urine pooling/urovagina, 773
uterine inertia, 780
uterine torsion, 781–782
vaginal prolapse, 785
vaginitis and vaginal discharge, 786
vitrification of equine embryos, 800–801
vulvar conformation, 802–803
Thiabendazole, for eyelid ringworm, 300
Thiamine
  for ionophore toxicosis, 427
  for lead toxicosis, 446
  for neonatal maladjustment syndrome, 507
Thoracic trauma, 740–741
Thoracocentesis
  in aspiration pneumonia, 91
  in pneumothorax, 600
  in thoracic trauma, 740
Thoracostomy tube
  for pneumothorax, 600
  for thoracic trauma, 741
Thoroughbred
  agammaglobulinemia, 399
  angular limb deformity, 67
  anhidrosis, 69
  congenital ocular problems, 451, 524, 717
  cryptorchidism, 195
  dorsal metacarpal bone disease, 231
  dynamic collapse of upper airways, 236
  enterolithiasis, 260
  eosinophilic enteritis, 263
  epiglottic entrapment, 266

rectal tears, 652–653
respiratory acidosis, 22
rib fractures in foals, 665
scrotal enlargement, 9, 10
thoracic, 600, 740–741
Tremorgenic mycotoxin toxicosis,
751–752
TRH. (*See* Thyroid-releasing hormone)
Triamcinolone
for distal and proximal interphalangeal
joint disease, 228
for distal tarsitis, 229
for habronemiasis, 182, 221
for heaves, 358
for metacarpo-(metatarso-)phalangeal
joint disease, 487
for navicular syndrome, 503
for osteoarthritis, 542
for osteochondrosis, 544
for pastern dermatitis, 553
for stress fractures, 721
for tendonitis, 734
Trichlorfon, for habronemiasis, 300, 562
Trichography, 47
Trichophyton equinum, 213–214
Trichorrhexis nodosa, 46
Trichosporum beigelii, 46
Trichothecenes, 325
Tricuspid atresia, 173–174, 178–179
Tricuspid regurgitation, 753–754
in atrial septal defect, 99, 100
Tricyclic antidepressants
for fearful behavior, 304
for locomotor stereotypic behaviors,
461
for narcolepsy and cataplexy, 502
for self-mutilation, 683
Triethylenethiophosphoramide, for
hematuria, 585
Trifluorothymidine, for viral (herpes)
keratitis, 797
Trifolium hybridum (alsike clover)
toxicosis, 749, 755
Trigeminal nerve sensitization, 354
Triiodothyronine (T$_3$), 224–225
Trimethoprim–sulfadiazine
for *Corynebacterium pseudotuberculosis,*
190
for mastitis, 477
Trimethoprim–sulfamethoxazole
for acute epiglottiditis, 27
for aspiration pneumonia, 91
for *Bordetella bronchiseptica,* 120
for chronic/recurrent colic, 169
for contagious equine metritis, 184
for *Corynebacterium pseudotuberculosis,*
190
for duodenitis–proximal jejunitis, 235
for fungal pneumonia, 324
for guttural pouch tympany, 353

for hemospermia, 364
for herpesvirus types 1 and 4, 374
for idiopathic colitis/typhlitis, 393
for internal abdominal abscesses, 420
for Tyzzer disease, 763
Trimethoprim–sulfonamides
for anaerobic bacterial infections, 54
for clostridial myositis, 160
for hepatic abscess and septic
cholangiohepatitis, 366
for leukocytoclastic pastern vasculitis,
456
for malabsorption, 475
for pastern dermatitis, 553
for postpartum metritis, 612
for seizures in foals, 681
for temporohyoid osteoarthropathy,
732
for urinary incontinence, 770
for urinary tract infection, 772
Tripelennamine hydrochloride, for
anaphylaxis, 56
Tris-EDTA, for endometritis, 256–257
Trocarization, for abdominal distention,
2
Trombiculidiasis, 246–247
Tropane alkaloids toxicosis, 756
Tropicamide, for mydriasis, 523
Truncus arteriosus, 178–179
Trypanosoma equiperdum, 232–233, 757,
758
Trypanosomiasis, 757–758
Trypsin, 52
Tuberculosis, 759
Tumors. (*See* Neoplasia)
Tumors of the respiratory system, 760
Twin pregnancy, 761–762
spontaneous abortion in, 16, 17
Typhlitis, idiopathic, 392–393
Tyzzer disease (*Clostridium piliforme*),
763

U

Ulcerative keratomycosis, 764–765
Ulcerative lymphangitis, *Corynebacterium
pseudotuberculosis,* 189–190
Ultrasonography
in abdominal distention, 2
in abdominal hernia, 4
in acute colic, 26
in acute kidney injury, 30
in aflatoxicosis, 35
in anuria/oliguria, 74
in aortoiliac thrombosis, 81
in artificial insemination, 83, 85
in arytenoid chondropathy, 86
in aspartate aminotransferase increase,
90
in azotemia and uremia, 103

in cervical lesions, 142
in cholelithiasis, 149
in chronic diarrhea, 151
in chronic kidney disease, 153
in chronic/recurrent colic, 168
in clitoral enlargement, 158
in coccidioidomycosis, 166
in colic in foals, 171
in conception failure in mares,
175–176
in *Corynebacterium pseudotuberculosis,*
189
in cryptorchidism, 195
in dynamic collapse of upper airway,
236
in early embryonic death, 241
in embryo transfer, 248
in endometritis, 255, 256
in febrile horses, 312
fetal assessment, 308–309, 375, 376
fetal sexing, 617–618
in gastric dilation/distention, 328–329
in gastric impaction, 330
in hemospermia, 364
in hepatic abscess and septic
cholangiohepatitis, 366
in hernias (umbilical and inguinal),
370
in hydrops allantois/amnion, 380
in icterus, 391
in impaction, 404
in increased peritoneal fluid, 6
in infectious arthritis, 407
in inspiratory dyspnea, 416
in intra-abdominal hemorrhage, 423
in large ovary syndrome, 440
in lymphosarcoma, 470
in neonatal diarrhea, 217
in neonatal septic arthritis, 684
in neonatal septicemia, 686
in omphalophlebitis, 526
in pericarditis, 564
in placental insufficiency, 592
in placentitis, 593
in pleuropneumonia, 597
in pneumothorax, 600
in postpartum metritis, 611
pregnancy diagnosis, 617
in premature placental separation, 620
in prolonged pregnancy, 632
in pyometra, 644
in rib fractures in foals, 665
in right and left dorsal displacement of
the colon, 666
in right dorsal colitis, 668
in sand impaction and enteropathy,
674
scrotal, 9, 11
in small intestinal obstruction, 697
in stress fractures, 720